TEXTBOOK OF
ADULT EMERGENCY MEDICINE

THIRD EDITION

EDITED BY

Peter Cameron MB BS MD FACEM
Professor of Emergency Medicine, Department of Epidemiology and Preventive Medicine, Monash University,
The Alfred Hospital, Melbourne, Victoria, Australia

George Jelinek MB BS MD DipDHM FACEM
Professor of Emergency Medicine, University of Western Australia, Sir Charles Gairdner Hospital, Nedlands,
Western Australia, Australia

Anne-Maree Kelly MD MClinED FACEM
Director, Joseph Epstein Centre for Emergency Medicine Research at Western Health and the University of
Melbourne, Footscray, Victoria, Australia

Lindsay Murray MB BS FACEM
Emergency Physician and Clinical Toxicologist, Sir Charles Gairdner Hospital, Nedlands, Western Australia,
Australia

Anthony FT Brown MBChB FRCP FRCS FACEM FCEM
Professor of Emergency Medicine, University of Queensland. Senior Staff Specialist, Department of Emergency
Medicine, Royal Brisbane and Women's Hospital, Brisbane, Queensland, Australia

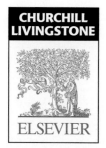

CHURCHILL
LIVINGSTONE

ELSEVIER

EDINBURGH   LONDON   NEW YORK   OXFORD   PHILADELPHIA   ST LOUIS   SYDNEY   TORONTO   2009

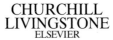

CHURCHILL LIVINGSTONE
ELSEVIER

First edition 2000
Second edition 2004
Third edition 2009
   Reprinted 2009, 2010

ISBN 9780443068195

British Library Cataloguing in Publication Data
A catalogue record for this book is available from the British Library

Library of Congress Cataloging in Publication Data
A catalog record for this book is available from the Library of Congress

Notice
Knowledge and best practice in this field are constantly changing. As new research and experience broaden our knowledge, changes in practice, treatment and drug therapy may become necessary or appropriate. Readers are advised to check the most current information provided (i) on procedures featured or (ii) by the manufacturer of each product to be administered, to verify the recommended dose or formula, the method and duration of administration, and contraindications. It is the responsibility of the practitioner, relying on their own experience and knowledge of the patient, to make diagnoses, to determine dosages and the best treatment for each individual patient, and to take all appropriate safety precautions. To the fullest extent of the law, neither the publisher nor the editors assume any liability for any injury and/or damage to persons or property arising out of or related to any use of the material contained in this book.

The Publisher

ELSEVIER
your source for books,
journals and multimedia
in the health sciences
www.elsevierhealth.com

Working together to grow
libraries in developing countries
www.elsevier.com | www.bookaid.org | www.sabre.org

ELSEVIER   BOOK AID International   Sabre Foundation

The
Publisher's
policy is to use
**paper manufactured
from sustainable forests**

Printed in China

TEXTBOOK OF
ADULT EMERGENCY MEDICINE

DATE DUE

For Elsevier

Commissioning Editor: Timothy Horne
Development Editor: Helen Leng
Project Manager: Camilla Cudjoe
Designer/Design Direction: Sarah Russell
Illustration Manager: Merlyn Harvey
Illustrator: Ethan Danielson

Preface to the first edition

Emergency Medicine has developed into the most exciting area of medical practice. Apart from the immediacy and unpredictability of managing acutely ill patients, emergency practice allows the clinician to use a broad range of skills and work in a team environment.

New treatments for respiratory and cardiovascular disease, new systems of care for trauma and psychiatric disorders, necessitate highly sophisticated healthcare at the 'front door'. Attempts to restrain healthcare costs by better use of hospital beds also demand trained professionals to assess emergency patients on arrival. The community now expects immediate access to skilled personnel in emergencies. The recent emphasis on continuity of care for patients from community to hospital and back into the community underlines the importance of Emergency Medicine in new healthcare systems.

Emergency Medicine has grown from the Emergency Room to the Emergency Department. In Australasia, it is the fastest growing medical specialty with more than 800 trainees. The UK has seen a similar rapid expansion. In the United States it has the most popular residency training programmes. Doctors working in Emergency Medicine in Europe and Asia are finally achieving specialist status.

The genesis of this book was the need for a definitive textbook of adult emergency medicine, based on current practice in Australia, New Zealand and the United Kingdom. Many areas of Emergency Medicine are changing rapidly and it is likely that at the time of publication, practice will have developed further. Not all subjects are covered with equal emphasis. This is deliberate in that, for example, there are excellent texts on fracture management. In other areas such as trauma management, we have tried to give basic principles, together with references for further reading.

The layout of the sections has been carefully designed to make it easy to use, with essential information summarized in a clear and concise way. The inclusion of a section on controversies aims to highlight areas of varying practice, change or ongoing research.

The book is aimed principally to meet the needs of doctors in training in Emergency Medicine. In addition, it will be an important resource for general practitioners, specialist emergency and critical care nurses, residents and medical students rotating through an emergency term.

This text is a collaborative effort, involving 113 contributors from Australia, New Zealand, the United Kingdom and the United States of America. Individual contributions have been edited to conform with a consensus style and approach. Material within the text should therefore follow current management in the United Kingdom, New Zealand and Australia. It is anticipated that this book will help develop a common management approach to emergency patients and promote the specialty of Emergency Medicine.

Many people have been involved in the production of this work; the Editors are extremely grateful to them all. We would particularly like to thank our partners, children and friends who have endured the long months of the hard work involved in the development of this book. For their excellent secretarial assistance and manuscript preparation, we thank Mimi Morgan, Celina Everton, Lien Wright and Janet Carr. We are very grateful to the individual contributors for the enthusiasm with which they embraced the task and their generosity in giving their time. Finally, we would like to thank the production staff at Harcourt Brace, particularly Janice Urquhart.

P. C.   2000
G. J.
A-M. K.
L. M.
J. H.
A. B.

Preface to the third edition

Since the first edition of this text in 2000, emergency medicine practice has changed enormously. The role of emergency physicians as principal specialists has increased around the globe with more than 20 countries now recognizing the specialty and many more developing specialty societies. This expansion has been driven by the self evident notion that specialized emergency medicine practitioners are a cornerstone of modern medical systems of care.

The concept that it is important to manage patients expertly from the time of accessing the health system, as opposed to a 'leisurely review' the following day in an inpatient bed, is hard to refute. With patients requiring resuscitation, this is even more evident. This means that frontline paramedics, nursing staff and doctors must be well drilled in the recognition and treatment of common and high-risk emergency conditions. Clearly, unsupervised rotating junior staff are not going to manage these situations well.

Ensuring that emergency presentations are admitted appropriately and have evidence-based treatment plans from the time of admission makes a significant difference to hospital bed usage and efficiency. The advent of short stay units, hospital in the home and other initiatives to limit inpatient stays has further increased the importance of emergency medicine practice in supporting the health system.

Advances in the science of resuscitation and emergency medical treatment of many conditions mean that there are many patients who can suffer adverse consequences from delayed or inadequate initial treatment. Common examples include acute myocardial infarction, antibiotic treatment in pneumonia and evacuation of traumatic intracranial haemorrhage. The promotion of 'care bundles', such as in 'early goal directed therapy' for sepsis, represents a new and exciting way to ensure early appropriate treatment. Trauma systems of care have been around for many years; however, the benefits are difficult to quantify and uptake has been limited on a global basis. The system of care approach is being developed in other disciplines such as stroke and cardiac care. Despite the enthusiasm, there are many questions regarding the best way of promoting and evaluating these concepts, and emergency medicine must be at the forefront of this new system-based approach.

Emergency medicine practice is likely to change even more dramatically over the next few years, with the necessity of providing a more flexible workforce to ensure an expert presence 24 hours per day seven days per week. Nurse practitioners, emergency physician assistants and paramedic practitioners are just some of the new providers. The best workforce model will no doubt develop over time and according to need. It is essential that clinicians in emergency medicine focus on the aim of emergency medicine – to provide the right care to the right person in the shortest possible time.

The purpose of this text is to provide the basic knowledge necessary to guide emergency clinicians in an evidence-based approach to managing emergency patients. The format is standardized and easy to read. For many areas where good evidence is lacking, current consensus on the topic is explained.

This comprehensive text received input from many contributors around the world and we are thankful for their expertise. The forbearance of partners, children, family and friends during the months of development is particularly appreciated. The production has involved significant contributions from many people, particularly Rosalie Clementson and Mimi Morgan.

P. C.   2009
G. J.
A-M. K.
L. M.
A. B.

Contributors

Jonathan Abrahams BSc MPH
Assistant Director Policy, Emergency
Management Australia, Dickson,
Australian Capital Territory,
Australia

Nicholas Adams MB BS FACEM
Staff Specialist, Emergency Department,
The Alfred Hospital, Prahran, Victoria,
Australia

Sam Alfred MBBS FACEM Dip Tox
Emergency Medicine Consultant and
Toxicology Fellow, Royal Adelaide Hospital,
Malvern, South Australia, Australia

Sylvia Andrew-Starkey MB BS FACEM
Emergency Department, Caboolture
Hospital, Caboolture, Queensland,
Australia

Philip Aplin MB BS FACEM
Senior Staff Specialist, Emergency
Department, Flinders Medical Centre,
South Australia, Australia

Michael W Ardagh MBChB DCH
FACEM PhD
Professor of Emergency Medicine,
University of Otago
Christchurch, New Zealand

Sean Arendse AKC BSc MB BS FACEM
Staff Specialist, Emergency Department,
The Alfred Hospital, Prahran, Victoria,
Australia

Jason Armstrong FACEM
Emergency Physician and Clinical
Toxicologist, Emergency Medicine,
The University of Western Australia,
Sir Charles Gairdner Hospital, Perth,
Western Australia, Australia

Richard Ashby MB BS BHA FRACGP
FRACMA FACEM FIFEM
Executive Director Medical Services,
Royal Brisbane and Women's Hospital,
Herston, Queensland,
Australia

Michael Augello FACEM
Emergency Physician, Emergency
Department, St Vincent's Hospital,
Fitzroy, Victoria,
Australia

Ashis Banerjee MS FRCS Eng & Ed MS FCEM
DTM&H
Consultant in Emergency Medicine, Chase
Farm Hospitals NHS Trust,
London, Honorary Senior Lecturer,
University College London Medical School,
London, United Kingdom

Simon Baston RGN RMN
Mental Health Liaison Nurse, Liaison
Psychiatry, Accident and Emergency
Department, Northern General Hospital,
Sheffield, United Kingdom

Shomoresh Bhattacharjee MB BS
Rheumatology and General Medicine
Registrar, Alfred Hospital,
Department of Rheumatology,
Melbourne, Victoria, Australia

Anthony J Bell MBBS G Cert BA FACEM
Director of Emergency Medicine,
Queen Elizabeth II Jubilee Hospital,
Coopers Plains, Queensland,
Australia

Stephen Bernard MD FACEM FJFICM
Staff Specialist, The Intensive Care Unit,
Alfred Hospital, Melbourne, Victoria,
Australia

Shom Bhattacharjee MB BS
Rheumatology Registrar and Monash
University Assistant Lecturer,
Central and Eastern Clinical School,
The Alfred Hospital, Prahran, Victoria,
Australia

David Bradt MD MPH FACEM FAFPMH
FAAEM DTM&H
Staff Specialist, Department of Emergency
Medicine, Royal Melbourne Hospital,
Parkville, Victoria, Australia

George Braitberg MB BS FACEM FACMT
Departments of Medicine and Emergency
Medicine, University of Melbourne,
Austin and Repatriation Medical
Centre, Heidelberg, Victoria, Australia

Victoria Brazil MBBS FACEM MBA
Staff Specialist, Department of Emergency
Medicine, Royal Brisbane Hospital,
Brisbane, Queensland, Australia

Richard J Brennan MBBS MPH FACEM
FIFEM
Senior Health Director,
International Rescue Committee,
New York, United States of America

Edward Brentnall MB BS
Dip Obstetrics (RCOG) FACEM
Retired Emergency Physician
Melbourne, Victoria, Australia

Anthony FT Brown MBChB FRCP FRCS
FACEM FCEM
Professor of Emergency Medicine,
University of Queensland,
Senior Staff Specialist, Department of
Emergency Medicine, Royal Brisbane and
Women's Hospital, Brisbane, Queensland,
Australia

Sheila Bryan MB BS BSc FACEM MRACMA
Dip Venereology
Staff Specialist,
Department of Emergency Medicine,
Danenong Hospital, Victoria,
Australia

Michael Bryant MB BS MBus MRACMA
FACEM
Clinical Director, Department of Emergency
Medicine, Western Hospital,
Footscray, Victoria, Australia

Nick Buckley MD FRACP
Associate Professor in Medicine,
Medical Professorial Unit,
POW Hospital Clinical School,
University of New South Wales,
New South Wales, Australia

Simon Byrne BA MBBS FRANZCP
Consultant Psychiatrist,
Departments of Psychiatry and Emergency
Medicine, Sir Charles Gairdner Hospital,
Nedlands, Western Australia,
Clinical Senior Lecturer,
University of Western Australia,
Australia

Adam Bystrzycki MBBS FACEM
Staff Specialist, Emergency Department,
The Alfred Hospital, Prahran, Victoria,
Australia

Mike Cadogan MA MB CHB FACEM
Clinical Senior Lecturer (UWA), Staff
Specialist in Emergency Medicine,
Department of Emergency Medicine,
Sir Charles Gairdner Hospital,
Nedlands, Western Australia, Australia

Peter Cameron MBBS MD FACEM
Professor Emergency Medicine,
Department of Epidemiology and
Preventive Medicine,
Monash University, Alfred Hospital,
Melbourne, Victoria, Australia

Antonio Celenza MBBS MClinEd FACEM
FCEM
Associate Professor of Emergency Medicine,
University of Western Australia,
Crawley, Western Australia, Australia

Betty Chan MB BS FACEM Phd
Emergency Physician & Clinical
Toxicologist, Prince of Wales Hospital,
Randwick, New South Wales,
Australia

Kim Chai Chan MB BS FRCS FAMS
Emergency Medicine, Tan Tock Seng
Hospital, Singapore

Rabind A Charles MBBS FRCS FCEM
Consultant and Residency Director,
Emergency Medicine, Singapore General
Hospital, Singapore
Honorary Fellow, Emergency Medicine,
The Alfred Hospital, Prahran, Victoria,
Australia

Raymond Chi Hung Cheng MRCSEd
FHKCEM FHKAM (Emergency Medicine)
Associate Consultant, Accident and
Emergency Department, Shatin NT,
Prince of Wales Hospital,
Honorary Clinical Assistant Professor,
Chinese University, Hong Kong, SAR,
China

Matthew WG Chu MB BS FACEM
Director of Emergency Medicine,
Canterbury Hospital, Sydney South West
Area Health Service, Campsie,
New South Wales, Australia

Chin Hung Chung MB BS FRCS FACS FCSHK
FHKCEM FHKAM FIFEM
Chief-of-Service, Accident & Emergency
Department, North District Hospital,
New Territories, Hong Kong,
China

Flavia Cicuttini MBBS PhD MSc DLSHTM
FRACP FAFPHM
Head, Musculoskeletal Unit DEPM, Head
Rheumatology Unit, Alfred Hospital,
Department of Epidemiology and
Preventive Medicine, Monash University,
Alfred Hospital, Melbourne, Victoria,
Australia

Michael Coman MB BS FACEM
Emergency Department, Sunshine
Hospital, St Albans. Victoria

Geoff Couser FACEM Grad Cert ULT
Emergency Physician, Royal Hobart
Hospital, Hobart, Tasmania, Australia,
Clinical Senior Lecturer, Discipline of
Medicine, Faculty of Health Science,
University of Tasmania, Australia

Roslyn Crampton MB BS
Staff Specialist in Emergency Medicine,
Director of Clinical Training, Westmead
Hospital, Wentworthville, NSW,
Australia

Frank Daly MB BS FACEM
Emergency Physician and Clinical
Toxicologist, Royal Perth Hospital,
Perth, Western Australia, Australia

Suresh S David MS(Surg) MPhil FACEM(Hon)
Professor, Emergency Department,
Christian Medical College Hospital,
Vellore, India

The late Andrew Dent MBBS FRCS FACEM
MPH
Formerly, Clinical Associate Professor,
Formerly, Director, Emergency Medicine,
St. Vincent's Health, Fitzroy, Victoria,
Australia

Stuart Dilley MBBS FACEM
Emergency Physician, St Vincent's Hospital,
Senior Fellow, Department of Medicine,
Dentistry and Health Sciences,
University of Melbourne, Victoria,
Australia

Jenny Dowd MD BS FRANZCOG
Specialist, Royal Women's Hospital,
Carlton, Victoria, Australia

Robert Dowsett BM BS FACEM
Senior Staff Specialist of Emergency
Medicine and Clinical Toxicologist,
Westmead Hospital, Westmead,
New South Wales, Australia

Martin Duffy MBBS MMed (Clin Epi) FACEM
Emergency Physician, Department of
Emergency Medicine, St Vincent's Hospital,
Sydney, New South Wales, Australia

Robert Dunn MB BS FACEM
Associate Professor & Director of
Emergency Medicine, Royal Adelaide
Hospital, Adelaide, South Australia,
Australia

Linas Dziukas MB BS MD FRACP FACEM
Emergency Physician, The Alfred
Hospital, Prahran, Victoria,
Australia

David Eddey MB BS DipRACOG FACEM
Director of Emergency Medicine, The
Geelong Hospital, Geelong,
Victoria, Australia

Robert Edwards MB BS FACEM
Staff Specialist in Emergency Medicine,
Westmead Hospital, Wentworthville, New
South Wales, Australia

Tor Ercleve BSc MB CHB
Senior Registrar, Department of Emergency Medicine, Sir Charles Gairdner Hospital, Nedlands, Perth, Western Australia

Karen Falk MB BS FRACR
Radiologist, Sydney X-Ray, Randwick CT and MRI, Randwick, New South Wales, Australia

Daniel M Fatovich MBBS FACEM
Associate Professor of Emergency Medicine, Centre for Clinical Research in Emergency Medicine, Western Australian Institute for Medical Research; University of Western Australia Centre for Medical Research; University of Western Australia, Royal Perth Hospital, Perth, Western Australia

Mark Fitzgerald ASM MB BS FACEM MRACMA
Director of Emergency Services, The Alfred Hospital, Prahran, Victoria, Australia

Peter Freeman MB ChB FRCS FCEM FACEM
Director of Emergency Medicine, Wellington Hospital, Wellington, New Zealand

James Galbraith MB BS FRANZCO FRACS
Ophthalmology Department, Royal Melbourne Hospital, Parkville, Victoria, Australia

G Michael Galvin BSC MB BS DTM&H FACEM
Emeritus Consultant in Emergency Medicine, Fremantle Hospital, Fremantle, Western Australia

Peter Garrett BSC MBBS FACEM FJFICM
Senior Lecturer University of Queensland, Senior staff specialist intensive care, Nambour Hospital, Sunshine Coast and Cooloola Health Service District, Nambour, Queensland, Australia

Michael Gingold MB BS BMEDSC
Rheumatology Registrar, Monash Medical Centre, Clayton, Victoria, Australia

Corinne Ginifer MB BS DipRACOG DA(UK) FACEM
Staff Specialist, Emergency Medicine, North West Regional Hospital, Burnie, Tasmania, Australia

Robert Gocentas MB BS FACEM
Emergency Department, The Alfred Hospital, Prahran, Victoria, Australia

Neil Goldie MB BS(Hons) FACEM
Emergency Physician, St Vincent's Hospital, Fitzroy, Victoria, Australia

Steve Goodacre MB ChB MRCP FCEM MSc PhD
Professor of Emergency Medicine, University of Sheffield, Medical Care Research Unit, Sheffield, United Kingdom

Adrian Goudie MB BS FACEM DDU
Emed Ultrasound, Wahroonga, NSW, Australia

Colin A Graham MB ChB MPH MD FRCS FCEM FHKCEM
Professor, Accident and Emergency Medicine Academic Unit, Trauma and Emergency Centre, Chinese University of Hong Kong, Prince of Wales Hospital, Shatin NT, Hong Kong SAR, China

Andis Graudins MB BS PHD FACEM
Senior Lecturer, Department of Medicine, University of New South Wales; Consultant Emergency Physician and Clinical Toxocologist, Prince of Wales Hospital, Randwick, New South Wales, Australia

Tim Gray MB BS FACEM
Staff Specialist, Emergency Department, The Royal Melbourne Hospital, Parkville, Victoria, Australia

Digby Green FACEM
Registrar in Emergency Medicine and Clinical Toxicology, Prince of Wales Clinical School, Prince of Wales Hospital, Randwick, NSW, Australia

Naren Gunja
Deputy Medical Director, NSW Poisons Information Centre, Clinical Toxicologist and Emergency Physician, Department of Emergency Medicine, Westmead Hospital, Sydney, New South Wales, Australia
Director of Emergency Ultrasound & Senior Staff Specialist in Emergency Medicine, Liverpool Hospital, Liverpool, New South Wales

Andrew Haig MBBS FACEM FCEM DDU
Director of Emergency Ultrasound & Senior Staff Specialist in Emergency Medicine Liverpool Hospital, Liverpool, New South Wales, Australia

Lim Swee Han
Senior Consultant and Head, Department of Emergency Medicine, Singapore General Hospital, Singapore General Hospital, Singapore

Richard D Hardern MB ChB FRCP(Ed) FCEM
Consultant & Honorary Clinical Lecturer, Emergency Medicine, University Hospital of North Durham, Durham, United Kingdom

Roger Harris MB BS FACEM
Emergency Physician, Royal North Shore Hospital, University of Sydney, St Leonards, New South Wales, Australia

James Hayes MB BS FACEM
Staff Specialist, The Northern Hospital, Epping, Victoria, Australia

Wayne Hazell DipObs FACEM
Head of Emergency Medicine Education and Research, Middlemore Hospital, Clinical Senior Lecturer, Auckland University, Auckland, New Zealand

Kenneth Heng MBBS FRCS (Edin), FAMS
Consultant, Emergency Medicine, Tan Tock Seng Hospital, Singapore

Ruth Hew MB BS FACEM
Staff Specialist, Department of Emergency Medicine, Sunshine Hospital, St Albans, Victoria, Australia

Rosslyn Hing MBBS FACEM
Emergency Physician, Department of Medicine, Royal Prince Alfred Hospital, Camperdown, New South Wales, Australia

Anna Holdgate MBBS (Hons) FACEM MMed
Director, Emergency Medicine Research Unit, Liverpool Hospital, Liverpool New South Wales, Australia

CONTRIBUTORS

Craig Hore MBBS FACEM FJFICM
Senior Staff Specialist, Intensive Care Unit,
The Wollongong Hospital, NSW,
Australia

Sue Ieraci MB BS FACEM
Senior Staff Specialist Emergency Medicine,
Bankstown Hospital, Bankstown,
New South Wales, Australia

Geoff Isbister BSc MB BS FACEM MD
Clinical Toxocologist and Emergency
Physician, Calvary Mater Hospital,
Newcastle, New South Wales,
Australia

Trevor Jackson MBBS FACEM
Emergency Physician, Sir Charles
Gairdner Hospital, Nedlands WA,
Australia

George Jelinek MB BS MD MD DipDHM
FACEM
Professor of Emergency Medicine,
University of Western Australia,
Sir Charles Gairdner Hospital,
Nedlands, Western Australia,
Australia

Daryl A Jones BSC MB BS
Intensive Care Specialist,
Intensive Care Unit, Austin Hospital,
Honorary Research Fellow,
Department of Epidemiology and
Preventative Medicine, Monash University,
Victoria, Australia

Anthony P Joseph MB BS FACEM
Emergency Physician, Royal North Shore
Hospital, University of Sydney,
St Leonards, New South Wales,
Australia

David Kaufman FRACS FRANZCO
Ophthalmology Department,
Royal Melbourne Hospital,
Parkville, Victoria, Australia

Anne-Maree Kelly MD MClinEd FACEM
Director, Joseph Epstein Centre for
Emergency Medicine Research,
Western Health, Professional Fellow,
University of Melbourne, Victoria,
Australia

Fergus Kerr MB BS FACEM MPH
Emergency Physician and Clinical
Toxicologist, Emergency Department,
Austin Hospital, Heidelberg,
Victoria, Australia

Diane King MBBS FACEM
Director, Emergency Services,
Southern Adelaide Health Service,
South Australia,
Australia

Jonathan C Knott MB BS FACEM
Head of Education and Research,
Emergency Department,
Royal Melbourne Hospital, Parkville,
Victoria, Australia

Ian Knox MB BS FACEM
Specialist in Emergency Medicine,
The Wesley Hospital, Toowong,
Queensland, Australia

Zeff Koutsogiannis MBBS FACEM G Cert
CLIN TOX
Emergency Physician, Department of
Emergency Medicine, Western Hospital,
Footscray, Victoria, Australia

Sashi Kumar MBBS DLO FACEM
Senior Staff Specialist,
Department of Emergency Medicine,
The Canberra Hospital, ACT,
Australia

Marian Lee MB BS DCH FACEM MHA
Emergency Physician, Senior Staff
Specialist, Director of Emergency Medicine
Training, Prince of Wales Hospital,
Randwick, New South Wales,
Australia

Julie Leung MBBS FACEM
Emergency Physician, Department of
Emergency Medicine, St Vincent's Hospital,
Sydney, New South Wales, Australia

David Lightfoot MB BS FACEM
Staff Specialist, Emergency Department,
Monash Medical Centre, Clayton,
Victoria, Australia

Mark Little MB BS FACEM MPH&TM
DTM&H
Emergency Physician and Clinical
Toxicologist, Director Department of
Emergency Medicine, Caboolture Hospital,
Caboolture Queensland,
Australia

David McCoubrie MB BS FACEM
Emergency Physician and Clinical
Toxicologist, Sir Charles Gairdner
Hospital, Nedlands, Western Australia,
Australia

Alastair McGowan OBE FRCP FRCS FRCA
FFAEM
Consultant in Emergency Medicine,
St James's University Hospital,
Leeds, United Kingdom

Lewis Macken MBBS FACEM FJFICM
Senior Staff Specialist, Intensive Care Unit,
Royal North Shore Hospital,
St Leonards, New South Wales,
Australia

Hamish Maclaren MA BSC MBChB MRCGP
FACEM
Honorary Senior Lecturer in Emergency
Medicine and Distance Learning,
University of Auckland, New Zealand,
Rural Practitioner, Aberfoyle Medical
Centre, Aberfoyle, UK

Andrew Maclean MB BS FACEM
Director, Emergency Services,
Box Hill Hospital, Box Hill, Victoria,
Australia

John E Maguire MB BS DipObs RACOG
FACEM
Assistant Director, Division of Emergency
Medicine, John Hunter Hospital,
New Lambton, New South Wales, Australia

Shin-Yan Man MMedSc FRCSEd FHKCEM
FHKAM
Associate Consultant, Accident and
Emergency Department, Prince of Wales
Hospial, Shatin, NT Hong Kong SAR,
China

Paul Mark MB BS DipRACOG FACEM
DipDHM MRACMA AFCHSE
Acting Executive Director,
Royal Perth Hospital,
Western Australia, Australia

Suzanne Mason MB BS FRCS FFAEM MD
Reader in Emergency Medicine,
Health Services Research Section,
School of Health and Related Research,
University of Sheffield, Sheffield,
United Kingdom

Dev Mitra MB BS
Emergency Department, The Alfred
Hospital, Prahran, Victoria, Australia

Mark P. Monaghan MBBS FACEM
Emergency Physician and Clinical
Toxocologist, Fremantle Hospital, Nedlands,
Western Australia,
Australia

Vanessa Morgan MBBS FACD
Dermatology Department, Royal
Melbourne Hospital, Parkville,
Victoria, Australia

Alfredo Mori MB BS FACEM
Emergency Department, The Alfred
Hospital, Prahran, Victoria,
Australia

Francis P Morris MBBS MRCP
Consultant, Emergency Department,
Northern General Hospital, Sheffield,
United Kingdom

David Mountain MB BS FACEM
Associate Professor, University of Western
Australia, Sir Charles Gairdner Hospital,
Nedlands, Western Australia,
Australia

Venita Munir MBBS(Hons) FACEM
Staff Specialist Emergency Physician,
Emergency Department, St Vincent's
Hospital, Fitzroy, Victoria, Australia,
Honorary Fellow (Lecturer),
University of Melbourne, Parkville,
Victoria, Australia

Lindsay Murray MB BS FACEM
Emergency Physician and Clinical
Toxicologist, Sir Charles Gairdner Hospital,
Nedlands, Western Australia,
Australia

Sandra Neate MBBS DipROCOG DA
FACEM
Emergency Physician, Emergency
Department, St Vincent's Hospital,
Fitzroy, Victoria, Honorary Fellow,
Department of Medicine, University of
Melbourne, Victoria, Australia

Debra O'Brien MB BS FACEM
Director, Emergency Medicine,
Sir Charles Gairdner Hospital, Nedlands,
Western Australia, Australia

Marcus Eng Hock Ong MBBS MPH FAMS
Consultant, Director of Research and Senior
Medical Scientist, Department of
Emergency Medicine, Singapore General
Hospital, Adjunct Associate Professor,
Duke-NUS Graduate Medical School,
Office of Research, Singapore

Ken Ooi MB BS FACEM
Director of Emergency Medicine,
The Queen Elizabeth Hospital,
Woodville South, South Australia

Shirley Beng Suat Ooi MBBS(S'pore) FRCSE
(A&E) FAMS(Emerg Med)
Clinical Associate Professor, Chief/Senior
Consultant, Emergency Medicine
Department, National University Hospital,
Singapore

Gerard M O'Reilly MBBS FACEM MPH
MBiostat
Emergency Staff Specialist, Director of
International Programs, Emergency
and Trauma Centre The Alfred Hospital,
Prahran, Victoria, Australia

Debbie Paltridge BappSc(Phyt)
MHlthSc(Ed)
Education Consultant, Health Education
Innovative Solutions,
Carindale, Queensland, Australia

Helen Parker MB BS FACEM DMJ(Clin)
Staff Specialist, Department of Emergency
Medicine, Western Hospital,
Footscray, Victoria, Division of Clinical
Forensic Medicine, Victorian Institute of
Forensic Medicine, Southbank,
Victoria, Australia

John Pasco MB BS FACEM DA(UK) Dip RACOG
BSc(Hons) DipEd
Emergency Department, The Geelong
Hospital, Geelong, Victoria,
Australia

Georgina Phillips MB BS FACEM
Emergency Physician, Emergency
Department, St Vincent's Hospital,
Fitzroy, Victoria, Australia

Stephen Priestley MB BS FACEM
Director, Department of Emergency
Medicine, Sunshine Hospital,
St Albans, Victoria,
Australia

Mark Putland MBBS
Emergency Physician, Yeronga,
Queensland, Australia

Timothy Rainer MD BSC MRCP
Professor, Chinese University of Hong Kong,
Director, Accident and Emergency
Medicine Academic Unit, Chief of Service,
Department of Accident and Emergency
Medicine, Trauma and Emergency
Centre, Prince of Wales Hospital,
Shatin, NT Hong Kong SAR,
China

Drew Richardson MB BS(Hons) FACEM
Emergency Department, The Canberra
Hospital, Garran, ACT, Australia

Darren M Roberts MBBS PhD
South Asian Clinical Toxicology Research
Collaboration, University of Peradeniya,
Sri Lanka, Department of Clinical
Pharmacology and Toxicology,
The Canberra Hospital, ACT, Australia

Ian Rogers MB BS FACEM
Director of Post Graduate Medical
Education and Research, Associate
Professor of Emergency Medicine,
University of Western Australia,
Sir Charles Gairdner Hospital, Nedlands,
WA, Australia

Pamela Rosengarten MB BS FACEM
Associate Professor
Monash Medical Centre, Clayton Victoria,
Australia

John M. Ryan FRCS Ed(A&E) FFAEM DCH
DipSportsMed
Consultant in Emergency Medicine, St
Vincent's University Hospital, Dublin,
Ireland

Eillyne Seow MBBS FRCS(Edin) FAMS
Head/Senior Consultant, Divisional
Chairman, Ambulatory & Diagnostic
Medicine, Emergency Medicine, Tan Tock
Seng Hospital, Singapore

Andrew Singer MBBS FACEM
Principal Medical Adviser, Australian
Government Department of Health and
Ageing, Senior Specialist in Emergency
Medicine, The Canberra Hospital, Garran,
ACT, Australia

David Smart BMedSci MBBS (Hons-1) MD
(UTAS) FACEM FIFEM FAICD FACTM Dip DHM
Medical Co-director, Department of Diving
and Hyperbaric Medicine, Royal Hobart
Hospital, Hobart, Tasmania, Australia

David Spain MBBS FRACGP FACEM
Deputy Director, Department of Emergency,
Gold Coast Hospital, Southport,
Queensland, Australia

Peter Sprivulis MBBS PHD FACEM FACHI
Clinical Associate Professor, Department
of Emergency Medicine, University of
Western Australia, Crawley,
WA, Australia

Liz Steel MBChB BMedSci MRCP FJFICM
Staff Specialist, Intensive Care Medicine,
Royal North Shore Hospital, Sydney,
Australia

Helen E Stergiou BSc MSc MBBS FACEM
Acting Director, Emergency Department,
Northern Hospital, Epping, Victoria,
Australia

Alan C Street MB BS FRACP
Deputy Director, Victorian Infectious
Disease Service, The Royal Melbourne
Hospital, Parkville, Victoria, Australia

Janet Talbot-Stern BA MA MD FACEM
FACEP
Senior Staff Specialist, Royal Prince Alfred
Hospital, Sydney: Clinical Senior Lecturer,
Department of Surgery, University of
Sydney, New South Wales, Australia

Gim Tan MBBS MRACMA FACEM
Staff Specialist, Director of Emergency
Medicine Training, Emergency and Trauma
Centre, The Alfred Hospital, Melbourne,
Australia

David McD Taylor MD MPH DRCOG FACEM
Director of Emergency Medicine Research,
Royal Melbourne Hospital, Parkville,
Victoria, Australia

James Taylor MB BS FACEM
Emergency Department, Sandringham &
District Memorial Hospital, Sandringham,
Victoria, Australia

Wee Siong Teo MBBS(NUS) MMed FRCP(Edin)
FACC FHRS
Senior Consultant and Director,
Electrophysiology and Pacing,
Department of Cardiology, National Heart
Centre, Singapore

Graeme Thomson MB BS FACEM
Department of Emergency Medicine,
Monash Medical Centre, Clayton,
Victoria, Australia

Gino Toncich MB BS(Hons) Dip Anaes MBA
FACEM
Staff Specialist, Emergency Department,
The Alfred Hospital, Prahran, Victoria,
Australia

Greg Treston BMedSci MBBS DTMH
DIMCRCS FACRRM FACEM
Staff Specialist, Emergency Medicine,
Redcliffe Hospital, Queensland,
Australia

Steven Troupakis MB BS DipRACOG FACEM
Staff Specialist, Emergency Medicine,
Monash Medical Centre, Clayton, Victoria,
Australia

Anthony Tzannes MBBS
Senior Registrar, Department of Emergency
Medicine, Sir Charles Gairdner Hospital,
Perth, Australia

Edward Upjohn MBBS MMed FACD
Dermatology Surgery Fellow, University of
Texas Southwestern, Dallas, Texas, USA

George Varigos MBBS PhD FACD
Dermatology Department, Royal
Melbourne Hospital, Parkville, Victoria,
Australia

John Vinen MB BS MHP FACEM FIFEM
Senior Staff Specialist, Blue Mountains
District Anzac Memorial Hospital,
Katoomba, New South Wales, Australia

Abel Wakai MD FRCSI FCEM
Emergency Medical Services (EMS) Fellow,
Division of Emergency Medicine,
Sunnybrook Health Sciences Centre,
Toronto, Canada

Andrew Walby MB BS DipRACOG FACEM
Staff Specialist, Department of Emergency
Medicine, Western Hospital, Footscray,
Victoria, Australia

Mark J Walland MB BS FRANZCO FRACS
Ophthalmology Department, Royal
Melbourne Hospital, Parkville, Victoria,
Australia

Richard Waller MB BS BMedSci FACEM
Staff Specialist, Emergency Department,
The Royal Melbourne Hospital, Parkville,
Victoria, Australia

Lee A Wallis MBChB MD FRCSEd FCEM FCEM
(SA)
Head: Division of Emergency Medicine,
University of Cape Town, Head: Emergency
Medicine, Provincial Government of the
Western Cape, Rondebosch, South Africa

Bryan G Walpole MB BS FRCS FACEM DTM&H
Senior Lecturer in Emergency Medicine,
University of Tasmania, Australia

The late Jeff Wassertheil CStJ MB BS
FACEM MRACMA MACLM Cert IV Workplace
Assess&Train
Director of Emergency Medicine, Peninsula
Health, Frankston, Victoria, Australia

Garry J Wilkes MB BS FACEM
Director of Emergency Medicine, WA
Country Health Service, Bunbury, Medical
Director, St John Ambulance WA, Belmont,
Clinical Associate Professor, Rural Clinical
School, University of Western Australia
Adjunct Associate Professor, Edith Cowan
University, Perth, Western Australia,
Australia

Aled Williams MBChB MRCGP FACEM
MPH&TM
Staff Specialist, Department of Emergency
Medicine, Sir Charles Gairdner Hospital,
Nedlands, Western Australia,
Australia

Simon Wood MB BS DipPaed(NSW) FACEM
Director of Emergency Medicine,
Joondalup Health Campus, Joondalup,
Western Australia,
Australia

Peter Wright MB BS FACEM
Staff Specialist, Maroondah Hospital,
Ringwood East, Victoria, Australia,
Australia

Kim Yates MBChB MMedSc FACEM
Emergency Medicine Specialist, North
Shore Hospital, Takapuna, North Shore City,
New Zealand

Anusch Yazdani MB BS FRANZCOG
Staff Specialist Gynaecology, Mater
Hospitals Complex, South Brisbane,
Queensland, Australia

Simon Young MB BS FACEM
Director Emergency Department, Royal
Children's Hospital, Parkville, Victoria,
Australia

Allen Yuen MB BS(Hons) FRACEP FACEM
Associate Professor, Monash University,
Director of Emergency Medicine,
Epworth Hospital, Richmond,
Victoria, Senior Examiner ACEM, Australia

Allen Yung MB BS OAM FRACP
Specialist in Infectious Diseases,
Royal Melbourne Hospital,
Parkville, Victoria,
Australia

Salomon Zalstein MB BS BMed Sc FACEM
Director of Emergency Medicine,
Bendigo Hospital, Bendigo,
Victoria, Australia

Contents

CONTENTS

CONTENTS

CONTENTS

RESUSCITATION

Edited by *Anthony F. T. Brown*

SECTION 1

1.1 Basic life support

Stephen Bernard

ESSENTIALS

1 The patient with sudden out-of-hospital cardiac arrest requires a bystander to institute the 'Chain of Survival', including an immediate call to emergency medical services and the initiation of cardiopulmonary resuscitation.

2 Recent evidence suggests that for patients in cardiac arrest of primary cardiac cause external chest compressions alone may be superior to external chest compressions plus expired air resuscitation.

3 Early defibrillation is essential in ventricular fibrillation, and should be regarded as a part of basic life support.

4 Earlier defibrillation may be provided using co-responders to ambulance services, such as firefighters.

5 Early defibrillation may be also delivered by untrained or minimally trained bystanders (public access defibrillation).

Introduction

The patient with sudden out-of-hospital sudden cardiac arrest requires a bystander to initiate a number of actions in rapid sequence for any hope of a successful resuscitation. These steps are known as the 'Chain of Survival'.[1]

Chain of survival

The first step is a call to the emergency medical services (EMS) system. The bystander then needs to institute basic life support (BLS) while awaiting the arrival of EMS. The BLS procedures may be undertaken by personnel with little or no training. For the latter, most EMS dispatch centres are able to provide bystander CPR instructions via the telephone.

BLS generally includes interventions that involve minimal use of ancillary equipment, but may now include the application of a semi-automatic external defibrillator (SAED) if one is available close to the site of the cardiac arrest.

This chapter describes the current approach to BLS delivered by the bystander while awaiting the arrival of EMS or medical expertise that will be able to provide advanced life support (ALS) skills (see Ch. 1.2).

Development of protocols

The guidelines for BLS must be evidence based and consistent across a wide range of providers. Many countries have established national committees to advise community groups, ambulance services and the medical profession on appropriate BLS guidelines. Table 1.1.1 shows the national associations that make up the International Liaison Committee on Resuscitation (ILCOR). This group meets every 5 years to review the BLS guidelines and to consider the scientific evidence that may lead to changes.

The most recent revision of the BLS guidelines occurred in 2005 and consisted of a comprehensive evaluation of the scientific literature for each aspect of BLS. Evidence evaluation worksheets were developed (available at www.c2005.org) and were then considered by ILCOR. The final recommendations were published in late 2005.[2]

Australian Resuscitation Council (ARC) BLS guidelines

Subsequently, each national committee endorsed the guidelines, with minor regional variations to take into account local practices. The recommendations of the Australian Resuscitation Council (ARC) on BLS were published in 2006.[3–6]

1

Table 1.1.1 Membership of the International Liaison Committee on Resuscitation (ILCOR)
American Heart Association
Australian Resuscitation Council
European Resuscitation Council
Heart and Stroke Foundation of Canada
Inter-American Heart Foundation
New Zealand Resuscitation Council
Resuscitation Council of Southern Africa

New Zealand Resuscitation Council (NZRC) BLS guidelines

The New Zealand Resuscitation Guidelines were also endorsed in 2006 (available at http://www.nzrc.org.nz/).

Initial evaluation: DR ABCD approach

A flowchart for the initial evaluation of the collapsed patient is shown in Figure 1.1.1.

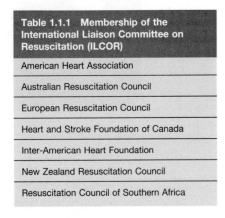

Basic life support flow chart

D — Check for **danger**

Hazards/risks/safety?

R — **Responsive?** (unconscious?)

If not, call for help
Call 000/Resuscitation team

A — Open **airway**
Look for signs of life

B — Give 2 initial **breaths**, if not breathing normally

C — Give 30 chest **compressions** (almost 2 compressions/second) followed by 2 breaths

D — Attach **AED** as soon as available and follow its prompts

Continue **CPR** until qualified personnel arrive or signs of life return

No signs of life = unconscious, unresponsive, not breathing normally, not moving
AED = automated external defibrillator

Fig. 1.1.1 Basic life support (BLS) flowchart algorithm.

It includes checking for danger, assessing responsiveness, then opening the airway, giving breaths and cardiac compressions, and attaching an automated defibrillator as soon as possible. This is known as the 'DR ABCD' approach. CPR is continued until qualified personnel arrive or signs of life return.[6]

The process commences with the recognition that a patient has collapsed and is unresponsive. The initial steps are as follows.

Check for dangers

As the patient is approached, the bystander should immediately consider any dangers that may be associated with the collapse of the patient. For example, the patient may have been electrocuted and there could be injuries to bystanders if the power source is not switched off prior to patient contact.

There may be a significant danger from collision with a passing vehicle in the case of a motor-vehicle accident where a patient is unconscious, as well as the potential risk of fire. Therefore, unless they are trapped, unconscious patients should be carefully removed from the vehicle prior to the arrival of emergency medical services, taking care to minimize movement of the neck unless they are trapped. It is considered that the risk of injury from fire or explosion exceeds the risk of moving an unconscious patient prior to immobilization of the cervical spine with a neck collar.

In the case of a patient who has collapsed in a confined space, the possibility of poisoning with a toxic gas such as carbon monoxide should be considered. Do not enter the scene until it can be made safe by emergency services, usually the fire brigade.

Finally, in current times of potential terrorist attack, if multiple victims are present, consider the possibility of the use of a chemical agent such as an organophosphate causing collapse and cardiac arrest. In this setting bystanders should immediately leave the area and await the arrival of EMS and a specialist hazardous agent team.

Check for response

The patient who has collapsed must be rapidly assessed to determine whether there is unconsciousness, indicating possible cardiac arrest. This is assessed by a gentle 'shake and shout' and observation of the patient's response.

Suspect cardiac arrest if the patient is unresponsive to the 'shake and shout', and immediately telephone the emergency medical services ('call first'). Alternatively, if the collapse is due to suspected airway obstruction (choking) or inadequate ventilation (drowning, hanging etc.), then commence resuscitation focusing on the airway for approximately 1 minute before calling the emergency medical services ('call fast').

Airway and breathing

Make an assessment of the airway and breathing if a patient has collapsed and is apparently unconscious.[3,4] Place the patient supine, check the airway by visual inspection, and open the airway with a head-tilt and/or a chin-lift manoeuvre.

Adequate respiration is assessed by visually inspecting the movement of the chest wall and listening for upper airway sounds. Occasional deep (agonal) respirations may continue for some minutes after the initial collapse in cases of cardiac arrest. These respirations are often mistaken for adequate breathing by untrained bystanders.

Cardiopulmonary resuscitation (CPR) will be required if the patient is found to have inadequate or absent breathing on initial assessment. On the other hand, when the initial assessment of an unconscious patient reveals adequate respiration, turn the victim on his/her side and maintain in the semi-prone recovery position. Make constant checks to ensure continued respiration while awaiting the arrival of the EMS.

Circulation

It was traditionally recommended that a bystander should attempt to palpate a pulse in order to diagnose cardiac arrest and, if absent, commence external cardiac compressions (ECC). It is now currently recommended that untrained bystanders do *not* attempt to palpate for a pulse,[5] as there is good evidence that the pulse check is inaccurate in this setting.[7] Therefore, cardiac arrest may instead be presumed if breathing is absent, and is highly likely if breathing is inadequate.

Management

Airway obstruction

Make a careful sweep with a finger if inspection of the airway reveals visible foreign material or vomitus in the upper airway. Take particular care not to be bitten, not to cause pharyngeal trauma, and not to propel material down into the lower airway.

There are a number of manoeuvres proposed to clear the airway if it is completely obstructed by a foreign body. In many countries abdominal thrusts (the Heimlich manoeuvre) are endorsed as the technique of choice. However, this technique is associated with potential complications such as intra-abdominal injury. In Australia the recommended techniques for clearing an airway that is obstructed by a foreign body are back blows and/or chest thrusts. As there is insufficient evidence to recommend one treatment over another, it is recommended that each be tried in succession until the obstruction is relieved.

Cardiopulmonary resuscitation (CPR)

The bystander should immediately commence cardiopulmonary resuscitation (CPR) if cardiac arrest is diagnosed and the EMS has been summoned, using both expired air resuscitation (EAR) and ECC until a defibrillator arrives.[6]

Expired air resuscitation (EAR) or 'rescue breathing'

Since the first description in 1958, EAR has become the standard in BLS for patients who have absent or inadequate respirations. It is now more often referred to as 'rescue breathing'. Two breaths should be delivered initially, followed by chest compressions (see later). Subsequently, deliver two breaths for every 30 chest compressions. However, there is often considerable reluctance by bystanders to perform EAR owing to the perceived difficulty of the procedure, the possibility of cross-infection and its disagreeable aesthetics.

Bystander ECC without EAR

Animal models show that some ventilation occurs during chest compressions, and it has been proposed that EAR may be withheld in adult patients who have a witnessed out-of-hospital cardiac arrest. A recent Japanese observational study (SOS-KANTO) compared the outcome of adult patients with a witnessed out-of-hospital cardiac arrest who received ECC only by bystanders with that of patients who received both EAR and ECC 'conventional CPR', as well as patients who received no bystander CPR.[8] There was a favourable neurological outcome in 6.2% of patients who received ECC only, compared to a 3.1% favourable neurological outcome in the patients who received EAR plus ECC ($P = 0.0195$). Only 2.2% of patients who received no bystander CPR had a favourable neurological outcome. Therefore, a strong case may be made that bystanders perform only ECC and not EAR.[9] However, this recommendation has not currently been endorsed by the Australian Resuscitation Council (ARC).

Simple airway adjuncts in medical facilities

Simple airway equipment may be used as an alternative to EAR when cardiac arrest occurs in a medical facility, such as mouth-to-mask ventilation and bag/valve/mask ventilation, with or without an oropharyngeal Guedel airway. This equipment has the advantage that there is often familiarity and no risk of cross-infection, although prior training in the use of these devices is required.

Whatever technique of assisted ventilation is used, an adequate tidal volume is assessed by the rise of the victim's chest, and by listening and feeling for air being exhaled from the patient's mouth. Also observe whether there is any distension of the stomach. Cease chest compressions briefly to allow ventilation in the absence of an advanced airway device such as an endotracheal tube.

The use of supplemental oxygen is increasingly considered part of BLS airway and breathing management. Although there are few data on outcome, it is intuitive that supplemental oxygen during CPR would increase the oxygen content of the blood and hence oxygen delivery to the brain and heart.

External cardiac compressions (ECC)

Place the patient supine on a firm surface such as a backboard, firm mattress or even the floor to optimize the effectiveness of chest compressions. Perform compressions that allow equal time for the compression and relaxation phases, with compression being approximately 50% of the cycle. Depress the lower sternum at least 4–5 cm in the adult, with complete recoil of the chest after each compression. Perform ECC at a rate of 100 compressions per minute, to ensure the delivery of a minimum of about 80 compressions per minute when accounting for the period spent on ventilations.[5] Recommendations are essentially to *push hard, push fast, allow complete release and minimize interruptions*.

'Thoracic pump' mechanism

There is still debate as to whether ECC generates blood flow via a 'cardiac pump' mechanism or a 'thoracic pump' mechanism. The thoracic pump theory is supported by transthoracic echocardiography performed during CPR demonstrating that the cardiac valves remain open during the relaxation phase of ECC. Also, forceful coughing during CPR has been observed to result in sufficient blood flow to maintain consciousness. The changes in intrathoracic pressure are presumed to lead to forward blood flow, with valves in the venous system preventing back flow.

'Cardiac pump' mechanism

However, more recent studies of transoesophageal echocardiography during ECC in humans found that during the compression phase the left ventricle is compressed, the mitral valve remains closed, and the aortic valve opens only at the end of compression. During the relaxation phase the mitral valve opens and the left ventricle fills. These findings suggest that blood flows during ECC as a result of cardiac compression.

Whatever the predominant mechanism of blood flow, ECC results in only about 20% of cardiac output in the adult, mainly owing to the relative rigidity of the chest wall. Consequently, there is a progressive metabolic acidosis due to inadequate oxygen delivery during CPR. Few adults survive a cardiac arrest when ECC has been given for more than 30 minutes. Thus, most EMS allow paramedics to cease resuscitation if a patient in cardiac arrest has failed to respond to CPR and advanced life support measures after 30 minutes, provided there are no extraordinary circumstances such as hypothermia or drug overdose. See also Ch. 1.2 on Advanced Life Support.

Defibrillation

Semi-automatic external defibrillation (SAED)

The semi-automatic external defibrillation (SAED) is now considered part of BLS. SAED devices are extremely accurate in diagnosing ventricular fibrillation or ventricular tachycardia, and are relatively simple for bystanders to use with minimal training. After switching the device on and applying the pads, the SAED will request confirmation of coma and absent respirations, and advise the bystander to 'stand clear'. The bystander is then advised to manually press a button to deliver a shock.

Most SAEDs have an algorithm that initially requests the delivery of three countershocks if ventricular fibrillation persists. As the recent ILCOR guidelines now recommend a single shock followed by 1 minute of CPR (except when using a manual defibrillator at a witnessed arrest), it is expected that SAEDs will progressively have their electronics upgraded to follow the new recommendations.[2]

Non-medical personnel and the SAED

Other first responders

A range of situations is proposed where non-medical personnel might use a SAED. Thus, the SAED may be used by first responders such as fire services, who co-respond with ambulance services. In Canada, the state of Ontario implemented an extensive programme to introduce rapid defibrillation across the state.[10] The use of fire department first responders resulted in 92.5% of cardiac arrest patients being defibrillated in under 8 minutes, compared to 76.7% under the previous system ($P<0.001$). Survival to hospital discharge improved from 3.9% (183/4690 patients) to 5.2% (85/1614 patients) ($P = 0.03$). This study demonstrates that an inexpensive, multifaceted, optimized systems approach to rapid defibrillation can lead to significant improvements in survival after cardiac arrest.

A study of a fire-service first-responder programme in Melbourne, Australia, found

that the time to defibrillation was reduced from a mean of 7.1 minutes for ambulance services to 6.0 minutes for a combined approach.[11] However, this study was not powered to assess the impact on patient outcome.

Public area SAED

Alternatively, the SAED may be placed in a public area for use by designated personnel, such as security staff who undergo a short training programme. This approach has been shown to be effective in places with large at-risk populations, such as casinos.[12]

Public-access SAED

The SAED may be placed in a public area for use by personnel with no previous training at all in their use. At Chicago airport defibrillators were placed in strategic locations, with signs advising on their correct use.[13] Over a 2-year period there were 21 patients with cardiac arrest, of whom 18 had an initial rhythm of ventricular fibrillation. A defibrillator was applied by a 'good Samaritan' bystander in 14 of these 18 patients and 11 were successfully resuscitated. Ten patients were alive and well 1 year later.

Shopping centres and apartment buildings

In a larger study,[14] SAEDs were placed in 993 sites such as shopping centres and apartment buildings. More patients survived to hospital discharge when the units were assigned to volunteers trained in CPR *plus* using an AED (30 survivors among 128 arrests) than when the units were assigned to have volunteers trained in CPR only (15 among 107; $P = 0.03$). However, as most cardiac arrests occur at home or when 'out and about', the widespread implementation of this approach to all public areas would be costly and result in relatively few lives saved.[15]

Home SAED

Finally, a SAED may be placed in the home of a patient who is at increased risk of sudden cardiac arrest, for use by a relative who might witness the event. However, a recent study that enrolled 7001 patients concluded that survival rates from sudden cardiac arrest at home were not increased when a defibrillator was available in the home.[16]

Implantable defibrillator insertion

Clearly, patients at highest immediate risk of unexpected cardiac arrest should have an implantable defibrillator inserted. Although most patients with an implanted defibrillator remain conscious during defibrillation, CPR should be commenced if the patient fails to respond to the device's countershocks and becomes comatose. In such cases, intermittent firing of the implanted defibrillator presents no additional risk to the bystanders or medical personnel.

BLS summary

Basic life support for a patient with sudden cardiac arrest has been described in terms of a 'Chain of Survival'. This includes recognition of cardiac arrest, a call to emergency medical services, the performance of cardiopulmonary resuscitation and, when available, early defibrillation using a semi-automatic external defibrillator.

Changes to BLS

The main recent change to basic life support is the so-called DR ABCD approach: the performance of chest compressions at a rate of 100 per minute, with 30 compressions followed by two ventilations, or '30:2', with no pause to determine the presence or absence of a pulse.[16] The exceptions to this are resuscitation of the newborn (use a 3:1 ratio of 90 compressions and 30 inflations to achieve 120 'events' per minute); and endotracheally intubated victims (use a ratio of 15:1 in adults and 15:2 in children). Also pulse checks and recovery checks are no longer performed, and CPR is only interrupted when signs of a return of spontaneous circulation are present.[17]

BLS controversies

- External cardiac compressions *without* expired air resuscitation/rescue breathing

- How external cardiac compressions cause blood to circulate

- The role of public access SAEDs, with or without first-responder training

---

References

1. Cummins RO, Ornato JP, Thies WH, Pepe PE. Improving survival from sudden cardiac arrest: The 'chain of survival' concept. A statement for health professionals from the advanced cardiac life-support subcommittee and the emergency cardiac care committee, American Heart Association. Circulation 1991; 83: 1832–1847.
2. International Liaison Committee on Resuscitation 2005. International consensus on cardiopulmonary resuscitation and emergency cardiovascular care science with treatment recommendations. Resuscitation 2005; 67: 181–341.
3. Australian Resuscitation Council. Airway: Australian Resuscitation Council Guideline 2006. Emergency Medicine Australasia 2006; 18: 325–327.
4. Australian Resuscitation Council. Breathing: Australian Resuscitation Council Guideline 2006. Emergency Medicine Australasia 2006; 18: 328–329.
5. Australian Resuscitation Council. Compressions: Australian Resuscitation Council Guideline 2006. Emergency Medicine Australasia 2006; 18: 330–331.
6. Australian Resuscitation Council. Cardiopulmonary resuscitation: Australian Resuscitation Council Guideline 2006. Emergency Medicine Australasia 2006; 18: 332–334.
7. Bahr J, Klingler H, Panzer W, et al. Skills of lay people in checking the carotid pulse. Resuscitation 1997; 35: 23–26.
8. SOS-KANTO study group. Cardiopulmonary resuscitation by bystanders with chest compression only (SOS-KANTO): an observational study. Lancet 2007; 369: 920–926.
9. Ewy GA. Cardiac arrest – guideline changes urgently needed. Lancet 2007; 369: 882–884.
10. Stiell IG, Wells GA, Field BJ, et al. Improved out-of-hospital cardiac arrest survival through the inexpensive optimization of an existing defibrillation program. Journal of the American Medical Association 1999; 281: 1175–1181.
11. Smith KL, McNeill JJ, Emergency Medical Response Steering Committee. Cardiac arrests treated by ambulance paramedics and fire fighters. Medical Journal of Australia 2002; 177: 305–309.
12. Valenzuela T, Roe TJ, Nichol G, et al. Outcomes of rapid defibrillation by security officers after cardiac arrests in casinos. New England Journal of Medicine 2000; 343: 1206–1209.
13. Caffrey SL, Willoughby PJ, Pepe PE, Becker LB. Public use of automated external defibrillators. New England Journal of Medicine 2002; 347: 1242–1247.
14. Hallstrom AP, Ornato JP, Weisfeldt M, et al. Public-access defibrillation and survival after out-of-hospital cardiac arrest. New England Journal of Medicine 2004; 351: 637–646.
15. Pell JP, Sirel JM, Marsden AK, et al. Potential impact of public access defibrillators on survival after out of hospital cardiopulmonary arrest: retrospective cohort study. British Medical Journal 2002; 325: 515–520.
16. Bardy GH, Lee KL, Mark DB, et al. Home use of automated external defibrillators for sudden cardiac arrest. New England Journal of Medicine 2008; 358: 1793–1804.
17. Wasserthiel J. Australian Resuscitation Guidelines: Applying the evidence and simplifying the process. Emergency Medicine Australasia 2006; 18: 317–321.

1.2 Advanced life support

John E. Maguire

ESSENTIALS[1,2]

1 Follow the advanced life support resuscitation guidelines developed by, or based on, those of the International Liaison Committee on Resuscitation (ILCOR).

2 Perform cardiopulmonary resuscitation (CPR) without interruption for patients with no pulse, except when performing essential advanced life support (ALS) interventions.

3 Defibrillate ventricular fibrillation (VF) and pulseless ventricular tachycardia (VT) until the rhythm has reverted to a stable, perfusing pattern.

4 Obtain, maintain and protect the airway and provide adequate oxygenation and ventilation.

5 Obtain vascular access and give boluses of epinephrine (adrenaline).

6 Correct reversible causes of cardiac arrest – the '4 Hs and 4 Ts'.

Introduction

The patient in cardiac arrest is the most time-critical medical crisis an emergency physician manages. The interventions of basic life support (BLS) and advanced life support (ALS) have the greatest probability of success when applied immediately, but become less effective with the passage of time, and after only a short interval without treatment are ineffectual.

Larsen et al., in 1993, calculated the time intervals from collapse to the initiation of BLS, defibrillation and other ALS treatments, and analysed their effect on survival from out-of-hospital cardiac arrest.[3] When all three interventions were immediately available the survival rate was 67%. This figure declined by 2.3% per minute of delay to BLS, by a further 1.1% per minute of delay to defibrillation, and by 2.1% per minute to other ALS interventions. Without treatment, the decline in survival rate was the sum of the three coefficients, or 5.5% per minute.

Chain of survival

The importance of rapid treatment for cardiac arrest has led clinicians to develop a systems management approach, represented by the concept of the 'Chain of Survival', which has become the widely accepted model for the emergency medical services (EMS) systems.[4] The Chain of Survival concept implies that more people survive sudden cardiac arrest when a cluster or sequence of events is set up as rapidly as possible. This Chain of Survival sequence includes:

- early access to the EMS system
- early BLS
- early defibrillation
- early advanced care.

All the links must be connected, as weakness in any link of the chain reduces the probability of patient survival. ALS involves the continuation of BLS as necessary, but with the addition of manual defibrillation, advanced invasive airway and vascular access techniques, and the administration of pharmacological agents.

Aetiology and incidence of cardiac arrest

Aetiology

The commonest cause of sudden cardiac arrest in adults is ischaemic heart disease.[1,2,5] Other causes include respiratory failure, drug overdose, metabolic derangements, trauma, hypovolaemia, immersion and hypothermia.

Incidence

The population incidence of sudden cardiac death (within 24 hours of the onset of any symptoms) has been estimated as 1.24:1000/year in the USA.[6] The incidence of cardiac arrest notified to ambulances in western metropolitan Melbourne, Australia, in 1995 was approximately 0.72:1000/year.[7] From among 20 communities in developed nations worldwide a population average of 0.62:1000/year received attempted resuscitation after out-of-hospital cardiac arrest.[6]

Advanced life support guidelines and algorithms

The most exciting and clinically relevant advance in ALS over the last decade has been the development of widely accepted universal guidelines and algorithms including scientifically proven therapies that have substantially simplified the management of cardiac arrest.

International Liaison Committee on Resuscitation (ILCOR)

In 2000, the American Heart Association, in collaboration with the International Liaison Committee on Resuscitation (ILCOR), convened the International Guidelines 2000 Conference on CPR and Emergency Cardiac Care (ECC). This was the first international assembly gathered specifically to produce international resuscitation guidelines, where the International Guidelines 2000 for CPR and ECC were developed and then published.[8] These guidelines represented a consensus of expert individuals and resuscitation councils and organizations across many countries, cultures and disciplines. The underlying principle guiding decision-making was that additions to existing guidelines had to pass a rigorous evidence-based review. Revisions or deletions occurred because of:

- lack of evidence to confirm effectiveness, and/or
- additional evidence to suggest harm or ineffectiveness, and/or
- evidence that superior therapies had become available.[8]

Researchers from the ILCOR member councils continued to apply and develop the above evidence evaluation process, which culminated in the publication in 2005 of the *Consensus on Science and Treatment Recommendations* (CoSTR).[1]

Consensus on Science and Treatment Recommendations (CoSTR)

Each ILCOR member body has used the CoSTR documents to develop its own guidelines for local use. Thus in 2006 both the Australian Resuscitation Council (ARC)[5] and the New Zealand Resuscitation Council (NZRC)[9] published their local guidelines. The ARC guideline on Adult Advanced Life Support[2] includes an Adult Cardiorespiratory Arrest algorithm (Fig. 1.2.1). This is clear, concise, and easy to memorize and adapt into poster format, and is readily applied clinically.

However, resuscitation knowledge is still incomplete, and some of the ALS techniques currently in use are not supported by the highest levels of scientific rigour. Thus strict adherence to any guidelines should be guided by common sense. Individuals with specialist knowledge may modify them according to the level of their expertise and the specific clinical situation or environment in which they practise.[10]

Initiation of ALS

The ARC guidelines and algorithm qualify the commencement of BLS with the statement *'if appropriate'*.[2] This is because BLS is only a temporary and inefficient substitute for normal cardiorespiratory function. ALS interventions are almost always necessary to produce the return of spontaneous circulation (ROSC).

Electrical defibrillation is the fundamental tenet of the treatment for VF and pulseless VT. However, the likelihood of defibrillation restoring a sustained, perfusing cardiac rhythm, and of a favourable long-term outcome, exists for as little as 90 seconds after the onset of cardiac arrest. The chances of survival to hospital discharge decline rapidly thereafter, as myocardial high-energy phosphate stores are consumed. Therefore, minimizing the time to defibrillation is the priority in resuscitation from sudden cardiac arrest. The purpose of BLS is to support the patient's cardiorespiratory status as effectively as possible until equipment – particularly a defibrillator – and drugs become available.[1,2]

The point of entry into the ALS algorithm depends on the circumstances of the cardiac arrest. In many situations, such as out-of-hospital cardiac arrest, BLS will already have been initiated and should be continued while the defibrillator/monitor is being prepared. Diagnosis must be swift and the defibrillator attached without delay when the patient is being monitored at the time of a cardiac arrest.[1,2]

Attachment of the defibrillator/monitor and rhythm recogniton

Automated external defibrillator

Apply the self-adhesive pads in the standard anteroapical positions for defibrillation (see below) using an automated external defibrillator (AED). An internal microprocessor analyses the ECG signal and, if VF/VT are detected, it causes the AED to display a warning and then either deliver a shock (automatic) or advise the operator to do so (semi-automatic).[2,11,12]

Manual external defibrillator

The critical decision for the rescuer after applying the self-adhesive pads or paddles of a manual external defibrillator is whether or not the cardiac rhythm is VF/VT.[1,2] Up to 70% of patients with an out-of-hospital cardiac arrest will be in VF/VT at the time of arrival of EMS personnel and a monitor/defibrillator.[11] The vast majority of cardiac arrest survivors come from this group.[1,2,4]

Rhythm recognition

Ventricular fibrillation (VF)

VF is a pulseless, chaotic, disorganized rhythm characterized by an undulating, irregular pattern that varies in amplitude and morphology, with a ventricular waveform of more than 150/minute.[1,2]

Ventricular tachycardia (VT)

Pulseless VT is characterized by broad, bizarrely shaped ventricular complexes associated with no detectable cardiac output. The rate is more than 100/minute by definition, and is usually in excess of 150.[1,2]

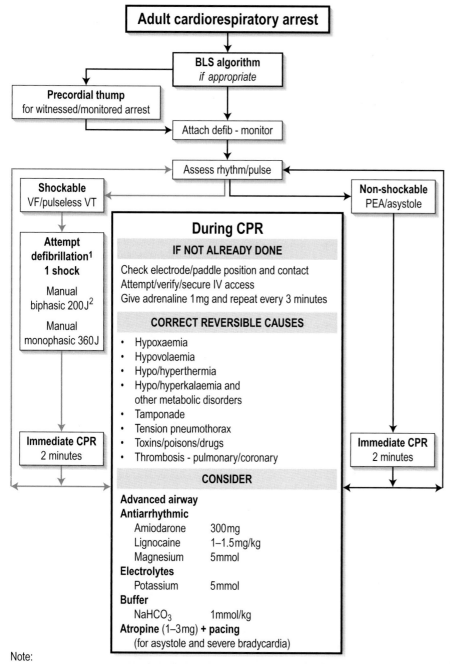

Adult cardiorespiratory arrest

BLS algorithm
if appropriate

Precordial thump
for witnessed/monitored arrest

Attach defib - monitor

Assess rhythm/pulse

Shockable
VF/pulseless VT

Non-shockable
PEA/asystole

Attempt defibrillation[1]
1 shock

Manual biphasic 200J[2]

Manual monophasic 360J

Immediate CPR
2 minutes

Immediate CPR
2 minutes

During CPR

IF NOT ALREADY DONE

Check electrode/paddle position and contact
Attempt/verify/secure IV access
Give adrenaline 1mg and repeat every 3 minutes

CORRECT REVERSIBLE CAUSES

- Hypoxaemia
- Hypovolaemia
- Hypo/hyperthermia
- Hypo/hyperkalaemia and other metabolic disorders
- Tamponade
- Tension pneumothorax
- Toxins/poisons/drugs
- Thrombosis - pulmonary/coronary

CONSIDER

Advanced airway
Antiarrhythmic
| | |
Amiodarone | 300mg
Lignocaine | 1–1.5mg/kg
Magnesium | 5mmol
Electrolytes
Potassium | 5mmol
Buffer
NaHCO$_3$ | 1mmol/kg
Atropine (1–3mg) + pacing
(for asystole and severe bradycardia)

Note:
1. For witnessed arrest, when using a manual defibrillator, give up to 3 stacked shocks at first defibrillation attempt. If further shocks are required these should be single shocks.
2. Default biphasic energy.

Fig.1.2.1 Algorithm for management of adult cardiorespiratory arrest. (Reproduced with permission from the Australian Resuscitation Council.)

Pulseless electrical activity (PEA) or electromechanical dissociation (EMD)

The absence of a detectable cardiac output in the presence of a coordinated electrical rhythm is called pulseless electrical activity (PEA), also known as electromechanical dissociation (EMD).[1,2]

Asystole

Asystole is identified by the absence of any electrical cardiac activity on the monitor. Occasionally it is incorrectly diagnosed ('apparent asystole') on the ECG monitor because:

❶ **The ECG lead may be disconnected or broken.** Look for the presence of electrical artefact waves on the monitor during external chest compression, indicating that the ECG leads are connected and intact. A perfectly straight line suggests lead disconnection or breakage.

❷ **Lead sensitivity may be inappropriate.** Increase the sensitivity setting to maximum. The resulting increase in the size of electrical artefact will confirm that the sensitivity selection is functioning.

❸ **VF has a predominant axis.** Even coarse VF may cause minimal undulation in the baseline if the axis is at right-angles to the selected monitor lead, and thus resemble asystole. Select at least two leads in succession before asystole is diagnosed, preferably leads at right-angles, such as II and aVL.

Defibrillation

The only proven effective treatment for VF and pulseless VT is electrical defibrillation.[1,2,10,12] The defibrillator must be brought immediately to the side of the person in cardiac arrest and, if the rhythm is VF/VT, defibrillation attempted without delay.

Placement of pads or paddles

Pads or paddles are often identified as 'sternum' and 'apex', or 'anterior' and 'posterior', which is of *no* relevance for emergency transthoracic defibrillation. It simply allows detection by the pads/paddles of the correct orientation of certain perfusing cardiac rhythms prior to synchronized cardioversion.[1,2,11,12,13]

Anteroapical pad or paddle position

There are two accepted positions for the defibrillation pads or paddles to optimize current delivery to the heart. The most common is the anteroapical position: one pad/paddle is placed to the right of the sternum just below the clavicle, and the other is centred lateral to the normal cardiac apex in the anterior or midaxillary line (V5–6 position).

Anteroposterior pad or paddle position

An alternative is the anteroposterior position: the anterior pad/paddle is placed over the praecordium or apex, and the posterior pad/paddle is placed on the patient's back in the left or right infrascapular region.

Do not attempt defibrillation over ECG electrodes or medicated patches, and avoid placing pad/paddles over significant breast tissue in females. Also the pad/paddles should be placed at least 12–15 cm away from the module and pulse generator, if the patient has respectively an implanted pacemaker or a cardioverter–defibrillator. Arrange to check the function of any pacemaker or cardioverter–defibrillator as soon as practicable after successful defibrillation.[1,2,11,12]

Timing of shocks

Three stacked shocks

The Australian Resuscitation Council (ARC) guidelines recommend that if the cardiac arrest is witnessed by a rescuer with a manual defibrillator, up to three stacked shocks should be used as the first defibrillation attempt. The pads or paddles should remain on the chest wall and the defibrillator immediately recharged after each shock, up to a total of three. Check the rhythm after each defibrillation attempt and repeat the shock if VF/VT persists. A total of three shocks should be delivered within 30–40 seconds. Any delay over 20 seconds between shocks is unacceptable and should lead to abandonment of the stacked shocks and immediate recommencement of CPR.[2]

Single shocks

Only deliver a single shock when the cardiac arrest has not been witnessed by the rescuer, or when additional shocks are required after the first three stacked shocks, followed immediately by CPR for 2 minutes. Do not delay recommencing CPR to assess the rhythm or to look for signs of life.[2]

The New Zealand Resuscitation Council (NZRC) guidelines and the ILCOR Universal Cardiac Arrest Algorithm do not recommend stacked shocks, but use the single shock regimen exclusively.[1,9]

Waveform and energy of shocks

Two main types of waveform are available from cardiac defibrillators.

Monophasic sinusoidal waveform

Older defibrillators use a damped monophasic sinusoidal waveform, which is a single pulse lasting for 3–4 ms. Set the energy level at the maximum when using a monophasic defibrillator in adults, which is usually 360 joules (J) for all shocks.[1,2,9]

Biphasic waveforms

Modern defibrillators using biphasic waveforms with impedance compensation should now be considered the 'gold standard'. These biphasic (bidirectional) truncated transthoracic shock defibrillators are as effective at lower energies as standard damped sine-wave shock defibrillators, and result in fewer post-defibrillation ECG abnormalities.[1,2,11–13]

Set the level at 200 J for all shocks when using a biphasic defibrillator in adults. Other energy levels may be used if the relevant clinical data for that defibrillator suggest an alternative energy level provides comparable success to the 'default' energy level of 200 J.[1,2,9]

Optimizing transthoracic impedance

A critical myocardial mass must be depolarized synchronously for defibrillation to be successful. This interrupts the fibrillation and allows recapture by a single pacemaker. Thus the transthoracic impedance must be minimized in order to maximize the probability of success.[1,2,11–13]

Reduction of transthoracic impedance

- Use pads/paddles 10–13 cm in diameter for adults. Smaller paddles/pads allow too concentrated a discharge of energy that may cause focal myocardial damage.[11,12] Larger pads/paddles do not make good chest contact over their entire area, and/or may allow current to be conducted through non-myocardial tissues.[11,13]
- Use conductive pads or electrode paste/gel. This reduces impedance by 30%.[11] Take care to ensure that there is no electrical contact between the pads or paddles, either directly or through electrode paste, as this results in current arcing across the chest wall.[11–13]
- Apply a pressure of about 5 kg to the paddle when adhesive pads are not being used.[11]
- Perform defibrillation when the chest is deflated, i.e. in expiration.[13]

- Deliver stacked shocks with a short interval between (some algorithms only).[11,13]

Current-based defibrillation

Conventional defibrillators are designed to deliver a specified amount of energy measured in joules. Depolarization of myocardial tissue is accomplished by the passage of electrical current through the heart; clinical studies have determined that the optimal current is 30–40 amperes (A).[11,13] The current delivered at a fixed energy is inversely related to the transthoracic impedance, so a standard energy dose of 200 J delivers about 30 A to the average patient. The current generated may be inadequate in patients with greater than average impedance, whereas patients with smaller transthoracic impedance may sustain myocardial damage from excessive current flow.[11–13]

Some newer current-based defibrillators automatically measure transthoracic impedance and then predict and adjust the energy delivered to avoid inappropriately high or low transmyocardial current. These devices have defibrillation success rates comparable to those of conventional defibrillators while cumulatively delivering less energy. The reduced energy should result in less myocardial damage and may reduce post-defibrillation complications.[11–13]

Automated external defibrillators (AED)

AEDs were first introduced in 1979 and have become standard equipment in EMS systems for use outside hospital, as well as within hospital in many circumstances.

AEDs are highly accurate, some models demonstrating 100% specificity and 90–92% sensitivity in correctly identifying coarse VF.[12] Their precision is less for fine VF and least for VT, but overall accuracy is comparable to that of an experienced cardiologist.[11] EMS systems equipped with AEDs are able to deliver the first shock up to 1 minute faster than when using conventional defibrillators. Rates of survival to hospital discharge are equivalent to those achieved when more highly trained first responders use manual defibrillators.[4]

The major advantage of AEDs over manual defibrillators is their simplicity, which reduces the time and expense of initial training and continuing education, and increases the number of persons who can operate the device.[4,11-12] Members of the public have been trained to use AEDs in a variety of community settings, and have demonstrated that they can retain skills for up to 1 year.[4] Encouraging results have been produced when AEDs have been placed with community responders such as firefighters, police officers, casino staff, security guards at large public assemblies and public transport vehicle crews.[4,11]

The Australasian College for Emergency Medicine recommends that all clinical staff in healthcare settings should have rapid access to an AED or a defibrillator with AED capability.[14]

Technical problems

Whenever attempted defibrillation is not accompanied by skeletal muscle contraction take care to ensure good contact, and that the defibrillator is turned on, charged up, develops sufficient power and is not in synchronized mode. The operational status of defibrillators should be checked regularly, and a standby machine should be available at all times. The majority of defibrillator problems are due to operator error or faulty care and maintenance.[12]

Complications of defibrillation

- Skin burns may occur, which are usually superficial and can be minimized by ensuring optimal contact between the defibrillator pad/paddle and the patient.
- Myocardial injury and post-defibrillation dysrhythmias may occur with cumulative high-energy shocks.[11,12]
- Skeletal muscle injury or thoracic vertebral fractures are possible, albeit rare.
- Electrical injury to the healthcare provider may occur as a result of electrical contact with the patient during defibrillation. These range from paraesthesiae to deep partial-thickness burns, and cardiac arrest in the healthcare provider is possible. The defibrillator operator must ensure that all rescue personnel are clear of the patient before delivering a shock. Ensure that the patient, rescuers and equipment are dry before defibrillation is ever attempted in wet conditions, such as outdoors or around a swimming pool area.[11,12]

The CPR 'Code Blue' process

Immediate defibrillation is of paramount importance for VF/pulseless VT, although periods of well-performed CPR help maintain myocardial and cerebral viability and may improve the likelihood of success with subsequent shocks.[1,2] Current ALS guidelines recommend that, after delivering a single shock, CPR should be resumed immediately and continued for 2 minutes. Only after this period of CPR should the rhythm and pulse be reassessed and further treatment initiated as necessary.[1,2,9]

Rationale for resumption of CPR

The rationale for this is that after one defibrillator shock there is typically a delay of several seconds before a diagnostic-quality ECG trace is obtained. Additionally, even when defibrillation is successful, there is often a temporary impairment of cardiac function from seconds to minutes, associated with a weak or impalpable pulse. Thus waiting for a recognizable ECG rhythm or palpating for a pulse that may not be present anyway after successful defibrillation will unnecessarily delay the recommencement of CPR. This is detrimental to the patient who does not yet have ROSC.[1,2]

Algorithm loops

Pay attention to each of the following, either continuously or after each loop of the algorithm:[1,2]

- Minimize any interruption to CPR during ALS interventions.
- Attempt to secure an advanced airway with ventilation technique, but do not interrupt CPR for more than 20 seconds.
- Obtain vascular access.
- Administer epinephrine as recommended in the algorithm.
- Administer other drugs or electrolytes as indicated for individual circumstances (see the 4Hs and 4Ts below).
- Correct potentially reversible conditions that may have precipitated the cardiac arrest and/or reduced the chances of successful resuscitation. These are listed in Figure 1.2.1 and are conveniently recalled under the headings of the 'Four Hs and Four Ts'.

'4Hs'
Hypoxaemia
Hypovolaemia
Hypo-/hyperthermia
Hypo-/hyperkalaemia and other metabolic disorders.

'4Ts'
Tamponade
Tension pneumothorax
Toxins, poisons, drugs
Thrombosis: pulmonary or coronary.

Even the best-trained team will be unable to complete all of these management aspects within a single loop of the algorithm, but further opportunity will be present if subsequent cycles are necessary.[1,2]

PEA or asystole

Reassess the ECG rhythm after 2 minutes of CPR and, when appropriate, the pulse. Give a single shock without delay if VF/pulseless VT persist.[1,2,9] However, when PEA or asystole are present on ECG rhythm and/or pulse assessment, do not defibrillate as it may be deleterious.[1,2,11,12]

The prognosis for PEA or asystole is much worse than for VF/VT, and unless there are potentially reversible causes (4Hs and 4Ts), the application of other ALS interventions (see below) is indicated, but seldom of value.[1,2]

Other ALS interventions

Not one ALS intervention other than defibrillation has been proved to improve patient outcome.[1,2,10,15] Some clinicians maintain that ALS has an incremental benefit compared to defibrillation alone,[4,15,16] but although some data support this, it remains impossible to prove.[10] Cardiac pacing does not improve survival from asystole, either pre-hospital or in the emergency department (ED) setting.[1,2]

Advanced airway management

Endotracheal intubation is considered the best technique for airway management during cardiac arrest and is recommended in the ARC guidelines.[2] However, no randomized controlled study exists that shows an improved outcome with endotracheal intubation compared to basic airway management.[1,2,10,15,16] Other advanced airway devices studied during CPR as alternatives to the endotracheal tube include the laryngeal mask airway (LMA), and the oesophageal–tracheal combitube (Combitube). None is definitely superior to basic airway management during cardiac arrest in terms of consistently improved survival.[1,2]

Advanced airway techniques

The optimal technique for airway management depends on the equipment available, the circumstances of the cardiac arrest and the training and experience of the resuscitation team.[1,2]

Endotracheal intubation: advantages

One technical benefit of an advanced airway such as endotracheal intubation is that no interruption to chest compressions is necessary for ventilations during CPR. Also, an endotracheal tube isolates and protects the airway and allows suction, and the administration of drugs in the absence of vascular access.[1,2,16,17]

Endotracheal intubation: disadvantages

The main disadvantages of endotracheal intubation are the interruption to chest compressions during tube insertion, which should never exceed 20 seconds, and unrecognized oesophageal tube placement.[1,2] Once an endotracheal tube has been inserted, correct placement *must* be verified by direct vision of the tube passing between the vocal cords, or by the success of chest ventilation as demonstrated by an oesophageal detector device (ODD) and/or by end-tidal CO_2 recording, which will only register when there is ROSC.[1,2]

Ventilation and oxygenation

Cardiac arrest and CPR cause an increase in dead space and a reduction in lung compliance that compromise gas exchange. Therefore, a fractional inspired oxygen concentration (F_IO_2) of 1.0 (100% oxygen delivery system) is essential in cardiac arrest to optimize oxygen delivery.[1,2,17]

Minute volume

Carbon dioxide (CO_2) production and delivery to the pulmonary circulation are limited by the markedly reduced cardiac output achieved during cardiopulmonary resuscitation. As a consequence, a relatively low minute volume of 3.5–5.0 L is sufficient to achieve adequate CO_2 excretion and prevent hypercapnia. This situation will be altered if a CO_2-producing buffer such as sodium bicarbonate is administered. A small increase in minute ventilation is then required to prevent the development of a respiratory acidosis.[1,2]

Ventilation rate and tidal volume

A ventilation rate of 8–10 per minute without pausing during chest compressions and a tidal volume of 400–500 mL (5–6 mL/kg) are sufficient to clear CO_2 during most cardiac arrest situations, when an advanced airway is in place. This should cause a visible rise and fall of the patient's chest.[17] A self-inflating bag/valve/mask system and/or an airway intubation device remain the mainstay of advanced airway and ventilation management in ALS.[1,2,17]

Vascular access and drug delivery

Intravenous (i.v.) route

The ideal route of drug delivery should combine rapid and easy vascular access with quick delivery to the central circulation. The intravenous (i.v.) route is preferred. This is most easily performed by inserting a cannula into a large vein in the upper limb or into the external jugular vein. Avoid lower limb veins because of their poor venous return from below the diaphragm during CPR, as well as immediate or inexperienced central line insertion which can have fatal consequences, such as pneumothorax or arterial laceration.

Drug delivery

Give a 20–30 mL i.v. fluid flush following any administered drug and/or raise the limb to facilitate delivery to the central circulation.[1,2] Central venous cannulae deliver drugs rapidly to the central circulation and should be used when already in place. Otherwise, as stated above, their insertion during CPR requires time and technical proficiency and interferes with defibrillation and the CPR process, which is unacceptable.[1,2]

Intraosseous (IO) route

The intraosseous (IO) route is also acceptable for drug delivery in adults as well as children.[1,2] Suitable sites of insertion include above the medial malleolus or the proximal tibia, but practice is needed to perfect the technique.

Intratracheal route

The intratracheal instillation of drugs is an alternative during cardiopulmonary resuscitation, especially when tracheal intubation precedes venous access. Epinephrine (adrenaline), lignocaine (lidocaine) and atropine may be safely administered through the endotracheal tube if there is a delay in achieving vascular access.

The ideal dose and dilution of drugs given by this route are unknown, but recommendations include using 3–10 times the standard i.v. drug dose diluted in 10 mL of water or normal saline. The drug should be delivered via a catheter or quill placed beyond the tip of the endotracheal tube, and followed by ventilations to aid dispersion.[1,2,18]

Fluid therapy

Crystalloid solutions are used as standard for the i.v. delivery of drugs during CPR. Glucose-containing solutions are avoided during CPR as they may contribute to post-arrest hyperglycaemia, which reduces or impairs cerebral recovery.[18]

Drug therapy in ALS

Not one drug used in resuscitation has been shown to improve long-term survival in humans after cardiac arrest.[1,2,10,15] Despite this, a number of agents continue to be employed based on theoretical, retrospective or anecdotal evidence of their efficacy.[1,2,10]

Epinephrine (adrenaline)[1,2,9,10,15,16]

The putative beneficial actions of epinephrine in cardiac arrest relate to its α-adrenergic effects, which result in an increased aortic blood pressure with increased perfusion of the cerebral and coronary vascular beds, and reduced blood flow to splanchnic and limb vessels. Epinephrine is considered the 'standard' vasopressor in cardiac arrest.

Indications

- Cardiac arrest due to VF/pulseless VT when there is no ROSC after the initial attempts at defibrillation
- Asystole and PEA as initial treatment.

Adverse effects

- Tachyarrhythmias
- Severe hypertension after ROSC
- Tissue necrosis after extravasation.

Dosage

The standard adult dose is 1 mg i.v. every 3 minutes. The NZRC guidelines recommend every second loop, i.e. 4–5 minutes. Higher doses have not been shown to improve long-term outcome.

Amiodarone[1,2]

Amiodarone has some benefit in refractory VF/VT in the setting of out-of-hospital cardiac arrest. Additionally, studies show an improvement in defibrillation response when amiodarone is given in VF or haemodynamically unstable VT. Consider amiodarone for refractory VF/VT.

Indications

- Persistent VF/pulseless VT following failed defibrillation and adrenaline administration.
- Prophylaxis of recurrent VF/VT.

Adverse effects

- Hypotension, bradycardia, heart block, QTc prolongation with proarrhythmic effects.

Dosage

The initial bolus of amiodarone is 300 mg or 5 mg/kg, followed by a further 150 mg if necessary.

Atropine[1,2]

Atropine has no consistent benefits in cardiac arrest, but may be considered in certain circumstances.

Indications

- Asystole
- Severe bradycardia.

Adverse effects

- Tachycardias
- Central nervous system (CNS) excitement and delirium; hyperthermia.

Dosage

Atropine is given as a bolus of at least 1 mg, repeated up to 3 mg (= 0.04 mg/kg), which is considered the vagolytic dose.

Calcium[1,2]

Calcium is *only* indicated when the cardiac arrest is caused or exacerbated by the specific conditions listed below.

Indications

- Hyperkalaemia
- Hypocalcaemia
- Poisoning by calcium-channel blocking drugs.

Adverse effects

- Increase in myocardial and cerebral injury mediated by cell death.
- Tissue necrosis with extravasation.

Dosage

The initial dose is 5–10 mL of 10% calcium chloride, or 15–30 mL of 10% calcium gluconate (three times the dose of calcium chloride).

Lignocaine (lidocaine)[1,2]

The antiarrhythmic properties of lignocaine in cardiac arrest are inconsistent. Its continued use is based purely on familiarity and historical precedent. The role of lignocaine in the prophylaxis of VF/VT is also unclear and at best equivocal.

Indications

- Cardiac arrest due to VF/pulseless VT refractory to defibrillation and adrenaline, when amiodarone is not available.
- Prophylaxis of recurrent VF or VT, if used during CPR.

Adverse effects

- Hypotension, bradycardia, heart block, asystole.
- CNS excitation with anxiety, tremor and convulsions, followed by CNS depression with coma.

Dosage

The initial dose is 1–1.5 mg/kg, with an additional bolus of 0.5 mg/kg after 5–10 minutes if indicated.

Magnesium[1,2,10]

Magnesium is indicated when the cardiac arrest is caused or exacerbated by the specific conditions listed below. There is no support for its routine use at present.

Indications

- *Torsades de pointes* (polymorphic VT). This is often associated with a prolonged QT interval due to ischaemia, hypokalaemia, hypomagnesaemia, hypocalcaemia, and drugs such as the phenothiazines, butyrophenones, tricyclic antidepressants, macrolide antibiotics, class 1A and 1C antiarrhythmics, and some antifungals and antihistamines.
- Hypokalaemia
- Hypomagnesaemia
- Digoxin toxicity
- Cardiac arrest due to VF/VT refractory to defibrillation and epinephrine.

Adverse effects

- Muscle weakness and paralysis if excessive quantities administered.

Dosage

The initial dose is a 5 mmol bolus (1.25 g or 2.5 mL of a 49.3% solution) repeated if indicated, and followed by an infusion of 20 mmol (5 g or 10 mL of a 49.3% solution) over 4 hours.

Sodium bicarbonate[1,2]

Sodium bicarbonate is only indicated when the cardiac arrest is caused or exacerbated by the specific conditions listed below. There is no support for its routine use in cardiac arrest.

Indications

- Hyperkalaemia
- Severe metabolic acidosis
- Poisoning by tricyclic antidepressants
- Protracted cardiac arrest beyond 15 minutes.

Adverse effects

- Metabolic alkalosis, hypernatraemia, hyperosmolality
- Production of CO_2 causing paradoxical intracellular acidosis, which may be partly ameliorated by adequate ventilation in CPR.

Dosage

The initial dose is 1 mmol/kg (1 mL/kg of 8.4% sodium bicarbonate) over 2–3 minutes, then as guided by the arterial blood gases.

Vasopressin[1,2,19]

Vasopressin is an alternative vasopressor to epinephrine. There is currently insufficient evidence to support or refute its use either alone or in combination with adrenaline in any cardiac arrest rhythm.

Consider administration for

- Vasopressor effects as an alternative to epinephrine.

Adverse effects

- Cerebral oedema or haemorrhage after ROSC.
- Persistent vasoconstriction following ROSC, which may exacerbate myocardial ischaemia and interfere with left ventricular function.
- Procoagulant effect on platelets.

Dosage

The dose is a single i.v. bolus of 40 U administered once during the episode of cardiac arrest.

Haemodynamic monitoring during CPR

End-tidal CO_2 (ETCO$_2$)[1,2,10,20]

Animal and clinical studies indicate that measuring ETCO$_2$ is an effective and informative technique for determining progress during CPR, particularly if there is ROSC.

ETCO$_2$ typically falls to less than 10 mmHg at the onset of cardiac arrest. It can rise to between one-quarter and one-third of normal with effective CPR, and rises to normal or supranormal levels over the next minute following ROSC. The changes in ETCO$_2$ parallel similar proportionate increases in cardiac output.

Changes in ETCO$_2$

An ETCO$_2$ of less than 1% during attempted resuscitation from cardiac arrest is an indication of ineffective CPR. This may be as a result of inadequate ventilation due to airway obstruction or even oesophageal intubation; or due to minimal cardiac output because of poor technique or underlying causes such as hypovolaemia, pulmonary embolism or pericardial tamponade (part of the 4Hs and 4Ts). Conversely, a sharp rise in ETCO$_2$ may be the first indication of ROSC.

ETCO$_2$ may also have a prognostic value, as patients who are eventually successfully resuscitated have higher ETCO$_2$ values during CPR than those who never have ROSC. Remember to exercise caution when interpreting ETCO$_2$ following the administration of epinephrine, as this causes a decrease in ETCO$_2$ which does not necessarily indicate a poorer prognosis.

Current ALS guidelines advise that ETCO$_2$ monitoring is a safe and effective non-invasive indicator of cardiac output during CPR, and is an early indicator of ROSC in intubated patients.

Arterial blood gases[1,2]

Arterial blood gas (ABG) monitoring during cardiac arrest is a useful indicator of oxygenation and the adequacy of ventilation, but is not an accurate measure of tissue acidosis. An increase in PaCO$_2$ may indicate improved tissue perfusion during CPR or with ROSC, if ventilation is constant. The measurement of ABGs should not interfere with the overall performance of good CPR.

When to discontinue ALS

The vast majority of patients who survive out-of-hospital cardiac arrest have ROSC before arrival at the ED. Only 33 of 5444 patients (0.6%) in 18 studies between 1981 and 1995, who were transported to an ED still in cardiac arrest after unsuccessful pre-hospital resuscitation, survived to hospital discharge.[21] Twenty-four of the surviving patients arrived in the ED in VF, and 11 of these had their initial cardiac arrest in the ambulance en route to hospital, or had temporary ROSC before arrival. Thus virtually all patients arriving at an ED still in asystole from out-of-hospital cardiac arrest die without leaving hospital.

Ceasing CPR pre-hospital

A recommendation made in 1993 for out-of-hospital cardiac arrest in the normothermic patient was that resuscitation should cease if there was no ROSC after 25 minutes of ALS.[22] Two important exceptions to this guide are:

- The cardiac arrest occurs in the presence of ambulance personnel.
- The patient has persistent VF.

These recommendations were applied and considered valid in a prospective study in that same year.[23]

In-hospital cardiac arrest outcomes

There are no early absolute predictors of futility in the resuscitation of patients with in-hospital cardiac arrest. Some variables are, however, associated with a greater or lesser chance of survival to discharge. Better outcomes are linked to ventricular tachyarrhythmias, the commencement of resuscitation within 5 minutes of collapse, and ROSC within 15 minutes of CPR.

In-hospital cardiac arrest with a poor outcome

A poor outcome is linked to pre-existing conditions such as cardiogenic shock, metastatic cancer, renal failure, sepsis and an acute cerebrovascular accident. Age is not an independent predictor of outcome, either in hospital or for out-of-hospital cardiac arrest.[24,25]

Outcome of prolonged ALS

ALS resuscitation efforts lasting more than 30 minutes without ROSC at any stage are so uniformly unsuccessful that resuscitation should be abandoned, except in certain special circumstances such as hypothermia, possibly some drug overdoses, and following thrombolysis in suspected massive pulmonary embolism (PE).[10,25] The return of spontaneous circulation at any time during the resuscitation process resets the clock to time zero.[1,5]

Prognosis for survival after cardiac arrest

The best prospect of neurologically intact long-term survival after a cardiac arrest occurs when:

- the victim is witnessed to collapse
- CPR is commenced immediately
- the cardiac rhythm is VF or pulseless VT

- defibrillation is performed as soon as possible, ideally within 2–3 minutes of collapse.[3,4,9]

Out-of-hospital cardiac arrest

Some variation in survival after an out-of-hospital cardiac arrest is due to differences in EMS systems, as well as to differing research methodology and data reporting. In a 1996 meta-analysis of 36 articles published between 1973 and 1992 describing 41 EMS systems in six countries,[26] survival varied from 0% to 21%, with an overall mean survival of 8%.

In-hospital cardiac arrest

The prognosis for survival from in-hospital cardiac arrest is only marginally better, with survival to discharge averaging 13.8% of 12961 patients described in reports published between 1961 and 1984.[24] However, in a further seven reports published between 1978 and 1989 this dropped to 11% of 1804 patients.[25]

Uniform reporting in cardiac arrest research

Cardiac arrest research and the interpretation of available data have been hampered by inconsistent methodology and reporting. An important initiative is recognizing the need for uniform, internationally recognized definitions and guidelines for the reporting of cardiac arrest data. A number of templates have been developed that include the most relevant variables for describing and comparing cardiac arrest research results. These are referred to as Utstein-style guidelines or templates, after Utstein Abbey, near Stavanger, Norway, where expert researchers and clinicians gathered in 1990.[27]

ALS controversies

❶ Acceptance of a universal algorithm

❷ The lack of a demonstrated role for any drug used in ALS

❸ When ALS should not be started

❹ When ALS should be ceased

References

1. International Liaison Committee on Resuscitation. 2005 International Consensus on Cardiopulmonary Resuscitation and Emergency Cardiac Care. Science with Treatment Recommendations. Resuscitation 2005; 67: 181–303.
2. Australian Resuscitation Council. Adult Advanced Life Support: Australian Resuscitation Guidelines 2006. Emergency Medicine Australasia 2006; 18: 337–356. [Also online http://www.resus.org.au/. Accessed 26 Oct 2007].
3. Larsen MP, Eisenberg MS, Cummins RO, et al. Predicting survival from out-of-hospital cardiac arrest: a graphic model. Annals of Emergency Medicine 1993; 22: 1652–1658.
4. Cummins RO, Ornato JP, Thies WH, Pepe PE. Improving survival from sudden cardiac arrest: the 'chain of survival' concept: a statement for health professionals from the Advanced Cardiac Life Support Subcommittee and the Emergency Cardiac Care Committee, American Heart Association. Circulation 1991; 83: 1832–1847.
5. Australian Resuscitation Council. ARC Guidelines 4–7, 9, 11–12. Emergency Medicine Australasia 2006; 18: 325–371. [Also online http://www.resus.org.au/. Accessed 26 Oct 2007.]
6. Becker LB, Smith DW, Rhodes KV. Incidence of cardiac arrest: a neglected factor in evaluating survival rates. Annals of Emergency Medicine 1993; 22: 86–91.
7. Bernard S. Outcome from prehospital cardiac arrest in Melbourne Australia. Emergency Medicine (Fremantle) 1998; 10: 25–29.
8. The American Heart Association in collaboration with the International Liaison Committee on Resuscitation. Guidelines 2000 for cardiopulmonary resuscitation and emergency cardiovascular care – an international consensus on science. Resuscitation 2000; 46: 1–447.
9. New Zealand Resuscitation Council. Level 1–7 Guidelines 2006. Available online http://www.nzrc.org. nz/. Accessed 26 Oct 2007.
10. Maguire JE. Advances in cardiac life support: sorting the science from the dogma. Emergency Medicine (Fremantle) 1997; 9: 1–21.
11. Truong JH, Rosen P. Current concepts in electrical defibrillation. Journal of Emergency Medicine 1997; 15: 331–338.
12. Bossaert LL. Fibrillation and defibrillation of the heart. British Journal of Anaesthesia 1997; 79: 172–177.
13. Kerber RE. Electrical treatment of cardiac arrhythmias: defibrillation and cardioversion. Annals of Emergency Medicine 1993; 22: 296–301.
14. Australasian College for Emergency Medicine. Statement on early access, defibrillation. ACEM July 2005; S1: 1. Available online http://www.acem.org.au/. Accessed 26 Oct 2007.
15. Pepe PE, Abramson NS, Brown CG. ACLS – Does it really work? Annals of Emergency Medicine 1994; 23: 1037–1041.
16. Ornato JP, Paradis N, Bircher N, et al. Future directions for resuscitation research. III. External cardiopulmonary resuscitation advanced life support. Resuscitation 1996; 32: 139–158.
17. Gabbott DA, Baskett PJF. Management of the airway and ventilation during resuscitation. British Journal of Anaesthesia 1997; 79: 159–171.
18. Gonzalez ER. Pharmacologic controversies in CPR. Annals of Emergency Medicine 1993; 22: 317–323.
19. Barlow M. Vasopressin. Emergency Medicine (Fremantle) 2002; 14: 304–314.
20. Ornato JP. Hemodynamic monitoring during CPR. Annals of Emergency Medicine 1993; 22: 289–295.
21. Brennan RJ, Luke C. Failed prehospital resuscitation following out-of-hospital cardiac arrest: are further efforts in the emergency department warranted? Emergency Medicine (Fremantle) 1995; 7: 131–138.
22. Bonnin MJ, Pepe PE, Timball KT, et al. Distinct criteria for termination of resuscitation in the out-of-hospital setting. Journal of the American Medical Association 1993; 269: 1457–1462.
23. Pepe PE, Brown CG, Bonnin MJ, et al. Prospective validation of criteria for on-scene termination of resuscitation efforts after out-of-hospital cardiac arrest. Annals of Emergency Medicine 1993; 22: 884–885.
24. McGrath RB. In-house cardiopulmonary resuscitation after a quarter of a century. Annals of Emergency Medicine 1987; 16: 1365–1368.
25. Jastremski MS. In-hospital cardiac arrest. Annals of Emergency Medicine 1993; 22: 113–117.
26. Nichol G, Destsky AS, Stiell IG, et al. Effectiveness of emergency medical services for victims of out-of-hospital cardiac arrest: a meta-analysis. Annals of Emergency Medicine 1995; 27: 700–710.
27. Dick WF. Uniform reporting in resuscitation. British Journal of Anaesthesia 1997; 79: 241–252.

1.3 Ethics of resuscitation

Michael W. Ardagh

ESSENTIALS

1 Ethical deliberation may be aided by considering the four principles of: respect for patient autonomy; beneficence; non-maleficence, and justice.

2 During deliberation, if the ethical principles seem to be competing, the relative benefits and harms of the application of each should be considered.

3 During resuscitation, urgency and the impaired competence of the patient conspire against adequate consideration of these principles, especially in regard to non-maleficence and respect for patient autonomy.

4 Resuscitation can be harmful in a number of ways. This should be considered when assessing the balance of benefit and harm of any resuscitation endeavour.

5 All medical interventions, including resuscitation, need some form of consent despite the urgency and the impaired competence of the patient. Presumed consent is the one most commonly employed of the consent options available. Presumed consent using professional substituted judgement is a model that best respects patient autonomy.

6 Living Wills (personal statements) and Not for Resuscitation orders (institutional statements) are useful prior determinations of the patient's likely wishes, which greatly aid decision making when the patient is no longer able to communicate. However, care needs to be taken in both the development and the interpretation of these statements, so that the decision that ensues does represent, as best it can, the patient's true autonomous wish.

7 The practice of resuscitation procedures on the newly dead, particularly endotracheal intubation, is common and possibly of value. However, some form of consent is required for this to occur, although currently there is no suitable model. Presumed consent would be appropriate if the practice was explicit and the public well informed. In so doing, those who would not consent are protected by the opportunity to decline. Until then, practising on the newly dead is ethically wrong.

Introduction

Medical ethics

This chapter discusses the ethical issues surrounding resuscitation. A working definition of ethics is 'the study of morality'. It is reasonable to describe moral behaviour as that which is 'the right thing to do'. Thus, medical ethical deliberation is the process of determining what is the right thing to do, when considering any of the dilemmas that arise in medical practice.

The law

The law also considers 'what is the right thing', but in a different way. Statutes and precedents (that is, previous decisions) can be applied to a given case, and particularly to the detailed events of that case, so that a definitive determination of 'right' can be made. The law is most useful when applied retrospectively, because of the application of different legal perspectives to the specifics of a case. In contrast, ethics has less well defined parameters for differentiating right from wrong (for example principles), and thus may struggle to come to a definitive determination.

Ethics and the clinician

However, owing to the relative simplicity of its tools (principles) and their general applicability, ethics is better suited to the prospective consideration of 'the right thing to do' by a clinician with a patient in front of them. In addition, ethics is more internationally applicable, whereas the law will vary from state to state and from country to country. Therefore, ethics (rather than the law) is generally what clinicians use when deciding what is the right thing to do.

Some guidance about legal issues related to resuscitation in an Australasian context may be accessed in publications such as those from the Australian Resuscitation Council Guidelines[1] and in the summary statement from the Medical Council of New Zealand.[2]

Philosophical models

The approach to ethical dilemmas may vary according to the philosophical perspective adopted.[3] Although there are a variety of models describing moral decision making, only a pragmatic overview will be given here. In general terms, a utilitarian approach may be adopted which values the positive balance of good over bad brought about by any action; or, alternatively, a deontological approach, which values actions that adhere to overriding moral principles. However, moral philosophers have recognized that moral principles may compete against each other when specific actions are considered. Moral principles should be honoured, but when they are competing in a given circumstance, we should then consider the relative balance of good and bad that ensues from the application of each principle. Thus, we have a composite philosophy wherein both the principles and the consequences of their application may be considered.

The principles of Beauchamp and Childress

Beauchamp and Childress[4] developed this further into a practical framework for medical ethical deliberation. They described four principles that should be honoured in medical decision making, and when these principles compete, the relative balance of good and bad should be considered. These four principles are:

- respect for patient autonomy
- beneficence
- non-maleficence
- justice.

Respect for patient autonomy

Autonomy is the patient's moral right to determine his or her own destiny and is a principle that has grown in stature in recent years. Recognition of the importance of informed consent is a consequence of this recognition.

Although the principle of respect for patient autonomy remains sound, there are many occasions in resuscitation medicine when the patient's competence is impaired. This is when he or she is unable to receive information, undertake rational deliberation, and/or express a decision free from coercion. Although we still endeavour to respect the patient's autonomy, we struggle to define what their autonomous wishes would be if they were not impaired. This will be further discussed later in the chapter.

Beneficence

Beneficence is the principle of acting in a way that benefits the patient. Historically, this and non-maleficence have been the overriding governing principles in medical practice. When these principles are enforced without due consideration of, or in contradiction to, the patient's perceived or expressed wishes, the action is termed 'paternalistic'.

When the principle of respect for patient autonomy is not honoured, the patient is deprived of a fundamental right and is treated as less worthy, by being reduced to a position where he or she is considered incapable of self-governance. This harm to the patient needs to be recognized when the relative benefits and harms of any action are considered.

Non-maleficence

Non-maleficence, or the principle of avoiding harm in therapeutic endeavours, is an established maxim attributed to Hippocrates. Although this is an obvious and commonsense principle, some harm will commonly be tolerated, for example when

delivering chemotherapy for cancer, or undertaking surgery that is known to have certain complications, this is because consideration of the other principles tells us our actions are right.

The principles of beneficence and non-maleficence risk being poorly considered because they 'go without saying'. However, the benefits and harms of our interventions should be reasonably certain before they may be considered right. For example, the performance of gastric lavage on a non-consenting patient after a trivial overdose several hours earlier is ethically unjustifiable, as there is insufficient benefit to override the principles of respect for autonomy and non-maleficence. In order to consider the benefits and harms, information is required regarding the outcomes of our interventions, and to this end research becomes an ethical necessity to provide the evidence upon which to judge competing principles.

Justice

The principle of justice is an essential balance to the first three principles, which apply primarily to the individual. Justice, or the concept of fairness, is best addressed by questioning whether there are others who might be adversely affected by a particular action. For example, in a mass casualty incident the performance of a hopeless resuscitation may be unjust, in addition to harming the patient, as it deprives another person with a greater chance of survival of those resuscitation facilities.

Application of the principles of Beauchamp and Childress to resuscitation medicine

There are two components of resuscitation medicine that conspire against adequate consideration of the principles outlined by Beauchamp and Childress. The first of these is urgency, and the second is the impaired ability of the patient to make reasonable autonomous decisions.

Urgency

Urgency may be a barrier to the application of these principles in any given case. It is often appropriate to perform resuscitation

assuming these deliberations might take place more fully when time permits, rather than withhold resuscitation on the basis of limited deliberation.

Impaired competence

The impaired competence of patients undergoing resuscitation complicates the principle of respect for autonomy, as the patient is commonly impaired in his or her ability to receive information, comprehend it, consider it in context, and then make a rational decision on the basis of that consideration. It is common practice not to seek or to ignore the wishes of the patient, and instead to presume that resuscitation is the right thing to do, based on arguments of beneficence and non-maleficence.

Thus, it is generally perceived that consent is not required for resuscitation because resuscitation brings benefit and prevents harm, and because the patient is not in a position to give or withhold consent. Although this approach usually does not mean that bad things are done, from an ethical perspective it is flawed. Resuscitation may be harmful in a number of ways, and some form of consent must be obtained, just as for any other medical intervention.

The harms of resuscitation

The benefits of resuscitation include the avoidance of death and the restoration of good health. The harms of resuscitation may be of the following five types:[5]

- **Unnecessary** The first harm is if resuscitation is unnecessary because the patient's condition is insufficiently serious to justify it. As a consequence, the harm includes pain and other discomfort to the patient, iatrogenic illness and unnecessary use of limited resources, thereby depriving others in greater need of those resources. The extent of overtreatment may be difficult to predict in resuscitation medicine, as it is hard to know whether the patient would survive intact without treatment. The most promising way of minimizing this harm is to have senior staff present during a resuscitation to draw upon their experience.
- **Unsuccessful** The second harm of resuscitation is if it is unsuccessful owing

to the patient's condition being too far advanced or without hope. When resuscitation will not produce the desired effect because the patient is too sick, there is the potential for a great number of harms to the patient, family, staff and the community. These include physical discomfort, loss of dignity, a prolonged death, and survival with an unacceptable quality of life. Harms to the family include the psychological discomfort of surrogate pain and loss of dignity, unfulfilled hope, loss of control of a loved one's destiny, the cost of lost earnings while at the bedside, and the cost of supporting a disabled survivor. The harms to health workers include frustration and sadness at lack of success, guilt at inflicting harm, and the cost of being unable to treat others waiting for resources. The harms to the community include the loss of resources to treat others, the deception that resuscitation offers hope, and the worry that death must be preceded by a loss of dignity.

- **Unkind** The third harm of resuscitation is if it is unkind because it brings about an outcome with which the patient or their family is unhappy. Resuscitation may condemn the patient to a quality of life below that considered acceptable. This is potentially a tragic harm, with an ongoing burden from which the patient and their carers may have no means of escape.
- **Unwise** The fourth harm of resuscitation is if it is unwise, as it diverts finite resources from alternative healthcare activities that would bring more benefit to other patients. Resuscitation is a significant user of resources and will cause significant harm if it is futile and beneficial healthcare activities cannot proceed for lack of resources.
- **Unwanted** Finally, resuscitation is harmful if it is against the patient's wishes. A preconceived 'Do Not Resuscitate' order written by or negotiated with the patient, or consent declined by a competent patient, must be honoured, in keeping with the ethical principle of respect for autonomy. However, a preconceived order (often called an Advance Directive, or 'Living Will') must be carefully considered, as it only relates to the situation in which the patient finds him or herself. For example, a written signed and witnessed Advance Directive statement declining resuscitation from cardiac arrest means that the patient should not be resuscitated from cardiac arrest. However, it does not mean that the patient has declined resuscitation from haemorrhagic shock. Similarly, a 'No Intensive Care' directive does not mean the patient has declined aggressive treatment for pulmonary oedema with a nitrate infusion and continuous positive airway pressure ventilation. Thus such directives may occasionally apply specifically to the patient's illness, but on other occasions they may not.

Advance directives

In the setting of some form of an advance directive, three questions should be considered:

❶ Did the patient make this decision based on well informed deliberation?
❷ Is the context they find themselves in now what they had in mind when they made the decision? If not, how closely does it relate to what they had in mind?
❸ Is there any indication that they might have changed their mind since they made this decision?

If the answers to any of these questions suggest some doubt as to how applicable the Advance Directive is to the resuscitation at this time, then it should be considered an indication of the patient's wishes, rather than morally binding.

Considering the harms

The harms of resuscitation must be considered when weighing the relative merits of the principles of respect for patient autonomy, beneficence, non-maleficence and justice. An ill-considered approach will lead to underrepresentation of patient autonomy in these deliberations, and an inadequate appreciation of the extent of harm that may ensue from resuscitation efforts.

Futility

The concept of futility has been widely discussed in the medical literature, with particular emphasis on resuscitation medicine.[6]

Regrettably, discussions of the harms of resuscitation have become stalled by failed attempts to define futility.

Deriving futility

The word futile is derived from the Latin *futilis*, meaning 'that which easily pours or melts'. The current usage stems from the story in which the daughters of the King of Argos murdered their husbands and were then condemned to collect water for eternity in leaking buckets. To arrive at your destination with an empty bucket when the intention of the journey was to bring water is undoubtedly a futile endeavour. However, futility in medicine is much more difficult to define.

Defining futility

Some emphasize physiological futility, meaning the inability to produce a physiological outcome objective, for example if CPR produces no pulse, or transfusion produces no blood pressure. The proponents of this definition suggest that it has the least risk of unilaterally imposed physician value judgements.

Others consider futility in terms of quantitative or qualitative measures. A quantitative estimate of futility is one in which an intervention is considered futile if it has failed in, for example, the last 100 attempts. The qualitative component describes futility if the patient's resultant quality of life falls below a threshold considered minimal by general professional judgement. It is unlikely that there will ever be agreement as to what physiological measure or quality of outcome measures are most appropriate, and what threshold measure separates futility from benefit. Although these arguments are interesting, it is unfortunate that they have taken on more importance than they merit.

The balance of benefit and harm

Futility defines the absence of acceptable benefit for any given intervention, whereas reasonable ethical deliberation demands that we consider the ratio of benefit to harm. If there is no benefit, any harm at all would make the benefit:harm ratio unfavourable. However, even if the endeavour is not futile and brings about measurable benefit, this does not necessarily mean that the endeavour is the right thing to do, as the amount of harm that ensues, as defined above, may outweigh any benefit. It is the benefit:harm balance, as assessed by considering the four ethical principles and the five types of harm described above, that has the most relevance in determining whether to start or to stop a resuscitation.

Consent, withholding and withdrawing resuscitation

Consent must be obtained for any medical intervention, including resuscitation. Informed consent, as is appropriate for elective surgery, may be inappropriate during resuscitation owing to the urgency of the treatment and the impaired competence of the patient. However, if informed consent is not relevant, other forms of consent still are. The two most common forms of consent used in resuscitation scenarios, where there is both urgency and impaired patient competence, are presumed consent and proxy consent.

Presumed consent

Presumed consent uses the concept that a reasonable patient under similar circumstances – or this patient if he or she were able to – would consent to the resuscitation endeavours proposed. This form of consent has merit and is commonly employed, but occasionally attracts criticism from bioethicists as being a form of medical paternalism, in that it may be perceived to be respecting the principle of beneficence, as the resuscitators perceive it, while ignoring respect for patient autonomy.

Proxy consent

Proxy consent involves obtaining consent for resuscitation from a family member or other person who is perceived to be able to speak on behalf of the patient. Proxy consent avoids the criticism of medical paternalism as the decision is taken out of the physician's hands, but it suffers as a model as the decision maker may be unable to adequately receive information, understand it, and deliberate over it during a hurried and rapidly evolving resuscitation.

In addition, the proxy may not reflect the views of the patient. There may be occasional circumstances where the proxy declines resuscitation because of some

financial or other benefit that would accrue from the patient's death. More commonly, proxies have a tendency to demand more resuscitation than the patient would have wanted, for fear of becoming responsible for their death. When this form of consent is used there is greater scope for the harms of resuscitation.

Proxy consent with substitued judgement

A modification of proxy consent that better addresses the issue of respect for patient autonomy is proxy consent with substituted judgement. This involves not asking what the proxy would want done for the patient, but instead what the proxy thinks the patient would want done. In other words, it attempts to see the resuscitation from the patient's perspective, as viewed by the proxy.

Presumed consent using professional substituted judgement

A modification of presumed consent is presumed consent using professional substituted judgement.[7] This means the resuscitators gather as much information about the patient as they possibly can to attempt to understand how the patient would view this decision. This usually involves speaking with the patient's loved ones. Then, with some knowledge of the likely outcome of the proposed resuscitation, based on previous experience and a knowledge of the medical literature, they can exercise their moral imagination by asking *Would I want this treatment if I was this patient?* In this way the patient's autonomy is as best respected as it can be under difficult circumstances, by combining a knowledge of the harms and benefits of the resuscitation with an appreciation of this balance from the patient's perspective.

The resuscitation cannot proceed if presumed consent using professional substituted judgement is employed and the answer to the question is *'No'*. To resuscitate without regard for the patient's explicit or perceived wishes is a harmful disrespect for their autonomy.

Often, and appropriately, a decision to proceed will be made on the basis of a perceived marginal benefit over harm. This balance is made more appealing by the

alternative of certain death if resuscitation is not undertaken. However, the balance is dynamic, with a clearer view of the likely benefits and harms only emerging as the patient responds or not to the resuscitation. All concerned should be willing to minimize the ongoing harms of resuscitation by withdrawing treatment if that treatment does not procure the hoped-for benefits, as the balance becomes more unfavourable.

Withholding and withdrawing treatment

The concept of withholding and withdrawing treatment is somewhat misdirected in that it implies a need for permission to stop the intervention, whereas the precedent in medicine is to obtain permission to proceed. It is wrong to withhold a resuscitation endeavour because of the concern that the life-saving treatment cannot be withdrawn at a later date if things are not going well. When resuscitation is withheld, a small but significant number of patients may miss out on the opportunity for a good outcome had the resuscitation been offered to them. Similarly, it is wrong to be unable to withdraw treatment because of the ill-conceived concept that once resuscitation has begun it must continue.

The resuscitators should recognize when the balance of benefit and harm becomes unfavourable from the patient's perspective, by employing professional substituted judgement. At this point they have a moral obligation to withdraw resuscitation, as they can no longer presume the patient's consent. The harms of resuscitation medicine will be minimized by appreciating the benefits and harms of resuscitation, the use of professional substituted judgement to view these from the patient's perspective, and by a commitment to stop resuscitation when the patient's consent cannot be presumed.

'Not For Resuscitation' (NFR) orders

A patient's written predetermination of whether to consent to resuscitation, in the form of an 'Advance Directive' or 'Living Will', has already been discussed. However, most people who become our patients have not made explicit and accessible determinations of their wishes. Many who need resuscitation are already in hospital or another healthcare institution, or have been in the recent past. Consequently, there is great opportunity for decision making during resuscitation to be aided by careful, documented, prior consideration of whether the resuscitators have 'permission to proceed'. Such documentation, when recorded in a patient's notes, is called a Not For Resuscitation (NFR) or Do Not Resuscitate (DNR) order.

The content of NFR orders

Most large Australasian hospitals have a policy about NFR orders and an increasing number use standardized forms to record the resuscitation status of patients. In addition, many provide information leaflets for patients and relatives explaining the NFR process and status.[8] Local policy, including the completion of standardized forms, should be followed.

Usually the NFR form will include the patient's diagnosis, the reasons for an NFR order, the date of issue, the date when it should be reviewed, the nature of the discussion with the patient and/or the relatives, or reasons why such a discussion did not occur. In addition, it should record exactly what is intended by the NFR status (for example, not for cardiopulmonary resuscitation in the event of cardiac arrest, or not for intensive care), including clarification that all other care will be provided as required. There is some evidence that those who have NFR orders may be denied other care owing to a perception that there is 'nothing more to offer them'.[9] It is most important that an ethically sound decision about resuscitation not being what the patient wants does not lead to an immoral neglect to provide good care. The nature of what care can and should still be delivered – for example analgesia, intravenous fluids, non-invasive ventilation etc. – should be clearly documented.

Establishing an NFR order

The process of establishing NFR status includes a consideration of the beneficence and non-maleficence of the resuscitation interventions in question, and then a determination that the patient does not consent to them. The NFR order should be completed with them if the patient has the capacity to make decisions, analogous to any informed consent process. However, the nature of this consent process has added difficulties. Patients need careful information about the poor prognosis of resuscitation interventions such as cardiopulmonary resuscitation, and about the often unappreciated harms that might ensue. Great care needs to be taken to ensure the patient does not perceive the discussion to be a message of impending death (if this is not the case), and they should be reassured that all other care will be delivered, including ensuring that they are kept comfortable.

There is some debate about having an NFR order without discussion with the patient, and some suggest that there should be a presumption of resuscitation for all who have not agreed to an NFR.[10] This view is counter to the arguments discussed above, which propose that some form of consent needs to be obtained for resuscitation to proceed, just as it is needed for all other medical interventions. There will be occasions when discussion with the patient is not undertaken, particularly if the patient is without decision-making capacity, or resuscitation is clearly without benefit. No rational person would consent to an intervention that is clearly more harmful than beneficial, and so lack of consent can be presumed, as discussed above. These details should be recorded.

Keeping an NFR order current

Like 'Advance Directives' or 'Living Wills', an NFR order may lose validity if the patient's condition changes, or they have a change of mind. An old NFR order (for example one made during a previous admission) will be influential to decision making, but is not binding if it is perceived that the patient would now consent. Consequently, NFR orders should be updated regularly, particularly if circumstances change.

Practising resuscitation procedures on the newly dead

Practising resuscitation procedures – most commonly endotracheal intubation – on patients who have died after an unsuccessful resuscitation is common in many parts of the world.[11] However, some view this with a repugnance that may be rationally argued. Others would propose that the benefit of this practice to subsequent patients outweighs any repugnance felt by others who witness it, or any harm done to the recently deceased.

Consent for practising resuscitation procedures on the newly dead

Practising resuscitation procedures on the newly dead requires permission before it may proceed, just like all other interventions in medicine. Informed consent may be obtained from the terminally ill for permission to perform procedures after they die, but this has limited relevance to the practice as it occurs in many emergency departments.

Implied consent argues that consent is implicit in the fact that the patient used the emergency services and therefore agreed to all that this entails, including being used for teaching. Implied consent criteria are commonly used for those who present of their own volition for non-invasive medical care. However, patients who die in the emergency department most often do not present of their own volition, but instead are brought in by others – usually ambulance staff – in a state of impaired competence. Furthermore, implied consent confers the right to administer treatment that the patient would reasonably expect at the time of presentation. Therefore, if a patient's attendance is involuntary, with impaired competence or with ignorance of the procedure, he or she cannot imply consent and medical staff cannot infer it.

'Construed consent' is a modification of implied consent, suggesting that if consent was obtained for a certain procedure it can be construed for a related procedure. If it is conceded that a form of consent (presumed consent, as suggested above) is obtained to intubate a patient during resuscitation, can it be construed that consent also applies to intubation after death? There is a superficial logic to this, as to perform the same procedure on the same patient with the same equipment one minute before, and one minute after, death seems a continuum of the same therapeutic relationship. However, on close analysis there is a sufficiently significant difference as to render previous consent null and void. The consent to resuscitate is based on a contract between medical staff and the patient dedicated to helping the patient. When the objective is no longer to help the patient, the previous contract is irrelevant and a new one must be entered into. Intubating the deceased under the old contract is a violation of the trust inherent in the previously formed therapeutic relationship. An appreciation of this violation contributes to the repugnance towards the procedure.

Presumed consent is appropriate when impaired competence renders the patient unable to give informed consent. Although it is likely that most would consent to postmortem procedures for the benefit of medical staff and subsequent patients, presumed consent does disadvantage the minority who would not. Formal application of a presumed consent rule for performing procedures on the recently dead mandates that the community should be well informed, so that individuals have the opportunity to explicitly decline consent if they so desire.

Proxy consent has also been argued in relation to this procedure. However, when proxy consent rules have been enforced the procedure tends not to take place, because staff are uncomfortable about obtaining consent in this way, or because relatives decline consent in an effort to protect their loved one from further harm.

May endotracheal intubation be practised on the newly dead?

The value of practising endotracheal intubation and other procedures on the newly dead is well argued, and therefore if it is disallowed there is a cost. However, the current pervading policy of 'don't ask, don't tell' is ethically unjustifiable. If a patient's consent is presumed and not sought, we are obliged to tell. The significant minority who would not consent are thereby protected by an opportunity to decline. Therefore, to proceed with presumed consent there must be a well-informed public, and preferably a statute to formalize consent.

An extrapolation of this, which is the most convincing solution, is called 'mandated choice', which proposes a process whereby, as a matter of public policy, individuals must choose on a variety of issues, with these choices being recorded on, for example, their driving licence. This process informs and honours individual choice, gives the significant minority the opportunity to decline, and avoids deception. However, in the absence of a suitably informed public from whom consent can be presumed, or a mandated choice, we do not have permission to proceed with postmortem resuscitation practice. Therefore, to do so is ethically wrong.

Conclusions

Emergency medicine abounds with clinical dilemmas requiring ethical deliberation. Such deliberation may be influenced by theories regarding the consequences of action, theories based on moral principles, or some combination of these two. Beauchamp and Childress[4] present a model for deliberation based on the principles of respect for autonomy, non-maleficence, beneficence and justice. Although this model frequently will not provide an answer that is beyond dispute, it does allow a rational examination of the important issues so that our subsequent actions will at least be better directed than they might otherwise have been.

Resuscitation medicine demands such deliberation despite the pressure of urgency and the common impairment of patient competence. Patient autonomy must be respected by employing a suitable consent process, such as the use of presumed consent using professional substituted judgement. In this way we can attempt to honour the patient's autonomy by viewing the benefits and harms of resuscitation from their perspective. Often, particularly in the early stages of resuscitation, the relative benefits and harms may be difficult to establish and the patient's perspective may be difficult to formalize. It is appropriate to continue with resuscitation until these

variables become more clear. However, the resuscitators have a moral obligation to stop resuscitation as soon as there is a negative answer to the question 'Would I want this done if I was this patient, knowing what I know about the patient, and knowing what I know about the likely outcome?'.

Controversies

❶ Performing resuscitation procedures where a poor outcome is expected or where there may be reason to suspect that the patient does not wish to be resuscitated.

❷ Withholding resuscitation procedures on the basis of an argument of futility.

❸ Establishing a 'Not For Resuscitation' status for a patient, without discussion with that patient.

❹ Practising procedures on the newly dead.

References

1. Australian Resuscitation Council. Adult advanced life support: Australian Resuscitation Council Guidelines 2006. Emergency Medicine Australasia 2006; 18: 337–356.
2. Medical Council of New Zealand. A doctor's duty to help in a medical emergency. August 2006. http://www.mcnz.org.nz/portals/0/Guidance/Doctors duties in an emergency.pdf (Accessed, August 2007).
3. Beauchamp TL. Philosophical ethics. An introduction to moral philosophy, 2nd edn. New York: McGrawHill, 1991.
4. Beauchamp TL, Childress JF. Principles of biomedical ethics, 5th edn. Oxford: Oxford University Press, 2001.
5. Ardagh M. Preventing harm in resuscitation medicine. New Zealand Medical Journal 1997; 110: 113–115.
6. Ardagh MW. Futility has no utility in resuscitation medicine. Journal of Medical Ethics 2000: 26: 393–396.
7. Ardagh MW. Resurrecting autonomy during resuscitation: the concept of professional substituted judgement. Journal of Medical Ethics 1999; 25: 375–378.
8. Sidhu NS, Dunkley ME, Egan MJ. 'Not for resuscitation' orders in Australian public hospitals: policies, standardized order forms and patient information leaflets. Medical Journal of Australia 2007; 186: 725.
9. Shepardson LB, Younger SJ, Speroff T, Rosenthal GE. Increased risk of death in patients with do-not-resuscitate orders. Medical Care 1999; 37: 727–737.
10. Ebrahim S. Do not resuscitate decisions: flogging dead horses or a dignified death? British Medical Journal 2000; 320: 115–156.
11. Ardagh M. May we practise endotracheal intubation on the newly dead? Journal of Medical Ethics 1997; 23: 289–294.

CRITICAL CARE

Edited by **Anthony F. T. Brown**

2.1 Airway and ventilation management

Stephen Bernard

ESSENTIALS

1 Respiratory failure is a common presentation to the emergency department and ventilatory support may be required.

2 Non-invasive assisted ventilation is appropriate for many patients, with endotracheal intubation and mechanical ventilation reserved for cases where non-invasive ventilation is unsuccessful or contraindicated.

3 Endotracheal intubation performed in the emergency department usually requires the use of sedative drugs plus muscle relaxants to facilitate tube placement.

4 Clinical checks of endotracheal tube position may be unreliable. Capnography and/or an oesophageal detector device should always be used to confirm tracheal placement.

5 A 'failed intubation drill' should be initiated immediately if visualization of the vocal cords at laryngoscopy is difficult or impossible, to avoid patient hypoxaemia.

6 Mechanical ventilation parameters in the ED should follow evidence-based guidelines, particularly the use of limited tidal volumes to avoid barotrauma in patients with acute lung injury.

Introduction

Assessment and management of the airway is the first step in the resuscitation of a critically ill patient in the emergency department (ED). Evaluation of the airway commences with a *'look, listen, feel'* approach to detect partial or complete airway obstruction. If airway compromise is suspected, initial basic airway manoeuvres include the jaw thrust, chin lift and head tilt (providing there is no suspicion of cervical spine injury), and placement of an oropharyngeal airway such as the Guedel (see Chapter 1.1 on Basic Life Support).

Gentle direct inspection of the upper airway using a laryngoscope may be necessary to detect a foreign body, which may be removed using a suction catheter and/or Magill's forceps for solid material. Once the airway is cleared, supplemental oxygen by face mask is commenced while consideration is given to the breathing status.

Reasons for endotracheal intubation

Endotracheal intubation is performed for one or more of the following four reasons: to create an airway; to maintain an airway; to protect an airway; and/or to provide for mechanical ventilation. Thus patients in respiratory arrest require immediate bag/valve/mask (BVM) ventilation while preparations are made for endotracheal intubation (ETI) and mechanical ventilation, and patients with a reduced conscious state and/or depression of the cough reflex may require early ETI for airway protection. Also, ETI may be indicated as part of sedative anaesthesia in the combative patient who requires imaging and/or a practical procedure, or for mechanical ventilation in patients with respiratory failure. However, in the latter a trial of non-invasive ventilation (NIV) should be considered.

Non-invasive ventilation

Many patients in respiratory failure with hypoxaemia and/or hypercapnia may benefit from a trial of non-invasive ventilation.[1] The use of NIV involves administration of a controlled mixture of oxygen and air delivered at a set positive pressure via a tightly sealed face mask. The pressure is maintained between 5 and 10 cmH$_2$O during both inspiration and expiration. This continuous positive airways pressure (CPAP) recruits lung alveoli that were previously closed, improving the ventilation/perfusion ratio and helping to correct hypoxaemia. There is also a reduction in the work of breathing as a result of an increase in pulmonary compliance. More recently, NIV machines have become available that administer positive pressure (i.e. 5–20 cmH$_2$O) above the elevated baseline pressure during inspiration, known as bilevel NIV. This additional inspiratory support is thought to further reduce the work of breathing.

Clinical indications for non-invasive ventilation in the ED
Patients who present with severe acute pulmonary oedema (APO) should receive CPAP to improve cardiac and pulmonary function while medical therapy with nitrates and diuretics is initiated.[2] However, the use of bilevel NIV in patients with APO gives no additional benefit and may increase the rate of myocardial infarction. On the other hand, patients who present with an exacerbation of chronic obstructive pulmonary disease (COPD) do benefit from bilevel NIV rather than CPAP alone.[3]

There is also some evidence to support the use of NIV in patients with respiratory failure due to other common ED conditions, such as community-acquired pneumonia[4] or asthma.[5] Thus it is common ED practice to now administer a trial of NIV in many patients with respiratory failure, prior to instituting ETI and mechanical ventilation. Contraindications to NIV include comatose or combative patients, poor tolerance of a tight-fitting face mask, and the lack of familiarity or lack of trained medical staff to institute and monitor the NIV.

Endotracheal intubation

Endotracheal intubation provides secure, definitive airway management and allows assisted mechanical ventilation. Patients with respiratory failure who are either ineligible for NIV or fail a trial of NIV should receive ETI and mechanical ventilation.

There are additional challenges to emergency endotracheal intubation in the ED compared to elective ETI in the operating theatre. There is often inadequate time for a complete clinical assessment of the upper airway or thorough consultation with the patient and/or family, and details of current medications, previous anaesthetics and allergies may not be available. Also, the status of the cervical spine in patients with an altered conscious state following trauma is unknown, even if initial plain imaging and even CT scanning appear normal.

There are a number of possible techniques for ETI, which are reviewed below. The selection of the appropriate technique depends on physician preference, experience and the clinical setting.

Rapid sequence induction (RSI) intubation
Unless the patient is deeply comatose or in cardiac arrest, upper airway reflexes will be present and ETI will require the use of sedative and neuromuscular blocking drugs to facilitate laryngoscopy and the placement of the endotracheal tube. Rapid sequence induction (RSI) of anaesthesia or rapid sequence intubation (the preferred North American RSI term) involves the simultaneous administration of sedation and a short-acting muscle relaxant in predetermined doses, and is the technique of choice when definitive emergency airway management is required in the ED.

Precautions and relative contraindications
Precautions and relative contraindications to the performance of RSI include patients with upper airway obstruction; distorted facial anatomy; likely difficult or impossible intubation, for example due to micrognathia or an ankylosed neck; and lack of appropriate operator skill or experience. An alternative intubation technique such as awake intubation under local anaesthesia, or an awake surgical airway such as a cricothyroidotomy or even a tracheostomy, may be preferred.

Preparation for RSI
Careful preparation is essential on each and every occasion RSI is required. If time and patient status allow, seek a history of

current medications, allergies and time of the last meal. Make a careful examination of the upper airway looking for anatomical features that may predict difficult intubation.

Intubation process
The conscious patient should receive explanation and reassurance. Pre-oxygenate with 100% oxygen to prevent oxygen desaturation during the procedure. Ideally, administer NIV with 100% oxygen for a 3-minute period.[6] If this is not possible, then breathing through a tight-fitting oxygen mask circuit using 15 L/min oxygen flow is an alternative way to pre-oxygenate the patient. Position the patient in the 'sniffing the morning air' position with the neck flexed and the head extended, using a pillow under the head. If the patient has suspected spinal column injury, immobilize the neck in the anatomically neutral position. Ensure there is reliable intravenous access, as well as equipment for suctioning the airway and a tipping trolley.

Monitoring during RSI
Arrange appropriate monitoring, including a continuous ECG trace and pulse oximetry. Measure the blood pressure either non-invasively using an automated monitoring device, or invasively using an intra-arterial cannula. Prepare waveform capnography for end-tidal carbon dioxide (ETCO$_2$) measurement following RSI.

Drugs used in RSI
The drugs required will depend on physician preference and the clinical situation. Common choices for induction include propofol at 1–2 mg/kg,[7] a narcotic such as morphine 0.15 mg/kg with a benzodiazepine such as midazolam 0.05–0.1 mg/kg, followed by a rapid-onset depolarizing neuromuscular blocking drug such as suxamethonium 1.5 mg/kg (Table 2.1.1). An alternative when suxamethonium is contraindicated is the rapid acting non-depolarizing drug rocuronium 1 mg/kg. Contraindications to suxamethonium include known allergy, hyperkalaemia or risk of from burns, spinal cord injury or crush injury (not in the acute setting), and a history of malignant hyperthermia (rare).[8] Details of the indications, dosages and side effects of all the commonly used drugs for RSI intubation are shown in Table 2.1.1.

Table 2.1.1 Common intravenous drugs for rapid sequence induction (RSI) intubation

Drug	Dose	Action	Onset (min)	Duration (min)
Premedication agents				
Atropine	0.02 mg/kg	Vagal blockade	1	30
Lidocaine	1.5 mg/kg	Decreases ICP	1	30
Fentanyl	1.5 µg/kg	Analgesic	2	30
Morphine	0.15 mg/kg	Analgesic	4	120
Midazolam	0.05 mg/kg	Anxiolytic	2	30
Vecuronium	0.01 mg/kg	Defasciculation	2	10
Induction agents				
Thiopentone	1–5 mg/kg	Rapid-onset sedation Reduces ICP	0.5	10
Propofol	1–2 mg/kg	Sedation	1	10
Fentanyl	10–20 µg/kg	Sedation, analgesic	1	20
Midazolam	0.05–0.1 mg/kg	Rapid-onset sedation	2	10
Diazepam	0.1 mg/kg	Rapid-onset sedation	2	20
Ketamine	1 mg/kg	Dissociative state	2	20
Muscle relaxants				
Suxamethonium	1.5 mg/kg	Depolarizing MR	0.5	5
Vecuronium	0.2 mg/kg	Non-depolarizing MR	2	40
Rocuronium	1.0 mg/kg	Non-depolarizing MR	1	30
Atracurium	0.5 mg/kg	Non-depolarizing MR	3	30
Pancuronium	0.1 mg/kg	Non-depolarizing MR	3	40

Preparation of equipment and personnel prior to RSI

All drugs must be drawn up and checked in advance, and the syringes clearly labelled. A spare laryngoscope must be available in case of failure of the first, and the appropriate size of endotracheal tube (ETT) opened, lubricated and the cuff checked. Another ETT (one size smaller) should be immediately available. Finally, an introducer and a gum-elastic or plastic bougie must be ready to hand.

At least two assistants will be required, one to assist the operator with the drugs and equipment, and another to provide cricoid pressure following the induction of sedation and muscle relaxation.[9] An additional person is required to provide in-line manual immobilization in the case of RSI for the trauma patient with possible spinal column injury. Additional equipment in case of difficult or failed intubation should be readily available, ideally kept together in a 'Difficult Airway Kit' containing the items necessary for a failed intubation protocol (Fig. 2.1.1).

Endotracheal tube insertion

When all preparations are complete, including pre-oxygenation, give the sedative drugs and, as consciousness is lost, the muscle relaxant (usually suxamethonium), with gentle cricoid pressure applied via the cricoid ring cartilage. Following

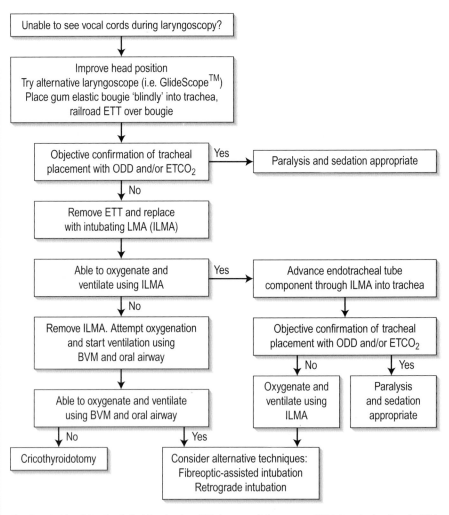

Fig. 2.1.1 Algorithm for failed intubation. ICP, intracranial pressure; BVM, bag/valve/mask; LMA, laryngeal mask airway; ILMA, intubating laryngeal mask airway; ODD, oesophageal detector device; ETCO₂, end-tidal carbon dioxide.

fasciculations and the loss of muscle tone, firm cricoid pressure is applied and the laryngoscopy performed. If the larynx is sighted, the endotracheal tube is placed through the vocal cords into the trachea, the cuff inflated and the ETT secured with tapes. Cricoid pressure must be maintained until the position of the tube is checked and secured, and the intubator indicates that he or she is happy with this.

Ensuring optimal tracheal position
Clinical methods of ensuring optimal tracheal position include sighting the passage of the ETT through the vocal cords, misting of the ETT during exhalation, and auscultation of breath sounds in the lung fields. However, when visualization of the vocal cords has been difficult, these clinical tests may be misleading and confirmatory tests are essential. The characteristic appearance of waveform capnography is regarded as the gold standard for confirmation of tracheal placement in patients with a palpable pulse.[10] However, during cardiac arrest there may be inadequate delivery of carbon dioxide to the lungs and hence a false negative reading. In this setting, the use of an oesophageal detector device (ODD) may be more appropriate.[11]

After successful endotracheal intubation, insert an orogastric or nasogastric tube and arrange a chest X-ray to confirm correct positioning of the tip of the ETT in the trachea at the level of the aortic knuckle, and not down the right main bronchus. It also allows confirmation of correct placement of the orogastric or nasogastric tube in the stomach.

Maintenance of sedation and paralysis
As the drugs used for sedation and muscle relaxation wear off, further drugs for the maintenance of sedation and paralysis will be required. Appropriate monitoring of vital signs, pulse oximetry and capnography with visual and audible alarms must be maintained at all times. Humidification of the inspired oxygen is desirable using a disposable heat and moisture filter. When the patient is placed on mechanical ventilation, the $PaCO_2$ should be checked to ensure adequate ventilation and to confirm correlation with the $ETCO_2$. The unconscious patient requires eye care, pressure area

care, temperature control and catheterization of the urinary bladder.

Complications of RSI intubation
Hypotension following endotracheal intubation is common and must be addressed promptly. The causes include the vasodilator and/or negative inotropic effects of the sedative drug(s) given, and/or the reduction in preload from positive-pressure ventilation decreasing venous return and cardiac output. Treatment consists of administration of a fluid bolus of 10–20 mL/kg and/or inotrope, depending on the clinical setting. Alternatively, in the setting of bronchospasm hypotension may be due to gas trapping, with dynamic hyperinflation from excessive ventilation and the development of auto-PEEP (positive end-expiratory pressure), or even to a tension pneumothorax occurring after the commencement of positive-pressure ventilation. Hypertension usually indicates inadequate sedation and should be treated with supplemental sedation.

The following additional measures need to be considered during intubation in patients with severe head injury. An assistant must hold the head in the neutral position as there is the possibility of cervical spine instability, which increases the difficulty of visualizing the larynx. Also, laryngoscopy may raise intracranial pressure, although the benefit of pretreatment with lignocaine (lidocaine) 1.5 mg/kg is uncertain.[12] Thiopentone or propofol must be used cautiously in patients with shock, or with severe head injury and possible hypovolaemia, as precipitate and prolonged hypotension may occur. Doses as small as one-tenth of normal may be necessary, e.g thiopentone 0.5 mg/kg or propofol 0.2 mg/kg.

The technique of RSI is not recommended for patients with a grossly abnormal upper airway, and/or impending upper airway obstruction. In this setting, the larynx may not be visualized and ventilation of the apnoeic patient may become impossible, leading to the extreme emergency of the 'can't intubate, can't ventilate' situation. An initial awake technique, such as using local anaesthesia, or a fibreoptic assisted intubation, should be performed in these patients. Alternatively, an inhalational anaesthetic agent or a short-acting intravenous agent such as propofol is used, as the sedative effects will rapidly reverse and spontaneous

respirations resume if intubation and ventilation prove impossible.

The difficult intubation
Endotracheal intubation under direct vision may be easy or difficult, depending on the view of the larynx during laryngoscopy. This view has been classified by Cormack and Lehane[13] into grades 1–4.

Cormack and Lehane laryngoscopy view
A Cormack and Lehane grade 1 laryngoscopy shows a clear view of the entire laryngeal aperture. A grade 2 laryngoscopy shows only the posterior part of the larynx visible. In a grade 3 laryngoscopy only the epiglottis is visualized, and in grade 4 only the soft palate is seen. A difficult intubation is defined as a grade 3 or 4 view at laryngoscopy.

Difficult intubation may be anticipated in the presence of pathological facial and upper airway disorders that may be congenital or acquired, such as maxillofacial and airway trauma, airway tumours and abscesses, or cervical spine immobility. There may also be anatomical reasons for a Cormack and Lehane grade 3–4 laryngoscopy, such as micrognathia or microstomia, poor mouth opening and/or a large tongue. A range of clinical tests have been proposed that may predict difficulty in visualization of the larynx, including relative size of the tongue to the pharynx, atlanto-occipital joint mobility, and a thyromental distance <6 cm. However, these are not always clinically useful in the emergency setting.[14]

Failed intubation drill
Attempts at blind placement of the ETT down the trachea when the larynx is not visualized are unlikely to be successful, and repeated attempts may result in direct pharyngeal or laryngeal trauma (making the situation even more difficult) and hypoxaemia. In this situation a failed intubation drill must be initiated.[15] A failed intubation algorithm suitable for use in the ED is shown in Figure 2.1.1. Depending on local hospital staffing and resources, an urgent call for assistance from another physician with additional experience should also be made.

Simple initial manoeuvres to improve visualization of the larynx include adding a second pillow to further flex the neck (unless cervical spine injury is suspected), the use of a straight Mackintosh laryngoscope blade, and 'backward/upward/rightward external pressure' (BURP) on the thyroid cartilage. A new approach to laryngoscopy using the GlideScope Video Laryngoscope (GVL) (Verathon, Bothell, WA, USA) provides a real-time view of the larynx on a colour monitor, which has been shown in a large case series to convert a Cormack and Lehane grade 3–4 view to a grade 1–2 view 77% of the time.[16] In the absence of a GlideScope, and if the larynx still cannot be visualized, blind placement of a gum-elastic bougie and subsequent insertion of the ETT by railroading it over the bougie should be attempted as the preferred next manoeuvre.[17] Rotating the ETT through 90° in an anticlockwise direction may be helpful if resistance to its passage occurs at the larynx.

If these initial steps are unsuccessful, adequate oxygenation must be maintained using a bag/mask with an oral airway at all times. Alternative equipment suitable for use in the ED should be prepared.[18] A summary of these devices for a failed intubation drill is given below (see Fig. 2.1.1). However, if oxygenation can not be maintained during the attempted use of these devices, immediate cricothyroidotomy is indicated. Make sure additional help has also been summoned.

Laryngeal mask airway

The laryngeal mask airway (LMA) is now used routinely for airway management during elective general anaesthesia. During a failed intubation drill, the LMA may be superior to a bag/mask and oral airway for oxygenation and ventilation.[15,17] However, the LMA has had a limited role in the ED, for two reasons. First, if pulmonary compliance is low or airway resistance is high, there will be a leak around the cuff of the LMA when peak inspiratory airway pressures exceed 20–30 mmHg. Second, there is the potential risk of aspiration pneumonitis as the airway remains unprotected. The LMA ProSeal (Vitaid Ltd, Toronto, Ontario, Canada) modification of the standard LMA minimizes this

risk, and includes a double cuff to improve the seal and a distal drainage tube to provide access for suctioning the upper oesophagus. The LMA may also be used to assist in orotracheal intubation, using either a 6 mm ETT passed blindly through the LMA, or an ETT placed over a fibreoptic bronchoscope which is then passed through the LMA into the trachea.

Intubating laryngeal mask airway

The 'intubating LMA' (ILMA) is a modification of the standard LMA that incorporates a rigid, anatomically curved airway tube with handle, and a special modified endotracheal tube and extender specifically made to pass blindly through the ILMA into the trachea. This appears to have a high success rate even with inexperienced operators, both in managing patients with a difficult airway in hospital[19] and in the pre-hospital setting.[20] The ILMA is placed and ventilation commenced, and once oxygenation is assured, the ETT component is passed through the ILMA. Once sited, the ETT cuff is inflated and the position confirmed using capnography and then chest X-rays.

Fibreoptic bronchoscope-assisted intubation

A fibreoptic bronchoscope assists in the intubation of the patient when RSI fails or is contraindicated. In particular, fibreoptic bronchoscope-assisted intubation (FBI) is the technique of choice in suspected traumatic injury to the larynx, and in the obstructed airway, particularly with distorted anatomy such as with an upper airway burn or tumour. The FBI may diagnose the severity of the laryngeal injury or pathology and the possible requirement for surgery. However, it requires considerable training and should only be performed by an experienced operator. Equipment sterilization, maintenance and checking procedures must also be in place (see later).

Intubation procedure

If the patient is awake, apply topical anaesthetic to the nasal passage and upper airway as for blind nasotracheal intubation

(BNTI – see later). Initially, introduce a well-lubricated ETT nasally and pass to the posterior pharynx. Then insert the bronchoscope through the ETT to visualize the vocal cords. The suction port of the bronchoscope may be used to clear any secretions, and also to administer further local anaesthesia into the airway. Advance the bronchoscope through the larynx and railroad the ETT over it and down the trachea. Administer further sedation at this time. Ventilate the patient with oxygen following removal of the bronchoscope. If a LMA has been used during a failed intubation drill and is in place to provide ventilation, this may be utilized to guide the bronchoscope (with the ETT already placed over it) into the larynx. Removal of the LMA then requires placement of a gum-elastic bougie; the ETT and LMA are removed, then the ETT is replaced over the bougie.

The use of a fibreoptic bronchoscope in the ED is limited by several factors. The bronchoscope and light source must be immediately available during a failed intubation drill. The technique requires considerable practice for skills maintenance, yet its use is rare in ED practice. The larynx may be difficult to visualize in the presence of blood, vomitus or copious secretions. Finally, the equipment is expensive to purchase and maintain.

Retrograde intubation

When other techniques fail the technique of retrograde intubation may occasionally be used in the ED if time permits.[21] The cricothyroid membrane is punctured by a needle/cannula and a guide-wire is passed through the cannula, directed cephalad. The wire is then brought out through the mouth using Magill's forceps. There are a number of techniques used to then guide the ETT over the wire and back into the larynx, such as a proprietary device (Cook, Cook Medical Inc, Bloomington, IN, USA), or the introducer of a Minitrach II kit (Portex Ltd, Hythe, Kent, UK).[22] Alternatively, the wire may be passed inside the end of the ETT and then out through the 'Murphy eye'. Resistance may be felt when the ETT reaches the larynx, and some anticlockwise rotation may be required to facilitate passage into the larynx. When the level of

CRITICAL CARE

the cricothyroid is reached, the guide-wire is removed and the ETT passed further down the trachea. The technique of retrograde intubation takes time and experience to perform and is usually unsuitable in a critical airway emergency.

Blind nasotracheal intubation

Blind nasotracheal intubation (BNTI) is a technique that is now rarely used in the operating theatre, but may occasionally be useful in the ED, either as the initial technique of choice or as part of a failed intubation drill once spontaneous respirations have resumed. Contraindications include a fractured base of skull or maxillary fracture, a suspected laryngeal injury, coagulopathy or upper airway obstruction.

High-flow oxygen is administered by mask and the nasal passages are inspected to assess patency. The larger nasal passage is prepared with a pledget soaked in local anaesthetic and vasoconstrictor, such as 5 mL lignocaine (lidocaine) 2% with epinephrine 1:100 000. After several minutes the pledget is removed and sterile lubricant applied. Local anaesthetic may also be sprayed into the upper airway, and/or intravenous sedation may be administered if required and clinically appropriate. An ETT one size smaller than the predicted oral size is passed via the nose to the pharynx and advanced slowly towards the larynx, with the operator listening for breath sounds.

The head may need to be flexed, extended or rotated to facilitate entry into the larynx, the ETT rotated clockwise through 90°, and/or a suction catheter used to guide the ETT. When the tube passes into the trachea, louder spontaneous respirations heard from the ETT, or the onset of coughing down the tube, confirm successful placement. However, there are significant complications with BNTI, including epistaxis,[23] injuries to the turbinates, perforation of the posterior pharynx, laryngospasm and injury to the larynx. In addition, an already jeopardized airway may be made worse, leaving the situation impossible to then control.

Cricothyroidotomy

Cricothyroidotomy is an essential skill for all emergency physicians and must be considered immediately in the situation of *'can't intubate, can't ventilate'*. There are several possible techniques for emergency cricothyroidotomy.

Techniques for emergency cricothyroidotomy

First, there are proprietary kits that allow a cricothyroidotomy tube to be placed using the Seldinger technique. In this approach, the cricothyroid membrane is punctured with a needle mounted on a syringe; free aspiration of air confirms placement in the airway. A guide-wire is passed through the needle down the trachea. The needle is then removed and a dilator passed along the wire, then a 4.5–6 mm cricothyroidotomy tube is mounted on a guide and passed along the wire and into the trachea. The position of the cricothyroidotomy tube must be carefully checked, as it is easy to misplace it anterior to the trachea. However, if the cricothyroidotomy tube is uncuffed, interpretation of a capnograph waveform can be difficult as much of the exhaled gas may pass into the upper airway, and not through the cricothyroidotomy tube during exhalation, resulting in a false-negative end-tidal CO_2 trace.

Surgical cricothyroidotomy

Alternatively, perform a surgical cricothyroidotomy by making a small vertical incision over the cricothyroid membrane. Use artery forceps for blunt dissection to the cricothyroid membrane, which is incised and the cricothyroid membrane opened horizontally with artery forceps. Pass a size 6 mm cuffed ETT or tracheostomy tube through the opening into the trachea, inflate the cuff and commence bag/valve ventilation. This technique is usually faster to perform than a guide-wire technique, although physicians with limited surgical experience may prefer the Seldinger approach.[24]

Longer-term placement of a larger tube (>6 mm) through the cricothyroid membrane is unsatisfactory because of the possibility of stricture occurring at the level of the cricoid ring. Therefore, the cricothyroidotomy is converted to either an oral endotracheal intubation or a tracheostomy when it is safe and convenient to do so.

Tracheostomy

Compared with cricothyroidotomy, a surgical tracheostomy is time-consuming and difficult to perform in the ED. Pre-tracheal dissection requires adequate lighting, instruments and diathermy, because the thyroid isthmus may be anterior to the trachea. Distorted anatomy and bleeding make the technique more complex. However, percutaneous dilatational tracheostomy is commonly performed in the ICU, and can be rapidly performed by an experienced operator in the ED, although there is little published experience with this technique outside the ICU. In addition, some techniques use a second operator visualizing correct tube placement via a bronchoscope.

Mechanical ventilation

Once intubation has been achieved, the patient is connected to a mechanical ventilator to provide continued ventilatory support. Because ventilated patients may initially be managed for some time in the ED, it is important that recommendations for optimal mechanical ventilation are implemented in the ED.

Recommendations for optimal mechanical ventilation

A tidal volume of 10 mL/kg and a respiratory rate of 10–14 breaths per minute are considered safe for most patients. However, patients with acute lung injury may have reduced pulmonary compliance and hence elevated peak inspiratory pressures. These patients should receive a 'protective lung strategy'.[25] This involves limiting the tidal volume to 6 mL/kg, with the respiratory rate setting increased to 16–20 breaths per minute to prevent excessive hypercapnia. Deliberate hyperventilation using a respiratory rate of 16–20 breaths per minute may also be indicated to provide hypocapnia in other situations, such as in patients with severe metabolic acidosis, and in patients with raised intracranial pressure, in whom transient hypocapnia of 30–35 mmHg (4.0–4.7 kPa) may temporarily reduce intracranial pressure while other treatments for intracranial hypertension are being implemented.

Conversely, patients with severe airways obstruction such as asthma or COPD should receive a standard tidal volume of 10 mL/kg, but a decreased respiratory rate from 4 to 8 breaths per minute to allow sufficient time for adequate passive exhalation.[26] This reduces the risk of pulmonary hyperinflation, with the development of auto-PEEP leading to hypotension, even electromechanical dissociation. Thus when ventilating a critical asthmatic the $PaCO_2$ level will rise (known as 'permissive hypercapnia'), with the aim being to initially concentrate only on oxygenation.

Extubation in the emergency department

Increasingly, patients who are intubated 'in the field' by paramedics or by a physician in the ED may be considered for planned extubation in the ED, after investigation and treatment have excluded a requirement for admission to the ICU. Examples include patients with a drug overdose, or those requiring brief general anaesthesia for a procedure.

Prediction of successful extubation

Prediction of successful extubation is problematic in the ICU,[27] and there are even fewer published data to guide successful elective ED extubation. In general, patients should be awake, able to follow commands and cough, pass a trial of spontaneous breathing with the ventilator set to a continuous positive airways pressure (CPAP) of 5 cmH_2O, with minimal pressure support of 5–10 cmH_2O, and who require only modest supplemental oxygen, that is, < 50% inspired oxygen (FiO_2 < 0.5). Ideally, the

stomach should be emptied via an orogastric or nasogastric tube prior to extubation.

Controversies

- Choice of drugs used in RSI intubation, and the role of premedication agents.

- Training and skills maintenance of airway management techniques in the ED.

- The optimal 'Difficult Airway Kit'.

- Practising the failed intubation drill in the ED, including the role of simulation.

References

1. Hill NS, Brennan J, Garpestad E, Nava S. Noninvasive ventilation in acute respiratory failure. Critical Care Medicine 2007; 35: 2402–2407.
2. Peter JV, Moran JL, Phillips-Hughes J, et al. Effect of non-invasive positive pressure ventilation (NIPPV) on mortality in patients with acute cardiogenic pulmonary oedema: a meta-analysis. Lancet 2006; 367: 1155–1163.
3. Ram FS, Lightowler JV, Wedzicha JA. Non-invasive positive pressure ventilation for treatment of respiratory failure due to exacerbations of chronic obstructive pulmonary disease. Cochrane Database Systematic Review 2004; (1): CD004104.
4. Keenan SP, Sinuff T, Cook DJ, et al. Does non-invasive positive pressure ventilation improve outcome in acute hypoxemic respiratory failure? A systematic review. Critical Care Medicine 2004; 32: 2516–2523.
5. Ram FS, Wellington S, Rowe B, et al. Non-invasive positive pressure ventilation for treatment of respiratory failure due to severe acute exacerbations of asthma. Cochrane Database Systematic Review 2005; (3): CD004360.
6. Baillard C, Fosse JP, Sebbane M, et al. Noninvasive ventilation improves preoxygenation before intubation of hypoxic patients. American Journal of Respiratory and Critical Care Medicine 2006; 174: 171–177.
7. Wilbur K, Zed PJ. Is propofol an optimal agent for procedural sedation and rapid sequence intubation in the emergency department? Canadian Journal of Emergency Medicine 2001; 3: 302–310.
8. Sluga M, Ummenhofer W, Studer W, et al. Rocuronium versus succinylcholine for rapid sequence induction of anesthesia and endotracheal intubation: a prospective, randomized trial in emergent cases. Anesthesia and Analgesia 2005; 101: 1356–1361.
9. Ellis DY, Harris T, Zideman D. Cricoid. Pressure in emergency department rapid sequence tracheal

10. intubations: a risk-benefit analysis. Annals of Emergency Medicine 2007; 50: 653–665.
10. Deiorio NM. Continuous end-tidal carbon dioxide monitoring for confirmation of endotracheal tube placement is neither widely available nor consistently applied by emergency physicians. Emergency Medicine Journal 2005; 22: 490–493.
11. Schaller RJ, Huff JS, Zahn A. Comparison of a colorimetric end-tidal CO_2 detector and an esophageal aspiration device for verifying endotracheal tube placement in the prehospital setting: a six-month experience. Prehospital and Disaster Medicine 1997; 12: 57–63.
12. Robinson N, Clancy M. In patients with head injury undergoing rapid sequence intubation, does pretreatment with intravenous lignocaine/lidocaine lead to an improved neurological outcome? A review of the literature. Emergency Medicine Journal 2001; 18: 453–457.
13. Cormack RS, Lehane J. Difficult intubation in obstetrics. Anaesthesia 1984; 39: 1105–1111.
14. Shiga T, Wajima Z, Inoue T, Sakamoto A. Predicting difficult intubation in apparently normal patients: a meta-analysis of bedside screening test performance. Anesthesiology 2005; 103: 429–437.
15. Henderson JJ, Popat MT, Latto IP, et al. Difficult Airway Society. Difficult Airway Society guidelines for management of the unanticipated difficult intubation. Anaesthesia 2004; 59: 675–694.
16. Cooper RM, Pacey JA, Bishop MJ, McCluskey SA. Early clinical experience with a new videolaryngoscope (GlideScope) in 728 patients. Canadian Journal of Anaesthesia 2005; 52: 191–198.
17. Jabre P, Combes X, Leroux B, et al. Use of gum elastic bougie for prehospital difficult intubation. American Journal of Emergency Medicine 2005; 23: 552–555.
18. Bair AE, Filbin MR, Kulkarni RG, et al. The failed intubation attempt in the emergency department: analysis of prevalence, rescue techniques, and personnel. Journal of Emergency Medicine 2002; 23: 131–140.
19. Ferson DZ, Rosenblatt WH, Johansen MJ, et al. Use of the intubating LMA-Fastrach in 254 patients with difficult-to-manage airways. Anesthesiology 2001; 95: 1175–1181.
20. Timmermann A, Russo SG, Rosenblatt WH, et al. Intubating laryngeal mask airway for difficult out-of-hospital airway management: a prospective evaluation. British Journal of Anaesthesia 2007; 99: 286–291.
21. Weksler N, Klein M, Weksler D, et al. Retrograde tracheal intubation: beyond fibreoptic endotracheal intubation. Acta Anaesthesiologica Scandinavica 2004; 48: 412–416.
22. Slots P, Vegger PB, Bettger H, et al. Retrograde intubation with a Mini-Trach II kit. Acta Anaesthesiologica Scandinavica 2003; 47: 274–277.
23. Piepho T, Thierbach A, Werner C. Nasotracheal intubation: look before you leap. British Journal of Anaesthesia 2005; 94: 859–860.
24. Sulaiman L, Tighe SQ, Nelson RA. Surgical vs wire-guided cricothyroidotomy: a randomised crossover study of cuffed and uncuffed tracheal tube insertion. Anaesthesia 2006; 61: 565–570.
25. Girard TD, Bernard GR. Mechanical ventilation in ARDS: a state-of-the-art review. Chest 2007; 131: 921–929.
26. Shapiro JM. Management of respiratory failure in status asthmaticus. American Journal of Respiratory and Critical Care Medicine 2002; 1: 409–416.
27. Meade M, Guyatt G, Cook D, et al. Predicting success in weaning from mechanical ventilation. Chest 2001; 120: 400S–424S.

2.2 Oxygen therapy

David R. Smart

ESSENTIALS

1 Oxygen is the most commonly used drug in emergency medicine.

2 Oxygen-delivery systems may be divided into variable performance (delivering a variable concentration of oxygen) and fixed performance (delivering a fixed concentration of oxygen, including systems that deliver 100% oxygen).

3 Controlled-dose oxygen therapy is required when treating patients with chronic obstructive pulmonary disease (COPD), commencing with 24–28%. Response to therapy in these patients should be monitored with arterial blood gases measurements.

4 Oxygen should never be abruptly withdrawn from patients in circumstances of suspected CO_2 narcosis.

5 Fixed-performance systems are essential where precise titration of oxygen dose is required, such as with COPD, or where 100% oxygen is required.

6 In attempting to deliver 100% oxygen, free-flowing circuits are least efficient. A reservoir or demand system improves efficiency, and a closed-circuit delivery system is most efficient.

7 Pulse oximetry provides valuable feedback regarding the appropriateness of oxygen dose provided to individual patients.

Introduction

Oxygen was first discovered by Priestley in 1772 and was first used therapeutically by Beddoes in 1794. It now forms one of the cornerstones of medical therapy.

Oxygen (O_2) constitutes 21% of dry air by volume. It is essential to life. Cellular hypoxia results from a deficiency of oxygen, regardless of aetiology. Hypoxaemia is a state of reduced oxygen carriage in the blood. Hypoxia leads to an anaerobic metabolism that is inefficient, and may lead to death if not corrected. A major priority in acute medical management is correction of hypoxia, hence oxygen is the most frequently administered and important drug in emergency medicine. There are sound physiological reasons for the use of supplemental oxygen in the management of acutely ill and injured patients.

Uses of supplemental oxygen

- To correct defects in the delivery of inspired gas to the lungs. A clear airway is essential.
- Where there is inadequate oxygenation of blood due to defects in pulmonary gas exchange.
- To maximize oxygen saturation of the arterial blood (SaO_2) where there is inadequate oxygen transport by the cardiovascular system.
- To maximize oxygen partial pressure and content in the blood in circumstances of increased or inefficient tissue oxygen demand.
- To provide 100% oxygen where clinically indicated.
- To titrate oxygen dose in patients with impaired ventilatory response to carbon dioxide.

Physiology of oxygen

Oxygen transport chain

Oxygen proceeds from inspired air to the mitochondria via a number of steps known as the oxygen transport chain. These steps include:

❶ Ventilation
❷ Pulmonary gas exchange
❸ Oxygen carriage in the blood
❹ Local tissue perfusion
❺ Diffusion at tissue level
❻ Tissue utilization of oxygen.

Ventilation

The normal partial pressure of inspired air oxygen (P_IO_2) is approximately 20 kPa (150 mmHg) at sea level. If there is a reduction in the fraction of inspired oxygen (F_IO_2), as occurs at altitude, hypoxia results. This is relevant in the transport of patients at 2400 m in commercial 'pressurized' aircraft, where ambient cabin pressures of 74.8 kPa (562 mmHg) result in a P_IO_2 of 14.4 kPa (108 mmHg).

Hypoxia can result from inadequate delivery of inspired gas to the lung. The many causes include airway obstruction, respiratory muscle weakness, neurological disorders interfering with respiratory drive (seizures, head injury), disruption to chest mechanics (chest injury), or extrinsic disease interfering with ventilation (intra-abdominal pathology). These processes interfere with the maintenance of an adequate alveolar oxygen partial pressure (P_AO_2), which is approximately 13.7 kPa (103 mmHg) in a healthy individual.

Alveolar gas equation An approximation of the alveolar gas equation permits rapid calculation of the alveolar oxygen partial pressures:

$$P_AO_2 = F_IO_2 \times (\text{barometric pressure} - 47) - PaCO_2/0.8$$

Pulmonary gas exchange

Oxygen diffuses across the alveoli and into pulmonary capillaries, and carbon dioxide diffuses in the opposite direction. The process is passive, occurring down concentration gradients. Fick's law summarizes the process of diffusion of gases through tissues:

$$\dot{V}O_2 \propto A/T \times Sol/\sqrt{MW} \times (P_AO_2 - P_{pa}O_2)$$

where $\dot{V}O_2$ = rate of gas (oxygen) transfer, $\propto$ = proportional to, A = area of tissue, T = tissue thickness, Sol = solubility of the gas, MW = molecular weight, P_A = alveolar partial pressure, and P_{pa} = pulmonary artery partial pressure.

In healthy patients oxygen passes rapidly from the alveoli to the blood, and after 0.25 seconds pulmonary capillary blood is almost fully saturated with oxygen, resulting in a systemic arterial oxygen partial pressure (P_AO_2) of approximately 13.3 kPa (100 mmHg). The difference between the P_AO_2 and the PaO_2 is known as the alveolar to arterial oxygen gradient (A–a gradient). It is usually small and increases with age.

Expected A–a gradient The expected A–a gradient when breathing air approximates to: age (years) ÷ 4 + 4. An approximation of the actual value may be calculated as follows:

A–a O_2 gradient = 140 − (PO_2 + PCO_2).

There is a defect in pulmonary gas exchange if the calculated value exceeds the expected value. The A–a O_2 gradient is increased if there is a barrier to diffusion, such as pulmonary fibrosis or oedema, or a deficit in perfusion such as a pulmonary embolism. An increased A–a gradient also reflects widespread ventilation–perfusion mismatch. In circumstances of impaired diffusion in the lung, raising the F_IO_2 assists oxygen transfer by creating a greater pressure gradient from the alveoli to the pulmonary capillary. The increase in F_IO_2 may not be as helpful when lung perfusion is impaired as a result of increased intrapulmonary shunting.

Oxygen carriage in the blood

Three steps are required to deliver oxygen to the periphery:

❶ Uptake of oxygen by haemoglobin (Hb).
❷ Generation of a cardiac output to carry the oxygenated haemoglobin to the peripheral tissues.
❸ Dissociation of oxygen from haemoglobin to allow diffusion from blood to cell.

The haemoglobin–oxygen (Hb–O_2) dissociation curve The haemoglobin-oxygen (Hb–O_2) dissociation curve is depicted in Figure 2.2.1, which also summarizes the factors that influence the position of the curve. If the curve is shifted to the left, this favours the affinity of haemoglobin for oxygen. These conditions are encountered when deoxygenated blood returns to the lung. A shift of the curve to the right favours unloading of oxygen and subsequent delivery to the tissues.

A number of advantages are conferred by the shape of the Hb–O_2 dissociation curve that favour uptake of oxygen in the lung and delivery to the tissues:[1]

• A flat upper portion of the curve allows some reserve in the P_AO_2 required to keep the haemoglobin fully saturated; a reduction in P_AO_2 of 20% will have minimal effect on the oxygen loading of Hb.
• The flat upper portion of the curve also ensures that a large difference remains between P_AO_2 and the pulmonary capillary oxygen partial pressure ($P_{pc}O_2$), even when much of the haemoglobin has been loaded with oxygen. This pressure difference favours maximal Hb–O_2 loading.

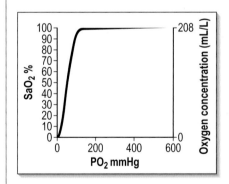

Fig. 2.2.1 The haemoglobin–oxygen dissociation curve.

• The lower part of the curve is steeper, which favours offloading of oxygen in peripheral tissues with only small falls in capillary PO_2. This maintains a higher driving pressure of oxygen, facilitating diffusion into cells.
• The right shift of the Hb–O_2 curve in circumstances of increased temperature, fall in pH, increased PCO_2 and increased erythrocyte 2,3-DPG assists in further offloading of oxygen, even when the driving pressure has fallen and PO_2 has reached 5.3 kPa (40 mmHg), i.e. venous blood which is still 75% saturated with oxygen.

Oxygen is carried in the blood as dissolved gas and in combination with haemoglobin. At sea level (101.3 kPa), breathing air (F_IO_2 = 0.21), the amount of oxygen dissolved in plasma is very small (0.03 mL oxygen per litre of blood for each 1 mmHg PaO_2). This dissolved component assumes greater significance in a hyperbaric situation, where at 284 kPa and F_IO_2 = 1.0 up to 60 mL oxygen can be carried in the dissolved form per litre of blood.

Haemoglobin carries 1.34–1.39 mL oxygen per gram when fully saturated. Blood with a haemoglobin concentration of 15 g/L carries approximately 200 mL oxygen per litre.

Oxygen flux The total amount of oxygen delivered to the body per minute is known as oxygen flux.[1]

Oxygen flux = (oxyhaemoglobin + dissolved O_2) × cardiac output
= (1.39 × Hb × S_aO_2/100 + 0.03 × PAO_2) × Q

where Hb = haemoglobin concentration g/L; S_aO_2 = arterial oxygen saturation (percentage); PaO_2 = partial pressure of arterial oxygen (mmHg); Q = cardiac output (L/min).

A healthy individual breathing air transports approximately 1000 mL oxygen per minute to the tissues, with a cardiac output of 5 L/min; 30% or 300 mL/min of this oxygen is not available, because at least 2.7 kPa (20 mmHg) driving pressure is required to allow oxygen to enter the mitochondria, and therefore approximately 700 mL/minute are available for use by peripheral tissues. This provides a considerable reserve above the 250 mL/min consumed by a healthy resting adult.

In illness or injury this reserve may be considerably eroded. Factors that reduce oxygen flux include a fall in cardiac output of any aetiology (including shock states), anaemia or a reduction in functional haemoglobin (carbon monoxide poisoning) and a drop in the S_aO_2. These situations are frequently encountered in emergency medicine. Supplemental oxygen is required in addition to specific therapy such as volume replacement, transfusion, and measures to improve cardiac output.

Local tissue perfusion and diffusion

Cellular hypoxia results if there is impairment of perfusion to local tissues. Oedema associated with medical illness or local injury increases the diffusion distance between blood and cell, thus mandating a higher PaO_2 to ensure adequate tissue oxygen delivery.

Tissue utilization of oxygen

Increased oxygen flux is required if:

- Tissue demands for oxygen are higher than normal, or
- Tissue utilization of oxygen is impaired.

Elevation of cardiac output increases oxygen flux in these circumstances, but frequently this too is significantly impaired by the disease state.

Tissue demands for oxygen increase by 7% for each degree Celsius elevation in body temperature, and considerably greater increases in demand occur in seizures, sepsis, severe dyspnoea, restlessness and shivering.[2]

Tissue extraction of oxygen is impaired in sepsis, and by poisons such as carbon monoxide or cyanide. In all cases, oxygen therapy must be combined with general measures such as reduction of fever and specific treatment of the primary disease process.

Oxygen delivery systems

Oxygen delivery systems are classified into three groups (Table 2.2.1):

❶ Variable-performance systems
❷ Fixed-performance systems
❸ One hundred per cent oxygen systems.

Table 2.2.1 Oxygen delivery systems
Variable-performance systems
Nasal cannulae
Hudson mask +/− reservoir
T pieces and Y connectors
Fixed-performance systems:
Venturi mask
Oxygen blenders
100% Oxygen systems
Non-rebreathing circuits
– Free-flowing circuits
– Self-refilling circuits
– Soft reservoir bags
– Oxygen-powered resuscitators
Partial-rebreathing circuits
Closed circuit systems

Definitions

Variable-performance oxygen delivery systems

These systems deliver a variable F_IO_2 to the patient that is altered by the inspiratory flow rate, the minute volume of the patient, and the physical characteristics of the delivery system.

Fixed-performance oxygen delivery systems

These systems deliver a specified F_IO_2 to the patient that is not altered by changes in ventilatory pattern, volume or inspiratory flow rate.

One hundred per cent (100%) oxygen systems

This is a subgroup of fixed-performance systems wherein 100% oxygen is delivered to the patient.

General principles

In most Australasian emergency departments the oxygen source consists of a wall-mounted flowmeter capable of delivering oxygen up to 15 L/min. Most available oxygen delivery systems connect to this apparatus. The 15 L/min flow rate limits the delivery of high F_IO_2 to adults for the following reasons:

- A quietly breathing adult has a peak inspiratory flow rate (PIFR) of approximately 30–40 L/min, which exceeds the oxygen supply. Hence a free flowing system such as a Hudson mask must entrain air into the system in order to match the patient's PIFR, with a

resultant reduction in F_IO_2 to a maximum of 0.6.[3]

- A quietly breathing adult has a respiratory minute volume of 4–8 L; in a child this value is approximately 150 mL/kg. Oxygen is stored during expiration by incorporating a reservoir into the circuit for use during inspiration, with a considerable improvement in the economy of oxygen use. This system is limited by the patient's minute volume. If the minute volume exceeds 15 L there is a danger of the patient asphyxiating due to insufficient gas supply, or if safety valves allow air into the system, the F_IO_2 falls.

Multiple-port oxygen supply outlets can overcome the above limitations of inspiratory flow rate and minute volume. The use of 'Y' connectors and 'T' pieces enable 30, 45 or 60 L per minute to be delivered to the patient to achieve an F_IO_2 of very nearly 1.0. Extra source oxygen flow may cause variable-performance systems such as the Hudson mask to become fixed-performance systems. Hence the terms 'variable performance' and 'fixed performance' are loosely applied and are largely dependent on whether or not the flow of gas delivered to the patient is sufficient to match their ventilatory requirements.

A fine example of this is in paediatric oxygen delivery. A high F_IO_2 can be delivered using a standard 15 L/min oxygen source because the child's ventilatory requirements are smaller in proportion to the available oxygen supply.

The oxygen delivery systems available for use in emergency medicine are broadly summarized in Table 2.2.1. They can be further subdivided according to economy of oxygen use and whether or not the system can be used to ventilate the patient manually. Figures depicting the various systems have been published elsewhere.[3]

Variable performance systems

The F_IO_2 delivered by these systems is summarized in Table 2.2.2. Options available for use in emergency medicine include:

- Nasal cannulae
- Face masks with air inlets
- T pieces and Y connectors.

Table 2.2.2 Variable-performance oxygen delivery systems

Apparatus	Oxygen flow (L/min)	Oxygen concentration (%)
Nasal catheters	1–4	24–40
Semi-rigid mask	6–15	35–60
Semi-rigid mask + double O_2 supply	15–30	Up to 80
Semi-rigid mask + reservoir bag	12–15	60–90

Nasal cannulae

The system must be used at flow rates 4 L/min or less to avoid painful drying of the nasal mucosa, although a flow rate of 2 L/min or less is insufficient to create a nasopharyngeal reservoir during the expiration pause, for inspiration with the next breath.

The inspired oxygen concentration is a function of the patient's inspiratory flow rate, and is usually in the vicinity of 22–28%. At flow rates of 2–4 L/min the nasopharynx acts as a partial reservoir during the expiratory pause, resulting in an increased F_IO_2. The delivered F_IO_2 is then influenced by the pattern of breathing (mouth or nose) and the positioning of the nasal cannula.[4]

Nasal cannulae provide a higher F_IO_2 in paediatric patients and nose breathers. They are less effective in dyspnoeic patients because of the greater amounts of air inspired through the mouth. They are frequently used in patients with stable COPD because of the absence of dead space that prevents CO_2 rebreathing. However, fluctuations in F_IO_2 make nasal cannulae less than ideal in the management of patients who rely on hypoxic respiratory drive, and they are second choice after Venturi masks in the emergency management of these patients. Advantages for home therapy include the ability to eat and drink, less noise than masks, and economy of oxygen use.

Face masks (e.g. Hudson, Edinburgh, Medishield)

A small reservoir of oxygen is provided by these masks, but this has little effect on F_IO_2. The small increase in dead space created by the mask necessitates a flow rate greater than 6 L/min to prevent rebreathing of CO_2. Two factors influence the F_IO_2 provided by this system:

❶ The patient's inspiratory flow rate
❷ The source oxygen supply flow rate.

At flow rates of 6–14 L/min, the delivered F_IO_2 varies from 0.35 to 0.6. This will be less in a dyspnoeic patient because of the higher inspiratory flow rate, and greater in a child because the converse applies. If the PIFR increases, greater amounts of air will be entrained into the mask, diluting the oxygen. During expiration, the exhaled gas and excess oxygen are vented through the side perforations.

Attaching a reservoir bag to this mask improves the economy of oxygen use by storing this vented gas during the expiratory phase. This increases the delivered F_IO_2, but this may be at the expense of increased CO_2 rebreathing. Commercially available reservoir bags have a volume of 750 mL to 1 L, which is inadequate for a dyspnoeic patient. The author recommends a minimum flow rate of 12 L/min to avoid CO_2 retention.

Using a source oxygen supply of 15 L/min, the maximum F_IO_2 delivered via a Hudson mask to a quietly breathing adult is 0.6.[3] By attaching another source of oxygen using a 'T' piece or 'Y' connector, the resultant flow rate of 30 L/min can deliver an F_IO_2 up to 0.8. With even greater flow rates the mask may be converted into a fixed-performance system delivering an F_IO_2 of almost 1.0. Then the ability to deliver 100% oxygen is limited by the mask's 'fit'.

The Medishield mask is stated to be more efficient than the Hudson because dead space is reduced by bringing the oxygen supply closer to the mouth, allowing more effective entrainment during inspiration. An F_IO_2 of 0.75 may be obtained with a gas flow rate of 15 L/min.

T pieces and Y connectors

The term 'T piece' has been used to describe a number of different oxygen delivery systems, including the 'T piece' for supplying humidified oxygen to patients with a tracheostomy, and the 'Ayre's T piece' which is the Mapleson E circuit. The use of 'T pieces' or 'Y connectors' in emergency medicine is to supplement an existing oxygen supply with:

- extra oxygen
- nebulized medication
- humidification.

The disadvantage of the system is that several oxygen ports are necessary, which is untidy and may restrict the patient's mobility. There is loss of economy of oxygen use because of higher flow rates. T pieces allow a higher F_IO_2 to be delivered to severely dyspnoeic patients.

Fixed-performance systems

Two systems are available for use in emergency departments:

❶ High-flow Venturi masks
❷ Oxygen blenders.

High-flow Venturi mask

Oxygen flow through a Venturi system results in air entrainment with delivery of a fixed concentration of oxygen to the patient. The masks deliver F_IO_2 values from 0.24, 0.28, 0.35, 0.40 and 0.50 to 0.60, using different colour-coded adaptors, or by varying the position of a dial on the mask. Many studies have assessed their accuracy.[5–8] It is generally considered that the patient receives the stated F_IO_2 provided the total flow rate exceeds 60 L/min or is 30% higher than the patient's PIFR.[9,10] As the patient's PIFR increases, the system's performance becomes variable.

In supplying an F_IO_2 of 0.24 using 6 L/min flow rate, the total flow rate delivered to the patient is 120 L/min. This falls to 30 L/min total flow for $F_IO_2 = 0.6$ using 15 L/min oxygen supply.[3] This is just equal to the PIFR of a quietly breathing adult, and unlikely to be sufficient to provide consistent performance in delivery of the stated F_IO_2. In severe dyspnoea these masks may not deliver the stated F_IO_2.[6] Increasing the oxygen flow rate above the manufacturer's recommendations will increase the total gas flow to the mask, while maintaining the stipulated F_IO_2.[8] At very high flow rates, however, turbulence is likely to reduce the performance of the system.

Venturi masks provide the best means of managing patients with chronic obstructive airways disease in the ED, because they provide a predictable F_IO_2 and the air entrained is more humid than fresh oxygen (see below). The entrained gas mixture can be further heated and humidified to assist with sputum clearance. High gas flows minimize rebreathing of CO_2 and claustrophobia, but cause problems with sleeping due to noise.

Oxygen blenders

Air is blended with oxygen from a number of inlet ports to supply a fixed F_IO_2 to the patient. It is a high-flow system, and fine-tuning of F_IO_2 from 0.21 to 1.0 is possible. The resultant mixture can then be channelled to the patient through systems such as continuous positive airways pressure, or humidifiers. Lack of portability and high cost are disadvantages. Oxygen blenders are best suited to the resuscitation room and critical-care settings.

100% oxygen delivery systems

These systems vary in their economy of oxygen use, and are summarized in Table 2.2.3. The least economical is the free-flowing system, because it can only deliver 100% oxygen if the flow rate exceeds the patient's PIFR. Incorporating a reservoir and unidirectional valves into the circuit enables greater economy of oxygen use by storing oxygen during expiration ready for the inspiratory phase.

Devices incorporating a reservoir into the circuit are capable of delivering 100% oxygen only when the total oxygen flow equals or exceeds the patient's respiratory minute volume (RMV), plus there are no leaks in the system. The reservoir volume must exceed the patient's tidal volume, otherwise storage of oxygen is inefficient, fresh gas loss occurs when the reservoir is full, and there is the risk of asphyxia during inspiration.

A demand valve system delivers precisely the patient's minute volume without the added bulk and problems of a reservoir. It is able to cope with changes in RMV provided fresh gas flow always exceeds the patient's PIFR. Closed-circuit systems are the most economical in oxygen consumption. Carbon dioxide is absorbed by soda lime, and low-flow fresh oxygen replaces that consumed during metabolism, which is approximately 250–1000 mL/min, which is considerably less than the patient's minute volume.

Classification

One hundred per cent oxygen-delivery systems available for use in emergency medicine are summarized in Table 2.2.3.

Free-flowing circuits

In order to provide 100% oxygen using a free-flowing system, flow rates in excess of the patient's PIFR are required. This necessitates the use of multiple oxygen ports. The system may not deliver 100% oxygen, is wasteful of oxygen and may be untidy, restricting patient mobility for investigations. Sophisticated free-flowing systems using oxygen blenders and humidification are available, but restrict the ability to move the patient.

Soft reservoir circuits

These are non-rebreathing systems incorporating unidirectional valves to channel fresh oxygen to the patient and exhaled gas to the atmosphere. With one oxygen supply port the system delivers 100% oxygen, provided the patient's minute volume is less than 15 L/min. Two oxygen supply ports enable delivery of up to 30 L/min. Fresh gas flow is titrated to the patient's minute volume by watching the reservoir bag. This should be fully distended at the start of inspiration, and more than one-third full when inspiration is complete.

The reservoir bag has a minimum volume of 3 L, and for optimal performance the patient's tidal volume should not exceed 2 L. A soft silicone mask is strapped to the head to ensure a firm but comfortable fit without leaks. The system cannot be used to ventilate patients manually, and may be hazardous if the patient has an impaired conscious state owing to the risk of aspiration if they vomit, and asphyxiation if there is a fall in fresh gas flow or a sudden rise in minute volume. Complications can be avoided with careful clinical vigilance, and the use of safety valves to entrain air if the oxygen supply ceases.

Self-refilling, non-rebreathing resuscitators (Air viva and Laerdal systems)

Most Australasian emergency departments possess at least one type of these self-refilling systems. They can be used to ventilate patients manually as well as allowing spontaneous ventilation. The Laerdal system has three sizes for adults, children and infants, whereas the Air viva system has one size for adults only (Table 2.2.4).

Table 2.2.3 Classification of 100% oxygen systems				
System	Rebreathing of gases	Fresh gas flow to deliver 100% O_2	Use for spontaneous and/or manual ventilation	Comments
Free-flowing systems	Non-rebreathing	45–90 L/min	Spontaneous	High fresh gas flow prevents CO_2 rebreathing.
Soft reservoir bag circuit	Non-rebreathing	7–15 L/min	Spontaneous	Can increase to 15–30 L/min with Y connectors to maintain $F_IO_2 = 1.0$
Self-refilling resuscitators (Laerdal, Air viva)	Non-rebreathing	15 L/min	Spontaneous/ manual	Manual ventilation possible with air if no oxygen available $F_IO_2 < 1.0$ if minute volume exceeds O_2 flow
Demand valve system (Oxy viva III)	Non-rebreathing	Delivers up to 120 L/min for inspiration only Usual RMV = 7–15 L/min	Spontaneous/ manual	Actual delivered volume of O_2 equals minute volume
Mapleson circuits	Partial rebreathing	15–40 L/min	Spontaneous/ manual	Fresh gas flow must be at least double minute volume to avoid CO_2 build-up
Oxy resuscitator	Closed circuit rebreathing	0.5–2 L/min	Spontaneous/ manual	Requires intermittent purging of reservoir to remove exhaled nitrogen from functional residual capacity

Table 2.2.4 Self-refilling, non-rebreathing resuscitators

	Self-refilling bag volume (mL)	Reservoir bag volume
Air viva	1700	2300
Laerdal (Adult)	1600	2600
Laerdal (Child)	500	2600
Laerdal (Infant)	240	600

Advantages

- Self-inflation and hence the ability to ventilate patients with air if oxygen supply is exhausted.
- Low resistance unidirectional valves prevent rebreathing of CO_2.
- Use in spontaneously ventilating patients and for manual ventilation.
- Provided fresh gas flow exceeds minute volume and the reservoir bag is attached, the system is capable of delivering F_1O_2 = 1.0. Without the reservoir bag, a maximum F_1O_2 of 0.6 is obtainable.
- A safety valve entrains air into the system to prevent asphyxiation if there is a sudden rise in minute volume, but this is at the expense of F_1O_2.
- Over-pressure valves are incorporated into the Laerdal paediatric and infant apparatus to prevent barotrauma in these patients.
- The addition of positive end-expiratory pressure (PEEP) to the system is possible by attaching a PEEP valve to the expiratory limb. Close apposition of the mask to the face, or endotracheal intubation, is required for this to be effective.

Disadvantages

- A reduction in F_1O_2 occurs when minute volume exceeds fresh gas flow. Dual oxygen supply ports can minimize this problem, especially in very dyspnoeic patients.
- The unit is bulky, and disconnections sometimes occur.
- There is less 'feel' during manual ventilation than with soft bag circuits, and inflation of the stomach is more likely during bag/mask ventilation, especially if there is airway obstruction or reduced pulmonary compliance.

Oxygen-powered resuscitators

Examples of this type of system include the Oxy viva, Laerdal, and DAN demand valve systems. High-pressure oxygen is fed to a demand valve which delivers high-flow oxygen to the patient. The system can be used in spontaneously breathing patients, and for manual ventilation by depressing a manual override button. Spontaneously ventilating patients initiate an oxygen flow of up to 120 L/min by generating a negative pressure of 0.3 kPa (2.25 mmHg) at the start of inspiration. Fresh gas flow is delivered at a pressure of up to 5.3 kPa (40 mmHg).

Advantages

- Portability, as it is easy to attach to an oxygen cylinder and take to the field. There are no bulky reservoir bags attached.
- Economy of oxygen use, as the patient's minute volume is precisely delivered at sufficient flow rates to match the PIFR. Provided there are no leaks, the system delivers F_1O_2 = 1.0.

Disadvantages

- Increased work of breathing for spontaneous ventilation because negative pressure must be generated to initiate oxygen flow.
- The system cannot function when fresh gas supply is exhausted.
- During manual ventilation it is almost impossible to judge ventilatory volume except by observing the patient's chest. The safety over-pressure valve may not prevent barotrauma, especially in children. Lack of 'feel' during manual ventilation may lead to over-inflation of the stomach if there is airway obstruction or reduced pulmonary compliance.

Mapleson circuits

A detailed description of these circuits has already been published.[11] Partial rebreathing of gases occurs with all of the circuits, and CO_2 retention can be avoided if fresh gas flow exceeds minute volume by a ratio of 2–2.5:1.

Mapleson circuits are still used in some emergency departments. The most commonly used versions are the Mapleson B and the Mapleson F, which are covered under paediatric considerations. Mapleson A, C, D and E circuits will not be discussed further.

Advantages of the Mapleson B circuit

- Use for both spontaneous and manual ventilation. Its performance is similar in both circumstances.
- The soft bag has excellent 'feel' for manual ventilation, and it is easy to monitor spontaneous ventilation by observing the filling and emptying of the reservoir bag.

Disadvantages

- Carbon dioxide build-up with lower oxygen flow rates. This can be avoided with higher flow rates, or by intermittently purging the reservoir bag.
- The system cannot function without a fresh gas supply.
- It may be difficult to use when ventilating patients manually using a mask.
- The valve assembly may occasionally 'stick'.

Closed-circuit systems

An example is the MD Oxyresuscitator. The circuit is the same as the Boyle's anaesthetic circle system. A soda lime canister absorbs exhaled CO_2, and a low-flow oxygen supply replaces oxygen consumed by metabolism at approximately 0.5–2 L/min. Considerable economy of oxygen use is thus achieved by rebreathing from the circuit.

Advantages

- Economy of oxygen use. More than 6 hours of oxygen can be provided by a 'C' sized oxygen cylinder at 1 L/min. This markedly exceeds the endurance of the cylinder using other systems.
- It can be used for spontaneous or manual ventilation. A soft reservoir bag provides excellent 'feel' for ventilation.
- The pressure on the system is controlled by the operator during manual ventilation. This minimizes gastric distension.
- It is portable and can easily be taken to the field.

Disadvantages

- The circuit ceases to function when fresh gas flow is exhausted.
- Exhaled nitrogen from the patient's early breaths may enter the circuit and reduce F_IO_2 below 1.0. This can be prevented by intermittent purging of the reservoir.
- CO_2 may accumulate if the soda lime canister is old or stops functioning.
- Incorrect packing of the soda lime canister may result in inhalation of soda lime dust (this is extremely rare).
- The reservoir bag is remote from the patient mask and the system may be cumbersome to operate.

Helium and oxygen mixtures

Over the last decade there has been interest in adding helium to oxygen (maximum 30% oxygen, also known as 'Heliox'). Heliox has a lower density than air and the potential to reduce airway resistance and hence the work of breathing, when treating disease processes such as COPD and asthma.

Helium (He_2, MW = 4) is much lighter than nitrogen and therefore significantly lowers the density of the gas mix when combined with oxygen in the range of $F_IO_2 = 0.2$–0.4. This advantage is lost when $F_IO_2 > 0.4$. Despite lower density, the viscosity of Heliox is not significantly lower than that of air. Its main theoretical advantage is if there is turbulent gas flow that is density dependent. This may occur with COPD, where there is a combination of small and medium airways disease. Early studies also suggested that Heliox may enhance nebulizer particles in the lung; however, greater flow rates may be required to drive the nebulizer.[12] Despite the potential advantages, the clinical evidence for use in COPD is not strong.

Two Cochrane reviews of the topic concluded that there is insufficient evidence to support the routine use of Heliox to treat COPD exacerbations, or exacerbations of asthma.[13,14] However, the review of adults and children with asthma did conclude that Heliox may improve pulmonary function when there is more severe obstruction. Most of the studies of Heliox for asthma have assessed it as a driver of nebulizer therapy, rather than for continuous administration. Of the two studies of Heliox therapy for COPD assessed in the Cochrane review, only one study included acutely decompensated patients in the ED.[15] This study failed to show a benefit from Heliox when it was used to drive nebulized β-agonist therapy. There is a need for further randomized studies using Heliox in asthma and COPD, both continuously and as a driver for nebulizer therapy, with hard endpoints such as physiological parameters, response to nebulized β agonists, need for non-invasive ventilation or intubation, and admission rates.

Measurement of oxygenation

Clinical assessment of oxygenation is unreliable, and the time-honoured sign of cyanosis varies with the level of haemoglobin, skin pigmentation, perfusion and external light.[1,16,17] Arterial blood gases and pulse oximetry provide an objective measurement of oxygenation and enable precise titration of oxygen therapy to the clinical situation.

Pulse oximetry

Pulse oximetry has become the most frequently used indicator of oxygenation in emergency medicine, as it is non-invasive.[18,19] It is colloquially known as the 'fifth vital sign', and provides continuous real-time assessment of a patient's oxygenation and response to therapy. It has a proven role in emergency medicine and is an excellent clinical tool, provided the limitations are understood. The principles behind pulse oximetry have been described elsewhere.[20,21]

A detailed knowledge of the haemoglobin–oxygen dissociation curve is required to interpret pulse oximetry, as well as the factors that influence readings obtained by this equipment. These factors are summarized in Table 2.2.5.

Paediatric considerations in oxygen therapy

The general principles of oxygen therapy and its indications apply equally well for children as for adults, but there are a number of important differences in relation to body size, psychology and oxygen toxicity.

Body size

Children are smaller than adults both anatomically and physiologically, so that any increases in equipment dead space will significantly increase CO_2 retention. Children are less able to tolerate increased resistance to ventilation, particularly if negative pressure must be generated to open valves in the apparatus.

Peak inspiratory flow rate and respiratory minute volume are lower; hence a given

Table 2.2.5 Factors that influence pulse oximetry readings[16,17,20,21]	
Factor	**Cause**
Signal interference	High-intensity external light source Diathermy Shivering/movement of digit
Reduced light transmission	Dark coloured nail polish Dirt (NB: melanin pigment/jaundice have no effect)
Reduction in plethysmographic volume	Peripheral vasoconstriction (shock, hypothermia)
Inaccurate readings due to abnormal haemoglobin	COHb causes over-estimation as is not distinguished from O_2Hb
	Methaemoglobin > 10% causes oximeter to read 85% saturation, regardless of O_2 saturation
	Profound anaemia – insufficient haemoglobin for accurate signal
Falsely low readings	Intravenous dyes with absorption spectra near 660 nm, e.g. methylene blue
	Stagnation of blood flow

oxygen supply flow rate will produce a higher F_IO_2 in a child than in an adult. A Hudson mask at 8 L/min may supply a F_IO_2 of 0.8 in a young child.[2] Reservoir bags are not required to deliver F_IO_2 values near 1.0 to children weighing less than 15 kg because available supply flow rates (maximum 15 L/min) exceed the child's PIFR.

Appropriately sized equipment is essential: many sizes of oxygen masks, oximeter probes, laryngoscopes and endotracheal tubes must be available to manage children of different ages, as serious barotrauma may result from the use of excessive volume during manual ventilation. Resuscitator bags are available with paediatric-sized reservoirs. The Laerdal system has both paediatric and infant sizes. These units also have a pressure relief valve designed to prevent barotrauma. Pressure rapidly rises as the child's lung reaches full inflation.

A smaller Mapleson circuit, the Jackson-Rees (Mapleson F) circuit, is available to ventilate children. It can be used for both spontaneous and manual ventilation. Rebreathing of carbon dioxide does not occur provided fresh gas flow is 2–3 times minute volume, and the bag is separated from the patient by a tube of internal volume greater than the patient's tidal volume. The overall relationship between fresh gas flow, minute volume and $PaCO_2$ is complex.[11] The principal advantages over the Laerdal system are that the operator can observe bag movement in spontaneous respiration, and has a better 'feel' for airway obstruction in manual ventilation. However, considerable skill and experience are required to use the system safely.

Psychological considerations

Gaining the trust and confidence of an ill child is an art learnt with experience. They frequently respond with fear when oxygen therapy is administered, so it is helpful to obtain assistance by asking their parents to nurse the child during treatment. A tight-fitting mask is less important in a child because source flow rate more closely approximates PIFR. Parents may assist by holding the oxygen mask close to the child's face, or by directing high-flow oxygen straight at the child's mouth using a tube only. A cupped hand with the oxygen tube held between middle and ring fingers can serve as a surrogate oxygen 'mask'.

Oxygen toxicity

Prolonged administration of oxygen at F_IO_2 > 0.6 for longer than 24 hours may be toxic to infants. This toxicity may not become apparent during their acute stay in the emergency department, but the oxygen dose received there contributes to the cumulative toxicity. Appropriate monitoring using pulse oximetry ensures administration of the correct dose and minimizes the risk of toxicity. However, supplemental oxygen should never be withheld because of fear of toxicity.

Transfer of patients on oxygen therapy

Supplemental oxygen therapy is a vital part of transporting the ill patient, and is especially important for air travel, where lower ambient P_IO_2 may exacerbate hypoxia already present as a result of the patient's disease process. The partial pressures of oxygen at various altitudes have been summarized elsewhere.[22] Patients with decompression illness or arterial gas embolism should not be transported at cabin pressures lower than 101.3 kPa (1 atmosphere absolute, ATA) because lower ambient pressure exacerbates their disease process by increasing bubble size. A number of factors must be considered for successful oxygen therapy during transport of a patient.[23]

Knowledge of the oxygen delivery apparatus and its maximum rate of delivery is essential for estimating transport oxygen requirements. These estimates must take into account current oxygen consumption, duration of transport (including delays), oxygen required in the event of deterioration, and a safety factor of at least 50%.

The sizes of oxygen cylinders available in Australasia, their filling pressures and approximate endurances are summarized

in Table 2.2.6. The most economical circuit for prolonged transport with $F_IO_2 = 1.0$ is a closed circuit with a CO_2 absorber, and the least economical is a free-flowing circuit.

Monitoring during transport should be of the same standard as that initiated in the emergency department. Pulse oximetry is an essential tool to detect hypoxia during transport, and should include audible and visual alarms. Oxygen therapy can be titrated against SaO_2, and this is particularly important in air travel, where P_IO_2 varies with ascent and descent. All the usual clinical parameters must also be monitored.

Oxygen therapy in specific circumstances

Asthma

Hypoxia in asthma results from ventilation–perfusion mismatch created by bronchospasm, secretions, and airway inflammation and oedema. Supplemental oxygen should be titrated to provide a SaO_2 >90% (preferably 94%), and must be continued during the interval between doses of inhaled bronchodilators.

Initial management should include a Hudson mask at 8 L/min flow rate. SaO_2 should be monitored continuously by pulse oximetry. The oxygen dose should be rapidly increased up to 100% if the patient remains hypoxic. Bronchodilator therapy should be administered proportionate to the severity of the attack, using oxygen to drive the nebulizer. Oxygen should not be withheld or administered in low doses because of fear of respiratory depression. Hypercapnia is an indication of extreme airway obstruction, and its presence mandates aggressive therapy and/or mechanical ventilation.

Table 2.2.6 Oxygen cylinder sizes for patient transport					
Cylinder size	Water capacity (kg)	Volume at 15000 kPa 15°C (L)	Approximate endurance at		
			8 L/min	15 L/min	30 L/min
C	2.8	420	52 min	28 min	14 min
D	9.5	1387	173 min	92 min	46 min
E	23.8	3570	446 min	238 min	119 min
G	48	7200	900 min	480 min	240 min

Mechanical ventilation in asthma

Mechanical ventilation requires an $F_1O_2 = 1.0$, high inspiratory flow rate (100 L/min), low tidal volume (6–8 mL/kg), a prolonged I:E ratio of at least 1:3 and a low ventilation rate (6–10 breaths/min or less), to reduce the risks of progressive dynamic hyperinflation and the development of auto-PEEP (iPEEP) reducing venous return and hence preload, and of barotrauma with the development of a pneumothorax. Permissive hypercapnia is accepted with mechanical ventilation.

Occasionally patients with asthma become hypoxic during nebulizer therapy because the oxygen flow rates driving the nebulizer (6–8 L/min) are lower than the flow rate required to maintain $SaO_2 > 90\%$. In these circumstances, extra oxygen may be supplied to maintain SaO_2 via a T piece or Y connector during the nebulizer therapy.

Chronic obstructive pulmonary disease

Most patients with chronic obstructive pulmonary disease (COPD) possess a degree of acute respiratory failure that has caused their emergency presentation. This may be due to infection, bronchospasm, retention of secretions, coexistent left ventricular failure, worsening right heart failure, pulmonary embolism, pneumothorax or sedation. Clues to the degree of severity and chronicity of the COPD may be obtained from the patient's history, past clinical records, emergency department blood gases and the response to initial oxygen therapy.

Clinical indicators of patients at risk of CO_2 retention include a housebound patient, $FEV_1 < 1$ L, polycythaemia, a warm vasodilated periphery and cor pulmonale. In the acutely unwell patient, treatment may be required before the history can be obtained.

COPD groups

In terms of management, patients with COPD fall into two groups, although this classification is still a source of debate.[24–26]

- Patients with a normal ventilatory response to CO_2 ('can't breathe' is the most common). Gas exchange and air flow into the lungs are impaired, but ventilatory drive is normal.

- Patients with impaired ventilatory response to CO_2 ('won't breathe' is less common). Ventilation does not increase in response to hypercapnia and acidosis.

There is an overlap between the advanced stages of illness. The aims of oxygen therapy are targeted to produce an SaO_2 of 88–90%, and to identify the second group of patients so that the oxygen dose can be titrated to achieve an acceptable clinical response, without excessive elevation of $PaCO_2$. Serial arterial blood gas analysis is an essential tool in the management of these patients.

The majority will have a normal ventilatory response to CO_2. Hypercapnia indicates that ventilatory failure is developing, and there may be a danger of respiratory arrest if the patient's disease is severe and progressive. This may also result from uncontrolled oxygen therapy and failure to monitor the patient's clinical status and arterial blood gases. Any patient with impaired consciousness due to respiratory failure should be manually ventilated while they are being clinically assessed and treated.

Controlled titration of oxygen dose in COPD

One of the foundations of successful management of the cooperative patient with COPD is controlled titration of oxygen dose. Variable-performance oxygen masks do not have a role in the emergency management of COPD. It is reasonable to use a consistent initial approach to oxygen therapy for conscious patients with advanced COPD because at the time of presentation their ventilatory response to CO_2 is unknown. In most patients the administration of 24–28% oxygen by Venturi mask will improve their oxygenation, with a target SaO_2 of about 88–92%.[27]

Below 90% saturation the Hb–O_2 dissociation curve is steep, and unless a pulmonary shunt is present even these small increments in oxygen will make a positive difference.[1] The patient's response to initial oxygen therapy ($F_1O_2 = 0.24$–0.28) will direct further oxygen dose changes and identify any patients not already known to be suffering chronic hypercapnia. A repeat ABG sample should be taken after 10 minutes of breathing $F_1O_2 = 0.24$–0.28. The

$PaCO_2$ may rise slightly because of the 'Haldane effect'.[1,25] If this rise is excessive (>1–1.3 kPa [8–10 mmHg]), it is consistent with an impaired ventilatory response to CO_2. The F_1O_2 should then be adjusted downwards in steps to achieve a satisfactory pulse oximetry reading that is compatible with acceptable CO_2 levels.

Arterial blood gas sampling in COPD

Arterial blood gas (ABG) samples taken during the initial assessment of these patients (breathing air or controlled oxygen) will assist management. If the bicarbonate level is >30 mmol/L or is elevated by more than 4 mmol/L for each 1.3 kPa (10 mmHg) rise in $PaCO_2$ above normal (5.3 kPa, 40 mmHg), this provides strong evidence of chronic hypercapnia, provided there is no other cause of metabolic alkalosis.[28]

Management considerations in COPD

Patients with a normal ventilatory response to CO_2 will not exhibit a significant elevation of $PaCO_2$ in response to oxygen therapy. If hypoxaemia persists and the $PaCO_2$ remains stable, then the oxygen dose may be increased incrementally until the desired oxygen saturation is achieved. A lower than normal SaO_2 (~88%) and PaO_2 (~56 mmHg) may be acceptable provided the patient remains conscious and cooperative.

Non-invasive positive-pressure ventilation is indicated if the patient remains hypoxic, or becomes progressively more hypoxic and the elevation of $PaCO_2$ persists or worsens, or their conscious state deteriorates.[27] Intubation and ventilation may be required, but this should be regarded as a last resort. Supplemental oxygen should never be abruptly withdrawn from patients with COPD because a catastrophic fall in PaO_2 will occur. All reductions in controlled oxygen dose should be in a stepwise manner.

In the majority of cases an acceptable balance between PaO_2 and $PaCO_2$ can be achieved, whereas both hypoxia and hypercarbia are reversed by specific therapy. Treating the cause of the ventilatory failure is a high priority and is covered in other chapters.

A pilot study[29] showed that the administration of bronchodilators using oxygen-driven nebulizers in the acute management of chronically hypercapnic patients may be safe. Caution is advised, however, because a recent Australian study[30] suggested that COPD is still poorly managed in the emergency department with respect to oxygen dose. Interestingly, the authors of that paper offered only limited practical advice on the titrated use of oxygen in the acute management of COPD, and did not differentiate between COPD patients with an acute elevation of CO_2 and those with chronic elevation.

Complications of oxygen therapy

These can be classified into three categories:

❶ Equipment-related complications
❷ Carbon-dioxide narcosis
❸ Oxygen toxicity.

Equipment-related complications

These are entirely preventable with careful monitoring and many have been dealt with in the discussion of each individual apparatus. Tight-fitting masks may cause asphyxia if there is insufficient oxygen reservoir or flow, and aspiration of vomitus may occur if the patient has depressed airway reflexes. Use of appropriate oxygen flow rates with rebreathing circuits prevents CO_2 accumulation.

During mechanical ventilation barotrauma can be prevented by the use of appropriate volumes and pressures, although it may be difficult to avoid when there is reduced lung compliance, as in the moribund asthmatic. Knowledge of potential equipment complications enables prompt intervention should they arise. When investigating a sudden deterioration in the patient's condition, a thorough check of the equipment in use is mandatory.

Carbon-dioxide narcosis

This can be prevented by controlled oxygen therapy titrating the F_iO_2 against SaO_2, arterial blood gases and conscious state (see above). Unconscious patients should be intubated and manually ventilated using high F_iO_2, preferably 100% oxygen. Patients with deteriorating conscious state and respiration due to CO_2 narcosis need

to be vigorously stimulated and encouraged to breathe, whilst F_iO_2 is reduced in a stepwise manner. Oxygen should never be suddenly withdrawn, because this precipitates severe hypoxia. Reversible causes of respiratory failure should be treated, and non-invasive ventilation instituted.[27,30]

Oxygen toxicity

Oxygen is toxic in high doses and this is a function of P_iO_2 and duration of exposure. The toxicity is thought to occur by the formation of free radicals and toxic lipid peroxides, inhibition of enzyme systems, and direct toxic effects on cerebral metabolism.[31] Toxicity is mainly restricted to the respiratory system and central nervous system (CNS), although it may affect other regions such as the eye. Premature infants develop retrolental fibroplasia after prolonged exposure to high F_iO_2. CNS oxygen toxicity manifested by neuromuscular irritability and seizures (Paul Bert effect) is restricted to hyperbaric exposures.

Pulmonary oxygen toxicity (Lorraine–Smith effect) is of the greatest relevance to emergency medicine, although exposures of 0.6–1 ATA for more than 24 hours are required to produce it.[31] Acute changes such as pulmonary oedema, haemorrhage and proteinaceous exudates are reversible on withdrawal of oxygen. Longer durations of high P_iO_2 may lead to permanent pulmonary fibrosis and emphysema. Physicians should be alert to acute symptoms of cough, dyspnoea and retrosternal pain, although these are non-specific symptoms of oxygen toxicity. A progressive reduction in vital capacity may be demonstrated. As with all drugs, oxygen dose should be monitored and carefully titrated against SaO_2 and clinical effect. However, oxygen therapy should never be withheld acutely because of fear of toxicity.

Special delivery systems

Oxygen humidification

This may be desirable when prolonged use (>6 hours) of supplemental oxygen is required, as oxygen is totally dry, possessing no water vapour. Humidification is particularly necessary in patients ventilated

with an endotracheal tube because the natural humidification that occurs in the nose, mouth and nasopharynx is bypassed. Patients with COPD and retained secretions benefit from humidification.

Additional heat is required to provide effective humidification by vaporization of water. Various systems are available to humidify inspired gas, and ideally they should be able to deliver inspired gas to the trachea at 32–36°C with low resistance and at greater than 90% humidity. These devices should be simple to use, and able to maintain temperature and humidity at varying gas flows and F_iO_2. There should also be safety alarms monitoring temperature and humidity.[28]

Humidification of warmed inspired gas also enables heat transfer to hypothermic patients, and is essential in treating the pulmonary complications of near drowning. Dry oxygen will exacerbate hypothermia. The Fischer and Paykel apparatus provides more effective humidification by using a heating coil with a large surface area for contact with inspired gas.

Continuous positive airways pressure

This topic has been reviewed in detail in the literature.[32] Continuous positive airways pressure (CPAP) has a role in the management of pulmonary oedema, pneumonia, bronchiolitis, respiratory tract burns and acute respiratory failure.[33–37] Benefit to the patient is achieved as a result of increasing functional residual capacity and reduced pulmonary compliance. Hypoxaemia is reversed by reduction in intrapulmonary shunting, and the work of breathing is reduced.[32]

Circuit designs for CPAP

Circuit designs usually consist of a reservoir based on the Mapleson D circuit, or a high-flow turbine system.[33] Humidification can be added to the system, and is considered essential for long-term use (>6 hours). Use of an oxygen blender enables variable F_iO_2 to be administered. CPAP has a proven role in the emergency department in the acute management of cardiogenic pulmonary oedema. Reduced requirements for endotracheal intubation have been demonstrated when CPAP is used for severely ill patients.[33] Complications of CPAP include aspiration and pulmonary barotrauma. It may elevate intracranial pressure, and precipitate hypotension by reducing venous return to the thorax.

Hyperbaric oxygen treatment

Hyperbaric oxygen (HBO) treatment consists of administering oxygen at pressures greater than 1 ATA, usually in the range of 2.0–2.8 ATA. This requires a hyperbaric chamber that is pressurized with air while the patient breathes $F_IO_2 = 1.0$ from various delivery systems for periods of 2–7 hours. The high P_IO_2 results in PaO_2 of up to 267 kPa (2000 mmHg) if 2.8 ATA treatment pressure is used. This is beneficial, as there is increased dissolved oxygen in the plasma (up to 300 mL oxygen may be carried to the periphery each minute in the dissolved form), which maintains oxygen flux even if haemoglobin is non-functional, for instance in carbon monoxide poisoning. Increased P_IO_2 enables more rapid elimination of toxic gases from the body, for example carbon monoxide or H_2S.

Uses of hyperbaric oxygen

The increased PO_2 also creates a greater driving pressure of oxygen into ischaemic tissues in problem wounds, and reduces swelling by vasoconstriction in crush injuries. HBO treatment has a number of benefits in treating gas embolism and decompression illness (DCI). It provides extra oxygen to tissues rendered ischaemic by nitrogen bubbles, and the increased pressure reduces bubble size and enhances nitrogen removal from the body. HBO treatment is also of benefit in anaerobic infections by being bacteriostatic to anaerobes, inhibiting clostridial α toxin, and stimulating host defences via granulocyte function. Recognized indications for acute referral to a hyperbaric facility for HBO treatment are summarized in Table 2.2.7[31] (see also Chapter 28.3).

Table 2.2.7 Indications for acute treatment with hyperbaric oxygen[31]

Decompression illness
  Air or gas embolism
  Carbon monoxide poisoning

Gas gangrene and anaerobic fasciitis   Necrotizing soft tissue infections
Acute crush injury with compartment syndrome
Acutely compromised skin flaps or grafts, due to injury or post surgery

References

1. West JB. Respiratory physiology – the essentials, 6th edn. Baltimore: Lippincott, Williams & Wilkins, 1999.
2. Oh TE, Duncan AW. Oxygen therapy. Medical Journal of Australia 1988; 149: 141–146.
3. Smart DR, Mark PD. Oxygen therapy in emergency medicine. Part 1. Physiology and delivery systems. Emergency Medicine (Fremantle) 1992; 4: 163–178.
4. Bethune DW, Collins JM. An evaluation of oxygen therapy equipment. Thorax 1967; 22: 221–225.
5. Campbell EJM. A method of controlled oxygen administration which reduces the risk of carbon dioxide retention. Lancet 1960; 2: 10–11.
6. Hill SL, Barnes PK, Hollway T, Tennant R. Fixed performance oxygen masks: an evaluation. British Medical Journal 1984; 288: 1261–1263.
7. Fracchia G, Torda TA. Performance of Venturi oxygen delivery devices. Anaesthesia and Intensive Care 1980; 8: 426–430.
8. Friedman SA, Weber B, Briscoe WA, et al. Oxygen therapy. Evaluation of various air-entraining masks. Journal of the American Medical Association 1974; 228: 474–478.
9. Goldstein RS, Young J, Rebuck AS. Effect of breathing pattern on oxygen concentration received from standard face masks. Lancet 1982; 27: 1188–1190.
10. Woolner DF, Larkin J. An analysis of the performance of a variable Venturi-type oxygen mask. Anaesthesia and Intensive Care 1980 8: 44–51.
11. Dorsch JA, Dorsch SE. The breathing system. II. The Mapleson systems. In: Dorsch JA, Dorsch SE, eds. Understanding anaesthesia equipment. Construction, care and complications, 2nd edn. Baltimore: Williams & Wilkins, 1984.
12. Hess DR. Heliox and non-invasive positive-pressure ventilations: a role for Heliox in exacerbations of chronic obstructive pulmonary disease? Respiratory Care 1999; 51: 640–650.
13. Rodrigo G, Pollack C, Rodrigo C, et al. Heliox for nonintubated acute asthma patients. Cochrane Database of Systematic Reviews 2006, Issue 4. Art No.: CD002884. DOI: 10.1002/14651858. CD002884.pub2.
14. Rodrigo G, Pollack C, Rodrigo C, et al. Heliox for treatment of exacerbations of chronic pulmonary disease. Cochrane Database of Systematic Reviews 2007, Issue 1. Art No.: CD003571. DOI: 10.1002/14651858. CD003571.
15. deBoisblanc BP, DeBleiux P, Resweber S, et al. Randomized trial of the use of heliox as a driving gas for updraft nebulization of bronchodilators in the emergency treatment of acute exacerbations of chronic obstructive pulmonary disease. Critical Care Medicine 2000; 28: 3177–3180.
16. Morgan-Hughes JO. Lighting and cyanosis. British Journal of Anaesthesia 1968; 40: 503–507.
17. Hanning CD. "He looks a little blue down this end". Monitoring oxygenation during anaesthesia. British Journal of Anaesthesia 1985; 57: 359–360.
18. Jones J, Heiselman D, Cannon L, Gradisek R. Continuous emergency department monitoring of arterial saturation in adult patients with respiratory distress. Annals of Emergency Medicine 1988; 17: 463–468.
19. Lambert MA, Crinnon J. The role of pulse oximetry in the Accident and Emergency Department. Archives of Emergency Medicine 1989; 6: 211–215.
20. Adams AP. Capnography and pulse oximetry. In: Atkinson RS, Adams AP, eds. Recent advances in anaesthesia and analgesia. Edinburgh: Churchill Livingstone, 1989; 155–175.
21. Phillips GD, Runciman WB, Ilsley AH. Monitoring in Emergency Medicine. Resuscitation 1989; 18: 21–35.
22. Hackett PH, Roach RC, Sutton JR. High altitude medicine. In: Auerbach PS, Geehr EC, eds. Management of wilderness and environmental emergencies, 2nd edn. Missouri: CV Mosby, 1989; 1–34.
23. Saunders CE. Aeromedical transport. In: Auerbach PS, Geehr EC, eds. Management of wilderness and environmental emergencies, 2nd edn. Missouri: CV Mosby, 1989; 359–388.
24. Stradling JR. Hypercapnia during oxygen therapy in airways obstruction: a reappraisal. Thorax 1986; 41: 897–902.
25. Aubier M, Murciano D, Milic-Emili J, et al. Effects of the administration of oxygen on ventilation and blood gases in patients with chronic obstructive pulmonary disease during acute respiratory failure. American Review of Respiratory Disease 1980; 122: 747–754.
26. Sassoon CSH, Hassell KT, Mahutte CK. Hyperoxic induced hypercapnia in stable chronic obstructive pulmonary disease. American Review of Respiratory Disease 1987; 135: 907–911.
27. McKenzie DK, Frith PA, Burdon JGW, et al. The COPDX Plan: Australian and New Zealand Guidelines for the management of chronic obstructive pulmonary disease 2003. Medical Journal of Australia 2003; 178: S1–S39.
28. Bersten A, Soni M. Oh's intensive care manual, 5th edn. Oxford: Butterworth–Heinemann, 2003.
29. Cameron P, Coleridge J, Epstein J, Teichtahl H. The safety of oxygen driven nebulisers in patients with chronic hypoxaemia and hypercapnia. Emergency Medicine (Fremantle) 1992; 4: 159–162.
30. Joosten SA, Xiaoning Bu, Smallwood D, et al. The effects of oxygen therapy in patients presenting to an emergency department with exacerbation of chronic obstructive pulmonary disease. Medical Journal of Australia 2007; 186: 235–238.
31. Feldmeier JJ. Indications and results. The Hyperbaric Oxygen Therapy Committee Report. Kensington, Maryland USA Undersea and Hyperbaric Medicine Society, 2003.
32. Duncan AW, Oh TE, Hillman DR. PEEP and CPAP. Anaesthesia and Intensive Care 1986;14: 236–250.
33. Bersten AD, Holt AW, Vedig AE, et al. Treatment of severe cardiogenic pulmonary oedema with continuous positive airway pressure delivered by face mask. New England Journal of Medicine 1991; 325: 1825–1830.
34. Taylor GJ, Brenner W, Summer WR. Severe viral pneumonia in young adults. Therapy with continuous airway pressure. Chest 1976; 69: 722–728.
35. Beasley JM, Jones SEF. Continuous positive airways pressure in bronchiolitis. British Medical Journal 1981; 283: 1506–1508.
36. Venus B, Matsuda T, Copiozo JB, et al. Prophylactic intubation and continuous positive airways pressure in the management of inhalation injury in burn victims. Critical Care Medicine 1981; 9: 519–523.
37. Katz JA, Marks JD. Inspiratory work with and without continuous positive airway pressure in patients with acute respiratory failure. Anesthesiology 1985; 63: 598–607.

2.3 Haemodynamic monitoring

Liz Steel • Craig Hore

ESSENTIALS

1 Haemodynamic monitoring involves observation of the complex physiology of blood flow with the aim of providing data that can be used to improve patient management and outcomes.

2 Numerous methods are available that should be considered in a stepwise fashion, from simple clinical assessment to highly technical, invasive procedures such as the pulmonary artery catheter.

3 Effective use of haemodynamic monitoring devices requires a good understanding of cardiovascular physiology.

4 Currently there is a move away from simple blood pressure measurements towards targeting end-organ perfusion and the adequacy of cardiac output.

5 Use of all monitoring technology in the emergency department needs to take into consideration the time associated with its introduction, the skill levels needed and the clinical benefits that may be provided.

6 No monitoring modality improves outcome unless it is linked to a treatment protocol.

7 The pulmonary artery catheter was for many years considered the 'gold standard' of haemodynamic monitoring, but current evidence suggests no improvements in patient outcome. It should therefore not be used in the emergency department.

8 Less invasive devices have been developed in recent years. Their role in the emergency department is yet to be fully elucidated.

9 Further developments will probably result in greater use of less invasive methods for haemodynamic monitoring and an increased ability to monitor at a microcirculation and/or cellular level, with better correlation between observed events and final diagnosis.

Introduction

Haemodynamics is concerned with the physiology of blood flow and the forces involved within the circulation.[1] *Haemodynamic monitoring* involves studying this complex physiology using various forms of technology to understand these forces and put them into a clinical context that can be used to direct therapy.[2] The utility of basic monitoring is universally accepted. However, the maxim that *'not everything that counts can be counted and not everything that can be counted counts'* (Albert Einstein, 1879–1955) should be borne in mind.[3] This is particularly salient in the emergency department (ED), where the pressure of work and the diversity of patients do not allow the unlimited use of complex and expensive monitoring systems.

This chapter provides an outline of current approaches to the various technologies available for haemodynamic monitoring and their applicability in the ED. Many methods are available which should be thought of in a stepwise progression from simple clinical assessment to invasive, highly technical methods and sophisticated devices.

Historical background

As recently as 100 years ago, only temperature, pulse and respirations were measured and used to manage patients. The technology for auscultatory blood pressure measurement was available, but did not come into regular use until the 1920s.

Intensive care as a medical/nursing specialty evolved in tandem with the electronic revolution of the 1960s.[4] At the same time, increasingly sophisticated haemodynamic and laboratory techniques vastly improved diagnosis, and provided a way to further evaluate therapy. Despite these major advances in the ability to monitor multiple physiological variables, there is little evidence to suggest that they have resulted in tangible improvements in patient outcome.[5]

The practical use of any monitoring device must be appropriate to the individual clinical environment. Thus, it may be reasonable to insert a pulmonary artery catheter in the intensive care unit (ICU) where the necessary time can be taken, yet impractical and potentially unsafe in a busy ED.[2] Another consideration is that haemodynamic monitoring should only be used when the clinical outcome can be influenced and potentially improved. Once irreversible cellular damage has occurred, current evidence suggests that no benefit will occur no matter how far therapy is maximized.[6] Further, haemodynamic monitoring may not improve patient outcome unless linked to a clinical protocol or 'goal-directed therapy'.[7–9] Improvements in morbidity and mortality have been shown when such protocols are utilized.[6,10,11]

Clinicians should only introduce monitoring equipment that will have a direct influence on their choice of therapy, as the use of invasive monitoring carries potential risks of harm to the patient. The injudicious use of physiologically based treatment protocols has been shown to cause harm and lead to worse outcomes.[12] All monitored variables must be evaluated and applied in a manner proven to lead to benefit, in terms of both the diagnosis and the management.[13]

Overview of cardiovascular physiology

It is beyond the scope of this chapter to go into a detailed discussion of cardiovascular physiology, but one possible reason that haemodynamic monitoring has not been associated with improvements in outcome is an inability to understand and manipulate patients' physiology effectively.

The circulatory model

Haemodynamic data are traditionally considered in the context of a circulatory model. This model varies, but usually consists of a non-pulsatile pump, and a hydraulic circuit with discrete sites of flow resistance, alongside the Frank–Starling mechanism with its concepts of preload, contractility and afterload.[14]

Cardiac output

Cardiac output (CO) is the volume of blood pumped by the heart per unit of time, usually expressed in litres per minute (L/min).[15] The heart operates as a pump and ejects a bolus of blood known as the *stroke volume* (SV) with each cardiac cycle. CO is the product of SV and heart rate (HR).

A complex set of interrelated physiological variables determines the magnitude of CO, including the volume of blood in the heart (*preload*), the downstream resistance to the ejection of this blood (*afterload*) and the *contractility* of the heart muscle.[16] However, it is the *metabolic requirements* of the body that are the most potent determinant of cardiac output.[4]

The regulation of CO is therefore complex. A single measurement represents the interaction of many interacting physiological processes. Basal CO is related to body size and varies from 4 to 7 L/min in adults.[16] The value can be divided by the body surface area to enable comparison between patients with different body sizes, giving the *cardiac index* (CI).

Although CO can be measured, this does not mean it should be done routinely. Indeed, misuse of CO data may worsen outcomes.[18] The International Consensus Conference on Haemodynamic Monitoring in Shock (2007)[17] suggested that monitoring

of CO is only of value if it guides therapies to improve outcome.

Cardiac index (CI)

CI measurement scores over simple blood pressure recording as it describes the total volume of blood flow in the circulation per unit of time, and hence serves as an indicator of oxygen delivery to the tissues. The CI is also useful for understanding and manipulating the pump activity of the heart.

Role of haemodynamic monitoring in the emergency department

The role of haemodynamic monitoring in the ED is even less well defined. Given the plethora of devices but the lack of a 'gold standard', there are insufficient data to recommend any one method over another.[17]

Recent advances in the management of sepsis include haemodynamic optimization with early goal-directed therapy (EGDT) during the pre-intensive care period, especially in the ED.[19] The Surviving Sepsis Campaign guidelines published in 2004[20] emphasized that resuscitation of a patient with severe sepsis should begin as soon as the diagnosis is made, and should not be delayed until ICU admission. The use of such an approach based on strict treatment protocols has been shown to reduce morbidity and mortality[6] (see Chapter 2.5).

Although widely accepted, the application of this strategy in clinical practice is far from common. Obstacles include a lack of skills to perform the initial procedures, and difficulties in providing the required higher level of care due to ED overcrowding.[19] However, with a potential stay in the ED of >24 hours,[21] and approximately 15% of critical care being provided in this setting,[22] it is necessary to address this issue in education terms and by improved use of available haemodynamic monitoring. This will improve the recognition of therapeutic opportunities in the ED that may be missed.[19]

Clinical assessment

Current guidelines on haemodynamic monitoring recommend frequent measurement

of blood pressure and physical examination variables, including signs of hypoperfusion such as reduced urine output and abnormal mental status.[17] Clinical examination is 'low risk' yet may yield much important information, but the sensitivity and specificity are low, even when individual elements are interpreted in isolation. Also, clinical assessment of the circulatory state can be misleading.[23]

Clinical assessment still has an important role in the initial assessment of a critically ill patient,[24] particularly as the use of some invasive methods leads to poorer outcomes.[13]

Paradoxically, the development of haemodynamic measuring devices was driven by the poor ability to assess the critically ill patient clinically,[25,26] yet those patients managed simply by clinical assessment may do better than those managed with invasive, complex devices.[13]

Clinical markers of cardiac output

The underlying issue may not be what a patient's CO *is*, but rather whether this CO is *effective* for that particular patient.[27] Trends are more important than specific, single-point values in guiding therapy. An effective CO should need no compensation, and therefore a patient should have warm toes simultaneously with a normal blood pressure and heart rate.[28,29] One of the advantages of *clinical endpoints* is that they remain the same whatever the phase of the illness.[27]

Clinical endpoints that are important in the management of septic shock were set out by the American College of Critical Care Medicine (ACCM) in 1999,[30] and again in 2007 by an International Consensus Conference.[17] These are essentially markers of perfusion and include skin temperature, urine output and cerebral function.

Physiological measurements and clinical endpoints should be viewed as complementary. Physiological measurements combined with clinical examination may provide a numeric target for a management strategy.[27] Measurements also provide a universal language for information exchange.

Sound clinical evaluation in the ED in terms of markers of effective CO aid the early diagnosis and implementation of EGDT.[19] Abnormal findings also suggest the need for more invasive haemodynamic monitoring, and the need to involve the ICU team early in the patient's management.

Blood pressure monitoring

The pressure under which blood flows is related to the force generated by the heart and the resistance to flow in the arteries.[32] Measurement of mean arterial pressure (MAP) is a more reliable measure of blood pressure than either the systolic or diastolic pressures. It is least dependent on the site or method of measurement, least affected by measurement damping, and it determines the actual tissue blood flow.[14]

Traditionally, low blood pressure was used to reflect shock and haemodynamic instability. This approach is being challenged as more reliance is placed on concepts of global tissue hypoxia, and the measurement of CO and its adequacy.[19]

Non-invasive blood pressure measurement

Non-invasive blood pressure (NIBP) measurements using a sphygmomanometer and palpation were first proposed in the late 1800s before Korotkoff introduced the auscultatory method in 1905.[32] Originally, routine blood pressure measurements were not a regular part of clinical patient assessment. Today, non-invasive or indirect blood pressure measurement is the most common method used in the initial assessment of cardiovascular status.[31] Although there are significant differences between direct (i.e. invasive) and indirect measurements,[33] non-invasive measurements should rightly form part of every patient's assessment and management in the ED.[17]

Non-invasive blood pressure devices

Non-invasive measurement techniques use blood flow within a limb to measure pressure. Automated oscillometric devices are now the standard, with manual methods (using either palpation or auscultation) becoming increasingly obsolete in clinical ED practice.

The cuff width should be about 40% of the mid-circumference of the limb. Failure to use the appropriate size of cuff leads to inaccurate and misleading measurements.

The cuff is inflated until all oscillations in cuff pressure cease, then the occluding pressure is gradually reduced and proprietary algorithms compute mean, systolic and diastolic pressures.

The 95% confidence limits in the normotensive range are ±15 mmHg, but in states of hypotension and hypertension oscillometry tends to respectively over- and underestimate the pressures.[14] Complications are unusual, although repeated measurements could cause skin bruising, oedema and even ulceration.

Invasive blood pressure measurement

Arterial cannulation allows continuous blood pressure measurement, beat-to-beat waveform display and repeated blood sampling.[14] A cannula inserted into an artery is connected via fluid-filled, non-compliant tubing <1 m in length to a linearly responsive pressure transducer. The system is then zeroed with reference to the phlebostatic axis (the midaxillary line in the fourth intercostal space). Modern transducers are precalibrated, and therefore no further calibration is needed.[34]

Sites and safety of arterial cannulation

The most common site for cannulation is the radial artery,[35] as this is easy to access during placement and subsequent manipulations, the wrist has a dual arterial supply,[31] and there is a low complication rate.[35–38] Temporary occlusion of the artery may occur, and in a small number of cases this may be permanent.[35] Other complications include haematoma formation,[39] bleeding,[40] cellulitis,[41] and those associated with the catheter itself.[42] Alternative arterial cannulation sites are femoral, axillary and brachial, but all have similar complications. Arterial cannulation is a safe procedure if the optimal site for insertion is selected carefully for each patient.[35] The preference in the ED is for the radial and femoral sites.

Use of invasive blood pressure monitoring

Invasive blood pressure monitoring should be used in all haemodynamically unstable patients and when vasopressor or vasodilator therapy is used.[17] Relying on external NIBP

monitoring to guide therapy and diagnosis does not provide sufficient diagnostic data, especially in sepsis.[6] Additional methods of haemodynamic monitoring may be considered in these patients, with early involvement of the intensive care department.

The remainder of this chapter discusses some of the supplementary methods available to assess various physiological measures considered important to guide the management of haemodynamically unstable patients.

Other non-invasive monitoring methods for cardiac output

The ideal device has yet to be developed for the non-invasive measurement of CO and other related variables in the ED setting. Devices that are available do not compare reliably with invasive methods, and are not suited to all patient cohorts and/or may be too elaborate or time-consuming for a busy ED.

Ultrasonic cardiac output monitor (USCOM)

This device was developed in Australia and introduced for clinical use in 2001. It provides non-invasive transcutaneous measurement of CO based on continuous-wave Doppler ultrasound.[43] An ultrasound transducer is used to obtain a Doppler flow profile (velocity–time graph) from either the aortic (suprasternal notch) or the pulmonary (left of sternum, below the second intercostal space) window. The transducer is manipulated to obtain the best flow profile and audible feedback. CO is calculated from the product of the velocity–time integral (vti) and the cross-sectional area of the target valve.[44]

The device appears to perform well in terms of the time taken to become a competent operator, and the reproducibility of its readings.[45,46] It appears to be a rapid and safe measure of CO and may assist in the prompt starting of EGDT by emergency physicians, even during a medical retrieval out of hospital.[47] The correlation of USCOM with standard measures of CO, such as by thermodilution using a pulmonary artery catheter, has been reported as good.[43]

Some concerns were raised that reliability is affected by patient pathology and the severity of their illness.[46]

More work is needed to clearly define the utility of USCOM in the ED. The device can be used as part of the overall clinical assessment, but probably should not be used in isolation. It may be best for looking at responses to treatment and diagnosis, such as changes in CO associated with a fluid bolus.

Oesophageal Doppler

Measurement of CO using various Doppler-based techniques has been extensively studied.[48] The main difficulties are an inability to obtain acceptable flow signals with the transthoracic approach, and problems in the measurement of the cross-sectional area using flow.[49] The transoesophageal approach has been found to be more reliable than the transthoracic.[50]

The oesophageal Doppler device requires minimal training, and volume challenge protocols may be developed so that nursing staff can use them at the bedside.[14] However, this technique is not well tolerated in awake patients[43] and thus has limited application in the ED.

Echocardiography

Echocardiography may be used to determine left ventricular size, thickness and performance.[52] Recently, it has also been reported to accurately identify patients who require fluids.[53] The use of echocardiography has increased as the technology has improved, and as the utility of non-invasive techniques has become more accepted. There is a move towards training for the majority of intensive care specialists in this technique, and there is no reason why ED physicians should not also learn. Effective treatment decisions can be based on what is seen on the screen, and in subsequent assessment of left ventricular function.[51]

The major criticisms regarding the use of echocardiography for haemodynamic monitoring is that it cannot be done continuously.[51] Other problems include the lack of skilled operators and the need to reassess variables after changes to patient management regimens. Thus, although promising, the usefulness of echocardiography for

haemodynamic monitoring in the ED is uncertain at present.

Invasive devices

Central venous pressure monitoring

Central venous access was first performed in Germany in the late 1920s,[54] but it was not until the 1950s, with the work of Brannon[55] and Zimmerman,[56] that the utility of the process was really appreciated. This ultimately led to the development of cardiac angiography, central blood oxygenation determination and pressure recordings.[57] The technique, management and clinical relevance of continuous central venous pressure (CVP) monitoring were first described in 1962.[58] This first step in bedside invasive cardiac monitoring allowed direct determination of right heart function and assessment of intravascular volume status.

However, correlation with left heart function was found to be unpredictable and unreliable in the critically ill.[57] Hence the physiological meaning of the values obtained and their role in patient management are not clear. Problems may result from errors in measurement and failure to correctly understand the physiology involved.[59]

Central venous access is obtained in the ED by inserting a catheter into a peripheral or central vein. Central venous access is defined by the position of the catheter tip: to be central the tip should be positioned at the junction of the proximal superior vena cava and right atrium.[60]

There is no ideal insertion site. Selection depends on the experience of the operator, and patient factors such as body habitus, injuries sustained and coagulation profile.[57] The main routes used are the internal jugular, subclavian and femoral veins.[14]

Indications for central venous access

Indications for the establishment of central access include fluid and electrolyte replacement; drug therapy where peripheral use is contraindicated, such as vasopressor; monitoring of the CVP to guide management; sampling of central venous blood to monitor central venous oxygen saturation; venous access for insertion of a pulmonary

artery catheter or transvenous pacemaker; and a lack of an accessible peripheral vein.

Complications related to insertion can be divided into early and late. The most relevant early complications in the ED setting include pneumothorax, haemothorax, dysrhythmias and injury to surrounding structures, including arterial puncture, and nerve and tracheal injury. Late complications include catheter-related sepsis, superior vena cava erosion with cardiac tamponade, and thrombosis.[14]

The CVP is often used as a marker of preload and is considered an estimate of right atrial pressure (RAP).[2] The normal CVP in the spontaneously breathing supine patient is 0–5 mmHg, whereas 10 mmHg is considered an upper limit of normal in those being mechanically ventilated.[14] The CVP also correlates with left ventricular end-diastolic pressure (LVEDP) in a patient with normal heart and lungs. However, in disease states this relationship is frequently abnormal.[57] Thus the CVP is only a rough guide to right ventricular preload, with emphasis on dynamic changes rather than absolute values.[2,14]

The Rivers' study

The Rivers' study[6] demonstrated that in cases of septic shock, early aggressive resuscitation guided by CVP, MAP and continuous central venous oxygen saturation (ScvO$_2$) monitoring reduced 28-day mortality rates from 46.5% to 30.5%. ScvO$_2$ is measured on blood taken via the central venous catheter and reflects the balance between oxygen delivery and oxygen consumption.[19] Normally oxygen extraction is about 25–30% and a ScvO$_2$ >65% reflects an optimal balance.[63,64] ScvO$_2$ correlates well with mixed venous saturations (SvO$_2$) obtained via a pulmonary artery catheter.[65,66] Current guidelines recommend instituting goal-directed therapy in septic shock, especially when the ScvO$_2$ is below 70%.[17] The ScvO$_2$ has also been shown to be significant in postoperative surgical patients in the ICU, with levels <70% being independently associated with a higher rate of complications[61] and increased length of hospital stay.[62]

Continuous measurement of ScvO$_2$ is feasible in the ED setting[67] where central venous catheterization is commonly performed, and where the alternative of pulmonary artery insertion is not practical.[19]

Pulse contour techniques for cardiac output

The use of pulse contour techniques to obtain a continuous CO by analysis of the arterial waveform dates back over 100 years.[2] Erlanger and Hooker[68] first proposed a correlation between stroke volume and changes in arterial pressure, and suggested there was a correlation between CO and the arterial pulse contour. Advances in computer technology have since led to the development of complex algorithms relating the arterial pulse contour and CO.

The appeal of arterial waveform monitoring is that it can now be performed using a minimally invasive technique, with at least four companies currently producing devices that take measurements from an arterial line. The PiCCO system (Pulsion Medical Systems, Munich, Germany) is discussed as one example. However, given the rapid pace of technological development in this area, alternative systems are likely to arise in the near future that may be of particular use in the ED.

PiCCO system of arterial waveform monitoring

The PiCCO system uses pulse contour analysis to provide a continuous display of CO according to a modified version of Wesseling's algorithm.[69,70] The patient requires a central line sited in either the internal jugular, the subclavian or the femoral veins, and an arterial catheter with a thermistor placed in one of the larger arteries, such as the femoral or axillary artery.[71] The femoral site is preferable as it requires only one sterile field for both lines, but does require a 50 cm long venous line.

The PiCCO system combines the pulse contour method for continuous CO measurement and a transpulmonary thermodilution technique to offer complete haemodynamic monitoring.[72] Transpulmonary thermodilution works on the principle that a known volume of thermal indicator (cold 0.9% NaCl) is injected into a central vein. The injectate rapidly disperses both volumetrically and thermally within the pulmonary and cardiac volumes. This volume of distribution is termed the intrathoracic

volume. When the temperature signal reaches the arterial thermistor, a temperature difference is detected and a dissipation curve is generated. The Stewart Hamilton equation is applied to this curve and CO is calculated.

This transpulmonary thermodilution also gives measures of preload in terms of global end-diastolic blood volume (GEDV) as well as intrathoracic blood volume (ITBV).[73] The extravascular lung water (EVLW) is also calculated and has been shown to be a sensitive indicator of pulmonary oedema.[74] The technique of transpulmonary thermodilution has been compared to pulmonary artery thermodilution and confirmed to be as accurate.[75] Following calibration by thermodilution the PiCCO continually quantifies various parameters.[71]

PiCCO parameters quantified

- Pulse-induced contour cardiac output (CO)
- Arterial blood pressure
- Heart rate
- Stroke volume (SV)
- Systemic vascular resistance (SVR)
- Intrathoracic blood volume (ITBV)
- Extravascular lung water (EVLW)
- Cardiac function index (CFI).

The last three parameters are relatively new, and the manufacturer has devised decision trees to guide their use in the clinical setting. The ITBV has been found to be a potentially more reliable and superior indicator of cardiac preload than pulmonary artery wedge pressure (PAWP)[76] and has also been shown to be helpful in guiding fluid therapy.[77]

EVLW correlates with extravascular thermal volume in the lungs[71] and with mortality. One study found that patients with an EVLW of up to 8–10 mL/kg had a mortality of 25%, which increased significantly to 75% if the EVLW was >10 mL/kg.[78] The EVLW may also be used to guide fluid management, especially in those already known to have pulmonary oedema.[79,80]

The Cardiac Function Index (CFI) aids in evaluation of the contractile state of the heart and hence overall cardiac performance. It is a preload-independent variable and reflects the inotropic state of the heart. The CFI has the potential to become a routine parameter of cardiac performance.[71]

The main advantage of the PiCCO system is that it is less invasive than a pulmonary artery catheter, requiring only a central line and an arterial line, which most critically ill patients already have. This in turn leads to fewer complications.[75] The data collected are also extensive and allow manipulation of haemodynamics using reliable parameters.

There are contraindications to using the PiCCO, for example when access to the femoral artery is restricted, such as in burns. The PiCCO may also give inaccurate thermodilution measurements in the presence of intracardiac shunts, an aortic aneurysm, aortic stenosis, pneumonectomy, and during extracorporeal circulation.[71]

The use of the PiCCO system in the ED is plausible. The technique is relatively non-invasive and uses access lines that are already used in the management of the critically ill. The device can both aid diagnosis and provide a monitoring tool for clinical decision making regarding fluid replacement.[81]

Pulmonary artery catheter

The pulmonary artery catheter (PAC) or Swan–Ganz catheter has long been considered the 'gold standard' method of monitoring the unstable circulation.[2] Since its introduction in the 1970s, it was assumed that the extra information provided improved patient outcomes. However, various observational studies have now shown that its use does not improve outcome and may even be associated with a worse outcome.[13] Hence, the use of the PAC without targeting specific endpoints confers no benefit to the patient. Conversely, the insertion of the PAC does not necessarily confer any disadvantage to the patient, except for the time, expertise and skill required to use it competently.[7–9]

Disadvantages of pulmonary artery catheters

The insertion of a PAC is time-consuming and requires skill and experience. The technique also has complications and the data generated are difficult to interpret.[13] Current guidelines recommend that the PAC is *not* used routinely in the management of shock,[17] and therefore its use in the ED should *not* be considered.

Conclusion

The real challenge in emergency medicine is to select those haemodynamic monitoring methods and technologies that are best suited to the clinical environment, and which are able to positively influence both the diagnosis and the subsequent management to improve patient outcome. Currently, the best approach is to begin with sound clinical assessment, and then to increase the invasiveness of monitoring in tandem with the patient's suspected diagnosis and response.

Future developments

- Interest in the microcirculation and metabolic assessment at a cellular level. Methods to assess these include near infrared spectroscopy (NIRS) and NADPH fluorescence. Both methods may have a role in the management of shock.[82,83]
- Other developing technologies include the direct assessment of the microcirculation using videomicroscopy.

Controversies

- The use of the PAC, and whether it confers any benefit to outcome.
- Whether the PAC data are actually of value but interpretation of them is lacking, or whether the detailed haemodynamic data cannot ultimately be translated to the benefit of the patient.
- Whether any monitoring technology taken in isolation, rather than in an evidence-based protocol, influences patient outcome, either beneficially or detrimentally.[2]
- The best haemodynamic monitoring devices to use and what physiological variables are important to measure.

References

1. Gattinoni L, Valenza F, Carlesso E. Adequate haemodynamics: a question of time? In: Pinsky MR, Payen D, eds. Functional haemodynamic monitoring. Heidelberg: Springer Verlag, 2005; 69–86.
2. Wilson J, Cecconi M, Rhodes A. The use of haemodynamic monitoring to improve patient outcome. In: Vincent JL, ed. Yearbook of intensive care and emergency medicine. Berlin: Springer, 2007; 471–478.
3. Young D, Griffiths J. Clinical trials of monitoring in anaesthesia, critical care and acute ward care: a review. British Journal of Anaesthesia 2006; 97: 39–45.
4. Darovic GO, Stratton KL. Introduction to the care of critically ill and injured patients. In: Darovic GO, ed. Haemodynamic monitoring, invasive and noninvasive: clinical application. St. Louis: WB Saunders, 2002; 3–8.
5. Bellomo R, Pinsky MR. Invasive haemodynamic monitoring. In: Tinker J, Browne D, Sibbald EJ, eds. Critical care: standards, audit and ethics. London: Edward Arnold, 1996; 82–105.
6. Rivers E, Nguyen B, Havstad S, et al. Early goal-directed therapy in the treatment of severe sepsis and septic shock. New England Journal of Medicine 2001; 345: 1368–1377.
7. Rhodes A, Cusack RJ, Newman PJ, et al. A randomized, controlled trial of the pulmonary artery catheter in critically ill patients. Intensive Care Medicine 2002; 28: 256–264.
8. Richard G, Warszawski J, Anguel N, et al. Early use of the pulmonary artery catheter and outcomes in patients with shock and acute respiratory distress syndrome: a randomized control trial. Journal of the American Medical Association 2003; 290: 2713–2720.
9. Harvey S, Harrison DA, Singer M, et al. Assessment of the clinical effectiveness of pulmonary artery catheters in management of patients in intensive care (PAC-Man): a randomized controlled trial. Lancet 2005; 366: 472–477.
10. Boyd O, Grounds RM, Bennett ED. A randomized clinical trial of the effect of deliberate perioperative increase of oxygen delivery on mortality of high-risk surgical patients. Journal of the American Medical Association 1993; 270: 2699–2707.
11. Pearse R, Dawson D, Fawcett J, et al. Early goal-directed therapy after major surgery reduces complications and duration of hospital stay. A randomized, controlled trial. Critical Care 2005; 9: R687–693.
12. Dos Santos CC, Slutsky AS. Protective ventilation of patients with acute respiratory distress syndrome. Critical Care 2004; 8: 145–147.
13. Connors AF, Speroff T, Dawson NV, et al. The effectiveness of right heart catheterization in the initial care of critically ill patients. SUPPORT Investigators. Journal of the American Medical Association 1996; 276: 889–897.
14. Morgan TJ. Haemodynamic monitoring. In: Bersten AD, Soni N, eds. Oh's intensive care manual, 5th edn. Oxford: Butterworth–Heinemann, 2003; 10: 79–94.
15. Rushmer R. The cardiac output. In: Rushmer RF (ed) Cardiovascular dynamics. Philadelphia: WB Saunders, 1961.
16. Bowdle TA, Freund PR, Rooke GA. Cardiac output. Issaquah: Spacelab's Medical 1993.
17. Antonelli M, Levy M, Andrews PJD, et al. Haemodynamic monitoring in shock and implications for management. International Consensus Conference, Paris, France, April 2006. Intensive Care Medicine. 2007; 33: 575–590.
18. Hayes MA, Timmins AC, Yau EH, et al. Elevation of systemic oxygen delivery in the treatment of critically ill patients. New England Journal of Medicine 1994; 330: 1717–1722.
19. Nguyen HB, River EP. The clinical practice of early goal-directed therapy in severe sepsis and septic shock. Advances in Sepsis 2005; 4: 126–131.
20. Dellinger RP, Carlet JM, Masur H, et al. Surviving Sepsis Campaign guidelines for the management of severe sepsis and septic shock. Critical Care Medicine 2004; 32: 858–872.
21. McCaig LF, Burt CW. National hospital ambulatory medical care survey: 2002 Emergency Department Summary. Advance Data 2004; 340: 1–34.
22. Nelson M, Waldrop RD, Jones J, et al. Critical care provided in an urban emergency department. American Journal of Emergency Medicine 1998; 16: 56–59.
23. Linton RA, Linton NW, Kelly F. Is the clinical assessment of the circulation reliable in postoperative cardiac surgical patients? Journal of Cardiothoracic and Vascular Anaesthesia 2002; 16: 394–400.
24. Stephan F, Flahault A., Dieudonne N, et al. Clinical evaluation of circulating blood volume in critically ill patients. British Journal of Anaesthesia 2001; 86: 754–762.
25. Rackow EC, Connors AF. Controversies in pulmonary medicine. Invasive measurements are required for assessing haemodynamic status in critically ill patients. American Review of Respiratory Disease 1988; 138: 1070–1072.
26. Eisenberg PR, Jaffe AS, Schuster DP. Clinical evaluation compared to pulmonary artery catheterization in haemodynamic assessment of critically ill patients. Critical Care Medicine 1984; 12: 549–553.
27. Palazzo M. Editorial I. Circulating volume and clinical assessment of the circulation. British Journal of Anaesthesia 2001; 86: 743–746.
28. Joly HR, Weil MH. Temperature of the great toe as an indication of the severity of shock. Circulation 1969; 39: 131–138.
29. Palazzo M, Soni N. Critical care studies: redefining the rules. Lancet 1998; 352: 1306–1307.
30. Task Force of the American College of Critical care Medicine SoCCM. Practice parameters for haemodynamic support of sepsis in adult patients with sepsis. Critical Care Medicine 1999; 27: 639–660.
31. Nara AR, Burns MP, Downs WG. Blood pressure. Issaquah: Spacelab's Medical 1989.
32. Darovic GO. Arterial pressure monitoring. In: Darovic GO, ed. Haemodynamic monitoring, invasive and noninvasive: clinical application. St. Louis: WB Saunders, 2002; 133–160.
33. Cohen JN. Blood pressure measurement in shock. Mechanism of inaccuracy in auscultatory and palpatory methods. Journal of American Medical Association 1997; 199: 118–122.
34. Gardner R, Hollingsworth K. Optimizing the electrocardiogram and blood pressure monitoring. Critical Care Medicine 1986; 14: 651–658.
35. Scheer BV, Perel A, Pfeiffer UJ. Clinical review: Complications and risk factors of peripheral arterial catheters used for haemodynamic monitoring in anaesthesia and intensive care medicine. Critical Care Medicine 2002; 6: 198–204.
36. Bedford RF. Long-term radial artery cannulation: effects on subsequent vessel function. Critical Care Medicine 1978; 6: 64–67.
37. Weiss BM, Gattiker RI. Complications during and following radial artery cannulation: a prospective study. Intensive Care Medicine 1986; 12: 424–428.
38. Sfeir R, Khoury S, Khoury Gh, et al. Ischaemia of the hand after radial artery monitoring. Cardiovascular Surgery 2003; 4: 456–458.
39. Davis FM, Stewart JM. Radial artery cannulation: a prospective study in patients undergoing cardiothoracic surgery. British Journal of Anaesthesia 1980; 52: 41–47.
40. Soderstrom CA, Wasserman DH, Dunham CM, et al. Superiority of the femoral artery for monitoring. A prospective study. American Journal of Surgery 1982; 144: 309–312.
41. Lindsay SL, Kerridge R, Collett B-J. Abscess following cannulation of the radial artery. Anaesthesia 1987; 42: 654–657.
42. Tuck M. Arterial catheter failure. Anaesthesia and Intensive Care 1996; 24: 119–120.
43. Tan HL, Pinder M, Parsons R, et al. Clinical evaluation of USCOM ultrasonic cardiac output monitor in cardiac surgical patients in intensive care unit. British Journal of Anaesthesia 2005; 94: 287–291.
44. USCOM Ltd. Ultrasonic cardiac output monitors. 2005. USCOM Ltd, Sydney, NSW 2000.
45. Dey I, Sprivulis P. Emergency physicians can reliably assess emergency department patient cardiac output using the USCOM continuous wave Doppler cardiac output monitor. Emergency Medicine Australasia 2005; 17: 193–199.
46. Steel L, Carroll R, Murgo M, et al. Non invasive ultrasonic cardiac output (USCOM): assessment of ease of use and inter-operator reproducibility. Poster presentation, 31st Australian and New Zealand Annual scientific Meeting on Intensive Care, Hobart, Tasmania, 2006.
47. Knobloch K, Hubrich V, Rohmann P, et al. Feasibility of preclinical cardiac output and systemic vascular

resistance in HEMS in thoracic pain – the ultrasonic cardiac output monitor. Air Medical Journal 2006; 25: 270–275.

48. Brown JM. Use of echocardiography for haemodynamic monitoring. Critical Care Medicine 2002; 30: 1361–1364.

49. Morrow WR, Murphy DJ, Fisher DJ, et al. Continuous wave Doppler cardiac output: use in paediatric patients receiving inotropic support. Pediatric Cardiology 1988; 9: 131–136.

50. Vandenbogaerde JF, Scheldewaert RG, Rijckaert DL, et al. Comparison between ultrasonic and thermodilution cardiac output measurements in intensive care patients. Critical Care Medicine 1986; 14: 294–297.

51. Viellard-Baron A. The meaning of hemodynamic monitoring in patients with shock: role of echocardiography. In: Vincent JL, ed. Yearbook of intensive care and emergency medicine. Berlin: Springer, 2007; 493–500.

52. Darovic GO. Monitoring patients with pulmonary disease. In: Darovic GO, ed. Haemodynamic monitoring, invasive and noninvasive: clinical application. St. Louis: WB Saunders, 2002; 421–469.

53. Combes A, Arnoult F, Trouillet JL. Tissue Doppler imaging estimation of pulmonary artery occlusion pressure in ICU patients. Intensive Care Medicine 2004; 30: 75–81.

54. Forssmann W. The catheterization of the right side of the heart. Klinische Wochenschrift 1929; 8: 2085.

55. Brannon ES, Weens HS, Warren JV. Atrial septal defect. Study of hemodynamics by the technique of right heart catheterization. American Journal of Medical Science 1945; 210: 480–492.

56. Zimmerman HA, Scott RW, Becker NO. Catheterization of the left side of the heart in man. Circulation 1950; 1: 357–362.

57. Kumar A, Darovic GO. Establishment of central venous access. In: Darovic GO, ed. Haemodynamic monitoring, invasive and noninvasive: clinical application. St. Louis: WB Saunders, 2002; 161–175.

58. Wilson JN, Grow JB, Demong CV, et al. Central venous pressure in optimal blood volume maintenance. Archives of Surgery 1962; 85: 55–61.

59. Dellinger RP. Central venous pressure: A useful but not simple measurement. Critical Care Medicine 2006; 34: 2224–2227.

60. Whiteman ED. Complications associated with the use of central venous access devices. Current Problems in Surgery 1996; 33: 331–340.

61. Pearse R, Dawson D, Fawcett J, et al. Changes in central venous saturation after major surgery, and association with outcome. Critical Care 2005; 9: R694–R699.

62. Boyle M, Steel E, Murgo M, et al. Incidence of low ScvO$_2$ after standard post-operative intensive care management. Poster presentation, 27th International Symposium on Intensive Care and Emergency Medicine, Brussels, Belgium, 2007. Critical Care 2007; 11: S123.

63. Orlando R. Continuous monitoring of mixed venous oxygen saturation in septic shock. Journal of Clinical Monitoring 1987; 3: 213–214.

64. Krafft P, Stelzer H, Hiemayr M, et al. Mixed venous oxygen saturation in critically ill septic patients. The role of defined events. Chest 1993; 103: 900–906.

65. Ladakis C, Myrianthefs P, Karabinis A, et al. Central venous and mixed venous saturation in critically ill patients. Respiration 2001; 68: 279–285.

66. Reinhart K, Kuhn HJ, Hartog C, et al. Continuous central venous and pulmonary venous saturation monitoring in critically ill. Intensive Care Medicine 2004; 30: 1572–1578.

67. Rivers EP, Anders DS, Powell D. Central venous oxygen saturation monitoring in the critically ill patient. Current Opinion in Critical Care 2001; 7: 204–211.

68. Erlanger J, Hooker DR. An experimental study of blood pressure and of pulse pressure in man. Johns Hopkins Hospital Records 1904; 12: 145–378.

69. Wesseling KH, Jansen JRC, Settels JJ, et al. Computation of aortic flow from pressure in humans using a nonlinear, three-element model. Journal of Applied Physiology 1993; 74: 2566–2573.

70. Rodig G, Prasser C, Keyl C, et al. Continuous cardiac output measurement: pulse contour analysis vs. thermodilution technique in cardiac surgical patients. British Journal of Anaesthesia 1999; 82: 525–530.

71. Cottis R, Magee N, Higgins DJ. Haemodynamic monitoring with pulse-induced contour cardiac output (PiCCO) in critical care. Intensive Care Critical Care Nursing 2003; 19: 301–307.

72. Belda FJ, Aguilar G, Perel A. Transpulmonary thermodilution for advanced cardiorespiratory monitoring. In: Vincent JL, ed. Yearbook of intensive care and emergency medicine. Berlin: Springer, 2007; 501–510.

73. Salukhe TV, Wyncoll DLA. Volumetric haemodynamic monitoring and continuous pulse contour analysis – an untapped resource for coronary and high dependency care units? British Journal of Cardiology 2002; 9: 20–25.

74. Schnidt SS, Westhoff TH, Hofmann C, et al. Effect of the venous catheter site on transpulmonary thermodilution measurement variables. Critical Care Medicine 2007; 35: 783–786.

75. Sakka SG, Meier Hellmann A, Reinhart K. Assessment of intrathoracic blood volume and extravascular lung water by single transpulmonary thermodilution. Intensive Care Medicine 2000; 26: 180–187.

76. Bindels AJGH, Van der Hoeven JG, Graafland AD, et al. Relationship between volume and pressure measurements and stroke volume in critically ill patients. Critical Care 2000; 4: 193–199.

77. Buhre W, Weyland A, Buhre K, et al. Effects of the sitting position on the distribution of blood volume in patients undergoing neurosurgical procedures. British Journal of Anaesthesia 2000; 84: 354–357.

78. Strum JA. Development and significance of lung water measurement in clinical and experimental practice. In: Lewis FR, Pfeiffer UJ, eds. Practical applications of fibreoptics in critical care monitoring. Berlin: Springer-Verlag, 1990; 129–139.

79. Mitchell JP, Schuller D, Calandrino FS, Schuster D. Improved outcome based on fluid management in critically ill patients requiring pulmonary artery catheterization. American Review of Respiratory Disease 1992; 145: 990–998.

80. Bindels AJGH, Van der Hoevan JG, Meinders AE. Pulmonary artery wedge pressure and extravascular lung water in patients with acute cardiogenic pulmonary oedema requiring pulmonary oedema. American Journal of Cardiology 1999; 84: 1158–1163.

81. Hofer CK, Ganter MT, Matter-Ensner S, et al. Volumetric assessment of left heart preload by thermodilution: comparing the PiCCO-VoLEF system with transoesophageal echocardiography. Anaesthesia 2006; 61: 316–321.

82. Soller BR, Cingo N, Puyana JC, et al. Simultaneous measurement of hepatic tissue pH, venous oxygen saturation and haemoglobin by near infrared spectroscopy. Shock 2001; 15: 106–111.

83. Ince C, Sinaasappel M. Microcirculatory oxygenation and shunting in sepsis and shock. Critical Care Medicine 1999; 27: 1369–1377.

2.4 Shock overview

Peter Garrett

ESSENTIALS

1 The broad categories of shock include disorders of intravascular volume, vascular resistance, cardiac rhythm and the myocardial pump. Overlapping aetiologies are commonly encountered in the difficult management case.

2 Hypotension, only one characteristic of shock, should be considered a late and concerning finding.

3 Interventions in all forms of shock are simple and initially directed at the physiological deficit, and should be seen as a test of the clinical hypothesis. Continuous reappraisal is required.

4 Hypovolaemia, and hence the need for volume resuscitation, should be considered in every patient with shock.

5 Common errors in the management of shock are late diagnosis; inadequate control of, or not considering a primary problem; inadequate fluid loading; delayed ventilatory assistance; and excessive reliance on vasopressors and inappropriate adjuncts.

6 The mortality following cardiogenic shock is improved by revascularization strategies and cardiothoracic surgical intervention. Thrombolysis alone has no proven benefit, but lysis supplemented with intra-aortic balloon counterpulsation may be a bridge to recovery or revascularization.

7 There are currently no adjunctive therapies of benefit in septic shock over adequate fluid resuscitation, judicious inotropes/vasopressors, appropriate antibiotics or timely surgery.

Introduction

Shock is a clinical syndrome where tissue perfusion, and hence oxygenation, is inadequate to maintain normal metabolic function of the cells and organ. Although the effects of inadequate perfusion are reversible initially, prolonged oxygen deprivation leads to generalized cellular hypoxia and the disruption of critical biochemical processes, eventually resulting in cell membrane ion pump dysfunction, intracellular oedema, inadequate regulation of intracellular pH and cell death.

Traditional texts classify and manage shock according to the aetiology, but a more common approach in practice is based on urgently attending to the cardiovascular physiological abnormalities, with assessment of the response used to adjust the working diagnosis, and with later attention to the underlying diagnosis.

Recognizing shock may be difficult, particularly at the extremes of age. Pre-existing disease and the use of medications modify the compensatory mechanisms that safeguard perfusion of vital organs. Consider the possibility of inadequate tissue perfusion ('shock') in any emergency presentation with clinical signs or physiological indications of abnormal function of multiple organs. Remember that early, aggressive and effective treatment of shock is associated with improved outcomes.

Aetiology and epidemiology

Shock is due to malfunction of any of the components of the cardiovascular system, and there may be more than one contributing mechanism. If the aetiology is recognized, classification based on the aetiology, such as hypovolaemic, cardiogenic and septic, neurogenic or anaphylactic shock,

can guide therapy. When the aetiology is unclear, or the shock fails to respond to usual therapy, the following physiologically based classification may assist in decision making.

Reduced return to the heart – reduced preload

- Volume loss – 'empty tank' (Table 2.4.1)
- Altered venous capacitance – 'inappropriately sized tank' (Table 2.4.2)

Table 2.4.1 Examples of volume loss contributing to shock

Intravascular compartment
Blood loss
External bleeding
trauma
gastrointestinal tract bleeding
Internal (concealed) bleeding
haemothorax
haemoperitoneum (ruptured abdominal aortic aneurysm, ruptured ectopic pregnancy)
retroperitoneum (ruptured abdominal aortic aneurysm, pelvic trauma)
Loss of plasma
Burns
Sweating/dehydration
Pancreatitis
Ascites (peritonitis, liver disease)
Toxic epidermal necrolysis (TEN), erythroderma, pemphigus
Gastrointestinal tract
Vomiting
Diarrhoea
Bowel obstruction
Renal tract
Adrenal insufficiency (aldosterone deficiency)
Diabetes mellitus (polyuria)
Diabetes insipidus (polyuria)
Diuretics
Polyuric intrinsic renal disease

Table 2.4.2 Examples of shock resulting from altered venous capacitance and/or reduced vascular tone
Septic shock
Anaphylactic shock
Neurogenic shock
Vasoactive drugs
Vasodilators, sedatives, or toxins
Adrenal insufficiency (cortisol deficiency)
Thyrotoxicosis/thyroid storm
Liver failure
Systemic inflammatory response syndrome (SIRS) e.g. pancreatitis, trauma, burns
Prolonged shock from any cause ('Decompensated shock')

Reduced total peripheral resistance – reduced afterload (Table 2.4.2)

- Arterial vasodilation
- Capillary leak
- Fistula

Pump dysfunction (Table 2.4.3)

- Reduced contractility – systolic dysfunction
- Inadequate filling – diastolic dysfunction and pericardial problems
- Abnormal cardiac rate or rhythm
- Forward flow failure – valvular dysfunction.

Neither classification is exhaustive, and contributory causes may feature in more than one category.

Pathophysiology

The heart is a relatively simple piece of machinery, and hence preload (the volume of blood in the left ventricle at the end of filling, or the amount of stretch of the left ventricle) determines stroke volume (SV) until disease states intervene. The heart's output (cardiac output) is dependent on this stroke volume and the heart rate (HR):

$$SV \times HR = CO$$

Most tissues and organs have the capacity to autoregulate, or adjust the flow through

Table 2.4.3 Examples of myocardial dysfunction resulting in shock
Reduced contractility (systolic dysfunction)
Ischaemia (acute myocardial infarction)
Cardiac contusion
Cardiomyopathy
Myocarditis (infectious, hypersensitivity)
Toxins/drugs
Inadequate filling
Pericardial tamponade and other pericardial disease*
Diastolic dysfunction
Right ventricular infarction
Pulmonary hypertension (large pulmonary embolus, chronic pulmonary hypertension)*
Atrial myxoma and left atrial mural thrombus*
Tension pneumothorax*
Arrhythmias
Bradycardia (heart block, drugs)
Atrial fibrillation (when cardiac output is dependant on atrial priming)
Sustained ventricular tachycardia
Failure of forward flow
Ruptured ventricular septum or free wall
Critical mitral or aortic stenosis
Mitral or aortic regurgitation
Post myocardial infarction chordae tendineae rupture or papillary muscle dysfunction
Prosthetic valve thrombus/dysfunction

*Usually thought of as causes of obstructive shock, as the myocardial pump itself is normal

them according to metabolic demand, as long as there is an adequate flow. This flow is dependent on a gradient between an area of higher pressure (mean arterial pressure, MAP) and the lower-pressure side of the venous system (represented by a central venous pressure, CVP). The mean arterial pressure may fail if the cardiac output is reduced, or if the total peripheral resistance (TPR) in the arterial tree falls:

$$CO \times TPR = MAP$$

Relaxation of the arterial and venous tone by vasoactive mediators or lack of vasotonic mediators will result in reduced resistance and increased capacitance, and lower

pressures in both the arterial and venous systems. Any injury to the endothelium will result in loss of volume, as well as failure of vascular autoregulation. Additionally, if there is a defective valve causing regurgitation of blood and re-pumping, or a fixed narrow orifice, there is a failure in forward flow.

Compensatory mechanisms are provoked by the combination of lowered pressure and inadequate perfusion of tissues, and these contribute to the symptoms and signs of shock. Neurohumeral stimulation produces increased circulating catecholamines, angiotensin, aldosterone and vasopressin, manifesting clinically with anxiety, thirst, restlessness, tachycardia, diversion of blood from the skin bed, and a reduction in urinary output and urinary sodium. Blood flow to the brain and heart is maintained at the expense of renal, splanchnic, skin and muscle blood flow.[1] Significant fluid shifts occur from the interstitium to the intravascular compartment, which can falsely maintain haematocrit.

The ultimate consequences of shock in the event that tissue perfusion is not returned by compensatory measures or resuscitation are inadequate regeneration of adenosine triphosphate (ATP), causing failure of membrane ion pumps to maintain the function and structural integrity of the cell. This cellular dysfunction manifests in the myocardium as systolic contractile dysfunction (also due in part to reduction in sensitivity to catecholamines and circulating myocardial depressant factors), and impaired ventricular relaxation (lusiotropy). This myocardial failure, along with failure of vascular beds despite the increased circulating catecholamines, contributes to what is described as 'decompensated shock'.

Clinical features in the initial diagnosis of shock

The clinical features are due to the inadequate perfusion of tissues and resulting multiorgan dysfunction of the body's compensatory mechanisms. The emergency physician should not wait for physical observations to trigger a preconceived limit before considering shock, but should actively consider and look for signs of inadequate perfusion in any patient presenting with abnormal organ function.

- The mental state may reflect reduced cerebral perfusion, and may range from anxiety or confusion to coma.

- The patient may describe thirst, coldness or impending doom, and may have presyncopal symptoms including nausea, yawning and preferring to lie down.
- In retrospect, the patient may have been difficult to assess, the vital signs difficult to elicit or variable, and venepuncture or IV access challenging.
- The peripheral circulation reveals venoconstriction, with decreased peripheral temperature, pallor and mottling. Capillary return may be prolonged beyond 4 seconds. Peripheral mottling or central cyanosis are late signs. However, in vascular failure such as spinal, anaphylactic, neurogenic shock and sepsis the skin may be warm and dry, and capillary refill indeterminate as a consequence of vasodilatation.
- Hypotension is a cardinal clinical sign, defined as a systolic blood pressure <90 mmHg or a reduction of >30 mmHg in a previously hypertensive patient. It is important to note that shock can occur despite elevations in blood pressure, and low systolic blood pressure may not be associated with other signs of shock. A low systolic blood pressure should be considered a highly significant, if not late, finding in shock. Increasingly, mean arterial pressure (MAP) is considered a more relevant and accurate measured parameter.[2] Tachycardia is frequently present, but may be masked by drugs or advanced age. The trend with serial observation is more significant than absolute values. Bradycardia may occur such as in younger patients with catastrophic haemorrhage from a ruptured ectopic pregnancy, or following an inferior myocardial infarction (MI), related to a neurocardiogenic mechanism (Bezold–Jarish reflex).
- Tachypnoea is regarded as a sensitive but non-specific predictor of deterioration, and may also be part of the shock syndrome.[3]
- Core temperature may be low, normal or elevated, and will be affected by age, environment, volume status, coexisting disease, drug therapy and pre-hospital interventions.
- Urine output is likely to be reduced, and levels below 0.5 mL/kg/h suggest underperfusion.

Initial emergency management of the shocked patient

A structured framework such as that advocated by EMST (ATLS) or ACLS promotes both effective therapy and a systematic survey to occur simultaneously. General measures based on an initial working diagnosis can be later modified by the observed responses to initial therapy, and the results of investigations. Frequent reassessment of status and adequacy of response is vital. Once shock is recognized as being present this implies a high chance of death, so escalation to management by a multidisciplinary team in a monitored resuscitation area is preferable, with an effective team leader and communicator being vital.[4,5]

Primary survey

- Assess and support the airway and ventilation. Give supplemental high-flow oxygen to ensure maximal arterial oxygen saturation. Consider tracheal intubation and mechanical ventilation in the significantly shocked patient for additional reasons to the standard indications of airway protection and intractable hypoxaemia: to divert needed cardiac output to other hypoperfused organs, reduce oxygen consumption from respiratory musculature, maximize arterial oxygenation, manage respiratory acidosis, facilitate invasive monitoring procedures, and guard against sudden catastrophic respiratory decompensation. The role of non-invasive ventilation is unproven in this setting. Positive-pressure ventilation and anaesthesia will have a significant effect in the setting of inadequate preload, so prior fluid resuscitation is vital (see Chapter 2.1).
- Control external haemorrhage immediately with direct (manual) pressure. Obtain and secure intravenous access in more than one site with short, large-bore peripheral cannulae, within the skill level of the operator. Central venous access is rarely required in an emergency and may increase delay and morbidity. Consider a supine position and elevation of the legs if tolerated.[6]
- Draw blood for investigations, with priority for a bedside glucose level and arterial blood gases at this point.

- Infuse fluid as the initial mainstay of correction of shock with hypotension. Hypovolaemia and hence the need for volume resuscitation should be assumed in every patient with shock, until proven otherwise. Close observation of the responses to the fluid boluses will guide further boluses.
- The commonest choice of initial fluid is isotonic normal saline or Hartmann's (lactated Ringer's) solution.
- Use immediately available blood products (O-negative or group specific) warmed by a cartridge warming device for haemorrhagic shock, or where haemoglobin may fall to a point where oxygen carriage may be compromised (<100 g/L).
- Add an effective inotrope/vasopressor such as epinephrine (adrenaline) by infusion if, despite ongoing rapid fluid volume resuscitation, hypotension and inadequate perfusion persist (see Goals of Treatment). This may, however, achieve an adequate blood pressure at the expense of correct assessment of fluid volume replenishment.

Secondary survey

- Review vital signs and any available history obtained, followed by a directed physical examination. Continuous cardiac rhythm and pulse oximetry (SaO$_2$) should be monitored. All the observations, including temperature, should be recorded regularly.
- Perform a chest X-ray, ECG and other emergency investigations at this point, which in most cases will point to the aetiology. Focused abdominal sonography technique (FAST) ultrasound may be diagnostic.
- Place an indwelling urinary catheter in all shocked patients. When occult gastrointestinal bleeding is suspected a nasogastric tube may assist the diagnosis.
- An important role of the resuscitation team leader is to anticipate complications and interventions, and organize definitive care and disposal. Liaise with surgeons, radiologists and other specialists early. The complications of hypothermia, coagulopathy,

hypoglycaemia, hypokalaemia and decompensation of breathing should be actively prepared for, sought and prevented. The need to move the patient to imaging or theatre should be anticipated and communicated to team members to allow for preparation of the patient and the monitoring system.

Guidance for interventions and treatments

A key goal of the treatment of shock during and after the initial resuscitation is the correction of the underlying problem. Methods used to guide resuscitation are discussed below.

Emergency department observations

The presence and progress of shock may be detected in the emergency department (ED) by careful recording of vital signs and *frequent and repeated* clinical assessment.

- The 'vital signs' – pulse, respirations, blood pressure and temperature – should be measured frequently and observed for absolute values, the trend, and adequacy of response to therapy. Accuracy and frequency of temperature measurement can be facilitated by an indwelling catheter with a temperature probe.
- ECG monitoring provides an assessment of heart rate and ST segment changes suggesting inadequate myocardial perfusion if calibrated.
- Continuous pulse oximetry provides assessment of hypoxaemia, as the management of shock necessitates the adequate delivery of oxygen to tissues.
- Non-invasive oscillometric blood pressure (NIBP) measurement is convenient and can be set to frequent automated measurement. Accuracy is affected by cuff size, age, movement, some disease states, and when the blood pressure (BP) is abnormally low or high. Mean arterial pressure (MAP) is more accurately and reliably measured than systolic.[2,7]
- Urine output is the most apparent bedside monitor of the adequacy of end-organ perfusion. Levels below 0.5 mL/kg/h suggest underperfusion of the renal bed. Diuretics can both confuse and exacerbate the shock state.

Emergency department investigations

- Bedside tests should include blood sugar level to exclude concomitant hypoglycaemia, which will compromise resuscitation efforts.
- Arterial or venous blood gas measurements are rapidly available and may contain information to assess the cause (e.g. haemoglobin level), guide the interventions required (hyperkalaemia correction, assisted ventilation), and monitor the adequacy of tissue perfusion by tracking lactate or base deficit changes with resuscitation.
- Lactate measurements are an objective marker of the presence and severity of shock. Normal levels are <2 mmol/L, and levels of >4 mmol/L are associated with increased mortality. Lactate and base deficit (BD) may be used to assess the adequacy of resuscitation, and have been used to predict mortality, transfusion requirements, the need for ICU and the length of stay.[8,9]
- Full blood count, coagulation profile, electrolytes, liver function tests and troponin, along with a chest X-ray and electrocardiogram, will usually be enough to assist in diagnosing the aetiology of shock states.
- Urinary sodium in most forms of shock is low (< 20 mmol/L). High levels may indicate adrenal insufficiency (see Adrenal Shock).
- Bedside focused ultrasound (FAST), or formal echocardiogram if available, is now incorporated into many resuscitation algorithms. FAST can be used in most hands to assess for free abdominal fluid and exclude pericardial tamponade. More advanced ultrasound skills allow assessment for intrathoracic free fluid, aortic diameter, and assessment of cardiac function: ventricular cavity dimensions (adequate filling), ventricular ejection fraction, regional wall motion abnormalities indicating ischaemia, and valvular dysfunction.

Invasive monitoring

Invasive monitoring in the ED may include:

- Intra-arterial blood pressure monitoring. This gives more reliable arterial pressures and detects hypotension earlier than intermittent non-invasive tonometry (NIBP).[2]
- Systolic pressure variation or the 'swing' of the arterial waveform baseline during respiration (usually with mechanical ventilation) is reported to be at least as sensitive as CVP or pulmonary artery (PA) wedge pressure as a marker of the need for more fluid.[10]
- Stroke volume variation is the difference between the maximal and minimal systolic blood pressure values during one (mechanical) breath, and 'delta down' is the component of this variation from apnoea to minimal SBP. A magnitude of greater than 5 mmHg suggests fluid responsiveness.[11]
- CVP monitoring via the subclavian or internal jugular veins. Response and trends in CVP may be followed in response to volume loading.
- End-tidal CO_2 in ventilated patients may be compared to arterial PCO_2. A difference of more than a few mmHg may suggest a shunt due to inadequate lung perfusion, and has been used to track the adequacy of resuscitation.[12]
- Central venous reflectance oximetry uses an oximeter incorporated into a central line to give central venous haemoglobin saturation. Normal levels are about 70–75%, and lower or higher levels than this suggest inadequate tissue perfusion.
- Pulse contour analysis devices (e.g. Flowtrac, Edwards Lifesciences) use the arterial pulse wave contour and an algorithm to present a cardiac output and other derived parameters which may be used to track responses in resuscitation.
- Pulmonary artery catheterization, peripheral invasive cardiac output monitors (PiCCO), gastric tonometry, sublingual capnometry, transoesophageal echocardiography, Doppler cardiac output studies and other more sophisticated investigations are best performed in an intensive care environment.

'Goal-directed' resuscitation

Several authors have promoted the concept of aiming for specific levels of cardiac output measured on invasive monitoring devices by manipulating haemoglobin concentration, inotropes, vasopressors, vasodilators and fluid volumes. Initial hypotheses suffered from mathematical linkage error, and balanced studies showed that aiming for excessive oxygen delivery or 'supranormal' cardiac outputs was not beneficial in undefined groups or trauma.[13,14]

More recently one landmark study proposed that in severe sepsis in the ED, a resuscitation algorithm guided by CVP, MAP and central venous saturation 'goals' led to an improvement in survival. The commonest intervention change was an increase in fluid resuscitation volume. This study was done in a single centre and so may not be applicable to other ED models.[15]

Having clear clinical goals communicated during resuscitation does allow the team to focus together. These targets can be physiological, time or intervention based.

Interventions in shock

Fluid therapy

Choice of fluid

A sensible maxim remains: Replace that which is lost, at the rate at which it is lost.

- There is no convincing evidence to say that one fluid type is superior in undifferentiated shock, so the commonest choice in the emergent situation remains 'isotonic' 0.9% normal saline. There is retrospective evidence to say that hypotonic fluids and glucose-containing fluid may be detrimental in the critically ill.[16] The SAFE study investigators influenced the crystalloid versus colloid debate by demonstrating that there was no difference in outcome, or any clinically significant measure, between those resuscitated with saline versus human albumin solution.[17,18]
- Albumin is not recommended in the initial resuscitation of burns.[4] Hartmann's (lactated Ringer's, or strong ion 'balanced') solution reduces the risk of hyperchloraemic acidosis from normal saline use, but this appears to be clinically irrelevant.[19] The theoretical advantages of hypertonic saline have not been demonstrated.[20]
- When blood is lost, or diluted by large volumes of fluid, attention needs to be paid to maintaining both oxygen carriage and coagulation activity. Retrospective

studies on transfusion triggers and a prospective randomized controlled multicentre trial suggest that Hb levels of 70–80 g/L are appropriate in patients without ischaemic heart disease, and levels of 100 g/L are tolerated by those patients.[21,22] More practically, creating a reserve is sensible in those who are shocked due to active bleeding, and aiming for a higher target Hb (>100 g/L or HCt > 0.4) may be suitable.

- Dilutional coagulopathy should be considered when coagulopathy is recognized as being present or may be compromising, and either sought for, or proactively avoided by administering fresh frozen plasma (FFP). Clinical coagulopathy may be present before laboratory parameters alter.

Fluid administration

Most publications describe aliquots of 10–40 mL/kg (averaging 20 mL/kg or a 1-L bolus) at free flow or *stat*. Smaller boluses should be given equally rapidly if the heart is suspected of having abnormal compliance or possibly being too 'full', and the clinical response then more closely observed.

In the emergency situation hand-pump infusion lines, or gravity or pressure bag-driven infusion, will deliver larger volumes. Cannulae sized 16 and 20 gauge may achieve flow rates of 1 L over 5 and 10 minutes, respectively.[23] Ward-type volumetric infusion pumps or lines should *not* be used in resuscitation, as the maximum rate of 1 L/h is inadequate, and alarm features may delay infusion. Pressure infusion pumps can achieve very high rates, but at a significant risk of complications.[24]

Route of fluid therapy

Large volumes can be delivered by any route, but central lines, smaller peripheral inserted catheters and intraosseous needles may require a driving pressure. The latter may fail unless carefully supervised. The antecubital, saphenous and femoral veins are reliably accessed with few complications. Consider ultrasound-guided access or venous cut-down in difficult cases.

Targets to titrate fluid therapy

Defining a target for 'how much is enough' is problematic, as each shock scenario has a different aetiology, clinical features and

monitoring requirements. Traditionally, the return of physiological variables towards normal and set perfusion targets are used (see below), but more practically decisions should be made using multiple inputs: preferably use a technique of fluid challenge and review the response to that challenge.

Traditional physiological targets

- Return of systolic BP to > 90 mmHg or to normal for that person
- MAP > 65 mmHg
- Pulse rate < 100/min
- CVP > 10 mmHg
- A sustained rise of CVP >7 mmHg in response to fluid.

Perfusion targets

- Urine output of > 0.5 mL/kg/h
- Lactate of less than 2 mmol/L
- Resolving base deficit
- Central venous oximetry levels of 70–80%
- Capillary refill times < 4 s
- Clinical impression of improved skin perfusion and peripheral pulses.

Invasive measurement targets

- Cardiac index of > 2.5 L/min/m^2
- Pulmonary artery occlusion pressure of > 15 mmHg
- Echocardiogram assessment of left ventricular end-diastolic volume and cardiac output (Table 2.4.4)
- Mixed venous oximetry of 70–75%.

Complications of fluid therapy

- Hypothermia is likely after infusing large volumes of fluid, and ED staff should all be aware of the potential for hypothermia and monitor core temperature. The ED should have a proactive strategy which includes a warmed environment, warmed fluid and blanket stores, and active warming devices. Consider using a commercial warming cartridge for all resuscitations anticipated above a certain volume, or when chilled blood products are used.
- Coagulopathy can be due to dilution, sepsis, or hypothermia and acidosis. Fresh frozen plasma will not resolve the latter pathologies. Hypocalcaemia is rarely an issue.
- Tissue oedema is common and usually clinically irrelevant, but may exacerbate

Table 2.4.4 Target physiological, perfusion and more invasive parameters in the management of shock states

Physiological

Return of systolic BP to > 90 mmHg
or to normal for that person
MAP > 65 mmHg
Pulse rate < 100 min
CVP > 10mmHg
A sustained rise of CVP of more than
7 mmHg in response to fluid

Perfusion

Urine output of > 0.5 mL/kg/h
Lactate of less than 2 mmol/L
Resolving base deficit
Central venous oximetry levels of
70–80 %
Capillary refill times < 4 s
Clinical impression of improved skin perfusion
and peripheral pulses

More invasive

Cardiac index of > 2.5 L/min/m^2
Pulmonary artery occlusion pressure
of > 15 mmHg
Echocardiogram assessment of left ventricular
end-diastolic volume and cardiac output

Note: changes in values and the overall patient response are as important as single figures.

limb and abdominal compartment syndromes.

- Pulmonary oedema is just as likely to be due to the inflammatory process that accompanies significant shock as to excessive preload, and can be managed by either positive-pressure ventilation or diuresis if appropriate. Respiratory failure or the requirement for ventilation does not affect mortality in most ICU studies on outcome, but renal failure, and infarction of the myocardium, brain and gut, are all major risk factors for death.
- Failure to recognize that ongoing fluid requirements are due to an unresolved primary process may cause later deterioration.
- Dilutional or 'hyperchloraemic' acidosis is common but clinically insignificant.
- Anaphylaxis to synthetic colloids or blood products does occur and will complicate the management of shock.

Inotropes and vasopressors

Choice of inotrope

- The drugs that are described as inotropes and vasopressors overlap considerably in activity, and traditional descriptions using receptor-based categories can confuse.

Personal familiarity, institutional preference, and awareness of the clinical effects and side effects, both desired and undesired, should influence their choice. Avoid choosing unfamiliar drugs from 'textbook recipes'.

- An 'inotrope' increases the velocity and force of myocardial muscle fibres and should result in increased contractility. This increased contractility, if combined with adequate preload/filling, will increase the stroke volume and hence cardiac output, and hopefully raise the blood pressure. This will require increase in oxygen consumption which may not be desirable, such as in myocardial ischaemia.
- A 'vasopressor' affects the venous or arterial vascular tone, and should raise total peripheral resistance and hence mean arterial driving pressures, as well as reducing venous capacitance and increasing preload/filling. Other vasoregulatory drugs affect the responsiveness of the vasculature to endogenous and infused vasopressors, including vasopressin and steroids.
- The effects of inotropes and vasopressors are mediated by cAMP-dependent processes through serpentine-receptor associated G proteins (adrenergic and dopaminergic); or by inhibiting phosphodiesterase (as with aminophylline and milrinone); or by cAMP-independent processes such as raising calcium levels (as with digoxin and calcium), or finally by sensitizing troponin C to calcium (as with levosimendan).
- The clinical effects desired from an inotrope or vasopressor are an increase in venous and arterial vascular tone to increase preload and mean systemic pressure, and an increase in contractility, and to achieve a heart rate that is adequate but not excessive. The commonest drugs used in the ED are norepinephrine, epinephrine, dobutamine and dopamine. Isoprenaline and salbutamol are not routinely used in shock. Dopexamine, levosimendan and the older phosphodiesterase inhibitors are rarely used in routine ED practice, and have not been convincingly proved to improve outcomes in either undifferentiated or cardiogenic shock.[25]

They may be used in specific and carefully monitored situations, such as shock with right ventricular (RV) failure, or shock with excessive β-blockade.

- Table 2.4.5 summarizes the clinical effects of the commonly used drugs recognized as inotropes or vasopressors. All those shown have a positive effect on cardiac output and blood pressure, except for dobutamine, which can reduce arterial pressure dramatically when there is hypovolaemia or vascular failure.
- There are expert opinion-based recommendations to guide the choice of inotrope/vasopressor in septic shock,[26] neurogenic shock and anaphylactic shock (discussed below). There are few prospective controlled multicentre trials with patient-centred or clinically meaningful outcomes comparing different inotropes and vasopressors.[27,28]
- Dopamine appears inferior to other catecholamines in shock.[29] Its use to prevent or ameliorate the development of renal failure does not work.[30]
- Although dobutamine is frequently recommended in older texts, its frequently deleterious effect on blood pressure means it should be avoided in hypotension, used in combination with norepinephrine, or guided by invasive monitoring.
- Uncertainty in the diagnosis and perceived severity of shock may suggest the addition of an inotrope/vasopressor, which may achieve an adequate blood pressure at the expense of correct assessment of fluid volume replenishment.

Administration

- Norepinephrine, epinephrine (salbutamol and isoprenaline) can be made up as 6 mg in 100 mL (or 3 mg in 50 mL) and given by volumetric infusion pump into a central vein. This dose dilution gives an infusion rate of 1 mL/h to equate to 1 μg/min (or for a 60 kg person a concentration of 1 μg/kg/h).
- Dobutamine and dopamine are presented as 250 mg and 200 mg ampoules, and may be made up as weight (kg) × 6 mg in 100 mL, or weight (kg) × 3 mg in 50 mL to then give a dose dilution where an infusion rate of 1 mL/h equates to 1 μg/kg/min.

Table 2.4.5 Clinical effects of inotropes and vasopressors

Drug infused	Clinically observed		Measured		Calculated			'Classic' receptor activity
	Blood pressure (BP)	Heart rate (HR)	Cardiac contractility (stroke volume)	Cardiac output (CO)	Arterial vascular tone	Venous capacitance	Diastolic relaxation (lusitropy)	
Adrenaline	++	++	++	++	+	+	+	$\beta1$ $\beta2$ $\alpha1$ ($\alpha2$)
Noradrenaline	++	0	++	+	+	++	-	$\beta1$, $\alpha1$ ($\beta2$, $\alpha2$)
Dopamine	+	++	+	+	+	+	-	$\beta1$ β $\alpha1$ dopA1
Dobutamine	-	+	++	++	-	-		$\beta1$ $\beta2$ (dopA1)
Metaraminol	++	0	0	0	+	++	0	$\alpha1$
Isoprenaline	-	++	+	+	-	-	0	$\beta1$ β
Levosimendan	+/-	+	++	++	0	0	+	Sensitizes troponin to Ca^{2+}
Vasopressin	+	0	0	0	++	+	0	V_1 V_2

Route

- In emergency situations inotropes/ vasopressors may be administered into a large peripheral vein with fast-flowing crystalloid. The clinical effect may be variable, and thrombophlebitis can occur.
- Dedicated lines and lumina without side injection ports should be used to avoid inadvertent boluses.
- Placement of central venous lines (CVL) or peripherally inserted central catheters (PICC) is best performed under strict asepsis in the appropriate setting, but may be required early in the ED for inotrope/ vasopressor infusions, although they are rarely vital for fluid management.

Targets to titrate inotropes/ vasopressors

- The use of inotropes/vasopressors without adequate preload is associated with worse outcomes,[31,32] so volume infusion should always precede the commencement of inotropes, unless unequivocal evidence exists that the heart is 'too full'. Even in cardiogenic shock, judicious boluses of fluid with close monitoring may result in improved cardiac output.
- Add an effective inotrope if, despite ongoing rapid fluid volume resuscitation, cardiac output markers such as MAP are low (see Goals of Treatment), and titrate rapidly upwards until an effect is noted. Subsequently wean the inotrope/ vasopressor as further volume infusion

allows, or evidence develops that the heart is over-full. Reassess frequently to judge whether further fluid is needed.
- The upper level of the infusion is titrated to effect, and limited only by the development of undesired side effects or recognition of lack of any effect. Published upper limits are not based on evidence. Thus an infusion rate is simply 'titrated to desired effect and monitored for undesired effect'.

Complications

- Undesired effects may include excessive tachycardia, excessive hypertension, tremor, anxiety and raised intracranial pressure (if monitored). Conversely, watch for disconnection or failure to infuse, when parameters unexpectedly fall.
- Epinephrine may cause metabolic effects including hyperglycaemia, hypokalaemia and lactic acidosis (usually clinically irrelevant).
- Increased myocardial oxygen consumption may worsen myocardial ischaemia and precipitate cardiac arrhythmias.
- Peripheral digit and skin infarction described in the past is probably due to endothelial injury from prolonged shock or the underlying primary cause, with no evidence that it was due to a vasoconstrictor effect.
- Splanchnic or myocardial infarction described in the past is more likely to be due to inadequate resuscitation and

hypotension rather than vasoconstriction, as these vessels are poorly reactive.
- Too large, too concentrated or too rapid a bolus will cause severe hypertension and risks sequelae such as intracranial haemorrhage and myocardial damage (particularly with epinephrine).

Other interventions

- The use of corticosteroids in shock should be reserved for adrenal insufficiency, or if the patient is already receiving corticosteroids. There is no evidence to support their use in anaphylactic shock (see Chapter 28.7).
- Corticosteroids in physiological dosages can improve some haemodynamic parameters in severe septic shock, but two controlled multicentre trials[33,34] found that corticosteroids have no effect on mortality. Steroids are still recommended in subsets of patients with meningitis.[35] Some spinal injury centres recommend high-dose methylprednisolone for 24–48 hours in spinal cord injury, but the data are unconvincing.[36]
- Military anti-shock trousers (MAST) or pneumatic anti-shock garments (PASG) wrap the legs and abdomen in inflatable compressive compartments. They are thought to reduce the venous capacitance in the lower body, thereby 'auto-transfusing' blood into the upper body, and also to raise peripheral resistance. There is no evidence to

support that their use reduces mortality, length of hospitalization or length of ICU stay in trauma patients, and it is possible that it may increase these.[37] They are not recommended in the ED.

The effects of shock on other interventions

- Hypoperfusion of tissues will affect the delivery of drugs, particularly orally and subcutaneously administered drugs, and affects the pharmacokinetics with a reduced clearance of drugs. Unpredictable delivery and efficacy may require dose changes or use of alternate routes. Carefully titrated intravenous doses given centrally are advisable.
- Sedative, analgesic and anaesthetic drugs, particularly thiopentone, midazolam, propofol and even ketamine (when the sympathetic ganglia are exhausted of catecholamine), may have adverse effects on vascular tone and cause worsening of shock. These drugs may also have a delayed circulation time and appear not to work.
- Catecholamines may be less efficacious in severe acidosis states, hence one theoretical but unproven use for sodium bicarbonate in severe metabolic acidosis.
- Endotracheal intubation and positive-pressure ventilation reduce venous return and may further reduce cardiac output and systolic blood pressure. Minimal initial tidal volume and PEEP settings may reduce this effect. Physiological dead space may be increased by positive-pressure ventilation reducing lung perfusion, and so the arterial PCO_2 may rise. 'Normalization' of PCO_2 may then lead to an apparent worsening of compensated metabolic acidosis.
- Inotropes are arrhythmogenic, and this complication is increased in the setting of hypokalaemia, acidosis and poorly perfused myocardium.
- The stress response and some inotropes may cause or exacerbate hyperglycaemia.
- Infused fluids will eventually redistribute to all tissues and produce widespread oedema. An example is the burns victim who may have minimal airway burns, but

after 22 L of crystalloid may have a compromised oedematous airway.

The management of specific shock syndromes

The following shock syndromes are discussed briefly here, and in further chapters in the book.

- Hypovolaemia (absolute)
- Hypovolaemia (relative)
- Neurogenic shock (see Chapter 3.3)
- Anaphylactic shock (see Chapter 28.7)
- Hypoadrenal shock (see Chapter 11.3)
- Cardiogenic shock (see Section 5 Cardiovascular)
- Septic shock (see Chapter 2.5)

Absolute hypovolaemia

Clinical features
The history and examination may point to fluid loss from vessels, gut, kidneys or evaporation. Bleeding needs to be excluded in all hypovolaemia (see Table 2.4.1). In addition to those described previously, the clinical signs will include signs of reduced preload, with flat neck veins as a consequence of low central venous pressure.

Investigations relevant to diagnosis
Where hypovolaemia is due to bleeding, haemostasis is the most effective intervention, meaning direct surgical or specialist intervention, and may parallel resuscitation and precede investigations. If initial resuscitation allows, investigations such as formal ultrasound, CT with or without contrast angiography, may identify the site of bleeding. Radiographic intervention such as angiography with embolization may be life-saving, for instance in severe pelvic trauma.

Therapy
- Initial resuscitation as described previously, and ensure all efforts are made to avoid hypothermia.
- Passive leg elevation is more effective in hypovolaemic shock than the Trendelenburg (head lower than the pelvis body position) in increasing left ventricular end-diastolic volume, stroke volume and cardiac output, but these effects are transient.[6]

- External haemorrhage is controlled with firm, direct manual pressure. Tourniquets are associated with morbidity, but may be useful in the short term.[38]
- Application of the pneumatic anti-shock garment (PASG or MAST suit) has no place in the management of hypovolaemic shock.[37]
- Surgical consultation is urgently required. Efforts to return the systolic blood pressure to 'normal' in bleeding trauma patients may be counterproductive and occasionally harmful, particularly in penetrating truncal trauma. This suggests that surgical haemostasis should take priority, and over-resuscitation should be avoided, adopting a 'minimal-volume' approach. Thus patients with uncontrolled haemorrhage following penetrating truncal trauma, who are in close proximity to facilities capable of definitive care, should undergo minimal-volume or 'hypotense' fluid resuscitation pending prompt surgical intervention.[39] 'Minimal volume' is interpreted variously as fluid sufficient to keep the line open, or small (250 mL) boluses titrated to palpable radial pulse or conscious level. Essentially, aim to keep the brain and heart perfused, although any minimal-volume approach is contraindicated when traumatic brain injury is associated with hypotension, as the cerebral perfusion pressure is dependent on maintaining the MAP.
- Infuse packed red cells in major blood loss, where oxygen delivery is known to be impaired or Hb is less than 70 g/L. Recognition or anticipation of coagulopathy will need fresh frozen plasma and platelets. Patients with lesser amounts of blood loss or controlled bleeding, or non-haemorrhagic hypovolaemic shock, can be managed with warmed crystalloid.[18]
- Hypertonic saline 3% or 7% was considered to improve outcome in a subgroup of patients with shock and traumatic brain injury, but this has not been proved. Despite this, hypertonic saline has been recommended as the initial fluid of choice in haemorrhaging battlefield casualties.[40]
- There are no current definitive recommendations concerning the use of

blood substitutes such as modified haemoglobin or non-blood perfluorocarbons.

- Other causes of impaired preload or contractility, such as tension pneumothorax, cardiac tamponade and myocardial contusion, should always be considered in the hypotensive trauma patient. Increased preload is still beneficial in these settings, and all trauma patients should be assumed to be hypovolaemic until proven otherwise. Urgent ultrasound is essential.

Relative hypovolaemia (anaphylaxis, addisonian crisis, neurogenic shock, drug or toxin effect)

Anaphylaxis (see Chapter 28.7)
The mainstay of treatment in shock is the physiological antagonist epinephrine, plus oxygen and fluid, with the patient supine and the legs raised.

Adrenal shock (see Chapter 11.3)
Hypotension due to hypoadrenalism is uncommon, but should be suspected in the acutely unwell patient with exposure to past or current steroid use, or when hypotension occurs with relative polyuria. Primary adrenal failure is less common now, but causes include abrupt cessation of long-term steroid therapy, autoimmune disease, retroperitoneal haemorrhage, HIV-associated infections, azole antifungal drugs and surgical removal of the adrenals.

Treatment includes initial resuscitation with crystalloid, and intravenous administration of steroids with mineralocorticoid effect. Dexamethasone 10 mg or hydrocortisone 50 mg tds, have adequate mineralocorticoid effect at those doses.

Investigations relevant to diagnosis
- Urinary sodium level is normally low (<10 mmol/L) in shock with hypotension. Consider hypoadrenalism if the urinary sodium is inappropriately high (> 20 mmol/L) in an initial urine sample; or diuretic use, excessive sodium administration and cerebral salt-wasting syndromes.
- Random free cortisol should be > 500 nmol/L in stressed shocked states.

A formal short Synachthen test is rarely done in the ED, but if dexamethasone (a synthetic steroid) is given, it allows for a short Synachthen test to be done later.

Neurogenic shock (see Chapter 3.3)
Neurogenic shock is manifested by the triad of hypotension, bradycardia and hypothermia in the setting of an acute spinal cord injury, related to the loss of sympathetic nerve tone. 'Spinal shock' is a term used to describe the state of transient physiological (rather than anatomical) reflex depression of all spinal cord function below the level of an injury, associated with the loss of all sensory and motor function. It may be transient and the term should never be used to describe final functional outcome.[41] Arterial hypotension may or may not be part of such phenomena. Thoracic lesions result in loss of lower extremity and splanchnic sympathetic tone, with subsequent venous pooling. Cervical lesions additionally result in the absence of cardiovascular sympathetic tone.

One in four patients with a complete cervical-cord injury may require haemodynamic support for their hypotension.[42] The presence of hypotension has no implications regarding the degree of completeness of cord injury or prognosis.

Clinical features
- Neurogenic shock is a diagnosis of exclusion in the trauma patient. Hypotension should be accompanied by flaccidity and areflexia distal to the suspected level of the lesion. There should be no compensatory tachycardia or peripheral pallor, sweating or vasoconstriction.
- Other causes of hypovolaemia or shock in the trauma patient should be actively sought, such as concealed bleeding, tension pneumothorax and cardiac tamponade, which need active exclusion with investigations such as abdominal ultrasound, or CT scanning.

Therapy
- The airway must be specifically assessed for compromise due to an altered level of consciousness, regurgitation or cervical haematoma.

- The adequacy of minute ventilation and the ability to clear secretions should be measured by clinical assessment, serial arterial blood gas, and spirometry. Anticipate respiratory failure in high spinal cord injuries, but note that hypoxaemia is a late sign.
- Support the circulation in neurogenic shock with hypotension:
  - If bradycardia and symptomatic hypotension are present, give atropine 0.5–1 mg to a maximum of 3 mg to counter unopposed parasympathetic vagal tone.
  - Relative hypovolaemia is likely and should be assessed with a fluid challenge: give 500–1000 mL aliquots of fluid, and follow the clinical response.
  - Consider pharmacological vasoconstriction if the above measures fail to return blood pressure and measurable signs of perfusion to normal. Give ephedrine 5–10 mg i.v., or phenylephrine 0.2–1 mg i.v. urgently. Norepinephrine or dopamine titrated to response can be used, provided other treatable causes of hypotension such as haemorrhage, tamponade, pneumothorax, etc. have been excluded.
- Monitoring is best done by markers of adequate tissue perfusion such as urine output and lactate.

Cardiac causes of shock: cardiogenic shock
Cardiogenic shock is the inability of the heart to deliver sufficient blood to the tissues to meet resting metabolic demands, and is clinically defined as a systolic blood pressure of <90 mmHg or ≥30 mmHg below basal levels for at least 30 minutes; an alternative definition is a significant arteriovenous oxygen difference and a cardiac index of <2.2 L/min/m^2 where pulmonary capillary wedge pressure is >15 mmHg. Failure to respond to correction of hypoxaemia, hypovolaemia, arrhythmias and acidosis is a requirement for the diagnosis.[43] There is clinical evidence of poor tissue perfusion in the form of oliguria, cyanosis and altered mentation.

Aetiology

The commonest cause of cardiogenic shock is myocardial infarction (MI) or ischaemia (see Table 2.4.3). Cardiogenic shock complicates 6–7% of patients with acute myocardial infarction and has a mortality as high as 56–74%. It is the commonest cause of in-hospital death post-infarction.[43,44] Only 10% of these patients develop the shock in the ED, but this subgroup has a higher mortality.[44]

Other cardiac causes of shock include valvular rupture or degeneration, critical stenosis, septal or free wall rupture and atrial myxoma. Cardiac tamponade or a large pulmonary embolus are better considered as obstructive causes of shock, as the myocardial pump is unaffected initially.

Older patients with anterior AMI, previous MI, diabetes, angina or congestive heart failure are at greatest risk of cardiogenic shock. There is a higher prevalence in patients with multivessel disease (e.g. diabetes) and involving the left main coronary artery.[45] Patients with persistent occlusion of the left anterior descending artery are at the highest risk of developing shock.[46] Only aggressive revascularization by coronary artery bypass grafting (CABG) within 12 hours of symptom onset makes any difference to these patients.

Pathophysiology

The activation of the sympathetic nervous and renin–angiotensin systems contributes to an increase in myocardial oxygen demand, which contributes to an increase in infarct size and further decreases in contractility, cardiac output and coronary perfusion pressure. Systolic dysfunction results in an increase in end-systolic volumes and reductions in ejection fraction, stroke volume and cardiac output. Diastolic dysfunction is also present.

Pulmonary oedema exacerbates hypoxia and systemic tissue hypoperfusion, and selective vascular redistribution leads to organ failure and metabolic acidosis.

Clinical features

The clinical signs in cardiogenic shock in addition to those described previously are:

- Profound effects due to catecholamine outflow, such as tachycardia, pallor, poor capillary refill and low cardiac output with a decreased urine output and raised lactate.
- Classic signs of left heart failure with a third heart sound gallop rhythm and basal crackles from pulmonary oedema, and/or a raised jugular venous pressure (JVP), hepatic congestion and peripheral oedema from right ventricular failure. These may occur alone in right ventricular infarction, usually associated with an inferior myocardial infarction and found by noting ST elevation in a right-sided V4 chest lead (V4R).
- Precordial examination may demonstrate a dyskinetic apex beat. A 'gallop' or additional heart sound suggests reduced ventricular compliance (fourth) and increased ventricular diastolic pressure (third). Loud murmurs or thrills in systole may be due to mitral regurgitation or critical aortic stenosis, and rarely, rupture of the ventricular septum.
- Blood pressure may initially remain within normal limits as a result of compensatory mechanisms, which also produce tachycardia and narrowed pulse pressure.

Investigations relevant to therapy

- Twelve-lead ECG may define territory and need for reperfusion therapy. Leads V4R and V7–9 are indicated in suspected right ventricular and posterior myocardial infarction, respectively.
- Troponin I or T levels, or serial CK (creatine kinase), CK-MB (creatine kinase, muscle–brain).
- Chest X-ray may show pulmonary oedema and enlarged cardiac silhouette. Bedside echocardiography should be available to all patients who remain with undiagnosed shock, as an extension of the physical examination. Pericardial effusion or cardiac tamponade are excluded and global systolic function, filling and regional wall motion abnormalities assessed.
- Transoesophageal echocardiography may additionally diagnose loculated cardiac tamponade, a haemodynamically significant pulmonary embolus, and obscure valvular lesions.

Therapy

- Initial care and monitoring should be provided as described earlier, with management of the myocardial infarct according to local policy. When cardiogenic shock is recognized, immediate discussion regarding revascularization should be made with a referral centre; also if echocardiogram defines a mechanical cause of shock.
- Tracheal intubation and ventilation should be considered early for cardiac 'respite', and CPAP or non-invasive ventilation with BIPAP for selected patients. Intra-arterial blood pressure monitoring is recommended.[47]
- Arrhythmias considered contributory to the presence of cardiogenic shock should be treated according to standard ACLS principles. See Chapter 22.3 for procedural sedation requirements.
- Hypovolaemia must be sought and corrected in all patients; 250 mL aliquots of fluid should be given as a bolus and the response assessed. Further boluses may be indicated. Volume loading to maintain higher right atrial filling pressures is important in inferior MI with right ventricular involvement, and all drugs that reduce preload avoided, including nitrates, diuretics and excess opiates. CVP monitoring may be indicated, although it is difficult to interpret in the presence of high right-sided pressures.
- Targets that may be more relevant are perfusion targets such as urine output, lactate, and clinical signs of improved skin perfusion and resolution of pulmonary oedema. An MAP of 60 mmHg is considered as allowing coronary autoregulation.
- Persistence of the shock state following adequate fluid challenge in the presence of end-organ dysfunction is an indication for intra-aortic balloon pump (IABP) and or inotropic support.[45]
- Intra-aortic balloon counterpulsation increases aortic root diastolic pressure (and hence coronary perfusion) and duration of apparent systole (and hence MAP), with no increase in oxygen demand. Complications include leg ischaemia, arterial dissection, thromboembolism and thrombocytopenia.[49]
- Early revascularization by either percutaneous coronary intervention (PCI) or CABG is recommended for patients less than 75 years old with ST elevation

or new left bundle branch block (LBBB) who develop cardiogenic shock within 36 hours of acute MI, and who are suitable for revascularization that can be performed within 18 hours of shock onset.[47] Early transfer and revascularization confers a survival advantage in patients with MI plus cardiogenic shock.[43–45]

- Initial therapy with thrombolysis should be given to patients who present to a facility without primary PCI capability or IABP, followed by urgent transfer, to reduce mortality.[45,46]
- Where an IABP is available, thrombolysis *and* IABP should be instituted early, as mortality is further improved with this combination.[48]
- The use of inotropes and vasopressors in cardiogenic shock has not been shown to improve survival.[47–49] Dobutamine and levosimendan have inotropic and vasodilator effects, but are not recommended when hypotension is present. Dopamine was commonly used, but the tachycardia limits its efficacy by increasing myocardial oxygen demand. Norepinephrine is increasingly used, allowing the later introduction of a vasodilator. There is no evidence for a reduction in mortality with the use of any of the newer inodilators, such as dopexamine, milrinone or levosimendan.[25,50]
- Vasodilators can be added when blood pressure has been restored but fails to improve peripheral end-organ perfusion. Glyceryl trinitrate is the vasodilator of choice in myocardial ischaemia, in a dose range of 0.5–2.0 µg/kg/min, to a maximum of 10 µg/kg/min. Angiotensin-converting enzyme inhibitors (ACEI) can be given early if titrated gradually, although precipitate hypotension may occur.
- Consider referral for emergency cardiac transplantation in younger patients.
- In summary, those patients with large infarctions, a resting tachycardia and signs of poor tissue perfusion should be identified early and managed aggressively as above. There should be early discussion with a cardiac referral centre, and if the patient is unstable or unsuitable for transfer, an IABP

considered with a lower threshold for thrombolysis, if not contraindicated. Inotropes are a temporizing measure.

Pericardial tamponade

Pericardial (cardiac) tamponade causes a failure of filling of the right atrium as a result of increased pericardial pressure. The right ventricle, and subsequently the left ventricle, has limited stroke volume and cardiac output. Tachycardia and raised peripheral resistance are compensatory mechanisms. Coexistent hypovolaemia may mask one of the classic clinical signs of tamponade, a full JVP rising on inspiration (Kussmaul's sign). Cardiac tamponade should be excluded by echocardiography.

Pericardial tamponade can be a fatal consequence of aortic dissection. Risk factors for aortic dissection include hypertension (particularly malignant), Marfan's or Ehlers–Danlos syndrome, aortic coarctation, Ebstein's anomaly, pregnancy hypertension and cocaine use. The presence of pericardial tamponade should also be suspected when there is unexplained shock with:

- Blunt or penetrating cardiac trauma
- Pericarditis due to infection, radiation, connective tissue disorders or malignancy
- Anticoagulant use
- Iatrogenic injury, e.g. CVP insertion.

Management

Volume loading will raise right-sided filling pressures and volumes. Tachycardia should be preserved. Vasopressor support will maintain MAP until pericardiocentesis under echo guidance or surgical pericardiotomy are performed.

Septic shock (see Chapter 2.5 for a detailed definition, management and discussion)

Septic shock is sepsis accompanied by hypotension (systolic BP <90 mmHg or 40 mmHg or more below normal baseline), and perfusion abnormalities such as elevated lactate (> 5 mmol/L), despite adequate fluid resuscitation (> 20 mL/kg).[51]

Clinical presentation

The presence and degree of shock in sepsis can be misinterpreted as the patient may have few signs of inadequate perfusion, and the physiological abnormalities may

be attributed to fever. Early signs may include tachypnoea, tachycardia, high or low temperature, oliguria, altered mental state and peripheral vasodilatation. Later signs may include reduced capillary refill, skin mottling, hypotension, further altered mental status, a reduction in urine output, evidence of myocardial dysfunction and a metabolic acidosis with raised lactate.

Therapy

- Initial resuscitation is provided as outlined previously in the primary survey.
- Removal of infection (source control) and appropriate antibiotics.
- There is no preferred fluid. A post-hoc analysis of the SAFE study suggests that albumin may have a survival advantage.[18]
- Persistent hypotension and/or signs of organ hypoperfusion despite ongoing rapid fluid resuscitation are indications for vasopressor/inotrope support. The early use of norepinephrine is recommended when the hypotension is severe and response to fluids or other inotropes is suboptimal.26 Vasopressin 0.04 units/min i.v. may be used as a vasopressor-sparing agent, although there is no evidence to date of effects on survival.[52]
- Corticosteroids improve some haemodynamic parameters, but trials have found no overall effect on mortality.[32–34]
- High-volume haemofiltration can improve the haemodynamic status in septic shock, possibly by removing various cytokines and other mediators.[53] No other ancillary treatments have been accepted as of benefit in septic shock.

Conclusion

The aetiology of shock in patients presenting to the emergency department is varied. Interventions in all forms of shock are simple and initially directed at the physiological deficit, and should be seen as a test of the clinical hypothesis. Continuous reappraisal is required. Hypovolaemia should be sought in all cases, although further specific management will depend on the underlying cause(s).

References

1. Dutton RP. Current concepts in hemorrhagic shock. Anesthesiology Clinics 2007; 25: 23–34, viii.
2. Pickering TG, Hall JE, Appel LJ, et al. Recommendations for blood pressure measurement in humans and experimental animals. Part 1: Blood pressure measurement in humans: a statement for professionals from the Subcommittee of Professional and Public Education of the American Heart Association Council on High Blood Pressure Research. Circulation 2005; 111: 697–716.
3. Fieselmann JF, Hendryx MS, Helms CM, Wakefield DS. Respiratory rate predicts cardiopulmonary arrest for internal medicine inpatients. Journal of General Internal Medicine 1993; 8: 354–360.
4. American College of Surgeons Committee on Trauma. Advanced Trauma Life Support for doctors. Instructors' course manual 1997. Chicago: ACS, 1997.
5. Jones AE, Aborn LS, Kline JA. Severity of emergency department hypotension predicts adverse hospital outcome. Shock 2004; 22: 410–414.
6. Terai C, Anada H, Matsushima S, et al. Effects of Trendelenburg versus passive leg-raising autotransfusion in humans. Intensive Care Medicine 1996; 22: 613–614.
7. Bur A, Herkner H, Vlcek M, et al. Factors influencing the accuracy of oscillometric blood pressure measurement in critically ill patients. Critical Care Medicine 2003; 31: 793–799.
8. Bakker J, Coffernils M, Leon M, et al. Blood lactate levels are superior to oxygen derived variables in predicting outcome in human septic shock. Chest 1991; 99: 956–962.
9. Davis JW, Parks JN, Kaups KL, et al. Admission base deficit predicts transfusion requirements and risk of complication. Journal of Trauma 1996; 41: 769–774.
10. Lamia B, Chemla D, Richard C, Teboul JL. Clinical review: interpretation of arterial pressure wave in shock states. Critical Care 2005; 9: 601–606. Epub 2005 Oct 26.
11. Tavernier B, Makhotine O, Lebuffe G, et al. Pressure variation as a guide to fluid therapy in patients with sepsis-induced hypotension. Anesthesiology 1998; 89: 1313–1321.
12. Jin X, Weil MH, Tang W, et al. End-tidal carbon dioxide as a noninvasive indicator of cardiac index during circulatory shock. Critical Care Medicine. 2000; 28: 2415–2419.
13. McKinley BA, Kozar RA, Cocanour CS, et al. Normal versus supranormal oxygen delivery goals in shock resuscitation: the response is the same. Journal of Trauma 2002; 53: 825–832.
14. Kern JW, Shoemaker WC. Meta-analysis of hemodynamic optimization in high-risk patients. Critical Care Medicine 2002; 30: 1686–1692.
15. Rivers E, Nguyen B, Havstad S, et al. and the Early Goal-Directed Therapy Collaborative Group. Early goal-directed therapy in the treatment of severe sepsis and septic shock. New England Journal of Medicine 2001; 345: 1368–1377.
16. American Heart Association Guidelines for Cardiopulmonary Resuscitation and Emergency Cardiovascular Care 2005. Circulation 2005; 112.
17. Finfer S, Bellomo R, Boyce N, et al. A comparison of albumin and saline for fluid resuscitation in the intensive care unit. New England Journal of Medicine 2004; 350: 2247.
18. The Albumin Reviewers (Alderson P, Bunn F, Li Wan Po A, et al.). Human albumin solution for resuscitation and volume expansion in critically ill patients. Cochrane Database of Systematic Reviews 2004, Issue 4. Art. No. CD001208.
19. Waters JH, Gottlieb A, Schoenwald P, et al. Normal saline versus lactated Ringer's solution for intraoperative fluid management in patients undergoing abdominal aortic aneurysm repair: an outcome study. Anesthesia and Analgesia 2001; 93: 817–822.
20. Bunn F, Roberts I, Tasker R. Hypertonic versus near isotonic crystalloid for fluid resuscitation in critically ill patients. Cochrane Database of Systematic Reviews 2004, Issue 3. Art. No. CD002045.
21. Hebert PC, Wells G, Blajchman MA, et al. A multicenter, randomized, controlled clinical trial of transfusion requirements in critical care. New England Journal of Medicine 1999; 340: 409–417.
22. Clinical Practice Guidelines on the use of Blood Components of National Health and Medical Research Council (NHMRC) & Australian and New Zealand Society of Blood Transfusion.
23. Becton Dickinson product information. Becton Dickinson Pty Ltd, Eight Mile Plains, QLD 4113.
24. Mendenhall ML, Spain DA. Venous air embolism and pressure infusion devices. Journal of Trauma 2007; 63: 246.
25. Mebazaa A. The SURVIVE-W Trial: Comparison of dobutamine and levosimendan on survival in acute decompensated heart failure. Paper presented at Program and abstracts from the American Heart Association Program and abstracts from the American Heart Association Scientific Sessions 2005.
26. Dellinger RP, Carlet JM, Masur H, et al. Surviving Sepsis Campaign guidelines for management of severe sepsis and septic shock. Critical Care Medicine 2004; 32: 858.
27. Myberg JA. An appraisal of selection and use of catecholamines in septic shock – old becomes new again. Critical Care Resuscitation 2006; 3: 353–360.
28. Müllner M, Urbanek B, Havel C, et al. Vasopressors for shock. Cochrane Database of Systematic Reviews 2004, Issue 3. Art. No. CD003709.
29. Sakr Y, Reinhart K, Vincent JL, et al. Does dopamine administration in shock influence outcome? Results of the Sepsis Occurrence in Acutely Ill Patients (SOAP) Study. Critical Care Medicine 2006; 34: 589.
30. Bellomo R, Chapman M, Finfer S, et al. Low-dose dopamine in patients with early renal dysfunction: A placebo-controlled randomized trial. Australian and New Zealand Intensive Care Society (ANZICS) Clinical Trials Group. Lancet 2000; 356: 2139–2143.
31. Beale RJ, Hollenberg SM, Vincent JL, et al. Vasopressor and inotropic support in septic shock: an evidence-based review. Critical Care Medicine 2004; 32: S455–465.
32. Nordin AJ, Makisalo H, Hockerstedt KA. Failure of dobutamine to improve liver oxygenation during resuscitation with a crystalloid solution after experimental haemorrhagic shock. European Journal of Surgery 1996; 162: 973.
33. Annane D, Sebille V, Charpentier C, et al. Effect of treatment with low doses of hydrocortisone and fludrocortisone on mortality in patients with septic shock. Journal of the American Medical Association 2002; 288: 862–871.
34. Lipiner-Friedman D, Sprung CL, Laterre PF, et al. Corticus Study Group. Adrenal function in sepsis: the retrospective Corticus cohort study. Critical Care Medicine 2007; 35: 1012–1018.
35. van de Beek D, de Gans J, McIntyre P, Prasad K. Corticosteroids for acute bacterial meningitis. Cochrane Database of Systematic Reviews 2007, Issue 1. Art. No. CD004405.
36. Bracken MB. Steroids for acute spinal cord injury. Cochrane Database of Systematic Reviews 2002, Issue 2. Art. No. CD001046.
37. Roberts I, Blackhall K, Dickinson K. Medical anti-shock trousers (pneumatic anti-shock garments) for circulatory support in patients with trauma. Cochrane Database of Systematic Reviews 1999, Issue 4. Art. No. CD001856
38. Lee C, Porter KM, Hodgetts TJ. Tourniquet use in the civilian prehospital setting. Emergency Medicine Journal 2007; 24: 584–587.
39. Bickell WH, Wall MJ Jr, Pepe PE, Martin RR. Immediate versus delayed fluid resuscitation for hypotensive patients with penetrating torso injuries. New England Journal of Medicine 1994; 331: 1105–1109.
40. Alam HB, Rhee P. New developments in fluid resuscitation. [Review] Surgical Clinics of North America 2007; 87: 55–72, vi.
41. Maynard FM, Bracken MB, Creasey G, et al. International standards for neurological and functional classification of spinal cord injury. Spinal Cord 1997; 35: 266–274.
42. Guly HR, Bouamra O, Lecky FE, on behalf of the Trauma Audit and Research Network. The incidence of neurogenic shock in patients with isolated spinal cord injury in the emergency department. Resuscitation 2007; 76: 57–62.
43. Califf RM, Bengston JR. Cardiogenic shock. Current concepts. New England Journal of Medicine 1994; 330: 1724–1730.
44. Webb JG, Sleeper LA, Buller CE, et al. Implications of the timing of onset of cardiogenic shock after acute myocardial infarction: a report from the SHOCK Trial Registry. SHould we emergently revascularize Occluded Coronaries for cardiogenic shocK? Journal of the American College of Cardiology 2000; 36: 1084.
45. Goldberg RJ, Gore JM, Thompson CA, et al. Recent magnitude of and temporal trends (1994–1997) in the incidence and hospital death rates of cardiogenic shock complicating acute myocardial infarction: The second National Registry of Myocardial Infarction. American Heart Journal 2001; 141: 65.
46. Wong SC, Sanborn T, Sleeper LA, et al. Angiographic findings and clinical correlates in patients with cardiogenic shock complicating acute myocardial infarction: a report from the SHOCK Trial Registry. SHould we emergently revascularize Occluded Coronaries for cardiogenic shocK?. Journal of the American College of Cardiology 2000; 36: 1077.
47. Antman EM, Anbe DT, Armstrong PW, et al. ACC/AHA guidelines for the management of patients with ST-elevation myocardial infarction. Available at: www.acc.org/qualityandscience/clinical/statements.htm (Accessed August 2006).
48. French JK, Feldman HA, Assmann SF, et al. Influence of thrombolytic therapy, with or without intra-aortic balloon counterpulsation, on 12-month survival in the SHOCK trial. American Heart Journal 2003; 146: 804.
49. Prieto A, Eisenberg J, Thakar RK. Non-arrhythmic complications of acute myocardial infarction. Emergency Medical Clinics of North America 2001; 19: 397–415.
50. Mebazaa A, Nieminen MS, Packer M, et al. Levosimendan vs dobutamine for patients with acute decompensated heart failure: the SURVIVE Randomized Trial. Journal of the Americal Medicine Association 2007; 297: 1883.
51. Levy MM, Fink MP, Marshall JC, et al. 2001 SCCM/ESICM/ACCP/ATS/SIS International Sepsis Definitions Conference. Critical Care Medicine 2003; 31: 1250–1256.
52. Dyke PC 2nd, Tobias JD. Vasopressin: applications in clinical practice. Journal of Intensive Care Medicine 2004; 19: 220.
53. Ronco C, Bellomo R, Homel P, et al. Effects of different doses in continuous veno-venous haemofiltration on outcomes of acute renal failure: a prospective randomised trial. Lancet 2000; 356: 26–30.

2.5 Sepsis and septic shock

Anna Holdgate

ESSENTIALS

1 Early intervention in the emergency department reduces mortality in patients with sepsis and septic shock.

2 Aggressive haemodynamic resuscitation with fluids, vasopressors and inotropes should begin as soon as possible.

3 Systemic blood pressure, serum lactate levels and urine output should be monitored closely to determine the effectiveness of treatment.

4 Broad-spectrum antibiotics should be administered within 1 hour of recognition of sepsis.

Introduction

Septic shock is the extreme end of the spectrum of septic syndromes. Globally, septic shock is associated with a mortality rate of up to 46%. In Australia and New Zealand the reported mortality is substantially lower (27.6%) for septic patients admitted from the emergency department (ED) to intensive care.[1] Each year approximately 1500 septic patients are admitted to Australasian ICUs from the ED, and this incidence has been steadily rising over the past decade.[1] ED management of the septic patient is crucial, as early intervention in several facets of care has been shown to reduce mortality.

Aetiology and pathophysiology

Approximately 95% of identified causative organisms are bacterial, with Gram-positive organisms (mostly *Staphylococcus aureus*, coagulase-negative staphylococci, enterococci and streptococci) now slightly more common than Gram-negative species (particularly *Escherichia coli*, *Klebsiella pneumoniae* and *Pseudomonas aeruginosa*). The remaining 5% are caused by fungi, mostly *Candida*, with the incidence of fungal sepsis increasing threefold in the last 20 years.[2] Pathogens are identified in approximately 70% of patients from blood or other tissue cultures. The primary source of infection is most commonly respiratory (36%), bloodstream (20%), intra-abdominal (19%), urinary tract (13%) and skin/other soft tissue (7%).[3]

Pathogenic mechanisms

The pathogenic mechanisms in sepsis are initiated by a variety of host responses to the infecting organism. Inflammatory mediators such as tumour necrosis factor α (TNF-α) and the interleukins are produced by the host, resulting in activation of neutrophils, direct injury to the endothelium with increased vascular permeability, and release of nitric oxide resulting in vasodilatation. Modification of the coagulation cascade causes an increase in procoagulant factors and lower levels of the anticoagulant factors protein C, protein S and antithrombin III. These proinflammatory and procoagulant responses lead to reduced vascular resistance, relative hypovolaemia, loss of vasoregulatory control in microvascular beds, reduced myocardial contractility, acute lung injury and renal dysfunction. These changes further impair oxygen delivery and consumption at a tissue level, resulting in tissue hypoxia and worsening organ dysfunction. Anaerobic metabolism results in a rising lactate, when oxygen delivery cannot meet tissue oxygen demands, and central venous oxygen saturations ($S_{cv}O_2$) will generally be low (<70%) as the peripheral tissues extract a higher percentage of oxygen, resulting in less oxygen in venous blood returning to the central circulation.[4,5]

The progression of sepsis to septic shock is associated with an inability to contain the infection, owing either to compromised patient immunity or to characteristics of the infection itself, such as highly virulent organisms, a high burden of infection and antibiotic resistance.

Clinical features

Infection associated with systemic illness results in a spectrum of clinical syndromes based on clinical signs.[6]

Clinical syndrome definitions

Systemic inflammatory response syndrome (SIRS)
This is defined as a patient presenting with two or more of the following criteria:

- Abnormal body temperature (>38°C or <36°C)
- Tachycardia >90 bpm
- Tachypnoea (respiratory rate >20/min or PCO_2<32 mmHg)
- Abnormal white cell count (>12 000/uL or <4000/uL or > 10% immature (band) cells)

Sepsis
This is defined as SIRS plus a documented infection site (positive culture for organisms from that site, although blood cultures do *not* need to be positive).

Severe sepsis
This is sepsis associated with hypoperfusion, characterized by hypotension or an elevated lactate.

Septic shock
This refers to severe sepsis with persistent hypotension despite adequate fluid resuscitation. Important components of the clinical history include the patient's immune status, assessment of acute respiratory, abdominal or urinary symptoms, and identification of potential sources for infection, such as recent procedures and prosthetic devices, including stents and indwelling catheters.

Physical examination

On physical examination the septic patient will have features of the inflammatory response outlined above, and may have other signs of end-organ dysfunction, such as acute confusion and oliguria. Examination should include a top-to-toe assessment, including the oropharynx, skin, joints and pelvic area. In addition to fluid depletion due to vomiting and third-space sequestration, septic patients are relatively hypovolaemic due to peripheral vasodilatation. The patient with severe sepsis may classically have warm peripheries and a bounding pulse due to mediator-driven vasodilatation, though in the later stages they are more usually peripherally shut down as a result of cardiovascular collapse.

Clinical investigations

Investigations are important in determining the nature of the underlying infection and the severity of sepsis. Basic blood pathology may identify potential causes such as biliary obstruction, and will quantify end-organ dysfunction such as renal failure, hypo-/hyperglycaemia and coagulopathy. Arterial blood gases should be measured early to assess both the degree of lactic acidosis and the adequacy of ventilation. Elevated lactate levels are associated with a higher mortality and may help identify patients at risk.[7,8]

The search for the underlying source should include urine microscopy, chest X-ray, culture of any open wounds, aspiration of superficial collections, and blood cultures both peripheral and from indwelling lines. In the absence of an identified focus, abdominal CT scanning and, particularly if there is an altered mental state, lumbar puncture are usually warranted, if not contraindicated by the patient's clinical status.

Treatment (see also Chapter 2.4)

The principles of treatment in sepsis are haemodynamic resuscitation, supportive measures to maximize tissue oxygen delivery, early antibiotic therapy and source control. The international Surviving Sepsis Campaign consensus guidelines have been developed to promote a more uniform 'bundle of care' for the acute management of patients with sepsis, aimed at reducing mortality.[9] These guidelines incorporate the concept of early goal-directed therapy (EGDT), with specific targeted endpoints to guide sequential treatment.

The use of standardized ED guidelines focused on haemodynamic resuscitation and early, appropriate antibiotic therapy improves compliance with recommended treatment and reduces mortality.[10,11]

Haemodynamic resuscitation and supportive care

Early goal-directed therapy

The components of EGDT are adequate volume replacement followed by vasopressor and inotropic therapy aimed at maintaining mean arterial pressure (MAP) $\geq$65 mmHg, urine output $\geq$0.5 mL/kg/h and, in some settings, $S_{CV}O_2$ $\geq$70%.[9] Whereas measurement of MAP and urine output is straightforward, measurement of $S_{CV}O_2$ requires either frequent blood gas sampling from a standard central venous catheter or continuous measurement using a commercial central venous catheter with a specialized fibreoptic module.

Fluid resuscitation

Fluid resuscitation begins with 500 mL boluses of normal saline. Patients who remain hypotensive, acidotic or oliguric after 2000 mL of crystalloid usually warrant central venous pressure (CVP) and invasive arterial pressure monitoring to guide further therapy.[9,12] Fluid resuscitation should continue to a CVP of 8–12 mmHg in the absence of pulmonary oedema.

Vasopressor therapy

Vasopressor therapy with norepinephrine or dopamine is indicated concurrently with fluid resuscitation in the presence of profound hypotension, or if fluid resuscitation fails to restore tissue perfusion (as indicated by normalization of MAP, lactate levels and urine output). Norepinephrine is the more potent agent and increases blood pressure predominantly by direct vasoconstriction, with a smaller increase in heart rate and stroke volume than with dopamine. Thus it has been the preferred agent in patients with profound hypotension.

Epinephrine has not been recommended as a first-line agent as it has been shown to cause greater splanchnic ischaemia than norepinephrine or dopamine.[9,12] However, a recent multicentre clinical trial showed no difference in clinical outcomes when epinephrine was compared with norepinephrine with or without dobutamine.[13] All vasopressor agents need to be administered via a central venous catheter and the infusion rate titrated to MAP, urine output and cerebral perfusion.

The measurement of $S_{CV}O_2$ has been advocated as a further endpoint to guide ongoing therapy. In the EGDT study by Rivers et al.[11] red cell transfusion to a haemocrit $\geq$30% and dobutamine infusion to improve cardiac output were used in patients who failed to achieve $S_{CV}O_2$ $\geq$70% with fluids, vasopressors and ventilatory support. Patients who received EGDT had a lower mortality than patients receiving 'standard' therapy.[11] However, other studies have not demonstrated a survival benefit with liberal blood transfusion and dobutamine usage, and there may be potential harm in critically ill patients.[14,15] Also, reported mortality rates for sepsis in Australasian patients are substantially lower than in the Rivers' study, hence the applicability of Rivers' EGDT in the Australasian setting is unclear.[1] International guidelines currently recommend the use of adjuvant dobutamine in patients with a low cardiac output despite fluids and vasopressors. Blood transfusion is recommended only to a haemoglobin level of 7–9 g/dL, except in patients with acute haemorrhage or significant coronary artery disease.[9]

Maximizing oxygen delivery

As sepsis is associated with increased oxygen consumption, oxygen delivery should be maximized via a high-flow face mask at the beginning of resuscitation. Endotracheal intubation and mechanical ventilation with appropriate sedation and paralysis will minimize oxygen consumption and should be considered early in patients with respiratory acidosis, hypoxia or persistent haemodynamic compromise. Low tidal volume ventilation (6 mL/kg) with peak inspiratory pressures maintained <30 cmH$_2$O are recommended to minimize further acute lung injury.[9,11]

Antibiotic therapy

The early instigation and selection of appropriate antibiotic therapy is an essential component of management of the septic patient in the ED. Antibiotic administration within 1 hour of onset of hypotension is associated with increased survival. In the first 6 hours after the onset of hypotension the mortality rate rises by nearly 8% for each additional hour of delay in commencing antibiotics.[16] Thus antibiotics should be administered as soon as possible after appropriate cultures have been collected, and should be started within 1 hour for patients with severe sepsis or septic shock.[9,12]

The choice of antibiotic depends on a number of criteria, including the likely source of infection, local bacterial sensitivities, and patient factors such as allergies, immunocompetence and renal function. The initial choice should be broad enough to cover all potential pathogens, as inadequate antibiotic treatment is associated with increased mortality.[17,18] Antibiotic therapy can be more specifically targeted when the causative organism and its sensitivities are known, but this is rarely appropriate in the ED.[19] Table 2.5.1 outlines one approach to initial antibiotic choice.

Empiric monotherapy with a third- or fourth-generation cephalosporin has been shown to be as effective as dual therapy with a β-lactam and an aminoglycoside. However, most of this evidence is derived from patients with febrile neutropenia, and only a few smaller studies have been conducted in immunocompetent patients with severe sepsis or septic shock. Many practitioners still prefer dual therapy on the basis that this may confer synergistic effects that enhance antibacterial activity and reduce the incidence of bacterial resistance. These potential benefits must be weighed against the increased risk of nephrotoxicity and ototoxicity associated with the use of aminoglycosides.[2]

Empirical treatment with glycopeptides such as vancomycin is only recommended in patients with known MRSA colonization, severe penicillin hypersensitivity, or in institutions with high levels of MRSA.[2] Empirical antifungal treatment with amphotericin or fluconazole is only recommended in patients at high risk for invasive candidiasis, such as those who have been treated with prolonged broad-spectrum antibiotics, are immunosuppressed and have had *Candida* isolated from multiple sites.[20]

Source control

Source control refers to physical measures to control or contain the focus of infection by drainage, debridement or anatomical repair. In principle, the removal of an infected nidus will help minimize the inflammatory response, but the size and site of the infective source will determine the feasibility and timing of source control. The focus in the ED is on identifying the likely source of infection and determining, in consultation with radiological, surgical and other specialties, the best method of drainage or containment.

Localized collections may be amenable to percutaneous drainage with or without radiological guidance. This is often appropriate for hepatic and other intra-abdominal abscesses and other soft tissue collections. Immediate debridement of infected and necrotic tissue is mandatory for soft tissue infections such as necrotizing fasciitis, but more deep-seated necrosis, such as pancreatitis, may need delayed debridement as early operative intervention in difficult-to-access areas is associated with significant morbidity.[21,22] Gastrointestinal perforation with leakage of luminal contents usually requires early surgical repair, except for contained perforations in diverticulitis. Biliary tract obstruction with associated infection requires early decompression with percutaneous cholecystostomy or endoscopic retrograde cholangiopancreatography (ERCP). Urinary sepsis with shock in association with ureteric obstruction should be managed by urgent percutaneous nephrostomy.

The best approach for sepsis associated with indwelling devices is removal of the device. However, this needs to be balanced against the risks of removal and the ongoing medical need.[9,22] Infected intravascular devices can be exchanged by 'rewiring' over a guide-wire, provided there are no signs of infection at the insertion site.[23] Alternatively, a combination of antibiotics and thrombolysis may be effective.[22]

Other therapies

Give patients who are on regular steroids 100 mg hydrocortisone i.v. as soon as possible in their ED care. Activated protein C infused over 36 hours has been shown to reduce mortality in some septic patients with organ dysfunction, and is recommended

Table 2.5.1 Empirical initial intravenous antibiotic recommendations based on likely source of infection in patients with severe sepsis[19]

Source of infection	Antibiotic regimen
Unknown	Flucloxacillin 2 g 4–6-hourly PLUS Gentamicin 4–6 mg/kg daily (subsequent doses adjusted to renal function) If mild penicillin hypersensitivity, substitute flucloxacillin with cephalothin 2–6-hourly. If severe immediate penicillin hypersensitivity, substitute flucloxacillin with vancomycin 25 mg/kg (max 1 g) 12-hourly If neutropenic, use ceftazidime 2 g 8-hourly and add vancomycin 25 mg/kg (max 1 g) 12-hourly if shocked or high-risk MRSA
Biliary/gastrointestinal	Ampicillin 2 g 6 hourly (substitute with ceftriaxone for mild penicillin hypersensitivity and vancomycin for severe penicillin hypersensitivity) PLUS Gentamicin 4–6 mg/kg daily (subsequent doses adjusted to renal function) PLUS Metronidazole 500 mg 12-hourly
Respiratory	Azithromycin 500 mg daily PLUS Ceftriaxone 1 g daily If severe immediate penicillin hypersensitivity, substitute ceftriaxone with moxifloxacin 400 mg daily
Urinary tract	Ampicillin 2 g 6 hourly PLUS Gentamicin 4–6 mg/kg daily (subsequent doses adjusted to renal function)
Skin	Flucloxacillin 2 g 6 hourly If severe immediate penicillin hypersensitivity, substitute with clindamycin 450 mg 8 hourly If high-risk MRSA, use vancomycin

CRITICAL CARE

in patients at high risk of death (multiorgan dysfunction or APACHE >25) but low risk of bleeding or need for surgery.

Following initial stabilization, tight glycaemic control should be maintained with a continuous infusion of insulin. Intravenous steroids have been shown to improve survival in patients with septic shock and relative adrenal insufficiency. However, the role and timing of steroids in septic patients without proven adrenal insufficiency remains controversial. Pragmatically, most of these interventions are usually administered within the first 24 hours of care in an intensive care unit, rather than in the first few hours of ED management.[9,24]

Controversies

- The role of early goal-directed therapy has not been established in the Australasian environment, where mortality rates are relatively lower than international figures.

- The routine measurement of central venous oxygen saturations as an endpoint for goal-directed therapy is currently not widely used in Australia or New Zealand.

- The use of dobutamine and liberal blood transfusion to attain designated endpoints of goal-directed therapy has not been universally accepted, and there is

evidence in some critically ill patients that these strategies might be potentially harmful.

- The role and timing of steroids in septic patients without proven adrenal insufficiency.

References

1. ARISE i, ANZICS. The outcome of patients with sepsis and septic shock presenting to emergency departments in Australia and New Zealand. Critical Care and Resuscitation 2007; 9: 8–18.
2. Bochud P-Y, Bonten M, Marchetti O, et al. Antimicrobial therapy for patients with severe sepsis and septic shock: An evidence-based review. Critical Care Medicine 2004; 32: S495–S512.
3. Bochud P-Y, Glauser M, Calandra T. Antibiotics in Sepsis. Intensive Care Medicine 2001; 27: S33–S48.
4. Russell J. Management of sepsis. New England Journal of Medicine 2006; 355: 1699–1713.
5. Rivers E, McIntyre L, Morro D, Rivers K. Early and innovative interventions for severe sepsis and septic shock: taking advantage of a window of opportunity. Canadian Medical Association Journal 2005; 173: 1054–1065.
6. Bone R, Balk R, Cerra F, et al. Definitions for sepsis and organ failure and guidelines for the use of innovative therapies for sepsis. Chest 1992; 101: 1644–1655.
7. Bakker J, Coffernils M, Gris P, et al. Blood lactate levels are superior to oxygen-derived variables in predicting outcome in human septic shock. Chest 1991; 99: 956–962.
8. Shapiro N, Howell M, Talmor D, et al. Serum lactate as a predictor of mortality in emergency department patients with infection. Annals of Emergency Medicine 2005; 45: 524–528.
9. Dellinger R, Carlet J, Masur H, et al. Surviving sepsis campaign guidelines for management of severe sepsis and septic shock. Critical Care Medicine 2004; 32: 858–873.
10. Micek S, Roubinian N, Heuring T, et al. Before-after study of a standardized hospital order set for the management of septic shock. Critical Care Medicine 2006; 34: 2707–2713.
11. Rivers E, Nguyen B, Havstad S, et al. Early goal directed therapy in the treatment of severe sepsis and septic shock. New England Journal of Medicine 2001; 345: 1368–1377.
12. Sessler C, Perry J, Varney K. Management of sepsis and septic shock. Current Opinion in Critical Care 2004; 10: 354–363.
13. Annane D, Vignon P, Renault A, the CATS Study Group. Norepinephrine plus dobutamine versus epinephrine alone for management of septic shock: a randomised trial. Lancet 2007; 370: 676–684.
14. Hayes M, Timmins A, Yau E, et al. Elevation of systemic oxygen delivery in the treatment of critically ill patients. New England Journal of Medicine 1994; 330: 1717–1722.
15. Hebert P, Wells G, Blajchman M, et al. A multicenter, randomized, controlled clinical trial of transfusion requirements in critical care. New England Journal of Medicine 1999; 340: 409–417.
16. Kumar A, Roberts D, Wood K, et al. Duration of hypotension before initiation of effective antimicrobial therapy is the critical determinant of survival in human septic shock. Critical Care Medicine 2006; 34: 1589–1596.
17. MacArthur R, Miller M, Albertson T, et al. Adequacy of early empiric antibiotic treatment and survival in severe sepsis: experience from the MONARCS trial. Clinical Infectious Diseases 2004; 38: 284–288.
18. Kollef M, Sherman G, Ward S. Inadequate antimicrobial treatment of infections: a risk factor for hospital mortality among critically ill patients. Chest 1999; 15: 462–474.
19. Antibiotic Guidelines Version 13: Severe Sepsis. Therapeutic Guidelines Limited. Available at: http://www.tg.com.au/ip/complete/. Accessed July 2007.
20. Rex J, Walsh T, Sobel J, et al. Practice Guidelines for the Treatment of Candidiasis. Clinical Infectious Diseases 2000; 30: 662–678.
21. Hsaio G, Chang C, Hsaio C, et al. Necrotizing soft tissue infections. Surgical or conservative treatment? Dermatologic Surgery 1998; 24: 247–248.
22. Marshall J, Maier R, Jiminez M, Dellinger E. Source control in the management of severe sepsis and septic shock: an evidence-based review. Critical Care Medicine 2004; 32: S513–S526.
23. Cook D, Randolph A, Kernerman P, et al. Central venous catheter replacement strategies: a systematic review of the literature. Critical Care Medicine 1997; 25: 1417–1424.
24. Osborn T, Nguyen H, Rivers E. Emergency medicine and the Surviving Sepsis Campaign: an internation approach to managing severe sepsis and septic shock. Annals of Emergency Medicine 2005; 46: 228–231.

2.6 Arterial blood gases

Robert Dunn

ESSENTIALS

1 Acid–base disorders are classified according to the major abnormality (acidosis or alkalosis) and its origin (metabolic or respiratory). Mixed disorders are common.

2 Calculation of the 'anion gap' may be useful in determining the origin of a metabolic acidosis.

3 Lactic acidosis is the most common cause of metabolic acidosis.

4 Treatment of acidosis is directed toward correction of the underlying cause; administration of $NaHCO_3$ is indicated in only a limited number of situations.

5 Metabolic alkalosis in the emergency department is usually secondary to prolonged vomiting, and its management is directed towards rehydration with normal saline and correction of the underlying cause.

6 The alveolar gas equation allows comparison of arterial and alveolar partial pressures of oxygen. A higher than expected value is indicative of a ventilation-perfusion defect (high A–a gradient).

Introduction

Acid–base disorders are commonly encountered in the emergency department (ED), and their recognition may aid the diagnosis, assessment of severity and monitoring of many disease processes. Although these disorders are usually classified according to the major metabolic abnormality present (acidosis or alkalosis) and its origin (metabolic or respiratory), acid–base disorders of a mixed type are common and their recognition and assessment is more complex.

Normal values

Familiarity with the concept of pH and awareness of the normal ranges for pH, PCO_2, and HCO_3^- are essential to interpret acid–base disorders. The pH is the log $[H^+]$ and may be derived from formulae such as:

$$pH = 6.1 + log[HCO_3^-]/(0.03 \times PCO_2)$$

or

$$pH = pK + log[A^-]/[HA]$$

(the Henderson–Hasselbalch equation).[1]

Serum pH is normally maintained between 7.35 and 7.45, which represents an $[H^+]$ of approximately 40 nmol/L. The normal range of arterial PCO_2 is between 35 and 45 mmHg, and the arterial $[HCO_3^-]$ is between 22 and 26 mmol/L.

Venous HCO_3^- has a normal range of 24–28 mmol/L and is higher than that of arterial blood owing to the exchange of HCO_3^- for Cl^- (the 'chloride shift') that occurs as a result of CO_2 transport by haemoglobin from the tissues. Haemoglobin-oxygen saturation may be directly measured by co-oximetry or calculated from the PO_2, assuming that the oxygen-haemoglobin dissociation curve is in a 'normal' position. This calculation may be inaccurate in the presence of chronic hypoxia, where increased levels of 2,3-DPG will alter the position of the curve. Measurement by co-oximetry is the gold standard, but it is not used by many bedside or portable blood gas analysers.

Definitions and conventions

The PO_2 and PCO_2 are the partial pressures of oxygen and carbon dioxide, and the site to which this refers is denoted by various prefixes. The symbol 'i' indicates inspired gas, 'a' indicates arterial blood and 'A' indicates alveolar gas. Where no prefix is used, it is usually assumed that the value relates to arterial blood.

The base excess is defined as the number of mmol of acid needed to be added to 1 L of whole blood (at standard temperature and pressure – STP) to return the pH to 7.4. The standard base excess is the number of mmol of acid needed to be added to 1 L of whole blood with a PCO_2 of 40 mmHg (at STP) to return the pH to 7.4.

Venous gas correlation

In the majority of cases arterial blood sampling is not required to provide the information needed regarding the patient's acid–base status. If an arterial blood sample is difficult to obtain, or the determination of PO_2 or PCO_2 is not important, the measurement of venous pH and HCO_3^- is an acceptable alternative and less invasive.[2–4] Sampling of 'arterialized' capillary blood (e.g. from a warmed earlobe) can provide accurate information regarding PO2 and PCO_2; however, the accuracy of capillary samples is reduced in the shocked adult.[5]

In the absence of shock, the venous pH is approximately 0.05 less than the arterial pH. Venous blood for pH determination should be obtained from as close as possible to the central venous system.

Arterial blood gas specimen collection

When attempting to collect arterial blood gas specimens the non-dominant limb should be used if possible. There should be no signs of overlying infection, and the arterial pulse of the vessel to be cannulated must be palpable unless ultrasound guidance is used. The radial artery at the wrist is the most commonly used site for specimen collection in adults, as it is easily accessible with the patient sitting upright. This is particularly useful in patients with respiratory distress.

Allen's test

An Allen's test should be performed before performing radial arterial puncture. The aim of this is to determine whether the supply from the ulnar artery is sufficient to maintain the viability of the hand, should flow through the radial artery be compromised by a complication of vascular puncture. The patient is asked to elevate the selected arm and make a tight fist while both the radial and ulnar arteries are occluded by the examiner's thumbs using firm pressure. After a few minutes the arm is lowered to waist level and the patient opens the hand. The pressure over the ulnar artery is then released, but pressure over the radial artery is maintained. In a negative test normal skin colour returns to the palm within 2 seconds. In a positive test the hand remains white for longer than 2 seconds. If the test is positive an alternative site for arterial puncture should be used.

Radial arterial puncture

The forearm should be in full supination with the wrist extended 45° for radial arterial puncture. The hand and forearm should be immobilized. Following skin preparation with antiseptic, a needle attached to a heparinized syringe is inserted along the line of the artery. The needle is directed along the long axis of the artery while the tip of the index finger of the operator's non-dominant hand palpates the pulse. The needle is inserted at an angle of 45° to the skin away from the direction of blood flow, with the bevel pointing upwards. The operator should aim to position the tip of the needle in the radial artery directly below the palpating finger.

This technique is used to maximize the area of the needle inlet exposed to arterial blood flow, and hence to facilitate syringe filling. A 25 G needle is the preferred size in the well-perfused patient, as it causes significantly less pain and vascular trauma than larger needles. Flow may be inadequate to fill the syringe using this size of needle in patients with poor perfusion, and a 23 G needle should be used. Once in the artery, arterial blood should fill the syringe passively against gravity. Some syringes require the barrel to be withdrawn to the desired amount prior to commencing sample collection. Suction should *not* be applied to the barrel, as this may alter the partial pressures of the gases in the solution.[6]

Interruption of filling after it has commenced is most commonly due to insertion of the needle too far, and is corrected by gently withdrawing the needle slightly. Slow filling in the well-perfused patient suggests incorrect needle position and sampling of an accompanying vein. Once at least 0.25 mL – and preferably 0.5 mL – of blood has been collected, the needle is removed quickly and direct pressure applied over the puncture site for at least 2 minutes in patients with normal coagulation, and up to 5 minutes in patients with significant coagulation abnormalities.

All air bubbles should be expelled from the syringe prior to capping it with an airtight stopper. The specimen should be transported as soon as possible to the point of analysis. The temperature of the patient should be noted for entry into the analyser. The specimen should be packed in ice and obtained using a glass syringe if a delay in analysis of more than 15 minutes is likely, or if an arterial lactate measurement is required.[7]

The brachial artery at the cubital fossa may be used if the radial artery is not suitable. This approach requires the elbow to remain extended throughout the procedure. The femoral artery is an acceptable alternative, particularly in the patient with extremely poor perfusion who may have no other palpable peripheral pulses. The close proximity of the femoral head to the femoral artery in infants makes this a less desirable site in this age group. The patient must be supine and the needle should be at least 4 cm long to perform femoral arterial puncture. Localization of the relevant vessel is assisted by the use of ultrasound.

Obtaining a sample through an arterial line requires withdrawal and discarding of three times the dead space volume of the arterial line system. The dead space of a 20 G arterial catheter and pressure transducer is approximately 1.2 mL, thus around 4 mL should be discarded.[8]

Complications of arterial puncture

Complications are rare following a single small-bore needle arterial puncture. They include local or generalize sepsis, arterial thrombosis and distal tissue ischaemia.

An arterial catheter should be inserted if repeated arterial or venous punctures are required, invasive blood pressure monitoring indicated, or as access for arteriovenous haemofiltration.

Indwelling arterial catheter insertion

The approaches used for arterial catheter insertion are the same as those for arterial puncture, and Seldinger or non-Seldinger techniques can be used. Whenever possible, prolonged femoral artery catheterization should be avoided because of the high incidence of infective and thromboembolic complications. Local anaesthesia should be used prior to arterial catheter insertion, and the catheter should be sutured in place and connected to a line pressurized to 250–300 mmHg. The appropriate catheter sizes are 18–20 G for the radial artery, 16 G for the femoral artery and 12 G for arteriovenous haemofiltration.

Arterial blood gas interpretation

Detecting a venous sample

This should usually be suspected by slow filling of the syringe at the time of obtaining the sample. An arterial PO_2 of 40 mmHg is suspicious of a venous sample. However, as there is no infallible method of differentiating venous from arterial samples on the basis of interpretation of the normally measured parameters, a repeat sample should be obtained when there is doubt about the correct source.

Alveolar gas equation

This equation is commonly used in emergency medicine practice despite its significantly limited utility. The equation is represented as follows:

$$P_{alveolar}O_2 = P_iO_2 - (P_ACO_2/R)$$

where R = respiratory quotient (usually 0.8), P_ACO_2 is approximated by P_aCO_2 and P_iO_2 = (atmospheric pressure − partial pressure of water vapour) × FiO_2.

At sea level the partial pressure of water vapour is 47 mmHg, and if breathing room air (at an FiO_2 of 0.21) then $P_iO_2 = 150$ mmHg.

Elevated A–a gradient

The purpose of the alveolar gas equation is to allow comparison of the measured P_AO_2 with the calculated alveolar value, the alveolar–arterial (A–a) gradient. Elevation of the A–a gradient indicates an abnormal ventilation–perfusion relationship in the lungs. The PaO_2 falls progressively as shunt fraction increases, but the $PaCO_2$ remains constant until the shunt fraction exceeds 50%. The normal range of the alveolar–arterial gradient in the erect patient is age (in years)/4. The usefulness of the equation for the detection of pulmonary disease is reduced if the patient is supine or the FiO_2 is > 0.21, as the normal A–a gradient increases by only 6 mmHg for every 0.1 increase in FiO_2 due to loss of regional hypoxic vasoconstriction in the lungs.

In addition, the respiratory quotient varies with the composition of the patient's diet, approaching 0.95 in a high-carbohydrate diet and as low as 0.6 if the diet is high in fat or ethanol. The results of the alveolar gas equation should be interpreted with caution, as the exact composition of the patient's diet is rarely known in the emergency setting. In addition, adjustment should also be made for the changes in inspired P_iO_2 due to changes in barometric pressure from altitude (above and below sea level), meteorological effects and diurnal variation.

Rules for complex acid–base disorders

Comparison of actual and calculated values of pH, PCO_2 and HCO_3^- may be of some use in determining the presence of more than one type of acid–base abnormality. These calculations are based on the assumption that 'normal' pH is 7.4, PCO_2 = 40 mmHg and HCO_3^- (arterial) = 24 mmol/L. They are more of theoretical interest than of significant practical value.

Simple metabolic acidosis

In the presence of a simple metabolic acidosis of >24 hours' duration, the expected PCO_2 should equal 1.5 × HCO_3^- + 8 (±5), with the lower limit of compensation being 10 mmHg.[1] In addition, the PCO_2 should equal the last two digits of the pH in a pH range between 7.4 and 7.1.

Simple metabolic alkalosis

In the presence of a simple metabolic alkalosis the PCO_2 should equal 0.7 × HCO_3^- + 21, and the PCO_2 should equal the last two digits of the pH in a pH range between 7.4 and 7.6.[1] As a compensatory mechanism, the PCO_2 will not increase to more than 60 mmHg.

Simple respiratory acidosis

In the presence of a simple respiratory acidosis, for every 10 mmHg increase in PCO_2 the HCO_3^- should increase by 1 mmol/L within 10 minutes, and if sustained, by 3–4 mmol/L by 4 days.

Simple respiratory alkalosis

In the presence of a simple respiratory alkalosis each 10 mmHg decrease in PCO_2 should reduce HCO_3^- by 1 mmol/L within 10 minutes and, if sustained, by up to 2 mmol/L by 4 days. In addition, the PCO_2 will only compensate to partial pressures between 10 and 60 mmHg, and the HCO_3^- will only compensate for a chronic respiratory acidosis to concentrations between 18 and 45 mmol/L.

Clinical use of blood gases in the seriously ill patient

Detection of hypoxia

An arterial blood gas is indicated if hypoxia is suspected and pulse oximetry has an unreliable signal or shows a value of < 90%. If a reliable oximeter trace is present and the systolic blood pressure is > 80 mmHg, one study[9] estimated that there is less than a 1:20 chance of a difference of 5% or more between the haemoglobin measured by blood gas analysis and pulse oximetry.

Electrolyte and haemoglobin measurement

Virtually all blood gas analysers also measure haemoglobin, sodium and potassium concentrations, and more sophisticated machines also measure calcium (ionized and non-ionized) and carboxy-, met- and sulphaemoglobin concentrations. Bedside analysers are usually accurate enough for clinical decisions to be made based on these results. For example, haemoglobin measured by point-of-care blood gas analysers is usually accurate to within 0.5 g/dL of that measured by a Coulter counter.[10] The majority of benefit from blood gas analysis is derived from the immediate measurement of items other than those related to acid–base status. These benefits are greatest when the history is limited and physical findings are non-diagnostic, such as:

- hypoglycaemia and altered mental state
- hyperglycaemia and dehydration
- hyperkalaemia and cardiac arrhythmias
- haemoglobin and blood loss
- hyponatraemia or hyperkalaemia and repeated seizures.

Chronic obstructive airways disease (COAD)

Determination of PCO_2, PO_2 and pH is often useful in the management of acute exacerbations of COAD, in deciding the optimum inspired oxygen concentration and whether, for instance, therapy with BiPAP should be commenced. Approximately 20% of patients with COAD requiring hospital treatment are at risk of suppression of ventilatory drive by higher than normally experienced arterial oxygen concentrations.[5] As clinical features of mild to moderate hypercarbia are non-specific, determination of PCO_2 may be useful. A venous PCO_2 of <45 mmHg can also reliably exclude the presence of arterial hypercarbia, and avoids arterial sampling in approximately 30% of cases.[11] A pH of < 7.25 in the presence of hypercarbia is an indication for the commencement of BiPAP.

Asthma

Arterial blood gases are far too commonly measured in many patients with asthma, as they only provide useful information in severe disease that does not respond to initial aggressive treatment. An elevation of $PaCO_2$ usually indicates that the peak expiratory flow rate (PEFR) is < 25% of predicted, whereas in less severe exacerbations $PaCO_2$ is usually low. Blood gas analysis is not indicated for mild or moderate exacerbations of asthma.

Pulmonary embolism

There is no combination of arterial blood gas values that can reliably exclude pulmonary embolism.[12] This is due to the large number of pulmonary vessels available for recruitment and the limitations in measuring the A–a gradient. It is estimated that a PaO2 < 80 mmHg on room air has a sensitivity of approximately 70% and a specificity of 25–50% in unselected patients with suspected pulmonary embolism. However, an elevation of the A–a gradient of > 20 mmHg in the absence of radiologically apparent airspace opacification on plain chest X-ray is highly suggestive of significant pulmonary embolism.

Mesenteric ischaemia

Blood gas analysis is commonly performed in patients with suspected mesenteric ischaemia. However, it is neither sensitive nor specific enough to be useful in clinical practice. Once serum lactate is sufficiently elevated to cause a significant metabolic acidosis, the prognosis from mesenteric ischaemia is already poor.

Poisoning

Detection of carboxyhaemoglobin, sulphaemoglobin and methaemoglobin can be made by blood gas analysis if the analyser uses co-oximetry. However, there are nearly always additional clinical findings to suggest the presence of significant sulphaemoglobinaemia or methaemoglobin toxicity, hence the utility of blood gases is greatest for the diagnosis of carbon monoxide poisoning, where these are lacking.

The presence of an unexplained anion gap metabolic acidosis may also indicate the presence of poisoning with ethylene glycol or methanol. It should be noted that the elevated anion gap associated with toxicity from these compounds may take a few hours to develop, thus its absence early on does not exclude significant toxicity. Acute ethanol, paracetamol, salicylate, NSAID, iron and isoniazid toxicity may also produce a significant raised anion gap metabolic acidosis.

Shock

The presence of an anion gap metabolic acidosis is the hallmark metabolic feature of shock. However, blood gas analysis is usually of reduced help in cases of obvious poor perfusion, compared with patients in whom physical features of shock may be less obvious.

Diabetic ketoacidosis (DKA)

Blood gas analysis is frequently performed in suspected diabetic ketoacidosis, its most useful role being the monitoring of serum potassium and pH early in resuscitation. The pH rises and the potassium falls in response to treatment with insulin and fluid therapy, and the timing of initiation of potassium replacement therapy is usually determined by values obtained from a blood gas analysis. In addition, the insulin infusion is usually stopped when the serum pH and base deficit return to normal, later in the resuscitation. A venous blood gas sample should be used unless it is important to measure arterial PCO2 or PO2. Despite the widespread use of blood gases in the management of diabetic ketoacidosis their utility is low, with one study estimating that they alter diagnosis and disposition in only 1% and treatment in 3.5% of cases.[4]

Detection of non-clinically suspected serious disease

There are no studies comparing blood gas analysis with clinical assessment in the detection of serious underlying disease. In the author's experience a reasonably common feature that may alert the clinician to the presence of unsuspected serious disease is the presence of a low venous bicarbonate, and/or an elevated anion gap. As a low serum bicarbonate correlates highly with the base deficit, the presence of this abnormality without explanation warrants careful re-evaluation of the patient.[13]

References

1. Kellum JK. Determinants of blood pH in health and disease. Critical Care 2000; 4: 6–14.
2. Kelly AM, McAlpine R, Kyle E, et al. Venous pH can safely replace arterial pH in the initial evaluation of patients in the emergency department. Emergency Medicine Journal 2001; 18: 340.
3. Kelly AM, McAlpine R, Kyle E. Agreement between bicarbonate measured on arterial and venous blood gases. Emergency Medicine Australasia 2004; 16: 407–409.
4. Kreshak A, Chen EH. Arterial blood gas analysis: are its values needed for the management of diabetic ketoacidosis? Annals of Emergency Medicine 2005; 45: 550–551.
5. Murphy R, Thethy S, Raby S, et al. Capillary blood gases in acute exacerbations of COPD. Respiratory Medicine 2006; 100: 682–686.
6. Woolley A, Hickling K. Errors in measuring blood gases in the intensive care unit: effect of delay in estimation. Journal of Critical Care 2003; 18: 31–37.
7. Knowles TP, Mullin RA, Hunter JA, et al. Effects of syringe material, sample storage time, and temperature on blood gases and oxygen saturation in arterialized human blood samples. Respiratory Care 2006; 51: 732–736.
8. Rickard CM, Couchman BA, Schmidt SJ, et al. A discard volume of twice the deadspace ensures clinically accurate arterial blood gases and electrolytes and prevents unnecessary blood loss. Critical Care Medicine 2003; 31: 1654–1658.
9. Hinkelbein J, Genzwuerker HV, Fiedler F. Detection of a systolic pressure threshold for reliable readings in pulse oximetry. Resuscitation. 2005; 64: 315–319.
10. Ray JG, Post JR, Hamiele C. Use of a rapid arterial blood gas analyzer to estimate blood hemoglobin concentration among critically ill adults. Critical Care 2002; 6: 72–75.
11. Kelly AM, Kerr D, Middleton P. Validation of venous pCO2 to screen for arterial hypercarbia in patients with chronic obstructive airways disease. Journal of Emergency Medicine 2005; 28: 377–379.
12. Maloba M, Hogg K. Diagnostic utility of arterial blood gases for investigation of pulmonary embolus. Emergency Medicine Journal 2005; 22; 435–436.
13. Martin MJF, Elizabeth S, Ali B, et al. Use of serum bicarbonate measurement in place of arterial base deficit in the surgical intensive care unit. Archives of Surgery 2005; 140: 745–751.

2.7 Cerebral resuscitation after cardiac arrest

Stephen Bernard

ESSENTIALS

1 Anoxic neurological injury is common following out-of-hospital cardiac arrest and carries a high rate of morbidity and mortality.

2 Successful resuscitation and reperfusion of the ischaemic brain results in biochemical cascades to further cell death, mediated largely by calcium influx into cells.

3 Therapeutic hypothermia (33 °C) after resuscitation from cardiac arrest is an effective treatment for anoxic neurological injury and is now recommended by the Australian Resuscitation Council (ARC) for 12–24 hours after resuscitation from cardiac arrest due to ventricular fibrillation.

4 There are no pharmacological interventions that improve neurological outcome after global ischaemia. However, treatment with minocycline has shown promise in preliminary studies in patients with focal ischaemia.

5 There is some evidence that hypotension and/or hyperglycaemia are deleterious to the injured brain, and these should be promptly treated.

Introduction

Out-of-hospital cardiac arrest is common and a leading cause of death in patients with heart disease. Prolonged cardiac arrest causing global cerebral ischaemia may lead to permanent neurological injury, despite effective cardiopulmonary resuscitation. Many patients who are initially successfully resuscitated from out-of-hospital cardiac arrest remain comatose in the emergency department (ED) because of the anoxic neurological injury. This injury results in considerable morbidity and mortality following hospital admission.[1] This chapter discusses the pathophysiology of anoxic neurological injury and current cerebral resuscitation therapies.

Definition

Cerebral resuscitation involves the use of pharmacological or other strategies to minimize injury to the brain following a prolonged ischaemic insult.[2]

Pathophysiology of cerebral ischaemia

The brain is highly dependent on an adequate supply of oxygen and glucose for metabolism. When cerebral oxygen delivery falls below 20 mL/100 g brain tissue/minute, aerobic metabolism changes to anaerobic glycolysis, with a marked decrease in the generation of adenosine triphosphate (ATP).[3]

After several minutes of cerebral ischaemia the supply of ATP is exhausted and cellular metabolism ceases. The failure of the sodium/potassium transmembrane pump leads to a shift of sodium into the cell, with cell swelling. In addition, hydrogen ions are generated and the resulting intracellular metabolic acidosis is toxic to intracellular enzyme systems. This acidosis is partly dependent on the concentration of glucose, with hyperglycaemia contributing to an increase in the intracellular acidosis.

Reperfusion injury

Additional injury occurs following resuscitation and reperfusion of the brain with oxygenated blood.[4] The intracellular levels of glutamate, an excitatory neurotransmitter released from presynaptic terminals, increase dramatically during reperfusion. Glutamate activates calcium ion channel complexes, and these shift calcium from the extracellular fluid to the intracellular fluid. The calcium influx into cells initiates multiple biochemical cascades, leading to the production of so-called free radicals and the activation of degradative enzymes.

Intracellular iron also plays an important role in free-radical production. Iron is usually maintained in the ferric state and is sequestered to intracellular proteins. During ischaemia, iron is reduced to the soluble ferrous form and reacts with peroxide, generating damaging hydroxyl free radicals.

There are also effects on leukocytes, endothelium and platelets. The generation of free radicals activates an upregulation of molecules that mediate leukocyte adhesion and extravasation into brain parenchyma. Also, occlusion of microvessels with leukocyte–platelet complexes leads to increased cerebral ischaemia.

Ischaemia and reperfusion are also a stimulus for nitric oxide synthase activation, which generates nitric oxide, a potent mediator of injury. The nitric oxide may combine with superoxide to form peroxynitrite radicals, which are potent activators of lipid peroxidation. Other proposed actions of nitric oxide include DNA damage, increased glutamate release and microvascular vasodilatation.

Finally, some neurons that survive the initial anoxic insult proceed to programmed cell death, known as apoptosis.[5] After reperfusion, this delayed neuronal death may occur at different rates, varying from 6 hours for neurons in the striatum to 7 days for hippocampal CA1 neurons. Apoptosis is characterized by cellular and nuclear shrinkage, chromatin condensation and DNA fragmentation.

Cerebral haemodynamics after reperfusion

Cerebral haemodynamics may remain abnormal for some hours after resuscitation and the restoration of a spontaneous circulation.[6] In animal models there is an initial hyperaemia after resuscitation, followed by reduced cerebral blood flow despite normal mean arterial blood pressure (MAP). Owing to the inflammatory processes described above, the cerebral metabolic rate for oxygen increases slightly. Thus, there may be a mismatch of cerebral oxygen delivery and demand for 12–24 hours following resuscitation from prolonged cardiac arrest. Cerebral oxygen delivery and/or demand is also adversely affected by arterial hypoxaemia, raised intracranial pressure, fever and/or seizure activity.

Pharmacological interventions

There has been considerable interest and research into pharmacological interventions that might reduce reperfusion injury, as much of the neurological injury seen following ischaemic injury occurs after reperfusion.[1,4]

A number of drugs that showed promise in animal models of global cerebral ischaemia have undergone large randomized, controlled human trials. These include thiopentone,[7] a corticosteroid,[8] lidoflazine,[9] nimodipine,[10] magnesium[11] and diazepam.[11] However, not one of these showed improved neurological or overall outcome.

Neuroprotective agents in stroke

Lysis of the blood clot causing ischaemia also results in a reperfusion injury in focal cerebral ischaemia or stroke. Most clinical trials of neuroprotective agents in stroke patients have been negative to date, except for one agent that did show some benefit. In an open-label preliminary study[12] the antibiotic minocycline 200 mg was administered orally for 5 days to patients between 6 and 24 hours of having a stroke. There were 152 patients included in the study, with 74 receiving minocycline and 77 receiving placebo. The NIH Stroke Scale and modified Rankin Scale were significantly lower in the minocycline-treated patients at 90 days. However, larger trials are required to confirm this preliminary finding.

Therapeutic hypothermia

Therapeutic hypothermia (TH) has been demonstrated to benefit patients who remain comatose after resuscitation from cardiac arrest. It is thought that the hypothermia reduces cerebral oxygen demand without also reducing cerebral oxygen supply. Also, TH reduces the reperfusion injury by reducing the production of oxygen free radicals after reperfusion.

Two prospective controlled human studies suggested improved outcome using moderate TH in comatose survivors of pre-hospital cardiac arrest.[13,14] In one study[13] 43 patients were randomized to TH (33°C for 12 hours) and 34 were maintained at normothermia. Hypothermia was induced in the ED using surface cooling with ice-packs. At hospital discharge, 21 of the 43 (49%) in the TH group had a good outcome, compared to 9 of 34 (26%) in the control group ($P=0.046$). Following multivariate analysis for differences at baseline, the odds ratio (OR) for a good outcome in the hypothermic group was 5.25 (95% confidence intervals (CI) 1.47–18.76; $P=0.011$). There were no adverse effects of TH apparent, such as sepsis, lactic acidosis or coagulopathy.

A second clinical trial of TH after cardiac arrest was conducted in Europe.[14] This study enrolled 273 comatose survivors of pre-hospital cardiac arrest, with 136 undergoing TH (33°C for 24 hours), and 137 maintained at normothermia. Hypothermia was induced in the ED and intensive care unit using a refrigerated air mattress. Six months after the cardiac arrest 55% of the TH patients had a good outcome, compared to 39% of the normothermic controls (OR 1.4, 95% CI 1.08–1.81). The complication rate did not differ between the two groups.

Australian Resuscitation Council (ARC) recommendation

These two trials formed the basis of the recommendation by the Australian Resuscitation Council (ARC) that therapeutic hypothermia (33°C for 12–24 hours) should be induced in patients who remained comatose after cardiac arrest due to ventricular fibrillation.[15]

Techniques and timing of therapeutic hypothermia

Current research in this area has focused on the techniques and timing of therapeutic hypothermia. Surface cooling in the clinical trials cited above had significant limitations. First, there was a relatively slow decrease in core temperature at 0.9°C/h using ice packs[13] and 0.5°C/h using forced cold air cooling.[14] Second, covering the patient with ice packs or cooling blankets during resuscitation is inconvenient and impractical for medical and nursing staff.

Another simple technique for rapid induction of TH is to use a large volume (40 mL/kg) of ice-cold (4°C) intravenous fluid.[16,17] A rapid intravenous infusion of large-volume 30 mL/kg lactated Ringer's solution at 4°C in an ED study of 22 patients resuscitated from out-of-hospital cardiac arrest was an effective and safe technique to induce mild hypothermia. This cooled crystalloid therapy reduced the core temperature by 1.7°C over 25 minutes, with improvements in mean arterial blood pressure as well as acid–base and renal function. There were also no apparent complications, such as pulmonary oedema.

In a pre-hospital study, Kim et al.[17] randomized 125 patients who were comatose following resuscitation from cardiac arrest to receive either standard care or intravenous cooling using large-volume (2000 mL) ice-cold (4°C) saline. Sixty-three patients received an infusion of 500 – 2000 mL of 4°C normal saline before hospital arrival which caused a decrease in temperature of 1.24°C, whereas 62 patients having standard care had an increase in temperature of 0.10°C. There was a trend towards an improved outcome in the patients randomized to in-field cooling who had the initial cardiac rhythm of ventricular fibrillation. Early cooling by paramedics is currently undergoing larger clinical trials to determine whether there is additional benefit from such earlier induced hypothermia therapy.

Other interventions

Other non-pharmacological strategies to reduce reperfusion injury are also undergoing evaluation. In newborns, resuscitation with air rather than 100% oxygen has been studied in a number of trials[18] on the assumption that normoxic (air) resuscitation might reduce the generation of oxygen free radicals. Currently, in adult patients with cardiac arrest there are insufficient data to recommend normoxic or hyperoxic resuscitation.

Animal studies of anoxic brain injury have also suggested that outcome may be improved if an elevated blood pressure is maintained in the post-resuscitation period.[19] The current recommendation of the Australian Resuscitation Council (ARC) is that blood pressure should be maintained at a systolic pressure of 100 mmHg or 'normal' for that patient.[15] Also, hyperglycaemia is associated with a worse outcome following cerebral ischaemia, and should be corrected using an intravenous insulin infusion.[20]

Outcome prediction

The early prediction of outcome is important after a severe anoxic neurological injury. Once a poor prognosis is reliably established, then decisions concerning limitations of costly advanced treatments may be made. Currently, the clinical examination at day 3 is regarded as the most accurate predictor of expected outcome.[21] Investigations such as brain computed tomography (CT), magnetic resonance imaging (MRI) and/or electroencephalography (EEG) are relatively insensitive and/or non-specific for the early prediction of neurological outcome. Although absent somatosensory responses bilaterally reliably predict a poor outcome after anoxic brain injury, this investigation is not available in many hospitals.[22]

Summary

Neurological injury is common in patients resuscitated from prolonged cardiac arrest. In addition to the usual supportive measures, such as endotracheal intubation and blood pressure correction, patients who remain comatose should undergo cerebral resuscitation with the rapid induction of therapeutic hypothermia. This may be most readily achieved using a rapid intravenous infusion of large-volume 40 mL/kg, ice-cold crystalloid. The therapeutic hypothermia should be maintained for 12–24 hours, as well as a normal or slightly elevated mean arterial blood pressure. Hyperglycaemia, if present, should be promptly corrected with intravenous insulin therapy. Because out-of-hospital cardiac arrest in adults often occurs in the setting of an acute ischaemic coronary syndrome, coronary artery reperfusion therapy may also be required.

Admission to an intensive care unit is required for most patients with anoxic brain injury following resuscitation for out-of-hospital cardiac arrest in order to maintain hypothermia and general supportive care. The prediction of a poor outcome cannot be reliably made for at least 3 days.

References

1. Fridman M, Barnes V, Whyman A, et al. A model of survival following pre-hospital cardiac arrest based on the Victorian Ambulance Cardiac Arrest Register. Resuscitation 2007; 75: 311–322.
2. Popp E, Böttiger BW. Cerebral resuscitation: state of the art, experimental approaches and clinical perspectives. Neurology Clinics 2006; 24: 73–87.
3. Ebmeyer U, Katz LM. Brain energetics after cardiopulmonary cerebral resuscitation. Current Opinion in Critical Care 2001; 7: 189–194.
4. Pan J, Konstas AA, Bateman B, et al. Reperfusion injury following cerebral ischemia: Pathophysiology, MR imaging, and potential therapies. Neuroradiology 2007; 49: 93–102.
5. Ferrer I. Apoptosis: future targets for neuroprotective strategies. Cerebrovascular Diseases 2006; 2: 9–20.
6. Oku K, Kuboyama K, Safar P, et al. Cerebral and systemic arteriovenous oxygen monitoring after cardiac arrest: Inadequate cerebral oxygen delivery. Resuscitation 1994; 27: 141–152.
7. The Brain Resuscitation Clinical Trial Study Group. Randomized clinical study of thiopentone loading in comatose survivors of cardiac arrest. New England Journal of Medicine 1986; 314: 397–410.
8. The Brain Resuscitation Clinical Trial Study Group. Glucocorticoid treatment does not improve neurologic recovery following cardiac arrest. Journal of the American Medical Association 1989; 262: 3427–3430.
9. Brain Resuscitation Clinical Trial II Study Group. A randomized clinical study of a calcium-entry blocker (lidoflazine) in the treatment of comatose survivors of cardiac arrest. New England Journal of Medicine 1991; 324: 1225–1231.
10. Roine RO, Kaste M, Kinnamen A, et al. Nimodipine after resuscitation from out-of-hospital ventricular fibrillation: A placebo-controlled double-blind randomized trial. Journal of the American Medical Association 1990; 264: 3171–3177.
11. Longstreth WT Jr, Fahrenbruch CE, Olsufka M, et al. Randomized clinical trial of magnesium, diazepam, or both after out-of-hospital cardiac arrest. Neurology 2002; 59: 506–514.
12. Lampl Y, Boaz M, Gilard R, et al. Minocycline treatment in acute stroke: an open-label, evaluator-blinded study. Neurology 2007; 69: 1404–1410.
13. Bernard SA, Gray TW, Buist MD, et al. A randomized, controlled trial of induced hypothermia in comatose survivors of prehospital cardiac arrest. New England Journal of Medicine 2002; 346: 557–563.
14. The Hypothermia after Cardiac Arrest Study Group. Mild therapeutic hypothermia to improve the neurological outcome after cardiac arrest. New England Journal of Medicine 2002; 346: 549–556.
15. Morley PT, Walker T. Australian Resuscitation Council: Adult advanced life support (ALS) guidelines 2006. Critical Care Resuscitation 2006; 8: 129–131.
16. Bernard SA, Buist M, Monteiro O, Smith K. Induced hypothermia using large volume, ice-cold intravenous fluid in comatose survivors of out-of-hospital cardiac arrest: A preliminary report. Resuscitation 2003; 56: 9–13.
17. Kim F, Olsufka M, Longstreth WT Jr, et al. Pilot randomized clinical trial of prehospital induction of mild hypothermia in out-of-hospital cardiac arrest patients with a rapid infusion of 4 degrees C normal saline. Circulation 2007; 115: 3064–3070.
18. Tan A, Schulze A, O'Donnell CP, Davis PG. Air versus oxygen for resuscitation of infants at birth. Cochrane Database Syst Rev 2005; Apr 18 (2): CD002273.
19. Safar P, Kochanek P. Cerebral blood flow promotion after prolonged cardiac arrest. Critical Care Medicine 2000; 28: 3104–3106.
20. Longstreth WT, Inui TS. High glucose levels on hospital admission and poor neurologic recovery after cardiac arrest. Annals of Neurology 1984; 15: 59–63.
21. Kaye P. Early prediction of individual outcome following cardiopulmonary resuscitation: systematic review. Emergency Medicine Journal 2005; 22: 700–705.
22. Wijdicks EF, Hijdra A, Young GB, et al. Quality Standards Subcommittee of the American Academy of Neurology. Practice parameter: prediction of outcome in comatose survivors after cardiopulmonary resuscitation (an evidence-based review): report of the Quality Standards Subcommittee of the American Academy of Neurology. Neurology 2006; 67: 203–210.

TRAUMA

Edited by **Peter Cameron**

3.1 Trauma overview

Peter Cameron • Gerard O'Reilly

ESSENTIALS

1 Trauma remains the leading cause of death in those from 1 to 40 years of age in Australasia, UK, and the USA.

2 Globally, by 2020 road trauma will rank third on the list of lives lost to death and disability.

3 Improvements in trauma care systems have resulted in fewer patients dying from avoidable factors.

4 Initial management of trauma patients involves a team approach. A primary survey (ABCDE) is followed by a secondary survey involving head-to-toe examination.

5 Airway management requiring endotracheal intubation should be performed using a rapid sequence induction technique.

6 Classic concepts regarding clinical signs in traumatic shock may underestimate blood volume loss.

7 Sedation should not be used in agitated major trauma victims unless the airway is adequately protected.

8 Audit of trauma systems is essential to improve outcomes.

Introduction

Trauma is the leading cause of death from 1 to 44 years of age in developed countries such as the USA and Australia.[1,2] It is an even greater problem in developing countries, where the majority of death and disability occurs.[3,4] Trauma deaths peak between the ages of 15 and 44, and therefore contribute significantly to the number of years of life lost in the population.[1,2] Deaths from unintentional injury are much more common than suicide or homicide, even in the USA.[1] However, in the USA, homicide causes more deaths than suicide in the 15–24-year age group;[1] this differs from other developed countries. Suicide now causes more deaths than motor vehicle accidents (MVAs) in regions such as Australasia and the UK.[2,5]

Morbidity due to injury affects a much larger group. For every death there are at least 15 serious non-fatal injuries, many causing long-term morbidity. The economic and social costs are great, as most victims are young and are major contributors to society through their work, family and organizational involvement.

In most developed countries there have been significant reductions in mortality and morbidity due to injury as a result of a systematic approach to trauma care. The majority of these reductions have resulted from prevention strategies, including seatbelt legislation, drink–driving legislation, improved road engineering, motor cycle and cycle helmet use, and road safety and workplace injury awareness campaigns. Changes in both trauma system configuration and individual patient management have brought about improvements in the survival rate of those who are seriously injured, although the impact has not been as great as that of injury prevention.

Civilian interest in injury morbidity and mortality was initially most evident in the USA because of the high incidence of urban violence and road trauma. Research into systems of trauma care began with epidemiological work by Trunkey and others examining trauma deaths,[6] who developed the concept of a trimodal distribution of trauma deaths. Trunkey proposed that about 50% of deaths occurred within the first hour as a result of major blood vessel disruption or massive CNS/spinal cord injury. This could only be improved by prevention strategies. A second more important group (from the therapy perspective) accounted for about 30% of deaths and included patients with major truncal injury causing respiratory and circulatory compromise. The remaining 20% of patients were said to die much later from adult respiratory distress syndrome, multiple organ failure, sepsis and diffuse brain injury. Trunkey initially identified the second group as most likely to benefit from improvements in trauma system organization, and it is a tribute to the effectiveness of such schemes that the number of patients dying from avoidable factors within the first few hours of injury has generally declined. In some systems it is reported to be as low as 3%, but generally is probably nearer to 10–15%.[7,8] Improvements in trauma system provision have resulted in a redistribution of the three groups proposed by Trunkey, and it is now generally accepted that far fewer than 30% are included in the second group. In fact, more recent studies have shown that complications such as multiple organ failure (MOF) and acute respiratory distress syndrome (ARDS) have decreased to such an extent, with improved initial management, that in mature trauma systems even the third peak is now minimal, with the vast majority of deaths occurring in the first 1–2 hours from major head injury and massive organ disruption.[33]

Trauma care systems have been developed to ensure a multidisciplinary approach and a continuum of care, from the roadside through hospital care to rehabilitation. Whereas initial work focused on the need for centres of expertise and trauma management, it is now accepted that the pre-hospital phase is of critical importance. Accurate triage of the patient to the closest most

appropriate facility is essential. High-risk patients should be taken to a hospital capable of managing critically ill trauma patients.[9] Table 3.1.1 lists some predictors of life-threatening injury. Using these as a triage tool without modification will result in significant over-triage: that is, many more patients with non-threatening injuries will be triaged. Over-triage is minimized if abnormal vital signs and overt major injury are used as the triage criteria. Sensitivity is still greater than 85%.[10] If mechanism is used as a triage tool then documented high speed and prolonged extrication time appear to be the most significant factors.[11]

Identifying weaknesses in such a system is always difficult because of the delay between cause and effect. Inappropriate management does not usually lead to immediate death: for example, a period of hypoxia may result in organ failure many hours later. Another difficulty is the relatively low incidence of death. Although this is of course to be welcomed, it does make statistical analysis more difficult when the 'adverse event' occurs uncommonly. Careful audit of the entire trauma process and accurate measurement of 'input' (i.e. injury severity) and 'output' (i.e. death or quality of survival) is essential if the process of trauma care is to be reviewed.

Initial management

Seamless integration with the pre-hospital personnel should ensure that the hospital is 'on standby' to receive the major trauma victim. The trauma team should be in attendance in the resuscitation area and the patient

brought directly to a prepared bay, the layout of which is illustrated in Figure 3.1.1. The general approach is to perform a primary survey to secure the airway/cervical spine, breathing and circulation. This is followed by a brief assessment of disability (neurological) and complete exposure of the patient. Life-threatening problems are thus identified and managed immediately. This is followed by a secondary survey involving a head-to-toe examination.

In most departments, parallel processing of the patient will occur simultaneously with management of ABCDE problems. The doctor and nurse team charged with protecting the airway immediately set about their task while the team leader obtains a brief history from the ambulance personnel and, if possible, the patient. The cervical spine is carefully controlled while the airway is being secured. The procedure doctor and the nurse team attend to intravenous access, blood tests, urinary catheter and other procedures. At this early stage of assessment and resuscitation the general philosophy should be to assume the worst and protect against all possible adverse events. Treatment is therefore designed to protect the patient against unforeseen consequences of the injury, rather than focusing on evident abnormalities. It is, however, important that this 'better safe than sorry' approach is not taken to extremes. Senior staff must be able to assess risk and avoid a situation where inexperienced personnel keep uninjured patients aggressively splinted for hours on end, so that the treatment itself becomes a cause of further injury.

The role of the various team members is shown in Table 3.1.2. In some facilities all

Table 3.1.1 Major trauma victims at high risk of life-threatening injury	
Vital signs	**Mechanism**
Glasgow Coma Score ≤13 or systolic blood pressure <90 or respiratory rate <10 or >29 Trauma score <14	Evidence of high-speed impact Falls 6 m or more Crash speed 60 kph or more 50 cm deformity of automobile Rearward displacement of front axle Passenger compartment intrusion 40 cm on patient side of car – 50 cm on opposite side of car Ejection of patient Rollover Death of same-car occupant Pedestrian hit at 30 kph or more
Injury	
Penetrating injury to chest, abdomen, head, neck and groin Some significant injury to two or more body areas Severe injury to head/neck or trunk Two or more proximal long bone fractures Burns of >15% or face or airway	
	Demographics
	Age <5 or >55 Known cardiac or respiratory disease (lower the threshold of severity resulting in trauma centre care)

RESUSCITATION BAY FLOOR PLAN

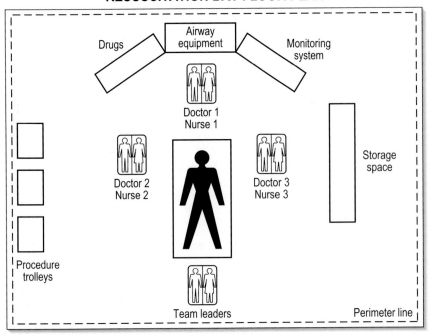

Fig. 3.1.1 The layout of a typical trauma resuscitation bay. (Reproduced with permission from Myers CT, Brown AF, Dunjey SJ, et al. Trauma teams: order from chaos. Emergency Medicine 1993; 5: 34.)

these functions may have to be performed by one or two personnel, in which case a sequential rather than a parallel process will take place.

Table 3.1.2 Team roles
Team leader
Overview
Resuscitation
Assessment
Communication
Ambulance
Referrals
Investigations
Other team members
Primary survey
Secondary survey
Airway doctor
Control of airway
Inline immobilization of cervical spine
Ventilation
Gastric tube
Procedure doctor
Intravenous access/bloods
Intercostal catheter
Urinary catheter
ABG/Art line
Nurses
Airway nurse
Procedure nurse
Scout nurse
Documentation/coordinator
Relatives
Radiographer

Airway

It should be assumed that hypoxia is present in all patients who have sustained multiple injuries. Early expert airway intervention is essential. Every patient should receive initial supplemental oxygen via a well-fitting face mask. This includes those few patients who might later be found to have chronic obstructive airways disease. Concerns regarding pre-existing dependence on hypoxic drive can be addressed once the initial trauma resuscitation has been completed.

If the airway is clear and protected, the neck should be immobilized with a semi-rigid collar, but if airway manoeuvres are necessary it is often better to use manual inline immobilization without a collar, ensuring minimal neck movement with constant vigilance. The management of an obstructed airway in a trauma patient should be undertaken by an experienced senior clinician with significant anaesthetic experience. The first priority is to clear the upper airway by direct visualization, suction, and removal of any foreign bodies. Insertion of an oropharyngeal or nasopharyngeal airway and the jaw thrust manoeuvre are usually successful in clearing an upper airway obstruction. Insertion of a nasopharyngeal airway can be hazardous in patients with a fracture of the cribriform

plate. The direction of insertion (backwards not upwards) is important. Chin lift is not recommended because it may cause additional movement of the cervical spine.

Early endotracheal intubation should be undertaken if the patient is apnoeic, has an unrelieved upper airway obstruction, has persistent internal bleeding from facial injuries, has respiratory insufficiency due to chest or head injuries, or the potential for airway compromise (airway burns, facial instability, coma or seizures). Intubation may also be necessary for procedures such as CT scanning, or for the management of confused or disturbed patients.

The following course of action is recommended for the emergency intubation of the major trauma victim:

- Skilled personnel (anaesthetist or emergency physician with appropriate anaesthetic experience)
- A fully equipped resuscitation area (suction, oxygen, drugs, monitoring equipment)
- The following sequence is suggested:
  - Pre-oxygenate with bag/valve/mask using 100% oxygen
  - Sedation
  - Manual immobilization (without cervical collar)
  - Cricoid pressure
  - Suxamethonium (1.5 mg/kg)
  - Visualize cords by direct laryngoscopy
  - Insert endotracheal tube (ETT) (using introducer if necessary)
  - Monitor gas exchange using pulse oximeter and capnograph
  - Once endotracheal tube position is confirmed give non-depolarizing muscle relaxant and sedation.

Any operator undertaking emergency intubation of major trauma victims (MTVs) should be prepared for a difficult intubation. When there is a high risk of difficult intubation and there is sufficient time, other techniques may be used, such as fibreoptic intubation. These are not appropriate as first-line emergency techniques. If the cords cannot be visualized and the ETT inserted within 30 seconds (try holding your breath for 30 seconds), then bag/mask ventilation should be resumed. If ventilation is possible then there is no urgency; if ventilation is not possible, a second attempt at ETT insertion should be made. If this is unsuccessful then a surgical airway using a cricothyroidotomy should be created. A laryngeal mask airway may also be useful as a temporary measure. The intubating laryngeal mask has also proved useful. Gum-elastic bougie and fibreoptic techniques may be helpful for difficult airways.

Cricothyroidotomy is the surgical airway of choice in an emergency because it is a relatively easy technique compared to tracheostomy, can be performed in a matter of seconds, has a low complication rate in adults, and requires only a scalpel, forceps and ETT. A cricothyroidotomy using a large-bore needle may be used as a temporary measure, especially in children, but will not allow adequate ventilation in adults, as it results in CO_2 accumulation. A number of proprietary kits are available. It must be emphasized that a needle cricothyroidotomy does not protect the airway from aspiration.

Ventilation
Once the airway is secure the patient should be ventilated to optimize oxygenation and maintain normocapnia. There is evidence that severe hypocarbia (<32 mmHg) may be harmful to the cerebral circulation by causing cerebral vasoconstriction.[12,13] Conversely, hypercarbia will produce cerebral vasodilatation with a resultant increase in intracranial pressure (ICP). Although modest hypocarbia was advocated until relatively recently, it has been found that this does not confer any significant benefit. The objective should be to maintain normocarbia. Arterial blood gases should be monitored closely, but capnography should only be used as a guide as there are frequently gross discrepancies. Ventilatory rates should be approximately 10–14 breaths per minute, with a tidal volume of 10 mL/kg (lean mass).

Paralysing agents
Suxamethonium (1.5 mg/kg) is the drug of choice for intubation because of its fast onset, short duration and relative guarantee of complete relaxation. Because it is a depolarizing muscle relaxant it has the disadvantage of transiently increasing ICP and intraocular pressure. It will also cause release of potassium from damaged tissues (e.g. burns/crush injury), but this is not an issue in the first 24–48 hours of injury. Experimentally, it has been shown that the rise in ICP caused by suxamethonium

is short-lived and not as significant as that caused by prolonged attempts at intubation and gagging. The rise in ICP can be lessened if adequate sedation (e.g. midazolam) is used.

The use of a non-depolarizing agent for intubation has never gained favour, mainly because of the slow onset. Newer agents such as rocuronium have a much faster onset (60 seconds), but are still not as good. For ongoing paralysis non-depolarizing agents such as cisatracurium are used.

Sedation
Sedation may be necessary in the MTV for the following reasons:

- Preparation for endotracheal intubation
- In the agitated patient
- In association with analgesics for pain relief.

A major risk with these agents is that in patients with hypovolaemia the loss of sympathetic drive and relaxation of vascular smooth muscle may result in sudden hypotension. Of the commonly used sedative drugs, thiopentone is the most likely to cause hypotension; however, if titrated (50 mg aliquots), it may be used successfully. It is effective in reducing ICP rises associated with intubation, and has a very short duration of action. Midazolam may cause hypotension even with small doses (0.5 mg), but it is also useful in reducing ICP. Fentanyl is not as effective in sedating the patient and reducing ICP, but may be used in relatively high doses (100–500 μg) without causing hypotension. Etomidate (0.2–0.3 mg/kg) is used in the USA and Asian centres such as Hong Kong because of the rapid onset, short duration and minimal haemodynamic effects. Ketamine should not be used in the head-injured patient because of its potential to cause a rise in ICP. It is very effective in producing a dissociative state in patients without neurotrauma, which may allow fracture manipulation and other procedures. Pain or discomfort (such as a distended bladder) may be expressed as agitation in the obtunded patient, and giving sedatives alone will increase the problem. It is therefore important to assess the cause of agitation/anxiety before treatment is given.

Circulation
Shock is a clinical syndrome in which the perfusion of vital organs is inadequate to maintain function. Blood loss is the major cause of shock in the MTV. Other less common causes of shock also need to be considered:

- Tension pneumothorax. This will cause rapid and severe disruption to the circulation.
- Cardiogenic shock. This may be pre-existing (e.g. AMI causing accident, drugs causing reduced cardiac compensation and hypovolaemia) or secondary to injury, i.e. myocardial contusion, valvular/septal injury or pericardial tamponade.
- Neurogenic shock. This results from loss of sympathetic tone. It may be caused by central brainstem injury and vasomotor instability, or spinal cord injury and interruption of descending sympathetic tracts. It is characterized by bradycardia, but this may also occur in profound hypovolaemic states (see below).
- Anaphylactic shock and septic shock may coexist with hypovolaemic shock.

Clinical presentation

The initial stages of hypovolaemia are difficult to detect. Although four stages of blood loss have been described, the distinction made on blood pressure and pulse is usually not clear cut. The cardiovascular response to simple haemorrhage is modified by the presence of tissue injury. Although most major trauma victims have a combination of both, it should be appreciated that those who present with pure blood loss (for example after a stab wound) will often have maintained their blood pressure but may have a bradycardia despite blood loss due to a vagal response. Tissue injury will result in a tachycardia. Hence a normal blood pressure and pulse may be found in patients who have lost a significant amount of blood through a mixture of tissue injury and major blood vessel disruption. Of course, once a very large amount of blood has been lost (30–40% of blood volume), the blood pressure and pulse will become abnormal. An intravenous infusion of even a relatively small amount of fluid to such a patient may bring the recordings back to normal despite persisting hypovolaemia. The picture is further complicated in older patients, and particularly in those who are receiving vasoactive drugs. The absolute values are less important than the trends.

Monitoring

All patients who have sustained an injury that could be associated with significant blood loss, however remote the possibility, must be carefully monitored. In the initial phase, measurement of the clinical parameters will give some information about vital organ perfusion. However, more invasive monitoring will be required if hypovolaemia is severe or sustained. Central venous pressure can be useful to detect changes in venous capacitance, and the response of the CVP to a fluid challenge may be a useful test. Blood pressure is most accurately measured by an indwelling arterial catheter. The acid–base status should be checked frequently.

Management

Venous access

It is essential to gain good venous access at the earliest phase in resuscitation. This is usually via two large-bore (>16 G) peripheral cannulae. In the absence of accessible arm veins, central venous access may be indicated. The recommended site (subclavian, jugular or femoral) depends on a number of factors. The subclavian vein is reliable in terms of patency, but the ease of access to the femoral vein is offset by its potential futility in major truncal haemorrhage. The internal jugular veins can be difficult to access in the immobilized trauma patient. Cut-downs of the saphenous veins and cubital fossa may also be used.

Fluids

Patients with class I and II haemorrhage, where there is no hypotension, can usually be managed without blood transfusion, unless there is ongoing blood loss. Initial treatment is with crystalloid. The Cochrane Collaboration has reviewed the choice of fluid in the trauma patient and favours the use of crystalloids over colloids.[14–16]

Given that there have been reported adverse events associated with colloid infusion, there is growing consensus that crystalloids should be the fluid of first choice. Hypertonic crystalloid has also been suggested, but the available data are inconclusive and more research is required.[17]

For class III and IV haemorrhage, where there is hypotension and tachycardia, blood transfusion should commence immediately, initially using O-negative blood and changing to group-specific or cross-matched blood as it becomes available. There is no evidence that whole blood is superior to packed cells and replacement of clotting factors, unless the blood is fresh (less than 1–2 days old). The availability of fresh blood is extremely limited.

Filters

Micropore blood filters slow the transfusion and do not appear to reduce complications from blood transfusion in the MTV.

Hypothermia

This is common in MTVs because of exposure and the use of cold intravenous fluids. Crystalloid infusions are usually administered at room temperature, although some centres prewarm fluids in blanket cupboards and microwave ovens. It is important to monitor this, as temperatures can fluctuate wildly. Blood is stored at 4°C and it is important to warm it; however, traditional blood warmers are cumbersome and slow to set up unless this can be done in anticipation. The use of the more expensive rapid infusion blood warmers is justified in trauma reception centres. There is growing consensus that a mild degree of hypothermia is probably not harmful and may well be cerebroprotective. Rapid active rewarming may cause worse outcomes in the context of isolated severe head injury.[18] However, hypothermia < 32°C will interfere with coagulation, reduce myocardial contractility and predispose to arrhythmias.

Coagulation factors

There is little evidence for the use of clotting factors if the total haemorrhagic loss is less than 5 L. In the clinical situation, where there is evidence of ongoing blood loss after the replacement of five to six units, clotting factors should be replaced, as a blood loss of twice this volume would be anticipated.

Coagulopathy is frequently present on arrival and may be secondary to mediators released as a result of direct tissue injury. Worsening coagulopathy is usually dilutional, but pre-existing problems such as liver disease and warfarinization should be looked for. Platelets should also be given if more than 10 units of blood are transfused. Although controversial, it is reasonable to give four units of fresh frozen or freeze-dried plasma for every six units of blood transfused. The use of cryoprecipitate is also recommended if fibrinogen levels are low. Haematologists have traditionally asked for evidence of coagulopathy before issuing clotting factors; however, in a rapidly deteriorating MTV requiring massive transfusion there is little logic in waiting for a coagulation result that reflects the situation 30–60 minutes previously. The place of Factor rVIIa in massive haemorrhage following trauma is still uncertain. At this stage there is little evidence of improved outcomes, although preliminary trials suggest a reduction in blood loss.[19] It should be seen as a potential rescue therapy after reversible factors such as surgical bleeding, hypothermia, acidosis and clotting factor replacement have been rectified.[20]

MAST suit

Once popular, these devices are now very rarely used. A number of complications have been reported and, importantly, no therapeutic benefit has been demonstrated.[21] There may be some value in applying the MAST suit to patients who have an unstable pelvic fracture associated with massive internal bleeding, but the advent of external fixators and specific pelvic binders that can be applied either prehospital or in the resuscitation area of the ED has largely removed this last indication.

Hypotensive resuscitation

In the last decade, increasing attention has been paid to the potential harm in overaggressive resuscitation of patients prior to definitive treatment of the cause of the bleeding. A number of studies have shown that in major trauma victims with penetrating injuries to the trunk, vigorous fluid resuscitation prior to operation actually results in a worse outcome.[22,23] This concurs with vascular surgical protocols, where it is acknowledged that outcomes are improved by limiting fluid resuscitation prior to the repair of leaking aneurysms. Logically, if the blood pressure is higher, more blood loss will occur. Therefore, more dilution of clotting factors, increased usage of blood products for replacement, hypothermia, coagulopathy, ARDS, sepsis etc. will result. Conversely, if there is no perfusing pressure to vital organs then irreversible injury to those organs may occur.

The essential point in this debate is that the most important determinant of outcome in MTVs is the time to definitive surgery. There is certainly no point in delaying surgery 'to normalize the intravascular volume'. The relevance of penetrating injury studies to blunt trauma is unclear. However, where there is a cause of bleeding that can be ligated, this should be done as soon as possible. This principle applies to bony injury (using fixation) as well as spleen, liver and other sources of bleeding. If there is no surgically remediable bleeding point, the physiological status should be returned to normal as soon as possible to prevent long-term complications from prolonged ischaemia to bowel and other organs.

Next steps

By this stage the trauma patient will have been received into a well-organized resuscitation area and the first life-saving procedures will have been initiated by an integrated and skilled team of doctors and nurses. Any immediately life-threatening conditions can be expected to have been identified and dealt with. Constant vigilance and reassessment are essential. Other occult injuries may be present in those patients identified with serious injuries.

While the trauma team leader continues to review the situation in the light of a constantly changing clinical scenario, and hopefully the provision of more biomechanical data from the site of the incident, he or she should also be beginning to consider the next steps. The first of these is the calling in of other experts. Whereas it will have been clear that an airway doctor will be an essential part of the initial resuscitation team, it may be some minutes before it is known which other skills are required. Usually

orthopaedic surgeons and neurosurgeons are near the top of the list. General surgery is not required as often as is commonly supposed,[24] although general surgeons are often useful in coordinating ongoing care. Whichever specialty is required, the patient's emergency problems demand experience, therefore, 'if in doubt, refer'.

Radiographs are required at this stage. The initial films should be limited to those that will have a direct bearing on immediate management, including a chest AP view and a pelvis AP view.

Lateral X-ray of the cervical spine is no longer mandatory at this stage of assessment. Cervical immobilization is routine, and it is not possible to exclude cervical injury with a lateral cervical spine X-ray. Therefore, a cervical X-ray does not alter initial management. Its utility at this stage would be to confirm an irretrievable injury, i.e. craniocervical dislocation.

Ideally, the resuscitation room should have an integrated X-ray facility, but if this is not available portable films should be obtained. It is not appropriate to transfer a multiply injured unstable patient to a separate X-ray facility.

Other forms of imaging have become popular in localizing the source of haemorrhagic shock. The increasing availability of FAST (focused abdominal sonogram in trauma) has superseded diagnostic peritoneal lavage (DPL) as the bedside adjunct for detecting intraperitoneal haemorrhage. Subsequent chapters deal with individual trauma problems, but it is essential that throughout the patient's stay in hospital a single clinician has overriding responsibility for his or her care. In the resuscitation area this is the 'team leader', who may be from any discipline. Handover to the clinician responsible for ongoing care must be comprehensive, timed, and well documented.

Trauma audit

Trauma kills people in a variety of ways, hence no one department in a hospital will see a large number of deaths. Many trauma victims die before they reach hospital, some in the ED, and others scattered through the inpatient specialties and in intensive care. Hence from any one clinician's perspective, trauma is not an outstanding problem.

However, when looked at from a public health perspective it is clearly a major issue, not least because some of the deaths are avoidable. Identifying these, and the much more difficult-to-define group of patients who survive but whose outcome is not as good as expected, is a major problem.

The most important variables to measure are the extent of the anatomical injury, the degree of physiological derangement that results, age, and the previous wellbeing of the patient. All these have a direct effect on outcome, and must therefore be measured before any comment can be made about the process of care. Outcome itself must also of course be measured. This is relatively easy in terms of mortality: the general accepted definition is death within 31 days of the incident. However, disability is a much more difficult issue, and currently there are no universally accepted measurement tools. The functional independence measure used in MTOS,[25] the Glasgow Outcome Scale,[26] GOSE[27] and the SF36[28] (Short Form – 36 Questions) are the best available tools. As 90% of MTVs survive their injury in a mature trauma system, it is important to measure disability and quality of life following major trauma when comparing outcomes.[29]

Trauma audit was first formalized by Champion at the Washington Hospital Centre in the 1970s. The TRISS[30] system is now widely used, but there have been many proposals for its modification.

Most current trauma systems are now audited using some variation of the TRISS methodology. This combines measurement of anatomical injury using the Abbreviated Injury Scale and the Injury Severity Score, together with the Revised Trauma Score to measure physiological derangement, with an adjustment made for age. A probability of survival can be calculated by reference to large databanks with known outcomes that contain a range of these scores. Perhaps more importantly, the comparative performance of hospitals, or the change in a single hospital's performance over time, can be determined by bringing together the probability of survival of a number of patients and comparing them with the actual survival. Anonymous league tables can then be developed with the objective of identifying features of the best hospitals associated with high survival rates (and vice versa).

Trauma in developing countries

On an international scale, trauma has become a major issue. According to the World Health Organization, by 2020 road trauma will rank third on the list of lives lost to death and disability.[1] That is, after cardiovascular disease and mental illness, road trauma causes the greatest loss of life when using the scale of DALYs (Disability-Adjusted Life Years).[3,4]

Globally, national governments are beginning to recognize the burgeoning human and economic cost of trauma, particularly road trauma. The public health achievements of the developed countries (seatbelts, helmets, alcohol and speed restrictions) are being implemented,[3,4,31] and similarly, governments of developing countries are looking to implement trauma systems.[31,32]

Research in developing countries reinforces the benefits of trauma systems previously described in countries with established EMS systems. For example, evidence indicates that people with life-threatening but potentially treatable injuries are up to six times more likely to die in a country with no organized trauma system than in one with an organized, resourced trauma system.[32] Trauma system development requires trauma outcome measurement. As such, developing countries are likely to adopt trauma registries over the next several decades, in an attempt to track the burden of trauma and the impact of system-wide interventions.

As developing countries embark upon trauma system development, it is becoming increasingly important to access standardized trauma care education through intensive short-courses. Advanced Trauma Life Support (ATLS) has been widely used. Other courses (such as Primary Trauma Care (PTC)) have also become popular in the developing world. Such courses are often less expensive and more flexible than ATLS.

Controversies

- The number of MTVs necessary for a hospital to maintain high-quality trauma care.

- The degree to which potential MTVs should be over-triaged to ensure that patients with major trauma are received at major trauma centres. There may be a greater risk in bypassing hospitals to take patients to a trauma centre, depending on distance and injury type. There is also the issue of deskilling of personnel from non-trauma centres, and what effect this has on overall system outcomes.

- The degree to which MTVs should be managed by protocol rather than clinical judgement. Clinicians are increasingly being asked to follow protocols in these critical situations. This prevents some adverse outcomes but may cause over-investigation and treatment.

- The role of hypotensive resuscitation in blunt trauma has not been defined. Where victims have prolonged delays to theatre, or the bleeding is not surgically correctable, then hypotensive resuscitation may cause more complications.

- The role of controlled hypothermia in head-injured patients.

References

1. Centre for Disease Control and Prevention, National Center for Injury Prevention and Control: WISQARS Atlanta, http://cdc.gov/ncipc/osp/charts, accessed 22 December 2007.
2. Australian Bureau of Statistics, http://www.abs.gov.au/austats, accessed 22 December 2007.
3. Nantulya WM, Reich MR. The neglected epidemic: road traffic injuries in developing countries. British Medical Journal 2002; 324: 1139–1141.
4. World Health Organization. World report on road traffic injury prevention. Geneva: WHO, 2004.
5. World Health Organization. Global burden of disease estimates. http://who.int/healthinfo/bodestimates/en/index, accessed 22 December 2007.
6. Trunkey DD. Trauma. Scientific American 1983; 249: 28–35.
7. Cales RH, Trunkey DD. Preventable trauma deaths. A review of trauma care systems development. Journal of the American Medical Association 1985; 254: 1059–1063.
8. Roy PD. The value of trauma centres: a methodologic review. Canadian Journal of Surgery 1987; 30: 17–22.
9. Eastman AB, Lewis FR, Champion HR, et al. Regional trauma system design: critical concepts. American Journal of Surgery 1987; 154: 79–87.
10. Mulholland SA, Gabbe BJ, Cameron P. Victorian State Outcomes Registry and Monitoring Group (VSTORM). Is paramedic judgement useful in prehospital trauma triage? Injury 2005; 36: 1298–1305.
11. Palanca S, Taylor D, Bailey M, et al. Mechanisms of motor vehicle accidents that predict major injury. Emergency Medicine Australasia 2003; 15: 423–428.
12. Pickard JD, Czosnyka M. Management of raised intracranial pressure. Journal of Neurology, Neurosurgery and Psychiatry 1993; 56: 845–858.
13. Fortune JB, Feustel PJ, Graca L, et al. Effect of hyperventilation, mannitol, and ventriculostomy drainage on cerebral blood flow after head injury. Journal of Trauma, Injury, Infection and Critical Care 1995; 39: 1091–1099.
14. Roberts I, Alderson P, Bunn F. Colloids versus crystalloids for fluid resuscitation in critically ill patients (Cochrane Review). In: The Cochrane Library (4), 2004.
15. The SAFE Study Investigators. A comparison of albumin and saline for fluid resuscitation in the intensive care unit. New England Journal of Medicine 2004; 350: 2247–2256.
16. The SAFE Study Investigators. Saline or albumin for fluid resuscitation in patients with traumatic brain injury. New England Journal of Medicine 2007; 357: 874–884.
17. Bunn F, Roberts I, Tasker R. Hypertonic versus near isotonic crystalloid for fluid resuscitation in critically ill patients (Cochrane Review). In: The Cochrane Library (3). 2004.
18. Clifton GL, Miller ER, Sung RN, et al. Lack of effect of induction of hypothermia after acute brain injury. New England Journal of Medicine 2001; 344: 556–563.
19. Boffard KD, Riou B, Warren B, et al. Recombinant factor VIIa as adjunctive therapy for bleeding control in severely injured trauma patients: two parallel randomized, placebo-controlled, double-blind clinical trials. Journal of Trauma, Injury, Infection and Critical Care 2005; 59: 8–15.
20. Cameron P, Phillips L, Balogh Z, et al. The use of recombinant activated Factor VII in trauma patients: experience from the Australian and New Zealand Haemostasis Registry. Injury 2007; 38: 1030–1038.
21. Mattox KL, Bickell W, Pepe I, et al. Prospective MAST study in 911 patients. Journal of Trauma 1989; 29: 1102–1112.
22. Bickell WH, Wall MJ, Pepe PE, et al. Immediate versus delayed fluid resuscitation for hypertensive patients with penetrating torso injuries. New England Journal of Medicine 1994; 331: 1105–1109.
23. Civil IDJ. Resuscitation following injury: an end or a means? Australian and New Zealand Journal of Surgery 1993; 63: 921–926.
24. Cameron PA, Dziukas L, Hadj A. Patterns of injury from major trauma in Victoria. Australian and New Zealand Journal of Surgery 1995; 65: 830–834.
25. Champion HZ, Copes WS, Sacco WJ, et al. The Major Trauma Outcome. Study establishing natural norms for trauma care. Journal of Trauma 1990; 30: 1356–1365.
26. Jennett B, Bond M. Assessment of outcome after severe brain damage. Lancet 1975; 1: 480–484.
27. Teasdale GM, Pettigrew LE, Wilson JT. Analysing outcome of severe head injury: a review and update on advancing the use of the Glasgow Outcome Scale. Journal of Neurotrauma 1998; 15: 587–597.
28. Garratt AM, Ruta DA, Abdulher MI. The SF36 Health Survey Questionnaire: an outcome measure suitable for routine use within the NHS? British Medical Journal 1993; 306: 1440–1444.
29. Willis CD, Gabbe BJ, Cameron PA. Measuring quality in trauma care. 2007; Injury 38: 527–537.
30. Boyd CR, Tolson MA, Copes WS. Evaluating trauma care. The TRISS method. Journal of Trauma 1987; 27: 370–378.
31. Fitzgerald M, Dewan Y, O'Reilly G. India and the management of road crashes – towards a national trauma system. Indian Journal of Surgery 2006; 68: 237–243.
32. Mock CN, Adzotor KE, Conklin E. Trauma outcomes in the rural developing world: comparison with an urban level 1 trauma center. Journal of Trauma 1993; 35: 518–523.
33. Pang JM, Civil I, Ng A, et al. Is the trimodal pattern of death after trauma a dated concept in the 21st century? Trauma deaths in Auckland 2004. Injury 2008; 39: 102–106. Epub 2007 Sep 18.

Further reading

American College of Surgeons. ATLS: Advanced Trauma Life Support for Doctors: Student Course Manual, 7th edn. 2004 Chicago.
Driscoll P, Skinner D, Earlam R. ABC of major trauma, 3rd edn. London: BMJ Publishing, 1999.

3.2 Neurotrauma

Lee Wallis • Peter Cameron

ESSENTIALS

1 Neurotrauma is associated with the majority of trauma deaths.

2 A detailed history of the mechanics of the trauma experienced is invaluable.

3 Secondary brain injury is a major and potentially preventable cause of mortality and long-term morbidity.

4 Cerebral cellular dysfunction secondary to trauma is a result of both primary and secondary mechanisms and involves sodium, calcium and potassium shifts across the cell membrane, the development of oxygen free radicals, and lipid peroxidation.

5 There are two features of prime importance to resuscitation in patients suffering neurotrauma: maintenance of airway/ventilation, and maintenance of cerebral perfusion pressure.

6 Inline stabilization of the cervical spine during rapid sequence induction and orotracheal intubation is the preferred method for gaining definitive airway control in the head-injured patient.

7 Current emergency department and neurosurgical practice involves the use of CT scanning to investigate mild, moderate and severe head injury.

Introduction

Neurotrauma is a common feature in the presentation of multisystem trauma, particularly when associated with motor vehicle accidents and falls. Over 50% of trauma deaths are associated with head injury. The implications for the health system are enormous, with an annual rate of admission to hospital wards associated with head trauma approaching 300 per 100 000 population,[1] and twice this in the elderly.[2] The long-term sequelae of moderate and severe neurotrauma are a major health resource drain, and the morbidities associated with mild brain injury are becoming clearer.

Advances in preventative strategies, trauma systems, resuscitative therapies and rehabilitation management have improved outcomes. However, neurotrauma remains a serious health issue, predominantly affecting the productive youth of society.

Pathogenesis

Primary brain injury occurs as a result of the forces and disruptive mechanics of the original incident: this can only be avoided through preventative measures, such as the use of bicycle helmets.

Secondary brain injury is due to a complex interaction of factors and typically occurs within 2–24 hours of injury.[3] A principal mechanism of secondary injury is cerebral hypoxia due to impaired oxygenation or impaired cerebral blood flow. Cerebral blood flow is dependent on cerebral perfusion pressure (CPP), mean arterial systemic blood pressure (MAP) and intracranial pressure (ICP).

$$CPP = MAP - ICP$$

Intracranial pressure may be raised as a result of the mass effect of the haemorrhage, or by generalized cerebral oedema. Cerebral vasospasm further reduces cerebral blood flow in patients in whom significant subarachnoid haemorrhage has occurred.

Cellular dysfunction is a result of both primary and secondary mechanisms and involves sodium, calcium, magnesium and potassium shifts across the cell membrane, the development of oxygen free radicals, lipid peroxidation and glutamate hyperactivity. Excessive release of excitatory neurotransmitters and magnesium depletion also occur.[4]

Classification of primary injury in neurotrauma

Primary injuries are classified as:

- Skull fracture
- Concussion
- Contusion
- Intracranial haematoma
- Diffuse axonal injury
- Penetrating injury.

Skull fracture

The significance of skull fracture is not related to the specific bony injury but rather the associated neurotrauma. Fractures in the region of the middle meningeal artery in particular may be associated with acute extradural haemorrhage. Fractures involving the skull base and cribriform plate may be associated with CSF leak and the risk of secondary infection. Depressed skull fractures may compress underlying structures, cause secondary brain injury and require surgical elevation. Injury to underlying structures may result in secondary epilepsy.

Concussion

Concussion is a transient alteration in cerebral function, usually associated with loss of consciousness and often followed by rapid and complete recovery. The proposed mechanism is a disturbance in the function of the reticular activating system. Post-concussive syndromes, including headache and mild cognitive disturbance, are not uncommon.[5,6] Symptoms, particularly headache, are usually short-lived but may persist. 'Second-impact syndrome' describes a greater risk of significant reinjury following an initial injury causing a simple concussion. It is likely to be due to diffuse cerebral swelling.[7] In animal models concussion may be associated with modest short-term increases in intracranial pressure and disturbances in cerebral cellular function.[8]

Contusion

Cerebral contusion is bruising of the brain substance associated with head trauma. The most common mechanism is blunt trauma. Forces involved are less than those required to cause major shearing injuries, and often occur in the absence of skull fracture. Morbidity is related to the size and site of the contusion, and coexistent injury. Larger contusions may be associated with haematoma formation, secondary oedema or seizure activity. The most common sites for contusions are the frontal and temporal lobes.[9]

Intracranial haematoma

Extradural Extradural haematoma (EDH) is uncommon but classically associated with fracture of the temporal bone and injury to the underlying middle meningeal artery. Haemorrhage subsequently occurs, stripping the dura from the skull and expanding to cause a rise in intracranial pressure and eventually uncal herniation and death. Haemorrhage may be from vessels other than the middle meningeal artery (e.g. brisk arteriolar or venous bleeding). Signs will depend on the site of the haematoma.

Subdural Subdural haematomata (SDH) may have an acute, subacute or chronic course. It generally follows moderate head trauma with loss of consciousness. In the elderly, SDH may be associated with trivial injury, and in children with shaking (abuse) injury. Haemorrhage occurs into the subdural space, slowly enlarging to cause a space-occupying collection whose functional implications will vary according to location. Acute subdural haemorrhage carries a high mortality (>50%), similar to acute EDH. Subacute and chronic SDH is associated with a degree of cerebral dysfunction, headache or other symptomatology, and is associated with a significantly lower mortality (up to 20%).[10]

Intracerebral As with cerebral contusion, the most common sites of intracerebral haemorrhage associated with trauma are the temporal and posterior frontal lobes. Functional expression is variable, depending on site. Intracerebral haemorrhage may progress from an initial contusion or be secondary to altered vascular characteristics. Symptom development and complications may be delayed as the size of the haemorrhage increases over time.

Subarachnoid and intraventricular haemorrhage Subarachnoid blood is relatively common after major head injury.

Intraventricular haemorrhage may also be evident. As in non-traumatic settings, the presence of subarachnoid blood may lead to cerebral vasospasm and secondary ischaemic brain injury.

Diffuse axonal injury

Diffuse axonal injury (DAI) is the predominant mechanism of injury in neurotrauma, occurring in up to 50% of patients.[11] Shearing and rotational forces on the axonal network may result in major structural and functional disturbance at a microscopic level. Disturbance to important communicative pathways sometimes results in significant long-term morbidity, despite non-specific or minimal changes on CT scanning. The exact pathogenesis of diffuse axonal injury is incompletely understood. Specific injury in the regions of the corpus callosum and midbrain has been proposed; however, DAI is believed to be the mechanism for persistent neurological deficits seen in head-traumatized individuals with normal CT scans.[12]

Penetrating injury

Penetrating neurotrauma is characterized by high levels of morbidity and mortality. This is especially true of gunshot wounds. Exposure of cerebral tissue through large compound wounds, or through basilar skull structures, is associated with a dismal outlook. Penetrating injury in the periorbital and pernasal regions is associated with high risk of infection.

Epidemiology

Neurotrauma is commonest in the young and the old: under 5 and over 80 years of age. In young children the majority of injuries are, fortunately, mild (although a significant proportion are the result of non-accidental injury). It is the leading cause of trauma deaths in under 25s.[13]

Common causes include motor vehicle accidents (including vehicle versus pedestrian and bicycle collisions), falls, assault and firearms. In young males, alcohol is often involved.

Prevention

Primary prevention of neurotrauma depends on the cause. Most preventative strategies are directed at vehicular traffic, and include speed-calming measures, in-car safety devices, and bicycle helmets. Improving roadside lighting and enhancing pedestrian visibility contribute to reduction of injury in this group.

Prevention of secondary injury involves maintenance of cerebral perfusion and oxygenation, and is addressed under clinical management.

Clinical features

Definition

Neurotrauma may be classified according to severity as minimal, mild, moderate or severe (Table 3.2.1).[14] Such a classification allows for directed investigation and management, but there is clearly a continuum of injury within the spectrum of neurotrauma.

History

A detailed history of the mechanics of the trauma is essential. This should be followed by consideration of time courses, pre-hospital care, pre-sedative and pre-relaxant neuromuscular function, and episodes and duration of hypotension or other decompensation. A history of previous health problems, allergies, medications and social setting is desirable.

Primary survey

As with all trauma patients, the initial assessment and therapy must be directed at

Table 3.2.1 Neurotrauma severity
Minimal
No loss of consciousness, and Glasgow Coma Score (GCS) 15, and Normal alertness and memory, and No neurological deficit, and No palpable depressed fracture or other sign of skull fracture
Mild
Brief (<5 minutes) loss of consciousness, or Amnesia for event, or GCS 14, or Impaired alertness or memory No palpable depressed fracture or other sign of skull fracture
Moderate or potentially severe
Prolonged (>5 minutes) loss of consciousness, or Persistent GCS <14, or Focal neurological deficit, or Post-traumatic seizure, or Intracranial lesion on CT scan, or Palpable depressed skull fracture

maintenance of airway, ventilation and circulatory adequacy along standard ATLS principles. Early assessment of neurological disturbance is important: the use of the formal Glasgow Coma Score (GCS) can be difficult in the primary survey, and this assessment may be reliably undertaken with the AVPU scale (Alert: GCS 14–15; response to Verbal stimuli: GCS 9–13; response to Painful stimuli: GCS 6–8; or Unresponsive: GCS 3–5). Simultaneous protection of the cervical spine by immobilization is fundamental. This management should commence in the pre-hospital setting and the level of care be maintained.

Inline stabilization of the cervical spine during rapid-sequence induction and orotracheal intubation is the preferred method for gaining definitive airway control in the head-injured patient.

The greatest risks to the patient with a moderate to severe head injury are hypoxic injury and deficient cerebral perfusion due to systemic hypotension.

Secondary survey

A full secondary survey, including log-roll, should follow.

Clinical assessment of the neurological status of head-injured patients commences with formal documentation of the GCS (Table 3.2.2). The maximum score is 15 and the minimum 3. The GCS has been incorporated into other assessment scales in trauma (Trauma Score, Revised Trauma Score) and in TRISS estimation of probability of survival.

Table 3.2.2 Glasgow coma score	
Best motor response	
Obeys command	6
Localizes to pain	5
Withdraw to pain	4
Abnormal flexion to pain	3
Abnormal extension to pain	2
Nil	1
Best verbal response	
Oriented	5
Confused	4
Uses inappropriate words	3
Incomprehensible sounds	2
Nil	1
Eye opening	
Spontaneously	4
To verbal command	3
To pain	2
Nil	1

Coma may be defined in terms of the GCS, in which patients have a total score of 8 or less:

- Fail to show eye opening in response to pain (Eye-opening response = 1)
- Fail to obey commands (Best motor response = 5)
- Make at best only incomprehensible sounds (Best verbal response = 2).

Examination of pupillary responses, particularly in the unconscious patient, is important as an indicator of increasing intracranial pressure; a non-responsive dilated pupil indicating ipsilateral herniation. However, a more common cause of abnormal pupil reactions in head injury is the presence of direct ocular trauma.

A general neurological examination, including reflexes and funduscopy, should be performed, the degree to which cooperation is possible and lateralization of signs being particularly important to document. Consideration of the pre-injury mental state is important, particularly where drug or alcohol intoxication is possible.

Clinical investigation

Minimal–mild head injury

In head injury associated with loss of consciousness or amnesia and a GCS of 14–15, CT scanning will demonstrate a relevant positive scan (i.e. cerebral contusion, haematoma, oedema, pneumocephalus) in 7–12%, and a subsequent craniotomy rate of 1–3%.[15–18]

On the weight of research evidence current ED investigation of mild head injury should include CT scanning in all patients in this group.[14,19–22] Despite considerable research in this area, reliable risk stratification is difficult. Stratification of high-risk discriminators within the GCS 14–15 group has not been definitively achieved. Certain high-risk groups, such as the intoxicated, the elderly (>65 years), anticoagulated or demented patients, warrant CT scanning after minor, presumed or possible head injury.

The Canadian Head Rules detail five high-risk criteria for neurosurgical intervention in patients with GCS 13–15 and mild head injury (see Table 3.8.4).[23]

However, there are a plethora of rules, all of which have a good evidence base to support them. The NICE head injury rules were based in part on the Canadian rules;[24] the NEXUS II[25] investigators showed that development of a simple head injury CT rule that is both sensitive and specific is extremely difficult. There have been conflicting results as to which has the best predictive power in adults and children; however, all produce an increase in the frequency of CT scanning and each has its critics for over-scanning.[26,27]

Although coagulation disturbance was not included, it is advisable to have a reduced threshold for scanning those on aspirin, warfarin or with a coagulopathy.

Cervical spine X-ray is indicated if the patient has neck pain, neurological abnormality, altered conscious state, intoxication or significant distracting injury.

Moderate–severe head injury

Urgent CT scanning is the investigation of choice in moderate-to-severe neurotrauma; however, other investigations and therapy may take priority in the patient with multisystem trauma, particularly in the presence of unresponsive haemorrhagic shock.

In the absence of a CT scan, consultation with a neurosurgeon or early transfer to an appropriate facility is essential.

Cervical spine X-ray is indicated in all patients with moderate to severe neurotrauma. A significant proportion of patients with severe head injury will have cervical spine fractures.

Treatment

Minimal–mild head injury

All patients with mild head injury must be counselled appropriately and discharged with written advice in the care of a responsible adult. Specific advice must be provided regarding expected duration of symptoms, possible risks or delayed complications, and reasons for re-presentation to the ED (Table 3.2.3). Information should also be given about the second-impact syndrome and exclusions from sporting activity.

Follow-up by a local medical officer should be arranged, and neuropsychological assessment may be warranted for high-risk groups. Patients should be cautioned about making

---

Table 3.2.3 Patient advice

General advice following head injury

The patient should read and understand these instructions.
* Rest comfortably at home in the company of a responsible adult for the next 12–24 hours.
* Resume normal activity after feeling recovered.
* Drink clear fluids and consume a light diet only for the first 6–12 hours (a normal diet may be commenced as desired after that).
* Mild pain killers (such as paracetamol) may be taken for headache as directed by the doctor.
* Following head injury a small number of patients develop ongoing symptoms, such as recurrent mild headache, concentration difficulties, difficulty with complex tasks, mood disturbance, etc. If you notice such problems, consult your local doctor for appropriate referral.
* Avoid exposure to activities that may create risk of further head injury within the next 2 weeks.
* If you do not understand these instructions and advice, check with emergency department staff before your discharge or consult your local doctor.
* If you require a certificate for work please make this clear to emergency department staff.

Report immediately the following problems

* Persistent vomiting (more than twice).
* Persistent drowsiness – unable to be woken up completely.
* Confusion or disorientation or slurred speech.
* Increased headache (not relieved by standard doses of paracetamol).
* Localized weakness or altered sensation or incoordination.
* Blurred or double vision.
* Seizures, fits or convulsions.
* Neck stiffness.

---

major life, occupational and financial decisions until they are free of post-concussive symptoms.

In minimal and mild head injury a normal CT scan and the absence of neurological abnormality are reasonable criteria for patient discharge.[3] It is essential to assess for ongoing post-traumatic amnesia (PTA), as this is frequently overlooked in the ED. A simple screen to use is the modified Westmead PTA scale.[6] In the presence of these criteria the persistence of mild symptoms (e.g. mild headache, nausea, occasional vomiting) is common, and patients should be advised accordingly. In adults, such symptoms may be treated with mild analgesics (paracetamol, aspirin) and antiemetics (metoclopramide, prochlorperazine) and the patient discharged when comfortable. Advising patients that there will be problems with post-concussive symptoms (including short-term memory and information processing) and providing them with written material has been shown to improve outcomes at 3 months.[6]

Currently there is no drug to treat the primary pathology in mild and minor head injury.[28]

Moderate–severe head injury

Priority in the management of moderate to severe neurotrauma is given to maintenance of the airway and an adequate cerebral perfusion pressure (CPP). Hypotension (SBP < 90) and hypoxia ($PaO_2 < 60$ [8 kPa]) should be corrected immediately.[29]

Control or modification of intracranial pressure (ICP) has a place in the emergency management of neurotrauma. Avoidance of secondary brain injury and associated cerebral swelling is the mainstay of such therapy, and the use of the head-up position, mannitol and hyperventilation is indicated in some situations.

Intracranial pressure monitoring is generally indicated in patients with severe head injury (GCS < 8) who remain comatose. Institutional variability exists in methods for measurement, as do specific indications for monitoring. Elevation of the head of the bed to 30° will reduce ICP modestly without altering CPP.

Mannitol (0.5–1.0 g/kg i.v. and hyperventilation to induce hypocapnia (30–35 mmHg [4–4.7 kPa]) may both produce a short-term reduction in ICP. Mannitol causes an osmotic dehydration, which is non-selective. Complications of mannitol therapy include fluid overload, hyperosmolality, hypovolaemia and rebound cerebral oedema. Contraindications to mannitol therapy include pre-existing hypovolaemia, serum osmolarity > 320 mmol/L and renal failure. Mannitol may be used as a temporizing measure to enable a patient with a surgically remediable lesion to get to theatre.

Hypocarbia reduces cerebral blood flow (and ICP) through vasoconstriction which, if extreme, may reduce CPP to the point of exacerbation of secondary brain injury.[30] Routine use of hyperventilation in head injury is contraindicated. Both osmotic

diuresis and hyperventilation should be used with care, and preferably in consultation with neurosurgeons.

Anticonvulsant prophylaxis (phenytoin 15–18 mg/kg i.v. over 30–60 minutes) is indicated for the prevention of seizures within the first week after injury.[31] Seizures are managed acutely using standard therapies and guidelines (including benzodiazepines and phenytoin). The use of barbiturates, endotracheal intubation and mechanical ventilation may be indicated for status epilepticus or seizures that are refractory to therapy.

Antibiotic prophylaxis is indicated for compound fractures (flucloxacillin 1 g 6-hourly i.v. or cephalothin 1 g 6-hourly i.v.). Tetanus immunoprophylaxis is given as part of routine wound care. Steroid therapy has had varied support but is not recommended;[32] in 2005, the CRASH collaborators reported conclusively that intravenous corticosteroids should not be used in the treatment of head injury.[33]

There has been considerable interest and experimental endeavour with regard to cerebral protection and salvage therapies. Examples include the use of adrenocorticotrophic hormone analogues, the calcium antagonist superoxide dismutase, glutamate antagonists, free radical scavengers and ciclosporin A.[34] There is also interest in the use of early decompressive craniectomy for patients with significant rises in intracranial pressure, and a large trial is currently being undertaken. Definitive outcomes of trials are awaited. General supportive therapy, including maintenance of thermoregulation, hydration, pressure care and nutrition, must be addressed.

Resuscitation in neurotrauma

There are two features of prime importance to resuscitation in patients suffering neurotrauma:

* Maintenance of airway and ventilation
* Maintenance of cerebral perfusion pressure.

With elevation of intracranial pressure and loss of autoregulation of cerebral circulation, relatively higher systemic blood pressures are required. The practice of minimal-volume resuscitation has no place in the patient with serious neurotrauma. Standard approaches to the management of hypovolaemia in head-injured patients should be adopted. The use of hypertonic solutions in resuscitation (including hypertonic saline) has been adopted in some centres, with favourable outcomes for head-injured patients.[35] The only randomized controlled trial performed with hypertonic saline showed no improvement in outcome.[36] Albumin has also been shown to have detrimental effects in severe traumatic brain injury.[37]

Indications for intubation and ventilation of the neurotrauma patient are inadequate ventilation or gas exchange (hypercarbia, hypoxia, apnoea); inability to maintain airway integrity (protective reflexes); a combative or agitated patient; and the need for transport where the status of the airway is potentially unstable (between hospitals, to CT, to angiography, etc.).

Disposition

In patients with minimal–mild head injury, recommendations with regard to a 'safe' period of observation, need for hospital admission or predictive value of injury mechanism are not consistent. Rural and isolated settings present logistic difficulties in the management of this group. Careful observation for a prolonged period is a reasonable alternative, and early neurosurgical consultation, together with a low threshold to transfer to a neurosurgical centre, is prudent.

Patients with moderate to severe neurotrauma require hospital admission, preferably under the care of a neurosurgeon in a specialized neurosurgical unit or ICU. Rehabilitation and social readjustment is a focus of therapy from early in the clinical course.

Inter-hospital transfer of patients with significant neurotrauma requires the attendance of skilled transfer staff and the maintenance of level of care during transfer. Airway management must anticipate the potential for the patient to deteriorate en route. The presence of pneumocephalus precludes unpressurized (high) altitude flight. The use of teleradiology and neurosurgical consultation will be of value in the management of the remote head-injured patient.

Prognosis

The level of residual neurological impairment is a function of the severity of the degree of trauma and quality of care. Worse outcome is associated with prolonged pre-hospital time, delay of transfer to the appropriate facility, admission to an inappropriate facility, and delay in definitive surgical treatment.

Overall mortality in severe head injury is of the order of 35%. A lower GCS at presentation is associated with a worse outcome. Approximately half the patients who remain comatose with GCS < 9 for longer than 6 hours will die.[12] Acute subdural haematoma and diffuse axonal injury producing persistent coma are associated with the vast majority of neurotrauma deaths. Early neurological abnormalities are, however, not reliable prognostic factors, and an initial period of maximally aggressive therapy is indicated in patients with closed neurotrauma.

Controversies

- Intracranial pressure monitoring has not been shown to improve outcome from major head injury.

- The role of CT scanning in minor head injury has become more widespread. Although it is increasingly accepted that CT is indicated, the timing or urgency of the investigation is controversial. Further studies are required to define discriminators and high-risk markers as guides to the most rational application of this investigation.

- Consideration should be given to referral of patients with minor or worse head injury with persistent post-concussive symptoms for neuropyschological assessment in order to facilitate recovery and resumption of normal activities.

References

1. Tennant A. Admission to hospital following head injury in England: Incidence and socioeconomic associations. BMC Public Health 2005; 5: 21–29.
2. Jamieson LM, Roberts-Thomson KF. Hospitalised head injuries among older people in Australia 1998/1999 to 2004/2005. Injury Prevention 2007; 13: 243–247.
3. Kay A, Teasdale MB. Head injury in the United Kingdom. World Journal of Surgery 2001; 25: 1210–1220.
4. Morris JA, Limbird TJ, MacKenzie E. Rehabilitation of the trauma patient. In: Moore EE, Mattox KL, Feliciano DV, eds. Trauma, 2nd edn. Norwalk: Appleton & Lange, 1991; 815.
5. Lahaye PA, Gade GF, Becker DP. Injury to the cranium. In: Moore EE, Mattox KL, Feliciano DV, eds. Trauma, 2nd edn. Norwalk: Appleton & Lange, 1991; 247.
6. Ponsford J, Willmott C, Rothwell A, et al. Factors influencing outcome following mild traumatic brain injury in adults. Journal of the International Neurological Society 2000; 6: 568–579.
7. McCory P. Does second impact syndrome exist? Clinical Journal of Sport Medicine 2001; 11: 144–149.
8. Goldman H, Hodgson V, Morehead M, et al. A rat model of closed head injury. Journal of Neurotrauma 1990; 8: 129.
9. Javid M. Head injuries. New England Journal of Medicine 1974; 291: 890.
10. Povlishock JT. Pathobiology of traumatically induced axonal injury in animals and man. Annals of Emergency Medicine 1993; 22: 980.
11. Meythaler JM, Peduzzi JD, Eleftheriou E, et al. Current concepts: Diffuse axonal injury-associated traumatic brain injury. Archives of Physical Medicine and Rehabilitation 2001; 82: 1461–1471.
12. Statham PF, Andrews PJ. Central nervous system trauma. In: Baillière's Clinical Neurology 1996; 5: 501.
13. Sosin DM, Sniezek JE, Waxweiler RJ. Trends in death associated with traumatic brain injury, 1979–1992. Journal of the American Medical Association 1995; 273: 1778.
14. Stein S, Ross S. Minor head injury: a proposed strategy for emergency management. [Editorial] Annals of Emergency Medicine 1993; 22: 1193–1196.
15. Shackford S, Waid S, Ross SE, et al. The clinical utility of computed tomographic scanning and neurological examination in the management of patients with minor head injuries. Journal of Trauma 1992; 33: 385–394.
16. Stein S, Ross SJ. Mild head injury: a plea for routine early CT scanning. Trauma 1992; 33: 11–13.
17. Richards KA, Lukin WG, Jones P. Minor head injuries. (Royal Brisbane Hospital, personal communication. Unpublished data, 1997).
18. Lenninger BE, Kreutzer JS, Hill MR. Comparison of minor and severe head injury emotional sequelae using the MMPI. Brain Injury 1991; 5: 199–205.
19. Newcombe R, Merry G. The management of acute neurotrauma in rural and remote locations: A set of guidelines for the care of head and spinal injuries. Journal of Clinical Neuroscience 1999; 6: 85–93.
20. Victorian Road Trauma Committee. Report of the Consultative Committee on Road Traffic Fatalities. Victorian Institute of Forensic Pathology, Royal Australasian College of Surgeons, 1997.
21. McAllister TW. Neuropsychiatric sequelae of head injuries. Psychiatric Clinics of North America 1992; 15: S395–S413.
22. Bullock R, Chesnut RM, Clifton G, et al. Guidelines for the management of severe head injury. European Journal of Emergency Medicine 1996; 2: 109–127.
23. Steil I, Wells G, Vandenheem K, et al. The Canadian CT rule for patients with minor head injury. Lancet 2001; 357: 1391–1396.
24. National Institute for Clinical Excellence. Clinical Guideline number 4. Head Injury. London: NICE, 2003.
25. Mower W, Hoffman J, Herbert M, et al. Developing a clinical decision instrument to rule out intracranial injuries in patients with minor head trauma: methodology of the NEXUS II investigation. Annals of Emergency Medicine 2002; 40: 504–514.
26. Smits M, Dippel DW, De Haan GG, et al. External validation of the Canadian CT Head Rule and the New Orleans Criteria for CT scanning in patients with minor head injury. Journal of the American Medical Association 2005; 294: 1519–1525.
27. Dunning J, Daly JP, Malhotra R, et al. The implications of NICE guidelines on the management of children presenting with head injury. Archives of Diseases of Children 2004; 89: 763–767.
28. McCrory P. New treatments for concussion: The next millennium beckons. Clinical Journal of Sport Medicine 2001; 11: 190–193.
29. Chesnut RM, Marshall LF, Klauber MR, et al. The role of secondary brain injury in determining outcome from severe head injury. Journal of Trauma 1993; 34: 216–222.
30. Fortune JB, Feinstel PJ, Graca L, et al. Effect of hyperventilation, mannitol and ventriculostomy drainage on cerebral blood flow after head injury. Journal of Trauma, Injury, Infection and Critical Care 1995; 39: 1091–1099.

31. Temkin NR, Dikmen SS, Wilensky AJ, et al. A randomised, double blind study of phenytoin for the prevention of post-traumatic seizures. New England Journal of Medicine 1990; 323: 497–502.
32. Clausen T, Bullock R. Medical treatment and neuroprotection in traumatic brain injury Current Pharmaceutical Design 2001; 7: 1517–1532.
33. Edwards P, Arango M, Balica L, et al. Final results of a randomised placebo controlled trial of intravenous

corticosteroid in adults with head injury – outcomes at 6 months. Lancet 2005; 365: 1957–1959.
34. Atkinson L, Merry G. Advances in neurotrauma in Australia 1970–2000. World Journal of Surgery 2001; 25: 1224–1229.
35. Vassar MJ, Fischer RP, O'Brien PE, et al. A multicenter trial for resuscitation of injured patients with 7.5% sodium chloride. The effect of added dextran 70. The Multicenter Group for the Study of Hypertonic Saline in Trauma Patients. Archives of Surgery 1993; 128: 1003–1011.

36. Cooper JD, Myles PS, McDermott FT, et al. Prehospital hypertonic saline resuscitation of patients with hypotension and severe traumatic brain injury. Journal of the American Medical Association 2004; 291: 1350–1357.
37. Myburgh J, Cooper J, Finfer S, et al. Saline or albumin for fluid resuscitation in patients with traumatic brain injury. New England Journal of Medicine 2007; 357: 874–884.

3.3 Spinal trauma

Jeff Wassertheil

ESSENTIALS

1 Cervical spine injury can be confidently eliminated in conscious, clear-headed patients using clinical examination criteria alone.

2 Physical examination alone does not assist in the diagnosis of unstable vertebral injury unless the deformity is gross.

3 A lack of neurological symptoms and signs does not eliminate spinal column injury or spinal cord at risk.

4 A patient can be ambulant and still have a major vertebral injury, even a potentially unstable one.

5 Spinal cord injury may not be associated with a vertebral injury as seen on plain X-ray. This situation is termed a SCIWORA (spinal cord injury without radiological abnormality) and is more common in children.

6 The natural history of spinal cord injury may lead to progressively increasing symptoms commencing some hours after the incident.

7 Magnetic resonance imaging is evolving as the imaging modality of choice in patients with neurological signs.

8 The likelihood of significant vertebral injury in unconscious trauma victims is 10%; 2% of all trauma victims with significant altered conscious state have a spinal cord injury.

9 Although spinal immobilization is a standard of care for protecting the spine, the use of these devices can have adverse clinical effects.

Introduction

Spinal cord injury is one of the most disabling, causing major and irreversible physical and psychological disability to the patient and permanently affecting their lifestyle. The emotional, social and economic consequences affect the individual, family, friends and society in general.

Approximately 2% of adult victims of blunt trauma suffer a spinal injury, and this risk is tripled in patients with craniofacial injury.[1]

Motor vehicle collisions, falls and sporting injuries – notably diving and water sports – are the major causes of acute spinal cord injury in Australia.[2–5] Road traffic accidents account for about half of all spinal injuries. Despite the work to minimize spinal injuries in contact sports such as rugby, serious spinal cord injuries still occur.[2,3] Spinal injuries occur mostly in young people, but minor falls in the elderly or low-impact injuries in people with pre-existing bony pathology can also cause spinal cord damage.[4] Spinal cord injury due

to pathological vertebral fractures may be the first presentation of malignancy.

Observations from two studies[6,7] suggest that possibly preventable neurological deterioration may be due to one or more of the following:

- The injury not being recognized initially, e.g. not being specifically examined for, occult, or masked by other injuries.
- The onset of the secondary effects of the spinal cord injury involving oedema and/ or ischaemia.
- Aggravation of the initial spinal cord lesion by inadequate oxygenation and/ or hypotension.
- Aggravation of the initial spinal cord lesion by inadequate vertebral immobilization.

Pathophysiology

Level of vertebral injury

The level of neurological injury in patients who sustain spinal injuries is variously reported. In studies from Victoria and New South Wales,[7,8] the distribution of the level of injuries was cervical 60%, thoracic 30%, lumbar 4% and sacral 2%.

Spinal cord injuries occur most commonly at the level of the 5th, 6th and 7th cervical vertebrae, largely because of the greater mobility of these regions. The C5–6 and C6–7 levels account for almost 50% of all subluxation injury patterns in blunt cervical spinal trauma.[9]

Associated injuries

There are three noteworthy observations[6,8] from associated injuries in patients with spinal injury:

- Approximately 8–10% of patients with a vertebral fracture have a secondary fracture of another vertebra, often at a distant site. These secondary fractures are usually associated with the more violent mechanisms of injury, such as ejection or rollover. Secondary injuries are usually relatively minor and stable, e.g. fractures of the vertebral processes, but occasionally they may be major and may also be associated with neurological damage. Therefore, when 'thinking spine', it is important to 'think whole spine' and, in particular, to attempt to avoid rotation of the vertebral column.
- Owing to the mechanism of injury, many patients with spinal injuries often have other associated injuries, including head, intrathoracic or intra-abdominal injuries, which may modify management priorities.[4,8]
- Patients may complain of pain from other injuries, and hence a back or neck injury may go unnoticed. Pain may often not be a significant feature despite severe vertebral column damage. Furthermore, spinal pain may take some time to become apparent because of other pathological processes modifying pain, such as swelling and inflammation.

Neurological injuries

Primary spinal cord damage
(Fig. 3.3.1)

Transverse spinal cord syndrome
The spinal cord is completely damaged transversely across one or more adjacent spinal segments. No motor or autonomic information can be transmitted below the damaged area, and ascending sensory stimuli from below the damaged spinal segments are blocked. The manifestations are: total flaccid paralysis, total anaesthesia, total analgesia, and usually areflexia below the injured segment.

The transverse cord syndrome can be incomplete, with partial paralysis, reduced sensation and pain sensibility below the injured part.

The term 'sacral sparing' implies that some sensibility with or without motor activity in the areas supplied by the sacral segments is preserved in an otherwise complete transverse cord syndrome. The presence of sacral sparing implies an

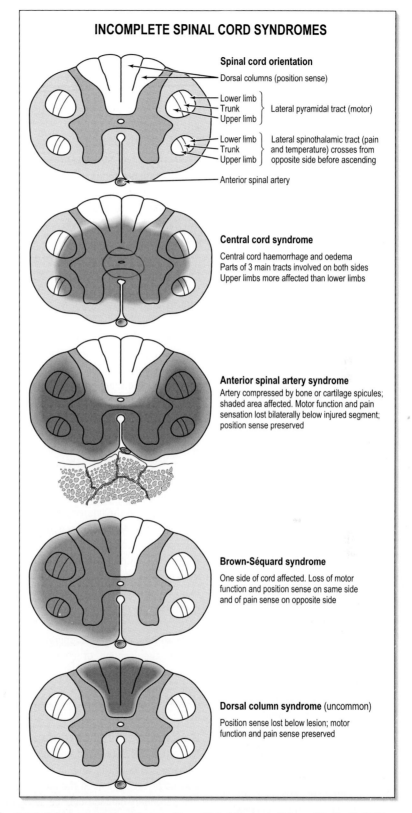

Fig. 3.3.1 Spinal core and syndromes. (From Clinical Symposia Volume 34, No. 2. 1998. Comprehensive Management of Spinal Cord Injury, Plate 11 p.17. Redrawn with permission of Novartis Pty Ltd, Basel, Switzerland.)

incomplete injury, as some neurological transmission through the injured segments is preserved. It will be recalled that spinothalamic and corticospinal transmission to and from sacral segments are located in the outermost parts of the spinal cord, and are therefore immediately adjacent to the origin of the spinal cord's blood supply.

Acute central cervical cord syndrome

The central part or grey matter of the spinal cord is injured. Transmission in the outer rim of the spinal cord is essentially intact but impaired. The signs of this injury are:

- Motor function: there will be weakness in both upper and lower limbs, with weakness marked in the upper limbs.
- Sensation: there is sensory loss in both upper and lower limbs, which is more severe in the upper limbs.
- Reflexes are variable.

This is frequently caused by a hyperextension injury and is typically seen in older patients with cervical spondylosis. In this situation the cord is compressed between posterior osteophytes and the intervertebral disc in front and the ligamentum flavum behind.

Acute anterior cervical cord syndrome

The anterior half of the spinal cord – the region supplied by the anterior spinal artery – is damaged. There is motor loss or paralysis below the level of the injured segment(s). Spinothalamic transmission is impaired and thus there is analgesia with loss of temperature sensation and coarse touch. As the dorsal columns are relatively intact there is some preservation of joint position, vibration sense and fine touch. In the context of an acute cord injury the patient may not interpret dorsal column preservation in terms of joint position sense or light touch. Dorsal column function may be manifested as preservation of vague and poorly localized sensation in the extremities.

These injuries are frequently the result of flexion–rotation or vertical compression injuries.

Brown-Séquard syndrome

This syndrome is a functional cord hemisection with dissociated sensory loss. One half of the cord is damaged. In a pure Brown-Séquard lesion ipsilateral motor function is impaired, as are light touch, joint position sense and vibration. Contralateral spinothalamic sensation – that is, pain and temperature – is impaired, whereas ipsilateral sensation is relatively preserved. Reflexes are variable.

Posterior cord syndrome

This is an uncommon injury that causes contusion or disruption to the dorsal columns, leading to impaired or disrupted proprioception, vibration and fine touch sensation.

This syndrome is usually the result of penetrating trauma to the back or a hyperextension injury in association with fractures of the vertebral arch.

Spinal cord concussion

This diagnosis implies a temporary cessation of spinal cord neurological function. In this instance there is a near full recovery of cord function within 48 hours. The patient will be first assessed as suffering from either a complete or an incomplete spinal cord injury, and will then recover within the above period. The patient has suffered an injury to the spinal cord that has been enough to temporarily cease electrical activity in the injured spinal segment, with no – or very little – mechanical or anatomical injury to the cord, such as haemorrhage or contusion. It is the pattern of recovery over a day or two that allows the diagnosis to be made. Unfortunately, this constitutes less than 1% of all spinal cord injuries.

In all the incomplete spinal cord syndromes the location of cord pressure or damage varies in terms of incompleteness and segmental level(s) of cord injury, and so will the range of symptoms and signs.

Secondary spinal cord damage

It is often believed that most spinal cord damage occurs at the time of injury, but it may occur subsequent to the initial injury.[9] This secondary damage may be caused by:

- Inappropriate manual handling.[7,8] Subsequent mishandling causes significant movement at the site of the primary vertebral injury, leading to spinal cord damage. This can be prevented by careful handling of the patient. It is important to be aware of the possibility of a spinal cord injury and protect the spine until the diagnosis has been excluded. This involves standard cervical inline immobilization, whole-spine immobilization using a spine board, or a Jordan frame and 'log roll' for moving the patient.
- Hypoxia and hypotension.[11,12] These aggravate the primary injury, causing progressive neurological deterioration by mechanisms similar to those that cause secondary brain damage in head injury.
- Acute response to injury.[11,12] Intrinsic metabolic changes in the previously undamaged spinal cord at the region of the initial vertebral injury may also cause secondary deterioration due to oedema, haemorrhage, and the release of metabolically active substances from damaged neurons. The culmination of the pathophysiological processes leads to cord ischaemia and oedema, thereby promoting further neurological damage.

The oedema and haemorrhage tend to resolve within 10–14 days,[13-15] with some improvement in neurological function. Resolving oedema results in local segmental recovery. However, residual ischaemic change in secondarily affected spinal cord adjacent to the primarily injured segments does occur, producing permanent neurologic deficit.

Autonomic nervous system effects of spinal cord damage

The whole of the sympathetic nervous system and the pelvic parasympathetic outflow is transmitted in the spinal cord. In an injury higher than the upper thoracic vertebrae there is significant impairment of total body sympathetic and pelvic parasympathetic functions. The extent and severity of autonomic dysfunction is dependent on the segmental level(s) and the extent or completeness of the neurological insult.

Direct effects

Direct effects include manifestations related to the cardiovascular, gastrointestinal, urogenital and thermoregulatory systems.

Cardiovascular effects

In complete quadriplegia sympathetic denervation causes relaxation of resting vasomotor tone, resulting in generalized systemic vasodilatation. It is recognized by dry extremities with variable warmth and colour during initial assessment. In males there may be penile engorgement or priapism. Owing to the peripheral vasodilatation there is a drop in total peripheral resistance, with consequent hypotension (neurogenic shock). Under normal circumstances this would result in a baroreceptor response in order to achieve compensation. However, as the effector arm of the sympathetic nervous system is paralysed, the normal compensatory effects of tachycardia and vasoconstriction do not occur. The vagus nerve carrying parasympathetic supply to the heart is unopposed, with resultant bradycardia. The higher and more complete the spinal cord injury, the more extensive the autonomic dysfunction.

The usual symptoms and signs of the shock process in response to hypovolaemia cannot occur, as tachycardia and vasoconstriction are mediated by the sympathetic nervous system, which has been interrupted by the high spinal cord lesion.

Gastrointestinal effects

Following spinal cord injury a paralytic ileus develops. This is usually self-limiting and recovers over 3–10 days. Paralysis of sphincters occurs at the lower end of the oesophagus and at the pylorus; as a consequence, passive aspiration of the stomach contents, especially of fluid, is a potential problem. Furthermore, owing to thoracic and abdominal wall muscle paralysis, the capacity to cough and hence clear the airway is diminished. In quadriplegia and high paraplegia, occult fluid aspiration due to passive regurgitation of retained gastric content may not be recognized. The airway therefore requires close observation and active protection. A nasogastric tube must be inserted and gastric contents drained.

Urinary effects

Urinary retention is partly the consequence of acute bladder denervation and, in the early post-injury phase, due to spinal shock. Catheter insertion is required to prevent over-distension of the bladder in order to optimize recovery. It also permits measurement of urinary output.

Thermoregulatory effects

Following cervical or upper thoracic spinal cord injury, the spinal patient effectively becomes poikilothermic. In a cold environment they are unable to vasoconstrict to conserve heat, or shiver to generate heat. The patient is already peripherally vasodilated, which promotes loss of heat and lowering of body temperature. In the warm environment, although the patient is already peripherally vasodilated, the capacity to sweat is sympathetically controlled and therefore lost.

Spinal shock[10,15–17]

Spinal shock is often confused with the neurogenic shock of sympathetic interruption. They are different entities. Complete separation of the spinal cord from the brain abolishes voluntary movement and sensory perception and causes changes in cord physiology and reflex activity. Acute cord confusion is a simple explanation of the resulting pathophysiology. Spinal shock is manifested by the transient cessation of cord activity in the normal cord below the injury. The cord distal to the injury is unable to function as one would expect from a newly created upper motor neuron lesion. Spinal shock may last for a few hours to several weeks, depending on the segmental level and extent of the cord injury. During this period both somatic and autonomic reflexes below the injured segments disappear. Spinal shock has been attributed to the sudden loss of descending facilitatory impulses from higher centres. Recovery from spinal shock is heralded by the return of the Babinski response, followed by the perineal reflexes. In quadriplegia and high paraplegia, as the cord recovers from spinal shock, either recovery of function (depending on the degree of injury resolution at the injury site) occurs or – more commonly – spasticity develops. If the cord injury is at the conus medullaris or the cauda equina, unless recovery occurs, a lower motor neuron pattern with areflexia remains.

Vertebral injury[2,10,13–20]

Cervical spine fractures

Cervical spine injuries may result from one or more combinations of the following mechanisms:

- Hyperflexion
- Hyperextension
- Flexion–rotation
- Vertebral compression
- Lateral flexion
- Vertebral compression
- Lateral flexion
- Distraction.

Hyperflexion

Hyperflexion produces the following injuries:

- A simple, stable wedge fracture
- A fracture with an anterior teardrop
- Bilateral anterior subluxation
- Clay shoveller's fracture
- Bilateral facet dislocation.

Radiographs may demonstrate an associated anterior disc space narrowing and a widened interspinous distance. Bilateral dislocations are evidenced by a displacement of more than 50% of a vertebral body's width of the vertebrae above over the vertebrae below. Oblique views of the cervical spine provide better visualization of the facet joints.

Flexion injuries can cause a vertebral body fracture with an anteroinferior extrusion teardrop fracture. This is often associated with retropulsion of a vertebral body fracture fragment or fragments into the spinal canal.

The clay shoveller's fracture is a particular spinous process fracture produced by a sudden load on a flexed spine, with resulting avulsion of the C6, C7 or T1 spinous processes.

Hyperextension

On X-ray, anterior widening of disc spaces, prevertebral swelling, avulsion of the anteroinferior corner of a vertebral body by the anterior longitudinal ligament, subluxation and crowding of the spinous processes are features of the hyperextension injury. Encroachment on the canal by an extruded disc or a posterior osteophyte may occur in patients with osteoarthritis of the cervical spine.

Flexion–rotation

This is responsible for unilateral facet dislocation or forward subluxation of the cervical spine. On lateral films this injury should be suspected when the vertebra above is displaced on the vertebra below by up to 25%. The injury is functionally stable by virtue of the locked facet and an intact contralateral facet joint. On the AP projection this injury is suggested by angulation of the spine at the level of injury of 11° or more, with the vertebrae above the injury angled towards the locked facet. This appears as a step in spinous process alignment.

Vertical compression

This is the mechanism responsible for burst fractures. The intervertebral disc is disrupted and driven into the vertebral body below. In addition, disc material may be extruded anteriorly into prevertebral tissues and posteriorly into the spinal canal. The vertebral body may be comminuted to varying degrees, with fragments being extruded anteriorly and posteriorly into the spinal canal.

Lateral flexion

This may produce uncinate fractures, isolated pillar fractures, transverse process injuries and lateral vertebral compression.

Distraction

These injuries may result in gross ligamentous and intervertebral disc disruption. The hangman's fracture may also occur by combined distraction and hyperextension mechanisms.

C1 – the atlas

Fractures of the atlas comprise 4% of cervical spine injuries. Mechanisms of injury generally involve hyperextension or compression. Around 15–20% of fractures may be associated with a C2 injury, and 25% may be associated with a lower cervical injury. The Jefferson fracture is a blowout fracture of the ring. Other fractures include isolated injuries of the posterior arch, the anterior arch and the lateral mass.

C2 – the axis

Axis fractures comprise 6% of cervical spine injuries, with an association with concurrent C1 injury in the majority of cases.

X-rays are examined for odontoid subluxation. This diagnosis is suggested when the space between the anterior arch of the atlas and the odontoid is greater than 5 mm. Three types of odontoid fracture are described:

- Type 1 is an avulsion of the odontoid tip. It is generally a stable injury and accounts for 5–8% of odontoid fractures.
- Type 2 injury is a fracture through the base of the dens and is generally unstable. It comprises 55–70% of odontoid injuries. In younger children the epiphysis may be present and be confused with a type 2 fracture.
- Type 3 is a subdental fracture of the odontoid extending into the vertebral body. It comprises 30–35% of odontoid fractures.

Other fractures of the odontoid include avulsion fractures of the lower anterior margin of the body due to a hyperextension injury. A hangman's fracture is a bilateral neural arch fracture of C2. It is a hyperextension injury and is associated with prevertebral soft tissue swelling, anterior subluxation of C2 on C3, and avulsion of the anteroinferior corner of C2.

C3–C7

Examination of the lateral cervical spine film is as previously described. In particular, attention should be directed to the prevertebral soft tissue shadow, which should have a thickness less than 5 mm at C3 and less than one vertebral body's width at C6. Children normally have a prevertebral space thickness two-thirds of the C2 body width. As this distance varies with ventilation, lateral cervical films should be taken in inspiration.

Fractures are defined as unstable when:

- The anterior and all of the posterior elements are disrupted.
- There is more than 3 mm overriding of the vertebral body above over the vertebral body below.
- The angle between two adjoining vertebrae is greater than 11°.
- The height of the anterior border of a vertebral body is less than two-thirds of the posterior border.

Fractures of thoracic spine

Hyperflexion is the principal mechanism of injury to the thoracic spine, with resultant wedging of vertebral bodies. Owing to the rigidity of the thoracic cage and the associated costovertebral articulations, most thoracic spine injuries are stable. However, internal stabilization may be necessary where kyphosis is pronounced.

Thoracolumbar spine

Fractures of the thoracolumbar spine comprise 40% of all vertebral fractures responsible for neurologic deficit. Most are flexion or hyperflexion–rotation injuries. Similar findings to those described in cervical spine injuries may be evident on X-ray. Plain films may demonstrate facet joint disruption, evidence of interspinal ligament disruption, posterior bony fragments protruding into the spinal canal, and burst fragments at the superior surface of the vertebral body. These fractures are generally unstable.

Lumbar spine

Injuries similar to those previously described do occur in the lumbar spine. Three specific injuries of the lumbar spine merit further discussion and are broadly considered posterior distraction injuries of the vertebral arch. They constitute a group known as seatbelt injuries, produced when a hyperflexion force is applied to a person wearing a lap-only type seatbelt.[19] In unrestrained persons a flexion injury generally flexes the spine around a point through the anterior spinal column, typically causing a wedge compression fracture of the body. In the restrained person the point of flexion is moved forward to the anterior abdominal wall. This change in momentum forces converts the hyperflexion mechanism to one of distraction. These injuries are caused by deceleration from high speed, as seen in head-on road traffic accidents or aircraft crashes.

Plain film radiology remains the first-line imaging study. Suggestive findings include:

- A vacant or empty appearance of the vertebral body on the AP film.
- Discontinuity in the cortex of the pedicles or spinous processes on the AP view.
- Fracture, with or without dislocation in the lateral view, which may be subtle.

Computed tomography (CT) or magnetic resonance imaging (MRI) are of value in further delineating architectural disruption. However, the exact nature of the fracture complex may be difficult to delineate on axial images, as the fractures are often orientated parallel to the scanning plane. Three-dimensional reconstruction of multi-slice CT images has greatly improved spinal injury imaging.

These injuries are often associated with concurrent intra-abdominal visceral injuries.

Chance fractures

These are characterized by an oblique or horizontal splitting of the spinous process and neural arch, extending the superior posterior aspect of the vertebral body into and damaging the intervertebral disc.

Horizontal fissure fracture

This fracture is very similar to the chance fracture, with the exception of the fracture line, which extends horizontally through the vertebral body to its anterior aspect.

Smith fracture

This spares the posterior spinous process. The fracture line involves the superior articular processes, the arch, and a small posterior fragment of the superior posterior aspect of the vertebral body. Although the spinous process is intact, the posterior ligaments are disrupted.

Spinal cord injury management

Patients presenting with a potential spinal cord injury are managed in keeping with the approach for any major trauma patient. Therefore, a standard approach of primary survey,[22] resuscitation, secondary survey and definitive management is adopted.

Primary survey

Airway

Assessment of the airway is vital in the management of suspected spinal cord injury, especially when the cervical spine is involved. Passive regurgitation and aspiration of fluid stomach contents may occur as a result of blunting or absence of cough, gag and vomiting responses. This is especially the case with higher cervical injuries. Therefore, the insertion of a nasogastric tube is of vital importance in minimizing the likelihood of aspiration. In quadriplegia and high paraplegia, unopposed vagal action owing to functional total or near-complete sympathectomy predisposes the patient to bradycardia on vagal stimulation of the pharynx. It is important that such patients have ECG monitoring and that atropine be immediately available to block these effects. Pretreatment with atropine prior to manipulation of the upper airway is a consideration.

Breathing

Ventilation may be affected by the level of cord injury, aspiration and primary lung injury. In the absence of major airway obstruction and flail chest the presence of paradoxical breathing is considered highly suggestive of cervical spine injury. Paradoxical breathing occurs because of loss of motor tone and paralysis of thoracic muscles innervated by thoracic spinal segments. Diaphragmatic action results in a negative intrapleural pressure. As a consequence of chest wall paralysis the tendency is for the soft tissues of the thorax to 'cave in', producing paradoxical chest wall movement. The diaphragm needs to undertake the full work of breathing, including overcoming added resistance to ventilation caused by paradoxical chest wall movement. In addition to standard respiratory status assessment, continuous pulse oximetry and assessment of vital capacity is necessary. Early intubation should be considered if vital capacity is inadequate or falling.

Ventilation may be reduced for several reasons:

- The diaphragm may simply fatigue and require assisted ventilation.
- A progressively ascending spinal cord injury owing to either further primary damage or secondary ascending spinal cord oedema may encroach upon the third to fifth cervical segments.
- The same segments may be involved with the initial injury, and thus the diaphragm may itself be partially paralysed.
- The consequences of coexisting chest trauma must also be taken into consideration, as respiration may be embarrassed by the natural progression of thoracic cage, pulmonary or intrapleural injuries.

Circulation

The impact of functional sympathectomy will depend upon the level and completeness of the neurological injury. Complete injuries above T1, and perhaps T4, can be expected to have clinically significant manifestations of neurogenic shock. The clinical signs are bradycardia due to unopposed vagal action, peripheral vasodilatation, and cessation of sweating. Peripheral vasodilatation is responsible for variable cutaneous manifestations. Initially, flushing can be expected; however, the skin may be pale or cyanosed, and its temperature elevated, reduced or within normal limits. The state of the above signs is dependent on perfusion pressure, adequacy of oxygenation and the ambient temperature.

Priapism in a trauma patient is due to penile vasodilatation and is regarded as a highly suggestive sign of spinal cord injury.

Circulatory status is best assessed by conscious state, urine output and venous pressure monitoring. In the early phases of management, close urine output monitoring is of major importance. Early insertion of the urinary catheter allows measurement of urine output, may assist in identifying occult renal tract injury, and also prevents undesirable bladder overdistension.

Volume resuscitation in the resuscitative phase of the primary survey is undertaken in keeping with usual practices. With the exception of perhaps diving injuries, hypotensive trauma victims should be considered as intravascular volume depleted and bleeding until proved otherwise. Standard initial volumes of resuscitation fluid will not adversely affect the haemodynamic welfare. Owing to peripheral vasodilatation, these patients are relatively intravascular volume depleted, and therefore volume preloading is appropriate. However, unnecessary volume overloading in an attempt to substantially raise systolic blood pressure will lead to acute pulmonary oedema.

Disability

Spinal cord injury has an association with significant head trauma.[28] In patients with altered conscious state due to head trauma, the early brief assessment of mental state and pupillary reflexes is important. All trauma victims with altered conscious state require spinal immobilization until spinal cord or unstable vertebral injury is excluded on physical examination and investigation.

In patients with injuries at or above T4 bilateral Horner's syndrome may be present, with relative pupillary constriction.

Exposure

As a spinal cord injury may be one of several injuries, the patient should be fully exposed in keeping with a routine approach to patients with multisystem trauma.

The secondary survey

The definitive diagnosis of a spinal cord injury is made from the findings on secondary survey. Two specific injury entities need to be considered: skeletal and neurological.

A head-to-toe clinical examination is conducted in keeping with the standard conventions used in examining any victim of major trauma. The following outlines the specific points of clinical examination pertinent to spinal injury.

Head and neck

An examination of the cervical spine is conducted while maintaining the patient immobile. Palpation of the spine posteriorly may demonstrate generalized tenderness owing to diffuse muscular spasm. However, the point of maximal tenderness should be determined. In hyperextension injuries the prevertebral and paravertebral muscles are often contused. This is a helpful sign when evaluating hyperextension–hyperflexion injuries in patients who were in stationary vehicles hit from behind. Longitudinal pressure to the head increases cervical pain. Such patients should be considered to have a higher likelihood of a significant vertebral injury.

The neck should be examined for swelling and bruising. Deformity will be noted if there is a dislocation with significant displacement. It should be remembered that significant bony and soft tissue injury frequently occurs without any major findings on external examination.

As prolonged immobilization of the cervical spine with rigid pre-hospital rescue collars and other rigid immobilization devices may unnecessarily add to patient discomfort, complications from the application of splinting devices and the need for ongoing spinal nursing, it is important to determine whether immobilization devices can be removed early during the assessment and treatment phases of management. Reasons for lengthy periods of immobilization include times to definitive radiological assessment and waiting for windows of opportunity to ensure vertebral stability. (Also see Spinal Immobilization and Clearing the Spine.)

An examination of the upper airway is required. A prevertebral haematoma can cause obstruction; the gag reflex may be blunted; airway protection may be embarrassed owing to paralysis of muscles below the neck, resulting in inefficient gag and cough. The patient will have gastric stasis and is at considerable risk of fluid aspiration.

The torso

The patient should either be lifted or rolled on to the side using a formal spinal-lifting technique, so that the back can be examined. The spine is examined for alignment, swelling, bruising and abrasion. Deformity is generally not a feature, except in the presence of major dislocation or disruption.

The rise and fall of the chest is noted. Paradoxical movement is a sign of thoracic cage muscular paralysis, and will be more pronounced the higher the segmental level of injury. Careful examination of the thorax, abdomen and pelvis is required. In both quadriplegia and high paraplegia serious injury may be masked by the use of analgesia and anaesthesia. Significant vertebral injury to the thoracic and lumbar spines is associated with major injuries to the thoracic, abdominal and pelvic organs.

The abdomen is specifically assessed for an evolving paralytic ileus.

Neurological assessment

A thorough examination of the peripheral nervous system is required. It is strongly recommended that both motor and sensory examinations be undertaken in accordance with the following convention. Examine motor, sensory and reflex components independently. Examination begins at the head, and then progresses across the shoulders. The upper limbs are then examined. The torso evaluation begins from just below the clavicles, extending inferiorly to the groins; each lower limb is then assessed. Finally, the saddle area and pelvic floor are assessed.

This approach reduces the likelihood of an incorrect diagnosis of paraplegia by finding a 'pseudo' neurological level of injury just below the clavicles when upper limbs have not been examined. It is therefore important that the upper limbs be assessed before examining the torso.

Motor function

Muscle power is assessed in terms of neurological segments and not muscle groups. Muscle power in each segment is graded from 0 to 5 in the following manner.

Power grade	Clinical finding
Grade 0/5	No movement
Grade 1/5	Flicker
Grade 2/5	Movement present, but not a full range against gravity
Grade 3/5	Full range of movement against gravity with no added resistance
Grade 4/5	Full range of movement against gravity with added resistance but with reduced power
Grade 5/5	Normal power

It is often impossible to assess power grades in certain segments owing to the patient's injuries. The upper limbs are the most easily examined. The strength of a cough provides some information as to the state of thoracic and abdominal musculature.

In the emergency setting the state of the pelvic muscles is determined through a rectal examination by assessing rectal tone and requesting the patient to tighten the sphincter on the examiner's gloved finger.

Sensory function

Dorsal column sensation is assessed using a piece of cotton wool and testing for light touch. Spinothalamic sensation is assessed using a pin or sharp object. Although proprioception, vibration and temperature can be assessed, these are not essential and add little to the emergency examination. When testing with a sharp object a hypodermic injection needle or a trocar stylet must not be used: these are engineered to stab the skin as painlessly as possible, therefore they cause trauma and are unreliable.

The general convention described below should be followed. Sensory examination begins on the face which, as it is supplied by the trigeminal nerve and bypasses the spinal cord, thus acts as a reference point. It is an important axiom based on anatomy that 'in the absence of head injury or local facial injury, sensation to the face is always normal in pure spinal cord injury' (the trigeminal nerve comes from above the spinal cord). It is recommended that examination of the head, neck and upper torso is performed as follows. Start by examining the C2 dermatome laterally on the neck behind the mandible and beneath the ear. Extend examination on to the top of the shoulder, thus assessing the C3, C4 and C5 dermatomes. In the upper limbs examine the dermatomes in segmental order. This should include T2 on the upper medial aspect of the arm. Then carry on examining the torso in the midclavicular plane or at the outer border of the surface marking of the rectus sheath.

Reflexes

Reflexes are examined in keeping with usual examination practices. Superficial abdominal reflexes should be noted. The anal and bulbocavernosus reflexes are important in assessing sacral segments.

Documentation conventions

Two of the pitfalls in the management of any neurological injury are terminology and documentation. The following convention is recommended.

Motor function is recorded either using segmental terminology in written format, or on a muscle chart (Fig. 3.3.2). It will be impossible to chart every segment accurately, but motor power in the upper and lower limbs should be able to be confidently recorded. Power should be graded using the 0–5/5 system.

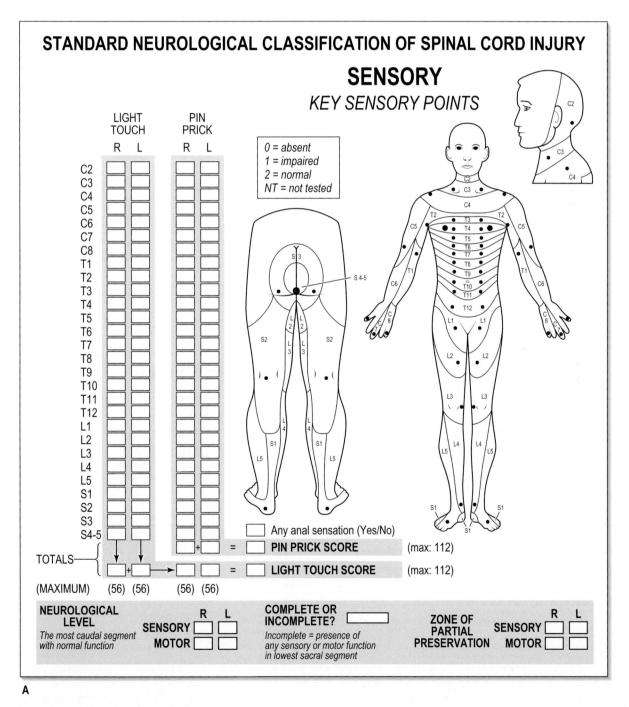

Fig. 3.3.2 Documentation of neurological injury.

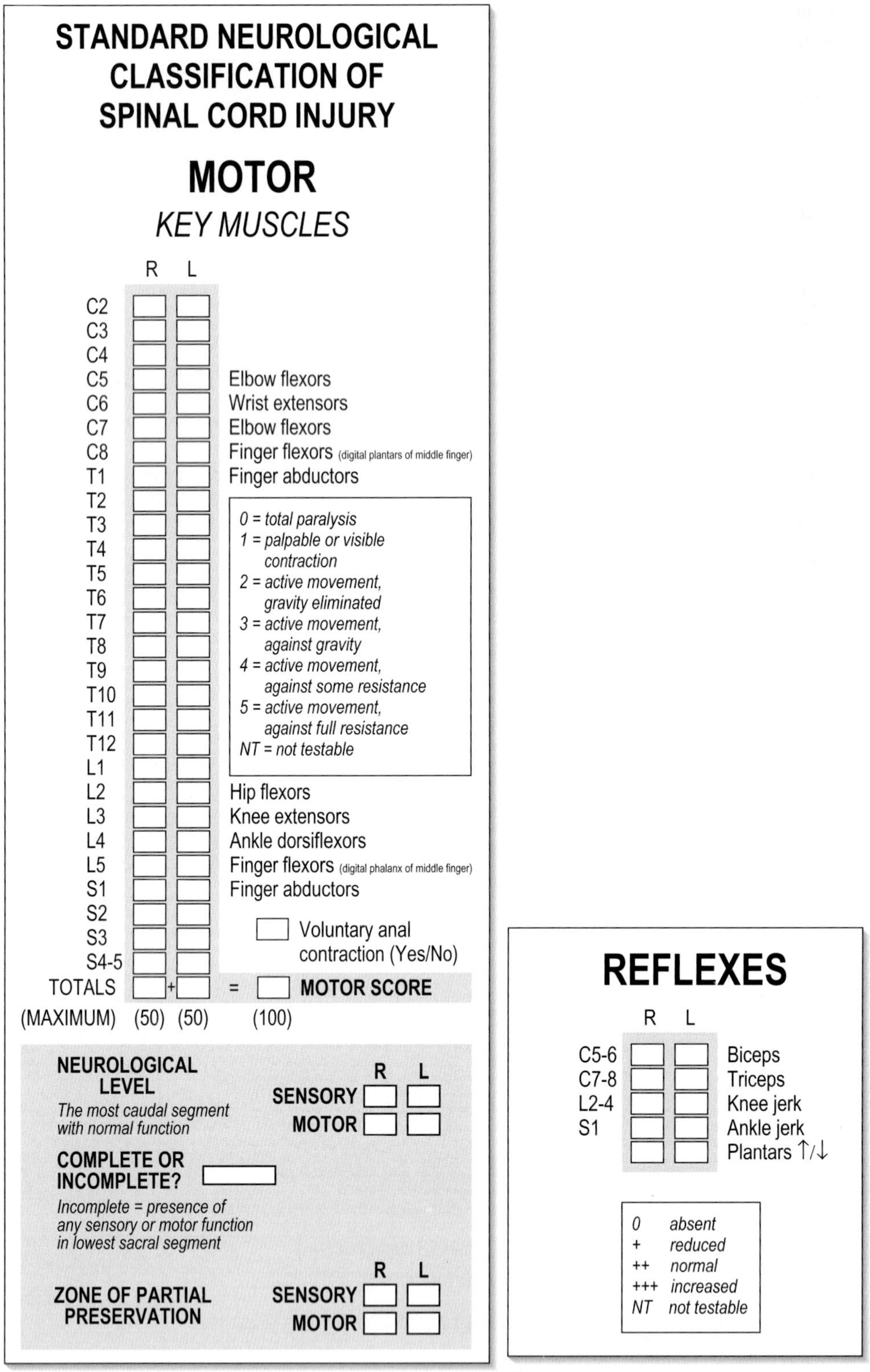

STANDARD NEUROLOGICAL CLASSIFICATION OF SPINAL CORD INJURY

MOTOR

KEY MUSCLES

	R	L	
C2	☐	☐	
C3	☐	☐	
C4	☐	☐	
C5	☐	☐	Elbow flexors
C6	☐	☐	Wrist extensors
C7	☐	☐	Elbow flexors
C8	☐	☐	Finger flexors (digital plantars of middle finger)
T1	☐	☐	Finger abductors
T2	☐	☐	
T3	☐	☐	
T4	☐	☐	
T5	☐	☐	
T6	☐	☐	
T7	☐	☐	
T8	☐	☐	
T9	☐	☐	
T10	☐	☐	
T11	☐	☐	
T12	☐	☐	
L1	☐	☐	
L2	☐	☐	Hip flexors
L3	☐	☐	Knee extensors
L4	☐	☐	Ankle dorsiflexors
L5	☐	☐	Finger flexors (digital phalanx of middle finger)
S1	☐	☐	Finger abductors
S2	☐	☐	
S3	☐	☐	
S4-5	☐	☐	

0 = total paralysis
1 = palpable or visible contraction
2 = active movement, gravity eliminated
3 = active movement, against gravity
4 = active movement, against some resistance
5 = active movement, against full resistance
NT = not testable

☐ Voluntary anal contraction (Yes/No)

TOTALS ☐ + ☐ = ☐ **MOTOR SCORE**
(MAXIMUM) (50) (50) (100)

NEUROLOGICAL LEVEL

The most caudal segment with normal function

	R	L
SENSORY	☐	☐
MOTOR	☐	☐

COMPLETE OR INCOMPLETE? ☐

Incomplete = presence of any sensory or motor function in lowest sacral segment

ZONE OF PARTIAL PRESERVATION

	R	L
SENSORY	☐	☐
MOTOR	☐	☐

B

REFLEXES

	R	L	
C5-6	☐	☐	Biceps
C7-8	☐	☐	Triceps
L2-4	☐	☐	Knee jerk
S1	☐	☐	Ankle jerk
	☐	☐	Plantars ↑/↓

0 absent
+ reduced
++ normal
+++ increased
NT not testable

C

Fig. 3.3.2—cont'd.

Sensation is recorded more descriptively. Normaesthesia, hyperaesthesia, hypoaesthesia and anaesthesia are the descriptors for dorsal column function and testing for light touch. Normalgesia, hyperalgesia, hypoalgesia and analgesia are used in describing pain perception. These are recorded on sensory charts or described according to the following two examples.

In a patient with a transverse spinal cord syndrome, incomplete below C6 and complete below T1, the sensation is described as:

- Normaesthesia and normalgesia to C5
- Hypoalgesia and hypoaesthesia below C5
- Anaesthesia and analgesia below T1.

In a patient with an acute central cervical cord syndrome below C6, with total segmental paralysis in the C6–C8 segments and with some involvement of C5, the sensation might be described as:

- Normaesthesia and normalgesia to C4
- Hypoalgesia and hypoaesthesia below C4
- Anaesthesia and analgesia below C5
- Hypoalgesia and hypoaesthesia below T1.

Unconscious patients

As previously mentioned, the definitive diagnosis of spinal cord injury is a secondary survey consideration and hence identified primarily from symptoms and physical findings. There is no pathognomonic sign of a spinal cord injury in an unconscious patient. The following should alert the examiner to the possibility of a coexisting spinal cord injury in an unconscious trauma victim: [10,15–17]

- Paradoxical breathing or chest wall movement (diaphragmatic breathing) in the absence of a major airway obstruction, stove-in or large flail chest suggests a cervical cord injury.
- Priapism in the unconscious trauma victim suggests quadriplegia or high to mid-thoracic paraplegia.
- Preserved facial grimace in the absence of a response to painful stimuli in the limbs.
- Lower limb flaccidity in the presence of normal upper limb tone suggests paraplegia.
- Observed upper limb movement in the absence of lower limb movement suggests paraplegia.

- The combination of the persistent bradycardia and hypotension despite volume challenge.
- Where this is accompanied by a flaccid rectal sphincter there is an increased likelihood of spinal-cord injury.

Investigation

General investigations are those for multisystem trauma and are tailored to the patient's needs, as determined from primary and secondary surveys (see Chapter 3.8, Radiology in Trauma). The following summarizes key points in medical imaging of spinal trauma (see Tables 3.8.5 and 3.8.6):

- Initial evaluation must include a supine cross-table lateral film. The sensitivity of this is reported as varying between 65% and 85%.
- In the early phase of management, the cervicothoracic junction must be displayed in at least one of a lateral, swimmer's lateral or, if necessary, 30° oblique views.
- Bony definition is best demonstrated by CT. CT demonstrates detail of bony injury, extent of spinal canal embarrassment by displacement of fracture fragments, and dislocated or subluxated vertebrae. CT is indicated in patients with abnormal or inadequate plain films requiring further evaluation, or normal films but unexplained traumatic neck pain in circumstances when there is an increased risk for fracture or cord injury.[23,24,26]
- The role of MRI in spinal injury continues to evolve. It is the investigation of choice in the presence of neurological signs or if clinical concern or other imaging modalities are suggestive of significant subluxation due to ligamentous disruption without fracture. In addition to bony detail, MRI clearly demonstrates the cause of compression, the extent of cord injury and oedema. It provides valuable information on the integrity of ligamentous and soft tissue structures, the state of intervertebral discs, the integrity of vascular supply and the extent of extradural haematoma (Fig. 3.3.4). It is indicated as the investigation of choice in evaluating spinal cord injury without radiological

abnormality (on plain X-ray) or SCIWORA. Although MRI is limited by its availability outside major trauma services, by the logistics of access and by resuscitation needs, it has allowed decisions to be made without the need for other invasive modalities (see Fig. 3.3.3).[24–27]

Management

General

The general management is in keeping with the approach to any victim of major trauma.

Analgesia and medications Owing to the variable physiology of the peripheral circulation due to vascular tone denervation and sympathetic efferent interruption, the absorption of subcutaneous and intramuscular medications is unreliable. It is recommended that analgesia be provided by continuous intravenous infusion, with careful monitoring of vital signs. For similar reasons and where possible, all other medications are administered by the intravenous route.

Specific

Temperature In complete quadriplegia the patient has been rendered poikilothermic by the interruption of efferent sympathetic activity. Attention is directed to ensuring that the core temperature remains within the normal range. Such patients will demonstrate a core body temperature in keeping with changes in ambient temperature.

Immobilization Patients should remain in immobilization devices until spinal trauma has been excluded and splinting of specific injuries can be effected. However, they do not need to be left in the devices applied by pre-hospital care providers: these are structured to provide rigid immobilization for initial stabilization and transport. Nor should they be left tied to spine boards or wrapped in extrication devices, as these are uncomfortable and can cause unwanted cutaneous pressure injuries. Tight webbing and wraps can interfere with respiratory excursion. In general the pre-hospital devices are removed and replaced with more appropriate ones for the emergency department environment.

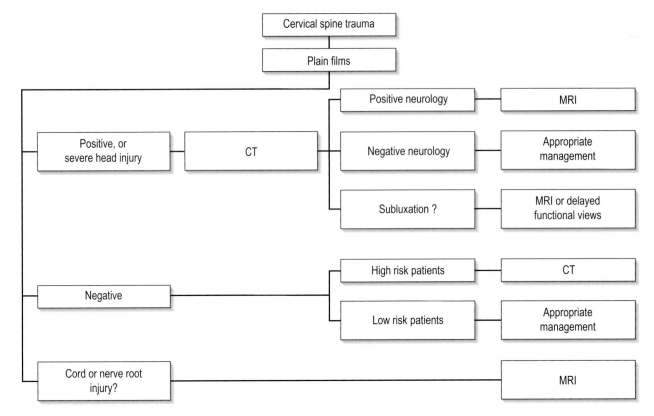

Fig. 3.3.3 Suggested radiological algrorithm for cervical spine trauma.

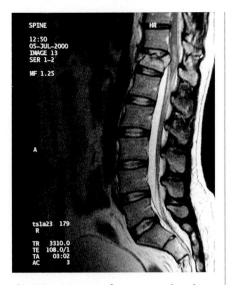

Fig. 3.3.4 MRI scan of acute central cord syndrome.

Corticosteroids–methylprednisolone

The benefit of steroids in spinal cord injury is considered borderline and questionable. Despite this, their use remains a treatment option and several centres prefer to use high-dose methylprednisolone[29–39] in the early management of patients with neurological injury. In Australia, spinal cord injury is not listed as an indication for high-dose methylprednisolone. Therefore, the decision to use high-dose corticosteroids should be made in conjunction with the specialist services, either the major trauma service or spinal injuries service that will be managing continuing care. If used, treatment must be commenced within 8 hours from the time of injury. The total treatment period should be for 24 hours if treatment is commenced within 3 hours of injury, and 48 hours if commenced between 3 and 8 hours.

The use of methylprednisolone is not without complications. It is contraindicated in patients with heavily contaminated open injuries, other heavily contaminated situations such as perforated bowel, and established sepsis. It is relatively contraindicated in diabetes mellitus. Prophylactic measures, such as for acute peptic ulceration and monitoring of blood glucose, should be instituted.

A guideline for the use of methylprednisolone in acute spinal cord injury is presented in Figure 3.3.5.[40]

Advanced airway management Early endotracheal intubation and assisted ventilation should be considered in patients with quadriplegia and high paraplegia. Regular assessment of respiratory status is undertaken and includes continuous pulse oximetry and frequent vital capacity measurement, in order to detect fatigue.

Blind nasal or endoscopic-assisted intubation under local anaesthetic is the preferred mode of non-emergency intubation. The use of suxamethonium is acceptable for a rapid-sequence intubation in the emergency setting. The hyperkalaemia associated with denervation is a concern in injuries more than 10–12 hours old (see Chapter 2.1, Airway and ventilation management).

Intravenous fluids After resuscitation fluids have been administered, haemorrhage controlled, ongoing losses replaced and fluid required for oedema responses to injury considered, routine maintenance fluids are all that is needed.

Paralysis of the sympathetic nervous system, and hence the compensatory mechanisms for intravascular volume depletion, necessitates a heightened suspicion of

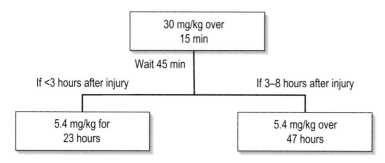

These doses may be approximated to the nearest 0.5 g. For example, a 70 kg patient requiring 24 hours of treatment would need:

Calculation
30 (mg/kg) x 70 (kg) = 2100 mg
followed by;
5.4 mg/kg/h x 70 (kg) = 8694 mg

Actual Dose
2g (1 x 2g or 2 x 1g or 4 x 500 mg vials)
followed by;
8.5g (4 x 2g + 1 x 500mg or 8.5 x 1g or 17 x 500mg vials) over 23 hours

Fig. 3.3.5 Methylprednisolone for acute spinal cord injury.

ongoing bleeding, the signs of which may be dramatic or subtle. Progressive hypotension is a key sign. Paradoxically, the heart rate may rise progressively from a bradycardia of 50–60 beats per minute to more normally acceptable rates. It is uncertain by which mechanism this pseudo or relative tachycardia of quadriplegia occurs. One thought is that with progressive hypotension and brainstem hypoperfusion the vagal effects are switched off by the brain stem, thus allowing the heart rate to rise towards a more normal or denervated range. The skin may develop patchy or blotchy cyanosis. This is due to a sluggish peripheral circulation and hence locally elevated levels of deoxygenated or desaturated haemoglobin.

Inotropic support is often unnecessary.[8,13] However, satisfactory cerebral perfusion is essential. In the patient with a previously normal Mini Mental State examination, deterioration may suggest intracranial hypoperfusion due to either intracranial trauma or the neurogenic shock process. Chronotropic and vasoconstrictor agents are occasionally required. These are more likely to be necessary in older patients, or those suffering from hypertension who are now relatively hypotensive despite volume loading. Chronotropic agents are occasionally required for patients prescribed β-blocker, peripheral and central vasodilator drugs. Likewise, patients with established cerebrovascular disease may require higher perfusion pressures than the resting pressure of the quadriplegic.

The degree of these physiological effects on the circulation will depend on the site and completeness of the injury. Spinal-cord injury below the sympathetic outflow will have little effect on the circulation; complete spinal-cord injury above the thoracic outflow will produce a total body sympathectomy. A complete spinal-cord injury in the mid-thoracic segments should result in preserved vasomotor function in the head, neck and upper limbs. Cardiac reflexes should also be relatively well preserved. Vasomotor tone to the abdominal cavity, pelvis and lower limbs will be paralysed. Likewise, incomplete lesions will have a varying affect depending on the site and completeness of the injury. Careful establishment of the segmental level and degree of spinal cord injury on secondary survey will assist in anticipating the likely extent of autonomic dysfunction.

The denervated lung is intolerant of volume overloading. Therefore, careful monitoring of fluid balance, including urine output and, in circumstances of low urine flow, central venous pressure, is required.

Skin protection Pressure areas and decubitus ulceration are difficult problems to manage. Pressure relief and protection of bony prominences are important concerns from the outset. Hourly pressure lifts should be implemented as soon as practicable: patients should not remain on hard, unpadded surfaces for longer than necessary.

Referral–disposition

Patients with a spinal cord injury should be referred to a centre with facilities for optimal management as soon as practicable. Specific treatments such as immobilization, specific therapy and transport considerations should be discussed with the continuing care provider or spinal injuries unit prior to transfer. If transport is delayed, it is appropriate that the spinal injuries unit be involved and contribute to the patient's initial management, especially in areas of specific management, as soon as possible, even if transfer is to be delayed by several days.

Other treatments

The use of hyperbaric oxygen, naloxone and tirilazad in minimizing spinal injury has been considered in the acute management of spinal cord injuries. Naloxone and tirilazad have no place in management.[29,36] The value of hyperbaric oxygen therapy is at present uncertain and logistically difficult.

The best outcomes in patients with a potential spinal cord injury are optimized by suspecting the injury in trauma victims and preventing secondary injury.

Clearing the spine

Prolonged immobilization of the spine with rigid pre-hospital rescue collars and other rigid immobilization devices may unnecessarily add to patient discomfort, complications of the immobilization devices and the need for ongoing spinal nursing.

Although various algorithms exist for clearing the spine of significant injures and compliance with such clearing algorithms is high,[41] none have been validated for clinical effectiveness. Most incorporate the elements of either the United States National Emergency X-Radiography Utilization Study (NEXUS) or the Canadian Cervical Spine Rules (Canadian C-Spine Rules) thus restricting evidence based decision rules to the cervical spine[42] (see Tables 3.8.5 and 3.8.6).

The need for imaging of the cervical spine can be safely determined by applying the criteria of NEXUS and/or the Canadian C-Spine Rules. The application of one or both of these two clinical tests essentially clears a number of patients of significant

TRAUMA

3

cervical spine injury. Applied during the early phase of the clinical examination, use of these screening clinical examination criteria alone can facilitate early removal of cervical spine immobilization devices without the need for cervical spine radiology.

The fundamental differences between the two tests are that the Canadian C-Spine Rules incorporate mechanism of injury, circumstances and examination findings of active movement of the cervical spine.

Both are sensitive yet non-specific. The NEXUS criteria have a sensitivity of 99% (95% CI 98.0–99.6%) and specificity of 12.9% (95% CI 12.8–13.0%). The Canadian C-Spine Rules have a sensitivity of 100% (95% CI 98–100%) and a specificity of 42.5% (95% CI 40–44%). Reduction in cervical spine imaging was 12.6% with NEXUS and 15.5% with Canadian C-Spine Rules. A comparison of the two methods found in favour of the Canadian C-Spine Rules.[43]

The lateral shoot-through view of the cervical spine is part of routine trauma imaging series in victims of major trauma. Although traditional and considered a standard of care, it is of limited value. Despite the test's high negative predictive value and accuracy, its sensitivity is variably reported to be between 70% and 85%. Therefore, it is a poor screening investigation, missing at least 15% of injuries. Although it can be considered useful in settings where more formal imaging is unavailable, a full imaging series must be performed.

There is little information available to provide evidence-based guidelines for clearing the thoracic, lumbar and sacral spine. The investigation and injury exclusion strategy is based on appropriate clinical reasoning and an understanding of the effectiveness and limitations of medical imaging options, in both logistics and effectiveness. All patients with significant mechanisms of injury and pain or tenderness along the thoracic, lumbar and sacral spine should be imaged. Additionally patients with multiple injuries and high risk mechanisms should be routinely imaged.[44]

Immobilization

Immobilization of the spine continues to be a standard of care. However, the effectiveness of common techniques is largely unproven and there are side effects from unnecessary immobilization. The Cochrane Collaboration failed to infer a potential for good, in spite of the fact that splinting any suspected bony injury is universally considered standard management.[45]

Although failure to detect and immobilize cervical spine injury in hospitalized patients is associated with a 7–10-fold risk of secondary neurological injury,[46,47] it is unclear whether the secondary injuries occur in the out-of-hospital setting and can be prevented by spinal immobilization devices.[48] Despite this, there is some evidence that suggests that not immobilizing the cervical spine is not asssociated with an increase in neurological injury.[49] The weight of opinion is in favour of splinting devices until spinal injury can be eliminated. Therefore, immobilization and the use of splinting devices remains commonplace in clinical practice.

Several types of devices exist and are used either alone or in combination. The common combination in out-of-hospital spine care comprises a cervical collar, spine board and associated padding to ensure a normal curvature of the spine. Other devices, such as extrication devices, not primarily designed as spinal immobilizers, have been used to splint the spine in special circumstances.[50]

The various devices and techniques are variably effective and do not completely immobilize.[51–53] However, they have generally been tested on uninjured subjects with normal muscular tone and posture.

Spinal immobilization can be harmful. Standard spinal immobilization applied to otherwise healthy subjects resulted in significant spinal pain in 100% of subjects.[54] Spinal immobilization can mask life-threatening injuries.[55] Cervical collars have been shown to increase intracranial pressure.[56,57] Spinal immobilization restricts pulmonary function in healthy adults and children.[58,59] Prolonged immobilization of the cervical spine with rigid pre-hospital rescue collars and other immobilization devices may unnecessarily add to patient discomfort and the need for ongoing spinal nursing. This predisposes to pressure area problems and problematic decubitus ulceration.[60]

Controversies

- The best intubation technique in critically ill trauma patients with probable cervical spine injury. Rapid-sequence induction with inline spinal immobilization is preferred in this situation.

- The role of corticosteroids in preventing secondary injury from spinal cord trauma. There are varying protocols in different countries. Although used, spinal cord injury is not listed as an indication for steroid therapy in Australia. Because of this some centres recommend that patients be given the option and formally consent to receive high-dose methylprednisolone. In the case of a patient who is unable to make a decision, a family member should be approached if practicable.

References

1. Lowery DW, Wald MM, Browne BJ, et al. Epidemiology of cervical spine injury victims. Annals of Emergency Medicine 2001; 38: 12–16.
2. Rotem TR, Lawson JS, Wilson FW, et al. Severe spinal cord injuries related to rugby union and league football in New South Wales, 1984–1996. Medical Journal of Australia 1998; 168: 379–381.
3. Yeo JD. Rugby and spinal injury: what can be done? Medical Journal of Australia 1998; 168: 372–373.
4. Lowery D, Marlena M, Browne B, et al. Epidemiology of cervical spine injury victims. Annals of Emergency Medicine 2001; 38: 12–16.
5. O'Connor P. Spinal cord injury, Australia 1999–00. Injury Research and Statistics Series. Adelaide: Australian Institute Of Health And Welfare (cat no. INJCAT 40), 2001.
6. Seleki BR, et al. Experience with spine injuries in NSW. Australian and New Zealand Journal of Surgery 1986; 56: 567–576.
7. Toscano J. Prevention of neurological deterioration before admission to a spinal cord injury unit. Paraplegia 1988; 26: 143–150.
8. Superspeciality Service Subcommittee of the Australian Health Ministers Advisory Council. Guidelines for acute spinal cord injury services. Australian Institute of Health, AGPS, 1990.
9. Goldberg W, Mueller C, Panacek E, et al. Distribution and patterns of blunt cervical spine injury. Annals of Emergency Medicine 2001; 38: 12–16.
10. Swain A, Dove J, Baker H. Trauma of the spine and spinal cord. ABC of major trauma. London: BMJ Publishing, 1991; 38–44.
11. Young W. Secondary injury mechanisms in acute spinal cord injury. Journal of Emergency Medicine 1993; 11: 13–22.
12. Anderson DK, Hall ED. Pathophysiology of spinal cord trauma. Annals of Emergency Medicine 1993; 22: 987–992.
13. Cloward RB. Acute cervical spine injuries. CIBA Clinical Symposia 1980; 32(1).
14. Donovan WH, Bedbrook G. Comprehensive management of spinal cord injury. CIBA Clinical Symposia 1982; 34(2).

15. Grundy D, Swain A. 2001 ABC of Spinal Cord Injury, 4th edn British Medical Journal Publishing, London.
16. American College of Surgeons. Spine and spinal cord trauma. Advanced trauma life support student manual. Chicago: American College of Surgeons: 2004; 177–189
17. Trauma Committee, Royal Australasian College of Surgeons. Spine and spinal cord trauma. Early management of severe trauma course manual. Melbourne: Royal Australasian College of Surgeons, 1992; 157–168.
18. Chandramohan K. The emergency care of spinal trauma. Emergency Medicine 1992; 203–214.
19. Domeier RM, Rawden WE, Evans MD, et al. Prehospital clinical findings associated with spinal injury. Prehospital Emergency Care 1997; 1: 11–15.
20. Schwartz GR, Wright SW, Fein JA, et al. Paediatric cervical spine injury sustained in falls from low heights. Annals of Emergency Medicine 1997; 30: 249–252.
21. Rogers LF. The roentgenographic appearance of transverse or Chance fractures of the spine: the seat belt fracture. Australian Journal of Radiology 1971; 111: 844–848.
22. Holley J, Jorden R, Jackson M. Airway management in patients with unstable cervical spine fractures. Annals of Emergency Medicine 1989 18: 1237–1239.
23. Blackmore CC, Emerson SS, Mann FA, et al. Cervical imaging in patients with trauma: determination of risk to optimise use. Radiology 1999; 211: 759–765.
24. Royal Australian and New Zealand College of Radiologists. Imaging Guidelines, 4th edn. RANZCR, 2001. Melbourne, Australia.
25. Demiatridias D, Charakambides K, Chahwan S, et al. Nonskeletal cervical spine injuries: epidemiology and diagnostic pitfalls. Journal of Trauma 2000; 48: 724–727.
26. Labattaglia MP, Cameron PA, Santamaria M, et al. Clinical outcomes of magnetic resonance imaging in blunt cervical trauma. Emergency Medicine Australasia 2007; 19: 253–261.
27. Cervical spine trauma. In: Lau L, ed. Imaging Guidelines, 4th edn. Royal Australian and New Zealand College of Radiologists, 2001; 45–47.
28. Neifeld GL, Keene JG, Hevesy G, et al. Cervical injury in head trauma. Journal of Emergency Medicine 1988; 6: 203–207.
29. Bracken MB, Shepard MJ, Collins WFJ, et al. A randomised controlled trial of methylprednisolone or naloxone in the treatment of acute spinal cord injury. Results of the second National Acute Spinal Cord Injury Study. New England Journal of Medicine 1990; 322: 1405.
30. Bracken MB, Collins WF, Freeman DF, et al. Efficacy of methylprednisolone in acute spinal cord injury. Journal of the American Medical Association 1984; 251: 45–52.
31. Bracken MB. 1998 Steroids for acute spinal cord injury. Cochrane Database of Systematic Reviews (1): CD001046. DOI: 10.1002/14651858.CD001046.
32. Himmelseher S, Büttner J, Baethmann A, et al. Management of acute spinal cord injury with corticosteroids. Anasthesiol Intensivmed Notfallmed Schmerzther 1999; 10: 716–726.

33. Nesathurai S. Steroids and spinal cord injury: revisiting the NASCIS 2 and NASCIS 3 trials. Journal of Trauma 1998; 45: 1088–1093.
34. Colemann WP, Benzel D, Cahill DW, et al. A critical appraisal of the reporting of the national acute spinal cord injury studies (II and III) of methylprednisolone in acute spinal cord injury. Journal of Spinal Disorders 2000; 13: 185–199.
35. Bracken MB, Shepard MJ, Holford TR, et al. Administration of methylprednisolone for 24 or 48 h or tirilazad mesylate for 48 h in the treatment of acute spinal cord injury. Results of the Third National Acute Spinal Cord Injury Randomized Controlled Trial. National Acute Spinal Cord Injury Study. Journal of the American Medical Association 1997; 28: 1597–1604.
36. Bracken MB, Shepard MJ, Holford TR, et al. Methylprednisolone or tirilazad mesylate administration after acute spinal cord injury: 1-year follow up. Results of the third National Acute Spinal Cord Injury Randomized Controlled Trial. Journal of Neurologic Surgery 1998; 89: 699–706.
37. Hulbert RJ, Moulton R. Why do you prescribe methylprednisolone for acute spinal cord injury? A Canadian perspective and position statement. Canadian Journal of Neurological Sciences 2002; 29: 236–239.
38. Short D. Is the role of steroids in acute spinal cord injury now resolved? Current Opinion in Neurology 2001; 14: 759–763.
39. Section on Disorders of the Spine and Peripheral Nerves of the American Association of Neurological Surgeons and the Congress of Neurological Surgeons. Guidelines for management of acute cervical spinal injuries. Chapter 9. Pharmacological therapy after acute cervical spinal cord injury. Neurosurgery 2002; 50: S63–72.
40. Brown D. Guidelines for the use of methylprednisolone in acute spinal cord injury. Melbourne: Victorian Spinal Cord Service Austin & Repatriation Medical Centre, 2000.
41. Ackland HM. The Alfred Spinal Clearance Management Protocol. Melbourne: The Alfred Hospital, 2006.
42. Hoffman JR, Mower W, Wolfson AB, et al. Validity of a set of clinical criteria to rule out injury to the cervical spine in patients with blunt trauma. New England Journal of Medicine 2000; 343: 94–99.
43. Stiell, IG, Wells, GA, Vandemheen KL, et al. The Canadian C-Spine Rule for radiography in alert and stable trauma patients. Journal of the American Medical Association 2001; 286: 1841–1848.
44. Stiell IG, Clement CM, McKnight RD, et al. The Canadian C-spine rule versus the NEXUS low-risk criteria in patients with trauma. New England Journal of Medicine 2003; 349: 2510–2518.
45. Kwan I, Bunn F, Roberts I, on behalf of the WHO Pre-Hospital Trauma Care Steering Committee. Spinal immobilization for trauma patients. Cochrane Database of Systematic Reviews (2), 2001.
46. Reid DC, Henderson R, Saboe L, Miller JD. Etiology and clinical course of missed spine fractures. Journal of Trauma 1987; 27: 980–986.

47. Davis JW, Phreaner DL, Hoyt DB. The etiology of missed cervical spine injuries. Journal of Trauma 1993; 34: 342–346.
48. First Aid Science Advisory Board. Part 10 First Aid Circulation. 2005; 112: 115–125.
49. Hauswald M, Ong G, Tandberg D. Out-of-hospital spinal immobilization: its effect on neurologic injury. Academic Emergency Medicine 1998; 5: 214–219.
50. Markenson DG. Foltin G, Tunik M, et al. The Kendrick extrication device used for paediatric spinal immobilization. Prehospital Emergency Care 1999; 3: 66–69.
51. Chandler DR, Nemejc C, Adkins RH, et al. Emergency cervical-spine immobilization. Annals of Emergency Medicine 1992; 21: 1185–1188.
52. Mazolewski P, Manix TH. The effectiveness of strapping techniques in spinal immobilization. Annals of Emergency Medicine 1994; 23: 1290–1295.
53. Walton R, DeSalvo JF, Ernst AA, et al. Padded vs unpadded spine board for cervical spine immobilization. Academic Emergency Medicine 1995; 2: 725–728.
54. Chan D, Goldberg R, Tascone A, et al. The effect of spinal immobilization on healthy volunteers. Annals of Emergency Medicine 1994; 23: 48–51.
55. Barkana Y, Stein M, Scope A, et al. Prehospital stabilization of the cervical spine for penetrating injuries of the neck – is it necessary? Injury 2000; 31: 305–309.
56. Kolb JC, Summers RL, Galli RL. Cervical collar-induced changes in intracranial pressure. American Journal of Emergency Medicine 1999; 17: 135–137.
57. Hunt K, Hallworth S, Smith M. The effects of rigid collar placement on intracranial and cerebral perfusion pressures. Anaesthesia 2001; 56: 511–513.
58. Bauer D, Kowalski R. Effect of spinal immobilization devices on pulmonary function in the healthy, nonsmoking man. Annals of Emergency Medicine 1988; 17: 915–991.
59. Schafermeyer RW, Ribbeck BM, Gaskins J, et al. Respiratory effects of spinal immobilization in children. Annals of Emergency Medicine 1991; 20: 1017–1019.
60. Ackland H, Cooper JD, Malham GM, et al. Factors predicting cervical collar-related decubitus ulceration in major trauma patients. Spine 2007; 32: 423–428.

Further reading

Burke DC, Burley HY, Ungar GH. Data on spinal injuries. Part Collection and analysis of 325 consecutive cases. Australian and New Zealand Journal of Surgery 1985; 55: 3–12.
Taskforce on Appropriateness Criteria for Imaging and Treatment Decisions. Appropriateness criteria for imaging and treatment decisions. Musculoskeletal injury. Cervical spine trauma. American College of Radiology 1995; MS 2.1–2.9.

3.4 Facial trauma

Lewis Macken

ESSENTIALS

1 Facial trauma is a common problem in the emergency department, usually as an isolated injury, often after an assault. It may also occur after multisystem injury.

2 Facial injuries that do not threaten the airway or risk life-threatening haemorrhage can usually be assessed and managed as part of the secondary survey.

3 Early diagnosis of facial injuries is important, as late diagnosis may lead to compromised function and an unsatisfactory cosmetic outcome.

4 CT scanning has largely replaced plain radiography for delineation of facial fractures.

5 Penetrating trauma to the face is rarely fatal, but may result in significant morbidity. Attention to early airway intervention is vital after penetrating injuries, especially in patients with gunshot wounds to the face.

Introduction

Facial trauma is defined as injury to the facial soft tissues (including the ear) and bony skeleton. This covers a wide spectrum of injuries.[1] Patients with facial trauma are usually male, between the ages of 20 and 25 years, and have usually sustained their injuries as a result of blunt trauma. Isolated facial injury after an assault accounts for most injuries, with motor vehicle injuries, contact sports and falls accounting for most of the remainder.[2] Up to 20% of patients with facial injuries as part of multisystem injury will have associated life-threatening injuries.[3–5]

Management of blunt and penetrating trauma to the face can be challenging. Life-threatening facial injuries are those that result in airway compromise or ongoing haemorrhage. At the same time, attention must be given to preserving long-term cosmesis and the normal functions of sight, speech and mastication. After immediate resuscitation and stabilization, management of facial injuries requires a knowledge of clinical and radiographic anatomy, the injuries commonly associated with facial injury, and an awareness of treatment methods for the differing injuries to the face.[6,7] Consultation should be sought when the injury threatens the restoration of normal function or appearance. Non-accidental injury should always be considered, as some studies report that over 20% of head, neck and facial injuries in women are the result of domestic violence.[8]

History

The evaluation should commence with the history, with emphasis given to the mechanism of injury. The velocity of force directed to the face determines the degree of facial fracture.[9] Respiratory and haemodynamic observations, and quantification of pre-hospital blood loss, are important components of the history.

Examination

The physical examination involves evaluation of all facial areas by inspection, palpation and assessment of function. Inspection of the face may reveal deformity, loss of normal symmetry, changes in contour, and localized areas of swelling. Skull-base fractures may be suggested by periorbital or postauricular bruising, and the ears must be inspected to exclude haemotympanum or CSF otorrhoea. Gentle systematic palpation of the facial skeleton should follow, assessing for tenderness, and feeling for asymmetry, bony margin irregularities, abnormal motion or crepitus. Specific attention should be given to the supraorbital and infraorbital margins, the zygomas, nasal bones, maxilla and mandible.[1] Mobility associated with midfacial maxillary fractures is assessed by grasping the anterior maxilla with the thumb and index finger of one hand, while stabilizing the forehead at the nasal bridge with the other.[6] Ophthalmological evaluation includes inspection for enophthalmos or exophthalmos, and globe injury, and assessment of pupillary responses, visual acuity, visual fields, extraocular movements, and inquiry for diplopia. Although eye injury is an infrequent complication of blunt trauma, subjective impairment in visual acuity remains the most sensitive single predictor of eye injury,[10] and examination that reveals the presence of an afferent pupillary defect or a non-reactive pupil is the most important factor in predicting the severity of eye injury.[11] The nose should be inspected for the presence of any septal deviation, haematoma (more common in children) or CSF rhinorrhoea. Oral examination is necessary to look for loose, broken or missing teeth, malocclusion of dentition, soft tissue lacerations and contusions.[12] Examination of the mandible includes assessment of the temporomandibular joint in the open and closed positions.

Assessment of the function of facial structures is the final component of the examination of the face. Malocclusion, often identified by the presence of a new gap between the occlusal surfaces of the teeth when the patient closes their jaws, is a good indicator of maxillary or mandibular fracture. Similarly, pain on biting on a tongue depressor, loss of bite strength and limitation of jaw movement are strongly suggestive of a fracture; the patient should be asked if the bite has subjectively changed.[13,14] Motor function of the facial nerve should be assessed, and all three branches of the trigeminal nerve should be evaluated. Commonly encountered symptoms and signs are hypoaesthesia or paraesthesia of the upper lip or upper alveolar margin, suggesting fracture of the maxilla causing injury to the alveolar branches of the infraorbital nerve. Sensory changes in the lower lip and lower alveolar margin suggest fracture through the mandibular canal, causing inferior alveolar nerve injury (a branch of the mandibular nerve).[13]

Radiographic examination

Depending on the mechanism of injury and the severity of the patient's associated injuries, plain radiography may be the initial screening study of choice. The most useful X-ray views for facial bones are Water's (occipitomental) view, which allows visualization of the maxilla, maxillary sinuses, inferior margins and floors of the orbits, and zygomatic bones; posteroanterior (PA) view of the face and skull, which shows the outline of the mandible, but superimposition of the zygoma and mastoid processes obscures the heads of the mandibular condyles; Towne's view (PA view of the mandible) shows the ascending rami and subcondylar regions; submentovertex ('jughandle') views demonstrate the zygomatic arches; and true lateral views. The best X-ray for suspected fracture of the mandible is the OPG (orthopantomogram) view. Aspiration of teeth or fractured dental segments should be excluded by review of a chest X-ray. X-rays should also be considered to help determine the presence of retained radio-opaque foreign bodies within the wounds.[1,6]

In interpreting facial X-rays the examiner should look for signs of loss of bony integrity, which, except for zygomatic arch fractures, will show as a disturbance of the continuity of the bony margins, rather than as a complete fracture line. Also, indirect signs suggestive of anatomical disruption should be sought: opacity or an air–fluid level within the sinuses, herniation of orbital soft tissue, and subcutaneous air.[1,6]

With increasing frequency, computed tomography (CT) is the initial imaging modality of choice. CT will be required for patients with clinically obvious complex facial injuries, especially of the upper and middle thirds of the face, and for patients with multisystem injuries.[15] CT offers the advantages of: clearly displaying soft tissues and showing their relation to the bony skeleton; allowing axial, coronal and sagittal views and three-dimensional reconstruction; showing the degree of skeletal distortion, displacement and comminution; assisting with surgical planning; and allowing other injured areas to be imaged at the same time for multitrauma patients.[6]

Immediate management in the emergency department

It is important to prioritize injuries in the management of the patient with facial trauma because facial injuries that do not threaten the airway or risk life-threatening haemorrhage can usually be assessed and managed as part of the secondary survey. Proper attention should be given to potentially more significant head, chest and abdominal injuries before a non-life-threatening facial injury is thoroughly evaluated, no matter how impressive and disfiguring the facial injury appears.[16] The association of facial injury with cervical spine or cord injury is questionable, especially if vehicular trauma was not the cause.[17] Patients with clinically significant head injuries (especially Glasgow Coma Score (GCS) < 9) are at greater risk of having cervical spine injuries than those with evidence of facial trauma;[18–21] intracranial injuries are more frequently associated with facial fractures than are cervical spine injuries.[22]

Airway management
Asphyxia due to upper airway obstruction is the major cause of death from facial trauma. The airway must be rapidly assessed, respiratory obstruction relieved and an adequate airway established. Signs of partial airway obstruction include tachycardia, tachypnoea, restlessness, fighting to sit up, noisy respirations, stridor, and supraclavicular and intercostal retractions. This may lead to complete obstruction. An unobstructed airway in the presence of facial trauma should be closely monitored because increasing oedema and persistent bleeding may later compromise airway patency.[7,16]

Fractures of the mandible and maxilla with posterior or inferior displacement, together with displaced soft tissues, blood, secretions or other foreign material, may lead to airway embarrassment. Simple airway measures such as chin lift and jaw thrust should be performed, and the mouth immediately examined. Any loose foreign material, such as food, broken dentures or teeth, or bone fragments, should be removed and blood clots suctioned. If anterior traction on the fractured mandible or on the mobile segment of the maxilla (performed by inserting two fingers behind the soft palate and lifting the middle third of the face forwards and upwards) fails to relieve posterior pharyngeal obstruction and does not establish unobstructed ventilation, a definitive airway must be placed.[7] Distorted facial anatomy may make bag and mask ventilation difficult. Rapid-sequence orotracheal intubation can usually be performed. Awake fibreoptic intubation is an option, but the presence of persistent bleeding makes the procedure technically difficult. Standard drills for anticipated intubation difficulties should be at hand, and equipment for performing a cricothyroidotomy and transtracheal jet ventilation should be available. A surgical airway may be life-saving when anatomical disruption makes intubation difficult. A tracheostomy performed under local anaesthesia in the operating theatre is often the safest option in a stable patient with significant midfacial injuries in whom airway difficulties are expected.[23]

Control of haemorrhage
Traumatic facial haemorrhage can be massive, difficult to manage, and potentially life-threatening in approximately 5% of patients with midfacial fractures.[24] Bleeding from midface trauma mainly originates from branches of the external carotid artery (with branches of the internal carotid artery also supplying the nose). Most haemorrhage can be controlled with direct pressure, anterior nasal packs, and double balloon catheters providing anterior and posterior nasopharyngeal tamponade (the placement of 12–14 G Foley catheters with 10 mL balloons inflated and taped under tension to the side of the face is an alternative).[25] Care must be taken with nasal instrumentation: the incidence of associated skull-base fractures is more common with orbital wall or

rim fractures than with more inferiorly located facial fractures. Also, a skull-base fracture is more likely in the presence of multiple facial fractures (the presence of three or more facial fractures is associated with an incidence of skull-base fracture of up to 33%).[26] Attempts to clamp bleeding vessels in the emergency department (ED) should be avoided because of the associated risks of damaging important structures, such as the facial nerve, parotid duct or lacrimal apparatus.[1] If simple measures fail to arrest the bleeding, operative reduction of the fractures, especially of the maxilla, and possible ligation of bleeding vessels should be undertaken, with angiography and selective embolization considered if other measures fail.

Disposition

After initial stabilization, immediate treatment of most facial injuries is mainly supportive. Fractures requiring operative management are often dealt with on a delayed basis, when soft tissue swelling is resolving. The need for antibiotics for patients with facial trauma depends on the mechanism of injury, the extent of the injury, and the immune status of the patient. Prophylactic antibiotics should be considered if there is extensive soft tissue injury, a contaminated wound, open fractures, or fractures communicating with the intranasal or intraoral or intrasinus spaces. Specific antibiotic choices include amoxicillin–clavulanate or cephalexin. However, the evidence to support or refute the use of prophylactic antibiotics in facial trauma is weak.

Most patients with isolated facial injuries not requiring immediate surgical repair can be managed as outpatients, with arrangements made for specialty review within 1 week of the injury.

Thorough documentation of injuries is important for medicolegal reasons, as facial injuries are frequently due to personal assault, and so later litigation is often likely.

Specific injuries

Soft tissue injuries

Soft tissue injuries include abrasions, contusions, lacerations, avulsions and burns. The aim of treatment is to preserve appearance and function. The management of soft tissue facial injuries involves consideration of how the wound should be repaired, and whether it should be repaired in the ED.[1] Possible reasons for delayed wound closure are more urgent coexisting injuries, severe crush injuries, the presence of a foreign body, severely contaminated wounds, and an underlying fracture. In these cases the wound should be irrigated, haemostasis achieved, and the wound covered with normal saline-soaked gauze.

Soft tissue injuries that usually require repair in the operating theatre include ocular or significant eyelid injury; parotid gland or duct injury; facial nerve injury (injuries to the cheek between the tragus of the ear and a line drawn vertically through the pupil may be associated with damage to the facial nerve, parotid gland or duct); nasolacrimal apparatus injury; alveolar process wounds and significant tooth injuries; lacerations with significant tissue loss or contamination or requiring exact anatomical closure; or where difficulties with patient cooperation are expected.[1] Careful consideration is required before areas of special concern are repaired in the ED, e.g. the lips and perioral area; tongue and oral cavity; nose; ears; periorbital structures; and eyebrows. If the wound is closed in the ED, careful attention must be given to thorough cleansing. This can be effectively achieved with pulsatile wound irrigation with normal saline, and abrasions containing dirt or other foreign bodies must be scrubbed to prevent traumatic tattooing of the dermis. If the wound is gaping, or if structures deeper than the skin and the subcutaneous layer are involved, then multiple-layer repair is usually advisable. This helps to prevent deep tissue space collections and may produce a better cosmetic result, with less scar depression or widening. Systemic antibiotics are not required for most facial wounds. However, antibiotics should be given for bites and grossly contaminated wounds; wounds that extend into the oral cavity, nose and paranasal sinuses; wounds with exposed nasal or ear cartilage; crush wounds and wounds with considerable oedema; and for immunologically compromised patients.[12] Tetanus immunity should be assessed.

Facial fractures

The facial skeleton is constructed to allow applied force to be dispersed via a series of small bone fractures, thereby protecting the skull and intracranial contents. The maxilla and mandible require three times the amount of applied force to cause a fracture as do the nasal bones.[1,27] Diagnosis of a facial fracture involves a combination of inspection, palpation and radiographic examination. Fractures other than undisplaced fractures of the nose, zygomatic arch or maxilla will usually require acute maxillofacial surgical review. All fractures should be managed initially with elevation of the patient's head, if associated injuries allow this, and the application of ice.

Mandible

The horseshoe shape of the mandible disperses applied force, which leads to fractures occurring at vulnerable sites regardless of the point of impact, and a high incidence of multiple fractures. Common sites of fracture are the condylar neck and angle, and the body at the level of the first or second molar.[28,29] Fractures of the mandibular body usually demonstrate point tenderness, malocclusion and abnormal range of motion, and interference with normal mastication. The integrity of the dental arch must be assessed. The application of a soft cervical collar may offer symptomatic relief by providing mandibular support.

Radiographic diagnosis is most easily made with a panoramic view, as this demonstrates the condylar region more clearly than other facial views. Antibiotics should be given when there is a suggestion of a compound fracture with extension into the oral cavity. Most fractures will require some form of internal fixation. Complications of mandibular fractures include chin paraesthesia or hypoaesthesia, delayed union, non-union, infection and malocclusion.[30]

Zygomatic arch

Isolated fractures of the zygomatic arch are uncommon and are more commonly part of a more extensive zygomatic complex fracture. An isolated fracture may be evidenced by a depression over the arch, point tenderness, and limited or painful mouth opening owing to impingement on the coronoid process of the mandible by the fractured arch. Surgical reduction is required for cosmetic reasons, or to correct restricted mandibular range of motion.

Zygomatic complex

Blunt trauma to the zygoma more commonly results in fractures at the articulations of the zygomatic bones with the frontal bone, maxilla and zygomatic process of the temporal bone. Separation at the zygomaticofrontal suture, the zygomaticotemporal suture, and at the zygomaticomaxillary suture or infraorbital rim produces the tripod or tripartite fracture. Frequently, the lateral wall of the maxillary sinus and the lateral and central portions of the orbital floor (not to be confused with the orbital blowout fracture) will also fracture as part of the zygomaticomaxillary complex fracture.

Clinical signs of a tripod fracture include flattening of the cheek initially (owing to depression of the fracture segment); this is best seen by standing behind and above the patient, but it is soon replaced by significant swelling. Other signs are hypo-/hyperaesthesia or paraesthesia in the distribution of the infraorbital nerve; asymmetry of the ocular levels; a palpable step defect of the inferior orbital margin; and circumorbital and subconjunctival ecchymoses.[1,13] Diplopia is often also present, and 10–20% of these fractures are accompanied by an ocular injury.[31] A maxillary antrum air–fluid level or evidence of herniation of the orbital contents is often present on X-ray. CT evaluation of these injuries is usually necessary, and all patients will require referral.

Orbital fractures

Fracture of the orbital floor may occur as part of a zygomaticomaxillary fracture, or as an isolated injury – the less common orbital blowout fracture. This is a fracture of the orbital floor without fracture of the orbital margin. An increase in intraorbital pressure, as delivered by a fist or a small ball, is transmitted to within the orbit and the relatively weak orbital floor is disrupted, with possible herniation of the contents into the maxillary sinus.[1] Very rarely a supraorbital rim fracture may be part of a frontal sinus fracture, or a lateral orbital wall fracture may be associated with

a fracture of the zygoma, or a medial orbital wall fracture may occur with a nasoethmoidal fracture. Clinical examination in cases of fracture of the orbital floor may reveal enophthalmos, a difference in pupillary levels, diplopia and impairment of upward gaze, and infraorbital hypo-/hyperaesthesia or paraesthesia.[7] An irregular edge to the orbital rim may be evident on palpation. The integrity and function of the eye should be documented to exclude associated injury. Radiographic examination may show emphysema of the orbit, displaced bony fragments in the maxillary sinus, or the 'hanging drop' sign of herniated contents within the maxillary sinus.[1,32] CT scanning is necessary to define these fractures fully. Orbital apex fractures are uncommon, but clinical or radiological signs of optic nerve compression (e.g. retrobulbar haematoma or bone fragment impingement) necessitate urgent surgical referral.[33] All patients with orbital margin or floor fractures require referral. Complications of surgical treatment of orbital floor fractures include persistent diplopia, hypo-/hyperaesthesia or paraesthesia, ectropion and epiphora.[34]

Maxillary fractures

Fractures of the maxilla include fractures of the alveolar ridge of the maxilla, fracture of the anterolateral wall of the maxillary sinus, and the Le Fort fractures. Isolated maxillary fractures are rare.

In Paris in 1901 Le Fort described a classification of patterns of midface fractures, following cadaveric experiments:[35] Le Fort I (horizontal maxillary fracture) involves only the maxilla at the level of the nasal fossae; Le Fort II (pyramidal fracture) is the most common midface fracture and involves the maxilla, nasal bones and medial aspect of the orbit; Le Fort III (craniofacial dysjunction) separates the midfacial skeleton from the base of the cranium, with the fracture extending through the base of the nose and ethmoid region and across the orbits and zygomatic arches bilaterally.[36]

Most midface fractures are combination injuries, with different Le Fort patterns on each side of the face.[1] Le Fort II and III fractures may require urgent reduction in the ED to improve airway compromise and to arrest ongoing haemorrhage. They may

demonstrate midface mobility and are associated with skull-base fractures, leading to CSF rhinorrhoea. All patients require a complete eye examination, and these injuries necessitate referral.

Nasal fractures

These are common facial fractures. Diagnosis is largely clinical, plain X-rays are unreliable and usually unnecessary, and the major concerns for the emergency physician are control of epistaxis and exclusion of a septal haematoma. Displaced fractures should be reduced within 7–10 days.

Nasoethmoidal fractures are more complicated and are caused by trauma to the bridge of the nose. Disruption of the medial canthal ligaments may produce rounding of the palpebral fissures or widening of the intercanthal distance (telecanthus).[13] Persistent epistaxis and CSF rhinorrhoea may also be evident. Referral is necessary for these patients.

Temporomandibular joint dislocation

Dislocation of the temporomandibular joint may follow trauma to the face or may occur as a result of simply opening the mouth widely. Patients complain of inability to close the mouth and moderate discomfort. X-rays should be performed to confirm that no fracture is present, and dislocation will be evidenced by the appearance of the condyle anterior to the articular eminence of the fossa. A directed history will exclude extrapyramidal dystonia mimicking a dislocation. Reassurance, sedation and firm downward pressure of the physician's thumbs on the patient's posterior teeth, with upward tilting of the symphysis, is usually successful in relocating the mandibular condyles. Post-reduction X-rays are not always necessary. Analgesia and a soft diet should be prescribed and the patient warned to avoid wide opening of the mouth in the short term.[37]

Penetrating injuries to the face

Penetrating trauma to the face from gunshot, shotgun and stab wounds, and impaling foreign bodies is often dramatic at the time of presentation. It is rarely fatal, but may result in significant morbidity. The wounding capability of penetrating projectiles (bullets and pellets) is proportional to the energy imparted to the tissue;[38–40] therefore, the mass of the slug, its velocity and design, and the density of the body tissue penetrated determine the amount of tissue destruction.[41]

Early aggressive airway management is necessary in patients with gunshot wounds to the face, as respiratory decompensation may be rapid: approximately one-third of patients will require emergency airway intervention.[42] Shotgun and stab wounds are less likely to require an emergency airway, although the presence of a significant vascular injury or oedema remains a universal indication for airway intervention, and patients with mandibular entry sites are more likely to require an emergency airway than those with midfacial entry sites. Orotracheal intubation can usually be achieved, with cricothyroidotomy the preferred alternative if necessary. Central nervous system injuries are common, and CT scans of the head and/or cervical spine should be performed at the same time as the facial CT scan.[41–43]

Arterial injury is suggested by evidence of active bleeding and an expanding haematoma; angiography (carotid and vertebral arteries), which is required in approximately 35–40% of cases,[42,43] should be performed when the bullet trajectory suggests proximity to major vessels or the skull base, or where the knife or foreign body is in close proximity to a major vascular structure.[41,43–46]

Peripheral nerve injuries, especially of the facial nerve and the mandibular branch of the trigeminal nerve, are also frequently present.[43] Careful eye examination is necessary because ocular trauma is the most common overall complication of penetrating facial trauma.[41]

Antibiotics and tetanus prophylaxis are indicated, and wounds are managed with conservative debridement, closed reduction of facial fractures, and early repair of palatal injuries. Open facial fracture reduction is usually delayed.[42]

Conclusion

Facial trauma is common in the ED, encompasses many types of injury, and after rapid exclusion of life-threatening complications requires thorough patient evaluation to exclude other more urgent injuries. The aim of management of isolated facial injuries is the maintenance of normal function and appearance.

Controversies

- Consideration of an immediate surgical airway, rather than attempted oral intubation, in a patient with significant facial trauma and a compromised or deteriorating airway.

- The role of angiography and selective embolization in the management of patients with significant haemorrhage from blunt and penetrating trauma.

- Consideration of early intubation in the presence of midface fractures with ongoing haemorrhage in the supine patient with other system injuries.

References

1. Cantrill SV. System injuries: face. In: Marx JA, Hockberger RS, Walls RM, eds. Rosen's emergency medicine – concepts and clinical practice, 5th edn. St Louis, Mosby Year Book, 2002; 314–329.
2. Hogg NJ, Stewart TC, Armstrong JE. Epidemiology of maxillofacial injuries at trauma hospitals in Ontario, Canada, between 1992 and 1997. Journal of Trauma 2000; 49: 425–432.
3. Tung T, Tseng WS, Chen CT. Acute life-threatening injuries in facial trauma patients: a review of 1025 patients. Journal of Trauma 2000; 49: 420–424.
4. Davidoff G, Jakubowski M, Thomas D. The spectrum of closed-head injury in facial trauma victims: incidence and impact. Annals of Emergency Medicine 1988; 17: 6–9.
5. Back CPN, McLean NR, Anderson PJ. The conservative management of facial fractures: indications and outcomes. Journal of Plastic, Reconstructive and Aesthetic Surgery 2007; 60: 146–151.
6. Hasan N, Colucciello SA. Maxillofacial trauma. In: Tintinalli JE, ed. Emergency medicine: a comprehensive study guide, 6th edn. New York: McGraw-Hill, 2004; 1583–1590.
7. Carithers JS, Koch BB. Evaluation and management of facial fractures. American Family Physician 1997; 55: 2675–2682.
8. Ochs HA, Neuenschwander MC, Dodson TB. Are head, neck and facial injuries markers of domestic violence? Journal of the American Dental Association 1996; 127: 757–761.
9. Rhee JS, Posey L, Yoganandan N. Experimental trauma to the malar eminence: fracture biomechanics and injury patterns. Otolaryngology Head and Neck Surgery 2001; 125: 351–355.
10. Dutton GN, al-Qurainy I, Stassen LFA, et al. Ophthalmic consequences of mid-facial trauma. Eye 1992; 6: 86–89.
11. Joseph E, Zak R, Smith S, et al. Predictors of blinding or serious eye injury in blunt injury. Journal of Trauma 1992; 33:19–24.
12. Hunter JG. Paediatric maxillofacial trauma. Pediatric Clinics of North America 1992; 39: 1127–1143.
13. Lynham AJ, Hirst JP, Cosson JA, et al. Emergency department management of maxillofacial trauma. Emergency Medicine Australasia 2004; 16: 7–12.
14. Alonso LL, Purcell TB. Accuracy of the tongue blade test in patients with suspected mandibular fracture. Journal of Emergency Medicine 1995; 13: 297–304.
15. Russel JL, Davidson MJ, Daly BD, Corrigan AM. Computed tomography in the diagnosis of maxillofacial trauma. British Journal of Oral and Maxillofacial Surgery 1990; 28: 287–291.
16. American College of Surgeons Committee on Trauma. Advanced Trauma Life Support for Doctors. Chicago: American College of Surgeons, 2001.
17. Davidson JS, Birdsell DC. Cervical spine injury in patients with facial skeletal trauma. Journal of Trauma 1989; 29: 1276–1278.
18. Hills MW, Deanne SA. Head injury and facial injury: is there an increased risk of cervical spine injury? Journal of Trauma 1993; 34: 549–553.
19. Williams J, Jehle D, Cottington E, Shufflebarger C. Head, facial, and clavicular trauma as a predictor of cervical spine injury. Annals of Emergency Medicine 1992; 21: 719–722.
20. Lalani Z, Bonanthaya KM. Cervical spine injury in maxillofacial trauma. British Journal of Oral and Maxillofacial Surgery 1997; 3: 18–21.
21. Adams C, Januszkiewicz J, Judson J. Changing patterns of severe craniomaxillofacial trauma in Auckland over 8 years. Australia and New Zealand Journal of Surgery 2000; 70: 401–404.
22. Sinclair D, Schwartz M, Gruss J. A retrospective review of the relationship between facial fractures, head injuries, and cervical spine injuries. Journal of Emergency Medicine 1988; 6: 109–112.
23. Taicher S, Givol N, Peleg M. Changing indications for tracheostomy in maxillofacial trauma. Journal of Oral and Maxillofacial Surgery 1996; 54: 292–295.
24. Ardekian L, Samet N, Shoshani Y. Life-threatening bleeding following maxillofacial trauma. Journal of Craniomaxillofacial Surgery 1993; 21: 336–338.
25. Murakami WT, Davidson TM, Marshall LF. Fatal epistaxis in craniofacial trauma. Journal of Trauma 1983; 23: 57–61.
26. Slupchynskyj OS, Berkower AS, Byrne DW. Association of skull base and facial fractures. Laryngoscope 1992; 102: 1247–1250.
27. Luce EA, Tubb TD, Moore AM. Review of 1000 major facial fractures and associated injuries. Plastic and Reconstructive Surgery 1979; 63: 26–30.
28. Halazonetis JA. The 'weak' regions of the mandible. British Journal of Oral Surgery 1968; 6: 37–48.
29. Dongas P, Hall GM. Mandibular fracture patterns in Tasmania, Australia. Australian Dental Journal 2002; 47:131–137.
30. Winstanley RP. The management of fractures of the mandible. British Journal of Oral and Maxillofacial Surgery 1984; 22: 170–177.
31. Larian B, Wong B, Crumley RL, et al. Facial trauma and ocular/orbital injury. Journal of Craniomaxillofacial Trauma 1999; 5:15–24.
32. Pathria MN, Blaser SI. Diagnostic imaging of craniofacial fractures. Radiology Clinics of North America 1989; 27: 839–853.
33. Linnau KF, Hallam DK, Lomoschitz FM. Orbital apex injury: trauma at the junction between the face and the cranium. European Journal of Radiology 2003; 48: 5–16.
34. Whitaker LA, Yaremchuk MJ. Secondary reconstruction of posttraumatic orbital deformities. Annals of Plastic Surgery 1990; 25: 440–449.
35. Le Fort R. Experimental study of fractures of the upper jaw. Revue Chirurgie Paris 1901; 23: 208–227, 360–379. (Reprinted in Plastic and Reconstructive Surgery 1972; 50: 497–506).
36. Manson PN, Hoopes JE, Su CT. Structural pillars of the facial skeleton: an approach to the management of Le Fort fractures. Plastic and Reconstructive Surgery 1980; 66: 54–61.
37. Luyk NH, Larsen PE. The diagnosis and treatment of the dislocated mandible. American Journal of Emergency Medicine 1989; 7: 329–335.
38. Khalil AF. Civilian gunshot injuries to the face and jaws. British Journal of Oral Surgery 1980; 18: 205–211.

39. Cole RD, Browne JD, Phipps CD. Gunshot wounds to the mandible and midface: evaluation, treatment, and avoidance of complications. Otolaryngology Head and Neck Surgery 1994; 111: 739–745.
40. Stiernberg CM, Jahrsdoerfer RA, Gillenwater A, et al. Gunshot wounds to the head and neck. Archives of Otolaryngology Head and Neck Surgery 1992; 118: 592–597.
41. Chen AY, Stewart MG, Raup G. Penetrating injuries of the face. Otolaryngology Head and Neck Surgery 1996; 115: 464–470.
42. Kihitir T, Ivatury RR, Simon RJ. Early management of civilian gunshot wounds to the face. Journal of Trauma 1993; 35: 569–575.
43. Dolin J, Scalea T, Mannor L. The management of gunshot wounds to the face. Journal of Trauma 1992; 33: 508–514.
44. Hollier L, Grantcharova EP, Kattash M. Facial gunshot wounds: a 4-year experience. Journal of Oral and Maxillofacial Surgery 2001; 59: 277–282.
45. Kreutz RW, Bear SH. Selective emergency arteriography in cases of penetrating maxillofacial trauma. Oral Surgery, Oral Medicine, and Oral Pathology 1985; 60: 18–22.
46. Doctor VS, Farwell DG. Gunshot wounds to the head and neck. Current Opinion in Otolaryngology and Head and Neck Surgery 2007; 15: 213–218.

3.5 Abdominal trauma

Garry J. Wilkes

ESSENTIALS

1 One in 10 deaths from trauma is due to abdominal injuries.

2 Abdominal injuries are often occult, overshadowed by more apparent external and orthopaedic injuries, and may be missed initially.

3 Detection of intra-abdominal injuries requires a high index of suspicion to avoid preventable morbidity and mortality.

4 CT scanning provides organ-specific diagnosis but requires sufficient stability for transfer from the resuscitation area.

5 Bedside investigations such as FAST and DPL assist in the evaluation of suspected intra-abdominal trauma but have limitations.

6 Intra-abdominal trauma frequently coexists with other system trauma. Evaluation and disposition are greatly enhanced by early involvement of senior trauma surgeons.

Introduction

One in 10 deaths from trauma is due to abdominal injuries. These may be difficult to detect initially, as the abdominal cavity cannot be viewed with the naked eye, plain radiography is insensitive to intra-abdominal bleeding and solid organ injury, and signs and symptoms of blood loss may be attributed to more obvious injuries. It is therefore not surprising that missed abdominal injuries are a major cause of preventable death in trauma patients. A high index of suspicion should be maintained for this important cause of morbidity and mortality.

A stepwise approach to the management of the multiply injured patient will address the possibility of significant intra-abdominal injury. The principles of initial management are to identify the presence or otherwise of such injury and to determine the need for surgery and the most appropriate timing of interventions. This process requires the presence of an experienced clinician at the earliest possible stage to direct and coordinate the trauma team. Ideally, the trauma surgeon should be present at the initial resuscitation.

The initial resuscitation, history, examination and specific investigations will be reviewed in turn.

Primary and secondary surveys

The abdomen does not normally form part of the primary survey. The unstable patient requiring continued fluid resuscitation without other sources of haemorrhage must be considered to have ongoing intra-abdominal bleeding. Specific points to remember are to expose the patient fully, including an examination of the back as well as the rectum and vagina.

History

The history and knowledge of the mechanism of injury will provide vital clues to the increased likelihood of significant intra-abdominal trauma (Table 3.5.1). Ambulance personnel will be able to provide valuable details of the incident. It is important to remember that trauma does not skip body regions, and that significant intra-abdominal injuries frequently occur in the absence of external signs of abdominal trauma. Other important aspects of focused history are summarized by the acronym AMPLE: Allergies; Medications; Past medical history; Last ate and drank; Events associated with the trauma incident.

Abdominal examination

Penetrating injuries are overt and dramatic. Blunt trauma is more common and more difficult to assess on clinical grounds. Bruising and abrasions are associated with intra-abdominal pathology. The spleen and liver are the most commonly injured organs, with different patterns of injury seen in blunt and penetrating injuries (Table 3.5.2).[1] Marks from lap-type

Table 3.5.1 Risk factors for intra-abdominal injury in trauma patients
High-speed vehicular collisions
Pedestrian struck by vehicle
Fall from greater than standing height
Hypotension or history of hypotension (systolic BP < 100 mmHg) at any time
Presence of significant chest or pelvic injuries
Significant injuries on physically opposing sides of the abdomen

Table 3.5.2 Organ injuries associated with blunt and penetrating trauma[1]

	Blunt trauma (%)	Stabbing (%)	Gunshot (%)
Spleen	40–55	–	–
Liver	35–45	40	30
Retroperitoneal haematoma	15	–	–
Small bowel	–	30	50
Diaphragm	–	20	–
Colon	–	15	40
Abdominal vascular structures	–	–	25

Table 3.5.3 Indications for laparotomy

Immediate

Evisceration
Gunshot wound
Stab wound with peritoneum breached
Haemodynamic instability despite correction of estimated blood loss from extra-abdominal sites
Frank peritonism (initially or on repeat examination)
Free gas on plain radiography
Ruptured diaphragm

Emergent

Positive trauma ultrasound
Positive DPL

seatbelts carry a high association with Chance fractures (T12/L1), small bowel injury and pancreatic injury. Palpation of the abdomen may reveal local/generalized tenderness and evidence of peritonism, but is less reliable in detecting retroperitoneal injury and in the presence of altered sensorium. Auscultation is rarely useful; however, the absence of bowel sounds should increase the suspicion of intra-abdominal injury.

Rectal examination may demonstrate frank blood from injured bowel, a high-riding or mobile prostate from urethral rupture, and may allow direct palpation of fractures or breaches of bowel wall integrity. Vaginal examination is important for similar reasons, and may detect an unrecognized gravid uterus. The examination of the abdomen is not complete until the back, buttocks and perineum have been fully exposed.

Although unexplained hypotension suggests intra-abdominal haemorrhage, not all patients with significant blood loss will display the typical pattern of hypotension and tachycardia.[2] This is especially true of the younger patient. Less than one-third of patients with significant blood loss will have both hypotension and tachycardia.[3] More important are changes in pulse and blood pressure with time and in response to fluid resuscitation. Continuing falls in blood pressure and rises in pulse rate indicate ongoing haemorrhage which, if no other source is identified, must be assumed to be intra-abdominal. Abdominal distension does not occur until several litres of blood have been sequestered, and can initially be confused with obesity.

Once the patient has been examined a urinary catheter should be inserted, unless there is suspicion of a urethral injury. Blood at the urethral meatus, scrotal haematoma and a high-riding or mobile prostate are suggestive of urethral injury, and a urological opinion should be sought before attempting to insert a catheter. In these circumstances a suprapubic catheter may be preferable. Patients with a suspicion of abdominal injury also require a gastric catheter. Nasogastric catheterization is more comfortable for the patient than the oral route, but is contraindicated by evidence of basilar skull fracture. Gastric decompression may be both diagnostic and therapeutic. Penetration of the stomach or proximal small bowel will produce a bloodied aspiration. Aspiration of air will relieve gastric tamponade, which is occasionally an unrecognized cause of hypotension from impaired venous return. Urinary and gastric catheterization is mandatory prior to diagnostic peritoneal lavage (DPL).

A penetrating object, such as a knife protruding from the abdomen, should be left in situ unless it is an immediate threat to life. It is tempting to remove such objects when the patient appears stable in order to examine the patient and the wound tract, but following this impulse can lead to disastrous consequences if the object is adjacent to or penetrates vascular structures. The sudden release of a tamponade may kill the patient in a very short time. The only place to remove a knife or other penetrating object is in an operating theatre, with staff on hand capable of dealing with all possible complications.

Investigations

In the initial resuscitation of all trauma patients blood is drawn for full blood count, urea and electrolytes, blood sugar determination, cross-matching, arterial blood gases (if available) and a trauma radiology series. There is little place for plain radiology of the abdomen.

The indications for immediate laparotomy are listed in Table 3.5.3. Gunshot wounds can produce secondary missiles, are unpredictable in their path, and all require laparotomy. Stab wounds that have penetrated the peritoneum may also require laparotomy and need immediate assessment by an experienced trauma surgeon. In cases where immediate laparotomy is indicated the patient should be escorted to theatre with no further investigations. Further investigations such as trauma ultrasound or DPL may assist in determining the need for or timing of laparotomy if other urgent procedures are also required. The final order is determined by the surgeons concerned.

Unstable patients require surgical intervention as soon as possible. Stable patients can be investigated further, allowing better planning of further management. The difficulty arises in the common situation where there are multiple injuries and only a suspicion – not confirmation – of significant intra-abdominal pathology. Some patients are at risk of abdominal injury but cannot be assessed on clinical grounds. These include those with head, chest and spinal injuries, intoxicated or sedated patients, and those who will be inaccessible while undergoing lengthy operations on other body regions. For these patients it is important to make a further assessment of the presence or otherwise of intra-abdominal injury. Additional investigations of benefit are DPL, computed tomography (CT) and ultrasound. Each has advantages and disadvantages (Table 3.5.4). They may also be

Table 3.5.4 Comparison of abdominal CT, DPL and ultrasound for investigation of abdominal trauma

Abdominal CT	DPL	Ultrasound
Advantages		
Anatomical information	Rapid, cheap, sensitive	Rapid, portable, repeatable
Non-invasive	Minimal training	Non-invasive
Visualizes retroperitoneum	Ideal in unstable patients	Ideal in unstable patients
Also views chest, pelvis	Can be done in resus. room	Can be done in resus. room
		Also views chest, pelvis
Disadvantages		
Not suitable for unstable patients	Not organ specific	Requires specific training
Requires transport from resus. room	False negative	Operator dependent
Patient safety	Retroperitoneal injuries	False negative
Inaccessible while scanning	Hollow viscus injury	Retroperitoneal injuries
Time	Diaphragm injury	Hollow viscus injury
Cost	Iatrogenic injury	Diaphragm injury
False negative	Fluid and gas introduced	False positive
Hollow viscus injuries	during the procedure interfere	Ascites
IV contrast reactions	with subsequent imaging	

consecutive and complementary, thereby minimizing the disadvantages of each individually. Areas poorly imaged by all modalities are hollow organ injuries, such as small bowel rupture and vascular compromise. Serial clinical examination is essential to detect these injuries, even if investigation results are normal.

DPL was first described by Root et al. in 1965.[4] Several modifications of the technique have been described, including open, semi-open and closed techniques, with and without pressure infusion of lavage fluid. Experienced operators can complete lavage in less than 4 minutes.[5] A positive lavage is indicated by aspiration of frank blood, exit of lavage fluid out of other catheters (e.g. intercostal), drainage of intestinal material or bile, or sufficient bloodstaining of the lavage fluid to prevent the reading of standard newspaper print. Additional tests on lavage fluid, such as red cell count, white cell count and amylase levels, have been suggested. The time taken to obtain these results, as well as deciding what constitutes a significant result, limits these other investigations.[6] For example, the most widely accepted cut-off point for significance in red cell count is 100 000 mm^{-3}.[1] Others have suggested a lower level of 10 000 mm^{-3} for penetrating trauma, and levels as low as 1000 mm^{-3} have been suggested in the presence of other injuries.[7] Despite these limitations, a specificity of 99% and accuracy of 95% have been achieved for intra-abdominal haemorrhage, which, when combined with clinical assessment, reduce the

non-therapeutic laparotomy rate to <5% in the presence of systolic hypotension.[8] DPL can also be performed in the operating theatre if desired. DPL does not exclude retroperitoneal injury. The final disadvantage is the lack of organ specificity: only the presence of an intraperitoneal injury is determined, not its location.

Abdominal CT

Abdominal CT is non-invasive and provides precise anatomical details of intra-abdominal pathology. The major disadvantages are associated with the use of intravenous contrast and the need for the patient to be transported from the resuscitation area to the CT scanner, where they are not accessible during the procedure. Intravenous contrast may rarely produce allergic reactions and can precipitate or exacerbate renal impairment, particularly in higher doses and in the presence of renal hypoperfusion and hypofunction. Although modern machines complete scans in a single breath-hold, time is still required to load and unload the patient. Transport and transfer are times of maximum patient risk and minimum monitoring. Therefore, only stable patients are suitable for transfer for CT scanning. Unstable patients require further resuscitation, or operative intervention if this is unsuccessful. The definition of stable is not agreed. The final decision can only be made by the most experienced physician available, although a systolic pressure of at least 90 mmHg

and no requirement for additional fluids after correction of estimated losses would be minimum requirements.

Focused trauma ultrasound

Focused ultrasound is a skill now practised by many clinicians involved in acute trauma management. Abdominal ultrasound is non-invasive, may be done at the bedside, and can be repeated as needed. The technique of focused assessment by sonography in trauma (FAST) can be easily learnt by clinicians and completed in less than 5 minutes without interfering with the function of a trauma resuscitation team.[9-12] Ultrasound combines the advantages of being rapid, accurate and non-invasive, and can be performed at the bedside. It is at least as accurate as DPL, and in experienced hands has similar results to CT in determining the presence of intraperitoneal injury. As a decision-making tool for identifying the need for laparotomy in hypotensive patients (systolic BP <90), FAST has a sensitivity of 100%, specificity of 96% and negative predictive value (NPV) of 100%.[13] Interest and experience in this technique continue to grow with established credentialling.[14] It is the bedside investigation of choice if an experienced operator is available.

Laparoscopy

Laparoscopy has been investigated in some centres, but the skills required and the time needed for a thorough examination limit the widespread usefulness of this modality in acute blunt trauma. However, it is useful in excluding peritoneal penetration in abdominal stab wounds.

Penetrating injuries

Penetrating injuries produce a different pattern of injury (see Table 3.5.2) and are managed in a different manner from blunt injuries (Figs 3.5.1 and 3.5.2). The potential for gunshot wounds to produce secondary missiles and cause widespread injury mandates formal laparotomy in all cases. Stab wounds with haemodynamic compromise or other indications should also proceed to laparotomy without delay for other investigations. Local exploration of stab wounds by

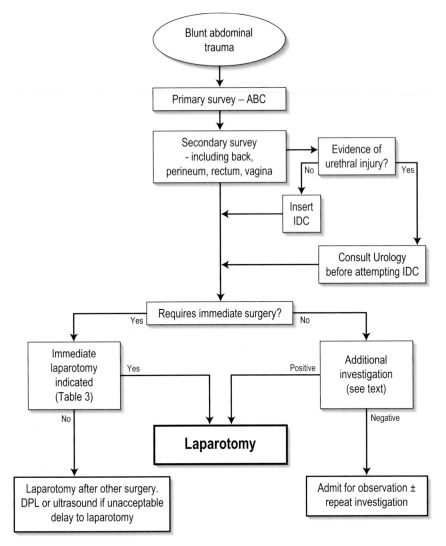

Fig. 3.5.1 Initial management of blunt abdominal trauma.

Disposition

Disposition decisions may be difficult in the less seriously injured patient or those with suspected injury. Every patient suspected or at significant risk of intra-abdominal injury should be admitted for observation and serial examinations, ideally by the same individual. Injuries to the bowel wall or intestinal blood supply may not be evident on initial clinical examination or investigation, and may take 24 hours to declare themselves. A higher index of suspicion is required for patients who cannot be assessed clinically. Unconscious, intubated, head-injured and spinally injured patients are all at increased risk of abdominal injuries and less able to declare them. Serial investigations and clinical vigilance are vital.

Future directions

The difficulty in managing abdominal trauma is determining the presence, location and details of intra-abdominal injury. Current imaging techniques have their disadvantages and limitations. The refinement of modalities such as ultrasound and portable CT will provide more detailed information at the bedside in the resuscitation area rapidly, without the need for invasive techniques. The other area of development will be in non-operative management of injuries using radiological or minimally invasive surgical techniques, thereby reducing the need for laparotomy.

More recently clotting factors such as Factor VIIa have been reported to be of benefit in massive, uncontrolled intra-abdominal haemorrhage. However, cost and prothrombotic effects limit this modality to the category of an investigative agent at this time.

experienced surgeons in patients without evidence of internal injury may be useful, as up to one-third of wounds do not breach the peritoneum. Selected patients may then be managed conservatively.

Controversies

- Haemodynamic stability is not dictated by a single reading of pulse or blood pressure. The need for ongoing fluids in order to maintain adequate perfusion indicates instability even in the presence of normal vital signs.

- In the multiply injured patient there is often difficulty in deciding whether to operate first on the head, chest, abdomen or limbs. All surgeons concerned must discuss the decision.

- Perhaps the most difficult decision is which is the most appropriate investigation in the otherwise stable patient? Each modality – CT, DPL and FAST – has inherent strengths and weaknesses.

- The role of newer pharmacological treatment such as clotting factors is promising and requires further evaluation. At present the most important therapy is early surgery for injury with ongoing bleeding.

- Stopping bleeding early is now recognized in the training of trauma surgeons with the advent of 'damage control laparotomy'. This involves immediate attempts to stop the bleeding, either by ligation or by tamponade, and the realization that definitive surgery can be delayed until the patient is stabilized.

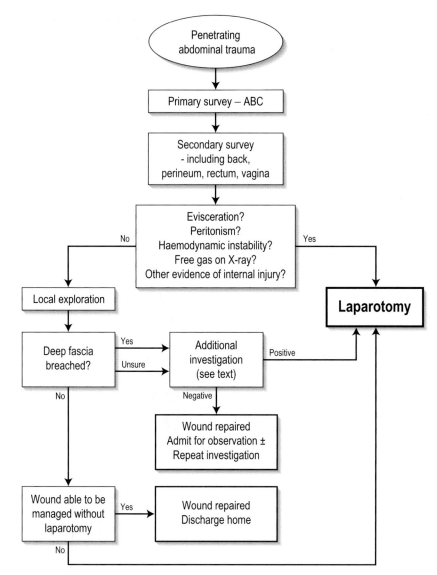

Fig. 3.5.2 Initial management of penetrating abdominal trauma.

References

1. American College of Surgeons Committee on Trauma. Advanced trauma life support student manual, 7th edn. Chicago: ACS, 2004.
2. Wilkes GJ, McSweeney PA. The diagnosis of traumatic intra-abdominal haemorrhage in patients with normal vital signs. Emergency Medicine 1996; 8: 19–23.
3. Grant RT, Reeve EB. Clinical observations on air-raid casualties. British Medical Journal 1941; 2: 293–297.
4. Root HD, Hauser CW, La Fave JW, et al. Diagnostic peritoneal lavage. Surgery 1965; 57: 633–637.
5. Sugrue M, Seger M, Gunning K, et al. A modified combination technique for performing diagnostic peritoneal lavage. Australian and New Zealand Journal of Surgery 1995; 65: 604–606.
6. Feliciano DV, Bitondo Dyer CG. Vagaries of the lavage white blood cell count in evaluating abdominal stab wounds. American Journal of Surgery 1994; 168: 680–683; discussion 683–684.
7. Feliciano DV, Rozycki GS. The management of penetrating abdominal trauma. Advances in Surgery 1995; 28: 1–39.
8. Day AC, Rankin N, Charlesworth P. Diagnostic peritoneal lavage: integration with clinical information to improve diagnostic performance. Journal of Trauma 1992; 32: 52–57.
9. Rozycki GS, Feliciano DV, Davis TP. Ultrasound as used in thoracoabdominal trauma. Surgical Clinics of North America 1998; 78: 295–310.
10. Shackford SR. Focused ultrasound examinations by surgeons: the time is now. Journal of Trauma 1993; 35: 181–182.
11. McGahan JP, Rose J, Coates TL, et al. Use of ultrasonography in the patient with acute abdominal trauma. Journal of Ultrasound Medicine 1997; 16: 653–662; quiz 663–664.
12. Shackford SR, Rogers FB, Osler TM, et al. Focused abdominal sonogram for trauma: the learning curve of nonradiologist clinicians in detecting hemoperitoneum. Journal of Trauma 1999; 46: 553–562.
13. Focused Assessment with Sonography for Trauma (FAST). http://www.trauma.org/index.php/main/article/214/ Updated July 2006. Accessed August 2007.
14. ACEM Policy on Credentialling for ED Ultrasonography: Trauma Examination and Suspected AAA. http://acem.org.au/media/policies_and_guidelines/P22_Credentialling_for_ED_Ultrasonography.pdf Updated July 2006. Accessed August 2007.

3.6 Chest trauma

Mark Fitzgerald • Robert Gocentas

ESSENTIALS

1 Less than 10% of blunt chest trauma patients require thoracic surgery.

2 Radiographs do not reliably exclude rib fracture or other complications.

3 Multislice CT is a useful screening and diagnostic tool for intrathoracic injuries in 'stable' high-risk patients.

4 Adequate analgesia is essential to prevent complications from chest-wall injury.

5 Needle thoracocentesis is an unreliable means of decompressing the chest of an unstable patient and should only be used as a technique of last resort.

6 Blunt dissection and digital decompression of the pleura is the essential first step for pleural decompression. Drainage and insertion of a chest tube is a secondary priority.

7 Pleural decompression and chest tube insertion during resuscitation is a procedure with a low complication rate.

8 Resuscitative thoracotomy should be restricted to those patients likely to benefit. There is clearly a role for resuscitative thoracotomy in shocked patients with sonographic evidence of cardiac tamponade.

Introduction

Thoracic trauma is responsible for 25% of all trauma deaths and contributes to a further 25%. In Australasia and the UK 90–95% of chest trauma is secondary to blunt injury.

The majority of chest trauma patients may be managed non-operatively. Only 10% of blunt thoracic trauma patients will require thoracotomy, the remainder requiring supportive care, including pleural decompression and drainage.

Supportive care, in particular resuscitation, is often suboptimal. Delayed or inadequate ventilatory resuscitation, inadequate shock management, insufficient monitoring of arterial blood gases, and delay or failure to perform pleural decompression and drainage remain identifiable problems that contribute to preventable morbidity and mortality.[1,2] Recently controversy has developed regarding the place of aggressive fluid resuscitation in penetrating chest trauma, which may exacerbate uncontrolled intrathoracic bleeding. It is certainly not a substitute for early operative intervention.[3]

Thoracic injuries evolve. Flail chest, pulmonary contusion, thoracic aortic transection, pneumothorax, haemothorax, pericardial tamponade, respiratory insufficiency secondary to rib fractures and ruptured hemidiaphragm are life-threatening injuries that may not be apparent on initial presentation. These diagnoses need to be pursued and actively excluded. Multislice CT is a useful screening and diagnostic test for 'stable' patients at high risk of potential life-threatening injuries, in additional to the initial supine chest X-ray.[4]

Patients with underlying airways disease and the elderly with diminished compliance are at particular risk.

Anatomically the thorax may be divided into:

- Chest wall and diaphragm
- Pleura
- Lung parenchyma
- Bronchi and trachea
- Mediastinum, including heart, great vessels and oesophagus
- Vertebral column and spinal cord.

When dealing with chest trauma a systematic approach should consider injury in each of these anatomical areas.

Chest wall injury

Fractured ribs

Fractured ribs are a common sequela of focal trauma. Fractured ribs cause pain, which may then interfere with ventilation and coughing, causing ventilatory impairment and atelectasis. This impairment may not be manifest for hours and occasionally days after the injury.

Underlying structures are often injured concomitantly, particularly the lungs, pleura and intercostal vessels. Fractures of the lower left ribs are associated with splenic injury, the lower right with hepatic injury, and the lower posterior ribs with renal injury. The first and second ribs are stronger and less easily injured, and when fractured are usually indicative of significant force to the upper mediastinum. Although first and second rib fractures have been traditionally associated with thoracic aortic injury, the positive predictive value of this association has been questioned.[5]

Rib fracture is essentially a diagnosis based on the clinical findings of local tenderness with or without deformity and crepitus. Up to 50% of fractured ribs are not apparent on the initial chest X-ray. A follow-up film is recommended to improve sensitivity.[6] Reliance on the X-ray to diagnose fractured ribs inevitably results in under-diagnosis. This may lead to delays in diagnosis and therapy and an adverse outcome, particularly with elderly patients and those with coexisting airways disease.

The management of rib fractures centres on pain relief, minimizing pulmonary sequelae and actively excluding associated injury. Oral analgesics usually provide adequate pain relief for single rib fractures. Local anaesthetic intercostal blocks, epidural analgesia and narcotic infusions improve ventilation when impaired by pain, and are often required for multiple rib fractures, particularly in the elderly. Breathing exercises, coughing and incentive spirometry minimize subsequent atelectasis.

Fractured sternum

This is a clinical diagnosis confirmed on lateral chest X-ray. As with rib fractures, concern centres on associated intrathoracic injuries, specifically myocardial and other mediastinal injuries.

The possibility of underlying injury has been related to the mechanism of injury. For example, in North America it is reported that up to 66% of patients with sternal fractures have associated injuries. It is believed that low seatbelt usage results in sternal fractures secondary to impact against the steering wheel. In Australasia, where seatbelt usage is high, sternal fracture is more often caused by the restraining belt. Therefore, comparatively lower deceleration forces are evident, resulting in a reduced association with underlying injury.[6-8]

For isolated sternal fractures admission for analgesia is usually required, although this may be only necessary for 1-2 days. Monitoring is not required unless the mechanism or subsequent investigations suggest underlying mediastinal injury.

Flail chest

Flail chest may occur where the continuity of the bony skeleton of the chest wall is disrupted in two places. It is characterized by paradoxical movement of the associated unanchored chest wall segment. Because of muscular spasms and splinting this segment may not be apparent initially, and may flail some time after the accident. Clinical features of a flail segment may also be masked by positive-pressure ventilation, which splints the chest wall internally. Elderly patients have a less compliant chest wall and are at greater risk of developing a flail segment.

Flail chest is often associated with ventilatory insufficiency. Ventilatory disturbance is caused by hypoventilation of the affected hemithorax due to the mechanical disruption and associated pain, compounded by the underlying pulmonary contusion. Therapy centres on maintaining oxygenation, ventilation and euvolaemia. Adequate analgesia should be supplemented with intercostal nerve blocks or epidural analgesia. In general, patients with a significant flail, which impairs ventilation, will require intubation and positive-pressure ventilation or pressure support. The use of malleable reabsorbable splints for the flail segment is a new approach undergoing clinical investigation.

Ruptured hemidiaphragm

Diaphragmatic rupture may be difficult to diagnose. High-velocity injuries with lateral torso trauma or thoracoabdominal crush injuries should alert the clinician to the possibility of underlying diaphragmatic injury. Associated injuries, such as lateral rib fractures, penetrating left upper quadrant wounds and fractured pelvis, are associated with an increased incidence of diaphragmatic disruption. There may be respiratory compromise, with diminished air entry in the involved hemithorax. Placement of a radio-opaque nasogastric tube will facilitate the diagnosis of left hemidiaphragmatic disruption on chest X-ray. Although gross rupture may be apparent initially, the classic radiological findings of viscera in the thoracic cavity, the nasogastric tube coiled in the thoracic cavity, or marked hemidiaphragm elevation are present only 50% of the time, with no intrathoracic pathology seen on 15% of occasions.[9] Thus many diaphragmatic injuries present late, with complications of diaphragmatic hernias. Spiral CT scan will display gross disruption but may miss small defects. Diagnostic yield may be better with multislice CT or MRI.[10] Occult diaphragmatic lacerations are associated with penetrating injuries of the thoracoabdominal region, and should be actively excluded by laparoscopy, thoracoscopy or open surgery.

The treatment of diaphragmatic disruption is surgical repair.

Pleural injury

Open pneumothorax

Open pneumothorax presents an immediate threat to life. An open chest wall defect disrupts the generation of a negative inspiratory pressure. If the opening is approximately two-thirds the diameter of the trachea, air will pass preferentially through the defect (a 'sucking' chest wound) and respiratory failure will occur.[11]

Initial management includes covering the defect with a sterile dressing and taping it on three sides to achieve a flutter-valve effect, prior to placement of an intercostal catheter and sealing of the defect. Definitive surgical closure is required.

Pneumothorax

Simple pneumothorax is characterized by a visceral pleural rent and pleural air preventing expansion of the associated lung. Although small (< 20%) pneumothoraces may be managed conservatively, larger ones mandate pleural decompression and drainage. There is no evidence that needle thoracotomy is a reliable means of pleural decompression (Fig. 3.6.1). The technique should be avoided during hospital trauma reception and resuscitation and used only as a technique of last resort. Blunt dissection and digital decompression of the pleura should be the technique of first choice. Once successfully performed, it reduces the urgency of the situation and allows time for the subsequent placement of a chest tube.[12]

Intercostal catheters with underwater seal or flutter-valve drainage should also be inserted for pneumothoraces if positive-pressure ventilation is anticipated or has been commenced. If small traumatic pneumothoraces are not drained, the patient should be followed closely with repeat chest X-rays. Intercostal catheters should be placed if the patient is to be airtransported to another facility. Clinicians should be aware of common problems with chest drain placement (Fig. 3.6.2).

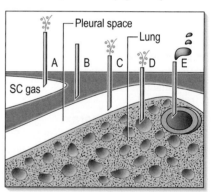

Fig. 3.6.1 Possible positions of needle thoracocentesis (NT). (A) False positive – as needle decompresses subcutaneous emphysema. (B) False negative – as needle does not reach pleural space. (C) Correct position of NT with decompression of tension pneumothorax. (D) False positive – with needle intrapulmonary in bulla or bronchial tree. If the tension pneumothorax is loculated due to pulmonary adhesions and missed by NT a false-negative result may occur with intrapulmonary placement. (E) True negative – with needle in a major vessel or the heart. This may be mis-interpreted as a false positive for haemothorax. Only C will decompress a tension pneumothorax. A, B, D and E have all been associated with failure to decompress the pleural space and fatal outcomes. From 'Fitzgerald M, Mackenzie CF, Marasco S, Hoyle R, Kossmann T. 'Pleural Decompression and Drainage during Trauma Reception and Resuscitation'. Injury 2008 Jan:39; 9–20.

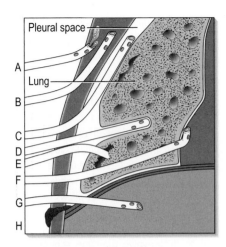

Fig. 3.6.2 Possible positions and complications of tube thoracostomy (TT). (A) Trauma to the intercostal neurovascular bundle. (B) Extrapleural placement. (C) Correct position in pleural space. (D) Intrafissural placement. (E) Intrapulmonary placement. (F) Mediastinal impingement or penetration. (G) Trans-diaphragmatic placement. (H) Infection. From 'Fitzgerald M, Mackenzie CF, Marasco S, Hoyle R, Kossmann T. 'Pleural Decompression and Drainage during Trauma Reception and Resuscitation'. Injury 2008 Jan:39; 9–20.

Thoracic CT scanning will demonstrate pneumothoraces that may not be apparent on plain radiographs.[13] This should prompt intercostal catheter placement in ventilated patients.

Tension pneumothorax

Tension pneumothorax occurs with the formation of a 'one-way valve' from the lung through disrupted visceral pleura. Air collects under tension in the hemithorax, collapsing the lung and displacing the mediastinum, impairing ventilation and obstructing venous return. Tension pneumothorax is more commonly associated with positive-pressure ventilation. It is essentially a clinical diagnosis, characterized by tachypnoea, tracheal deviation away from the affected hemithorax, diminished ipsilateral breath sounds, diminished compliance, oxygen desaturation and hypotension.

If clinically suspected, the affected hemithorax should be immediately decompressed and an intercostal catheter subsequently inserted. Needle thoracocentesis using a 14 G needle inserted anteriorly in the second intercostal space, in the midclavicular line, is the currently recommended initial approach.[14] There should be no attempt to delay chest decompression in favour of a chest X-ray.

Some thoracic trauma patients, after intubation and ventilation, demonstrate air under tension and subcutaneous emphysema on initial chest X-ray, without a pneumothorax being visible. This should prompt immediate chest tube placement, as this is a precursor of ipsilateral tension pneumothorax. The subcutaneous tissues in communication with the air leak offer less initial resistance and display air under pressure, prior to tension developing within the pleural space.

Haemothorax

Blood may accumulate within the pleural space after lung laceration or laceration of a chest-wall vessel and, less commonly, after mediastinal injury. It is indicated by diffuse opacification of a hemithorax on supine chest X-ray, or blunting of the costophrenic angle on an upright film. Once digital pleural decompression has occurred the haemothorax is best drained via placement of a 32 Fr or larger intercostal catheter, positioned in the fifth intercostal space just anterior to the midaxillary line on the affected side. The use of suction (20 cmH$_2$O) facilitates drainage. If haemorrhage is ongoing the blood can be collected in a suitable closed system and may then be autotransfused.

Bleeding is usually self-limiting following drainage. Drainage of more than 1500 mL following initial intercostal catheter insertion, or a sustained loss of more than 200 mL/h for more than 2 hours, are indications for thoracotomy.[15] Large blood losses frequently come from intercostal arteries.

Clamping the intercostal catheter in an attempt to tamponade bleeding and 'buy time' for an intubated and ventilated, unstable patient with a massive and ongoing hemithorax could be considered if delays to thoracotomy arise. However, this technique is yet to be validated in a controlled trial.

Lung injury

Pulmonary contusion

Pulmonary contusion follows focal pulmonary trauma and is characterized by the leakage of blood into the alveoli and pulmonary interstitium, culminating in consolidation and atelectasis. Associated hypoxia may be profound and is evident on arterial blood gases. Tachypnoea with rales is a common clinical finding. The initial chest X-ray

may not demonstrate the severity of injury. Pulmonary contusion may take some time to be radiologically apparent, with 21% of experimentally incurred contusions still not visible on chest X-ray 6 hours after injury.[16]

CT scans provide the most sensitive test for gauging the extent of pulmonary contusion, although arterial blood gases provide the best measure of physiological derangement requiring intervention. Therapy is based on ensuring adequate oxygenation, ventilatory support and fluid restriction. Ventilation should involve low-volume, low-pressure techniques to reduce barotrauma and secondary injury. Steroids have not been shown to improve outcome.[14]

Tracheobronchial injury

Injuries to the trachea and bronchi are rare, accounting for less than 1% of injuries after blunt chest trauma.[17] Eighty per cent of injuries occur near the carina, with mediastinal and cervical emphysema resulting. A persistent air leak should alert the clinician to the possibility of a tracheobronchial injury. Fibreoptic bronchoscopy is the investigative modality of choice. Persistent air leaks often require operative repair.

Mediastinal injury

Myocardial contusion

Although myocardial contusion is common, significant sequelae are rare. Cardiac failure and hypotension are uncommonly associated with myocardial contusion. Although the ECG is used as a predictor of myocardial contusion, it is non-specific and poorly portrays the right ventricle – the area most commonly injured. Cardiac enzyme elevation does occur but is non-predictive and unhelpful. Echocardiography may demonstrate dyskinesis of the ventricular wall. Patients with hyperacute ECG changes or conduction defects should be admitted and monitored for dysrhythmias.

Myocardial laceration and cardiac tamponade

Precordial penetrating injury is associated with myocardial laceration. Bedside echocardiography is useful in demonstrating myocardial injury and pericardial collections. Patients presenting with signs of pericardial tamponade (hypotension, diminished heart sounds, jugular venous distension) require urgent surgical intervention.

Patients who acutely deteriorate into cardiac arrest yet who had signs of life en route to hospital or on arrival require a resuscitative thoracotomy in the emergency department.[18] Outcome for blunt trauma patients without initial signs is very poor (< 2%), but penetrating injury has a higher survival rate. This procedure should only be undertaken judiciously because of the infection risks to personnel. Prolonged (> 9 minutes) external cardiac massage is futile in these patients.[18]

Tension pneumopericardium

Tension pneumopericardium, albeit much less common than tension pneumothorax, is thought to arise via a similar 'one-way valve' mechanism, particularly after the institution of positive-pressure ventilation. It is characterized by raised jugular/central venous pressure and hypotension, and requires urgent pericardiocentesis.[19]

Thoracic aortic transection

Eighty-five per cent of patients with transection of the thoracic aorta die before reaching hospital. Of the survivors, 50% die within the next 48 hours if not operated upon. Sixty-five per cent of injuries are to the proximal descending aorta.

A mechanism of injury involving violent/ high deceleration forces should alert the physician to the possibility of thoracic aortic injury. Lateral- as well as frontal-impact motor vehicle crashes contribute to aortic transection.[20]

Clinical signs, such as pulse deficits, upper body hypertension, unequal blood pressures bilaterally or dysphonia, are uncommon findings. The initial chest X-ray may demonstrate mediastinal widening, loss of the aortic knuckle, loss of the paraspinal stripe, massive haemothorax, and tracheal or oesophageal deviation from the midline.

When blunt thoracic aortic injury was studied prospectively, mediastinal widening was demonstrated in 85% of cases.[21] Mediastinal widening on chest X-ray is 90% sensitive and 10% specific for aortic transection. This means that approximately 10% of patients with aortic transection have a normal mediastinum on the initial chest X-ray. Associated fractures of the thoracic spine

also cause mediastinal widening and make interpretation difficult. There is no thoracic skeletal injury that is a clinically useful predictor of acute thoracic aortic transection.[6]

At present, angiography remains the imaging gold standard. Conventional CT has been shown to be diagnostic in 75% of cases and transoesophageal echocardiography (TOE) in 80%.[21] CT will reliably demonstrate mediastinal haematoma and is therefore a useful screening test. If aortic injury is not apparent and mediastinal haematoma is evident on conventional CT, the patient should undergo angiography. However, better definition with new multislice CT scans is increasing the diagnosis of intimal injury. This newer modality is replacing the need for angiography compared to when conventional CT is used. However, aortography may still be indicated for selected cases when the diagnosis of aortic injury on multislice CT is equivocal.[4]

TOE accuracy is operator dependent. It has been used as a screening tool for aortic tears[22] and is useful for patients in theatre or those unable to be moved to angiography.[23,24]

Multicentre studies of aortic transection demonstrate three patient populations: those in extremis, those who are unstable, and a third, more 'stable', group.[25] Patients in extremis from aortic transection rarely survive. In unstable patients (systolic BP < 90 mmHg) surgical repair is indicated, although overall mortality is greater than 85%. Recent research suggests that in 'stable' patients (systolic BP > 90 mmHg) blood pressure control with β-blockade is indicated prior to surgical repair. Blood pressure control reduces shearing forces at the site of aortic transection, increasing the likelihood of containment within the mediastinal haematoma prior to operative repair. 'Stable' patients with coronary artery disease and 'stable' patients aged over 55 may fare worse with immediate operative repair, and non-operative management or endoluminal graft placement should be considered.[25]

Recent data support the use of endovascular stent placement as a treatment for blunt thoracic aortic injury. To date, the safety and efficacy of endoluminal stenting appear to be comparable to or possibly better than for primary aortic repair.[26–30]

Oesophageal perforation

Oesophageal rupture after blunt chest trauma is rare. The lower third of the oesophagus is the commonest site of rupture, presumably secondary to a forced Valsalva manoeuvre. Mediastinitis is a subsequent development. Retrosternal pain is common and mediastinal air may be seen on chest X-ray.

A Gastrografin swallow and CT scanning is the study of choice. Mortality is directly related to time to operative repair.[31]

Gunshot injuries across the truncal midline more commonly involve mediastinal and spinal structures and therefore have a much greater mortality than unilateral injuries.[32] It is important to exclude oesophageal injury early with penetrating and transmediastinal wounds, as it constitutes significant morbidity and mortality in those patients who survive to hospital.

Vertebral column and spinal cord injury

Exclusion of thoracic spine fractures and spinal-cord injury forms part of the routine work-up of the chest trauma patient. Occult injuries are common, and unstable injuries in ventilated patients require skilled nursing. Such injuries are easily overlooked.

Indications for emergency thoracotomy[33]

Although more than 90% of chest trauma patients may be managed non-operatively, the following categories warrant surgical intervention:

- Cardiac tamponade
- Acute deterioration – cardiac arrest in patients with penetrating truncal trauma
- Vascular injury at the thoracic outlet
- Traumatic thoracotomy (loss of chest-wall substance)
- Massive air leak from chest tube
- Massive or continuing haemothorax
- Mediastinal traversing penetrating injury
- Endoscopic or radiographic demonstration of oesophageal injury
- Endoscopic or radiographic demonstration of tracheal or bronchial injury

- Radiographic evidence of great vessel injury
- Thoracic penetration with industrial liquids (especially coal tar products).

Resuscitative thoracotomy

Left anterolateral thoracotomy as a resuscitative manoeuvre allows direct access to the heart and pericardial decompression for patients who have lost output following cardiac lacerations. Myocardial wounds can then be directly controlled. Right atrial catheterization facilitating IV fluid administration, pulmonary hilar clamping, cross-clamping of the descending aorta and open cardiac massage are adjunctive procedures performed if indicated.

Survival rates of better than 40% have been reported in some subgroups of penetrating trauma arrest, specifically precordial stab wounds. Survival was dependent on resuscitative thoracotomy performed within 10 minutes of arrest secondary to penetrating chest trauma and an organized cardiac electrical rhythm being present.[34-37] Left anterolateral thoracotomy allows pericardial decompression[17] in patients who have lost output following penetrating injury to the heart. Myocardial wounds can then be directly controlled. The role of resuscitative thoracotomy in blunt trauma arrest is more controversial, with a relatively low survival rate (< 3%).[38]

Focused assessment with sonography in trauma (FAST) is an important triage tool in determining the presence of cardiac tamponade. Immediate use of ultrasonography can establish the diagnosis of haemopericardium, and prompt repair of the injury may improve overall survival. Unresponsive hypotension with a systolic blood pressure of less than 70 mmHg and a FAST positive for pericardial tamponade is a consensus-based indication for immediate resuscitative thoracotomy. For patients with severe hypotension or in extremis, the treatment of choice is resuscitative thoracotomy, decompression of the pericardium and control of the cardiac injury.

Given the widespread availability of ultrasound, arguments about resuscitative thoracotomy for blunt trauma should include the important decision support provided by sonography. There is clearly a role for resuscitative thoracotomy in shocked patients with cardiac tamponade following blunt trauma.

Conclusion

Less than 10% of blunt thoracic trauma patients will require thoracotomy, the remainder requiring supportive care, including chest decompression and drainage. Indications for immediate chest decompression are ventilatory or respiratory compromise (Fig. 3.6.3). The significance and severity of chest trauma may not be obvious on initial examination. Patients with underlying airway disease and elderly patients with diminished compliance are at particular risk. Delayed or inadequate ventilatory resuscitation, inadequate shock management, insufficient monitoring of arterial blood gases, and delay or failure to perform pleural decompression and drainage remain identifiable problems in emergency departments.

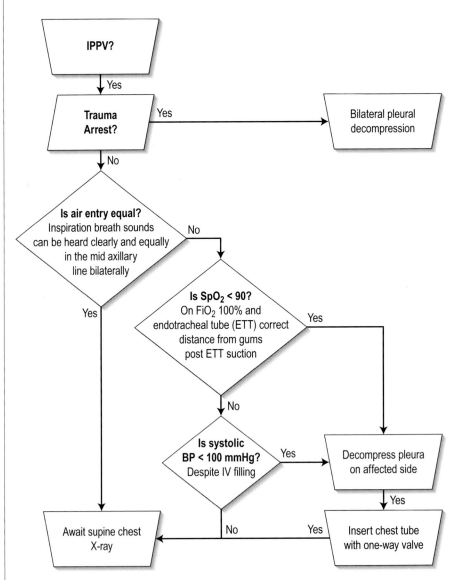

Fig. 3.6.3 Initial binary decision tree for pleural decompression. From 'Fitzgerald M, Mackenzie CF, Marasco S, Hoyle R, Kossmann T.'Pleural Decompression and Drainage during Trauma Reception and Resuscitation'. Injury 2008 Jan:39; 9–20.

References

1. McDermott F. Severe chest injuries: problems in Victoria. Issues and controversies in the early management of major trauma. Melbourne: Alfred Hospital and Monash University Department of Surgery, 1994.
2. Danne P, Brazenor G, Cade R, et al. The Major Trauma Management Study: an analysis of the efficacy of current trauma care. Australian and New Zealand Journal of Surgery 1998; 68: 50–57.
3. Civil I. Resuscitation following injury: an end or a means? Australian and New Zealand Journal of Surgery 1993; 63: 5–10.
4. Mirvis SE. Imaging of acute thoracic injury: The advent of MDCT screening Seminars in Ultrasound, CT and MRI 2005; 26: 305–331.
5. Lee J, Harris JH, Duke JD, Williams JS. Noncorrelation between thoracic skeleton injuries and traumatic aortic tear. Journal of Trauma 1997; 43: 400–404.
6. Hehir MD, Hollands MJ, Deane SA. The accuracy of the first chest X-ray in the trauma patient. Australian and New Zealand Journal of Surgery 1990; 60: 529–532.
7. Brookes JG, Dunn RJ, Rogers IR. Sternal fractures: A retrospective analysis of 272 cases. Journal of Trauma 1993; 35: 46–54.
8. Hills MW, Delprado AM, Deane SA. Sternal fractures: associated injuries and management. Journal of Trauma 1993; 35: 55–60.
9. Brasel KJ, Borgstrom DC, Meyer P. Predictors of outcome in blunt diaphragm rupture. Journal of Trauma 1996; 41: 484–487.
10. Mirvis SE. Diagnostic imaging of acute thoracic injury Seminars in Ultrasound, CT and MRI 2004; 25: 156–179.
11. American College of Surgeons Committee on Trauma. Advanced trauma life support student manual. Chicago: American College of Surgeons 2004;105.
12. Fitzgerald M, Mackenzie C F, Marasco S. Pleural decompression and drainage during trauma reception and resuscitation. Injury 2008; 39; 9–20.
13. Blostein P, Hodgman CG. Computed tomography of the chest in blunt thoracic trauma: results of a prospective study. Journal of Trauma 1997; 43: 3–18.
14. American College of Surgeons Committee on Trauma. Advanced trauma life support student manual. Chicago: American College of Surgeons, 1997;153.
15. American College of Surgeons Committee on Trauma. Advanced trauma life support student manual. Chicago: American College of Surgeons, 2004;109.
16. Cohn S. Pulmonary contusion: review of the clinical entity. Journal of Trauma 1997; 42: 973–979.
17. Mulder DS, Barkun JS. Injuries to the trachea, bronchus and oesophagus. In: Moore EE, Mattox KL, Feliciano DV, eds. Trauma. Norwalk: Appleton & Lange, 1991; 345–355.
18. Jorden RC. Penetrating chest trauma. Emergency Medicine Clinics of North America 1993; 11: 97–106.
19. Fitzgerald MC, Foord K. Tension pneumopericardium following blunt trauma. Emergency Medicine 1993; 5: 74–77.
20. Katyal D, McLellan B, Brenneman F, et al. Lateral impact motor vehicle collisions: a significant cause of traumatic rupture of the thoracic aorta. Journal of Trauma 1997; 45: 769–772.
21. Fabian T, Richardson JD, Croce MA, et al. Prospective study of blunt aortic injury: multicenter trial of the American Association for the Surgery of Trauma. Journal of Trauma 1997; 42: 374–383.
22. Cohn SM, Burns, GA, Jaffe C, Milner KA. Exclusion of aortic tear in the unstable trauma patient: the utility of transoesophageal echocardiography. Journal of Trauma 1995; 39: 1087–1090.
23. Ben-Menachem Y. Assessment of blunt aortic-brachiocephalic trauma: should angiography be supplanted by transoesophageal echocardiography? Journal of Trauma 1997; 42: 969–972.
24. Mattox K. Red River anthology. Journal of Trauma 1997; 3: 353–368.
25. Camp PC, Shackford SR and the Western Trauma Association Multicenter Study Group. Outcome after blunt thoracic aortic laceration: identification of a high-risk cohort. Journal of Trauma 1997; 43: 413–422.
26. Lebl DR, Rochelle AD, Spain DA, et al. Dramatic shift in the primary management of traumatic aortic rupture Archives Surgery 2006; 141: 177–180.
27. Andrassy J, Weidenhagen R, Meimarakis G. Stent versus open surgery for acute and chronic traumatic injury of the thoracic aorta: a single center experience. Journal of Trauma 2006; 60: 765–772.
28. Hoornweg LL, Maarten KD, Goslings CJ. Endovascular management of traumatic rupture of the thoracic aorta: a retrospective multicenter analysis of 28 consecutive cases in The Netherlands 2006. Journal of Vascular Surgery 2006; 43: 1096–1102.
29. Neschis DG, Moaine S, Gutta R. Twenty consecutive cases of endograft repair of traumatic aortic disruption: lessons learned. Journal of Vascular Surgery 2007; 43: 487–492.
30. Reed AB, Thompson JK, Crafton CJ, et al. Timing of endovascular repair of blunt traumatic aortic transection Journal of Vascular Surgery 2006; 43: 684–688.
31. Jackimczyk K. Blunt chest trauma. Emergency Medicine Clinics of North America 1993; 11: 81–96.
32. Hirshberg A, Or J, Stein M, Walker R. Transaxial gunshot injuries. Journal of Trauma 1996; 41: 460–461.
33. Pickard LR, Mattox KL. Thoracic trauma and indications for thoracotomy In: Mattox KL, Moore EE, Feliciano DV, eds. Trauma. Norwalk: Appleton & Lange, 1988; 315–320.
34. Tyburski JG, Astra L, Wilson RF. Factors affecting prognosis with penetrating wounds of the heart. Journal of Trauma – Injury Infection & Critical Care 2000; 48: 587–591.
35. Battistella FD, Nugent W, Owings JT. Field triage of the pulseless trauma patient. Archives of Surgery 1999; 134: 742–746.
36. Renz BM, Stout MJ. Rapid right atrial cannulation for fluid infusion during resuscitative emergency department thoracotomy. American Surgeon 1994; 60: 946–949.
37. Mattox KL, Feliciano DV. Role of external cardiac compression in truncal trauma. Journal of Trauma 1982; 22: 934–936.
38. Aihara R, Millham FH, Blansfield J, et al. Emergency room thoracotomy for penetrating chest injury: effect of an institutional protocol. Journal of Trauma – Injury Infection & Critical Care 2001; 50: 1027–1030.

3.7 Limb trauma

Alfredo Mori

ESSENTIALS

1 Fractures are soft tissue injuries with loss of bone continuity.

2 Skin under pressure over a fracture is an orthopaedic emergency.

3 Fracture management consists of reduction, immobilization and rehabilitation.

4 Optimal trauma resuscitation and fracture management will reduce limb and life-threatening complications.

5 Specific limb trauma assessment is part of the secondary survey.

Introduction

Limb trauma accounts for most trauma-related presentations to emergency departments (EDs). It may present in isolation, or as part of a multitrauma complex. Fracture fixation is a major part of the operative workload of trauma centres. Limb trauma and splints may distract the clinician caring for the multi-trauma patient from other more immediate threats to life. A full primary and secondary survey should be performed on all patients.

Ensuring a haemodynamically stable patient, with attention given to the specific complications of open fractures and crush injury, will reduce the life-threatening complications of fractures, i.e. bleeding, crush syndrome and hyperkalaemia, and sepsis.

The only immediate threat to life from fractures is hypovolaemic shock. Limb trauma may pose a therapeutic challenge in trauma resuscitation by limiting available vascular access. Deformed or injured limbs should, as a rule, be avoided when placing intravenous cannulae, and patients with multiple injured limbs may require early central venous access. Estimates of blood loss, in addition to external scene and ED blood loss, include:

- 1200–1500 mL for femoral fracture
- 500–1000 mL for tibial fracture
- 500 mL for humeral fracture.

The immediate goal of management in the multitrauma patient, then, is control of haemorrhage, followed by limb salvage. The overall aim of limb trauma care is a return to full pain-free function and good cosmesis. The function of the upper limb is to communicate a person's will to the external world. The function of the lower limbs is independent ambulation. Rehabilitation plays an essential part in recovery, and must be considered early with regard to the role of splints from the outset of trauma care.

A fracture is a soft tissue injury with loss of bone continuity. The soft tissue component is often underestimated. Tense or white skin over a closed fracture is an orthopaedic emergency requiring urgent reduction, even before imaging. Ischaemic skin over bone, such as in the area of the anterior tibia, has a high rate of necrosis and a poor response to skin grafting. This may result in the disastrous complication of limb amputation.

All transferred patients should have splints removed and the underlying tissues carefully assessed. No splint should remain over skin for more than 8 hours without removal and reassessment. Discharged patients should have clear instructions for returning should there be an increase in pain, tightness under a plaster or splint, or numbness and pain in the limb distal to the fracture. Timed follow-up is essential.

Fractures where the overlying skin is intact are closed. Open or compound fractures are defined by their being exposed to the environment. Compound fractures may be classified as follows:

- Grade 1: wound < 1 cm punctured from below (fracture fragment).
- Grade 2: wound up to 5 cm long with no contamination, crush, skin loss or necrosis.
- Grade 3: Large laceration with associated contamination or crush (closed after debridement). Periosteal stripping of bone (will require skin flap for closure).
- Grade 4: total or subtotal amputation.

Patients at high risk of fracture complications from single limb trauma include the elderly, the immunocompromised, alcoholics (from repeated falls and poor follow-up), and patients with peripheral vascular disease. High-risk mechanisms in limb injury from multiple trauma include falls from over 3 m, pedestrians, motorcyclists, and high-speed motorists. Haemodynamically unstable patients, those with open fractures, with delayed (> 6 hours) presentation times, and the severely head-injured also form a group of associated injuries at high risk of complications. Severely head-injured patients are prone to coagulopathy, further increasing fracture bleeding. Clinical assessment of limb trauma is affected by poor feedback from a head-injured conscious state, or sedation and intubation.[1–5]

Presentation

History and examination
Injury history and pre-hospital care should be presented in the MIST format on arrival at hospital:

- Mechanism.
- Injuries identified or suspected. Specifically, attention to external blood loss, limb deformity (and correction) or amputation.
- Symptoms and signs: in particular vital signs, whether the patient mobilized at the scene, areas of limb weakness or numbness, and pale or pulseless limbs.
- Treatments commenced and the response to them: a note should be made of all splints placed, and their type (hard, soft or anatomic).

The general history should also include patient's normal state of health, medications and allergies, hand dominance, tetanus prophylaxis, and fasting state. The history should be presented at the same time as the primary survey commences. Only when this is completed may a meticulous secondary survey start to exclude and treat limb trauma. All splints should be removed for limb trauma assessment, especially in patients transferred between hospitals, given the often long intervals before definitive assessment and treatment.

The assessment of limbs for trauma includes:

- Looking for deformity, bruising, open fractures, bleeding, skin blistering (which denotes soft tissues under pressure), and white or pressured skin. Comparison should always be made with the other limb.
- Feeling for local pain, crepitus or deformity. All peripheral pulses should be examined for and their absence investigated further.
- Active (patient controlled) and passive (examiner controlled) movement. Joints with a full active range of movement are almost never dislocated. Full active movement of the elbow may exclude an elbow fracture, and straight leg raising a major pelvic fracture. Passive movement should include an assessment of ligament stability, especially around the knee.
- Peripheral vascular assessment includes pulses and capillary refill.
- Peripheral neurological assessment includes motor power and sensation. The most accurate indicator of sensory function is two-point discrimination.
- Vascular injury should be suspected in elbow and knee dislocations, regardless of whether the peripheral vascular examination is normal after reduction. Abnormal peripheral vascular signs include absent or decreased distal pulses, prolonged capillary refill, pale peripheries unilaterally, ongoing wound bleeding, or an expanding haematoma.

Investigations

Plain radiographs
Plain X-rays are the investigation of choice in the diagnosis of limb fracture. They may be performed in the trauma bay where available, or in the radiology area once the patient is stable for transfer.

Two views in two planes are required for accurate diagnosis and planning of reduction. The joints above and below the injury site should also be imaged.

Other indicators of injury that may alter management include the presence of air or foreign bodies around injury sites and joints, and soft tissue swelling such as the sail sign in distal humerus fractures. Joint injury may be indicated by soft tissue swelling and lipohaemarthroses (radio-opaque effusions), which may indicate an underlying fracture.

Joints and fractures should be X-rayed again after reduction. Timed repeated X-rays may be used in injuries where there is doubt about the presence of a fracture (for example the scaphoid in peripheral wrist injuries).

The multitrauma patient may have over 30 X-rays as part of the diagnostic and specific radiological screen. Such large numbers of X-rays, or where there is any doubt about the presence of a fracture, should be reviewed in conjunction with a radiologist or other senior clinician.

Ultrasound

Ultrasound is now commonplace in trauma centres and many EDs, and is increasingly being used in the pre-hospital setting. Also, many emergency physicians and registrars are becoming proficient in its use. Bedside ultrasonography is cheap, reliable, safe, non-invasive and easily repeatable. Its role in major trauma is to exclude traumatic cardiac tamponade and haemoperitoneum. Doppler scanning may be used to identify peripheral pulses.

The role of ultrasound in limb trauma is less well defined, but includes the diagnosis of muscle or tendon ruptures (the rotator cuff and the Achilles tendon, respectively), and soft tissue foreign bodies or free fluid. Therapeutically, ultrasound may aid in peripheral and central line placement in the patient with limb trauma.

Angiography

The role of angiography in limb trauma may be both diagnostic and therapeutic. Angiograms may be performed in the trauma centre, in the angiography suite, or in theatre.

Diagnostic angiography is indicated in:

- All dislocations or disruptions of the knee joint, as tears of the media of the popliteal artery may not be otherwise safely excluded.
- All limb injuries with vascular compromise distally, in particular high-velocity injuries such as firearm wounds.

Angiography may have a role therapeutically in limb amputation with uncontrolled or difficult-to-control haemorrhage.

Specialist staff, such as radiologists, must be alerted early, as angiography suites may require some time to staff and prepare. In major trauma centres this may take up to an hour in out-of-hours scenarios. This, and the preparation of a transfer team, should be the role of the trauma team leader.

Manometry

Pressure manometry is used specifically in the measurement of compartment pressures. Tools such as the Stryker manometer, or a peripheral cannula connected to a blood pressure or arterial line manometer, may be used repeatedly in the ED.

Computed tomography (CT)

CT scans have a limited role in the acute management of fractures. Indications may include further imaging and quantification of tibial plateau fractures, particularly the posterior component of the tibial plateau, and carpal and tarsal injuries that may by difficult to assess on plain X-ray. CT has been used in the diagnosis of suspected femoral neck fractures in the elderly.

Magnetic resonance imaging (MRI)

The indications for emergency MRI do not include limb trauma. Compartment syndromes may be identified using MRI, but this is of limited value in the acute setting. The role of MRI is usually limited to acute spinal injury with neurological deficits.

Bone scan

There is no place for bone scans in the early management of limb trauma. Bone scans are most reliable 3 days after injury in the diagnosis of occult fractures. They may also be used in the diagnosis and assessment of osteomyelitis as a complication of fractures.

Management

Resuscitation and the primary survey take precedence in limb trauma. Splints and limb injuries may distract the team or clinician from this process. Limb trauma may impede or limit the placement of peripheral cannulae. In the primary survey, limb trauma assessment is limited to control of visible haemorrhage by external pressure.

Open wounds should be covered with sterile dressings, and fractures splinted in the initial phase of care.

All rings, bracelets and other constricting foreign bodies, such as clothing, should be removed from the affected limbs.

Tetanus prophylaxis should be provided. Severely contaminated wounds should receive tetanus immunoglobulin and urgent debridement in theatre.

There is very good evidence that early systemic antibiotics reduce infection rates in open fractures, with a number needed to treat (NNT) of 13 in a recent Cochrane Review.[6] Antibiotics are not a substitute for good wound care, which includes decontamination, irrigation and early surgical debridement. Crushed, penetrating and macerated injuries should receive antibiotic prophylaxis against *Staphylococcus aureus, Streptococcus pyogenes, Clostridium perfringens*, and aerobic Gram-negative bacteria. Recommended antibiotic combinations include flucloxacillin, gentamicin and metronidazole, or cephalothin and metronidazole.[7] Cephazolin is also commonly used.

Gentamicin and benzylpenicillin are indicated in severely soiled wounds, severe tissue damage, or devitalized tissue, to cover against Gram negatives and *Clostridium perfringens*, respectively.

Compound wounds should be protected from secondary injury and decontamination by gentle washing with normal saline, and a sterile moist dressing placed over the wound. A Polaroid photograph may be taken of the wound and placed over the dressing until definitive care is provided.

Pain, even in the sedated or intubated patient, may cause life-threatening arrhythmias or emergent hypertension, especially in the multitrauma patient. Analgesia may be pharmacological or non-pharmacological. Non-pharmacological measures include splinting and fracture reduction.

Pharmacological analgesia may be general or local. General agents include narcotics, which should be titrated to comfort and physiological response. The use of ketamine is increasingly widespread in the pre-hospital transport of injured patients, and in reduction of fractures and dislocation in the ED. It should be used by experienced clinicians in monitored, selected patients. Some procedures, such as reduction of disrupted joints, or in the uncooperative, intoxicated or polytrauma patient, may require general intravenous anaesthesia and intubation.

Local nerve blocks may prove useful. Specifically, in splinted femoral shaft fractures the femoral nerve block is very useful in reducing quadriceps muscle spasm.

The role of splints

Splinting is almost universal in limb trauma management, being used in every stage of care, from scene to long-term rehabilitation.

The role of splints includes communication, analgesia, haemorrhage control, tissue protection, immobilization, facilitating transport, and perhaps, reduction of fat embolism. All splinted areas should be treated as fractured till proved otherwise. All splints should be noted and removed when possible, and a full inspection made of the whole limb. Pain relief is assisted by less movement of injured tissue. Splinted, reduced injuries have less local bleeding and oedema. Definitive bone apposition will reduce fracture bleeding. Injured tissues may be protected during transport until definitive assessment and care. Immobilized limbs are less painful, and bleed less. Patient immobilization may facilitate safe and efficient transfer to definitive care. Fat embolism may be reduced, though the role of early splinting is controversial and based on poor historical evidence.

Splints may be classified by area (general splints such as spine boards, or local such as cervical spine collars) or type (anatomical, such as the unaffected leg, soft, rigid, air, or slings).

All splints are foreign bodies, with consequent complications: they may be distracting to other injuries, or cause local skin pressure and necrosis, compartment syndromes, loss of limb function and distal hypoperfusion. A limb cannot be adequately assessed while a splint is in place.

The definitive management of fractures and dislocations is reduction, immobilization and rehabilitation. Ideally, all deformed, injured limbs should be splinted to an anatomically neutral position. Early reduction offers pain relief by distracting fracture edges and pressure on local innervated tissue. It also facilitates patient transport. Pressure on the overlying skin and nearby neurovascular structures is also reduced. Limb deformities with overlying skin under pressure are true orthopaedic emergencies which should be reduced before imaging. Any suspect penetrating joint injury should be reviewed under anaesthesia for assessment and lavage.

Injured limbs should be immobilized in the pre-hospital setting in the anatomical, or neutral, position where possible. The joints above and below an injured area should be immobilized. Some specific injuries, such as femoral shaft fractures, will require traction immobilization to overcome local muscle spasm. Common devices include the Donway splint and variations of the Thomas splint. Once applied, all distal areas of splinted limbs should be neurovascularly reassessed.

Rehabilitation of limb trauma commences in the ED. Early movement of uninjured limbs should be encouraged. Supervised practice with crutches and the removal and care of slings will improve outpatient independence and reduce complications from these devices. Timed follow-up of all fractures, complicated wounds, and patient groups otherwise at risk of complications is essential. Patients should be discharged home from the ED when limb and life-threatening injuries have been excluded, when they are safely ambulant, are tolerating food and drink, have adequate oral analgesia, and have planned follow-up arranged.

Compound fractures and contaminated wounds are time-critical emergencies. There is a paucity of evidence regarding the ideal time to theatre, but ethically, the sooner these injuries are definitively attended, the better the expected outcome. Time to theatre is related to infection rates and necrosis of overlying soft tissue.

Wound management

The role of wound irrigation agents in the acute setting is controversial. There is no evidence to support the use of full-strength povidone–iodine, and if used, it should be diluted to less than 1%. Povidone–iodine has been shown to delay wound healing and increase infection rates in chronic wounds. Shaving of wounds should be avoided as it promotes local inflammation.

Gross contamination should be removed, and the wound irrigated using normal saline. The efficacy of normal saline is related to the irrigation pressure. Pulsatile pressure at 7–10 psi (48–69 kPa) removes debris and bacteria without further dissemination of micro-organisms in the tissue. This pressure may be produced with a 20 mL syringe and a 19 G needle with a splash guard. There is no evidence that high-pressure irrigation offers any benefit. Reviews of the techniques and materials used in wound irrigation recommend normal saline.[8–10]

Tense haemarthroses (joint swelling from acute bleeding) should be assessed and drained. This may be diagnostic in revealing a lipohaemarthrosis and thereby increase the suspicion of an underlying fracture, will facilitate joint assessment by increasing range of movement, and is therapeutic in providing pain relief by reducing local joint pressure. A sterile field and an aseptic technique performed by experienced staff is essential to prevent iatrogenic septic arthritis.

Disposition

The ED is a critical care area, not a final disposition. Patients will be discharged home, admitted to a general or trauma ward, taken to theatre or admitted to the intensive care unit. In the interim, some patients may require transfer for angiography, CT scanning or MRI. Patients who have been completely managed in the ED may be discharged home with a written care plan, and timed follow-up at their GP, an injury or fracture clinic, or the ED. Elderly patients with splints should be assessed for mobilization safety, and appropriate aids provided by an expert team. Adequate oral analgesia should be prescribed for at least a week, with specific care taken to cover weekend and holiday periods. Nonsteroidals (NSAIDs) should be avoided, particularly in the elderly, as they offer no benefit and may cause harm. Sleep with injured limbs may be interrupted and difficult. Slings should be removed during rest periods, and adequate replacements, such as cushions, planned for. Minor sedatives may be prescribed in some cases.

Patients with a plaster should have documented evaluation of the plaster, the affected limb(s), and use of any splints or walking aids, such as crutches. Upper limb slings should have cushioned supports where they come in contact with the neck, especially at the site of any securing knot. All injured limbs should be elevated for the first 48 hours, preferably in a splint such as a sling, or with specific instructions, such as elevation of the leg above the height of the hip when sitting or lying. Patients should be instructed to return if their injury becomes too painful to cope with, even with discharge analgesia, if the distal area becomes numb, painful to move, or pale or blue in colour. All initial plasters should be reviewed at 24 hours, and removed at 1 week or earlier should they become tight, wet or damaged, the injury and the patient reassessed.

Operating theatre

Urgent transfer to the operating theatre specifically for limb injury is indicated in:

- Uncontrollable haemorrhage
- Severely contaminated wounds or open fractures
- Limbs ischaemic for over 6–8 hours
- Crushed limbs requiring amputation as a life-saving procedure
- Infected limbs requiring amputation as a life-saving procedure.

In patients with complex polytrauma, patients in extremis with an otherwise high intraoperative mortality risk, or in departments in which the surgical workload will overload theatre resources, damage control surgery may be indicated. In the 1970s early fixation of fractures resulted in a dramatic fall in fat embolism syndrome and so became standard practice. Damage control orthopaedic surgery is the initial temporary fixation of fractures in patients in whom the overall burden of definitive surgery may be too great, with a definitive secondary procedure planned for a later date. The aims of damage control surgery are to control haemorrhage, contamination and wound swelling, and reduce the potential risk of skin necrosis and fat embolism syndrome. The patient is then usually transferred to an intensive care unit for haemodynamic stabilization and correction of gross physiologic derangements.[11–13]

General or trauma ward

Patients transferred to a general or trauma unit ward should have the same documented attention as discharged patients. Specific issues include fasting status, fluid requirements, mobilization restrictions, analgesia with particular stress on systemic analgesia for breakthrough pain, or pain after wound care on the ward. Considerable care should be given to adequate sighting, labelling, and communication of any procedures planned. Other general care issues include bladder and bowel care, pressure care, and elevation of injured limbs in splints or on pillows.

Hyperbaric oxygen therapy

The role of hyperbaric therapy (HBOT) in acute limb injuries is controversial and remains unresolved. Theoretically, it enhances oxygen delivery to areas affected acutely by hypoxia and at risk of such by cellular and tissue oedema. This may reduce the number of cells at risk from delayed ischaemia and necrosis from local oedema. Animal and human case studies have demonstrated benefit in crush injury, compartment syndrome and malunited or non-united fractures. The US Hyperbaric Society lists crush injury and compartment syndrome as indications for hyperbaric therapy. However, recent systematic reviews have failed to demonstrate any evidence for hyperbaric therapy in acute wound care, citing a paucity of prospective trials. Clinicians should be aware of their region's recommendations and practice. There are currently prospective randomized controlled trials of HBOT in the care of acute compound fractures.[14–16]

Complications

Arterial injury

Arterial injury is a limb- and potentially life-threatening emergency. Ischaemic times of 4–6 hours may result in permanent damage to tissues. Peripheral circulation and distal pulses must always be assessed, and sides compared. All splints in transferred patients should be removed and underlying tissues and distal circulation assessed. High-risk patients include those that have been transferred by air with air splints in situ, unconscious patients and shocked patients, as the shock state may mask local limb ischaemia.

There may be a role for hypotensive resuscitation in complete arterial injury, whereby a reduced, controlled perfusion pressure may leave intact a clot formed as a result of complete arterial laceration. Aggressive fluid resuscitation in these patients, where not otherwise indicated, or inadequate analgesia, may cause a rise in mean arterial pressure, dislodgement of the clot at the site of injury, and resumption of arterial bleeding.

The presence of a distal pulse does not exclude arterial injury, which may be incomplete. Other signs to consider in this diagnosis include the presence of a dislocation, limb deformity or open fracture in that limb, brisk bleeding from an open wound, reduced pulses compared to the other side (either clinically or on Doppler), and an expanding wound haematoma. Delayed signs include a false aneurysm or the presence of a bruit on examination.

Sites at specific risk of arterial injury include:

- Brachial artery in the upper limb.
- Popliteal artery around the knee and adductor canal of the medial distal femur.
- Deep femoral artery at the trochanter level of the femur.
- The anterior tibial artery in the tibia.

Angiography is the investigation of choice.

Nerve injury

Nerve injury in limb trauma may be a direct result of laceration by foreign bodies or fracture fragments. Nerves may be crushed, bruised or stretched. Ischaemia must be excluded as a cause for neurological deficits. Nerve injury from penetrating injury ideally should be explored in the operating theatre.

Nerve injuries may be classified as:

- Neuropraxia. This is a transient change in conduction. It usually follows crush or contusion or stretching of a nerve. There is usually some return of function within days and complete return of function within 8 weeks.
- Axonotmesis. Complete denervation with an intact nerve sheath, usually as a result of blunt trauma causing severe bruising and stretching. Regeneration takes place over months along the intact nerve sheath.

- Neurotmesis. Complete division of a nerve and its sheath. Spontaneous regeneration is not expected and surgical repair is required.

The neurovascular status of the injured limb should be assessed and documented before and after any manipulation and relocation. Specific nerve injury presentations include:

- Wrist drop from radial nerve injury of the middle or distal third of the humerus.
- Foot drop from peroneal nerve injury to the proximal fibula.
- Shoulder skin numbness from axillary nerve injury in shoulder dislocation.
- Lower limb numbness and weakness from sciatic nerve injury due to posterior dislocations of the hip.
- Hand numbness and weakness from median nerve injury in distal fractures of the wrist and dislocations of the carpal bones.
- Hand numbness and weakness from ulnar nerve injury in injuries to the medial forearm or humerus.

Acute limb compartment syndrome

Acute limb compartment syndrome (ALCS) is a limb- and occasionally life-threatening complication of limb trauma. It is caused by bleeding or oedema in a closed muscle compartment surrounded by fascia, interosseous membrane and bone. The syndrome leads to muscle and nerve ischaemia and the release of potentially lethal potassium and hydrogen ions and myoglobin. Untreated compartment syndrome leads to muscle necrosis, limb amputation, and, if severe in large compartments, acute renal failure and death.

Clinical suspicion, elevation with local ice packs, occasional compartment pressure measuring, and surgical decompression with fasciotomy are the mainstay of treatment.

Clinically the outstanding sign is ischaemic muscle pain. That is, pain that is difficult to control and greater than expected for the injury seen. This may be brought on by passive flexion or extension of the distal digits. Peripheral pulses are usually present, and their loss is a very late sign as mean arterial pressure is usually adequately maintained. Affected muscle compartments are firm, tense and tender on palpation.

Causes of compartment syndrome include crush injuries, closed fractures, injections or infusions into compartments, reperfusion of arterial ischaemia, snakebite, electric shock, burns, exercise, and hyperthermia. Splinting of suspected limbs and removal of any circumferential casts, splints or dressings is essential so as not to increase compartment pressure further.

Areas in which ALCS occurs most commonly are the leg (anterior, lateral, superficial and deep posterior compartments), thigh (quadriceps), and forearm (volar and dorsal compartments). Less commonly it may also occur in the buttocks (gluteals), the hand (interosseous muscles) and the arm (biceps and triceps).

The investigation of choice is compartment pressure monitoring. The use of this modality is controversial, although some centres advocate continuous monitoring. Normal compartment pressure is 4–8 mmHg. The pressure mandating fasciotomy remains controversial, but most departments would agree on an orthopaedic review with a view to fasciotomy for any pressure above 40 mmHg. Compartment pressure may be monitored with commercial devices such as the Stryker pressure monitor, or by insertion of an intra-arterial pressure monitor and cannula.

Patients who should have compartment pressure measured include all those with tense compartments whose contralateral limbs cannot be clinically compared, patients with distracting injuries such as compound fractures, and severely intoxicated or intubated patients.

The definitive management of compartment syndrome is surgical decompression with fasciotomy.[17,18]

Fat embolism syndrome

Fat embolism – the passage of fat from one area of the body to another via the vascular system – is a normal consequence of long bone fractures and was first described in 1862. Fat embolism syndrome (FES), the life-threatening multiorgan syndrome affecting the lungs, brain cardiovascular system, and skin, is very rare, occurring in perhaps less than 1% of all long bone fractures. The exact incidence is difficult to measure, given that FES may be subclinical, or masked by other syndromes such as acute respiratory distress syndrome (ARDS), and its investigative diagnosis non-specific and inconsistent. It usually follows 6–48 hours after long bone fracture. Other causes include closed cardiac massage, severe burns, liver injury, bone marrow transplantation and liposuction.

Clinically, patients deteriorate with hypoxaemia, chest X-ray changes, skin petechiae and an altered conscious state. The respiratory syndrome is similar to ARDS. There may be petechiae on the skin and conjunctivae.

Investigations are useful only in the exclusion of other causes such as ARDS, pulmonary contusion or pulmonary embolism. Some tomographic changes may be more specific for FES, and these are thought to represent the fat emboli themselves and the systemic inflammatory response to them. Treatment is both prophylactic and supportive. General ICU management includes adequate oxygenation and ventilation, haemodynamic stability, and prophylaxis for DVT and stress-related upper gastrointestinal bleeding. FES is self-limiting,

Studies support early fixation of fractures to prevent recurrent FES. There is controversy regarding the role of reaming with intramedullary nails the fractures of long bones such as the femur and tibia, as by the nature of this technique relatively large amounts of fat are released into the systemic circulation.[19–26]

Crush syndrome

Crush syndrome is a life-threatening systemic manifestation of muscle damage resulting from pressure or crushing. Crush syndrome was first described in the early 20th century following the Messina earthquake of 1906, and work in Germany in World War 1, and by Beals and Bywater in London in 1941. Following the Armenian earthquake of 1988, the International Society of Nephrology established the Renal Disaster Relief Task Force in direct response to the overwhelming demand for dialysis of crush injury survivors in these earthquakes. Specific protocols for the prevention and management of renal failure due to crush syndrome have been established.

Crush syndrome is a result of both external pressure on muscles, and time. Crushed or compressed muscle cells may immediately burst due to overwhelming external compressive force, releasing potassium, hydrogen ions (causing hyperkalaemia and acidosis respectively) and myoglobin, oxygen free radicals and phosphate ions (causing acute renal injury and death from renal failure). The release of the above may occur in cells not initially crushed but at risk of cell wall breakdown from local ischaemia, as in compartment syndrome, or cell membrane damage without disruption from external compressive force. The toxic metabolites listed above are initially usually restricted to the local tissue environment as venous return is impeded by the crush injury itself. Creatinine kinase (CK) is also released and may be a measure of myoglobin load, predicting renal injury and dialysis. Hence the release of crushed tissue from a compressive environment and the re-establishment of local blood flow may release all of the above systemically. Therefore, pre-hospital fluids may be able to pre-empt renal injury and death before a limb is released from crush injury.

Diagnosis is from the history of a crush injury. Apart from earthquake survivors, other groups at risk include trapped motor vehicle accident victims, IV drug users who collapse unconscious on a limb or limbs, and elderly collapsed patients who remain unattended for some time (for example after a hip fracture). Other causes of rhabdomyolysis are the destruction of skeletal muscle, heat stroke, severe exertion, cocaine and amphetamine use, serotoninergic syndrome and snake bites.

As with compartment syndrome, clinically patients may exhibit tense, hard, tender muscles, with overlying skin that may be bruised or blistered due to high interstitial pressure. They may be hypothermic and shocked due to prolonged exposure and inadequate fluid intake. The urine is dark (like machinery oil, or black tea) and reflects the presence or myoglobin and other toxic haem proteins. The bedside investigation of choice is an ECG to exclude the consequences of life-threatening hyperkalaemia. Blood tests may initially only demonstrate hyperkalaemia, but in time will reflect metabolic acidosis and worsening acute renal failure. The CK is often raised above 5000 in significant crush injury. A CK over 75 000 is predictive of acute renal failure and death.

Early deaths from crush syndrome are due to arrhythmias from hyperkalaemia, and hypovolaemic shock. At 3–5 days after injury death is from renal failure, coagulopathy and haemorrhage (DIC), and sepsis. Treatment is aimed at stabilizing the cardiac milieu against hyperkalaemia, aggressive volume therapy to prevent shock and renal failure, enhancing haem protein elimination, and limiting haem protein cytotoxicity.

Trapped patients should have aggressive fluid loading with normal saline before extraction. They may also receive calcium gluconate or bicarbonate intravenously to counter ensuing hyperkalaemia. In severe crush injury, fluid requirements in addition to baseline needs average 12 L in the first 48 hours to prevent renal failure.

Once in the ED, patients should be monitored and, given the large fluid load expected intravenously and the brisk diuresis desired, have an arterial line placed, and an indwelling catheter and a central line considered.

Once urine flow is established an alkaline–mannitol diuresis is recommended, aiming for 2 mL/kg/h output. Mannitol increases renal tubular blood flow, is a renal vasodilator and free radical scavenger. It is also an osmotoic diuretic. It may have an effect on compartment pressures, though compartment syndrome should be treated by fasciotomy, as mentioned. Urine pH should be maintained at over 5, at which myoglobin is over 50% soluble and thus prevented from precipitating into the renal tubules. Bicarbonate at 50 mmol/h after the first 3 L of normal saline will help achieve this. Clinicians should be aware that, if safe to do so, intravenous potassium may be given in addition to bicarbonate to further alkalinize urine.

Dialysis may be indicated in oligoanuric patients with refractory hyperkalaemia or acidosis, or in fluid overload and pulmonary oedema. Local management of affected limbs and assessment as outlined above is mandatory.[14,27–36]

Immobilization

It is worth reminding clinicians that, by definition, an injured limb will result in some loss of function of that limb until fully recovered. Some patients may therefore require prolonged periods of immobilization, usually in hospital, but also in rehabilitation facilities or at home. The consequences of prolonged immobilization include pressure sores and skin breakdown, muscle atrophy and weakness (with an increased risk of falls subsequently), postural hypotension, dependent-lung atelectasis and secondary pneumonia, constipation, insomnia, social isolation and depression. Management plans that are well communicated and documented should prevent and manage many of these complications.

Controversies

- The type of fluid and technique for the irrigation of contaminated wounds.

- The role of limb compartment pressure monitoring, in particular continuous pressure monitoring.

- The role of early splinting in preventing fat embolism syndrome in long bone fractures.

- The role of hyperbaric therapy in the management of acute limb trauma.

- The timing of early fracture fixation and reduction to prevent fat embolism syndrome and skin necrosis.

References

1. Deitch EA, Dayal SD. Intensive care unit management of the trauma patient. Critical Care Medicine 2006; 34: 2294–2301.
2. Sagraves SG, Toschlog EA, Rotondo MF. Damage control surgery – the intensivist's role. Journal of Intensive Care Medicine 2006; 21: 5–16.
3. Perron AD, Brady WJ. Evaluation and management of the high-risk orthopedic emergency. Emergency Medicine Clinics of North America 2003; 21: 159–204.
4. Tintinalli J, Gabor D, Stapczynski J (eds) Emergency medicine: a comprehensive study guide. McGraw Hill, 2003.
5. Rosen P, Barkin (eds) Emergency medicine: concepts and clinical practice. Mosby Year Book, 1997.
6. Gosselin RA, Roberts I, Gillespie WJ. Antibiotics for preventing infection in open limb fractures. Cochrane Database System Reviews (20041): CD003764.
7. Victorian Drug Usage Advisory Committee. Antibiotic Guidelines. Melbourne, 1999.
8. Crowley DJ, Kanakaris NK, Giannoudis PV. Irrigation of the wounds in open fractures. Journal of Bone and Joint Surgery 2007; 89B: 580–585.
9. Chatterjee JS. A critical review of irrigation techniques in acute wounds. International Wound Journal 2005; 2: 258–265.
10. Moreira ME, Markovchick VJ. Wound management. Emergency Medicine Clinics of North America 2007; 25: 873–899, xi.
11. Noonburg GE. Management of extremity trauma and related infections occurring in the aquatic environment.

Journal of the American Academy of Orthopaedic Surgeons 2005; 13: 243–253.

12. Okike K, Bhattacharyya T. Trends in the management of open fractures. A critical analysis. Journal of Bone and Joint Surgery 2006; 88A: 2739–2748.

13. Houston M, Hendrickson RG. Decontamination. Critical Care Clinic 2005; 21: 653–672, v.

14. Buettner MF, Wolkenhauer D. Hyperbaric oxygen therapy in the treatment of open fractures and crush injuries. Emergency Medicine Clinics of North America 2007; 25: 177–188.

15. Butler J, Foex B. Best evidence topic report. Hyperbaric oxygen therapy in acute fracture management. Emergency Medicine Journal 2006; 23: 571–572.

16. Bennett MH, Stanford R, Turner R. Hyperbaric oxygen therapy for promoting fracture healing and treating fracture non-union. Cochrane Database System Reviews (2005)1: CD004712.

17. Salcido R, Lepre SJ. Compartment syndrome: wound care considerations. Advances in Skin and Wound Care 2007; 20: 559–565; quiz 566–567.

18. Gourgiotis S, Villias C, Germanos S, et al. Acute limb compartment syndrome: a review. Journal of Surgical Education 2007; 64: 178–186.

19. Taviloglu K, Yanar H. Fat embolism syndrome. Surgery Today 2007; 37: 5–8.

20. Husebye EE, Lyberg T, Roise O. Bone marrow fat in the circulation: clinical entities and pathophysiological mechanisms. Injury 2006; 37: S8–18.

21. Habashi NM, Andrews PL, Scalea TM. Therapeutic aspects of fat embolism syndrome. Injury 2006; 37: S68–73.

22. White T, Petrisor BA, Bhandari M. Prevention of fat embolism syndrome. Injury 2006; 37: S59–67.

23. Giannoudis PV, Tzioupis C, Pape HC. Fat embolism: the reaming controversy. Injury 2006; 37: S50–58.

24. Van den Brande FG, Hellemans S, De Schepper A, et al. Post-traumatic severe fat embolism syndrome with uncommon CT findings. Anaesthesia and Intensive Care 2006; 34: 102–106.

25. Pape HC, Krettek C. [Management of fractures in the severely injured – influence of the principle of 'damage control orthopaedic surgery']. Unfallchirurgie 2003; 106: 87–96.

26. Dunham CM, Bosse MJ, Clancy TV, et al. Practice management guidelines for the optimal timing of long-bone fracture stabilization in polytrauma. patients: the EAST Practice Management Guidelines Work Group. Journal of Trauma 2001; 50: 958–967.

27. James T. Management of patients with acute crush injuries of the extremities. International Anesthesiology Clinics 2007; 45: 19–29.

28. Vanholder R, van der Tol A, De Smet M, et al. Earthquakes and crush syndrome casualties: lessons learned from the Kashmir disaster. Kidney International 2007; 71: 17–23.

29. Sever MS, Vanholder R, Lameire N. Management of crush-related injuries after disasters. New England Journal of Medicine 2006; 354: 1052–1063.

30. Gonzalez D. Crush syndrome. Critical Care Medicine 2005; 33: S34–41.

31. Garcia-Covarrubias L, McSwain NEJ, Van Meter K, Bell RM. Adjuvant hyperbaric oxygen therapy in the management of crush injury and traumatic ischemia: an evidence-based approach. American Surgeon 2005; 71: 144–151.

32. Greensmith JE. Hyperbaric oxygen therapy in extremity trauma. Journal of the American Academy of Orthopaedic Surgeons 2004; 12: 376–384.

33. Smith J, Greaves I. Crush injury and crush syndrome: a review. Journal of Trauma 2003; 54: S226–230.

34. Better OS, Rubinstein I, Reis DN. Muscle crush compartment syndrome: fulminant local edema with threatening systemic effects. Kidney International 2003; 63: 1155–1157.

35. Greaves I, Porter K, Smith JE. Consensus statement on the early management of crush injury and prevention of crush syndrome. Journal of the Royal Army Medical Corps 2003; 149: 255–259.

36. Eknoyan G. The Armenian earthquake of 1988: a milestone in the evolution of nephrology. Advances in Renal Replacement Therapy 2003; 10: 87–92.

3.8 Radiology in major trauma

Tony Joseph • Karen Falk • Roger Harris

ESSENTIALS

1 The trauma team leader should supervise the primary and secondary surveys and the initial trauma series X-rays.

2 The trauma team should be mindful of the risks of radiation and wear adequate protection.

3 Evaluation of facial trauma requires an adequate clinical and radiological examination.

4 Evaluation of the cervical spine by computed tomography (CT) will identify most bony cervical spine abnormalities.

5 Injuries to the thoracolumbar spine should be evaluated by sagittal reconstruction of axial CT scans of the chest/abdomen/pelvis or by plain X-rays.

6 Injury to the carotid or vertebral arteries should be suspected clinically and investigated by CT angiography.

7 Chest CT is a useful screening test for mediastinal or large vessel injury.

8 Pelvic CT is invaluable for the classification of pelvic fractures and angiography/embolization should be part of the treatment algorithm for haemodynamically unstable patients with pelvic fractures.

Emergency department reception

The reception of the major trauma patient requires planning and organization. There should be timely notification of the impending arrival of the trauma patient, and the ambulance personnel should provide the following information: Mechanism and time of injury, Injuries suspected, vital Signs and Treatment given (MIST). The initial trauma X-rays usually consist of lateral cervical spine, chest and pelvic films.

Hazards of radiation

Exposure of both trauma team members and patients to ionizing radiation should be minimized and staff should wear protective lead gowns and thyroid shields. These garments have been shown to protect against ionizing radiation within recommended occupational limits.[1]

The number of X-rays taken in the resuscitation area should be kept to a minimum. As radiation exposure decreases inversely with the square of the distance from the source, staff should position themselves at a maximum distance from X-ray equipment in use whenever possible. The use of permanent lead barriers should be considered.

The radiation dose from various diagnostic imaging examinations may be calculated as an 'effective dose' for the purpose of comparison and quantification of risk. Effective dose, evaluated in millisieverts (mSv), refers to the radiation dose from an examination averaged over the entire body, and accounts for the relative sensitivities of the different tissues exposed.[1-3]

A single CT scan sequence gives tissue doses in the range of 10–30 mSv. Tissue doses in the range 50–200 mSv have been shown to cause an increase in cancer risk among atomic bomb survivors, and the risk is higher for lower age at exposure.[4-6] The United States Food and Drug Administration estimates that CT examination with an effective dose of 10 mSv may carry a 1:2000 lifetime risk of inducing fatal cancer.[7] Table 3.8.1 gives typical whole-body effective doses for selected radiological examinations.

Typical values cited for radiation dose should be considered as estimates, as they may vary with the size of the patient, the type of procedure and equipment and the operational technique used. This is particularly relevant for CT, where estimates of effective dose can vary widely.

Table 3.8.1 Whole-body effective doses (mSv)	
Examination	*Radiation dose (mSv)*
CXR[1]	0.02
PXR[1]	0.44
SXR[1]	0.07
Cervical spine X-ray	0.2
CT head[2]	1.7–4.9 (Av 2)
CT chest[2]	3.8–26 (Av 9.3)
CT abdomen[2]	3.6–26.5 (Av 10.1)
CT pelvis[2]	3.5–15.5 (Av 9.0)
CT abdo/pelvis[2]	7.3–31.5 (Av 16.3)
Background[3]	3

The trauma series

The initial 'trauma series' of X-rays should consist of the lateral cervical (Cx) spine, AP chest (CXR) and AP pelvic X-rays (PXR). The lateral cervical spine X-ray should be taken with a team member exerting gentle traction on the arms in order to pull down the shoulders and expose the lower cervical spine to the C7–T1 junction (Fig. 3.8.1).

Systematic examination of this film includes assessment of alignment, bony structures, cartilage and soft tissue (ABCS) (Table 3.8.2, Fig. 3.8.2). Some trauma centres have abandoned the lateral cervical spine X-ray if the patient requires a CT brain scan and will perform a CT of the cervical spine with axial cuts plus coronal and sagittal reconstructions. This approach gives more information than the lateral cervical spine film, which poorly visualizes both the occipitoatlantal junction and the cervicothoracic junction.

The CXR performed is usually a supine (AP) rather than an erect (PA) film owing to the inability to sit the patient up until the spine is cleared. The CXR should include both clavicles, ribs, lung fields, mediastinum and diaphragm. If there is

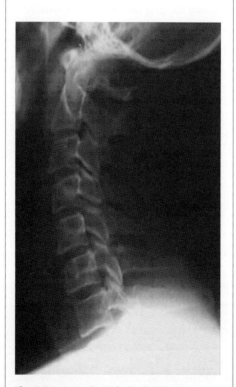

Fig. 3.8.1 Lateral cervical spine X-ray.

Table 3.8.2 Radiological examination of the lateral cervical spine	
A	Alignment
B	Bony structures
C	Cartilage spaces
S	Soft tissue

adequate penetration, the thoracic spine may be seen. The mediastinum may be falsely enlarged owing to the frontal nature of the film, and this should be taken into account. The CXR will exclude life-threatening injuries such as massive haemothorax or pneumothorax, and may show signs of major vessel injury indicated by a widening of the mediastinum (Fig. 3.8.3).

The pelvic X-ray will include all the bony pelvic components and the hip joints (Fig. 3.8.4).

Specific regional radiology

Head

Head trauma is responsible for 50–75% of the mortality associated with major trauma.[8] The spectrum of head injury ranges from mild concussion to diffuse axonal injury incompatible with life, and includes all causes of intracranial haemorrhage.

A CT brain scan is the investigation of choice for all but minor head injuries (see Table 3.8.3 for CT indications in serious head injury). A non-contrast CT brain scan with bone windows is adequate for the detection of intracranial haematoma, cerebral oedema with or without midline shift, and skull vault fractures (Fig. 3.8.5).

The Canadian CT Head Rule[9] for patients with minor head injury also provides guidance for CT brain scanning in patients with minor head injury (GCS 13–15).

The authors have found that the presence of any of the high-risk factors (Table 3.8.4) was 100% sensitive for predicting the need for neurological intervention. They also found that the presence of medium-risk factors was 97.2% sensitive for detecting clinically important brain injury.

There are very few indications for a skull X-ray in a trauma patient if a CT scanner is available.

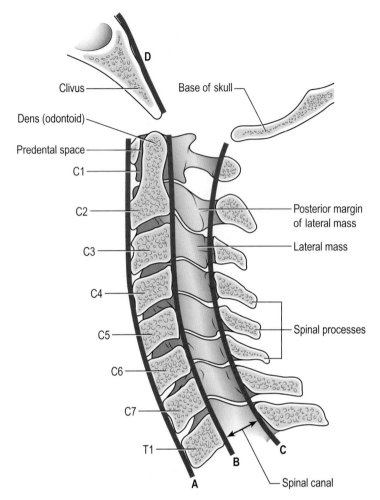

Fig. 3.8.2 Normal cervical spine lateral X-ray. (A) Anterior vertebral line; (B) Posterior vertebral line; (C) Spino-laminar line.

Table 3.8.3 Indications for a CT brain scan in significant head injury
Glasgow Coma Score (GCS) <9 after resuscitation
Neurological deterioration of 2 or more GCS points
Drowsiness or confusion (GCS 9–13) that persists for longer than 2 hours
Persistent headache or vomiting
Focal neurological signs (e.g. pupillary abnormalities or focal neurological signs)
Skull fracture known or suspected
Penetrating injury known or suspected
Age over 50 years with a suspicious mechanism of injury
Any head injury in a patient on anticoagulation therapy

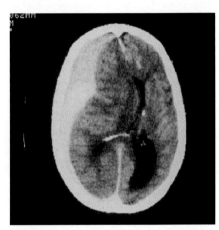

Fig. 3.8.5 CT brain right SDH with midline shift.

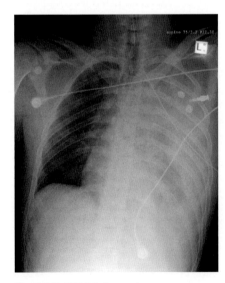

Fig. 3.8.3 CRX left haemothorax.

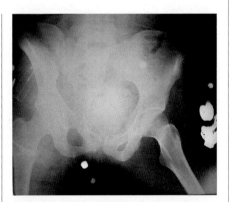

Fig. 3.8.4 Pelvic X-ray lateral compression fracture.

Table 3.8.4 CT Head Rule is only required for patients with minor head injuries with any one of the following:
High risk (for neurological intervention) • GCS score <15 at 2 h after injury • Suspected open or depressed skull fracture • Any sign of basal skull fracture (haemotympanum, 'racoon' eyes, cerebrospinal fluid otorrhoea/rhinorrhoea, Battle's sign) • Vomitting ≥ two episodes • Age ≥65 years
Medium risk (for brain injury on CT) • Amnesia before impact >30 min • Dangerous mechanism (pedestrian struck by motor vehicle, occupant ejected from motor vehicle, fall from height >3 feet or five stairs) Minor head injury is defined as witnessed loss of consciousness, definite amnesia or witnessed disorientaion in a patient with a GCS score of 13–15.

If a compound or depressed fracture of the skull is suspected clinically, a CT brain scan should be performed. A compound depressed skull fracture is considered a neurosurgical emergency because of the increased risk of infection, such as meningitis or brain abscess.

There are no current indications for MRI scan of the brain in acute neurotrauma owing to the technical difficulties associated with the presence of patient monitoring and life support equipment, which interferes with the MRI.

Neck injury

If there is a clinical suspicion of a traumatic dissection, occlusion or tear of either the carotid or vertebral arteries (head or neck pain, increasing cervical haematoma, Horner's syndrome or abnormal neurological signs) then vascular imaging should be performed. Four-vessel digital subtraction angiography (DSA) is the reference standard for diagnosing vascular injury, but it is invasive and requires transfer of the patient to the DSA suite. CT angiography (CTA) is a valuable screening tool for vascular injury that combines high diagnostic accuracy with clinical practicability.[10] Doppler studies may provide some relevant information with regard to vascular status in the carotid or vertebral arteries if the patient is haemodynamically unstable for a CT angiogram to be performed, but has reduced sensitivity compared to CTA or DSA.

Figure 3.8.6 shows a dissection of the right internal carotid artery due to blunt trauma.

Facial injury

Facial trauma may range from relatively trivial undisplaced nasal bone fractures to the life-threatening problems of airway protection and haemorrhage associated with midfacial (Le Fort) fractures. There may also be underlying cerebral injury associated with frontal bone fractures.

The commonest injury to the midface is the blowout fracture caused by a direct blow to the orbit, which results in a fracture of the orbital floor or the medial wall of the orbit in the region of the paper-thin lamina papyracea (Fig. 3.8.7). There may be tenderness over the fractured bone associated

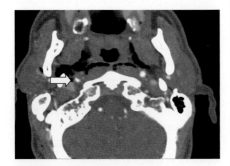

Fig. 3.8.6 Right internal carotid artery dissection on axial CT scan.

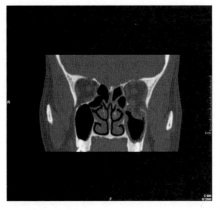

Fig. 3.8.7 Coronal CT scan of facial bones with blowout fracture left orbital floor with orbital contents extruding into left maxillary antrum.

with diplopia due to entrapment of orbital contents, or (less commonly) visual disturbance due to globe or optic nerve injury. These fractures are best seen on CT scans with multiplanar reconstructions. Blowout fractures with entrapment of orbital contents require surgical elevation.

Mandibular fractures are usually obvious clinically because of pain, malocclusion and drooling. Mandibular fractures may be difficult to demonstrate on standard PA and oblique views. A panoramic view or orthopantomogram (OPG) is more useful, but CT of the mandible provides optimal demonstration of mandibular fractures, including those involving the mandibular neck, condyle and temporomandibular joint (TMJ) (Fig. 3.8.8).

Fractures of the zygoma are classified as (a) tripod fractures and (b) isolated fractures of the zygomatic arch. The tripod fracture or zygomaticomaxillary fracture separates the malar eminence of the zygoma from its frontal, temporal and maxillary attachments. Tripod fractures are usually caused by a significant force to the body of the zygoma or the malar eminence. The three fractures that constitute the tripod fracture are located in the inferior orbital margin, the lateral orbital margin or the zygomaticofrontal suture and the zygomatic arch. These fractures are best viewed on CT scans (Fig. 3.8.9).

The Le Fort fractures are caused by direct trauma to the midface. The Le Fort 1 fracture involves the maxilla at the level of the nasal floor and will allow mobility of the palate. Le Fort 2 passes through the

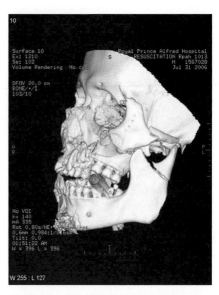

Fig. 3.8.8 Left mandibular ramus fracture as seen on 3D reconstruction (associated with mandibular body and zygomatic fractures). (Courtesy of Dr Richie Maher.)

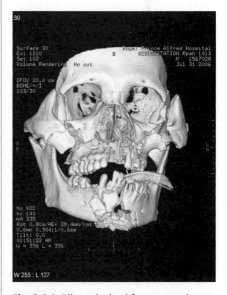

Fig. 3.8.9 Bilateral tripod fractures and mandibular fracture seen on 3D CT reconstruction. (Courtesy of Dr Richie Maher.)

nasal bones, as well as the medial, inferior and lateral walls of the maxillary antrum. The Le Fort 3 involves the nasal bones, the medial and lateral orbital walls, and the zygomatic arch.

Some facial fractures are unable to be classified owing to marked fragmentation of the bones and are termed as 'central facial smash'. These fractures are best viewed by axial CT scans with multiplanar reformatting.

Frontal sinus fractures commonly occur as a result of direct force and are often compound, with the risk of associated intracranial infection. There may be an associated intracranial haematoma or cerebral contusion. A CT scan will best evaluate these fractures, and determine the involvement of the posterior sinus wall. These fractures often require surgical exploration for debridement and repair.

Spine

Cervical spine

Cervical spine injuries can be classified into those with:

- fractures and no neurological deficit
- fractures associated with neurological deficit
- a small group of patients with cord injuries associated with contusion, haemorrhage or oedema without bony injury.

The cervical spine can be evaluated radiologically by plain X-rays, CT and MRI.

The cervical spinal column is the most frequently injured part of the spinal canal (60%)[11] owing to its flexibility and exposure. Any patient with significant blunt trauma and some who have penetrating injuries are at risk for cervical spine fracture.[12]

Patients who sustain blunt trauma have an estimated overall incidence of cervical spine fracture of 3–8%.[12] There is also an increased incidence of cervical spine fractures with an injury above the clavicles, as well as with any head injury.[13]

Ryan et al.[14] found that, if there was a fracture of C1–C2, there was a 9% chance of a cervical fracture below C3; hence the importance of imaging the entire cervical spine to the cervicothoracic junction. Unconscious patients with a significant mechanism of injury should have full spinal precautions until there is the opportunity for clinical and radiological evaluation of the spinal column and its contents.

Absolute indications for radiology of the cervical spine include patients who present with signs of cord injury and those with an altered level of consciousness where a clinical assessment of the spinal column and cord cannot be made.

There are established criteria for identifying patients with a low risk for cervical

Table 3.8.6 Low-risk criteria for radiological clearance of the cervical spine in a multitrauma patient (NEXUS criteria)
Disturbed conscious state e.g. head injury, intoxication for any reason
Any neurological motor or sensory signs
Midline cervical tenderness
Other major distracting injuries in a multitrauma patient

spine injury who do not require imaging, as derived from the NEXUS Study (National Emergency X-Radiography Utilization Study)[15] (Table 3.8.6). The NEXUS study was a large validation study that identified 818 spinal injuries out of 34 000 patients, and identified patients as low risk for cervical spine injury if all four high-risk clinical findings were absent. If the above criteria were met, there was no need for any imaging or further immobilization of the cervical spine. The results were 99.6% sensitive for clinically important cervical spine injuries. However, the specificity was only 12.9%, which led to some concern that the use of cervical X-rays may actually increase.

The NEXUS study also found that cervical spine X-rays missed up to one-third of secondary spinal injuries where it was thought there was a single non-significant spinal injury, and up to 25% of those missed injuries were non-contiguous with the original injury.[16] These findings have led to increased use of CT in full evaluation of the cervical spine.

The Canadian C-Spine Rule for radiography in alert and stable trauma patients[17] may be more valuable clinically and is well validated in a prospective cohort study (Table 3.8.5). This rule demonstrated 100% sensitivity and 42.5% specificity for clinically important cervical spine injuries, and there was good interobserver agreement for each variable, with κ value > 0.6 and a strong association with outcome (spinal injury) $P < 0.05$.

The above clinical decision rules should be applied with caution in the elderly or the very young (< 2 years). Owing to the relative immobility of the cervical spine or to pre-existing spinal disease the elderly may sustain cervical spine fractures even in the presence of a seemingly trivial injury.[12]

If the cervical spine cannot be cleared clinically, then a radiological examination must be performed.

Cervical spine X-ray The trauma series for cervical spine clearance consists of lateral, anteroposterior and open-mouth odontoid process (peg) views.

The lateral view must be adequate (to the C7–T1 junction) and show appropriate *alignment* of the three lines (see Fig. 3.8.2). As well as alignment and adequacy, one should inspect the bones (for fractures), cartilage and soft tissues.

Inspection of *alignment and adequacy* on the lateral cervical spine X-ray (see Fig. 3.8.1) should include the four lordotic lines: anterior and posterior vertebral lines, the spinolaminar line, and the line linking the tips of the spinous processes. In adults up to 1.0 mm of anterior subluxation (and up to 3 mm in children) may be normal in a true lateral film taken at 1.8 m.

True pseudosubluxation is commonest in children up to the age of 8 years, but may be seen up to age 18.[18] It commonly occurs between C2 and C3, and less commonly at the C3–4 and C4–5 levels. The key radiological feature is the preservation of the spinolaminar line in flexion/extension views of the lateral cervical spine.[16]

Angulation of up to 11° between adjacent vertebrae may be normal.[19] The sagittal (AP) diameter of the spinal canal should be measured. At the C2 level the lower limit radiographic measurement of the AP diameter of the spinal canal is 14 mm, and the upper limit of the cord AP measurement is 11 mm. At the C7 level the lower limit of the AP canal diameter is 12 mm and the upper limit of the cord measurement is 9 mm.[20]

Bony canal All the cervical vertebrae should be systematically examined, including vertebral body, pedicles, facet joints, laminae and spinous processes and the interspinous distance.

The 'ring' of increased radiodensity formed by the odontoid process and the facet joints of C1–C2 is known as the 'Harris ring'. This ring should be intact anteriorly, superiorly and posteriorly, indicating an intact odontoid process and facet joints of C1–2. A type 2 fracture of the odontoid process through the body may be visible on the lateral cervical spine X-ray.

Table 3.8.5 The Canadian C-Spine rule

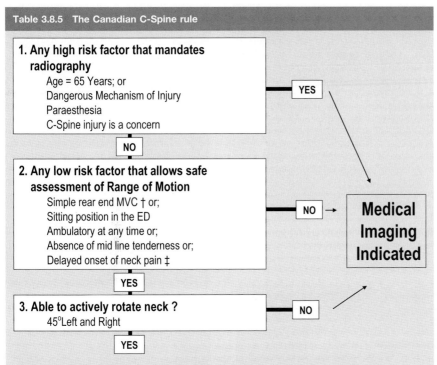

1. Any high risk factor that mandates radiography
Age = 65 Years; or
Dangerous Mechanism of Injury
Paraesthesia
C-Spine injury is a concern

NO

2. Any low risk factor that allows safe assessment of Range of Motion
Simple rear end MVC † or;
Sitting position in the ED
Ambulatory at any time or;
Absence of mid line tenderness or;
Delayed onset of neck pain ‡

YES

3. Able to actively rotate neck ?
45°Left and Right

YES

YES → **Medical Imaging Indicated** ← NO

NO

The Canadian C-Spine Rule for alert (Glasgow Coma Scale score = 15) and stable trauma patients where cervical spine injury is a concern

From Stiell IG, Wells GA, McKnight RD, et al. Canadian C-Spine Rule study for alert and stable trauma patients: I. Background and rationale. *CJEM* 2002;4(2):84-90

Canadian C-spine Rules – Key

Inclusion Criteria
Alert (GCS=15)
Stable (BP.90, RR>12, HR: 50-140)
C-Spine injury is a concern

* Dangerous Mechanism
Fall from a height > 1 metre / stairs
Axial load to head (eg diving)
Motorised recreational vehicles
Bicycle collision

† Simple Rear End MVC excludes:
Pushed into oncoming traffic
Hit by bus or large truck
Rollover
Hit by high speed vehicle

≠ Delayed
Not immediate onset of pain

Atlanto-occipital and atlantoaxial bony injuries

Atlanto-occipital dislocation is usually associated with a fatal injury, whereas atlanto-occipital subluxation is radiologically subtle and the patients usually survive.

The diagnosis is made by recognizing an abnormal basion–axial interval and/or an abnormal basion–dental interval. Normally neither should exceed 12 mm,[22] and this is best seen on the lateral cervical spine X-ray or the sagittal CT scan of the cervical spine (Fig. 3.8.10).

The space between the odontoid and the anterior arch of C1 measured at its most inferior margin should not exceed 3 mm in adults, and may be up to 5 mm in children. If this distance is exceeded there may be a rupture of the transverse atlantal ligament of the dens.

Occipital condyle[23] and C1–C2 fractures are often missed on the lateral cervical spine X-ray, with the only indication of a fracture being an increase in soft tissue swelling in this area. The initial lateral cervical spine X-ray should be accompanied by an open-mouth (odontoid process) and an AP view.

The open-mouth (odontoid) view should be inspected for alignment of the lateral

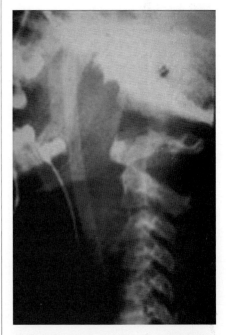

Fig. 3.8.10 Imaging of the cervical spine atlanto-occipital dislocation.

Cartilage All the spaces between adjacent vertebrae should be inspected for equality.

Soft tissue The prevertebral soft tissue should be inspected. A distance greater than 7 mm at C2 and 22 mm at C6 in the adult indicates the presence of a prevertebral haematoma.[21] If this is present, then a fracture or ligamentous disruption must be excluded. In children the upper prevertebral space may be larger than in adults owing to the presence of increased nasopharyngeal lymphoid tissue, and it may also increase in infants during crying.

masses of C1–C2, which is abnormal in the Jefferson fracture, fracture of the odontoid process (types 1–3) and rotatory subluxation of C1 on C2. Rotation of the head can simulate pathological malalignment in this region. The AP view of the cervical spine should be checked for alignment of the articular pillars and vertebral bodies. The spinous processes should be centred, and deviation of these from the midline may indicate a unilateral facet dislocation. Widening of the interspinous distance may indicate subluxation or dislocation. Fractures and dislocations may cause malalignment or compression of the vertebral bodies.

CT scan cervical spine

Many trauma centres now routinely perform limited plain X-rays and a CT scan of the entire cervical spine from occipital condyles down to and including T4–5 (Table 3.8.7). There is now a limited role for swimmer's and oblique views of the cervical spine, given the widespread use of CT scan (Figs 3.8.12–16).

Indications for MRI of the cervical spine include:

- patients with complete or incomplete neurological deficit
- deteriorating neurological status
- suspected ligamentous or intervertebral disc injury.

MRI will provide clear and concise pictures of all structures, particularly the spinal cord, intervertebral discs and soft tissues. Bony structures are also demonstrated, but fine bony detail is best seen on a CT scan. A MRI scan may show abnormalities in different planes and will highlight solid/fluid structures depending on the weighting of

Table 3.8.7 Imaging of patients with major trauma (Spinal Clearance Management Protocol, 30.6.05, Helen Ackland, The Alfred Hospital, Melbourne, Australia)
Plain AP and lateral X-rays cervical spine
MSCT* 1 mm cuts C0–C3 (axial + sagittal and coronal reformats)
MSCT 3 mm cuts C2–T 4/5 (axial + sagittal reformats)

*Multislice CT scans

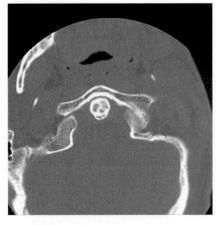

Fig. 3.8.11 CT of normal cervical spine axial view CI and odontoid process.

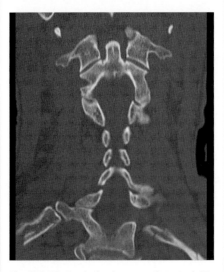

Fig. 3.8.12 Cervical spine normal coronal CT view.

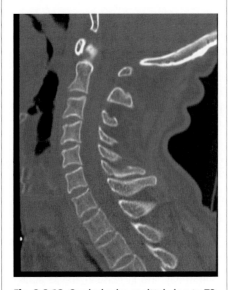

Fig. 3.8.13 Cervical spine sagittal view to T3.

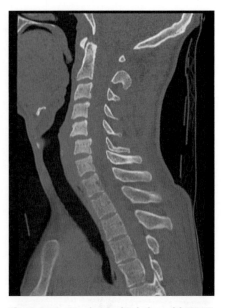

Fig. 3.8.14 CT spine sagittal view with C5/6 subluxation.

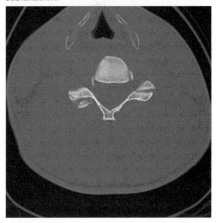

Fig. 3.8.15 CT cervical spine axial view C5-6 right unilateral facet fracture dislocation.

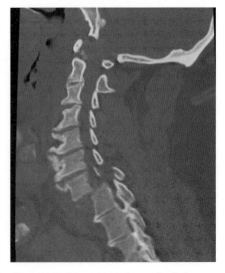

Fig. 3.8.16 CT cervical spine sagittal view bifacet dislocation C7/T1.

the images (Table 3.8.8). There is a small group of patients who will be unsuitable for an MRI scan (Table 3.8.9). An MRI scan also provides information regarding spinal cord injury patterns, such as central cord syndrome, which have been previously unavailable with other imaging modalities (Fig. 3.8.17).

Indications for flexion/extension films include ongoing pain or tenderness of the cervical spine in a patient who is neurologically intact and fully alert, looking for evidence of ligamentous instability. The patient must be able to flex and extend his or her neck voluntarily, and these X-rays

Table 3.8.8 Spinal abnormalities seen on the MRI scan
Spinal cord injury (haemorrhage or oedema)
Disc herniation
Epidural haematoma
Epidural abscess
Bone fracture/dislocation
Ligamentous rupture

Table 3.8.9 Conditions unsuitable for MRI scan
Metallic components, e.g. bullets, aneurysm clips
Haemodynamically unstable patients
Patients requiring ventilation and extensive physiological monitoring

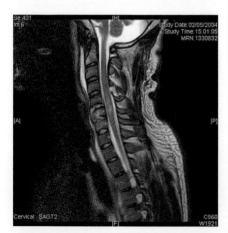

Fig. 3.8.17 MRI sagittal view C6 fracture + cord contusion.

should be supervised by the medical officer who ordered the investigation.

In the unconscious patient there is controversy as to the best approach for clearing the cervical spine, as there is a clear need to remove the hard collar in order to prevent the development of scalp pressure areas.

Dynamic flexion/extension X-rays in unconscious patients have a poor sensitivity for detecting cervical instability, have high rates of inadequacy, are not cost-effective and are potentially dangerous.

Hospitals which receive trauma victims should have agreed guidelines for clearing the cervical spine in unconscious patients which involves multislice CT (MSCT) and plain X-rays. If there is any abnormality seen on CT (such as misalignment of the vertebrae or a high cervical fracture), then MRI is performed to exclude ligament, disc or atlanto-occipital/atlantoaxial disruption. If the imaging is normal, the cervical spine is cleared. The patient can then be nursed without the cervical collar, and care should be taken to avoid extreme cervical spine flexion or extension until a clinical examination can be made. (See Spinal clearance Management Protocol, for further information).

Vertebral artery dissection

Any fracture of the cervical spine that involves the vertebral foramina may involve the vertebral artery, and consideration should be given to assessing this artery for acute dissection by CT angiography. Vertebral artery dissection may result in brainstem ischaemia or infarction.

Thoracolumbar spine

The second most frequently injured area of the spinal column after the cervical spine is the thoracolumbar junction (T11–L2). Cord injuries in this region comprise about 20% of all spinal cord injuries.[11] The main reasons for the susceptibility of this vertebral region are the abrupt transition from the rigidly fixed thoracic spine to the more mobile lumbar spine, and the fact that the spinal canal in the thoracic region is smaller in diameter than the cervical or lumbar spinal canals, resulting in increased risk to the cord.

An important concept used for interpreting thoracolumbar injuries is the 'three-column' theory described by Denis.[24] This is a widely accepted concept which divides a vertebra into three columns: the anterior column, which consists of the anterior longitudinal ligament and the anterior part of the vertebral body; the middle column, which includes the posterior part of the vertebral body and the posterior longitudinal ligament; and the posterior column, which includes all the bony and ligamentous structures posterior to the posterior longitudinal ligament. Fractures involving the anterior column are considered stable, whereas fractures involving the anterior and middle columns or all three columns are considered unstable.

It is also of note that injuries in the T1–T10 region comprise 16% of cord injuries, and lumbosacral injuries such as cauda equina lesions comprise approximately 4% of spinal neurological injuries.[11]

As it is often difficult to obtain satisfactory images of the upper thoracic spine, particularly the T1–T4 region, multislice CT with multiplanar reconstructions is currently the most effective method of establishing the extent of bony injury. It is the practice of many trauma centres to routinely perform a CT of the cervical spine to T4–5 with multiplanar reconstructions.

Classification of thoracolumbar spine injuries

- Stable fractures, which include transverse process fractures, spinous process fractures, pars interarticularis fractures, and wedge compression fractures involving the anterior two-thirds only of the vertebral body.
- Unstable fractures/dislocations, which include compression fractures with middle and/or posterior column disruption, the 'Chance' fracture, the burst fracture and flexion/distraction injuries.

Fractures in the fused thoracic spine (ankylosing spondylitis, diffuse interstitial spinal hypertrophy (DISH) (see Fig. 3.8.16) and advanced degenerative disc disease with bridging osteophytes) constitute a unique subset. These injuries are typically a result of hyperextension, usually involve three columns, and are therefore unstable. Cord damage is common in this type of fracture.

If a patient is unable to be examined clinically because of pain or tenderness of the thoracolumbar spine, or is unconscious, this area must be imaged. If a CT scan of the chest and abdomen/pelvis is performed, then sagittal and coronal reconstructions of the thoracolumbar (TL) spine can be done.

If CT of the torso is not performed, then plain X-rays of the thoracolumbar spine should be taken, with limited CT of any areas difficult to visualize or where there is clinical suspicion (Fig. 3.8.18).

The Chance fracture is an example of a distraction or seatbelt injury, with the lap belt as the axis of rotation and failure of the spinal column in its posterior ligamentous and bony elements. This fracture is horizontal through the entire bony column, including vertebral body, pedicles, laminae and spinous processes, and is by definition unstable. This fracture may also be associated with injuries to the abdominal contents, e.g. pancreas or duodenum.

Fractures of the lower lumbar spine and sacrum may involve the cauda equina and associated sacral nerve roots. There may be bladder, bowel and sexual dysfunction, as well as variable motor and sensory deficit in the lower limbs. There is often significant neuralgia that is disabling and difficult to treat. Plain X-rays will give some indication of the severity of the bony injury, but CT scanning is required for definitive information if surgical fixation is required.

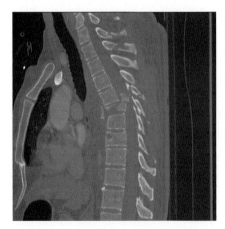

Fig. 3.8.18 CT sagittal view fracture T6 burst fracture with retropulsion of the bony fragments into the spinal canal.

Coccygeal fractures are due to direct blows and are both treated and diagnosed clinically. Radiology is not usually necessary for diagnosis, which is best made by CT scanning. There may be an associated rectal injury that requires operative repair, but otherwise analgesia only is required.

Chest trauma

The chest X-ray has a key role in the investigation of multiple trauma involving the thorax. There remains controversy, however, regarding the roles of chest CT, digital subtraction angiography (DSA) and transoesophageal echo (TOE). Investigations other than CXR may be decided to some extent by the availability of the above modalities at different institutions. The CT chest scan has become more accessible in recent years, whereas the use of TOE and angiography remains confined to the major centres. It is important that the trauma team leader has a clear understanding of the advantages, disadvantages and limitations of each investigation so that he/she can carefully choose the most appropriate investigation available at each institution.

A recent study by Traub and colleagues[25] found that chest CT was more effective than X-rays in detecting lung contusions, pneumothoraces and mediastinal haematoma, as well as fractured ribs, scapula, sternum and vertebrae. The authors found that it was more likely than CXR to provide further diagnostic information in the presence of chest wall tenderness, reduced air entry and/or abnormal respiratory rate.

The trauma room CXR should ideally be performed in the erect position with a nasogastric tube in situ. However, because it is often impossible to clear the cervical or thoracolumbar spine in the trauma room, the CXR is frequently taken in the supine position. This can create a number of difficulties in interpretation of the results. The AP projection of the X-ray beam will magnify the mediastinal structures and, when the patient is supine, the thoracic veins will passively distend and add to this appearance of mediastinal widening. Small pneumothoraces and haemothoraces are also difficult to detect on the supine CXR because the air distributes as a thin film

anteriorly[26] and blood as a thin homogeneous layer posteriorly. A haemothorax of 200–300 mL will normally be visible on a good-quality erect CXR, whereas it will usually require 800–1000 mL to produce the 'fuzzy' appearance of a haemothorax seen on the supine CXR.[27]

Examination of the CXR will often begin with a review of the bones and soft tissues. The CXR is a poor diagnostic aid for rib fractures as it will miss up to 50% of anterior and lateral fractures;[25] instead, the assessment should be directed more towards the complications of rib fractures, such as pneumothorax or haemothorax. It is also important to remember that the clavicles and scapulae are visible on the CXR. Fractures of these bones, along with fractures of the first and second ribs, are indicators of significant blunt thoracic trauma and should prompt a careful examination for underlying visceral and vascular injuries.

Sternal fractures may be seen on a lateral CXR but are best seen on CT. The significance of sternal fractures will largely direct the examination towards underlying mediastinal injuries. Brookes et al.,[27] in a retrospective study, found a 2% incidence of sternal fractures associated with motor vehicle accidents. These patients had a very low incidence (1.5%) of cardiac arrhythmias due to cardiac muscle contusion requiring treatment, and a mortality rate of less than 1%. The authors found that those at risk of cardiac arrhythmias requiring treatment were over 65 years of age and either had preexisting ischaemic cardiac disease or were on digoxin treatment. They recommended that cardiac monitoring was not required unless the patient fulfilled the above criteria. They also found that the 12-lead ECG was not predictive for the development of arrhythmias requiring treatment.

In a prospective study of 333 patients with significant blunt thoracic trauma, Velmahos et al.[28] found that the combination of normal ECG and troponin I both at admission and 8 hours later ruled out the diagnosis of significant blunt cardiac injury. Significant blunt cardiac injury was defined as the presence of cardiogenic shock, arrhythmias requiring treatment and post-traumatic structural deficits.

In cases of penetrating chest trauma, a foreign body may be evident on the CXR.

AP and lateral projections with appropriate skin markers will normally be required to help locate the position of the foreign object. In cases where the foreign object is embedded close to or in a pulsatile thoracic structure, the object may appear blurred on the film, indicating the proximity of the foreign body to the vessel.

Subcutaneous emphysema may be seen on the CXR and may result from injury to the lung, the tracheobronchial tree, the larynx, pharynx and oesophagus. Subcutaneous emphysema should prompt a careful examination for evidence of a pneumothorax and pneumomediastinum. Subcutaneous emphysema and pneumothorax are common findings in traumatic injury to the lung, and also occur in tracheobronchial injury.

In cases of suspected tracheal laceration, where the patient has been intubated, the appearance of the endotracheal tube on the CXR should be carefully examined. The normal position of the balloon is 2.5 cm proximal to the tip of the endotracheal tube (Table 3.8.10).

If a pneumothorax is suspected but not visible on the supine CXR, a CT scan is the definitive investigation.

In cases of penetrating chest trauma, the development of a detectable pneumothorax may be delayed and so it is recommended that check CXR be performed at 6 and 12 hours.[26]

The lung fields may become opacified by contusion, aspiration, pulmonary fat embolism and either cardiogenic or non-cardiogenic pulmonary oedema. Lung contusions will usually develop rapidly within 6 hours of an injury, whereas the changes of aspiration and pulmonary infarction are often delayed for 12–24 hours. Rib fractures are frequently associated with pulmonary contusions, although in paediatric patients and young adults the ribs are more compliant and may bend in, causing a contusion without fracture.

Diaphragmatic injuries are more frequent in penetrating than in blunt trauma. In blunt trauma, however, 80% of diaphragmatic injuries occur on the left side because the liver and its ligamentous attachments protect the right side (Table 3.8.11).

If a nasogastric tube is in situ, it may be seen to pass down into the abdomen and back up into the chest contained within the herniated stomach. Lower rib fractures are often seen in association with injuries to the diaphragm.

Thoracic aortic injury

Ninety per cent of injuries occur in the region of the aortic isthmus, i.e. that part of the proximal descending aorta between the origin of the left subclavian artery and the site of attachment of the ligamentum arteriosum (1.5 cm in length). The ascending aorta is involved in only 5% of cases.[29]

As previously described, the supine AP CXR magnifies the mediastinal silhouette. Superior mediastinal widening is a common finding in cases of both penetrating and blunt trauma to the great thoracic vessels. The mediastinal width is measured at the top of the aortic knob. A width greater than 8.0–8.5 cm in a supine film or 6 cm in an erect film is suggestive of a mediastinal haematoma.[26]

The sensitivity of a widened mediastinum on CXR for the detection of thoracic aortic injuries has been estimated at 90% and the specificity 10%, but approximately 7% of patients with aortic rupture have a normal chest radiograph[30] (Fig. 3.8.19; Table 3.8.12).

Injuries to the oesophagus may occur in association with both blunt and penetrating chest trauma. The predominant X-ray finding in oesophageal injury is pneumomediastinum, and this may be associated with subcutaneous emphysema, pneumothorax, a left pleural effusion or a widened mediastinum.

Thoracic CT scan

Thoracic MSCT has become a common diagnostic aid in investigating the multitrauma patient with chest injuries. The

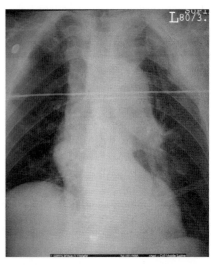

Fig. 3.8.19 CXR with widened mediastinum.

Table 3.8.10 Chest X-ray signs of tracheal laceration
Subcutaneous emphysema
Mediastinal emphysema
Pneumothorax
Deviation of the endotracheal tube tip to the right relative to the tracheal lumen
Distension of the endotracheal tube balloon
Migration of the endotracheal tube balloon distally towards the tube tip

Table 3.8.11 Signs of diaphragmatic injury on CXR
Elevated hemidiaphragm
Abnormal or indistinct contour of the diaphragm
Collapse of the lower lung fields
Inhomogeneous mass in the relevant hemithorax
Displacement of the mediastinum away from the injury

Table 3.8.12 Signs of aortic disruption on chest X-ray [29]

Widened mediastinum
  >6 cm in erect PA film
  >8 cm in supine AP film

Deviation of the oesophagus/NG tube to the right of T4 spinous process
Obliteration of aortic knob
Opacification of the aortopulmonary window
Deviation of the trachea to the right of the T4 spinous process
Depression of the left main bronchus to below 40° from the horizontal
Increased right paratracheal stripe (>4 mm)
Increased left paravertebral stripe (>5 mm)
Left apical cap

increasing speed and greater clarity of the MSCT scan gives a reliable and rapid means of screening for most intrathoracic injuries. The strength of CT lies in its ability to distinguish mediastinal haematoma from other causes of mediastinal widening detected on initial chest radiographs, e.g. magnification, mediastinal fat and tortuous vessels.

Chest CT is also a sensitive test for detecting pneumothorax, pneumomediastinum, pulmonary contusion and haemothorax and, with intravenous contrast, may demonstrate an intimal tear or pseudoaneurysm of the traumatized aorta.

Mediastinal haematoma is an indirect sign of aortic injury and appears as a soft tissue density around mediastinal structures,[30] or in acute aortic dissection a false lumen may be seen.

As a screening tool a conventional chest CT will detect a mediastinal haematoma, which will then require formal vascular imaging to exclude either a traumatic aortic rupture or dissection of the aorta or one of its branches. If no mediastinal haematoma is detected on CT, the probability of a significant aortic injury is very low and angiography is generally not needed. If direct signs of aortic injury are identified on CT, the patient may be taken to angiography, or occasionally directly to surgery.

If mediastinal major vascular injury is initially suspected a CT angiogram is the preferred screening investigation; however, conventional angiography or DSA remain the gold standard. CT angiography with 2–3 mm slices using injections of 100–150 mL contrast may be reconstructed in multiple planes to produce detailed images of the aorta. Studies have shown that CT angiography is sensitive for traumatic aortic injury (83–100%) with a high negative predictive value (NPV) of 99–100%[28,30] (Fig. 3.8.20).

A 3D spiral CT scan of the chest with contrast, but not performed as a CT angiogram, may overlook an intimal flap in the thoracic aorta.

Angiography

Transfemoral angiography is widely accepted as the gold standard for the diagnosis of major thoracic vascular injuries, particularly those involving the aorta and great vessels.[30] This investigation is not

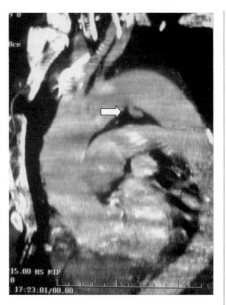

Fig. 3.8.20 CT angiogram showing small traumatic aortic rupture (arrow).

free from complications, although the morbidity and mortality are low. Significant complications such as rupture at the site of injury during contrast injection are rare, but have been reported.[31]

At most institutions, aortography is performed on patients who have suffered rapid deceleration injury, and who have a widened mediastinum or obscured aortic knuckle and descending aorta on CXR, or who have direct or indirect signs of aortic injury detected by CT.

At least two projections must be obtained, usually the left anterior oblique and the anteroposterior views. Arch angiography is more expensive than CT chest scans, especially when used as a screening tool for the exclusion of aortic injury, but the CT scan is less invasive and will show other traumatic chest injuries. Hunink[32] calculated that the cost per life saved was $2 million when CXR and angiography alone were used, compared to $500,000 per life saved when CT was introduced into the screening algorithm for low-to-moderate risk of aortic rupture.

Digital subtraction angiography (DSA)[33] offers some advantages over conventional angiography, being less expensive, with shorter examination times and requiring smaller amounts of contrast. The sensitivity, specificity and diagnostic accuracy of DSA are equivalent to those of conventional angiography.

Angiography remains the key investigation for the stable patient with penetrating injury to the thorax and lower neck. However, in one small study[34] angiography displayed a sensitivity of 67% and a specificity of 98%, whereas transoesophageal echocardiography (TOE) was accurate in predicting the presence or absence of an aortic injury with both a sensitivity and a specificity of 100%.

Transoesophageal echocardiography (TOE)

TOE has many supporters of its value as both a screening and a diagnostic test in the investigation of suspected mediastinal haematoma. Some authors[34,35] suggest that TOE is more accurate than angiography in detecting aortic injuries, although it is acknowledged that interpretation is operator dependent.

The advantages of TOE are that it can be performed quickly in the resuscitation area, it is minimally invasive, and it has a low rate of complications such as aspiration and oesophageal perforation. It can demonstrate myocardial, pericardial and valvular injuries. Disadvantages are that it may require sedation and intubation in the trauma patient, and may provide limited information about the distal ascending aorta, the aortic arch and the arch vessels.[35] Although the incidence of injury to the arch and major branch vessels is low, angiography is required when injury to these vessels is suspected.

The role of intravascular ultrasound is limited, but it may be of use to confirm subtle angiographic changes in the descending aorta.[36]

MRI is generally not practical for the diagnosis of traumatic aortic rupture.

Oral contrast studies

Oral contrast provides useful information in the investigation and diagnosis of oesophageal and diaphragmatic injuries. In cases of oesophageal perforation, Gastrografin is the preferred contrast medium, as it is less irritant than barium should there be a leak into the surrounding mediastinal tissues. A Gastrografin swallow is mandatory in the evaluation of suspected penetrating injuries of the oesophagus. If there is a risk of aspiration, Gastrografin should not be used as it produces a severe pneumonitis. In these circumstances contrast designed for intravenous use can be administered orally in order to demonstrate oesophageal perforation.

Flexible or rigid oesophagoscopy may also be used to exclude oesophageal perforation.

Abdomen/pelvis

Abdominal X-ray

The role of the plain abdominal X-ray (AXR) in the investigation of abdominal trauma is extremely limited. In cases of penetrating injuries it may be useful in the detection and localization of foreign bodies, and in the detection of free air under the diaphragm in hollow viscus rupture. An erect CXR may show free gas under the left hemidiaphragm more commonly than on the right. In cases of duodenal perforation, free retroperitoneal air may be seen as pockets of gas along the right psoas line (shadow) on a supine AXR. Both blunt and penetrating abdominal trauma may result in an ileus, seen as dilated bowel loops containing fluid levels on both erect and lateral decubitus films. Dilated small bowel can form a 'stepladder'-like appearance of the small intestine as it forms multiple loops lying one on top of the other.

Abdominal CT scan

Abdominal CT is usually performed with both oral and intravenous contrast. However, as most multitrauma patients have delayed gastric emptying, the bulk of oral contrast tends to remain in the stomach and upper gastrointestinal tract. This phenomenon has led some authors to suggest that oral contrast is of little use in this setting.[37] The increased speed of the helical CT scanner has resulted in excellent resolution for the detection of vascular injuries involving the liver, spleen and kidneys after intravenous contrast. In stable patients with possible intra-abdominal injuries, the abdominal CT has become the investigation of choice because, as well as being non-invasive, it reliably identifies intraperitoneal fluid, solid organ injury, retroperitoneal injuries and spinal and pelvic fractures. The use of intravenous contrast will also give some indication of both renal perfusion and function, as contrast is excreted into the ureters and bladder. One of the main limitations of abdominal CT is

that the investigation must be carried out in the radiology department, and so is inappropriate for any unstable patient. Injuries that may be missed on abdominal CT include upper intestinal perforation as well as injury to the diaphragm, pancreas and bladder[37] (Fig. 3.8.21).

Focused assessment by sonography for trauma (FAST) examination

Since the introduction of the focused ultrasound examination for trauma in the early 1990s in North America and in the late 1990s in Australasia, there has been some debate regarding the sensitivity, specificity and accuracy of the examination compared to diagnostic peritoneal lavage (DPL). In those centres that use FAST on a regular basis there has been a markedly reduced requirement for DPL. One of the criticisms of DPL has been its low specificity, resulting in an excessive non-therapeutic laparotomy rate of up to 30% in some centres.[38,39] The main utility of the FAST examination has been shown in the unstable trauma patient with intra-abdominal haemorrhage who requires urgent surgery,[40] and it has replaced DPL as the diagnostic modality of choice in these patients.

FAST requires the examination of four areas (Table 3.8.13). Its limitations include:

- It requires training.
- It cannot differentiate between fluids (blood vs ascites vs urine).
- Poor-quality images in obesity, subcutaneous emphysema and dilated bowel loops.[41]

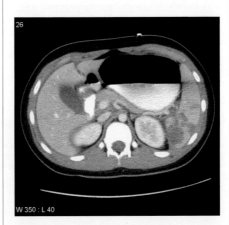

Fig. 3.8.21 CT abdomen with splenic laceration and associated haemoperitoneum.

Table 3.8.13 The FAST examination
1. The right upper quadrant (Morison's pouch)
2. The left upper quadrant (splenorenal recess)
3. The subxiphoid area (pericardium)
4. The suprapubic area (pouch of Douglas/ rectovesical pouch)

The FAST examination can be completed in 2–5 minutes, is non-invasive and is repeatable. It is very poor at detecting specific solid organ or hollow viscus intra-abdominal injuries, but if abdominal haemorrhage is ruled out and the patient is haemodynamically stable, then abdominal CT is indicated.

Tiling et al.[42] reported that FAST could consistently detect 200–250 mL of blood. Many studies have consistently reported a sensitivity of 80–100% and a specificity of 88–100% for the detection of intraperitoneal blood. It has also been consistently reported that FAST will not detect hollow viscus injuries, lacerations in the intra-abdominal solid organs, retroperitoneal or diaphragmatic injuries.

More recently there has been the development of contrast-enhanced ultrasound, which involves the intravenous injection of a small amount of microbubbles filled with substances such as perfluorocarbon which show a strong response when a low acoustic pressure is applied.[43] This technique can detect solid organ injuries and may enable non-operative treatment and avoid excessive use of radiation.

There is also some evidence that FAST is of value in penetrating trauma. Boulanger et al.[44] found that the routine use of FAST in penetrating trauma was useful for the detection of pericardial and peritoneal fluid. However, they cautioned that a negative FAST did not exclude hollow viscus or diaphragmatic injuries.

Many centres have introduced FAST into the algorithm for the routine assessment of victims of trauma. Boulanger et al.[45] have demonstrated in a prospective study that a FAST-based algorithm for blunt abdominal injury was more rapid, less expensive, and as accurate as an algorithm that used CT or DPL only. Hence there is a growing body of evidence showing that the only indication for DPL (when no FAST is available) is for suspected bowel perforation, which is usually diagnosed either by clinical examination or by CT.

There is also ample evidence in the literature that both emergency physicians[40,46] and surgeons[47] can learn to perform the FAST examination with clinically acceptable sensitivity, specificity and accuracy after a relatively short introductory course and hands-on practical supervision, combined with a supervised period of clinical scanning.

Radiology in pelvic trauma

In addition to plain radiology, pelvic CT scanning and angiography are becoming increasingly important in the diagnostic and therapeutic work-up of pelvic trauma. The trauma room AP X-ray of the pelvis should include all the bony pelvic components as well as both hip joints and the proximal femora, including greater and lesser trochanters.

Most anterior pelvic fractures are seen on the AP film, but up to 30% of posterior fractures involving the sacrum and sacroiliac joints will not be seen on the plain radiology. These fractures will be best seen on a two-dimensional or reformatted 3D CT scan of the pelvis (Fig. 3.8.22).

Acetabular fractures are often difficult to visualize on AP views and a CT scan of the pelvis may be required.

There are a number of radiological classifications of pelvic fractures that must be interpreted in association with the clinical impression of the fracture and associated complications. The greater the AP disruption of the pelvic ring and hence the greater the pelvic cavity volume, the more the potential for severe haemorrhagic shock and visceral damage.

A useful current classification is that by Young and Resnik (Table 3.8.14),[48] which is a modification of the Pennel and Tile classification[49] of pelvic fractures. This classifies fractures by mechanism of injury into AP compression, lateral compression, vertical shear and a combination; and takes into consideration rotational and/or vertical instability of the pelvic ring. If the pelvic ring is fractured anteriorly and posteriorly, stability is usually lost, with disruption of the posterior ligaments (sacroiliac, sacrotuberous and sacrospinous), and there will be widening of the sacroiliac joint(s) on the AP view. The classification provides a graded probability of bleeding related to the fracture, the development of haemorrhagic shock and associated organ damage.

CT scan of the pelvis

CT and plain X-rays are complementary modalities in the evaluation of pelvic fractures. Patients with pelvic fractures associated with haemodynamic instability are not suitable for placing in the CT scanner.

If the patient with pelvic fractures is haemodynamically unstable, it is important to ascertain whether there is intra-abdominal bleeding or not. If the FAST examination excludes intra-abdominal bleeding, then the patient should proceed to angiography if this is available.[50]

In stable patients CT is useful for demonstrating posterior fractures involving the sacrum and sacroiliac joints, as well as sacroiliac joint diastasis. Reformatted 3D images are particularly useful for the assessment of acetabular and pubic bone fractures.

More recently the speed and definition of MSCT scanners have meant that contrast-enhanced MSCT is a highly accurate, non-invasive way of identifying ongoing arterial bleeding.[51]

Pelvic angiography

Pelvic fractures that disrupt the posterior aspect of the pelvic ring have the potential to cause considerable arterial and/or venous injury. 'Open-book' or AP compression pelvic ring fractures are more likely to have venous rather than arterial bleeding, and compression of the pelvic ring by external fixation should help to minimize this blood loss, although this practice has not been validated by prospective, randomized controlled trials.

There remains considerable controversy regarding the role of angiography and arterial embolization in pelvic trauma, although with recent advances treatment options are becoming clearer. Factors such as age > 65, absence of long bone fractures and haemodynamic instability necessitating urgent angiography have been identified as predicting the likelihood of arterial bleeding in pelvic fractures.[48] Recent studies of the efficacy of angiographic embolization in select groups of haemodynamically unstable patients with pelvic fractures suggesting success rates for controlling bleeding in excess of 90% have led to a shift towards early radiographic intervention.[52–54]

The femoral artery is catheterized and angiography of both internal iliac arteries performed. If arterial bleeding is identified, then the vessels can be selectively embolized using coils, or the entire internal iliac

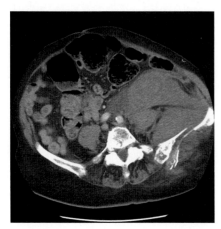

Fig. 3.8.22 Axial CT pelvis showing left pelvic fracture with large haematoma.

Table 3.8.14   Young and Resnick classification of pelvic fractures
AP compression
Type 1: Disruption of the symphysis pubis with less than 2.5 cm diastasis; no significant posterior pelvic injury
Type 2: Disruption of the symphysis pubis of more than 2.5 cm with tearing of the anterior sacroiliac, sacrospinous and sacrotuberous ligaments
Type 3: Complete disruption of the pubic symphysis and posterior ligament complexes, with hemipelvic displacement.
Lateral compression
Type 1: Posterior compression of the sacroiliac joint without ligament disruption; oblique pubic ramus fracture
Type 2: Rupture of the posterior sacroiliac ligament; pivotal internal rotation of the hemipelvis on the anterior SI joint with a crush injury of the sacrum and an oblique pubic ramus fracture
Type 3: Findings as in Type 2 injury with evidence of an AP compression injury to the contralateral hemipelvis.
Vertical shear
Complete ligament or bony disruption of a hemipelvis associated with hemipelvis displacement.

This classification does not take into consideration isolated fractures outside the bony pelvic ring or acetabular fractures.

vessels may be occluded with a Gelfoam slurry. There is a rich vascular supply to the pelvic viscera and major ischaemic complications are rare following pelvic embolization, but other problems such as impotence may occur.

Contrast studies

The main contrast studies used in pelvic fractures are the urethrogram and cystogram. Rupture of the membranous urethra may occur in association with pelvic fractures, particularly those involving distraction of the pubic symphysis or fractures involving both superior and inferior pubic rami. If there is clinical and radiological suspicion of potential urethral damage, an urethrogram should be performed. This is done by inserting a soft catheter into the urethral meatus and injecting contrast while screening with an image intensifier. The urethral passage, if patent, will be visualized and it may be possible to catheterize the urethra. If there is obstruction to the passage of dye or a false track is identified, a suprapubic catheter will be required. Further contrast is then injected into the bladder and PA and oblique views taken to assess for extravasation of contrast suggesting bladder rupture.

Extremities

Missed injuries occur in about 2–6% of blunt trauma patients. One retrospective study[55] found that musculoskeletal injuries and spinal fractures featured highly (6%) among the injuries not found after the initial primary and secondary surveys. The musculoskeletal injuries comprised mainly fractures and a small number of soft tissue injuries. Among the factors contributing to the missed injuries were the presence of closed head injury and intoxication. In comparison, one study[56] found the rate of abdominal missed injuries to be 2%.

A careful clinical examination of all joints and limbs looking for swelling, deformity and crepitus must be made in order to direct radiological investigation. Fractures, dislocations and ligamentous instability are more likely to be missed in the smaller, peripheral bones. As these injuries may be a source of ongoing disability due to late diagnosis, they may also be a potential source of litigation. Dislocations of joints

such as the anterior shoulder and elbow should be readily obvious, but less so are posterior shoulder and lunate/perilunate dislocation in the wrist. AP and lateral X-rays should be taken of any joint considered abnormal on examination during the secondary survey. In the lower limb, posterior dislocation of the hip and knee joints may cause serious sciatic nerve and popliteal artery damage, respectively, and require urgent reduction. If the viability of the limb or skin is threatened, a dislocation (e.g. knee or ankle) should be immediately reduced on clinical grounds, and X-ray performed after reduction to check for position and bony fractures.

Bony fractures in the upper limb which are commonly missed include medial or lateral epicondylar fractures, and supracondylar fractures of the elbow in children. In the adult, fractures of the carpal bones, in particular the scaphoid and triquetrum, may be missed unless carefully looked for, and these injuries may result in significant disability. Fractures and dislocations involving the metacarpals and phalanges are also easily missed in the multitrauma patient. The skier's (or gamekeeper's) thumb[57] is an acute sprain or rupture of the ulnar collateral ligament at the metacarpophalangeal joint caused by forceful abduction of the thumb. This injury may be missed unless the joint is specifically examined for stability, and stress views taken if indicated.

In the lower limb, fractures of the tibial plateau and calcaneus, which may occur as a result of a fall, may be missed unless sought both clinically and radiologically. Appropriate AP and lateral X-rays should be taken of these areas. In the foot, loss of Boehler's angle (normal 25–40°) may indicate a depressed fracture of the subtalar part of the calcaneus. Falls in general, and calcaneal fractures in particular, may be associated with fractures of the upper lumbar spine.

CT scans of complex fractures and dislocations may assist the orthopaedic surgeon in planning appropriate fixation. Joints where this may be helpful include large joints such as shoulder, hip and knee, e.g. tibial plateau fractures. Calcaneal fractures are often not clearly seen on plain X-rays and require a CT scan for a more accurate view. MRI is the investigation of choice for ligamentous or meniscal injuries in the knee.

Angiography is required when there is suspected or clinically obvious vascular compromise to either upper or lower limb. The axillary or brachial arteries may be damaged or transected in blunt or penetrating injuries to the upper limb. The brachial plexus can also be damaged in trauma around the shoulder joint, and should be actively looked for in these injuries. The commonest serious vascular injury to the lower limb may be associated with posterior dislocation of the knee and intimal disruption of the popliteal artery. Angiography will give accurate information regarding the degree of arterial damage and the state of the collateral flow.

Conclusion

Radiology in the multitrauma patient requires judicious decision making and interpretation of X-rays and other specialized modalities such as CT, MRI and ultrasonography. There is less reliance on plain X-rays and more emphasis on CT scans to rule in or out serious injury in the head, spine, chest and abdomen. Radiation exposure should be considered for all CT scans, especially in younger trauma patients. The use of the FAST examination has replaced DPL in the abdominal assessment, particularly if the patient is haemodynamically unstable. Missed injuries that are not diagnosed in the first 24–48 hours often contribute significantly to patient morbidity and mortality. These injuries may involve the musculoskeletal system in the form of limb or spinal fractures, and must be actively sought and excluded by appropriate clinical and radiological examination.

Controversies

- Clearance of the cervical spine in obtunded trauma patients can be made on the basis of fine cuts in a multislice CT scan, and MRI is not usually indicated. Flexion/extension X-rays should only be performed on awake and cooperative patients.

- CT angiography is invaluable in the investigation of blunt vascular injury to the neck, and should also be performed if there is cervical spine injury at the intervertebral foramen.

- Chest CT is the investigation of choice to exclude significant intrathoracic injury.

- The FAST examination is now part of the accepted trauma assessment and the indications for DPL are very few, e.g. exclusion of ruptured intra-abdominal viscus in an unstable patient.

- Pelvic angiography and embolization should be part of the resuscitation protocol in haemodynamically unstable patients with major pelvic fractures.

References

1. Tan GA, Van Every B. Staff exposure to ionizing radiation in a major trauma centre. ANZ Journal of Surgery 2005; 75: 136–137.
2. Wall BF, Hart D. Revised radiation doses for typical X-ray examinations. British Journal of Radiology 1997; 70: 437–439.
3. Aldrich JE, Bilawich AM, Mayo JR. Radiation doses to patients receiving computed tomography examinations in British Columbia. Canadian Association of Radiology Journal 2006; 57: 79–85.
4. http://www.radiologyinfo.org/en/safety/index.cfm?pg=sfty_xray&bhcp=1
5. Pierce DA, Shimizu Y, Preston DL, et al. Studies on the mortality of atomic bomb survivors. Report 12, Part 1, Cancer: 1950–1990. Radiation Research 1996; 146; 1–27.
6. Thompson DE, Mabuchi K, Ron E, et al. Cancer incidence in atomic bomb survivors. Part 11, Solid tumours. 1958–1987. Radiation Research 1994; 137: S17–S67.
7. http//www.pueblo.gsa.gov/cic_text/health/fullbody-ctscan/risks.htm
8. Valadka AB, Narayan RK. Injury to the cranium. In: Feliciano DV, Moore EE, Mattox KL, eds. Trauma, 3rd edn. Stamford CT: Appleton and Lange, 1996; 267–278.
9. Stiel IG, Wells GA, Vandemheen K, et al. The Canadian CT Head Rule for patients with minor head injury. Lancet 2001; 357: 1391–1396.
10. Zengel D, Rademacher G, Hanson B, et al. Screening for blunt cerebrovascular injuries: The essential role of computed tomography angiography. Seminars in Ultrasound CT and MRI 2007; 28: 101–108.
11. Satisky E, Votey S. Emergency department approach to acute thoracolumbar spine injury. Journal Emergency Medicine 1997; 15: 49–59.
12. Bell RM. Clearing the cervical spine. Personal communication 2000.
13. Williams J, Jehle D, Cottington E, et al. Head, facial and clavicular trauma as a predictor of cervical-spine injury. Annals of Emergency Medicine 1992; 21: 719–722.
14. Ryan MD, Henderson J. The epidemiology of fractures and fracture-dislocations of the cervical spine. Injury 1992; 23: 38–40.
15. Hoffman JR, Mower WR, Wolfson AB, et al. Validity of a set of clinical criteria to rule out injury to the cervical spine in patients with blunt trauma. National Emergency X-Radiography Utilisation Study Group. New England Journal of Medicine 2000; 343: 94–99.
16. Barrett TW, Mower WR, Zucker MI, et al. Injuries missed by limited computed tomographic imaging of patients with cervical spine injuries. Annals of Emergency Medicine 2006; 47: 129–133.
17. Stiell IG, Wells, GA, Vandemheen K, et al. The Canadian C-Spine Rule for Radiography in alert and stable trauma patients. Journal of the American Medical Association 2001; 286: 1841–1848.
18. Berquist TH. Cervical spine trauma. In: Kricum ME, ed. Imaging of sports injuries. Aspen Publications, 1992; 31–64.
19. Murphy MD, Batnizsky MD, Bramble JM. Diagnostic imaging of spinal trauma. In: Sartoris DJ. Ed. Musculoskeletal trauma. Radiology Clinics of North America 1989; 27: 855–872.
20. Lusted LB, Keats TE. The spine. In: Atlas of roentgenographic measurement, 2nd edn. Chicago: Yearbook Medical Publications, 1967; 101–103.
21. Keene JG, Daffner RH. Spinal trauma. In: Rosen P, Doris PE, Barkin RM, et al., eds. Diagnostic radiology in emergency medicine. St Louis: Mosby-Year Book, 1992; 210–270.
22. Harris JH. The cervicocranium: its radiographic assessment. Radiology 2001; 218: 335–337.
23. Noble EF, Smoker WRK. The forgotten condyle: The appearance, morphology, and classification of occipital condyle fractures. American Journal of Neuroradiology 1996;17: 507–513.
24. Denis F. The three column spine and its significance in the classification of acute thoracolumbar spinal injuries. Spine 1983; 8: 817–831.
25. Traub M, Stevenson M, McEvoy S, et al. The use of chest computed tomography versus chest X-ray in patients with major blunt trauma. Injury 2007; 38: 43–47.
26. Wilson RF. Thoracic trauma. In: Tintinalli JE, Ruiz E, Krone RC, eds. Emergency medicine. A comprehensive study guide. American College of Emergency Physicians, 4th edn. McGraw-Hill 1996; 1156–1182.
27. Brookes JG, Dunn RJ, Roger IR. Sternal fractures: A retrospective analysis of 272 cases. Journal of Trauma 1993; 35: 46.
28. Velmahos G, Karaiskakis M, Salim A, et al. Normal electrocardiography and serum troponin I levels preclude the presence of clinically significant blunt cardiac injury. Journal of Trauma 2003; 54: 45–51.
29. Sammett EJ. Aorta, trauma www.emedicine.com/radio/topic44.htm 2003.
30. Creasy JD, Chiles C, Routh WD, et al. Overview of traumatic injury of the thoracic aorta. Radiographics 1997; 17: 27–45.
31. Holtzman SR, Bettmann MA, Casciani T, et al. Expert Panel on Cardiovascular Imaging. Blunt chest trauma-suspected aortic injury. [online publication]. Reston (VA): American College of Radiology (ACR), 2005.
32. Hunink MGM, Bos JJ. Triage of patients to angiography for detection of aortic rupture after blunt chest trauma: cost-effectiveness analysis of using CT. American Journal of Neuroradiology 1995; 165: 27–36.
33. Mirvis SE, Pais SO, Gens DR. Thoracic aortic rupture: advantages of intra-arterial digital subtraction angiography. American Journal of Roentgenology 1986; 146: 987–991.
34. Keaney PA, Wesley Smith D, Johnson SB, et al. Use of transoesophageal echocardiography in the evaluation of traumatic aortic injury. Journal of Trauma 1993; 34: 696–703.
35. Smith MD, Cassidy JM, Souther S, et al. Transoesophageal echocardiography in the diagnosis of traumatic rupture of the aorta. New England Journal of Medicine 1995; 332: 356–362.
36. Williams DM, Dale MD, Bolling SF, et al. The role of intravascular ultrasound in acute traumatic aortic rupture. Seminars in Ultrasound, CT and MRI 1993; 14: 85–90.
37. Tsang BD, Panacek EA, Brant WE, et al. Effect of oral contrast administration for abdominal computed tomography in the evaluation of acute blunt trauma. Annals of Emergency Medicine 1997; 30: 7–13.
38. Ross SE, Dragor GM, O'Malley KF, et al. Morbidity of negative celiotomy in trauma. Injury 1995; 26: 393–394.
39. Henneman PL, Marx JA, Moore EE, et al. Diagnostic peritoneal lavage: Accuracy in predicting necessary laparotomy following blunt and penetrating trauma. Journal of Trauma 1990; 30: 1345.
40. Hsu JM, Joseph AP, Tarlinton LJ, et al. The accuracy of focused assessment with sonography in trauma (FAST) in blunt trauma patients: Experience of an Australian major trauma service. Injury. International Journal of Care of the Injured 2007; 38: 71–75.
41. Melanson SW, Heller M. The emerging role of bedside ultrasonography in trauma cases. Emergency Medical Clinics of North America 1998; 16: 165–189.
42. Tiling T, Bouillon B, Schmid A, et al. Ultrasound in blunt abdomino-thoracic trauma. In: Border JR. Allgoewer M, Hansen ST, et al., eds. Blunt multiple trauma: comprehensive pathophysiology and care. New York: Marcel Dekker, 1990; 415–433.
43. Valentino M, Serra C, Pavlica P, Barozzi L. Contrast-enhanced ultrasound for blunt abdominal trauma. Seminars in Ultrasound, CT and MRI 2007; 28: 130–140.
44. Boulanger BR, Kearney PA, Tsuei B, et al. The routine use of sonography in penetrating torso injury is beneficial. Journal of Trauma 2001; 51: 320–325.
45. Boulanger BR, McLellan BA, Brenneman FD, et al. Prospective evidence of the superiority of a sonography-based algorithm in the assessment of blunt abdominal injury. Journal of Trauma 1999; 47: 632–637.
46. Mandevia DP, Aragona J, Chan L, et al. Ultrasound training for emergency physicians – a prospective study. Academic Emergency Medicine 2000; 7: 1008–1014.
47. Shackford SR, Rogers FB, Osler TM, et al. Focused abdominal sonogram for trauma: the learning curve of nonradiologist clinicians in detecting haemoperitoneum. Journal of Trauma 1999; 46: 553–564.
48. Gill Cryer H, Johnson E. Pelvic fractures. In: Feliciano DV, Moore EE, Mattox KJ, eds. Trauma, 3rd edn. Stamford: Appleton and Lange, 1996; 635–659.
49. Pennel GF, Time M, Waddell JP, et al. Pelvic disruption: assessment and classification. Clinical Orthopedics 1980; 151: 12.
50. Martin J, Heetveld, Harris I, et al. Management of unstable patients with pelvic fractures. (Practice Guidelines, Liverpool Hospital NSW, July 2003.) http://www.swsahs.nsw.gov.au/livTrauma.
51. Stephen DJ, Kreder HJ, Day AC, et al. Early detection of arterial bleeding in acute pelvic trauma. Journal of Trauma 1999; 47: 638–642.
52. Velmahos GC, Toutouzas KG, Vassiliu P, et al. A prospective study of the safety and efficacy of angiographic embolization for pelvic and visceral injuries. Journal of Trauma 2002; 52: 303–308.
53. Miller PR, Moore PS, Mansell E, et al. External fixation or arteriogram in bleeding pelvic fracture: Initial therapy guided by markers of arterial haemorrhage. Journal of Trauma 2003; 54: 437–443.
54. Fangio P, Asehnoune K, Edouard A, et al. The epidemiology of fractures and fracture-dislocations of the cervical spine. Journal of Trauma 2005; 58: 978–984; discussion 984.
55. Kremli MK. Missed musculoskeletal injuries in a University Hospital in Riyadh: types of missed injuries and responsible factors. Injury 1996; 27: 503–506.
56. Sung C, Kim KH. Missed injuries in abdominal trauma. Journal of Trauma 1996; 41: 276–278.
57. Musharafieh RS, Bassim YR, Atiyeh BS. Ulnar collateral ligament injury in the emergency department. Journal of Emergency Medicine 1997; 15: 193–196.

3.9 Trauma in pregnancy

Steven Troupakis

ESSENTIALS

1 Trauma in pregnancy is the most common cause of non-obstetric maternal death, with most of the mortality due to head injury and haemorrhagic shock.

2 Fetal death occurs far more often than maternal death and is dependent on the severity of the maternal injuries. Placental abruption and direct fetal trauma cause most deaths.

3 Common causes of trauma are motor vehicle collisions, falls and assaults.

4 Important sequelae are bruising, fractures, premature labour, placental abruption, disseminated intravascular coagulopathy, fetomaternal haemorrhage, intra-abdominal injuries, uterine rupture and haemorrhagic shock.

5 The physiological changes that occur with pregnancy, such as the relative hypervolaemia and the gravid uterus, can make clinical assessment of the patient difficult.

6 Continuous cardiotocographic monitoring for at least 4 hours is the best predictor of placental abruption and fetal distress. Ultrasound and CT are also useful, especially in assessing intra-abdominal organs and for intraperitoneal fluid.

7 Maternal resuscitation remains the best method of fetal resuscitation.

Introduction

Trauma during pregnancy presents a unique set of challenges for the emergency department (ED), as the anatomical and physiological changes that occur during pregnancy will influence the evaluation of the patient. An appreciation of these changes is important. Aggressive resuscitation of the mother remains the best treatment for the fetus. Early obstetric consultation will help improve the outcome of these patients.

Anatomical and physiological changes in pregnancy

Cardiovascular

Blood volume increases by about 45% by the end of the third trimester.[1] With relative hypervolaemia the patient may lose up to 35% of her blood volume before signs of haemorrhagic shock appear. Maternal cardiac output increases by 1–1.5 L/min in the first 10 weeks. The resting heart rate increases by 15–20 beats/min by the end of the third trimester. Systolic and diastolic blood pressure fall by 10–15 mmHg during the second trimester, but rise again towards the end of the pregnancy. ECG changes may occur with the cephalic displacement of the heart, such as left axis deviation by 15°, T-wave inversion or flattening in leads III, V1 and V2, and Q waves in III and AVF.[2] After 20 weeks' gestation, supine positioning may cause inferior vena cava (IVC) obstruction by the gravid uterus, leading to a fall in cardiac output.

Haematological

A dilutional anaemia occurs with a fall in haematocrit (31–35% by the end of pregnancy). Pregnancy induces a leukocytosis, with levels up to 18 000/mm^3 in the third trimester. The erythrocyte sedimentation rate (ESR) is elevated by the third trimester (average 78 mm/h). Coagulation factors increase (fibrinogen, Factors VII, VIII, IX, X), increasing the risk of venous thrombosis. The buffering capacity of the blood is reduced.[3]

Respiratory

The diaphragm is elevated by about 4 cm. Tidal volume increases by 40% and the residual volume falls by about 25%. A respiratory alkalosis results, with a fall in PCO_2 to 30 mmHg. The anteroposterior diameter of the chest is increased, and the mediastinum is widened on chest X-ray.

Gastrointestinal

Cephalic displacement of intra-abdominal structures and delayed gastric motility increase the risk of aspiration. The intestines are displaced to the upper part of the abdomen and may be shielded by the uterus. The peritoneum is stretched by the gravid uterus, which may make signs of peritonism less reliable.[3] Alkaline phosphatase levels may triple because of placental production.

Urinary

Dilatation of the renal pelvis and ureters occurs from the 10th week of gestation. The bladder becomes hyperaemic and is displaced into the abdomen from the 12th week, making it more susceptible to trauma.

Uterine

There is a massive increase in uterine size. Blood flow to the uterus increases from 60 to 600 mL/min by the end of the pregnancy.

Epidemiology

The incidence of trauma during pregnancy is approximately 7%, the causes being similar to those in the general population.[4] Blunt trauma is the commonest injury, with motor vehicle accidents, falls and assaults being the other common causes in that order. Penetrating injuries are less common and usually the result of domestic violence. Stab wounds have a better prognosis for the fetus than do projectile wounds. Most trauma is of a minor nature, resulting in bruising, minor fractures and threatened premature labour. Maternal death from trauma is rare, but is the leading non-obstetric cause of death, with most fatalities due to head injuries and haemorrhage from internal injuries. Younger (age<20) and older (age>35) multiparous women at gestational ages of less than 28 weeks have a higher risk of adverse outcomes.[5] Women who are discharged undelivered continue to have delayed morbidity, with increased rates of placental abruption, low-birthweight infants and a ninefold increase in thrombotic events.[6] Fetal death occurs in about 1–2% of cases and is dependent on the gestational age and the pattern and severity of maternal injury. Most fetal deaths are due to placental abruption or direct trauma. High-speed (>80 km/h) and broadside motor vehicle accidents have a higher incidence of placental abruption and fetal and maternal death than do frontal collisions.[7] Similarly, ejection from a vehicle, and motorcycle and pedestrian collisions are associated with poor fetal outcome.[8] Maternal hypotension and vaginal bleeding are associated with increased fetal loss.[9] In one trauma series, pregnant patients with an Injury Severity Score (ISS) ≥12 had a fetal death rate of 65%; those with an ISS <12 had no fetal deaths.[10] Other studies have shown pregnancy loss with low ISS.[7,11]

Specific injuries

Pelvic fracture

Pelvic fracture is often the result of a high-speed motor vehicle accident. Massive haemorrhage can occur from the uterus, as well as bladder, urethral and ureteric lacerations. Retroperitoneal haemorrhage occurs and may be difficult to diagnose. Direct fetal skull fractures can lead to fetal death. The most common type of pelvic fracture involves the pubic rami of one half of the pelvic rim.[12] The majority of patients with a pelvic fracture can be delivered vaginally.

Placental abruption

Placental abruption complicates 1–5% of patients with minor trauma and between 20 and 50% of cases with major trauma.[13] The placenta separates from the underlying decidua because of shearing forces between the relatively inelastic placenta and the more elastic uterus. This leads to fetal hypoxia and death. Thromboplastin release may lead to the development of disseminated intravascular coagulopathy (DIC).

Uterine rupture

Uterine rupture is rare but leads to considerable haemorrhage and almost 100% fetal mortality. It should be suspected when there is maternal shock, fetal death, difficulty defining a uterus, easily palpable fetal parts and a positive peritoneal lavage.[14]

Fetomaternal haemorrhage

Fetomaternal haemorrhage is the transplacental spread of fetal blood into the maternal circulation. It occurs in approximately 8–30% of trauma cases, and may lead to Rhesus sensitization of the mother, neonatal anaemia, fetal cardiac arrhythmias and fetal death.[3] The Kleihauer–Betke test is used to identify and quantify fetomaternal haemorrhage. This test relies on the principle that fetal cells are stable in acid (pH 3.2), whereas adult haemoglobin is eluted from maternal red cells. Microscopy will identify fetal red blood cells on blood smear.

Presentation

History

Questions should be directed to determining the severity and type of trauma, as well as an obstetric history. In a motor vehicle accident, high speed, side collisions, ejection from the vehicle, and improper use of seatbelts and lap belts alone are associated with a greater likelihood of serious injuries.[7] Direct trauma to the abdomen is more likely to cause fractures, splenic and liver injuries, whereas indirect trauma via shearing forces is more likely to cause placental abruption. Pelvic pain, uterine contractions and vaginal bleeding may indicate placental abruption. An obstetric history is essential. The gestational age (>22 weeks) is the main determinant for fetal viability. Lack of fetal movements may indicate fetal death.

Primary survey

The airway should be assessed and cleared. Intubation may be difficult because of the aspiration risk, breast enlargement and cervical trauma. Breathing should be assessed and the patient given supplemental oxygen to improve both maternal and fetal oxygenation. If the patient is more than 20 weeks pregnant she should be placed on her side (preferably the left) to relieve any caval compression. If spinal immobilization is necessary, wedges can be placed underneath a spinal board, or alternatively the uterus pushed to the left manually. The blood pressure and circulation can then be assessed, remembering that signs of shock may present late because of relative hypervolaemia.

A quick assessment of conscious level and any major neurological deficits should be made. The patient should be adequately exposed for a thorough examination, but protected from a drop in temperature.

Secondary survey

The sequence of the secondary survey is the same as in the non-pregnant patient, but with an obstetric examination included in the abdominal examination. The uterus should be assessed for fundal height, tenderness, contractions, fetal heart tone, fetal movements and position. A Doppler ultrasound, stethoscope or fetoscope should be used to assess the fetal heart rate. An obstetrician should perform the pelvic examination, looking for trauma to the genital tract, cervical dilation, fetal presentation and station relative to the ischial spines. Nitrazine paper can be used to test for the presence of amniotic fluid: it turns blue in the presence of the alkaline fluid. Rectal examination and urinalysis are essential.

Investigations

Blood tests

Routine blood tests, such as full blood count, electrolytes, coagulation studies, group and hold, should be performed looking for evidence of anaemia and disseminated intravascular coagulopathy (DIC).[2] A Kleihauer–Betke test will indicate the necessary dose of Rhesus immunoglobulin in Rh-negative patients, but has proved unreliable in predicting fetal outcome.[4]

X-rays

In severe trauma it is necessary to take cervical spine, chest and pelvic films. The abdomen should be shielded and repetition of films avoided. There has been no increased risk to the fetus when radiation exposure has been limited to less than 0.1 Gy, and after 20 weeks' gestation radiation is unlikely to cause abnormalities.[2,15] A standard pelvic film delivers less than 0.01 Gy.

Ultrasonography

Ultrasonography is useful in determining gestational age, placental position and fetal well-being, and estimating amniotic fluid volume.[16] It can be used to diagnose placental abruption and uterine rupture, but this is dependent on the expertise of the operator. Rapid ultrasonography in the ED can indicate the presence of intra-abdominal fluid, especially in patients too unstable for CT.[17] Ultrasonography will detect only 40–50% of placental abruptions.[18] Cardiotocography (CTG) has proved more sensitive in diagnosing placental abruption.[8,19]

Cardiotocography

CTG monitoring beyond the 20th week of pregnancy has proved a sensitive way of diagnosing placental abruption early. It should be instituted early and continuously for at least 4 hours.[3,20] Frequent uterine contractions and fetal distress are suggestive of placental abruption. In one study no placental abruptions were missed if CTG monitoring remained normal for the first 4 hours.[13]

Computed tomography

Computed tomography (CT) is an accurate and non-invasive way of assessing uterine and retroperitoneal structures, but it is time-consuming and involves a higher radiation dose than normal X-rays, with exposure generally between 0.05 and 0.1 Gy.[2]

Diagnostic peritoneal lavage

Diagnostic peritoneal lavage (DPL) is highly sensitive in indicating significant intra-abdominal trauma.[12] However, it does not indicate which organ is involved, or if there is a retroperitoneal injury. It is safe and accurate in pregnancy as long as the operator is experienced in using an open technique, with the incision above the fundus.[2]

Management

Maternal resuscitation is the best method of fetal resuscitation. If the injuries are severe the patient should be in a resuscitation area, with a team approach to management and early surgical and obstetrical consultation. Attention to adequate oxygenation, proper positioning and aggressive fluid replacement is important. Oximetry, ECG, blood pressure monitoring and cardiotocography should be started early. A nasogastric tube should be inserted to reduce the risk of aspiration, as should an indwelling catheter for urinalysis and to allow better assessment of the uterus. X-rays as indicated should be performed as well as CT, DPL and ultrasound as necessary, to evaluate abdominal injuries. The choice between the three depends on the injuries suspected, the experience of the staff and the stability of the patient. If the patient remains unstable with hypotension or continued bleeding, laparotomy is indicated.[1] Ultrasound is particularly useful in the resuscitation phase to assess fetal heart rate and uterine bleeding.

The presence of vaginal bleeding, abdominal tenderness or pain, hypotension, absent fetal heart sounds, fetal distress on CTG and amniotic fluid leakage requires an urgent obstetric opinion and possibly a caesarean section.

Premature labour can be treated with tocolytic agents such as intravenous salbutamol. However, salbutamol causes maternal and fetal tachycardia, which may mask symptoms of hypovolaemia. Magnesium sulphate is recommended as an alternative tocolytic in abdominal trauma.[18,21]

Disseminated intravascular coagulopathy may develop as a result of placental abruption, amniotic fluid embolism and fetal death. Clotting factors may need to be replaced.

Anti-D immunoglobulin should be administered to all Rhesus-negative mothers.[22]

In general, penetrating injuries should be explored by laparotomy, especially if they involve the upper abdomen, where there is a high possibility of bowel perforation. Some authors argue that stab wounds over the uterus can be treated conservatively if there is no evidence of visceral injury, the entrance wound is below the fundus, the patient is stable and the missile is within the uterine cavity.[14]

Postmortem caesarean section should be considered within the first 4 minutes of the mother's arresting. There have been many cases of fetal survival up to 20 minutes after maternal death. The fetuses who have the best chance of surviving neurologically intact are those delivered within 5 minutes of the maternal arrest, who weigh more than 1000 g, and are of more than 28 weeks' gestation.[2,12]

Disposition

Patients who are haemodynamically unstable and who have extensive head or chest injuries will require surgical intervention and intensive-care support. Patients who are stable but show signs of fetal distress should undergo caesarean section. All patients with minor injuries who are more than 20 weeks pregnant should have CTG monitoring for at least 4 hours, preferably in a labour ward.

Prognosis

Most women who sustain trauma during pregnancy suffer few complications.[12,23] There is greater maternal and fetal mortality in pregnant women with higher Injury Severity Scores. Placental abruption can still occur as a result of minor trauma 24–48 hours after the accident, but 4 hours of CTG monitoring should detect this group of patients.[3]

Prevention

Properly worn seatbelts reduce both maternal and fetal mortality. In one study of serious motor vehicle accidents maternal mortality following ejection from the vehicle was 33%, compared to only 5% in those who were not ejected: fetal mortality was 47% and 11%, respectively.[14] A three-point seat bar system should be used, with the lap portion as low as possible, preferably over the thighs, and with the shoulder portion passing between the breasts and above the gravid uterus.

In a small series it appears that side airbags do not increase the risk of injury to pregnant women as long as other three-point restraints are used as well.[24]

Controversies

- The duration of CTG monitoring: most authors agree 4 hours should be enough to predict placental abruption, although some argue that 24–48 hours may be needed.

- Exploration of penetrating wounds to the abdomen: some authors argue for a conservative approach to a wound below the uterine fundus, whereas others argue that all such wounds should be explored.

References

1. American College of Surgeons. Advanced Trauma Life Support. Chicago, Illinois: American Chemical Society, 1993.
2. Esposito TJ. Trauma during pregnancy. Emergency Medicine Clinics of North America 1994; 12: 167–199.
3. Pearlman MD, Tintinalli JE, Lorenz RP. Blunt trauma during pregnancy. New England Journal of Medicine 1990; 323: 1609–1613.
4. Connolly A, Katz VL, Bash KL, et al. Trauma and pregnancy. American Journal of Perinatology 1997; 14: 331–336.
5. El Kady D, Gilbert WM, Anderson J, et al. Trauma during pregnancy: An analysis of maternal and fetal outcomes in a large population. American Journal of Obstetrics and Gynecology 2004; 190: 1661–1668.
6. El Kady D, Gilbert WM, Xing G, Smith LH. Association of maternal fractures with adverse perinatal outcomes. American Journal of Obstetrics and Gynecology 2006; 195: 711–716.
7. Aitokallio-Tallberg A, Halmesmaki E. Motor vehicle accident during the second or third trimester of pregnancy. Acta Obstetrica Gynecologica Scandinavica 1997; 76: 313–317.
8. Curet MJ, Schermer CR, Demarest GB, et al. Predictors of outcome in trauma during pregnancy: Identification of patients who can be monitored for less than 6 hours. Journal of Trauma 2000; 49: 18–25.
9. Baerga-Varella Y, Zietlow SP, Bannon MP, et al. Trauma in pregnancy. Mayo Clinic Proceedings 2000; 75: 1243–1248.
10. Ali J, Yeo A, Gana TJ, McLellan BA. Predictors of fetal mortality in pregnant trauma patients. Journal of Trauma 1997; 42: 782–785.
11. Schiff MA, Holt VL. The Injury Severity Score in pregnant trauma patients: predicting placental abruption and fetal death. Journal of Trauma 2002; 53: 946–949.
12. Kuhlmann RS, Cruikshank DP. Maternal trauma during pregnancy. Clinical Obstetrics and Gynaecology 1994; 37: 274–293.
13. Pearlman MD, Tintinalli JE, Lorenz RP. A prospective controlled study of outcome after trauma during pregnancy. American Journal of Obstetrics and Gynecology 1990; 162: 1502–1510.
14. Vaizey CJ, Jacobson MJ, Cross FW. Trauma in pregnancy. British Journal of Surgery 1994; 81: 1406–1415.
15. Goldman SM, Wagner LK. Radiological management of abdominal trauma in pregnancy. American Journal of Roentgenology 1996; 166: 763–767.
16. Bode PJ, Niezen RA, Van Vugt AB, Schipper J. Abdominal ultrasound as a reliable indicator for conclusive laparotomy in blunt abdominal trauma. Journal of Trauma 1993; 34: 27–31.
17. Stone IK. Trauma in the obstetric patient. Obstetric and Gynecology Clinics of North America 1999; 26: 459–467.
18. Henderson SO, Mallon WK. Trauma in pregnancy. Emergency Medicine Clinics of North America 1998; 16: 209–228.
19. Goodwin TM, Breen MT. Pregnancy outcomes and fetomaternal haemorrhage after noncatastrophic trauma. American Journal of Obstetrics and Gynecology 1990; 162: 665–671.
20. Connolly A, Katz VL, Bash KL, et al. Trauma in pregnancy. American Journal of Perinatology 1997; 14: 331–336.
21. Pak LL, Reece EA, Chan L. Is adverse pregnancy outcome predictable after blunt abdominal trauma? American Journal of Obstetrics and Gynecology 1998; 179: 1140–1144.
22. Warner MW, Salfinger SG, Rao S, et al. Management of trauma during pregnancy. Australian and New Zealand Journal of Surgery 2004; 74: 125–128.
23. Shah KH, Simons RK, Holbrook T, et al. Trauma in pregnancy: maternal and fetal outcomes. Journal of Trauma 1998; 45: 83–86.
24. Asterita DC, Feldman B. Seat belt placement resulting in uterine rupture. Journal of Trauma 1997; 42: 738–740.

3.10 Wound care and repair

Richard Waller • Gim Tan

ESSENTIALS

1 Good cosmesis can be achieved in the emergency department with conservative treatment, thorough debridement and accurate apposition of everted skin edges.

2 Choose a suture that is monofilament, causes little tissue reactivity, and retains tensile strength until the strength of the healing wound is equal to that of the suture.

3 Dirty, contaminated, open wounds should generally be cleansed, debrided and closed within 6 hours to minimize the chance of infection.

4 Suspected tendon injuries require examination of the full range of movement of joints distal to the wound while observing the tendon in the base of the wound for breaches. This is often done under anaesthesia.

5 The success of a tendon repair (as measured by function) relates in large part to the postoperative care and therapy, not simply to the suture and wound closure.

6 Appropriate splinting and elevation of limb wounds at risk of infection takes precedence over antibiotics in the postoperative prevention of infection.

7 If prophylactic antibiotics are used, they should be given intravenously prior to wound closure to achieve adequate concentrations in the tissues and haematomas that may collect. There is no need for antibiotics with simple lacerations not involving tendon, joint or nerves.

8 Wounds that breach body cavities, such as the peritoneum and joints, or involving flexor tendons, nerves and named arteries, should be referred to a specialist for consideration of repair and inpatient care.

9 Foreign bodies such as clay chemically impair wound healing.

10 Puncture wounds such as bites may be managed by either second-intention healing after thorough lavage, or better still by excisional debridement, lavage, antibiotics and atraumatic closure, if less than 24 hours old (preferably less than 6 hours).

Introduction

Open wound injury comprises a significant component of emergency department (ED) workload. Data from the Victorian Injury Surveillance System[1] showed that 72% of all ED presentations for unintentional cutting and/or piercing injury that did not require admission were open wounds. In addition, open wounds may accompany other injuries such as fractures. Of open wounds that occur in the home, 19% are in the paediatric age group (0–14 years), 62% occur in people under 35, and less than 10% in the over-65s. Overall, 65% of patients are male.

Location data show that more than 53% of these wounds occur in the home,[1] mostly during activity described as leisure. The three major causes are falls up to 1 m; contact with cutting or piercing objects; or having been struck or collided with. Most are unintentional and only 3% are due to an assault. Injuries to the face, head and neck comprise 12%, and the upper extremity is involved in 62%. Eighty-eight per cent of all presentations are repaired in the ED and the patient is discharged home. Almost half are referred to GPs and specialists for review. It is those wounds suitable for ED repair that will be further discussed.

Clinical presentation

An initial general assessment of the patient is important as it defines the likely mode of repair and the injured structures, and identifies factors for complications. The assessment includes the traditional history, examination and investigation of the patient.

It is important in the history to identify the time and mechanism of injury, the likely presence of foreign bodies, and the patient's tetanus immunization status. Past medical history; allergies to agents such as local anaesthetics, antibiotics, preparation solutions and tapes; and current medications such as warfarin or cytotoxics all have a bearing on management. For example, there is a greater risk of infection and poor wound healing in diabetic patients with extremity wounds of the lower limbs sustained in a crush injury. Other relevant general conditions, particularly in the setting of dirty wounds such as bites, include prior mastectomy, and other causes of chronic oedema of the affected region, prior splenectomy, liver dysfunction, immunosuppression, or autoimmune disease such as systemic lupus erythematosus (SLE). Smokers have impaired collagen production in healing wounds.[2]

The general examination comprises a search for all injuries sustained and concurrent medical illness that may have a bearing on the results of repair, such as poor circulation in patients with peripheral vascular disease. The patient needs to be recumbent (beware of syncope) and any clothing that may obstruct a thorough examination removed. Constricting rings or other jewellery that encircle the injured body part should also be removed. A general examination is performed, followed by a local examination of the wound coupled with initial cleansing. Function and nerve or vessel injury are then examined for. A detailed examination of the depth of the wound, which usually requires good anaesthesia, is then performed. A surface wound caused by the entrance of a foreign body does not necessarily mean that the foreign body has remained in the vicinity. A decision is made regarding the requirement for further investigations, which include radiographs for fractures and some foreign bodies, or ultrasound for radiolucent foreign bodies.

An injury to a tendon in the base of the wound may only be apparent when the joints over which it acts are in a particular position, reflecting the position of the limb at the time of injury. At other positions the tendon injury may slide out of view. Marked pain with use may be a clue to a partial tendon injury.

Any tendon injury or other factors such as nerve damage indicate the need for referral to a plastic surgeon.

Wound cleansing

To provide optimum conditions for healing without infection it is essential to remove all contaminants, foreign bodies and devitalized tissue prior to wound closure.

Universal precautions, including eye protection (goggles or similar), clothing protection (gown) and gloves, must be taken for all wound care and repair. Gloves should be powder free to avoid adding starch as a foreign body to the wound, which will delay healing and produce granulomas.[3] One must be aware of the risk of latex allergy to both the glove wearer and the patient.[3]

If necessary, hair can be removed by clipping 1–2 cm above the skin with scissors. Shaving the area with a razor damages the hair follicle and is associated with an increased infection rate. Scalp wounds closed without prior hair removal heal with no increase in infection.[4]

The skin surface should be cleaned using sterile normal saline. This has the lowest toxicity and there is no benefit in using antiseptic.[5]

Recent studies have shown that the use of tap water in the cleaning of simple lacerations is as effective as normal saline.[6]

A wide variety of cleansing solutions is available (Table 3.10.1), with differing attributes.

Anaesthesia is necessary for wounds to be cleansed adequately. Extensive wounds, or particularly heavily contaminated wounds that need vigorous scrubbing, such as road debris tattooing, may require general anaesthesia. Local anaesthetic may be given by local infiltration or as a regional nerve blockade. Needles introduced through the wound cause less pain, but may theoretically track bacteria into the tissues, although this has not been demonstrated to be a problem clinically. After anaesthesia, irrigation with a pressure of at least 8 psi (55 kPa)[7,8] is required to dislodge bacteria and reduce the incidence of infection. This can be achieved with a 19 G needle, a 25–50 mL syringe, a three-way tap and a flask of fluid such as sterile saline (Fig. 3.10.1).[9] High-pressure irrigation (>20 psi, 138 kPa) may cause tissue damage.[10]

Radio-opaque foreign bodies, such as gravel, metal, pencil lead and glass >2 mm in size,[11] may be identified using X-rays. A radio-opaque marker such as a paperclip can be placed at the wound to help identify the position of the foreign body.[12] This is not sensitive for plastic or wood, however,[13] which may be detectable with ultrasound if larger than 2.5 mm. However, if there is gas due to an open wound, this will make ultrasound less sensitive.

Table 3.10.1 Preparation solutions and their properties				
Solution	Properties	Mechanism of action	Uses	Disadvantages
Normal saline	Isotonic, non-toxic	Simple washing action	In wound for irrigation	No antiseptic action
Chlorhexidine 0.1% w/v – aqueous	Bacteriostatic	Antibacterial and washing action	Cleanse skin surrounding wound	Not near eyes (causes keratitis), perf. ear drum or meninges
Chlorhexidine 0.1% w/v + cetrimide 1% w/v	Bacteriostatic	Antibacterial and soap action, removes sebum, 'wetting' the skin	Cleanse skin surrounding wound	Not near mucous membranes, eyes (causes keratitis), perf. ear drum or meninges
H_2O_2 3%	Bactericidal to anaerobes	Forms superoxide radicals	Severely contaminated wounds with anaerobic type pathogens	Obstruction of wound surface capillaries and subsequent necrosis
Povidone-iodine 10% w/v	Bactericidal fungicidal viricidal sporicidal	Releases free iodine	On surrounding skin, or in severely contaminated wounds (dilute 1% w/v)	Use on/in large wounds may cause acidosis due to iodine absorption[28]

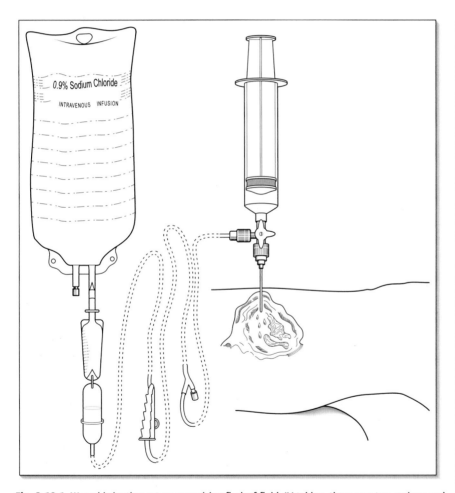

Fig. 3.10.1 Wound irrigation set-up comprising flask of fluid, IV tubing, three-way tap, syringe and 19 G needle designed to deliver fluid at at least 8 psi (55 kPa). (From an original drawing by Elaine Wheildon.)

Adequate debridement of devitalized tissue has always been a tenet of surgical practice. More recently, there has been a change in emphasis from radical to meticulous debridement. If the skin is devitalized it should be removed using a scalpel blade. Viable tissue will bleed when cut, and viable muscle will contract when stimulated. If viability is in doubt it may be better to wait for demarcation over the following days, with regular close observation. Fat and fascia are relatively avascular, and if semi-viable, in contaminated wounds, should be removed. Semi-viable muscle can usually be preserved when well drained.[13] Nerves, major vessels and tendons should not be debrided in the ED. Lavage and debridement should be continued until the wound is clean. Organic material and anionic soils such as clay pose the greatest risk of infection if not removed. The highly charged clay particles directly affect leukocytes, preventing phagocytosis of bacteria. They also react chemically with antibiotics, limiting their action.

Once the wound is clean the decision to close immediately or later is made.

Guidelines for delayed closure may include:

- Puncture wounds, such as with a tooth or a knife.
- Wounds unable to be adequately debrided.
- Contaminated wounds more than 6 hours old.
- Too much tension in the wound, particularly with crush injury.

In some cases, such as thoroughly lavaged puncture wounds, it may be prudent to allow healing by secondary intention. If in doubt, consult with a plastic surgeon. When repair in the ED may be delayed, it is prudent to have nursing staff perform a preliminary preparation of the wound along the lines shown in Table 3.10.2.

Table 3.10.2 Preliminary wound preparation procedure instructions for nurses
Explain the procedure to the patient
Identify any allergies, especially to iodine-like products and adhesive tapes
Medicate the patient prior to the irrigation, as needed for pain control
Protect patient clothing from soiling by the irrigation solution or wound drainage
Position the patient so that irrigating solution can be collected in a basin, depending on the wound's location
Maintain a sterile field during the irrigation procedure as appropriate
Irrigate wound with appropriate solution, using a large irrigating syringe and set-up (see Fig. 3.10.1)
Instill the irrigation solution at 8 psi (55 kPa), reaching all areas
Avoid aspirating the solution back into the syringe
Cleanse from cleanest to dirtiest areas of the wound
Continue irrigating the wound until the prescribed volume is used or the solution returns clear
Position the patient after the irrigation to facilitate drainage
Cleanse and dry the area around the wound after the procedure
Dispose of soiled dressing and supplies appropriately
Lightly pack the wound with well wrung-out, saline soaked lint-free sterile gauze, or an alginate dressing
Apply a sterile dressing as appropriate until repair is performed

Antibiotics are only necessary in wounds involving joints, tendons, nerves, vessels, significant crush injury or if due to human or animal bites.[36]

Tetanus prophylaxis

The risk of tetanus is greatest in the very young and the very old, with an overall death rate of 1:10 in Australia,[14] so prevention is all important. An average of 10 cases per year occur in Australia,[13] usually in older adults who have not been immunized or who have allowed immunization to lapse. The anaerobic bacterium *Clostridium tetani* is present in soil and animal faeces. After incubation of 3–21 days after inoculation into a wound, the toxin produced by the bacteria causes severe muscle spasm and convulsions. Death occurs commonly as a result of respiratory failure. The types of wound at risk are listed in Table 3.10.3, but tetanus may occur after apparently trivial wounds.

Tetanus immunoglobulin is given into the opposite limb to the tetanus toxoid in patients with inadequate protection against tetanus (see Table 3.10.4), providing passive protection.

Table 3.10.3 Wounds that are prone to tetanus
Compound fractures
Deep penetrating wounds
Wounds containing foreign bodies, e.g. wood splinters, thorns
Crush injuries or wounds with extensive tissue damage, e.g. burns
Wounds contaminated with soil or horse manure
Wound cleansing delayed more than 3–6 hours

Wound-healing mechanisms

Wounds never gain more than 80% of the strength of intact skin.[15]

There are three phases of healing. Days 1–5 are the initial lag phase (inflammatory), where there is no gain in the strength of the wound. Days 5–14 are a period of rapid increase in wound strength, associated with fibroplasia and epithelialization. The wound has only 7% of its final strength at day 5. Wound maturation progresses from day 14 onwards, with production, cross-linking and remodelling of collagen.

The surgical maxim that wounds heal from side to side is only partly true: if left to heal by itself the entire wound will contract around its margin prior to epithelialization. This has been termed secondary closure or healing by second intention. Allowing the wound to close without intervention relies on healing up from the base and from the edges, and often results in unsightly scars. Primary closure involves the apposition of wound edges, preferably within 6 hours of injury, with sutures, staples, tissue adhesive glue, etc. After a delay of 6 hours or more the chance of a wound infection increases. Delayed primary closure is performed 4–5 days after injury, when it is clear there is no infection. This may be used for contaminated wounds that present more than 6 hours post injury.

Factors that affect the rate of wound healing include:

- Technical factors of the repair
- Anatomic factors (intrinsic blood supply etc.)
- Drugs (steroids, cytotoxics etc.)
- Associated conditions and diseases (diabetes, vitamin C, zinc deficiency etc.)
- The general nutritional state of the patient.

Suture types

Wounds may be closed with tape, staples, sutures or tissue adhesive.

Purpose-made commercial tapes reinforced with rayon provide an excellent means of closure. The adherence of tapes (Fig. 3.10.2) may be improved by the application of adhesive adjuncts, such as tincture of benzoin, or gum mastic paint.[16] These adhesives must not be allowed to enter the wound,[17] as they potentiate infection and cause intense pain. The rates of infection with tapes and staples are lower than with conventional sutures.[18]

Staples have the advantage of rapid insertion and wound closure, particularly for extensive wounds. They are applied using a staple gun and must be removed using the appropriate device, which may be a problem with follow-up arrangements.

Table 3.10.4 Tetanus vaccination schedule for acute wound management (Adapted from Lammers R. Foreign bodies in wounds. In: Singer AJ, Hollander JE, eds. Lacerations and acute wounds: an evidence-based guide. Philadelphia: FA Davis, 2003; 147)

History of tetanus vaccination	(CDT) Td	Type of wound	DTP, DT (ADT)* or tetanus toxide as appropriate	Tetanus immunoglobulin
3 doses or more	If less than 5 years since last dose	All wounds	no	no
	If 5–10 years since last dose	Clean minor wounds	no	
		All other wounds	yes	no
	If more than 10 years since last dose		yes	no
		All wounds		
Uncertain, or		Clean minor wounds	yes	no
less than 3 doses		All other wounds	yes	yes

*DTP, diphtheria, tetanus, pertussis for children before 8th birthday.
DT, child diphtheria tetanus (CDT) if pertussis is contraindicated.
Td, adult diphtheria tetanus (ADT) for children after their 8th birthday.

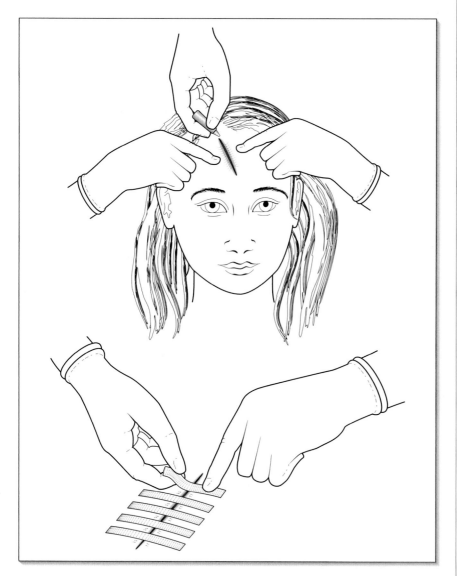

Fig. 3.10.2 Steristrips and glue are typically used for children in most simple split lacerations, thereby avoiding the use of needles. (From an original drawing by Elaine Wheildon.)

From horsehair in World War Two[19] to today's soluble monofilament plastics with prolonged tensile strength, necessity has seen the development of many different suture materials (Fig. 3.10.3) of different grades and using different types of needles. The ideal suture is monofilament, causes no tissue reaction, does not promote infection, is completely absorbed, and yet has a tensile strength and secure knots that last until tissue strength has equalled that of the suture. It should stretch to accommodate wound oedema, recoil to its original length, and be inexpensive. However, as yet no such suture exists.

A key factor in choosing absorbable suture is the length of time over which it retains adequate strength. The inflammatory phase of healing lasts for 7 days. Catgut prolongs this phase and is removed by enzymatic action, whereas absorbable plastics simply hydrolyse. Braided sutures produce greater tissue reaction than monofilaments. Braided and catgut sutures should be avoided in contaminated wounds,[20] as the interstices provide a haven for bacteria from phagocytes. Traditional absorbable sutures have included Vicryl and Dexon, both braided multifilament. Extensive studies have shown new monofilament absorbable sutures to have superior strength both initially and at 4 weeks; less interference with bacterial clearance; more secure knots requiring fewer throws; and lower drag forces through tissue, compared to the braided absorbable types.[21]

Tissue adhesive agents such as Histoacryl (enbucrilate; B. Braun Surgical GmbH) – 'superglue' – have been developed particularly with the minor superficial paediatric wound in mind. The results can be excellent, provided good wound edge apposition is achieved prior to application of the glue on the surface (see Fig. 3.10.2).

In the future, biological tissue adhesive agents such as fibrin sealant[19] for use in the wound may replace sutures as the means of wound closure. As yet these are experimental in sterile, surgically created wounds.

Needles

Early surgical needles had eyes like traditional sewing needles and caused tissue trauma as the bulk of folded-back thread

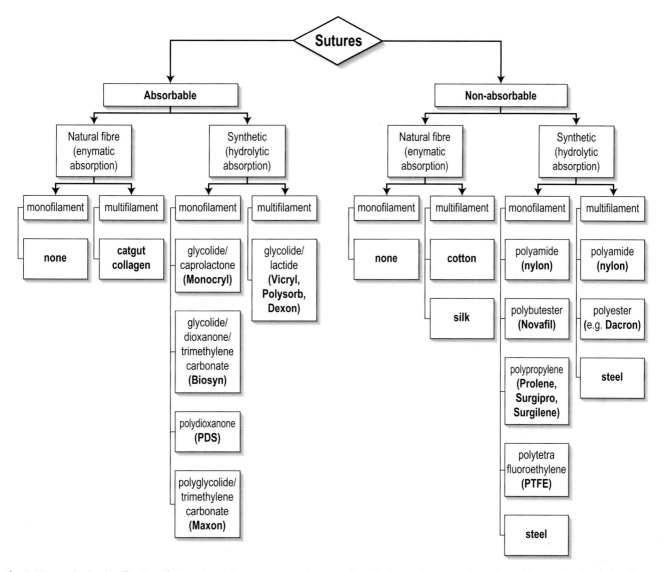

Fig. 3.10.3 A simple classification of suture types in current usage. (Adapted from Van Winkle W Jnr, Hastings JC. Considerations in the choice of suture material for various tissues. Surgery, Gynecology and Obstetrics 1972;135: 113–126.)

and needle passed through the tissues. The first swaged needles were invented over 100 years ago, and modern disposable swaged needles have largely replaced the reusable eyed needles. There are three parts to a needle: the swage, the body and the point (Fig. 3.10.4).

Advances in metallurgy have allowed the production of nickel stainless steel wire, from which needles are cut. They may be straight, or curved in arcs of varying degrees to produce portions of a circle, such as 90°, 135°, 180° and 225° parts. A compound curved needle comprises two different arcs, limiting the amount of supination necessary to pass it through tissue. Skin repair usually requires half-circle needles. The points of surgical needles may be tapered, cutting,

or a combination. Taper-point needles are generally round or oval bodied and are not suitable for skin as they are difficult to pass through the tightly bundled collagen fibres of the dermis. Their role is in repair of soft tissues such as fascia, blood vessels and bowel, etc. Cutting needles are for skin, and have a triangular point with sharp cutting edges to facilitate tissue penetration. Conventional cutting needles have the apex of the triangle towards the concavity of the curved needle (see Fig. 3.10.4). Reverse cutting needles have the apex on the convexity of the needle. This style of needle and suture will not cut out when the needle is passed through tissue, or once the knotted suture is resting against a block of tissue rather than a cut. Such needles

are structurally stronger.[22] Combination cutting at the point and taper for the remainder of the body are for slightly denser tissues such as tendon or aponeurosis. Needle holders are generally used with curved needles, and straight needles are handheld. The risk of needle-stick injuries with handheld needles makes their use hazardous.

Basic suture technique

Prior to closure, prophylactic antibiotics (see Chapter 9.10) should be given intravenously if required. This ensures that any haematoma that collects in the wound after or during closure will contain antibiotic.

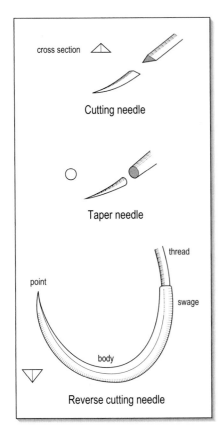

Fig. 3.10.4 Surgical needle characteristics and types. (From an original drawing by Elaine Wheildon.)

Table 3.10.5 Surgical instruments required for wound repair	
Contents of a typical simple suture tray	*Contents of a typical 'plastics' suture tray*
1 × Nelson Hegar needle holder 61/2 in	2 × Mosquito forceps curved
1 × Curved artery forceps	2 × Mosquito forceps straight
1 × Gillies dissectors	1 × Hegar needle holder 5.5 in
1 × McIndoe dissectors	1 × Gillies needle holder
2 × Small bowls	1 × Straight Mayo scissors
1 × Kidney dish autoplas 255 mm	1 × Curved Mayo scissors
1 × Fenestrated drape	1 × Vein straight scissors
1 × Huck towel	1 × Vein curved scissors
1 × McIndoe dissectors	
1 × Adson dissectors	
1 × Gillies toothed dissectors	
2 × Skin hooks	
2 × Catspaw refractors	
1 × Bard–Parker handle no. 3	
1 × Bard–Parker handle no. 4	
1 × Vein hook Alcot	
1 × Rampley sponge holder	
3 × Gallipots	
1 × Kidney dish	
3 × Towel clips	
4 × Huck towel	

Having prepared a sterile field with the contents of a suture tray (Table 3.10.5) laid out, the wound anaesthetized and cleaned, and the sterile drapes placed around the wound, repair can begin. A very contaminated wound should be anaesthetized, lavaged and cleansed before re-preparing with antiseptic and draping for formal debridement, further lavage and repair.

One should choose the thinnest possible suture that will tolerate the tissue tensions and provide adequate strength. The needle holder must grasp the needle in the body, usually two-thirds of the length from the tip of the needle, rather than over the swage where the metal is relatively weak. Stretching the suture in the hands, supporting it at the needle swage, will remove its 'memory', making handling easier. The needle holder should be held in the palm of the hand and controlled with the index finger, using a supination/pronation action in the arc of the needle (Fig. 3.10.5). The placement of the first suture varies with the wound: in a small linear wound it may be convenient to simply suture from one end to the other. In longer wounds without good corresponding landmarks on either side it is helpful to subdivide the wound serially, to ensure that one does not finish up with a 'dog-ear'. If an assistant is available, stretching the wound is helpful (Fig. 3.10.5). In more irregular complex wounds it is helpful to approximate corresponding landmarks first: for example, the apex of a flap is best stitched first (Fig. 3.10.6).

After wound contraction has occurred, the wound edge has a natural tendency to inversion, resulting in a shallow crater. To prevent this, the edges must be everted at closure. To do this the skin near the wound edge is depressed (Fig. 3.10.7) or lifted with a skin hook or forceps, so that the needle enters and exits perpendicularly to the skin in both running and interrupted sutures. The sutures so placed may be interrupted with separate tied closed loops or continuous loops passing through tissue, tied at either end. Vertical mattress sutures (Fig. 3.10.8) and horizontal mattress sutures (Fig. 3.10.9) are designed to evert wound edges that are difficult to maintain in eversion with simple sutures.

Knots are the weakest link in the suture, particularly for continuous sutures, where the failure of a knot will release the whole suture along the length of the wound. The knots may be tied with instruments or by hand. One must be careful, when using instrument ties, not to damage the suture by either crushing with the serrated jaws of a needle holder or tearing on the edges of the jaws. A reef knot with a snug third throw produces the best results for nylon or polypropylene. Synthetic monofilament sutures require several twists in the first and second throws to prevent unknotting (see Fig. 3.10.5). It is important that the

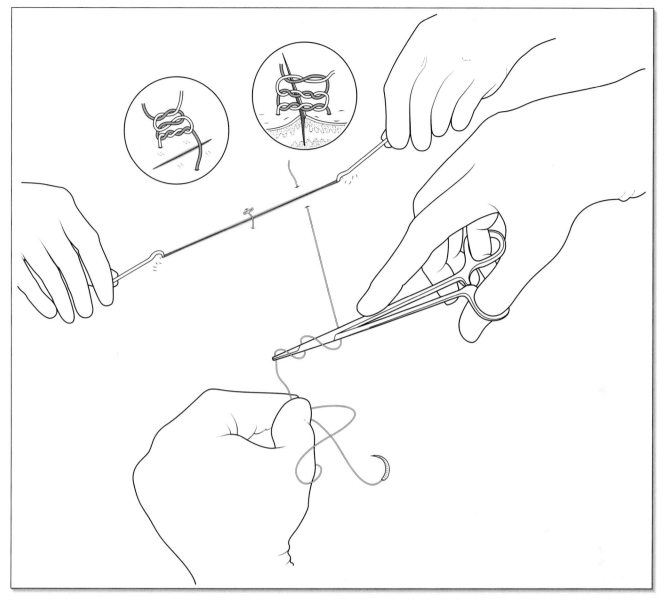

Fig. 3.10.5 The basic technique of how to hold a needle driver, put the wound on the stretch, and suture a long wound in halves using surgical knots. For synthetic sutures the reef knot with the third throw requires several twists, as illustrated, to prevent loosening. (From an original drawing by Elaine Wheildon.)

wound be closed without excessive tension on the sutures.

Interrupted sutures have the advantage of individual removal to allow drainage of an infected wound, or for cosmetic reasons to limit the time a suture stays in while retaining some sutures for wound strength; however, there is a trade-off in the time it takes to close a wound using multiple knots. Sutures tied too tightly, exacerbated by oedema in the wound and from the trauma created by the needle's passage, will cause suture marks due to local ischaemia on the skin surface. An individual

suture that is strangling tissue will continue to do so until it is cut. One way to avoid tissue strangulation is to use a loop throw in an interrupted suture[15] (Fig. 3.10.10).

Studies have shown no increase in wound infection or reduction in wound strength with the use of continuous sutures,[23] which may be placed rapidly in long linear wounds, distributing tension evenly. However, if one knot fails or the stitch is cut they will loosen along the length of the wound. Continuous sutures may be percutaneous or intradermal (subcuticular). If intradermal, they should surface every 3 cm to facilitate removal.[24]

Intradermal sutures are most appropriate for surgical wounds. Monofilament polypropylene has a very low surface coefficient of friction and is thus easiest to remove in the setting of continuous percutaneous or subcuticular closure.[25] One should ensure that the suture glides easily through each segment and is not looped, otherwise removal may become very difficult. Recently, absorbable monofilament such as glycolide caprolactone – Monocryl (Ethicon Inc.) – has supplanted polypropylene for continuous subcuticular suture as it does not have to be removed.

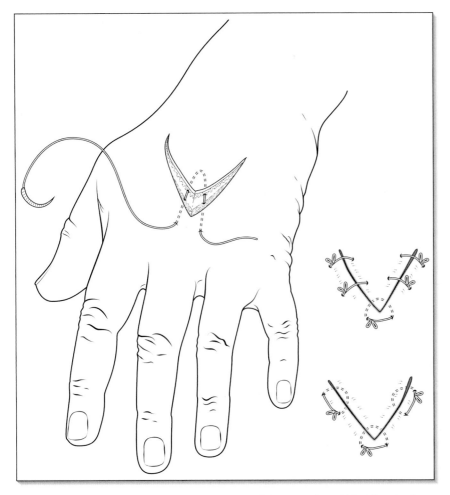

Fig. 3.10.6 Closure of a flap requires an initial suture of the apex, after which either simple or horizontal mattress sutures may be used. (From an original drawing by Elaine Wheildon.)

Historically, Halstead[26] considered it important to 'obliterate with the greatest care all of the dead spaces of a wound'. In 1974 it was demonstrated that suture closure of dead space increases the incidence of infection secondary to the foreign body (the suture) in the wound, thereby eliminating the benefits of dead space closure.[27] Some authors[15] stress the importance of using buried sutures to obtain wound edge eversion and dead space closure. Modern hydrolysable monofilament sutures allow this. The long-term maintenance of dermal edge apposition, either with or without deep sutures, is the key to obtaining the narrowest possible scar. Techniques have been developed to encourage this and to avoid leaving buried sutures, with their attendant risk of wound infection. To allow the removal of a deep space-obliterating suture without disrupting the

wound some creative methods have been devised (Fig. 3.10.11).[28]

Wounds that slice obliquely through thick skin, such as on the back, can be trimmed with a scalpel blade perpendicular to the skin or sutured with a vertical mattress to prevent one bevelled edge sliding over the other. If necessary to prevent a wound edge step, adjustments in the height of the wound edges can be achieved by exiting the needle superficially on the high side and deeper on the low side, using either continuous or interrupted sutures.[15]

Special sites and situations

Scalp lacerations may be closed using the 'hair braiding' technique,[34,35] either on its own or combined with tissue adhesive. In this technique, four to five strands

of hair from opposite sides are brought together, twisted once and tissue adhesive applied.

The face, particularly with dirty wounds such as bites, requires early repair to achieve good cosmesis. Delay for up to 24 hours is acceptable, prior to definitive debridement and repair in the operating theatre, provided interim wound care is of a good standard. To enable adequate cleansing, local nerve blocks should be used.

A field block is generally required for ears. Ear cartilage must be aligned and skin coverage achieved to prevent perichondritis.

Injuries involving the eyelid need a good examination of the underlying globe to exclude scleral and conjunctival lacerations; also, canaliculi may be torn. A lacerated canaliculus should be microsurgically repaired and stented within 24 hours. Accurate apposition of eyebrows and vermilion border is essential. Never shave an eyebrow.

Damaged facial muscle must be repaired in the interests of facial symmetry. In cheek injuries, the facial nerve and parotid duct must be checked for intactness: The nerves are generally deep in the cheek. Terminal repair of nerves medial to the midpupillary line is unnecessary.

Tattooing should be removed within 12 hours to avoid tissue fixation. Use a sterile brush and magnification and be meticulous. It is useful to have sterile toothbrushes available in the ED for this. After 12 hours a formal dermabrasion and/or debridement may be needed.

Complications of facial wounds are numerous and provide some special problems (Table 3.10.6).

Special suture techniques

Techniques for relieving the tension in a wound include limited undermining, and the use of horizontal mattress sutures (see Fig. 3.10.9). Very rarely should skin flaps be raised in acute trauma. These may be advancement (e.g. V-Y advancement), rotation or transposition in design. It is usually better to apply a split skin graft to heal the wound primarily and perform later scar revision or reconstruction. In some settings V-Y flaps can be advanced or retreated, depending on the direction of tension (Fig. 3.10.12).

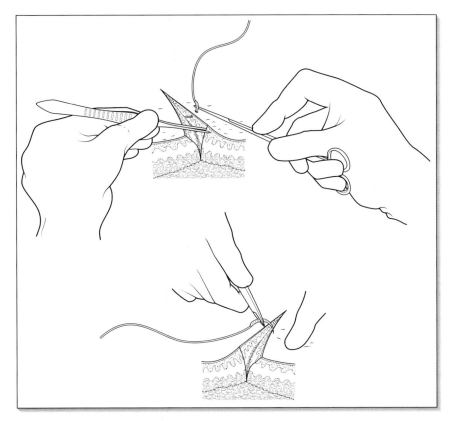

Fig. 3.10.7 Everting the wound edge using Gillies tissue forceps or digital pressure when placing a suture improves the cosmetic result. (From an original drawing by Elaine Wheildon.)

The 'dog-ear'

The term 'dog-ear' refers to a conical pucker of redundant skin that may collect at the end of a wound towards the end of closure (Fig. 3.10.13), particularly in wounds with an elliptical area of skin defect. In order to avoid a 'dog-ear' the wound should be sutured in halves, placing each new stitch between the previous ones (see Fig. 3.10.5). There are several ways to remove a dog-ear.[29]

- The direct overlap excision technique involves drawing the redundant skin from one side across the wound and excising along the line of the wound. Any remaining redundant skin is drawn across the wound from the other side, and excised along the line of the wound (Fig. 3.10.13).
- Unilateral dog-ears are best removed by elevating the redundant skin with a skin hook in the centre, followed by incising along the edge of the fold and then allowing the created flap to fall back along the line of the sutures, where it is trimmed off. This results in a J-shaped repair (Fig. 3.10.13).

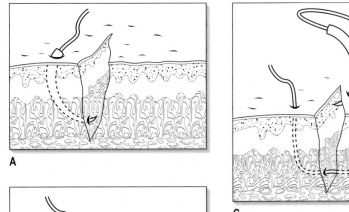

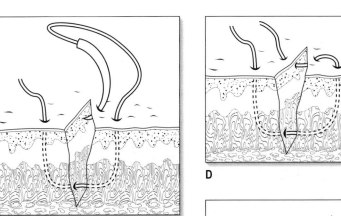

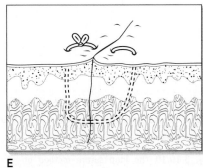

A

B

C

D

E

Fig. 3.10.8 The vertical mattress suture technique is useful to evert wound edges with a natural tendency to roll inward despite correctly placed simple sutures. (From an original drawing by Elaine Wheildon.)

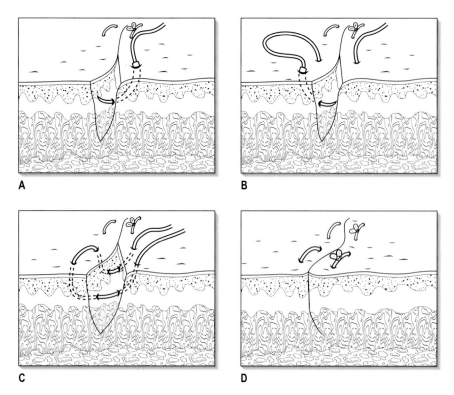

Fig. 3.10.9 The horizontal mattress suture redistributes tension and everts wound edges. (From an original drawing by Elaine Wheildon.)

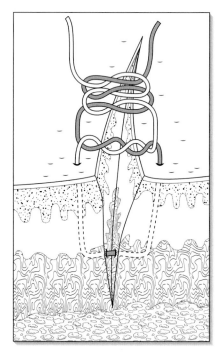

Fig. 3.10.10 The loop suture method of avoiding excessive tension on a stitch.[15] (From an original drawing by Elaine Wheildon.)

- An elliptical excision of the dog-ear in line with the closure can excise the defect (Fig. 3.10.13), but this also lengthens the wound.
- In very large dog-ears a V-Y excision and closure will provide good closure.
- Thick dog-ears that are aligned perpendicularly to the original closure can be excised and closed in a T repair (Fig. 3.10.13).

Wound drainage

Fluid trapped within the closed wound predisposes to infection by:

- Progressive loss of opsonins.
- Interfering with access of phagocytes to bacteria.
- Providing a nutrient medium for bacterial growth.
- Putting pressure on adjacent vasculature, compromising blood supply.

Fluid also prevents the apposition of healing tissues. The build-up of fluid can be prevented by immobilization, preventing shearing forces between tissue planes; firm but not tight dressings; and drainage. The indications for drainage are:

- Dead-space elimination to prevent fluid accumulation (with an active suction drain or a compressive dressing with a passive drain).
- Removal of established fluid collections.

Suction drains are superior to passive drains, which rely on gravity; however, blockage of drain holes and of the drain tube lumen can be a problem. There are many commercial closed suction systems on the market. A simple suction drain can be constructed from a 'butterfly' cannula and a vacuum blood specimen tube (Fig. 3.10.14)[7] by cutting off the syringe adapter and fenestrating the tubing prior to placement through a stab incision into the wound. The vacuum tube can be changed as necessary. Clamp the tube before changing it to prevent the ingress of contaminants into the wound via the drain. Patients with drains will need regular review, either in the ED or by the local doctor. Drains are generally removed at 48 hours unless they are draining copiously.

Dressings

It has long been recognized that the dressing and subsequent wound care are as important as the operative technique.[30] The depths of the wound must be moist for healing, but the skin surface must not become macerated.

The appropriate style of dressing for abrasions is still debated. The 'moist' versus 'dry' debate revolves around saline packs, sterile paraffin, solugel, seaweed preparations, occlusive plastic film dressings and various foam preparations.

In covering the sutured wound, the dressing aims to keep the primarily apposed skin edges dry, wicking away any ooze, haemorrhage or exudate. It should only be changed if its capacity to absorb fluid is exceeded, and ideally it should stay on until the time for suture removal. Where this is not possible, the wound may be bathed or showered 24 hours after closure, provided it is thoroughly dabbed dry and not

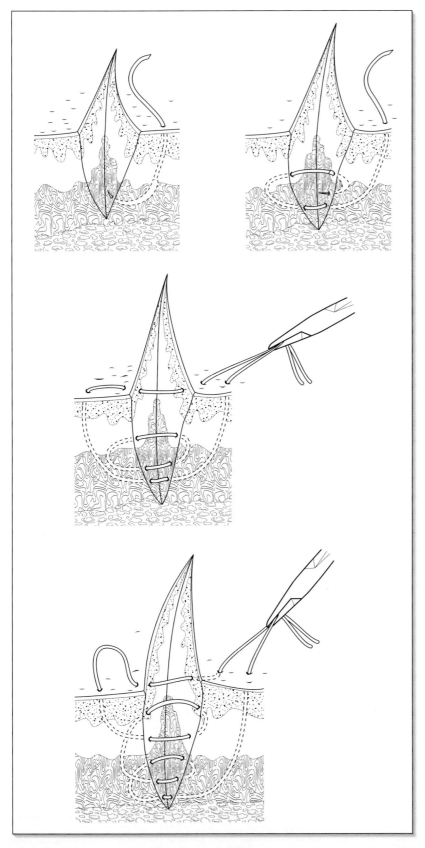

Fig. 3.10.11 A deep closure method utilizing a variable number of loops, adapted from a Mayo Clinic stitch.[28] (From an original drawing by Elaine Wheildon.)

immersed and soaked in water. In the case of scalp wounds this allows showering and hair washing, and avoids the problem of fixing a dressing to hairy skin. Wounds that are contaminated and at high risk of infection need review and re-dressing at 48 hours.

Immobilization

Wounds that traverse joints or which occur on highly mobile skin, such as in the hand, require immobilization. Splinting with plaster slabs is a cheap, traditional and reliable method. Apart from protecting and stabilizing the wound to allow healing, the splint also reduces the likelihood of infection. If practicable, potentially infected wounds of the upper limbs should be in a sling, elevated to reduce oedema. Lower limbs may be rested using crutches, and elevated whenever possible.

Disposal/removal

Despite an apparently good cosmetic result at the time (Table 3.10.7) of suture removal (5–14 days) in head and neck wounds, there is evidence of a poor correlation with wound appearance 6–9 months later.[31] The degree to which different factors, such as wounding mechanism, wound repair technique and patient host factors, have a role remains to be determined. Keloid or hypertrophic scarring is more common in negroid and Asian races, and in wounds located over the deltoid muscle or sternum.

All percutaneous stitches will cause needle marks if left in situ longer than 8 days, as epithelium migrates down the needle track. Removal too early predisposes to wound dehiscence (Fig. 3.10.15); however, the wound may be supported by skin tapes. If tapes were the primary method of closure they may be left on for at least 10 days, or until they fall off, provided the skin is not sensitive to the adhesive, as evidenced by erythema or bulla formation.

Suture removal technique is also important. To avoid tissue trauma and additional scarring, stitches should be cut at the knots with iris scissors after gentle washing with saline to remove the eschar, and the suture gently pulled through. So-called suture scissors are actually too big for the task.

Table 3.10.6 Complications of facial wounds	
Complication	**Notes**
Infection with the brain	Potentially fatal owing to the valveless venous communication
AV fistulae	Due to profuse vascularity – uncommon
Scarring	Producing facial asymmetry and cosmetic implications
Deformity	Due to unrecognized fractures, such as of the nose or malar bone
Facial palsy	Due to damaged facial nerves
Epiphora damage	With tissue loss or scarring everting the lower lid, or canaliculus
Salivary fistula	After disruption of the parotid duct
Drooling	With tissue loss, scar contracture or local nerve damage
Corneal exposure	With tissue loss, scar contracture or local nerve damage

Inelastic paper tape can be used to support a wound and help stop the scar from stretching until such time as the collagen is near maturation, beyond 3 months. Paper tape is also useful in the setting of keloid scarring in an attempt to provide pressure and encourage remodelling. In some cases silicone gel pads and even pressure garments are required to control keloid scarring.

If the wound suppurates then the sutures will need to be removed, either partly or completely, to allow the egress of pus.

Controversies

- Drainage will remove fluid and haematoma that potentiate infection, but the drain itself may predispose to infection. This is less the case with suction drains.

- Interrupted dermal sutures will close dead space, thereby reducing haematoma and wound infection, but may lead to infection in contaminated wounds. Their major role is to reduce skin tension, and they should be used in large clean wounds.

- The degree of debridement required for a dirty wound has moved from radical to conservative but meticulous, with an emphasis on preservation of viable skin to improve cosmesis.

- Povidone–iodine packs, which are tissue toxic, are used by some surgeons in the setting of open wounds over compound fractures while the patient awaits transfer to the operating theatre for definitive repair.

- Opinions as to the appropriate dressings for abrasions range from moist, such as plastic film, to dry, such as mercurochrome paint and dry gauze.

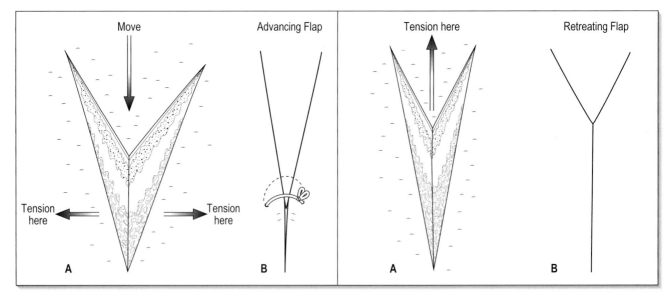

Fig. 3.10.12 The V-Y flap advancement or retreat is useful to redistribute and reduce tension across a wound. (From an original drawing by Elaine Wheildon.)

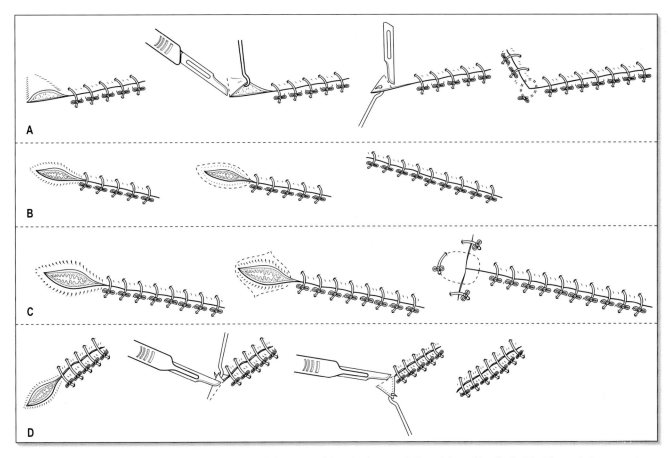

Fig. 3.10.13 Various methods of dealing with a dog-ear. (A) Hockey-stick or back-cut technique; (B) Double elliptical incision technique; (C) Perpendicular elliptical T-repair technique; (D) Direct overlap excision technique. (From an original drawing by Elaine Wheildon)

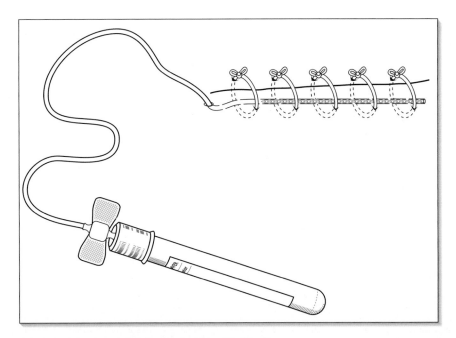

Fig. 3.10.14 A simple suction drain. (From an original drawing by Elaine Wheildon.)

Table 3.10.7 Guide to time for removal of sutures (Adapted from Gusman D. Wound closure and special suture techniques. Journal of the American Podiatric Medical Association 1995; 85: 2–10)

Location	Days to removal
Scalp	6–8
Face (incl. ear)	4–5
Chest/abdomen	8–10
Back	12–14
Arm/leg*	8–10
Hand*	8–10
Fingertip	10–12
Foot	12–14

*Add 2–3 days for lacerations crossing extensor surfaces of joints and if early motion is required for rehabilitation, e.g. post flexor tendon repair.

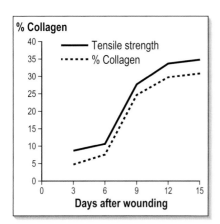

Fig. 3.10.15 The relationship between tensile strength and collagen deposition. (From an original drawing by Elaine Wheildon.)

References

1. Clark B, Cassell E, Ashby K, et al. Hazard. Edition No 52, Spring 2002, Victorian Injury Surveillance and Applied Research System.
2. Jorgensen LN, Kallenhave F, Christensen E, Siana JE. Less collagen production in smokers. Surgery 1998; 123: 450–455.
3. Ellis H. Hazards from surgical gloves. Annals of the Royal College of Surgeons of England 1997; 79: 161–163.
4. Howell JM, Morgan JA. Scalp laceration repair without prior hair removal. American Journal of Emergency Medicine 1988; 6: 7.
5. Dire DJ, Welch AP. A comparison of wound irrigation solution used in the Emergency Department. Annals of Emergency Medicine 1996; 19: 704.
6. Bansal BC, Weike RA, Perkins SD, Abramo TJ. Tap water irrigation of lacerations. American Journal of Emergency Medicine 2002; 20: 469.
7. Rodeheaver GT, Pettry D, Thacker JG, et al. Wound cleansing by high pressure irrigation. Surgery, Gynecology and Obstetrics 1975; 141: 357–362.
8. Brown LL. Evaluation of wound irrigation by pulsatile jet and conventional methods. Annals of Surgery 1978; 187: 170.
9. Gfeller RW, Crow DT. The emergency care of traumatic wounds: current recommendations. Veterinary Clinics of North America 1994; 24:1249–1274.
10. Wheeler CB, Rodeheaver GT, Tracker JG, et al. Side-effects of high pressure irrigation. Surgery, Gynecology and Obstetrics 1976; 143: 775–778.
11. Lammers R. Foreign bodies in wounds. In: Singer AJ, Hollander JE, eds. Lacerations and acute wounds: an evidence-based guide. Philadelphia: FA Davis, 2003; 147.
12. Wyn T, Jones J, McNinch D, et al. Bedside fluoroscopy for the detection of foreign bodies. Academic Emergency Medicine 1995; 2: 979–982.
13. Fackler MI, Breteau JP, Courbil CJ, et al. Open wound drainage versus wound excision in treating the modern assault rifle wound. Surgery 1989; 105: 576–584.
14. National Health and Medical Research Council. The Australian Immunisation Handbook, 9th edn. Canberra: NHMRC, 2008.
15. Moy RL, Lee A, Zalka A. Commonly used suturing techniques in skin surgery. American Family Physician 1991; 44: 1625–1634.
16. Moy RL, Quan MB. An evaluation of wound closure tapes. Journal of Dermatology, Surgery and Oncology 1990; 16: 721–723.
17. Panek P, Prusak MP, Bolt D. Potentiation of wound infection by adhesive adjuncts. American Surgeon 1972; 38: 343–345.
18. Edlich RF, Becker DG, Thacker JG, Rodeheaver GT. Scientific basis for selecting staple and tape skin closures. Clinics in Plastic Surgery 1990; 17: 571–578.
19. Spotnitz WD, Falstrom MA, Rodeheaver GT. The role of sutures and fibrin sealant in wound healing. Surgical Clinics of North America 1997; 77: 651–669.
20. Van Winkle W Jnr, Hastings JC. Considerations in the choice of suture material for various tissues. Surgery, Gynecology and Obstetrics 1972;135: 113–126.
21. Rodeheaver GT, Beltran KA, Green CW, et al. Biomechanical and clinical performance of a new synthetic monofilament absorbable suture. Journal of Long-Term Effects of Medical Implants 1996; 6: 181–198.
22. Bendel LP, Trozzo LP. Tensile and bend relationships of several surgical needle materials. Journal of Applied Biomaterials 1993; 4: 161–167.
23. Mclean NR, Fyfe AH, Flint EF, et al. Comparison of skin closure using continuous and interrupted nylon sutures. British Journal of Surgery 1980; 67: 633–635.
24. Drake DB, Gear AL, Mazzarese PM, et al. Search for a scientific basis for continuous suture closure: a 30 year odyssey. Journal of Emergency Medicine 1997; 15: 495–504.
25. Pham S, Rodeheaver GT, Dang MC, et al. Ease of continuous dermal suture removal. Journal of Emergency Medicine 1990; 8: 539–543.
26. Halstead WS. The treatment of wounds with especial reference to the value of blood clot in the management of dead spaces. Bulletin of the Johns Hopkins Hospital 1990–91; 2: 255.
27. De Holl D. Potentiation of infection by suture closure of dead space. American Journal of Surgery 1974; 127: 716–720.
28. Arnold PG. Space obliterating skin suture. Plastic and Reconstructive Surgery 1997; 100: 1506–1508
29. Gusman D. Wound closure and special suture techniques. Journal of the American Podiatric Medical Association 1995; 85: 2–10.
30. Ivy RH, et al. (eds) Manual of standard practice of plastic and maxillofacial surgery. Philadelphia: WB Saunders, 1943.
31. Hollander JE, Blasko B. Poor correlation of short and long-term cosmetic appearance of lacerations. Academic Emergency Medicine 1995; 2: 983–987.
32. Pietsch J, Meakins JL. Complications of povidone-iodine absorption in topically treated burns patients. Lancet 1976; 1: 280–282
33. Trott AT. Wounds and lacerations: emergency care and closure, 2nd edn. St Louis: Mosby Year Book, 1997.
34. Aoki N, Oikawa A, Sakai T. Hair braiding closure for superficial wounds. Surg Neurol 1996; 46: 150.
35. Hock M, Ooi SBS, Saw SM, Lim SH. A randomised controlled trial comparing the hair apposition technique with tissue glue to standard suturing in scalp lacerations (HAT) study. Annals of Emergency Medicine 2002; 40: 19.
36. Spicer WJ, Garland S, Christiansen K, et al. Skin and soft tissue infection. In: Therapeutic guidelines antibiotic version 13. Melbourne: Therapeutic Guidelines Limited 2006; 230–232.

3.11 Burns

Tim Gray • Gerard O'Reilly

ESSENTIALS

1 Advances in treatment of severely burned patients, including fluid resuscitation, control of sepsis, early excision and use of skin substitutes, have made previously lethal burns survivable.

2 Signs of laryngeal oedema should prompt early intubation.

3 Burn resuscitation formulas should be considered as a guide only.

4 Meta-analysis suggests that resuscitation with colloid, as opposed to crystalloid, does not improve survival.

5 Extensive or complicated burns should be managed in a specialized burns unit.

6 Chemical burns, after decontamination and specific antidotes, are treated in similar fashion to thermal burns.

Introduction

Advances in burn management over the last three decades have significantly reduced mortality and improved quality of life for victims. With vigorous fluid resuscitation, in addition to early debridement and the appropriate use of antibiotics, hypovolaemia and sepsis are no longer the major contributors to mortality in burns. Multiorgan failure is the most likely event leading to death, whereas age, burn surface area and inhalational injury are the major contributors to a poor outcome.[1–3]

Pathophysiology

The skin is the largest organ of the body. Its most important functions are:

- To act as a vapour barrier to prevent water loss from the body.
- To present the body's major barrier against infection.
- Temperature regulation.

The skin consists of two main layers. The epidermis is stratified squamous epithelium that acts as the major barrier to passive water loss from the body. The dermis contains the adnexal structures, namely sweat glands, hair follicles and sebaceous glands, as well as pain and pressure receptors, and the cutaneous blood vessels, which play a major role in temperature regulation by controlling radiant heat loss (Fig. 3.11.1).

The adnexae are embryologic downgrowths of the epidermis. Following burn injury, the epithelial cells of these structures undergo metaplastic change to stratified squamous epithelium, proliferate, and gradually cover the wound. Thus burns that partially or completely spare these structures will usually heal without scarring. Deeper burns involve greater loss of adnexal cells, resulting in poorer epithelial coverage and hence greater scarring.

Burned skin undergoes coagulative necrosis with three distinct zones of injury. A central zone of coagulation, in which irreversible cell death occurs, is surrounded by a zone of stasis, in which vasoconstriction and intravascular coagulation contribute to local ischaemia. A zone of hyperaemia surrounds the wound. In the early stages of the burn, evolution of these zones results in a progressive deepening of the wound, which may be minimized by appropriate early treatment.[4,5]

Classification

Burns may be classified according to their depth as superficial, partial thickness or full thickness.

Superficial burns involve only the epidermis. Pain and swelling usually subside within 48 hours and the superficial epidermis peels off within a few days. Healing occurs by proliferation of undamaged cells of the germinal layer of the epidermis and is usually complete within 7 days.

Partial thickness burns involve destruction of the epidermis and superficial dermis. They are characterized by blister formation and may be further classified into superficial and deep partial thickness. Healing is dependent on the amount of intact epithelium in the adnexae.

Superficial partial thickness burns are typically bright red with a moist surface, are exquisitely sensitive to stimulus and heal in 2–3 weeks, generally with minimal scarring. Deep partial-thickness burns are typically dark red or yellow-white and take longer than 3 weeks to heal, as few epithelial elements survive. Hypertrophic scarring usually occurs.

Full-thickness burns involve the epidermis and dermis, including the epidermal appendages. Clinically they appear charred or pearly white in appearance, and are usually insensate. Because loss of epidermal adnexae is complete, full-thickness burns only heal by scarring or skin grafting.

THERMAL BURNS

Presentation

History

History may be obtained from the patient, from witnesses and from fire or ambulance personnel. Details of the nature of the injury are important, especially the nature

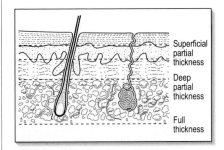

Fig. 3.11.1 Diagram of skin layers.

Superficial partial thickness

Deep partial thickness

Full thickness

of the burning materials, duration of exposure, whether the patient was trapped in an enclosed space or lost consciousness, or whether there was an associated fall, vehicular accident or blast injury.

A history of altered consciousness or confinement in a burning environment suggests the likelihood of carbon-monoxide poisoning. Past medical history, current medications, allergies, and tetanus status should also be obtained.

Examination

The initial examination should be directed to identifying signs suggestive of airway burns as well as the presence of other injuries. Early haemodynamic compromise is

rarely due to burn injury alone and should prompt a search for other causes.

Facial and oral burns, singed nasal hairs, carbonaceous sputum, tachypnoea and wheeze are clinical signs suggesting an increased risk of inhalation injury; however, in the absence of laryngeal oedema, inhalation injury may not become clinically evident for 12–24 hours.[6,7]

Signs of laryngeal oedema, namely hoarseness, brassy cough or stridor, indicate the need for early endotracheal intubation as oedema formation may rapidly distort the anatomy, necessitating a surgical airway.

The adequacy of peripheral circulation should be assessed, particularly in the setting of circumferential limb burns.

Evaluation of burn area

The extent and depth of the burn must be assessed as accurately as possible. Representation of the burn area diagrammatically on a body chart aids assessment. The simplest method is the 'Rule of nines' where the adult body is divided into anatomical regions that represent 9% of the total body surface area.

In infants and young children, the Lund and Browder chart is used to correct for proportional variation at different ages: for instance, an infant's head is approximately 18% of the total body surface area, compared to 9% in an adult (Fig. 3.11.2).

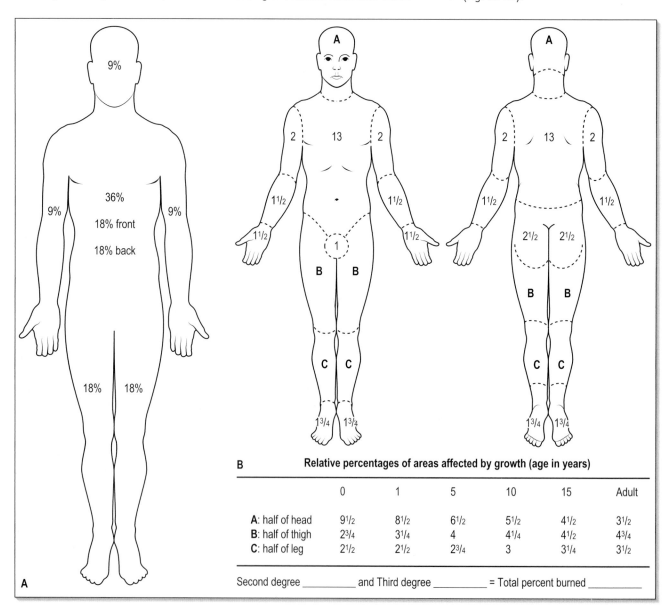

Relative percentages of areas affected by growth (age in years)

	0	1	5	10	15	Adult
A: half of head	9½	8½	6½	5½	4½	3½
B: half of thigh	2¾	3¼	4	4¼	4½	4¾
C: half of leg	2½	2½	2¾	3	3¼	3½

Second degree _____ and Third degree _____ = Total percent burned _____

Fig. 3.11.2 (A) 'Rule of nines' diagram. (B) Lund and Browder chart.

Investigations

Blood should be taken for baseline full blood examination, serum electrolytes, creatinine and creatinine kinase.

There is no test to quantify the severity of inhalational injury. Chest X-ray and blood gases should be obtained to assess alveolar function, but these may be normal initially.

Carboxyhaemoglobin levels extrapolated to the time of injury may give an estimate of the severity of exposure. An admission carboxyhaemoglobin level >15% suggests significant smoke inhalation.[4] If the patient requires intubation, then bronchoscopy may be used to assess the degree of inhalational injury.[3]

Management

Pre-hospital

Pre-hospital care of the burned patient should be directed at stopping the burning process, assessing and stabilizing the airway, breathing and circulation, and rapidly transferring the patient to hospital. Where possible, major burns should be triaged to a burn centre[8] (Table 3.11.1).

En route to hospital recent burns should be covered with a clean dressing (e.g. Melolin), soaked in cool water so as to limit the depth of burn by dissipation of heat. After this cooling process, or if it is not required, the burns can be covered with a clean dry dressing. Cling wrap is used for interhospital transfers. Prolonged exposure to cool water should be avoided, and ice should

Table 3.11.1 Patients who fulfil the following criteria should be considered for transfer to a specialist burns unit
Partial-thickness burns >20% in all age groups, or >10% in the under 10 and over 50 age groups
Full-thickness burns >5% in any age group
Burns involving face, eyes, ears, hands, feet, genitalia, perineum or a major joint
Inhalation burns
Electrical burns, including lightning injury
Burns associated with other significant injuries
Smaller burns in patients with pre-existing disease that could complicate management

never be applied directly to the wound as it may increase the depth of burn.

The patient should be kept warm, supplemental oxygen administered, and where prolonged transport times are anticipated, intravenous fluid therapy should be instituted.

Emergency department

Initial management

Supplemental oxygen should be administered, and cardiac and oxygen saturation monitoring instituted.

Stabilization of the airway and treatment of life-threatening injuries take priority over management of the burn wound itself. As previously discussed, signs of laryngeal oedema indicate the need for early endotracheal intubation, particularly if the patient is to be transferred. Intravenous fluid resuscitation with crystalloid solution as outlined below should be started in any patient with burns of more than 20% total body surface area (TBSA). A urinary catheter should be inserted to assess the adequacy of fluid resuscitation.

Subsequent management

Having stabilized the patient and initiated fluid resuscitation, a careful secondary survey should be performed, looking for associated injuries.

Adequate analgesia is an important facet of management. Small burns may be managed with a combination of cool compresses and oral analgesia; larger burns will require parenteral analgesia.[8] Opiates will generally be the first option; an infusion of ketamine can be useful for continuous analgesia where there are extensive burns.

Tetanus immunoglobulin should be given if the burn is grossly contaminated or more than 6 hours old, or if the patient has not had a tetanus booster during the preceding 5 years.[8]

A nasogastric tube should be inserted in patients with major burns to avoid gastric dilatation.

Escharotomy may occasionally be necessary in the setting of circumferential limb burns with circulatory compromise, or circumferential chest burns with respiratory compromise.

Extensively burned limbs should be elevated early, and frequent observations of pulse strength, capillary return and

sensation – particularly two-point discrimination – must be performed. Escharotomy may be necessary even when pulses are present; however, the receiving unit should be consulted before escharotomies are performed.[1]

Fluid resuscitation[7]

There are many formulae for the fluid resuscitation of burns victims. Although considerable debate continues, the general principles of fluid resuscitation are:

- In the first 24 hours, isotonic salt solution should be used to replace the large volumes lost to tissue oedema, with about half the fluid given in the first 8 hours after injury, coincident with the period of most rapid oedema formation.
- The administration of colloid is unnecessary for patients with burns of less than 40% TBSA and during the first 8 hours. Meta-analysis of previous studies suggests that resuscitation with colloid does not result in improved survival.[9]
- Fluid resuscitation formulae are a guide only, and the patient's haemodynamic status must be monitored by cardiovascular parameters and hourly urine volume measurement. Increased resuscitation fluid volume (per kg) is required in children weighing less than 30 kg, in high-voltage electrical injuries, if resuscitation is delayed, and in the presence of inhalation injury.

Most burn formulae use between 2 and 4 mL of crystalloid per kg body weight per cent TBSA burned. It is felt that the latter rate allows a more rapid correction of shock.

The Parkland formula allows for 4 mL/kg/% TBSA burned over 24 hours, with half the total fluid requirement to be given in the first 8 hours. In children under 30 kg, the above fluid should be given in addition to calculated maintenance fluid.[1]

Haemodynamic status may be difficult to evaluate in the severely burned patient. Parameters that imply adequacy of resuscitation are urinary output of 50 mL per hour in adults and 1 mL/kg/h in children, normalization of haemodynamic parameters, and correction of metabolic acidosis.

Patients generally receive more fluid than the Parkland's formula dictates, and this appears to be associated with better outcomes than historical data.[10,11]

Notwithstanding this, strategies have been proposed to reduce the total volume of resuscitation fluid. These have included the use of colloid and hypertonic salt solutions. The generalized increase in capillary permeability that occurs with major burns results in the loss of plasma protein, particularly albumin, from the circulation. There is a coincident reduction in hepatic albumin production post burn. Colloid administration helps maintain oncotic pressure, but does not reduce tissue oedema in the first 8 hours and has not been shown to improve clinical outcome compared to crystalloid.[12]

Hypertonic saline solution would appear to be useful in patients with limited cardiopulmonary reserve; however, there is considerable debate over the safety of this technique, and again, there is no evidence of outcome benefit compared to isotonic solution.[6,7,13]

Management of the burn injury

The development of effective topical antimicrobial agents has minimized the incidence of early burn wound infection.

Infecting organisms are most likely to originate from the patient's own gastrointestinal tract. The most important primary infecting agents are the Gram-negative bacteria, particularly *Pseudomonas aeruginosa*, *Proteus*, *Klebsiella* and *Escherichia coli* species. β-Haemolytic streptococci, *Staphylococcus aureus* and *Candida* spp. are also important pathogens.[4]

Until recently, silver sulfadiazine (SSD) cream has been the topical antimicrobial agent traditionally used and is relatively free from side effects, apart from rashes, transient leukopenia, and occasionally serum hyperosmolarity. It may have a role where there is a considerable delay (>6 hours) before presentation to a burns centre, or where the burns are clearly infected. Drawbacks include the need for daily application and the obscuration of the burn wound. More recently, silver-impregnated occlusive dressings (e.g. Acticoat) have provided at least the same antibacterial effect, with the convenience of less frequent dressing changes.[14,15]

Burn shock

The pathophysiology of burn shock is complex and involves a combination of haemodynamic and local tissue factors.

The early post-burn period – i.e. within the first 8 hours – is marked by the rapid formation of tissue oedema, predominantly in the wound itself, but also in non-burned tissue. Factors contributing to this fluid accumulation are not fully understood, but include local release of inflammatory mediators, particularly prostaglandins and leukotrienes. These increase capillary permeability both locally and systemically, in addition to increasing regional blood flow. Increased interstitial osmotic pressure in burned tissue due to the release of osmotically active cellular components and partial degradation of collagen also contributes to tissue oedema.[4,7,16]

Major evaporative loss from burned skin due to loss of epithelial integrity significantly adds to fluid losses. In addition to the fluid shifts, cardiac output may fall by 30–50% in major burns, possibly due to a circulating myocardial depressant factor.[4]

Inhalation injury

The presence of inhalation injury has a considerable negative impact on prognosis in the burns patient.[3,17] Direct thermal trauma below the larynx is rare, except in the case of steam inhalation.

Pulmonary complications are largely due to inhalation of toxic products of combustion, particularly in house or vehicular fires. Smoke consists of a particulate fraction – predominantly carbon – and a gaseous fraction, which may include carbon dioxide, carbon monoxide, oxides of nitrogen and sulphur, hydrogen cyanide and PVC, depending on the materials being burnt. These agents adhere to the moist respiratory mucosa, forming corrosive compounds that cause inflammation, hypersecretion and mucosal sloughing, resulting in airway obstruction and atelectasis. Smoke inhalation also triggers the release of thromboxane, resulting in increased pulmonary artery pressures.[3,6]

Disposition

Patients with major burns as outlined in Table 3.11.1 should be managed in a specialist burns unit. The patient should be discussed with the receiving unit prior to transfer, so that appropriate measures may be undertaken to stabilize them. Plastic cling wrap applied directly over the burn provides a good non-adherent dressing that will reduce heat and fluid loss. As noted previously, silver sulfadiazine (SSD) cream should not be applied to these burns as it interferes with subsequent evaluation. At the burns centre, burns will be dressed with a silver-impregnated, non-adherent, occlusive dressing (e.g. Acticoat).

Current management of full- and deep partial-thickness burns involves early excision and autologous skin grafting. In extensive burns, excision and autologous grafting may need to be staged, allowing sufficient skin to regenerate.[6,7]

Less extensive burns (i.e. not meeting the criteria for burns centre transfer) may be admitted to a general or plastic surgery service. Loose skin and broken blisters should always be debrided. Blisters may otherwise be initially left intact, although some would advocate that all blisters be deroofed.[8] A moist silver-impregnated dressing (e.g. Acticoat) may then be applied to areas of epithelial loss.

Superficial or partial-thickness burns involving less than 10% TBSA may be suitable for outpatient management subject to the criteria in Table 3.11.1, and depending on the social and psychological status of the patient. The choice of dressings for outpatient management depends on the depth of the burn, the extent and size of blisters, and the amount of exudate from the burn surface.[4,8]

Superficial burns can also be covered with a moist ointment (e.g. paraffin-based Dermeze), or moist dressing (e.g. Burnaid, which contains melaleuca-derived local anaesthetic properties). Superficial partial-thickness burns involve loss of epithelium with considerable exudate and hence are prone to infection. After gentle cleansing and debridement of loose tissue, a moist, non-adherent dressing such as Bactigras should be applied. These patients will need to be reviewed the next day, at which time the dressing will be changed. A silver-impregnated occlusive dressing is also an option to minimize crusting and dressing adherence.

Epithelialization commences at 7–10 days, by which time the burn surface should be drying out. At this stage the more convenient hydrocolloid or film dressings may be used until epithelialization is complete.

If healing is not well established by 10–14 days, the patient should be referred for specialist opinion, as excision and grafting may be required.

CHEMICAL BURNS

A wide range of products available in both the industrial and domestic environments can lead to burns. Although the mechanism is different, chemical burns demonstrate a similar spectrum of injury to thermal burns. Superficial burns are associated with itching, burning or pain; partial-thickness burns are associated with tissue oedema and the formation of bullae; and full-thickness burns are associated with damage extending through the dermis. The extent of tissue damage in chemical burns is determined by the nature and concentration of the chemical, as well as the extent and duration of contact.

In addition to the burn itself, toxicity may occur as a result of systemic absorption.

The majority of chemical burns are caused by acids and alkalis. Acids cause coagulation, with the formation of a tough eschar that may limit further tissue damage. Alkalis cause liquefactive necrosis, allowing deeper penetration. Many other types of chemical cause burns, but distinguishing them by mechanism of action is not relevant to the clinician as their management, apart from a few exceptions, is similar.

General principles

Chemical agents continue to damage tissue until they are removed or inactivated. Therapy then is directed to decontamination and, where appropriate, the use of specific antidotes as well as recognition and treatment of systemic toxicity.

Adequate protection of medical personnel to prevent secondary contamination is essential. Copious irrigation is the cornerstone of therapy, but contaminated garments should be removed and dry chemical particles brushed away before irrigation commences. Adherent or oily compounds may need to be removed with mild soap and a scrubbing brush, and nails, hair and intertriginous areas should be carefully checked.

The duration of irrigation depends on the agent. Alkali in particular may require prolonged lavage owing to its tissue penetration. The use of litmus paper to determine wound pH may guide the duration of irrigation in acid and alkali burns.

Other than decontamination and treatment of systemic toxicity, management is similar to that for thermal burns.

Disposition

Most patients with chemical burns can be treated on an outpatient basis. Indications for admission include:

- Partial-thickness burns >15% TBSA
- All full-thickness burns
- Burns involving hands, feet, eyes, ears or perineum
- Evidence of or potential for systemic toxicity
- Significant associated injuries or complicating medical conditions.

Specific chemicals

Hydrofluoric acid

Hydrofluoric acid is a relatively weak acid used in glass etching, electronics and oil-refining industries. It is also a component of many industrial and domestic rust removers. In strong solution it causes corrosion of tissue owing to the release of hydrogen ions; however, its major toxicity is caused by the dissociated fluoride ion that complexes calcium and magnesium to form insoluble salts. Cell destruction associated with severe pain results. In severe burns, hypocalcaemia and hypomagnesaemia may occur.

Contact with strong solution (> 50%) causes immediate pain and tissue destruction; however, exposure to weaker solutions, particularly <20%, may cause little or no pain initially. Thus it may take up to 24 hours for the burn to become apparent. Once apparent, the burn causes excruciating pain that is difficult to control even with parenteral narcotics.

After irrigation, specific therapy is aimed at precipitation and hence neutralization of free fluoride ions. Methods depend on the severity and location of the burn. Calcium gluconate gel, made by mixing calcium gluconate with a water-soluble lubricant to make a 2.5–10% solution, should be applied directly to the affected area.

Relief of pain is the marker of adequate treatment. If pain is not relieved, or recurs, parenteral therapy is required. Generally this consists of subcutaneous injection of calcium gluconate, aiming for 0.5mL of 10% solution per square centimetre. Hand and digital burns pose a problem, as vascular compromise may occur if too much fluid is injected. Alternatives include intra-arterial injection of calcium gluconate, or regional perfusion using Bier's technique.[18]

References

1. Wolf SE, Rose JK, Desai MH, et al. Mortality determinants in massive paediatric burns. Annals of Surgery 1997; 225: 554–569.
2. Miller SF, Schurr MJ, Jeng JC, et al. National burn registry 2005: a ten year review. Journal of Burn Care and Research 2005; 27: 411–436.
3. Fraser JF, Mullany D, Traber D. Inhalational lung injury in patients with severe thermal burns. Contemporary Critical Care 2007; 4: 1–12.
4. Shaw A, Anderson J, Hayward A, Parkhouse N. Pathophysiological basis of burn management. British Journal of Hospital Medicine 1994; 52: 583–587.
5. Singh V, Dengan L, Bhat S, Milner SM. The pathogenesis of burn wound conversion. Annals of Plastic Surgery 2007; 59: 109–115.
6. Nguyen TT, Gilpin DA, Meyer NA, Herndon DN. Current treatment of severely burned patients. Annals of Surgery 1996; 233: 14–25.
7. Monafo WW. Initial management of burns. New England Journal of Medicine 1996; 335: 1581–1586.
8. Reed JL, Pomerantz WJ. Emergency management of paediatric burns. Paediatric Emergency Care 2005; 21: 118–129.
9. Roberts I, Alderson P, Bunn F, et al. Colloids versus crystalloids for fluid resuscitation in critically ill patients. Cochrane Database of Systematic Reviews 2004, Issue 4.
10. Mitra B, Fitzgerald M, Cameron P, Cleland H. Fluid resuscitation in major burns. Australia and New Zealand Journal of Surgery 2006; 76: 35–38.
11. Freiburg C, Igneri P, Sartorelli K, Rogers F. Effects of differences in percent total body surface area estimation on fluid resuscitation of transferred burn patients. Journal of Burn Care and Research. 2007; 28: 42–48.
12. Alderson P, Bunn F, Li Wan Po A, et al. Human albumin solution for resuscitation and volume expansion in critically ill patients. Cochrane Database of Systematic Reviews 2004, Issue 4.
13. Bunn F, Roberts I, Tasker R. Hypertonic versus near isotonic crystalloid for fluid resuscitation in critically ill patients. Cochrane Database of Systematic Reviews 2004, Issue 3.
14. Caruso DM, Foster KN, Blome-Eberwein SA, et al. Randomized clinical study of hydrofiber dressing and silver or silver sulfadiazine in the management of partial thickness burns. Journal of Burn Care and Research 2006; 27: 298–309.
15. Peters DA, Verchere C. Healing at home: comparing cohorts of children with medium-sized burns treated as outpatients with in-hospital applied Acticoat to those children treated as inpatients with silver sulfadiazine. Journal of Burn Care and Research 2006; 27: 198–201.
16. Demling RH. The burn edema process: current concepts. Journal of Burn Care and Rehabilitation. 2005; 26: 207–227.
17. Ipaktchi K, Arbabi S. Advances in burn critical care. Critical Care Medicine 2006; 34: 239–244.
18. Bretolini JC. Hydrofluoric acid: A review of toxicity. Journal of Emergency Medicine 1992; 10: 163–168.

4.1 Injuries of the shoulder

Anne-Maree Kelly

ESSENTIALS

1 Most clavicular fractures heal despite displacement, therefore reduction is not necessary.

2 Injuries to the shoulder region may also involve injury to local neurovascular structures.

3 Acromioclavicular joint injuries and fractures of the scapula are usually treated conservatively.

4 Posterior sternoclavicular dislocations require reduction.

5 In dislocation of the shoulder, careful examination of the axillary (circumflex) nerve, brachial plexus and axillary artery is mandatory both before and after reduction.

6 In anterior dislocation of the shoulder, surgical repair of the capsule is recommended for recurrent dislocators and first-time dislocators who are young and engaged in high-risk sports.

Fractures of the clavicle

Fractures of the clavicle account for 2.6–5% of all fractures and usually result from a direct blow on the point of the shoulder, but may also be due to a fall on the outstretched hand. The most common site of fracture is the middle third of the clavicle, which accounts for 69–82% of clavicular fractures. There are varying degrees of displacement of the fracture ends, with overlapping fragments and shortening being common. Owing to the strategic location of the clavicle, injury to the pleura, axillary vessels and/or brachial plexus is possible, but fortunately these complications are rare.

The clinical signs of clavicular fracture are a patient supporting the weight of their arm at the elbow and local pain and tenderness, often accompanied by deformity.

In non-displaced or minimally displaced fractures, treatment consists of an elbow-supporting sling (e.g. broad arm sling) for 2–3 weeks. For comfort, this may be worn under clothes for the first few days. The sling may be discarded when local tenderness has subsided. Note that clinical union precedes radiological union by weeks. Early shoulder movement should be encouraged within the limits of pain. Non-union is rare.

Midshaft fractures with complete displacement, comminution or fractures in the elderly or women with osteoporosis, have a higher rate of non-union and poorer functional outcome. Recent evidence suggests that this group may benefit from surgical stabilization with either plate-and-screw fixation or intramedullary devices. Fractures of the outer third of the clavicle may involve the coracoclavicular ligaments. If so, surgical management should be considered. This may be performed by open or arthroscopic techniques.

Late complications include shoulder stiffness and a local lump at the site of fracture healing, which is rarely of cosmetic significance.

Acromioclavicular joint injuries

Acromioclavicular (AC) joint injuries usually result from a fall where the patient rolls onto his/her shoulder. The degree of the injury relates to the number of ligaments damaged. The clavicle is attached to the scapula by acromioclavicular, trapezoid and conoid ligaments. In sprains and subluxations, only the AC ligament is damaged; in dislocations, the conoid and trapezoid ligaments are also ruptured and displacement may be severe.

On clinical examination of the standing patient, the outer end of the affected clavicle may be prominent and there will be local tenderness over the AC joint. The degree of damage can be ascertained by taking standing X-rays of both shoulders with the patient holding weights in both hands (stress X-rays) and by ultrasound. Stress X-rays may be normal in mild strains, but dynamic ultrasonographic techniques may better define the injury.

Treatment is with a broad arm sling. For minor sprains 1–2 weeks is usually sufficient; dislocations may require 4–6 weeks of immobilization. If there is gross instability, surgery should be considered.

Sternoclavicular subluxation and dislocation

Sternoclavicular injuries are uncommon and usually due to a fall on the outstretched hand or a blow to the front of the shoulder. Subluxation is more common than dislocation, with the affected medial end of the clavicle displaced forwards and downwards. Dislocations may be anterior or, rarely, posterior. In the latter case, the great vessels or trachea may be damaged.

Clinical features include local tenderness and asymmetry of the medial ends of the clavicles. The diagnosis is essentially clinical. X-rays can be difficult to interpret. They are not necessary for subluxations, but may be helpful to confirm major dislocations. CT scanning may assist in identification.

Subluxations should be treated in a broad arm sling for 2–3 weeks. Anterior sternoclavicular joint instability should also be treated conservatively; however, there is a significant risk of ongoing instability that is usually well tolerated and of little, if any, functional impact. For patients with posterior dislocation expeditious diagnosis and treatment are important. Closed reduction, performed under general anaesthesia, is usually stable and the joint can then be managed in a brace or sling for 4–6 weeks. Operative stabilization is required if closed reduction is unsuccessful or there is persistent instability.

Fractures of the scapula

Fractures of the scapula are uncommon, accounting for less than 1% of all fractures. They typically occur after high-energy trauma, and up to 90% of patients have other associated injuries.

Fractures of the blade of the scapula are usually due to direct violence. Clinical features are local tenderness, sometimes with marked swelling. Healing is usually rapid, even in the presence of comminution and displacement, with an excellent functional outcome. Treatment is non-operative, with a broad arm sling and early mobilization.

Fractures of the scapula neck are often comminuted and may involve the glenoid. Swelling and bruising of the shoulder may be marked. Clinical examination and X-rays should ensure that the humeral head is enlocated. Computed tomography (CT) scans may be useful in defining the anatomy and the degree of involvement of the glenoid, including any steps in the articular surface. Surgery is often indicated for fractures involving the scapular neck or glenoid.

The 'floating shoulder' is an uncommon injury pattern. Although it is usually defined as an ipsilateral fracture of the clavicle and scapular neck, recent studies suggest that ligamentous disruption

associated with a scapular neck fracture can give the functional equivalent of this injury pattern, with or without an associated clavicle fracture. Because the degree of ligament disruption is difficult to assess, indications for non-surgical and surgical management are not well defined. Minimally displaced fractures typically do well with conservative management. The degree of fracture displacement and ligament disruption that results in poor outcome with conservative management is not well defined and the indications for surgery are controversial, as is choice of surgical technique. Options include fixation of the clavicular fracture, which often indirectly reduces the scapular fracture, or fixation of both fractures.

Rotator cuff injuries

Rotator cuff injuries become more common with advancing age as degeneration weakens the cuff. Indeed, the presence of asymptomatic partial or complete tears identified on ultrasound or MRI may be as high as 40% in patients aged over 50.

Symptomatic injuries may follow minor trauma or the sudden application of traction to the arm. Many are acute on chronic in nature, rather than truly acute, and this can be defined with ultrasound or MRI if required. The clinical features of a strain include a painful arc of abduction centred at 90° of abduction, and tenderness under the acromion. If the tear is complete, no abduction at the glenohumeral joint will occur, although some abduction to 45–60% is possible by scapular rotation. In both cases there is a full passive range of abduction.

Treatment of rotator cuff strains is conservative, usually including analgesia and physiotherapy. Local injection of hydrocortisone may be useful if symptoms persist. Treatment of rotator cuff tears is controversial, with no clear evidence guiding the choice of operative versus non-operative therapy or the components or duration of non-operative treatments. Most experts would still recommend a trial of non-operative therapy before considering surgery. An exception to this may be the patient with a previously asymptomatic shoulder who sustains trauma with resultant weakness (after the pain from the injury subsides) in whom imaging studies indicate an acute full-thickness tear.

Dislocation of the shoulder

Dislocation of the shoulder results in the humeral head lying anterior, posterior or inferior to the glenoid. Of these, anterior dislocation is the most common.

Anterior dislocation

Anterior dislocation of the shoulder is most often due to a fall resulting in external rotation of the shoulder, for example the body rotating internally over a fixed arm. It is most common in young adults, often being related to sports. There is inevitable damage to the joint capsule (stretching or tearing), and there may be associated damage to subscapularis and the greater trochanter of the humerus. Complications may include damage to the axillary (circumflex) nerve (resulting in inability to contract deltoid and numbness over the insertion of deltoid) and, rarely, the axillary vessels and the brachial plexus.

Clinical features include severe pain, reluctance to move the shoulder, and the affected arm being supported at the elbow, often in slight abduction. The contour of the shoulder is 'flattened off' and there is a palpable gap just under the acromion where the humeral head usually lies. The displaced humeral head may be palpable anteriorly in the hollow behind the pectoral muscles. Dislocation is confirmed by X-ray. The dislocation may be evident on the AP film but cannot be ruled out on a single view. Additional views (e.g. an axial lateral, translateral, tangential lateral) are required. These may reveal an associated fracture of the greater trochanter, but this does not influence initial management.

The principles of management are the provision of adequate analgesia as soon as possible (ideally, this should take the form of titrated intravenous opioid), reduction of the dislocation, and immobilization followed by physiotherapy. There are more than 20 described methods for the reduction of anterior dislocations, with reported success rates ranging from 60% to 100%. These include the Spaso technique, the modified Kocher's manoeuvre, the Milch technique and scapular rotation techniques. There is no high-quality evidence to assist in selecting the most effective. That said, the Hippocratic method is not recommended as the traction involved may damage neurovascular structures. Gravitational traction, having the patient lie face down with a weight strapped to the limb, is occasionally successful and may be worthwhile if there will be a delay until reduction by another method. All reduction methods require adequate analgesia. Intra-articular local anaesthetic may also be useful. Sedation, in an appropriately controlled environment, may be of assistance in augmenting analgesia and providing a degree of muscle relaxation and amnesia. Failure of reduction under analgesia/sedation is rare and mandates reduction under general anaesthesia.

Spaso technique

The patient is placed in the supine position. The affected arm is held by the forearm or wrist and gently lifted vertically, applying slight traction. While maintaining vertical traction, the shoulder is externally rotated, resulting in reduction.

Modified Kocher's manoeuvre

While applying traction to the arm by holding it at the elbow, the shoulder is slowly externally rotated, pausing if there is muscle spasm or resistance. External rotation to about 90° should be possible, and reduction often occurs during this process. The elbow is then adducted until it starts to cross the chest, and then internally rotated until the hand lies near the opposite shoulder.

Scapular rotation

This technique is traditionally performed with the patient prone, but can be performed on a seated patient. For both variations, the scapula is manipulated by adducting (medially displacing) the inferior tip using thumb pressure while stabilizing the superior aspect with the other hand.

Post-reduction X-rays confirm reduction, and neurovascular status must be rechecked. The arm should be immobilized in a sling under clothes for several days and the patient advised not to abduct or externally rotate the arm. This should be followed by an external broad arm sling and physiotherapy. The duration of immobilization and the timing of physiotherapy are controversial.

If there is an associated fracture of the greater trochanter, it usually reduces when the shoulder is reduced. If it remains displaced, open reduction and internal fixation may be required.

Primary surgery, usually by arthroscopic techniques, is recommended for patients having suffered recurrent dislocations and should be considered for first-time dislocators, especially those who are young, as surgery has been shown to significantly reduce the risk of recurrent dislocation.

Recurrence is rare in the elderly, but approaches 50% in younger patients.

Posterior dislocation

Posterior dislocation is frequently mentioned in medicolegal reports as it is easy to miss, especially in the unconscious. It may result from a fall on the outstretched or internally rotated hand, or from a blow from the front. It is also associated with seizures and electrocution injuries, where it is not uncommonly bilateral. The dislocation is usually not apparent on an AP film, so additional views are required. Reduction is performed by traction on the limb in the position of 90° abduction, followed by external rotation. Aftercare is the same as for anterior dislocation.

Posterior dislocation is prone to recurrence. Good functional outcomes are associated with early detection and treatment, a small osseous defect, and stability following closed reduction. Poor prognostic factors include late diagnosis, a large anterior defect in the humeral head, deformity or arthrosis of the humeral head, an associated fracture of the proximal part of the humerus and the need for an arthroplasty. The indications for surgery are controversial.

Inferior dislocation

This type of dislocation is rare and usually obvious, as the arm is held in abduction. Neurovascular compromise is a significant risk requiring careful examination and prompt reduction. Reduction is by traction in abduction followed by swinging the arm into adduction. Aftercare is the same as for anterior dislocation.

Controversies

- The role of surgery for midshaft clavicular fractures.

- Timing of mobilization after dislocation of the shoulder.

- The role of surgery in rotator cuff tears.

- The best technique for reduction of anterior dislocation of the shoulder.

- Surgery for first dislocations of the shoulder.

Further reading

Bicos J, Nicholson GP. Treatment and results of sternoclavicular injuries. Clinical Journal of Sport Medicine 2003; 22: 359–370.

Canadian Orthopaedic Trauma Society. Non-operative treatment compared with plate fixation of displaced midshaft clavicular fractures. A multi-center randomized clinical trail. Journal of Bone and Joint Surgery 2007; 89A: 1–10.

Kuhn JE. Treating the initial anterior shoulder dislocation – an evidence-based medicine approach. Sports Medicine and Arthroscopy Review 2006; 14: 192–198.

Miljesic S, Kelly AM. Reduction of anterior dislocation of the shoulder: the Spaso technique. Emergency Medicine 1998; 10: 173–175.

Oh LS, Wolf BR, Hall MP, et al. Indications for rotator cuff repair: a systematic review. Clinical Orthopaedics and Related Research 2007; 455: 52–63.

Zlowodzki M, Bhandari M, Zelle BA, et al. Treatment of scapula fractures: systematic review of 520 fractures in 22 case series. Journal of Orthopaedic Trauma 2006; 20: 230–233.

4.2 Fractures of the humerus

Timothy Rainer • Raymond Chi Hung Cheng

ESSENTIALS

1 Fractures of the proximal humerus occur primarily in the elderly, whereas distal humerus fractures occur more often in children.

2 Falls producing fractures in elderly patients are often precipitated by an underlying medical problem that should be sought and managed.

3 Most proximal humeral fractures do not require surgical intervention.

4 The aim of treatment is to minimize pain, to maximize the return of normal function as soon as possible, and to achieve acceptable cosmesis.

5 Humeral shaft fractures, displaced distal humeral fractures and fractures associated with neurovascular compromise require early orthopaedic review.

6 Low-force fractures, especially in the elderly, suggest the presence of osteoporosis. 'At-risk' patients not already identified as having osteoporosis should be referred for bone density scans and vitamin D testing and treatment.

Introduction

The function of the upper limb depends on an intact shoulder girdle that is in turn affected by the integrity of muscles, tendons and ligaments, bones, joints, blood vessels and nerves. Fractures of the humerus severely limit efficient function of the upper limb, and may be divided into proximal (neck), middle (shaft) and distal (supracondylar) segments.

Fractures of the proximal humerus

Patterns of injury

Fractures of the proximal humerus represent 5% of all fractures presenting to emergency departments (ED) and 25% of all humeral fractures. The fracture typically occurs as a result of an indirect mechanism in elderly, osteoporotic patients who fall on their outstretched hand with an extended elbow. These injuries are important to understand, as the majority do not require surgical intervention and may initially be treated in the ED. A subset with non-viable humeral head requires early surgical intervention, and it is therefore important to identify this group. Fractures of the humerus may also occur in patients with multiple injuries or in the elderly with associated fractures of the neck of femur.[1]

Clinical assessment

History and examination

Patients typically present soon after injury holding their arm close to the chest wall. They complain of pain, and exhibit swelling and tenderness of the shoulder and upper arm. Although crepitus and bruising may occur, the former should not be elicited because it causes excessive and unnecessary pain. Bruising is usually delayed, occurring several days after injury. It appears around the lower arm rather than at the fracture site as a result of gravity and blood tracking distally.

A neurovascular examination is essential as the axillary nerve, brachial plexus and/or axillary artery may be damaged. The axillary nerve is the most commonly injured, and presents with altered sensation over the badge area (insertion of the deltoid) and reduced deltoid muscle contraction (which may be hard to assess because of pain). The axillary artery is the commonest vessel to be injured and may present with any combination of limb pain, pallor, paraesthesia, pulselessness, poor limb perfusion and paralysis.

As these injuries frequently occur in elderly patients, careful attention must be paid to the reason for the fall, as an underlying acute medical condition may have precipitated the event and require management in its own right.

Investigations
Three radiographic views – anteroposterior, lateral and axillary – will allow most proximal humeral fractures to be correctly diagnosed.

Fracture classification
Although the majority of these fractures are easily managed in the ED, the challenge is to differentiate these from the minority that require orthopaedic intervention.

Neer classification system
In this system, fractures are classified first according to four anatomical sites (anatomical and surgical necks, greater and lesser tuberosities); second, according to the number of fragments (one to four parts); and third, according to the degree of fracture displacement, defined as 1 cm separation or $>45°$ angulation (Figs 4.2.1 and 4.2.2).

One-part fracture One-part fractures account for 80% of proximal humeral fractures. Any number of fracture lines may exist, but none are significantly displaced.

Two-part fracture Two-part fractures account for 10% of proximal humeral fractures, and usually one fragment is significantly displaced. Two-part fractures of the humerus may involve the anatomical neck (Fig. 4.2.1a), the surgical neck (Fig. 4.2.1b), the greater tuberosity (Fig. 4.2.1c) or the lesser tuberosity (Fig. 4.2.1d).

Three- and four-part fracture Three- and four-part fractures account for the remaining 10% of proximal humeral fractures, with two or three significantly displaced fragments (Fig 4.2.2a–c).

Management
One-part fractures (both displaced and undisplaced) and undisplaced two-part fractures can be treated with a collar and cuff sling, adequate analgesia and follow-up. Early mobilization is important, and the prognosis is good.

Definitive management of displaced two-part fractures may include open (intra-operative) or closed reduction depending upon neurovascular injury, rotator cuff integrity, associated dislocations, likelihood of union and function. Early orthopaedic assessment is recommended.

For undisplaced three- and four-part fractures, the consensus is for open reduction and internal fixation. However, recent reviews suggest that there is little evidence that surgery is superior to the non-operative approach.[2]

For displaced proximal humeral fractures, surgical management remains varied and controversial.[3] Small randomized controlled trials suggest that external fixation may confer some benefit over closed manipulation,[4] and that conservative treatment is better than tension band osteosynthesis.[5] A recent study shows that the decision should be made according to the viability of the humeral head. Locking plate technology may also provide better outcomes in patients with unstable displaced humeral fractures having a viable humeral head.[6] Other small-scale studies suggest that some bandaging styles may be better than others,[7] that early physiotherapy may improve functional outcome, but that pulsed high-frequency electromagnetic energy gives no additional benefit.[8]

Special cases

Fracture of the anatomical neck and articular surface
Fractures at these sites are uncommon, but are important to recognize as they have a high incidence of compromised blood supply to the articular segment, may result in avascular necrosis and may require a humeral hemiarthroplasty.

Fracture dislocations
Fractures of the greater tuberosity accompany 15% anterior glenohumeral dislocations and may be associated with rotator cuff tears. Although the fracture may be grossly displaced, reduction of the dislocated shoulder usually also reduces the fracture. In patients who require the full

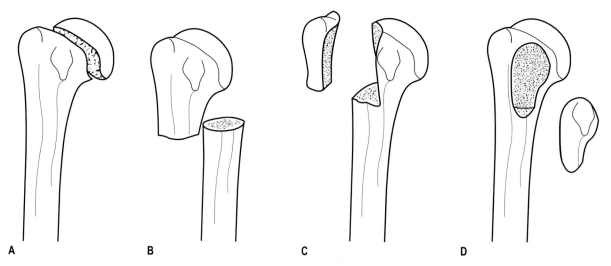

Fig. 4.2.1 Neer classification with two-part fractures of (a) the anatomical neck, (b) the surgical neck, (c) the greater tuberosity and (d) the lesser tuberosity.

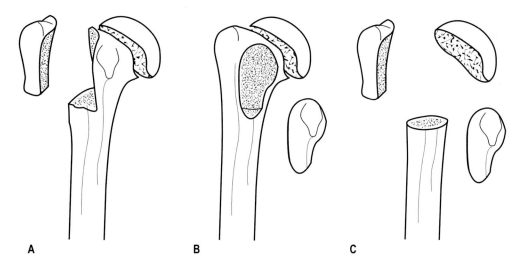

Fig. 4.2.2 Neer classification with three-part fractures of (a) the greater tuberosity and anatomical neck, (b) the lesser tuberosity and anatomical neck, and (c) four-part fracture involving the anatomical neck, greater tuberosity and lesser tuberosity.

range of movement of their shoulders, surgical repair of the cuff may be required.

Fractures of the lesser tuberosity are associated with posterior glenohumeral dislocations.

Disposition

Most patients with undisplaced one- and two-part fractures may be discharged from the ED with a collar and cuff sling, analgesia, early mobilization and appropriate follow-up. High-risk cases, including displaced three- and four-part fractures, all open fractures, and the special proximal humeral fractures described above, require orthopaedic consultation and admission, as do those with medical problems requiring investigation or treatment.

Low-energy fractures, especially in the elderly, suggest the presence of osteoporosis. 'At-risk' patients not already identified as having osteoporosis should be referred for bone density scans and vitamin D testing and treatment.

Fractures of the shaft of humerus

Patterns of injury

Fractures of the humeral shaft commonly occur in the third decade (active young men) and in the seventh decade of life (osteoporotic elderly women). The commonest site is the middle third, which accounts for 60% of humeral fractures. The close

proximity of the fracture to the radial nerve and brachial artery commonly leads to neurovascular deficits.

Direct blows tend to produce transverse fractures, whereas falls on the outstretched hand produce torsion forces and hence spiral fractures. Combinations of the two mechanisms may produce a butterfly segment. Pathological fractures are also common, most resulting from metastatic breast cancer.

The angle and degree of displacement of the fracture depends on the site of injury and its relationship to the action and attachment of muscles on either side of the injury (Fig. 4.2.3).

Clinical assessment

History and examination
Patients typically present complaining of pain and supporting the forearm of the injured limb, flexed at the elbow, held close to the chest wall. Examination of the limb reveals tenderness, swelling, shortening and possibly deformity. The skin should be assessed for tension or disruption, and particular attention should be paid to the shoulder and elbow regions for associated fractures or dislocations. Initial and post-reduction assessments of the brachial artery and vein, and ulnar, median and radial nerves are essential.

The commonest complication is radial nerve injury resulting either from injury or reduction of the fracture, and evidenced

by wrist drop and altered sensation in the first dorsal web space. A recent systemic review reported that radial nerve injury occurs in 11% of mid-shaft humerus fractures.[9]

Investigations

Two radiographic views – anteroposterior and lateral – will allow the correct diagnosis in most cases.

Fracture management and disposition

Uncomplicated, closed fractures account for the majority of injuries and may be treated by immobilization, analgesia, a functional brace such as a hanging or U-shaped cast (Fig. 4.2.3), and a broad arm or collar and cuff sling. The acceptable deformity is 20° anterior/posterior angulation, and 30° valus/valgus deformity.[10] The union rate is usually higher than 90%. Early specialist follow-up is recommended.

Some departments may prefer a humeral brace rather than U-shaped plaster for immobilization, as the former may permit greater functional use without affecting healing or fracture alignment.[11] For oblique/spiral fractures some orthopaedic surgeons prefer an operative approach for a better functional outcome.[12]

Open fractures and complications affecting the vessels require surgical repair. Although the majority of radial nerve injuries are neuropraxia and recover without surgical intervention, each case should be

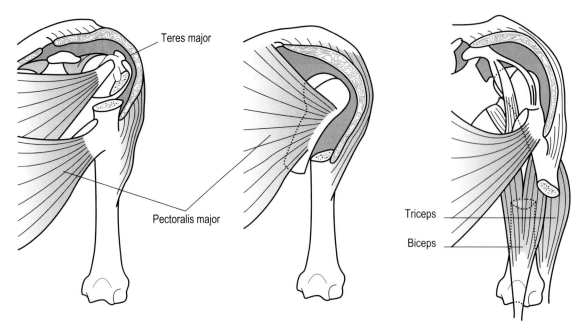

Fig. 4.2.3 Relationships between humeral fracture site and the actions of inserting muscles determine bony angulation and displacement.

considered individually by an orthopaedic surgeon with a view to possible operative exploration.

Fractures of the distal humerus

Classification and patterns of injury

Unlike in children, fractures of the distal humerus in adults are very uncommon and patterns of injury tend to reflect the anatomical two-column construction (condyles) of the humerus. Several classification methods have been used, such as the Riseborough and Radin, Mehne and Matta classifications, but the simplest and most commonly used are the AO/ASIF classifications.[13] These classify injuries into three categories: type A are extra-articular fractures, type B are partial articular, and type C are complete articular fractures. Practically, distal humeral fractures may be classified into supracondylar, intercondylar and other types. Supracondylar fractures lie transversely, whereas intercondylar T or Y fractures include an additional vertical extension between the condyles.

Mechanisms of injury usually involve a direct blow to the flexed or extended elbow. In the former, the olecranon is driven upwards, thereby either splitting the condyles apart producing a T or a Y pattern, or shearing off one condyle.

Clinical assessment

History and examination

Patients typically present with a swollen, tender, deformed elbow. As very little subcutaneous or other tissue separates the bone from skin, any disruption of the skin should be carefully examined for the possibility of a compound fracture. Distal neurological and vascular injury must be assessed carefully, as the possibility of nerve injury has been reported to be as high as 12–20%.[14]

Investigations

Two radiographic views – anteroposterior and lateral – should be obtained. Some authors suggest that an internal oblique view may improve the diagnostic accuracy.[15] Pain and inability to extend the elbow often result in poor-quality radiographs. Although high-quality radiographs are essential for operative planning, repeat films should not be attempted in the ED as they rarely provide the desired result. When there is any suspicion of severe injury, either from the history or from gross soft tissue swelling, early CT scanning should be considered to give better detail, especially of intra-articular fractures.

Undisplaced fractures may not be visible on radiography but may be suggested by posterior or anterior fat pad signs, which result from fat displaced by an underlying haemarthrosis. Ultrasonography, CT and MRI may all improve diagnostic precision. They alter management and improve outcome in patients with occult fractures, mostly of intra-articular type.

Fracture management and disposition

Uncomplicated, undisplaced, closed fractures with minimal swelling should be immobilized for 3 weeks in 90° flexion with an above-elbow cast and a broad arm sling, followed by active mobilization.

Patients with severe swelling, compound fractures, displaced fractures or neurovascular compromise require orthopaedic intervention.

Controversies

Guidance for management is based primarily on experience rather than rigorous research evidence.

- For humeral shaft fractures, it is unclear whether hanging plasters are better than U-shaped plasters for pain relief, fracture healing and position.

- Small-scale studies suggest that bracing may yield better functional results than U-shaped plaster immobilization for fractures of the humeral shaft.

- Low-intensity pulsed ultrasound may be useful in the treatment of non-union. Whether it may enhance normal fracture healing is not known.[16]

- The role of magnetic resonance imaging in the diagnosis of bone bruising and humeral fracture has not been studied.

References

1. Mulhall KJ, Ahmed A, Khan Y, Masterson E. Simultaneous hip and upper limb fracture in the elderly: incidence, features and management considerations. Injury 2002; 33: 29–31.
2. Handol HHG, Madhok R. Interventions for treating proximal humeral fractures in adults. Cochrane Database Systematic Review (4): 2003. CD000434. DOI: 0.1002/14651858.CD000434.
3. Weber E, Matter P. Surgical treatment of proximal humerus fractures – an international multicenter study [In German]. Swiss Surgery 1998; 4: 95–100.
4. Kristiansen B, Kofoed H. Transcutaneous reduction and external fixation of displaced fractures of the proximal humerus. A controlled clinical trial. Journal of Bone and Joint Surgery 1988; 70: 821–824.
5. Zyto K, Ahrengart L, Sperber A, Tornkvist H. Treatment of displaced proximal humeral fractures in elderly patients. Journal of Bone and Joint Surgery 1999; 79: 412–417.
6. Vallier HA. Treatment of proximal humerus fractures. Journal of the Orthopaedic Trauma 2008; 21(7): 469–476.
7. Rommens PM, Heyvaert G. Conservative treatment of subcapital humerus fractures. comparative study of the classical Desault bandage and the new Gilchrist bandage. Unfallchirurgie 1993; 19: 114–118.
8. Livesley PJ, Mugglestone A, Whitton J. Electrotherapy and the management of minimally displaced fracture of the neck of the humerus. Injury 1992; 23: 323–327.
9. Shao YC, Harwood P, Grotz MRW, et al. Radial nerve palsy associated with fractures of the shaft of the humerus: A systematic review. Journal of Bone and Joint Surgery 2005; 87-B: 1647–1652.
10. Klenerman L. Fractures of the shaft of the humerus. Journal of Bone and Joint Surgery 1966; 48B: 105–111.
11. Camden P, Nade S. Fracture bracing the humerus. Injury 1992; 23: 245–248.
12. Ring D, Chin K, Taghinia AH, Jupiter JB. Nonunion after functional brace treatment of diaphyseal humerus fractures. Journal of Trauma 2007; 62: 1157–1158.
13. Diana JN, Ramsey ML. Decision making in complex fractures of the distal humerus: current concepts and potential pitfalls. Orthopaedic Journal 1998; 11: 12–18.
14. Ramachandran M, Birch R, Eastwood DM. Clinical outcome of nerve injuries associated with supracondylar fractures of the humerus in children, the experience of a specialist referral centre. Journal of Bone and Joint Surgery 2006; 88B: 90–94.
15. Song KS, Kang CH, Min BW, et al. Internal oblique radiographs for diagnosis of nondisplaced or minimally displaced lateral condylar fractures of the humerus in children. Journal of Bone and Joint Surgery 2007; 89A: 58–63.
16. Nolte PA, van der Krans A, Patka P, et al. Low-intensity pulsed ultrasound in the treatment of nonunions. Journal of Trauma 2001; 51: 693–702.

Further reading

McRae R (ed) Practical fracture treatment. Edinburgh: Churchill Livingstone, 1994; 99–127.
Uehara DT, Rudzinski JP. Injuries to the shoulder complex and humerus. In: Tintinalli JE, Kelen GD, Stapczynski JS, eds. Emergency medicine. A comprehensive study guide. New York: McGraw-Hill, 2000; 1783–1791.
Willet K. Upper limb injuries. In: Skinner D, Swain A, Peyton R, Robertson C, eds. Cambridge textbook of accident and emergency medicine. Cambridge: Cambridge University Press, 1997; 601–617.

4.3 Dislocations of the elbow

Raymond Chi Hung Cheng • Timothy Rainer

ESSENTIALS

1 Elbow dislocations are the third most common large joint dislocation.

2 Surgical intervention is rarely required for simple elbow dislocations.

3 Surgical intervention may be required when fractures of the radius, ulnar and humerus are associated with elbow dislocation, or when neurovascular injury occurs.

4 The commonest neurovascular complication involves the ulnar nerve.

5 After reducing elbow dislocations, it is important to reassess joint stability and potential neurovascular complications.

Introduction

Elbow dislocation, along with glenohumeral and patellofemoral joint dislocations, is one of the three most common large joint dislocations.[1] The elbow joint is a hinge-like articulation involving the distal humerus and proximal radius and ulna. Owing to its strong muscular and ligamentous supports, the joint is normally quite stable and rarely requires operative intervention, even for acute instability after dislocation.

Elbow dislocations can be classified as either anterior or posterior. Posterior dislocation is the most common type and can be further divided into posteromedial or posterolateral. It usually results from a fall on the outstretched hand with some degree of flexion or hyperextension at the elbow. The radius and ulna commonly dislocate together. Similarly, anterior dislocation can also be divided into anteromedial or anterolateral. This type is less common and is usually due to a direct blow to the dorsal side of the elbow.

Uncommonly, the radius or ulna alone may dislocate at the elbow. In such cases there is always a fracture of the other bone. One common example is in Monteggia fractures, where anterior or posterior radiohumeral dislocation occurs alongside a fracture of the ulna shaft (Fig. 4.3.1). A rarer example is a posterior ulna–humeral dislocation with fracture of the radial shaft. So, although elbow dislocations may appear to be isolated, it is essential to look for associated intra-articular or shaft fractures.

Clinical assessment

History and examination

Patients typically present holding the lower arm at 45° to the upper arm and with swelling, tenderness and deformity of the

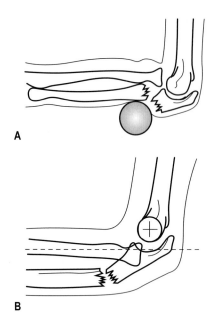

Fig. 4.3.1 Monteggia fracture dislocation. Fracture of the ulnar shaft may be associated with (a) anterior radiohumeral dislocation or (b) posterior radiohumeral dislocation.

elbow joint. The three-point anatomical triangle of olecranon, medial and lateral epicondyles should be assessed for abnormal alignment, as this strongly suggests dislocation.

The commonest neurovascular injury involves the ulnar nerve, reported in 10–15% of elbow dislocations,[2] but the median and radial nerves, and the brachial artery may also be affected.

The differential diagnosis is a complex distal humerus fracture which, in a swollen elbow, may be hard to differentiate clinically from an elbow dislocation.

Investigations

Anteroposterior and lateral radiographic views should be obtained and scrutinized for associated fractures of the coronoid process, radial head, capitellum and olecranon.

Magnetic resonance imaging (MRI) characterizes bony injury more accurately than radiography in children with elbow injuries, but its potential role for diagnosis and guiding management in adults has not been well evaluated.[3] Duplex Doppler ultrasound can be use to identify early brachial artery injury.[4]

Management

Simple dislocation can be reduced using a closed method. With adequate sedation, gentle traction and counter-traction, the joint relocates quite easily. Medial and posterolateral dislocations may also require sideways correction. Dislocation of the stable elbow joint produces severe soft tissue injury and resultant instability, therefore, after reduction, signs and symptoms of compartment syndrome should be sought along with an assessment of joint instability. The reduced elbow joint should move smoothly. Any crepitation or resistance, particularly during the mid-range, suggests incongruent reduction or soft tissue interposition, which is commonly associated with coronoid process or epicondylar fractures. Inability to fully flex or extend the elbow suggests a loose bone or cartilaginous fragment, or a capsular tear. Post-reduction films should be assessed, not only for correct joint relocation, but also for associated fractures. After successful reduction the elbow should be placed in a posterior plaster slab in 90° of flexion. Cylinder casts are contraindicated because of the likelihood of severe soft-tissue swelling.

There is little evidence that surgical intervention improves outcome in patients with medial or lateral elbow instability after dislocation. One small randomized controlled trial showed no evidence that surgical ligamentous repair produced better results than conservative management.[5] Another small study, a case series of patients with humeral medial condyle fracture, suggested good results after surgical management using absorbable implants compared to removal of the bony fragment.[6] Current practice is to treat all Monteggia fractures by early reduction and stabilization of the ulnar facture. The majority could be treated very well with close reduction and percutaneous intramedullary K-wire fixation of the ulnar fracture.[7] All late cases require open reduction and internal fixation; 45% of these cases are associated with complications and poor long-term functional outcome.[8]

Ulnar nerve injuries can occur both before and after closed reduction. The reported rate varies between 10% and 15%. Most of them are neuropraxia and will recover with conservative measures. The most sensitive sign and symptoms are numbness over the little fingers.

Compound fracture dislocation should be reduced by the open method.

Patients with irreducible dislocations, neurovascular complications, associated fractures or open dislocations require orthopaedic intervention.

Disposition

Current practice is that most patients may be discharged from the emergency department (ED) with analgesia, plaster slab support and a broad arm sling with appropriate follow-up. A recent prospective, randomized French study[9] suggested that early mobilization is superior to plaster immobilization in terms of functional recovery, without any increased instability or a recurrence of dislocation for patients with uncomplicated posterior dislocations, so the duration of immobilization is controversial. Patients with irreducible dislocations, neurovascular complications, associated fractures or open dislocations require admission.

Controversies

- There are no large-scale randomized studies comparing operative and non-operative management of elbow dislocation. It is therefore unclear whether one method may produce better outcomes than another.

- Early mobilization may be superior to plaster immobilization after reduction of uncomplicated posterior dislocations.

- The epidemiology of elbow injury including dislocation in patients presenting to emergency departments has not been well described, and requires further studies.

- Roles for ultrasound, computerized tomography and magnetic resonance imaging in evaluating elbow injury and influencing management require further study.

References

1. Uehara DT, Chin HW. Injuries to the elbow and forearm. In: Tintinalli JE, Kelen GD, Stapczynski JS (eds) Emergency medicine. A comprehensive study guide. New York: McGraw-Hill, 2000; 1763–1772.
2. Robert S, David R. Current concepts review: the ulnar nerve in elbow trauma. Journal of Bone and Joint Surgery 2007; 89A: 1108–1116.
3. Griffiths JF, Roebuck DJ, Cheng JCY, et al. Comparison of radiography and magnetic resonance imaging in the detection of injuries after paediatric elbow trauma. American Journal of Roentgenology 2001; 176: 53–60.
4. Ergunes K, Yilik L, Ozsoyler I, et al. Traumatic brachial artery injuries. Texas Heart Institute Journal 2006; 33: 31–34.
5. Josefsson PO, Gentz CF, Johnell O, Wendeberg B. Surgical versus non-surgical treatment of ligamentous injuries following dislocation of the elbow joint. A prospective randomized study. Journal of Bone and Joint Surgery 1987; 69: 605–608.
6. Partio EK, Hirvensalo E, Bostman O, Rokkanen P. A prospective controlled trial of the fracture of the humeral medial epicondyle – how to treat? Annales Chirurgiae Gynaecologiae 1996; 85: 67–71.
7. Lam TP, Ng BKW, Ma RF, Cheng JCY. Monteggia fractures in children – a review of 30 cases. Journal of the Japanese Pediatric Orthopedic Association 2004; 13: 193–195.
8. Reynders P, De Groote W, Rondia J, et al. Monteggia lesions in adults. A multi-centre Bota study. Acta Orthopaedica Belgica 1996; 62: 78–83.
9. Rafai M, Largab A, Cohen D, Trafeh M. Pure posterior luxation of the elbow in adults: immobilization or early mobilization. A randomized prospective study of 50 cases. Chirurgie de la Main 1999; 18: 272–278.

Further reading

McRae R. Practical fracture treatment. Edinburgh: Churchill Livingstone, 1994.
Willet K. Upper limb injuries. In: Skinner D, Swain A, Peyton R, Robertson C, eds. Cambridge textbook of accident and emergency medicine. Cambridge: Cambridge University Press, 1997;601–617.

4.4 Fractures of the forearm and carpal bones

Peter Wright

ESSENTIALS

1 Forearm fractures are among the most common fractures seen in the ED.

2 When assessing the need for, or success of, reduction the external appearance of the limb is a key feature.

3 Median nerve function must be assessed before and after reduction of all distal radial fractures.

4 Splinting or functional bracing may be sufficient for stable fractures. Early movement and load bearing aids functional recovery.

5 General indications for orthopaedic referral include fractures which are compound, unstable, associated with intra-articular or neurovascular injury, and those that have failed reduction in the ED.

6 Displaced, isolated fractures of the ulna or radius may be associated with a dislocation of the radius or ulna respectively (Monteggia and Galeazzi fracture-dislocations). These should be carefully sought, as there is high risk of long-term disability.

7 Significant or persistent symptoms with the absence of a visible fracture on plain X-ray may be due to an undetected fracture or significant soft-tissue injury. A high index of suspicion and review in 1 or 2 weeks are recommended. Further investigation with CT, MRI or repeat X-ray may be indicated.

Radial head fractures

Clinical features

History

Patients have usually had a fall onto their outstretched hand or received a direct blow to the lateral side of the elbow, and present with pain and restricted movement at the elbow.

Examination

Usually there is swelling and tenderness over the radial head. Sometimes, with more subtle injuries, rotating the forearm while palpating the radial head may be necessary to elicit tenderness. Elbow extension and forearm rotation are limited. Severely comminuted fractures may have proximal displacement of the radius, which can be associated with disruption of the interosseous membrane and subluxation of the distal radioulnar joint (Essex–Lopresti fracture-dislocation).

Imaging

Anteroposterior (AP) and lateral X-rays of the elbow are required. A radiocapitellar view may be necessary if the fracture is subtle. The presence of an anterior fat pad sign alone on X-ray is associated with an underlying radial head or neck fracture in up to 50% of patients. In this case a fracture should be assumed to be present if there is an appropriate mechanism and local signs. A follow-up X-ray or CT scan is indicated only in the presence or persistent pain, stiffness or locking.

Classification

Radial head fractures may be described as hairline, marginal (displaced and undisplaced), segmental (displaced and undisplaced) or comminuted. They may also be classified into four types (Fig. 4.4.1). Fractures of the radial neck may be undisplaced or have various degrees of lateral tilting.

Management

Type I and minor type II radial head fractures without mechanical block may be managed with a bandage and sling. If there is severe pain, aspiration of the fracture haematoma, intra-articular bupivacaine or a back slab may be useful. Mobilization

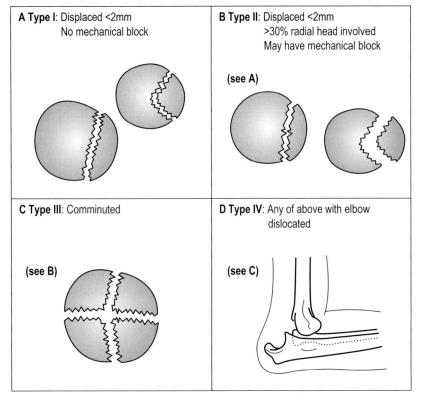

A Type I: Displaced <2mm
No mechanical block

B Type II: Displaced <2mm
>30% radial head involved
May have mechanical block

(see A)

C Type III: Comminuted

(see B)

D Type IV: Any of above with elbow dislocated

(see C)

Fig. 4.4.1 Mason–Hotchkiss classification of radial head fractures.

can occur after 1–2 days depending on symptoms. Prognosis is good, but full extension may not be possible for many months.

All type III and those type II fractures with the presence of a mechanical block to movement require surgical intervention. Mechanical block can be difficult to assess acutely due to pain. Intra-articular injection of bupivacaine may assist early assessment, or assessment may be deferred until pain has settled. Surgical options include open reduction and internal fixation, and excision of the radial head with or without implantation of a prosthesis.

Radial neck fractures with up to 20° tilts can be managed conservatively. More severe tilt can be reduced using intra-articular bupivacaine. The forearm is pronated until the most prominent part of the radial head is felt. Then traction is applied to the forearm and pressure applied to the radial head. Open reduction is indicated if closed methods fail or displacement is gross.

Complications

Neurovascular complications and compartment syndrome are uncommon. Most complications relate to disturbance of the relationships of the proximal radioulnar and radiocapitellar articular surfaces causing limitation of movement. This is uncommon with minor fractures and often responds to radial head excision.

Shaft fractures

History

This type of injury requires great force, typically from a motor-vehicle accident, a fall from a height or a direct blow. These fractures are commonly open and nearly always displaced.

Examination

The forearm is swollen and tender and may be angulated and rotated. Examination looking for an open wound, local neurovascular compromise, compartment syndrome or musculotendinous injury is required. Given the mechanism of injury, other injuries should also be sought.

Imaging

AP and lateral X-rays of the forearm, including the wrist and elbow joints, are needed. Displacement and angulation are easily determined, but torsional deformity may be subtle. Because the ulna and radius are rectangular in cross-section rather than circular, a change in bone width at the fracture site indicates rotation. The radial and ulnar styloid processes normally point in opposite directions to the bicipital tuberosity and coronoid process, respectively. A change in this alignment also suggests torsion.

Management

Adult forearm fractures are less stable than those in children, and lack of remodelling limits tolerance to incomplete reduction. Undisplaced fractures may be managed with an above-elbow cast, but must be reviewed at 1 week for displacement and angulation. Most fractures, however, are displaced and require open reduction and internal fixation.

Complications

Early complications include wound infection, osteomyelitis, neurovascular injury and compartment syndrome. Later, non-union, malunion, reduced forearm rotation and reflex sympathetic dystrophy are possible complications.

Isolated fracture of the ulnar shaft

These fractures are due to a direct blow to the ulna, often when raised in defence; hence they are also known as 'nightstick' fractures. Patients present with localized pain and swelling. AP and lateral X-rays delineate the location of the fracture and degree of angulation. Look for associated dislocation of the radial head if displacement is present (Monteggia fracture-dislocation).

Fractures displaced less than 50% of the ulna width heal well with a non-union rate of 0–4%. Traditional treatment involves fixing the forearm in mid-pronation with a plaster cast, extended above elbow if the middle or proximal thirds of the ulna are fractured. The cast is removed once union occurs, usually in 6–8 weeks. Other proven options include a below-elbow plaster (BEPOP) for proximal fractures, early mobilization with bandage after 1–2 weeks in BEPOP, or functional bracing after 3–5 days, which allows movement at wrist and elbow.

Fractures with more than 10° of angulation or displaced more than 50% of the diameter of the ulna require surgical intervention.

Monteggia fracture-dislocation

This is a rare fracture of the proximal ulna with dislocation of the radial head. It occurs either through a fall onto the outstretched hand with hyperpronation or through a force applied to the posterior aspect of the proximal ulna. Patients present with pain, swelling and reduced elbow movement. The forearm may appear shortened and the radial head may be palpable in the antecubital fossa. Associated posterior interosseous nerve injury is common.

On X-ray the fracture is obvious, but the dislocation is commonly missed. Check that a line through the radial shaft bisects the capitellum on both views. Dislocation is anterior in 60%, but may be anterolateral or posterolateral.

All Monteggia fractures require open reduction and internal fixation. Common complications include malunion and non-union of the ulnar fracture and an unstable radial head.

Isolated radial shaft fracture

Isolated fractures of the proximal two-thirds of the radial shaft are uncommon and are usually displaced. Rare undisplaced fractures can be treated similarly to isolated ulnar shaft fractures. Displaced fractures require open reduction and internal fixation.

Galeazzi fracture-dislocation

Fractures of the distal third of the radial shaft occur as a result of a fall onto the outstretched hand or a direct blow. There may be an associated subluxation or dislocation of the distal radioulnar joint (DRUJ), known as the Galeazzi fracture-dislocation. Patients have pain and swelling at the radial fracture site. Those with a Galeazzi injury will also have pain and swelling at the DRUJ and a prominent ulnar head.

X-rays show the radial fracture, which is tilted ventrolaterally. Widening of the DRUJ space on the AP and dorsal displacement of the ulnar head on the lateral are seen (Fig. 4.4.2). An ulnar styloid fracture is seen in 60% of cases.

AP view wrist

(see A Fig. 4.4.1)

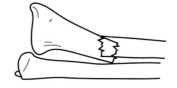

(see B Fig. 4.4.1)

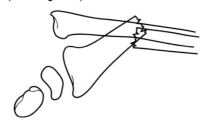

Fig. 4.4.2 The Galeazzi fracture-dislocation.

All Galeazzi fracture-dislocations require surgical management. Complications include malunion or non-union of the radial fracture and subsequent instability of the DRUJ.

Fractures of the distal radius and ulna

Fractures of the distal radius and ulna are common, particularly in children, young men and elderly women. Fractures in the latter group are indications for evaluation of bone-mineral density.

Clinical features

History and examination

Fractures usually occur after a fall onto the outstretched hand resulting in bending, shearing or impaction forces being applied to the distal metaphysis; or from a direct blow. Patients present with pain, tenderness and variable degrees of swelling and deformity. It is important to examine for associated injuries to carpals, radial and ulnar shafts, elbow and shoulder joints, for median nerve injury, vascular compromise, and for extensor tendon injury.

Imaging

Anteroposterior and lateral X-rays of the wrist demonstrate most injuries. For patients with significant symptoms or signs and a normal X-ray, consider an occult undisplaced fracture or ligamentous injury.

Although this chapter uses eponymous names, it is important to be aware that orthopaedic circles have moved to more formal classification systems for distal radial fractures. Several have been proposed and are beyond the scope of this text. The author recommends being familiar with anatomical descriptions and fracture features associated with need for reduction, instability of reduction, and indications for operative intervention.

Management

Prompt attention to analgesia, splinting and elevation is essential while awaiting X-rays.

Reduction is indicated in the following circumstances to improve long-term function:

- Visible deformity of the wrist.
- Loss of volar tilt of the distal radial articular surface beyond neutral.
- Loss of >5° of the radial inclination of the distal radius (normally approximately 20°).
- Intra-articular step of >2 mm.
- Radial shortening >2–3 mm.

Greater deformity can be accepted in low-demand, elderly patients.

Anaesthetic options for reduction include intravenous anaesthesia with Bier's block, haematoma block, and procedural sedation. Reduction is traditionally maintained with an encircling plaster cast moulded to oppose displacement forces from volar metacarpal crease to proximal forearm for 6 weeks. Displaced or comminuted fractures at high risk of swelling, especially in the elderly or coagulopathic patients, are immobilized with non-encircling splints.

Factors associated with instability of the distal fragment and failure to maintain reduction include:

- Comminution > two-thirds to three-quarters of metaphyseal width on lateral X-ray.
- Shearing fractures (Barton-type).
- The magnitude of the initial displacement.

Weekly X-rays for 2–3 weeks with orthopaedic follow-up are recommended for all displaced fractures, those with intra-articular extension and potentially unstable fractures.

ORTHOPAEDIC EMERGENCIES

4

Stable, undisplaced, extra-articular fractures can be managed more conservatively with splinting and referral to a family doctor for early mobilization after 4 weeks.

Indications for operative management are debated, but should be considered for:

- Comminuted, displaced, intra-articular fractures.
- Open fractures.
- Associated carpal fractures.
- Associated neurovascular or tendon injury.
- Failed conservative treatment (failed reduction or unstable after reduction).
- Bilateral fractures/impaired contralateral extremity.

Complications

Median nerve injury may occur acutely due to the injury, as a result of reduction, or later due to pressure effects from the plaster. Median nerve function must be documented before and after reduction.

Loss of reduction may require delayed surgical intervention.

Malunion with chronic wrist pain, arthritis and secondary radioulnar and radiocarpal instability are associated with intra-articular extension of the fracture.

Delayed ruptures of the extensor pollicis longus can occur.

Colles' fracture

First described in 1814, the Colles' fracture is a metaphyseal bending fracture. The wrist has a classic 'dinner-fork' appearance, often with significant swelling of the soft tissues. This appearance is reflected in the radiographs (Fig. 4.4.3). There is often associated damage to the radioulnar fibrocartilage. There may be comminution, commonly dorsally, which can extend into the radiocarpal or radioulnar joints.

Management

The aim of reduction is to restore radial length, volar tilt and radial angulation. A minimum of 0° tilt is acceptable if full reduction is not possible. Reduction is achieved by first disimpacting the fracture with traction in the line of the forearm. If this fails, traction in extension or hyperextension should be tried. Volar tilt is then restored with volar pressure over the dorsum of the distal fragment while traction

AP view wrist

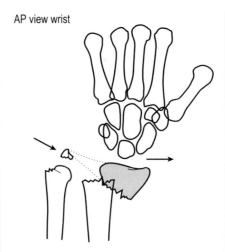

Lateral view wrist

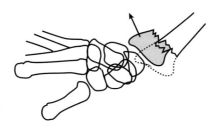

Fig. 4.4.3 Colles' fracture. A fracture of the distal radial metaphysis with six classic deformities. The lateral view shows anterior angulation, dorsal displacement and impaction. The AP view reveals radial displacement, ulnar angulation and an ulnar styloid fracture.

is maintained. Lastly, correct radial tilt and radial displacement with ulnar pressure over the radial side of the distal fragment. Reduction is successful in 87%, but almost two-thirds lose reduction over 5 weeks, most of this occurring during cast immobilization.

The commonly accepted cast immobilization position is with the wrist joint in 10° flexion, full ulnar deviation and pronation. However, some evidence suggests better outcomes are achieved with the wrist in dorsiflexion and mid-supination. The cast must be carefully moulded over the dorsum of the distal fragment and the anteromedial forearm. Functional bracing allowing wrist movement has also shown good outcomes.

Smith's fracture

This metaphyseal bending fracture of the distal radius occurs through a direct blow or fall onto the back of the hand or a fall backward onto the outstretched hand in supination.

AP and lateral X-rays of the wrist show a 'reverse Colles' fracture' with a similar AP appearance, but with volar displacement and tilt on the lateral X-ray view.

Closed reduction to achieve anatomical radial length and volar tilt should be attempted. Traction is first applied to restore length, followed by dorsal pressure over the volar surface of the distal radius to reverse displacement and angulation. A full above-elbow cast is applied with the wrist in supination and fully dorsiflexed to prevent loss of reduction.

Barton's fracture

Barton's fractures are dorsal or volar intra-articular fractures of the distal radial rim (Fig. 4.4.4). The mechanisms of injury are similar to those seen with Colles' and Smith's fractures, respectively. There is often significant soft-tissue injury and the carpus is usually dislocated or subluxed along with the distal fragment. These fractures are complicated by arthritis of the radiocarpal joints and carpal instability.

Minimally displaced fractures involving less than 50% of the joint surface and without carpal displacement may be reduced along the lines of a Colles' or Smith's fracture. Immobilization should occur with wrist flexed for dorsal Barton's and extended for volar Barton's. However, most fractures are unstable and potentially disabling, requiring

Dorsal Barton's

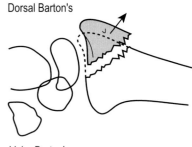

Volar Barton's

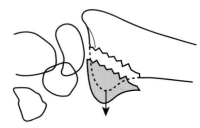

Fig. 4.4.4 Barton fractures demonstrated on lateral views of the wrist.

AP view wrist

(see A Fig. 4.4.1)

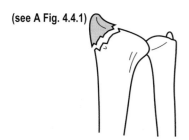

Fig. 4.4.5 Radial styloid (Hutchison or chauffeur) fracture.

early operative management, especially in younger patients. Early orthopaedic follow-up is mandatory.

Radial styloid (Hutchison or chauffeur's) fracture

This oblique intra-articular fracture of the radial styloid is caused by a direct blow or fall onto the hand. Displacement is associated with carpal instability and long-term arthritis. The fracture is seen best on AP X-rays of the wrist (Fig. 4.4.5). Undisplaced fractures can be treated with a cast for 4–6 weeks. Displaced fractures should be referred to an orthopaedic surgeon for anatomical reduction and fixation.

Ulnar styloid fracture

An isolated fracture can occur through forced radial deviation, dorsiflexion, rotation, or a direct blow. If displaced there may be associated damage to the triangular radio-ulnar fibrocartilage with subsequent DRUJ instability. Fractures should be treated with a splint or cast with the wrist in ulnar deviation, and referred to an orthopaedic surgeon to assess DRUJ stability.

Carpal fractures and dislocations

Carpal fractures account for 18% of hand fractures. The bones in the proximal carpal row are more commonly involved (scaphoid 70%, triquetral 14%). Isolated fractures of other carpal bones are rare. Management depends on the degree of displacement and damage and stability. Generally, undisplaced fractures with minimal comminution can be managed by cast immobilization. Given the importance of wrist function, early orthopaedic review

should be sought for patients with displaced or comminuted fractures, or where instability or an associated carpal dislocation is suspected.

Scaphoid fracture

The most common mechanism of injury is a fall on the outstretched hand. Clinical features include wrist pain and local tenderness over the scaphoid, palpated dorsally or via the anatomical snuffbox. Imaging with AP, lateral and scaphoid views will often identify the fracture.

Fractures of the scaphoid are classified by their location (proximal third, waist, distal third or tubercle) and by their stability. Stable fractures are undisplaced with little comminution, and unstable fractures are displaced with considerable comminution. Stable fractures are treated with a below-elbow cast for 10–12 weeks. Unstable fractures require surgical intervention. Complications include non-union and avascular necrosis of the proximal segment.

A cohort of patients have clinical features suggestive of scaphoid fracture without confirmatory X-ray evidence. In the past, cast immobilization for 1–2 weeks followed by repeat X-ray was advocated. Although this is still advocated by some, a number of alternative approaches have been suggested, including bandaging with clinical review at 7–10 days followed by CT if clinical features persist or early primary CT. Both have been shown to be effective and avoid the wrist stiffness that often results from casting. MRI is advocated as an additional imaging modality if required.

Dislocations of the wrist

Dislocations involving the wrist usually result from high-energy falls on the outstretched hand (such as from a height) that result in forced hyperextension. The distal row of carpal bones is commonly displaced dorsal to the proximal row as a result of a scaphoid fracture, a scapholunate dislocation, or a perilunate dislocation. Trans-scaphoid perilunate fracture-dislocation is slightly more common than perilunate dislocation. Clinical features include mechanism of injury, wrist pain, swelling and tenderness, and possibly reduced grip strength. Imaging requires PA and lateral X-rays. The normal PA view should show two rows of carpal bones in a

normal anatomic position with uniform joint spaces of no more than 1–2 mm. No overlap should be seen between the carpal bones or between the distal ulna and the radius. On the lateral film, a longitudinal axis should align the radius, the lunate, the capitate, and the third metacarpal bone.

Radiographic features include:

- Lunate dislocation: On the usual PA image, the lunate has a triangular shape rather than its usual trapezoidal shape. On the lateral film, the lunate has a 'C' or 'half-moon' shape. The rest of the carpal bones are in a normal anatomic position in relation to the radius.

- Perilunate dislocation: On the lateral film, the lunate is in a normal anatomic position with respect to the radius with and the rest of the carpal bones displaced dorsally. On the PA film crowding is evident between the proximal and distal carpal bones.

- Scapholunate dislocation: On a PA radiograph, the scapholunate space is greater than 4 mm (also known as the Terry-Thomas sign). The scaphoid rotates, producing the classic signet-ring sign. Associated carpal fractures, especially of the scaphoid, may be evident. All wrist dislocations require orthopaedic consultation and prompt reduction.

Controversies

- Optimal immobilization for distal radial fractures.

- The role of splints and functional braces versus traditional plaster casts.

- Duration of immobilization for undisplaced fractures.

- Operative versus non-operative management of distal radial fractures, particularly in the elderly.

- Optimal management strategy for suspected scaphoid fracture with normal initial X-rays.

Further reading

Barton's fracture/dorsal shearing fracture. In: Wheeless III CR. Wheeless' textbook of orthopaedics. http://www.wheelessonline.com/ortho/dorsal_bartons_fracture_dorsal_shearing_frx. Accessed Jan 2008.

Connolly JF. Nonoperative fracture treatment. In: Bucholz RW, Heckman JD, Court-Brown C, et al., eds. Rockwood and Green's fractures in adults, 6th edn. Baltimore: Lippincott Williams & Wilkins, 2005.

Geiderman JM, Magnusson AR. Humerus and elbow. In: Rosen P, Barker, eds. Emergency medicine, 4th edn. St. Louis: Mosby-Year Book, 1998.

Closed reduction of distal radius fractures. In: Wheeless III CR. Wheeless' textbook of orthopaedics. http://www.wheelessonline.com/ortho/closed_reduction_of_distal_radius_fractures. Accessed Jan 2008.

Cruikshank J, Meakin A, Braedmore R, et al. Early computerized tomography accurately determines the presence or absence of scaphoid and other fractures. Emergency Medicine of Australasia 2007; 19: 223–228.

de Beaux AC, Beattie T, Gilbert F. Elbow fat-pad sign: implications for clinical management. Journal of the Royal College of Surgeons of Edinburgh 1992; 37: 205–206.

Distal Radial Frx: position of immobilization. In: Wheeless III CR. Wheeless' textbook of orthopaedics. http://www.wheelessonline.com/ortho/distal_radius_frx_position_of_immobilization. Accessed Jan 2008.

Eisenhauer MA. Wrist and forearm. In: Rosen P, Barker R, eds. Emergency medicine, 4th edn. St. Louis: Mosby-Year Book, 1998.

Ferris BD, Thomas NP, Dewar ME, Simpson MA. Brace treatment of Colles' fracture. Acta Orthopaedica Scandinavica 1989; 60: 63–65.

Hanel DP, Jones MD, Trumble TE. Wrist fractures. Orthopaedic Clinics of North America 2002; 33: 35–57.

Irshad F, Shaw NJ, Gregory RJ. Reliability of fat-pad sign in radial head/neck fractures of the elbow. Injury 1997; 28: 433–435.

Kouros GJ, Schenck RR, Theodorou SJV. Carpal fractures. http://www.emedicine.com/orthoped/topic36.htm. Accessed Jan 2008.

Kuntz DG Jr, Bararz ME. Fractures of the elbow. Orthopaedic Clinics of North America 1999; 30: 37–61.

Mackay D, Wood L, Rangan A. The treatment of isolated ulnar fractures in adults: a systematic review. Injury 2000; 31: 565–570.

McRae R. Practical fracture treatment, 3rd edn. London: Churchill Livingstone, 1994.

Uehara DT, Chin HW. Injuries to the elbow and forearm. In: Tintinalli JE Kelen GD, Stapcznski JS, et al., eds. Emergency medicine, 5th edn. New York: McGraw Hill, 2000.

Radial inclination of distal radius frx. In Wheeless' Textbook of Orthopaedics. http://www.wheelessonline.com/ortho/radial_inclination_of_distal_radius_frx. Accessed Jan 2008.

Ruch DS. Fractures of the distal radius and ulna. In: Bucholz RW Heckman JD, Court-Brown C, et al., eds. Rockwood and Green's fractures in adults, 6th edn. Baltimore: Lippincott Williams & Wilkins, 2005.

Sarmiento A, Latta L. The evolution of functional bracing for fractures. Journal of Bone and Joint Surgery 2006; 88B: 141–148.

Smith's fracture. In: Wheeless III CR. Wheeless III CR. Wheeless' textbook of orthopaedics. http://www.wheelessonline.com/ortho/smiths_fracture. Accessed Jan 2008.

Szabo RM. Extra-articular fractures of the distal radius. Orthopaedic Clinics of North America 1993; 24: 229–237.

Uehara DT, Chin HW. Wrist injuries. In: Tintinalli JE, Kelen GD, Stapczynski JS, et al., eds. Emergency medicine, 5th edn. New York: McGraw Hill, 2000.

Van Glabbeek F, Van Riet R, Verstreken J. Current concepts in the treatment of radial head fractures in adults. A clinical and biomechanical approach. Acta Orthopaedica Belgica 2001; 67: 430–441.

Villarin LA Jr, Belk KE, Freid R. Emergency department evaluation and treatment of elbow and forearm injuries. Emergency Medicine Clinics of North America 1999; 17: 843–858.

Volar Barton's fracture. In: Wheeless III CR. Wheeless' Textbook of Orthopaedics. http://www.wheelessonline.com/ortho/volar_bartons_fractures. Accessed Jan 2008.

4.5 Hand injuries

Peter Freeman

ESSENTIALS

1 A comprehensive knowledge of hand anatomy and function is essential for appropriate initial management of the injured hand.

2 Hand injuries are common and most carry a good prognosis if treated early and competently.

3 Aftercare and rehabilitation are essential for return to normal function.

Introduction

Five to 10% of emergency department (ED) attendances involve injury to the hand. Presentations may be due to wounds (~35%), contusions (~20%), fractures (~20%), sprains (~10%) or infections (~5%).[1] Males injure their hands more than females. The effect of hand injury on an individual cannot be overestimated. Apart from the initial pain and trauma, occupational and psychological concerns play a major role in the aftermath of these injuries. Even a relatively minor fingertip injury can result in an individual being away from work for several days, with consequent loss of earnings and concerns for long-term function and appearance. It is therefore essential that initial assessment and management are appropriate. Complications of traumatic wounds account for the highest number of medicolegal actions against emergency physicians in the United States.

Clinical features

History

Time taken eliciting an accurate history of the mechanism of injury is never more important than in cases of hand injury. Key questions include: When did the injury occur? What was the position of the hand at the time? Was the hand injured with a sharp implement such as glass, or crushed in a machine? Incised wounds caused by sharp implements tend to damage structures such as nerves and tendons, whereas crush injuries may cause fractures and lacerations. Was there brisk bleeding, and does any part of the hand feel numb? These symptoms are important, as in the fingers the digital arteries lie adjacent to the nerves. What was the environment of the injury? Is it likely that the wound is contaminated or contains foreign material? Glass is radio-opaque to a varying degree, and if there is any doubt it is best to assume the wound contains glass and X-ray will confirm or otherwise. Is the patient right or left handed, and what are their occupation and leisure activities? It is also important to ascertain medications and allergies, to guide analgesia and antibiotic choice and tetanus prophylaxis status.

Examination

The injured hand must be examined in a well-lit area. Temporary dressings may need to be soaked off if they have been allowed to dry out and become adherent. At triage an initial moist dressing is ideal, with firm pressure and elevation if there is significant haemorrhage.

Hand and finger injuries are painful and suitable analgesia must be given to allow full examination. Local infiltration of lignocaine without epinephrine (adrenaline) around a wound or as a digital nerve block will allow examination of all aspects except sensation, which must be tested and recorded prior to anaesthesia. A wrist block is useful when some or all of the hand needs to be anaesthetized (Fig. 4.5.1), and longer-acting local anaesthetic is generally used to prolong the effect.

Testing sensation is achieved by light touch or two-point discrimination in the distribution of the three main nerves that supply the hand (Fig. 4.5.2). The median nerve supplies the palmar aspect of the thumb, index, middle and half of the ring finger, extending to supply the fingertip and nailbed. The ulnar nerve supplies both palmar and dorsal aspects of the other half of the ring finger and the little finger. The radial nerve supplies the radial dorsum of the hand, thumb, index, middle and radial aspects of the ring finger. If the patient is unable to describe sensation because they are too young or unconscious, it is useful to remember that the digital nerves also carry the sympathetic supply to the fingers, and that division will cause a dry finger in the distribution of the digital nerve.

The hand examination should be holistic and not just concentrate on the obvious injury. Inspection of the hand will provide information about the perfusion of the tissues, local swelling and position of wounds. The resting position of the hand may be a clue to tendon injury, as the normal uninjured position is held with the fingers in increasing flexion from the index to the little finger (Fig. 4.5.3a). A pointing finger may indicate a flexor tendon injury (Fig. 4.5.3b). Obvious bone or joint deformity should be recorded.

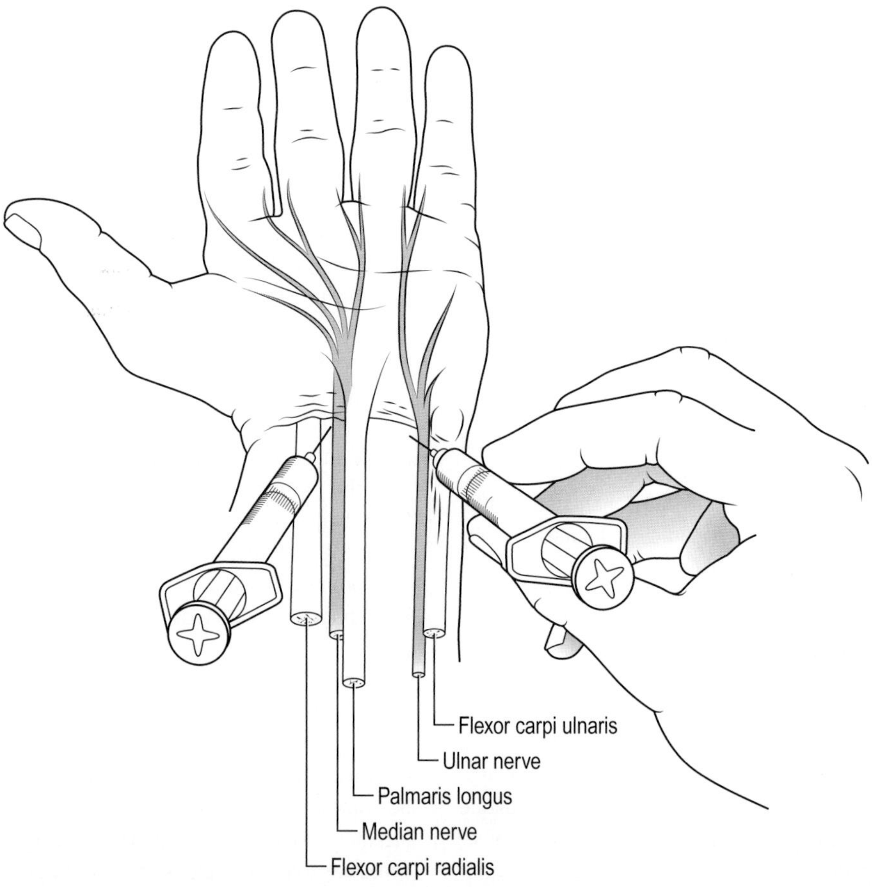

Palpation of the hand will elicit any local tenderness, and the metacarpals and phalanges are all easily palpable subcutaneously.

Functional testing should be performed for all injured hands. Tendon function is tested by asking the patient to perform specific movements. Some tendon injuries may be obvious, such as mallet finger injuries and the pointing finger; however, two flexor tendons supply each finger, and simply asking the patient to flex the finger will not exclude a divided flexor digitorum superficialis tendon. The profundus tendon flexes the distal interphalangeal joint and is tested by asking the patient to flex the tip of each finger in turn while the examiner holds the proximal interphalangeal joint. The superficialis tendon is tested by asking the patient to flex each finger individually, while the examiner holds the other fingers straight. The extensor tendons to the fingers are tested by asking the patient to extend the fingers as much as possible. It is important to remember that the interconnections between the extensor tendons make it possible to extend to near neutral in the presence of a divided tendon. Partial tendon injuries may still exist despite normal functioning of the fingers. The functioning hand should allow full extension of all fingers and comfortable flexion of the fingers into the palm.

Displaced fractures or dislocations may be apparent as deformity. More subtle rotational deformity will be detected by a finger crossing its neighbour when flexed.

Flexor carpi ulnaris
Ulnar nerve
Palmaris longus
Median nerve
Flexor carpi radialis

Fig. 4.5.1 Palmar wrist block. (Reproduced with permission from American Society for the Surgery of the Hand. The hand, 2nd edn. Boston, MA: Churchill Livingstone, 1990.)

Investigations

Most information will be obtained from a full history and examination. Radiology of the hand and fingers will be necessary if bone/joint deformity or tenderness is elicited. Dislocations should always be X-rayed prior to manipulation, however trivial they may seem. Radiography can

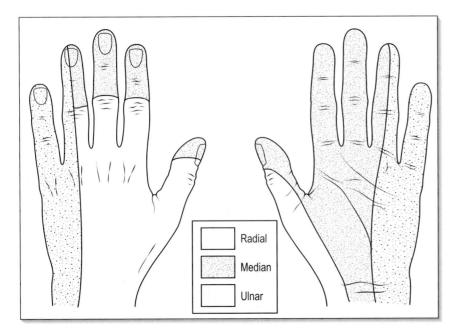

Fig. 4.5.2 The nerve supply to hand.

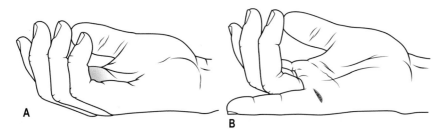

Fig. 4.5.3 The normal resting hand (a). The pointing finger (b). (Reproduced with permission from American Society for the Surgery of the Hand. The hand, 2nd edn. Boston, MA: Churchill Livingstone, 1990.)

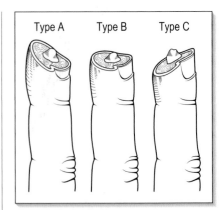

Fig. 4.5.4 Classification of fingertip amputations.

also reveal radio-opaque glass in a wound. Organic foreign bodies and infections can often be detected by ultrasound imaging using a small-parts soft tissue probe.

Blood investigations are rarely of use in the acutely injured hand.

Magnetic resonance imaging (MRI) is useful in selected injuries as it shows the soft tissues of the hand clearly, but it is relatively unavailable acutely and should be reserved for conditions where clinical examination requires supplementary information about the integrity of the soft structures in the hand, e.g. tendon injury.

Treatment

Appropriate analgesia should be provided as previously described. Rings should be removed from injured fingers to prevent subsequent compromise of circulation as the finger swells. Elevation is essential after hand injury to reduce swelling. Minor injuries can be successfully managed in the ED, but more significant injuries usually require specialist repair.

Fingertip injuries

The fingertips have an excellent blood supply and will usually heal if given the correct environment. Fingertip avulsions are classified as type A when the skin loss is oblique dorsal, type B when the loss is transverse, and type C when the loss is oblique volar (Fig. 4.5.4).

The most complex to manage is type C, as there is loss of palmar skin. When there is a type A or B injury involving less than 50% of the nailbed, conservative treatment is often the best option. Care of the fingertip initially is likely to require haemostasis followed by an occlusive dressing. There is good evidence that this kind of dressing promotes healing by being non-adherent and allowing fast re-epithelialization of the fingertip.[2] The dressing is also quick to apply, easily removed, and comfortable for the patient. Most other dressings adhere to the wound and pull epithelial cells off when removed. Alternatives to conservative dressings include skin grafts to the fingertips, advancement flaps and cross-finger flaps. These should be performed by surgeons trained in the specialist techniques, and reserved for injuries involving large areas of skin loss.

Major amputations of the fingertip or crush injuries may require terminalization of the finger. This should be fully discussed with the patient, who may be prepared to forgo finger length in exchange for early healing. Small tuft fractures of the underlying terminal phalanx are stable and will be supported by the dressing or nailbed repair.

Occasionally patients will bring amputated pieces of the injured fingertip with them into the ED. This tissue may be useful for harvesting full-thickness skin and must be thoroughly defatted before use. No attempt should ever be made to resuture avascular tissue. If there is any doubt about the viability of fingertip tissue the patient should be referred to a specialized hand service.

Digital nerve injuries

Nerve repairs distal to the distal interphalangeal joint are rarely rewarding. More proximal injuries may be repaired under magnification by an experienced surgeon. Salvage of the digital nerve will depend on the extent of local tissue damage.[3] Good results are achieved with early repair of digital nerves when the ends can be approximated without tension using a fine (>8/0) suture. The return of protective sensation depends on the level of repair and axon regeneration.

Nailbed injuries

These injuries are frequently underestimated, often because of a reluctance to remove the nail. An underlying fracture or growth-plate slip of the terminal phalanx will usually be associated with nailbed disruption. A subungual haematoma larger than 25% of the area of the nail mandates removal of the nail itself. Small painful subungual haematomas can be released using a hot paperclip or trephine burr. Often damage to the nailbed results in spontaneous separation of the nail, preceded by new nail growth which pushes the damaged nail off. Assuming the nail root is intact, a new nail will grow back at a rate of 1 mm per week; thus full growth of a new nail takes approximately 80 days. Removal of the damaged nail is achieved under digital nerve block using blunt dissection with a pair of fine forceps or scissors. The nail should be retained for use as a dressing later. Underlying fractures should be reduced with pressure, and fracture haematoma irrigated away to achieve anatomical approximation of the bone ends. Fractures distal to the insertion of the profundus tendon are stable. Repair of the fragmented nailbed should be performed with fine (6/0 or 7/0) absorbable suture on an atraumatic needle. Care needs to be taken not to cut out with the needle as the nailbed is extremely friable. Haemostasis can be achieved with the prior application of a finger tourniquet or firm pressure. Ideally, the nail is trimmed and reapplied as an organic splint and dressing.

Terminalization

Terminalization of a finger is sometimes necessary when fingertip damage precludes reconstruction. Occupation and leisure activities must be considered before embarking on this course, and informed patient consent obtained. This procedure can be performed under digital nerve/ring block anaesthesia, but requires skill as removal of the nail root and fashioning of the stump are vital for a good cosmetic result.

The terminal phalanx should be nibbled down short enough to allow loose closure. Ideally, the insertion of the profundus tendon into the base of the terminal phalanx should be preserved, but often this needs to be sacrificed to achieve skin closure. Terminal vessels and digital nerves should be cauterized with bipolar diathermy. Loose closure of the skin should be performed with 5/0 or 6/0 non-absorbable monofilament suture, being careful to avoid 'dogears'. The skin flaps must be observed to ensure adequate perfusion. Postoperatively the hand should be elevated and analgesia provided.

Distal interphalangeal joint injuries

Acute flexion injuries of the terminal phalanx may either rupture the extensor tendon at the level of the distal interphalangeal (DIP) joint or avulse its insertion into the terminal phalanx. This produces an acute flexion deformity of the DIP joint, known as a mallet finger. An X-ray of the finger should be taken, as an intra-articular fracture involving more than one-third of the joint surface may require internal fixation. Small avulsion fractures and tendon ruptures are best treated by the application of a correctly fitting mallet splint, which should not be removed for 8 weeks. Persisting mallet finger deformity after treatment or late presentations is often best treated conservatively as the finger is still functional despite the deformity.

Avulsion fractures resulting from hyperextension of the fingertip are unstable owing to the detachment of the profundus tendon and require internal fixation.

Simple dislocations of the distal interphalangeal joint are easily reduced and rarely cause long-term instability. However, prior radiography should be performed to differentiate dislocation from the more complicated intra-articular fractures.

Middle phalangeal injuries

The middle phalanx takes the insertion of the superficialis tendon slips through which passes the profundus tendon. Fracture of the middle phalanx can disrupt the fibrous tunnel of the profundus tendon and cause adhesions. These fractures need to be accurately reduced and may require internal fixation. They are usually unstable owing to the pull of the tendons. Palmar wounds at this level are likely to divide the profundus tendon or digital nerves and should be explored by a specialized hand service if these injuries are suspected on clinical grounds.

Proximal interphalangeal joint injuries

This is the joint that causes most long-term complications, owing to stiffness and joint contracture. The proximal interphalangeal (PIP) joint is mechanically complex and is supported dorsally by the extensor apparatus, whereas on the palmar aspect is the strong fibrous volar plate. Lateral stability is provided by the collateral ligaments. Rupture of either the volar plate or the extensor apparatus will result in joint instability and potential long-term disability. Tears in the extensor apparatus may result from relatively minor trauma. Dislocations of the proximal interphalangeal joint invariably displace both structures. Occasionally, the central slip of the extensor tendon or the volar plate avulses a small fragment from the middle phalanx which will be visible on lateral finger X-ray. Reduction of dislocations should be followed by extension splinting and early follow-up. The boutonnière deformity (flexion of the PIP joint accompanied by hyperextension of the DIP joint) is a hand surgeon's nightmare and ideally should be prevented, as long-term results from reconstructive surgery are poor. These injuries should not be underestimated, and ultrasound can be used to aid in early diagnosis.

Proximal phalangeal injuries

Both flexor tendons pass along the palmar aspect of the proximal phalanx, and therefore fractures of this bone tend to be unstable. Rotational deformity is particularly disabling and may not be noticeable with the finger held straight. These fractures usually require internal fixation. The lateral X-ray will often be the most useful in determining the degree of angulation or displacement. Wounds may damage digital nerves or either or both of the flexor tendons. Examination of the finger should detect these injuries, and referral to a specialized hand service will be required.

Metacarpophalangeal joint injuries

Subluxation of the metacarpophalangeal (MCP) joint may occur in the older patient after relatively minor trauma. The clinical appearances are subtle and the injury is easy to miss on X-ray. The clue is the inability of the finger to extend fully. In recent injuries reduction is achieved by traction on the finger, although once the displacement is established reduction becomes difficult even with open procedures.

MCP joint injuries relating to forced contact between a fist and a tooth are common and should be assumed to be infected. The extensor tendon may be divided and X-ray may show fracture of the metacarpal head. These injuries should be treated aggressively by joint irrigation, splinting and antibiotics.

The ulnar collateral ligament rupture (gamekeeper's or skier's thumb) results from an abduction injury of the thumb and, when complete, results in MCP joint instability. The ligament when completely ruptured may become folded back outside the adductor aponeurosis. X-rays must be taken to identify avulsion fractures of the base of the proximal phalanx. Stress X-ray views will confirm joint instability. Early repair

gives superior results to conservative splinting when complete rupture is diagnosed.

Metacarpal injuries

These injuries are caused by punching, crush injury or falls on to the closed fist. The commonest injury is fracture of the neck of the fifth metacarpal, which is usually best treated conservatively. Correction of significant angulation will only be achieved by open reduction and internal fixation. Spiral fractures of the shaft of a metacarpal will result in shortening of the bone and loss of the contour of the knuckle. Conservative management of these fractures should involve splinting the hand in intrinsic plus (Fig. 4.5.5) with the metacarpophalangeal joint flexed to 70%. The fingers must be splinted straight, with support to the fingertip. Abduction injuries of the thumb may cause a Bennett's fracture, which is an intra-articular fracture of the base of the thumb metacarpal. Bennett fractures, when displaced, should be referred for internal fixation.

Dorsal hand injuries

Wounds on the dorsum of the hand may divide the extensor tendons, which are relatively superficial. Division may be apparent by loss of full extension, but the extensor tendons have extensive cross-insertions, and therefore visualization of the intact tendon throughout its range of movement is the only safe way to exclude damage. Repair of these tendons is relatively straightforward, if there are suitable facilities and equipment.

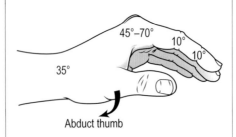

Fig. 4.5.5 Intrinsic plus – recovery position. (Reproduced with permission from American Society for the Surgery of the Hand. The hand, 2nd edn. Boston, MA: Churchill Livingstone, 1990.)

Good exposure of the tendon is required, and haemostasis may be achieved using an ischaemic arm block. Good approximation of the tendon ends is required, using interrupted slowly absorbable sutures. Splinting of the hand in extension will be required for 3 weeks, followed by guarded active flexion. Aftercare must be provided, with access to occupational therapy or physiotherapy during rehabilitation.

Palmar hand injuries

Penetrating wounds on the palm of the hand are likely to divide flexor tendons or main digital nerves. These injuries should be detected by examination. Briskly bleeding wounds proximal to an area of anaesthesia are a clue to digital nerve injury because of coexisting damage to both neurovascular structures. Neurovascular and tendon damage will require referral for specialist repair.

Foreign bodies in the hand can be notoriously difficult to find, and damage to other structures can result from injudicious exploration. The best results are achieved in a bloodless field with full anaesthesia. Nail-gun injuries require an X-ray prior to removal of the nail to establish its location with respect to bone, and to see whether the nail has barbs that will make removal difficult. High-pressure grease- or paint-gun injuries result in extensive tissue penetration and should never be underestimated. Wide exposure and decompression of the tract will require the care of a specialist hand service.

Disposition

Many hand injuries can be well managed in an appropriately equipped ED ambulatory care area. No attempt should be made to operate surgically on a hand without good instruments, adequate lighting and assistance, and fine sutures. After treatment the hand should be elevated in a high arm sling and suitable analgesia provided. Some injuries will require access to a specialized plastic or orthopaedic hand service. When in doubt, early consultation with a specialist hand service is mandatory.

Prognosis

Hand injuries recover best with early definitive treatment, as badly managed injuries can be very difficult to salvage at a later date. Stiffness and loss of function can be avoided if good surgical principles of wound management are adhered to. Appropriate initial splinting and guarded mobilization are the cornerstones of rehabilitation. The injured hand recovers best when splinting has been in a functional position. Whenever possible, the hand should be immobilized with the fingers straight and the MCP joints flexed to 70°. This can be achieved in even the most swollen hand by careful application of a volar plaster slab. Early referral for definitive surgery and subsequent rehabilitation will be essential for severe or complicated injuries. An explanation to the patient of the need to prevent joint stiffness is important when the finger requires dressings for more than 3 weeks.

Prevention

Hand and finger injuries can be prevented. Strategies for prevention involve providing data for public awareness, identifying strategies (e.g. safety equipment, machinery modification) to prevent occupational injuries, and lobbying officials to legislate for sensible measures to prevent injury.

Controversies

- Emergency physicians should keep an open mind to new dressings. There is good evidence that a sterile moist environment for wound healing is beneficial and promotes re-epithelialization. There is no doubt that dressings that adhere to wounds are uncomfortable to remove, damage new epithelial cells, and delay healing.

- Emergency departments have long used sterile solutions to cleanse wounds. There is no evidence that using tap water results in more infected wounds and is cost effective.

- Foreign body removal from the hand can range from being entirely straightforward to being excessively difficult and damaging. A judgement needs to be made on the likely ease of removal and the facilities available. The first attempt is usually the easiest. Wood and glass can be very difficult to find in the tissues without precise localization and a bloodless field.

- To suture or not? Injudicious suture of an acutely injured finger can compromise circulation and confer a secondary injury. Skin closures may be used to bring the skin edges together or, where there is gross swelling, dressings may be used to maintain the anatomy of the finger. The application of a non-adherent dressing may be sufficient or allow secondary closure a few days later.

- Antibiotics have no role in the initial management of hand injuries. The exception to this is the grossly contaminated injury and those known to be caused by bites. Open fractures of the hand bones will need to be admitted for surgical debridement.

References

1. Angermann P, Lohmann M. Injuries to the hand and wrist. Journal of Hand Surgery 1993; 18B(5): 642–644.
2. de Boer P, Collinson PO. The use of silver sulphadiazine occlusive dressings for fingertip injuries. Journal of Bone and Joint Surgery 1981; 63B(4): 545–547.
3. Jabaley M. Technical aspects of peripheral nerve repair. Journal of Hand Surgery 1984; 9: 9–14.

Further reading

American Society for the Surgery of the Hand. The Hand – primary care of common conditions, 2nd edn. Boston, MA: Churchill Livingstone, 1990.
Atasoy E, Ioakimidis E, Kasdan ML, et al. Reconstruction of the amputated finger tip with a triangular volar flap. Journal of Bone and Joint Surgery 1970; 52A: 921–926.
Hart RG, Kleinert HE. The hand in emergency medicine. Emergency Medicine Clinics of North America 1993; 11: 755–756.
Quinn J, Cummings S, Callaham M, Sellers K. Suturing versus conservative management of lacerations of the hand (RCT). British Medical Journal 2002; 325: 299–300.
Stewart C. Hand injuries. Emergency Medicine Reports 1997; 18: 223–234.

4.6 Pelvic injuries

Michael Cadogan

ESSENTIALS

1 Pelvic fractures constitute 3% of skeletal fractures.

2 Understanding the mechanism of injury and observing the pelvic fracture pattern on X-ray provides insight into the potential for complications such as associated neurovascular or urogenital injuries.

3 Fractures are either stable or unstable. Unstable fractures are associated with considerable mechanical forces and result in concomitant injuries, with a significant overall mortality.

4 Isolated stable pelvic fractures are usually treated conservatively.

Anatomy

The pelvic ring is formed by the two innominate bones and the sacrum. The innominate bones are made up of the ileum, ischium and pubis, and are joined anteriorly at the symphysis pubis and posteriorly at the left and right sacroiliac joints.

The lateral surface of the innominate bone forms a socket, the acetabulum, contributed to by the ileum, ischium and pubis. Stability of the pelvic ring is dependent on the strong posterior sacroiliac, sacrotuberous and sacrospinous ligaments. Disruption of the ring can result in significant trauma to the neurovascular and soft tissue structures it protects.

Classification of pelvic fractures

Pelvic fractures may be open or closed, major or minor, stable or unstable depending on the degree of ring disruption, and may be associated with haemodynamic compromise and/or hollow viscus injury.

The Young and Resnik classification outlined in Chapter 3.8 classifies pelvic fractures by the mechanism of injury and the direction of the causative force. It does not include isolated fractures outside the bony pelvic ring, or acetabular fractures, which are discussed later in this chapter.

Young and Resnik pelvic fracture classification

Most pelvic fractures result from lateral compression, anteroposterior compression or vertical shear forces. These injuries may be suggested by the history and are confirmed radiographically.

Lateral compression injuries

Lateral compression accounts for 50% of pelvic fractures and commonly occurs when a pedestrian or motor vehicle occupant is struck from the side. Most of these injuries are stable, but as a result of the considerable forces involved there is a high potential for associated injuries. This mechanism of injury can produce several fracture patterns involving anterior and posterior pathology.

Anteriorly there is always a transverse fracture of at least one set of pubic rami. These fractures can be unilateral or bilateral, and may include disruption of the pubic symphysis. The posterior element of lateral compression fractures is important, but may be overlooked by the emergency physician concentrating on the anterior findings. However, it is critical in determining the functional stability of the pelvic ring and defining associated injuries.

Type 1 fractures Type 1 fractures are the most common, and involve a compression injury to the sacrum posteriorly and oblique pubic rami fractures anteriorly.

These injuries occur on the side of impact and are usually stable, involving impaction of the cancellous bone of the sacrum without ligamentous disruption. X-rays confirm discontinuity of the sacral foramina posteriorly.

Type 2 fractures Type 2 fractures result from greater lateral compressive forces. The iliac wing is fractured posteriorly, with the fracture line often extending to involve part of the sacroiliac joint. This leaves part of the ileum firmly attached to the sacrum. Anteriorly there are associated fractures of the pubic rami. Stability is determined by the degree of sacroiliac joint disruption, and mobility of the anterior hemi-pelvis involved. These fractures are usually stable to external rotation and vertical movement, but are more mobile to internal rotation.

Type 3 fractures Type 3 fractures usually occur when one hemi-pelvis is trapped against the ground and a lateral force rolls over the mobile hemi-pelvis. This produces a lateral compression injury to the side of primary impact and an unstable anteroposterior compressive injury to the contralateral sacroiliac joint.

Anteroposterior compression injuries

Anteroposterior compression injuries of the pelvis account for 25% of pelvic fractures. They result from anterior forces applied directly to the pelvis or indirectly via the lower extremities to produce an open-book type injury.

Type 1 injuries Type 1 injuries result from low-energy forces that stretch the ligamentous constraints of the pelvic ring. The pubic symphysis is disrupted anteriorly, but with less than 2.5 cm diastasis observed radiographically. These fractures are stable and there is usually no significant posterior pelvic injury.

Type 2 injuries Type 2 injuries classically cause an open-book fracture. They involve rupture of the anterior sacroiliac, sacrospinous and sacrotuberous ligaments posteriorly and disruption of the pubic symphysis anteriorly. There is widening of the anterior sacroiliac joint with diastasis of the pubic symphysis by more than 2.5 cm on radiology, and occasionally avulsion of the lateral border of the lower sacral segments. Considerable force is involved to disrupt these ligaments, and neurovascular injuries and complications are common. The pelvis is unstable to external rotation, and external compression will 'spring' the pelvis.

Type 3 injuries Type 3 injuries occur when an even greater force is applied and involve disruption of all the pelvic ligaments on the affected side. Rupture of the posterior sacroiliac ligaments leads to lateral displacement and disconnection of the affected hemi-pelvis from the sacrum. They are completely unstable and are associated with the highest rate of neurovascular injury and haemorrhage (see Fig. 4.6.1).

Vertical shear injuries (Malgaigne fracture)

These injuries account for only 5% of pelvic fractures. They usually occur following a fall from a height or during a motor vehicle accident when the victim reflexly extends their leg against the brake pedal before impact. These mechanisms force the hemi-pelvis in a vertical direction and result in complete ligamentous or bony disruption, with cephaloposterior hemi-pelvis displacement.

Anterior disruption occurs through the pubic symphysis or pubic rami. Posteriorly, dissociation usually occurs through the sacroiliac joint, but may occur vertically through the sacrum. These fractures are usually unilateral, but may be bilateral and may be associated with significant intra-abdominal injury.

Clinical assessment

It is essential that a standard trauma management protocol is adhered to in the multitrauma patient, with attention being paid initially to the airway, breathing and circulation (ABCs) in the primary survey and resuscitation phases of care.

General examination

The back is examined to assess for injury to the lumbar spine, sacroiliac regions and coccyx. Abdominal, rectal, vaginal and perineal examinations are required. The rectal examination includes observation for fresh blood, assessment of anal sphincter tone, and the position and tenderness of the prostate. A thorough neurovascular examination must be performed.

The pelvis is examined during the secondary survey phase. The suprapubic, pelvic and urogenital regions are examined for signs of bruising, abrasions, open wounds and obvious deformity. In males the urethral meatus is inspected for the presence of frank blood and the scrotum for bruising. Flank bruising may indicate retroperitoneal haemorrhage.

Palpation of the pelvic ring

Palpation of the pelvis commences at the anterior superior iliac spines. Evidence of internal rotation is assessed by compressing the spines towards each other, and external rotation is tested by pulling both the spines outwards. The pelvic compression test does not always correlate with the significance of the injury, and in the haemodynamically unstable patient this examination should only be performed once, to avoid exacerbating haemorrhage by dislodging any clots.

Radiology

The AP pelvic X-ray will usually reveal anterior fractures, although posterior fractures are often difficult to visualize. Further plain X-rays or a CT scan may be warranted.

Injuries associated with pelvic fractures

Haemorrhage

Haemorrhage is the most significant complication of pelvic fractures. It may result from bleeding at fracture sites, local venous or arterial tears, and disruption of major vessels. Catastrophic bleeding may result from disruption of the internal iliac arteries, their tributaries and accompanying veins as they pass over the anterior aspect of the sacroiliac joint.

Severe hypovolaemia due to persistent haemorrhage without major vessel disruption is a significant cause of mortality. Up to 4 L of blood can be lost into the retroperitoneal space before tamponade occurs. Anteroposterior type 3 injuries and vertical shear injuries disrupt the sacroiliac joint and are associated with significant haemorrhage.

Treatment to minimize or stop the haemorrhage associated with pelvic fractures requires urgent interventional radiology with angiography and embolization, external fixation, and/or open reduction with internal fixation. A multidisciplinary team approach is essential.

Genitourinary and bladder injuries

Pelvic fractures are associated with injury to the lower urinary tract in up to 16% of cases. They are more prevalent in males, who sustain a much higher rate of urethral

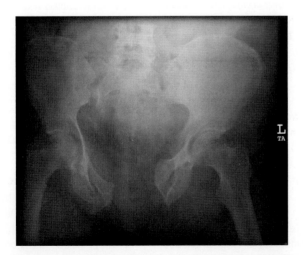

Fig. 4.6.1 'Open-book' pelvic fracture, with pubic symphysis diastasis and sacroiliac disruption, following an anteroposterior compression injury.

ORTHOPAEDIC EMERGENCIES

injury. Pelvic trauma may also result in bladder rupture. The bladder is normally protected by the pelvis, and rupture usually indicates significant disruption of the pelvic ring.

Almost 90% of blunt trauma patients with bladder rupture have an associated pelvic fracture. Patients are usually hypotensive with frank haematuria, although gross haematuria is a non-specific sign of genitourinary trauma, and is not necessarily indicative of bladder rupture. Therefore, a retrograde urethrogram is performed to delineate any urethral trauma prior to performing retrograde cystography.

Urethral and genital injuries

Urethral rupture is rare in females. Rupture of the urethra secondary to blunt trauma commonly occurs in the anterior bulbous urethra just distal to the urogenital diaphragm. It is associated with bilateral fractures of the pubic rami, pubic symphysis disruption and vertical shear injuries.

Suspect a urethral rupture in the adult male with a pelvic fracture, blood at the urethral meatus, a high-riding prostate, perineal haematoma and urinary retention. However, not all these 'classic' signs may be present. A retrograde urethrogram is diagnostic, and must be performed prior to urethral (Foley) catheterization when indicated clinically.

Injury to the female genitalia is uncommon but often overlooked. Vaginal lacerations are associated with pelvic fractures in 4% of cases. They normally present with bleeding, but may be occult. A bimanual pelvic examination is necessary in women with a pelvic fracture. This may necessitate anaesthesia because of patient discomfort. Complications such as abscess formation and sepsis can be severe.

Management of unstable pelvic fracture

The mainstay of pelvic fracture management in the ED is to identify and assess the degree of pelvic injury, provide adequate fluid resuscitation to minimize life-threatening haemorrhage, and provide pain relief. Early identification of the potential for major pelvic trauma with mobilization of general surgical, orthopaedic, vascular,

interventional radiology and intensive care specialists is essential.

Fluid resuscitation

Start fluid resuscitation with intravenous crystalloid in the hypotensive patient with pelvic trauma using two large-bore peripheral intravenous cannulae. Include blood products if the patient remains hypotensive despite intravenous fluids. The average blood transfusion requirement for anteroposterior compression fractures is 15 units, for vertical shear injuries is 9 units, and for lateral compression injuries is 3.5 units.

Pelvic immobilization

Pelvic sling or sheet

Immobilization of the pelvis with attempted reapproximation of the bony fragments creates a tamponade effect that reduces the risk of continuing haemorrhage prior to definitive treatment. This may be achieved initially by simply bracing the pelvis in a sheet and supporting it laterally with sandbags. Alternatively, use a proprietary radiolucent pelvic sling device with a pulley mechanism to effectively apply compression pressure.

Pneumatic anti-shock garment

The efficacy of the pneumatic anti-shock garment (PASG) in the ED is unproven, but they may still be used in the pre-hospital setting to provide stabilization and immobilization during transport. The PASG reduces haemorrhage from anteroposterior compression fractures, but conversely may increase fracture displacement with lateral compression injuries. Other complications of their use include catastrophic hypotension on sudden injudicious removal, compartment syndrome, and reduced access to the lower limbs.

External fixation

External fixation is a rapid and simple procedure designed to stabilize and immobilize the pelvis in the ED to reduce pelvic haemorrhage prior to definitive treatment. Three pins are placed through each iliac crest and then clamped to an external frame to reduce the displaced pelvic ring injury. The advantages of external fixation are that it is quick, effective, and can proceed in the ED without delaying the

continued management of the multiply injured patient. The disadvantages include the lack of support for the posterior component of the pelvic ring fracture, difficulty of placement in the obese patient, and reduced pelvic surgical access in the event of laparotomy being required.

Embolization

Life-threatening arterial haemorrhage is estimated to occur in 5–20% of patients with blunt pelvic fracture. Emergency angiography is both diagnostic and therapeutic to control primary haemorrhage. Early recognition of this subset of patients, organizing transfer to a hospital with angiography capabilities and mobilizing an interventional radiologist, reduces mortality but is logistically challenging. The procedure is operator dependent, time-consuming, and does not address venous blood loss, which still requires appropriate replacement of blood and blood products.

Open pelvic fractures

Open pelvic fractures are rare and associated with increased morbidity and mortality. Open fractures with pelvic ring disruption lose any tamponade effect by virtue of an enclosed space and can result in massive and fatal haemorrhage.

Management

Control of haemorrhage is a priority in open pelvic injury, with attempts to avoid early infection. Sterile gauze packed into the wounds applies a direct pressure tamponade. Urgent operation to repair associated open bowel and bladder injuries and to debride bleeding wounds is paramount, with stabilization of the pelvic fracture as the last step in treatment.

Stable fractures of the pelvis

Isolated avulsion fractures

These are often sustained by young adults following acute stress to the muscular and ligamentous insertions onto the bony pelvis. They include anterior superior iliac spine fracture, anterior inferior iliac spine fracture and ischial tuberosity fracture.

Anterior superior iliac spine fracture
The anterior superior iliac spine may be fractured in jumping activities due to powerful contraction of the sartorius muscle. Such injuries cause pain on weightbearing, with local tenderness and swelling at the fracture site. Active flexion and abduction of the thigh reproduces the pain. There is usually minimal displacement of the avulsed fracture on the AP film of the pelvis.

Anterior inferior iliac spine fracture
Forceful contraction of the rectus femoris muscle in sports that involve kicking may avulse the anterior inferior iliac spine. These patients complain of a sharp pain in the groin and are unable to actively flex the hip. The fracture is usually evident on plain AP pelvic views, with the fragment being displaced distally.

Ischial tuberosity fracture
Fracture of the ischial tuberosity is rare and occurs with forceful contraction of the hamstrings, usually in young adults whose apophyses are not fully united. They are associated with hurdling and other jumping activities. Pain may be reproduced by local palpation and by active flexion of the hip with the knee extended. Plain X-rays of the pelvis reveal minimal displacement of the apophysis from the ischium.

Isolated pubic ramus fractures
These injuries are commonly seen in the elderly with direct trauma following a fall. The patient has difficulty in weightbearing, and local pain and tenderness in the groin. They should be carefully looked for in any patient unable to bear weight with a suspected hip fracture, when X-ray of the hip is normal.

Pain is usually reproduced with the FABER test. The ipsilateral foot is placed on the contralateral knee, forcing the ipsilateral hip to be Flexed, ABducted and Externally Rotated, causing typical pain to exacerbate. Pelvic radiographs confirm non-displaced isolated fractures of the pubic rami.

Iliac wing fracture (Duverney fracture)
Direct lateral trauma may result in an isolated iliac wing fracture. Patients complain of severe pain on weightbearing and walk with a waddling gait. Localized tenderness and bruising occur over the site of injury, associated with abdominal guarding, ileus, and lower quadrant tenderness. These fractures are usually minimally displaced, rarely comminuted, and are easily visualized on AP pelvic X-rays.

Coccyx fractures
These fractures are more frequent in women and are caused by a falls onto the buttocks with both hips flexed. Patients have difficulty in mobilizing and have local pain, swelling, bruising and tenderness over the lower sacral region. Radiographic confirmation is unnecessary if physical examination confirms an isolated injury.

Management of isolated stable fractures
Avulsion fractures, pubic ramus fractures and iliac wing fractures are treated conservatively with non-steroidal anti-inflammatory drugs (NSAIDs) and non-weightbearing crutches for 10 days. Slow mobilization and physiotherapy allow resumption of normal activities in 3–4 weeks. Coccygeal fractures require rest, analgesia and stool softeners. Sitting is painful, and a doughnut-ring foam cushion is helpful.

Acetabular fractures
Acetabular fractures account for 20% of pelvic fractures and are usually associated with lateral compression forces. They also occur with posterior forces applied distally through the femur. Their classification is complex.

Clinical features
Acetabular fractures are caused by direct impaction of the femoral head that may be associated with a central hip dislocation. These fractures are associated with sciatic and femoral nerve injury, depending on the position of the hip dislocation. A thorough neurovascular examination is mandatory. In addition, these fractures are often associated with other pelvic injuries, knee injury, hip fractures and dislocations, which should all be looked for separately.

Management
Standard radiographs of the hip and pelvis are useful in defining the fracture, but a CT scan is essential to show the anterior and posterior fragments and the involvement of ilioischial and iliopubic columns. All fractures should be referred for inpatient orthopaedic management.

Controversies
- Optimal multidisciplinary management in the emergency department of the hypotensive pelvic trauma patient; who to call and when; and who takes charge.
- The role of external pelvic fixation devices in the emergency department.
- The optimum timing of embolization to control primary haemorrhage.

Further reading
Blackmore CC, Cummings P, Jurkovich G, et al. Predicting major hemorrhage in patients with pelvic fracture. Journal of Trauma 2006; 61: 346–352.
Burgess AR, Eastridge BJ, Young JW, et al. Pelvic ring disruptions: effective classification system and treatment protocols. Journal of Trauma 1990; 30: 848–856.
Dalal SA, Burgess AR, Siegel JH, et al. Pelvic fracture in multiple trauma: classification by mechanism is key to pattern of organ injury, resuscitative requirements, and outcome. Journal of Trauma 1989; 29: 981–1002.
Fallon B, Wendt JC, Hawtrey CE. Urological injury and assessment in patients with fractured pelvis. Journal of Urology 1984; 131: 712–714.
Gokcen EC, Burgess AR, Siegel JH, et al. Pelvic fracture mechanism of injury in vehicular trauma patients. Journal of Trauma 1994; 36: 789–796.
Kellam JF. The role of external fixation in pelvic disruptions. Clinical Orthopaedics and Related Research 1989; 241: 66–82.
Mattox KL, Bickell W, Pepe PE, Mangelsdorff AD. Prospective randomized evaluation of antishock MAST in post-traumatic hypotension. Journal of Trauma 1986; 26: 779–786.
Pennal GF, Tile M, Waddell JP et al. Pelvic disruption: assessment and classification. Clinical Orthopaedics and Related Research 1980 151: 12–21.
Rothenberger DA, Velasco R, Strate R, et al. Open pelvic fracture: a lethal injury. Journal of Trauma 1978 18: 184–187.
Sarin EL, Moore J, Moore E, et al. Pelvic fracture pattern does not always predict the need for urgent embolization. Journal of Trauma 2005; 58: 973–977.

4.7 Hip injuries

Michael Cadogan

ESSENTIALS

1 Trauma to the hip is a major cause of morbidity and mortality, with a huge impact on healthcare and resources.

2 Hip injuries are frequently a pathological disease of the elderly. However, there has been an increased incidence of hip fractures and dislocations in young people sustaining high-energy trauma.

3 Avascular necrosis of the femoral head is a complication of intracapsular femoral neck fractures.

4 Extracapsular neck of femur fractures are associated with significant haemorrhage.

5 The hip joint is least stable when flexed and adducted and prone to dislocation. Posterior hip dislocations are an orthopaedic emergency as they are associated with sciatic nerve injury and avascular necrosis.

6 Anterior hip dislocations are associated with femoral neurovascular injury and occult hip joint fractures.

Anatomy

The hip joint is a large ball and socket articulation encompassing the acetabulum and proximal femur. The hip joint provides a high degree of stability and mobility.

Blood supply

The head and intracapsular portion of the femoral neck receive the majority of their blood supply from the extracapsular arterial ring, the trochanteric anastomosis, with a minor supply arising from the obturator artery via the ligamentum teres, known as the foveal artery. Retinacular arteries from the extracapsular ring pass under the reflection of the hip capsule to supply the femoral neck and head in a retrograde manner. Intracapsular fractures disrupt this 'distal to proximal flow' and so may result in avascular necrosis of the femoral head.

Avascular necrosis (AVN)

Avascular necrosis in the context of hip injuries refers to ischaemic bone death within the femoral head following compromise to its blood supply. Increased bone density of the femoral head is the radiographic feature of AVN, but may take up to 6 months to become manifest.

AVN results primarily from the disruption of the trochanteric anastomosis in femoral neck fractures, and is the commonest early complication of these fractures.

Traumatic haemarthrosis, with or without a fracture, may result in intracapsular tamponade. AVN can occur if the intracapsular pressure exceeds the diastolic blood pressure.

The risk of AVN with posterior dislocations is related to the degree of trauma and the length of time the femoral head is out of the joint. Early management is an orthopaedic emergency.

Chronic pancreatitis, alcohol abuse, sickle cell anaemia, vasculitis, irradiation, decompression illness (DCI) and the prolonged use of corticosteroids may also result in AVN.

Classification of hip fractures

Hip fractures are either intracapsular or extracapsular. Intracapsular fractures involve the femoral neck or head. Extracapsular fractures include intertrochanteric, trochanteric and subtrochanteric types, and are four times more common than intracapsular fractures.

The incidence of hip fractures increases exponentially with age, as the fracture rate doubles for every decade over 50 years. Hip fractures occur most frequently in white postmenopausal women, as 50% of 65-year-old women, and 100% of women over the age of 85, have a bone mineral content below fracture threshold level.

Intracapsular fractures

Femoral head

Femoral head fractures are uncommon and are usually associated with dislocations of the hip. They often occur in young patients, 75% of cases being associated with motor vehicle accidents.

Classification Fractures of the superior aspect of the femoral head are usually associated with anterior dislocations, whereas inferior femoral head fractures occur with posterior dislocations. Fractures may involve a single fragment (type 1) or comminution (type 2).

Clinical evaluation The symptoms and signs of femoral head injuries are usually those of the associated dislocation rather than the fracture itself. Femoral head fractures are not always picked up on initial X-rays. In the absence of abnormality on plain radiographs further radiological imaging with CT should be performed in the presence of persistent pain following reduction of a hip dislocation.

Management Orthopaedic consultation is essential as prompt reduction of the dislocation and appropriate stabilization of the fracture reduce the risk of AVN, increasing the chances of a full return of mobility. The prognosis is related to the severity of the initial trauma, time to definitive reduction, and the number of failed closed relocation attempts.

Complications AVN occurs in 15–20% of cases, post-traumatic arthritis in 40%, and myositis ossificans in 2%.

Femoral neck fractures

Intracapsular fractures are four times more common in females than males. There are four main causes of this type of injury:

- Elderly, with minimal trauma following a fall onto the greater trochanter (pathological fracture).
- Elderly, with torsion or twisting injury prior to fall (pathological fracture).
- Young persons involved in high-energy trauma (excessive loading).
- Repetitive stress or cyclical loading injuries (stress fracture).

Classification The Garden classification system is commonly used to describe intracapsular neck of femur fractures.

Garden I Incomplete, impacted or stress fractures that are stable. Trabeculae of the inferior neck are still intact and, although they may be angulated, they are still congruous.

Garden II Undisplaced fracture across the entire femoral neck. The weightbearing trabeculae are interrupted, without displacement. These fractures are inherently unstable and must be fixed.

Garden III Complete femoral neck fracture with partial displacement. There is associated rotation of the femoral head, with non-congruity of the head and acetabular trabeculae.

Garden IV Complete subcapital fracture with total displacement of fracture fragments. There is no congruity between proximal and distal fragments, but the femoral head maintains a normal relationship with the acetabulum.

These fractures may be further simplified into non-displaced (Garden I and II) and displaced (Garden III and IV).

Clinical assessment and management

Non-displaced fractures Non-displaced fractures include stress fractures, Garden I and Garden II fractures. Stress fractures are usually the result of repetitive abnormal forces on normal bone in fit, active young people such as military recruits or marathon runners, but may occur with repetitive normal stresses on abnormal bones, such as in rheumatoid arthritis or patients taking long-term steroids.

They present with pain that is gradual in onset and worse after activity, radiating from the groin to the medial aspect of the knee. Patients walk with a limp and often present late. Physical examination reveals no obvious deformity, although there is mild discomfort on passive movement at the extremities of motion and percussion tenderness over the greater trochanter.

Additional radiological examination with a bone scan and/or MRI is indicated when initial X-rays are normal but there is persistent pain. MRI is the investigation of choice, being more sensitive than bone scans in the first 24 hours, but is of similar accuracy to bone scans in fracture assessment at 72 hours.

Stress fractures and Garden I impacted fractures are considered stable and may be treated conservatively under close orthopaedic supervision. Garden II fractures, although non-displaced, are inherently unstable and must be fixed internally.

Displaced fractures Elderly patients with displaced fractures usually present with pain in the hip area and markedly reduced hip movement. The lower limb is shortened, abducted and externally rotated distal to the fracture, albeit less than with intertrochanteric fractures. X-ray reveals the fracture and the degree of posterior comminution of the proximal fragment. Systemic analgesia and a femoral nerve block reduce discomfort. Skin traction will also reduce pain and helps preserve femoral head vascularity.

Traumatic femoral neck fractures in the young adult are uncommon and usually involve normal bone. These fractures are outside of the Garden classification. They follow a large degree of force and have up to a 35% risk of AVN and up to a 57% risk of non-union.

Complications

Mortality Femoral neck fractures are associated with a mortality of 14–36% in the first year after injury, the rate returning to the pre-fracture level after this. Mortality is increased threefold in those who were institutionalized prior to the fracture, with risk factors of male gender, increased age, malnutrition, multiple medical problems and end-stage renal failure also increasing the mortality.

Morbidity AVN is the most common complication despite optimal treatment. Non-union, postoperative infection and osteomyelitis are also common.

Extracapsular femur fractures

Intertrochanteric femur fractures

Fractures of the proximal femur that occur along a line between the greater and lesser trochanters are referred to as intertrochanteric. They are usually pathological, occur in the elderly, and have a female preponderance.

Mechanism A simple fall with a direct force applied to the greater trochanter in the elderly is enough to cause an intertrochanteric femoral fracture. In young adults they are associated with high-speed motor vehicle accidents or falls from a height.

Clinical assessment Patients sustaining an intertrochanteric fracture are unable to bear weight and have significant pain on hip movement. There is often a large haematoma overlying the greater trochanter, owing to the highly vascular bone that has been fractured without any intracapsular containment. Examination reveals a markedly shortened, abducted, significantly externally rotated lower limb.

X-ray confirms the fracture in most cases. However, internal rotation of the hip on the AP view prevents rotation of the greater trochanter, which may obscure the fracture. The lateral view depicts the size, location and degree of comminution of the fracture fragments and determines stability.

Classification Numerous classification systems are available for intertrochanteric fractures, the simplest of which is by Evans. This divides intertrochanteric fractures into stable and unstable. However, for the emergency physician an anatomical description of the fracture detailing the degree of comminution, subtrochanteric extension and the presence of displaced posterior fragments is adequate (Fig. 4.7.1).

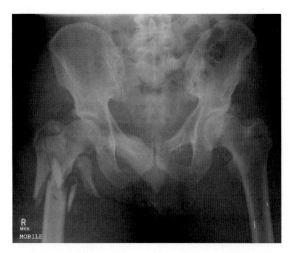

Fig. 4.7.1 Unstable comminuted intertrochanteric fracture with subtrochanteric extension.

Management A complete evaluation is essential to formulate an early treatment plan, as intertrochanteric fractures occur most frequently in the elderly. Patients may lose up to 1.5 L of blood from comminuted fractures and are often dehydrated, malnourished and in significant pain on arrival in the emergency department (ED). Systemic analgesia and fluid resuscitation are important in preparation for theatre.

Skin traction or immobilization with sandbags prevents further soft tissue damage and bony comminution, and reduces blood loss. Full preoperative evaluation requires a search for associated injuries such as rib fractures, distal radial fractures and vertebral compression fractures at the level of T12 and L1.

An ECG, bloods, and chest X-ray help to elucidate the cause of the fall and may indicate the need for associated medical treatment.

Treatment aims to return the patient to their pre-fracture status. Open reduction with internal fixation (ORIF) produces better anatomical alignment, a shorter hospital stay, and improved function with reduced mortality than does conservative management.

Complications Survival is directly related to the patient's age and pre-existing medical factors.

Greater trochanteric fracture

Mechanism Isolated fractures of the greater trochanter are uncommon. They usually occur between 7 and 17 years of age and involve true epiphyseal separation secondary to indirect trauma. Forceful muscular contraction by the gluteus medius causes avulsion of the apophysis. The displaced, non-comminuted fragment may be separated by up to 6 cm.

Greater trochanteric fractures in adults are rare and usually result from direct trauma, causing a comminuted fracture whose fragments are rarely displaced and usually involve only part of the trochanter.

Clinical assessment Patients with a greater trochanter injury are tender to palpation over the area of avulsion or comminution, but bruising is uncommon. There is often an associated flexion deformity of the hip as a result of pain and muscle spasm, and weightbearing produces a limp.

Management The prognosis after these fractures is good. Most are treated with bed rest for 3 days, followed by non-weightbearing crutches for 4 weeks. Open reduction and internal fixation are needed when there is marked separation of the bony fragment.

Lesser trochanteric fracture

Isolated fractures of the lesser trochanter usually occur in children and young athletes, with 85% occurring before the age of 20.

Mechanism Lesser trochanter fractures are usually an apophyseal avulsion secondary to the forceful contraction of iliopsoas.

Clinical assessment Patients complain of pain on flexion and internal rotation of the hip. Examination reveals tenderness in the femoral triangle. The patient is unable to flex the hip and raise the foot off the ground in a seated position (Ludloff sign).

Radiology is often inconclusive, as there may not be complete separation of the bony fragment and comparison views may be required.

Management Ten days of bed rest and slow mobilization result in a full recovery. Open reduction and internal fixation are not indicated, even with wide apophyseal separation.

Subtrochanteric femoral fractures

The subtrochanteric region of the femur lies between the lesser trochanter and a point 5 cm distally. Fractures in this region are termed subtrochanteric. They account for 11% of hip fractures and occur in the elderly with osteoporosis, bone metastases or end-stage renal failure. High-energy injuries in young adults with normal bone are less common.

Mechanism Ninety per cent of these fractures are as a result of blunt trauma, either from a simple fall in the elderly or following a high-speed MVA or fall from a height in young adults. In the USA up to 10% are due to high-energy gunshot wounds.

Classification A variety of classification systems are available, but none is widely used. As with intertrochanteric fractures, it is best to describe the location, presence of comminution and the position of the lesser trochanter proximal or distal to the fracture line.

Clinical assessment In the elderly subtrochanteric fractures are usually isolated. However, as substantial force is required, in young adults the presence of other injuries must be actively sought. The limb distal to the fracture is usually held in abduction, flexion and external rotation. Haemorrhage from a comminuted subtrochanteric fracture may be up to 2 L. Assess the patient's circulatory status and commence fluid resuscitation to prevent hypovolaemic shock.

Management The affected limb should be immobilized in a splint following parenteral analgesia. Suitable splints include proprietary splints such as the Donway or Hare, and fluid resuscitation started as required. The older, more laborious Thomas splint is rarely now used. Orthopaedic referral is necessary for open reduction and internal fixation of these fractures.

Complications There is up to a 20% mortality associated with these fractures in the first year, mainly in the elderly. Subtrochanteric bone is cortical, unlike the cancellous bone involved in intertrochanteric fractures, therefore these fractures often lack the vascularity for adequate new bone growth and repair. They are associated with a higher rate of non-union and implant failure. The further down the shaft of femur the fracture line is located, the greater the degree of non-union and implant failure.

Hip dislocation

The hip joint is inherently stable and considerable force is required to produce a dislocation. Associated injuries must always be sought.

Hip dislocations are classified anatomically into anterior and posterior, depending on the final position of the femoral head relative to the acetabular rim.

Non-prosthetic hip dislocations are an orthopaedic emergency, as the femoral head's blood supply is precarious, and also because of the proximity of the sciatic nerve. Failure to reduce a hip dislocation within 6 hours dramatically increases the risk of AVN and sciatic nerve ischaemia.

Posterior dislocation

Mechanism
Posterior dislocations represent 85–90% of traumatic hip dislocations. Classically, a direct distal force applied to the flexed knee, with the hip in varying degrees of flexion, causes a posterior dislocation of the hip, as when seated in the front of a car. The hip and knee are usually flexed to 90° and the hip adducted, which is the least stable position for the hip to be in. The force applied by the dashboard in a head-on collision to a seated individual may produce a simple posterior dislocation. The abducted and partially flexed hip in the same scenario is more stable, and if the force of impact is great enough will result in a posterior dislocation with displaced acetabular fracture.

Clinical assessment
Examination of the affected limb will reveal shortening, adduction, internal rotation and some degree of flexion. A single AP pelvis radiograph is usually adequate to confirm a posterior dislocation. However, as up to half of these dislocations are associated with an acetabular, femoral head or femur fracture, further radiological imaging is essential. Judet views, AP hip with internal rotation and AP and lateral femoral views will reveal these associated fractures.

Neurological examination is important in posterior dislocations, particularly with marked internal rotation, which may compress the sciatic nerve and its branches. This results in neurological deficits, particularly in the peroneal nerve distribution. Associated injuries such as ipsilateral knee ligament disruption with a posterior cruciate rupture must be looked for at the same time.

Management
The orthopaedic team should be consulted early. A thorough search for associated periarticular and distal limb injuries, neurological evaluation and adequate imaging are essential in the ED.

Closed reduction
Closed reduction of posterior hip dislocations may be performed in the ED under procedural sedation, unless there is immediate access to an operating theatre (see Chapter 22.3).

There are numerous methods of relocation, many requiring significant physical strength. The most common is the Allis manoeuvre, whereby the patient lies supine with assistants on either side stabilizing the pelvis with downward pressure on anterior superior iliac spines. The operator forcefully distracts the lower leg with the hip and knee in 90° of flexion. Other techniques include the lateral traction–countertraction method and the Whistler technique.

Complications
The risk of developing AVN is directly proportional to the length of time the hip remains dislocated, and increases dramatically if the dislocation is not reduced within 6 hours of injury. Sciatic nerve neuropraxia may occur in 15% of cases but is usually relieved by reduction. Permanent ischaemic changes with neurological deficit secondary to pressure necrosis have been reported in up to 3% of cases, usually in the peroneal nerve distribution. Missed knee injuries occur in up to 15% of cases, as well as patellar, tibial plateau and posterior cruciate injuries.

Anterior dislocation
Anterior dislocations account for 10–15% of traumatic hip dislocations, and are associated with femoral neurovascular injury and occult hip joint fractures. They usually result from a direct blow to the abducted and externally rotated hip. When the hip is in abduction, the femoral neck or greater trochanter impinges on the rim of the acetabulum. A direct force applied distally can lever the head out of the acetabulum and tear the anterior capsule of the hip.

Classification
Anterior dislocations may be superior or inferior. Type I or superior dislocations occur when the hip is extended at the time of injury. These are also known as iliac dislocations. Type II or inferior dislocations occur when the hip is flexed at the time of injury, and are also known as obturator dislocations. They may be further subclassified as simple dislocation, associated femoral neck fracture, or associated acetabular fracture.

Clinical assessment
The superior type of injury causes an extended, externally rotated and slightly abducted distal limb. The distal limb in the inferior type of dislocation is externally rotated, abducted, and in flexion. The femoral head may be palpated around the anterior superior iliac spine in superior types and in the obturator foramen in inferior types.

A neurovascular examination is essential in anterior dislocations, particularly the superior type, where trauma to the femoral artery, vein and nerve is common. Hip and pelvis radiographs must be studied carefully for associated fractures of the acetabulum and femoral head. Further imaging with CT is indicated for persistent post-reduction pain.

ORTHOPAEDIC EMERGENCIES

4

Management

A thorough general examination looking for associated life-threatening injuries is essential, as these injuries are usually associated with high-energy trauma. Orthopaedic consultation is mandatory because of the high probability of vascular injury and the need for closed reduction under general anaesthesia.

Complications

Early complications in superior dislocations result from direct pressure on the femoral vessels, with the potential for distal neurovascular compromise. Late complications include post-traumatic arthritis and AVN. Recurrent dislocation is common when anterior capsular healing is incomplete following inadequate immobilization after reduction.

Controversies

- The efficacy of applying skin traction and immobilization to reduce extracapsular femoral fractures in the emergency department.

- The early use of CT and MRI to evaluate the reduced non-prosthetic hip may reduce (missed) associated morbidity.

- Whether the hip reduction should take place in the emergency department or in the operating theatre, as it is essential to treat hip dislocations early.

Further reading

Dahners LE, Hundley JD. Reduction of posterior hip dislocations in the lateral position using traction–countertraction: safer for the surgeon? Journal of Orthopaedic Trauma 1999; 13: 373–374.

Garden RS. The structure and function of the proximal end of the femur. Journal of Bone and Joint Surgery 1961; 43B: 576–589.

Hirasawa Y, Oda R, Nakatani K. Sciatic nerve paralysis in posterior dislocation of the hip. Clinical Orthopedics 1977; 126: 172–175.

Holmberg S, Conradi P, Kalen R, Thorgren KG. Mortality after cervical hip fracture: three thousand two patients followed for six years. Acta Orthopaedica Scandinavica 1986; 57: 8–11.

Jazayeri M. Posterior fracture dislocations of the hip joint with emphasis on the importance of hip tomography in their management. Orthopedic Review 1978; 7: 59–64.

Keller CS, Laros GS. Indications for open reduction of femoral neck fractures. Clinical Orthopedics 1980; 152: 131–137.

Walden PD, Hamer JR. Whistler technique used to reduce traumatic dislocation of the hip in the emergency department setting. Journal of Emergency Medicine 1999; 17: 441–444.

4.8 Femur injuries

Michael Cadogan

ESSENTIALS

1 Early femoral fracture reduction and immobilization in traction reduces mortality.

2 Haemorrhagic shock is a major complication, with a closed femoral fracture having an average blood loss of 1200 mL.

3 Femoral shaft fractures are associated with other significant injuries, which should be sought.

Femoral shaft fracture

Mechanism

Considerable force is required to break the adult femur in the absence of a pathology such as osteoporosis or metastatic disease. The majority of femoral shaft injuries occur in young adults following road traffic accidents, falls from a height or gunshot wounds.

Classification

The description of a femoral shaft fracture is important, but no universally accepted classification system exists. A precise description of the fracture provides the orthopaedic specialist with an indication of the potential for blood loss and the urgency of definitive management.

Femoral fractures are either open or closed and may be transverse, oblique, spiral or segmental. They may occur within the proximal third, midshaft or distal third of the femur. The degree of fracture comminution, soft tissue involvement and neurovascular status should also be described.

The majority of fractures occur in young adults with healthy bones and are transverse fractures. Greater mechanical force usually results in comminution (Fig. 4.8.1). Minimal force with pathological bone tends to produce metaphyseal fractures with propagation into the shaft.

Stress fractures of the femoral shaft are becoming increasingly common. They occur when repetitive mechanical forces are applied to the femur, such as in marathon running or military recruits. They are associated with pain in the mid-thigh and apparently normal X-rays, although a bone scan will detect the fracture, and low-impact training such as cycling is used in rehabilitation. They are rarely displaced.

Clinical evaluation

The clinical diagnosis of femoral shaft fracture is usually straightforward. The thigh is shortened and externally rotated, with the hip held in slight abduction. Palpation reveals tenderness over the fracture site and extreme pain on attempted movement. Neurovascular injuries are rare, but the distal pulses, capillary refill and distal sensation must be carefully examined.

Vascular damage is usually limited to rupture of the profunda femoris perforating branches in closed fractures. The resulting tense, swollen haematoma is limited to the thigh and is not associated with distal circulatory compromise. However, penetrating trauma and open fractures may cause femoral artery disruption with distal circulatory

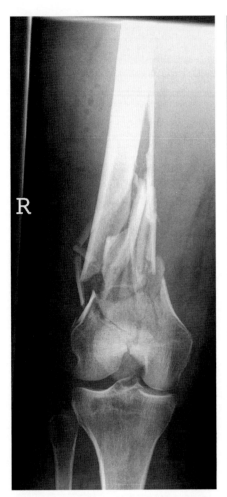

Fig. 4.8.1 Comminuted femoral fracture.

compromise, so repeated vascular evaluations are important. Any evidence of an expanding haematoma or diminished distal pulses requires further investigation with Doppler imaging or arteriography.

Associated injuries

Commonly associated injuries include fractures of the pelvis, the femoral head and neck, dislocation of the hip, and soft tissue disruption of the knee. Up to 50% of closed femur injuries are associated with meniscal and collateral ligament injuries in the knee, although it is usually impossible to evaluate these injuries reliably in the acute setting.

Up to 1.5 L of blood may extravasate into the surrounding soft tissues.

Management

The treatment of any associated head, neck, thoracic or pelvic injury must take priority in the setting of multiple trauma. The administration of analgesia, fluid resuscitation and femoral shaft fracture reduction and immobilization are indicated prior to X-ray of the lower limb.

Analgesia

Adequate pain relief is essential in the ED. Intravenous opioid analgesia is necessary, titrated to effect. A femoral nerve block is an important adjunct that should be considered prior to fracture reduction (see Chapter 22.2).

Reduction and immobilization

Early fracture reduction and immobilization in traction reduces overall mortality and pain, limits blood loss and reduces the risk of fat embolism. Fractures are reduced to near anatomic alignment using longitudinal traction, following appropriate analgesia with the knee in extension.

Proprietary splints such as the pneumatic Donway or Hare traction splints have replaced the skin traction Thomas splint in the ED. These provide smooth and gentle traction with minimal discomfort to the patient, and have the additional benefit of reducing blood loss by direct pressure and tamponade of haematoma formation.

Traction is only an interim procedure prior to definitive management, as it cannot maintain a constant force of sufficient magnitude to maintain the length and alignment of adult femur fractures.

Fluid resuscitation

Haemorrhagic shock is a major complication with an average blood loss from a closed femoral fracture of 1200 mL. All patients must be resuscitated with intravenous fluid, cross-matched for blood, kept fasted, and an indwelling catheter inserted to monitor fluid balance.

Orthopaedic management

Early operative fixation is indicated in adults within 8 hours, typically intramedullary nailing. Open fractures require immediate operative debridement with antibiotic cover, followed by delayed intramedullary nailing.

Complications

Complications include fat embolus syndrome, haemorrhagic shock and adult respiratory distress syndrome, with a higher incidence in comminuted fractures. Long-term complications of shortening, malalignment and non-union may result in post-traumatic arthritis. Early mobilization following intramedullary nailing greatly reduces those complications associated with prolonged immobilization. Patients older than 60 years with closed femoral fractures have a mortality rate of 17% and a complication rate of 54%.

Controversies

- Indications for arteriography, particularly in distal third femoral fractures following proximity penetrating trauma, even in the absence of initial vascular compromise.

Further reading

Provost R, Morris J. Fatigue fracture of the femoral shaft. Journal of Bone and Joint Surgery 1969; 51A: 487–498.

Russell RH. Fracture of the femur. A clinical study (Abridged by Peltier LF). Clinical Orthopedics 1987; 224: 4–11.

Taylor M, Banerjee B, Alpar E. Injuries associated with a fractured shaft of the femur. Injury 1994; 25: 185–187.

Vanganess C, DeCampos J, Merritt P. Meniscal injury associated with femoral shaft fractures. An arthroscopic evaluation of incidence. Journal of Bone and Joint Surgery 1993; 75: 207–209.

West H, Turkovich G, Donnell C. Immediate prediction of blood requirements in trauma victims. Southern Medical Journal 1989; 82: 186–189.

ORTHOPAEDIC EMERGENCIES

4.9 Knee injuries

Michael Cadogan

ESSENTIALS

1 The knee is the most commonly injured joint in the body.

2 Knee injuries often occur in the young, usually associated with sport.

3 The mechanism of injury is an essential part of the history, and examination must include the hip and ankle joint.

4 Anterior cruciate ligament disruption is associated with meniscal and collateral ligament injuries in 50% of cases.

5 Lateral tibial plateau fractures are associated with anterior cruciate and medial collateral ligament disruption, whereas medial tibial plateau fractures are associated with posterior cruciate and lateral collateral ligament disruption.

6 Knee dislocations require urgent reduction followed by angiography, and so represent time-critical orthopaedic emergencies.

Anatomy

The knee is the largest, most complicated joint in the body. It is a synovial, complex hinge joint comprising the patellofemoral and tibiofemoral joints. Movement ranges from 10° of extension to 140° of hyperflexion, with up to 12° of rotation present through the full arc.

The ligaments of the knee are classified as extracapsular or intracapsular. The main extracapsular ligaments are the medial and lateral collaterals (MCL and LCL). The main intracapsular ligaments are the anterior and posterior cruciate ligaments (ACL and PCL), which are extrasynovial. The collateral ligaments provide lateral stability and stability in extension, whereas the cruciate ligaments provide knee stability in flexion.

Knee stability is further enhanced by muscular extensions such as the vastus medialis giving patella stability, the fibrous extension of vastus lateralis and medialis (the patellar retinaculum) strengthening the knee anteriorly, and the iliotibial tract strengthening the knee in slight flexion.

Clinical assessment

An exact history of the mechanism of injury, degree of force, presence of immediate swelling and the ability to bear weight immediately after injury are essential to diagnose soft tissue injuries. Injury may be due to direct or indirect trauma, and may involve valgus or varus stress.

Comprehensive knee physical examination

Always examine both legs with the patient undressed and lying supine on a trolley (never sitting). Visual inspection may reveal swelling, bruising, erythema, deformity and associated wounds.

Swelling appearing within the first few hours of trauma is usually associated with a haemarthrosis due to a vascular response to subchondral, bone or synovial injury. Swelling developing gradually over several hours to days is more likely due to an effusion from a synovial reaction.

Palpation is started away from the point of trauma to detect warmth, swelling, crepitus, muscle mass and neurovascular status, and is then used to localize the areas of maximal tenderness to define the underlying pathology. It is important to assess the insertion points of the quadriceps tendon, patellar tendon, collateral ligaments and the medial and lateral joint lines, as well as the bony structures of the knee joint.

Assess active and passive movements of the knee joint, noting the degree of flexion, extension, and internal and external rotation. Always test for the ability to straight leg raise while supine, to assess for potential damage to the extensor mechanism of the knee.

Anterior and posterior drawer tests

The examination is completed with an assessment of the knee's functional stability. The stability of the anterior and posterior cruciate ligaments may be crudely determined with the anterior and posterior drawer tests. Ligamentous laxity decreases with age, so comparison with the opposite knee is more important than absolute laxity. The patient must be supine with the hip flexed at 45°, the knee flexed at 90° and the hamstrings relaxed. The examiner sits on the patient's foot to stabilize the limb and attempts to demonstrate abnormal forward movement of the tibia on the femoral condyles (positive anterior drawer test), and/or abnormal backward movement of the tibia on the femoral condyles (positive posterior drawer test). However, the accuracy of the anterior drawer test, as defined by subsequent arthroscopy, is only 56% for rupture of the ACL, whereas posterior displacement of the tibia by more than 5 mm is indicative of PCL ruptures, with a sensitivity of 85%.

Lachman's test

In the acute setting, Lachman's test is a more sensitive manoeuvre for testing ACL integrity, especially in the presence of a haemarthrosis. The operator supports the distal femur with one hand with the knee in 20–30° of flexion, and uses the other hand to draw the tibia forwards on the femoral condyles. Increased anterior displacement of the proximal tibia compared to the unaffected limb indicates a positive test.

Collateral laxity

The collateral ligaments are assessed by applying varus or valgus stress to the knee in 0° and 30° of flexion. The degree of ligamentous laxity is determined by the amount of movement produced between the tibia and fibula, compared to the normal side.

McMurray's test

McMurray's test is used to demonstrate a meniscal injury. The patient lies supine and the knee is passively flexed and extended. One hand is placed over the knee to feel for crepitus while the other hand rotates the tibia on the femur. Internal rotation tests the lateral meniscus, and external rotation tests the medial meniscus. Pain and crepitus at the extremes of movement indicate a positive test.

Apley's test

Apley's test is also used to demonstrate a meniscal injury. This is performed with the patient lying prone with the knee flexed to 90°. The tibia is rotated on the femur with downward pressure on the heel. Meniscal tears are associated with pain on downward pressure at the extremes of movement, relieved by the release of pressure.

Radiology

Clinical decision rules to determine the requirement for knee radiography have been published that aim to reduce emergency department (ED) radiographs, waiting times and costs. At present, as none have gained wide acceptance, all knee injuries associated with significant pain, inability to bear weight, suspected haemarthrosis or joint line tenderness should be X-rayed.

Standard knee X-ray evaluation includes AP and lateral views. AP views assess for the integrity of the medial and lateral joint spaces and the femoral tibial angle. They also show the size, position and integrity of the patella.

Lateral views may identify a lipohaemarthrosis effusion, seen as a horizontal line demarcating darker, more radiolucent fat floating on lighter, more radiodense blood. It is indicative of an intra-articular fracture and is most helpful when the actual injury is hard to see, such as with an undisplaced condylar fracture, patellar or tibial spine fracture.

Oblique X-rays are helpful in elucidating tibial plateau fractures. The tunnel view enhances the intercondylar region.

Skyline X-rays are taken to further evaluate the patella and patellofemoral joint, particularly following reduction of a patellar dislocation. They can identify undisplaced vertical fractures of the patella and

subtle subluxation not seen on the conventional views.

Computed tomography

Computed tomography (CT) is important to define fractures such as those of the tibial plateau. Magnetic resonance imaging (MRI) is reserved for evaluation of complex soft tissue knee injuries, unless arthroscopy is preferred.

Fractures around the knee joint

Distal femur

Distal femoral fractures account for 4% of femoral fractures. They are usually associated with high-energy injuries secondary to a fall or a direct blow to the femur in a motor vehicle accident.

Classification

Distal femoral fractures are divided anatomically into supracondylar, intercondylar and isolated condylar fractures. Supracondylar fractures are extra-articular and occur immediately above the femoral condyles. Intercondylar fractures involve separation of the femoral condyles. Although the fracture line may extend through the supracondylar region, in general they are treated as intra-articular fractures. Isolated condylar fractures are uncommon and occur when a varus or valgus force is applied to a weightbearing, extended knee. The tibial eminence is driven into the femoral intercondylar notch, creating an intra-articular fracture associated with significant ligamentous disruption.

Clinical assessment

Patients with injuries to the distal femur are in significant pain and are unable to bear weight. Examination may reveal swelling, deformity, rotation and shortening. The joint is tender to palpate along the medial or lateral joint lines, and an acute haemarthrosis secondary to associated ligamentous injury or intra-articular involvement is common.

The whole lower limb should be examined to exclude ipsilateral hip dislocation, associated tibial fractures and quadriceps damage. Neurovascular deficit is assessed, including loss of sensation in the web space between the first and second toes due to deep peroneal nerve injury.

Anteroposterior and lateral X-rays of the femur and knee reveal the fracture and its degree of displacement or comminution. A pelvic X-ray is necessary to exclude an associated proximal femur fracture or hip dislocation.

Management

Administer adequate analgesia and apply a splint in the ED to prevent excessive motion at the fracture site. Cast immobilization is usually sufficient for undisplaced or impacted fractures without joint involvement.

Fractures with joint incongruity usually require open reduction and internal fixation.

Early orthopaedic consultation is required

Distal femoral fractures are a complex orthopaedic problem and long-term complications of malunion, quadriceps adhesion and osteoarthritis are common.

Tibial plateau fracture

The tibial plateaus are the superior articulating surfaces of the medial and lateral tibial condyles. They are covered by hyaline cartilage and a fibrocartilaginous meniscus, and their integrity is vital for knee alignment, articulation and stability.

Mechanism

Tibial plateau fractures account for 1% of all skeletal fractures and are commonest in the elderly. They occur when a valgus or varus deforming force is applied to the weightbearing knee. Lateral tibial plateau fractures are twice as common as medial injuries, but both tibial plateaus are involved in 10–30% of cases. Anterior fractures occur when the knee is in extension, and posterior fractures when the knee is flexed.

Classification

Fracture classification is complex owing to the varying degrees of comminution, displacement and compression of the plateaus. The most widely used system is that of Schatzker, which divides the factures into six different types. Fracture types 1, 2 and 3 involve the lateral tibial plateau with increasing articular depression (Fig. 4.9.1). Type 4 involves the medial plateau. Fracture types 5 and 6 involve both

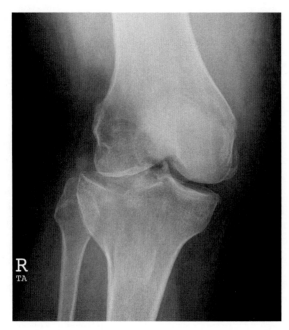

Fig. 4.9.1 Schatzker type 3 tibial plateau fracture.

tibial plateaus with increasing comminution and joint instability.

Segond fracture

Tibial plateau avulsion fractures at the site of lateral capsular ligament insertion are called Segond fractures. They are associated with excessive internal rotation and varus stress to the flexed knee, and are usually associated with sporting injuries. These fractures are important markers of ACL disruption with rotatory instability.

Clinical assessment

Patients are usually unable to bear weight and present with a painful, swollen knee. Pain and haemarthrosis limit active and passive movements of the knee. Focal tenderness is palpated at the fracture site and over any associated collateral ligament tears.

Distal circulatory compromise may be present secondary to compression of the popliteal artery by comminuted subcondylar fragments. Peroneal nerve neuropraxia and paralysis may complicate displaced lateral condylar fractures, resulting in foot drop. Soft tissue injuries occur in up to 35% of injuries. Generally, lateral tibial plateau fractures are associated with ACL and MCL disruptions, whereas medial plateau fractures are associated with PCL and LCL disruptions.

Radiology

Most tibial plateau fractures are evident on standard knee X-rays, although oblique views may be required to elucidate subtle fractures and to further classify fractures. CT is important to further evaluate non-displaced and comminuted fractures, although MRI is preferred to quantify the degree of any associated ligamentous damage.

Management

Orthopaedic consultation is essential. Many fractures may be treated conservatively with closed reduction and casting, but comminuted fractures with articular surface disruption require open reduction and internal fixation.

Common complications include undiagnosed neurovascular injuries, compartment syndrome and osteoarthritis.

Fractures of the tibial spine and intercondylar eminence

The tibial spine separates the medial and lateral tibial condyles and is divided into anterior and posterior areas by the intercondylar eminence. These areas provide flat surfaces for the attachment of the ACL and PCL, respectively. The intercondylar eminence is divided into a medial and a lateral tubercle visible on anteroposterior X-rays, although nothing actually attaches to these tubercles.

Mechanism

Most tibial spine and intercondylar eminence fractures occur in children, as the cruciate ligaments are stronger than the skeletal physeal plates. Considerable force is required for these fractures to occur in adults. The tibial spine is usually fractured during violent twisting knee movements. The anterior tibial spine fractures 10 times more frequently than the posterior. Intercondylar eminence fractures are associated with severe hyperextension or hyperflexion injuries.

Clinical assessment

The patient usually complains of severe pain, immediate swelling of the knee and inability to bear weight. The knee is usually held in slight flexion and cannot be fully extended. Examination confirms the presence of an acute haemarthrosis and limited knee movement. An associated ACL disruption may be confirmed with a positive Lachman's or anterior drawer test, although pain may prevent these.

Radiology

AP and lateral X-rays plus tunnel or oblique views are used to confirm the diagnosis. MRI is preferred to quantify the degree of any associated ligamentous damage.

Management

Most injuries are treated conservatively, but refer displaced fractures with marked ligamentous injury for open reduction and internal fixation.

Patellar fracture

The patella is the largest sesamoid bone in the body and lies within the quadriceps tendon. It improves the stability, strength and mechanical advantage of the extensor mechanism, and offers some protection to the femur.

Mechanism

Patellar fractures account for 1% of skeletal injuries and occur predominantly in males between the ages of 20 and 50 years as a result of direct or indirect trauma. Direct trauma to the anterior aspect of the patella results in incomplete, stellate, comminuted or vertical patellar fractures. These commonly occur in motor vehicle accidents when the knee strikes the dashboard. There is usually little or no separation of the bony fragments, as the medial and lateral quadriceps expansions remain intact.

Indirect trauma usually occurs when stumbling or falling forwards. The combination of powerful quadriceps contraction proximally and the strong patellar insertion distally overcomes the intrinsic strength of the patella and leads to a transverse fracture. These fractures account for up to 80% of patellar fractures, and occur mainly in the central and lower third of the patella. The extent of the fragment separation is dependent on the degree of quadriceps expansion tear.

Clinical assessment

Physical examination reveals pain, swelling and bruising over the patella. The ability to walk and actively extend the knee is dependent on the type of fracture, and is important when considering surgical repair. Test for the ability to perform a straight leg raise while in a supine position, to confirm the integrity of the knee extensor mechanism. Patients with non-displaced fractures may be ambulatory and able to demonstrate active knee extension against gravity. Patients with displaced transverse patellar fractures are unable to extend the knee actively.

Management

Fractures with fragment displacement of more than 3 mm are associated with disruption of the extensor mechanism and require referral to an orthopaedic specialist for open reduction and internal fixation with tension band wiring. Treat non-displaced patella fractures with an intact extensor mechanism conservatively with a long-leg cast in full extension for 6 weeks.

Dislocations around the knee joint

Dislocation of the knee

Knee dislocations are rare and usually occur in males in their third decade. They are orthopaedic emergencies associated with vascular damage that require urgent reduction.

Mechanism

Tibial femoral knee dislocation usually involves rupture of both cruciate ligaments and one collateral ligament. Such injuries are associated with high-velocity injuries such as from a motorcycle accident. They are described with respect to the displacement of the tibia in relation to the femur. Anterior dislocations are the most common.

Evaluation

Examination usually reveals gross distortion of the knee, with the clinical deformity being easily palpable. Knee dislocations are associated with a high rate of peroneal nerve and popliteal artery injury, and so a careful neurovascular assessment is essential. Compression and distortion of the posteriorly placed popliteal artery and vein may cause distal vascular compromise, although 10% of vascular injuries are associated with normal pedal pulses. Peroneal nerve dysfunction is present in up to 50% of patients suffering knee dislocation, causing foot drop and sensory impairment of the lateral border of the foot.

Radiology

Immediate plain X-rays confirm the dislocation, but must never delay reduction.

Management

Prompt consultation with the orthopaedic and vascular teams is essential, with early reduction under procedural sedation in the ED if necessary. The risk of developing a compartment syndrome and/or needing amputation is considerably increased when reduction is not performed within 6 hours.

Failed reduction secondary to buttonholing of the femoral condyle is uncommon and necessitates open reduction under general anaesthesia. Angiography is essential following every reduction to assess for any vascular injury.

Patella dislocation

Traumatic patellar dislocation is common and may become recurrent, with further patellar subluxation or dislocation. The majority of dislocations occur in the setting of patellofemoral dysplasia, or malalignment syndromes secondary to hypoplastic vastus medialis, a shallow trochlear groove or genu valgum. Lateral dislocations are overwhelmingly the most common, usually caused by a direct blow to the anterior or medial surface of the patella. The medial retinaculum is disrupted by being stretched in subluxations or torn in dislocations.

Clinical assessment

Patients complain of the knee suddenly 'giving way', accompanied by immediate pain and swelling. They are unable to bear weight or extend the knee. Palpation reveals an anterior defect, a laterally deviated patella, swelling, and medial joint line tenderness.

Standard AP and lateral X-rays confirm the diagnosis, and are important to exclude an associated osteochondral fracture. However, particularly in recurrent dislocations, X-rays may follow immediate reduction.

Management

Some dislocations reduce spontaneously or are reduced prior to arrival at the ED. Closed reduction is performed following suitable analgesia or conscious sedation. Apply anteromedial pressure to the lateral aspect of the patella with gentle knee extension. Immobilize the knee in extension for 3–6 weeks after post-reduction X-rays, to allow the medial retinaculum time to heal.

Complications

Recurrent dislocation occurs in over 15% of cases and may require surgical repair. However, up to 50% of patients suffer symptoms of instability or anterior knee pain following traumatic dislocation.

Proximal tibiofibular joint dislocation

Mechanism

The proximal tibiofibular joint is supported by a capsule anteriorly, the popliteus muscle posteriorly and the LCL superiorly. Tibiofibular joint dislocation is rare and only possible when the LCL support is relaxed, with the knee in flexion. Thus they occur mainly in violent athletic twisting injuries, such as during the shot put.

Clinical assessment

The patient holds the knee flexed at 20–30° and is able to bear weight with difficulty, with point tenderness over the fibula head. Common peroneal nerve neuropraxia is unusual.

Radiology

AP and lateral comparison views reveal the dislocation, which is usually anterolateral.

Management

Reduction is by firm pressure over the head of fibula towards the centre of the knee, under procedural sedation. Success is associated with a satisfying 'click'. Surgical intervention is rarely needed.

Soft tissue injuries

Collateral ligaments

Medial collateral ligament

The medial collateral ligament (MCL) complex comprises a long superficial ligament with a distal point of insertion and a short deep ligament attached to, and stabilizing, the medial meniscus. The MCL provides medial stabilization to the knee joint in conjunction with the capsule and semimembranosus, resisting valgus laxity and medial rotational instability.

MCL injuries are the most common isolated knee ligament injury. They occur when an excessive valgus force is applied to the knee, usually by a direct blow to the lateral aspect. The greater the degree of the valgus deforming force, the greater the risk of an associated ACL disruption.

Lateral collateral ligament

The lateral collateral ligament (LCL) is the phylogenetically degenerate part of peroneus longus. It is a cord-like ligament running from the lateral epicondyle of the femur to the head of the fibula. It is separated from the lateral meniscus by the popliteal tendon. The LCL is the major lateral stabilizer of the knee, providing the main resistance to varus deforming forces, especially when the knee is extended.

LCL injuries are less common, but more debilitating, than MCL injuries. The lower incidence of LCL injuries is a result of the lateral ligament's mobility and the protective effect of the opposite leg. They result from a direct blow to the medial aspect of the knee. Associated injuries to the insertion of biceps femoris and to the common peroneal nerve at the fibular head must also be excluded.

Clinical evaluation of the collateral ligaments

Medial and lateral ligament damage is often associated with sporting events. Examine for point tenderness at the site of injury, demonstrable laxity and a haemarthrosis. Stress the affected ligament complex to duplicate the pain, especially with partial tears. Complete rupture of the ligament complex is associated with instability, and stress testing causes the joint line to open up on the affected side.

The MCL is tested in 0° and 30° of flexion. Pressure is applied to the lateral joint line with one hand while the other hand creates a valgus stress by gently pushing the medial malleolus laterally. At 0° the medial complex is reinforced by the ACL, but at 30° the testing is specific for MCL rupture.

Lateral instability is assessed with pressure applied to the medial joint line with one hand, and by a varus stress performed by moving the lower leg medially.

Radiology

Standard X-rays can only reveal collateral ligament injury when there has been a bony avulsion. Calcification at the origin of the MCL occurs in chronic injuries (Pellegrini–Stieda). MRI helps delineate the degree of ligamentous disruption and highlights associated injuries in complex cases.

Management

Treat all isolated collateral ligament injuries conservatively, provided damage to the ACL and PCL complexes has been excluded. Discomfort is reduced by immobilizing the knee in a proprietary splint such as a three-panel Velcro knee immobilizer, or by an elastic knee support, with ice massage and anti-inflammatory drugs. Quadriceps strengthening exercises are essential to aid recovery and early return to movement using a hinged splint.

Cruciate ligaments

The cruciate ligaments are the primary stabilizers of the knee in flexion and extension.

Anterior cruciate ligament

The anterior cruciate ligament (ACL) extends from the medial aspect of the lateral femoral condyle to the anterior intercondylar area of the tibia. It prevents backward displacement of the femur on the tibial plateau and limits extension of the lateral condyle of the femur. It helps control the rotation of the knee in twisting and turning activities, and is much more commonly injured than the PCL.

Mechanism The ACL is commonly injured during sporting activities such as skiing and rugby, with patients readily able to define the causative mechanism. Injury results from direct trauma as the tibia is forcefully displaced anteriorly on the femur or the femur posteriorly on the tibia, or by indirect injury when the flexed knee suffers a sudden twisting movement with the foot firmly planted on the ground.

Clinical assessment ACL injuries are classically associated with sudden severe pain and an audible 'pop', with an acute haemarthrosis and inability to bear weight. Immediate swelling of the knee indicates serious intra-articular pathology.

The anterior drawer test or Lachman's test is used to assess ACL integrity. ACL disruption is associated with meniscal and collateral ligament injuries in 50% of cases, with the most common combination involving the triad of ACL and MCL disruption, with a lateral meniscal tear.

Radiology X-rays may show avulsion of the anterior tibial spine, although an MRI scan is necessary to determine ACL rupture with any certainty, having over 90% sensitivity and specificity.

Management Arthroscopy is the gold standard in assessing the integrity of the ACL and has the advantage of allowing simultaneous debridement and repair. Arthroscopic repair or reconstruction is usually performed on young, active patients after 2–3 weeks to allow the initial swelling to subside.

Posterior cruciate ligament

The posterior cruciate ligament (PCL) extends from the lateral aspect of the medial femoral condyle to the posterior intercondylar area of the tibia. It prevents excessive forward displacement of the femur on the tibia and is essential in providing mechanical support when walking downhill or down stairs, as it is the only stabilizing structure in the flexed, weightbearing knee.

Mechanism PCL rupture is normally caused by a posteriorly directed force on the proximal tibia, such as with falls onto the tibial tubercle, knee dislocations and dashboard injuries. It is less commonly associated with sporting injuries than ACL ruptures.

Clinical assessment Immediate pain and swelling are common with PCL rupture, which unlike the ACL, rarely causes any popping or tearing sensations. Stability is usually adequate to allow partial weight-bearing. Isolated PCL ruptures result in posterior 'sag' of the tibia compared to the unaffected limb, with the posterior drawer test performed to asses PCL integrity. Associated MCL and ACL disruptions are common and must be actively sought.

Radiology X-rays may reveal avulsion of the posterior tibial spine, but as with ACL injuries, MRI is indicated to demonstrate over 90% sensitivity and specificity for PCL rupture.

Arthroscopy Arthroscopic PCL examination is less reliable than MRI examination.

Management The treatment of isolated PCL rupture is largely non-operative and focuses initially on pain management and non-weightbearing immobilization. Operative intervention within 2 weeks is more usual when PCL injuries are combined with other ligamentous injuries.

Patellar tendon rupture

The patellar tendon is the final connection of the extensor mechanism from the inferior pole of the patella to the tibial tuberosity. Rupture usually occurs under the age of 40 years, often associated with a previous history of patellar tendonitis or steroid injections. Injury is associated with stressful sporting activity and occurs with forceful quadriceps contraction. It causes significant pain.

Examination reveals a palpable defect, which may be masked by significant swelling. Comparison lateral X-ray views of both knees may reveal a high-riding patella. MRI is indicated in complex cases to differentiate partial and complete tears. Partial tears are treated non-operatively with cast immobilization in extension for 6 weeks. Complete tears of the patellar tendon should be referred to the orthopaedic specialist for surgical intervention.

Quadriceps tendon injury

The quadriceps tendon is a trilaminar junction of the quadriceps muscle. Rupture is commonest in the older age groups as the tendinous blood supply declines. Young persons usually suffer a muscular disruption. Rupture occurs three times more commonly than patellar tendon rupture, and is usually due to a direct blow to the knee or a hyperextension injury. It is associated with intense pain, and the patient is unable to walk without assistance.

Examination reveals a tender, palpable defect more apparent on attempted knee extension. Swelling secondary to a haemarthrosis and bruising are usually present.

The straight leg raise is impossible in complete rupture, whereas extension of the knee from a flexed position cannot be performed in a partial tear. Comparison lateral knee X-rays may demonstrate a low-lying patella in the affected knee. In doubtful cases MRI is indicated to distinguish between a partial and a complete rupture.

Management

Partial tears are treated non-operatively, but a complete rupture requires early surgical intervention for the best results.

Patellar and quadriceps tendonitis (jumper's knee)

Both these extensor tendons are susceptible to tendonitis secondary to repetitive overloading. Patellar tendonitis is more common than quadriceps tendonitis. Patients present with anterior knee pain with point tenderness over the inferior or superior pole of the patella, commonly in athletes who participate in running and jumping activities.

Inflammation and pain in patellar tendinitis at the insertion point of the patella tendon into the patella is six times more common than at the insertion to the tibial tuberosity. Patellar tendonitis may be associated with fragmentation of the inferior pole of the patella on X-ray.

Initial treatment involves rest, ice and anti-inflammatory medication. Longer-term recovery and prevention requires conditioning and training of the extensor musculature.

Meniscal injury

The menisci are semilunar fibrocartilaginous structures found on the medial and lateral sides of the superior aspect of the tibia. They enhance the fluidity of articulation between the femoral and tibial condyles and increase the stability of the tibiofemoral articulation. The medial meniscus is immobile, being firmly attached to the deep portion of the medial collateral ligament and joint capsule. The lateral meniscus has a uniform thickness and a larger tibial area than the medial. It has no attachment to the LCL and is more mobile than the medial meniscus, making it more prone to injury.

Mechanism

Meniscal injuries are usually associated with collateral or cruciate ligament injury, which should be sought when examining the acutely injured knee. Chronic degenerative processes account for only a small percentage of injuries. The menisci are uncommonly injured in isolation, but suspect an isolated meniscal injury in the young athlete sustaining a violent twisting or rotational injury to the weightbearing knee.

Clinical assessment

The patient is able to partially bear weight following meniscal injury and usually complains of medial or lateral joint line pain. Delayed swelling, intermittent locking and a sensation of the knee 'giving way' with sudden loss of stability are clues to meniscal damage.

Examination usually confirms the presence of an effusion and joint line tenderness, especially in the extremes of flexion and extension. McMurray's test may be positive, but is not pathognomonic, and in the acute setting pain often prevents adequate hyperflexion for the test to be accurate.

The 'locked' knee is held in 30° of flexion and a springy block to extension on examination with associated pain. Bucket-handle meniscal tears are classically associated with a true 'locked' knee. They are longitudinal tears, usually of the medial meniscus, and frequently associated with ACL disruption.

Radiology

Routine X-rays do not show any direct evidence of meniscal damage but are useful to exclude commonly associated bony injuries.

MRI may determine both meniscal and ligamentous injuries in complex cases.

Management

Arthroscopy is used to evaluate and treat meniscal injuries, revealing the extent of damage and determining whether resection of the torn cartilage or meniscectomy is required.

Controversies

- Evaluating and validating further clinical decision tools for the use of radiographs in acute knee injuries.

- Replacing cylindrical plaster cast treatment of patellar fractures and some soft tissue injuries with three-panel Velcro knee immobilizer splints and hinged supports.

- The role of CT scans in condylar and tibial plateau knee injuries.

- The role of MRI over arthroscopy in complex soft tissue knee injuries.

Further reading

Bachmann LM, Steurer J, Ter Riet G, et al. The accuracy of the Ottawa knee rule to rule out knee fractures: A systematic review. Annals of Internal Medicine 2004; 140: 121–124.

Bandyk DF. Vascular injury associated with extremity trauma. Clinical Orthopedics 1995; 318: 117–124.

Kendall NS, Hsu SY, Chan KM. Fracture of the tibial spine in adults and children. Journal of Bone and Joint Surgery 1992; 74B: 848.

Kode L, Lieberman JM, Motta AO, et al. Evaluation of tibial plateau fractures: Efficacy of MR imaging compared with CT. American Journal of Roentgenology 1994; 163: 141.

Roberts DM, Stallard TC. Emergency department evaluation and treatment of knee and leg injuries. Emergency Medical Clinics of North America 2000; 18: 67–84.

Schatzker J. Fractures of the tibial plateau. In: Schatzker J, Tile M, eds. Rationale of operative fracture care. New York: Springer Verlag, 1987; 279.

Seaburg DC, Yealy DM, Lukens T, et al. Multicenter comparison of two clinical decisions rules for the use of radiography in acute, high-risk knee injuries. Annals of Emergency Medicine 1999; 32: 8–13.

Wascher DC, Dvirnak PC, Decoster TA, et al. Knee dislocation: initial assessment and implications for treatment. Journal of Orthopedic Trauma 1997; 11: 525–529.

4.10 Tibia and fibula injuries

Stuart Dilley • Michael Cadogan

ESSENTIALS

1 Tibial shaft fractures are the commonest long bone fracture, and the subcutaneous nature of the tibia leaves it vulnerable to open fracture.

2 Neurovascular injury and compartment syndrome are a risk in tibial shaft fractures.

3 Proximal fibula fractures are associated with common peroneal (lateral popliteal) nerve injury.

4 Tibial tubercle injuries range from apophysitis to acute fracture.

Anatomy

The tibia is the weightbearing strut of the lower leg. Proximally, the tibia articulates with the femoral condyles and distally the bony extension provides medial stability to the ankle joint. Its shaft is triangular in cross-section and is subcutaneous anteromedially.

The fibula head is proximal and connects to the fibular shaft by the neck. Distally the fibula is palpated subcutaneously as the lateral malleolus.

The tibia and fibula are connected by superior and inferior tibiofibular joints, and a dense interosseous membrane. Distally this union is strengthened by a syndesmosis, which enhances the stability of the ankle mortise.

Lower leg fascial compartments

The lower leg is divided into four compartments by bone and fascia. Each compartment contains a sensory nerve and muscles with specific functions. Increased pressure within a compartment is readily evaluated clinically by impaired function according to the functional anatomy.

The anterior compartment contains the tibialis anterior and the long toe extensor muscles that dorsiflex the ankle and foot. The deep peroneal nerve supplies these muscles and the first web space of the foot. The anterior tibial artery is contained within the compartment down to the ankle, where it becomes the dorsalis pedis artery.

The lateral compartment contains the peroneus longus and peroneus brevis which evert the foot, and the superficial peroneal nerve that supplies sensation to the dorsum of the foot. The superficial posterior compartment contains the gastrocnemius, plantaris and soleus muscles, which plantarflex the ankle. The sural nerve lies in this compartment before piercing the fascia to supply the lateral side of the foot and distal calf.

The deep posterior compartment contains the tibialis posterior and long toe flexor muscles that plantarflex the toes. The tibial nerve is within the compartment and supplies sensory function to the sole of the foot. The posterior tibial and peroneal arteries also lie in this compartment (Table 4.10.1).

Fractures of the tibia

Tibial shaft fracture

Tibial shaft fractures are the most common long bone fracture and are usually easily

Table 4.10.1 AO Classification of tibial shaft fractures

Type A (simple)	1	Spiral
	2	Oblique (angle > 30°)
	3	Transverse (angle < 30°)
Type B (multifrag wedge)	1	Spiral wedge
	2	Bending wedge
	3	Fragmented wedge
Type C (multifrag complex)	1	Spiral wedge
	2	Segmental
	3	Irregular

recognized. They are also the commonest open fracture, owing to the subcutaneous nature of the tibial shaft.

A considerable amount of direct or indirect energy is needed for the tibial shaft to fracture. Direct injuries may occur secondary to bending forces or a direct blow. Direct violence such as in a motor vehicle accident or when a pedestrian is struck cause deformation at the site of contact, resulting in transverse or comminuted, usually open, fractures. High-energy injuries have an increased degree of displacement, comminution, soft tissue injury and fibular involvement. They are associated with marked vascular, interosseous and bony involvement and are unstable, with a high risk of compartment syndrome.

Indirect torsional forces applied to the tibia produce spiral fractures as the body rotates about a fixed foot. Such injuries are common in skiing accidents and have increasing degrees of comminution depending on the amount of energy applied.

Classification

The description of the fracture must be clear and concise in relation to the following (AO Classification of tibial shaft fractures[1,2] (Table 4.10.1)).

- Skin integrity: open or closed.
- Anatomical site: proximal, middle or distal third.
- Fracture type: transverse, oblique, spiral or comminuted.
- Angulation of the distal fragment in relation to the proximal fragment,

expressed in degrees and direction (anterior, posterior, varus or valgus).
- Degree of displacement and rotation.
- Involvement of the fibula.

Clinical assessment

At the site of the fracture pain is usually severe. The patient is unable to bear weight, and inspection reveals swelling and deformity of the leg. The skin should be checked for integrity and to identify areas of pressure caused by displaced fragments. The neurovascular status of the lower leg and foot must be assessed as a matter of urgency, including skin colour, capillary refill, and the distal dorsalis pedis and posterior tibial pulses.

Contusion of the peroneal nerve may occur in high-energy injuries with proximal fibular fractures, although direct peroneal nerve injury may occur rarely in closed tibial shaft fractures. The motor function of the deep peroneal nerve is tested by active ankle and toe dorsiflexion, and the sensory function is tested in the first dorsal web space. The motor function of the superficial peroneal nerve is tested by active foot eversion, and the sensory function is tested over the dorsal lateral aspect of the foot. Associated injuries of the ipsilateral femur, hip, knee, foot and pelvis must be excluded.

Radiology

AP and lateral views of the lower leg must include the entire tibia and fibula from the knee to the ankle, to document tibial shaft fractures, identify associated fibula fractures, the fracture pattern, any degree of comminution and/or displacement (Fig. 4.10.1). The knee and ankle joint are X-rayed to look for associated joint involvement.

Management

Pain management is the first priority. This usually requires intravenous opiates, followed by reduction of displaced and/or compound fractures, and immobilization of the lower leg as early as possible.

Compartment syndrome

Emergency department (ED) documentation of the neurovascular status is essential to exclude acute neurovascular injury,

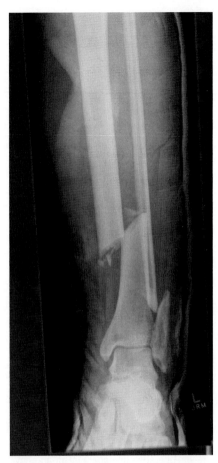

Fig. 4.10.1 Open, oblique, distal third tibia fracture with displaced varus deformity and fibula involvement.

as well as to detect actual or potential compartment syndrome development. Development of a compartment syndrome may occur in up to 20% of closed injuries and may take up to 24 hours to appear. It is less common in compound injuries.

Increasing pain despite reduction and casting may be an early indicator of compartment syndrome. It should be suspected if there is weakness of muscle action, pain on passive movement, and diminished sensation over the distal sensory nerve territory. Pulses may still be present, and a strong pedal pulse does *not* exclude the presence of a compartment syndrome. The deep posterior compartment is most commonly affected, followed by isolated elevation of pressure in the anterior compartment.

If there is any concern, compartment pressures should be measured. A compartment syndrome may occur if the compartment pressure is found to be

> 30 mmHg or within 30 mmHg of mean arterial pressure.

Open wounds are assessed for depth and associated soft-tissue damage, then dressed to avoid further contamination. Reduce displaced, rotated and angulated fractures in the ED under appropriate analgesia and procedural sedation (see Chapter 22.3). Reduction aims to stop local swelling, release the tension of any skin 'tented' over a displaced fracture, and reduce associated soft tissue damage. Exposed bone is returned under the skin after appropriate decontamination. Check the tetanus status and give parenteral antibiotics such as dicloxacillin 2 g 6-hourly i.v., or cephalothin 2 g 6-hourly i.v.

Immobilize the leg following reduction with 20° of knee flexion and take post-reduction films to confirm the position. Re-check the neurovascular status of the lower leg and foot and document this.

Definitive orthopaedic management

There are various options for definitive management, including conservative, closed reduction, open reduction and internal fixation (ORIF), and intramedullary rods.

Non-operative management in an above-knee plaster of Paris (POP) cast is appropriate for low-energy fractures without significant comminution, shortening or displacement.[3] Conservative management may also be appropriate for fractures with > 50% cortical contact, < 5–10° of varus/valgus angulation, < 10–15° of anterior or posterior bowing, < 5–7° of rotation and no more than 10–15 mm of shortening.[4]

Operative management is considered for patients with high-energy displaced fractures, compound fractures, or who have failed closed treatment. Intramedullary nailing results in shorter hospital stays, fewer outpatient visits and earlier return to work.[4] ORIF is also considered for displaced intra-articular fractures of the tibia involving the knee or ankle.

Tibial tubercle fracture

The tibial tubercle lies proximally on the anterior border of the shaft of the tibia. It is readily palpable beneath the infrapatellar bursa, and receives the insertion of the patellar tendon. Fractures of the tubercle are uncommon and occur in adolescents, typically as a result of indirect injury.

Avulsion fractures of the tubercle are usually the result of violent flexion of the knee against tightly contracted quadriceps muscle.

Three grades of injury were described by Watson-Jones. In type I injuries the tubercle is hinged upwards without displacement; type II injuries involve avulsion of a small portion of the tubercle proximally; and type III injuries are intra-articular. The fragment is displaced and may be comminuted.

Examination reveals pain and tenderness over the anterior aspect of the knee and proximal tibia. There may be a haemarthrosis and loss of active extension, depending on the severity of the injury.

Plain X-rays confirm the diagnosis. The lateral tibial view reveals the avulsion fragment, its degree of displacement and comminution.

Management is dependent on the degree of displacement and the presence of joint involvement. Watson-Jones type I and II injuries are treated with cylindrical long leg casts until healed. Type III injuries require open reduction and internal fixation with tension band wiring and fixation screws.[5]

Osgood–Schlatter's disease (traction apophysitis of the tibial tubercle)

The commonest differential diagnosis of tibial tuberosity fracture is Osgood–Schlatter's disease. This condition is traction apophysitis of the tibial tubercle caused by repeated microtrauma to the growing tubercle during adolescence. It is chronic and associated with repetitive activity, and unlike tubercle fractures is never accompanied by a haemarthrosis. Active knee extension is possible, albeit painful. Treatment is conservative with rest, ice and compression. A return to full mobilization follows rehabilitation and strengthening of the quadriceps complex.

Tibial stress fractures

Tibial stress fractures are common, affecting the proximal third of the tibia in adolescents and the junction of middle and distal thirds of the tibia in runners. Clinically, there is point tenderness over an area of induration. X-rays may appear negative early, or may show periosteal reaction. A bone scan or MRI may detect these injuries earlier. The differential diagnosis includes

'shin splints' (see below), fascial hernias and exertional compartment syndrome. Management is usually conservative, reducing activity and impact on the tibia. Symptoms may persist for over 12 months.

Shin splints

Shin splints is also known as 'medial tibial stress syndrome', which is characterized by exercise-induced pain in the midsection of the leg with tenderness noted along the posteromedial border of the middle and distal thirds of the tibia. Tenderness is usually more diffuse than the localized tenderness of a stress fracture. There may be periostitis near the origin of the soleus and flexor digitorum longus muscles. It is rare in children under 15 years of age.

Fractures of the fibula

Proximal fibula fractures may occur in isolation or in association with tibial and ankle injuries.

Associated tibial shaft fracture

Most fibula fractures are associated with fractures of the tibial shaft and are managed as for tibial fractures. The pattern of the associated fibular fracture indicates the degree of energy imparted. Severe comminution of the fibula or tibiofibular diastasis implies disruption of the interosseous membrane and indicates an unstable fracture. The fibula usually heals well with whatever treatment is selected for the tibia, and with a better rate of union. Complications of fibula fractures associated with tibial shaft fractures are rare.

Isolated proximal fibula fractures

Isolated proximal fibula or fibula shaft fractures are less common. They are usually associated with a direct blow to the lateral aspect of the leg, with symptoms of local tenderness, swelling, bruising, and difficulty walking. A neurovascular assessment is important, as the common peroneal nerve passes around the neck of fibula and may be contused or disrupted in these isolated injuries. Rarely, thrombosis of the anterior tibial artery may occur.

Full-length AP and lateral X-rays of the tibia and fibula, including the ankle and knee joints, will confirm the fracture pattern.

Non-displaced fractures associated with little pain are treated with ice, compression bandage, analgesia and non-weightbearing crutches for 3 weeks. Weightbearing is advanced progressively as tolerated. Mildly displaced fractures or those with significant pain may require a long leg cast for up to 6 weeks. Severely displaced fractures, or those associated with peroneal nerve deficit such as foot drop, require orthopaedic consultation and consideration for fixation.

Maisonneuve fracture

A medial malleolus or distal tibial fracture associated with a proximal fibula fracture is termed a Maisonneuve fracture. These fractures occur when an external rotatory force is applied to the ankle, resulting in partial or complete disruption of the syndesmosis, and are unstable. Palpation of the proximal fibula following complex ankle injuries is therefore essential to assess for this fracture. Refer all such fractures to the orthopaedic team for operative fixation.

Controversies

- The use and value of compartment pressure monitors in the emergency department.

- Which clinical features or actual compartment pressure require urgent active management.

References

1. Muller ME, Nazarian S, Koch P. The AO Classification of Fractures. New York: Springer-Verlag, 1988.
2. South Australian Orthopaedic Registrar's Notebook. http://som.flinders.edu.au/FUSA/ORTHOWEB/notebook/home.html (Accessed August 2007).
3. Hooper G, Keddell R, Penny I. Conservative management or closed nailing for tibial shaft fractures: A randomized prospective trial. Journal of Bone and Joint Surgery 1991; 73B: 83–85.
4. Wheeless' Textbook of Orthopaedics. http://www.wheelessonline.com/ortho/ (Accessed August 2007).
5. Balmat P, Vichard P, Pem R. The treatment of avulsion fractures of the tibial tuberosity in adolescent athletes. Sports Medicine 1990; 9: 311–316.

Further reading

Roberts D, Stallard T. Emergency department evaluation and treatment of knee and leg injuries. Emergency Medical Clinics of North America 2000; 18: 67–84.

4.11 Ankle joint injuries

Stuart Dilley • Michael Cadogan

ESSENTIALS

1 Ankle injuries are common and occur as isolated injuries, or related to high-energy multitrauma.

2 The Ottawa Ankle Rules (OAR) are used to determine the need for imaging of the ankle (or foot) in adults with isolated acute ankle injuries.

3 Lateral malleolar fractures are the most common ankle fracture.

4 The Henderson (Potts) classification is the most simple for describing ankle fractures.

5 Ankle sprains should be mobilized early.

6 The calf-squeeze test (Thompson or Simmond's test) is used to confirm the diagnosis of Achilles tendon rupture.

Anatomy

The ankle joint is a complex hinge joint that permits articulation between the tibia, fibula and talus, providing a stable but mobile support for the body. It helps absorb the forces of ambulation, maintain an upright posture, and allows for uneven terrain.

The stability of the ankle joint relates to the bony architecture, the joint capsule and the ligaments. The bones and ligaments are best visualized as a ring structure centring on the talus, which provides the stability. This ring is made up of the tibial plafond, the medial malleolus, the medial (deltoid) ligament, calcaneus, lateral collateral ligaments, lateral malleolus and the syndesmotic ligaments. The joint becomes unstable when more than one element of this ring structure is disrupted.

The lateral malleolus of the distal fibula, the medial malleolus of the distal tibia and the distal tibial plafond form the bony mortise of the joint. This provides intrinsic bony stability constraining the wedge-shaped talus distally. The medial ligament of the ankle or deltoid ligament fans out from the tip of the medial malleolus to attach to the tuberosity of the navicular, the medial aspect of the talus and the sustentaculum tali of the calcaneus. The lateral ligament comprises three discrete parts, the anterior and posterior talofibular ligaments and the calcaneofibular ligament.

Most ankle joint injuries are as a result of abnormal movement of the talus within the mortise. Movement causes stress to the encompassing ring of structures of the ankle joint, and instability arises when disruption of the malleoli or their associated ligaments results in distraction of the talus within the mortise.

Clinical assessment

Injuries around the ankle include fractures to the ankle and adjacent tarsal bones, ligamentous sprains, dislocations and tendon ruptures. All these need to be considered when assessing the patient with an ankle injury.

History

Inability to bear weight and the presence of swelling immediately following an injury imply significant pathology. Additional essential information includes the circumstances surrounding the injury, the position of the foot at the time, and the magnitude and direction of loading forces applied, particularly rotational. A history of inversion injury should prompt the examiner to also assess the base of the fifth metatarsal.

Examination

Give the patient analgesia, and rest, ice and elevate the affected limb. Examination of the ankle includes the entire lower leg, and begins with a comparison between the injured and non-injured sides. Note the integrity of the skin and the presence of bruising, swelling or deformity. Palpation for point tenderness may localize ligament, bone or tendon injury, and should commence at a site away from the area of obvious injury. The entire length of the tibia and fibula, as well as the base of the fifth metatarsal, calcaneus and Achilles tendon, must be examined. Palpation of the posterior aspects of the malleoli should commence 6–10 cm proximally and include both ends of the collateral ligament attachments. The anterior plafond and the medial and lateral aspects of the talar dome are then palpated in plantarflexion.

Then assess the range of active and passive movement at the ankle joint, including inversion, eversion, dorsiflexion and plantarflexion. A soft tissue injury is likely when there is a significant difference between the active and passive ranges of movement.

Finally, the foot should always be checked for motor or sensory impairment, capillary return, the presence of dorsalis pedis and posterior tibial pulses, and injury to the base of the fifth metatarsal.

Stress tests for ligamentous instability of the acutely injured ankle, and an evaluation of weightbearing ability, should only proceed if clinical suspicion of a fracture is low. The talar tilt test assesses the calcaneofibular ligament by applying a gentle inversion stress to the calcaneum. The anterior and posterior drawer tests assess

the anterior and posterior talofibular ligaments by gentle forward traction on the heel, although all require appropriate analgesia for evaluation.

Radiology and the Ottawa Ankle Rules

Standard radiography of the acutely injured ankle includes anteroposterior, lateral and mortise views. All patients with obviously deformed fractures or dislocations should undergo immediate X-ray following analgesia. The need for imaging of the ankle or mid-foot in patients with less obvious injuries may be determined using the Ottawa Ankle Rules (OAR). When used on a competent patient, the OAR are more than 98% sensitive for detecting clinically relevant ankle fractures in adults[1,2] and 98% sensitive in children.[3,4] These rules specify that an ankle X-ray series is only required if there is any pain in the malleolar region and any one of:

- Bone tenderness over the posterior aspect or inferior tip of the distal 6 cm of the lateral malleolus.
- Bone tenderness over the posterior aspect or inferior tip of the distal 6 cm of the medial malleolus.
- Inability to bear weight for at least four steps, both immediately after the injury and at the time of emergency department (ED) evaluation.

The OAR also include indications for foot X-ray in suspected mid-foot fractures; these are described elsewhere (see Foot Injuries, Chapter 4.12).

Further imaging

Computed tomography (CT) may be used to further evaluate complex fractures, and MRI for difficult or recalcitrant ligamentous injuries. Bone scans may delineate osteochondral and stress fractures.

Ankle fracture classification

Several classification systems are used to describe ankle fractures and dislocations, some more complicated than others.

Henderson or pott's classification

The Henderson or Pott's classification is a simple system based on radiographic findings:

- Unimalleolar fractures affecting the lateral or medial malleolus. The stability of these fractures is dependent on the integrity of contralateral ligaments and the inferior tibiofibular joint.
- Bimalleolar fractures affecting the medial and lateral malleoli, which are usually unstable.
- Trimalleolar fractures involving the medial, lateral and posterior tibial plafond, which are always unstable.

Weber classification

The Weber classification system divides ankle fractures into three types, based on the level at which the fibula fractures. The more proximal the fibula fracture, the greater the associated syndesmosis disruption and potential for ankle instability.

Type A fractures involve the distal fibula below the level of the tibial plafond; type B involve an oblique or spiral fracture at the level of the syndesmosis; and type C occur when the fibula is fractured above the level of the syndesmosis.

The original Weber classification system does not take into account medial or posterior malleolar fractures. The AO system applies three subdivisions to each Weber fracture type to account for these injuries and to further define ankle stability.[5]

Fracture management

Minimally displaced avulsion fractures of the distal fibula less than 3 mm in diameter which are not associated with medial ligament disruption should be treated as sprains.

Grossly displaced fractures are reduced and splinted promptly in the ED, with appropriate analgesia and or procedural sedation, prior to imaging if distal ischaemia is identified or skin integrity is compromised (see Fig 4.11.1).

Extra-articular or non-displaced fractures with an intact mortise joint on X-ray may be treated non-operatively in a below-knee plaster of Paris (POP) cast in a neutral position, that is, with the ankle at 90° with no inversion or eversion to maintain the correct anatomical position of the talus. Refer these injuries for orthopaedic follow-up, with advice that fracture movement may occur and that operative intervention may still be required. Displaced and potentially unstable fractures require early orthopaedic

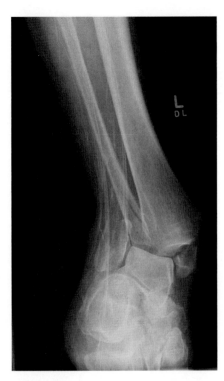

Fig. 4.11.1 Unstable bimalleolar ankle fracture.

consultation, including all bimalleolar and trimalleolar fractures and those unimalleolar fractures with contralateral ligamentous injuries. The majority of these injuries will require operative intervention (ORIF).

Pilon fractures

Pilon fractures involve the distal tibial metaphysis and result from high-energy injuries directed through the talus into the distal tibia, with tibial plafond disruption. Their frequency has increased with the greater numbers of motor vehicle accidents and falls from heights, and are usually associated with multiple other injuries. They are also often open, comminuted, and associated with massive soft tissue deformity.

The fracture is reduced and splinted under appropriate analgesia and procedural sedation to reduce the potential for massive soft tissue swelling and conversion of a closed fracture to an open one as a result of overlying skin necrosis. Treatment usually requires operative fixation.

Maisonneuve fracture

The Maisonneuve fracture is a fracture of the proximal end of the fibula associated with a medial malleolus fracture or disruption of the medial (deltoid) ligament. The proximal fibula fracture is associated with disruption of the interosseous membrane from the tibiofibular syndesmosis up to the proximal fibular head. They are unstable and require operative fixation.

Ankle dislocations

Ankle dislocations are frequently associated with a fracture, but do occur in isolation, and may be open or closed. They require considerable energy, such as when an external force is directed against the plantarflexed foot, squeezing the talus out of the mortise. The direction of the initial loading force determines the final position of the dislocation. Posterior dislocations are the most common.

Closed dislocations

Closed dislocations are associated with marked soft tissue disruption and skin tethering, although neurovascular compromise is uncommon. Dislocations should be reduced promptly in the ED to minimize any associated soft tissue injury, using gentle manipulation, appropriate analgesia and procedural sedation, just as for grossly displaced fractures. Despite the potential for ligamentous disruption, they usually have an excellent outcome following immobilization for 8 weeks.

Open dislocations

Open dislocations may be associated with disruption of the dorsalis pedis and posterior tibial vessels. They require surgical debridement in theatre, but again should initially be reduced and splinted with POP in the emergency department. Open injuries are associated with more long-term complications than closed, in particular traumatic arthritis and reduced mobility.

Soft tissue injuries

Ligamentous injuries

Ankle sprains are one of the most common injuries presenting to the ED: 75% of injuries to the ankle are sprains, and 90% of these affect the lateral ligament complex, predominantly the anterior talofibular ligament. Typically, injuries to the lateral ligament proceed from anterior to posterior as increasing force is applied. Medial ligament disruption is more frequently associated with lateral malleolar fractures or Maisonneuve-type injuries involving the proximal fibula and syndesmosis disruption.

Lateral ligament injuries are graded according to the degree of fibre disruption, and reflect the progression of injury from anterior to posterior as well as subsequent stability of the ankle joint:

- Grade I: Partial tear, usually of the anterior talofibular ligament. Patients are usually able to bear weight with minimal swelling and normal stress testing.
- Grade II: Partial tear, usually extending to the calcaneofibular ligament. Patients have pain at rest, difficulty weightbearing, significant swelling and mild to moderate joint instability.
- Grade III: Complete tear of two or more elements of the lateral ligament. Patients are unable to bear weight, with severe pain, immediate swelling and marked joint instability.

Grade I and most grade II injuries are treated conservatively with rest, ice, compression, elevation and non-steroidal anti-inflammatory drugs for 48 hours. Current evidence suggests that early functional treatment is probably better than immobilization in the treatment of lateral ligament injuries.[6–9]

Operative intervention for grade III lateral ligament injuries is controversial, although direct repair is usual for athletes. Conservative treatment involving cast immobilization for 6–8 weeks with orthopaedic follow-up is appropriate in the rest. Delayed surgical repair or reconstruction has similar results to early intervention.

Achilles tendon rupture

Achilles tendon rupture is traditionally associated with sedentary middle-aged individuals during a burst of unaccustomed strenuous physical activity, although young, fit athletes have also sustained this condition. Predisposing medical conditions include rheumatoid arthritis, systemic lupus erythematosus (SLE), chronic renal failure, gout, hyperparathyroidism and long-term steroid or ciprofloxacin use. The segment of the Achilles tendon particularly prone to rupture lies 2–6 cm proximal to the tendon's insertion into the calcaneus. The blood vessels that supply this area are prone to atrophy, and the resultant reduction in collagen cross-linking leads to a reduced tensile strength in the tendon.

History

Rupture usually occurs while pushing off with the weightbearing foot, but may occur with sudden dorsiflexion or direct trauma. The sensation of a direct blow to the back of the ankle and even an audible 'pop' are followed by difficulty in walking. The patient often states that they thought they had been hit from behind.

Examination

Examination may reveal a visible and palpable deficit in the tendon, but swelling around the tendon sheath may rapidly mask these signs. Some degree of plantarflexion of the ankle joint is preserved by the other long flexors of the ankle, foot and toes, and should not be used as a sign that the Achilles tendon is intact, although the patient cannot stand on tiptoe.

The calf-squeeze test (Thompson or Simmond's test)

There is loss of normal plantarflexion when lying prone compared with the unaffected side. The calf-squeeze test (Thompson or Simmond's test) confirms the diagnosis. Perform this with the patient kneeling on a chair with the feet hanging free over the edge. Alternatively, it is often more comfortable for the patient to lie prone with the feet and ankles extended beyond the end of the examination couch and hanging freely. Demonstrate normal plantarflexion initially on the unaffected calf, as it is gently squeezed just distal to its maximal girth. Absence of plantarflexion in the affected limb confirms Achilles rupture. Ultrasound is useful if the diagnosis is in doubt, and can demonstrate partial or full-thickness tears of the tendon.

Management

The choice of operative or non-operative treatment is controversial.[10] Surgery is usually recommended for younger patients and those who are diagnosed early. Operative risks include fistula formation, skin necrosis and infection. However, the procedure has a lower rate of muscle atrophy, a lower re-rupture rate, and allows an earlier resumption of physical activity.

Non-operative management includes applying a POP cast to the ankle in an equinus position to bring the two ends of the ruptured tendon into apposition. One regimen involves a cast for 4 weeks in equinus, 4 weeks in partial plantarflexion, and then 2 weeks in the neutral position. Complications of non-operative management include a higher re-rupture rate requiring surgical intervention.

Controversies

- Are physiotherapy and early mobilization the treatment of choice for low-grade sprains, as lengthy periods of immobilization and crutches are still employed?

- Should the enhanced stability and early return to mobilization of operative intervention be offered to all patients, rather than just for grade III sprained ankles as is currently reserved for elite athletes?

- Operative versus conservative management of Achilles tendon.

References

1. Stiell I, Greenberg G, McKnight R, et al. Decision rules for the use of radiography in acute ankle injury. Refinement and prospective validation. Journal of the American Medical Association 1993; 269: 1127–1132.
2. Bachmann L, Kolb E, Koller M, et al. Accuracy of Ottawa ankle rules to exclude fractures of the ankle and midfoot: systematic review. British Medical Journal 2003; 326: 417–423.
3. Libetta C, Burke D, Brennan P, et al. Validation of the Ottawa ankle rules in children. Journal of Accident and Emergency Medicine 1999; 16: 342–344.
4. Plint A, Bulloch B, Osmond M, et al. Validation of the Ottawa ankle rules in children with ankle injuries. Academic Emergency Medicine 1999; 6: 1005–1009.
5. Muller ME, Nazarian S, Koch P. The AO Classification of Fractures. New York: Springer-Verlag, 1988.
6. Jones M, Amendola A. Acute treatment of inversion ankle sprains: Immobilization versus functional treatment. Clinical Orthopaedics and Related Research 2007; 445: 169–172.
7. Karlsson J, Eriksson BI, Sward L. Early functional treatment for acute ligament injuries of the ankle joint. Scandinavian Journal of Medicine and Science in Sports 1996; 6: 341–345.
8. Van Dijk C. Management of the sprained ankle. British Journal of Sports Medicine 2002; 36: 83–84.
9. Bukata R. Contemporary treatment of ankle sprains Part II. Emergency Medicine and Acute Care Essays 2000; 24: 1.
10. Cetti R, Christensen S, Ejsted R. Operative versus non-operative treatment of Achilles tendon rupture: a prospective randomized study and review of the literature. American Journals of Sports Medicine 1993; 21: 791–799.

Further reading

Borrer R, Famo-Salek M, Totten V, et al. Managing ankle injuries in the emergency department. Journal of Emergency Medicine 1999; 17: 651–660.
Wedmore I, Charette J. Emergency department evaluation and treatment of ankle and foot injuries. Emergency Medical Clinics of North America 2000; 18: 85–113.

4.12 Foot injuries

Stuart Dilley • Michael Cadogan

ESSENTIALS

1 Standard radiological imaging includes AP, lateral and 45° internal oblique projections of the foot.

2 Most calcaneal fractures are intra-articular, and are associated with a Bohler's salient angle of less than 20°.

3 Major talar fractures have a significant risk of subsequent avascular necrosis.

4 Navicular body fractures may require internal fixation.

5 Fractures of the base of the second metatarsal are pathognomic of Lisfranc injury (Fleck sign).

Anatomy

The foot is composed of 28 bones with 57 articular surfaces. It may be divided into three anatomical regions: the hindfoot containing the talus and calcaneum; the midfoot containing the navicular, cuboid and cuneiforms; and the forefoot containing the metatarsals and phalanges.

The subtalar joint collectively describes the three articulations of the inferior aspect of the talus with the calcaneus. It allows inversion and eversion of the hindfoot. The midtarsal joints incorporate the talonavicular and calcaneocuboid joints. They connect the hindfoot and midfoot and allow abduction and adduction of the forefoot. The five tarsometatarsal joints (Lisfranc joints) connect the midfoot and forefoot and form an arch, which lends stability to the foot.

Clinical assessment

History

Injury to the foot occurs as a result of direct or indirect trauma. Indirect trauma from a twisting injury usually results in minor avulsion-type injuries. Direct trauma is often associated with considerable soft tissue swelling and fracture. Record any pain, swelling, loss of function, reduced sensation and deformity or associated ankle injuries.

Examination

Commence inspection with the patient lying on a bed with both lower limbs exposed. Comparison with the unaffected limb helps identify bruising, swelling, deformity, skin wounds, pallor or cyanosis. Start gentle and careful palpation over the entire foot away from the area of maximal pain. Point tenderness or crepitus may be elicited at the site of fracture. Specific sites to be palpated include the Achilles tendon, calcaneus, base of the fifth metatarsal and the area under the head of the second metatarsal.

Ask the patient to demonstrate active foot movements before performing gentle passive movements and comparing with the other foot. Subtalar motion is evaluated with the foot in a neutral position, with one hand on the lower leg and the other holding the heel. The heel is inverted and everted and should attain 25° of motion.

Midtarsal motion is assessed with one hand stabilizing the heel while the other hand grasps the forefoot at the bases of the metatarsals. The forefoot is pronated, supinated, adducted and abducted. Finally, forefoot motion is evaluated by individually flexing and extending the metatarsophalangeal (MTP) and interphalangeal (IP) joints.

Ask the patient to stand and walk if no obvious focus of the pain is found during the initial examination, to assess gait and the ability to bear weight. Then assess the circulation of the foot by observing capillary refill, skin colour, and the presence of dorsalis pedis and posterior tibial pulses.

The posterior tibial pulse is palpable behind the medial malleolus unless there is excessive swelling or damage to the artery. The dorsalis pedis is more variable, being too small or absent in 12% of the population. Doppler may be needed to determine the presence of flow if there is doubt. Neurological assessment includes motor and sensory function.

Radiology

Standard radiological imaging includes AP, lateral and 45° internal oblique projections. The lateral view visualizes the hindfoot and soft tissues, whereas oblique and AP projections provide the best images of the midfoot and forefoot. An axial calcaneal view is best to visualize the hindfoot, if calcaneal fracture is suspected with pain around the heel or there is a history of a fall from a height.

The Ottawa Ankle and Foot Rules

The Ottawa Ankle and Foot Rules[1,2] include indications for X-ray for suspected midfoot fractures. All patients with obvious deformities should have X-rays. However, if clinical findings are more subtle, a foot X-ray is only required if there is pain in the midfoot region and any one of:

- Bone tenderness over the navicular.
- Bone tenderness over the base of the fifth metatarsal.
- The patient was unable to bear weight for at least four steps, both immediately after the injury and at the time of emergency department (ED) evaluation.

These rules do not apply to suspected hindfoot or forefoot fractures.

Other investigations

Bone scans are indicated when a stress fracture is suspected and may become positive 2–3 weeks before conventional radiographs demonstrate a fracture. Computed tomography (CT) is an excellent modality for imaging the calcaneum, subtalar joint and Lisfranc joint complex in more difficult injuries, or when a fracture is strongly suspected but plain X-rays are inconclusive.

Hindfoot injuries

Calcaneal fractures

The calcaneus is the largest bone in the foot and is the most commonly fractured tarsal bone. The calcaneus forms the heel of the foot, provides vertical support for the body's weight, and functions as a springboard for locomotion. Fractures of the calcaneus occur as a result of direct axial compression during falls from a height. Seven percent are bilateral. Lower-extremity injuries are present in 25% of cases, and vertebral compression fractures are found in 10%.

Classification

Seventy-five per cent of calcaneal fractures are intra-articular. Fractures may be non-displaced, displaced or frequently comminuted, owing to cancellous bone in the calcaneus and the magnitude of force associated with these fractures (Fig. 4.12.1).

Clinical assessment

Patients usually present following a fall with direct trauma to the heel. The patient may be able to walk, but weightbearing on the heel is impossible. Examination reveals pain, swelling and tenderness over the heel, with bruising that may extend over the sole of the foot. Associated fractures are common, and examination of the vertebral column, pelvis, affected lower extremity and opposing calcaneus is essential, as 10% of patients have additional cervical or lumbar crush fractures.

Radiology

Standard X-rays are usually sufficient to reveal most comminuted calcaneal fractures, whereas more subtle fractures are visualized with the aid of specific calcaneal (Harris or axial) views. The AP view highlights the anterosuperior calcaneus and calcaneocuboid joint. The lateral view may reveal compression fractures of the body and posterior facet. Bohler's salient angle normally ranges from 20° to 40° measured on the lateral X-ray. A compression fracture is likely if Bohler's angle is less than 20°.[3] A CT scan is necessary to define complex fractures and is useful in preoperative planning.

Management

Calcaneal fractures are notoriously difficult to manage and frequently have a poor outcome, with up to 50% suffering chronic pain and functional disability. Intra-articular, displaced and comminuted fractures are prone to gross swelling of the foot and have a risk of compartment syndrome. Admit patients with these fractures for elevation, further imaging and consideration of surgical intervention.

Operative intervention may be indicated in younger patients and those with greater degrees of Bohler's angle disruption.[4] Extra-articular fractures are usually non-displaced and are treated conservatively in a posterior non-weightbearing cast for 6 weeks.

Talar fractures

The talus provides support for the body when standing, and bears more weight per surface area than any other foot bone. It has no muscular attachments and is held in place by the malleoli and ligaments, and comprises a head, neck and body. The head has articulations with the navicular and calcaneus, and the body articulates with the tibia, fibula and calcaneus. The neck joins the head and body and is extra-articular. The blood supply to the talus arises from an anastomotic ring from the peroneal, posterior and anterior tibial arteries, and is tenuous and easily disrupted, leading to avascular necrosis.

Mechanism and classification

Talar fractures are the second most common tarsal fracture, and are either major or minor. Minor fractures are caused by inversion injuries to the plantar- or dorsi-flexed foot, often from minimal trauma, and may present as an apparent ankle sprain.

Major talar fractures follow significant force, such as a motor vehicle accident, or involve axial loading in a fall from a height (when they are associated with calcaneal fracture).

Hawkins classification of talar neck fractures

Talar neck fractures account for 50% of major talar injuries and are related to extreme dorsiflexion injuries. The Hawkins classification is commonly used to describe these fractures. Type I fractures are non-displaced with the fracture line entering the subtalar joint between the middle and

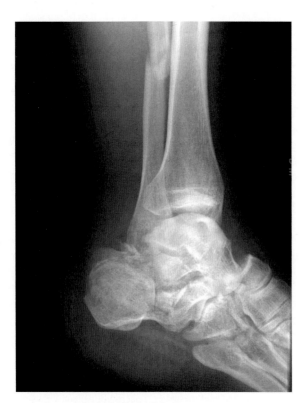

Fig. 4.12.1 Intra-articular comminuted calcaneal fracture.

posterior facets. The risk of avascular necrosis (AVN) in these injuries is < 10%.

Type II fractures are identified by any degree of displacement or subtalar subluxation, and have an incidence of AVN of 30%. Type III injuries involve displaced talar neck fractures with dislocation from both the subtalar and ankle joints. The incidence of AVN is up to 90%. Commonly associated injuries include vertebral compression, calcaneal and medial malleolar fractures.

Talar dome fractures

Talar dome fractures are difficult to diagnose on plain films, though a large ankle joint effusion may be apparent. Specific plain X-ray talar views are necessary, although CT scans are frequently required to confirm the diagnosis. It is important to diagnose these fractures as they involve the weightbearing articular surface of the talus within the ankle joint.

Talar head fractures are uncommon and result from a compressive force applied to the plantarflexed foot, and are associated with disruption of the talonavicular joint, navicular fractures and anterior malleolar fractures. Talar body fractures are usually of the minor avulsion type. Lateral process fractures are being seen more frequently as snowboarding injuries.

Talar dome, lateral talar process and posterior talar process fractures are frequently missed and diagnosed as ankle sprains. A high index of suspicion is needed in order to identify these fractures and avoid long-term complications that might arise from a delay in diagnosis and treatment.[5]

Clinical evaluation

Minor talar fractures are usually subtle. The patient presents following an inversion injury with mild swelling around the ankle joint and is able to partially bear weight. Active plantar- and dorsiflexion are possible, but inversion and eversion at the subtalar joint is painful. Major talar fractures are associated with large compressive forces and cause considerable swelling and tenderness dorsally.

Radiology

Standard X-rays of the foot will reveal all but the most subtle avulsion fractures. CT scans are required when there is clinical suspicion of talar fracture, but plain films are inconclusive.

Management

Major talar fractures have a significant risk of subsequent avascular necrosis. Displaced fractures, especially if associated with neurovascular or cutaneous compromise, should be reduced in the ED under appropriate analgesia and procedural sedation by grasping the hindfoot and midfoot and applying longitudinal traction in plantarflexion. Apply a POP posterior splint with the ankle flexed at 90°.

Emergency closed reduction is used to improve fracture alignment and to reduce the risk of vascular compromise. Refer major fractures to an orthopaedic specialist for consideration of open reduction and internal fixation. Minor talar fractures are treated with a below-knee non-weightbearing posterior cast with orthopaedic follow-up.

Subtalar dislocation

Subtalar dislocations are rare and follow considerable deforming forces. Such injuries involve the simultaneous dislocation of the talonavicular and talocalcaneal joints, with preservation of the tibiotalar joint.

Mechanism and classification

Subtalar dislocations are often associated with motor vehicle accidents, but a significant number are incurred during sport, particularly basketball. They are described in terms of the final position of the foot in relation to the talus following dislocation. Medial dislocations account for 85% of these injuries and are caused by forceful foot inversion in plantarflexion. Ten per cent of subtalar dislocations are open, and 50% are associated with proximally located injuries.[6]

Clinical assessment

Subtalar dislocations are associated with obvious deformity, swelling, and tension of the skin over the opposing joint margin. Neurovascular status should be examined but is rarely compromised. Standard X-rays are difficult to interpret because of the distortion of the foot. The most helpful is the AP view, which confirms disruption of the talonavicular joint.

Management

Reduce closed subtalar dislocations in the ED under appropriate analgesia and procedural sedation to minimize the chance of the skin tented over the head of the talus becoming necrotic.

Closed reduction of a medial subtalar dislocation requires firm longitudinal traction applied to the foot, with countertraction on the leg with the knee flexed to relax the tension from the Achilles tendon on the calcaneum, thereby increasing the mobility of the hindfoot. The foot is initially inverted to accentuate the deformity, and then everted with digital pressure over the head of the talus to reverse the deformity. Eighty per cent of dislocations may be reduced non-operatively. Following reduction, the ankle is placed in a posterior POP splint in 90° of flexion. Orthopaedic consultation is required.

Midfoot fractures

The midfoot comprises the navicular, cuboid and cuneiform bones. It is inherently stable and is rarely injured. However, midfoot fractures are often associated with a delay in diagnosis owing to the difficulty in X-ray interpretation and poorly localized pain. The Ottawa Ankle Rules[1] are an accurate tool to assist in determining which patients with midfoot pain require imaging.

Navicular fractures

The navicular is a curved bone with extensive articulations. It has a tenuous blood supply and, like the talus, is susceptible to avascular necrosis.

Mechanism and classification

The navicular is the most commonly injured of the midfoot bones, although the overall incidence is rare. Fractures may involve the dorsal surface, the tuberosity or the body. Dorsal avulsion fractures are the most common. They occur in eversion injuries and are associated with deltoid ligament or talonavicular capsular injury. Tuberosity fractures also result from eversion injuries with avulsion of the posterior tibial tendon insertion. Body fractures from axial loading are rare and are frequently comminuted.

Clinical evaluation

Point tenderness is elicited over the dorsum and medial aspect of the midfoot.

Passive eversion and active inversion reproduce the pain. Standard X-rays usually reveal the fracture, but bone or CT scans may be required.

Management

Refer all intra-articular, displaced and comminuted fractures to the orthopaedic specialist in the ED, as they are frequently complicated by subsequent avascular necrosis. Dorsal avulsion and tuberosity fractures are treated conservatively in a walking cast for 6 weeks. Navicular body fractures may require internal fixation.

Cuboid fractures

Isolated cuboid fractures are rare, and are most commonly associated with Lisfranc-type injuries with lateral subluxation of the midtarsal joint, the 'nutcracker' fracture, and fractures of the posterior malleolus. They are best visualized with an oblique foot X-ray.

Management

Treatment ranges from weightbearing POP casts for undisplaced fractures to operative fixation for displaced and comminuted fractures. All cuboid fractures require orthopaedic consultation.

Cuneiform fractures

These fractures are extremely rare. They usually occur with direct trauma, and an associated Lisfranc injury should be excluded. Displaced fractures require orthopaedic intervention, but non-displaced fractures are treated conservatively in a cast.

Lisfranc fractures and dislocations

The Lisfranc joint includes the articulation of the first three metatarsal bases with their respective cuneiforms, and the fourth and fifth metatarsal bases with the cuboid. The second metatarsal is the most important structure within this complex as it holds the key to stability.

Mechanism and classification

Injury results from rotational forces applied to the fixed forefoot, axial loads and crush injuries. Although commonly associated with vehicular crashes, Lisfranc injuries may also occur in sports that involve fixation of the forefoot, such as horse-riding and rowing. They are classified by the direction of dislocation in the horizontal plane.

Divergent dislocations usually involve medial and lateral splaying of the first and second metatarsals. All five metatarsals are displaced in the same direction in ipsilateral injuries, either medially or laterally. In isolated dislocations, one or more of the metatarsals are displaced away from the others.

Lisfranc dislocations are usually associated with fracture of the metatarsals, especially the second metatarsal base, and with fracture of the midfoot in 40% of cases.[7] Although vascular compromise is uncommon, significant haemorrhage may occur with disruption of the dorsalis pedis branch to the plantar arch as it passes between the first and second metatarsal bases.

Clinical assessment

Lisfranc injuries should be suspected when midfoot fractures are present. They are associated with severe midfoot pain and an inability to bear weight on the toes. Examination may reveal deformity, swelling and bruising over the dorsum of the foot. Point tenderness over the joint, with pain on passive abduction and pronation, may also be present.

Radiology

Standard X-rays are sufficient to visualize most Lisfranc injuries. AP views identify Lisfranc fractures and oblique views determine their alignment. Lateral views demonstrate the soft tissues and identify the presence of dorsal or plantar displacement. Fractures of the base of the second metatarsal are pathognomic of a Lisfranc injury (Fleck sign).

Management

Refer all Lisfranc injuries for orthopaedic consultation. Most are treated with closed reduction and K-wire fixation, followed by non-weightbearing for 12 weeks. Despite aggressive management chronic pain, reflex sympathetic dystrophy and degenerative arthritis are common.

Forefoot fractures

Metatarsal shaft fractures

Metatarsal shaft fractures occur as a result of direct trauma or a rotational injury to the fixed forefoot. The second and third metatarsals are relatively fixed and are prone to stress fractures. Metatarsal fractures are associated with difficulty in weightbearing, and ill-defined tenderness and bruising over the plantar aspect of the foot. They are also commonly associated with Lisfranc injuries and phalangeal fractures. Standard X-rays will detect most fractures and determine their alignment, angulation and displacement.

Management

Undisplaced shaft fractures of the second to fifth metatarsals are treated in a below-knee walking cast for 3–4 weeks. Closed reduction and application of a non-weightbearing cast for 6 weeks is necessary when these fractures have more than 3 mm of displacement or 10° of angulation.

Injury to the great toe metatarsal requires more aggressive treatment because of its load-bearing function. Non-displaced fractures require 4–6 weeks in a non-weightbearing cast, whereas displaced fractures require operative treatment. Therefore, orthopaedic consultation is required for multiple or displaced fractures and all fractures of the great toe metatarsal.

Metatarsal head and neck fractures

These fractures are usually the result of direct trauma and are often multiple. Non-displaced fractures are treated with a walking cast for 4–6 weeks, and displaced fractures require closed reduction to maintain the integrity of the transverse arch.

Fractures of the base of fifth metatarsal

These are the most common of the metatarsal fractures, and there are two distinct types. The most common fracture is that of the fifth metatarsal tuberosity, which occurs when the plantarflexed foot undergoes sudden inversion. It is caused by avulsion of the lateral band of the plantar aponeurosis and is usually extra-articular.

Jones fracture

The second type of fracture is known as the Jones fracture[8] and is defined as a transverse fracture through the base of the fifth metatarsal from 15 to 31 mm distal to the proximal end of the bone. This fracture is intra-articular, as it involves the intermetatarsal articulation of the fourth and fifth metatarsals. Jones fractures occur when a load is applied to the lateral aspect of the foot without inversion. Activities such as jumping and dancing are typically associated with such injuries, which may also occur as 'stress-type' injuries due to repetitive strain.

The patient has difficulty weightbearing with both types of fracture, and there is point tenderness over the fifth metatarsal tuberosity and passive inversion is painful. Intra-articular fractures, which involve more than 30% of the articular surface or more than 2 mm of displacement, may require surgical fixation. Extra-articular tuberosity fractures heal well regardless of size or degree of displacement. They are treated symptomatically with either a compression bandage or, less commonly, a POP walking cast for 3 weeks. Non-displaced fractures are treated in a non-weightbearing cast for 6 weeks.

In children the normal growth plate at the base of the fifth metatarsal should not be confused with an acute fracture. Fracture lines usually pass transversely through the base of the fifth metatarsal, whereas growth plates run in a longitudinal or oblique direction.

Metatarsophalangeal (MTP) dislocations

MTP dislocations are uncommon. The fifth MTP joint is most commonly dislocated laterally when the little toe is snagged on an object. First or hallux MTP joint dislocations are usually dorsal and follow violent hyperextension injuries. They are usually obvious, with the metatarsal head palpable on the plantar surface. Other dislocations are usually more subtle.

Management

Most MTP joint dislocations are easily reduced with longitudinal traction under local anaesthesia. After reduction they are managed with a buddy strap. First MTP joint dislocations are more difficult to reduce and may require open reduction if there is buttonholing of the joint capsule. They should be treated in a POP walking cast with a toe-plate extension for 3 weeks.

Phalangeal fractures and dislocations

Phalangeal fractures are common and usually occur with direct trauma, most often involving the proximal phalanx. They are associated with pain, deformity and difficulty walking.

Management

Non-displaced fractures heal well and are 'buddy strapped' to reduce pain and prevent displacement. Place gauze between the splinted toes to prevent skin maceration. Pain may be expected for up to 3 weeks until the fracture is stabilized by callus.

Reduce displaced fractures with traction under digital nerve anaesthesia. Operative fixation may be indicated if the fracture is unstable, especially if it is intra-articular, involves the hallux or is rotated.

Interphalangeal dislocations are uncommon and usually involve the hallux. They are reduced with longitudinal traction under digital nerve anaesthesia. Those involving the great toe require a toe-plated walking cast for 3 weeks following reduction. All other interphalangeal dislocations are treated with a buddy strap once reduced.

Controversies

- Optimal use of nurse-initiated X-ray in lower limb injuries.

- Best imaging modality for osteochondral talar dome fractures.

- Role of the bone scan, CT and MRI in other foot injuries.

References

1. Bajammal S, Tornetta P, Sanders D, et al. Displaced intra-articular calcaneal fractures. Journal of Orthopaedics and Trauma 2005; 19: 360–364.
2. Bachmann L, Kolb E, Koller M, et al. Accuracy of Ottawa ankle rules to exclude fractures of the ankle and midfoot: systematic review. British Medical Journal 2003; 326: 417–423.
3. Chen M, Bohrer S, Kelly T, et al. Boehler's angle: A reappraisal. Annals of Emergency Medicine 1991; 20: 122–124.
4. Judd DB, Kim DH. Foot fractures frequently misdiagnosed as ankle sprains. American Family Physician 2002; 66: 785–794.
5. Lawrence S, Botte M. Jones' fractures and related fractures of the proximal fifth metatarsal. Foot and Ankle International 1993; 14: 358–365.
6. Merchan E. Subtalar dislocations: Long-term follow-up of 39 cases. Injury 1992; 23: 97–100.
7. Stiell I, Greenberg G, McKnight R, et al. Decision rules for the use of radiography in acute ankle injury. Refinement and prospective validation. Journal of the American Medical Association 1993; 269: 1127–1132.
8. Vuori J, Aro H. Lisfranc joint injuries: Trauma mechanisms and associated injuries. Journal of Trauma 1993; 35: 40–45.

Further reading

Heckman JD. Fractures and dislocations of the foot. In: Rockwood CA, Green DP, Bucholz RW, eds. Rockwood and Green's fractures in adults, 3rd edn. Philadelphia: JB Lippincott, 1991; 2267–2405.

ORTHOPAEDIC EMERGENCIES

4

CARDIOVASCULAR

Edited by **Anne-Maree Kelly**

5.1 Chest pain

Steve Goodacre

ESSENTIALS

1 Acute coronary syndrome (ACS) is common, life threatening and treatable, so identifying and treating ACS is fundamental to chest pain management.

2 Serious alternative causes, such as pulmonary embolus or aortic dissection, and extrathoracic causes, such as pancreatitis or peptic ulcer, should not be overlooked.

3 Anxiety-related chest pain is common, significantly impairs quality of life and is treatable, yet it is often ignored or dismissed.

4 Gastro-oesophageal pain should generally only be diagnosed in the emergency department after ACS has been ruled out.

5 A normal ECG does not rule out ACS.

6 Troponin predicts adverse outcome. Patients with a positive troponin may benefit from inpatient investigation and treatment. Patients with a negative troponin taken at least 6 hours after symptom onset are unlikely to benefit from inpatient care, although this does not rule out coronary heart disease.

7 Cardiac biomarkers should be judged on the basis of their specificity and prognostic value, not just sensitivity.

Introduction

Chest pain is one of the most common presenting complaints in emergency medicine. It is also associated with life-threatening pathology, so it is arguably the most important complaint faced by the emergency physician. It is certainly one of the most challenging. Failure to appropriately diagnose and manage patients with acute chest pain is a frequent cause of avoidable mortality and morbidity, and is a leading cause of malpractice litigation. It is therefore not surprising that physicians often err on the side of caution, but this can also have adverse consequences for the patient and society. Patient anxieties following unnecessary investigation are often unrecognized but may severely affect quality of life, and over-investigation and unnecessary hospital admission for chest pain waste millions of healthcare dollars each year.

Epidemiology

The incidence of acute chest pain presenting to the emergency department (ED) appears to be increasing. Awareness of the importance of early treatment for myocardial infarction has led to public information campaigns that increase ED attendances with chest pain. Meanwhile, general practitioners are increasingly being bypassed in favour of an emergency ambulance response. These changes in health service use have coincided in many developed countries with a reduction in the incidence of coronary heart disease. It therefore seems likely that patients presenting to the ED with acute chest pain have a decreasing prevalence of acute coronary syndrome (ACS) and an increasing prevalence of more benign conditions.

Differential diagnosis

The main differential diagnoses are outlined in Table 5.1.1. The most common causes of acute chest pain are ACS (unstable angina or myocardial infarction), musculoskeletal pain, anxiety, gastro-oesophageal pain and non-specific chest pain. The most serious causes (in terms of threat to life) are ACS, pulmonary embolism and aortic dissection. Because ACS is both common and life-threatening it is inevitably the primary focus of assessment. ACS is discussed in detail in Chapter 5.2, pulmonary embolus in Chapter 5.5 and aortic dissection in Chapter 5.10.

Musculoskeletal chest pain may be related to a precipitating episode, such as chest wall injury or physical overexertion. Alternatively, it may be caused by inflammation in chest wall structures. Tietze's syndrome (costochondritis) is most commonly seen in women and is characterized by tenderness of the costochondral cartilages. Epidemic myalgia (Bornholm disease) is due to inflammation of chest wall muscles and pleura occurring after viral infection, typically with Coxsackie

Table 5.1.1	Causes of acute chest pain
Musculoskeletal	Muscular strain Epidemic myalgia Tietze's syndrome
Cardiac	Myocardial infarction Unstable angina Stable angina
Pericardial	Pneumomediastinum Pericarditis
Gastro-oesophageal	Gastro-oesophageal reflux Oesophageal spasm
Psychological	Anxiety/panic attacks Hyperventilation Cardiac neurosis
Pleuritic	Pulmonary embolus Pneumothorax Pleurisy Pneumonia
Neurological	Cervical/thoracic nerve root compression Herpes zoster
Abdominal	Peptic ulcer Biliary colic/cholecystitis Pancreatitis
Mixed	Aortic dissection

B virus. Herpes zoster produces severe pain along the distribution of a thoracic nerve that may be misdiagnosed as musculoskeletal pain if the patient presents before any rash or vesicles have developed.

Gastro-oesophageal pain occurs when gastric contents reflux into the oesophagus or when the oesophageal muscles spasm. Pneumomediastinum can occur spontaneously after vigorous exercise, vomiting or an asthma attack, or may be associated with barotrauma from diving or inhalation during drug abuse. Pericarditis is most commonly caused by viral infection, but may be associated with systemic illness, such as uraemia or autoimmune disease, or follow myocardial infarction or cardiac surgery (Dressler's syndrome).

Anxiety-related chest pain is a common and frequently unrecognized cause of acute chest pain. It may also coexist with and be an important factor alongside other causes of chest pain. The patient with coronary heart disease and anxiety-related chest pain presents a particularly difficult diagnostic and management challenge. Anxiety may be related to a specific serious cause of chest pain and can be exacerbated by misguided efforts to provide reassurance through diagnostic testing. In extreme cases this can lead to 'cardiac neurosis', in which the patient's anxieties about cardiac disease cause more severe disruption to their daily activities and quality of life than would be expected from the pathology that worries them.

Pleurisy is typically caused by viral infection and produces pain that is worse on inspiration. It may be differentiated from pulmonary embolus by the presence of systemic features and the absence of breathlessness or risk factors for thromboembolism, although investigation for pulmonary embolism is often required. Pneumonia and pneumothorax can also cause pleuritic pain, but should be evident on chest radiography.

There are a number of serious abdominal complaints that may present as chest pain. These include biliary colic (acute biliary pain), cholecystitis, peptic ulcer disease and pancreatitis. Failure to take a careful history and examine the abdomen may lead to delayed diagnosis.

Finally, a substantial proportion of patients will be labelled entirely appropriately as 'non-specific chest pain' after ED evaluation.

These patients have pain that simply cannot be categorized into a clear diagnostic group. It is more honest to accept this than to apply an inaccurate diagnostic label.

Clinical features

Clinical assessment is primarily aimed at identifying patients with a significant risk of serious pathology who require further investigation and possibly inpatient care. The most common serious pathology is ACS, so clinical assessment is often focused on associated features; other serious conditions, however, such as pulmonary embolism and aortic dissection, should not be neglected.

ACS is classically associated with chest pain that is crushing, gripping or squeezing in nature and radiates to the left arm, but presenting features in the ED may be much more variable, particularly in patients with no past history of coronary heart disease and a non-diagnostic ECG. Table 5.1.2 shows the likelihood ratios of clinical features that may help to diagnose ACS. It is notable that pain radiating to the right arm or to both arms is a powerful predictor of ACS. Pain described as 'burning' or 'like indigestion' can be associated with ACS in ED patients, as is pain occurring on exertion. So the diagnoses of gastro-oesophageal reflux or stable angina should be made with great caution. Pain that is sharp or associated with inspiration or movement is less likely to be cardiac, but these findings alone do not exclude ACS. Risk factors for coronary heart disease should be routinely recorded, although they may have surprisingly little diagnostic value. This is perhaps because patients are aware of these risk factors and take them into account when deciding whether or not to seek help for episodes of chest pain. In this respect, social and cultural factors may have an importance influence upon patients' interpretation of their symptoms and health-seeking behaviour.

Clinical examination is of limited diagnostic value and aimed mainly at identifying non-cardiac causes of chest pain or complications of ACS, such as arrhythmia, heart failure or cardiogenic shock. Pain that can be reproduced by chest wall palpation is less likely to be cardiac, but this finding does not exclude the possibility of ACS.

Table 5.1.2 Likelihood ratios of clinical features useful for diagnosing acute myocardial infarction	
Useful for ruling in myocardial infarction	
Radiation to the right arm or shoulder	4.7
Radiation to both arms or shoulders	4.1
Described as burning or like indigestion	2.8
Association with exertion	2.4
Radiation to left arm	2.3
Associated with diaphoresis	2.0
Associated with nausea or vomiting	1.9
Worse than previous angina or similar to previous myocardial infarction	1.8
Described as pressure	1.3
Useful for ruling out myocardial infarction	
Described as pleuritic	0.2
Described as positional	0.3
Described as sharp	0.3
Reproducible by palpation	0.3
Inframammary location	0.8
Not associated with exertion	0.8

It is also important to determine specifically that chest wall palpation is reproducing the pain that led to presentation. Simply identifying chest wall tenderness has little value – everyone has a tender chest wall if you press hard enough!

Clinical assessment should not just focus on ACS, but should aim to positively identify other causes. Pulmonary embolism is diagnostically challenging. Suspicion should be raised by chest pain that is clearly pleuritic in nature, haemoptysis, associated breathlessness, features of deep vein thrombosis or risk factors for venous thromboembolism (immobilization, malignancy, recent trauma or surgery, pregnancy, intravenous drug abuse or previous thromboembolism). Clinical examination may reveal tachycardia, tachypnoea or features of deep vein thrombosis (see Chapter 5.5). Aortic dissection is characterized by severe pain radiating to the back with associated diaphoresis. Neurological symptoms or signs, sometimes transient, are common. Clinical examination may reveal a discrepancy between blood pressure in the right and left arms (see Chapter 5.10).

Clinical assessment of chest pain should always include examination of the abdomen to identify tenderness, guarding, rebound tenderness or a positive Murphy's sign.

Unnecessary investigation can be avoided if non life-threatening pathology can be confidently diagnosed by clinical assessment. Pain that is reproduced by chest wall palpation in a patient at low risk of coronary heart disease and with no significant risk factors for pulmonary embolus can be confidently diagnosed as musculoskeletal. A positive diagnosis is particularly valuable for the patient who is suffering primarily from anxiety-related symptoms. In this case pain is typically described as tightness around the chest and associated with a feeling of restricted breathing. Other features include palpitations (particularly awareness of the heartbeat), sweating, breathlessness, light-headedness, feelings of panic, or paraesthesia of the lips or fingertips.

Clinical investigation

The ECG is the most useful clinical investigation and should be performed on all patients presenting with acute non-traumatic chest pain. Table 5.1.3 shows the value of ECG features for diagnosing myocardial infarction. It is important to recognize that a normal ECG does not rule out myocardial infarction. ST segment elevation or depression, new Q-waves and new conduction defects are specific for acute myocardial infarction and

Table 5.1.3 Likelihood ratios of ECG features useful for diagnosing acute myocardial infarction	
New ST elevation >1 mm	5.7–53.9
New Q wave	5.3–24.8
Any ST-segment elevation	11.2
New conduction defect	6.3
New ST-segment depression	3.0–5.2
Any Q wave	3.9
Any ST-segment depression	3.2
T-wave peaking and/or inversion >1 mm	3.1
New T-wave inversion	2.4–2.8
Any conduction defect	2.7

predict adverse outcome. Patients with these features should be managed in a coronary care unit. Other changes associated with myocardial infarction are less helpful. T-wave changes are often non-specific and may be positional, or due to numerous other causes. ECG changes in pulmonary embolism are also non-specific.

A standard 12-lead ECG may be augmented by serial ECG recording or continuous ST-segment monitoring. These may detect evolving ECG changes or dynamic ST segment changes. However, these techniques may also identify non-specific false-positive changes, such as minor T-wave inversions, especially if they are used inappropriately in patients with a low risk of coronary heart disease. ST-segment monitoring was developed for the high-risk coronary care population. In low-risk ED patients with chest pain it has a very low yield of significant positive findings.

Like clinical examination, the chest radiograph is mainly intended to identify non-cardiac causes for chest pain, such as a pneumothorax or fractured rib, and complications of myocardial infarction, such as left ventricular failure. Although it is often routinely ordered it is also often unhelpful.

Biochemical cardiac markers are key investigations in acute chest pain and are a source of much heated debate. They are also a rapidly developing technology, so this chapter will focus on the principles that should guide their use.

Three key features determine the clinical value of a cardiac marker. The sensitivity tells us how good the marker is at identifying patients with disease, and thus how useful it is for ruling out myocardial ischaemia. The specificity tells us how good the marker is at identifying patients without disease, and thus how useful it is for ruling in myocardial ischaemia (i.e. a specific test that is positive suggests that the patient is very likely to have ischaemia). The prognostic value (often expressed as a relative risk) tells us how good the marker is at predicting future adverse events, such as death, myocardial infarction or life-threatening arrhythmia.

Intuitively, clinicians tend to be most concerned about sensitivity. If a marker lacks sensitivity then it may miss cases of myocardial infarction, leading to potentially catastrophic discharge home without appropriate treatment. However, sensitivity and specificity are often related and may be influenced by the threshold of the marker used to determine a positive test. The lower the threshold used for a positive test the higher the sensitivity and the lower the specificity. Many evaluations of new markers deliberately optimize sensitivity by selecting a low threshold and sacrificing specificity. This may be an acceptable trade-off in a high-risk population, but ED patients with no past history of coronary heart disease and a non-diagnostic ECG typically have a low prevalence of myocardial infarction (<10%). In these circumstances a test with low specificity will generate many false positive results, requiring hospital admission and investigation, as well as unnecessary anxiety for the patient.

The prognostic value of a marker is arguably even more useful than its diagnostic parameters, particularly if the marker can predict high-risk patients who will benefit from treatment. If a prognostically powerful marker is positive then we know the patient needs active intervention; if it is negative then we know that, even if further investigation is required to identify the exact cause of their chest pain, they are unlikely to benefit from hospital admission and treatment.

Prognostic considerations explain recent changes in the definition of myocardial infarction. The original World Health Organization (WHO) definition of myocardial infarction was based on creatinine kinase, a cardiac marker with limited sensitivity and specificity, and only weak evidence of an association with adverse prognosis. The new American Heart Association/European Society of Cardiology definition is based on troponin. Research has shown that the higher the troponin level in ACS the higher the risk of adverse outcome. Furthermore, there appears to be no threshold below which a detectable troponin level carries the same prognosis as no detectable troponin. This makes troponin the optimal cardiac marker for defining myocardial infarction. However, because troponin detects degrees of myocardial damage that are not detected by creatinine kinase, the adoption of troponin in the definition of myocardial infarction has created an apparent increase in the incidence of myocardial

infarction. This has led to problems in measuring the sensitivity and specificity of cardiac markers, as these parameters depend on the definition of myocardial infarction used.

Creatinine kinase is released by damaged myocardium, but is also released by muscle and liver, and is measurable in the blood in the absence of pathology. Its MB isoenzyme (CK-MB) is more cardiac specific but shares the same problems. Substantial myocardial damage is required to produce an elevated CK-MB, but CK-MB may also be elevated in the absence of myocardial injury. Its role in diagnosis is becoming increasingly limited, although there is some evidence that measuring the gradient of the CK-MB mass assay may allow early diagnosis of myocardial infarction.

There are two troponin assays, troponin I and troponin T, with little to choose between them in terms of diagnostic or prognostic performance. As mentioned above, any detectable troponin has prognostic significance and suggests pathology. This does not mean that troponin is perfectly specific for ACS. Troponin can be elevated in pulmonary embolus, sepsis, renal failure, congestive cardiac failure and a number of other illnesses. However, in the emergency setting it is reasonable to conclude that any detectable troponin suggests serious pathology that needs inpatient investigation and treatment. This makes troponin an excellent blood test for the ED. It can be used liberally to detect serious pathology with minimal risk of generating false positives.

The only major limitation of troponin is its lack of early sensitivity. It is estimated that troponin takes up to 12 hours after symptom onset to achieve optimal sensitivity. If it is used too early after symptom onset it may produce a false negative result. This has led to the widespread practice of delaying troponin measurement until at least 12 hours after symptom onset to achieve optimal sensitivity. This practice may not be ideal because:

- Most patients present a few hours after symptom onset, so enforcing a 12-hour delay will typically require hospital admission or use of observation facilities. If there is limited availability of such facilities, clinicians may feel under

pressure to discharge the patient without any testing. Thus a strategy intended to increase patient safety may paradoxically put patients at risk when applied in the real world.
- There is emerging evidence that newer, more sensitive troponin assays have good early sensitivity and, particularly when applied to low-risk patients, can reliably rule out myocardial infarction within 6 hours of symptom onset.

Myoglobin is released early after myocardial damage and may be useful for detecting myocardial infarction during the initial hours after symptom onset. It has very poor specificity, however, so most patients with chest pain and an elevated myoglobin will not have myocardial infarction. This limitation can be addressed to some extent by ignoring the absolute level of myoglobin and basing decision-making on the gradient rise between two measurements.

Markers of myocardial damage, such as troponin and CK-MB, tend to have limited early sensitivity because it takes time for these enzymes to be released from damaged myocardium and achieve detectable levels in the serum. Recent interest has therefore focused on biochemical markers that detect ischaemia, such as ischaemia-modified albumin and heart-type fatty acid-binding protein. These markers may have better early sensitivity than markers of myocardial damage and may identify patients with ischaemia but no infarction. Research is currently under way to define their role.

Many other biomarkers are being developed and emergency physicians can expect to see headline-grabbing publications extolling their virtues. However, they should be wary before indiscriminately using new markers in patients with chest pain. As described earlier, ED patients with chest pain are a heterogeneous population with a relatively low prevalence of ACS compared to the high-risk patients who usually comprise research study populations. Indiscriminate use of markers with limited specificity will lead to many false positive results and consequent patient anxiety, unnecessary investigation and waste of resources.

Provocative cardiac testing, usually using an exercise treadmill, is becoming a practical option in many EDs. Patients typically undergo a short period of observation and cardiac marker testing to rule out myocardial infarction before undergoing an exercise treadmill test. Concerns about the safety of this procedure have been addressed by data from a number of centres: however, it should be recognized that selection of low-risk patients plays a key role in ensuring safety. Performing an exercise test on a patient with ACS can be an alarming experience!

Exercise treadmill testing has limited sensitivity and specificity for coronary heart disease, but is prognostically useful and predicts the risk of adverse events over the months following attendance. It is therefore used to risk-stratify rather than to diagnose. A patient with a negative treadmill test may have coronary heart disease but can be reassured that they are at low risk of an adverse outcome.

The combination of observation and cardiac marker testing to rule out myocardial infarction, followed by provocative cardiac testing to risk-stratify, has been adopted in many hospitals in the form of a chest pain pathway or chest pain unit. These have a number of potential benefits for patients and health services, and some evidence to suggest that they reduce the probability of admission, reduce the risk of discharge with ACS, improve patient satisfaction and quality of life, and reduce health service costs. However, as an organizational intervention, the effect of the chest pain unit will depend heavily on local circumstances and may be influenced by staff attitudes, professional roles and local leadership. Furthermore, the presence of a chest pain unit may attract additional attendances with chest pain. Whether this represents identification of unmet demand or unnecessary work is a matter of opinion.

A variety of other methods of provocative cardiac testing and cardiac imaging may be used to evaluate patients with chest pain. These include echocardiography, radionuclide imaging, stress echocardiography, high-resolution CT scanning and coronary angiography. Their widespread use in the chest pain population is currently limited to the research setting. However, the development of CT as a practical way of providing non-invasive imaging of the coronary arteries raises the exciting possibility of this test being used to simultaneously evaluate for ACS, pulmonary embolism (PE) and aortic dissection.

This approach needs careful evaluation, and the caveats mentioned previously about extrapolating data from selected high-risk patients to the general chest pain population will need to be considered. The presence of coronary atheroma does not necessarily confirm that the patient's chest pain was cardiac.

A number of clinical risk scores have been developed to risk-stratify patients with suspected ACS. The Goldman algorithm and the Acute Cardiac Ischaemia Time Insensitive Predictive Instrument (ACI-TIPI) were developed and validated on large cohorts of patients with chest pain in the 1980s and 1990s. The Goldman algorithm uses a series of questions about the patient's age, clinical history and ECG findings to categorize patients into a low ($<7\%$) or high ($>7\%$) risk of myocardial infarction, based on the WHO definition used at the time. ACI-TIPI can be incorporated into a computerized ECG. The user enters the patient's age, gender, and whether chest or left arm pain is the primary symptom. The computer then uses these data and analysis of the ECG to generate a probability of acute cardiac ischaemia.

The Thrombolysis in Myocardial Infarction (TIMI) score has been developed and validated as a predictor of adverse outcome in patients with diagnosed ACS (see Chapter 5.2). Studies have evaluated the TIMI score in ED patients with suspected ACS and shown that higher scores are associated with a higher risk of adverse outcome. This has led to the TIMI score being used to risk-stratify patients with chest pain before a diagnosis of ACS has been confirmed.

Treatment

Treatment of acute chest pain is obviously directed at the specific cause. The treatment of acute coronary syndrome is outlined in Chapter 5.2, pulmonary embolus in Chapter 5.5, and aortic dissection in Chapter 5.10.

Musculoskeletal chest pain, whether due to muscular strain, chest wall injury, Tietze's syndrome or epidemic myalgia, should be treated with simple analgesia and the patient advised to see their general practitioner if the pain persists beyond a few weeks. It is also worth considering whether anxiety may be exacerbating the symptoms.

Gastro-oesophageal pain can be treated acutely with antacids, although the diagnostic value of observing relief of pain with the so-called 'GI cocktail' is debatable. ACS often presents as burning or indigestion-type pain and, pain being typically fluctuant, may ease coincidentally with the administration of an antacid. Gastro-oesophageal pain should be diagnosed with caution and ideally only after ACS has been investigated and ruled out. In these circumstances a course of treatment with a proton pump inhibitor is appropriate. Follow-up will depend on local practice along with the duration and severity of symptoms.

Anxiety-related symptoms range from simple chest wall muscular tension to panic attacks, hyperventilation syndrome and cardiac neurosis. Treatment should therefore be tailored to the patient's individual needs. In many cases anxiety will be an understandable reaction to concerns about heart disease or other serious pathology. The first step is therefore to provide clear and unequivocal reassurance. If diagnostic uncertainty makes this impossible then it may still be possible to provide reassurance by highlighting the excellent prognosis of patients with chest pain whose tests are negative. Patients with more severe symptoms may benefit from relaxation techniques, cognitive behavioural therapy or treatment with an antidepressant. These are best arranged through the patient's general practitioner.

Managing anxiety in the ED patient is often complicated by difficulties in satisfactorily ruling out serious physical illness. A diagnosis of anxiety may be considered likely, but until cardiac testing is complete (perhaps even involving coronary angiography) the treating physician may be reluctant to discuss treatment of anxiety with the patient. This is inappropriate. If the patient has significant anxiety-related symptoms then this will adversely affect their quality of life and should be addressed regardless of whether they ultimately also need treatment for cardiac disease.

Non-specific chest pain obviously presents a diagnostic challenge. With no clear diagnosis it is difficult to advise an appropriate treatment. However, patients can be advised that, although no clear diagnosis can be made, about half such patients presenting to the ED have no further episodes of pain over the following month.

Those who do suffer further episodes are unlikely to be troubled. Treatment is therefore unlikely to be required.

Finally, an acute episode of chest pain provides an opportunity to identify and manage cardiac risk factors at a time when the patient is likely to be most receptive to lifestyle advice. Smokers should be advised to use the episode as a stimulus to stop smoking, and referral to a smoking cessation service arranged. General dietary and exercise advice may also be helpful. Blood pressure, blood glucose and lipid profile may be requested as part of clinical assessment, although any abnormalities identified should preferably be referred to the patient's general practitioner, who will be best placed to provide overall cardiovascular risk assessment, intervention and long-term follow-up.

Prognosis

Prognosis will also depend upon the underlying pathology, and the prognoses of various causes of chest pain are discussed in the relevant chapters. Patients with no obvious diagnosis after clinical assessment and ECG have an excellent prognosis, with 6-month mortality less than 1%. There is some evidence that patients who attend the ED with chest pain have a higher risk of adverse cardiac events than the general population, even if cardiac disease is 'ruled out' at initial presentation, but this risk is not high enough to warrant active intervention beyond ensuring that any cardiac risk factors identified have been addressed.

Likely developments over the next 5–10 years

Chest pain is responsible for a substantial and growing number of emergency medical admissions in many countries. This is placing a major burden on healthcare systems. The value of hospital admission for ACS and pulmonary embolus is being questioned, and it is likely that there will be increasing efforts to develop outpatient care for people with acute chest pain. These efforts may be successful for younger patients with no comorbidities and a single potentially serious cause for their chest

pain, but may be difficult to implement among the growing population of older patients with comorbidities or multiple potentially serious causes for their pain.

A variety of new cardiac markers are being evaluated for the purpose of either identifying ACS at or shortly after attendance, or identifying troponin-negative patients who are at risk of subsequent cardiac events. Current evidence is not sufficient to support the routine use of these markers, but as these biomarkers become commercially available clinicians will have to make careful choices about which to use in their chest pain protocols.

Chest pain management is likely to be influenced by changes in health service policy, which are in turn likely to depend on local social, political and economic factors. These changes will be variable and may be unpredictable. On the one hand, public awareness of the medical significance of chest pain and policies aimed at increasing rapid access to care may lead to increased numbers of patients presenting with chest pain. On the other hand, reorganization of services and attempts to control costs may result in an opposite effect. Specifically, the development of primary angioplasty services may lead to centralization of chest pain services and patients bypassing facilities without primary angioplasty.

Controversies

- The role of clinical scores for acute coronary syndrome in the assessment of undifferentiated chest pain is unclear. The TIMI score was developed to predict future events in patients with acute coronary syndrome, but is often used for diagnostic assessment in patients with chest pain (i.e. estimating whether the patient has myocardial infarction at presentation).

- There is considerable debate regarding the optimal use of biochemical markers to rule out ACS, particularly the use of multiple cardiac markers and point-of-care testing.

- The use of immediate exercise treadmill testing. Advocates point to

a good safety record, prognostic value for cardiac events and reassurance value for patients. Sceptics raise concerns about limited sensitivity and specificity for coronary heart disease, and the impracticality of performing the test in the ED.

- The role of chest pain units.

- The role of multislice CT to identify coronary artery disease, and in investigation when PE and aortic dissection are viable alternative diagnoses.

Further reading

Antman E, Tanasijevic MJ, Thompson B, et al. Cardiac-specific troponin I levels to predict the risk of mortality in patients with acute coronary symptoms. New England Journal of Medicine 1996; 335: 1342–1349.
Chase M, Robey JL, Zogby KE, et al. 2006 Prospective validation of the thrombolysis in myocardial infarction score in the emergency department chest pain population. Annals of Emergency Medicine 48: 252–259.
Chun AA, McGee SR. Bedside diagnosis of coronary artery disease: a systematic review. American Journal of Medicine 2004; 117: 334–343.
Conway-Morris A, Caesar D, Gray S. TIMI risk score accurately risk stratifies patients with undifferentiated chest pain presenting to an emergency department. Heart 2006; 92: 1333–1334.
Fleet RP, Dupuis G, Marchand A, et al. Panic disorder, chest pain and coronary artery disease: literature review. Canadian Journal of Cardiology 1994; 10: 827–834.
Goodacre SW, Angelini K, Arnold J, et al. Clinical predictors of acute coronary syndrome in patients with undifferentiated chest pain. Quarterly Journal of Medicine 2003; 96: 893–898.
Goodacre S, Locker T, Arnold J, et al. Which diagnostic tests are most useful in a chest pain unit protocol? BioMed Central Emergency Medicine 2005; 5: 6.
Goodacre S, Nicholl J, Dixon S, et al. Randomised controlled trial and economic evaluation of a chest pain observation unit compared with routine care. British Medical Journal 2004; 328: 254–257.
Joint European Society of Cardiology/American College of Cardiology Committee. Myocardial infarction redefined – a consensus document of the Joint European Society of Cardiology/American College of Cardiology Committee for the Redefinition of Myocardial Infarction. European Heart Journals 2000; 36: 959–969.
McCord J, Nowak RM, McCullough PA, et al. Ninety-minute exclusion of acute myocardial infarction by use of quantitative point-of-care testing of myoglobin and troponin I. Circulation 2001; 104: 1483–1488.
Mitchell AM, Brown MD, Menown IBA, et al. Novel protein markers of acute coronary syndrome complications in low-risk outpatients: A systematic review of potential use in the emergency department. Clinical Chemistry 2005; 51: 2005–2011.
Panju AA, Hemmelgarn BR, Guyatt GH, et al. Is this patient having a myocardial infarction? Journal of American Medical Association 1998; 280: 1256–1263.
Swap CT, Nagurney JT. Value and limitations of chest pain history in the evaluation of patients with suspected acute coronary syndromes. Journal of the American Medical Association 2005; 294: 2623–2629.

5.2 Acute coronary syndromes

Steve Goodacre • Anne-Maree Kelly

ESSENTIALS

1 Every patient with possible ACS should receive a 12-lead ECG as soon as possible after arrival to identify whether they may benefit from reperfusion therapy. If interpretation is uncertain, then senior or specialist advice should be sought immediately.

2 Every patient with suspected ACS should be given aspirin, unless they have a contraindication.

3 Primary prevention of ACS involves overall cardiovascular risk assessment and is most appropriately undertaken in primary care.

4 Stable angina is not ACS, but patients do not usually attend the emergency department with stable angina.

5 The ECG can identify patients with ACS who are at high risk, but cannot rule out ACS.

6 Primary angioplasty is more effective than thrombolysis, but only if it can be delivered promptly by appropriately trained staff.

Introduction

Acute coronary syndrome (ACS) is the most common life-threatening condition in emergency medicine. Failure to identify and treat it promptly risks avoidable morbidity and mortality.

Aetiology, pathogenesis and pathology

ACS nearly always occurs as a consequence of atheroma in the coronary arteries, commonly known as coronary heart disease (CHD). Many people have coronary atheroma but are asymptomatic because it is not extensive enough to occlude coronary blood flow. Others have a degree of coronary occlusion that does not cause symptoms unless they exert themselves, or if myocardial oxygen demand is increased by some other mechanism, such as anaemia. Cardiac chest pain that only occurs on exertion and is rapidly relieved by rest is known as stable angina and is not classified as ACS.

ACS usually occurs when an atheromatous plaque ruptures or fissures. Haemorrhage may occur into the plaque, or thrombus may accumulate over the fissure. The type of ACS that results from this process depends on the extent of the rupture and degree of haemorrhage or thrombus formation. A gradually progressive occlusion will produce symptoms of unstable angina: progressive symptoms of myocardial ischaemia occurring on less exertion or at rest. A rapidly progressive occlusion may lead to myocardial infarction (MI), with severe pain at rest and the potential for serious complications such as arrhythmia, heart failure, cardiogenic shock or sudden cardiac death.

If coronary occlusion is minor or transient then the consequent myocardial ischaemia will not lead to myocardial damage. If coronary occlusion is severe or prolonged then myocardial necrosis will occur. Traditionally, biochemical cardiac tests (such as creatinine kinase (CK) and troponin) detect markers that are released during myocardial necrosis and are used to define the diagnosis of MI. Recently, alternative cardiac markers (such as ischaemia-modified albumin) have been developed that detect ischaemia without infarction.

Not all coronary artery occlusion is due to coronary atheroma. Prinzmetal angina describes a syndrome in which myocardial ischaemia is associated with coronary artery spasm, and is characterized by transient ST elevation on the ECG. Coronary angiography may show minor atheroma or normal coronary arteries. Uncommonly, coronary artery spasm may be severe enough to cause myocardial necrosis and an associated troponin rise.

Other rare causes of coronary artery occlusion include Kawasaki's disease, in which occlusion is due to inflammation in the coronary artery and aortic dissection that involves the coronary arteries.

ACS may involve occlusion of one or more of the coronary arteries, and the location of occlusion may determine the clinical presentation, ECG findings and likelihood of complications. Anterior or anteroseptal MI is the most common site and usually results from occlusion of the left anterior descending artery. It has a worse prognosis than other types of MI and complications are more common. Sudden cardiac death may result from total occlusion of the left anterior descending artery, giving a lesion in this location the grim sobriquet of 'widow-maker'. Lateral infarction is caused by occlusion of the circumflex artery or the diagonal branch of the left anterior descending artery. Inferior MI is caused by occlusion of the right coronary artery or the circumflex artery. It has a better prognosis than anterior infarction and ventricular dysfunction is less likely, although heart block due to involvement of the atrioventricular node is more common. Posterior infarction is usually due to occlusion of the right coronary artery or, less commonly, the circumflex artery in patients with dominance of the left coronary circulation. Posterior or inferior MI may result in right ventricular infarction leading to right ventricular failure.

ACS may be associated with a number of life-threatening complications. Myocardial ischaemia or infarction may lead to arrhythmia, such as atrial fibrillation, ventricular tachycardia and ventricular fibrillation. Supraventricular tachycardias are not usually associated with ACS. Heart block may occur with small infarcts affecting the nodal branch of the right coronary artery or larger septal infarcts. Infarction may lead to myocardial dysfunction, resulting in heart failure or cardiogenic shock. Massive MI may cause papillary muscle dysfunction and mitral regurgitation, ventricular septal defect or cardiac rupture. The probability of any of these complications occurring increases with the severity of myocardial damage incurred.

Epidemiology

Coronary heart disease is the leading cause of death in the world, with 8.1 million deaths in 2002. It is responsible for 6.8% of disability-adjusted life years (DALYs) lost through disease by men and 5.3% of DALYs lost by women. The global burden of CHD is expected to rise from 47 million DALYs in 1990 to 82 million in 2020. Most of this increasing burden will be in developing countries, where currently 60% of the burden of CHD is already felt. However, CHD mortality rates have dramatically decreased in many developed countries since the 1980s. Studies suggest that 50–75% of the falls in cardiac deaths can be attributed to population interventions, particularly those relating to smoking, hypertension and high cholesterol. The remaining 25–50% is due to treatments for patients with CHD, such as thrombolysis, aspirin, angiotensin-converting enzyme inhibitors, statins and coronary artery bypass surgery.

The main risk factors for CHD are well established and include smoking, diabetes, hypertension, hyperlipidaemia and a family history of CHD, while obesity and lack of exercise may play a contributory role. Age and gender are also important. CHD prevalence increases with age, and increases at an earlier age (40 to 50 years) in men than in women (over 60 years). Everyone over the age of 60 is effectively at risk of CHD. Conversely a history of CHD presenting in a relative when they were aged over 60 should not be considered a significant risk factor.

Patients presenting to the emergency department with chest pain in general, and ACS specifically, show a diurnal variation with a peak of attendances during the morning, although many of these attendances relate to symptoms occurring overnight. Presentation is more common on a Monday, when cardiovascular mortality appears to be higher. Cardiovascular mortality also increases during the winter months, particularly in colder climates.

Prevention

Prevention of ACS is achieved principally by preventing underlying CHD, although secondary prevention of ACS in patients with established CHD can be attempted by ensuring appropriate treatment with daily low-dose aspirin, β-blockers and lipid-lowering therapy.

Primary CHD prevention can take place at population or individual patient level by addressing the important coronary risk factors that are amenable to intervention. The most important modifiable risk factors at a population level are smoking, obesity and lack of exercise. These may be tackled by legislation and education, and by economic and social policy. Diabetes, hypertension and hyperlipidaemia can be addressed at an individual level. It is increasingly recognized that the importance of any one risk factor depends on the presence of other risk factors, and so cardiovascular risk is most appropriately assessed by a comprehensive assessment involving all risk factors, along with age and gender. Screening programmes should be based on overall cardiovascular risk assessment, rather than individual risk factors. Similarly, the decision to prescribe treatments for risk factors, particularly lipid-lowering therapy, should be based on overall cardiovascular risk.

This has implications for emergency medicine. It may be tempting to use the patient's attendance at the ED to undertake opportunistic screening by, for example, measuring blood pressure, blood sugar or lipids, even though they will not influence management of the presenting complaint. This approach is inappropriate because it does not involve overall cardiovascular risk assessment. Furthermore, it may be considered unethical because the patient is effectively being screened (with potential implications for health insurance) without the opportunity to make an informed choice about whether they wish to receive screening. For these reasons, coronary risk assessment for primary prevention is best left to primary care physicians.

Although opportunistic screening in the ED is best avoided, opportunistic patient education about risk factors may be very salient, particularly if the patient has presented with symptoms that could be related to CHD. An episode of chest pain, even if ultimately diagnosed as non-cardiac, may offer an ideal opportunity to promote smoking cessation.

Clinical features

Clinical assessment of suspected ACS is described in detail in Chapter 5.1. Chest pain is suggestive of MI if it radiates to either arm, both arms or shoulders; is described as burning, like indigestion, heavy, pressing or band-like; occurs on exertion; is associated with diaphoresis, nausea or vomiting; or is worse than previous angina or similar to previous MI. Chest pain is less likely to be MI if it is sharp, pleuritic, positional, reproduced by palpation, inframammary in location, or not associated with exertion.

Clinical assessment of cardiac pain is required to determine whether it is due to stable angina or ACS (unstable angina or MI). Stable angina is caused by a fixed narrowing of the coronary artery and is characterized by pain that is predictable, precipitated by exertion, relieved by rest or glyceryl trinitrate (GTN), and is not becoming more frequent or severe. Unstable angina is caused by a dynamic narrowing of the coronary artery and is characterized by pain that may be unpredictable, may occur at rest or minimal exertion, may not be immediately relieved by rest or GTN, or may be increasing in frequency or severity. The latter may also be described as crescendo angina.

Patients with stable angina do not typically present to the ED. They are often used to their symptoms and will not seek medical help unless something unexpected happens. If a patient presents with apparently stable angina the diagnosis should be considered carefully. It should be remembered that pain precipitated by exertion is known to be predictive of MI in ED patients. Stable angina should generally be diagnosed with caution in the ED.

CARDIOVASCULAR

5

Clinical examination is generally unhelpful in making the diagnosis of ACS, which should be based on clinical history and investigations. However, clinical examination is essential to identify complications of ACS. Heart failure may be identified by poor peripheral circulation, tachycardia, pulmonary crepitations, elevated jugular venous pressure and a third heart sound on cardiac auscultation. The additional finding of hypotension suggests cardiogenic shock. A systolic murmur raises the possibility of papillary muscle rupture or ventricular septal defect secondary to MI, although pre-existing aortic or mitral valve disease are much more common.

Differential diagnosis

Alternative diagnoses and their differentiation from ACS are described in Chapter 5.1. The most potentially serious alternative diagnoses are pulmonary embolus and aortic dissection. These should be considered in any patient with suspected ACS who is diaphoretic, tachycardic, tachypnoeic, hypotensive, or reports associated neurological symptoms but does not have definite ECG features of ACS.

Clinical investigation

The 12-lead ECG is an essential investigation and should be performed as soon as possible after arrival in any patient with the slightest suspicion of ACS. Pre-hospital ECGs can be obtained by some emergency medical services and may be used to prioritize patients and guide triage to high-dependency areas/cardiac catheter laboratories.

The critical decision upon reviewing an initial 12-lead ECG is to determine whether the patient has ACS that may benefit from rapid early reperfusion, i.e. has evidence of ST-elevation MI (STEMI) or MI with new bundle branch block. If there is any doubt about this element of ECG interpretation then senior or specialist advice should be sought immediately. Repeat ECG recording should only be planned if a senior clinician feels there is insufficient certainty to allow for an immediate decision.

Identifying new bundle branch block presents a challenge, especially if previous notes are not immediately available. A number of ECG features seen in association with left bundle branch block, known as the Sgarbossa criteria, suggest an increased likelihood of MI. These are ST-elevation of 1 mm or more that is concordant with (in the same direction as) the QRS complex; ST-depression of 1 mm or more in leads V1, V2, or V3; and ST-segment elevation of 5 mm or more that was discordant with (in the opposite direction to) the QRS complex. These may be used to help identify patients with a new MI, but their absence should not preclude reperfusion in patients who clearly have new bundle branch block or a history that is highly suggestive of an acute MI.

Other ECG changes may be useful in diagnosing AMI and are described in Chapter 5.1 and Table 5.1.3. Q waves typically follow ST elevation, but may appear as early as 4 hours after symptom onset. Their presence does not therefore preclude early reperfusion. Tall, upright T waves ('hyperacute' T waves) may be present in the very early stages of infarction. Deep (>3 mm) inverted T waves suggest a subendocardial MI and a troponin rise can be expected. Similarly, patients with significant (>1 mm) ST depression have an increased risk of adverse outcome and are likely to have a troponin rise. Unfortunately, despite suggesting an increased risk of adverse outcome, neither ST depression nor deep T-wave inversion is associated with benefit from thrombolytic therapy.

Other T-wave changes, such as small inversions (<3 mm), flat T waves and biphasic T waves, are common and non-specific. They may suggest ACS, but may also occur in patients with hypertension, patients who are hyperventilating, and in the normal population. If these changes are dynamic (i.e. they develop or resolve on subsequent ECGs) then the suspicion of ACS may be raised, but even quite dramatic T-wave changes can be induced by hyperventilation or changing patient position.

In addition to changes directly suggesting ACS, the ECG should be inspected for any concurrent pathology or evidence of complications. Cardiac rate and rhythm, and P-wave presence and morphology should be evaluated for evidence of arrhythmia or heart block. Tall R waves or S waves suggest ventricular strain or hypertrophy that may contribute to or be a consequence of ACS.

A subtle sign that can indicate ischaemia or ventricular dysfunction is poor anterior R-wave progression. Normally R waves progressively increase in size across leads V1 to V4. Small R waves across these leads suggest pathology.

Repeated 12-lead ECG recording or continuous ST-segment monitoring can help to identify transient or dynamic ECG changes. The development of significant (>1 mm) ST deviation provides clear evidence of ischaemia, identifies high-risk patients, and may facilitate rapid identification of patients requiring reperfusion. T-wave changes, by contrast, are non-specific and often arise as a result of hyperventilation or changes in patient position during monitoring. The incidence of significant ST changes decreases and the incidence of false positive T-wave changes increases in patients with a lower likelihood of significant ACS. Therefore, repeated ECG recording and ST-segment monitoring should be reserved for high-risk patients.

A normal or non-diagnostic ECG does not rule out ACS or necessarily stratify the patient to very low risk. In fact, most patients admitted with ACS do not have diagnostic ECG changes. Serial ECG recordings and ST-segment monitoring do not substantially increase the negative predictive value of the ECG or provide very useful prognostic data. Negative ECG recording therefore has limited value.

Biochemical markers are discussed in detail in Chapter 5.1. Their role in emergency medicine is principally diagnostic, in that they are used to identify patients with ACS from among those presenting with chest pain, and to rule out ACS if negative. However, it should be remembered that a negative cardiac marker, even if highly sensitive and performed at an optimal time after the worst symptoms, does not rule out CHD, or even necessarily ACS. Patients with negative markers will still require risk stratification and further cardiac testing if ACS is considered a likely diagnosis.

Biochemical markers (particularly troponin) have a valuable prognostic role. Any patient with an elevated troponin is at increased risk of adverse outcome and has the potential to benefit from hospital admission. If ACS is the likely cause of a troponin elevation then the patient should be admitted under the care of a cardiologist. As a general rule, the higher the troponin level the greater risk of adverse outcome. So patients with minor troponin elevations may be managed conservatively and possibly without ECG monitoring, whereas those with substantial troponin elevations should be managed on a coronary care unit and considered for early percutaneous coronary intervention (PCI), even if they have no significant ECG changes.

Provocative cardiac testing, such as exercise treadmill testing, is also described in Chapter 5.1. Its main role is to risk-stratify patients with chest pain who do not have ECG or biochemical changes suggesting ACS, and thus allow discharge home if negative. Provocative testing can be used to risk-stratify patients presenting with chest pain and known CHD. In these circumstances an early positive test will prompt rapid referral to cardiology for consideration of cardiac catheterization, whereas a late positive or negative test suggests that conservative treatment is appropriate. The use of provocative cardiac testing to risk-stratify patients with troponin-positive ACS is best left to the cardiologists.

As described in Chapter 5.1, radionuclide scanning and CT imaging may be used in some EDs to screen for significant CHD, but their use is not currently widespread and relates mainly to ruling out CHD in low-risk patients rather than risk-stratifying those with ACS.

Criteria for diagnosis

The term ACS covers a spectrum of disorders, including unstable angina, non-ST elevation MI (NSTEMI) and ST-elevation MI (STEMI). The diagnostic definition of MI has been a matter of intense debate in recent years and a consensus is gradually emerging. In contrast, the challenge of defining a diagnosis of ACS per se has been largely overlooked.

The original World Health Organization (WHO) diagnosis of MI is outlined in Table 5.2.1. It required an elevation of creatinine kinase to more than twice the upper limit of the normal range. With the development of troponins it became apparent that this definition failed to include a substantial number of patients with

---

Table 5.2.1 WHO criteria for definite acute MI (1970)

1. Definite ECG, or
2. Symptoms typical or atypical or inadequately described, together with probable ECG or abnormal enzymes, or
3. Symptoms typical with abnormal enzymes with ischaemic or non-codable ECG, or ECG not available, or
4. Fatal case with necropsy findings or MI or recent coronary occlusion

---

prognostically significant myocardial damage, as evidenced by a troponin rise. Therefore the American Heart Association and European Society of Cardiology (AHA/ESC) developed a new definition of MI, outlined in Table 5.2.2, which required a rise in serum troponin above the 99th percentile of the values for a reference control group.

The AHA/ESC definition has been widely adopted, despite a number of concerns and criticisms. Patients with ACS who fulfil this definition have a higher risk of adverse outcome than those who do not. However, patients with MI according to the AHA/ESC criteria alone have a lower risk of adverse outcome than those who fulfil both the AHA/ESC and WHO criteria. This has led to problems in maintaining consistent care over time, and some experts have suggested identifying a threshold level for troponin (for example troponin T >1 ng/mL) above which clinically important MI should be diagnosed. This controversy is unlikely to be completely resolved in the near future, particularly if newer and more sensitive biochemical markers are developed. However, the most important issue to recognize is that any detectable troponin is associated with an increased risk of adverse outcome, and the higher the troponin level the higher that risk.

MI can be usefully defined as STEMI or NSTEMI on the basis of the ECG. If there is evidence of significant ST elevation on any ECG (>2 mm in two consecutive chest leads, or >1 mm in two consecutive limb leads) then the patient has STEMI. These

---

Table 5.2.2 The AHA/ESC criteria for MI (2000)

Typical rise and fall of biochemical markers of myocardial necrosis with at least one of the following:
1. Ischaemic symptoms
2. Q waves
3. Ischaemic ECG changes
4. Coronary artery intervention

---

patients are likely to benefit from early reperfusion therapy. Patients without these changes but with evidence of myonecrosis based on cardiac markers are defined as having NSTEMI and do not benefit from reperfusion with thrombolytics, although PCI may be beneficial. NSTEMI and ACS without criteria for MI may be categorized together as non-ST elevation ACS. The terms STEMI and NSTEMI have largely replaced the terms Q wave and non-Q wave MI. ST elevation at presentation is usually associated with the subsequent development of Q waves on later ECGs, so the terms may be interchangeable. However, because STEMI and NSTEMI can be differentiated at presentation, when the key clinical decisions have to be made, they have much more practical value than definitions based on the development of Q waves.

The diagnosis of ACS can be made in the absence of a troponin rise if the patient has characteristic ECG changes, such as ST-segment deviation or deep T-wave inversion. However, significant ECG changes are usually associated with a troponin rise. This means that the clinical diagnosis of ACS without MI is usually based on the clinical history, possibly augmented by provocative cardiac testing, myocardial perfusion scanning or coronary artery imaging. As the clinical features are known to be unreliable for ACS (see Chapter 5.1) and many patients with suspected ACS do not receive further cardiac testing, differentiation between ACS and either stable angina or non-coronary pain may be uncertain. This fact is often overlooked when guidelines are developed for ACS. Identifying a patient with ACS or suspected ACS relies on clinical judgement that is often imperfect. This is an important issue because only a minority of patients admitted to hospital with ACS have diagnostic ECG changes.

Treatment

Some treatments are indicated for all ACS, whereas others have specific application to STEMI, NSTEMI and other ACS.

Treatments for all ACS

Analgesia
GTN and intravenous (i.v.) morphine are the analgesic agents of choice. Sublingual GTN

may be appropriate if pain is mild to moderate, but severe pain usually requires titrated i.v. morphine. Doses of up to 20 mg, in small increments, are sometimes required. If i.v. morphine fails to control pain and the clinical condition is suitable, i.v. GTN by infusion at a rate titrated to effect (20–200 μg/min) is indicated. If this is insufficient to control pain and the patient is tachycardic, control of rate with small increments of β-blocker may be beneficial. It is important to note that ongoing severe pain, particularly in the absence of ECG changes, should raise concerns about an alternative diagnosis, such as aortic dissection.

Oxygen

Although the basis for the recommendation is pathophysiological rather than outcomes based, there is consensus that oxygen should be administered to achieve SpO_2 >95%.

Aspirin

Aspirin 300 mg should be administered unless already given (e.g. by emergency services or GP) or contraindicated. The principal contraindication to aspirin is known allergy. A previous history of gastritis or indigestion is not a contraindication to the use of aspirin in ACS.

STEMI

Reperfusion

Patients with STEMI who present within 12 hours of symptom onset should have a reperfusion strategy implemented promptly. Reperfusion can be obtained by fibrinolytic

therapy, PCI, or rarely, with emergency coronary artery bypass grafting. The choice of reperfusion therapy will depend on time from symptom onset, availability of PCI, delay to fibrinolysis, contraindications to fibrinolysis, location and size of the infarct, and the presence or absence of cardiogenic shock.

PCI is the best available treatment if provided promptly. It is generally accepted that a delay of 90 minutes between presentation and balloon inflation is the maximum desirable. If this is not possible, fibrinolysis should be used. For patients presenting very early (symptom duration less than 1 hour) fibrinolytic therapy is highly effective, so the maximum tolerable delay to PCI is 1 hour from presentation. For patients aged less than 75 years with cardiogenic shock, PCI markedly improves outcomes.

Fibrinolytic agents include streptokinase and tissue fibrin-specific agents such as alteplase and tenecteplase. Available evidence suggests that fibrin-specific agents reduce mortality compared to streptokinase, despite an increased risk of intracranial bleeding. Note that streptokinase should not be given to patients who have been previously exposed to it (more than 5 days ago). There is also some evidence that it may be less effective in populations with high levels of exposure to streptococcal skin infections, such as Aboriginal and Torres Strait Islander peoples. Contraindications to fibrinolytic therapy are shown in Table 5.2.3.

Pre-hospital fibrinolysis should be considered when delay to PCI exceeds 90 minutes and transfer times to a fibrinolysis-capable facility exceed 30 minutes.

Clopidogrel

All patients undergoing PCI or fibrinolysis should receive clopidogrel. Current recommended doses are 600 mg for PCI and 300 mg for fibrinolysis.

Antithrombin therapy

Antithrombin therapy should be used in conjunction with PCI and fibrin-specific fibrinolytic agents. The use of antithrombin therapy with streptokinase is optional. Unfractionated heparin or low molecular weight heparin can be used, although there are evolving data that low molecular weight heparin may be more effective than unfractionated heparin for preventing recurrent MI in patients receiving fibrinolytic therapy.

When used with PCI, unfractionated heparin is administered i.v. and the dose will depend on the concomitant use of glycoprotein IIb/IIIa inhibitors (GP inhibitors). A recommended aim is to achieve an activated clotting time (ACT) of between 200 and 300 seconds if using GP inhibitors, or between 300 and 350 seconds if not using them.

When used with fibrinolysis, unfractionated heparin should be given in an initial i.v. bolus of 60 units/kg (maximum 4000 units) followed by an infusion of 12 units/kg/h (maximum 1000 units/h) titrated to an activated partial thromboplastin time (APPT) of 1.5–2 times control. Low molecular weight heparin can be used in patients under 75 years old provided they do not have significant renal dysfunction.

Newer agents such as fondaparinux (a factor Xa inhibitor) and bivalirudin (a direct thrombin inhibitor) have shown similar efficacy to the heparins with less bleeding. Their place in the management of ACS is evolving.

Glycoprotein IIb/IIIa inhibitors

The role of GP inhibitors is evolving and data are conflicting and complex. At this stage, some guidelines consider it 'reasonable' to use abciximab with primary PCI. The use of full-dose GP inhibitors with fibrinolysis should be avoided because of the increased bleeding risk, and the combination of GP inhibitors with reduced doses of fibrinolytic therapy is not recommended, as it

---

Table 5.2.3 Contraindications to fibrinolytic therapy in STEMI (Modified from Antman EM, Anbe DT, Armstrong PW, et al. Circulation 2004; 110: e82–292).

1. Absolute contraindications
- Active bleeding or bleeding diathesis (excluding menses)
- Significant head or facial trauma within 3 months
- Suspected aortic dissection (including new neurological symptoms)
- Any prior intracranial haemorrhage
- Ischaemic stroke within 3 months
- Known structural cerebral vascular lesion (e.g. AV malformation)
- Known malignant intracranial neoplasm (primary or secondary)

2. Relative contraindications
- Current use of anticoagulants: the higher the INR, the higher the risk of bleeding
- Non-compressible vascular punctures
- Major surgery within 3 weeks
- Traumatic or prolonged CPR (>10 minutes)
- Internal bleeding (e.g. gastrointestinal or urinary tract) within the last 4 weeks
- Active peptic ulcer disease
- History of chronic, severe, poorly controlled hypertension
- Severe uncontrolled hypertension at presentation (systolic >180 mmHg, diastolic > 110 mmHg)
- Ischaemic stroke more than 3 months ago, dementia or other known intracranial abnormality, not described previously
- Pregnancy

does not improve outcomes compared to full-dose fibrinolytic therapy and increases the bleeding risk.

Non-STEMI

Antiplatelet therapy
In addition to aspirin, patients should receive clopidogrel 300 mg loading dose and 75 mg/day unless they are likely to undergo emergency coronary bypass surgery or immediate coronary angiography.

Antithrombin therapy
Subcutaneous low molecular weight or unfractionated heparin should be given until angiography or for 48–72 hours. The dose of low molecular weight heparin should be reduced if there is renal impairment. The dose of heparin is as above.

Glycoprotein IIb/IIIa inhibitors
I.v. GP inhibitors are recommended in those patients is whom an early angiography/revascularization is planned and for those with ongoing ischaemia despite antiplatelet and antithrombin therapy. Tirofiban has been recommended for diabetic patients with NSTEMI.

β-Blockers
Initiation of a β-blocker is recommended unless contraindicated.

Invasive management
Patients with NSTEMI should have early coronary angiography (ideally within 48 hours), unless they have severe comorbidities.

Disposition

Disposition depends on the type of ACS. Patients with STEMI and NSTEMI require admission to hospital for further care. Those with STEMI should be admitted to a monitored bed in a cardiac care unit because of the small but significant risk of life-threatening arrhythmia. It is currently usual practice to also admit patients with NSTEMI to monitored beds, but this is being challenged on the basis that there are subgroups within this classification at very low risk of adverse events. Patients with ACS without ECG changes or cardiac marker elevations require a period of assessment in the ED/chest pain unit, and

disposition will depend on the risk identified during that process (see Chapter 5.1).

Complications

Arrhythmias and conduction disturbances (see Chapter 5.4)

Pericarditis (see Chapter 5.6)

Acute left ventricular failure and cardiogenic shock Most myocardial infarctions are accompanied by some degree of left ventricular failure, which may range in severity from asymptomatic to pulmonary oedema or cardiogenic shock. Mortality depends in part on the degree of left ventricular failure, with cardiogenic shock having a reported mortality of approximately 80%.

Management includes maintaining adequate oxygenation, correcting electrolyte imbalances and optimizing ventricular filling pressures. Patients with pulmonary oedema may require non-invasive ventilatory support (see Chapter 5.3). If there is hypotension or other evidence of inadequate perfusion in the presence of adequate intravascular volume, inotropes should be initiated early and aggressively. PCI has been shown to markedly improve outcome for patients with STEMI accompanied by cardiogenic shock. Left ventricular assist devices may bridge to recovery, cardiac surgery or transplantation in selected patients.

Thromboembolism
Thrombus can form on areas of hypokinetic myocardium due to relative stasis and the prothrombotic effects of local inflammatory changes. It is more common with large anterior infarctions with left ventricular aneurysm formation, where the incidence has been reported to be up to 10%. Echocardiography is used to confirm the presence of thrombus. Systemic anticoagulation is required to prevent embolic complications.

Mechanical defects
Mechanical defects may include:

- Ventricular aneurysm formation with the attendant risk of thrombus formation and embolization.
- Acute mitral insufficiency secondary to papillary muscle dysfunction/rupture.
- Ventricular septal defect.

- Cardiac rupture, which may present as sudden death or acute pericardial tamponade.

Prognosis

The prognosis of ACS varies substantially between patients, depending on age, comorbidities, risk factors, severity of coronary occlusion and myocardial necrosis, and the presence of complications. Treatment of ACS should be guided by prognosis: the worse the prognosis, the greater the potential impact of treatment. Prognostic scoring therefore has an important role to play in the management of ACS.

The Thrombolysis in Myocardial Infarction (TIMI) score has been developed and validated as a predictor of adverse outcome (mortality, life-threatening arrhythmia or subsequent myocardial infarction) in ACS. Patients are ascribed a score between zero (lowest risk) and seven (highest risk) by scoring one point for each factor listed in Table 5.2.4. Higher scores are associated with a higher risk of adverse outcome, as shown in Table 5.2.5. The TIMI score is simple to calculate and applicable to a wide range of patients. It can be used to predict which patients will benefit from early invasive management. Patients with a TIMI score of 3 or more appear to benefit from early invasive treatment, whereas those with a TIMI score of 2 or less do not. Patients with a TIMI score of 3 or more should therefore be considered high risk and receive early coronary angiography.

An alternative to the TIMI score is the Global Registry of Acute Coronary Events (GRACE) score, which uses the components

Table 5.2.4 Components of the TIMI score
Age ≥65 years
Previous coronary artery stenosis > 50%
Three or more risk factors for coronary heart disease
ST-segment deviation
Aspirin use in the preceding 7 days
Two or more anginal events in last 24 hours
Elevated cardiac biomarkers

Table 5.2.5 TIMI score and risk of death or MI at 14 days	
TIMI score	Risk of death or MI at 14 days (%)
0 or 1	3
2	3
3	4
4	6
5	11
6 or 7	19

Table 5.2.6 Components of the GRACE score
Age
Heart rate
Systolic blood pressure
Creatinine
Killip class
Cardiac arrest at presentation
ST-segment deviation
Elevated cardiac markers

outlined in Table 5.2.6. Each component is weighted to give an estimate of the probability of in-hospital and 6-month death or MI. The weighting process makes the GRACE score a little more difficult to calculate in the clinical setting, but allows for a more precise estimate of prognosis.

It is worth noting that ST-segment deviation on the ECG and elevated cardiac markers feature in both the TIMI and GRACE scores, and are powerful predictors of adverse events following ACS. A simple approach to prognostication and management would thus be that any patient with ST-segment deviation or significant troponin elevation requires early coronary angiography. Those with no ST-segment deviation or significant troponin elevation can be further risk-stratified with exercise testing, only proceeding to coronary angiography if this is positive.

Likely developments over the next 5–10 years

- Improved models of care to facilitate early primary angioplasty or thrombolysis for STEMI. The exact model for reperfusion will depend upon geography, local services and health service policy. It is likely that widely dispersed rural populations will benefit more from pre-hospital thrombolysis, whereas primary angioplasty is more likely to be feasible in densely populated urban areas where specialist services are within reach of a large population.
- New biochemical markers to assist in diagnosis of non-infarction ACS and to better diagnose and risk-stratify ACS. Of particular interest are markers of myocardial ischaemia, rather than necrosis, such as ischaemia-modified albumin (IMA) and heart-type fatty acid-binding protein (H-FABP). These markers may detect ischaemia in patients with unstable angina but no myocardial necrosis, and thus be useful for risk stratification of troponin-negative patients.
- Innovative models of care allowing safe, outpatient management of selected patients with non-STEMI ACS, perhaps similar to those developed for pulmonary embolism. Whether this becomes a reality in the next 5–10 years will depend on the degree to which barriers to outpatient care can be overcome.
- Further advances in pharmacotherapy for ACS.

Controversies

- Primary angioplasty for STEMI appears to be more effective than thrombolysis, provided both are rapidly available. However, whereas thrombolysis can be provided quickly by a wide range of health professionals, primary angioplasty requires an experienced cardiologist, support staff and a coronary catheterization laboratory. It has been estimated that primary angioplasty is only more effective than thrombolysis if the comparative delay between the provision of primary angioplasty and the provision of thrombolysis is less than 90 minutes. This target may be difficult to achieve and require a systems approach if this window of opportunity is to be met.
- The role of pre-hospital thrombolysis. Data from meta-analyses show that pre-hospital thrombolysis is more effective than in-hospital thrombolysis. However, the advantage is likely to be marginal in settings where the transport times to hospital are short and may not justify the resources, such as staff training and audit, required to support the service.
- Selective ECG monitoring of patients with ACS. ECG monitoring can be useful for facilitating rapid recognition of life-threatening arrhythmia in patients with ACS. However, if it is used indiscriminately in all patients with ACS it will provide a very low yield of significant positive findings. This has led some to argue that ECG monitoring should only be used in selected high-risk patients, and to develop risk-stratification rules to identify those who will benefit from monitoring.
- The role of glycoprotein IIb/IIIa inhibitors in the management of ACS.

Further reading

Antman E, Cohen M, Bernink P, et al. The TIMI risk score for unstable angina/non-ST elevation MI: A method for prognostication and decision-making. Journal of the American Medical Association 2000; 284: 835–842.
Aroney CN, Aylward P, Kelly A-M. Guidelines for the management of acute coronary syndromes. Medical Journal of Australia 2006; 184: S1–S30.
Braunwald E, Antman EM, Beasley JW, et al. ACC/AHA guidelines for the management of patients with unstable angina and non-ST-segment elevation myocardial infarction. Journal of the American College of Cardiology 2000; 36: 970–1062.
Fox KAA, Birkhead J, Wilcox R, et al. British Cardiac Society Working Group on the Diagnosis of Myocardial Infarction. Heart 2004; 90: 603–609.
Fox KAA, Dabdous OH, Goldberg RJ, et al. Prediction of risk of death and myocardial infarction in the six months after presentation with acute coronary syndrome: prospective multinational observational study (GRACE). British Medical Journal 2006; 333: 1091–1094.
Joint European Society of Cardiology/American College of Cardiology Committee. Myocardial infarction redefined – a consensus document of The Joint European Society of Cardiology/American College of Cardiology Committee for the redefinition of myocardial infarction. European Heart Journal 2000; 21: 1502–1513.
Keeley EC, Boura JA, Grines CL. Primary angioplasty versus intravenous thrombolytic therapy for acute myocardial infarction: a quantitative review of 23 randomised trials. Lancet 2003; 361: 13–20.
Mukherjee D, Eagle KA. The use of antithrombotics for acute coronary syndromes in the emergency department: considerations and impact. Progress in Cardiovascular Diseases 2007; 50: 167–180.

5.3 Assessment and management of acute pulmonary oedema

David Lightfoot

ESSENTIALS

1 Severe APO is associated with high morbidity and mortality.

2 APO is a pathophysiological state characterized by a maldistribution of fluid; most patients do not have fluid overload.

3 Therapy is aimed at maintaining oxygenation and cardiac output and reversing the underlying pathophysiology. Reversible causes should be sought and corrected.

4 Hypotensive patients require ventilatory and inotropic support.

5 For most patients, the mainstays of therapy are high-flow oxygen, nitrates and non-invasive ventilation (NIV).

6 NIV is safe and effective in APO. It has been shown to reduce rates of intubation, ICU admission and death.

Table 5.3.1 Causes of cardiogenic pulmonary oedema

Acute valvular dysfunction
Anaemia
Arrhythmias
Dietary, physical or emotional excess
Fluid overload – may be iatrogenic
Medication adverse effect
Medication non-compliance
Myocardial ischaemia/infarction
Myocarditis
Post cardioversion
Pulmonary embolus
Worsening congestive cardiac failure

Introduction

Acute pulmonary oedema (APO) occurs mainly in elderly patients and, if severe, is associated with a very poor long-term prognosis (1-year mortality approaching 40%).[1] It is a pathophysiological state characterized by fluid-filled alveolar spaces, with impaired alveolar gas exchange and reduced lung compliance. Acute dyspnoea, hypoxia, and increased work of breathing are the resultant symptoms and signs. APO occurs when increased pulmonary capillary pressure, reduced plasma oncotic pressure or pulmonary capillary permeability changes lead to plasma leaving the capillaries and building up in the pulmonary interstitium. When this occurs at such a rate that lymphatic drainage from the lung cannot keep up, flooding of the alveoli results.

Pathophysiology

The causes of APO can be divided into cardiogenic (the commonest cause in ED patients) and non-cardiogenic. In cardiogenic APO, an acute reduction in cardiac output associated with an increase in systemic vascular resistance (SVR) leads to back-pressure on the pulmonary vasculature, with resultant increased pulmonary capillary pressure. Once established, APO can lead to a downward spiral where decreasing oxygenation and increasing pulmonary vascular resistance (with its resultant increased right ventricular end-diastolic pressure) worsens left ventricular dysfunction and worsens pulmonary oedema.[2] In most cases the patient has a maldistribution of fluid rather than being fluid overloaded. They may, in fact, have a whole-body fluid deficit. This understanding has led to a change in the management of this condition, from the use of large doses of diuretics to a focus on vasodilators and non-invasive ventilation that reduce SVR and improve cardiac output. Some of the causes of cardiogenic pulmonary oedema are listed in Table 5.3.1.

In non-cardiogenic APO, the mechanism is thought to be increased pulmonary vascular permeability, brought about by an insult, leading to alveolar flooding. Injury to alveolar cells will also reduce their ability to clear this oedema fluid from the alveolar space (this may also play some role in cardiogenic APO). Some of the causes of non-cardiogenic pulmonary oedema are listed in Table 5.3.2.

Clinical assessment

History

As with all emergencies, the clinical assessment and management should take place in parallel. There is usually a history of sudden-onset severe dyspnoea. A focused history concentrating on the recent occurrence of chest pain, a past history of ischaemic heart disease or congestive heart failure, or other causative factor is sought. Details of current medication and compliance are also important.

Examination

Patients are pale or cyanosed, sweaty (sometimes profusely) and frightened. They strive to maintain an upright position at all costs, and may be unable to sit still. They may cough up pink or white frothy sputum, adding to their feeling of drowning. The respiratory rate is high, with use of the accessory muscles of respiration, and breathing is often noisy. Oxygen saturation is severely reduced, indicating hypoxia. Most patients are hypertensive or normotensive. Hypotension indicates cardiogenic shock and a very poor prognosis. There

Table 5.3.2   Causes of non-cardiogenic pulmonary oedema

Airway obstruction
Aspiration
Asthma
DIC
Eclampsia
Head injury, intracerebral haemorrhage
Hyperbaric oxygen treatment
Inhalation injury
Lung re-expansion, e.g. after treatment of a pneumothorax
Lung reperfusion
Near drowning/cold water immersion
Opiates and opiate antagonists (naloxone and naltrexone)
Pancreatitis
Pulmonary embolism (thrombus, fat, amniotic fluid, other)
Rapid ascent to high altitude
Renal/hepatic failure
SCUBA diving
Sepsis
Shock
Toxins
Trauma

may also be a raised jugular venous pressure (JVP), third heart sound or gallop rhythm, and signs of right heart strain. Signs of chronic heart failure should also be sought, as well as murmurs that may hint at the cause. The chest may be dull to percussion and fine crepitations, which are often extensive, will be heard on auscultation. Importantly, there may be other adventitial lung sounds, including wheeze – so-called 'cardiac asthma'.

Investigation

An ECG is required, looking for acute ischaemia, and a chest X-ray will show cardiac size (usually enlarged) and help differentiate APO from airways disease. The chest X-ray findings of pulmonary oedema reflect the changes in fluid distribution. Initially blood is diverted to the upper lobe veins, which become more prominent than normal. As the oedema worsens, interstitial oedema results in basilar and hilar infiltrates, which are hazy and more confluent than patchy, and interlobular oedema is seen as Kerley B lines. There is loss of vascular delineation. In severe APO widespread changes representing alveolar oedema appear. There may also be pleural effusions if the interstitial pressure exceeds pleural pressure. Changes associated with the underlying cause can also be seen, e.g. cardiomegaly and pleural effusions in cardiogenic APO. It is important to note that the X-ray changes may not be bilateral and may mimic consolidation from other causes, e.g. pneumonia.

Blood tests include haemoglobin, electrolytes, cardiac markers, or other cause specific bloods as indicated, e.g. lipase.

Brain or B-type natriuretic peptide (BNP) levels may be useful in distinguishing APO from other causes of acute dyspnoea.[3–5] BNP is a hormone secreted by ventricular myocytes in response to stretch. Plasma levels rise during acute heart failure and APO. In the setting of acute dyspnoea, levels of BNP <100 pg/mL make a diagnosis of acute heart failure and APO less likely. Conversely, when the levels are >500 pg/mL then acute heart failure is more likely. Unfortunately, levels between 100 and 500 are difficult to interpret. False positive results may result from such conditions as pulmonary embolism, sepsis and renal failure, as well as advancing age. In addition, false negative results may occur in the early phases of APO, owing to the delay prior to secretion of BNP, as well as in obese patients and those with valvular heart disease.[6] These aspects, as well as the high cost of the test, have limited its uptake among Australasian emergency physicians.

Oximetry (in some cases supplemented with arterial blood gases) will reflect severity, and help monitor the patient's response to therapy. Rarely, in some more severe cases invasive monitoring, including pulmonary artery catheterization, may be useful.

Management

In all patients with APO, management strategies should provide supportive care to maximize cardiac output and oxygenation, followed by treatment of the underlying cause.

Treatment of the patient with non-cardiogenic pulmonary oedema consists of removing the patient from the causative environment, supportive therapies aimed at maintaining oxygenation, including non-invasive and sometimes invasive, ventilation, and treating the underlying cause.

Most patients with APO in the ED have a cardiogenic aetiology. Therapy varies according to haemodynamic parameters.

Normotensive or hypertensive patients

The mainstays of treatment are reduction of preload and afterload with nitrates, and optimization of oxygenation, often with non-invasive ventilatory support. The patient should be managed sitting up. This posture reduces ventilation–perfusion mismatch and helps with the work of breathing.

Nitrates

Nitrates act to increase cyclic guanosine monophosphate (cGMP) in smooth muscle cells, leading to relaxation. In lower doses this predominantly causes venodilation and preload reduction. At higher doses the arterioles are also affected, leading to afterload and blood pressure reduction. In addition, coronary artery dilatation leads to increased coronary blood flow. Myocardial work and oxygen demands are reduced, and oxygen delivery is improved. Nitrates are therefore the ideal agents for treating APO by reversing the pathophysiological process. Their use is limited by their hypotensive effect and by the tachyphylaxis that occurs with prolonged use. Therefore, they should be titrated against the patient's haemodynamics and require careful monitoring. Nitrates are contraindicated in those patients who have taken sildenafil or its relatives within the previous 24 hours, owing to profound vasodilation and hypotension. They should also be used with caution in patients with fixed cardiac output (e.g. those with severe aortic stenosis or hypertrophic obstructive cardiomyopathy). Although nitrates may also be used topically or sublingually, in the patient with APO the i.v. route is preferred, as dosing can be titrated to effect and therapy ceased promptly if the patient becomes hypotensive. Topical or sublingual therapy is often used as a temporizing measure until i.v. access can be secured. The peak effect of i.v. nitrates occurs after

5 minutes,[7] which compares well with fruse-mide, which causes venodilatation after about 15 minutes.[8]

The usual dosing regimen is to begin the infusion at $5-10\,\mu g/min$ and increase the rate by $5\,\mu g/min$ every 3 minutes, titrated to clinical effect and limited by falling blood pressure. A reasonable blood pressure target is a systolic pressure of 110–120 mmHg. Some studies[9,10] have looked at using higher-dose bolus i.v. nitrates and have shown good efficacy and safety, with improved results over low-dose nitrates, fruse-mide and non-invasive ventilation. Patient numbers, however, have been small, and these dosing regimens are not currently widely used.

Angiotensin-converting enzyme inhibitors (ACEIs)

At lower doses nitrates predominantly reduce preload rather than afterload, and as mentioned, tolerance follows prolonged use. ACEIs effectively reduce afterload, and in cardiogenic pulmonary oedema can also improve pulmonary capillary wedge pressure and cardiac output. When added to standard therapy they can produce a more rapid improvement in haemody-namics and symptoms than placebo.[11] Their use in pulmonary oedema is also associated with reduced intubation rates and ICU length of stay.

Unfortunately, no i.v. or sublingual pre-parations are currently available in Austra-lia, and so the rapid onset of action that follows these routes of administration will not be seen. These agents should be used with caution in patients who have renal impairment or are hypotensive.

Frusemide

Frusemide has been the first-line treatment for patients with APO for many years. Its usefulness is due to venodilatory properties that lead to reduced preload as well as to its diuretic properties. The venodilation occurs before diuresis begins. It can, how-ever, lead to increased peripheral vascular resistance via reflex sympathetic and renin–angiotensin system actions.[12] As mentioned above, fluid overload is not usu-ally a contributing factor in acute heart fail-ure, and so diuresis is not a necessary endpoint of therapy. The obvious exception is in patients with APO of iatrogenic origin after i.v. fluid therapy.

Although it is an established therapy, there are no controlled studies that show benefit from the use of frusemide in APO. At least two studies[8,13] have shown that nitrates are more beneficial than frusemide in relation to haemodynamic and clinical outcomes. Nevertheless, a single dose of frusemide at 1–1.5 mg/kg is still com-monly recommended in the initial manage-ment of this illness.

Morphine

Morphine's main role is in the relief of chest pain that is resistant to nitrate therapy. Its other effects in APO result from central sympatholysis and anxiolysis. The resultant vasodilation with reduced heart rate, blood pressure and cardiac contractility causes reduced preload and myocardial oxygen demand. In addition, it may help alleviate some of the terror felt by patients with APO, but at the risk of reduced respiratory effort. Other negative aspects include its respiratory and central nervous system depressant effects, hence there must be close observation for any signs of narcosis. Patients with hypotension, an altered con-scious state or with respiratory depression should not be given morphine.

There have been no controlled studies looking at the role of morphine in the ED management of APO, and one retrospective analysis linked its use to increased rates on intubation and ICU admission.[14]

Morphine has been one of the major drugs used in the treatment of APO but its use is now controversial. If it is used, it should be in small, titrated i.v. doses with close observation.

Aspirin

The most common cause of APO in patients presenting to ED is myocardial ischaemia/infarction. Aspirin has been shown to reduce the risk of death and myocardial infarction in patients with myocardial ischaemia. Although it does not directly treat APO, when the cause is thought to be myocardial ischaemia, aspirin should be given.

Ventilatory support

All patients with APO should be given high-flow supplemental oxygen using an oxygen delivery system that can meet their minute volume needs, such as a Venturi system. They are hypoxic and, uncorrected, this will worsen APO through direct pulmonary vas-cular constriction and reduced myocardial oxygen delivery.

Patients with a severely reduced level of consciousness, agonal respirations, or respi-ratory arrest require endotracheal intuba-tion and mechanical ventilatory support. This should be accomplished using rapid-sequence intubation.

In recent years, non-invasive ventilation (NIV) using continuous positive airway pressure (CPAP) or bilevel positive airway pressure (Bi-PAP) has allowed many pati-ents to avoid endotracheal intubation. CPAP pressures of $5-10\,cmH_2O$ are used. When using Bi-PAP expiratory pressures are usually begun at $3-5\,cmH_2O$, with the inspiratory pressure 5–8 cm higher. The benefits of these therapies result from a number of effects. Oxygen concentration can be accurately controlled and higher percentages can be delivered than via a face mask. By using CPAP, functional capac-ity is increased by alveolar recruitment, with a resultant increase in gas exchange area, improved pulmonary compliance and reduced work of breathing. The addition of inspiratory pressure support with Bi-PAP further reduces the work of breathing, and may be more useful in hypercapnic or tiring patients. Cardiovascular effects result from positive intrathoracic pressures, with reduced venous return and reduced left ventricular transmural pressures. These pre-load and afterload effects improve cardiac output without increasing myocardial oxy-gen demand. In general these therapies have had few complications and are consid-ered safe. Complications that have been reported include nasal bridge abrasions, patient intolerance, gastric distension and aspiration, pneumothorax and air embo-lism. The last three potentially serious adverse events are extremely rare and appear to occur in selected populations with other underlying disease processes (e.g. pneumothorax in patients with *Pneu-mocystis carinii* pneumonia).[15]

A number of studies have compared CPAP and/or Bi-PAP both with each other and with conventional therapy in APO. They have been extensively reviewed else-where.[15–19] When CPAP was compared to standard medical therapy there were signif-icant improvements in oxygenation, venti-lation, respiratory rate and distress, and heart rates, without significant adverse events. There were also significantly reduced rates of endotracheal intubation, intensive care lengths of stay and, more importantly, reduced mortality.

The evidence for Bi-PAP is not so straightforward, and comes from a smaller number of low-powered trials. There is a clear reduction in the rate of intubation and ICU admission when using Bi-PAP compared to standard therapy. Although there appears to be a trend towards a mortality benefit, it does not reach significance. In the earliest trials of Bi-PAP in APO there appeared to be an unexplained increase in the rate of myocardial infarction among patients in the Bi-PAP groups. These trials involved very small numbers and had methodological issues. Subsequent trials and meta-analyses have not shown an increase in myocardial infarct rates among the Bi-PAP groups. When CPAP and Bi-PAP were compared with each other, there was no significant difference in intubation, myocardial infarction or death rates. As there is no convincing evidence of benefit of Bi-PAP over CPAP, and no proven mortality benefit of Bi-PAP over standard therapy, CPAP is currently the NIV method of choice in APO.

New agents

Levosimendan[20,21] Levosimendan is the first of a new class of drugs known as the calcium sensitizers, and is currently only available in Australasia via the special access scheme. It binds to troponin-C and stabilizes the molecule in its pro-contraction state, prolonging contraction. This occurs without impairment of diastolic relaxation and without increasing calcium concentration (with its concomitant risk of arrhythmia and cell death). Cardiac output increases and pulmonary capillary wedge pressures decrease without significantly increased oxygen demand. It also causes vasodilation (venous and arteriolar) via potassium channel opening, leading to reduced preload and afterload. Adverse effects include a small rise in heart rate, potential hypotension and headache. QTc may also increase.

A number of randomized controlled trials[20,22] have evaluated this drug in patients with acutely decompensated heart failure and have shown improved haemodynamics and survival compared to dobutamine

and/or placebo. As yet there are no trials examining its use in patients with acute pulmonary oedema.

Nesiritide This drug is currently available in the United States and some other regions, but not in Australia. It is a recombinant brain natriuretic peptide. Its actions are to cause arterial (including coronary) and venous vasodilation, and to suppress the renin–angiotensin–aldosterone and sympathetic nervous systems.[23] It has been shown to increase cardiac index and to reduce pulmonary capillary wedge pressure, vascular resistance, and self-reported dyspnoea in patients with decompensated heart failure. Adverse events include dose-related hypotension and bradycardia. There are also trends towards increased renal impairment and death in nesiritide-treated patients in some randomized controlled trials.[24]

Although its mechanism of action would suggest a benefit in patients with APO, significant questions have been raised regarding its actual clinical utility, lack of advantage over existing cheaper alternatives, and safety profile.[24,25] There are no studies using the drug only in APO, and so it cannot be recommended as first-line therapy at present.

Endothelin receptor antagonists Endothelin is a potent vasoconstrictor and modulator of the sympathetic nervous and renin–angiotensin–aldosterone systems. Tezosentan, an endothelin receptor antagonist, has been shown to increase cardiac index, reduce pulmonary capillary wedge and pulmonary arterial pressures, and reduce systemic vascular resistance in patients with moderate to severe heart failure.[26] One trial[27] has examined the use of this drug versus placebo (in addition to standard care) in patients with APO. There was no difference between the drug and placebo in the endpoints of death, recurrent APO, intubation or AMI. At higher doses, outcomes in patients receiving the drug were worse than those receiving placebo.

Hypotensive patients

In general, patients with APO who are hypotensive are at the most severe end of the disease spectrum, defined as cardiogenic shock. They require both ventilatory and haemodynamic support. Endotracheal intubation using rapid-sequence intubation

and ventilation maximize oxygen delivery and minimize oxygen utilization. A positive end-expiratory pressure of 5–10 cmH$_2$O may be useful. These patients may have a fluid deficit, and therefore cautious fluid bolus resuscitation should be titrated against haemodynamic parameters and clinical effect. Inotropic support is also required, with epinephrine (adrenaline) or dopamine being the first-line agents. These drugs will increase cardiac output, but do so at the expense of increased myocardial oxygen demand and increased arrhythmogenicity. Invasive monitoring may be most useful in this group, as it helps guide fluid and inotropic management. Some time may be bought by the use of invasive therapeutic manoeuvres such as an intra-aortic balloon pump. This device reduces myocardial oxygen demand via afterload reduction and increases coronary flow through diastolic augmentation. Reversible causes should be treated, e.g. reperfusion for acute myocardial infarction, surgical correction of acute valvular dysfunction.

Controversies

- The use of BNP as diagnostic aid.
- The use of standard-dose infusions versus high-dose bolus nitrates.
- The use and dosage of frusemide and morphine.
- The role of new agents such as levosimendan.

References

1. Adnet F, Le Toumelin P, Leberre A, et al. In-hospital and long-term prognosis of elderly patients requiring endotracheal intubation for life-threatening presentation of cardiogenic pulmonary edema. Critical Care Medicine 2001; 19: 891–895.
2. Cotter G, Kaluski E, Moshkovitz Y, et al. Pulmonary edema: new insight on pathogenesis and treatment. Current Opinion in Cardiology 2001; 16: 159–163.
3. Mattu A, Martinez JP, Kelly BS. Modern management of cardiogenic pulmonary edema. Emergency Medicine of Clinics of North America 2005; 23: 1105–1125.
4. Mayo DD, Colletti JE, Kuo DC. Brain natriuretic peptide (BNP) testing in the emergency department. Journal of Emergency Medicine 2006; 31: 201–210.
5. Chircop R, Jelinek GA. B-type natriuretic peptide in the diagnosis of heart failure in the Emergency Department. Emergency Medicine of Australia 2006; 18: 170–179.
6. Rogers RL, Feller ED, Gottlieb SS. Acute congestive heart failure in the emergency department. Cardiology Clinic 2006; 24: 115–123.

7. Morrison RA, Wiegand UW, Jahnchen E, et al. Isosorbide dinitrate kinetics and dynamics after intravenous, sublingual and percutaneous dosing in angina. Clinical Pharmacology and Therapeutics 1983; 33: 747–756.

8. Dikshit K, Vyden JK, Forrester JS, et al. Renal and extrarenal hemodynamic effects of furosemide in congestive heart failure after acute myocardial infarction. New England Journal of Medicine 1973; 288: 1087–1090.

9. Cotter G, Metzkor E, Kaluski E, et al. Randomised trial of high-dose isosorbide dinitrate plus low-dose furosemide versus high-dose furosemide plus low-dose isosorbide dinitrate in severe pulmonary oedema. Lancet 1998; 351: 389–393.

10. Sharon A, Shpirer I, Kaluski E. High-dose intravenous isosorbide dinitrate is safer and better than Bi-PAP ventilation combined with conventional treatment for severe pulmonary oedema. Journal of the American College of Cardiology 2000; 36: 832–837.

11. Hamilton RJ, Carter WA, Gallagher EJ. Rapid improvement of acute pulmonary edema with sublingual captopril. Academic Emergency Medicine 1996; 3: 205–212.

12. Francis GS, Siegel RM, Goldsmith SR, et al. Acute vasoconstrictor response to intravenous furosemide in patients with congestive heart failure. Annals of Internal Medicine 1985; 103: 1–6.

13. Nelson GI, Silke B, Ahuja RC, et al. Haemodynamic advantages of isosorbide dinitrate over frusemide in acute heart failure following myocardial infarction. Lancet 1983; 1: 730–733.

14. Sacchetti A, Ramoska E, Moakes ME, et al. Effect of ED management on ICU use in acute pulmonary edema. American Journal of Emergency Medicine 1999; 17: 571–574.

15. Pang D, Keenan SP, Cook DJ, et al. The effect of positive pressure airway support on mortality and the need for intubation in cardiogenic pulmonary edema. A systematic review. Chest 1998; 114: 1185–1192.

16. Cross AM. Review of the role of non-invasive ventilation in the emergency department. Journal of Accident and Emergency Medicine 2000; 17: 79–85.

17. Masip J, Roque M, Sánchez B, et al. Noninvasive ventilation in acute cardiogenic pulmonary edema. Systemic review and meta-analysis. Journal of the American Medical Association 2005; 294: 3124–3130.

18. Winck JC, Azevedo LF, Costa-Pereira A, et al. Efficacy and safety of non-invasive ventilation in the treatment of acute cardiogenic pulmonary edema – a systematic review and meta-analysis. Critical Care 2006; 10: R69.

19. Peter JV, Moran JL, Phillips-Hughes J, et al. Effect of non-invasive positive pressure ventilation (NIPPV) on mortality in patients with acute cardiogenic pulmonary

oedema: a meta-analysis. Lancet 2006; 367: 1155–1163.

20. Holley AD, Ziegenfuss M. Levosimendan. A new option in acute cardiac failure. Emergency Medicine of Australia 2006; 18: 505–509.

21. Innes CA, Wagstaff AJ. Levosimendan. A review of its use in the management of acute decompensated heart failure. Drugs 2003; 63: 2651–2671.

22. Collins SP, Hinchkley WR, Storrow AB. Critical review and recommendations for Nesiritide use in the Emergency Department. Journal of Emergency Medicine 2005; 29: 317–329.

23. Mebazaa A, Barraud D, Welschbillig S. Randomized clinical trials with Levosimendan. American Journal of Cardiology 2005; 96: 74G–79G.

24. Topol EJ. Nesiritide – not verified. New England Journal of Medicine 2005; 353: 113–116.

25. Kesselhelm AS, Fischer MA, Avorn J. The rise and fall of Natrecor for congestive heart failure: Implications for drug policy. Health Affairs 2006; 25: 1095–1102.

26. Cheng JWM. Tezosentan in the management of decompensated heart failure. Cardiology Review 2005; 13: 28–34.

27. Kaluski E, Kobrin I, Zimlichman R, et al. RITZ-5: randomized intravenous tezosentan (an endothelin-A/B antagonist) for the treatment of pulmonary edema. Journal of the American College of Cardiology 2003; 41: 204–221.

5.4 Arrhythmias

Marcus Eng Hock Ong • Swee Han Lim • Wee Siong Teo

ESSENTIALS

1 Cardiac arrhythmias require urgent attention, as some are life-threatening and can lead to sudden death.

2 The most important initial evaluation is for haemodynamic stability. Patients who are hemodynamically stable should have a 12-lead ECG, whereas unstable patients require preparation for immediate intervention.

3 The patient's underlying medical condition is very helpful in making a correct diagnosis of the arrhythmia.

4 Bradyarrhythmias should always be evaluated in the light of the patient's presenting symptoms as well as the ECG abnormality.

5 Patients with wide complex tachycardia should be considered to have ventricular tachycardia unless proved otherwise.

Introduction

Arrhythmia is the term used to describe an abnormal heart rhythm. The most common arrhythmia is atrial or ventricular ectopic beats. Tachycardia occurs when the heart rate is >100 beats per minute (bpm), and bradycardia is defined as a rate of <60 bpm. The management of cardiac arrhythmias depends on the presentation of the patient, haemodynamic stability, underlying heart disease (if any) and the exact type of the arrhythmia. Patients with asymptomatic stable arrhythmias with no underlying heart disease usually do not require emergency treatment, but patients with symptomatic arrhythmias, especially when associated with underlying heart disease, require more aggressive therapy. The key objective in a patient with haemodynamic instability is restoration of adequate cardiac output to maintain cerebral perfusion as well as a stable rhythm, using interventions least likely to cause harm.

Pathophysiology and pathogenesis

An understanding of cardiac arrhythmia requires knowledge of the normal conduction system (Fig. 5.4.1). In the normal heart, electrical impulses start from the sinoatrial (SA) node and conduct via the atria to the atrio-ventricular (AV) node. The electrical impulses then conduct down the bundle of His to the right and left bundle branches, and subsequently via the Purkinje fibres to the ventricular myocardium.

Different mechanisms, such as re-entry, enhanced automaticity and triggered activity, can result in arrhythmias. Abnormalities in the SA node, as in sick sinus syndrome, can result in failure of impulse formation. Abnormalities in the AV node can result in failure of electrical conduction from the atrium to the ventricles, resulting in various degrees of AV block. Ectopic impulses in the atria result in atrial ectopics or atrial tachycardia. Accessory pathways between the atrium and ventricle can result in supraventricular tachycardia.

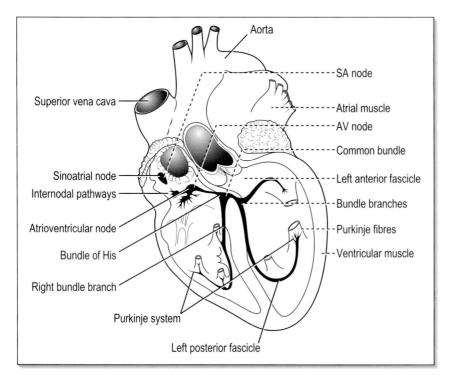

Fig. 5.4.1 Conducting system of the heart. (Reproduced with permission from Ganong WF. A review of medical physiology, 17th edn. Connecticut: Appleton & Lange, 1995.)

Abnormalities in ventricular conduction can result in bundle branch blocks or a variety of intraventricular conduction abnormalities. The most dangerous arrhythmias arise from the ventricles, as these, especially in the presence of underlying structural heart disease, may be associated with sudden death.

Re-entry

Re-entry occurs when a closed loop of conducting tissue transmits an electrical impulse around the loop and stimulates atrial or ventricular electrical activity with each pass around the circuit. Atrial and ventricular fibrillation and flutter are examples of micro re-entry, whereas paroxysmal supraventricular tachycardia is an example of macro re-entry.

Principles of assessment and management

Patients with arrhythmias may present with symptoms due to the arrhythmia, or may actually be asymptomatic and have the arrhythmia noticed during routine examination or investigations. All patients should initially be managed in an area where cardiac and other monitoring is available.

The urgency of treatment is dictated by the patient's clinical condition. For stable patients, the usual clinical process, including history, physical examination and investigations (particularly ECG), is appropriate. For the unstable patient urgent intervention is required, with restoration of a stable cardiac rhythm and cerebral perfusion being the priority. Clinical information, if promptly available, may be useful. For example, a patient with history of renal failure or heart failure taking spironolactone should raise the suspicion that a wide complex tachycardia is due to hyperkalemia.

Intravenous access would be obtained and blood can be drawn for investigations such as full blood counts, electrolytes and cardiac markers (if indicated). A 12-lead electrocardiogram (ECG) is essential, and a chest X-ray may be helpful. Other specific investigations, such as serum digoxin level, thyroid function tests and theophylline levels, may sometimes be indicated, depending on the arrhythmia and the clinical context.

The management of arrhythmias should begin with attention to the airway, breathing and circulation. Management of cardiac arrest is discussed in Section 1.

Bradyarrhythmias

Bradycardia is defined as a heart rate of less than 60 bpm. It is important to take into account the patient's underlying clinical state when treating bradyarrhythmias. ECG diagnosis of bradyarrhythmias can be simplified by the algorithm in Figure 5.4.2. Note that denervated transplanted hearts will not respond to atropine, and so if treatment is required, go at once to pacing, catecholamine infusion or both.

Sinus bradycardia

Physiological sinus bradycardia may be associated with good physical conditioning (e.g. marathon runners), drug effects (e.g. β-blockers, calcium antagonists) and vagal stimulation (e.g. vomiting). More serious causes include acute inferior myocardial infarction, raised intracranial pressure, hypothermia and hypothyroidism.

Clinical features

There are often no signs or symptoms. Symptoms may be related to the underlying cause.

ECG features

- Atrial rate equal to ventricular rates.
- Normal PR interval.
- Normal P-wave morphology.

Management

Special management is not usually required. Treat the underlying cause.

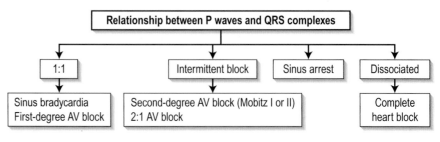

Fig. 5.4.2 Algorithm for ECG diagnosis of bradyarrhythmias.

If there is evidence of hypoperfusion, intravenous atropine 0.4–0.6 mg may be used while the cause is investigated. Physiological bradycardia does not require treatment. Disposition will depend on the cause.

Sick sinus syndrome (bradycardia–tachycardia syndrome)

This is most commonly found in elderly patients and results from fibrosis around the sinus node. It can also occur with congenital heart disease, rheumatic disorders, myocarditis, pericarditis, rheumatological disease, metastatic tumours, surgical damage, cardiomyopathies and ischaemic heart disease. It is a heterogeneous disorder that includes a wide variety of intermittent supraventricular tachycardias and bradyarrhythmias. Pathophysiologically, there is sinus bradycardia with intermittent failure of sinus node function, with the prolonged pause interrupted by a temporary escape rhythm. Drugs such as β-blockers, digoxin and antiarrhythmics, as well as conditions such as abdominal pain, thyrotoxicosis and hyperkalemia, can exacerbate the condition.

Clinical features

Typical features are syncope, light-headedness, palpitations, dyspnoea, chest pain, collapse and cerebrovascular accidents.

ECG features

- Sinus bradycardia.
- Intermittent cessation of P-wave activity.
- Long pauses interrupted by escape rhythms.
- Resumption of sinus node activity.

Management

Unstable patients should be managed with atropine 0.4–0.6 mg i.v. as a bridge to pacing. Transcutaneous pacing should be used if atropine is ineffective. Admission for emergency temporary pacing is required.

Drug treatment for tachyarrhythmia risks aggravating pre-existing AV block or sinus arrest and should be avoided until pacemaker insertion. These patients eventually require a permanent pacemaker.

Heart block

First-degree AV block

In first-degree AV block, conduction of the atrial impulse to the ventricle is delayed. A P wave precedes each QRS complex, but the PR interval is more than 0.2 seconds. Causes include drug effects, vagal stimulation, inferior myocardial infarction and high vagal tone (especially in young patients). Rarely it may be a sign of myocarditis (e.g. rheumatic myocarditis), digoxin toxicity, idiopathic fibrosis or aortic valve disease.

Clinical features There are no specific clinical features.

ECG features (Fig. 5.4.3)
- Every P wave is followed by a QRS.
- PR interval is constant but > 200 ms (five small squares on the ECG).

Management Usually no specific treatment is required. Unless associated with acute ischaemia, first-degree AV block is not itself an indication for hospital admission.

Second-degree AV block: Mobitz type I (Wenckebach)

In Mobitz type I AV block, conduction of the atrial impulses to the ventricles is intermittently blocked. This condition is due to impaired conduction in the AV node, and so the atrial rate is greater than the ventricular rate. There is a progressive increase in the PR interval until a dropped QRS complex occurs. After the dropped QRS, AV conduction recovers, resulting in a normal PR interval, and then the progressive increase in PR

interval starts again. Anatomically, this block is above the bundle of His in the AV node. It is thought to be due to prolongation of the refractory period of the AV node.

Causes include inferior myocardial infarction, digoxin toxicity and high vagal tone. The condition is nearly always benign and asymptomatic, but in the setting of acute ischaemia may progress to complete heart block.

Clinical features There are no specific clinical features.

ECG features (Fig. 5.4.4)
- Progressive increase in PR intervals until a dropped QRS complex occurs.
- First PR after dropped QRS is shorter.

Management No treatment is required for stable patients. Atropine or cardiac pacing may be indicated in the haemodynamically unstable patient.

Second-degree Mobitz type II AV block

Mobitz type II AV block is due to intermittent failure of conduction of atrial impulses to the ventricles. The PR interval remains constant, but there is regular intermittent failure of P-wave conduction. This is usually due to impaired conduction in the bundle of His or bundle branches (i.e. it is infranodal). Advanced second-degree block is the block of two or more consecutive P waves. This condition may be seen with acute coronary syndrome involving the left coronary artery, or less commonly, idiopathic fissure of the bundle branches.

Clinical features Although it may be asymptomatic, Mobitz type II AV block is more likely to be associated with stroke, Stoke–Adams attacks (syncope), a slow ventricular rate and sudden death.

ECG features (Fig. 5.4.5)
- Atrial rate > ventricular rate.
- Atrial rhythm is regular (Ps plot through).
- Some P waves are not followed by a QRS (more Ps than QRS).
- PR interval may be within normal limits or prolonged, but is constant for each conducted QRS.
- QRS complexes are dropped periodically. They may be narrow or widened.

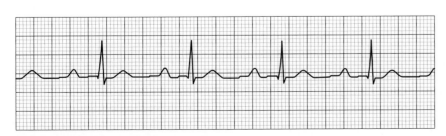

Fig. 5.4.3 Rhythm strip of first-degree AV block.

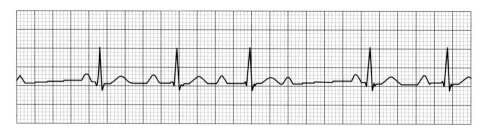

Fig. 5.4.4 Rhythm strip of second-degree AV block, Mobitz I.

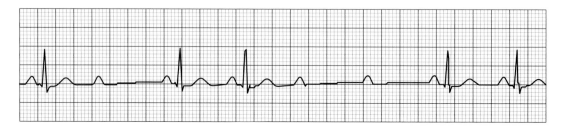

Fig. 5.4.5 Rhythm strip of second-degree AV block, Mobitz II.

Management   If the patient is haemodynamically unstable, atropine 0.4–0.6 mg i.v. and occasionally pacing may be needed. Patients with this condition should be admitted, as it can deteriorate to complete heart block.

Third-degree AV block

In third-degree or complete AV block, conduction of atrial impulse to the ventricles is completely blocked. Subsidiary pacemakers arise. If they are within the bundle of His, QRS complexes are narrow (Fig. 5.4.6). In contrast, if the block is infranodal, subsidiary pacemakers usually arise in the left or right bundle branches and the QRS complexes are wide (Fig. 5.4.7). The commonest cause of complete heart block is myocardial fibrosis; however, it is also seen in up to 8% of inferior myocardial infarctions, where it is often transient. Complete heart block is also associated with sick sinus syndrome, Mobitz II block and transient second-degree block with new bundle branch or fascicular block.

Clinical features   The patient may be asymptomatic. Syncope or near syncope is common. Clinically, cannon 'a' waves may be seen in the neck veins and the first heart sound may vary in loudness.

ECG features
- Complete dissociation of P waves and QRS complexes.

- Ventricular escape pacemaker is at 20–50 bpm.
- QRS may be wide or narrow.

Management   Haemodynamically compromised patients should have measures taken to increase ventricular rate to a level that results in adequate perfusion. Judicious use of atropine 0.4–0.6 mg i.v. may be helpful. If this is unsuccessful, dopamine or epinephrine (adrenaline) infusions, titrated to effect, may be effective. In ischaemic tissue epinephrine is preferred, as coronary perfusion is better maintained. External pacing may be required if these measures are ineffective. Admission is required and permanent pacing is often necessary.

   Never treat third-degree heart block with ventricular escape beats using lignocaine or any agent that suppresses ventricular escape rhythms, as this will suppress the already slow heart rate, resulting in reduced cardiac output.

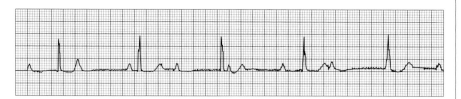

Fig, 5.4.6 Rhythm strip of narrow complex third-degree heart block.

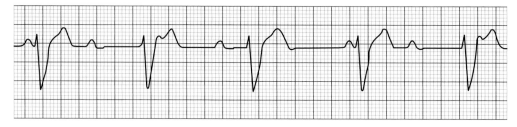

Fig. 5.4.7 Rhythm strip of third-degree heart block.

Tachyarrhythmias

There is a wide range of tachyarrhythmias. Immediate diagnosis and management may be considered on the basis of the width of the QRS complex and the regularity of the rhythm (Fig. 5.4.8).

Broad complex tachycardias

The differential diagnosis of a regular broad complex tachycardia includes ventricular tachycardia (VT) or supraventricular tachycardia (SVT) with aberrant conduction. Considerable research has been undertaken in an attempt to define ECG criteria that can reliably distinguish SVT from VT. Although relatively high sensitivities for some criteria have been reported, the high prevalence of VT in ED patients with broad complex tachycardia (approximately 80% in some studies) lowers the predictive value of those criteria. Features that increase the chance of a broad complex tachycardia being VT are shown in Table 5.4.1. It is usually safest to treat a broad complex tachycardia as VT unless there is very strong evidence to the contrary.

Ventricular arrhythmias

The proper identification of a ventricular arrhythmia is important in the evaluation of a patient. The management of ventricular arrhythmia depends on the correct identification of the rhythm, assessment of the risk–benefit ratio of antiarrhythmic drug therapy, and an awareness of non-pharmacological modes of treatment. The presence or absence of heart disease and left ventricular function (ejection fraction) also influence the management approach. Risk increases with the severity of structural heart disease and left ventricular dysfunction.

Ventricular tachycardia

Sustained VT is defined as a succession of ventricular impulses at a rate of > 100 per minute and lasting more than 30 seconds or resulting in haemodynamic compromise. If the patient is haemodynamically stable, a 12-lead ECG should be recorded to characterize morphology.

Clinical features Patients may be asymptomatic or complain of palpitations, dizziness or chest pain. Cannon 'a' waves may be seen in the neck veins. The patient may lose consciousness.

In the older patient with underlying ischaemic heart disease, syncope and hypotension, VT would be the most likely diagnosis.

ECG features (Figs 5.4.9 and 5.4.10)
- Wide QRS complexes > 140 ms.
- Rate > 100 bpm: commonly 150–200 bpm.
- Rhythm regular, although there is some beat-to-beat variability.
- Constant QRS axis, often with marked left axis deviation or northwest axis.
- AV dissociation.
- Fusion beats or capture beats.
- Deep S wave with r/S ratio < 1 in RBBB morphology VT.

Management VT should be managed according to current AHA/ACC guidelines. Management of pulseless VT is addressed in Section 1 of this book. All patients with VT require oxygen therapy and i.v. access, at which time blood for electrolyte and cardiac marker analysis is obtained. Electrolyte imbalances, particularly of potassium, should be corrected.

An unstable patient requires emergency cardioversion, with sedation as required. Caution is needed, especially as these patients usually have low blood pressure. The first recommended DC shock should be 100 J (synchronized). If this does not convert the rhythm, it can be increased to 150 J and then 200 J. This can be further increased to 360 J if required. The equivalent biphasic energy should be used for biphasic defibrillators (escalating 70 J, 120 J, 150 J, 170 J). Shock-resistant VT may respond after administration of amiodarone. Lignocaine, magnesium and procainamide are considered second-line adjuncts to cardioversion as there is less evidence to support their efficacy. An infusion of either amiodarone or lignocaine should be commenced after cardioversion. If the blood pressure is low, consider the use of inotropic support, for example with dopamine infusion.

Stable patients may be treated with:

- Intravenous amiodarone 150 mg slow bolus over 10 minutes. This can be repeated a second time if conversion has not been achieved.
- An alternative is i.v. procainamide 100 mg every 5 minutes to a maximum dose of 10–20 mg/kg body weight.

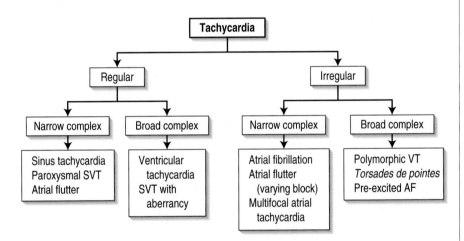

Fig. 5.4.8 Approach to tachyarrhythmias.

Table 5.4.1 Features that increase the chance of broad complex tachycardia being diagnosed as VT		
History	*Clinical features*	*ECG features*
Age >35 years	Cannon 'a' wave in JVP	AV dissociation
Smoker	Variable intensity of S1	Fusion beats
Ischaemic heart disease	Unchanged intensity of S2	Capture beats
Previous VT	QRS with >140 ms (<120 ms SVT)	
Active angina	Concordance of QRS vectors in pericardial leads	
Left axis variation >30° favours VT		
QRS morphology in V1		

If any doubt, treat as VT!

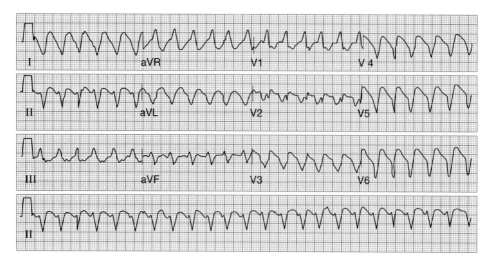

Fig. 5.4.9 Ventricular tachycardia (VT).

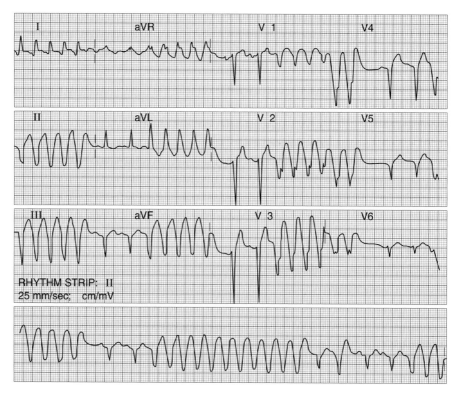

Fig. 5.4.10 Non-sustained VT.

- Intravenous lignocaine 50–100 mg i.v. push at a rate not more than 50 mg/min. This can be repeated a second time if conversion is not achieved. It should be noted, however, that lignocaine is relatively ineffective for terminating haemodynamically stable VT of unknown aetiology.

Sotolol 1 mg/kg may be considered a second-line agent. Following successful conversion, an infusion of the successful agent should be commenced for maintenance therapy. If pharmacological therapy is unsuccessful, cardioversion under sedation is indicated.

Polymorphic VT

VT with a continuously varying QRS morphology is called polymorphic VT. It is often associated with ischaemia and tends to be more electrically unstable than monomorphic VT.

Polymorphic VT includes a specific variant called *torsades de pointes*, which is associated with a prolonged QT. This is characterized by QRS peaks that twist around the baseline (Fig 5.4.11) and this occurs in the presence of repolarization abnormalities. Causes are summarized in Table 5.4.2.

Clinical features Syncope is the usual presenting symptom.

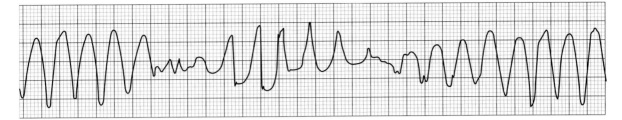

Fig. 5.4.11 *Torsades de pointes.*

Table 5.4.2 Causes of *torsades de pointes*
Hypomagnesaemia
Hypocalcaemia
Class I and class II antiarrhythmic drugs
Phenothiazines
Tricyclic antidepressants
Congenital prolonged QT syndrome
Organophosphates
Complete heart block
Drug interaction of terfenidine with erythromycin

ECG features
- Regular or irregular fast, wide QRS complexes.
- Continuously varying QRS morphology.

Management *Torsades de pointes* is very sensitive to magnesium. A bolus of 2 g over 1–2 minutes followed by an infusion will usually cause reversion. Cardioversion is recommended if the patient is haemodynamically compromised, but *torsades de pointes* can be resistant. Accelerating the heart rate, thereby shortening ventricular repolarization (e.g. by overdrive pacing to a rate of 90–120 bpm, or isoprenaline infusion titrated to similar effect) may be successful. Treatment of the underlying cause is essential as *torsades de pointes* is very difficult to control.

Idiopathic ventricular tachycardia
Idiopathic ventricular tachycardia is a monomorphic VT that occurs in the absence of structural heart disease. It is often exercise dependent and is named according to its site of origin. The QRS morphology during tachycardia can indicate the site of origin.

Idiopathic ventricular tachycardia presents as one of two subclasses:

- LBBB morphology VT due to right ventricular outflow tract ventricular tachycardia.
- RBBB morphology VT due to idiopathic left ventricular tachycardia.

Right ventricular outflow tract ventricular tachycardia
Right ventricular outflow tract ventricular tachycardia has a typical LBBB inferior axis morphology. The aetiology is believed to be cyclic-AMP (cAMP)-mediated triggered activity.

Clinical features This typically occurs in young patients and is slightly more common in females. There is usually no evidence of underlying structural heart disease.

ECG features
- QRS is broad (>120 ms) with a left bundle branch inferior axis morphology.
- AV dissociation is not usually seen as the tachycardia is often very rapid.
- Repetitive monomorphic forms may occur.

Management It is usually responsive to β-blockers, as it is catecholamine sensitive.

It is important to exclude underlying structural heart disease, especially arrhythmogenic right ventricular cardiomyopathy.

Idiopathic left ventricular tachycardia (ILVT)
Idiopathic left ventricular tachycardia is a fascicular ventricular tachycardia. The pathophysiology is a re-entrant phenomenon in the posterior fascicle of the left bundle branch.

Clinical features Fascicular VT occurs in young patients without structural heart disease.

ECG features (Fig. 5.4.12) QRS morphology is broad and shows a right bundle branch block pattern with left axis deviation. The duration of the QRS complex is 100–140 ms with an RS interval <80 ms. For ischaemic VT the duration of the QRS complex is usually >140 ms and the RS interval >100 ms.

ECG may also show capture beats or fusion beats.

Management The drug of choice is intravenous verapamil. Amiodarone and sotalol have been reported to be equally effective. Vagal manoeuvre and intravenous adenosine are ineffective in converting this arrhythmia. Lignocaine, which may used for ischaemic VT, is not effective for ILVT.

Pre-excited atrial fibrillation
Pre-excited atrial fibrillation (Wolff–Parkinson–White (WPW) AF) is a differential diagnosis for an irregular, wide complex tachycardia.

Clinical features The patient is usually young (age <50) with a previous history of palpitations, rapid heart rate, syncope or documented history of WPW.

ECG features (Fig. 5.4.13)
- Rapid ventricular response (>180 bpm; this response rate is much too rapid for conduction down the AV node).
- Broad and bizarre QRS complex, signifying conduction down the aberrant pathway.
- Occasionally, a narrow QRS can be seen, representing conduction through the AV node.
- Changing R-R intervals; a QRS complex that changes frequently.

During sinus rhythm, the ECG of patients with WPW shows a PR interval <0.12 seconds, a slurred R-wave upstroke (δ wave) and a wide QRS >0.10 seconds (Fig. 5.4.14).

Differential diagnosis Certain subtypes of polymorphic VT, such as *torsades de pointes*, present with an undulating baseline. In contrast, WPW AF usually has a stable electrocardiographic baseline with no alteration in the polarity of the QRS complexes.

CARDIOVASCULAR

5

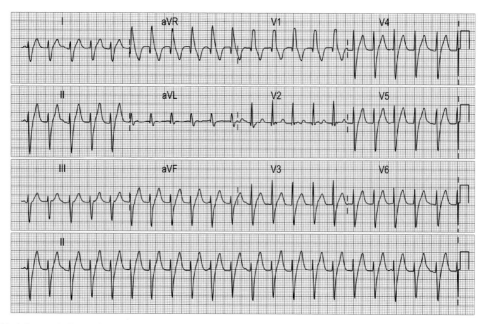

Fig. 5.4.12 Idiopathic left ventricular tachycardia (ILVT).

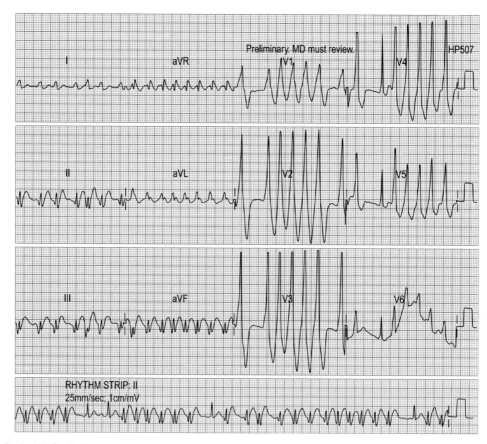

Fig. 5.4.13 Pre-excited atrial fibrillation.

Atrial fibrillation with aberrant conduction occurs when a patient with a pre-existing bundle branch block (or a rate-responsive bundle branch block) has a rapid ventricular response to AF. The ECG will show a wide complex tachycardia of irregular rate with stable beat-to-beat QRS configuration, contrasting with the variable beat-to-beat QRS configuration in WPW AF.

Management Haemodynamically unstable pre-excited AF is managed by immediate synchronized cardioversion. Haemodynamically stable pre-excited AF could be treated with:

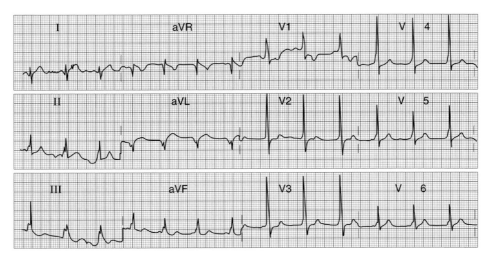

Fig. 5.4.14 Wolff–Parkinson–White syndrome: 12-lead ECG showing δ waves.

- I.v. procainamide (30 mg/min, maximum dose 17 mg/kg). Because of the potential for severe hypotension with rapid i.v. administration, procainamide requires a slow rate of infusion; it may not reach therapeutic blood levels for 40–60 minutes.
- I.v. ibutilide, a class III antiarrhythmic agent, can also be used. Dosage is 1 mg (0.01 mg/kg for patients <60 kg) over 10 minutes, repeated once after 10 minutes if needed. It has a very short half-life of 4 hours. Its dosing requires no concern for hepatic or renal function, and it is safe in elderly patients. It acts rapidly, with a mean conversion time of approximately 20 minutes.
- I.v. flecainide has been described as an alternative treatment.
- Amiodarone administration modifies sinus and AV node properties with little, if any, effect on fast-channel tissues (i.e. accessory pathways) and it is not effective in treatment of WPW with AF.

Narrow complex tachycardias

Sinus tachycardia Sinus tachycardia is defined as a heart rate >100 bpm. It not an arrhythmia per se, but rather an indication of an underlying disorder. Common causes include shock, hypoxia, cardiac failure, anaemia, drug effects, fever/infection, pain, anxiety, thyrotoxicosis and pregnancy.

Clinical features Patients may complain of palpitations, but are often asymptomatic. Clinical features would be those of the underlying cause.

ECG features
- Rate: 100–160 bpm
- Rhythm: regular
- P waves: uniform and upright in appearance, one preceding each QRS complex
- PR interval: 0.12–0.20 s
- QRS: <0.10 s.

Management Treat the underlying cause.

Paroxysmal supraventricular tachycardia

Paroxysmal supraventricular tachycardia (PSVT) originates from either an ectopic atrial focus or a re-entry circuit. Those caused by atrial flutter and fibrillation will be considered separately below.

Re-entry circuits are responsible for pre-excitation, which exists when whole or part of the ventricular muscle is activated earlier than anticipated. The majority of re-entry circuits involve the AV node. Retrograde conduction may also involve an AV bypass tract. WPW syndrome is the most common of these. It is characterized by an electrically conductive muscle bridge (bundle of Kent) connecting atria and ventricle and bypassing the AV node. ECG may show a PR interval of less than 0.12 s, a δ wave (slurred upstroke) and a wide QRS > 0.10 s (Fig. 5.4.14).

Clinical features Patients may have palpitations, chest pain or syncope.

ECG features (Fig. 5.4.15)
- Rate: 150–250 bpm.
- Rhythm: regular.
- P waves: atrial P waves differ from sinus P waves.
- P waves are usually identifiable at the lower end of the rate range but seldom identifiable at rates > 200 bpm.

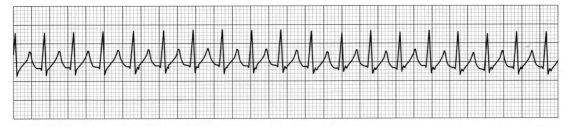

Fig. 5.4.15 Paroxysmal supraventricular tachycardia (PSVT).

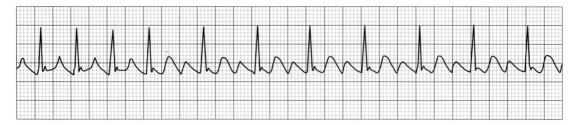

Fig. 5.4.16 Rhythm strip of atrial flutter.

- P waves may be lost in preceding T wave.
- PR interval: usually not measurable because the P wave is difficult to distinguish from the preceding T wave; if measurable, is 0.12–0.20 s.
- QRS: <0.10 s.

Management If the patient is haemodynamically unstable, cardioversion is indicated. Sedation is usually required.

If the patient is mildly symptomatic but blood pressure is >100 mmHg, vagal manoeuvres may be tried. If vagal manoeuvres are unsuccessful or inappropriate, the choice of drug therapy lies between adenosine (escalating 6 mg, 12 mg and 18 mg rapid boluses into a large vein) or verapamil (5 mg i.v. slowly, which may be repeated, or a continuous slow infusion of 1 mg/min to a maximum of 20 mg). There is scant evidence to show one is more effective than the other. Both have adverse effects. With adenosine, patients experience a transient sense of impending doom, chest discomfort and shortness of breath that can be very distressing. With verapamil hypotension may occur, hence the cautious administration. Concurrent use of β-blockers may potentiate this. Flecainide (2 mg/kg over 30–45 min) would be considered third-line therapy. Patients who are resistant to chemical cardioversion may require electrical cardioversion.

Atrial flutter

Atrial flutter rarely occurs in the absence of underlying heart disease. Causes include ischaemic heart disease, acute myocardial infarction, congestive cardiac failure, pulmonary embolism, myocarditis, chest trauma and digoxin toxicity.

Clinical features Patients may have palpitations and chest pain, or more commonly are asymptomatic.

ECG features (Fig. 5.4.16)
- Rate: atrial rate 250–350/min, flutter rate usually about 300/min.
- Ventricular rate variable, usually 150/min with 2:1 AV block. Rarely 1:1 or higher-degree AV block (3:1, 4:1).
- Rhythm: atrial rhythm regular; ventricular rhythm usually regular, but may be irregular.
- P waves: sawtoothed 'flutter waves'. Best seen in II, III, aVF.
- PR interval: not measurable.
- QRS: usually <0.10 s, but may be widened if flutter waves are buried in the QRS complex.

Management Treatment of the underlying illness is essential and will often result in spontaneous reversion. Haemodynamically unstable patients will usually respond to low-energy cardioversion (e.g. 50 J). Flecainide can be used for chemical reversion and verapamil for rate control, if required.

Atrial fibrillation

Atrial fibrillation (AF) is the result of chaotic atrial depolarization from multiple areas of re-entry within the atria. Thus, there is a lack of coordinated atrial activity. AF is characterized by an irregularly irregular rhythm without discrete P waves, and may be acute or chronic. Causes of AF seen in the ED are summarized in Table 5.4.3.

There are three variations of AF:

- Atrial fibrillation.
- Atrial fibrillation with slow ventricular response.
- Atrial fibrillation with regular ventricular response.

Clinical features Patients with acute episodes of AF often experience palpitations, dyspnoea, dizziness or angina. Those with chronic AF often have no specific

Table 5.4.3 Causes of AF seen in the emergency department
Cardiac
Ischaemic heart disease
Pericarditis
Hypertension
Rheumatic heart disease
Pre-excitation syndromes
Cardiomyopathy
Atrial septal defect
Atrial myxoma
Postoperative
Non-cardiac
Electrolyte imbalances
Sepsis
Pulmonary embolism
Drug and alcohol intoxication
Chronic obstructive airways disease
Thyrotoxicosis
Lung cancer
Intrathoracic pathology

symptoms, especially if their heart rate is <100 bpm. Clinically, the pulse is irregularly irregular and S1 varies in intensity.

Investigations Investigations will be guided by the clinical context. Patients with acute-onset AF should have electrolyte studies and thyroid function tests as well as consideration of cardiac marker levels. All patients with AF should have echocardiography, if not recently performed. This can be done as an outpatient procedure in those successfully treated in the ED.

ECG features (Fig. 5.4.17)

- Absent P waves.
- Chaotic irregular baseline – fibrillatory waves.
- Irregularly irregular RR cycles – fast or slow AF.
- Wide QRS due to aberrance may occur intermittently (Ashman's phenomenon).

Management Emergency management depends on the chronicity of the condition, the ventricular response rate,

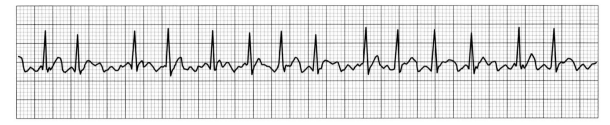

Fig. 5.4.17 Rhythm strip of atrial fibrillation.

haemodynamic stability, the presence of underling structural heart disease and any associated conditions.

The aim of treatment for patients with chronic AF is rate control and treatment of any associated illness. In patients with acute-onset AF the choice lies between cardioversion in the ED (electrical or pharmacological), rate control and anticoagulation with delayed elective electrical cardioversion, or rate control alone. The choice will be governed by the duration of the episode, the age of the patient, known structural heart disease, comorbidities and previous attempts at cardioversion. In general, a rhythm-control strategy is recommended for younger patients, those who are symptomatic, those presenting for the first time with lone AF, and those with AF secondary to a treatable/correctable precipitant. A rate-control strategy is recommended in patients aged over 65, those with coronary artery disease, those with contraindications to antiarrhythmic drugs, those unsuitable for cardioversion and those with congestive heart failure.

Haemodynamically stable patients where onset of AF is within 48 hours may be treated with either pharmacological or electrical cardioversion. Where AF is of a longer duration, a delayed elective cardioversion or rate control-only strategy is indicated. There is a case in otherwise well patients with very recent-onset paroxysmal AF in the absence of structural heart disease or other underlying condition for a period of observation, as up to 90% will revert spontaneously – usually within 24 hours.

For pharmacological cardioversion in patients without structural heart disease a class Ic agent such as flecainide (2 mg/kg over 20–30 min) or propafenone is recommended. Sotolol (1 mg/kg over 30 min) is an alternative. Where structural heart disease is present, amiodarone (2–3 mg/kg over 5–10 min, repeated if necessary) is

the drug of choice. Rate control can be achieved with β-blockers (e.g. metoprolol 5–10 mg i.v. over 2 min), verapamil (5–10 mg i.v. over 2–5 min), amiodarone or diltiazem. Digoxin is not recommended.

In patients with life-threatening haemodynamic instability, emergency electrical cardioversion should be attempted, irrespective of the duration of the AF. In patients with WPW syndrome, flecainide may be used as an alternative to attempt pharmacological cardioversion. Atrioventricular node-blocking agents (such as diltiazem, verapamil or digoxin) should not be used. In patients with known permanent AF where haemodynamic instability is caused mainly by a poorly controlled ventricular rate, a pharmacological rate-control strategy should be used. β-Blockers or rate-limiting calcium antagonists are the agents of choice or, where these are contraindicated or ineffective, amiodarone.

Multifocal atrial tachycardia

This rare arrhythmia is characterized by three or more atrial foci, a ventricular rate of more than 100 bpm, and variable PP, PR and RR intervals. It is associated with chronic obstructive lung disease, hypoxia, electrolyte disturbance, pulmonary embolus and digoxin toxicity. Treatment is directed at improving the underlying condition. Specific treatment of the arrhythmia is rarely required and often not helpful.

Unifascicular blocks

A unifascicular block is a conduction block that affects one of the major infranodal conduction pathways: right bundle branch block (RBBB), left anterior fascicular block (LAFB) or left posterior fascicular block (LPFB). Conduction blocks can be caused by ischaemia, cardiomyopathies, valvular disease, myocarditis, surgery, congenital disease and degenerative diseases (Lenegre or Lev disease).

Left anterior fascicular block

Clinical features There are no specific clinical features.

ECG features
- Left axis deviation.
- Normal QRS duration.

Management Usually no treatment needed. Treat the underlying cause.

Left posterior fascicular block

Clinical features There are no specific clinical features.

ECG features
- Right axis deviation.
- Normal QRS duration.

Management Usually no treatment needed. Treat the underlying cause.

Right bundle branch block

RBBB can be a normal variant. Other causes include pulmonary embolism, right ventricular hypertrophy, ischaemic heart disease, congenital heart disease and cor pulmonale.

Clinical features Clinical features will be those of the underlying cause.

ECG features (Fig. 5.4.18)
- rSR pattern, most noted in V1 and V2.
- Broad S wave in left ventricular leads.
- QRS > 120 ms in complete RBBB and ≤ 120 ms with incomplete RBBB.

Management Treat the underlying cause. If there is a new RBBB, the cause should be actively determined.

Combination blocks

A bifascicular block is a conduction block that affects two of the major infranodal

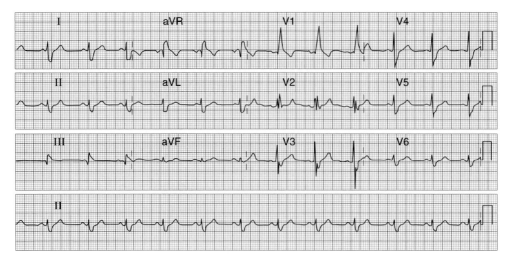

Fig. 5.4.18 Right bundle branch block.

conduction pathways. This may be a left bundle branch block (LBBB) or a combination of RBBB and LAFB or LPFB. Trifascicular block is a combination of conduction blocks of all three fascicles. Examples include:

- RBBB and LAFB with first-degree AV block.
- RBBB and LPFB with first-degree AV block.
- LBBB with first-degree AV block.
- Alternating RBBB and LBBB.

Blocks may be permanent or transient. In the setting of an acute myocardial infarction both bi- and trifascicular blocks may degenerate to complete heart block. Thus admission to a monitored bed is needed and pacemaker insertion considered.

Left bundle branch block

LBBB is usually pathological. Causes include myocardial infarction, ischaemic heart disease, left ventricular hypertrophy, congenital heart disease and left ventricular strain.

Clinical features Clinical features will be those of the underlying cause.

ECG features (Fig. 5.4.19)
- RR pattern, best seen in left ventricular leads V5 and V6.
- QRS > 120 ms.

Management Treat the underlying cause. If there is a new LBBB in the setting of myocardial ischaemia, management should be as for acute myocardial infarction.

Other disturbances of cardiac rhythm and conduction

Atrial ectopics

Atrial ectopics are mostly asymptomatic and may be precipitated by alcohol, nicotine and caffeine. They may be associated with atrial fibrillation, underlying heart disease or respiratory disease.

ECG features
- Usually earlier than normal (premature).
- P-wave morphology different from sinus P. May be lost or deformed.
- PR interval may be short or long.
- QRS usually normal unless aberrantly conducted.

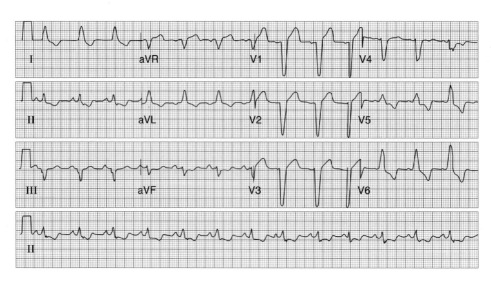

Fig. 5.4.19 Left bundle branch block.

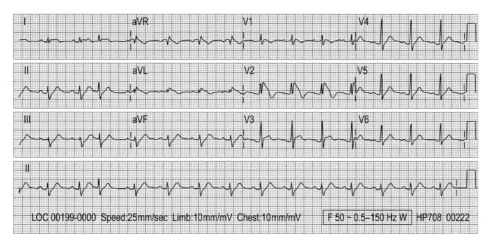

Fig. 5.4.20 Brugada syndrome.

- When early, may be blocked – blocked atrial ectopic.

Management Usually no treatment is necessary.

Junctional rhythm
A junctional rhythm is usually asymptomatic.

ECG features
- Rate is slower than sinus rhythm.
- Rhythm is regular.
- No preceding P wave.
- Infrequently P wave may precede or be just after the QRS (the P waves are inverted in II, III, aVF).
- QRS usually narrow unless aberrantly conducted.

Management Usually no treatment needed.

Brugada syndrome
The Brugada syndrome is a newly diagnosed syndrome with the ECG showing right bundle branch morphology and coved ST segment elevation in V1 and V2 with terminal T inversion (Fig. 5.4.20). The ECG pattern may be associated with sudden cardiac death from ventricular fibrillation. There may be a family history of sudden death. Occasionally the ECG pattern is seen only during fever or after taking antiarrhythmic drugs, especially class IC antiarrhythmics such as flecainide or propafenone. Patients with the Brugada pattern should be referred for further evaluation and risk stratification.

Controversies

- There is not much evidence for the use of many second-line antiarrhythmic drugs from randomized controlled trials.

- How safe is it to attempt immediate cardioversion for atrial fibrillation in the ED without formal echocardiography to exclude atrial thrombosis? Is 24 or 48 hours the safer cut-off duration?

- Is there a role for a period of observation for minimally symptomatic recent-onset paroxysmal AF?

- Is a slow-infusion calcium antagonist safer, more effective and more cost-effective than adenosine in converting supraventricular tachycardia?

Further reading

Atkins DC, Dorian P, Gonzalez ER, et al. Treatment of tachyarrythmias. Annals of Emergency Medicine 2001; 37: S91–S110.

Blaauw Y, Crijns HJ. Atrial fibrillation: insights from clinical trials and novel treatment options. Journal of Internal Medicine 2007; 262: 593–614.

Brugada P, Brugada J. Right bundle branch block, persistent ST segment elevation and sudden cardiac death: a distinct clinical and electrocardiographic syndrome. A multicenter report. Journal of the American College of Cardiology 1992; 20: 1391–1396.

Gorgels AP, van den Dool A, Hofs A, et al. Comparison of procainamide and lidocaine in terminating sustained monomorphic ventricular tachycardia. American Journal of Cardiology 1996; 78: 43–46.

National Collaborating Centre for Chronic Conditions. Atrial fibrillation. National clinical guideline for management in primary and secondary care. London (UK): Royal College of Physicians, 2006. http://www.guideline.gov/summary/summary.aspx?ss=15&doc_id=9629&nbr= 5149#s23. Accessed November 2007.

Sgarbossa EB, Pinski SL, Barbagelata A, et al. Electrocardiographic diagnosis of evolving acute myocardial infarction in the presence of left bundle-branch block. GUSTO-1 (Global Utilization of Streptokinase and Tissue Plasminogen Activator for Occluded Coronary Arteries) Investigators. New England Journal of Medicine 1996; 334: 481–487.

Sgarbossa EB, Pinski SL, Wagner GS. Left bundle-branch block and the ECG in diagnosis of acute myocardial infarction. Journal of the American Medical Association 1999; 282: 1224–1225.

Shah CP, Thakur RK, Xie B, et al. Clinical approach to wide complex tachycardias. Emergency Clinics of North America 1998; 16: 331–359.

Teo KK, Yusuf S, Furberg CD. Effects of prophylactic antiarrhythmic drug therapy in acute myocardial infarction. An overview of results from randomized controlled trials. Journal of the American Medical Association 1993; 270: 1589–1595.

Tzivoni D, Banai S, Schuger C, et al. Treatment of torsade de pointes with magnesium sulfate. Circulation 1988; 77: 392–397.

5.5 Pulmonary embolism

David Mountain • Peter Cameron

ESSENTIALS

1 Venous thromboembolic (VTE) disease has protean clinical manifestations and is a continuum from deep venous thrombosis to the main life-threatening complication of pulmonary embolus.

2 Patients with a diagnosis of pulmonary embolus (PE), left untreated, have a high mortality rate that is significantly reduced by anticoagulation.

3 Diagnostic and treatment decisions rely on good risk stratification to avoid excessive investigation, unnecessary therapy and, for those diagnosed with PE, to guide early discharge or aggressive management. The decision to treat is based on reaching a diagnostic threshold (about 70–80% chance of PE) where PE morbidity/mortality outweigh the risks of anticoagulation. The investigative algorithm involves ECG, chest X-ray (CXR) and measures of oxygenation (plus other investigations for alternative diagnoses) to stratify risk, guide radiological testing and look for alternative causes. Which validated combinations of D-dimer, lower limb ultrasound, V/Q scan and CT angiogram (± CT venography) are used to refine probability will depend on local resources.

4 The gold standard test of pulmonary angiography is not easily available. If it is available, it should be reserved for the small group of patients where the probability of PE is still indeterminate after exhaustive non-invasive investigations.

5 In massive PE transthoracic or, if available, transoesophageal echocardiography is the recommended initial investigation.

6 Low molecular weight heparin (although UFH is still considered adequate) is now recommended for treatment of deep-vein thrombosis and pulmonary embolus. It can safely be used on an outpatient basis in selected patients.

7 Thrombolysis (or embolectomy if thrombolysis is contraindicated) is indicated for haemodynamically unstable/shocked PE (limited RCT data). Stable patients with evidence of right ventricular strain (see below for definition) should be monitored more vigilantly with thrombolysis initiated urgently if they deteriorate.

Introduction

Pulmonary embolus (PE) is the third most common cardiovascular disease, and historical data suggest that, left untreated, it is associated with high hospital mortality. Treating PE with anticoagulation reduces the overall hospital mortality to 6–12%. Of these deaths, 4–9% are due to comorbidity and 1.5–5% directly to PE.[1, 2]

Many risk factors and conditions are proven to be associated with PE. However, 25–50% of PEs, particularly those presenting to the emergency department (ED), are idiopathic.[2,3] Most risk factors act via more than one of the processes in Virchow's triad (e.g. vessel wall injury, venous stasis or hypercoagulable states). The major risk factors associated with secondary (e.g. provoked) PE are surgery/trauma (particularly pelvic/lower limb and CNS) (15–30%); neoplasms (10–25%), systemic disease with immobilization, particularly heart disease and disabling strokes (5–15%), and a past history of DVT/PE (particularly unprovoked and recent).[4] Other provoking factors important in individuals (although not a common overall cause) are hypercoagulable states, e.g. antithrombin 111 deficiency, antiphospholipid syndrome, protein C and S deficiencies, hyperhomocysteinaemia, and many others both congenital and acquired.[2,3] Other associations include increasing age (particularly over 60), indwelling venous devices, the oral contraceptive pill, obesity, pregnancy, some vasculitic diseases with venous involvement, smoking, and probably long-haul air travel.[2,3]

The diagnosis and management of PE is difficult and relies on the estimation of probabilities rather than any definitive test. At all times the possibility of alternative serious conditions causing the symptoms/signs should be considered. In general, if the risk of PE is below 3–5% (e.g. low-risk emergency patients) then an alternative diagnosis should be sought. Indeed, in this population excessive investigation may find more false positive venous thromboembolism (VTE) than real PE or DVT. The threshold for diagnosing PE is around 70–80% probability of PE, so that the benefits of therapy outweigh the significant risks. These probabilities may vary for individual patients if the risks of PE are high (e.g. pre-existing lung/right heart disease) or bleeding risks are excessive (e.g. high risk of falls). The probability is based on history, examination and investigations, which may include chest X-ray, arterial blood gas analysis, ECG or other investigations looking for an alternative diagnosis. For those who are not experts, the estimate is best made using validated scoring systems. The best validated system and most widely disseminated is the Wells rule[5] (Table 5.5.1). Most institutions now use ventilation/perfusion (V/Q) scan and/or computed tomographic (CT) pulmonary angiography (CTPA) where necessary. Many diagnostic pathways also include D-dimer assay and venous ultrasound (or CT venography). Some centres may also use echocardiography for risk stratification or unstable cases. MRI has been investigated in some centres but is not routinely used (Fig. 5.5.1).

History

The history is the most important screen. Virtually all patients with PE will present with a

Table 5.5.1 Wells clinical criteria for PE	
Clinical signs of DVT	3.0
Pulse rate >100 (at rest)	1.5
Immobilized ≥3 days	1.5
Surgery < 4 weeks	1.5
Past history PE/DVT	1.5
Haemoptysis	1.0
Current/recent neoplasm	1.0
No alternative diagnosis more likely than PE*	3.0
Score	
Low	<2
Moderate	2–6
High	>6

*Including information from ECG, ABG, CXR and other tests for alternative diagnoses.

history of either recent-onset dyspnoea (particularly if rapid or recurrent episodic), chest pain or both (sensitivity 97%, specificity 10%).[6] Syncope with respiratory symptoms or signs (even if transient), or in patients at high risk of VTE, is a marker for severe PE. Symptoms of DVT should be asked for in all patients. Haemoptysis has some predictive value but is an uncommon symptom/sign.[5] Other symptoms are less important in the diagnosis of PE, but may help to suggest or exclude other causes. Associated risk factors (as described above) increase the probability of PE and should be documented and incorporated into the risk assessment. No single symptom or sign has the sensitivity or specificity to either establish or exclude the diagnosis.

Examination

Physical signs are occasionally useful in making the diagnosis of PE more likely. A persistent unexplained tachycardia at rest does increase the concern for PE. Leg (or arm) signs of DVT, particularly a swollen leg with pain in the venous distribution, or thrombophlebitis, significantly increase the risk of PE and require imaging for a complete work-up.[5] Other features found not infrequently are tachypnoea (50–80%), cough (10–20%), mild fever (<38.5 °C), wheeze and pleural effusion. They are not discriminatory for PE.[5] Occasionally, elevated jugular venous pressure

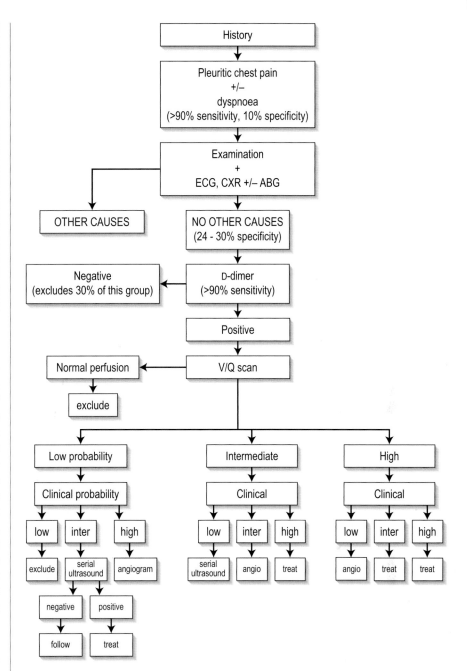

Hypoxaemic/haemodynamically unstable consider CT angiogram/TOE

Fig. 5.5.1 Investigation algorithm for pulmonary embolism.

(JVP), a loud S2 and a pulmonary systolic murmur may be found and are markers of right ventricular strain.

Investigations

The initial screening tests for PE are:

• CXR: A normal CXR with significant hypoxia is suggestive of PE. However, the

CXR is reportedly abnormal in 80–90% of patients diagnosed with PE. If definitely present, an enlarged descending pulmonary artery, pulmonary oligaemia or cut-off, a plump pulmonary artery and 'Hampton's hump' (a semicircular opacity with the base abutting the pleural surface) are all quite specific for PE (70–90%). However, these signs may be subtle and have poor sensitivity.[4,6] Pleural effusion, plate atelectasis, enlarged heart shadow and non-specific consolidation are seen commonly but do not occur more often in PE patients. The main role of CXR is in the identification of alternative causes for symptoms, and to decide on which radiological test is appropriate.

- ECG: At least 21 potential signs have been postulated, but they are relatively insensitive and most lack specificity. Some signs have significant specificity for PE with right ventricular strain. The most significant are tachycardias (particularly atrial), RBBB (including incomplete or transient patterns), right axis deviation (particularly S1–3), T-wave inversion (especially deep V1–V3) and S1Q3T3. The more features of right ventricular strain that are present on the ECG, the more suggestive it is for major PE. These changes have been associated with poorer outcome in PE.[7,8]

- Arterial blood gas (ABG): In recent years the role of ABG in the diagnosis of PE has been challenged. A $PaO_2 < 80$mmHg in the absence of another cause makes PE likely; however, 12% of patients with PE have $PaO_2 > 80$mmHg. An abnormal A-a gradient increases the likelihood of PE, but 20% of patients with PE will have a normal A-a gradient.[9] If there is coexisting pulmonary disease then a previous ABG is essential to interpret the result. In current clinical practice an oxygen saturation measurement is sufficient to exclude significant hypoxaemia (<92%). There is little to be gained in using ABG for routine screening for PE.

- D-dimer tests: these have been available clinically since the 1980s. They are now well validated in emergency practice and are recommended by most current guidelines, but only have adequate specificity when used in ED populations. They will reduce the need for further investigations in a reasonable number of patients (20–50%). D-dimers are only useful to exclude PE when negative, as in many conditions other than VTE they may be raised. To be used safely and efficiently, it is important that the following steps are used: they should be used as part of an agreed diagnostic process; patients must be adequately

stratified into either dichotomous low/ high or low/intermediate/high risk groups; patients with little chance of a negative D-dimer should be excluded (e.g. recent surgery, active cancer, late pregnancy or shocked). Patients with prolonged symptoms (over a week) are more likely to have false negative tests and should not be tested.[10]

The D-dimer test's diagnostic performance should be known. If it is a high-sensitivity test such as VIDAS© or one of the newer validated rapid latex tests, then it is safe to use in low/intermediate groups (< 30% chance of PE). Low-sensitivity tests such as Simpli-Red or most latex agglutination tests are only safe to use in low-risk patients (< 10% chance of PE). If the D-dimer is positive and no alternative diagnosis has become clear, further investigation is indicated. The test should not be used if PE is not a significant part of the differential diagnosis.[10]

Following screening tests, more definitive investigations, including V/Q scan, CTPA, US or CT venography, should be performed. V/Q or CTPA are the normal initial investigations. If both are available, decisions should be made according to patient-related issues (discussed below with each modality) and local logistics. Pulmonary angiography is now rarely available as most radiology departments have replaced CTPA with multislice scanners, but it gives a definitive result if it is available. In unstable patients echocardiography is the preferred initial test. MRI scanning may be used occasionally for patients where V/Q and CTPA are contraindicated or unavailable.[10]

V/Q scan

V/Q scanning is normally readily available in major hospitals, has a low complication rate, moderate radiation exposure, and can be used in patients with renal dysfunction. Problems are that potentially unwell patients may spend a long time in often distant nuclear medicine departments, and many do not provide 24-hour-a-day scanning. The major criticism of V/Q scanning is that the majority of scans are non-diagnostic (>50% in the PIOPED study),[11] requiring additional testing to adequately rule PE in or out. Because patients with obvious abnormalities on CXR (e.g. major collapse, pleural effusions or parenchymal

lung disease) or major lung disease are almost certain to have indeterminate V/Q scans, they should have CTPA if available.[10]

Two major studies (PIOPED[11] and McMaster[12]) have helped to define these probabilities and their combination with clinical risk assessment. Scans were defined as normal, low, intermediate and high probability, according to the number and size of lung segments not perfused, and matching with ventilation defects. The interobserver variability in the intermediate and low-probability interpretations was as high as 70% in the PIOPED study. Although variations on the definitions have occurred and some centres may report differently, the majority use the PIOPED reporting system. Most Australian centres now mostly use technetium rather than Xenon (used in PIOPED), because it gives better views. More recently it has been suggested that the number of segments may be less open to interpretation errors and just as accurate in predicting the probability of PE as the number and size of the segments.[13] Further management depends on the combination of clinical risk and V/Q results, as discussed below.

Normal/near-normal scan

A normal/near-normal perfusion scan excludes significant PE, but in PIOPED only 14% had a normal/near-normal scan. This rate is probably greater in ED populations and if patients with abnormal CXR are excluded.[11,12]

High probability

A high-probability scan was associated with a greater than 85% chance of PE, but only 13% had a high-probability scan. Also, 15% of patients treated on the basis of just a high-probability scan would be anticoagulated, or even thrombolysed, unnecessarily. However, the majority of those without PE are low-risk patients with a high probability scan (only 55% PE +ve). This group should have further investigations.[11,12]

Low/intermediate

The low- and intermediate-probability groups had a 15–30% and a greater than 30% chance, respectively, of having PE. Patients with a low clinical risk assessment and a near-normal/low-probability V/Q scan have a < 5% chance of PE. Most of these patients can be discharged (if other major diagnoses are excluded) but care, with consideration of further imaging, should be taken in patients with critical cardiorespiratory problems, as they may have high mortality from even small missed PE.[11,12,14]

There is much debate about how to manage patients with low/intermediate combinations of clinical risk and V/Q scan results. In PIOPED these combinations had rates of PE of 16%. However, a number of studies have shown that with serial or even single negative lower limb studies (US or venography) to exclude DVT there are low rates of recurrent PE or death.[10] Patients who are at high risk from small PE should be investigated more aggressively. Patients with dichotomous risk/V/Q results (low/high) or intermediate/intermediate results need further definitive investigation.[10,14]

Computed tomographic pulmonary angiography and venography (CTPA and CTV)

Multislice CTPA is increasingly available in many centres, and after-hours availability is frequently higher than for V/Q scanning. CT is preferable to V/Q in most patients with pre-existing lung disease. CT appears to be accurate in diagnosing main, lobar and segmental vessel emboli. Sensitivity for subsegmental emboli is low, but the prevalence

(6–30% reported) and clinical significance of this group of PEs is not known. Multislice CTPA has increased sensitivity for smaller PE, reported as 90–100% in some studies. It has good specificity for PE (93–99%).[14] However, the recent PIOPED2 study suggested that sensitivity may be as low as 85% for PE. When combined with CT venography (CTV), sensitivity was improved to 90%. The endpoints used in this study probably overestimated the true rate of PE, so that sensitivity was probably better than that reported.[15] Large numbers of patients have been followed up after negative CTPA and leg imaging, and the rates of recurrent PE/death are about 1–2/0.2–0.5%. These are similar to findings after negative PA or normal V/Q scans.[10,14,15] Many centres are now using CT and lower limb ultrasound (or CTV) to exclude significant PE. This is probably a safe strategy for excluding PE in all but high-risk patients without an alternative diagnosis. In patients initially at low clinical risk of PE a negative CTPA without leg imaging is a safe strategy[14,16] (Fig. 5.5.2).

A major advantage of CTPA is that other thoracic causes of chest pain can be imaged. In some series alternative diagnosis are seen in up to 60% of scans, with acute serious conditions in 20–30%.[16] Additionally, as

scanners become more powerful, data on right ventricular size and shape may assist in risk-stratifying PE. Finally, in some centres CTV using the dye from the CTPA during the run-off phase to image the venous system (legs to heart) can be used instead of ultrasound. Almost all of the additional yield (3–5% additional PE/DVT diagnosed in some studies) is from imaging leg veins, and radiation doses to the gonadal areas from pelvic/abdominal scanning can be avoided.[15,16]

CTPA has some significant problems in clinical practice. In some studies up to 15% of scans are technically inadequate. It requires a significant dye load, so patients with renal dysfunction or contrast/iodine allergies should have alternative investigations if possible. The radiation dosing in total is high. However, in males the scans are generally to radioinsensitive tissues, but in women under 40–45 proliferative breast tissues receive high radiation doses (2–4 Gy per breast), conferring a significant increased lifetime risk of breast cancer. V/Q scanning and ultrasound of the legs should be preferred in all young female patients, including pregnant women.[16]

Pulmonary angiography

Pulmonary angiography is a 'gold standard' in diagnosing PE. It has very good sensitivity (98–100%) and specificity (97–100%) in all but the smallest PE. At subsegmental level disagreements between radiologists are common. Because there are significant technical, logistical and clinical difficulties in its performance and a mortality of 0.3%/complication rate of 3%, it is now rarely used.[10,16]

Magnetic resonance imaging

Magnetic resonance imaging (MRI) techniques are improving rapidly. Sensitivity for central emboli is already > 90%, with high specificity. However, there is little place at this stage for MRI in the acute setting (unless CT/VQ are not available/contraindicated) because of access, cost and availability. The advantage of both MRI and CT is that they allow simultaneous imaging of other thoracic structures.[14]

Echocardiography – transthoracic or transoesophageal (TTE/TOE)

Echocardiography is a rapid and relatively accurate method of diagnosing massive PE with instability. It can exclude other causes of hypotension and raised venous pressure (such as tamponade, major valve or myocardial dysfunction), and in almost all cases of massive PE will demonstrate right heart

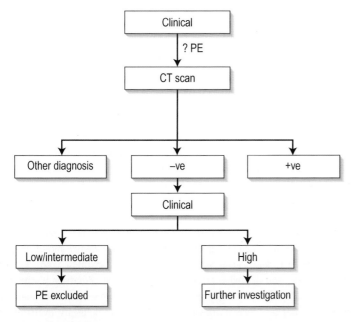

Fig. 5.5.2 Alternative algorithm.

dysfunction and sometimes pulmonary artery or atrial clot. Importantly, it can be performed in the resuscitation room and can guide thrombolytic treatment for the unstable patient.[10] It is not sensitive for peripheral emboli and is not part of the normal diagnostic strategy.[14] However, in the haemodynamically stable patient echocardiography gives useful information on right heart strain and in-hospital prognosis. Those with right heart strain are at much higher risk of a poor outcome (5–15% mortality vs 0–2% in those without).[10,16] If available, this information may affect management decisions after PE is diagnosed.

Management

General measures and risk stratification

The management of PE begins with prevention. Thromboembolic disease should be considered a continuum from DVT to PE. The greatest single preventable cause of DVT is surgery. Low-dose anticoagulation should be routine, and the introduction of low molecular weight heparin has made this safer and more effective for some groups. Venous stasis as a result of bed rest, cardiopulmonary disease and travel is a further important cause of PE. Mobilization techniques are important, and low-dose anticoagulation has been demonstrated to improve outcomes in medical patients admitted for bed rest.[17] This should be started as early as possible, and there is a role for emergency physicians to start thromboprophylaxis in high-risk patients in the ED.

Risk stratification

Patients diagnosed with PE need to be risk-stratified for prognosis during their hospital stay. This is because there are significant differences in both ongoing therapy and monitoring required for PE patients with a different prognosis from PE. In general, the features that determine prognosis are overt haemodynamic or respiratory failure (at any stage), features suggesting right ventricular overload or severe VQ mismatch, and severe underlying comorbidities.[14,18,19] Haemodynamic or respiratory instability should be clinically obvious, although the use of venous/arterial gases to expose unexpected lactic acidosis/hypoxia if a patient looks non-specifically unwell, is reasonable. In patients without obvious instability prognosis may be determined by looking at

historical features such as collapse/syncope/arrest or severe comorbidity; physical examination (e.g. borderline perfusion, BP, persistent tachycardia, signs of right ventricular failure/cor pulmonale); bedside/laboratory investigations, e.g. ECG – right ventricular strain patterns, particularly if multiple features, troponin rises (5–20% mortality), possibly raised BNP (>90 pg/mL) or hypoxia on oximetry (persistently < 95%) or by ABG on room air; echocardiography – with signs of right ventricular strain (5–20% mortality if present) or occasionally thrombus in transit (mortality 20–60%).[18,19] Other features that raise concerns for patients are a demonstration of a massive clot load (e.g. massive DVT), recurrent PE on adequate therapy, and serious cardiopulmonary comorbidity.

Treatment

General approach

Almost all patients with diagnosed PE need to have a combination of supportive care, including oxygen therapy, thromboprophylaxis, analgesia, and careful observation for an initial period while early prognosis is determined and heparin/warfarin therapy is initiated (unless there is an absolute contraindication). Thought should be given to taking a thrombophilia screen before heparin is started when there is an unprovoked PE, or if the PE is recurrent and thrombophilia has not been checked previously.[20] Heparin therapy can be given either as intravenous unfractionated heparin (UFH) or low molecular weight heparin. LMWH therapy has been shown to be at least as effective as (clinically and by cost) and probably safer than UFH for DVT and PE. The evidence for PE is weaker than for DVT, but the equivalence of the therapies is accepted and some authorities accept an overall benefit.[20] Dosing for enoxaparin is usually 1.5 mg/kg daily or 1 mg bd, but all LMWH will provide adequate therapy. Dosing must be reduced for those with poor renal function (reduced dose and frequency) and the morbidly obese (e.g. 100 kg maximum weight). The use of LMWH is particularly useful if early discharge from inpatient units or even home therapy is being contemplated. Home therapy is widely used in North America in low-risk PE, and in well-selected cases it seems to be safe.[21] It is recommended in some current guidelines, such as those of the British Thoracic Society (2003).[20]

However, this strategy is still controversial and relies on good risk stratification.[21] Warfarin should be started after initial heparin therapy is therapeutic and maintained for at least 3 months. The risk of anticoagulation causing major bleeding may be as high as 10% over 6 months in high-risk patients (probably 2–4% in well-controlled patients), with 1–3% intracranial haemorrhage rates in some registries and mortality from bleeding of 0.1–1% pa.[20,22] There are risk scores for assessing who is at high risk of bleeding. Clearly the elderly, hypertensive, falling, alcoholic or severely comorbid patients are at much higher risk. Although the overall in-hospital mortality from untreated PE may approach 30%, the risk of not treating low-probability scans (and therefore small PEs), particularly if the lower limbs are free of clot, and following the patient clinically, may be lower.

Patients at high risk of deterioration

Patients without cardiorespiratory stability but with features consistent with right ventricular strain or major PE (see above) should be considered for close observation and/or continuous monitoring in a high-dependency or critical care area. The reason for this is the high rate of deterioration/death in these patients, with up to 25% requiring inotropes, intubation or thrombolysis for instability, and mortality rates of up to 10% (e.g. similar to acute AMI).[16,18,19] A management plan should have been decided upon before transfer out of the ED, with criteria for (or at least further consultation about) initiation of thrombolysis/thrombectomy.

Unstable patients

Patients presenting with overt shock, deteriorating respiratory failure or a history of recovery from cardiorespiratory arrest should be resuscitated, stabilized, and in most cases given thrombolysis (or alternative treatments if thrombolysis is contraindicated; see below).[18,20] Severe hypoxaemia may require endotracheal intubation and ventilation. Haemodynamic instability requires gentle intravascular fluid loading with 250–500 mL bolus crystalloids, with no more than 1 L in total unless dehydration or hypovolaemia are clearly coexistent with PE. The reason for this is that in massive PE the right ventricle is already pressure overloaded and failing, and excessive fluids just overstretch a failing ventricle (Starlings' Law).

This treatment may be sufficient to maintain blood pressure. However, persistent hypotension will require inotropic support. There is little evidence to support the use of norepinephrine (noradrenaline) over epinephrine (adrenaline) as the inotrope of choice.[23] Patients requiring inotropes should not be treated with isoprenaline as this results in vasodilatation, reduced peripheral resistance and increased cardiac output, without an improvement in coronary perfusion.

Specific treatments in unstable patients

Thrombolysis

The widespread use of thrombolytic therapy for coronary disease has led to a reappraisal of thrombolytics in PE. There is definite evidence of reduced pulmonary artery pressures and improved right ventricular function after thrombolysis, which may persist following the acute episode.[24] One small randomized trial in shocked patients showed a clear mortality benefit for thrombolysis. In addition, some meta-analyses suggest that in the sickest patients with PE there is probably a mortality benefit.[20] Very few clinicians would withhold thrombolytics for massive PE. There is widespread use of thrombolytics in Europe for moderate-sized PE, with some registry evidence of improved mortality or reduced complications.[25,26] However, there seems to be less acceptance in the USA and Australia for this indication as the evidence is weak.

Tissue plasminogen activator (rTPA) appears to be the easiest and quickest to give and to have the fewest side effects (excepting ICH) compared to urokinase and streptokinase. rTPA has been used as an infusion of 100 mg over 2 hours.[24] Bolus reteplase (10 U/s + 10 U/s, separated by half an hour) or tenectaplase (weight-based short infusion) should be just as effective and easier to use, although they have not been properly studied in PE and do not have TGA approval for this indication.

Thrombolysis is associated with a major bleeding episode in up to 20% of patients, with ICH rates as high as 4% and death from bleeding in 0.3–2%.[20, 26]

Surgery

Patients with persistent haemodynamic instability or hypoxia with major contraindications to thrombolysis should be considered for thoracotomy and/or embolectomy.[20,26] Patients in this category are not necessarily at hospitals with facilities for cardiopulmonary bypass, and therefore alternative therapies have been developed. The use of mechanical clot disruption for massive PE has been reported in case studies, but controlled studies are difficult to design because of the infrequency of the event and the emergency nature of massive PE. By passing a standard pulmonary artery catheter J wire past the clot, sliding the catheter over this and withdrawing the catheter, the clot can be fragmented. Unlike other surgical techniques, the expertise and equipment for this procedure are readily available in most large hospitals. Pulmonary embolectomy without cardiac bypass has been used as a last resort for haemodynamically unstable patients, with a reported survival of more than 50%.[27] Following cardiac arrest survival rates are much lower, although survivors have been reported.

There is no evidence that mechanical removal of clot results in better outcome than does thrombolysis, and it may well be worse. In the pre-arrest or arrested patient the transfer to cardiopulmonary bypass may buy additional time. In general, hospitals should decide on thrombolysis versus thrombectomy as their preferred management of unstable PE to avoid confusion and unnecessary delays to management in shocked patients.

The use of caval interruption techniques should be considered in cases of recurrent PE despite coagulation, or where there is bleeding. It has also been recommended for massive PE or massive leg DVT with PE.[20,26] Fatal PE usually occurs as a result of further clot progressing along the inferior vena cava (IVC). Percutaneous IVC umbrellas may be inserted relatively easily and prevent further deterioration.

Prognosis

The prognosis is largely dependent on coexistent illness and the size of the initial PE. Patients with arrest/shock have mortality rates of 25–50% even with thrombolysis. Those with right ventricular strain but haemodynamic stability have mortality rates of 5–10%. In addition, they are at risk of developing chronic thromboembolism and persistent pulmonary hypertension.[19] Patients without significant comorbidity or signs of severity have very low rates of poor outcomes.[19–21] Even with anticoagulation, hospital mortality may still be high (2.5–12%). Recurrent PE occurs in 25% of patients by 8 years.[28]

Disposition

Patients with haemodynamic instability, post arrest or with significant hypoxia should be admitted to an ICU. Thrombolysis or surgical referral should be strongly considered for ongoing instability. Patients with right atrial emboli in transit should have emergency thrombolysis or thrombectomy, and will definitely require ICU admission. Most patients with stable PE can be admitted directly to the ward, with a high-dependency environment required for those with right ventricular strain. Early discharge with LMW heparin should be considered for those with small PEs and a low risk of complications.[19,20]

Conclusion

The diagnosis and management of PE is based on an estimate of the probability of diagnosis versus the risk of treatment. Nowhere else in medicine is the 'art' of medicine more in evidence.

Controversies

- Is multislice CTPA the new gold standard for PE, or does it still need to be combined with leg imaging for moderate to high-risk patients?

- Whether helical CT should replace V/Q scanning as the first imaging technique in PE.

- The role of thrombolysis: it is generally accepted for use in massive/shocked PE, but some have advocated thrombolysis for sub-massive PE with evidence of right ventricular strain or massive DVT to prevent long-term complications.

- Should all patients with PE have an echocardiogram (or equivalent investigations), and should all patients with right ventricular strain be monitored and/or considered for thrombolysis?

- In what situations should thrombectomy/mechanical embolectomy be preferred to thrombolysis?

- Outpatient treatment of PE with LMW heparin.

- How can we better risk-stratify patients with proven PE so that we can provide appropriate dispositions to home, ward or high-dependency areas?

References

1. Goldhaber SZ, Visani L, De Rosa M. Acute pulmonary embolism: clinical outcomes in the International Cooperative Pulmonary Embolism Registry (ICOPER). Lancet 1999; 353: 1386–1389.
2. White RH. The epidemiology of venous thromboembolism. Circulation 2003; 107: I4–I8.
3. Kroegel C, Reissig A. Principle mechanism underlying venous thromboembolism: epidemiology, risk factors, pathophysiology and pathogenesis. Respiration 2003; 70: 7–30.
4. Elliott CG, Goldhaber SZ, Visani L, et al. Chest radiographs in acute pulmonary embolism. Results from the International Cooperative Pulmonary Embolism Registry. Chest 2000; 118: 33–38.
5. Wells PS, Anderson DR, Rodger M, et al. Excluding pulmonary embolism at the bedside without diagnostic imaging: management of patients with suspected pulmonary embolism presenting to the emergency department by using a simple clinical model and D-dimer. Annals of Internal Medicine 2001; 135: 98–107.
6. Palla A, Putruzelli S, Donnamaria V, et al. The role of suspicion in the diagnosis of pulmonary embolism. Chest 1995; 107: 21–24.
7. Manganelli D, Palla A, Donnamaria V, et al. Clinical features of pulmonary embolism: doubts and certainties. Chest 1995; 107: 25–32.
8. Iles S, LeHeron CJ, Davies G, et al. ECG score predicts those with the greatest percentage of perfusion defects due to acute pulmonary thromboembolic disease. Chest 2004; 125: 1651–1656.
9. Stein PD, Goldhaber SZ, Henry JW. Alveolar-arterial oxygen gradient in the assessment of acute pulmonary embolism. Chest 1995; 107: 139–143.
10. Mountain, D. Diagnosing pulmonary embolism: A question of too much choice? Emergency Medicine 2003; 15: 250–262.
11. The PIOPED Investigators. Value of the ventilation/perfusion scan in acute pulmonary embolism. Journal of the American Medical Association 1990; 263: 2753–2759.
12. Hull RD, Hirsh J, Carter CJ, et al. Diagnostic value of ventilation-perfusion lung scanning in patients with suspected pulmonary embolism. Chest 1985; 88: 819–828.
13. Stein PD, Henry JW, Gottschalk A. The addition of clinical assessment to stratification according to prior cardiopulmonary disease further optimises the interpretation of ventilation/perfusion lung scans in pulmonary embolism. Chest 1993; 104: 1472–1476.
14. Roy PM, Colombet I, Durieux P, et al. Systematic review and meta-analysis of strategies for the diagnosis of suspected pulmonary embolism. British Medical Journal 2005; 30: 259.
15. Stein PD, Fowler SE, Goodman LR, et al. (PIOPED 2 investigators). Multidetector computed tomography for acute pulmonary embolism. New England Journal of Medicine 2006; 354: 2317–2327.
16. Mountain D. Multislice computed tomographic pulmonary angiography for diagnosing pulmonary embolism in the emergency department: Has the 'one-stop shop' arrived? Emergency Medicine of Australasia 2006; 18: 444–450.
17. Fletcher J, MacLellan D, Fisher C, et al. Prevention of venous thromboembolism: best practice guidelines for Australia and New Zealand, 3rd edn. Sydney: Health Education Management International (HEMI), 2005.
18. Goldhaber SZ. Cardiac biomarkers in pulmonary embolism. Chest 2003; 123: 1782–1784.
19. Kline JA, Hernandez-Nino J, Rose GA, et al. Surrogate markers for adverse outcomes in normotensive patients with pulmonary embolism. Critical Care Medicine 2006; 34: 2773–2780.
20. British Thoracic Society. Guidelines for the management of acute pulmonary embolism. Thorax 2003; 58: 470–484.
21. Aujesky D, Obrosky DS, Stone RA, et al. A prediction rule to identify low-risk patients with pulmonary embolism. Archives of Internal Medicine 2006; 166: 169–175.
22. Linkins LA, Choi PT, Douketis JD. Clinical impact of bleeding in patients taking oral anticoagulant therapy for venous thromboembolism: a meta-analysis. Annals of Internal Medicine 2003; 139: 893–900.
23. Tapson VF, Witty LA. Massive pulmonary embolism. Clinics in Chest Medicine 1995; 16: 329–407.
24. Goldhaber SZ, Haire WB, Feldstein MI, et al. Alteplase vs heparin in acute PE: randomised trial assessing right-ventricular function and pulmonary perfusion. Lancet 1993; 341: 507–511.
25. Konstantinides S, Geibel A, Olschewski M, et al. Association between thrombolytic treatment and the prognosis of hemodynamically stable patients with major pulmonary embolism: results from a multicenter registry. Circulation 1997; 96: 882–888.
26. Goldhaber S. Modern treatment of pulmonary embolism. European Respiratory Journal 2002; 19: 22S–27S.
27. Clarke DB, Abrams LD. Pulmonary embolectomy: 25 years' experience. Journal of Thoracic and Cardiovascular Surgery 1986; 92: 442–445.
28. Hirsch J, Hoak J. Management of deep vein thrombosis and pulmonary embolism (AHA medical/scientific statement). Circulation 1996; 93: 2212–2245.

CARDIOVASCULAR

5.6 Pericarditis, cardiac tamponade and myocarditis

James Hayes • Anne-Maree Kelly

PERICARDITIS

ESSENTIALS

1 Myocarditis is often associated with the clinical condition pericarditis. This has important clinical implications.

2 Pericarditis is most commonly diagnosed on ECG findings, but may ultimately be a purely clinical diagnosis.

3 The majority of cases of pericarditis have a presumed viral aetiology, and most run a benign course.

4 The correct distinction of pericarditis from myocardial infarction is essential, as the administration of thrombolytics in cases of pericarditis may result in life-threatening complications.

5 Longer-term follow-up is essential as a subacute or chronic course can develop, with further complications such as chronic constrictive pericarditis.

Introduction

Pericarditis may be acute, subacute or chronic. It is defined as inflammation of the pericardium. It should be noted, however, that the condition is better described as perimyocarditis. In the majority of cases there are variable degrees of associated 'epimyocarditis', which has important clinical implications. The causes of pericarditis are listed in Table 5.6.1.

Clinical features

History

Idiopathic or viral types may have a history of a recent viral illness, and the history should be directed towards the known causative pathologies. The pain is usually retrosternal, sometimes with radiation to the trapezius muscle ridges, but not generally to the arms. It may also be pleuritic in nature, worse with movement and respiration. It is typically worse when lying supine, and better when sitting up and leaning forward. True dyspnoea is not a feature, but respiration may be shallow because of pain.

Examination

With viral or idiopathic types, fever may be present. Sinus tachycardia is common. A pericardial friction rub may be heard, caused by rubbing between parietal and visceral pericardial layers or between parietal pericardium and lung pleura. The rub may therefore be heard despite the presence of a large effusion. It may be audible anywhere over the precordium, but is best heard with the diaphragm of the stethoscope over the lower left sternal edge, where the least amount of lung tissue intervenes, with the patient leaning forward in full expiration. The rub has a superficial scratching or 'Velcro-like' quality. Rubs may be difficult to detect, as they can be transient and migratory. The patient should be examined for any signs of a complicating cardiac tamponade. A search should also be made for any signs of an underlying causative condition.

Investigations

Blood tests

- FBC: leukocytosis is common.
- Serum biochemistry: may identify underlying renal failure.
- ESR or CRP provide confirmatory evidence of an inflammatory process, and can be used to follow treatment.
- Cardiac biomarkers may be elevated because of the associated myocarditis.
- Other blood tests will be dictated by the

Table 5.6.1	Causes of acute pericarditis
Idiopathic (about 25%)	Most of these are probably viral
Malignancy (about 25%)	Primary, e.g. sarcoma and mesotheliomas Secondary, e.g. haematological, breast, lung and melanoma
Infective	Viral, e.g. Coxsackie B, mumps, EBV, influenza, HIV Bacterial, e.g. staphylococcal, streptococcal, Gram-negatives and TB Mycotic, e.g. histoplasmosis
Autoimmune/connective tissue	Rheumatoid arthritis, systemic lupus erythematosis, sarcoidosis, scleroderma, Stevens–Johnson syndrome, inflammatory bowel disease
Trauma	Blunt or penetrating Post pericardiotomy syndrome Radiation injury
Myocardial infarction associated	Acute: days to weeks following transmural myocardial infarction Dressler's syndrome: weeks to months following myocardial infarction
Drugs	SLE-type syndromes, e.g. hydralazine Hypersensitivity syndromes, e.g. penicillin
Systemic illnesses	Uraemia Myxoedema
Other	Dissecting aneurysm

clinical assessment and the degree of clinical suspicion for any given causative pathology derived from this.

Chest X-ray

Chest X-ray does not confirm the diagnosis of pericarditis but will rule out other causes of pleuritic chest pain, and find evidence of a complicating pericardial effusion, or evidence of causative pathology such as malignancy.

ECG

The ECG is the most important investigation and will show abnormalities in 90% of patients with acute pericarditis. ECG changes are the result of the associated epimyocarditis. The pericardium is electrically neutral and of itself does not produce ECG changes. Therefore, in the occasional 'pure' case of pericarditis the ECG will be normal. It may follow the typical evolution of changes, but in a sizeable minority will not.

The typical pattern follows four stages:

- Stage 1: hours to days
  - diffuse concave upwards ST elevation; this may occur in all leads apart from AVR, and often V1.
  - PR-segment depression (reflecting subepicardial atrial injury); this may occur in all leads apart from AVR and V1. These two leads may in fact show PR-segment elevation.
- Stage 2: the PR and ST segments normalize, which can lead to a transiently normal ECG.
- Stage 3: days to weeks; T-wave inversion occurs.
- Stage 4: normalization of the ECG; over a period of up to 3 months, however, in some cases the T-wave changes may be permanent.

Atypical ECGs may include the following:

- A normal ECG in cases of 'pure' pericarditis (remembering that during stage 2 the ECG may also be transiently normal during a typical evolution).
- The PR-segment depression may occur in isolation, without any ST segment elevation.
- Stages 1 and 2 without progression to stage 3.
- Localized as opposed to diffuse ECG changes.

Echocardiography

This may give indirect evidence for pericarditis by showing the presence of an effusion or a thickened pericardium. High-quality echocardiograms are able to distinguish bloody from serous effusions. Transoesophageal echocardiography (TOE) is better at measuring thickness of the pericardium than transthoracic echocardiography (TTE). A normal echocardiogram does not rule out a diagnosis of pericarditis.

CT scan/magnetic resonance imaging (MRI)

CT and MRI have the advantages of a larger field of view and excellent imaging of anatomy that is not possible with echocardiography. They also have high soft tissue contrast. In most patients they provide excellent images of the pericardium, including thickness, the presence of effusions and any pericardial lesions.

Making the diagnosis

Stage 1 ST-segment deviations are virtually diagnostic of acute pericarditis when typically distributed among limb and precordial leads. However, a sizeable minority of ECGs will be atypical, and indeed in some cases may be normal. The diagnosis of pericarditis may therefore ultimately be a clinical one, based on the presence of typical pain and a rub heard on auscultation or the presence of an effusion on echocardiography. Cases where pain is typical but a rub is not heard present more difficulty and should be followed closely. If clinical suspicion is high, again an echocardiogram finding of an effusion in the presence of typical pain would be highly suggestive. Convenient diagnoses, such as 'muscular', 'fibrositis', 'costochondritis' and 'viral' should be avoided until more important conditions, such as pericarditis, pulmonary embolus and pneumothorax, are excluded. The most difficult clinical decision in the emergency department (ED) is differentiating between pericarditis, benign early repolarization (BER) and myocardial infarction. This is especially so when the decision to use thrombolytics is being considered. Thrombolytic therapy may result in life-threatening haemorrhagic cardiac tamponade in patients who have pericarditis. ECG features to assist in distinguishing between these diagnoses are summarized in Table 5.6.2.

Table 5.6.2 Pericarditis vs AMI vs BER			
ECG feature	**Acute pericarditis**	**AMI**	**BER**
ST segment morphology	Concave upwards ST elevation	Convex upwards ST elevation	Concave upwards ST elevation
ST segment elevation	Usually <5 mm	May be >5 mm, more suspicious	<5 mm the greater the elevation
ST segment changes distribution	Diffuse	Anatomic	Precordial only
Reciprocal changes	No, mild depressions only in AVR, V₁	Deep reciprocal changes opposite ST elevated segments	No
Q waves	No (unless associated with infarction)	Yes	No
PR segments	PR-segment depressions (may be elevated in AVR and V1)	No	No
T wave inversion	T-wave inversion after ST segments normalize	T waves may invert concurrently with elevation of ST segments	No
ST/T ratio	>0.25	N/A	<0.25
Usual pattern of evolution of changes	Days to weeks	Minutes to days	Stable over many years

CARDIOVASCULAR

Management

The symptoms of pericarditis are generally well controlled with non-steroidal anti-inflammatory agents (NSAIDs). Occasionally more severe symptoms of pain will require steroids. Rest is essential, as exercise may exacerbate an associated myocarditis. Complications such as arrhythmias are treated along conventional lines. If a significant effusion is suspected this should be confirmed on echocardiography and signs of early cardiac tamponade looked for. An underlying cause for the pericarditis should be sought and treatment directed at this, though the majority will be viral. In high-risk patients HIV should also be considered as a possible underlying aetiology.

Disposition

The clinical course really depends on the underlying pathology. Patients with pericarditis can usually be safely managed on an outpatient basis unless there are high-risk features such as temperature >38°C, a subacute onset, immunosuppression, a history of recent trauma, oral anticoagulant therapy, myopericarditis, a large pericardial effusion and/or cardiac tamponade.

The viral and idiopathic groups commonly follow a benign and self-limiting course over 10–14 days. Patients with severe symptoms should be admitted; some may require narcotic analgesia. Those in whom the diagnosis remains uncertain, especially when other serious conditions such as myocardial infarction cannot be ruled out, should also be admitted. Follow-up is also essential to monitor progress (particularly the development of features of myocarditis) and to identify the development of chronicity and constrictive pericarditis.

Controversies

- Whether all patients with pericarditis should be admitted. Although patients with usual pericarditis are at low risk of adverse events, clinical diagnosis is not always accurate.

NON-TRAUMATIC CARDIAC TAMPONADE

ESSENTIALS

1 Cardiac tamponade is a life-threatening condition.

2 The signs and symptoms of cardiac tamponade are non-specific and often not present, or at least difficult to elicit. A high index of suspicion is therefore essential to ensure that the condition is not missed.

3 The 'gold standard' investigation is echocardiography, as it is the most sensitive and the most specific.

4 The urgency and type of treatment will depend on the rapidity, as well as the degree, of accumulation of pericardial contents. It will also depend on the aetiology.

5 Needle pericardiocentesis is best reserved as a drainage procedure of last resort. The preferred method should be subxiphoid pericardiotomy if the clinical situation allows. In cases of myocardial rupture and aortic dissection, thoracotomy with drainage and definitive repair is the method of choice, rather than pericardiocentesis.

Introduction

Pericardial effusion is the accumulation of fluid (exudate, transudate, blood or chylus) within the pericardial cavity. Normally this cavity contains up to 35 mL of fluid. More than this can be accommodated in the short term, up to about 200 mL. In the longer term, if it accumulates slowly, up to 2 L can be accommodated with little clinical consequence. However, above these values the process of cardiac tamponade will occur, with lethal consequences if unrecognized.

Cardiac tamponade can be defined as an accumulation of pericardial fluid that inhibits the diastolic filling of the atria and ventricles and, if left unchecked, will lead to a clinical state of shock. It may be recognized by clinical signs in the late stages, but the diagnosis should be confirmed by echocardiography as these signs are non-specific. It is now recognized that the process of cardiac tamponade may occur before significant clinical signs develop. Echocardiography can diagnose this early 'compensated' stage of the process.

The best classification for cardiac tamponade is traumatic (dealt with elsewhere in

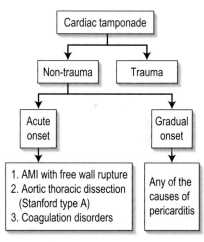

Fig. 5.6.1 Causes of pericardial effusion and cardiac tamponade.

this book) and non-traumatic (Fig. 5.6.1), as not only the aetiology, but the clinical course and approach to management are very different.

Clinical features

History

The symptoms and signs of cardiac tamponade are non-specific and their onset and course depend on whether the condition is acute or gradual. They are also inconsistent and sometimes difficult to elicit. A high index of suspicion for the condition must therefore be maintained, which requires thorough knowledge of the clinical settings in which tamponade can occur.

The commonest symptom of cardiac tamponade is dyspnoea (sensitivity 87–89%). Most other symptoms will relate to those of diminished cardiac output (e.g. faintness, dizziness, apprehension) or to the underlying disease process (e.g. pain of pericarditis).

Examination

Generally, signs are difficult to elicit and very non-specific. The classic signs are those of Beck's triad: hypotension, diminished heart sounds and elevated jugular venous pressure (JVP). It should be noted that cardiac tamponade may be present in the absence of an elevated JVP in conditions of significant hypovolaemia, and that diminished heart sounds are a very non-specific and subjective finding. Furthermore, the absence of hypotension does not rule out cardiac tamponade: indeed, in some cases hypertension may be present.

The clinical features found to occur in the majority of patients are dyspnoea (sensitivity 87–89%), tachycardia (sensitivity 77%), pulsus paradoxus >10 mmHg (sensitivity 82%) and elevated JVP (sensitivity 76%). Loss of the apical impulse or, if present, an area of cardiac dullness extending beyond the apical impulse, may give a clinical clue to the presence of an effusion but not cardiac tamponade. In the later stages of cardiac tamponade, tachypnoea is common. If cardiac function is otherwise normal the lung fields are typically 'clear'. There may be associated pleural effusions and signs of pericarditis (e.g. fever, pericardial rub). Pleuropericardial rubs may still be heard even in the presence of a large effusion.

Differential diagnosis

The differential diagnosis of cardiac tamponade is given in Table 5.6.3.

Table 5.6.3 The differential diagnosis of cardiac tamponade

Massive pulmonary embolism
Tension pneumothorax
Superior vena cava obstruction
Chronic constrictive pericarditis
Air embolism
Right ventricular infarct
Severe congestive cardiac failure/cardiogenic shock
Extrapericardial compression: haematoma, tumour

Investigations

Chest X-ray

Cardiomegaly on CXR has a reported sensitivity of 89%, but is a non-specific finding. It should be remembered that in cases of acute tamponade the cardiac silhouette may appear entirely normal. At least 250 mL of fluid must be present within the pericardial cavity before an increase in the cardiac silhouette can be appreciated.

ECG

This may provide clues to the presence of an effusion, with low voltages and electrical alternans, but again will not indicate whether tamponade is occurring.

Echocardiography

Echocardiography is the current 'gold standard' investigation for the diagnosis of cardiac tamponade. It is the most specific and sensitive investigation for the detection of effusion and of the process of tamponade. It can be performed rapidly and non-invasively (in the case of transthoracic echocardiography, TTE) in the emergency department (ED). In patients in whom a transthoracic study is difficult to perform or in whom the result is equivocal, then a transoesophageal (TOE) study may be performed. This technique may detect occult loculated effusions missed by TTE and can even be performed in the intubated patient during CPR. Echocardiography can provide valuable information about associated cardiac function and abnormalities. It may also detect the process of tamponade before significant clinical signs develop.

It is important to remember that clinically significant tamponade is a clinical diagnosis, and that 'echocardiographic signs of tamponade' are not in themselves an indication for acute intervention.

Computed tomography and magnetic resonance imaging

Computed tomography (CT) and magnetic resonance imaging (MRI) are sensitive and specific for the detection of pericardial fluid and are good alternatives if echocardiography is not available. They are much less reliable in determining whether tamponade is occurring, giving only indirect clues. Neither is suitable in the critically ill patient.

Haemodynamic monitoring

In the ICU setting, pulmonary artery catheter findings of 'equalization' of the right heart diastolic pressures (i.e. right atrial, right ventricular end-diastolic, diastolic pulmonary artery and pulmonary artery wedge pressures) suggest the diagnosis of cardiac tamponade.

Treatment

The treatment of cardiac tamponade is drainage of the pericardial fluid. Medical management aims to improve the clinical condition while arrangements for drainage are being made.

General measures

Oxygenation should be optimized. Fluid loading may provide some minor 'temporizing' support of the cardiac output. Inotropic agents are usually ineffective. Institution of mechanical ventilation may cause a sudden drop in blood pressure as the positive intrathoracic pressure further impairs cardiac filling.

Definitive measures

Drainage procedures

Pericardiocentesis is best performed in the cardiac catheter laboratory under fluoroscopic guidance. Recently bedside echocardiography-guided pericardiocentesis has also been shown to be safe and effective. Surgical drainage is required for purulent or recurrent effusions, and when tissue is required for diagnosis; a subxiphoid approach is preferred.

'Blind' needle pericardiocentesis should be considered a method of last resort. It is best reserved for the pre-arrest or just-arrested patient, as it can be technically difficult and has significant complications, especially when smaller volumes of fluid are involved. If it is to be carried out it is best followed up with the insertion of an indwelling 'pigtail'-type catheter for ready aspiration should the patient's condition deteriorate. It must be remembered that CPR in the arrested patient will not be effective in cases of cardiac tamponade, when immediate needle drainage followed in many cases by thoracotomy will be required.

Thoracotomy without attempts at drainage should be performed when definitive surgical repair of the causative pathology is necessary. Examples in this category include trauma, rupture of the myocardium, and dissecting thoracic aneurysm causing cardiac tamponade. Indeed, attempts at drainage before definitive repair in the case of dissecting aortic aneurysm may be positively detrimental.

Treatment must also be directed at the underlying pathology.

Disposition

Pericardial effusion may with time lead to cardiac tamponade. All cases of cardiac tamponade will lead to shock and death if left untreated, the rapidity of which will depend on the amount of fluid present, the rate at which it accumulated, and the compliance of the pericardium.

Patients with clinically 'compensated' non-traumatic cardiac tamponade should be admitted to a high-dependency area for close observation while a definitive drainage procedure is planned and organized. In cases of decompensated tamponade, urgent drainage is required and the choice of management will depend on the aetiology, clinical urgency and expertise available.

Controversies

- The distinction between clinical and echocardiographic tamponade with the advent of more sensitive imaging.
- The type and timing of drainage procedures in the critically ill.

MYOCARDITIS

ESSENTIALS

1 Myocarditis is most commonly caused by viral infection; the majority of cases run a benign course, with full recovery.

2 Occasionally acute fulminating episodes occur, giving rise to arrhythmias, cardiac failure and death. Survivors of these episodes may, however, make a full recovery with supportive treatment.

3 Diagnosis is difficult and is usually made on clinical grounds.

4 Myocarditis may present in a similar manner to myocardial infarction, including similar chest pain, ECG changes and elevation of cardiac enzymes.

5 Long-term follow-up is important in patients who have had myocarditis, as some cases may progress to a chronic form with the development of dilated cardiomyopathy.

Introduction

Myocarditis is myocardial inflammation and injury in the absence of ischaemia. It is frequently associated with pericarditis, resulting in a myopericarditis.

Epidemiology

Given its highly variable clinical presentation, the real incidence of myocarditis is unknown. It accounts for up to one-third of cases of dilated cardiomyopathy.

Pathogenesis and pathophysiology

Myocarditis is caused by a wide range of viral, fungal, bacterial, protozoal and parasitic pathogens, toxin and drugs, as well as immune-mediated disease. The more common of these are shown in Table 5.6.4.

The exact mechanism by which viral myocarditis and its longer-term complications develop is unknown. It probably involves the interplay of several factors, including direct damage due to the virus itself, damage in the acute and long term by the host's immune responses, and a genetic predisposition in an individual.

Clinical features

The clinical spectrum of myocarditis is variable. It may manifest as any of the following:

- Asymptomatic/subclinical.
- Fever with 'viral' illness, with minimal cardiac features.
- Acute myopericarditis.
- Unexplained arrhythmias, including conduction delays.

Table 5.6.4 Commoner causes of myocarditis	
Viral	Adenovirus Coxsackie B virus Cytomegalovirus HHV-6 HIV Influenza A Herpes simplex virus-1 Parvovirus Respiratory syncytial virus
Toxin or drug	Anthracyclines Trastuzumab Ethanol Clozapine Snake or scorpion bite Ionizing radiation
Immune mediated	Chagas' disease Sarcoidosis Scleroderma Systemic lupus erythematosus Alloantigen (heart transplant recipient) Kawasaki's disease
Bacteria	Rickettsia species Leptospira Coxiella burnetti Corynebacterium diptheriae Mycoplasma pneumoniae
Protozoa, fungi and parasites	Toxoplasma Cryptococcus species

- Unexplained cardiac failure, ranging from mild to cardiogenic shock.
- Sudden, unexpected cardiac death.
- Delayed (years later) dilated cardiomyopathy.

History

Many cases are asymptomatic. There may be a history of an antecedent viral illness. After a delay of 10–14 days symptoms relating to cardiac involvement develop, such as arrhythmias causing palpitations or dizziness, or cardiac failure causing shortness of breath. Pleuritic-type pain may be a feature owing to an associated pericarditis. Myocarditis may also present similarly to acute myocardial infarction, with chest pain, ischaemic ECG changes and elevated cardiac biomarkers. This presentation is more common in younger patients, with few cardiac risk factors, a preceding viral illness and subsequent normal coronary angiography.

Examination

On examination a fever may be present; however, patients are often afebrile. Sinus tachycardia is often found and is said to be 'out of proportion' to the degree of fever. Other arrhythmias may also be found. A pericardial rub due to an associated pericarditis may be present. There may be signs of heart failure, ranging from mild to pulmonary oedema or cardiogenic shock.

Investigations

A definitive diagnosis of acute viral myocarditis cannot be made in the ED and must in the first instance be presumptive. The commonest scenario will be the young patient who presents with cardiac failure, shock or arrhythmias for which there is no obvious aetiology. Testing may provide supportive evidence for the diagnosis.

Blood

A number of blood tests can give support to a diagnosis of myocarditis, but none is specific. These include elevation of the white cell count, elevation of the ESR and/or CRP. Cardiac biomarkers may also be elevated. These parameters can be used to assess response to treatment.

Chest X-ray

This may show cardiomegaly with changes of congestive failure in severe cases, but again is non-specific. The chest X-ray may also be normal.

ECG

In most cases the ECG will be abnormal; however, the changes are not specific for myocarditis. Sinus tachycardia is usually seen. The most common finding is non-specific ST-T-wave changes. Rhythm disturbances of any type may occur, including a significant proportion with conduction delays. Occasionally ST elevation may occur that is indistinguishable from myocardial infarction.

Echocardiography

This can give supportive evidence but is not diagnostic. Global wall motion abnormalities are a characteristic finding, but in some cases more regional abnormalities will be seen. An associated effusion may be found. Evidence of myocardial failure can be found with ventricular cavity dilation and reduced ejection fraction.

Nuclear medicine scanning

Antimyosin myocardial scintigraphy (indium-111 (^{111}I) antimyosin Fab) has a reported sensitivity of 83–100%, a negative predictive value of 92–100%, and specificity of 55% for myocarditis. It is no longer available for clinical use and is very costly.

Cardiac MRI

Cardiac MRI with early and late enhancement after gadolinium contrast injection is becoming an important diagnostic tool in suspected acute myocarditis, particularly to differentiate myocarditis from acute myocardial infarction.

Endomyocardial biopsy

This is currently the only way to make a definitive diagnosis. It is, however, not a gold standard, as the following problems may be encountered:

- Acute myocarditis may be patchy and diagnosis may be missed on a single specimen.
- False-positive results are possible.
- It may underestimate more minor cases of myocarditis.

There has long been debate about patient selection for endomyocardial biopsy, particularly after the negative results of the Myocarditis Treatment Trial. Molecular biological techniques, such as detection of viral genome by PCR testing, which can identify a group of patients with a poorer prognosis who might benefit from interferon therapy, has renewed interest in this test. That said, patient selection remains controversial. Complications include venous injury, arrhythmias and cardiac perforation.

Treatment and disposition

Treatment consists of traditional heart failure therapy and supportive care, progressing to implantable defibrillators, aggressive mechanical assist devices as bridging therapy and, in severe cases, heart transplantation.

Supportive treatment should attend to airway, breathing and circulation. Oxygenation is important, and in cases of pulmonary oedema non-invasive ventilatory support may be necessary. Analgesia will be required if pain is a significant feature. Strict bed rest is advised, as exercise has been shown to increase the degree of myocyte necrosis. Diuretic therapy, vasodilators and inotropic support are used to optimize cardiac filling and increase cardiac output. Angiotensin-converting enzyme (ACE) inhibitors and angiotensin II receptor blockers should be initiated early. Complicating arrhythmias are treated along conventional lines. In patients who develop cardiogenic shock, intervention should be early and aggressive. The use of inotropes, extracorporeal membrane oxygenation (ECMO) or ventricular assist devices is recommended as a bridge to transplant or recovery. In severe refractory cases cardiac transplantation may ultimately be required. Immunosuppression trials have to date been largely disappointing, with no randomized trial showing sustained clinical or mortality benefit. Preliminary data suggest that administration of interferon-β (INF-β) to patients with persistent depression of left ventricular ejection fraction (LVEF) and PCR-positive genome expression for enteroviral or adenoviral DNA may enhance viral clearance and improve LVEF. Confirmatory data are awaited.

Survivors of myocarditis must be followed carefully for the possible future development of dilated cardiomyopathy. Patients should not undertake any competitive sport for 6 months after the onset of clinical myocarditis. Athletes may return to training if left ventricular function, wall motion and dimensions return to normal, arrhythmias are absent, serum markers of inflammation have resolved and the ECG has normalized.

All patients with suspected acute myocarditis should be admitted to CCU/ICU.

Prognosis

Prognosis from acute myocarditis depends on severity of symptoms and signs, histological classification and biomarkers. Paradoxically, patients with more severe heart failure at presentation may have better overall survival. Clinical predictors of a fatal outcome include hypotension and elevated pulmonary wedge pressure. Biochemical markers associated with poorer outcome include serum Fas, Fas ligand, antimyosin autoantibodies and interleukin-10 (IL-10) levels. Increased tumour necrosis factor-α (receptor 1) expression and persistent viral genome expression for selected viruses have also recently been associated with progressive impairment/failure of recovery of LVEF.

Complications at presentation are usually the result of arrhythmias and heart failure; however, the majority of cases will run a benign course with a full recovery. Arrhythmias may include conduction delays with a potential for sudden death. Occasionally an acute fulminant course may occur, with intractable arrhythmias or, more often, with acute heart failure rapidly progressing to cardiogenic shock and death. Survivors of this fulminant course will often make a complete recovery.

The whole spectrum of asymptomatic through to fulminant cases may progress to a chronic course. Myocarditis is thought to be the cause of up to a third of cases of dilated cardiomyopathy. It may also explain some instances of recurrent unexplained arrhythmias and sudden unexpected cardiac death, especially in younger age groups. See Figure 5.6.2 for a summary of the natural history of myocarditis.

Controversies

- The role of immunosuppressive agents in the management of myocarditis.

- Optimal diagnostic strategy.

- The indications for endomyocardial biopsy in patients suspected of having viral myocarditis.

Further reading

Acker MA. Mechanical circulatory support for patients with acute fulminant myocarditis. Annals of Thoracic Surgery 2001; 71: S73–S76.

Allen KB, Faber LP, Warren WH, Shaar CJ. Pericardial effusion: subxiphoid pericardiostomy versus percutaneous catheter drainage. Annals of Thoracic Surgery 1999; 67: 437–440.

Ariyarajah V, Spodick DH. Acute pericarditis: diagnostic cues and common electrocardiographic manifestations. Cardiology Review 2007; 15: 24–30.

Brown J, MacKinnon D, King A, et al. Elevated arterial blood pressure in cardiac tamponade. New England Journal of Medicine 1992; 327: 463–466.

Coplan NL, Goldman B, Mechanic G, et al. Sudden haemodynamic collapse following relief of cardiac tamponade in aortic dissection. American Heart Journal 1986; 111: 406.

Ellis CR, Di Salvo T. Myocarditis: basic and clinical aspects. Cardiology Review 2007; 15: 70–77.

Feldman AM, McNamarra D. Myocarditis. New England Journal of Medicine 2000; 343: 1388–1398.

Fowler NO. Cardiac tamponade: a clinical or echocardiographic diagnosis? Circulation 1993; 87: 1738–1741.

Hayes JE. Cardiac tamponade. Emergency Medicine 1997; 9: 123–135.

Hoit BD. Pericardial disease and pericardial tamponade. Critical Care Medicine 2007; 35: S355–S364.

Kim JS, Kim HH, Yoon T. Imaging of pericardial diseases. Clinical Radiology 2007; 62: 626–631.

Little WC, Freeman GL. Pericardial disease. Circulation 2006; 113: 1622–1632.

Spodick DH, Greene TO, Saperia G. Acute myocarditis masquerading as acute myocardial infarction. Circulation 1995; 91: 1886–1887.

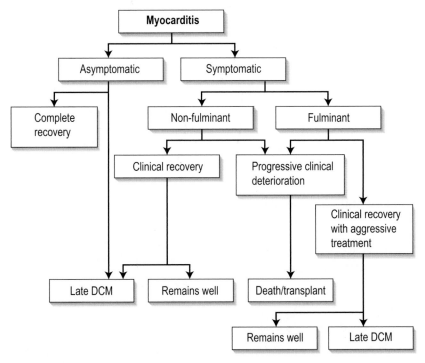

Fig 5.6.2 Natural history of myocarditis.

CARDIOVASCULAR

5.7 Heart valve emergencies

Marian Lee

ESSENTIALS

1 Infective endocarditis is effectively a multiorgan disease and is often missed.

2 There has been a shift in the predominant organism in infective endocarditis from *Streptococcus viridans* to *Staphylococcus aureus*, and nosocomial infections are becoming more common.

3 Degenerative heart disease and prosthetic valve are currently the high-risk factors in infective endocarditis in developed countries.

4 Antibiotic prophylaxis in patients with valvular or congenital heart disease is an important consideration in the appropriate clinical context.

5 The causes of acute deterioration in chronic valve lesions must be recognized and treated expeditiously to prevent life-threatening haemodynamic instability.

Introduction

Heart valve emergencies are a cause of sudden deterioration in cardiac function. The underlying cause depends on the valve involved.

Infective endocarditis

This is a commonly missed diagnosis. A high index of suspicion must be maintained, as a delay in diagnosis will increase the mortality and morbidity.

Epidemiology

The incidence of infective endocarditis is 3.6/100 000, of which prosthetic valve endocarditis (PVE) accounts for 20–30%. The male to female ratio is 2:1 and it is more common in the fifth and sixth decades of life.

In the developing countries, rheumatic heart disease is the commonest risk factor for infective endocarditis. Despite a fall in the incidence of rheumatic fever in developed countries, the prevalence of infective endocarditis has not fallen. In the developed world, the risk factors are:

- Host-related factors:
  - Poor oral hygiene
  - Intravenous drug use
  - Severe renal disease on haemodialysis
  - Diabetes mellitus
  - Mitral valve prolapse, particularly in the presence of valve incompetence or thickening of the leaflets
  - Degenerative valve sclerosis associated with age (mitral valve most common, then aortic, tricuspid and pulmonary valves, respectively).
- Procedure-related factors:
  - Infected intravascular device
  - Post genitourinary procedure
  - Post gastrointestinal procedure
  - Surgical wound infection.

Pathology and pathogenesis

In infective endocarditis, the interactions between host and organism are complex. Platelet–fibrin deposits form at sites of endothelial damage and are called nonbacterial thrombotic endocarditis. Invasion and multiplication by a virulent microbe lead to enlargement of these vegetations, which become infected. The consequences are the basis of the clinical complications of infective endocarditis. The vegetations can fragment and embolize, leading to distal foci of infection. Obstruction of vessels by these fragments can also result in tissue ischaemia and infarction. Seeding from the fragments perpetuates the bacteraemia. Local destruction of the valve may produce intracardiac complications such as rupture of the chordae tendinae, abscess of the valve annulus and conduction problems.

Staph. aureus, entering through a breach in the skin, has surpassed *Strep. viridans* as the commonest bacterial pathogen in both native valve endocarditis (NVE) and prosthetic valve endocarditis. This change reflects better dental care and an increased incidence of nosocomial infections. Note that in proven *Staph. aureus* bacteraemia the incidence of infective endocarditis is 13–25%.

Overall, three major pathogens account for more than 80% of cases: *Staph aureus*, *Streptococcus* species and *Enterococcus* species. Nosocomial infective endocarditis is defined as occurring after 72 hours of hospital admission or within 4–8 weeks of an invasive procedure performed in a hospital. Organisms responsible for nosocomial endocarditis are *Staphylococcus* species (>75%, mainly *Staph. aureus*) and *Enterococcus* species in genitourinary and gastrointestinal tract procedures. Organisms associated with particular host categories are shown in Table 5.7.1.

Fungal infections account for less than 10% of cases and are most common in intravenous drug users, the immunocompromised and those with prosthetic valves. The Gram-negative HACEK group (*Haemophilus* species, *Actinobacillus actinomycetemcomitans*, *Cardiobacterium hominis*, *Eikanlla corrodens*, *Kingella kingae*) are growing in importance and lead to large vegetations that may result in large vessel embolization or cardiac failure.

Prevention

The decision to administer procedural prophylactic antibiotic to at-risk patients depends on a risk assessment of the abnormal valve for endocarditis, coupled with the risk of bacteraemia of the procedure being undertaken. High-risk valve lesions are prosthetic valves, mitral valve prolapse with significant incompetence, and rheumatic heart disease in indigenous Australians. Procedural risk of bacteraemia is summarized in Table 5.7.2. Single dose preprocedural dosing is now recommended. Current recommendations should be checked in available local guides.

Table 5.7.1 Bacterial pathogens associated with host categories

IVDU	*Staph. aureus*; 80% of tricuspid valve involvement is due to this pathogen Streptococcal species *Pseudomonas aeruginosa* Fungi, especially *Candida* Multiple organisms
IVDU with HIV infection	Unusual organisms such as *Salmonella*, *Listeria*, *Bartonella*
Prosthetic heart valves, within 2 months of valve surgery	*Staph. epidermidis* *Staph. aureus* *Enterococcus* species
Prosthetic valves, more than 2 months post valve surgery	*Staph. aureus* *Strep. viridans*
Pre-existing malignancy or procedures involving the genitourinary or gastrointestinal tracts	*Enterococcus* species

Table 5.7.2 Procedural risk of bacteraemia

Periodontal surgery	88%
Tooth extraction	60%
Tooth brushing	40%
Genitourinary procedures	Up to 60%
Respiratory procedures	16%
Gastrointestinal procedures	<10% if no mucosal breach

Clinical features

Infective endocarditis should be considered a multisystem disease. The symptoms and signs are non-specific, compounding the difficulty of diagnosis. Symptoms usually occur within 2 months of the event responsible for the initiation of bacteraemia, although this may be difficult to identify. It is important to suspect infective endocarditis in patients with an unexplained fever and a predisposing factor.

The two most frequent systemic features are fever and malaise. Fever is present in 80–85% of cases: usually >38°C, but rarely >39.4°C. It can be absent in the severely debilitated, the elderly, and those with cardiac failure, chronic renal failure, liver failure, recent antibiotic use, and if the infection is by an organism with low virulence.

Malaise is reported in up to 95% of cases. Other symptoms are variable and non-specific, and may include headache, confusion, cough, chest pain (more common in IVDU), dyspnoea, abdominal pain, anorexia, weight loss and myalgia.

Other clinical features include immunological phenomena as well as those related to the lesion itself and embolizations. Immunological phenomena include glomerulonephritis, Osler's nodes, Roth's spots and an elevated rheumatoid factor.

With respect to cardiac features, a new or changed incompetent murmur may be found. However, in 70–95% of cases a murmur is pre-existent; hence the discovery of an acute murmur is an uncommon but highly significant finding. The absence of a murmur does not exclude the diagnosis of infective endocarditis. A new or a change of murmur is more likely in patients with a prosthetic valve or congestive cardiac failure.

Congestive cardiac failure may occur and is usually a result of infection-induced valvular damage. Involvement of the aortic valve is more likely to cause congestive cardiac failure than mitral valve damage. The other cause is extension of the infective process beyond the valvular annulus. Involvement of the septum produces atrioventricular, fascicular and bundle branch blocks. Cardiac rupture and tamponade have been reported but are rare. Pericarditis can result from extension into the sinus of Valsalva. Myocardial infarction as a result of infective embolism to the coronary arteries can also occur, but is rare.

Neurological manifestations, the result of embolic events from left-sided lesions, are present in approximately 15% of patients, and are more likely if the pathogen is *Staph. aureus*. These include meningoencephalitis, focal deficits, transient ischaemic attacks and stroke. Embolic stroke is the most frequent event, but intracranial haemorrhage may occur as a result of rupture or leak of a mycotic aneurysm, septic arteritis or bleeding into an infarct. The mortality is high.

Systemic embolization occurs in 40% of cases and gives rise to the peripheral manifestations of infective endocarditis. The embolization usually antedates the diagnosis. Its incidence falls with the administration of appropriate antibiotics. They may involve any organ, but skin, splenic, hepatic and renal emboli are most common. Notably, systemic emboli are absent in infective endocarditis of the tricuspid valve.

Petechiae are commonly found in the palpebral conjunctivae and are also present in the mucosal membranes. Splinter haemorrhages under the fingernails, Osler's nodes (painful tender swellings of the fingertips or toe pads), Janeway lesions (small haemorrhages with a slightly nodular character on the palms and soles) and Roth's spots (oval retinal haemorrhages with a clear pale centre) are uncommon.

Renal dysfunction may be due to altered renal haemodynamics, immune complex-mediated glomerulonephritis or nephrotoxicity from medications. Splenomegaly is present in 30% of cases. This is due to splenic abscesses arising from direct seeding from the bacteraemia or from an infective embolus. It leads to persistent fever, abdominal pain and diaphragmatic irritation. Tender hepatomegaly may also be present. Anaemia is common.

Diagnosis

The diagnosis of infective endocarditis requires an integration of data from various sources. This is due to the non-specific nature of the clinical manifestations. The Duke criteria for infective endocarditis are a useful diagnostic tool that has good specificity and a negative predictive value >92%. These combine patient risk factors, isolates from blood cultures, the persistence of bacteraemia, echocardiographic findings and other clinical and laboratory data (Fig. 5.7.1).

When fever is persistent and unexplained, infective endocarditis must be considered:

- In patients with acquired or congenital valvular heart disease, a pre-existing

Clinical criteria for infective endocarditis require:
- Two major criteria, or
- One major and three minor criteria, or
- Five minor criteria

MAJOR CRITERIA:

- **Positive blood culture for infective endocarditis**
  Typical micro-organism consistent with IE from 2 separate blood cultures, as noted below:
    - viridans streptococci, *Streptococcus bovis*, or HACEK or
    - community-acquired *Staphylococcus aureus* or enterococci, in the absence of a primary focus

  or

  Micro-organisms consistent with IE from persistently positive blood cultures defined as:
    - 2 positive cultures of blood samples drawn 12 hours apart, or
    - all of 3 or a majority of 4 separate cultures of blood (with first and last sample drawn 1 hour apart)

- **Evidence of endocardial involvement**
  Positive echocardiogram for IE defined as:
    - Oscillating intercardiac mass on valve or supporting structures, in the path of regurgitant jets, or on implanted material in the absence of an alternative anatomical explanation, or
    - abscess, or
    - new partial dehiscence of prosthetic valve

  or

  New valvular regurgitation (worsening or changing of pre-existing murmur not sufficient)

MINOR CRITERIA:

- **Predisposition:** predisposing heart condition or intravenous drug use
- **Fever:** temperature ? 38.0° C (100.4° F)
- **Vascular phenomena:** major arterial emboli, septic pulmonary infarcts, mycotic aneurysm, intracranial haemorrhage, conjunctival haemorrhages, and Janeway lesions
- **Immunological phenomena:** glomerulonephritis, Osler's nodes, Roth's spots and rheumatoid factor
- **Microbiological evidence:** positive blood culture but does not meet a major criterion as noted above or serological evidence of active infection with organism consistent with IE
- **Echocardiographic findings:** consistent with IE but do not meet a major criterion as noted above

---

Fig. 5.7.1 Duke criteria for the diagnosis of infective endocarditis. (Modified from Durack DT, Lukes AS, Bright DK. New criteria for diagnosis of infective endocarditis: utilization of specific echocardiographic findings. Duke Endocarditis Service. American Journal of Medicine 1994; 96: 200–209.)

prosthetic valve, hypertrophic cardiomyopathy, congenital heart disease (persistent ductus arteriosus, PDA; ventricular septal defect, VSD; coarctation of the aorta), intracardiac pacemakers, central venous lines or intra-arterial lines, or a new or changed cardiac murmur.

- In patients with known bacteraemia. In *Staph. aureus* bacteraemia the risk of infective endocarditis is higher if it is community acquired, there is no primary focus of infection, there is a metastatic complication and, in the context of an intravascular catheter being a possible focus of infection, if fever or bacteraemia is present for more than 3 days, despite removal of the catheter.
- If there has been a recent procedure likely to cause a bacteraemia, e.g. dental, bronchoscopy, gastrointestinal and genitourinary procedures.
- If there are features of an embolic event, especially if recurrent.
- In young patients with unexpected stroke or subarachnoid haemorrhage.
- In patients with a history of IVDU, especially if there are pulmonary features such as cough and pleuritic chest pain.
- When there is persistent bacteraemia or fever despite treatment, congestive cardiac failure, or new ECG features of atrioventricular heart block, fascicular block and bundle branch block.

Investigations

Blood cultures

Blood cultures are crucial to the diagnosis of infective endocarditis. If no antibiotics have been given, blood cultures are positive in 95–100% of cases, often in the first two sets. The major causes of culture-negative infective endocarditis are prior use of antibiotics (62%) and fastidious organisms. In the stable patient without evidence of complications, three sets of blood cultures should be collected from different vascular puncture sites at least 1 hour apart over a 24-hour period prior to the start of empirical antibiotics. The timing of venepuncture does not need to coincide with fever, as bacteraemia is continuous. An aerobic and an anaerobic medium is used in each set. Arterial and venous blood are equally likely to be infected. In unwell patients, empirical antibiotics should not be delayed and the timing between blood cultures can be truncated.

Full blood count

Anaemia is demonstrated in most patients. It is usually normochromic and normocytic. There is a leukocytosis in acute infective endocarditis, but this may be absent in sub-acute cases. Thrombocytopenia is rare.

ESR

The ESR is a non-specific test; however, it is raised in almost all patients to a magnitude of >55 mm/h. A normal ESR makes infective endocarditis unlikely.

Urinalysis

Urinalysis is abnormal in 50% of cases, with proteinuria and microscopic haematuria. Normal renal function may be maintained.

Echocardiography

Echocardiography provides morphological confirmation of the diagnosis by visualizing heart valves and vegetations, assessing haemodynamic impact and identifying complications (such as perivalvular involvement, abscesses). Two modes of echocardiography are used. In NVE, transthoracic echocardiography (TTE) has a specificity for vegetations of 98%, but a sensitivity of less than 60–70%. The reason for the low sensitivity is the technical problems in those with chest wall deformity, chronic airway limitation and obesity. In PVE, sensitivity of TTE for vegetations is 15–35% and it is especially poor for mitral valve vegetations. However, it has the benefit of being non-invasive. Transoesophageal echocardiography (TOE) is invasive and more difficult to obtain. It has a specificity of 85–98% and its sensitivity is 75–95% for vegetations. In particular, it is more likely to detect perivalvular lesions and abscesses. The indication for TTE in infective endocarditis is suspected NVE with no technical hindrance to imaging. If the result is negative and coupled with a low clinical suspicion, a subsequent TOE is not warranted. The indications for TOE in infective endocarditis are:

- Prosthetic valves.
- Suspected myocardial involvement.
- Unexplained Gram-negative coccus bacteraemia.
- Catheter-related *Staph. aureus* bacteraemia.
- Current intravenous drug use.
- Suspected perivalvular extension of disease.

Despite the virtues of TOE, a negative study does not exclude the diagnosis or the need to start treatment if clinical suspicion is high. The false-negative range is 6–18%, which decreases to 4–13% with a repeat study. There are a number of limitations of echocardiography: infectious vegetations cannot be distinguished from marantic lesions on native valves or thrombus on prosthetic valves, and healed lesions cannot be easily separated from active ones. Entities that may mimic vegetations are thickened valves, ruptured chordae or valves, calcifications and nodules.

Complications

Complications are summarized in Table 5.7.3.

Management

Management involves the use of antibiotics to eradicate the pathogen and other interventions to deal with the intracardiac and distal complications of the infections. Surgery may be required for the latter.

Antibiotic therapy

In the emergency department (ED) a microbiological diagnosis is not possible. Toxic patients must start empirical antibiotics after the collection of three sets of cultures from three separate vascular puncture sites. In septic patients these do not need to be separated in time.

Antibiotic penetration of vegetations is difficult as they are a mixture of fibrin, platelets and bacteria, and it is hard to achieve local bacteriocidal drug levels. The principles of antibiotic therapy are to use antibiotics in combination with empirical therapy determined by the most likely group of organisms in a given patient and a long duration of therapy, usually 4–6 weeks. Antibiotic choice is tailored once the pathogen and its sensitivities are known.

The current recommendations for empirical antibiotics in Australia are:

- For community-acquired NVE:
  - Benzylpenicillin 1.8 g i.v. 4-hourly with
  - Flucloxacillin 2 g i.v. 4-hourly with
  - Gentamicin 4–6 mg/kg i.v. daily.

Vancomycin (25 mg/kg up to 1 g i.v. 12-hourly) replaces penicillin in PVE, hospital-acquired infections, or where there is penicillin sensitivity.

Surgery

Native valve endocarditis Congestive cardiac failure, evidence of embolization to major organs and vegetations larger than 10 mm have been shown to have a poor outcome on medical management alone. The indications for surgery in haemodynamically unstable patients are:

- Cardiac failure, aortic incompetence or mitral incompetence.
- Complications of heart block, annular or aortic abscess, or the presence of perforating lesions, e.g. perforated valve leaflets.
- Virulent organisms resistant to treatment.
- Fungal endocarditis.

The indications in haemodynamically stable patients are less clear.

Prosthetic valve endocarditis The indications for surgery include cardiac failure, valve dehiscence, valve dysfunction (increased stenosis or incompetence) and complications such as abscess formation.

Anticoagulation Anticoagulation with aspirin or warfarin has not been shown to reduce the risk of embolic events and may contribute to an increased risk of bleeding, especially intracranial. They should only be used with caution where there is a clear indication for them distinct from endocarditis.

Prognosis

The overall mortality for native and prosthetic valve endocarditis is 20–25% at 1 year and 50% at 10 years. The major causes of death are haemodynamic deterioration and embolic complications of the CNS. Nosocomial endocarditis has an

Table 5.7.3 Complications of infective endocarditis	
Organ system	**Complications**
Cardiac	Congestive cardiac failure Valvular incompetence Arrhythmias Cardiac rupture/tamponade Pericarditis Myocardial infarction Cardiac fistulae
Renal	Immune-mediated glomerulonephritis
Neurological	Stroke or TIA Cerebral abscess Intracranial haemorrhage from aneurysm rupture Meningitis/encephalitis
Other	Mycotic aneurysm of any artery Emboli to any organ, e.g. spleen, liver, skin

inpatient mortality of 24–50% compared to community-acquired endocarditis (16–20%). In right-sided lesions in intravenous drug users the mortality is 10%. The most important determinant of mortality is congestive cardiac failure.

Mortality is also related to the organism isolated. It is greater than 50% in *Pseudomonas aeruginosa*, enterobacteriaciae or fungal infection. *Staph. aureus* infection has a mortality of 25–47%.

Relapse occurs usually within 2 months of stopping antibiotics. The rate of relapse in NVE is <2% for *Strep. viridans*, 11% for *Staph. aureus* and 8–20% for enterococci. In prosthetic valve endocarditis the relapse rate is 10–15%.

Long term, approximately 50% of cases require heart valve replacement.

Acute aortic incompetence

Aetiology and pathophysiology

The causes of acute aortic valve incompetence are infective endocarditis, proximal aortic dissection, blunt chest trauma, and spontaneous rupture of an abnormal valve. The result is an acute and progressive volume overload within the left ventricle that has not had time to compensate. The consequently elevated left ventricular end-diastolic pressure is transmitted to the left atrium and pulmonary venous bed, leading to pulmonary oedema. Cardiac output is diminished as the stroke volume is shared between forward and regurgitant flow into the left atrium. The compensatory mechanisms via the sympathetic nervous system result in positive inotropy and chronotropy. However, the rise in the systemic peripheral vascular resistance impedes left ventricular outflow and worsens the regurgitation. Ventricular oxygen demand is also increased and myocardial ischaemia is a real risk, even if coronary artery disease is not present.

Clinical features

Acute aortic incompetence is poorly tolerated. Severe congestive cardiac failure and hypotension are typical. Ischaemic chest pain may be reported. The diastolic murmur is soft and extends only to mid-diastole. The first heart sound is also of low intensity. The pulse pressure is large and tachycardia is almost always present.

Investigations

The CXR may reveal the underlying cause. Pulmonary congestion is often present without cardiac enlargement. Echocardiography is diagnostic and provides useful data, especially in the selection of timing for surgery. A TOE is required if aortic root dissection is thought to be the cause. Cardiac catheterization precedes surgery except under dire circumstances.

Management

Valve replacement is crucial to survival, as severe left ventricular failure is the commonest cause of death. Medical treatment with a positive inotrope (dopamine or dobutamine) and concurrent vasodilatation (with nitroprusside) is used, but serves only as a temporizing measure prior to surgery.

Intra-aortic balloon counterpulsation is contraindicated. β-Blockers should be used with caution as the compensatory tachycardia will be prevented.

Acute deterioration in chronic aortic incompetence

Pathophysiology

In chronic aortic valve incompetence the pathophysiology is dictated by the combination of pressure and volume overload. The initial stage of compensation is achieved by hypertrophy of the left ventricle. The left ventricular ejection fraction (LVEF) is never in the normal range even in the compensated stage. However, the patient can be asymptomatic for decades. This is followed by the uncompensated stage, where there is a significant reduction of the left ventricular ejection fraction, defined as 50% or less at rest. This results predominantly from volume overload. It is reversible initially, with full recovery of left ventricular function if aortic valve replacement is performed. The uncompensated phase eventually becomes irreversible with enlargement of the left ventricle. Symptoms become severe and reversal by surgery is then not possible.

Decompensation can be the result of decreased myocardial contractility due to progressive left ventricular dilatation or myocardial ischaemia or excessive volume overload.

Apart from abnormalities intrinsic to the aortic valve, aortic root dilatation from various causes must be considered.

Clinical features

The clinical features are those of cardiac failure and angina. The patient is usually hypertensive. Clinical findings of severe disease are a wide pulse pressure, a displaced apical impulse, a diastolic murmur in the left third/fourth intercostal space, a third heart sound and an Austin–Flint murmur.

Investigation

The aim of investigations is to identify those who will need surgery. Serial investigations are usually performed. The most important is the assessment of ejection fraction and left ventricular systolic and diastolic volumes by echocardiography. This also allows assessment of the aortic root.

Management

Medical

For symptomatic patients in the ED, medical management is aimed at improving left ventricular dysfunction as a temporizing measure prior to surgery. This is achieved by using vasodilators. The dose is titrated to the blood pressure, aiming to reduce it to a level tolerated by the patient. Medication options include sodium nitroprusside and hydralazine, both of which reduce end-diastolic volume and increase forward flow. Nifedipine, in a single dose, does not consistently produce this result, but may do so when used longer term.

Surgical

Indications for AV replacement are:

- Symptomatic patient: angina or significant dyspnoea.
- Asymptomatic patients with ejection fraction ≤50%.
- Asymptomatic patients with severe left ventricular dilatation and left ventricular end-systolic volume of >55 mm or LV end-diastolic volume >75 mm.

Prognosis

Patients with evidence of angina or cardiac failure have a poorer outcome. Mortality for those with angina is 10%/year and for those with cardiac failure approaches 20%/year.

Acute deterioration in critical aortic stenosis

Patients with severely stenosed aortic valves can remain asymptomatic for many years. Medical treatment can achieve a 5-year survival of 40% and a 10-year survival of 20%. The risk of sudden death in the asymptomatic patient is 2%, even when critical stenosis is present. With the development of syncope and angina, the survival falls to 2–3 years. When complicated by cardiac failure, 50% of patients will die within 18 months with no surgical intervention.

Pathophysiology

Aortic valve stenosis restricts left ventricular outflow and imposes a pressure load on the left ventricle. The latter is hypertrophied, with consequent poor compliance, and is at risk of ischaemia and dysrhythmia. Cardiac function is delicately balanced between preload and afterload. Preload on the hypertrophied ventricle is elevated to support the stroke volume, but not high enough to lead to pulmonary congestion. Systemic vascular resistance is elevated but does not cause an increase in the oxygen demand that cannot be met. The increased demand during exercise causes abnormal distribution of flow, leading to vulnerability of the subendocardium to ischaemia. The reserve margin is slim. A small and sudden alteration in any of these factors will precipitate pump failure.

Causes of aortic stenosis include:

- Congenital bicuspid valve.
- Calcification of a normal valve.
- Rheumatic heart disease, usually with associated mitral valve disease.

Causes

Causes of acute deterioration include:

- An acute fall in preload: hypovolaemia, excessive diuresis and vasodilatation.
- Atrial flutter or fibrillation. These are both uncommon and should raise suspicion of associated mitral valve disease.
- Acute afterload reduction. This leads to a reduction in coronary artery perfusion and places the hypertrophied left ventricle at risk of ischaemia. It does not

improve the left ventricular stroke volume as the problem lies in the stenotic valve and not the systemic vascular resistance.

Clinical features

Patients with aortic stenosis may be asymptomatic for many years. Presentations to the ED may be for angina, syncope or left ventricular failure (mild–severe) or hypotension. At its worst, acute decompensation will result in acute pump failure: shock and pulmonary oedema.

The murmur will have the expected features, including aortic area location, systolic timing and radiation to the carotids. It will be less impressive if cardiac output is poor. The most important finding consistent with critical stenosis is the paradoxical splitting of the second heart sound.

Investigations

ECG, chest X-ray and cardiac markers

Indications for these are dictated by the clinical presentation.

Echocardiography

Echocardiography confirms the diagnosis and allows assessment of transvalvular flow, transvalvular pressure gradients and the effective valve area.

Management

Medical therapy aims to relieve symptoms and optimize left ventricular function prior to definitive surgical management. Rapid reversal of the precipitant is essential.

Practice points

- Expedient treatment of atrial dysrhythmias may necessitate cardioversion. This helps by maximizing the contribution of atrial systole to left ventricular filling.
- Excessive reduction in preload will reduce stroke volume and hence cardiac output.
- Diuretics, digoxin and ACE inhibitors should only be used with caution.
- Sodium nitroprusside may be used for preload and afterload reduction, but only with the assistance of invasive haemodynamic monitoring.
- Angina treatment requires cautious use of nitrates and β-blockers.

Acute deterioration in mitral stenosis

Pathophysiology

The adult mitral orifice is 4–6 cm^2. Symptom onset occurs when the valve orifice is less than 2.5 cm^2, and critical stenosis occurs when this is reduced to 1 cm^2. That said, the patient may remain asymptomatic for years. A pressure load is imposed on the left atrium, with pulmonary congestion and pulmonary hypertension as the consequences. The major damage is incurred by the lungs and right ventricle.

The predominant cause of mitral stenosis is rheumatic carditis. Other causes include atrial myxomas, severe annular calcification and ball valve thrombi. Congenital malformations are rare.

Causes of acute deterioration

Acute deterioration can be precipitated in two ways. When the heart rate is increased, the ventricular filling time in diastole is reduced. The atrial pressure rises and is transmitted retrogradely to the pulmonary bed, leading to acute dyspnoea and pulmonary oedema. Atrial fibrillation with a rapid ventricular response is a common example of this. In addition, loss of atrial systole in atrial fibrillation leads to a 20% decrease in cardiac output. Therefore, major haemodynamic instability can occur.

The second cause of acute deterioration is related to flow across the stenosed valve. When the flow is increased, the transvalvular pressure gradient is increased by a factor equal to the square of the flow rate. The left atrial pressure rises and can precipitate pulmonary congestion. The common clinical contexts in which the transvalvular flow is increased are exercise, pregnancy, infection, hypervolaemia and hyperthyroidism.

Clinical features

Patients may be asymptomatic for many years, but will have an abnormal physical examination. Symptomatic patients present with dyspnoea, fatigue, a thromboembolic event, atrial fibrillation or pulmonary congestion/oedema. The onset of symptoms is usually followed by a period of minimal disability that may last many years. Pulmonary congestion, pulmonary hypertension or systemic or pulmonary emboli herald rapid deterioration. Auscultatory findings include a loud first heart sound, an opening snap and a mid-diastolic murmur with pre-systolic accentuation.

Signs of critical stenosis are small pulse pressure, soft first heart sound, early opening snap, long diastolic murmur, diastolic thrill and evidence of pulmonary hypertension (right ventricular heave and loud P2). Acute pulmonary oedema may be present. Atrial fibrillation with a rapid ventricular rate is frequently the cause. Evidence of systemic embolization of a left atrial thrombus should be sought.

Investigations

Chest X-ray and ECG
The CXR features are those of an enlarged left atrium, pulmonary congestion and pulmonary hypertension. The heart size is usually normal. Left atrial enlargement on the ECG is found in 90% of patients in sinus rhythm.

Echocardiogram
A detailed echocardiograph assessment will confirm the diagnosis, exclude other causes of mitral valve obstruction, identify associated or coexisting structural heart disease, determine the severity of mitral stenosis and estimate pulmonary artery pressure.

Management
Medical management aims to reduce symptoms and prevent complications. It does not change the course of mitral valve deterioration, which requires surgery for definitive management. This is usually indicated when symptom severity is at NYHA functional class III.

Medical management for pulmonary oedema is described in Chapter 5.3. If atrial fibrillation with rapid ventricular response is a contributing factor, rate control is the first priority, either with drugs or with cardioversion (see Chapter 5.4). Anticoagulation is indicated for patients in atrial fibrillation.

Prognosis
In asymptomatic or minimally symptomatic patients the average 10-year survival is more than 80%. In those with significant symptoms, 10-year survival is 0–15%. In untreated patients, mortality is due to pulmonary congestion, right heart failure, systemic emboli, pulmonary emboli and infective endocarditis.

Acute mitral incompetence

Pathophysiology
Acute volume overload into the left atrium by the regurgitant stream is the crucial factor in acute mitral incompetence. The left atrium has limited capacity to accommodate this insult, and pulmonary oedema occurs. There is an associated rise in the pulmonary vascular resistance. Right ventricular failure may result. Cardiac output is reduced owing to a low stroke volume. The consequent elevation in the systemic vascular resistance impedes cardiac output. Tachycardia occurs but confers no benefit, as the diastolic filling time is reduced.

Aetiology
The causes of acute mitral incompetence are:

- Infective endocarditis
- Papillary muscle disorder
  - ischaemia or infarction
  - trauma
  - infiltrative disease
- Rupture of the chordae tendinae
  - acute rheumatic fever
  - infective endocarditis
  - chest trauma
  - balloon valvotomy
  - myxomatous degeneration
  - spontaneous rupture
- Mitral leaflet disorder
  - infective endocarditis
  - myxomatous degeneration
  - atrial myxoma
  - systemic lupus erythematosus
  - trauma.

Clinical features
Acute mitral valve incompetence is poorly tolerated and patients are always symptomatic. There is reduced perfusion with concurrent acute pulmonary oedema. The blood pressure is variable, and can be normal or low. The precordial findings do not correlate with the severity of the pathology – in fact, a third heart sound may be the only finding. The apical mitral murmur is soft and occurs in early systole, and does not become pansystolic. It radiates to the axilla and is commonly accompanied by a short apical diastolic murmur.

Investigations

Chest X-ray and ECG
The CXR will show pulmonary oedema but not cardiomegaly. The ECG may show a recent infarct if this was the precipitant.

Echocardiography
Echocardiography is diagnostic and provides valuable information on left ventricular function. It demonstrates the lesion and assesses its severity. Both TTE and TOE may be required for adequate assessment.

Management
Surgery is urgently required. Medical treatment is usually only a temporizing step.

Medical treatment
The mortality in patients with severe left ventricular failure is high. Medical treatment is directed at reducing the regurgitant volume and thereby diminishing the pulmonary congestion. It also aims to improve the forward output of the left ventricle. The modalities used depend on the blood pressure.

In normotensive patients, sodium nitroprusside may achieve all of the above objectives. In hypotensive patients, a combination of sodium nitroprusside and an inotrope such as dobutamine is required. Aortic balloon counterpulsation may be required to improve left ventricular ejection volume and further assist in the reduction of the regurgitant volume.

In infective endocarditis, appropriate antibiotics are required.

Acute deterioration in chronic mitral incompetence

Pathophysiology
In chronic mitral valve incompetence the increased left ventricular end-diastolic volume leads to an increased left ventricular stroke volume and hence forward flow is preserved. The other factors that enable this are the increased preload on the left ventricle and the ability of the left ventricle to reduce afterload by backfilling into the left atrium. The result is enlargement of the left atrium and ventricle. In this compensated phase the patient is asymptomatic. This phase may last for years.

In the decompensated phase, left ventricular systolic dysfunction occurs as a result of contractile failure. This causes further left ventricular dilatation and increased left ventricular preload. A fall in forward outflow and pulmonary congestion may result. However, the factors are often still in favour of the left ventricle and the ejection fraction may be in the lower range of normal, i.e. 0.5–0.6.

Causes of chronic mitral incompetence include rheumatic carditis, ischaemic heart disease, mitral valve prolapse syndrome, collagen vascular disease and dilatation of the valvular annulus. Ischaemic causes have the worst prognosis, as myocardial dysfunction is often coexistent.

Clinical features

Features of decompensation may be subtle. A history of reduced exercise tolerance is an important clue. Symptoms are those of pulmonary congestion and reduced cardiac output. Examination findings indicating severe disease include displacement of the apical impulse and evidence of pulmonary congestion. A third heart sound is commonly found and is not necessarily evidence of left ventricular failure.

Investigations

CXR and ECG may provide useful information regarding cardiac size and heart rhythm. The most important test is echocardiography, which will confirm the diagnosis of mitral incompetence and document left ventricular and left atrial size. The integrity of the tricuspid valve is also important.

Management

Medical treatment

Atrial fibrillation is a common morbidity in chronic mitral valve incompetence; however, embolic risk is lower than for mitral stenosis with atrial fibrillation. AF is also an independent predictor of poor outcome after surgery. The ventricular rate requires control (Chapter 5.4). Anticoagulation is used as prophylaxis for embolic complications.

In functional mitral incompetence, preload reduction is beneficial if there is left ventricular dysfunction. Useful agents include ACE inhibitors and β-blockers, especially carvedilol.

Surgical treatment

Surgery is indicated for:

- Symptomatic patients in NYHA functional class II–IV with
  ○ left ventricular ejection fraction ≥ 0.30 or
  ○ left ventricular end systolic dimension ≤ 55 mm
- Asymptomatic patients with
  ○ left ventricular ejection fraction between 0.30 and 0.60
  ○ left ventricular end systolic dimensions ≥ 40 mm.

Prognosis

The risk of death is related to the degree of left ventricular decompensation.

Prosthetic valve complications

Prosthetic valve complications are common. As discussed previously, they are prone to infective endocarditis and so appropriate antibiotic prophylaxis is essential.

Antithrombotic therapy

This is given to prevent embolic complications. The risk is greater in mitral than in aortic prostheses, regardless of the type. It is also highest in the first few months, as the prosthesis has not been fully endothelialized. Warfarin is the anticoagulant of choice.

Mechanical valves

Target INR values for mechanical valves are summarized in Table 5.7.4.

Aspirin in the dose range of 80–100 mg/day may be used in addition to warfarin in patients with an embolic event where the INR is in the therapeutic range, with known vascular disease or with a susceptibility to hypercoagulability. This has been shown to reduce the risk of thromboembolism and

cardiovascular mortality. The data only refer to aspirin doses within this range.

Biological valves

The increased risk of thromboembolism is in the first 3 months, with the incidence at its greatest during the initial few days. After the 3-month period, the biological prosthetic valve can be regarded as a native valve.

Heparin therapy, followed later by warfarin, is started as soon as surgical bleeding is reduced. Warfarin is ceased in two-thirds of the patients at 3 months. The remaining one-third stay on lifetime treatment with an INR in the range of 2.0–3.0. Patients requiring lifetime warfarin therapy include those with atrial fibrillation, a past history of thromboembolism, a risk of hypercoagulability, and those with severe left ventricular dysfunction with a LVEF <0.3.

Controversies

- Anticoagulation in infective endocarditis.

- Indications for and timing of surgery for haemodynamically stable patients with infective endocarditis. The aim of early surgery would be to maximize salvage of the valvular apparatus and minimize the risk of endocardial complications.

Further reading

Bonow RO, Blase A, Carabello KC, et al. ACC/AHA 2006 Guidelines for the management of patients with valvular heart disease: A report of the American College of Cardiology/American Heart Association task force on practice guidelines. Circulation 2006; 114: e84–e231.

Endocarditis (revised 2006 June). In: eTG complete (Internet). Melbourne: Therapeutic Guidelines Limited; 2007 July. Online. Available: <http://www.tg.com.au/ip/complete/> Accessed Sept 2007.

Hill EE, Herijgers P, Herregods MC, et al. Evolving trends in infective endocarditis. Clinical Microbiology and Infection 2006; 12: 5–12.

Hoen B. Epidemiology and antibiotic treatment of infective endocarditis: an update. Heart 2006; 92: 1694–1700.

Karchmer AW. Infective endocarditis. In: Zipes DG, Libby P, Bonow R, et al., eds. Braunwald's heart disease: A textbook of cardiovascular medicine, 7th edn. Philadelphia: WB Saunders, 2005; 1633–1654.

Mylonakis E, Calderwood SB. Medical progress: infective endocarditis in adults. New England Journal of Medicine 2001; 345: 1318–1330.

Strom BL, Abrutyn E, Berlin JA, et al. Risk factors for infective endocarditis – oral hygiene and nondental exposures. Circulation 2000; 102: 2842.

Wang A, Athan E, Paul A, et al. Contemporary clinical profile and outcome of prosthetic valve endocarditis. Journal of the American Medical Association 2007; 297: 1354–1361.

Table 5.7.4 Target INR values for prosthetic valves		
Position	Valve	INR range
Aortic	Bi leaf of Medtronic Hall	2.0–30.
	Starr–Edwards or other discs	2.5–3.5
Mitral	Any	2.5–3.5

5.8 Peripheral vascular disease

Colin Graham

ESSENTIALS

1 The incidence of peripheral arterial and venous disease in the developed world continues to increase significantly with the continuing rise in the elderly population.

2 Claudication is the most important symptom of arterial disease in an extremity, although a well developed collateral circulation will delay the onset of symptomatic extremity ischaemia.

3 Acute arterial occlusion is usually associated with a number of classic symptoms and signs. It is a time-critical emergency requiring urgent access to an experienced vascular surgeon.

4 If venous thrombosis is suspected, detailed assessment is essential. Unfortunately, the presence or absence of signs and symptoms of deep venous thrombosis (DVT) does not correlate well with the presence or absence of actual venous clot. Homan's sign is non-specific and unreliable.

5 Optimal assessment for DVT consists of defining a pre-test probability of disease and then performing appropriate non-invasive investigations in the first instance.

6 Compression ultrasonography is the investigation of choice for the diagnosis of DVT.

7 Anticoagulation is the recommended treatment for DVT above the level of the popliteal vein. Treatment of below-knee DVT remains controversial, but evidence suggests that these patients should also receive anticoagulation treatment to prevent complications.

8 Extensive iliofemoral thrombus or thrombus of the upper limb may require early surgical and or thrombolytic treatment to minimize the risk of post-thrombotic syndrome.

ARTERIAL DISEASE

Introduction

Extremity ischaemia may be acute, chronic or acute on chronic. The onset and severity of symptoms may be modified by the development of collateral circulation.

Chronic arterial ischaemia

The prevalence of peripheral arterial disease increases with age (most symptomatic patients are aged over 60) and is twice as high in men as in women between the ages of 50 and 70 years, but almost identical after the age of 70.

Peripheral arterial disease is usually due to atherosclerosis of the lower abdominal aorta or the iliac, femoral and/or popliteal arteries. In common with carotid and coronary artery disease, the common disease processes that exacerbate peripheral arterial disease include diabetes mellitus, hypertension, smoking, hyperlipidaemia, and previous limb surgery or trauma. A significant collateral circulation is made up of pre-existing pathways arising from the distributing branches of large and medium-sized arteries. It develops over time when there is an increase in the velocity of flow through them secondary to arterial occlusion developing in a main vascular pathway. Collateral flow can usually provide an adequate supply to the resting limb, and sufficient additional requirements to sustain moderate exercise.

Clinical features

Presentation may be acute or chronic. Symptoms consist of pain, ulceration, or changes in appearance with swelling or discolouration. Lower limb ischaemia usually manifests as claudication – the most important symptom of extremity arterial occlusive disease. Chronic critical lower limb ischaemia is defined by either of the following two criteria:

- Recurring ischaemic rest pain persisting for more than 2 weeks and requiring regular analgesics. There should be an ankle systolic pressure of ≤ 50 mmHg, a toe systolic pressure of ≤ 30 mmHg, or both.
- Ulceration or gangrene of the foot or toes, with similar haemodynamic parameters.

The classic description of claudication is of pain in a functional muscle unit that occurs as a result of a consistent amount of exercise and is promptly relieved by rest. Limp may also be pronounced. The commonest site of occlusion leading to claudication is the superficial femoral artery, resulting in pain in the calf. This occurs on walking upstairs or slopes and is relieved by rest. Less commonly, aortoiliac disease produces symptoms of pain in the thigh or buttock. Night pain experienced in the foot, relieved by either dependency or, paradoxically, by walking around, implies a reduction in blood flow to a level below that required for normal resting tissue metabolism. Typically, rest pain tends to be distal to the metatarsals, severe, persistent, and worsened by elevation.

Detailed examination of the peripheral vascular system is essential. Abnormalities tend to be related to changes in the peripheral arteries and tissue ischaemia. Distal pulses may be absent or diminished in amplitude, and bruits (commonly femoral) may be present. Capillary return is usually reduced, atrophic changes are present and the foot is cool to the touch. Pallor may be apparent on exercise and is usually associated with pain. There may be pallor on elevation of the foot, with reactive hyperaemia on dependency: the more limited the elevation resulting in pallor, the greater the degree of stenosis (Buerger's test).

As ischaemia becomes more advanced the skin becomes shiny and scaly, with associated atrophy of the subcutaneous tissues and muscle. In advanced stages of ischaemia there may be red discolouration, caused by capillary blood stasis and high oxygen extraction. There may also be tissue necrosis and non-healing wounds or ulcers secondary to trauma, which may progress to gangrene.

Clinical investigations

Routine blood tests should be carried out to derive baselines for renal and hepatic function as well as to exclude anaemia, polycythaemia, hyperglycaemia, thrombocythaemia and hyperlipidaemia. The ankle–brachial pressure index (ABPI) should be measured to confirm the clinical diagnosis. This is calculated (for each leg) by dividing the highest systolic pressure recorded at the respective ankle by the highest systolic brachial pressure obtained in recordings from both arms. Resting ABPI is normally >1, and figures of <0.92 indicate arterial disease. Values between 0.5 and 0.9 may be associated with claudication and <0.5 with rest pain. Normal ABPI values may be recorded in diabetic patients, even though they have claudication, owing to the presence of medial arterial calcification. Angiography is required to identify the site and extent of lesions and their amenability to intervention.

Management

In patients with a chronic stable disease process, treatment is focused mainly on preventing progression of the disease process. This is usually coordinated by the patient's primary care physician and consists of regular exercise, control of associated medical diseases and cessation of smoking. Specific measures should be taken to address hyperlipidaemia, diabetes mellitus and hypertension. In more advanced progressive disease, strategies to minimize other complications, including lower limb

ulcers and gangrene, should also be considered. Patients presenting to the emergency department (ED) at this stage or with debilitating symptoms merit early referral for vascular surgical assessment with view to operative or radiological (endovascular) intervention.

Acute arterial ischaemia of the lower limb

Acute lower limb ischaemia, or 'limb-threatening' ischaemia, is associated with significant morbidity and mortality. Early recognition of the signs and symptoms is critical. The arterial occlusion will cause symptoms most obviously when there is inadequate collateral circulation. Causes may be embolic, thrombotic, traumatic, or iatrogenic in nature, of which emboli are the most common. Most arterial emboli originate in thrombus formation from the heart (85%), the vast majority of these from left atrial thrombus related to chronic atrial fibrillation. Other uncommon causes include arterial thrombosis due to endothelial injury or alterations in the blood flow to the limb. Iatrogenic causes may be secondary to intra-arterial cannulation, recent cardiac catheterization or ischaemic limb anaesthesia (such as a Bier's block).

Clinical features

Sudden occlusion of a previously patent artery is a dramatic event. Unfortunately, recognition can be difficult, particularly in elderly people with chronic confusional states, and careful examination is therefore essential. Occlusion may be portrayed by one or more of the classic signs of pulselessness, pain, pallor, paraesthesia and paralysis (the '5 Ps'). However, none of the above, either alone or in combination, is sufficient to definitely establish or exclude the diagnosis of an acute ischaemic limb. Loss of a palpable pulse in the symptomatic limb compared to the other side should raise significant concern.

The pain is a severe, constant ache which requires intravenous opiates for relief. The ischaemic periphery is pale, white or cadaveric in appearance, and feels cold to touch. Progression occurs with blotchy areas of cyanosis and further discolouration. Pain, tense swelling and acute tenderness of a

muscle belly are late findings. If these findings persist for longer than 12 hours, irreversible ischaemia with gangrene is highly likely.

Clinical investigation

Doppler ultrasound should be used in all patients where there is concern about the arterial circulation of a limb. A handheld Doppler probe will confirm the presence or absence of a pulse and give some quantification of flow. Other investigations, including basic haematology and biochemical profiles, as well as electrocardiography and chest radiography, help to identify other diagnostic possibilities (e.g. low cardiac output state, polycythaemia, aortic dissection) and other contributing factors (such as atrial fibrillation), and establish fitness for urgent surgical intervention.

Differential diagnosis

It is important (but can be difficult) to differentiate between an embolic event and acute progression of a thrombus. The embolic event will tend to be sudden in onset and exhibit some combination of the '5 Ps'. In-situ progression of thrombus will occur in patients who have long-standing significant peripheral arterial disease and a well-developed collateral circulation. Other diagnoses that must be considered include aortic dissection and phlegmasia cerulea dolens. The latter is a massive iliofemoral deep venous thrombosis. The initial symptom may be of an acutely swollen and painful leg. As the swelling continues there may be secondary arterial insufficiency. Acute embolus, however, tends to produce pallor and a sharp demarcation, whereas with phlegmasia cerulea dolens there is a large cyanotic-appearing limb.

It is important to consider other medical causes that can mimic acute embolism of the upper or lower limb. These include neurological disorders (spinal subarachnoid haemorrhage) and low-output states such as advanced sepsis, myocardial infarction or pulmonary embolus.

Management

The key to management is rapid diagnosis and access to definitive care. Irreversible changes begin to occur within 4–6 hours of symptom onset, and revascularization is reported to be less effective after 8–12 hours of ischaemia. Intravenous heparin should be given immediately (in the absence of any contraindication) and other correctable aggravating factors (dehydration, sepsis, arrhythmias, myocardial infarction) should be considered and addressed appropriately. Urgent surgical intervention is critical. Embolectomy using a Fogarty catheter, with or without a more definitive revascularization procedure, is the preferred option. Angiography is not necessary in such circumstances as it introduces unnecessary delay.

Ultrasound may be used to rapidly establish the level of arterial occlusion. Intra-arterial thrombolytic therapy has been used in selected cases but it can be time-consuming. Unfortunately, complications include partial clot lysis and further distal embolization. A Cochrane Review suggested that the risks of stroke, haemorrhage and distal embolization were higher in patients treated with thrombolysis rather than surgery, but survival was not affected. These risks will outweigh the benefits in many cases.

Acute arterial ischaemia of the upper limb

Symptomatic vascular disease of the upper limb is relatively rare compared to the lower limb. Presentation to the ED is usually due to coldness or colour changes in the upper limb or digits.

Acute arterial obstruction may arise secondary to emboli, or from penetrating, blunt or iatrogenic trauma. Less commonly, acute occlusion may be associated with thoracic aortic dissection. Emboli affecting the upper limb most frequently involve the brachial artery. Radial and ulnar artery emboli tend to arise from atherosclerotic plaques, aneurysms of the subclavian and axillary arteries, and from complications of thoracic outlet syndrome, rather than from a cardiac source. The diagnosis may be obvious (e.g. trauma) or suggested by the presenting history and clinical findings.

Acute occlusion of a digital artery results in profound ischaemia of the involved digit. Diagnosis is made on clinical grounds, with sudden onset of pain, pallor, coldness and numbness in the affected digit. A chest X-ray may identify a cervical rib. Referral to a vascular surgeon is indicated for further investigations to identify the cause.

Clinical features
Examination of the limb, comparing with the other side, palpation of the pulses and delayed capillary return, as well as detailed examination of the neck, may help localize the level of occlusion. Use of the handheld Doppler and ultrasound may negate the need for preoperative angiography.

Management
When emboli are the cause, embolectomy is the treatment of choice, usually under local anaesthesia; in some cases thrombolysis may be considered. In the presence of acute ischaemic symptoms of the forearm and hand due to trauma, urgent operative repair is mandatory. In the case of injuries to the radial or ulnar arteries, if only one vessel is damaged and collateral flow is satisfactory, the injured vessel may be ligated.

VENOUS DISEASE: LOWER LIMB

Introduction

In contrast to arterial disease, chronic peripheral venous disease most commonly gives rise to cosmetic concerns (varicose veins) only. However, thrombosis in the deep venous system is a life-threatening emergency requiring urgent treatment.

Pathology
It is important to understand that the venous drainage of the lower limb comprises superficial and deep systems connected by perforating veins. A complex system of valves and muscle pumps ensure that blood is carried up from the feet back to the heart. Venous pathology such as valvular destruction results in directional flow change and venous pooling.

Venous insufficiency and varicose veins

Primary varicose veins develop in the absence of deep venous thromboses (DVT).

The main underlying physiological defect in varicose veins is venous valvular incompetence. Varicose veins may also arise secondary to venous outflow obstruction plus valvular incompetence, or there may be primary venous outflow obstruction only.

Acute complications of varicose veins leading to ED attendance are uncommon. However, the skin overlying varices can become thin and erosion can occur spontaneously or with minor trauma alone, resulting in bleeding. The essentials of treatment include elevation of the limb and gentle digital pressure on the site. Ligation of the offending vein may be necessary. Surgical treatment or injection of the varicosities is usually required as a later procedure.

Superficial venous thrombosis

This is a benign, self-limiting disease in most cases. Exclusion of DVT is usually required, although occasionally the diagnosis is obvious. Patients usually present with pain, tenderness and induration along the course of the vein, which may feel firm, cord-like, and have associated erythema. There are usually no signs of impaired venous return. Underlying causes include varicose veins, surrounding cellulitis or a history of preceding trauma. In the upper limb, the commonest cause is intravenous cannulation.

Treatment depends on the extent, aetiology and symptoms. Superficial, mildly tender and well-localized thrombophlebitis may be treated with mild analgesics (usually non-steroidal anti-inflammatory agents (NSAIDs), topical NSAID creams, elastic supports and continued daily activity. More severe thrombophlebitis with marked pain, tenderness and erythema may require a period of rest and elevation of the limb. Antibiotics are not indicated. Anticoagulation is necessary only if the process extends into the deep venous system or approaches the saphenofemoral junction. The prognosis is usually good, and there is no associated tendency for the development of deep venous thrombosis. The process may take 3–4 weeks to resolve. If associated with a varicose vein, superficial thrombophlebitis may recur unless the varix is excised.

Deep venous thrombosis

Deep venous thrombosis (DVT) is a condition characterized by active thrombosis in the deep venous system of one or both lower limbs. Depending upon the thrombus load and the level of extension of the thrombotic process, embolism proximally into the central pulmonary circulation can lead to sudden collapse and death. Early recognition and treatment is therefore essential. The diagnosis and management of acute DVT has changed in recent years, with a move towards structured assessment, non-invasive investigations and more aggressive treatment for patients with distal clots.

Clinical features

Symptoms and signs vary, with one-third having no clinical signs at all. A small number may have classic manifestations. Pain may be located in the calf and/or the thigh, ranging from a dull ache to a tight sensation, and is sometimes related to exercise. Examination findings include calf swelling, calf tenderness, tenderness over the popliteal or femoral veins, and oedema, but may occasionally be entirely normal. Circumferential limb measurements may be helpful, but differences up to 1 cm occur naturally. Homan's sign is non-specific and unreliable. In addition, it is important to incorporate an objective assessment of risk factors for DVT.

One validated prediction model for assessment resulting in the generation of a pre-test probability of DVT has been developed and validated by Wells et al. One point is assigned for various risk factors for DVT (including a period of acute immobilization or paralysis (including lower limbs fractures in a plaster cast), previous DVT, presence of superficial collateral (non-varicose) veins, pitting oedema of the affected leg, calf swelling >3 cm than the non-affected side, swelling of the entire leg, localized tenderness of the deep venous system, recently bedridden for >3 days, recent major surgery (<12 weeks) and active cancer). Two points are then deducted for an alternative diagnosis (for example, cellulitis, ankle oedema due to heart failure, etc.). A pre-test probability score of ≥2 means that DVT is 'likely' and compression ultrasonography should be performed. If the score is less than 2, then DVT

is 'unlikely', and a D-dimer assay should be performed (see below).

Clinical investigation

If the derived pre-test probability of DVT is 'likely', compression ultrasonography is recommended. It is the imaging method of choice to diagnose DVT. Local protocols and expertise will determine whether this is done by a radiologist or an emergency physician. If necessary, patients who are haemodynamically stable and are otherwise fit for outpatient care can be given an injection of a low molecular weight heparin (LMWH) for the treatment of presumed DVT and allowed home, to return during office hours the following day for their compression ultrasound investigation. The overall sensitivity of ultrasound for any lower limb DVT is in the range of 95%, with >96% specificity. A negative ultrasound result in the setting of a likely DVT warrants repeat testing at 5–7 days. If this remains negative, but clinical suspicion remains high for DVT, venography should be considered, although this is now rarely performed because it has the disadvantages of being invasive, painful, expensive, inconvenient to perform, and associated with potential phlebitis, anaphylaxis and other complications. In most circumstances an alternative diagnosis is more likely at this stage.

If the pre-test probability is 'DVT unlikely', a D-dimer assay is performed to determine the need for imaging to exclude DVT. D-Dimers are degradation products of cross-linked fibrin blood clots, typical of those found in DVT. The level therefore rises in acute DVT, but it also rises in other acute conditions, such as infection and following trauma. Therefore a positive test does not rule in DVT, but a negative test has a high negative predictive value for DVT and can therefore rule out disease. The combination of a low pre-test probability of disease and a negative D-dimer effectively excludes DVT, and the patient can be safely discharged without the need for further investigation. However, D-dimer test characteristics vary greatly depending on whether the method used is an enzyme-linked immunosorbent assay (ELISA) or a variant of a whole blood latex agglutination study. Local expertise in the interpretation of these markers is essential in such circumstances. Local clinical protocols should therefore be followed to ensure that

patients who are discharged are being appropriately and safely screened for DVT.

Differential diagnosis

The prevalence of DVT in patients with suggestive symptoms attending the ED ranges from 16% to 30%. Other alternative diagnoses include cellulitis, superficial thrombophlebitis, a ruptured Baker's cyst, chronic leg oedema, chronic venous insufficiency, postoperative swelling and arthritis.

Management

The standard treatment for established DVT is anticoagulation. If clinical assessment suggests that DVT is likely, and there is any delay in confirming the diagnosis by compression ultrasonography, anticoagulation with LMWH should be instituted, provided there are no contraindications (e.g. active bleeding). The treatment of choice for DVT is now LMWH unless the patient has severe renal impairment, when unfractionated heparin should be used.

There is agreement that when a DVT is diagnosed in the popliteal vein and above, anticoagulation is indicated. In these circumstances, for most patients, LMWH can be administered on an outpatient basis.

Outpatient treatment is preferred by patients and appears to be cheaper. Hospital-based treatment is indicated if there is severe oedema of the whole of the lower limb, or if there is thrombus above the groin. The LMWH should be continued while oral warfarin treatment is started, and until the INR is above 2. The target range is between 2 and 3. Irrespective of the initial anticoagulation regimen employed, all patients require ongoing anticoagulation with warfarin for 3–6 months, although the optimal duration continues to be debated. Patient care should be continued by referral to a haematologist or vascular physician according to local practice.

For patients with an extensive iliofemoral thrombus consideration should be given to thrombolysis, especially if there are haemodynamic changes suggestive of multiple pulmonary emboli. Thrombectomy may be indicated if the vital functions of the lower limb are threatened, with the aim of reducing the risk of post-thrombotic syndrome. Occlusive lower extremity venous thrombi respond poorly to systemic thrombolysis, and the risks of bleeding may outweigh the justification of its use. Catheter-directed thrombolytic therapy, however, has been used to treat large symptomatic iliofemoral thrombi with some success.

Pregnant women with suspected DVT have not been extensively studied with respect to excluding DVT, so caution must be exercised when assessing these patients. In general, they should all undergo compression ultrasonography and there should be a low threshold for treatment with LMWH.

A dilemma arises when there is an isolated DVT below the level of the popliteal vein, or when there is an equivocal finding in the infrapopliteal area and negative findings above. Options include withholding anticoagulation and following the patient with serial ultrasound studies; performing venography in equivocal cases where there is a strongly suggestive history; or implementation of anticoagulation. In the setting of an infrapopliteal or calf-vein clot where anticoagulation is not commenced, repeat ultrasound at 5–7 days will determine with a high degree of sensitivity whether the clot has propagated above the knee. As the risk of pulmonary embolism from calf DVT is of the order of 5%, and given the safety of LMWH treatment, it is probably prudent to treat confirmed below-knee DVT and to further investigate equivocal cases with venography or serial ultrasound studies. Those patients with recurrent emboli, or who have contraindications for anticoagulation, should be referred for insertion of an inferior vena cava filter. See Chapter 5.5 for the diagnosis and management of pulmonary embolism.

VENOUS DISEASE: UPPER LIMB

Introduction

Thrombosis of the subclavian and axillary veins is much less common than thrombosis of the lower extremity veins. This occurs predominantly in males and often follows upper extremity exertion such as weightlifting – 'effort thrombosis'.

Clinical features

Patients present with swelling of the extremity, developing either rapidly or slowly over a period of weeks. Severe pain is uncommon: the usual symptoms are arm heaviness and discomfort exacerbated by activity and relieved by rest.

Clinical findings may include an increased prominence of hand and forearm veins, venous patterning over the shoulder and hemithorax, skin mottling or cyanosis, and non-pitting oedema. There may be tenderness to palpation of the axillary vein within the axilla. The ipsilateral internal jugular vein is not usually enlarged. If it is, the possibility of a superior vena cava obstruction should be considered.

Clinical investigation

Diagnosis may be made by Doppler assessment or ultrasound scanning.

Differential diagnosis

Thrombosis of the upper limb veins may also occur in association with heart failure, trauma, metastatic tumours of the mediastinum and breast, and central line placement, particularly in chemotherapy patients.

Management

Standard treatment consists of anticoagulation with heparin to prevent progression of thrombosis. Traditionally, unfractionated heparin has been used, but there are increasing reports of successful management of upper limb DVT with LMWH. Rest, heat and elevation of the arm in a sling give good symptomatic relief. A more multidisciplinary approach incorporating catheter-directed thrombolytic therapy, anticoagulation and possibly venous angioplasty may be more effective in restoring vein patency and reducing the risk of re-thrombosis. Thoracic outlet decompression should also be considered if appropriate.

The use of long-term anticoagulation may be justified in cases of late diagnosis. Axillary vein thrombosis secondary to local trauma associated with central venous cannulation may be treated conservatively, provided the patient is asymptomatic and there are no signs of propagation.

Likely developments over the next 5–10 years

- New developments in drug therapy are likely to change the management of venous disease further in the next decade.

- Further advances in the investigation and assessment of patients with suspected DVT will lead to streamlined protocols for emergency department care.
- The impact of statin therapy and other secondary prevention of vascular disease will lead to a reduction in the incidence of peripheral arterial disease in developed countries, and the increasing incidence of smoking and atherogenic dietary consumption in developing countries will lead to an increase in the incidence of arterial and cardiovascular disease there.

Controversies

- The role of systemic or intra-arterial thrombolysis for acute arterial occlusion.

- The optimum drug regimen and duration of anticoagulation therapy for DVT is still not clear.

- Anticoagulation for below-knee DVT.

- Investigative protocols and treatment algorithms for pregnant women have not been researched adequately, so the previous recommendations cannot be applied to pregnant women.

- The increasing use of central venous catheters, including peripherally inserted central lines, may lead to a higher incidence of upper limb venous thrombosis, and the management of these patients is not clear.

- Optimal treatment strategy for upper limb DVT.

Further reading

Alnaeb ME, Alobaid N, Seifalian AM, et al. Statins and peripheral arterial disease: potential mechanisms and clinical benefits. Annals of Vascular Surgery 2006; 20: 696–705.

Banerjee A. The assessment of acute calf pain. Postgraduate Medical Journal 1997; 73: 86–88.

Berridge DC, Kessel D, Robertson I. Surgery versus thrombolysis for initial management of acute limb ischaemia. Cochrane Database of Systematic Reviews (1) CD002784. DOI: 10.1002/14651858.CD002784. 2002.

Blinc A, Poredos P. Pharmacological prevention of atherothrombotic events in patients with peripheral arterial disease. European Journal of Clinical Investigation 2007; 37: 157–164.

Cesarone MD, Belcaro G, Agus G, et al. Management of superficial vein thrombosis and thrombophlebitis: Status and expert opinion document. Angiology 2007; 58: S7–S14.

Cogo A, Lensing AWA, Koopman MMW, et al. Compression ultrasonography for diagnostic management of patients with clinically suspected deep vein thrombosis: prospective cohort study. British Medical Journal 1998; 316: 17–20.

Comerota AJ, Gravett MH. Iliofemoral venous thrombosis. Journal of Vascular Surgery 2007; 46: 1065–1076.

Insall RL, Davies RJ, Prout WG. Significance of Buerger's test in the assessment of lower limb ischaemia. Journal of the Royal Society of Medicine 1989; 82: 729–731.

Khan NA, Rahim SA, Anand SS, et al. Does the clinical examination predict lower extremity peripheral arterial disease? Journal of the American Medical Association 2006; 295: 536–546.

Marshall SM, Flyvbjerg A. Prevention and early detection of vascular complications of diabetes. British Medical Journal 2006; 333: 475–480.

Marston WA, Davies SW, Armstrong B, Farber MA, Mendes RC, Fulton JJ, Keagy BA. Natural history of limbs with arterial insufficiency and chronic ulceration treated without revascularization. Journal of Vascular Surgery 2006; 44: 108-114.

Rodger MA, Gagné-Rodger C, Howley HE, et al. The outpatient treatment of deep vein thrombosis delivers cost savings to patients and their families compared to inpatient therapy. Thrombosis Research 2003; 112: 13–18.

Rutherford RB (ed) Vascular surgery, 5th edn. Vols 1 & 2. London: WB Saunders, 2000.

Scarvelis D, Wells PS. Diagnosis and treatment of deep-vein thrombosis. Canadian Medical Association Journal 2006; 175: 1087–1092.

Thomas IH, Zierler BK. An integrative review of outcomes in patients with acute primary upper extremity deep venous thrombosis following no treatment or treatment with anticoagulation, thrombolysis, or surgical algorithms. Vascular Endovascular Surgery 2005; 39: 163–174.

Wells PS, Anderson DR, Rodger M, et al. Evaluation of D-dimer in the diagnosis of suspected deep-vein thrombosis. New England Journal of Medicine 2003; 349: 1227–1235.

Wells PS, Owen C, Doucette S, et al. Does this patient have deep vein thrombosis? Journal of the American Medical Association 2006; 295: 199–207.

CARDIOVASCULAR

5.9 Hypertension

Marian Lee

ESSENTIALS

1 Hypertension is defined as a systolic blood pressure ≥ 140 mmHg and/or a diastolic blood pressure ≥ 90 mmHg.

2 Hypertensive emergencies are more likely to complicate inadequately controlled hypertension, including those that are undiagnosed.

3 The exact mechanism for the acute rise in blood pressure in hypertensive crisis is not well understood.

4 The pathophysiological consequences of hypertensive crisis are fibrinoid necrosis in arterioles followed by endothelial damage, platelet and fibrin deposition, loss of autoregulatory function, and microangiopathic haemolytic anaemia.

5 Management depends on the clinical syndrome, the presence of complications or coexisting conditions, and the risks of intervention.

6 Hypertensive encephalopathy mandates urgent control of the blood pressure.

7 There is insufficient evidence to support aggressive blood pressure control in the setting of acute stroke.

Introduction

Normal blood pressure is defined as <120/<80 mmHg. The spectrum of hypertension is shown in Table 5.9.1.

Hypertensive crises are uncommon and occur in 1–2% of the hypertensive population. They are defined by a diastolic BP >120 mmHg. However, some have argued that the absolute magnitude of the blood pressure is not important. Rather, the defining factor is the presence of end-organ dysfunction. The latter is uncommon when the diastolic BP is <130 mmHg.

Hypertensive crisis can be divided into two distinct clinical entities. Where the sudden rise in the systolic and diastolic BP is associated with end-organ dysfunction, this is a hypertensive emergency and reduction of blood pressure within 1–2 hours is vital to outcome. A hypertensive urgency is when there is no evidence of end-organ dysfunction. The risk of decompensation is, however, high, and blood pressure control within 24–48 hours is the goal. When a hypertensive crisis is present, it is crucial this it is recognized early and appropriate management undertaken.

Epidemiology

The current prevalence of hypertension in the Australian population is 11%, and hypertension is estimated to affect 1 billion people worldwide; 3% of the adult population develop hypertension each year. It is more common in males than in females, and the risk of developing hypertension increases with age. Australian indigenous peoples and African-Americans have a predisposition to hypertension.

It is estimated that 30% of hypertensive patients are undiagnosed, and 29% of patients with known hypertension are inadequately controlled.

Hypertensive emergencies

Aetiology and pathophysiology
Hypertensive emergencies can complicate both primary and secondary hypertension (Table 5.9.2), the former being more

Table 5.9.1	Spectrum of hypertension
Hypertension category	**Blood pressure range**
High normal	120–139/80–89 mmHg
Grade 1	140–159/90–99 mmHg
Grade II	160–179/100–109 mmHg
Grade III	>180/>110 mmHg
Isolated systolic hypertension	>140/<90 mmHg

Table 5.9.2 Causes of secondary hypertension

System	Specific pathology
Vascular	Aortic dissection
Renal disease (primary)	Renal artery stenosis Renal parenchymal disease IgA nephropathy
Endocrine	Thyrotoxicosis Cushing's syndrome Primary hyperaldosteronism Phaeochromocytoma Hyperparathyroidism
Drug-induced	Cocaine Amphetamines Selective serotonin reuptake inhibitors Monoamine oxidase inhibitors when taken with tyramine-containing foods
Drug withdrawal	Clonidine β-Blockers Angiotensin-converting enzyme inhibitors
Other	Autonomic hyperactivity

common. The majority of hypertensive emergencies occur in patients with pre-existing hypertension. The pathophysiology of hypertensive crisis remains incompletely deciphered. The actual magnitude of the blood pressure is not a dependable guide to the likelihood of end-organ damage.

The chronicity of the underlying pathology means that adaptive vascular mechanisms are present. Hence end-organ damage occurs at a higher pressure than in patients with recent-onset hypertension. For instance, a previously well patient with an acute rise in blood pressure as a result of acute glomerulonephritis will have end-organ dysfunction at a lower blood pressure than a patient with long-standing hypertension.

The actual precipitant of an acute increase in vascular tone is unknown, but the result is the release of humoral vasoconstrictors. The consequent increase in blood pressure leads to:

- Mechanical stress on endothelium, with local release of vasoconstrictors perpetuating hypertension, activation of platelets and the coagulation cascade and, ultimately, fibrinoid necrosis of small vessels.
- Natriuresis and consequent volume depletion results in activation of the renin–angiotensin–aldosterone system, thereby perpetuating vasoconstriction

and increasing plasma volume. The consequent systemic vasoconstriction impairs target organ perfusion, culminating in ischaemia.

Clinical syndromes

The essential clinical features of hypertensive emergencies are symptom complexes reflecting the target organ concerned. Target organs of particular interest are the brain, heart, kidney and large arteries. Target organ dysfunction is uncommon at diastolic BP <130 mmHg.

The recognized hypertensive emergencies are:

- Hypertensive encephalopathy
- Hypertension with stroke
- Acute pulmonary oedema
- Acute myocardial ischaemia
- Acute aortic dissection
- Acute renal dysfunction
- Pre-eclampsia (see Obstetric section).

Hypertensive encephalopathy

This is an acute organic brain syndrome resulting from a failure of cerebral vascular autoregulation. Autoregulation occurs between a mean arterial pressure (MAP) of 60 and 120 mmHg, and cerebral blood flow is constant between this range. As BP rises, there is compensatory vasoconstriction to prevent hyperperfusion. The upper limit of the compensatory mechanism is a MAP of 180 mmHg. When this point is reached vasodilatation occurs, resulting in cerebral oedema (due to endothelial damage) and, less commonly, cerebral haemorrhage. The magnitude of the MAP at which hypertensive encephalopathy is manifested depends on the chronicity of the hypertension. In previously normotensive patients this can occur at a BP of 160/100, i.e. MAP of 120 mmHg. In patients with known hypertension, encephalopathy may not occur until the blood pressure is much higher, probably because of a shift in the cerebral autoregulation range.

The classic clinical triad is severe hypertension, altered level of consciousness (confusion, coma, seizures) and retinopathy (retinal haemorrhages, exudates, papilloedema). Symptoms may include headache of gradual onset and blurring of vision.

If unrecognized, cerebral haemorrhage, oedema and death result. Patients at

higher risk include those with untreated or inadequately controlled hypertension, renal disease, thrombotic thrombocytopenic purpura, pre-eclampsia and eclampsia, and those on medications such as erythropoietin and certain immunotherapy treatments.

Accelerated malignant hypertension is an entity referring to severe hypertension with retinal changes, including flame haemorrhages and soft exudates but without encephalopathy. Papilloedema may or may not be present. It is found in patients with long-standing hypertension. Headache and blurred vision are common (85% and 55%, respectively).

Acute pulmonary oedema and myocardial ischaemia

An acute and severe rise in the blood pressure can cause an acute myocardial ischaemia syndrome and acute pulmonary oedema without obstructive coronary arteries disease. However, in patients who have pre-existing hypertension, coronary artery disease may already be present and the risk of myocardial dysfunction is increased. An acute blood pressure rise leads to increased mechanical stress on the left ventricular wall and consequently a rise in myocardial oxygen demand.

In patients presenting with symptoms and signs consistent with acute pulmonary oedema and myocardial ischaemia, the magnitude of the blood pressure will identify those with a hypertensive emergency.

Acute aortic dissection

This is the most rapidly deteriorating hypertensive emergency. It is also the most devastating, and the mortality remains high. It should be suspected in the setting of hypertension associated with chest pain. This is discussed in detail in Chapter 5.10.

Acute renal failure

An acute and severe elevation in blood pressure may lead to deterioration in renal function, which is usually unsuspected. Acute and severe hypertension is more likely to be the result of renal disease than the cause of renal dysfunction, thus it is essential to look for evidence of underlying renal disease. Urinalysis may be abnormal. In acute severe hypertension there is severe proteinuria, haematuria and cellular sediments. In chronic hypertension, mild proteinuria without haematuria is more usual.

Additionally, renal insufficiency may itself be the cause of the hypertensive emergency. This creates a vicious cycle of deterioration in renal function leading to an elevation of the blood pressure, which in turn compounds the renal dysfunction. Risk groups include patients with chronic renal failure, especially those requiring dialysis, and patients who have had a renal transplant, especially if taking corticosteroids and ciclosporin.

Clinical evaluation

History is focused on determining the cause of hypertension, whether it has been previously diagnosed, and if so, the type of treatment and compliance, a drug history, and a search for symptoms of target organ dysfunction.

Examination concentrates on BP measurement, a careful cardiovascular examination (peripheral pulses, cardiac failure, renal bruits), neurological examination and funduscopy. The finding on funduscopy of retinal haemorrhages, microaneurysms and exudates is associated with a high risk of subsequent stroke.

Investigations

The objectives of the investigations are to detect the presence of end-organ dysfunction as well as to identify the underlying cause of the hypertension.

Bedside tests

- ECG, particularly in the setting of chest pain and hypertension. ECG is abnormal in ~22% of asymptomatic patients with diastolic BP >110 mmHg, although the clinical significance of this is unclear.
- Urinalysis: for haematuria and proteinuria.
- Urine drug screen: if sympathomimetic drugs are suspected.

Blood tests

- Full blood examination to detect anaemia and haemolysis.
- Renal function tests.
- Serum electrolytes may reveal a secondary cause for hypertension.

Imaging

- CXR: A routine chest X-ray is of little diagnostic value.
- Cerebral CT: if evidence of neurological impairment. This will rule out haemorrhagic stroke and may show the characteristic posterior leukoencephalopathy indicative of hypertensive encephalopathy.

Other investigations will be dictated by the clinical presentation.

Management

General

Management depends on the clinical syndrome, the presence of complications or coexisting conditions, and the potential risks of intervention. The aim of treatment is to stop progressive deterioration of target organ function. The risk in treatment is iatrogenic target organ hypoperfusion from an overshoot in blood pressure reduction. In general, the aim is to reduce mean arterial pressure by no more than 25%, as a higher reduction risks organ hypoperfusion, especially in those with chronic underlying hypertension. The goal is to achieve this within 1–2 hours in order to halt progressive damage – the exception being aortic dissection, where BP control within 5–10 minutes is desirable. If the BP is to be manipulated pharmacologically this should take place in a resuscitation area with intra-arterial BP monitoring. Volume depletion is common secondary to pressure natriuresis. Volume replacement with normal saline to restore organ perfusion may prevent a precipitous fall in blood pressure and its consequences.

It should be recognized that large clinical trials looking at the optimum therapy in hypertensive emergencies are not available. The design and interpretation will be confounded by the heterogeneity of the clinical manifestations. Hence the specific treatments discussed below are largely not evidence based but supported by consensus.

Specific conditions

Hypertension and acute stroke Management of hypertension is determined by the type of stroke. In ischaemic stroke, reduction in BP is always at the risk of causing hypoperfusion of the peri-ischaemic area, which may result in an extension of the stroke. In ischaemic stroke, hypertension is usually transient and has not been shown to adversely affect the clinical course. In fact, there is some evidence that patients with higher mean arterial pressures have better outcomes. In the absence of other end-organ dysfunction or intention to treat with thrombolysis, current AHA (American Heart Association) guidelines recommend treatment if the systolic BP >220 mmHg and/or the diastolic BP >120 mmHg. Australian guidelines agree regarding the systolic cut-off but recommend treatment if the diastolic BP >110 mmHg. For patients suitable for thrombolysis, treatment is required to achieve systolic BP <180 mmHg or diastolic BP <105 mmHg. If there is evidence of other organ dysfunction, treatment should be tailored to reduce damage to that organ while balancing the risk of further cerebral ischaemia.

In haemorrhagic stroke/primary intracranial haemorrhage, hypertension is part of the reflex response to the resultant intracranial hypertension and is usually transient. The rationale for treatment of BP is that this would reduce further bleeding and hence haematoma expansion. This has not been proven for primary intracranial haemorrhage, and evidence to support treatment of hypertension in this clinical scenario is lacking. It has been shown that isolated systolic BP <210 mmHg is not associated with intracranial haemorrhage expansion or neurological deterioration, and that reduction of mean arterial pressure by 15% is not associated with neurological deterioration. Recommendations regarding treatment of intracranial haemorrhage-associated hypertension are largely based on consensus and vary around the world. As a general indication, recommendations in Australia are to treat if the systolic BP >180 mmHg or the diastolic >110 mmHg. The stated target BP is 160/90.

Myocardial ischaemia (see Chapter 5.2) The aim is to reduce myocardial work and promote coronary blood flow and thus reduce ischaemia. The agent of choice is i.v. glyceryl trinitrate. β-Blockers, especially metoprolol, may be a useful adjunct.

Acute pulmonary oedema (see Chapter 5.3) Glyceryl trinitrate is preferred because of its vasodilatory effect on coronary arteries as well as preload and afterload reduction. Diuretics should be reserved for patients who are volume overloaded, as they may exacerbate pressure-induced natriuresis and increase stimulation of the renin–angiotensin system.

Hypertensive encephalopathy The divide between the risks and benefits of treatment in hypertensive encephalopathy is small. The clinical manifestation may be reversible; however, the risks of treatment are ischaemia and infarction due to too rapid a fall in the mean arterial pressure. The consensus is a fall in mean arterial pressure by 20–25% or to a diastolic blood pressure of 100–110 mmHg, whichever value is greater, over 2–4 hours. Vigilant monitoring is essential, as any deterioration of clinical status must result in reduction or cessation of the drug used, irrespective of the magnitude of the reduction in BP.

Centrally acting drugs that can affect mental status are not used. The preferred agent is sodium nitroprusside (SNP). Possible alternatives are intravenous labetalol and glyceryl trinitrate The dose range for sodium nitroprusside is 0.5–10 μg/kg/min. SNP requires normal hepatic and renal function for its metabolism and excretion and hence cannot be used in patients with renal or hepatic impairment. Labetolol, an α- and β-adrenergic blocker, is given as an infusion of 1–2 mg/min.

Aortic dissection (see Chapter 5.10)

Acute renal insuffiency In patients with chronic renal failure an acute elevation in BP with subsequent worsening of renal function may require a combination of treatment targeting volume imbalance (e.g. by dialysis) as well as blood pressure (e.g. with sodium nitroprusside). Diuretic use should be judicious, as in the absence of hypervolaemia it may be deleterious. In patients with de novo acute renal insufficiency, sodium nitroprusside is the agent of choice. Emergency ultrafiltration may be required in cases refractory to medical treatment.

Hypertensive urgency

The appropriate management of hypertensive urgency relies on an accurate assessment of the presence or absence of end-organ dysfunction. In the asymptomatic patient it can be difficult to determine whether the dysfunction is acute or pre-existing. Past history and laboratory results are extremely useful to provide a comparison. It may be that this decision cannot be made and treatment is started without a clear distinction between emergency and urgency. The importance of the clinical assessment in hypertensive urgency is to identify the subset most likely to progress to a hypertensive emergency. The features suggestive of this are a first presentation of severe hypertension, a history of poorly controlled hypertension, ischaemic heart disease or cerebrovascular disease.

The treatment goal in this group is a reduction of the blood pressure over 24–48 hours using an oral antihypertensive. The aim is to reduce the mean arterial pressure by 20% over this period. The patient should be admitted and an oral antihypertensive started if the diastolic BP remains above 120 mmHg 30–60 minutes after resting.

A wide range of oral antihypertensives is available. Angiotensin-converting enzyme (ACE) inhibitors are a reasonable first line in most patients. Note that the majority of patients are hypertensive due to poor or non-compliance with medications. In general, the disposition of the patient depends on the presence of significant comorbidities, response to treatment, and the availability and accessibility for outpatient follow-up within 24 hours of discharge.

Prognosis and disposition

Prognosis depends on the success of treatment to halt deterioration of target organs.

All patients with hypertensive emergencies should be admitted to an intensive care unit. The high-risk patient with hypertensive urgency requires hospital admission for observation and BP stabilization.

Developments in the next 5–10 years

Better understanding of the precipitants of hypertensive emergencies.

Controversies

- Reduction of the elevated BP in the acute phase of a stroke remains controversial. There is no consensus on the indication to treat or the timing of intervention. Each case should be considered individually, with careful consideration given to the risks and benefits of lowering the BP.

Further reading

Broderick J, Connolly S, Feldmann E, et al. Guidelines for the Management of Spontaneous Intracerebral Hemorrhage in Adults. 2007 Update. Guidelines from the American Heart Association/American Stroke Association Stroke Council, high blood pressure research council, and the quality of care and outcomes in research interdisciplinary working group. AHA/ASA Guidelines. Stroke 2007; 38: 2001–2023.

Cherney D, Straus S. Management of patients with hypertensive urgencies and emergencies – a systematic review of the literature. Journal of General Internal Medicine 2002; 17: 937–945.

Chobanian AV, Bakris GL, Black HR, et al. Seventh Report of the Joint National Committee on Prevention, Detection, Evaluation and Treatment of High Blood Pressure. Hypertension 2003; 42: 1206–1252.

Feldstein C. Management of hypertensive crises. American Journal of Therapeutics 2007; 14: 138–139.

Gray RO. Hypertension. In: Marx JA, et al., eds. Rosen's emergency medicine: concepts and clinical practice, 6th edn. Philadelphia: Mosby, 2006; 1314–1315.

Haas AR, Marik PE. Current diagnosis and management of hypertensive emergency. Seminars in Dialysis 2006; 19: 502–516.

Mansoor GR, Frishman WH. Comprehensive management of hypertensive emergencies and urgencies. Heart Disease 2002; 4: 358–371.

Marik PE, Varon J. Hypertensive crisis: challenges and management. Chest 2007; 131: 1949–1962.

National Heart Foundation Australia. Hypertension management guide for doctors. 2004 Available at http://www.heartfoundation.org.au/Professional_Information/Clinical_Practice/Prevention.htm. Accessed August 2007.

Patel HP, Mitsnefes M. Advance in pathogenesis and management of hypertensive crisis. Current Opinion in Pediatrics 2005; 17: 210–214.

Shayne PH, Pitts SR. Severely increased blood pressure in the emergency department. Annals of Emergency Medicine 2003; 41: 513.

Therapeutic Guidelines Ltd. Acute stroke treatment (revised Jan. 2007) in: eTG complete (Internet). http://www.tg.com.au/ip/complete/ Accessed August 2007.

Tisdale JE, Huang MB, Borzak S. Risk factors for hypertensive crisis: importance of out-patient blood pressure control. Family Practice 2004; 21: 420–424.

Underwood M, Lobo BL, Finch C, et al. Overuse of antihypertensives in patients with acute ischaemic stroke. Southern Medical Journal 2006; 99: 1230–1233.

Varon J, Marik PE. Clinical review: The management of hypertensive crises. Critical Care 2003; 7: 374–384.

Vaughan CJ, Delanty N. Hypertensive emergencies. Lancet 2000; 356: 4411–4417.

Waybill MM, Waybill PN. A practical approach to hypertension in the 21st century. Journal of Vascular Intervention Radiology 2003; 14: 961–975.

Wong TY, Mitchell P. Hypertensive retinopathy. New England Journal of Medicine 2004; 352: 2310–2317.

5.10 Aortic dissection

Michael Coman

ESSENTIALS

1 Untreated aortic dissection has a mortality rate of approximately 1% per hour for the first 48 hours and 90% at 3 months. Early diagnosis and aggressive management improve mortality rates to 20–40%.

2 Aortic dissection is a clinical diagnosis confirmed through focused investigation. A high index of suspicion is required.

3 Both false negative and false positive diagnoses of aortic dissection result in increased morbidity and mortality.

4 If available, transoesophageal echocardiography in the unstable patient and CT aortography or magnetic resonance imaging in the stable patient are the preferred imaging modalities for patients suspected of suffering aortic dissection.

5 Therapy aimed at reducing blood pressure and the force of ventricular contraction should commence as soon as the diagnosis is suspected.

6 Proximal dissections require emergency surgery, whereas distal dissections are generally treated medically, surgery offering no improvement in outcome for the majority of patients.

Introduction

Aortic dissection (AD) is an uncommon yet potentially lethal condition. A high index of suspicion is required to diagnose AD owing to the broad range of presenting signs and symptoms. Investigations must be carefully chosen and rapidly performed to confirm the diagnosis. It is imperative to institute emergency therapy as soon as the diagnosis is suspected, as if left untreated the mortality rate is approximately 1% per hour for the first 48 hours.[1]

AD is one of a number of conditions that constitute the acute aortic syndrome (AAS). AAS describes the acute presentation of patients with one of several life-threatening aortic pathologies, including AD, intramural haematoma (IMH), penetrating aortic ulcer and traumatic aortic transection with incomplete rupture resulting in AD or IMH.[2] All of the conditions that fall under the umbrella of AAS produce the same pathophysiological endpoint: separation of the aortic intima from the outer aortic layers, with resulting sequelae. There is considerable overlap in the signs, symptoms and principles of management of the conditions that constitute AAS.

Epidemiology

The annual incidence of AD is 5–10 patients/million/year.[1,3] One-third to half of all cases are diagnosed at autopsy.[4] Although the overall incidence is low, AD is the most common catastrophe of the aorta, being two to three times more common than rupture of the abdominal aorta.[1]

Most cases occur in males, particularly between the ages of 50 and 70. Proximal dissections have a peak incidence 10 years earlier than distal dissections.[4] Risk factors for AD are shown in Table 5.10.1. Hypertension is the single most important risk factor. The diagnosis of AD must be considered in any patient with a history of hypertension who presents with sudden severe chest, back or abdominal pain.

Pathophysiology

Arterial hypertension and degeneration of the aortic media are the two key elements of AD. Dissection occurs when blood is forced along a low-resistance pathway created by the diseased and weakened media.

Two pathophysiological processes have been proposed. The traditional explanation requires a breach in the intima (an intimal tear) to initiate the dissection process. The tear occurs at sites where hydrodynamic and torsional forces on the aorta are greatest, most commonly a few centimetres above the aortic valve (60–65%) or just beyond the insertion of the ligamentum arteriosum (30–35%).[1,5] A column of high-pressure aortic blood gains access to the media and, under pressure, dissects through the weakened tissue plane, creating a false lumen. The dissecting column of blood can extend in an antegrade or retrograde direction. The alternative proposed mechanism suggests that diseased or unsupported vasa vasorum within the media rupture as a result of medial degeneration, initiating AD.[5] A haematoma develops, which dissects through the media as it expands. The intima loses its support as dissection progresses, and is subjected to increased shearing forces during diastolic recoil of the aorta. Eventually – but not necessarily – this may lead to a tear in the intima. In this scenario, an intimal tear is a consequence of the dissection, not an initiating factor. An intimal tear is not identified in 12% of autopsies, suggesting that it is not a mandatory precursor for AD.[5,6]

Regardless of the primary process producing dissection, the sequelae are identical. As the

Table 5.10.1 Predisposing factors for aortic dissection
Major associations
Hypertension
Congenital cardiovascular disorders
Aortic stenosis
Bicuspid aortic valve
Coarctation of the aorta
Connective tissue disorders
Marfan's syndrome
Ehlers-Danlos syndrome
Other associations
Iatrogenic (post cardiac surgery or balloon angioplasty for coarctation)
Cocaine
Pregnancy
Inflammatory diseases
Giant-cell arteritis

dissection extends, any structures caught in its path may be affected. Branch vessels of the aorta may be distorted or occluded, resulting in signs and symptoms of ischaemia to the organs they supply. Proximal dissection may produce acute aortic valve incompetence, and continued proximal extension may enter the pericardial sac, tamponading the heart. The false lumen created by the dissection may also partially or completely obstruct the true lumen. It may end in a blind sac or rupture back into the true lumen at any point. The false lumen may also rupture outwards through the adventitia. If this occurs, rapid exsanguination will occur if the haematoma is not contained. Common sites of external rupture are into the left pleural cavity or mediastinum.

Once the dissection begins, its propagation is dependent on the blood pressure and the gradient of the arterial blood pressure wave, which is a function of the velocity of left ventricular contraction. Hence urgent pharmacological treatment is aimed at lowering arterial blood pressure and reducing the ventricular contractile force.

Classification

AD may be classified anatomically or pathophysiologically. The Stanford and De Bakey systems are the two anatomically based classification systems in use. Both describe the site of the dissection, providing information that is pivotal in determining patient management.

The Stanford system divides AD into two types (Fig. 5.10.1). Type A (65–70%) involves the ascending aorta, with or without the descending aorta. The presence or absence of an intimal tear, the site of the tear, and the extent of distal extension are not considered in this classification. Type B (30–35%) dissections involve the descending aorta only,[7] which by definition begins distal to the origin of the left subclavian artery. The Stanford system is simple, easy to remember, and reflects the two major management pathways of AD. Type A generally requires surgical repair, whereas type B is generally managed medically.

The De Bakey classification system divides AD into three types (see Fig. 5.10.1). Type I involves both the ascending and the descending aorta. Type II involves the ascending aorta only. Type III involves the

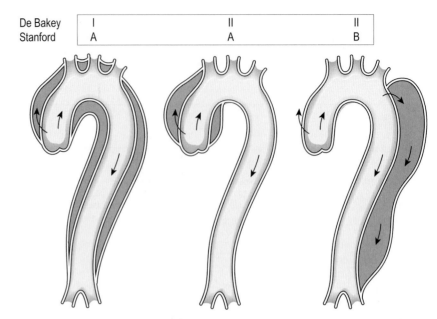

| De Bakey | I | II | II |
| Stanford | A | A | B |

Fig. 5.10.1 Anatomical classification of AD. (Reproduced with permission from Erbel R, Alfonso F, Boileau C, et al. Diagnosis and management of aortic dissection. European Heart Journal 2001; 22: 1642–1681.)

descending aorta only, and is subdivided into type IIIa, which is confined to the thoracic aorta, and type IIIb, which extends into the abdominal aorta.

AD is classified as acute if symptoms are present for fewer than 14 days, chronic if longer than 14 days. Note that the term 'dissecting thoracic aneurysm' is confusing and should be avoided, as dissections can and usually do occur in the absence of aneurysmal dilatation of the aorta.

Clinical features

History

Pain is the most common presenting symptom, occurring in 74–95% of patients.[1,4] Pain is classically described as severe, unremitting, tearing or ripping in nature, and maximal at onset.[1] It may be migratory, reflecting proximal or distal extension of the tear. The site of the pain may reflect the site of the dissection, with involvement of the ascending aorta typically producing anterior chest pain, whereas neck and jaw pain may suggest aortic arch dissection. Interscapular pain can occur with involvement of the descending aorta, and as distal dissection continues, the pain may migrate to the lower back or abdomen.[1]

Other symptoms of AD are related to the effects of major aortic side branch occlusion. Almost 20% of dissections present with coma, confusion or stroke.[1,7] This may signify carotid artery involvement, or may reflect end-organ hypoperfusion due to hypovolaemic shock from external rupture of the aorta, or cardiogenic shock caused by pericardial tamponade. Neurological symptoms often fluctuate. Lower limb paraplegia or paraesthesia (2–8%) may occur as spinal arteries are separated from the aortic lumen.[4] Syncope (18% type A and 3% type B) may suggest rupture into the pericardial sac.[4,7]

Symptoms may also be due to local compression from a contained rupture. These are uncommon, but may include superior vena cava syndrome, dysphonia, dyspnoea, dysphagia, upper airway obstruction and Horner's syndrome.[4]

A history of risk factors for AD should also be obtained (Table 5.10.1).

Examination

There is no single examination finding that will confirm the diagnosis of AD. It is common for patients to be acutely distressed, apprehensive, and for their pain to be resistant to narcotic analgesia.

Patients usually present with a tachycardia owing to a combination of pain, anxiety and possibly shock. Hypertension is seen in 50–78% of patients, especially those suffering from type B dissection. This may reflect an underlying history of hypertension or an acute response to pain and anxiety. Hypotension is an ominous sign, suggesting free rupture of the aorta or pericardial tamponade. Evidence of side branch occlusion may include stroke, limb ischaemia or neurological dysfunction, pulse deficits or a difference of 15 mmHg or more in manually taken blood pressures between the upper limbs.

Evidence of proximal extension to involve the aortic valve or pericardium may produce acute aortic incompetence, possibly with signs of acute left ventricular failure. A diastolic murmur indicative of acute aortic incompetence is a common finding in proximal dissection (50–68%). Pericardial tamponade may manifest with Beck's triad: hypotension, muffled heart sounds and raised jugular venous pressure. Pulsus paradoxus may be present, or a pericardial friction rub may be heard. Involvement of the renal arteries may result in oliguria or anuria.

Aortic rupture may present with shock or clinical signs of a haemothorax, usually left-sided. Frank haemoptysis or haematemesis in this clinical context also suggests aortic rupture. Compression of local structures by a contained haematoma, particularly within the mediastinum, may be evident.

Serial examination is very important, as signs may change as the dissection progresses.

Investigation

Specific investigations are required to confirm or exclude AD. There are, however, a number of initial investigations that may identify an alternative diagnosis or increase the clinical suspicion of AD. Routine haematological or biochemical investigations are of little value in the immediate diagnosis of AD, and at best provide baseline renal function and haemoglobin.

Electrocardiography

An electrocardiogram (ECG) should be performed on all patients with suspected AD, as acute myocardial infarction (AMI) is a major differential diagnosis. Ten to 40% of patients with AD will have ECG evidence suggestive of acute ischaemia.[8] Seven per cent of dissections involve the coronary arteries, yet only 0.9–2.4% of patients will have ECG changes in keeping with AMI.[4,7] Total

coronary artery occlusion is less common than partial occlusion, and the right coronary artery is more commonly involved than the left. The ECG may display voltage criteria for left ventricular hypertrophy, reflecting a long-standing history of hypertension.

Chest X-ray

A number of chest X-ray (CXR) abnormalities have been described in patients with AD (Table 5.10.2). The sensitivity and specificity of each individual finding is poor, and for this reason no single finding should be used in isolation for predictive purposes. Many findings are subtle and are best seen on a good-quality erect PA film. In reality, the clinical condition of the patient may only allow a supine, mobile AP film. Retrospective audits of plain radiographs of patients known to have dissection reveal abnormalities suggesting AD in 72–90% of cases; however, attempts to prospectively identify AD in blinded studies yield less reliable results (sensitivity of 81% and specificity of 82–89%).[9] Up to 20% of radiographs are normal in patients suffering dissection. At best, the CXR may increase the clinical suspicion of AD or identify alternative pathology. A normal-appearing CXR must never be used to exclude AD.

Table 5.10.2 Radiographic features suggesting dissection
Widening of the superior mediastinum (52–75%)
Dilatation of the aortic arch (31–47%)
Change in the configuration of the aorta on successive CXR (47%)
Obliteration of the aortic knob
Double density of the aorta (suggesting true and false lumina)
Localized prominence along aortic contour (38%)
Disparity of calibre between descending and ascending aorta (34–67%)
Displacement of the trachea or nasogastric tube to the right
Distortion of the left main stem bronchus
Calcium sign (>6 mm between the intimal calcium and the shadow of the outer aortic wall: 7–17%)
Pleural effusion, more common on the left (15–20%)
Cardiomegaly (21%)

Specific investigations

All patients in whom AD is suspected must have a diagnostic test performed without delay. Options include computed tomography (CT), echocardiography, aortography and magnetic resonance imaging (MRI). The aim is to determine whether a dissection is present, its site, the structures involved and the presence of complications. Unfortunately, no single test is ideal, and the most appropriate investigation may differ depending on the individual and the institution. Factors such as patient stability, test availability, operator availability and expertise, the physical location of the diagnostic equipment, and the variable institutional sensitivity and specificity of each test need to be taken into account. Each emergency department (ED) should have a prearranged imaging strategy for the diagnosis of suspected AD, factoring in the above variables.

CT

Technological advances over the past decade have revolutionized the amount and rate of information that can be acquired by CT. Helical CT with rapid administration of intravenous contrast can be timed to acquire data during peak contrast opacification of the aorta, effectively creating a CT aortogram. Images can be reconstructed in multiple planes, and motion artefact – once a problem with older and slower scanners – has been greatly reduced as data acquisition takes place during a single breath-hold. Increased availability, after-hours reporting via teleradiology, and the trend to position scanners in close proximity to EDs have made CT a good option for patients who are suitable to be transported. It is the preferred study, particularly in stable patients with a low-to-moderate index of suspicion for AD, as it may be effective in identifying alternative pathologies. Diagnosis is based on the demonstration of an intimal flap, shown as a low-attenuation linear structure within the aortic lumen. Secondary findings of AD include internal displacement of luminal calcification, and delayed contrast enhancement of the false lumen. Sensitivity and specificity for diagnosing arch vessel involvement are high (93% and 98%, respectively).[6] CT can identify complications of AD, including pericardial, mediastinal and pleural blood. Disadvantages include the requirement for intravenous contrast and patient transport. CT cannot provide a functional assessment of the aortic valve.

Recent advances in multislice CT, including CT coronary angiography, raise the possibility of diagnostic testing for both AD and coronary artery disease in one test, albeit with higher contrast and radiation loads. There are currently insufficient data to determine the safety or utility of this approach.

Echocardiography

Transthoracic echocardiography (TTE) is no longer considered a useful screening test in view of its low sensitivity and specificity (Table 5.10.3). TTE is particularly poor at imaging the transverse arch and the descending aorta, owing to interference from the airway.

Transoesophageal echocardiography (TOE) has emerged as an excellent diagnostic investigation for AD in centres where it is available. Ideal for critically ill patients, TOE can be rapidly and safely performed at the bedside and is highly sensitive and specific[9,10] (Table 5.10.3). In addition, TOE can give a functional assessment of the aortic valve and the left ventricle, and can identify other complications of AD, including the involvement of coronary arteries and the presence of pericardial blood. Disadvantages of TOE include the limited availability outside major centres and office hours, and the requirement for a skilled and available operator. TOE is invasive and patients may require sedation and airway protection to perform the test. It is contraindicated in patients with known oesophageal pathology, including varices, strictures or tumours. The diagnosis is confirmed by demonstrating the intimal flap separating the true and false lumina. The true lumen can be distinguished from the false lumen as it is usually smaller, expands during systole (compared to compression of the false lumen during systole), and is less commonly thrombosed.[11] Central displacement of luminal calcium may confirm the presence of AD in situations where the false lumen has thrombosed.

Aortography

Formerly the gold standard investigation for AD, aortography is now rarely performed owing to the development and refinement of less invasive, more sensitive and rapid alternatives.

Magnetic resonance imaging

MRI is highly sensitive and specific, providing excellent visualization of the site and extent of the dissection, and the complications of dissection, including side branch involvement. The availability of MRI is improving, and data acquisition is becoming more rapid. The major disadvantages relate to patient safety. Studies are still lengthy, patient accessibility is poor during the study, and patient monitoring is problematic due to the requirement for equipment that is compatible with the magnetic field. Additionally, MRI equipment is frequently located at a distance from resuscitation facilities. For these reasons, MRI is unsafe for unstable or potentially unstable patients despite the comprehensive information it can provide.

Biomarkers

Biomarkers for early detection of AD are attracting interest. An immunoassay of monoclonal antibodies to smooth muscle myosin heavy chain protein is being investigated. An early small trial claims a sensitivity of 90% and specificity of 97% at 12 hours.[12] D-Dimer assay has also been reported as having high sensitivity when studied in selected patient groups.[13,14] Clearly, biomarkers will need to rapidly attain a high sensitivity to be clinically useful. In time, this may eventuate and biomarkers may find a role in algorithms to confirm or exclude the diagnosis of AD.

Differential diagnosis

The diagnosis of AD is rarely straightforward, and there is a long list of differential diagnoses (Table 5.10.4) owing to the wide range of presenting symptoms and signs. The fear of misdiagnosing AD for acute myocardial infarction and the subsequent administration of a thrombolytic agent is a concern of many clinicians. The facts show this to be a rare occurrence. AMI is approximately 1000 times more common than AD,[15] and only a small percentage of patients suffering AD (0.9–2.4%)[4,7] have ECG changes suggesting AMI. CXR is sometimes advocated as a screening test to exclude dissection in this circumstance. However, based on the reported sensitivity of 81%, specificity of 89%[9] and an AD incidence of 0.26% in patients with a clinical diagnosis of AMI,[16] the positive predictive value of CXR is 1.9%. That is, 49 patients suffering AMI would be falsely labelled as potentially suffering AD for every true case identified. Delay in treatment of AMI while a definitive investigation is performed may result in an adverse outcome for these patients. Unless the clinical presentation suggests AD, routine CXR is an ineffective screening tool in patients with a clinical presentation suggesting AMI.

As thrombolysis for acute embolic stroke is gaining popularity, care must be taken to consider AD as a stroke mimicker prior to the administration of thrombolytic agents.

Treatment

Treatment must be started as soon as the diagnosis is suspected. Unstable patients require immediate resuscitation. Diagnostic

Table 5.10.4 Differential diagnosis of aortic dissection
Cardiovascular
Acute coronary syndrome with or without ST-segment elevation
Shock
Acute pulmonary oedema
Acute valvular dysfunction
Pericarditis
Acute extremity ischaemia
Pulmonary
Pulmonary embolus
Pneumothorax
Gastrointestinal
Pancreatitis
Peptic ulcer disease (including perforation)
Oesophageal spasm/reflux
Ischaemic bowel
Neurological
Stroke/transient ischaemic attack
Spinal cord compression
Renal
Renal colic

Table 5.10.3 Sensitivity and specificity of diagnostic investigations		
Investigation	Sensitivity (%)	Specificity (%)
CT	83–100[7]	90–100[7]
TTE	78–100[7]: type A 31–55[7]: type B 59–85[7]: all	63–96[7]
TOE	97–99[5]	97–100[5]
Aortography	81–91[7]	94[7,19]
MRI	95–100[20]	95–100[20]

investigations and management of life-threatening complications may need to take place simultaneously. Measures to minimize progression of the dissection need to be instituted rapidly, and early surgical referral is mandatory. Early diagnosis, control of blood pressure and heart rate, and early surgical repair are all associated with improved survival.

Patients with AD are usually in severe pain and require large doses of titrated i.v. narcotic analgesia, which should not be delayed or withheld. A secondary benefit from the relief of pain is a reduction in blood pressure and heart rate.

Pharmacological treatment is aimed at decreasing the pulsatile load ($\Delta p/\Delta t$) delivered by the left ventricle to the column of blood within the false lumen. This minimizes the likelihood of ongoing dissection.[6] The pulsatile load is determined by the systolic blood pressure and the velocity of blood ejected from the heart. Importantly, blood pressure must be lowered without increasing the velocity of ventricular contraction, which can occur if afterload is reduced prior to blocking the reflex tachycardia and increased contractile velocity of the heart that afterload reduction produces.

If there is no contraindication, β-blockade is the ideal first-line agent owing to its negative inotropic and chronotropic effects on the heart. Esmolol, a short acting β-blocker (half-life 9 minutes), which can be given by peripheral intravenous infusion and titrated to heart rate and blood pressure, is effective. A loading infusion of 0.5 mg/kg may be given by hand-held syringe over 1 minute. Following this, a maintenance infusion ranging from 50 to 200 μg/kg/min is commenced. If esmolol is unavailable, or experience in its use is limited, titrated i.v. boluses of metoprolol are equally effective. A heart rate of 60–80 bpm and a systolic blood pressure of 100–120 mmHg are commonly quoted target ranges,[6] but these figures are not absolute. Blood pressure must be titrated to the clinical condition of the patient, being modified if signs of end-organ hypoperfusion, or signs and symptoms of ongoing dissection, become evident. Intra-arterial monitoring is necessary for optimal blood pressure management.

If further BP reduction is required following β-blockade, a vasodilator may be added. Sodium nitroprusside reduces afterload via systemic vasodilatation. Delivered by i.v. infusion, it is effective, has a rapid onset and short duration of action, and can be readily titrated to effect. The usual infusion range is 0.5–10 μg/kg/min. Owing to the possibility of cyanide toxicity, the infusion should not continue beyond 24 hours. An alternative agent to reduce blood pressure is glyceryl trinitrate (GTN), a drug more commonly and confidently used by most clinicians. Delivered by peripheral i.v. infusion, GTN reduces both preload and afterload by relaxing vascular smooth muscle. Reflex tachycardia is a common side effect, and must be prevented by prior β-blockade. The infusion range is 5–50 μg/min, and it can be rapidly titrated to clinical effect.

Surgical intervention

Immediate surgery is the treatment of choice for acute proximal (type A) AD. The aim is to prevent rupture of the false lumen, re-establish blood flow to regions affected by occluded side branches, correct any associated acute aortic valve incompetence, and prevent pericardial tamponade. Usual practice is to excise the section of the aorta containing the intimal tear and replace this with a prosthetic interposition graft. Operative mortality ranges from 5% to 21%.[17] Without surgery, up to 90% of patients with acute type A dissection will die within 3 months.[17] With surgery, there is a 56–87% 5-year survival.[17]

The traditional treatment for type B dissections has been medical management, with survival rates approaching 80%. Surgical intervention in these cases is complicated by tissue friability, coagulopathy, the risk of spinal cord ischaemia and resulting paraplegia, renal failure, distal arterial embolization and infection. Despite these risks, there are circumstances where surgical management for type B dissections is indicated, usually when life-threatening complications develop or medical management has failed. These are listed in Table 5.10.5.

Recent advances in endovascular stent grafting have challenged the traditional management of type B dissections.[18] Expandable metal stents covered by a prosthetic fabric graft material are deployed percutaneously through the femoral artery. These stents may be seated over the intimal flap to occlude flow between the true and false lumina. In addition, stenting of occluded side branches of the aorta including visceral and renal arteries has been successfully performed, avoiding the need for high-risk surgery. Studies have reported success in restoring flow to side branches of the aorta occluded by AD in excess of 90%, with average 30-day mortality rates of 10%.[6]

All patients are discharged on lifelong β-blockers, regardless of initial medical or surgical treatment, or whether the patient is hypertensive or normotensive.[6] Serial MRI examinations are necessary for long-term surveillance of the aorta.

Prognosis

A dramatic improvement in survival has been observed over the past 30 years owing to advances in medical and surgical management of AD. One-year survival rates of 52–69% for type A and 70% for type B have been reported.[6] Eighty-six per cent of deaths from AD are due to aortic rupture, 70% of those rupturing into the pericardial sac.[7] Multiorgan failure is another major cause of death following medical or surgical therapy.

Table 5.10.5 Indications for surgical repair of type B aortic dissection
Leaking or ruptured aorta
Ischaemic compromise of vital organs
Marfan's syndrome
Extension of dissection despite appropriate medical therapy
Intractable pain
Intractable hypertension
Aortic dilatation (>5 cm)

Disposition

Those patients not eligible or stable enough for emergency surgery require admission to an intensive care area for monitoring and aggressive therapy aimed at minimizing propagation of their dissection. Patients in peripheral or regional centres will require transfer to a specialist cardiothoracic unit after their condition has been stabilized.

Controversies

- The role of intravascular ultrasound (IVUS). Sensitivities and specificities of close to 100% have been reported, but its practicality in the emergency department is unproven.

- Appropriate investigation. Lack of utility of CXR as a screening test. Choice of investigative modalities governed by availability of testing modalities and stability of patient.

- The role of biomarkers.

- Improved surgical/interventional outcomes in distal dissection challenge the dictum that these patients should be treated medically.

- Preventative therapy in Marfan's syndrome. Routine β-blockade is advocated. Elective grafting of the aortic valve and ascending aorta is being advocated in some patients considered at high risk.

References

1. Zappa MJ, Harwood-Nuss A. Recognition and management of acute aortic dissection and thoracic aortic aneurysm. Emergency Medicine Reports 1993; 14: 1–8.
2. Ahmad F, Cheshire N, Hamady M. Acute aortic syndrome: pathology and therapeutic strategies. Postgraduate Medical Journal 2006; 82: 305–312.
3. Chen K, Varon J, Wenker OC. Acute aortic dissection and its variants. Journal of Emergency Medicine 1997; 15: 859–867.
4. Spittel PC, Spittel JA, Joyce JW, et al. Clinical features and differential diagnosis of aortic dissection: experience with 236 cases. Mayo Clinic Proceedings 1993; 68: 642–651.
5. O'Gara PT, DeSanctis RW. Acute aortic dissection and its variants. Circulation 1995; 92: 1376–1378.
6. Erbel R, Alfonso F, Boileau C, et al. Diagnosis and management of aortic dissection. European Heart Journal 2001; 22: 1642–1681.
7. Richards KA. Emergency department recognition and management of dissecting thoracic aneurysm. Emergency Medicine 1995; 7: 99–105.
8. Bourland MD. In: Rosen P, Barkin RM, eds. Emergency medicine: concepts and clinical practice. Chicago: Mosby, 1992; 1384–1390.
9. Jagannath AS, Sos TA, Lockart SH, et al. Aortic dissection: a statistical analysis of the usefulness of chest pain radiographic findings. American Journal of Radiology 1986; 147: 1123–1126.
10. Weintraub AR, Erbel R, Gorge G, et al. Intravascular ultrasound imaging in acute aortic dissection. Journal of the American College of Cardiologists 1994; 24: 495.
11. Erbel R, Zamorano J. The aorta. Critical Care Clinics 1996; 12: 733–766.
12. Kamp TJ, Goldschmidt-Clermont PJ, Brinker, JA, et al. Myocardial infarction, aortic dissection, and thrombolytic therapy. American Heart Journal 1994; 128: 1234–1237.
13. Suzuki T, Katoh H, Watanabe M, et al. Novel biochemical diagnostic method for aortic dissection. Circulation 1996; 93: 1244–1249.
14. Akutsu K, Sato N, Yamamoto T, et al. A rapid bedside D-dimer assay (cardiac D-dimer) for screening of clinically suspected acute aortic dissection. Circulation Journal 2005; 69: 397–403.
15. Ohlmann P, Faure A, Morel O, et al. Diagnostic and prognostic value of circulating D-dimers in patients with acute aortic dissection. Critical Care Medicine 2006; 34: 1358–1364.
16. Wilcox RG, Olssen CG, Von der Lippe G, et al. Trial of tissue plasminogen activator for mortality reduction in acute myocardial infarction. Anglo-Scandinavian study of early thrombolysis (ASSET). Lancet 1988; 2: 525–530.
17. Kouchoukos NT, Dougenis D. Medical progress: surgery of the thoracic aorta. New England Journal of Medicine 1997; 336: 1876–1888.
18. Vlahakes GJ. Concise review: endovascular stent-graft placement in the treatment of aortic dissection. In: Braunwald E, Fauci AS, Isselbacher DL, et al., eds. Harrisons Online 2000. Accessed August 2007.
19. Erbel R, Daniel W, Visser C, et al. Echocardiography in the diagnosis of aortic dissection. Lancet 1989; i: 457–461.
20. Sarasin FP, Louis-Simonet M, Gaspoz JM, et al. Detecting acute thoracic aortic dissection in the emergency department: time constraints and choice of the optimal diagnostic test. Annals of Emergency Medicine 1996; 28: 278–288.

5.11 Aneurysms

Chin Hung Chung

ESSENTIALS

1 Patients with expanding or ruptured abdominal aortic aneurysm (AAA) may have pain located in the abdomen, flank, loin or groin. AAA should be excluded in elderly patients with a provisional diagnosis of unexplained abdominal pain, renal colic or back pain.

2 Elderly patients presenting with abdominal or back pain with unexplained hypotension should have AAA excluded with bedside ultrasonography. However, rupture cannot be reliably demonstrated by ultrasonography.

3 A hypotensive patient with a bedside diagnosis of AAA should be sent to the operating theatre immediately, without further delay for additional imaging studies.

4 Symptomatic aneurysms of any size should be considered an emergency, even if the patient's condition is stable.

5 Computed tomography has no role in the unstable hypotensive patient with suspected ruptured AAA.

6 All patients with ruptured AAA should be regarded as unstable, but the appropriate amount of fluid to be given is controversial.

7 Even though the risk of rupture increases with increasing aneurysm diameter, no 'safe' size exists and it is impossible to predict when any given aneurysm will rupture. All aneurysms discovered incidentally should be referred to a specialist for assessment and monitoring.

8 A high proportion of patients with aneurysm are asymptomatic.

9 The primary risk of central arterial aneurysms is rupture. Peripheral arterial aneurysms rarely rupture; instead, they are usually complicated by thrombosis or embolism.

10 Peripheral aneurysms tend to be multiple. All patients with a lower extremity aneurysm should be evaluated for the presence of other aneurysms.

Introduction

By definition, a true aneurysm is a permanent, localized or diffuse dilatation of an artery at least 1.5 times its normal diameter and involving all three layers of the vessel wall. The term ectasia is used when the dilation is less than 50%. Aneurysms are described as fusiform if the entire circumference of the vessel wall is dilated, or saccular if only part of the circumference is involved. True aortic aneurysms and aortic dissections are very different conditions, the latter still occasionally being called dissecting aortic aneurysms (see Section 5.10). A pseudoaneurysm (false aneurysm) is a localized collection of flowing blood that communicates with the arterial lumen but is contained only by the adventitia or surrounding soft tissue. Aneurysms can occur anywhere in the body, but the vast majority occur in the abdomen.

Aetiology, genetics, pathogenesis and pathology

Aneurysm growth is dictated by a combination of mural weakness and haemodynamic force. Traditionally, atherosclerotic degeneration has been regarded as the most common cause of aneurysms, but recent evidence suggests a multifactorial aetiology. Ageing results in degradation of collagen and elastin, fragmentation of elastic fibres and loss of elasticity, with weakening of the arterial wall and subsequent dilation. Other causes include aortic dissection, trauma, infection (e.g. mycotic, syphilitic), arteritis, connective tissue disorders and genetic disorders (e.g. Marfan's syndrome, Ehlers–Danlos syndrome). Risk factors include age, male gender, smoking, a positive family history, hypertension and chronic obstructive pulmonary disease. There is a 15–19% incidence of aneurysm among first-degree relatives of patients with aortic aneurysm.

Aneurysms caused by atherosclerosis progress slowly over years, affecting the elderly disproportionately. The incidence will continue to increase in line with our ageing population. Those caused by trauma or infection enlarge over days, weeks or months.

Central aneurysms

Central aneurysms include the aorta, iliac arteries, pulmonary artery, visceral arteries and cerebral arteries. The primary risk of central aneurysms is rupture – an emergency with a high risk of sudden death.

Abdominal aortic aneurysms (AAA)

As the average size of the adult infrarenal aorta is 2 cm, abdominal aortic aneurysms are usually defined by a diameter greater than 3 cm. AAA rarely presents before the age of 50, but the incidence increases sharply afterwards, with 5–10% of elderly men aged between 65 and 79 having an abdominal aortic aneurysm. The incidence is lower in women and there is ethnic variation. Rupture can occur once a diameter of 3 cm has been reached, but almost never before then. The mean expansion rate is exponential and the risk of rupture is proportional to the diameter. Most aortic aneurysms occur in the infrarenal segment (90–95%); rarely do they extend above the renal arteries, although extension into the common iliac arteries is fairly common. Most are due to atherosclerosis. The natural history of expansion and rupture can only be interrupted by elective repair. The mortality rate can be lowered by diagnosing asymptomatic aneurysms and referring the patients for elective repair before they rupture.

Clinical features

Abdominal aortic aneurysms present a significant diagnostic challenge. Unlike coronary artery, cerebrovascular and peripheral vascular diseases, most AAAs remain asymptomatic and undetected for years until they rupture. Abdominal examination may be insensitive in the detection of AAA, particularly in the obese. Most AAAs are discovered incidentally during unrelated imaging studies or routine physical examinations.

The most common and most important complication is rupture with life-threatening haemorrhage, which may be the first presentation of the disease. One to two-thirds of AAAs may eventually rupture if left untreated. The presentation of those with rupture who reach the emergency department (ED) may be dramatic or subtle, and misdiagnosis leading to delayed therapy is common. The characteristic manifestation of rupture is the classic triad of pain, hypotension and a pulsatile abdominal mass. This triad is present in approximately half of the cases reaching hospital, but many patients have only one or two of the components. The pain may be located in the abdomen, flank, loin or groin, and is commonly sudden, constant and excruciating. The presence of syncope or shock with back pain should strongly suggest the diagnosis. There may be non-specific constitutional symptoms such as nausea, vomiting and diaphoresis. Many patients however, do not present classically. Misdiagnosis is common, especially with haemodynamically stable patients. The presentation may be suggestive of renal colic or musculoskeletal back pain, or a more sinister diagnosis such as an 'acute abdomen' or acute myocardial infarction. Rarely, AAAs may rupture into the gastrointestinal tract (aortoenteric fistula) causing haematemesis or melaena, or into the inferior vena cava (aortocaval fistula) causing high-output congestive heart failure and distal ischaemia.

Symptoms may also occur from aneurysm expansion with pressure effects on adjacent structures, causing back pain, groin pain or bowel obstruction; from embolization of intramural thrombus resulting in the 'blue toe' or 'trash foot' syndrome; and from inflammation causing obstructive uropathy.

Symptomatic aneurysms of any size should be considered an emergency, even if the patient's condition is stable.

Investigations

Plain X-rays in the anteroposterior (AP) or lateral projection may show a calcified bulging contour – the classic eggshell appearance – or a paravertebral soft tissue mass. Calcification is more easily visualized on the lateral projection, as it is free from obscuration by the vertebral column. That said, a tortuous aorta may mimic an AAA unless calcification of both opposing aortic walls can be clearly seen. The classic eggshell finding is present in about half of cases and is a highly specific sign when present. On the other hand, plain X-ray cannot exclude the presence of an AAA.

Ultrasonography (US) should be the initial imaging modality for screening or when an asymptomatic, pulsatile abdominal mass is palpated. Rapid bedside ultrasound has been claimed to be 100% accurate if the entire abdominal aorta can be visualized.[1] It is ideal for the unstable patient with unexplained hypotension, demonstrating the presence of an AAA and measuring its diameter. Obesity or bowel gas may make the study difficult. Rupture however cannot be reliably seen. On the other hand, an unstable patient with an AAA demonstrated by ultrasonography should be presumed to have a ruptured aneurysm requiring immediate surgery, and should be sent to the operating room without further delay by other imaging studies.[1]

Computed tomography (CT) with intravenous contrast can demonstrate the anatomical details of the aneurysm and associated retroperitoneal haemorrhage, and is 100% accurate.[1,2] It is much more sensitive than ultrasonography in detecting retroperitoneal haemorrhage. However, it is appropriate only in haemodynamically stable patients.[1]

Angiography and magnetic resonance imaging (MRI), although highly accurate for elective cases, have no place in the emergent evaluation of suspected ruptured AAAs.[1]

Management and prognosis

Abdominal aortic aneurysms are repaired more often than any other aneurysms.[3] The indications for surgery are based on size, growth rate and symptoms. Currently, elective repair is recommended for aneurysms larger than 5.5 cm. The accepted mortality rate with elective conventional open surgical repair is less than 5%. Endovascular stent-graft placement is possible for about 40% of non-ruptured AAAs, with an even lower mortality rate. Life expectancy after elective repair is close to that of the general population.

Ruptured AAAs are uniformly fatal unless treated surgically. Many patients die before reaching hospital. The reported mortality rate for patients reaching hospital is 80%, and 50% for those undergoing emergency surgery. Hypotension is the strongest factor predicting a poor outcome, but survival has been reported in patients with preoperative cardiac arrest.

The principal aims in the care of the patient with acute rupture of an AAA are to make the diagnosis promptly, resuscitate actively and arrange surgery expeditiously. The patient should be managed in an appropriate resuscitation area and receive high-flow oxygen. Multiple large-bore intravenous access should be established. Blood should be sent for haematological and biochemical studies, coagulation profile, typing and cross-matching of 6–10 units of blood. A 12-lead electrocardiogram and chest X-ray should be performed if time permits. Narcotic analgesia should be given intravenously in small increments, titrated to response. A urethral catheter should be inserted before surgery if time permits.

The patient with a ruptured AAA is unstable, but the appropriate amount of fluid to be given is controversial.[2] No evidence exists that lowering the blood pressure is beneficial in patients with ruptured AAA, and these elderly patients tolerate hypotension poorly and are at risk of precipitous hypotension. On the other hand, overly aggressive fluid resuscitation may be harmful.[1,2]

Thoracic aortic aneurysms (TAA)

The average size of the thoracic aorta is 3.5 cm, and a diameter greater than 4.5 cm should be considered aneurysmal. Men are affected two to four times more frequently than women. Thoracic aortic aneurysms most often occur in the descending thoracic aorta, the most common cause being atherosclerosis. Up to 25% of patients with TAA also have an AAA.[4]

Thoracic aortic aneurysms are usually asymptomatic and discovered incidentally on chest X-ray or CT scan for other reasons. Symptoms appear when the aneurysm begins to expand or leak. The most common presenting symptom is pain. This may be acute, implying impending rupture or dissection, or chronic, suggesting compression or distension, and may be located in the anterior chest, neck, back or even the epigastrium. Symptoms may result from pressure on or erosion into the surrounding structures. Compression on the superior vena cava may cause distended neck veins. Stretching of the recurrent laryngeal nerve may result in hoarseness of voice. Compression on the trachea or bronchus may cause stridor, wheezing, dyspnoea or cough. Compression on the oesophagus may result in dysphagia. Erosion into surrounding structures may result in haemoptysis, haematemesis or haematochezia. Erosion into the vertebral column may cause back pain, spinal cord compression or thrombosis of spinal arteries, resulting in symptoms of paraparesis or paraplegia.

Thoracic aneurysms may be visible on plain chest X-ray and characterized by enlargement of the aortic knob, an enlarged mediastinal shadow, tracheal displacement, or calcification outlining the walls of the aneurysm. CT scan with contrast has become the most widely used diagnostic tool. Other investigations include transoesophageal echocardiography, MRI and aortography, all of which are also highly accurate.

The most common complications of TAA are acute rupture or dissection. Acute rupture occurs in 2–5% of cases. The natural history of expansion and rupture can be interrupted only by elective repair. For this reason, asymptomatic thoracic aneurysms larger than 5–6 cm and symptomatic aneurysms regardless of size should be considered for repair. Conventional surgical repair involves replacement with a Dacron graft. Descending TAA may be treated by open surgery or by endovascular stent-grafting. The operative mortality ranges from 4% to 10% for ascending aneurysms, 25% for arch aneurysms, 5–15% for descending aneurysms, and 1.5% for endovascular stent-grafting.

Cerebral aneurysms (see sections 8.2 and 8.3)

Visceral (splanchnic artery) aneurysms

The increasing use of diagnostic imaging studies has probably contributed to the increased awareness of visceral aneurysms, which may involve the splenic, hepatic, coeliac, superior mesenteric, renal, pancreaticoduodenal, gastroduodenal and other arteries. Visceral aneurysms result from abnormal haemodynamics, atherosclerosis or infectious causes. Most visceral aneurysms are asymptomatic and are detected incidentally on imaging studies. However, they should be considered in any patient with abdominal pain, a pulsatile mass (but rarely palpable), abdominal bruit, intra-abdominal bleeding or gastrointestinal bleeding. The diagnosis can be confirmed with CT, US, MRI or angiography. Up to 25% of visceral aneurysms may be complicated by rupture, and the mortality rate after rupture is between 25% and 70%.[3] Treatment should be considered in all patients with symptoms related to the aneurysm, if the aneurysm is more than 2 cm in diameter, if the patient is pregnant, or if there is demonstrated growth of the aneurysm.[3] The type of treatment depends on the clinical condition, the artery involved and the surgeon's preference, and can be open surgical ligation, prosthetic or venous graft reconstruction, percutaneous transcatheter metal coil embolization, endovascular stent-graft placement, and even organ removal.

Splenic artery aneurysms (SAA) account for 60% of all visceral arterial aneurysms. They are the only aneurysms that are more common in women, with a female-to-male ratio of 4:1. Multiple aneurysms are present in about 20–30% of patients. The more common causes are atherosclerosis and portal hypertension. Splenic artery aneurysms are usually an incidental discovery on abdominal X-rays as signet ring calcifications in the left upper quadrant, especially in elderly patients. Most are less than 2 cm in diameter. Symptoms include left upper quadrant or epigastric pain radiating to the left shoulder or subscapular area. Only 2% of splenic artery aneurysms result in rupture. Of those that do rupture, >95% occur in young women during the third trimester of pregnancy, with reported 35–75% maternal and 95% fetal mortality rates.[3] Symptomatic SAAs require immediate operative intervention, particularly in pregnant women or women of childbearing age. In asymptomatic patients, treatment is controversial but should be considered if the diameter of the aneurysm is larger than 2 cm. Ruptured SAA is usually treated by splenectomy. Other treatment options include open surgical ligation, bypass graft reconstruction, percutaneous transcatheter embolization with metal coils, and endovascular stent-graft placement.

Hepatic artery aneurysm constitutes 20% of visceral artery aneurysms and occurs most commonly in elderly men. Most are asymptomatic, and calcifications may be identified on abdominal X-ray. More than 50% present with right upper quadrant or epigastric abdominal pain radiating to the back. Rupture into the biliary tract may result in the classic triad of acute biliary pain, haemobilia and jaundice. Erosion of the aneurysm into the stomach or duodenum may lead to haematemesis or melaena. Extrinsic compression of the biliary duct may cause obstructive jaundice. Because of the high mortality rate associated with rupture, surgical resection or transarterial catheter occlusion is warranted.

Superior mesenteric artery aneurysms are the third most common visceral aneurysm (8%). More than 90% are symptomatic, presenting with upper abdominal pain, gastrointestinal bleeding or acute mesenteric ischaemia from thromboembolism. Around 50% have a pulsatile mass on physical examination.

Coeliac artery aneurysms (4%) may manifest as epigastric pain, upper gastrointestinal bleeding, or dysphagia due to oesophageal compression.

Renal artery aneurysms are very rare (<0.1%). They may present with hypertension, haematuria, thrombosis, embolism, arteriovenous fistula formation and rupture.

Peripheral aneurysms

Peripheral aneurysms tend to be multiple. Unlike central aneurysms, peripheral arterial aneurysms rarely rupture; instead, they are usually complicated by thrombosis or embolism, including claudication, rest pain, thromboembolism, 'blue toe' syndrome or even gangrene. Aneurysmal dilatation can cause nerve or venous compression, resulting in deep vein thrombosis, neuralgia or weakness. The diagnosis may be suspected if there is a pulsatile mass. Plain X-ray may show calcifications. Duplex ultrasonography, arteriography, CT or MRI can confirm the diagnosis. The conventional surgical approach is bypass graft with exclusion or ligation of the aneurysm. Endovascular repair may be advantageous in selected high-risk patients. Operative results are closely related to the presence of symptoms, the status of the distal arterial tree, and the type of conduit employed.

Lower extremity aneurysms

The overall prevalence of lower extremity aneurysms is less than 1%. They are usually atherosclerotic in origin. More than 95% of the patients are elderly men, commonly with hypertension. Non-atherosclerotic aneurysms may occur as a complication of inflammatory or collagen disorders, bacterial infection, entrapment syndromes, and blunt or penetrating trauma.

Over 70–85% of peripheral arterial aneurysms occur in the popliteal artery, followed by the femoral artery. The popliteal artery is considered aneurysmal if its external diameter exceeds 2 cm, and for the femoral artery 2.5 cm. It has been claimed that 35–40% of patients with popliteal aneurysm (PAA) have an aortic aneurysm and 50–60% have a contralateral PAA. The incidence of AAA is almost 80% in patients with bilateral PAA. On the other hand, only 1–2% of AAA are associated with PAA. Thus, all patients with a lower extremity aneurysm should be evaluated for the presence of other aneurysms.

Approximately 33–45% PAA are asymptomatic at the time of initial diagnosis. In contrast to AAA, patients with PAA usually present with acute or chronic limb ischaemia secondary to thrombosis or embolism, and rupture is rare. Rarely, pressure on nerves leads to pain or weakness; and compression on veins results in distal oedema or deep venous thrombosis. The risk of ischaemic complications from an asymptomatic popliteal aneurysm ranges from 8% to 100%. Hence, surgery is recommended in all symptomatic PAAs and asymptomatic ones larger than 2 cm. The conventional surgical approach is bypass graft with exclusion or ligation of the aneurysm. Endovascular repair may be advantageous in selected high-risk patients. Operative results are closely related to the presence of symptoms, the status of the distal arterial tree, and the type of conduit employed.

Upper extremity aneurysms

Upper extremity aneurysms are rare, usually the result of trauma, and may involve the innominate, subclavian, axillary, brachial, radial, ulnar and even the digital arteries. Subclavian artery and axillary artery aneurysms share the common complications of limb ischaemia, thromboembolism and central nervous system ischaemia by retrograde thromboembolism in the vertebral and carotid circulation. Expansion may result in a pulsating mass, and brachial plexus compression may cause pain. Rupture can cause death from exsanguination. Subclavian artery aneurysm may present as a superior mediastinal mass on chest X-ray. Because of their severe potential morbidity, these aneurysms should be surgically repaired promptly after diagnosis.

Ulnar artery aneurysm is caused by repeated trauma to the heel of the palm as a result of hammering, pushing or twisting objects. The patients are often industrial workers such as mechanics and carpenters.

Likely developments over the next 5–10 years

- Multidetector helical CT scanning is quickly replacing angiography as the diagnostic test of choice in many institutions.

- Endovascular stent-graft placement is applicable to increasing proportions of patients with non-ruptured AAA, visceral and peripheral aneurysms, allowing repair in high-risk patients who might not tolerate an operation under general anaesthesia.

- Screening for asymptomatic AAA may become popular.

Controversies

- No evidence exists that lowering the blood pressure is beneficial in patients with ruptured AAAs, and these patients are at risk of precipitous hypotension. On the other hand, overly aggressive fluid resuscitation may be harmful.

- Some patients may decline or be advised against elective repair of an aneurysm because of coexisting medical illness. However, they may subsequently opt for life-saving emergency repair after rupture, which has a tenfold higher mortality.

References

1. Bessen HA. Abdominal aortic aneurysms. In: Marx JA, Hockberger RS, Walls RM, eds. Rosen's emergency medicine: concepts and clinical practice, 6th edn. Philadelphia: Mosby, 2006; 1330–1341.
2. Johnson GA. Aortic dissection and aneurysm In: Tintinalli JE, Kelen GD, Stapczynski JS, eds. Emergency medicine: a comprehensive study guide, 5th edn. New York: McGraw-Hill, 2000; 412–416.
3. Pasha SF, Gloviczki P, Stanson AW, et al. Splanchnic artery aneurysms. Mayo Clin Proc 2007; 82: 472–479.
4. Nelson BP, Benzer TI, Isselbacher EM. Aneurysm, thoracic. eMedicine. (upated 30 Aug 2006). Online. Available: http://www.emedicine.com/emerg/topic942.htm Accessed 1 Jun 2007.

RESPIRATORY

Edited by **Anne-Maree Kelly**

6.1 Upper respiratory tract

Ken Ooi

ESSENTIALS

1 Airway management and the ABCs take precedence over the history, examination and specific treatment of upper airway obstruction.

2 Direct laryngoscopy can be an important technique for both investigation and management of upper airway obstruction.

3 The Heimlich manoeuvre (abdominal thrust) is a useful first aid technique in foreign body upper airway obstruction, albeit unproven.

4 Acute viral respiratory infections are a frequent reason for seeking medical attention. Over-prescribing of antibiotics continues to be a major problem.

5 Bacterial infections and collections are uncommon but may compromise the upper airway.

6 A high index of suspicion is needed to diagnose blunt traumatic injuries to the larynx and trachea.

7 Cervical spine injuries frequently accompany significant blunt laryngeal injuries.

Introduction

The upper respiratory tract extends from the mouth and nose to the carina. It comprises a relatively small area anatomically, but is of vital importance. Presenting conditions may be acute and potentially life-threatening, requiring immediate evaluation or treatment, although the majority of presentations are not life-threatening.

Urgent conditions requiring immediate attention or intervention are those likely to compromise the airway. Protection and maintenance of airway, breathing and circulation (the ABCs) take precedence over history taking, detailed examination or investigations. Possible causes of airway obstruction are listed in Table 6.1.1.

Non-urgent presentations include rash or facial swelling not involving the airway, sore throat in a non-toxic patient, and complaints that have been present for days or weeks with no recent deterioration. Pharyngitis and tonsillitis are common causes for presentation in both paediatric and adult emergency practice.

Triage and initial evaluation

Initial evaluation should be aimed at differentiating those patients needing urgent management to prevent significant morbidity and mortality, from those needing less immediate intervention. Triage must be based on the chief complaint and on vital signs, as the same clinical presentation may result from a range of pathophysiologies, e.g. stridor can be due to trauma, infection, drug reactions or anatomical abnormalities such as tracheomalacia.

Symptoms and signs of airway obstruction include dyspnoea, stridor, altered voice, dysphonia and dysphagia. Evidence of increased work of breathing includes subcostal, intercostal and suprasternal retraction, flaring of the nasal alae, as well as exhaustion and altered mental state. The presence of these signs may vary with age and accompanying conditions. Cyanosis is a late sign. Further examination will be

Table 6.1.1 Causes of upper airway obstruction

Altered conscious state

Head injury
CVA
Drugs and toxins
Metabolic: hypoglycaemia, hyponatraemia, etc.

Foreign bodies

Infections

Tonsillitis
Peritonsillar abscess (quinsy)
Epiglottitis
Ludwig's angina
Other abscesses and infections

Trauma

Blunt or penetrating trauma resulting in oedema or haematoma formation
Uncontrolled haemorrhage
Thermal injuries
Inhalation burns

Neoplasms

Larynx, trachea, thyroid

Allergic reactions

Anaphylaxis
Angio-oedema

Anatomical

Tracheomalacia: congenital or acquired (secondary to prolonged intubation)
Other congenital malformations

Acute on chronic causes

Patients with chronic narrowing of the airway (e.g. due to tracheomalacia) may present with worsening obstruction with an acute upper respiratory tract illness or injury

directed by the presenting complaint and initial findings and includes:

- General appearance – facial symmetry, demeanour.
- Vital signs – temperature, heart rate, respiratory rate, BP, pulse oximetry.
- Head and face – rash, swelling, mucous membranes, lymphadenopathy.
- Oropharynx – mucous membranes, dental hygiene, tongue, tonsils, uvula.

Upper airway obstruction

Upper airway obstruction may be acute and life-threatening or may have a more gradual onset. It is essential that the adequacy of the airway is assessed first. Any emergency interventions that are required to maintain the airway should be instituted before obtaining a detailed history and examination. This may range from relieving the obstruction to providing an alternative airway.

Obstruction may be physiological, with the patient unable to maintain and protect an adequate airway owing to a reduced conscious state. Mechanical obstruction may be due to pathology within the lumen (aspirated foreign body), in the wall (angio-edema, tracheomalacia) or to extrinsic compression (Ludwig's angina, haematoma, external burns). Obstruction may be due to a combination of physiological and mechanical causes. A summary of potential causes of upper airway obstruction is provided in Table 6.1.1. Despite the plethora of possible causes, the initial treatment to secure the airway is the same.

Investigation

Investigations are secondary to the assessment and/or provision of an adequate airway. Once the airway has been assessed as secure, the choice of investigations is directed by the history and examination.

Endoscopy

Direct laryngoscopy by an experienced operator is the single most important manoeuvre in patients with acute upper airway obstruction. It may concurrently form part of the assessment, investigation or treatment. By visualizing the laryngopharynx and upper larynx the cause of the obstruction can be seen. Any foreign bodies may be removed or, if necessary, a definitive airway such as an endotracheal tube introduced. In the case of the stable patient with an incomplete obstruction this should only be attempted when there are full facilities available for intubation and the provision of a surgical airway. It may be more appropriately deferred until expert airway assistance is available.

Bronchoscopy may be required to assess the trachea and distal upper airway, but is not part of the initial resuscitation. It is more appropriate to transfer the stable patient to the operating suite or ICU for this procedure.

Pathology

Some tests may be useful in guiding further management. These include full blood count, arterial blood gases, and throat swab and blood cultures. Those required will be guided by the clinical presentation. Initial treatment in the emergency department (ED) should not await their results.

Imaging

Neck X-rays

A lateral soft tissue X-ray of the neck is sometimes helpful once the patient has been stabilized. Metallic or bony foreign bodies, food boluses or soft tissue masses may be seen. A number of subtle radiological signs have been described in epiglottitis (Table 6.1.2).

Table 6.1.2 Radiological findings in adult epiglottitis

The 'thumb' sign	Oedema of the normally leaf-like epiglottis resulting in a round shadow resembling an adult thumb. The width of the epiglottis should be less than one-third the anteroposterior width of C4.
The vallecula sign	Progressive epiglottic oedema resulting in narrowing of the vallecula. This normally well-defined air pocket between the base of the tongue and the epiglottis may be partially or completely obliterated.
Swelling of the aryepiglottic folds	
Swelling of the arytenoids	
Prevertebral soft tissue swelling	The width of the prevertebral soft tissue should be less than half the anteroposterior width of C4.
Hypopharyngeal airway widening	The ratio of the width of the hypopharyngeal airway to the anteroposterior width of C4 should be less than 1.5.

Computed tomography

In the patient with a mechanical obstruction a computed tomography (CT) scan of the neck and upper thorax may be helpful in diagnosing the cause of the obstruction as well as the extent of any local involvement. It may aid in planning further management, especially if surgical intervention is indicated, for example for a retrothyroid goitre or a head and neck neoplasm.

Management

Management initially consists of securing the airway. This is discussed in more detail elsewhere in this book, but simple interventions include chin lift or jaw thrust and an oropharyngeal airway, or more sophisticated items such as the laryngeal mask, endotracheal tube or surgical airway. A surgical airway is rarely necessary in the ED, although it is important that equipment is always available and that the techniques have been practised. These include needle insufflation and cricothyrostomy. A number of commercial kits, such as the 'Mini-trach II' and the Melker Emergency Cricothyroidotomy Catheter Set, are available. Further management will depend on the underlying cause.

Trauma

Trauma to the upper airway may involve obstruction by a foreign body, blunt or penetrating trauma or thermal injury.

Foreign body airway obstruction

Foreign body aspiration is often associated with an altered conscious state, including alcohol or drug intoxication as well as cerebrovascular accident (CVA) or dementia. Elderly patients with dentures are at increased risk. Laryngeal foreign bodies are almost always symptomatic and are more likely to cause complete obstruction than foreign bodies below the epiglottis. If the obstruction is incomplete and adequate air exchange continues, care should be taken not to convert partial obstruction into a complete block by overzealous interference. Foreign bodies in the oesophagus are an uncommon cause of airway obstruction, but if lodged in the area of the cricoid cartilage or the tracheal bifurcation, can compress the airway, causing partial airway obstruction. Oesophageal foreign bodies may also become dislodged into the upper airway.

Management

The Heimlich manoeuvre or abdominal thrust is one recommended technique for dislodgement of a foreign body. The rescuer stands behind the patient, placing clenched fists over the patient's upper abdomen well clear of the xiphisternum. A short, sharp upward thrust is made to force the diaphragm up and expel the foreign body. There is a risk of injury to internal organs and so this should only be done by rescuers who have been trained in the technique. Chest thrusts may be more effective in obese patients if the rescuer is unable to encircle the patient's abdomen.

Chest thrusts are a similar technique that may be used in children or pregnant women, and back blows can be used in small children. Patients who are asymptomatic after uncomplicated removal of a foreign body should be observed for a time in the ED, and if they remain well may be discharged home.

In the unconscious patient direct laryngoscopy may be performed, with removal of the foreign body under direct vision with Magill forceps or suction.

Blunt trauma

Laryngotracheal trauma is rare, comprising 0.3% of all traumas presenting to an ED. The upper airway is relatively protected against trauma as the larynx is mobile and the trachea compressible, and because the head and mandible act as shields. Blunt trauma may be difficult to diagnose, as external examination may be normal and there may be distracting head or chest injuries.

Mechanism

'Clothesline injuries' involve cyclists or other riders hitting fences or cables. Direct trauma from assaults, sporting equipment or industrial accidents also occurs. Suicide attempts by hanging may cause traumatic injuries to the neck as well as airway obstruction due to the ligature. 'Dashboard injuries' occur when seatbelts are not worn, with sudden deceleration resulting in hyperextension of the neck and compression of the larynx between the dashboard and the cervical spine.

Pathology

The most common laryngeal injury is a vertical fracture through the thyroid cartilage. Fractures of the hyoid bone and cricoid cartilage also occur, and may be found in cases of manual or ligature strangulation. The cricothyroid ligament and the vocal cords may be ruptured and the arytenoids dislocated. Complete cricotracheal transection may occur. Mortality rates depend on the location of the injury, ranging from 11% for isolated fractures of the thyroid cartilage to 50% for injuries involving the cricoid cartilage, bronchi or intrathoracic trachea. Asphyxiation is the most common cause of death in blunt laryngeal trauma. Up to 50% of patients sustaining significant blunt airway trauma have a concurrent cervical spinal injury.

Clinical

Tracheal or laryngeal injury should be suspected if aphonia, hoarseness, stridor, dysphagia or dyspnoea occur. Patients may present with complete obstruction or may deteriorate rapidly after arrival. There may be minimal external evidence of injury or the larynx may be deformed or tender, and there may be subcutaneous emphysema. It is important to check for associated head, chest and cervical spine injuries.

Penetrating trauma

Mechanism

Penetrating injuries may be secondary to assault or to sporting or industrial accidents. A focused history is mandatory.

Clinical

Penetration of the airway should be suspected if there is difficulty breathing, a change in voice, pain on speaking, subcutaneous emphysema or bubbling from the wound. This is often associated with great vessel or pulmonary injuries, and the patient may require an emergency airway procedure. Uncontrolled haemorrhage is a potentially life-threatening condition. Other causes include head and neck malignancies eroding vascular structures, or following radiotherapy. Uncontrolled haemorrhage may lead to exsanguination as well as compromising the airway, and requires prompt surgical intervention.

Management of blunt and penetrating trauma

Airway management with protection of the cervical spine is essential. Fibreoptic bronchoscopic intubation is preferable to minimize complications such as laryngeal disruption, laryngotracheal separation or the creation of a false tracheal lumen. Cricothyrostomy is relatively contraindicated because of the altered anatomy. Emergency tracheostomy may even be required, ideally performed in the operating theatre. Early ENT involvement is important, and indications for surgical exploration include airway obstruction requiring tracheostomy, uncontrolled subcutaneous emphysema, extensive mucosal lacerations with exposed cartilage as identified on bronchoscopic or laryngoscopic examination, vocal cord paralysis, and grossly deformed, multiple or displaced fractures of the larynx, thyroid cartilage or cricoid cartilage.

Thermal injury

Pathology

Burns may affect the airway because of facial and perioral swelling, laryngeal oedema or constricting circumferential neck burns. Smoke inhalation occurs in about 25% of burn victims and may cause bronchospasm, retrosternal pain and impaired gas exchange.

Clinical

External examination may show evidence of burns. Carbonaceous material in the mouth, nares or pharynx suggests the possibility of upper airway thermal injury. If the patient presents with stridor or hoarseness, early intubation is essential because of the danger of increasing airway oedema. Smoke inhalation may be associated with carbon-monoxide poisoning, and in the setting of domestic or industrial fires cyanide poisoning should also be considered.

Investigations

Endoscopy

Endoscopy includes both laryngoscopy and bronchoscopy, performed in the operating theatre, as urgent surgical intervention

Table 6.1.3	Grading of blunt laryngeal injury
Grade	Endoscopic and radiological findings
I	Minor laryngeal haematoma without detectable fracture
II	Oedema, haematoma or minor mucosal disruption without exposed cartilage, or non-displaced fractures on CT
III	Massive oedema, tears, exposed cartilage, immobile cords

may be required. Fuhrman et al. (see Further reading) suggest a classification system for the severity of blunt upper airway injury based on endoscopic and radiological findings (Table 6.1.3).

Imaging

Plain X-ray

X-rays should only be considered if the patient is stable, with adequate ventilation. Lateral soft tissue X-rays of the neck may provide information about airway patency, subcutaneous or soft tissue emphysema, and fractures of the hyoid and larynx. Elevation of the hyoid bone indicates cricotracheal separation. Plain X-rays may also confirm the presence of a foreign body. Cervical spine X-rays should be considered because of the association between upper airway injuries and cervical spine injuries. Chest X-rays may show signs of trauma and subcutaneous or mediastinal emphysema.

CT

CT scans of the neck are useful in assessing the extent of injuries to the larynx, oesophagus, cervical spine and adjacent structures, but should only be considered in the stable patient.

Infections

Infections may involve the upper respiratory tract directly or affect adjacent structures. They range from the common and trivial to the rare and potentially life-threatening. Croup and epiglottitis usually occur in children, but may be seen in

adults. Acute respiratory infections are the most frequent reason for seeking medical attention in the USA, and are associated with up to 75% of total antibiotic prescriptions there each year. Unnecessary antibiotic use can cause a number of adverse effects, including allergic reactions, GI upset, yeast infections, drug interactions, an increased risk of subsequent infection with drug resistant *Streptococcus pneumoniae* and added costs of over-treating.

Non-specific upper airway infections

Upper airway infections are generally diagnosed clinically. Symptom complexes where the predominant complaint is of sore throat are labelled pharyngitis or tonsillitis, and where the predominant symptom is cough, bronchitis. Acute respiratory symptoms in the absence of a predominant sign are typically diagnosed as 'upper respiratory tract infections' (URTI). Each of these syndromes may be caused by a multitude of different viruses, and only occasionally by bacteria. Most cases resolve spontaneously within 1–2 weeks. Bacterial rhinosinusitis complicates about 2% of cases and should be suspected when symptoms have lasted at least 7 days and include purulent nasal discharge and other localizing features. Those at high risk for developing bacterial rhinosinusitis or bacterial pneumonia include infants, the elderly and the chronically ill. The antibiotic prescription rate for uncomplicated URTIs in the USA has been previously shown to be 52%, despite the fact that these infections are typically viral in origin and that antibiotic treatment does not enhance illness resolution nor alter the rates of these complications. Treatment should be symptomatic only.

Pharyngitis/tonsillitis

Sore throat is one of the top 10 presenting complaints to EDs in the USA. The differential diagnosis is large and includes a number of important conditions (Table 6.1.4). Pharyngitis has a wide range of causative bacterial and viral agents, most of which produce a self-limited infection with no significant sequelae. The major role for antibiotics in treating pharyngitis is for suspected group A β-haemolytic streptococcal infection (GABHS) or *Streptococcus pyogenes*. Timely use of appropriate antibiotics

Table 6.1.4 Differential diagnosis of sore throat in the adult

Infective pharyngitis
  Bacterial: Group A β-haemolytic streptococcus most common pathogen. Diphtheria should be considered in patients with membranous pharyngitis
  Viral: including EBV and HSV

Traumatic pharyngitis (exposure to irritant gases)

Non-specific upper respiratory tract infection

Quinsy (peritonsillar abscess)

Epiglottitis

Ludwig's angina

Parapharyngeal and retropharyngeal abscesses

Gastro-oesophageal reflux

Oropharyngeal or laryngeal tumour

reduces the duration of symptoms by an average of 8 hours but increases the rate of adverse effects. Antibiotic use also reduces the incidence of suppurative complications such as otitis media, quinsy and retropharyngeal abscess. If given in the first 9 days they prevent the development of acute rheumatic fever. Antibiotics have not been shown to reduce the incidence of post-streptococcal glomerulonephritis, which is related to the subtype of streptococcus. Antibiotic therapy is also recommended for patients from the following groups: patients with scarlet fever, with known rheumatic heart disease, or from populations with high incidence of acute rheumatic fever, including some Aboriginal populations in Central and Northern Australia.

Up to 50% of pharyngitis in children is caused by GABHS, but only between 5% and 15% of adult cases. The most reliable clinical predictors for GABHS are Centor's criteria. These include tonsillar exudates, tender anterior cervical lymphadenopathy or lymphadenitis, absence of cough and a history of fever. The presence of three or more criteria has a positive predictive value of 40–60%, whereas the absence of three or more has a negative predictive value of approximately 80%.

Rapid antigen tests are available which have sensitivities ranging between 65% and 97% but are not widely used. They may have a future role in deciding the need for antibiotics. Throat cultures take 2–3 days and may give false positive results

from asymptomatic carriers with concurrent non-GABHS pharyngitis. The Infectious Diseases Society of America recommends cultures for children and adolescents with appropriate clinical criteria but negative rapid antigen testing. In adults, because of the lower incidence of streptococcal infection and lower risk of rheumatic fever, a negative rapid antigen test is considered sufficient. Despite the availability of a number of guidelines, there are still wide variations in the management of pharyngitis. Serological testing is not useful in the acute treatment of pharyngitis but is useful in the diagnosis of rheumatic fever.

Neisseria gonorrhoeae is an uncommon cause of pharyngitis and may be asymptomatic. It is seen in persons who practise receptive oral sex. It is important to correctly diagnose *N. gonorrhoeae* pharyngitis, both for appropriate treatment and because of the need to trace and treat contacts. Ceftriaxone 125 mg i.m. as a single dose is the recommended treatment for uncomplicated pharyngeal gonorrhoea, and consideration should be given to concomitant treatment for chlamydia if this has not been ruled out. HIV is an unusual cause of pharyngitis but should be considered in high-risk populations. The acute retroviral syndrome may present with an Epstein–Barr virus (EBV) mononucleosis-like syndrome.

Most patients with pharyngitis are managed as outpatients. Airway compromise is rare, as the nasal passages provide an adequate airway. Some patients who are toxic or dehydrated may need admission for i.v. hydration and antibiotics. High-dose penicillin remains the drug of choice for streptococcal pharyngitis. The role of oral, i.m. or i.v. steroids remains controversial, but they may be useful in relieving airway obstruction and reducing the duration of symptoms.

Quinsy/peritonsillar abscess

Peritonsillar infections occur between the palatine tonsil and its capsule. Peritonsillar cellulitis may form pus and progress to abscess formation. Cellulitis responds to antibiotics alone, but differentiating between the two and identifying those that require drainage may be difficult clinically. Peritonsillar abscesses occur most commonly in males between 20 and 40 years of age. Symptoms include a progressively worsening sore throat, fever and dysphagia.

On examination the patient may have a muffled 'hot potato' voice, trismus, drooling, a swollen red tonsil with or without purulent exudate, and contralateral deviation of the uvula. Complications include airway obstruction and lateral extension into the parapharyngeal space. GABHS is the most common organism associated with quinsy, but others include *Staphylococcus aureus*, *Haemophilus influenzae* and anaerobic species such as fusobacterium, peptostreptococcus and bacteroides. Treatment generally requires admission for i.v. penicillin and metronidazole. Clindamycin may be used as an alternative. Needle aspiration in experienced hands can be useful, but has a 12% false negative rate and carries the risk of damaging the carotid artery. Formal surgical drainage may be necessary.

Ludwig's angina

Peripharyngeal space infections have become rare in the post antibiotic era but, of these, Ludwig's angina or cellulitis of the submandibular space remains the most common. It was first described by Wilhelm Fredrick von Ludwig in 1836, and at that time was usually fatal because of rapid compromise to the airway. With prompt treatment, including i.v. antibiotics, the mortality rate has declined to less than 5%. Clinical features include toothache, halitosis, neck pain, swelling, fever, dysphagia and trismus. Ludwig's angina is classically bilateral. Infection may spread rapidly into adjacent spaces, including the pharyngomaxillary and retropharyngeal areas and the mediastinum. Ludwig's angina is related to dental caries involving the mandibular molars, or it may be associated with peritonsillar abscess, trauma to the floor of the mouth or mandible, and recent dental work. Cultures are usually polymicrobial and include viridans streptococci (40.9%), *Staph. aureus* (27.3%), *Staph. epidermidis* (22.7%) and anaerobes (40%) such as bacteroides species. Treatment necessitates admission and careful airway management. This may include endotracheal intubation, as abrupt obstruction can occur. Surgical drainage is indicated if the infection is suppurative or fluctuant. The i.v. antibiotics of choice are high-dose penicillin plus metronidazole or clindamycin.

Other abscesses

Parapharyngeal abscesses involve the lateral or pharyngomaxillary space. Presentation and treatment are similar to those of Ludwig's angina, from which they may develop. As well as the complications of Ludwig's angina, including airway obstruction and spread to contiguous areas, there is the added risk of internal jugular vein thrombosis and erosion of the carotid artery, which has a mortality of 20–40%.

Retropharyngeal abscesses are more common in children under 5 years of age. In adults they often result from foreign bodies or trauma. Presenting symptoms and signs include fever, odynophagia, neck swelling, drooling, torticollis, cervical lymphadenopathy, dyspnoea and stridor. Lateral neck X-rays show widening of the prevertebral soft tissues and sometimes a fluid level. CT of the neck may help in determining the extent and in differentiating an abscess from cellulitis. MRI, if available, is more sensitive than CT in assessing soft tissue infections of the head and neck, but demonstrates cortical bone poorly. Treatment requires admission, airway management and i.v. antibiotics, and may include surgical drainage.

Epiglottitis

Epiglottitis is becoming an adult disease, although in adults there is significantly less risk to the airway than in children. The incidence of adult epiglottitis has remained relatively stable at 1–4 cases per 100 000 per year, with a mortality of 7%, but this may change over the next 10–20 years as vaccinated children grow into adolescents and adults. Acute adult epiglottitis is often referred to as supraglottitis because the inflammation is not confined to the epiglottis, but also affects other structures such as the pharynx, uvula, base of tongue, aryepiglottic folds and false vocal cords. *H. influenzae* has been isolated in 12–17% of cases, and the high rate of negative blood cultures may reflect viral infections or prior treatment with antibiotics in cases that present late. *Strep. pneumoniae, H. parainfluenzae* and herpes simplex have also been isolated. Epiglottitis may also occur following mechanical injury such as the ingestion of caustic material, smoke inhalation, and following illicit drug use (smoking heroin).

Sore throat and odynophagia are the most common presenting symptoms. Drooling and stridor are infrequent. Factors shown to be associated with an increased risk of airway obstruction include stridor, dyspnoea, sitting upright, and short duration of symptoms. A number of X-ray changes have been described in epiglottitis, which are listed in Table 6.1.2. Management requires admission and i.v. ceftriaxone or cefotaxime. The role of steroids and nebulized or parenteral epinephrine (adrenaline) is controversial. Chloramphenicol may be used in patients with cephalosporin sensitivity. Most adults can be treated conservatively without the need for an artificial airway.

Controversies

- The role of steroids in acute pharyngitis/tonsillitis and quinsy.

- Reaching a uniform approach to the use of antibiotics in adult pharyngitis.

- The role of intubation, steroids and nebulized or parenteral epinephrine (adrenaline) in adult epiglottitis.

Further reading

Alcaide ML, Bisno AL. Pharyngitis and epiglottitis. Infectious Disease Clinics of North America 2007; 21: 449–469.

American Heart Association. Guidelines for cardiopulmonary resuscitation and emergency cardiac care. Circulation 2005; 112: Supplement.

Ames WA, Ward WMM, Tranter RMD, et al. Adult epiglottitis: an under-recognized, life-threatening condition. British Journal of Anaesthesia 2000; 85: 795–797.

Atkins BZ, Abbate S, Fischer S, et al. 2004 Current management of laryngotracheal trauma: case report and literature review. Journal of Trauma 56: 185–190.

Atkins BZ, Abbate S, Fischer S, et al. Current management of laryngotracheal trauma: case report and literature review. Journal of Trauma 2004; 56: 185–190.

Bisno AL, Gerber MA, Gwaltney JM, et al. Infectious Diseases Society of America. Practice guidelines for the diagnosis and management of group A streptococcal pharyngitis. Clinical Infectious Disease 2002; 35: 113.

Centor RM, Witherspoon JM, Dalton HP, et al. The diagnosis of strep throat in adults in the emergency room. Medical Decision Making 1981; 1: 239–246.

Cicala RS. The traumatized airway. In: Benumof JE, ed. Airway management: principles and practice. St Louis: Mosby-Year Book, 1996; 736.

Cooper RJ, Hoffman JR, Bartlett JG, et al. Principles of appropriate antibiotic use for acute pharyngitis in adults: Background. Annals of Internal Medicine 2001; 134: 509–517.

Del Mar CB, Glasziou PP, Spinks AB. 2006 Antibiotics for sore throat. Cochrane Database of Systematic Reviews (4): CD000023. DOI: 10.1002/14651858.CD000023.pub3. Accessed December 2007.

Fuhrman GM, Stieg FH, Buerk CA. Blunt laryngeal trauma: Classification and management protocol. Journal of Trauma 1990; 30: 87–92.

Frantz TD, Rasgon BM, Quesenberry CP. Acute epiglottitis in adults. Journal of the American Medical Association 1994; 272: 1358–1360.

Gonzales R, Bartlett JG, Besseer RE, et al. Principles of appropriate antibiotic use for treatment of acute respiratory tract infections in adults: Background, specific aims, and methods. Annals of Emergency Medicine 2001; 37: 690–697.

Gonzales R, Bartlett JG, Besser, RE, et al. Principles of appropriate antibiotic use for treatment of nonspecific upper respiratory tract infections in adults: Background. Annals of Emergency Medicine 2001; 37: 698–702.

Gonzales R, Steiner JF, Sande MA. Antibiotic prescribing for adults with colds, upper respiratory tract infections and bronchitis by ambulatory care physicians. Journal of the American Medical Association 1997; 278: 901–904.

Howes DS, Dowling PJ. Triage and initial evaluation of the oral facial emergency. Emergency Medicine Clinics of North America: Oral-Facial Emergencies 2000; 8: 371–378.

Hurley MC, Heran MKS. Imaging studies for head and neck infections. Infectious Disease Clinics of North America 2007; 21: 305–353.

Linder JA, Chan JC, Bates DW. Evaluation and treatment of pharyngitis in primary care practice: the difference between guidelines is largely academic. Archives of Internal Medicine 2006; 166: 1374–1379.

McCollough M. Update on emerging infections from the centers for disease control and prevention: commentary. Annals of Emergency Medicine 1999; 34: 110–111.

Minard G, Kodak KA, Croce MA, et al. Laryngotracheal trauma. American Surgeon 1992; 58: 181–187.

Nemzek WR, Katzberg RW, Van Slyke MA, et al. A reappraisal of the radiologic findings of acute inflammation of the epiglottis and supraglottic structures in adults. American Journal of Neuro Radiology 1995; 16: 495–502.

Richardson MA. Sore throat, tonsillitis, and adenoiditis. Medical Clinics of North America: Otolaryngology for the Internist 1999; 83: 75–84.

Schamp S, Pokieser P, Danzer M, et al. Radiological findings in acute adult epiglottitis. European Radiology 1999; 9: 1629–1631.

Scott PMJ, Loftus WK, Kew J, et al. Diagnosis of peritonsillar infections: a prospective study of ultrasound, computerized tomography and clinical diagnosis. Journal of Laryngology and Otology 1999; 113: 229–232.

Stewart MH, Siff JE, Cydulka RK. Evaluation of the patient with sore throat, earache, and sinusitis: an evidence based approach. Emergency Medicine Clinics of North America: Evidence Based Emergency Medicine 1999; 17: 153–188.

Steyer TE. Peritonsillar abscess: diagnosis and treatment. American Family Physician 2002; 65: 93–96.

Thierbach AR, Lipp MDW. Airway management in trauma patients. Anesthesiology Clinics of North America 1999; 17: 63–82.

Victorian Medical Postgraduate Foundation. Therapeutic Guidelines: Antibiotic Version 12. 2006.

6.2 Asthma

Anne-Maree Kelly

ESSENTIALS

1 Asthma is a major health problem worldwide, resulting in significant morbidity and mortality.

2 Asthma is characterized by episodic bronchoconstriction and wheeze in response to a variety of stimuli.

3 Features suggesting an increased risk of life-threatening asthma include a previous life-threatening attack, previous intensive care admission with ventilation, and having required a course of oral corticosteroids within the previous 6 months. Behavioural and adverse psychosocial factors have also been implicated in life-threatening asthma, including non-compliance, obesity and psychiatric illness.

4 Attacks vary in severity from mild to life-threatening, and may develop over minutes.

5 Clinical features supported by bedside pulmonary function tests and pulse oximetry are reliable guides to the severity of attacks.

6 Oxygen, β-adrenergic agents and corticosteroids are the mainstay of therapy.

7 Hospital admission is essential if pretreatment PEFR or FEV_1 is less than 25% of predicted, or post-treatment levels are less than 40% of predicted.

Introduction

The prevalence of asthma varies significantly between regions across the world. In Australasia, New Zealand and the UK it is thought to affect about 20% of children and 10% of adults. Sufferers tend to present to emergency departments (ED) when their usual treatment plan fails to control symptoms adequately. The respiratory compromise caused can range from mild to severe and life-threatening. For these patients the main role of the emergency physician is therapeutic. Other reasons for patients with asthma to attend EDs include having run out of medication, having symptoms after a period of being symptom and medication free, and a desire for a 'second opinion' about the management of their asthma. For this smaller group the primary role is one of educating about the disease, of planning an approach to the current level of asthma symptoms, and of referral to appropriate health professionals, e.g. respiratory physicians or general practitioners.

Epidemiology

Asthma is a major health problem in many countries, resulting in significant morbidity and mortality. The cost in terms of long-term medications and lost school and work days is difficult to quantify, but would run to millions of US dollars annually. Australasia, the UK and North America have a greater prevalence of asthma than the Middle East and some Asian countries. There is also considerable geographical variation in severity, with Australasia reporting the highest proportion of severe disease. The reason for this geographical variation is unclear, but may relate in part to ethnicity, rural versus metropolitan environment, and air pollution. A number of epidemiological studies suggest that the prevalence and severity of asthma is slowly increasing worldwide.

Pathophysiology

Asthma is characterized by hyperreactive airways and inflammation leading to episodic, reversible bronchoconstriction in response to a variety of stimuli. Traditionally, it has been divided into extrinsic (allergic) and intrinsic (idiosyncratic) types.

Extrinsic asthma is initiated by a type I hypersensitivity reaction induced by an extrinsic allergen. IgE-mediated activation of mucosal mast cells results in the release of primary mediators (histamine and eosinophilic and neutrophilic chemotactic factors) and secondary mediators including leukotrienes, prostaglandin D_2, platelet-activating factor and cytokines. These result in bronchoconstriction via direct and cholinergic reflex actions, increased vascular permeability and increased mucous secretions.

In contrast, intrinsic asthma is initiated by diverse non-immune mechanisms, including respiratory infections (in particular viruses), drugs such as aspirin and β-blockers, pollutants and occupational exposure, emotion and exercise.

The morphological changes in asthma are over-inflation of the lungs, bronchoconstriction, and the presence of thick mucous plugs in the airways. Histologically there is thickening of the basement membrane of the bronchial epithelium, oedema and an inflammatory infiltrate in the bronchial walls, increased numbers of submucosal glands and hypertrophy of bronchial wall muscle.

Pathophysiologically the effects of acute asthma are:

- Increased physiological dead space.
- Respiratory muscle fatigue.
- Intrinsic positive end-expiratory pressure secondary to hyperventilation with air trapping.

There is increasing evidence that there are different phenotypes of both acute and chronic asthma. For acute asthma, a rapid onset may be closer to anaphylaxis in pathology, with minimal inflammation, and may respond more quickly to treatment.

Clinical assessment

History

Asthma is characterized by episodic short-ness of breath, often accompanied by wheeze, chest tightness and cough. Symptoms may be worse at night, which is thought to be due to variations in broncho-motor tone and bronchial reactivity. Attacks may progress slowly over days or rapidly over minutes.

Features in the history indicating a significant risk of life-threatening asthma include a previous life-threatening attack, previous intensive care admission with ventilation, requiring three or more classes of asthma medication, heavy use of β-agonist therapy, repeated ED attendances, and having required a course of oral corticosteroids within the previous 6 months. It has been identified that behavioural and psychosocial features increase the risk of life-threatening episodes of asthma. These include non-compliance with medications, monitoring or follow-up, self-discharge from hospital, psychiatric illness, denial, drug or alcohol abuse, obesity, learning difficulties, employment or income problems, domestic, marital or legal stressors and major tranquillizer use. These should be sought in order to more accurately assess risk and plan management.

Examination

Physical findings vary with the severity of the attack and may range from mild wheeze and dyspnoea to respiratory failure. Findings indicative of more severe disease include an inability to speak normally, use of the accessory muscles of respiration, a quiet or silent chest on auscultation, restlessness or altered level of consciousness, and cyanosis. Clinical features are a good guide to the severity of attacks. Features of the major severity categories are summarized in Table 6.2.1. Pulsus paradoxus has been abandoned as an indicator of severity.

Investigation

For mild and moderate asthma investigations should be limited to pulmonary

Table 6.2.1 Categorization of asthma severity based on clinical features. (Modified from Guidelines for Emergency Management of Adult Asthma, Canadian Association of Emergency Physicians, British Guideline on the Management of Asthma (SIGN) and Asthma Management handbook (NAC).)

Severity category	Features	Respiratory function
Near death	Exhaustion Confusion, coma Cyanosis Sweating Silent chest Inability to speak Reduced respiratory effort Dysrhythmia, bradycardia Hypotension	FEV_1/PEFR inappropriate SpO_2 <90% despite supplemental oxygen
Severe	Laboured respiration Sweating, restless Tachycardia, heart rate >120 Tachypnoea, respiratory rate >25/min Difficulty speaking: words or short phrases only	FEV_1/PEFR unable or <40% predicted SpO_2 <90% on air PEFR <200 L/min
Moderate	Dyspnoeic at rest Able to speak in short sentences Chest tightness Wheeze Partial or short-term relief with usual therapy Nocturnal symptoms	FEV_1/PEFR 40–60% predicted PEFR 200–300 L/min
Mild	Exertional symptoms Able to speak normally Good response to usual therapy	FEV_1/PEFR >60% predicted

function tests (PEFR or FEV_1) and pulse oximetry. A chest X-ray is only indicated if examination of the chest suggests pneumothorax or pneumonia. Arterial blood gases are not useful in this group of patients.

For severe asthma a chest X-ray is necessary, as localizing signs in the chest may be hard to detect. Arterial blood gas analysis is useful if the oxygen saturation is less than 92% on room air at presentation, if improvement is not occurring as expected, and if the patient appears to be tiring. For those with severe asthma, blood gases may show respiratory alkalosis and mild-to-moderate hypoxia (reflecting an increase in respiratory rate in an attempt to maintain oxygenation) or hypoxia and respiratory acidosis as the $PaCO_2$ rises with fatigue and air trapping. Blood gases may also be helpful if intubation is being considered. Otherwise, their impact taken early in management is minimal. They should never be considered 'routine'.

Full blood examination is usually not useful, as a mild to moderate leukocytosis may be present in the absence of infection. Electrolyte measurements may show a mild hypokalaemia, particularly if frequent doses of β-agonists have been taken.

Management

The emergency management of acute asthma varies according to severity, as defined by the clinical parameters above. The principles are to ensure adequate oxygenation, reverse bronchospasm and minimize the inflammatory response.

Mild asthma

Mild attacks are managed using inhaled β-adrenergic agonists such as salbutamol by metered dose inhaler (MDI) or spacer, the commencement of inhaled corticosteroids if the patient is not already taking them, and education about the disease and the proposed management and follow-up plan.

Moderate asthma

Patients with moderate attacks may require oxygen therapy titrated to achieve oxygen saturation in excess of 92%. The mainstays of therapy are inhaled β-adrenergic agents (by MDI with a spacer or nebulizer) and systemic corticosteroids. The dosage of salbutamol is 5–10 mg by nebulizer or eight puffs by MDI and spacer, every 15 minutes for three doses. Corticosteroids are equally effective given by the oral or intravenous routes. The usual dose is 50 mg prednisolone orally or 250 mg hydrocortisone intravenously. Reassessment, including repeat pulmonary function tests, should occur at least 1 hour after the last dose of β-agonist, with a view to the need for further therapy and decision on hospital admission. For patients who are discharged, oral corticosteroids at a dose of 0.5–1 mg/kg/day, in addition to inhaled steroids at standard doses, should be continued for at least 5 days or until recovery.

Severe asthma

Severe attacks require supplemental oxygen to achieve oxygen saturation in excess of 92%. Because of high respiratory rates it is important to ensure adequate gas flow by the use of either a reservoir-type mask or a Venturi system. High oxygen concentrations may be necessary. Patients should have continuous cardiac and oximetric monitoring, and should receive continuous β-agonist by nebulizer at the doses described above, plus oral or intravenous corticosteroids. The addition of nebulized ipratropium (500 μg 2-hourly) is recommended. If patients fail to respond, an intravenous β-agonist (e.g. salbutamol as a bolus of 250 μg followed by an infusion at 5–10 μg/kg/hour) and/or ventilation should be considered. Intravenous magnesium (1.2–2 g) may be beneficial (see below). Although pooled studies and meta-analyses fail to show benefit in adults, there is anecdotal evidence that selected, rare patients who fail to respond to the above treatment may benefit from i.v. aminophylline (5 mg/kg loading dose over 20 minutes, followed by 0.3–0.6 mg/kg/h). It should not be used without specialist input, and should be used with particular care in patients already taking oral xanthines at admission.

If ventilatory support is required for patients with an acceptable conscious state and airway protective mechanisms, non-invasive ventilation may be suitable. Continuous intensive monitoring is mandatory. If the patient is unsuitable or does not improve with non-invasive ventilation, endotracheal intubation and ventilation will be needed. Ketamine, which has been shown to be an effective bronchodilator, is the induction agent of choice. Care must be taken with ventilation, as severe air trapping results in markedly raised intrathoracic pressure

with cardiovascular compromise. A slow ventilation rate of 6–8 breaths/min with prolonged expiratory periods is recommended.

A number of other therapeutic modalities are outlined below.

Epinephrine (adrenaline)

Small studies have suggested that epinephrine administered by nebulizer and subcutaneously has a similar effect to nebulized salbutamol. These studies are limited by small sample size and the inclusion of patients with mild and moderate asthma.

Epinephrine may have advantages over salbutamol as a parenteral agent. This is based on the theoretical reduction of bronchial mucosal oedema by α-adrenergic mechanisms and inhibition of cholinergic neurotransmission. Anecdotes and small case series indicate that epinephrine is safe and effective, but no studies comparing epinephrine to more selective agents have been published.

Bicarbonate

The postulated mechanism of action of bicarbonate in severe asthma is the facilitation of adrenergic effects and the countering of acidosis, thereby improving respiratory muscle function. To date only small case series support this view, and the quality of evidence is poor. There are also concerns that its administration to patients with pure respiratory acidosis may have deleterious effects.

Non-invasive ventilation (NIV: CPAP and BIPAP)

In acute asthma, NIV has been shown to reduce airways resistance, bronchodilate, counter atelectasis, reduce the work of respiration, and reduce the cardiovascular impact of changes in intrapleural and intrathoracic pressures caused by asthma. It does not, when used alone, improve gas exchange. An unrandomized study of CPAP in combination with pressure support ventilation in patients with severe asthma found rapid correction of pH and improvement in ventilation at lower pressures than were necessary with mechanical ventilation. Other small studies also suggest that NIV may reduce the need for intubation in selected patients and result in faster improvement. NIV also appears to be associated with a lower risk of adverse events than endotracheal intubation. There are currently no guidelines governing the use of NIV in asthma; however, in suitable patients,

a trial of NIV under closely supervised conditions would seem reasonable.

Heliox

Heliox is a blend of 70% helium and 30% oxygen. It may have advantages in asthma because of its better gas flow dynamics. Small studies have had conflicting results. A recent Cochrane Review concluded that the existing evidence did not support the use of heliox in patients with acute severe asthma in the ED.

Ipratropium bromide

β-Agonists have been shown to be more effective bronchodilators than ipratropium bromide when these agents are used alone, but evidence about the impact of combined therapy is contradictory. A meta-analysis concluded that combination therapy resulted in a statistically significant additional improvement in FEV_1, but doubted the clinical significance of this difference. Prospective trials have conflicting results, but there is little if any benefit from the addition of ipratropium to nebulized salbutamol in mild or moderate asthma. Subgroup analysis suggests that there may be benefit from combination nebulized therapy in severe asthma (PEFR <200 L/min). Ipratropium may also have a place in patients who fail to respond adequately to standard initial therapy, particularly those taking long-acting β-agonists, in whom a degree of tolerance to bronchodilation with short-acting β-agonists can occur.

Ketamine

A potential benefit from cautious subinduction doses of ketamine in severe asthma has been suggested. The postulated mechanisms of action of ketamine in asthma are sympathomimetic effects, direct relaxant effects on bronchial smooth muscle, antagonism of histamine and acetylcholine, and a membrane-stabilizing effect. There is only one randomized trial investigating the role of ketamine in acute asthma. It showed that in doses with an acceptable incidence of dysphoria, ketamine did not confer benefit. For intubated patients, there is some preliminary evidence that ketamine infusion (bolus 1 mg/kg, followed by 1 mg/kg/h) may improve blood gas parameters. No outcome benefit has yet been demonstrated.

Magnesium

The postulated mechanisms of action of magnesium in acute asthma are a bronchodilator effect by impeding the uptake of calcium ions into smooth muscle cells, and an anti-inflammatory effect by attenuation of the neutrophil respiratory burst associated with asthma. Magnesium can be administered i.v. or by nebulizer.

With respect to i.v. magnesium, a Cochrane Review suggests that there is no benefit from its use (in addition to standard therapy) in mild or moderate asthma, but that for severe asthma ($FEV_1 < 25\%$ predicted) the addition of magnesium resulted in highly significant increases in FEV_1 and reduced admission rates. No serious adverse reactions were noted in any of the studies.

Regarding nebulized magnesium, doses used have varied from 125 mg as a single dose to 384 mg every 20 minutes for three doses. A Cochrane Review failed to find evidence of benefit over inhaled β-agonists in mild to moderate asthma, but concluded that nebulized inhaled magnesium, in addition to β-agonists, appears to have benefits with respect to improved pulmonary function in patients with severe asthma.

Racemic salbutamol

The salbutamol in common use comprises a racemic mixture of (R) and (S) isomers. The (R) isomer is responsible for the therapeutic effects. The (S) isomer has been shown to oppose the bronchodilatory effects of the (R) isomer and to be proinflammatory. It is also metabolized more slowly than the (R) isomer. The single isomer salbutamol preparation ((R) isomer, levalbuterol) has been postulated to be more potent with fewer side effects, but is much more expensive. A recent review concluded that current clinical trials do not provide evidence of a substantial advantage of levalbuterol over racemic albuterol, although the data are insufficient to determine whether subsets of the patient population might benefit from single isomer therapy.

Leukotriene inhibitors

Leukotriene receptor antagonists (e.g. montelukast) were developed in response to the finding that leukotrienes exhibit biological activity that mimics some of the clinical features of asthma and are found in increased amounts in patients with asthma, especially during exacerbations. They may have a role in the management of chronic asthma. There have been no ED-based studies of acute asthma investigating the potential role of these agents.

Disposition

Patients with severe or life-threatening asthma require admission to an intensive care or respiratory high-dependency unit. Patients with mild disease can usually be discharged after treatment and the formulation of a treatment plan. Those for whom admission or discharge may be in question are the moderate group. Bedside pulmonary function tests can be useful to guide these decisions. Hospital admission is mandated if pre-treatment PEFR or FEV_1 is < 25% of predicted, or post-treatment <40% of predicted.

For those with post-treatment pulmonary function tests in the 40–60% of predicted range, discharge may be possible if improvement is maintained over a number of hours. In addition, other factors should be considered in estimating the safety of discharge. These include history of a previous near-death episode, recent ED visits, frequent admissions to hospital, current or recent steroid use, sudden attacks, poor understanding or compliance, poor home circumstances, and limited access to transport back to hospital in case of deterioration.

All discharged patients should have an asthma action plan to cover the following 24–48 hours, with particular emphasis on what to do if their condition worsens. They should also have a scheduled review, either in the hospital or with a general practitioner within that time. A short course of oral steroids (e.g. 50 mg/day for 5–7 days) is usual.

Controversies

- The relative efficacy and safety of intravenous epinephrine compared to intravenous salbutamol.

- The role of intravenous and nebulized magnesium in severe asthma.

- The role of non-invasive continuous positive airway pressure as an alternative to intubation and mechanical ventilation.

Further reading

Beveridge RC, Grunfeld AF, Hodder RV. Guidelines for the emergency management of asthma in adults. CAEP/CTS Asthma Advisory Committee. Canadian Medical Association Journal 1996; 155: 25–37.

Blitz M, Blitz S, Beasley R, et al. Inhaled magnesium sulfate in the treatment of acute asthma. Cochrane Database System Review 2005 Oct. 19; (4): CD003898.

Fernandez MM, Villagra A, Blanch L. Non-invasive mechanical ventilation in status asthmaticus. Intensive Care Medicine 2001; 27: 486–492.

Haney S, Hancox RJ. Overcoming beta-agonist tolerance: high dose salbutamol and ipratropium bromide. Two randomized controlled trials. Respiratory Research 2007; 8: 19.

Kelly AM, Kerr D, Powell CVE, et al. Is severity assessment after one hour of treatment better for predicting the need for admission in acute asthma? Respiratory Medicine, 2004; 98: 777–781.

Kelly HW. Levalbuterol for asthma: a better treatment? Current Allergy and Asthma Reports 2007; 7: 310–314.

National Asthma Council Australia. Asthma Management Handbook. Melbourne: National Asthma Council Australia, 2006.

Parameswaran K, Belda J, Rowe BH. Addition of intravenous aminophylline to beta2-agonists in adults with acute asthma. Cochrane Database Systematic Reviews. 2000: (4) CD 002742.

Putland M, Kerr D, Kelly AM. Adverse events associated with the use of intravenous adrenaline in emergency department patients presenting with severe asthma. Annals of Emergency Medicine 2006; 47: 559–563.

Rodrigo G, Pollack C, Rodrigo C, et al. Heliox for nonintubated acute asthma patients. Cochrane Database System Review (4): CD002884, October 2006.

Rodrigo G, Rodrigo C, Pollack C, et al. Helium–oxygen mixture for nonintubated acute asthma patients. Cochrane Database Systematic Reviews (1) CD002884, 2001.

Scottish Intercollegiate Guidelines Network. British guidelines on the management of asthma. http://www.sign.ac.uk/guidelines/published/support/guideline63/download.html. Accessed 4 July 2007.

6.3 Community-acquired pneumonia

Mark Putland

ESSENTIALS

1 The term community-acquired pneumonia refers to a syndrome of acute lower respiratory tract infection with a new infiltrate on chest X-ray.

2 Scoring systems such as the Pneumonia Severity Index and the CURB-65 score have been developed to help identify low-risk cases for home treatment, but are poor at identifying high-risk cases that may need ICU care.

3 *Streptococcus pneumoniae* is the most common causative agent. Others vary with demographics, severity and epidemics. A knowledge of local organisms, susceptibilities and outbreaks will allow for better empirical prescribing.

4 β-Lactams and macrolides are the mainstay of antibiotic treatment. Respiratory fluoroquinolones have a role, but cost and emerging resistance may limit it.

5 Use of a locally adapted, structured guideline for management of community-acquired pneumonia is associated with improvement in mortality.

Introduction

Community-acquired pneumonia (CAP) represents a spectrum of disease from mild and self-limiting to severe and life-threatening. The great majority of cases are treated in the community with oral antibiotics, many without radiological confirmation. In the emergency department (ED) CAP is generally not a great diagnostic challenge, but rather represents a challenge of separating the serious cases that require inpatient treatment and supportive care from the mild cases that can be managed with minimal expense to the community and minimal inconvenience to the patient at home. Infrequently CAP presents with the need for urgent, life-saving interventions and critical care.

A great deal of work in recent years has focused on risk stratification of CAP cases and a number of scoring systems have been developed in an attempt to reduce unnecessary admissions and to identify severe cases for early critical care.

A recent change in CAP investigation is the addition of urinary antigen tests (UAT) to the standard work-up of X-ray, blood and sputum microbiology, serology and general tests. The role of routine blood cultures

has also increasingly been questioned in the literature. A rational approach to the use of pathology testing is required to avoid excess healthcare costs and to prevent inappropriate decisions based on spurious or misleading results.

Antibiotic management of CAP has changed little for some decades, but the recent development of new 'respiratory' fluoroquinolones such as moxifloxacin and levofloxacin, and the emergence of drug-resistant *Streptococcus pneumoniae* (DRSP) and community-acquired methicillin-resistant *Staphylococcus aureus* (CA-MRSA) present new challenges in management.

Recent years have seen the publication of comprehensive evidence-based guidelines from the British Thoracic Society (BTS) and the Infectious Diseases Society of America and the American Thoracic Society (IDSA/ATS), as well as similar documents from Japan, Sweden, Canada and other countries. The Australian Therapeutic Guidelines continues to provide up-to-date antibiotic guidelines for the Australian setting. There is mounting evidence that the use of a structured, guideline-based approach to CAP management improves mortality, and that such guidelines should be adapted to local conditions.

Pathogenesis and aetiology

Most cases of CAP result from the aspiration of flora from the upper respiratory tract. Certain organisms, such as *Legionella* spp. and *Mycobacterium tuberculosis*, may be aspirated directly in aerosolized droplets suspended in the atmosphere. Haematogenous spread to the lung also occurs, for example from right-sided endocarditis.

Large-volume aspiration of gastrointestinal and upper respiratory tract contents is normally prevented by a coordinated swallow and intact gag and cough reflexes; however, microaspiration occurs routinely in normal individuals during sleep. Any aspirated matter is generally quickly cleared by the mucociliary escalator and by periodic coughing.

Pathogens that lodge on the lower respiratory mucosa meet with a fine layer of mucus, rich in secreted IgA, that acts to prevent their adhesion and to activate other arms of the immune system, including macrophages, innate (natural killer) and specific (T and B cell) immune cells, the complement cascade, cytokines, neutrophil response and antibody production. These defences are still breached from time to time by the common organisms. Derangement of the defences allows 'opportunistic' organisms to cause infection, such as the Gram-negative rods, anaerobes, *Staphylococcus* spp. and fungi.

Estimates of the rates of occurrence of various organisms implicated in CAP are difficult for several reasons. Isolation of a causative organism occurs in only around 70% of cases in hospital-based studies, less so in community-based ones, and much less commonly in actual clinical practice (particularly in CAP treated in the community). The most common organism isolated in all settings and in all classes of CAP, *Streptococcus pneumoniae*, is one of the easiest to isolate, whereas *Chlamydophila pneumoniae* and *psitacii* (formerly *Chlamydia pneumoniae* and *psitaccii*) and the *Legionella* species present much greater difficulty, potentially skewing the data in favour of pneumococcus. There is a great deal of heterogeneity in the pneumonia studies with regard to underlying patient characteristics, setting, case definition, degree of diagnostic investigation and timing with relation to epidemics, which further complicates interpretation of the data.

Streptococcus pneumoniae

This encapsulated bacterium is isolated from around 30% of cases of CAP in the community, hospital wards and ICU (50–60% of cases where a cause is found) and more commonly when highly sensitive methods are used for its detection. It appears on Gram stain as a Gram-positive coccus in pairs or short chains. In about 25% of cases bacteraemia is identified, and in a few of these there are other foci of invasive disease (such as meningitis).

Traditionally this organism has been extremely sensitive to penicillin, but in recent years drug-resistant Strep. pneumoniae (DRSP) has emerged, with rates varying around the world. Sensitivity is generally described by the minimum concentration of antibiotic required to inhibit growth in vitro (MIC) with an MIC <0.1 mg/L representing a sensitive organism, MIC 0.1–1 mg/L representing intermediate sensitivity, and MIC ≥2 mg/L higher-level resistance. In Australia approximately 16% of isolates express intermediate sensitivity to penicillin, but only around 12% have high-level resistance, with considerable local variation. Invasive strains (isolated from blood or CSF) tend to be more susceptible: in Australia 5% are intermediate or highly resistant. Rates in the UK are lower, where less than 3% of pneumococcal bacteraemias are of intermediate or high penicillin resistance, whereas in Asia resistance is much more common, with 23% of isolates exhibiting intermediate sensitivity and 29% high-level resistance, again with marked local variation. Blood levels achieved by giving 1 g amoxicillin orally 8-hourly or 1.2 g benzyl penicillin i.v. 6-hourly, are sufficient to treat the sensitive and intermediate sensitivity strains. In fact, it is only strains with an MIC > 4 mg/L (<2% of Australian isolates, 3% in England and Wales and 6% in Canada) that present a significant likelihood of treatment failure at these doses.

Macrolide resistance ranges from 15% in the UK to 92% in Vietnam. Again, invasive strains are less commonly resistant than non-invasive ones.

Multiple drug resistance is a problem, with around 17% of Australian isolates demonstrating diminished sensitivity to two or more classes of antibiotic. Whereas respiratory fluoroquinolone resistance remains rare in Australia and the UK, in countries where levofloxacin or moxifloxacin have been more extensively used resistance is already becoming a problem.

Outbreaks occur in crowded institutions, but these make up a small percentage of cases.

Mycoplasma pneumoniae

These single-celled organisms are not strictly bacteria. They lack a cell wall and so are innately insensitive to β-lactams, but are treated by macrolides, tetracyclines and fluoroquinolones. They are fastidious in vitro, and so diagnosis is generally by serological or complement fixation testing. Pneumonia due to Mycoplasma is most common in 5–20-year-olds and is rare in the elderly and in the tropical north of Australia. A 4-yearly cycle of winter epidemics (with the number of reports varying by a factor of 6–7) is well demonstrated in the UK, and surveillance data from Australia suggests that the same phenomenon occurs. Mycoplasma accounts for perhaps 10–15% of cases of CAP. The disease is usually mild and probably self-limiting in adults, although patients with sickle cell disease or cold agglutinin disease are at risk of severe complications.

Legionella species

These organisms are aerobic Gram-negative bacilli which are fastidious in culture. They occur in sources of lukewarm water, probably hosted by fresh water amoebae, and are killed by temperatures above 60°C. Legionella pneumophila serogroup 1, L. pneumophila indeterminant serogroup and L. longbeachiae account for approximately equal shares of legionellosis in Australia. The genus causes a small percentage of cases of mild and moderate CAP (<5%) but is over-represented among severe cases, causing 17.8% of cases in UK intensive care units. Outbreaks occur

due to contaminated water in air conditioning cooling towers and water supplies, and are a significant public health issue. The disease tends to be severe and is often a multisystem illness. Patients on long-term oral steroids are more susceptible, but it is less common among the elderly.

Staphylococcus aureus

Staph. aureus appears on microscopy as clusters of Gram-positive cocci. It is a commensal on the skin and in the oro- and nasopharynx, and may reach the lung by aspiration or by haematogenous spread. It is over-represented in severe disease, accounting for 25% of ICU pneumonia in the UK, and is associated with a high mortality. It is almost universally resistant to penicillin, but most cases are sensitive to flucloxacillin and dicloxacillin. Community-acquired methicillin-resistant strains (CA-MRSA) are an emerging problem. Staphylococcal pneumonia classically occurs following influenza and complicates two-thirds of cases of influenza pneumonia in the ICU.

Mycobacterium tuberculosis

A comprehensive review of TB pathogenesis and treatment is beyond the scope of this chapter. This slow-growing obligate aerobe is able to survive intracellularly in macrophages. The classic pattern of disease is for inhalation of the bacillus to lead to a chronic inflammatory reaction, usually in the right lower lobe, producing a walled-off granuloma that contains surviving organisms and giant macrophages, which gradually becomes calcified. At some time in the future, often in the context of immunocompromise due to steroids, malignancy, HIV, malnutrition or old age, the disease reactivates and lobar pneumonia develops (typically in the right upper lobe). The disease is usually subacute in onset and relentless without treatment. The patient often suffers chronic cough, weight loss, fevers and fatigue. That said, TB presents in many and varied ways, and a high index of suspicion should be maintained. The patient with pulmonary TB and a productive cough presents a significant infection control and public health risk and respiratory isolation must be initiated while the diagnosis is confirmed.

Other important organisms

Non-typable *Haemophilus influenzae* is a rare cause of mild CAP and is uncommon in young patients. Although it is associated with exacerbations of chronic obstructive pulmonary disease (COPD), it is no more common as a cause of CAP in these patients than in the general population. It does, however, become more common with increasing severity of pneumonia and increasing age. Less than 25% of isolates are β-lactamase producing; others are susceptible to aminopenicillins (and somewhat less so to benzylpenicillin). *Moraxella catarrhalis* has similar antibiotic susceptibilities and is less common than *Haemophilus*. Second-generation cephalosporins, tetracyclines or the combination of amoxicillin and clavulanate is adequate if amoxicillin alone fails.

Chlamydophila (formerly *Chlamydia*) *pneumoniae* causes a mild illness and there is some doubt about its role as a pathogen at all. It is sensitive to macrolides and tetracyclines.

Burkholderia pseudomallei occurs in the soil in the tropical north of Australia and in South East Asia. Infection with it (melioidosis) typically causes a severe pneumonia (although any organ may be affected) and 50% of cases are bacteraemic. Bacteraemic melioidosis has been reported to have 50% mortality. It is a problem mainly during the wet season and risk factors include diabetes mellitus, renal failure, chronic lung disease, alcoholism, long-term steroid use and excess kava intake. It is somewhat sensitive to third-generation cephalosporins, although better treated with ceftazidime or carbapenems. It is intrinsically resistant to aminoglycosides. The Gram-negative rod *Acinetobacter baumanii* occurs in a similar area, time of year and group of people, and also causes severe pneumonia. It is generally treated with aminoglycosides. Expert consultation should be sought.

Influenza A and B are common causes of pneumonia in adults. Disease may be mild, moderate or severe. Coinfection with *Staph. aureus* is a well-described complication. Clinical and radiological differentiation from bacterial pneumonia is unreliable, and diagnosis is usually made with viral studies on nasopharyngeal or bronchial aspirates or on serological testing after convalescence.

Anaerobic organisms are generally aspirated in patients with poor dentition. Edentulous patients are thus protected, and these organisms are actually rare in aspiration pneumonia among nursing home patients.

The Gram-negative rods are a varied group of opportunistic agents which all carry a high risk of severe pneumonia and mortality. They are more common in nosocomial pneumonia than in CAP. They include *Pseudomonas aeruginosa*, *Serratia* spp., and *Klebsiella pneumoniae*. Emergence of antibiotic resistance during treatment is a particular problem with *Pseudomonas*, and antibiotics from two classes should be used concurrently if infection is proven or highly likely.

Epidemiology

Rates of pneumonia are difficult to estimate because of issues of case definition and the fact that the majority of cases occur unstudied in the community. However, data from around the world suggest that the incidence is around 5–11/1000/year in 16–59-year-olds in the community, and over 30/1000/year in those over 75. The incidence of CAP requiring hospitalization in the UK is less than 5/1000/year and comprises probably less than 50% of CAP cases. On the other hand, CAP accounts for 8–10% of medical admissions to intensive care units.

Rates of admission to ICU vary enormously around the world and probably represent resource availability and usage more than differences in disease severity. New Zealand studies report 1–3% of cases needing ICU, whereas in the UK it is around 5%. Much higher percentages are reported from the United States.

The mortality rate of CAP treated in the community is thought to be very low, probably <1%. Mortality among hospitalized patients varies depending on health service, but is around 5–10%. Mortality among patients admitted to ICU with CAP is much higher, but the statistics are much more varied, again depending on ICU admission criteria. In the UK, where almost all ICU patients require mechanical ventilation, mortality is 50%, but in Spain and France it is around 35%. Mortality obviously varies with severity of disease (see the section below on severity assessment) and also with organism. *Staph. aureus*, Gram-negative bacilli (especially *Pseudomonas*), *Burkholderia pseudomallei* and *Legionella* spp. all carry a higher than baseline mortality, whereas *Mycoplasma* and *Chlamydophila* spp. have lower mortality.

Influenza and pneumonia (ICD codes J10–J18) account for 2.3% of all deaths in Australia and are a contributing cause in 13.3%.

Associations between particular risk factors and particular organisms in CAP patients are weak, and it is important to remember that routine questioning about risk factors is likely to be misleading. For example, despite the well-known association between *Chlamydophila psittaci* and sick parrots, 80% of patients with psittacosis have no history of bird contact. Stronger associations are those between *Staph. aureus* and influenza, between *Staph. aureus* and intravenous drug use (IVDU), and between *Legionella* and travel. Workers in the animal handling and slaughtering industries are at risk of infection with *Coxiella burnetii* (Q fever). Awareness of any local epidemics is important (particularly outbreaks of *Mycoplasma* or legionellosis).

Prevention

Prevention of pneumonia in the developed world centres on vaccination for influenza and pneumococcus. In developing regions, the provision of adequate nutrition and housing is more important. Legionellosis is avoided by appropriate design and maintenance of air-conditioning and water supply systems in large buildings. It is worth noting that aspiration pneumonia is not prevented by the use of nasogastric or PEG feeding tubes.

Clinical features

Pneumonia should be suspected in patients with:

- Fever
- New cough
- Rigors
- Change in sputum colour
- Pleuritic chest pain
- Dyspnoea.

Many patients with these features, however, will not have pneumonia, and certain groups of patients (particularly the elderly) may have pneumonia with few or none of these features.

A normal chest examination makes pneumonia less likely but does not rule it out. The classically described progression of chest examination findings is from crackles and reduced air entry in the first days, to a dull percussion note and bronchial breathing which persists until resolution begins at around day 7–10, when crackles return. Fever is said to be persistent until a 'crisis', followed by resolution. Of course the actual clinical reality may bear little resemblance to this. The presence of classic findings in the chest may precede radiological abnormality by several hours, particularly in pneumococcal pneumonia.

Much has been made of the role of the clinical syndrome as a predictor of aetiology, but the evidence shows it to be unreliable. Previously 'typical' and 'atypical' pneumonia were differentiated clinically, but there is now a general consensus that these terms should be abandoned as they are misleading. The term 'atypical organism', however, has persisted as an umbrella term for the *Chlamydophila* spp., the *Legionella* spp. and *Mycoplasma*. With these caveats in mind, there are certain associations that should be considered (Table 6.3.1).

The term 'community-acquired pneumonia' is as opposed to hospital-acquired pneumonia,

which is generally defined as pneumonia occurring in a patient who has been an inpatient in hospital in the last 10 or 14 days. Patients with AIDS, cystic fibrosis, current chemotherapy or active haematological malignancy presenting with pneumonia should be considered to be presenting with a complication of their underlying condition rather than with CAP. The question of how to classify patients with pneumonia presenting from nursing homes remains unresolved. Nursing home patients have tended to be overlooked by authors of guidelines on CAP management, and the issue is clouded by ethical questions around care of the debilitated elderly. Nursing home status carries an increased mortality risk and an increased risk of both aspiration pneumonitis and infection with *Staph. aureus* and aerobic Gram-negative bacilli.

Differential diagnosis

The clinical syndrome of pneumonia is non-specific and the differential diagnosis is broad. CXR findings of a lobar infiltrate, however, narrow the possibilities significantly. Underlying malignancy should always be considered, especially in older smokers. Pulmonary embolus (PE) is less likely in the presence of a lobar infiltrate, but this should be differentiated from the wedge-shaped opacification of a pulmonary infarction due to PE. Bi-basal pneumonia can be very difficult to distinguish from left ventricular failure, especially in the elderly patient in whom clinical signs and white cell count can be unreliable. CXR changes may be pre-existing, such as in localized fibrosis due to radiotherapy, or when there has been a recent pneumonia with opacification yet to resolve. Aspiration pneumonitis should be differentiated from pneumonia as antibiotic therapy is less likely to be of benefit. The main indicators are on history (neurological deficit, loss of consciousness, choking while eating or vomiting in the patient with diminished airway reflexes) although most episodes go unwitnessed.

Complications

Pleural effusion is a fairly common occurrence in hospitalized patients with CAP, occurring in 36–57% of admitted patients. Effusion detectable on CXR is an indicator of severity, especially if bilateral. Persistent

fever raises the likelihood of an effusion. The majority of effusions resolve with antibiotic treatment, but empyema requires drainage. As effusion and empyema are radiologically indistinguishable, any significant effusion should be aspirated. Cloudy fluid, pus cells or organisms on Gram stain, or a pH of <7.2 indicate empyema and the need for drainage. Aspiration will also provide a specimen for aetiological diagnosis, although the yield is not high.

Lung abscess is a rare complication, most common in the alcoholic, debilitated or aspiration pneumonia patient. Some will respond to antibiotics, but drainage is often required. *Staph. aureus,* anaerobes and Gram-negatives are more likely culprits and polymicrobial infection is common. Tuberculosis should be considered in any patient with a cavitating lesion.

Severe sepsis syndromes are a relatively common occurrence in CAP. Approximately 40% of hospitalized patients develop non-pulmonary organ dysfunction, with 28% having evidence of it at presentation. Septic shock develops in 4–5% of cases and is manifest at presentation in just under half of these. The presence or absence of systemic inflammatory response syndrome (SIRS) criteria has little or no predictive value for death, severe sepsis or septic shock in CAP; however, the Pneumonia Severity Index (see below) does correlate with the likelihood of severe sepsis.

Respiratory failure is the most common reason for ICU admission in CAP. In patients with moderate to severe disease a widened A-a gradient can be detected, with PCO_2 being depressed as the patient increases minute volume to compensate for failure of gas exchange. As severity increases the PCO_2 will return to normal as the patient tires, and PO_2 will fall. Type II respiratory failure generally occurs late.

Renal failure may occur in any case of severe CAP but is particularly associated with legionellosis. Multiorgan failure may occur as a result of severe sepsis.

Investigation

Imaging

Chest X-ray

The presence of a new infiltrate on CXR remains central to the diagnosis of

---

Table 6.3.1 Clinical features associated with specific organisms

Streptococcus pneumoniae
- Increasing age
- High fever
- High acuity
- Pleurisy

Bacteraemic pneumococcal pneumonia
- Female
- Diabetic
- Alcoholic
- COPD
- Dry cough

Legionella spp.
- Young and previously healthy patient
- Smoker
- Multisystem illness (LFT abnormality, elevated CK, GIT upset, neurological disturbance)
- More severe illness

Mycoplasma
- Young and previously healthy patient
- Antibiotic use prior to presenting to hospital
- Isolated respiratory illness

Streptococcus aureus
- IVDU
- Severe illness
- History of influenza

Gram-negative rods
- Alcoholic
- Nursing home resident

pneumonia. Diagnosis without CXR is shown to be unreliable, although a normal chest examination makes the diagnosis unlikely.

CXR has proved to be an unreliable indicator of aetiology, but some clues may be found. *Mycoplasma* is less likely in the presence of homogeneous shadowing, but is suggested by lymphadenopathy. Multilobar infiltrates and pleural effusions make bacteraemic streptococcal pneumonia more likely, whereas a multilobar infiltrate with pneumatocoeles, cavitation and pneumothorax is suggestive of *Staph. aureus*. *Klebsiella* tends towards the right upper lobe, but the described association between this agent and a bulging horizontal fissure is unsupported by evidence.

Tuberculosis should always be considered in cases of an upper lobe infiltrate, especially in the presence of a Ghon focus or calcified nodule, usually found in the right lower lobe.

Clues to severity may be found on the CXR (see below).

The role of the repeat X-ray is unclear. The rate of improvement is quite variable. It is slower with increasing age, presence of comorbidity, multilobar infiltrates and streptococci (especially bacteraemic) or *Legionella* as pathogens. *Legionella*, in fact, is characterized by worsening radiological appearance after admission. The role of a convalescent film is likewise unclear. Rates of underlying lung cancer vary in studies of patients with pneumonia, and most cases are diagnosed on the acute film. Smokers over 50 are particularly at risk, and routine convalescent imaging should be considered in this group.

CT

CT currently has a limited role in diagnosis of pneumonia because of the cost, radiation dose and lack of a clear benefit over plain CXR. In some cases a diagnosis may be made on CT when another diagnosis is being excluded (e.g. CTPA for exclusion of pulmonary embolus).

General pathology

The roles of non-microbiological pathological testing in CAP are to help confirm the diagnosis, to assess severity, to identify complications and to screen for underlying or comorbid conditions. With this in mind, the majority of previously well young people with non-severe pneumonia are unlikely to benefit from routine tests.

Full blood count

The full blood count is routine in patients requiring hospitalization with pneumonia. Anaemia, thrombocytopenia, severe leukocytosis and leukopenia are all markers of severity (see below). Polycythaemia may indicate dehydration or underlying chronic hypoxia. A white cell count $>15\,000$ cells/mm^3 is suggestive of a bacterial cause (especially *Strep. pneumoniae*) but is insensitive and non-specific.

Urea and electrolytes

Urea, electrolytes and creatinine are also routinely measured in the hospitalized patient. Hyponatraemia (Na <130 mmol/L) and elevated urea (≥ 11 mmol/L) are proven markers of severe pneumonia. Acute renal impairment is a relatively common complication of severe pneumonia, whereas chronic renal failure is a risk factor for severe disease.

Liver function tests

Liver function tests frequently demonstrate some abnormality, although this may not change management. Chronic liver disease is a risk factor for severe pneumonia.

Blood gas testing

Measurement of arterial blood gases has been common practice in patients hospitalized with pneumonia. Recent evidence demonstrates that a venous blood gas is acceptable for assessment of acid–base status and may be a valid screening tool for hypercapnoea. Transcutaneous oxygen saturation measurement (SpO$_2$) is likewise an acceptable screening tool for hypoxia, although it becomes inaccurate when SpO$_2$ is $<90\%$.

Inflammatory markers

Measurement of CRP remains contentious. The recent British Thoracic Society guidelines update concluded that 'there is no clear consensus in the literature about value of CRP in differentiating between infective causes. There is no value of CRP in severity assessment'. At best, CRP may have a role in differentiation between exacerbation of COPD and pneumonia or non-infective causes and pneumonia in uncertain cases.

Both serum procalcitonin and D-dimer have been found to correlate with severity of pneumonia, but their discriminatory value and role, if any, remain undefined.

Testing for aetiology/microbiology

As discussed above, achieving an aetiological diagnosis in CAP is difficult, even in the research setting in tertiary referral centres. The advantages of doing so include the opportunity to tailor therapy, to detect outbreaks such as Legionnaire's disease, influenza or *Mycoplasma*, and to identify resistant organisms. An emerging concern in recent years is that of bioterrorism, which may be identified early due to reporting of aetiological diagnoses. A further consideration is the paucity of published data on the aetiology of pneumonia, particularly from Australia and New Zealand. Current knowledge depends heavily upon laboratory reports to surveillance authorities and 'accumulated knowledge' rather than scientific studies.

Disadvantages of an aggressive diagnostic approach are the cost compared to the low yield, the risk of inappropriate changes to therapy based on false positive results from contaminants, the long lag time to obtain a result (particularly from culture and paired serology), the potential to delay treatment while specimens are obtained, and the exposure of the patient to added unpleasant and invasive procedures (such as multiple venepunctures for blood culture). Moreover, it is uncommon for therapy to be streamlined despite a microbiological diagnosis, and the only randomized controlled trial comparing empiric to directed therapy found no benefit to a pathogen-directed approach, although there was a small mortality benefit found in the ICU subgroup.

Sputum

Sputum can be collected for microscopy and for culture. The two should be considered separately as they are very different tests and are likely to be valuable in different settings. The value of sputum collection has been debated, however. Unfortunately, many patients are unable to produce sputum, and waiting for them to do so may cause significant delays to antibiotic treatment.

Microscopy (generally with Gram stain, although Zeil–Neilsen stain for acid-fast bacilli should be requested if tuberculosis is suspected) can potentially provide useful guidance for empiric prescribing as well as an indication of whether the specimen is of sufficient quality for culture to be useful.

If a good specimen can be obtained, transport is prompt, the laboratory staff are experienced in its examination and antibiotics are yet to be given, then a negative Gram stain is strong evidence against *Staphylococcus*, *Pseudomonas* and Gram-negative rods. A sputum Gram stain showing Gram-positive cocci in clusters is an indication to include anti-staphylococcal treatment. Gram-positive diplococci or cocci in short chains are suggestive of *Strep. pneumoniae* infection, but this is less reliable.

Sputum culture has a higher sensitivity than Gram stain and provides more definite identification, typing and sensitivity data; however, results are not available when treatment is started and colonization may be hard to distinguish from infection, particularly if the Gram stain was negative or not performed. Special culture is indicated if *Legionella* or *M. tuberculosis* is to be identified.

The sensitivity of both microscopy and culture declines if antibiotic therapy has already started, and even under ideal conditions neither is highly sensitive or specific. Likewise, tuberculosis requires both special stains and culture media as well as prolonged culture time. The provision of good clinical details to the laboratory, including suspected organism, timing of specimen and use of antibiotics, is essential.

Blood culture

Blood cultures have traditionally been recommended for all patients admitted to hospital with suspected pneumonia. More recently the performance of blood cultures in admitted pneumonia patients has been linked to hospital accreditation in the USA. The most common non-contaminant organism isolated is *Pneumococcus*, which is generally covered by empiric treatment and yields are generally low (around 7% overall and 25% at most in pneumococcal pneumonia). Contaminants are found with similar frequency. That said, a positive result (other than coagulase-negative *Staphylococcus*) is highly specific for a microbiological aetiology.

A rational approach is to limit blood culture use to cases where yield is higher, the likelihood of a resistant or non-pneumococcal organism is higher, the consequences of inappropriate prescription are greatest, or where there is concern about a significant outbreak or epidemic.

Independent predictors of a positive blood culture in CAP include coexistent liver disease, systolic blood pressure <90 mmHg, temperature <35°C or ≥40°C, pulse ≥125/min, urea ≥11 mmol/L, Na <130 mmol/L, WBC <5000 cells/mm^3 or >20 000 cells/mm^3, and lack of prior antibiotic therapy. A prediction rule has been developed based on these variables, with the presence of two or more predictors associated with a 16% rate of positive blood culture. These indicators are also markers of severity, and it is patients with severe pneumonia who are most at risk of an adverse outcome if initial antibiotics are not sufficient. A positive pneumococcal urinary antigen test is associated with a higher yield from blood culture and may be an indication for performing blood culture to monitor community resistance rates.

Current British Thoracic Society guidelines indicate that blood cultures have little role in non-severe pneumonia, and the IDSA/ATS guidelines recommend blood cultures for ICU patients and those with cavitation, leukopenia, alcoholism, chronic liver disease, asplenia, a positive pneumococcal UAT or a pleural effusion.

Urinary antigen testing

A relatively new addition in the field of diagnostic testing for CAP is the urinary antigen test (UAT). The two commonly available are the *Legionella* and pneumococcal antigen tests. Both are fast and simple to perform, and minimally affected by the use of antibiotics. The pneumococcal UAT is 50–80% sensitive and >90% specific. False positives occur in children with chronic respiratory illness and colonization with pneumococcus, and in adults who have had CAP in the last 3 months. The *Legionella* UAT is probably highly sensitive and specific for *L. pneumophila* serogroup 1, is positive from day 1, and remains so for up to 3 weeks.

The precise role of these tests remains uncertain, however. CAP is assumed to be pneumococcal by default, and so a positive test provides little helpful information, whereas a negative test is of little predictive value. As discussed above, the UAT might be used as a triage tool to identify patients who will have a higher yield from blood cultures. The *Legionella* UAT identifies only *Legionella pneumophila* serogroup 1, which accounts for less than half of cases in Australia. It is currently unclear whether a positive *Legionella* UAT justifies streamlining to macrolide monotherapy in sick inpatients, or whether it mandates upgrading from oral to i.v. macrolides. A positive *Legionella* UAT is associated with ICU admission, perhaps because the higher antigen load in positive cases represents a greater infective burden. A negative *Legionella* UAT, however, does not rule out legionellosis, as other species and serogroups are not detected.

Other tests

Serology has little to offer the emergency management of CAP but has a public health role if an outbreak of viral or 'atypical' pneumonia is suspected. If symptoms have been ongoing for more than 7 days then a high titre of *Mycoplasma* or *Legionella* IgM is diagnostic, but otherwise paired serology weeks apart is required, with the diagnosis coming only after treatment is completed.

Influenza rapid point-of-care testing has a low sensitivity (50–70%) and cross-reacts with adenovirus. A positive test may be an indication for treatment with antivirals, where available, and may be useful in outbreak detection, although it is unlikely to be superior to physician judgement in this role. Influenza direct fluorescent antibody testing is more reliable but takes 2 hours and requires special laboratory skills. It is used for identification of specific strains of influenza (e.g. H5N1).

Severity assessment

A key clinical problem in patients with suspected CAP is assessment of severity. The great majority of CAP cases are mild and self-limiting, although antibiotic treatment shortens the illness. However, a significant minority of cases cause an acutely debilitating illness, and a small minority are life-threatening. Attempts at formalizing the process of severity assessment have focused on two aims: identifying those who can safely be managed at home, thereby reducing unnecessary admissions and unplanned readmissions; and identifying those who are likely to need ICU care, with the aim of reducing mortality and complications from delayed recognition of severe disease while avoiding overuse of ICU. Those seeking the former goal have met with a great deal of success, but the latter has remained elusive. A number of scoring systems have been developed and validated, including the Pneumonia Severity Index (PSI), the British Thoracic Society's BTS, modified BTS, CRB, CURB and CURB-65 scores, the American Thoracic Society's ATS, modified ATS (m-ATS) and revised ATS (r-ATS) scores, and the Spanish SEPAR score.

Proven markers of severity

The following have all been defined as markers of severity in various studies:

- Demographic factors
  - Increasing age
  - Residence in a nursing home or being bedridden
  - Male gender
  - Comorbidity
  - Congestive cardiac failure, diabetes mellitus, coronary artery disease, chronic lung disease, liver disease, cerebrovascular disease, chronic renal failure and neoplastic disease
- Examination findings
  - Respiratory rate >30/min or <6/min
  - Confusion (AMTS <8 or new disorientation to time, place or person)
  - Systolic BP < 90 mmHg, diastolic BP< 60 mmHg or septic shock requiring aggressive fluid resuscitation or vasopressors
  - Temperature <35°C or ≥40°C
  - Heart rate ≥125/min
- Haematological
  - Haematocrit <30%
  - White cell count <4000 cells/mm^3 or > 20 000 cells/mm^3
  - Platelets <100 000 cells/mm^3
- Biochemical
  - Urea elevated (cut-offs vary)
  - Sodium <130 mmol/L
  - Glucose >14 mmol/L
  - Arterial pH <7.35
  - Hypoxia (PaO$_2$ <60 mmHg, SpO$_2$ <92%, PaO$_2$:FiO$_2$ <250 mmHg)

- Radiological features
  - Bilateral or multilobar involvement
  - Effusions, especial bilateral
  - Worsening radiological changes after admission in the ICU patient
- Microbiological
  - Positive blood culture (not available at time of initial assessment)
  - Strep. pneumoniae, Gram-negative bacilli, Staph. aureus, and Ps. Aeruginosa.

The Pulmonary Severity Index (PSI)

The PSI was derived by retrospective chart review and validated both retrospectively and prospectively in separate groups of patients in the late 1980s and early 1990s. In all, over 54 000 patients and 275 hospitals from across the USA and Canada were involved in the study. The rule is a two-step process, with low-risk patients being identified on clinical grounds alone in the first step and then all other patients being further differentiated on the basis of age and 19 dichotomized and weighted clinical and investigation features into four further groups (Tables 6.3.2 and 6.3.3).

Despite its rigorous derivation and validation, criticisms have been levelled at the PSI. A major issue is its complexity. The large number of variables and their differing weights are difficult to remember and the score is complex to calculate. Also, the PSI is heavily weighted towards elderly patients. A young patient, compensating well early in an illness, might be significantly hypoxic and still be stratified into the lowest risk group. Social factors and the presence of unusual comorbidities are not accounted for, nor is the presence of bilateral or multilobar infiltrates on CXR. Moreover, the PSI has subsequently been used to stratify patients not only for discharge and admission but also for ICU care and for antibiotic regimen, purposes for which it was not originally intended.

In its favour, the variables used by the PSI are all available at the end of a typical work-up, particularly as there are data supporting the substitution of venous pH for arterial pH. PSI calculators are now readily available which makes calculation much easier.

Clinical judgement is recommended when using the PSI. The tool has been well validated for identifying patients who may be safely treated at home, but young patients, particularly if hypoxic (SpO$_2$ <94% on air), should be assessed with caution. A patient who is vomiting, homeless or unreliable should not be discharged on oral antibiotics from the ED, and some underlying conditions may warrant admission for relatively mild pneumonia, such as advanced neuromuscular disease and general frailty.

Patients likely to require ICU care are particularly poorly identified by the PSI and all other scoring systems. It is important to apply clinical judgement together with the PSI score and consider other markers of severity and the general clinical picture when deciding whether ICU might be needed in the patient with CAP.

Finally, the PSI was derived and validated in adult patients with no recent hospitalization who did not have HIV. Its use in immunocompromised patients has been investigated in one study and was found to perform well in patients with HIV, solid organ transplant or treatment with immunosuppressive drugs, and poorly in patients with haematological malignancy, on chemotherapy or after chest radiotherapy or bone marrow transplantation.

The CURB-65 score

The British Thoracic Society (BTS) currently recommends use of this score for stratification of CAP patients. The system stratifies patients on the basis of a scale of 0–6, with one point scored for each of:

- Confusion of new onset (AMTS <8 or new disorientation to time, place or person)
- Urea >7 mmol/L
- Respiratory rate ≥30/min
- Blood pressure <90 mmHg (systolic) or ≤ 60mmHg (diastolic), and
- Age ≥65 years.

Scores are correlated with risk of death and site of care is suggested (Table 6.3.4).

The CURB-65 score has the significant advantage of simplicity, and has been shown to perform as well as a previous two-stage BTS score. It is easy to remember and quick to calculate. It is worth noting, for community

Table 6.3.2   Calculating the PSI (After Fine MJ, Auble TE, Yealy DM, et al. A prediction rule to identify low-risk patients with community-acquired pneumonia. New England Journal of Medicine 1997; 336: 243–250.)

Step 1

The patient is Class I and needs no further investigation if they are ≤50 years old and have none of the following:

History
- Neoplastic disease
- Liver disease
- Renal disease
- Congestive cardiac failure
- Cerebrovascular disease

Examination
- Acutely altered mental state
- Respiratory rate ≥30/min
- Systolic BP <90mmHg
- Temperature <35°C or ≥40°C
- Pulse rate ≥125/min

Step 2

If the above is not satisfied then the PSI score need to be calculated as follows:

Factor	Score
Demographic	
• Age	• Age in years
• Sex	• 10 if female
• Nursing home (not hostel) resident	• +10
Coexisting illness	
• Neoplastic disease	• +30
• Liver disease	• +20
• Congestive cardiac failure	• +10
• Cerebrovascular disease	• +10
• Chronic renal disease	• +10
Signs on examination	
• Acutely altered mental state	• +20
• Respiratory rate ≥30/min	• +20
• Systolic blood pressure <90mmHg	• +20
• Temperature <35°C or ≥40°C	• +15
• Pulse rate ≥125/min	• +10
Investigations	
• Arterial pH <7.35	• +30
• Serum urea ≥11mmol/L	• +20
• Serum sodium <130 mmol/L	• +20
• Serum glucose ≥14mmol/L	• +10
• Haematocrit <30%	• +10
• PaO_2 <60mmHg or SpO_2<90%	• +10
• Pleural effusion on CXR	• +10

Table 6.3.3   Mortality and PSI class

Score	Class	30-Day mortality (%)
N/A	I	0.1
1–70	II	0.6
71–90	III	0.9
91–130	IV	9.3
>130	V	27

The CURB-65 score has been compared with the PSI as well as the various ATS scores in a number of studies. All perform similarly well, with the PSI generally gaining some increase in sensitivity and specificity for death and ICU admission at the expense of greater complexity. All are strong at identifying well patients who can be safely treated at home as long as clinical judgement is brought to bear, as discussed above. However, all are fairly poor at identifying patients at high risk of death, and should be used cautiously in this context.

At present no score is a substitute for regular review by a senior clinician during the hospital stay.

Treatment

Site of care

As discussed above, the PSI and the CURB-65 score are both useful for identifying patients who are well enough to be discharged home as long as oxygenation, psychosocial factors and the overall clinical picture are considered. Typically cases with of PSI class I or CURB-65 score of 0 can be treated at home with confidence, and cases with PSI class II or CURB-65 score of 1 are probably safe to discharge as well.

Cases of intermediate severity (PSI III or CURB-65 score 2) are likely to benefit from a short period of supervised hospital treatment to ensure that antibiotics are given effectively and to monitor for any deterioration. Emergency Observation Units or Short Stay Units are ideal for this purpose. Alternatively, a 'hospital in the home' service may be appropriate, particularly if it incorporates early medical review.

More severe cases should be treated in hospital, with early referral to ICU if appropriate.

General supportive care

For the patient being discharged to the community, general advice regarding rest, analgesia for chest wall pain and maintenance of adequate hydration and nutrition is appropriate. Physiotherapy is of no proven benefit. All discharged patients should undergo scheduled medical review within 24–48 hours in case of deterioration.

practitioners, that the CRB-65 score (CURB-65 without the urea measurement) performs similarly well, and that patients with a CRB-65 score of 0 are generally safely managed in the community whereas those with a score of 1 or more should be assessed at hospital. The CURB-65 score has been validated in thousands of patients from the UK and other countries, and is the result of a process of refinement of a series of other validated scoring systems.

Score	Risk of death or ICU admission (%)	Comments
0	0.7	Low risk. Non-severe pneumonia. May be suitable for
1	3.2	treatment at home
2	13	Increased risk of death. Consider for short inpatient or hospital-supervised outpatient treatment
3	17	High risk of death. Treat as inpatients with severe
4	41.5	pneumonia. Consider use of ICU
5	57	

Table 6.3.4 Mortality and the CURB-65 score

For the admitted patient similar measures will be required. Hydration may need to be supplemented with intravenous fluids, and in severe or prolonged illness nutritional support will be required. Oxygen should be provided to maintain $SpO_2 > 95\%$ ($PaO_2 > 60$ mmHg). A lower SpO_2/PaO_2 may be desirable in patients with severe COAD.

The role of non-invasive ventilatory support (NIV) in respiratory failure due to pneumonia is controversial. In patients with underlying COPD it is almost certainly of benefit. In other patients it has been shown to raise SpO_2 and reduce heart rate, but deterioration requiring intubation is common and patients intubated after a failure of a prolonged trial of NIV fare worse than those intubated early. At best it is probably a temporizing measure if intubation is not immediately possible, or if it is not immediately clear that intubation is appropriate.

Invasive ventilation should be low volume (6 mL/kg of ideal body weight) even if hypercapnia results. Severe sepsis syndrome and septic shock should be recognized and treated early and aggressively.

The use of structured guidelines for CAP management, covering a range of interventions, has been shown to reduce hospital mortality. The particular guidelines used seem less important than that they are locally appropriate (taking into account local patient demographics, comorbidity spectrum, social issues, organism prevalence and antibiotic resistance patterns). There is wide local variation noted in antibiotic resistance rates, both between and within countries.

Antibiotic treatment

Initial therapy in CAP is almost always empiric, with antibiotics selected to cover the likely organisms. *Strep. pneumoniae* is generally treated with a β-lactam. The 'atypical' organisms are generally covered with a macrolide, although a tetracycline is acceptable if oral therapy is being used. These also provide cover against *Legionella* spp. Addition of specific coverage for Gram-negative coliforms, *Staph. aureus*, *Pseudomonas aeruginosa*, *Burkholderia pseudomallei* and *Acinetobacter baumanii* are added when severity or the clinical or epidemiological picture warrant. Monotherapy with a fluoroquinolone is an alternative to the combination of β-lactam and macrolide in mild pneumonia, but emerging resistance is a problem.

Drug-resistant *Strep. pneumoniae* (DRSP) is a growing problem around the world, particularly in Asia, but it remains an uncommon cause of pneumonia in Australia and the UK. Macrolide resistance is common in vitro, but the significance of this has been questioned. Modern macrolides are concentrated at the site of infection, and until recently few cases of treatment failure with macrolide monotherapy had been reported. Recently, macrolide resistance among pneumococci has been recognized as a significant clinical problem.

Community-acquired MRSA (CA-MRSA) is another looming problem, although it has mainly been reported from paediatric skin infections rather than from CAP. It tends to be less broadly resistant than HA-MRSA. Ominously, the genes for drug resistance in CA-MRSA tend to be associated with the gene for Panton–Valentine leukocidin, which is associated with necrotizing pneumonia, respiratory failure and shock.

As discussed above, the clinical and radiological pictures are often unhelpful in assessing the microbiological aetiology of CAP. In the absence of a positive UAT or sputum Gram stain it is unlikely that initial treatment decisions will be made on data other than the clinical picture and a knowledge of local pathogens. With increasing severity of pneumonia antibiotic coverage is generally broadened for two reasons, as organisms other than *Strep. pneumoniae* become more likely and there is more to be lost by failure to cover the causative agent in the first instance.

Despite the widespread dissemination of antibiotic guidelines, over-prescribing of broad-spectrum antibiotics remains a problem. Pneumonia guidelines are often generalized to non-pneumonic lower respiratory tract infections such as bronchitis and exacerbations of COPD, and severe pneumonia tends to be over-diagnosed. Over-prescription of broad-spectrum antibiotics contributes to increases in antibiotic associated enteropathy and *Clostridium difficile* infection, in other side effects such as anaphylaxis, in healthcare costs, and in the spread of resistant organisms.

The PSI has been recommended by the *Australian Therapeutic Guidelines: Antibiotic* as a tool for selection of antibiotic coverage. It is to be noted that this is not directly supported by the available evidence, although it is in line with the principles discussed above.

Mild pneumonia

Oral therapy is preferred in patients well enough to be treated at home who are able to tolerate oral medications and are likely to be compliant with a treatment regimen. Given the known spectrum of pathogens as described above, whether to use a β-lactam alone or in combination with dedicated 'atypical cover' is debated. A Cochrane Review has found no benefit in the addition of 'atypical cover', although most of the studies examined compared fluoroquinolone monotherapy to β-lactam monotherapy. In the UK, where the 4-yearly cycle of *Mycoplasma* epidemics is well described, amoxicillin as a single agent is recommended, with erythromycin as an alternative, if tolerable, unless a *Mycoplasma* outbreak is known to be occurring. In the USA the practice of using macrolide monotherapy is well established but it can fail against DRSP. Australian guidelines recommend monotherapy with amoxicillin unless there is specific concern about atypical organisms.

The combination of a macrolide with amoxicillin has always been shown to be effective against DRSP, and the combination increases the likelihood of covering *H. influenzae* adequately. Cefuroxime is an alternative to amoxicillin as it has a similar spectrum, including moderate activity against *Haemophilus*. Monotherapy with a fluoroquinolone such as moxifloxacin is an alternative for mild pneumonia and is useful if immediate hypersensitivity to penicillins is suspected; however, these drugs remain expensive, and treatment failure due to resistance is starting to be reported in parts of the world. There is concern that use of these agents will increase resistance to important reserve agents such as ciprofloxacin.

In cases where a single dose of i.v. antibiotic is to be given before discharge from the ED benzylpenicillin is preferred to amoxicillin for its narrower spectrum of activity. Amoxicillin is preferred for oral treatment as oral phenoxymethyl penicillin is unlikely to reach adequate levels to cover intermediate resistant DRSP, and is of no value against *H. influenzae*.

Patients who prefer to be treated at home but who are unlikely to comply with oral therapy can be treated with i.m. procaine penicillin 1.5 g daily for 5 days, which can be supplemented by a supervised daily dose of oral azithromycin.

Moderate pneumonia

For patients requiring hospitalization, in light of the likely pathogens including atypicals which account for up to 20% of cases, the combination of benzylpenicillin or amoxicillin and a macrolide remains most appropriate. The β-lactam should be given intravenously to guarantee sufficient blood levels to treat intermediate-sensitivity *Strep. pneumoniae*. If non-immediate penicillin hypersensitivity is thought to be a problem then a third-generation cephalosporin should be used intravenously instead, and in cases of immediate hypersensitivity to penicillin a fluoroquinolone is indicated.

A sputum specimen should be sent for Gram stain if this service is available, and if Gram-negative bacilli are seen gentamicin can be added or a third-generation cephalosporin substituted for penicillin/amoxicillin.

Severe pneumonia

Although *Strep. pneumoniae* remains the most common pathogen, there is an over-representation of *Staph. aureus*, *Legionella* spp. and Gram-negatives in severe cases. Moreover, it is of greater importance in this group that initial therapy be adequate. Therefore, empiric cover needs to be broader than for the less severe cases. The most commonly recommended approach is to use a combination of a third-generation cephalosporin with an intravenous macrolide. Alternatively, the combination of benzylpenicillin, an aminoglycoside and an intravenous macrolide has also been recommended, although head-to-head studies demonstrating equivalence of this to the former, more established regimen are lacking. Staphylococcal pneumonia should always be considered in this group (see below).

Staphylococcal pneumonia

In all severe cases of pneumonia a sputum specimen should be examined if possible, but this should not delay therapy. If Gram-positive cocci in clusters are seen staphylococcal pneumonia is likely, and treatment should be instituted with flucloxacillin/dicloxacillin. It is important to be aware of local rates of CA-MRSA. In most places at present this is a rare cause of CAP, and it is not necessary to treat with vancomycin in the first instance in cases of moderate illness. In severely ill patients vancomycin should be used until susceptibilities are known. If the clinical or radiological picture is strongly suggestive of staphylococcal pneumonia then anti-staphylococcal cover should be instituted regardless of the sputum Gram stain findings.

Aspiration pneumonia

Most cases of aspiration do not result in any significant respiratory compromise, and of those that do, the majority are not infective pneumonia but non-infective chemical pneumonitis. Unfortunately, the two are very difficult to distinguish. Treatment recommendations vary and hard evidence is limited. If antibiotic therapy is to be used a β-lactam and metronidazole are an appropriate combination in most cases. In edentulous patients anaerobic cover is probably not required, but in certain patients (nursing home residents and alcoholics) Gram-negative cover with a third-generation cephalosporin should be considered.

Pneumonia in tropical areas

Patients in certain tropical areas are prone to infection with *Burkholderia pseudomallei* and *Acinetobacter baumanii*, while 'atypicals' such as *Mycoplasma* and *Legionella* are much less common. Mild pneumonia can generally be treated safely with a β-lactam alone. In moderate cases, if risk factors for these infections are present, a third-generation cephalosporin (for *Burkholderia*) and gentamicin (for *Acinetobacter*) should be used. In severe pneumonia in these regions, especially during the wet season, all patients should be treated with a carbapenem and macrolide.

Likely developments over the next 5–10 years

- Drug-resistant organisms will become an increasing problem, particularly multidrug-resistant pneumococcus.
- Increasing rates of HIV, increasing numbers of patients on long-term immunosuppression after organ transplant and on long-term chemotherapy and an ageing population are likely to alter the spectrum of CAP, with increasing frequency of opportunistic infection.
- Better transportation systems and increased movement of people around the world, coupled with an increasing population of immunocompromised patients, is likely to contribute to a resurgence in tuberculosis in the developed world, with multidrug-resistant strains becoming a particular problem.
- The emergency department short-stay unit may develop an increasingly important role in the management of mild-moderate pneumonia, in order to balance cost and risk-management concerns.

Acknowledgements

The author thanks Professor RM Robins-Browne, Department of Immunology and Microbiology, University of Melbourne, for advice on microbiological detail.

Controversies

- Optimal antibiotic therapy for mild pneumonia is not defined, particularly with regard to the need to treat for atypicals such as *Mycoplasma* and *Chlamydophila* spp.

- The value of an aggressive approach to aetiological investigation, given the expense. Pathogen-directed therapy has not been shown to have a mortality benefit over empiric treatment.

- The use of the PSI and other risk stratification tools to guide empiric antibiotic therapy and site of care.

- Prediction tools for identification of severe and life-threatening cases remain elusive.

- Antibiotics are commonly prescribed for aspiration episodes despite the fact that most of them do not involve infection. A reliable way of predicting cases that require antibiotics is not available.

- The role of fluoroquinolones given their cost, availability and emerging resistance.

- The optimal treatment for patients with severe pneumonia and immediate penicillin hypersensitivity is not clear.

Further reading

Antibiotic Expert Group. Community-acquired pneumonia. In: Therapeutic Guidelines: antibiotic, 13th edn. Melbourne: Therapeutic Guidelines Ltd, 2006.

Dremsizov T, Clermont G, Kellum JA, et al. Severe sepsis in community-acquired pneumonia: when does it happen, and do systemic inflammatory response syndrome criteria help predict course? Chest 2006; 129: 968–978.

Elliott JH, Anstey NM, Jacups SP, et al. Community-acquired pneumonia in northern Australia: low mortality in a tropical region using locally-developed treatment guidelines. International Journal of Infectious Diseases 2005; 9: 15–20.

Fine MJ, Auble TE, Yealy DM, et al. A prediction rule to identify low-risk patients with community-acquired pneumonia. New England Journal of Medicine 1997; 336: 243–250.

Gottlieb T, Collignon P, Robson J, on behalf of the Australian Group for Antimicrobial Resitance (AGAR). *Streptococcus pneumoniae* Survey 2005 Antibicrobial Susceptibility Report. Australian Group for Antibicrobial Resistance (AGAR) 2006. Accessed July 2007. http://www.agargroup.org/surveys/spneumo%2005%20cdi%20report.pdf

Johnson PDR, Irving LB, Turnidge JD. Community-acquired pneumonia. Medical Journal of Australia 2002;176: 341–347.

Kennedy M, Bates DW, Wright SB, et al. Do emergency department blood cultures change practice in patients with pneumonia? Annals of Emergency Medicine 2005; 46: 393–400.

Macfarlane JT, Boswell T, Douglas G, et al. BTS Guidelines for the Management of Community Acquired Pneumonia in Adults. Thorax 2001; 56: Supplement 4.

Macfarlane JT, Boswell T, Douglas G, et al. BTS Guidelines for the Management of Community Acquired Pneumonia in Adults - 2004 Update. British Thoracic Society (http://www.britthoracic.org.uk/c2/uploads/macaprevisedapr04.pdf) Accessed July 2007.

Mandell LA, Wunderink RG, Anzueto A, et al. Infectious Diseases Society of America/American Thoracic Society consensus guidelines on the management of community-acquired pneumonia in adults. Clinical Infectious Diseases 2007; 44: S27–72.

Metersky ML, Ma A, Bratzler DW, et al. Predicting bacteremia in patients with community-acquired pneumonia. American Journal of Respiratory Critical Care Medicine 2004; 169: 342–347.

Mylotte JM. Nursing home-acquired pneumonia. Clinical Infectious Disease 2002; 35: 1205–1211.

Shefet D, Robenshtok E, Paul M. Empiric antibiotic coverage of atypical pathogens for community acquired pneumonia in hospitalized adults. Cochrane Database Systematic Review 18(2): CD004418, 2005.

6.4 Influenza and emerging respiratory infections

Shin-Yan Man • Timothy H. Rainer

ESSENTIALS

1 Influenza causes up to 500 000 deaths per year.

2 Influenza is difficult to differentiate clinically from the common cold.

3 Avian influenza is a potential pandemic threat with a mortality of 50%.

4 Antiviral medication is unlikely to be effective.

5 Departmental preparedness is important.

6 Staff safety and morale are paramount in the fight against emerging and existing infectious diseases.

Introduction

Influenza, commonly known as 'flu', is an infectious disease that primarily affects the respiratory system of birds and mammals, including humans, swine, horses and dogs, and which is caused by an RNA virus of the family Orthomyxoviridae. Every year seasonal epidemics of influenza predictably cause between 250 000 and 500 000 deaths worldwide, primarily affecting the elderly, the immunocompromised and the undernourished. The global community is familiar with flu, its regularity and its effects, and so is generally unperturbed by its consequences. Of greater concern is the potential for a pandemic that could cause millions of fatalities. Lessons from pandemics of history and the emergence of two recent infections (namely SARS and avian flu), coupled with the potential for huge economic effects have focused interest in pandemic flu. Preparedness involves both individual case management and departmental organization. This chapter will summarize important aspects of the disease and epidemiological classification, and describe the clinical features, diagnosis and management. There is also a brief summary of principles and practice at a managerial/organizational level which are important to implement if staff are to be safely protected during a pandemic. These principles nevertheless need to be part of day-to-day activity and applied before a pandemic arises.

INFLUENZA

History

Symptoms compatible with human influenza were first described by Hippocrates in 412 BC, but there is considerable overlap with the presentation of other infectious diseases. The term 'influenza' allegedly originated from 15th century Italy and was thought to be caused by the *influences* of the stars. The term 'influenza di freddo', meaning 'influence of the cold' was coined to describe the illness. In some senses this confuses influenza with the common 'cold', which is not helpful as the aetiological agents causing the common cold and influenza, and the associated mortality of the two diseases, are distinctly different. However, in practice it is often difficult to differentiate the two conditions clinically, and 'influence of the cold' has a certain pragmatic reality about it.

The first recorded pandemic attributed to influenza A was in 1580 AD, which began in Asia and spread to Europe via Africa. In fact, many of the world's emerging infections appear to have originated in Asia. This may in part be due to the close proximity of highly numerous human and animal populations, coupled with poor hygiene and

climatic changes. Since the 16th century there have been five recorded pandemics, including the 'Asiatic' flu (H2N2) in 1890; another in 1900 (H3N8); the most famous and devastating outbreak, the Spanish flu (H1N1) which killed an estimated 40–100 million people in 1918; a fourth in 1957 (H2N2); and most recently the Hong Kong flu (H3N2) of 1968 which caused a million deaths.

The recent SARS outbreak was not caused by an influenza virus but rather by a coronavirus, a virus which causes the common cold. Nevertheless, within several weeks it had affected at least 8437 cases in over 30 countries worldwide, and had a 10% mortality. Travel advisories were issued by the WHO, hospitals and schools were closed, small companies collapsed and economies failed. Although the disease originated in the community, it appeared that health workers faced the greatest threat. More recently a new illness has emerged – avian influenza A (H5N1), otherwise known as avian flu. Although the illness has a mortality in excess of 50% there is no evidence of human-to-human transmission, so at the time of writing the number of cases is relatively few and a pandemic remains a potential threat rather than a present reality.

Epidemiology and pathology

Epidemiological definitions

It is important to understand the definitions of and hence the differences between endemic, epidemic and pandemic disease.

Endemic means *within people*. A disease is endemic when the infection is maintained within the population without the need for external input, and is usually in a steady state, e.g. chicken pox.

Epidemic is when a disease/infection appears as new cases in a given population, during a given period, at a rate that exceeds what is expected based on recent experience, and is not in a steady state but is increasing, e.g. rabies or SARS.

A pandemic is an epidemic that spreads across a large region and increases massively. Generally speaking, three conditions need to be met for a pandemic. First, the emerging disease is new to the population. Second, the agent infects humans, causing serious illness. Third, the agent spreads easily and sustainably. Avian flu meets the first

two criteria, but at the time of writing not the third.

Epidemic and pandemic spread

Again, generally speaking, three factors contribute to the global spread of infectious disease: wind patterns, migratory birds and air travel. The last certainly contributed to the spread of SARS and has led some to coin the anecdotal term 'aviation flu' for the next epidemic.

Influenza viruses are found in many different animals, and wild birds are the primary source of influenza A viruses. The range of symptoms in birds varies greatly depending on the viral strain. Some of the H5 and H7 virus subtypes are known to cause highly pathogenic forms of disease leading to widespread disease and death among wild and domestic birds. Pigs can be infected with both human and avian viruses, and the circulation of H5 and H7 virus in poultry allows the virus to mutate into a highly pathogenic form that may infect humans.

New viral strains are constantly being produced in two ways: antigenic drift and antigenic shift. Antigenic drift is a minor change in the antigenicity of haemagglutinin or neuraminidase by mutation, which enables the virus to evade immune recognition, causing most seasonal epidemics. Antigenic shift is a major change through genetic reassortment between different subtypes of influenza A during animal co-infection, which produces an entirely new antigen. A novel virus could cause a pandemic if it is able to spread among the non-immune population and cause illnesses that will result in millions of deaths.

Human influenza epidemics typically occur during the winter months, where the cold and dry weather enables the virus to survive longer outside the body. There are two peak flu seasons each year because of different winter times in the northern and southern hemispheres, and this explains why the there are two different vaccine formulations every year. The stages of an influenza epidemic are shown in Table 6.4.1.

Microbiological classification

The influenza viruses are classified into three types (A, B, C) based on their core proteins. Unlike influenza C, types A and B will cause epidemics. Influenza A is more virulent than the other two types and

Table 6.4.1 Stages of an influenza pandemic
Interpandemic period
No new influenza subtypes detected in humans
No new influenza subtypes detected in humans but an animal variant threatens human disease
Pandemic alert period
Human infections – new subtype; no human-to-human spread
Small clusters with limited human-to-human transmission
Large clusters but human-to-human spread still localized
Pandemic period
Increased and sustained transmission in general population

causes the most severe disease. Type A viruses are further divided into subtypes or strains based on two surface proteins, namely haemagglutinin H (H1–H16) and neuraminidase N (N1–N9). Haemagglutinin binds to the sialic acid receptors at the cell surface and mediates viral attachment and entry into the host cell. The specificity of this binding partly explains the species barrier between avian and human influenza viruses. Neuraminidase cleaves the binding between the host cells and viral particles, which in turn facilitates the spread of the virus. Both haemagglutinin and neuraminidase are targets for antiviral drugs. Influenza B is not divided into subtypes.

Incubation period and infectivity

The incubation period is typically 2 days (range 1–4 days) and transmission may be by one of three main modes:

- Large droplet spread by coughs and sneezes. This is the main route of transmission.
- Contact, either direct or indirect, with respiratory secretions.
- Transmission through droplet nuclei, i.e. airborne spread.

Sneezing, coughing and even talking can produce droplets of a wide variety of particle sizes that can facilitate droplet or droplet nuclei infection. An infected person can be infectious from the day before they develop symptoms until 5–7 days afterwards. The infection is easily confused with other viral respiratory infections such as the common cold, although influenza is usually a more serious illness. Infected persons with

minimal symptoms may still shed the virus and be infectious. Primary infection in young children is usually symptomatic, although up to 50% may be asymptomatic. Viral shedding occurs for approximately 3–5 days in adults, up to 3 weeks in young children, and for more than 3 weeks in severely immunocompromised persons. The amount of viral shedding correlates with the severity of illness and temperature elevation. Pre-existing antibodies against related influenza strains are partially protective, i.e. a higher infective inoculum is required with a lower likelihood of clinical illness.

Survival of the influenza virus outside the body varies with temperature and humidity. It generally survives 24–48 hours on hard, non-porous surfaces, 8–12 hours on cloth/paper/tissue, and 5 minutes on hands. Survival of the virus is enhanced under conditions of low humidity and in the cold. Most influenza strains can easily be inactivated by disinfectants and detergents.

Clinical features

Influenza viruses can cause disease in all age groups, but the mortality and complication rates are higher in the elderly, young children and any persons who have chronic medical conditions.

The clinical manifestations of influenza are diverse, ranging from asymptomatic to severe infection, and can lead to respiratory failure and death. Uncomplicated influenza illness is characterized by the abrupt onset of constitutional and respiratory symptoms and signs: fever, myalgia, headache, malaise, non-productive cough, sore throat and rhinitis. Gastrointestinal symptoms are more commonly seen in children than in

adults. In children, otitis media, nausea and vomiting are also commonly reported.

Symptoms typically resolve after a limited number of days in the majority of cases, although cough and malaise can persist for more than 2 weeks. In some people influenza can exacerbate underlying medical conditions (particularly pulmonary or cardiac disease), leading to secondary bacterial pneumonia, primary influenza viral pneumonia or coinfections with other viral or bacterial pathogens. Influenza infection has also been associated with encephalopathy, transverse myelitis, Reye's syndrome, myositis, myocarditis and pericarditis.

There are no pathognomonic signs and symptoms for influenza and it is difficult to distinguish influenza from other respiratory infectious disease. However, patients with symptoms of upper respiratory tract infections during an influenza outbreak are likely to have the infection. Some key similarities and differentiating features between influenza and the common cold are shown in Table 6.4.2.

Case definition in pandemic flu outbreaks

It is important to realize that the World Health Organization case definitions are primarily designed for public health surveillance and disease reporting, and not for early identification of disease. Emergency department (ED) staff will frequently have to make decisions based on the early presentation of illness when aspects of illness do not meet all the criteria for case definitions.

Case definitions are subcategorized into probable and confirmed cases. In view of the time required for laboratory confirmation of pandemic influenza infection, the

Table 6.4.2 Features differentiating influenza and the common cold	
Influenza	*Cold*
Flu virus	Corona virus
Fever, sore throat	Fever, sore throat
No runny nose	Runny nose
Myalgia, malaise, headache	Myalgia, malaise, headache
Pneumonia	No pneumonia
Days, severe	24 hours, mild
High mortality	Low mortality

probable case definition will be the working definition for operational considerations.

Persons are considered probable pandemic influenza cases when the following conditions are fulfilled:

- Abrupt onset of fever ≥ 38°C (except in persons aged ≥60 years), and
- Non-productive cough, and either
  - a positive epidemiological link (travel to a country with pandemic influenza or contact history with an infected person), or
  - a positive rapid test kit result, if available.
- Fever may often be absent in persons aged ≥60 years and in immunocompromised patients such as diabetics and patients on steroids or other immunosuppressants. Therefore, in the absence of fever, any of the following symptoms, in addition to non-productive cough, should raise a high index of suspicion for persons in this category:
  - malaise
  - chills
  - headache
  - myalgia.

Persons are considered confirmed pandemic influenza cases when there is laboratory confirmation of infection with pandemic influenza.

Assessment

Management decisions are based primarily on the disease severity and the identification of the 'at-risk' group. Patients with mild disease and a low risk of developing disease complications can be managed in the community. However, patients in the high-risk group or with severe illnesses should be assessed in hospital.

Investigations

Blood tests
Blood tests with full blood count may show a leukocytosis in patients with pulmonary involvement. Lymphopenia has been noted in severe H5N1 infection.

Imaging
A chest X-ray should be performed to exclude pulmonary involvement in high-risk patients. A thoracic CT scan or bronchoscopic examination may be required later, depending on clinical progress.

Microbiology
Laboratory confirmation will be required between annual influenza epidemics. Although the commercially available diagnostic test kits can detect influenza viruses from throat swabs and nasopharyngeal aspirate specimens within 30 minutes, they cannot distinguish human from avian influenza virus or their subtypes. Collecting clinical specimens for viral culture remains crucial to identifying the circulating influenza subtypes and strains. The information obtained helps to guide clinical decisions regarding influenza treatment, chemoprophylaxis and vaccine formulation.

Treatment

Most mildly infected people only require symptomatic treatment. Antibacterial agents are mainly used for preventing or treating secondary bacterial pneumonia.

General measures
Patients with flu should rest, keep well hydrated, and take antipyretics (e.g. paracetamol for fever and muscle aches). Antibiotics are not indicated unless there is clear evidence of a secondary bacterial infection in a previously healthy individual, or if there is a very high probability of bacterial illness in a patient with a strong history of proven secondary bacterial infection.

Seriously infected patients may require respiratory support and intensive care management.

Antiviral agents
Antiviral agents are a second line of defence in the prevention and treatment of influenza. The administration of antiviral agents before infection or during the early stage of the disease may help prevent the infection, reduce the duration of illness by approximately 24 hours, and reduce the disease complication rate.

There are two classes of antiviral agent: M2 inhibitors (adamantanes) and neuraminidase inhibitors. Adamantanes are less expensive antiviral drugs active against influenza A, but there is a high incidence of drug resistance which makes them less useful in treating influenza. Neuraminidase inhibitors (oseltamavir and zanamivir) are newer and more expensive agents. They inhibit viral neuraminidase and have activity against both influenza A and B infection. They have also been shown to be effective in treating animals infected with H5N1. They are currently considered the drugs of choice in treating influenza. Antiviral medications should be started within 2 days of symptoms onset, and should be prescribed for 5 days. They have not been shown to be effective if administered more than 2 days after onset. The major adverse effect of oseltamivir is nausea, which occurs in 10% of patients. Rare cases of transient neuropsychiatric events (self-injury or delirium) have been reported in Japan. Zanamivir is not recommended for persons with underlying airways disease.

The following points should be borne in mind when considering prescribing neuraminidases. They inhibit the spread of virus in the respiratory tract and are not useful unless given very early in the course of the illness. Usually viral reproduction precedes symptoms, and so neuraminidases tend to be prophylactic rather than therapeutic. They have only been tested in seasonal flu and limit the duration of the illness by 1 day at the most. They have no proven effect on mortality. Moreover, these antivirals are not equally effective against different subtypes of influenza virus, and therefore it is difficult to predict their usefulness in future pandemics.

Prevention

Although epidemics occur every year, their severity, duration and impact on society cannot be accurately predicted. Yearly vaccination remains the best effective method for preventing influenza and reducing the impact of epidemics. Provided there is a good match between vaccine antigens and circulating viruses, influenza vaccines can offer approximately 70–90% protection against clinical disease in healthy adults, reduce hospital admissions among the elderly by 25–39%, and reduce the overall mortality by 39–75%. Influenza vaccination is therefore useful in reducing both the healthcare costs and productivity losses associated with influenza epidemics.

The frequent changes in the viral surface antigens make the annual reformulation of vaccines necessary to match the circulating viruses. Annual 'flu' vaccination is highly recommended for children, the elderly, patients with chronic medical illness, nursing home residents, healthcare workers and pregnant women. Influenza vaccines should not be used in people with allergy to egg proteins.

Avian influenza

A highly pathogenic strain of H5N1, also known as 'avian influenza' normally only infects birds, but recently it has been reported to cause disease in humans. It was first noted in Hong Kong in 1997, when 18 people were infected, of whom six died. The virus then disappeared until 2003, when it reappeared in the human population. By May 2006 a total of 218 patients had been infected, of whom 124 had died, a mortality rate of 57%.

Unlike the mild disease seen in normal seasonal influenza, the disease caused by H5N1 has a poor prognosis and a high fatality rate. This virus is now considered endemic in some parts of Indonesia, Vietnam, Cambodia, China, Thailand and Lao People's Democratic Republic. At present, there is no evidence to suggest efficient human-to-human transmission of avian influenza virus. Most infected patients have had direct contact with poultry. However, the constantly changing avian virus may eventually develop an efficient human transmission mechanism to start a pandemic. Vaccines against H5N1 are under development in several countries; they are, however, not commercially available to the general public. Neuraminidase inhibitors could be used for both chemoprophylaxis and as therapeutic agent, but there is limited evidence to support hopes.

No-one is certain about the time, scale and impact of the next pandemic. Strategic actions should be aimed at strengthening national, hospital and departmental preparedness, reducing the emergence of a novel virus, improving the warning system, delaying the international spread of disease and expediting vaccine development.

Organizational issues

Emergency departments (ED) need to develop their own guidelines for an outbreak and regularly practise upgrading their systems. Such guidelines should cover:

- Clinical characteristics of pandemic flu and its initial management (see above).
- Alert criteria and their respective responses.
- Isolation and transfer to designated flu hospitals/health centres.
- Physical infrastructure and equipment in order to receive, manage and arrange for the appropriate disposition of potentially infected patients.
- Staff personal protection and hygiene.
- Education and training, audits, exercises, surveillance, prophylaxis and stockpiling.

Infection control in the emergency department

All EDs should have basic infection control measures that will need to be systematically enhanced as the world moves closer towards a pandemic flu situation. These routine measures should include the following:

- Screening of all patients at the entrance of the ED.
- Separate pathways for potential patients with and without fever or contact history.
- Isolation of all such patients screened as infectious in a separate area, preferably with its own separate negative-pressure ventilation system.
- Use of personal protective equipment (surgical mask, hospital scrubs) when attending to patients who are potentially infectious..
- Hand-washing or use of alcohol rubs before and after attending to any patient.
- Special isolation facilities for high-risk patients who require inpatient care.
- Screening surveillance. This provides an early warning of an impending infectious disease outbreak, and may also serve as a regular reminder to staff on the need to remain vigilant for such outbreaks.

Controversies

- The therapeutic value of antiviral medication is unclear. Pharmaceutical companies and investors stand to make huge gains from promoting their potential value.

- The degree of personal protection equipment required to protect healthcare workers is unclear.

Further reading

Avian influenza ('bird flu') fact sheet. WHO, February 2006. Retrieved on 2006–10–20. www.who.it.

Avian influenza: frequently asked questions. WHO (Revised 5 December 2005). Retrieved on 2007–12–20. www.who. it/csr/disease/influenza

Bartlett JG. Planning for avian influenza. Annals of Internal Medicine 2006; 145: 141–144.

British Infection Society. British Thoracic Society. Health Protection Agency. Pandemic flu: clinical management of patients with an influenza-like illness during an influenza pandemic. Provisional guidelines from the British Infection Society, British Thoracic Society, and Health Protection Agency in collaboration with the Department of Health. Thorax 2007; 62: 1–46.

Centre for Disease Control. The Influenza Viruses. Accessed at http://www.cdc.gov/flu/about/fluviruses.htm 2 January2008.

Eccles R. Understanding the symptoms of the common cold and influenza. Lancet Infectious Diseases 2005; 5: 718–725.

Influenza Antiviral Medications: Summary for Clinicians CDC. (last updated October 23, 2007) Retrieved on 2007–12–28. www.cdc.gov/flu

Key facts about seasonal influenza. CDC (last updated November 16, 2007). Retrieved on 2007–12–20. www. cdc.gov/flu

Liu JP. Avian influenza – a pandemic waiting to happen?. Journal of Microbiology Immunology and Infection 2006; 39: 4–10.

Moscana A. Neuraminidase inhibitors for influenza. New England Journal of Medicine 2005; 353: 1363–1373.

Questions and answers. Seasonal influenza. CDC (last modified November 08, 2006) Retrieved on 2007–12–17. www.cdc.gov/flu

Role of laboratory diagnosis of influenza. CDC (last updated September 26, 2006) Retrieved on 2007–12–28. www. cdc.gov/flu

The influenza (Flu) viruses. CDC (last modified October16, 2007) www.cdc.gov/flu Retrieved on 2007–12–17.

Webster RG, Govorkova EA H5N1 influenza – continuing evolution and spread. New England Journal of Medicine 2006; 355: 2174–2177.

Wilson JC, von Itzstein M. Recent strategies in the search for new anti-influenza therapies. Current Drug Targets 2003; 4: 389–408.

Wong SS, Yuen KY. Avian influenza virus infections in humans. Chest 2006; 29: 156–168.

World Health Organization. Epidemic and Pandemic Alert and Response. Influenza. Accessed at http://www.who. int/csr/disease/influenza/en/ on 2nd January 2008.

6.5 Chronic obstructive pulmonary disease

Julie Leung • Martin Duffy

ESSENTIALS

1 Chronic obstructive pulmonary disease is characterized by airflow limitation that is not fully reversible.

2 The majority of exacerbations of COPD are due to infection, but other important precipitants need to be excluded.

3 It is prudent to control oxygen flow rate to achieve an arterial oxygen saturation of approximately 90% to ensure correction of hypoxia while avoiding the complication of hyperoxic hypercapnia.

4 The use of non-invasive ventilation in acute respiratory failure is associated with reduced mortality, reduced rates of intubation and reduction in treatment failure.

5 Bronchodilators and systemic steroids are recommended for acute exacerbations.

Introduction

Chronic obstructive pulmonary disease (COPD) is a major public health problem causing chronic morbidity and mortality throughout the world. It is characterized by airflow limitation that is not fully reversible, is usually progressive, and is associated with an abnormal inflammatory response of the lung to noxious particles or gases. Small airway narrowing (with or without chronic bronchitis) and emphysema are the common conditions resulting in COPD. An acute exacerbation is an event in the natural course of the disease characterized by a change in the patient's baseline dyspnoea, cough and/or sputum that is beyond normal day-to-day variations, is acute in onset, and may warrant a change in regular medication in a patient with underlying COPD. COPD is important for two reasons: it may present as life-threatening respiratory failure, or it may be a significant comorbidity that can affect the management of other illnesses.

Aetiology, genetics, pathogenesis and pathology

The most important factor leading to the development of COPD is cigarette smoking.

Less common factors include genetic disorders such as α_1-antitrypsin deficiency, occupational exposures and exposure to air pollution. Why one patient with the above risk factors develops COPD and another with similar risk factors does not, remains unclear. For instance, only 10–15% of smokers develop clinically significant COPD, and almost two-thirds of those homozygous for α_1-antitrypsin deficiency have well-preserved pulmonary function.

The airflow limitation seen in COPD is due to a variable combination of luminal obstruction with mucus hypersecretion, disruption of alveolar attachments, and mucosal and peribronchial inflammation and fibrosis (obliterative bronchiolitis).

Epidemiology

Projections from the Global Burden of Disease Study suggest that COPD will be the fifth leading cause of disability-adjusted life-years lost worldwide by the year 2020. More than half a million Australians are estimated to have moderate to severe disease, and as the population ages, the burden of COPD is likely to increase. COPD ranks fourth among the common causes of death in Australian men and sixth in women. In New Zealand, it ranks third in men and fourth in women.

Clinical features

History

Most patients with COPD experience a slow, steady deterioration in their respiratory function. Most emergency department (ED) presentations are the result of a superimposed acute exacerbation. As the disease becomes more severe, the frequency of exacerbations also increases.

It is important to have a good understanding of the patient's baseline function. Questioning to determine this should include the following:

Background
- When did the patient first develop symptoms?
- When was the diagnosis first made?
- The presence of risk factors
- Is the patient a smoker: past or present?
- Maintenance therapy: short- and long-acting bronchodilators, inhaled glucocorticoids
- Use of oral steroids
- Normal level of activity
- Home monitoring, e.g. PEFRs
- Use of home oxygen therapy
- Record of hospitalizations, including ICU admissions.

Acute deterioration
- Fever
- Increased cough and sputum production
- Chest pain suggestive of a pulmonary embolus or pneumothorax
- Coexisting illnesses, e.g. ischaemic heart disease, congestive heart failure, diabetes
- Inhaler technique and compliance with medications
- Intercurrent use of inappropriate medications, e.g. β-blockers, sedatives.

Examination

In clinical practice there is usually a variety of presentations between the two classic descriptions of patients with COPD. The 'pink puffer' is usually a thin, barrel-chested patient with obvious dyspnoea, tachypnoea and pursed lip breathing, but no cyanosis.

Use of the accessory muscles of respiration is evidenced by the classic tripod posture, with both elbows resting on the patient's knees or other surfaces, as well as sternomastoid muscle hypertrophy. The 'blue bloater' is typically described as an overweight, oedematous cyanosed patient suffering from chronic cough and sputum production. Features of cor pulmonale may be present in later stages.

Clinical features strongly suggestive of airflow obstruction, with specificities of 98–99%, are the presence of wheezes, a barrel chest, reduced cardiac dullness, and a subxiphoid cardiac impulse. Unfortunately, the sensitivities of these features are extremely poor (8–15%), limiting their clinical usefulness.

The goal of the initial evaluation of a patient presenting with an exacerbation of COPD is to determine the severity of the attack, as well as to search for and treat any precipitating factors and complications.

Important precipitants and complications to search for include:

Precipitants of acute respiratory failure

- Infection – acute bronchitis, pneumonia
- Bronchospasm
- Sputum retention
- Air pollution
- Pneumothoraces and bullae
- Pulmonary embolism
- Trauma, e.g. rib fractures, pulmonary contusion
- Reduced respiratory drive, e.g. inappropriate sedative use
- Reduced respiratory muscle strength, e.g. metabolic or neuromuscular cause
- Increased metabolic demands – sepsis, fever
- Left ventricular failure.

Complications of COPD

- Pulmonary hypertension
- Right ventricular failure
- Secondary polycythaemia
- Loss of weight
- Medication adverse effects, e.g. complications secondary to long-term steroid use; tachyarrhythmias with β-agonists.

Classification of severity

The Global Initiative on Chronic Obstructive Lung Disease classifies COPD into four stages of severity, based on spirometry:

- Stage I: Mild COPD – characterized by mild airflow limitation (FEV_1/FVC < 0.70; FEV_1 ≥80% predicted); the individual is usually unaware that his or her lung function is abnormal.
- Stage II: Moderate COPD – characterized by worsening airflow limitation (FEV_1/FVC < 0.70; 50% ≤FEV_1 < 80% predicted); patients typically seek medical attention because of chronic respiratory symptoms or an exacerbation of their disease.
- Stage III: Severe COPD – characterized by further worsening of airflow limitation (FEV_1/FVC < 0.70; 30% ≤FEV_1 < 50% predicted), greater shortness of breath, reduced exercise capacity, fatigue, and repeated exacerbations that almost always have an impact on patients' quality of life.
- Stage IV: Very severe COPD – characterized by severe airflow limitation (FEV_1/FVC < 0.70; FEV_1 < 30% predicted or FEV_1 < 50% predicted plus the presence of chronic respiratory failure); quality of life is very appreciably impaired and exacerbations may be life-threatening.

The BODE Index, which includes assessment of weight (body mass index), airway obstruction (FEV_1), dyspnoea and exercise capacity, has been useful in assessing the risk of death and as a predictor of hospitalization. However, the above measures do not significantly affect the immediate management of COPD patients presenting acutely to the ED.

Clinical investigations

The following investigations may be used during the evaluation of a patient with COPD, but not all will be necessary in every situation. It is important to use tests that will have an impact on management decisions.

Tests performed at the bedside include:

- Pulse oximetry: Provides invaluable 'real-time' non-invasive evaluation of oxygenation, helping with the initial assessment of the patient and allowing observation of trends in response to therapy. The typical goal is a saturation of >90%. Oximetry does not provide information about carbon dioxide status and is inaccurate in the presence of poor peripheral circulation.
- Spirometry: Provides confirmation of obstruction – FEV_1 <80% of predicted and FEV_1/FVC <0.7. In the acute situation spirometry often cannot be performed by the patient, and it has little role in management decisions such as intubation.
- Electrocardiography (ECG): May detect arrhythmias such as multifocal atrial tachycardia or atrial fibrillation, or demonstrate evidence of intercurrent ischaemic heart disease. ECG evidence of pulmonary hypertension and right ventricular hypertrophy may be present, but is often insensitive and non-specific.

Tests that have results available within minutes include:

- Arterial blood gases: Provide information regarding acute versus chronic respiratory failure and may be used to monitor improvement or deterioration with several measurements. Acute hypercarbia can be distinguished from chronic hypercarbia by consideration of HCO_3 levels and pH. In the acute setting, an acidotic pH value in a patient with chronic carbon dioxide retention signifies superimposed acute decompensation. Although this information is useful, ABGs play little part in clinical decisions such as intubation.
- Chest radiograph: In the acute setting provides valuable information regarding the presence of coexisting illnesses which may be life-threatening and require specific interventions, e.g. pneumothorax, pneumonia, pleural effusions, heart failure. Studies have demonstrated that up to 23% of admitted patients may have a change in their management related to their CXR findings. Features of chronic airflow limitation may include hyperinflation, flattened diaphragms, bullae, increased retrosternal airspace, reduced vascular markings and a small heart.

Other useful tests (but which have a limited or no role in acute setting) are:

- Full blood examination: May reveal evidence of secondary polycythaemia or a raised white cell count due to infection, long-term steroid use or the hyperadrenergic stress response of the acutely ill patient.

- Electrolytes: Note potassium levels, hyponatraemia, glucose.
- Sputum culture: 50% of exacerbations of COPD may be due to bacteria, with *H. influenzae, Strep. pneumoniae* and *Moraxella catarrhalis* the predominant pathogens. Exacerbations complicated by pneumonia have similar pathogens. Patients with more compromised lung function have a higher frequency of infections with *Pseudomonas aeruginosa* and other Gram-negative bacteria than those less severely affected. Colonization of the respiratory tract can make interpretation of results difficult.
- Viral cultures and detection assays: 20% of acute exacerbations are due to viruses such as rhinoviruses, influenzae, parainfluenzae and coronaviruses. However, viral studies are usually not performed in the ED as they are expensive, have varying sensitivities and specificities, and rarely alter management.
- Theophylline level: Rarely required; note that a patient may be toxic despite having a measured level within the therapeutic range.
- Plasma brain natriuretic peptide (BNP) level: Adds to the current clinical and laboratory evaluation of patients with COPD presenting with worsening dyspnoea, although not widely available in Australia. A plasma BNP level < 100 pg/mL argues against heart failure playing a role in the clinical deterioration. A plasma level > 500 pg/mL points to decompensation of heart failure but does not exclude concomitant COPD exacerbation. Plasma BNP levels ranging from 100 to 500 pg/mL need to be interpreted in conjunction with clinical findings.
- Respiratory function tests: Demonstrate largely irreversible airflow obstruction with elevated lung volumes; reduced carbon monoxide uptake implies emphysema.
- High-resolution chest CT: Demonstrates air trapping and is thus useful in the diagnosis of emphysema, but of questionable value in the ED setting given the limited availability and as yet undetermined advance on other diagnostic modalities available for the assessment of most patients with COPD. CT pulmonary angiograms are useful for investigating possible pulmonary embolism, especially when the chest X-ray is abnormal.
- Cardiac studies: Echocardiography and gated nuclear scans may be required to determine the role of ventricular dysfunction in the clinical picture.

Treatment

The overall goals of treatment in COPD are to confirm the diagnosis and assess severity; optimize function (including use of long-acting bronchodilators to provide sustained relief of symptoms in moderate-to-severe COPD and the use of inhaled glucocorticoids in patients with a documented response or those who have severe COPD with frequent exacerbations); prevent deterioration; develop a support network and self-management plan; and manage exacerbations.

The following is a summary of the therapeutic modalities used to treat an acute exacerbation of COPD. The timing and level of intervention depends on the severity at the time of presentation. It is important to remember that management decisions for the patient in extremis are solely clinical – no further investigation is necessary to determine whether immediate intubation is required.

Oxygen therapy

Hypoxaemia must be corrected. Oxygen therapy for most patients with COPD will not produce clinically significant carbon dioxide retention, a multifactorial condition caused by changes in pulmonary blood flow, worsening V/Q mismatching and increasing dead space ventilation, not simply hypoventilation from loss of hypoxic drive. However, it is recommended that oxygen delivery be controlled, with a minimal acceptable saturation in most cases of 90%, corresponding to an arterial oxygen tension of 60–70 mmHg. There is an increased risk of morbidity and mortality in patients with hypercapnic respiratory failure when the arterial oxygen tension is increased above this level (>93–95%). The degree of hypoxaemia at presentation rather than the initial degree of hypercapnia is a better predictor of hyperoxic hypercapnia. For the mildly unwell patient an oxygen saturation of 90% may be achieved with the use of nasal prongs at 2 L/min. For patients with more severe disease the use of a Venturi mask with an appropriate fractional inspired oxygen concentration is more appropriate. In most cases these devices are of the fixed-performance type, i.e. the FiO_2 is independent of patient factors. However, in the severely dyspnoeic patient, peak inspiratory flow rate may exceed the peak flow rate of the device, leading to fluctuations in FiO_2. To avoid this, a circuit with a large reservoir will be necessary. Persisting hypoxia (SpO_2 <85%) necessitates a search for complicating factors such as pneumonia, pulmonary oedema, pulmonary embolus or pneumothorax, as well as consideration of ventilatory assistance.

Ventilatory assistance

Ventilatory assistance may be non-invasive (NIV) or invasive.

Non-invasive ventilation (NIV)

NIV has become the first line intervention in the management of acute respiratory failure in patients with COPD. Continuous positive airway pressure (CPAP) and bilevel positive airway pressure (BiPAP) are the two main modes of non-invasive positive-pressure ventilation.

The presence of dynamic hyperinflation and the development of intrinsic positive end-expiratory pressure (PEEPi) during an acute deterioration lead to an increased work of breathing. The application of CPAP or external PEEP at levels to overcome PEEPi, has been shown to reduce respiratory work. This has resulted in patients reporting less dyspnoea and laboratory evidence of better gas exchange.

BiPAP involves the use of both inspiratory and expiratory pressure support ventilation and has also proved an effective form of NIV in acute respiratory failure. Initiation of ventilation triggers the inspiratory positive airway pressure, which is limited to a predetermined level, usually 10–20 cmH_2O. Expiratory positive airway pressure of approximately 5 cmH_2O is predetermined and persists throughout expiration. The whole process thus reduces the work of breathing.

Numerous studies, using either a face mask or nasal mask and varying combinations of the above airway pressure manipulations, have shown significant reductions in the need for intubation. Brochard et al's prospective randomized study demonstrated that NIV in selected patients not only reduced the need for intubation, but also reduced length of hospital stay, complications and in-hospital mortality. A Cochrane Review of 14 randomized controlled studies of patients admitted to hospital with acute respiratory failure secondary to an exacerbation of COPD concluded that non-invasive positive-pressure ventilation in addition to usual medical care resulted in reduced mortality (NNT 10), reduced need for intubation (NNT 5) and a reduction in treatment failure (NNT 4). In addition, NIV was associated with rapid improvement in acidosis and respiratory rate within 1 hour of initiation, and complications associated with treatment and length of hospital stay were also reduced. Clinical practice guidelines from ACP-ASIM/ACCP and the Thoracic Society of Australia and New Zealand/Australian Lung Foundation (COPD-X plan) and evidenced-based management guidelines from the Global Initiative for Chronic Obstructive Lung Disease (GOLD) recommend that NIV should be considered early in the course of respiratory failure, before severe acidosis ensues.

Indications for NIV include moderate to severe dyspnoea with use of accessory muscles and paradoxical abdominal motion, moderate to severe acidosis and/or hypercapnia (PaCO$_2$ >45 mmHg) and respiratory rate >25 breaths per minute. Contraindications include respiratory arrest, cardiovascular instability (hypotension, arrhythmias, myocardial infarction), change in mental status or an uncooperative patient, high aspiration risk, viscous or copious secretions, recent facial or gastro-oesophageal surgery, craniofacial trauma and burns. However, there are no definite clinical predictors to identify which patients with respiratory failure will benefit from NIV. Patients who have a pH < 7.30 and > 7.25 appear to receive the greatest benefit. The chance of COPD patients with acute respiratory failure having a second episode of acute respiratory failure after an initial (first 48 hours) successful response to NIV is about 20%.

The concurrent delivery of nebulized β$_2$-agonists with NIV is an important therapeutic issue. Theoretical concerns of reduced drug delivery because of the rates of fresh gas flow required to effectively run CPAP circuits have been confirmed. However, these concerns were not of clinical significance in a group of stable asthmatic patients. Extrapolation to COPD patients with acute respiratory failure should be made with caution, but its use may be appropriate given the favourable effects of CPAP on respiratory mechanics and subsequent drug delivery.

Invasive ventilation

Endotracheal intubation with positive-pressure ventilation is used in patients who fail non-invasive ventilatory assistance or who have indications for intubation present at the outset, e.g. unprotected airway, respiratory arrest. The goal of mechanical ventilation is to prevent excessive work of breathing while maintaining a work of breathing that is sufficient to prevent respiratory muscle atrophy. The major problems with positive-pressure ventilation in this patient population are the risk of barotrauma and the production of PEEPi. Commonly recommended ventilation strategies include using tidal volumes of approximately 5–7 mL/kg, using a reduced respiratory rate, and using an inspiratory: expiratory ratio of 1:3. Most patients also usually require a bolus of intravenous fluids to counter the effects of positive-pressure ventilation on venous return and cardiac output. Patients who need mechanical ventilation have an inpatient mortality of 17–30%.

Concerns about subsequent ventilator dependence are often unfounded, with premorbid level of activity and FEV$_1$ being the best predictors of successful weaning.

Bronchodilators

Bronchodilators are used in the management of acute exacerbations because of the possibility of a small reversible component to the airflow obstruction. In the ED setting these drugs are usually given by nebulizer, though there is little evidence to support this route over metered-dose inhalers, particularly when used in conjunction with a spacer device. It is common practice to use the anticholinergic agents and β$_2$-agonists in combination.

Anticholinergic agents

A systematic review of randomized controlled trials comparing anticholinergic bronchodilators versus β$_2$-sympathomimetic agents for acute exacerbations of COPD found no significant difference in the degree of bronchodilation between the two agents, and the combination of the two did not appear to increase the effect on FEV$_1$ more than either agent used alone. However, the duration of action of short-acting anticholinergics is greater than that of short-acting β-agonists, and they also have a lower adverse effect profile.

The most commonly used agent in Australia is ipratropium bromide. The usual dose is 500 μg by nebulizer every 4 hours. Doses as frequent as every 20 minutes are used in clinical practice, albeit with little supporting evidence.

Tiotropium bromide is a long-acting anticholinergic agent that is used once daily and has been shown to produce significant improvements in lung function, symptoms and quality of life, as well as reducing exacerbations in chronic stable COPD. However, its role in the immediate management of a patient presenting with an acute exacerbation of COPD is yet to be established.

β$_2$-Agonists

Salbutamol is commonly used as a first-line agent in Australia. The usual dose is 5 mg via nebulizer, repeated as necessary. The dose equivalent to 5 mg of salbutamol delivered by nebulizer is 8–10 puffs of 100 μg salbutamol by metered-dose inhaler and spacer. Nebulized salbutamol is often used continuously in the severely ill patient. Occasionally in the patient with a severe exacerbation the intravenous route may be required, though evidence for this practice is lacking. Common side effects include tachycardia, tremor, and a reduction in potassium levels.

Long-acting β$_2$-agonists (e.g. salmeterol, eformoterol) cause prolonged bronchodilatation for at least 12 hours, and can thus be administered twice daily. They have been shown to produce statistically significant benefits in lung function, quality of life, use of 'reliever' short-acting bronchodilators and acute exacerbations. As with tiotropium, their role in the immediate management of a patient presenting with an acute exacerbation of COPD is not yet known.

Theophylline

Rarely used in the acute setting because of significant side effects and questionable efficacy.

Corticosteroids

Systemic corticosteroids have been shown to hasten recovery, reduce hospital stay and reduce early treatment failure in patients with acute exacerbations of COPD. It would be necessary to treat nine patients to avoid one treatment failure. Maximal improvement is usually gained within 2 weeks of therapy; prolonging treatment thereafter does not result in further benefit and long-term systemic corticosteroid use in COPD is not recommended. For acute exacerbations, the optimal initial dose is yet to be determined, but prednisolone 30–50 mg/day for 7–10 days is currently recommended. Evidence suggests that oral administration is just as effective as parenteral administration of steroids, except in conditions that preclude the oral route, such as vomiting. In these cases, 100–200 mg hydrocortisone may be administered i.v. Short courses have minimal side effects, whereas the complications of long-term use are myriad. The potential role of hypothalamopituitary–adrenal axis suppression complicating patient presentations needs to be remembered.

The effects of inhaled corticosteroids (beclomethasone, budesonide, fluticasone, ciclesonide) on the course of a COPD exacerbation are uncertain.

Antibiotics

Bacteria play a role in approximately 50% of exacerbations of COPD. In 30% of patients no clear cause can be found. Current evidence suggests that it would be necessary to treat eight patients with antibiotics to reduce mortality (95% CI 6–17), three patients to reduce treatment failure (95% CI 3–5) and eight patients to reduce sputum purulence (95% CI 6–17). An adverse effect such as diarrhoea occurred for every 20 patients treated (95% CI 10–100). The presence of increased dyspnoea, increased sputum purulence, increased sputum volume or fever/leukocytosis is a reasonable trigger for commencing antibiotic therapy. Patients with more severe exacerbations are more likely to benefit from antibiotic treatment than those with less severe exacerbations.

Drugs should cover *H. influenzae*, *S. pneumoniae* and *Moraxella catarrhalis*, depending on local sensitivities. A β-lactamase-resistant drug (e.g. ampicillin with clavulanic acid or doxycycline) is often required. The use of fluoroquinolones has increased, but they are expensive and have not been shown to be more effective than traditional antibiotics. The presence of an altered mental state, inability to swallow safely or a chest X-ray suggesting pneumonia may require the administration of intravenous antibiotics. The antibiotic treatment for pneumonia in COPD patients should follow the recommendations for initial treatment of community-acquired pneumonia. However, the results of recent sputum cultures may affect the final antibiotic regimen.

Heliox

There is currently little evidence to support the use of a helium–oxygen mixture in acute exacerbations of COPD. Theoretically the low density of heliox mixtures may reduce airway resistance and hence the work of breathing.

Chest physiotherapy

Chest physiotherapy, in the form of mechanical percussion in an attempt to improve mucus clearance, has been shown to be ineffective.

Other therapies

- Monitor fluid balance and nutrition.
- Correction of electrolyte abnormalities.
- Consider subcutaneous heparin for DVT prophylaxis.
- Identify and treat associated conditions.

Longer-term measures

- Smoking cessation
- Vaccinations (pneumococcal, influenza, Hib)
- Home oxygen therapy
- Lung volume reduction surgery
- Transplantation.

Prognosis

Acute exacerbations of COPD often require hospital admission for treatment of respiratory failure. Hospital mortality for such patients is about 10%, reaching 40% by 1 year after discharge, and is higher for

patients aged over 65. Whether the patient requires admission will depend on the severity of the present exacerbation, how easily correctable the precipitating factor is, and how well the patient responds to therapy.

Indications for hospitalization of patients with COPD include a marked increase in intensity of symptoms, inadequate response to initial medical management, inability to walk between rooms when previously mobile, inability to eat or sleep because of dyspnoea, inability to manage at home even with homecare resources, presence of high risk comorbidity conditions, altered mental status suggestive of hypercapnia, worsening hypoxaemia or cor pulmonale, newly occurring arrhythmia or diagnostic uncertainty.

Indications for ICU admission of patients with exacerbation of COPD include severe dyspnoea that responds inadequately to initial emergency therapy, changes in mental status (confusion, lethargy, coma), persistent or worsening hypoxaemia despite supplemental oxygen, worsening hypercapnia ($PaCO_2$ >70 mmHg) or severe or worsening respiratory acidosis, requirement for assisted mechanical ventilation and haemodynamic instability requiring vasopressors.

A decision to discharge the patient from the ED requires the presence of good home conditions, social supports and the organization of appropriate follow-up.

Controversies

- The role of point-of-care tests for diagnosis of infective exacerbations of COPD and as a guide to treatment with antibiotics. These can be used to rapidly diagnose influenza, pneumococcal infections, *Legionella* and respiratory syncytial virus infections. This may avoid the unnecessary use of broad-spectrum antibiotics and reduce the emergence of antibiotic-resistant organisms. However, they may not necessarily lead to better patient outcomes or financial savings.

- The role of home management for acute exacerbations of COPD.

- The role of neutrophil inhibitors and antioxidants.

Further reading

Aubier M, Murciano D, Fournier M, et al. Central respiratory drive in acute respiratory failure of patients with chronic obstructive pulmonary disease. American Review of Respiratory Disease 1980; 122: 191.

Bone RC, Pierce AK, Johnson RL. Controlled oxygen administration in acute respiratory failure in chronic obstructive pulmonary disease: a reappraisal. American Journal of Medicine 1978; 65: 896–902.

Brochard L, Mancebo J, Wysocki M, et al. Non-invasive ventilation for acute exacerbations of chronic obstructive pulmonary disease. New England Journal of Medicine 1995; 333: 817–822.

Celli BR, Cote CG, Marin JM, et al. The body-mass index, airflow obstruction, dyspnoea and exercise capacity index in chronic obstructive pulmonary disease. New England Journal of Medicine 2004; 350: 1005–1012.

Global Initiative for Chronic Obstructive Lung Disease (GOLD). 2006. URL: www.goldcopd.com. Accessed Sept 2007.

Holleman DR Jr, Simel DL. Does the clinical examination predict airflow limitation? Journal of the American Medical Association 1995; 273: 1334.

Jelic S, Jemtel T. Diagnostic usefulness of B-type natriuretic peptide and functional consequences of muscle alterations in COPD and chronic heart failure. Chest 2006; 130: 1220–1230.

Joosten SA, Koh MS, Bu X. The effects of oxygen therapy in patients presenting to an emergency department with exacerbation of chronic obstructive pulmonary disease. Medical Journal of Australia 2007; 186: 235–238.

Keenan SP, Kernerman PD, Cook DJ. Effect of noninvasive positive pressure ventilation on mortality in patients admitted with acute respiratory failure: a meta-analysis. Critical Care Medicine 1997; 25: 1685–1692.

Koh Y. Ventilatory management in patients with chronic airflow obstruction. Critical Care Clinics 2007; 23: 169–181.

McCrory DC, Brown CD. Anti-cholinergic bronchodilators versus beta2-sympathomimetic agents for acute exacerbations of chronic obstructive pulmonary disease. Cochrane Database System Review, CD 003900, 2003.

McKenzie D, Abramson M, Crockett AJ, et al. The COPD-X Plan: Australian and New Zealand Guidelines for the management of Chronic Obstructive Pulmonary Disease. 2007.

Moretti M, Cilione C, Tampieri A, et al. Incidence and causes of noninvasive mechanical ventilation failure after initial success. Thorax 2000; 55: 819–825.

Morris DG, Szekely LA, Thompson BT. Chronic obstructive pulmonary disease. In: Lee BW, Hsu SI, Stasiar DS, eds. Quick consult manual of evidence-based medicine. Philadelphia: Lippincott-Raven 1997; 222–244.

Ong KC, Earnest A, Lu SJ. A multidimensional grading system (BODE index) as predictor of hospitalization for COPD. Chest 2005; 128: 3810–3816.

Plant PK, Owen JL, Elliott MW, et al. Early use of noninvasive ventilation for acute exacerbations of chronic obstructive pulmonary disease on general respiratory wards: a multicentre randomized controlled trial. Lancet 2000; 355: 1931–1935.

Ram FSF, Picot J, Wedzicha JA. Non-invasive positive pressure ventilation for treatment of respiratory failure due to exacerbations of chronic obstructive pulmonary disease. Cochrane Database System Review Issue (3): CD004104. DOI: 10.1002/14651858. CD004104.pub3, 2004.

Ram FSF, Rodriguez-Rosin R, Granados-Navarette A. Antibiotics for exacerbations of chronic obstructive pulmonary disease. Cochrane Database Systematic Review CD 004403.pub2, 2006.

Snow V, Lascher S, Mottur-Pilson C, for the Joint Expert Panel on COPD of the American College of Chest Physicians and the American College of Physicians-American Society of Internal Medicine. The evidence base for management of acute exacerbations of COPD: Clinical Practice Guideline, Part 1 [special report]. Annals of Internal Medicine 2001; 134: 595–599.

Wood-Baker R, Gibson P, Hanney M, et al. Systemic corticosteroids for acute exacerbations of chronic obstructive pulmonary disease. Cochrane Database Systematic Review CD 001288, 2005.

6.6 Pneumothorax

Anne-Maree Kelly • Janet Talbot-Stern

ESSENTIALS

1 Pneumothorax can occur spontaneously, as a result of trauma, or iatrogenically. Spontaneous pneumothorax has been further subdivided into primary and secondary (related to underlying lung pathology). The utility of this distinction, as understanding of the pathology of pneumothorax evolves, is being challenged.

2 The diagnostic test of choice is a chest X-ray.

3 Treatment options include observation, aspiration, thoracotomy, and primary or delayed surgery. The evidence base to guide choice of therapy is weak.

4 Tension pneumothorax is rarely seen, particularly after spontaneous pneumothorax. It is, however, a life-threatening problem and must be managed immediately. It is a clinical, not a radiological, diagnosis.

Introduction

Pneumothorax is the presence of free air in the interpleural space which may occur spontaneously, as a result of trauma, or iatrogenically.

The most common form of pneumothorax is spontaneous. By definition, primary spontaneous pneumothoraces arise in otherwise healthy people without lung disease and without any apparent precipitating event. The reported incidence is 18–28/100 000 per year for men and 1.2–6/100 000 per year for women. Many patients do not seek medical advice for several days, with 46% waiting more than 2 days before presentation despite symptoms in one study.

Despite the absence of underlying pulmonary disease, subpleural blebs and bullae are likely to play a role in the pathogenesis, as they are found in up to 90% of cases at thoracoscopy or thoracotomy and in up to 80% of cases on CT scanning of the thorax. Primary spontaneous pneumothorax is more common in tall thin males aged 20–40 years who smoke.

Secondary spontaneous pneumothorax occurs as the result of underlying lung disease. It has a peak incidence at 60–65 years. Although chronic obstructive airways disease and asthma are the most common underlying conditions in developed countries, secondary pneumothorax may also be due to bacterial or tuberculous pneumonia, HIV with active *Pneumocystis* pneumonia, cancer, honeycomb lung disorders and cystic fibrosis. Secondary pneumothorax has also been seen in association those who abuse amphetamine, cocaine, Ecstasy, marijuana and nitrous oxide. Rarely, secondary pneumothorax can occur in women with pelvic endometriosis who may develop pneumothoraces (predominantly right-sided) within 72 hours of menstruation.

Iatrogenic pneumothorax may result from central line placement, intercostal blocks, thoracocentesis, lung biopsy, bronchoscopy and high pressures from artificial ventilation. Traumatic pneumothorax occurs in up to 15–20% of patients who sustain blunt chest trauma, and is usually secondary to fractured ribs. It may also be the result of penetrating wounds or barotrauma.

In most cases the air leak seals spontaneously, but in some the air continues to leak. In a subset of these a ball-valve effect can occur, with the development of tension pneumothorax. The trachea and mediastinal structures are pushed away from the collapsed lung and venous return to the heart may become obstructed. The result is severe respiratory compromise and hypotension. Emergent decompression is required. Tension is rare as a complication of primary spontaneous pneumothorax.

Clinical features

History

Symptoms of primary spontaneous pneumothorax often begin suddenly when the patient is at rest, but can be associated with deep inspiration, hyperventilation or coughing. It may also be precipitated by changes in atmospheric pressure that occur with flying and diving. Chest pain on the side of the pneumothorax is the most common presenting symptom (90% of cases). It can be sharp and pleuritic or dull, and may radiate to the back or neck. Dyspnoea occurs in up to 80% of patients but is generally not severe. Some patients, however, may be relatively asymptomatic or become asymptomatic after 24 hours. Many patients do not seek medical advice for several days, with up to 50% waiting more than 2 days despite symptoms. Chest pain is less common with secondary pneumothorax, dyspnoea being the predominant presenting complaint. These patients are more likely to be hypoxic, in part related to underlying lung pathology. Those with pneumothorax and pneumomediastinum related to drug abuse may also have neck pain, sore throat and dysphagia.

Examination

The classic signs of pneumothorax are reduced or absent breath sounds and hyper-resonance to percussion; however, at times the chest examination is unremarkable. Findings may be related to the size

of the pneumothorax. Less common findings include subcutaneous emphysema, unilateral enlargement of the chest, reduced excursion of the hemithorax with respirations, inferior liver displacement and Hamman's crunch (a noise heard with each heartbeat due to mediastinal emphysema). Patients who develop tension pneumothorax have evidence of air hunger, distended neck veins, tachycardia, hypotension and, classically, as a late sign, a deviated trachea.

Differential diagnosis

The differential diagnosis of this type of presentation includes costochondritis, pneumonia, pleurisy, pulmonary embolus, exacerbation of bronchospastic disease and myocardial ischaemia.

Investigations

No investigations are indicated for patients with suspected tension pneumothorax and cardiorespiratory compromise. It is a clinical, not a radiological diagnosis, and requires immediate treatment.

In stable patients with a suspected pneumothorax the investigation of choice is chest X-ray. Although traditionally expiratory chest X-rays have been used for the detection of pneumothoraces, presumably because of an assumption that expiration enhances contrast between lung parenchyma and pleural air, studies now suggest they do not increase detection of clinically relevant pneumothoraces. Findings include hyperlucency, lack of pulmonary markings and a fine line which represents the retraction of the visceral from the parietal pleura. There may also be blunting of the costophrenic angle. If the findings are not convincing, a lateral decubitus view may better reveal air. Large bullae or lung cysts may mimic a pneumothorax, and again a lateral decubitus view may be helpful, or a CT scan of the chest may be diagnostic.

If a supine X-ray is taken the only clue to a pneumothorax may be a deep sulcus sign on the affected side, an unusually distinct cardiac apex or increased hyperlucency of the upper abdominal quadrants. A cross-table lateral view should confirm the diagnosis. Thoracic ultrasound has recently been

advocated if X-ray is delayed. Associated pneumomediastinum is seen in 1.5% of pneumothoraces.

Current therapeutic guidelines divide pneumothoraces into small and large, although the details of the definitions vary. The British Thoracic Society defines 'small' as the presence of a visible rim of <2 cm between the lung margin and the chest wall on X-ray, but does not define where this measurement should be taken. The American College of Respiratory Physicians defines small pneumothoraces as those with less than 3 cm apical interpleural distance. The *Therapeutics Guidelines (Australia): Respiratory* divide pneumothoraces into 'large' and 'small' based on the rim of air surrounding the lung, similar to the British Thoracic Society guidelines. A 2 cm rim is said to approximate 50% collapse.

The patient's oxygenation is an essential component of assessment as, along with size, it is a key determinant of choice of management. Pulse oximetry is acceptable in most patients, but arterial blood gases may be necessary in sicker patients.

Role of CT

In addition to discriminating large bullae from pneumothoraces, CT scanning can identify dystrophic lung changes, primarily pulmonary blebs, in the affected and contralateral lung. The role of these findings in predicting recurrence, in defining which patients benefit from surgery and in defining the role of preventative surgery on an unaffected lung remains to be determined.

An ECG will often be part of the assessment, particularly if myocardial ischaemia is a differential diagnosis.

Management

General measures

Patients should initially receive supplemental oxygen, particularly if hypoxic. This increases the rate of pleural air absorption considerably, by reducing the partial pressure of nitrogen and increasing the gradient for nitrogen absorption. It is useful for both pneumothorax and pneumomediastinum.

The evidence base to guide choice of treatment for pneumothoraces is weak. Factors to be considered include the clinical condition of the patient, respiratory reserve, severity of symptoms, cause of pneumothorax and pneumothorax size. Most iatrogenic pneumothoraces can be treated conservatively or by aspiration. Many secondary and traumatic pneumothoraces require continuous catheter drainage because of low respiratory reserve or associated chest wall or lung injuries.

Emergency drainage

Patients who present in severe respiratory insufficiency or shock should be treated with immediate decompression. This involves the prompt placement of a large intravenous (e.g. 14 G) cannula or small-bore catheter by the Seldinger technique in the second intercostal space, midclavicular line (or the fifth intercostal space midaxillary line) with free drainage to air or to a Heimlich valve. Definitive therapy is then required.

Conservative management

Conservative treatment was the mainstay of management of primary spontaneous pneumothoraces until the 1940s. It was then largely rejected in favour of intercostal catheter drainage because it was believed that the latter resulted in a more rapid re-expansion of the lung and the assumption that this yielded a better outcome for the patient. This logic has been challenged, and there is now a move back towards the use of conservative management in selected cases. Conservative management is considered less appropriate for secondary and traumatic pneumothoraces.

It is been widely accepted that small primary spontaneous pneumothoraces in patients without respiratory compromise can be managed conservatively. It has been shown that 70–80% of pneumothoraces estimated as being smaller than 15% have no persistent air leak, and recurrence in those managed conservatively is less than in patients treated with intercostal tube drainage. There are very few data about outcome for patients with larger primary spontaneous pneumothoraces treated conservatively, but success rates of the order 90% have been reported.

The rate of resolution/reabsorption of primary spontaneous pneumothoraces was previously estimated as 1.25–1.8% of the volume of hemithorax every 24 hours. Recent data, based on CT volumetrics and a larger sample of patients, estimate the rate of re-expansion at 2.2%/day. Importantly, that study also found significant between- and within-patient variations in re-expansion rates, with a tendency for larger pneumothoraces to re-expand at a faster rate. Based on these data, a prudent follow-up strategy would be to repeat X-rays the next day (to detect deterioration) and then once or twice weekly until resolution. The patient needs to be given clear, specific written instructions about what to do if their symptoms worsen or their condition deteriorates.

The disadvantages of conservative treatment include the risk of unrecognized tension, the risk of deterioration, delay in the instigation of other therapy, interruption of employment/school in some patients, and potentially longer time to cessation of symptoms. The advantages of the conservative approach include the avoidance of the need for hospitalization and associated cost savings, minimal interruption to employment in selected candidates, avoidance of the risks and discomfort associated with some of the more invasive therapies, and good patient acceptance.

Most patients in this group who 'fail' conservative management and require intercostal tube drainage have secondary pneumothoraces.

Simple aspiration

Aspiration of pneumothoraces by placement of a needle – or more often a catheter – into the pleural space and aspiration of the pleural air is popular in some regions. The aim of this treatment is to convert a larger pneumothorax into one that can safely be managed conservatively. For primary spontaneous pneumothorax, successful re-expansion of the lung after simple aspiration is of the order of 50–83%. Available data suggest that rates for secondary pneumothoraces are lower. A recent randomized controlled trial showed that simple aspiration was as successful in treating first primary pneumothoraces as immediate intercostal tube drainage.

Successful aspiration has been shown to depend on age (under 50 years: 70–81% success; over 50 years: 19–31% success) and the size of the pneumothorax (<3 L aspirated: 89% success; >3 L: no success; >50% size on chest film: 62% success; <50% size on chest film: 77% success). There is a modest gain (up to 83% overall success) with a second or third attempt at aspiration. The question of whether patients who have undergone successful aspiration can be treated as outpatients is not settled. A period of observation of at least 4 hours to ensure that the pneumothorax does reaccumulate is required. Thereafter, disposition decisions should take into account the patient's underlying condition, proximity to assistance if required, their understanding of what to do if they deteriorate, and their wishes.

Few complications are reported to result from the use of aspiration, and all are minor: vasovagal reactions, local subcutaneous emphysema, and occasional problems with catheter kinking, blockage or dislodgement. It has been suggested that aspiration may carry a risk of empyema, but none has been formally reported. There are also no reported cases of lung laceration or of re-expansion pulmonary oedema.

Attempts to compare aspiration with intercostal catheter drainage have been scarce. A recent Cochrane Review found no significant difference between simple aspiration and intercostal tube drainage with regard to immediate success rate, early failure rate, duration of hospitalization, 1-year success rate and number of patients requiring pleurodesis at 1 year.

Intercostal catheter drainage

Intercostal catheters, traditionally between 10 and 40 Fr in size, may be inserted by an anterior, axillary or posteroapical approach. For practical and cosmetic reasons an axillary approach is currently the most favoured. Primary success rates of 66–97% have been reported. There is no evidence that the addition of suction improves outcome. Reported duration of hospital admission ranges from 7 to 9 days. All patients with intercostal catheters in situ should be admitted to hospital.

Potential disadvantages of intercostal catheters range from chest and abdominal visceral trauma from sharp trocars (now not favoured for insertion) to practical management issues such as the bulkiness of the underwater seal bottle system that must be kept upright. Available data suggest that the rate of aberrant placement is 4–9%, and empyema risk has been estimated at

1%. Other potential complications include bronchopleural fistulae, arteriovenous fistulae, perforation of the internal mammary artery, pulmonary or mediastinal blood vessels, focal lung infections, re-expansion pulmonary oedema and lung infarction. There are insufficient data to quantify the risk of these complications.

Pleural catheter options

In some centres, pleural catheters (usually 8–16 Fr) have been combined with the use of one-way valves (e.g. Heimlich valves) with good results. These allow the patient to ambulate and are easier to care for. One study has reported that small-bore pleural catheters were as effective as large intercostal catheters (ICC) in the initial resolution of primary spontaneous pneumothorax.

A variant of small-bore catheter drainage is the use of a pigtail catheter. A study comparing pigtail catheters to ICC reports that duration of drainage, mean hospital stay, evacuation rate and total cost were similar. Another reports success rates at 24 hours of 61% and at 1 week of 85%, with an average length of stay of 2.3 days. They also allow the possibility of outpatient management. This has been the subject of a number of case series and small studies, with reported success rates of 74–100%. Failure rate for outpatient treatment has been reported as 4.5%.

Surgery

Axillary thoracotomy with bullectomy, pleural abrasion and partial pleurectomy was, in the past, the routine surgical approach for recurrent pneumothoraces or failure of conservative treatment. The immediate problem is corrected and an attempt made to prevent recurrence by obliterating the pleural space. It has a low recurrence rate but is associated with significant morbidity. Since the 1990s, video-assisted thoracoscopic surgery (VATS) has increasingly been used for the treatment of primary pneumothoraces. Most authors recommend it for patients who continue to have an air leak after 3–7 days, recurrent pneumothoraces, airline pilots, frequent plane travellers and divers, contralateral or bilateral pneumothoraces, and failure of effectiveness of sclerosant through the chest tube. A range of techniques are used according to the findings, including pleurodesis with talc or scarification, blebectomy and/or bullectomy with electrocautery and stapling. It is not used routinely for secondary pneumothoraces.

Prognosis

Recurrence after the first pneumothorax is up to 50% for primary and secondary pneumothoraces, half of which occur within 4 months. This increases to 60–70% for subsequent recurrences.

Disposition

Patients with asymptomatic primary pneumothoraces and those with primary pneumothoraces successfully treated with simple aspiration may be discharged home, with close follow-up. All other patients require admission for either observation or definitive management.

As pneumothoraces will increase in size at altitude owing to changes in atmospheric pressure, flying with a pneumothorax is potentially dangerous. Current guidelines suggest that the pneumothorax should be fully resolved for at least 1 week (and preferably 1 month) before flying. Owing to the theoretical risk that higher barometric pressures associated with scuba diving may precipitate recurrence, patients having suffered a primary or secondary pneumothorax are advised not to dive in future. Whether this advice should apply to those who have had surgical interventions for pneumothorax is controversial, as recurrence is reduced but not eliminated. The absolute risks of recurrence and mortality are unknown, but CT scanning to identify dystrophic changes may help better define the risk.

Controversies

- The role of CT to identify pulmonary dystrophia with a view to predicting recurrence, in defining which patients benefit from surgery and in defining the role of preventative surgery on an unaffected lung.

- Choice of treatment for stable primary pneumothoraces.

- Could stable patients treated with small lumen/pigtail catheters be safely discharged home with Heimlich flutter valves?

- If patients fail conservative therapy, should they have an intercostal catheter placed or be referred for thoracoscopy?

- The place of primary VATS (without prior aspiration or intercostal catheter placement) in stable patients with recurrent pneumothorax.

- Advice regarding scuba diving for patients who have had surgical intervention for pneumothorax.

Further reading

Baumann MH, Strange C, Heffner JE, et al. Management of spontaneous pneumothorax: an American College of Chest Physicians Delphi consensus statement. Chest 2001; 119: 590–602.

Henry M, Arnold T, Harvey J. Pleural Diseases Group, Standards of Care Committee, British Thoracic Society. BTS guidelines for the management of spontaneous pneumothorax. Thorax 2003; 58: ii39–52.

Kelly AM, Loy J, Tsang AY. Estimating the rate of re-expansion of spontaneous pneumothorax by a formula derived from computed tomography volumetry studies. Emergency Medicine Journal 2006; 23: 780–782.

Kelly AM. Management of primary spontaneous pneumothorax: Is the best evidence clearer fifteen years on? Emergency Medicine Australasia 2007; 19: 303–308.

Therapeutic Guidelines: Respiratory. Therapeutic Guidelines Limited. Melbourne: 2005. Accessed at http://etg.hcn.net.au/ March on 31 May 2007.

Wakai A, O'Sullivan RG, McCabe G. Simple aspiration versus intercostal tube drainage for primary spontaneous pneumothorax in adults. Cochrane Database Systematic Review 1: CD004479, 2007.

6.7 Pleural effusion

Suzanne Mason

ESSENTIALS

1 In the vast majority of patients a posteroanterior and lateral chest X-ray will confirm and localize an effusion. Lateral decubitus films, ultrasound and CT scanning are more sensitive in diagnosing and localizing small effusions.

2 Pleural fluid analysis is the principal investigation to determine the underlying cause of the effusion. The key to management is the differentiation of transudates from exudates.

3 Pleural biopsy improves the diagnostic yield in the presence of TB and malignancy to 80% and 90%, respectively, when combined with pleural fluid analysis.

4 Treatment is dependent on the underlying disease. Large pleural effusions with cardiorespiratory compromise should be aspirated to provide symptomatic relief.

5 Transudates respond to treatment of the underlying condition. Exudates usually require further investigative procedures and specific local treatments.

Introduction

A pleural effusion is an accumulation of fluid in the pleural space caused by a disruption of the homoeostatic forces that control normal flow. Massive pleural effusions may produce significant cardiorespiratory compromise requiring urgent attention in the emergency department (ED). However, many are asymptomatic or produce minimal disturbance. In this latter group the role of the emergency physician assessment is to ascertain the aetiology of the effusion, as this dictates the most appropriate treatment. Much information regarding the likely cause can be obtained by a thorough history and physical examination. Important adjuvant investigations include chest X-ray, examination of pleural fluid and biopsies obtained during thoracocentesis. Bronchoscopy and thoracoscopy have a role to play in the small group of patients in whom the above procedures fail to establish a cause, but their use is beyond the scope of initial ED assessment and stabilization.

Pathophysiology

The pleural cavity is normally a small space bordered by the visceral and parietal pleura. It contains between 1 mL and 15 mL of clear fluid.[1] The pleura act as semipermeable membranes and fluid movement is determined principally by capillary pressure and plasma oncotic pressures and capillary permeability, governed by Starling's Law. Net flow is from parietal pleura to visceral pleura via the pleural cavity. Additional pleural fluid drainage occurs via pleurolymphatic communications or stomas, augmented by an active muscle pump. Overall absorptive capacity exceeds production by a factor of 10–20. Pleural effusions occur in one of the following:

- Disturbances in the hydrostatic–osmotic pressure gradients, resulting in a transudate.
- Pleural inflammation with loss of semipermeable membrane function, resulting in a protein-rich exudate.
- Lymphatic obstruction (usually producing a transudate).

Transudates are ultrafiltrates of plasma and arise as a result of a relatively small number of conditions. Exudates are produced by a wider variety of inflammatory conditions and often require more extensive investigation.

Aetiology

Table 6.7.1 lists the causes of transudative and exudative pleural effusions. The commonest causes are congestive cardiac failure, pneumonia and malignancy.[2]

Classification

Pleural effusions are classified according to their aetiology as transudates or exudates. Light[3] first proposed the criteria to differentiate the two. This involved measurement of both serum and pleural markers. An exudate is present if one or more of the following three are present:

- Ratio of pleural fluid–LDH level to serum LDH level >0.6.
- Pleural fluid–LDH level > two-thirds upper limit of normal for serum LDH level.
- Ratio of pleural fluid protein level to serum protein level >0.5.

If the fluid is found to be an exudate, then further tests are required to determine the underlying cause of disease.

Clinical features

History

The history will often identify the cause of a pleural effusion. Features suggestive of the common causes (congestive heart failure, pneumonia, malignancy and pulmonary embolism) should be sought. Specific questioning regarding previous occupational exposures, drug treatments, radiation therapy, trauma, tuberculosis exposure and collagen vascular disease may be rewarding. Pleural effusions rarely cause symptoms other than dyspnoea, although a mild non-productive cough is sometimes described. A more severe or productive cough suggests underlying pulmonary pathology. Chest pain in association with an effusion may indicate malignancy, pulmonary embolus or pleural inflammation. More unusually, a chest wall swelling may

Table 6.7.1 Causes of transudative and exudative pleural effusions

Effusion always transudative
Congestive cardiac failure
Cirrhosis
Nephrotic syndrome
Peritoneal dialysis
Hypoalbuminaemia
Urinothorax
Atelectasis
Constrictive pericarditis
Superior vena caval obstruction

'Classic' exudates that can be transudates
Malignancy
Pulmonary embolism
Sarcoidosis
Hypothyroidism

Exudates
Infectious
    Bacterial pneumonia
    Tuberculosis
    Parasites
    Fungal disease
    Atypical pneumonia
    Nocardia, actinomyces
    Subphrenic abscess
    Hepatic abscess
    Splenic abscess
    Hepatitis
    Spontaneous oesophageal rupture

Iatrogenic
Drug-induced (nitrofurantoin, dantrolene
sodium, methysergide maleate, procarbazine
HCl, methotrexate, medications causing drug-
induced lupus syndrome: procainamide HCl,
hydralazine HCl, quinidine)
Oesophageal perforation
Oesophageal sclerotherapy
Central venous catheterization
Enteral feeding

Malignancy
Carcinoma
Lymphoma
Mesothelioma

Leukaemia
Chylothorax

Other inflammatory disorders
Pancreatitis
Benign asbestos pleural effusion
Pulmonary embolisn
Radiation therapy
Uraemic pleurisy
Sarcoidosis
Post cardiac injury syndrome
Haemothorax
ARDS

Increased negative intrapleural pressure
Atelectasis
Cholesterol effusion

Connective tissue disease
Lupus pleuritis
Rheumatoid pleurisy
Mixed connective tissue disease
Churg–Strauss syndrome
Wegener's granulomatosis
Familial Mediterranean fever

Endocrine dysfunction
Hypothyroidism
Ovarian hyperstimulation syndrome

Lymphatic abnormalities
Malignancy
Yellow nail syndrome
Lymphangiomyomatosis

Movement of fluid from the abdomen to pleural space
Pancreatitis
Pancreatic pseudocyst
Meig's syndrome
Carcinoma
Chylous ascites
Urinothorax

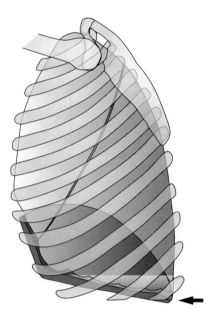

Fig. 6.7.1 Small pleural effusion detected on lateral chest X-ray (arrow indicates the effusion).

be due to metastatic cancer or an expanding empyema.

Patients may have myriad associated systemic symptoms due to the underlying pathological process, such as fever, weight loss, abdominal and joint pain.

Physical examination

Small effusions may be undetectable clinically. However, mild hypoxaemia is common, often associated with dyspnoea, which can be due to distortions of the diaphragm or chest wall during repsiration. The classic signs of pleural effusion are reduced chest wall expansion, stony dullness to percussion, absent breath sounds, diminished or absent vocal resonance and tactile fremitus on the affected side. In large unilateral effusions, tracheal displacement toward the unaffected side may be detected. In

addition, signs of underlying disease should be sought.

Investigations

Chest X-ray

In the majority of patients a posteroanterior (PA) and lateral chest X-ray will provide the required information to confirm and localize an effusion (Figs 6.7.1 and 6.7.2). The classic radiological features of effusion are of a gravity-dependent homogeneous opacity within the pleural cavity with a concave lateral air–fluid interface (meniscus sign). Effusions larger than 150 mL are seen as blunting of costophrenic angles on erect films (Fig. 6.7.2). Occasionally the collection may be subpulmonary. Signs suggestive of this include apparent elevation

of the diaphragm, abnormal diaphragmatic contour (lateral displacement of the apex on PA film, sharp angulation of apparent anterior diaphragm on lateral film), and more than a 2 cm space between the gastric bubble and the apparent left diaphragm. Very small and/or isolated effusions may not be seen on standard views. Lateral or lateral decubitus films are often helpful where a fluid level at least 1 cm deep indicates that the effusion is accessible by thoracocentesis (Fig. 6.7.1). If the fluid does not form a uniform level, this may indicate the presence of a loculated effusion, which requires more careful management. Chest ultrasound and computed tomography (CT) are more sensitive in diagnosing and localizing small effusions. CT can also be helpful in examining the lung parenchyma and mediastinum for associated pathology.

The chest X-ray can also provide other diagnostic clues to the aetiology of the effusion. Large effusions with lack of mediastinal shift indicate a bronchial obstruction, infiltration of the lung with tumour, mesothelioma or a fixed mediastinum (due to tumour or fibrosis). Bilateral effusions with an enlarged heart shadow are usually due to congestive cardiac failure. Pleural plaques and calcification may indicate asbestos exposure, and findings consistent

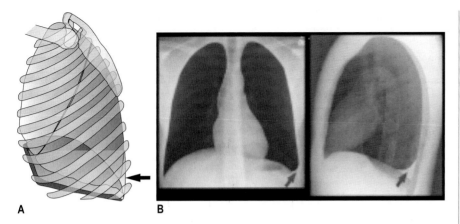

Fig. 6.7.2 Larger pleural effusion (A). This can be visible on both the lateral and PA chest views (B). (arrow indicates the effusion.)

with pneumonia or malignancy may indicate a cause for the associated effusion.

Thoracocentesis

If the diagnosis is known (e.g. congestive heart failure with recurrent effusions) further investigations need only be performed to aid management of the underlying problem. When the diagnosis is still uncertain the most useful investigation is diagnostic thoracocentesis. A variety of techniques have been reported, but the common underlying principle is the advancement of a needle, trocar or cannula into the pleural space under strict aseptic conditions, and the withdrawal of a volume of fluid for analysis. Fluid should be procured for biochemical, microbiological and cytological analysis in order to classify the effusion as outlined above and indicate an underlying cause (Fig. 6.7.3).[4]

The gross appearance of the pleural fluid can be helpful in diagnosis. Table 6.7.2 outlines the common differentials according to gross findings.

With respect to exudates, microscopy, Gram's stain and cytology should be performed. The diagnostic yield in malignant disease ranges from 50% to 80%[5] and is improved with larger-volume collections and repeated sampling. Pleural fluid pH may be helpful in diagnosis. In parapneumonic effusions, a pH < 7.2 indicates the need for urgent drainage, whereas a pH >7.3 suggests that treament with systemic antibiotics should be sufficient.[6] In malignant effusions, a pleural pH <7.3 indicates more extensive pleural involvement and shorter survival times.[7] A low pleural fluid pH also correlates well with glucose levels. Glucose <0.5 times serum is suggestive of bacterial infection, malignancy or rheumatoid arthritis. An elevated amylase in the pleural fluid suggests oesophageal rupture, effusion associated with pancreatitis, or malignancy. Pleural fluid antinuclear antibody and rheumatoid factor tests should be ordered when collagen vascular diseases are suspected.

There are no absolute contraindications to thoracocentesis, but relative contraindications include a bleeding diathesis or anticoagulation, small fluid volumes, mechanical ventilation, and cutaneous disease over the proposed puncture site.[8,9] The puncture location is chosen based on clinical examination and chest X-ray findings. Smaller effusions can often be located with ultrasound guidance.

Additional techniques

Two other procedures deserve consideration when thoracocentesis is not diagnostic. Percutaneous pleural biopsy involves obtaining a closed biopsy of the parietal pleura using either an Abrams or a Cope needle. It is relatively easy to perform and improves the diagnostic yield in the presence of tuberculosis and malignancy to 80% and 90%, respectively, when combined with pleural fluid analysis. The second is thoracoscopy, which involves pleural biopsy under direct visualization through a thoracoscope. Thoracoscopy has a very high yield for diagnosing both benign and malignant pleural disease; however, it requires general anesthesia and is usually employed only after other diagnostic procedures have proved non-diagnostic.

Management

If a pleural effusion is causing respiratory distress then it should be drained regardless of whether it is a transudate or an exudate (Fig. 6.7.3). Drainage of a relatively small volume of fluid can cause significant relief from symptoms. All patients undergoing this procedure should be well oxygenated, with oxygen saturations monitored and kept above 90%, as thoracocentesis may increase ventilation–perfusion mismatches.[10] Removal of large volumes (usually >1500 mL) may produce re-expansion pulmonary oedema, so large effusions should be drained in stages, with at least 12 hours between procedures.

All transudates should be managed by treating the underlying disease. Large-bore tube thoracostomy should be employed for empyema and traumatic haemothorax.

Table 6.7.2 Gross appearance of pleural fluid (Modified from Light RW. Pleural effusion. New England Journal of Medicine 2002; 346: 1971–1977.)		
Appearance of fluid	**Test indicated**	**Interpretation of result**
Bloody	Haematocrit	<1% non-sigificant 1–20% malignancy, pulmonary embolus, trauma >50% haemothorax
Cloudy or turbid	Centrifugation Triglyceride level	Turbid supernatant – high lipid levels >110 mg/dL chylothorax >50 mg/dL need lipoprotein analysis Chylomicrons chylothorax <50 mg/dL and cholesterol>250 mg/dL pseudochylothorax
Putrid odour	Gram stain and culture	Possible anaerobic infection

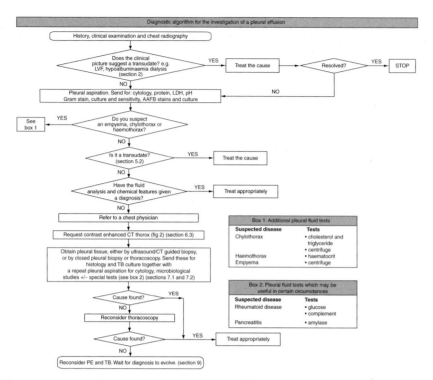

Fig. 6.7.3 Guidelines for the investigation of a unilateral pleural effusion in adults.[4]

Empyemas tend to loculate early, in which case 250 000 units of streptokinase may be instilled to dissolve the fibrin membranes. Should this fail, surgical drainage or decortication should be performed. Systemic organism-specific antibiotic therapy should also be instituted.

Malignant effusions can be managed by thoracostomy and tetracycline pleurodesis, thoracoscopy and talc poudrage, or pleuro-peritoneal shunt. Chylothoraces should be treated by pleuroperitoneal shunting, as long-term drainage may result in malnutrition and altered immunocompetence.

Complications

Pleural effusions can produce significant respiratory distress which is alleviated only through drainage. Other complications are those of the underlying pathological process, such as fever and toxicity in the case of parapneumonic effusions.

There are recognized complications associated with thoracocentesis, such as pain at the puncture site, cutaneous or internal bleeding, pneumothorax, empyema, and splenic or hepatic puncture.[8] Pneumothorax complicates around 12% of thoracocenteses. Risk factors include chronic obstructive or fibrotic pulmonary disease, previous chest irradiation, using larger thoracocentesis needles, multiple passes to obtain fluid and aspiration of air during the procedure.[11,12]

Disposition

The requirement for inpatient investigation and management will depend on the degree of respiratory compromise, the presence of coexisting or underlying disease, and the patient's wishes. In many cases chronic relapsing effusions in the otherwise stable patient may be managed on an outpatient basis.

Summary

Pleural effusion complicates many local and systemic illnesses. The vast majority can be detected with a good history, physical examination and a chest X-ray. The key to management is the differentiation of transudates from exudates. In general, transudates respond to treatment of the underlying condition. Exudates usually require further investigative procedures and specific local treatments.

References

1. Light RW. Diseases of the pleura, mediastinum, chest wall and diaphragm. In: George RB, Light RW, Matthay MA, et al, Chest medicine: essentials of pulmonary and critical care medicine, 3rd edn. Baltimore: Williams & Wilkins, 1995; 441–447.
2. Light RW. Pleural effusion. New England Journal of Medicine 2002; 346: 1971–1977.
3. Light RW, Macgregor MI, Luchsinger PC, et al. Pleural effusions: the diagnstoic separation of transudates and exudates. Annals of Internal Medicine 1972; 77: 507–513.
4. Maskell NA, Butland RJA, on behalf of the British Thoracic Society Pleural Disease Group, a subgroup of the British Thoracic Society Standards of Care Committee. BTS guidelines for the investigation of a unilateral pleural effusion in adults. Thorax 2003; 58: ii8–ii17.
5. Health and Public Policy Committee American College of Physicians. Diagnostic thoracocentesis and pleural biopsy. Position paper. Annals of Internal Medicine 1985; 103: 799–802.
6. Good JT Jr, Taryle DA, Maulitz RM, et al. The diagnostic value of pleural fluid pH. Chest 1980; 78: 55–59.
7. Sahn SA, Good JT Jr. Pleural fluid pH in malignant effusions: diagnostic, prognostic, and therapeutic implications. Annals of Internal Medicine 1988; 108: 345–349.
8. Sahn SA. State of the art: the pleura. American Review of Respiratory Diseases 1988; 138: 184–234.
9. Bartter T, Santarelli R, Akers SM. The evaluation of pleural effusion. Chest 1994; 106: 1209–1214. Erratum, Chest 1995; 107: 592.
10. Estenne M, Yernault JC, De Troyer A. Mechanism of relief of dyspnoea after thoracocentesis in patients with large pleural effusions. American Journal of Medicine 1983; 74: 813–819.
11. Doyle JJ, Hnatiuk OW, Torrington KG. Necessity of routine chest roentgenography after thoracocentesis. Annals of Internal Medicine 1996; 124: 816–820.
12. Raptopoulos V, Davis LM, Lee G. Factors affecting the development of pneumothorax aasociated with thoracocentesis. American Journal of Roentgenology 1991; 156: 917–920.

Further reading

Boutin C, Astoul P, Seitz B. The role of thoracoscopy in the evaluation and management of pleural effusions. Lung 1990; 168: 113–1121.
Burgess KR. MJA practice essential 3. The chest wall and pleural space. Medical Journal of Australia 1997; 166: 604–609.
Kosowsky J. Pleural disease. In: Rosen P, Barkin R, eds. Emergency medicine concepts and clinical practice, 3rd edn. Chicago: Mosby, 1992;

6.8 Haemoptysis

Stuart Dilley

ESSENTIALS

1 The majority of patients are stable and can be managed and investigated as outpatients.

2 Patients may have difficulty differentiating between haemoptysis and haematemesis.

3 Chest X-ray is normal in 20–30% of patients with haemoptysis.

4 Bronchoscopy is the specific investigation of choice if haemoptysis is thought to be due to a lesion in the bronchial tree.

5 In 30% of cases, no cause for haemopytysis will be found.

6 The priorities in massive haemoptysis are the maintenance of ventilation, circulatory support, and identification of the source of bleeding.

Introduction

Most patients who present with haemoptysis describe small amounts of blood mixed with sputum or saliva. The majority are stable and can be managed as outpatients. Rarely, patients present with massive haemoptysis where respiratory and circulatory systems are severely compromised, and death by asphyxiation can be quite rapid. These patients require urgent skilful management of the airway and circulation. Nonetheless, by obstructing an airway, a small blood clot may compromise ventilation just as effectively as a massive bleed that floods an entire lung.

Aetiology

The causes of haemoptysis are summarized below. In approximately 30% of cases no cause will be found (Table 6.8.1).

Clinical features

The relative importance of resuscitation, history, examination and investigation in patients presenting with haemoptysis depends very much on the degree of bleeding and respiratory compromise. Most patients do not have compromised respiratory or circulatory systems, so the emphasis is on clinical assessment.

Patients may have difficulty in differentiating between haemoptysis and haematemesis. Bronchial blood is usually bright red, frothy and alkaline, whereas gastrointestinal blood is usually darker, may be mixed with food particles, and is acidic. Haemoptysis also needs to be differentiated from upper airway bleeding, particularly posterior epistaxis. History and examination should be tailored to elicit information relevant to the common causes of haemoptysis, as listed above.

Clinical investigations

Imaging

Chest X-ray
Between 20% and 30% of patients with haemoptysis will have a normal chest X-ray. X-ray abnormalities tend to reflect pre-existing chronic lung disease rather than identifying a definitive cause for the bleeding. Evidence of infection, abscess formation, tuberculosis, bronchiectasis or tumours may be seen.

Computed tomography
Computed tomography (CT) of the chest may occasionally provide additional information not evident on chest X-ray, and is particularly useful in cases of bronchocarcinoma and bronchiectasis to further delineate anatomy.

Other
Ventilation–perfusion scan, CT angiography and other investigations may be indicated if the diagnosis is thought to be pulmonary embolism. Pulmonary and bronchial angiography may be useful if bleeding is ongoing and no source is found by other means.

Bronchoscopy
Bronchoscopy allows direct visualization of the bronchial tree and the source of bleeding, and is the specific investigation of choice in cases of haemoptysis thought to

Table 6.8.1 Causes of haemoptysis	
Pulmonary	*Extrapulmonary*
Pneumonia	Pulmonary embolism
Neoplasm	Coagulopathies
Bronchitis	Mitral stenosis
Lung abscess	Oral or pharyngeal blood
Bronchiectasis	Heart failure
Tuberculosis	Thoracic aortic aneurysm
Connective tissue disorder	Oesophageal carcinoma
Arteriovenous malformation	
Trauma	
Cystic fibrosis	

be due to abnormalities of the bronchial tree. In the case of massive haemoptysis, bronchoscopy should be performed early. It should also be performed on those patients diagnosed with pneumonia or bronchitis who continue to bleed or who do not respond to antibiotic therapy. In addition to direct visualization of the bronchial tree, bronchoscopy facilitates the gathering of sputum and cytological samples for further analysis.

Rigid bronchoscopy allows for more complete removal of blood and better ventilation in the case of massive haemoptysis, although upper lobe airways are not well visualized. The fibreoptic bronchoscope (FOB) is thinner and more flexible, and can be used to visualize areas of the bronchial tree not seen with the rigid bronchoscope. It cannot cope with the large volumes of blood that need suctioning in massive haemoptysis, but can be passed down the lumen of the rigid bronchoscope once the majority of blood has been removed.

Sputum

When the origin of haemoptysis is thought to be infective or neoplastic, sputum should be collected for bacteriological and cytological assessment, including Zeihl–Neelsen staining for acid-fast bacilli.

Other

Haemoglobin, platelet count and clotting studies should be undertaken but will usually be normal in an otherwise healthy individual. A raised white cell count may indicate the presence of infection. Assessment of oxygenation by pulse oximetry or arterial blood gas analysis is particularly important for the patient with respiratory distress and massive bleeding. Blood cross-matching may be needed in the case of massive haemoptysis.

Treatment

In most cases haemoptysis is mild and transient and is usually due to an infective process. Malignant disease also needs to be excluded. Patients can usually be discharged from the emergency department (ED), on appropriate antibiotics if appropriate, for outpatient or general practitioner follow-up of sputum studies, repeat chest

X-rays, CT scans and bronchoscopy as indicated. Those with respiratory compromise, pulmonary emboli or carcinoma should be managed accordingly.

Massive haemoptysis

Massive haemoptysis is rare, accounting for less than 2% of all cases of haemoptysis, but has a high mortality (up to 80% in some studies). It is not only frightening to the patient, but can also test the skill of the treating physician. Opinions vary as to the most appropriate course of management, an indication of the paucity of evidence-based literature on this topic.

Haemoptysis arises from the systemic pressure in bronchial arteries in 90% of cases, with only 5% arising from the low-pressure pulmonary circulation.[1] Massive haemoptysis has been arbitrarily defined by various authors as being as little as 100 mL to as much as 1000 mL of blood loss in 24 hours.[2] Others give a more useful definition as 'the volume that is life-threatening by virtue of airway obstruction or blood loss'.[3] Exsanguinating haemoptysis of more than 150 mL per hour and a loss of more than 1000 mL per day has a mortality of 75%.[4] Massive haemoptysis is usually due to tuberculosis, bronchiectasis or infections, including fungal infections. Bronchogenic carcinoma, albeit a common cause of haemoptysis, rarely causes massive bleeding.

The general principles of 'ABCs' apply as in all serious illness. The immediate threat to the patient is asphyxia. Patients may rapidly become severely hypoxic, restless and uncooperative, and immediate intubation may be necessary. The airway should be vigorously suctioned and supplemental oxygen administered. Blood should be collected for full blood count, cross-matching and arterial blood gases, and intravenous fluids or blood infused. Coagulation abnormalities should be corrected. Early consultation with respiratory and/or cardiothoracic specialties is essential.

Although it is customary to nurse the patient with the suspected bleeding lung dependent to prevent aspiration into the normal lung,[1,2] some have argued that this may increase the rate of bleeding.[5] The Trendelenburg position is also recommended to aid drainage of blood from the thorax.

The need to secure an airway provides a dilemma. A large-bore endotracheal tube (ETT) will permit ventilation but may not protect the lungs. However, it will allow the passage of a fibreoptic bronchoscope and large-bore suction catheter to both visualize the bronchial tree and remove blood. In extreme circumstances the ETT may be advanced into the right main-stem bronchus to protect the right lung if bleeding appears to be left-sided, but may lead to occlusion of the right upper lobe bronchus. The ETT can be used to guide a balloon occlusion catheter into the right main-stem bronchus to tamponade the right lung if bleeding appears to be right-sided, although the ETT will then need to be replaced so that circuit connections can still be made. Blindly advancing the ETT into the left main bronchus is a more difficult procedure. A bronchoscope may be directed into the left main bronchus, allowing the subsequent passage of an ETT to protect the left lung if bleeding is right-sided. Balloon catheters may also be more accurately placed under bronchoscopic guidance.[2]

Double-lumen tubes provide protection for the normal lung and a chance to suction or tamponade the bleeding lung. However, they may not be readily available and take considerably more skill to insert than a standard single-lumen ETT.[7] High rates of misplacement have been reported.[1] They are also too narrow to allow the passage of a fibreoptic bronchoscope, and hence limit further assessment of the bleeding source. They are perhaps best reserved for use after bronchoscopy has been performed.[6]

Urgent bronchoscopy should be performed in unstable patients with massive haemoptysis.[2] Bronchoscopy can help to localize the source of bleeding and may facilitate the passage of a balloon-tip catheter into the bleeding bronchus to tamponade the bleeding source. Angiography may also help identify the source of bleeding. However, there is significant anatomical variability in terms of number of bronchial arteries and their origins, and bleeding is not usually fast enough to show extravasation of contrast.

The place of surgical treatment in massive haemoptysis is controversial. Some authors advocate early surgical resection of the bleeding site and the adjacent lung. It may be difficult to identify the source of the bleeding, however, and most surgeons prefer to operate on a stable patient whose bleeding has ceased. Additionally, some patients will not have the pulmonary reserve to cope with a partial or full lobectomy. Other authors suggest a more conservative approach,[7,8] including airway management, suction, endobronchial balloon tamponade, antibiotics, iced saline lavage, topical epinephrine (adrenaline) and bronchial artery embolization, and report mortality rates of 0–25%. They suggest surgery should be reserved for patients who continue to suffer massive haemoptysis despite these measures.

Radiologically guided bronchial artery embolization is a useful procedure, halting bleeding in most patients. Twenty per cent of patients will re-bleed within 6 months, and 50 % will have significant bleeds in the longer term.[9] However, this procedure may buy some time to allow thoracotomy to be performed semi-electively. Significant complications such as spinal cord injury and arterial dissection, although rare, have been reported.

Other agents such as tranexamic acid and vasopressin have been tried, with mixed results. Vasoconstriction may hamper attempts at bronchial artery embolization, however. Direct instillation of antifungal agents in cases of massive haemoptysis due to mycetoma has shown greater promise than the use of systemic antifungal agents.[3]

Controversies

- What is the appropriate positioning for the patient with massive haemoptysis?

- Should CT or bronchoscopy be the investigation of choice following CXR?

- What method of endotracheal or endobronchial intubation is most appropriate for acute massive haemoptysis in the emergency department?

- Should rigid or flexible bronchoscopy be used to assess massive haemoptysis?

- Conservative versus operative management of massive haemoptysis.

References

1. Jean-Baptiste E. Clinical assessment and management of massive haemoptysis. Critical Care Medicine 2000; 28: 1642–1647.
2. Dweik R, Stoller J. Role of bronchoscopy in massive hemoptysis. Clinics in Chest Medicine 1999; 20: 89–105.
3. Lordan J, Gascoigne A, Corris P. The pulmonary physician in critical care, illustrative case 7: Assessment and management of massive haemoptysis. Thorax 2003; 58: 814–819.
4. Rudzinski JP, del Castillo J. Massive hemoptysis. Annals of Emergency Medicine 1987; 16: 561–564.
5. Patel U, Pattison CW, Raphael M. Management of massive haemoptysis. British Journal of Hospital Medicine 1994; 52: 74–78.
6. Goldman J. Hemoptysis: Emergency assessment and management. Emergency Medicine Clinics of North America 1989; 7: 325–338.
7. Haponik E, Fein A, Chin R. Managing life-threatening hemoptysis. Has anything really changed? Chest 2000; 118: 1431–1435.
8. Jones D, Davies R. Massive haemoptysis: Medical management will usually arrest the bleeding. British Medical Journal 1990; 300: 889–890.
9. Marshall T, Flower C, Jackson J. Review: The role of radiology in the investigation and management of patients with haemoptysis. Clinical Radiology 1996; 51: 391–400.

RESPIRATORY

7.1 Dysphagia

Graeme Thomson

ESSENTIALS

1 Dysphagia is a diagnostic challenge and a broad differential diagnosis should be considered. A carefully taken history will reveal the likely cause in most cases.

2 Dysphagia due to a pharyngeal or oesophageal disorder will increase the amount of food in the pharynx and may be complicated by aspiration. An assessment of that risk should be made before allowing the patient to take oral fluids or food.

3 Patients with moderate to long-term dysphagia may have significant fluid and electrolyte abnormalities and severe nutritional disturbances.

4 Emergency department investigations should be directed to the detection of high-grade obstructions and lesions causing significant risks from airway compromise, haemorrhage or sepsis.

5 Dysphagia is very rarely caused by a psychological disorder. There is nearly always a physical cause to be found.

Introduction

Dysphagia is a broad term encompassing the many forms of difficulty with deglutition (swallowing). The main issues are to determine the likely causes, to identify those patients at risk of significant complications, to treat those causes that are amenable to acute intervention, and to refer appropriately for further investigations and treatment.

Dysphagia may be associated with odynophagia (pain on swallowing). Globus is a related term that means the sensation of a lump in the throat. This is rarely of psychological origin. Since the advent of sophisticated investigative techniques it has been recognized that in the great majority of cases there is an identifiable physical cause.

Aetiology

Problems may occur with any of the three stages of swallowing: oral, pharyngeal or oesophageal. Oral and pharyngeal causes may be grouped as transfer dysphagia and oesophageal problems may be referred to as transport dysphagia.[1] The passage of food may be obstructed by a physical barrier such as a tumour or a disorder of muscle coordination such as a neurological deficit.

In addition to diseases, several drugs are recognized to induce dysphagia. They include tetracyclines, non-steroidal anti-inflammatory drugs, ascorbic acid, quinidine, ferrous sulphate and potassium chloride.

Clinical features

Symptoms may appear suddenly or develop insidiously. If insidious, there may be an acute precipitating event leading to presentation, often complete or partial obstruction owing to the impact of a food bolus in the oesophagus. This may present as pain, a feeling of a lump in the neck or central chest, severe retching, or drooling and an inability to swallow saliva. Patients may report increasing difficulty swallowing solids and then fluids, but in some cases there may be no previous history of dysphagia.

Where a neurological disorder is causing difficulty initiating swallowing there may be other neurological deficits. The voice may have changed. Regurgitation of food from the mouth or nose, coughing or frank aspiration may be evident when the patient eats. It should be assumed that patients with recent cerebrovascular events or bulbar dysfunction are dysphagic until formal assessment of swallowing and airway protection can be undertaken.

Examination should focus on testing of cranial nerve function plus careful examination of the mouth, neck, chest and abdomen.

Perforation may be suspected if there is a history of ingestion of a corrosive substance or sharp object, or if pain is a prominent feature. There may be evidence of surgical emphysema in the neck. If presentation is delayed there may be signs of sepsis.

Clinical investigation

Investigations are directed by the history and likely aetiology. For oropharyngeal and upper oesophageal lesions a lateral X-ray of the soft tissues of the neck may reveal a lesion impinging on the oesophagus. An impacted dense bone or other solid foreign body may also be seen. For suspected mid and lower oesophageal lesions, frontal and lateral chest radiographs may reveal a fluid level, a mediastinal tumour, tuberculous lesions or an aneurysm of the thoracic aorta. Oesophageal perforation may also be detected. If food bolus obstruction is suspected a Gastrografin swallow may reveal the site and degree of obstruction.

Computed tomography (CT) scanning and endoscopy may also be indicated, but in most cases they can be deferred and performed on a semi-elective basis. A videofluorographic swallowing study is the best semi-elective investigation.[2] It may reveal structural abnormalities as well as disorders

of muscular coordination. Manometry is less reliable.

Laboratory investigations are guided by likely aetiology and complications, but should include basic biochemistry and full blood examination looking for electrolyte disturbances and anaemia.

Treatment

Definitive treatment depends on the underlying cause and will rarely be completed in the emergency department (ED). The degree of oesophageal obstruction, the acuity of onset and the presence of complications dictate the need for emergency treatment. Patients with high-grade obstruction should have oral fluids and food withheld and should be given intravenous fluids if the obstruction persists for more than a few hours.

For food bolus obstruction, intravenous glucagon may relax the oesophageal muscles enough to allow a bolus to pass through.[3] This is less likely to be successful if the bolus is a piece of meat.[4] An initial dose of 1 mg may be followed by a 2 mg dose if necessary. Complications are rare, but include allergy, nausea and hypotension. Phaeochromocytoma is a contraindication to the use of glucagon. Sublingual glyceryl trinitrate may be used as an alternative to glucagon, but hypotension is more likely. After glucagon, a gas-producing substance may be given in an attempt to dilate the oesophagus. Aerated drinks are adequate for this purpose.[5] This technique should be used with great caution because a patient with upper oesophageal obstruction will be at greater risk of aspiration if given a foaming substance. This approach should be avoided if there is any suspicion of perforation. Endoscopic removal will be required in many cases, but this is usually attempted after a period of expectant treatment.

Bones or similar foreign bodies impacted in the pharynx can often be removed in the ED. Topical anaesthetic sprays may suppress the pharyngeal reflexes adequately to allow direct or indirect laryngoscopy and removal with forceps. Removal may immediately relieve the dysphagia, but symptoms due to local oedema or abrasions may persist.

Oesophageal or pharyngeal perforation is a serious complication requiring cover with broad-spectrum antibiotics and urgent surgical referral.

Odynophagia may be relieved by parenteral or topical analgesia. Oral administration of a viscous preparation of lidocaine will ease the pain caused by luminal inflammatory disorders. The maximum recommended dose is 300 mg and should be reduced in the elderly, who may be more affected by systemic absorption.

Other issues

Appropriate disposition depends on the likely aetiology and the presence of complications. Admission is indicated for patients at risk of airway compromise, severe haemorrhage, sepsis, or those with high-grade oesophageal obstruction. It will also be indicated when dysphagia is part of a broader disease process.

If a food bolus has passed spontaneously, the patient should be referred for semi-elective endoscopy.

Controversies

- Choice between flexible and rigid endoscopy for removal of a food bolus. In many departments referral patterns will be fixed; however, if there is a choice, rigid endoscopy is preferred for removal of an upper oesophageal bolus and flexible endoscopy for boluses impacted more distally. Overall, flexible endoscopy has a lower complication rate.[6]

- Observation unit management. There may be arguments for a period of observation of 12 hours or more before referral for endoscopy, as the majority of food bolus obstructions will resolve spontaneously.[7]

References

1. Mendelson MH. Dysphagia. In: Tintinalli JE, Kelen GD, Stapczynski JS, eds. Emergency medicine: a comprehensive study guide. New York: McGraw Hill, 2004; 509–510.
2. Palmer JB, Drennan JC, Baba M. Evaluation and treatment of swallowing impairments. American Family Physician 2000; 61: 2453–2462.
3. Glauser J, Lilja GP, Greenfeld B, et al. Intravenous glucagon in the management of oesophageal

food obstruction. Journal of the American College of Emergency Physicians 1979; 8: 228–231.

4. Sodeman TC, Harewood GC, Baron TH. Assessment of the predictors of response to glucagon in the setting of acute oesophageal food bolus obstruction. Dysphagia 2004; 19: 18–21.

5. Mohammed SH, Hegedus V. Dislodgement of impacted oesophageal foreign bodies with carbonated beverages. Clinical Radiology 1986; 37: 589–592.

6. Gmeiner D, von Rahden BH, Meco C, et al. Flexible versus rigid endoscopy for treatment of foreign body

impaction in the oesophagus. Surgical Endoscopy 2007; (Epub ahead of print).

7. Tsikoudas A, Kochillas X, Kelleher R, et al. The management of acute oesophageal obstruction from food bolus: Can we be more conservative? European Archives of Otorhinolaryngology 2005; 262: 528–530.

7.2 Approach to abdominal pain

Kim Chai Chan • Eillyne Seow

ESSENTIALS

1 Abdominal pain accounts for 5–10% of all emergency department visits. A significant proportion of these patients will require hospital admission.

2 Abdominal pain most frequently arises from pathologies in the gastrointestinal and the genitourinary systems; however it may also result from cardiovascular, pulmonary, metabolic, infective and toxic causes.

3 Special considerations should be given to four subgroups of patients: the elderly, the immunocompromised (including those with HIV infection), women of childbearing age and children. These patients require careful assessment to avoid missed diagnoses and poor outcomes.

4 In up to 25–40% of patients the exact cause of the abdominal pain may not be determined in the emergency department. After ruling out life-threatening causes, and with relief of symptoms, most of these patients may be discharged with appropriate advice.

5 Patients with abdominal pain should be given adequate analgesia (including the use of opioids). Adequate analgesia can aid diagnosis and does not conceal signs of an acute abdomen.

Introduction

The assessment of patients with abdominal pain is challenging because:

- The contact time with the patient is relatively short and diagnosis may be difficult, especially early on in the disease process.
- The patient's presentation may be atypical, especially for the very young, the immunocompromised and the elderly.
- The degree of pain may not be commensurate with the severity of the disease.
- The absence of abnormal vital signs cannot rule out a serious underlying condition.
- The absence of physical findings of an acute abdomen does not rule out a

surgical abdomen, e.g. serious conditions such as ischaemic colitis may have very non-specific physical findings.

- A large number of potential differential diagnoses may need to be considered.

The emergency department (ED) approach to acute abdominal pain emphasizes disposition over diagnosis: it is more important to recognize an acute abdomen than to identify the exact cause of the pain.[1]

Epidemiology

It has been estimated that abdominal pain accounts for approximately 5–10% of all ED visits.[2] A significant proportion (18–42%) of these patients will require admission.[1] The elderly (aged 60 and over) are

over-represented in the admitted patient group. In one study on elderly patients presenting with abdominal pain, at least 50% were hospitalized and about 30–40% eventually had surgery. Up to 40% of patients were initially misdiagnosed, and the overall mortality was about 10%.[3]

Pathophysiology and differential diagnosis

Abdominal pain may result from:

- Visceral pain: This pain is poorly localized, colicky, intermittent and recurrent in nature. Stimulation of autonomic nerves investing the visceral peritoneum causes visceral pain, e.g. when hollow organs are distended, or when capsules covering solid organs are stretched. Visceral pain localizes to the abdominal region that correlates with the embryonic segments of the viscera:
  - Foregut structures (stomach, duodenum, liver, biliary tract, pancreas) localize to the upper abdomen
  - Midgut structures (small bowel, proximal colon, appendix) localize to the periumbilical region
  - Hindgut structures (distal colon, genitourinary tract) localize to the lower abdomen.
- Somatic pain: This pain is well localized, and is often constant and intense. Somatic pain results from local irritation of the parietal peritoneum. It is localized more specifically to the area of pathology (Table 7.2.1). It is, however, important to recognize that the area of pain does not always correspond to the supposed

Table 7.2.1 Differential diagnosis of pain by location (list not exhaustive)

Right upper quadrant	Epigastrium	Left upper quadrant
Hepatobiliary pathology Duodenal ulcer, duodenitis Renal colic, pyelonephritis Retrocaecal appendicitis Pneumonia, pulmonary embolism	Gastritis, peptic ulcer Hepatobiliary pathology Pancreatitis Aortic aneurysm Early appendicitis Myocardial infarction	Gastritis, peptic ulcer Renal colic, pyelonephritis Splenic pathology Pancreatitis Pneumonia
Right lumbar or flank	**Midline or periumbilical**	**Left lumbar or flank**
Renal colic, pyelonephritis Aortic aneurysm Psoas abscess Appendicitis	Visceral pain from midgut structures Early appendicitis Aortic aneurysm	Renal colic, pyelonephritis Aortic aneurysm Psoas abscess
Right lower quadrant	**Suprapubic**	**Left lower quadrant**
Appendicitis Ectopic pregnancy, tubo-ovarian pathology, endometriosis, pelvic inflammatory disease Urinary tract infection, ureteric colic Diverticulitis Hernia Aortic aneurysm Testicular torsion, epididymo-orchitis	Cystitis, bladder pathology Urinary tract infection Prostatitis Ectopic pregnancy, tubo-ovarian pathology, endometriosis, pelvic inflammatory disease	Similar to causes for right lower quadrant pain except for appendicitis (very rarely left sided)
Pain radiating to the back		
Perforated peptic ulcer Acute pancreatitis Abdominal aortic aneurysm, aortic dissection		

Note: Pain from inflammatory bowel disease, diverticulitis, colitis, gastroenteritis, volvulus, intestinal obstruction, adhesions, ischaemic colitis and constipation may localized to any part of the abdomen.

anatomic location of the underlying pathology,[4] e.g. acute appendicitis may present as suprapubic or flank pain.

- Referred pain: Pain felt at a distance from the site of origin. It is thought that referred pain occurs because afferent pain fibres from areas of high sensory input (e.g. the skin) enter the spinal cord at the same level as nociceptive fibres from an area of low sensory input (e.g. the viscera). The brain, being more used to pain signals from the skin, wrongly interprets the pain signal from the viscera as that from the dermatome.

Both visceral and somatic pain may manifest as referred pain. Some examples are:

- Shoulder pain due to diaphragmatic irritation.
- Pain at the tip of the scapula due to gallbladder pathology.
- Epigastric pain due to acute myocardial infarction.

Causes of diffuse abdominal pain

Generalized diffuse pain that is poorly localized may be due to benign causes (e.g. gastroenteritis, constipation and menstrual cramps) or from life-threatening conditions (Table 7.2.2).

Extra-abdominal

There are a number of extra-abdominal causes for abdominal pain that must be considered along with abdominal causes (Table 7.2.3).

Table 7.2.2 Some potentially life-threatening causes of generalized, diffuse abdominal pain

Haemoperitoneum from any cause, e.g. ruptured abdominal aortic aneurysm, ruptured ectopic pregnancy, trauma
Mesenteric ischaemia
Perforated viscus
Peritonitis (any cause)
Pancreatitis
Bowel obstruction
Diverticulitis
Inflammatory bowel disease
Metabolic disorders (e.g. diabetic ketoacidosis), sickle cell crisis, typhoid fever

Adapted from Gray-Eurom K, Deitte L. Imaging in the adult patient with non-traumatic abdominal pain. Emergency Medicine Practice 2007; 9: 2.

Table 7.2.3 Extra-abdominal causes of abdominal pain

Thoracic
Myocardial infarction/unstable angina Pneumonia Pulmonary embolism Herniated thoracic disc (neuralgia)
Genitourinary
Testicular torsion
Systemic
Diabetic ketoacidosis Alcoholic ketoacidosis Uraemia Sickle cell disease Systemic lupus erythematosus Vasculitis Hyperthyroidism Porphyria Glaucoma
Toxic
Methanol poisoning Heavy metal poisoning Scorpion bite Black Widow spider bite
Abdominal wall
Muscle spasm Muscle haematoma Herpes zoster
Infections
Strep pharyngitis (more often in children) Mononucleosis

Adapted from Purcell TB. Nonsurgical and extraperitoneal causes of abdominal pain. Emergency Medicine Clinics of North America 1989; 7: 721.

Clinical features

Vital signs and general condition

During triage a rapid assessment is made by looking at the patient's general condition as well as vital signs. Obviously ill patients, those in severe pain or with abnormal vital signs should be given priority. However, one cannot rule out life-threatening causes of abdominal pain by the absence of abnormal vital signs. It has been estimated that up to 7% of patients with normal vital signs may have an underlying life-threatening process, and this percentage increases in the elderly.[5] Tachycardia may be absent in patients with autonomic dysfunction, in the elderly, and in patients on medications that may blunt the cardiac response to illness or volume loss.[6] The elderly, the immunocompromised, or those in severe septic shock may sometimes not mount a febrile response. Even in the immunocompetent, fever may not always accompany acute inflammatory conditions. In a study on patients with pathologically proven cholecystitis, only 32% had a documented temperature rise within 8 hours of arrival at the ED. The absence of fever was as likely in those below 60 as in those above.[7]

History

An accurate, focused history often provides the best clue to the possible aetiology of the abdominal pain. Clinical impression derived from the history will direct decisions regarding further diagnostic work-up.

Patient demographics and background history

- Age and gender: The likelihood of certain conditions is higher in patients of a specific age and gender (Table 7.2.4). For women of childbearing age it is important to ascertain the presence or absence of pregnancy.
- Background history: Key questions in the background history are:
  - Previous abdominal surgery
  - Use of tobacco, alcohol, or recreational drugs
  - Chronic illness, e.g. diabetes mellitus, hypertension, coronary artery disease, human immunodeficiency infection, systemic lupus erythematosus
  - Vascular, thrombotic and embolic risks e.g. atrial fibrillation, vasculitis, peripheral vascular disease
  - Medication history, e.g. use of non-steroidal anti-inflammatory drugs, pain medications, antibiotics, steroids, anticoagulants
  - History of recent trauma.

Pain attributes

The nature and time course of pain are key clues to diagnosis. The following attributes should be noted:

- Onset and progress of abdominal pain over time (Table 7.2.5): Acute vascular events and rupture of hollow viscus typically presents with maximal pain at the onset. Ureteric and biliary colic also often presents with severe pain in the early stages. This is in contrast to pain from inflammatory processes such as acute appendicitis, which tends to progress and 'mature' over hours.
- Location of pain (see Table 7.2.1), migration of pain, radiation of pain: Location of pain helps to localize the area of pathology, though occasionally this may be misleading, especially if the pain is referred. Migration of pain over time gives a clue to possible underlying aetiology, e.g. pain from appendicitis typically starts at the umbilicus or epigastrium and later localizes to the right iliac fossa.
- Radiation of pain may suggest specific conditions (Table 7.2.1), e.g. pain from acute pancreatitis and perforated peptic ulcers often radiates to the back.
- Severity of pain: Severity of pain experienced is dependent on a number of factors in addition to the underlying pathology, and is not always commensurate with the severity of the underlying illness. The elderly in particular often have a diminished sense of pain. Nonetheless, patients in severe pain should be assessed early and given pain relief. Pain scores may be used to record and monitor progress.
- Character of pain: Colicky abdominal pain results usually from obstruction of a hollow viscus. Constant non-colicky pain usually denotes an inflammatory or vascular process.
- Precipitating and relieving factors: Pain from peritonitis worsens with movement, deep breathing, coughing or sneezing. Pain from peptic ulcer disease classically increases with hunger and decreases with food, antacid or milk. Pain from

Table 7.2.5   Temporal characteristics of abdominal pain
Sudden maximal pain at or near onset
Perforated peptic ulcer
Ruptured abdominal aortic aneurysm
Ruptured ectopic pregnancy, ruptured ovarian cyst
Ovarian/testicular torsion
Mesenteric infarction
Pulmonary embolism
Acute myocardial infarction
Progression to maximal pain within minutes
Acute pancreatitis
Renal and ureteric colic
Biliary colic
Strangulated hernia
Volvulus
Intussusception
Gradual onset (increased pain over hours)
Appendicitis
Strangulated hernia
Inflammatory bowel disease
Chronic pancreatitis
Salpingitis/prostatitis
Cystitis

White MJ, Counselman FL. 2005 Troubleshooting acute abdominal pain Emedmag 2002 http://www.emedmag.com/html/pre/cov/covers/011502.asp.

Table 7.2.4 Common causes of abdominal pain according to age group and gender		
Causes	*Age group*	*Gender*
Biliary tract disease	Peak age 35–50; rare in those < 20	Female:male 3:1
Ruptured ectopic pregnancy	Childbearing ages	Female
Appendicitis	All ages and both genders, peak at young adulthood; higher risk of perforation in the elderly, women, and children	
Mesenteric ischaemia	Elderly, those with vascular, thrombotic or embolic risks	
Abdominal aortic aneurysm	Increased with advancing age	Men more common
Diverticulitis	Increased with advancing age	Men more common

biliary colic tends to occur after full or fatty meals. Pain from acute pancreatitis classically worsens with supine posture and is relieved by sitting up.

- Recurrent episodes of abdominal pain: This suggests chronic recurrent conditions, e.g. peptic ulcer, biliary colic, renal colic, diverticulitis. Mesenteric ischaemia and testicular torsion may also present with recurrent episodes.

Associated symptoms

Patients with abdominal pain often have other associated symptoms that may give a clue to the possible cause. These include:

- Constitutional symptoms, e.g. fever, chills, rigors, weight loss, arthralgia.
- Gastrointestinal tract symptoms, e.g. anorexia, nausea, vomiting, diarrhoea, constipation. Nausea and vomiting are non-specific symptoms which may result from intra- and extra-abdominal causes.

However, feculent vomitus is highly indicative of intestinal obstruction. Vomiting of fresh or altered blood, as well as the passage of black tarry stools, indicates gastrointestinal haemorrhage. Failure to pass stools and flatus over a 24–48-hour period suggests possible intestinal obstruction.

- Genitourinary tract symptoms, e.g. dysuria, frequency, urgency, haematuria, suggest urinary tract pathologies. A purulent discharge from the vagina suggests possible pelvic inflammatory disease.

Table 7.2.6 lists some of the historical high-yield questions in abdominal pain.

Physical examination

A careful, systematic, directed and thorough physical examination can help strengthen the clinical impression formed from the history or to uncover unexpected abnormalities.

Physical findings help to rule in, but not rule out, the underlying diagnosis.

General

Consider the general condition and the vital signs of the patient. Patients who look drowsy or unwell, or have abnormal vital signs, need urgent attention. The posture of the patient may give a clue to the possible underlying disease. Patients with renal colic typically roll about in pain, whereas those with peritonitis lie still to avoid movements that might aggravate the pain. Inspect for pallor, jaundice, hydration status, enlarged lymph nodes, and signs of chronic liver or renal disease.

The abdomen

This is carried out with the patient lying supine and the abdomen exposed from the costal margins to the pubic symphysis. Ideally the patient should be fairly relaxed, comfortable and cooperative; it is almost impossible to perform an abdominal examination in an uncooperative patient thrashing about in pain. Adequate pain relief should be given before examination if necessary. There is strong evidence that analgesia does not mask physical signs. Abdominal examination in an obtunded patient is unreliablem and other assessment modalities such as imaging have to be considered.

- Inspection: Look for movement with respiration, shape (e.g. distended or scaphoid), the presence of any surgical scars and external lesions (e.g. bruises, distended veins, hernias). Sometimes markedly enlarged organs (especially the liver or spleen) or distended bowels may be seen.
- Palpation and percussion: Palpation is usually the most informative part of the abdominal examination. Start with the abdominal region away from the area of pain. Perform light, followed by deep palpation systematically over all quadrants of the abdomen. Look for tenderness, guarding, rebound and masses. The area of abdominal tenderness helps to localize the pathology. The presence of involuntary guarding (or rigidity) and rebound indicates peritoneal irritation. Findings of abnormal abdominal masses may help point to the possible diagnosis. Finally,

Table 7.2.6 High-yield historical questions
1. How old are you? Advanced age means increased risk.
2. Which came first- pain or vomiting? Pain first is more likely to be caused by surgical disease.
3. How long have you had the pain? Pain for less than 48 hours is more likely to be caused by surgical disease.
4. Have you ever had abdominal surgery? Consider adhesion or obstruction in patients with previous abdominal surgery.
5. Is the pain constant or intermittent? Constant pain is more likely to be caused by surgical disease.
6. Have you had this before? A report of no prior episode is more likely to be caused by surgical disease.
7. Do you have a history of cancer, diverticulosis, pancreatitis, kidney failure, gallstones, or inflammatory bowel disease? All are suggestive of more serious disease.
8. Do you have human immunodeficiency virus (HIV)? Consider occult infection or drug-related pancreatitis.
9. How much alcohol do you drink per day? Consider pancreatitis, hepatitis, cirrhosis.
10. Are you pregnant? Test for pregnancy; consider ectopic pregnancy.
11. Are you taking antibiotics or steroids? These may mask infection.
12. Did the pain start centrally and migrate to the right lower quadrant? High specificity for appendicitis.
13. Do you have a history of vascular or heart disease, hypertension, or atrial fibrillation? Consider mesenteric ischaemia and abdominal aneurysm.

Adapted from Colucciello SA, Lukens TW, Morgan DL. Assessing abdominal pain in adults: A rational, cost-effective, and evidence-based strategy. Emergency Medicine Practice 1999; 1: 1.

DIGESTIVE

7

palpate and percuss for hepatosplenomegaly; palpate bimanually for renal masses, and examine for costovertebral angle tenderness (renal punch). Percussion for shifting dullness may be performed in patients with suspected ascites.

- Auscultation: This is performed to look for abnormal or absent bowel sounds, and for vascular bruits. In gastric outlet obstruction a succussion splash may be heard in the upper abdomen when the patient is shaken from side to side. Auscultation is the least rewarding aspect of physical examination: findings from auscultation have been found to be neither sensitive nor specific.[8] However, high-pitched, tinkling or absent bowel sounds have been found to be associated with acute small bowel obstruction, especially in the presence of abdominal distension.[8] Abnormal bowel sounds in the elderly may indicate serious underlying disease.[3]
- Specific abdominal signs (Table 7.2.7): Distinctive signs have been described that are associated with specific diagnoses. Some of these signs have not been studied and their sensitivity and specificity remain unknown.

Rectal examination

This is useful in cases of gastrointestinal haemorrhage, perianal or perirectal diseases, stool impaction, prostatic pathologies and rectal foreign bodies. Contrary to classic teaching, rectal examination does not provide additional input in suspected cases of appendicitis.[9]

Examination of hernia orifices

All hernias should be examined for signs of strangulation. Hernias are most commonly present in the inguinal or femoral area, along the midline, or arising from old surgical scars. Rarely, they may be present in the paramedian, lumbar or gluteal areas.

Examination of genitalia

In women, examination of the pelvic organs may yield important clues to possible gynaecologic or obstetric causes of abdominal pain. Testicular pathology needs to be considered in male patients with lower abdominal pain.

Limitations of the abdominal examination

A significant proportion of patients with serious intra-abdominal conditions, such as ruptured aortic abdominal aneurysm and mesenteric ischaemia, may present with non-specific abdominal findings. The area of tenderness does not always correlate to the anatomical location of the disease. For example, up to 20% of patients with surgically proven appendicitis have no right lower quadrant tenderness.[10] Signs of peritonism may not always be present, especially in the elderly and the immunocompromised.

Although involuntary guarding or rigidity increase the likelihood of peritonitis,[9] rebound tenderness has been shown to have no predictive value.[11]

Examination of extra-abdominal systems

Besides the abdomen, extra-abdominal systems, especially the cardiovascular and respiratory systems, should also be examined. Directed examination of extra-abdominal systems is important because:

- The cause of the abdominal pain may be extra-abdominal (Table 7.2.3).
- It may provide clues to the possible intra-abdominal pathology, e.g. the presence of atrial fibrillation or peripheral vascular disease suggests possible mesenteric ischaemia.
- There may be complications from the abdominal condition, e.g. associated chest infection.

Serial examination

Physical signs may often be non-specific in the early phases of the disease. Serial examinations over a period of hours can help to distinguish a surgical from a non-surgical abdomen and improve the diagnostic yield.

Investigations

Although the history and physical examination may give a clue to the possible underlying pathology, many patients with abdominal pain do not present 'classically'.

Sign	Description	Association
Murphy's sign	Inability of patient to perform deep inspiration due to pain on palpation of right hypochondrium	Acute cholecystitis (sensitivity 97%; specificity 50%)[30]
Kehr's sign	Severe left shoulder tip pain especially when the patient is lying supine	Haemoperitoneum, e.g. from ruptured spleen or ectopic pregnancy
Cullen's sign	Ecchymoses around the periumbilical area	Retroperitoneal haemorrhage (haemorrhagic pancreatitis, abdominal aortic aneurysm rupture)
Grey–Turner's sign	Ecchymoses of the flanks	Retroperitoneal haemorrhage (haemorrhagic pancreatitis, abdominal aortic aneurysm rupture)
McBurney's sign	Tenderness localized to a point at 2/3 distance on a line drawn from the umbilicus to the right anterior superior iliac spine	Appendicitis
Iliopsoas sign	Extension of right hip causes abdominal pain	Appendicitis (sensitivity 16%; specificity 95%)[10]
Obturator's sign	Internal rotation of the flexed right hip causes abdominal pain	Appendicitis
Rovsing's sign	Right lower quadrant (RLQ) pain with palpation of the left lower quadrant	Appendicitis
Heel-drop sign	RLQ pain on dropping heels on the ground after standing tiptoes; alternatively RLQ pain from forcefully banging the patient's heel with the examiner's hand	Appendicitis (sensitivity 93%)[31]
Cough test	Post-tussive abdominal pain	Peritonitis (sensitivity up to 95%)[32,33]

White MJ, Counselman FL. 2005 Troubleshooting acute abdominal pain Emedmag. 2002 http://www.emedmag.com/html/pre/cov/covers/011502.asp

Investigations may assist in determining diagnosis and disposition.

Bedside tests

- Urine pregnancy tests: Bedside urine tests are rapid and accurate. Most are able to detect β-hCG to a level as low as 25 mIU/mL of urine. It has been estimated that up to 1% of ectopic pregnancies are associated with β-hCG values lower than this.[12]
- Urine analysis: This provides useful early information for patients with suspected urinary tract infection and ureteric colic. However, it is important to interpret urine analysis results in the context of the patient's clinical presentation. About 30% of patients with acute appendicitis may present with blood and leukocytes in their urine;[13] about 30% of patients with ruptured aortic abdominal aneurysm may have haematuria.[14]
- Electrocardiogram (ECG): Acute coronary events may manifest as abdominal symptoms, e.g. epigastric pain, nausea and vomiting. ECG should be performed in cases where there is suspicion of ACS, especially in patients with cardiovascular risks or in the elderly. ECG may also suggest the possible cause of the abdominal pain in some cases, e.g. mesenteric ischaemia from atrial fibrillation, abdominal pain and vomiting from digoxin toxicity.
- Capillary blood sugar: Patients with diabetic ketoacidosis (DKA) may present with symptoms and signs mimicking an acute abdomen. Capillary blood sugar should be performed in all patients with known diabetes mellitus, or in cases where there are clinical suspicions of DKA (e.g. dehydration, Kussmaul breathing, ketotic breath).

Laboratory tests

Most laboratory tests do not aid in differentiating surgical from non-surgical causes of abdominal pain.[15]

- Full blood count: This most commonly ordered laboratory study does not add value to the assessment of patients with abdominal pain. A normal white count (including normal absolute neutrophil count) may lead to a false sense of security even though it does not rule out a surgical cause of pain. Ten to 60% of patients with surgically proven appendicitis have a normal initial white count;[1] only about 50% of patients with severe intra-abdominal pathology have an elevated white count.[16] On the other hand, an elevated white count may lead to further investigations which may not add to the information already gleaned from the history and physical examination.[17]
- Amylase and lipase: These tests are most useful in patients with suspected pancreatitis. Serum lipase has been found to be more accurate than serum amylase.[18] Both lipase and amylase may be normal in patients with CT-proven pancreatitis, especially in those with recurrent disease.
- Liver function test: This should only be ordered selectively, in cases where there is suspicion of hepatobiliary disease, or when urine tests detect the presence of urobilinogen.
- C-reactive protein (CRP): This has been found to be about 62% sensitive and 66% specific for appendicitis.[19] The sensitivity improved in patients with more than 12 hours of symptoms, and appendicitis is rare in those with two normal CRPs performed 12 hours apart.[20]

Imaging

Plain X rays

The value of plain radiographs for evaluation of patients with abdominal pain is limited. However, there is still a place for plain X-rays as a first-line investigation in patients with suspected bowel obstruction, bowel perforation and foreign body. A three-view series comprising the upright chest, supine and upright abdominal radiographs is recommended.[6] X-ray findings for bowel obstruction and perforation are fairly specific but not sensitive, i.e. they help to establish, but not exclude, these diagnoses.

Ultrasound

Ultrasound does not involve ionizing radiation, is rapid, non-invasive, and may be performed at the bedside. This makes it the ideal evaluation tool in unstable patients or those who are pregnant. Selective use of focused ultrasound in the appropriate clinical setting maximizes its diagnostic sensitivity. However, ultrasound is operator dependent and appropriate training is necessary to ensure competence. The sensitivity of ultrasound may also be reduced by technical limitations (e.g. obesity, bowel gas, subcutaneous emphysema). Focused bedside emergency ultrasound examination has significantly affected the diagnosis and management of the following life-threatening conditions:

- Abdominal aortic aneurysm (AAA): Ultrasound is a useful screening tool for the presence of AAA (defined as an aortic diameter >3 cm), especially when the patient is not suitable for transfer to a CT facility. Ultrasound cannot reliably identify rupture, but the detection of an AAA in a hypotensive patient with symptoms suggestive of rupture (abdominal pain, backache or flank pain) is an indication for urgent intervention.
- Ectopic pregnancy: In a patient with a positive pregnancy test, an empty uterus (especially in the presence of free intraperitoneal fluid) implies ectopic pregnancy until proven otherwise. Other ultrasound findings include detection of an adnexal mass, an extrauterine gestational sac, extrauterine blood clots and interstitial ectopic pregnancy. On the other hand, identification of intrauterine pregnancy (IUP) essentially reduces the risk of an ectopic pregnancy to < 1:5000 (1:50 for women undergoing assisted reproduction). Transvaginal ultrasound is more sensitive than transabdominal ultrasound in detecting early IUPs. Repeat examination in a stable patient may be needed if the study is inconclusive (e.g. a positive pregnancy test but no IUP and no adnexal mass).[1]
- Haemoperitoneum from abdominal trauma: The focused abdominal sonogram for trauma (FAST) examination is now considered to be an essential evaluation in unstable patients who have sustained abdominal trauma. The presence of free intraperitoneal fluid implies the development of haemoperitoneum. FAST is highly specific (99%), although its overall sensitivity is about 66% compared to CT. FAST is almost 100% sensitive in the hypotensive patient. The sensitivity of FAST improves with serial examination.

Ultrasound may also be used for evaluation of patients in the following conditions that may not be immediately life threatening:

- Assessment of suspected gallbladder disease: Ultrasound is the recommended imaging study of first choice for suspected gallbladder disease. Discretion should be applied to avoid over-interpretation, e.g. the mere presence of gallstones does not imply choleolithiasis as the cause of the abdominal pain.
- Tubo-ovarian pathologies: Ultrasound is the first-line investigation for patients with suspected pelvic inflammatory disease or tubo-ovarian pathology. Transvaginal ultrasound provides detailed visualization of the pelvic organs, and trans-abdominal ultrasound provides a complementary global view.
- Ureteric colic: Ultrasound combined with abdominal radiographs may be used to screen patients with suspected ureteric colic. The diagnostic sensitivity for nephrolithiasis is about 63–85%,[6] fairly similar to that for intravenous urography (IVU), which has a sensitivity of 64–90%. The advantages of this imaging technique over IVU are that the use of radiocontrast is avoided, and the radiation dose involved is much lower.
- Detection of free peritoneal fluid in non-traumatic abdominal pain: In the appropriate clinical context this may suggest the presence of ascites, intraperitoneal haemorrhage, pus or leakage of gut content.
- Appendicitis: Ultrasound may be used to evaluate for the presence of appendicitis if there are contraindications to CT (e.g. pregnancy) or if CT is unavailable. Ultrasound is not as sensitive as CT and helps to rule in but not rule out this diagnosis.

Computed tomography (CT)

With the advent of helical and multidetector scanning technology, CT has become the imaging modality of choice for evaluation of abdominal pain in the non-obstetric patient.

A survey of emergency physicians[21] ranked CT of the abdomen and pelvis as the most valuable diagnostic test in evaluating patients with non-traumatic abdominal pain. It has a high degree of accuracy, establishing

diagnoses in more than 95% of cases in one study.[22] In the elderly, CT resulted in changes to the management and disposition of significant proportion of patients.[23]

CT allows for detailed visualization of intra-, extra- and retroperitoneal structures. It identifies the exact site of disease, as well as its impact on the surrounding structures, thereby guiding further management. CT may be performed with or without intravenous and oral contrast agents. In the emergency setting, CT is useful for:

- Assessment in abdominal trauma.
- Detection of inflammatory lesions (e.g. appendicitis, pancreatitis, diverticulitis, abscesses).
- Detection of neoplastic lesions.
- Evaluation of vascular pathology (e.g. aortic aneurysm, aortic dissection, mesenteric ischaemia).
- Detection of intra-abdominal and retroperitoneal bleed or abscesses.
- Detection of pneumoperitoneum, obstruction of hollow organs, and abnormal calcifications, e.g. ureteric calculi.
- Assessment of the kidneys and urinary tracts.

The main limitations to CT are that the patient must be stable enough for transport to the scanning facility; ionizing radiation is involved; it may miss up to 20% of gallstones because the stones may be of the same radiographic density as bile; and it may miss up to 10–17% of traumatic small bowel perforations.[24]

The sensitivity of CT is not 100% for most conditions. Clinical decisions should not be based on CT results alone. If initial CT findings are negative but clinical suspicion is high, further observation, evaluation or even repeat scans may be needed.

Pitfalls

The elderly

In elderly patients presenting with abdominal pain, conditions requiring surgical intervention (e.g. cholangitis, intestinal obstruction), serious vascular pathologies (e.g. AAA, aortic dissection, mesenteric ischaemia) and intra-abdominal neoplasms are more common (Table 7.2.8). Unfortunately, abdominal pain is frequently misdiagnosed in the elderly because:

Table 7.2.8 Disease spectrum in those less than 50 years old vs those over 50		
Confirmed cause of acute abdominal pain	Acute abdominal pain in patient <50 (n=6317) (%)	Acute abdominal pain in patient ≥50 (n=2406) (%)
Biliary tract disease	6	21
Non-specific abdominal pain	40	16
Appendicitis	32	15
Bowel obstruction	2	12
Pancreatitis	2	7
Diverticular disease	<0.1	6
Cancer	<0.1	4
Hernia	<0.1	3
Vascular	<0.1	2

Adapted from deDombal FT. Acute abdominal pain in the elderly. Journal of Clinical Gastroenterology 1994; 29: 331–335.

- The elderly often present atypically or with non-specific complaints, e.g. poor appetite, lethargy, constipation, vomiting, loose stools, falls.
- Pain perception in the elderly may be blunted.
- Vital signs may be normal in spite of serious underlying illness.
- Signs of peritonism may not be present in cases of a surgical abdomen; physical findings may be non-specific or subtle.
- Laboratory tests such as full blood count may be normal.

Adverse outcomes in the elderly are more common as a result of missed or delayed diagnosis than in younger patients. This is because the elderly tend to seek treatment late in the disease process and complications tend to be more common, they have reduced physiological reserve, and often more comorbidities. It has been estimated that with each decade of life, diagnostic accuracy decreases while mortality increases, such that for the octogenarian diagnostic accuracy is about 30%, although the corresponding mortality rate is 70 times that of patients under 30.[25] Therefore, geriatric patients with abdominal pain need to be carefully evaluated and the threshold for imaging studies, surgical consultation and admission should be lowered.

The immunocompromised

Inflammatory responses are suppressed in the immunocompromised and abdominal signs from peritoneal irritation may be absent. Patients with human immunodeficiency virus (HIV) infection may develop unusual conditions such as opportunistic viral or bacterial enterocolitis (e.g. cytomegalovirus or *Mycobacterium avium intrecellulare* enterocolitis), AIDS-related cholangiopathy, lymphoma, or drug-induced pancreatitis. Patients on peritoneal dialysis or with advanced liver cirrhosis are at risk of developing spontaneous bacterial peritonitis.

Women of childbearing age

It is important to determine whether these patients are pregnant. Menstrual history, compliance with contraception, history of tubal ligation or claims of sexual abstinence cannot reliably exclude the possibility of pregnancy.

If the patient is pregnant, the possibility of ectopic pregnancy should be considered. In addition, pelvic conditions (e.g. pelvic inflammatory disease, ovarian pathology, pregnancy-related complications such as threatened or missed abortion) and urinary tract infections are relatively common.

For patients in the second or third trimester of pregnancy the gravid uterus may displace structures in the lower abdomen away from their usual position, e.g. the appendix may migrate to a higher position in the right hypochondrium or the right flank, changing symptoms and signs.

Dangerous mimics (Table 7.2.9)

Misdiagnosed patients are most commonly given the labels of gastroenteritis, constipation, gastritis, urinary tract infection, or pelvic inflammatory disease.[26]

Diagnosis versus disposition

In the ED management of patients presenting with abdominal pain, empirical management of acute conditions and proper disposition are more important than diagnostic accuracy. When the diagnosis is based only on clinical findings and basic laboratory investigations, overall diagnostic accuracy is about 50% (as high as 80% in young adults[27] and as low as 30% in the elderly[25]). Fortunately, the rate of inappropriate discharge from the ED is low (about 1% across all age groups), albeit slightly higher in the elderly (about 4%).[28]

General management

Resuscitation

Prompt resuscitation should take precedence over diagnosis in unstable patients. Patients may be in shock as a result of blood loss, fluid loss, sepsis, or from concurrent cardiovascular events. Appropriate fluid therapy and inotropic support should be instituted early to prevent further deterioration and end-organ dysfunction.

Symptom relief

Pain relief should be instituted as early as possible for patients presenting with abdominal pain. Relieving pain does not mask signs of peritonism or obscure the diagnosis.

Antibiotics

Antibiotics are indicated in suspected intra-abdominal sepsis. The antibiotics used should cover Gram-negative aerobes as well as anaerobes. Additional coverage for Gram-positive aerobes is required in patients with spontaneous bacterial peritonitis.

Surgical consultation

Early consultation should be the rule in cases of suspected surgical abdomen. Early surgical intervention is crucial in improving outcome for urgent conditions, e.g. ruptured abdominal aortic aneurysm, ruptured ectopic pregnancy, intraperitoneal haemorrhage and bowel perforation.

Disposition

Admission

The following patients need to be admitted:

- Patients with specific diagnoses that require inpatient management.
- Patients who are ill, unstable or with altered mentation.
- The elderly or the immunocompromised in whom diagnoses are unclear.
- Patients in whom potentially serious conditions cannot be excluded.
- Patients in whom symptoms (e.g. pain, vomiting) cannot be ameliorated.
- Patients who are unable to follow discharge instructions or who have poor social support.

In addition, the admission threshold should be lowered for patients returning to the ED for the same complaints, especially

Table 7.2.9 Dangerous mimics	
True diagnosis	*Initial misdiagnosis*
Appendicitis	Gastroenteritis, pelvic inflammatory disease (PID), urinary tract infection (UTI)
Ruptured abdominal aortic aneurysm	Renal colic, diverticulitis, lumbar strain
Ectopic pregnancy	PID, UTI, corpus luteum cyst
Diverticulitis	Constipation, gastroenteritis, non-specific abdominal pain
Perforated viscus	Peptic ulcer disease, pancreatitis, non-specific abdominal pain
Bowel obstruction	Constipation, gastroenteritis, non-specific abdominal pain
Mesenteric ischaemia	Constipation, gastroenteritis, ileus, small bowel obstruction
Incarcerated or strangulated hernia	Ileus, small bowel obstruction
Shock or sepsis from perforation, bleed and abdominal infection in the elderly	Urosepsis or pneumonia (in elderly)

From Colucciello SA, Lukens TW, Morgan DL. Assessing abdominal pain in adults: A rational, cost-effective, and evidence-based strategy. Emergency Medicine Practice 1999; 1: 1.

where the cause of the abdominal pain had not been fully elucidated.

Observation

Patients who do not meet admission criteria but have persistent pain may be observed over a period of hours in the ED. Serial examination over a period of 10 hours has been found to improve the diagnostic accuracy of appendicitis.[29]

The main aims of observing the patient with abdominal pain are to improve diagnostic yield with serial examination, to monitor progress after treatment, to detect the development of signs of acute abdomen, and for further diagnostic work-up if indicated.

Non-specific abdominal pain (NSAP)

A large proportion of stable patients with abdominal pain will not have a definitive diagnosis on discharge from the ED. In patients under 50 years of age, NSAP may be as high as 40%. This figure is lower in the elderly, at about 15% (see Table 7.2.8).

Most younger patients may be safely discharged from the ED once their symptoms have resolved with treatment and a period of observation. They should be clearly informed that the cause of their pain has not been discerned, and appropriate discharge advice, including to return to the ED if symptoms recur or worsen, should be given. Referral to a specialist for further evaluation may be indicated.

NSAP in younger patients tends to have a benign course. However, about 10% of the elderly labelled with NSAP are subsequently found to have an underlying malignancy. It is also important to rule out extra-abdominal causes in the elderly.

Discharge advice

It is important to give discharge advice, as the patient will have spent a relatively short time in the ED. The patient should be advised to return if:

- Pain is persistent (> 24 hours) or worsening.
- They develop incessant vomiting or are unable to retain fluids.

- Vague pain has become localized, e.g. to the right iliac fossa.
- The patient develops high fever or chills, or feels increasingly ill, weak or unwell.
- The patient develops fainting episodes.
- Abdominal distension develops.
- There is blood in the stools or vomitus.
- The patient develops new medical problems requiring urgent consultation.

Developments in the next 5–10 years

With the development of newer and fast MRI techniques, motion-related artefacts can now be eliminated and the use of MRI to image the abdomen is now possible.

The advantages of MRI over CT are that MRI offers better soft tissue visualization than CT, and no ionizing radiation is involved. MRI is able to provide increased information for hepatobiliary disease, pancreatitis and mesenteric ischaemia,[6] but is significantly more costly and takes longer to perform. MRI is contraindicated in patients with claustrophobia or implanted metallic devices.

Controversies

- Use of opioids for pain relief. Traditionally, it was thought that the use of opioids in patients with abdominal pain would lead to loss of abdominal signs, resulting in missed diagnosis. This widely held dogma has been disproved in many studies; in fact, the use of opioids in abdominal pain is not only safe, but actually aids diagnosis by facilitating physical examination and relaxing the abdominal musculature.[1] The dosage used should be titrated to the patient's response.

- Clinical scoring systems for abdominal pain. Various clinical scoring systems, e.g. the Alvarado score for acute appendicitis, have been proposed. These systems may involve relatively simple algorithms or may be 'computer-based'. They help to ensure a more systematic approach to the evaluation of a patient, but none has been shown prospectively to improve on the physician's judgment.

References

1. Colucciello SA, Lukens TW, Morgan DL. Assessing abdominal pain in adult: A rational, cost-effective, and evidence-based strategy. Emergency Medicine Practice 1999; 1: 1.
2. McCaig LG, Stussman BJ. National Hospital Ambulatory Medical Care Survey: 1996 Emergency Department Summary. Advance Data from Vital and Health Statistics: 1997; 293.
3. Marco CA, Schoenfeld CN, Keyl PM. Abdominal pain in geriatric emergency patients: variables associated with adverse outcomes. Academic Emergency Medicine 1998; 5: 1163–1168.
4. Yamamoto W, Kono H, Maekawa M. The relationship between abdominal pain regions and specific diseases. Journal of Epidemiology 1997; 7: 27–32.
5. Powers RD, Guertler AT. Abdominal pain in the emergency department: stability and change over 20 years. American Journal of Emergency Medicine 1995; 13: 301.
6. Gray-Eurom K, Deitte L. Imaging in the adult patient with non-traumatic abdominal pain. Emergency Medicine Practice 2007; 9: 2.
7. Gruber PJ, Silverman RA, Gottesfeld S. Presence of fever and leukocytosis in acute cholecystitis. Annals of Emergecy Medicine 1996; 28: 273–277.
8. Eskelinen M, Ikonen J, Lipponen P. Contributions of history-taking, physical examination, and computer assistance to diagnosis of acute small-bowel obstruction: a prospective study of 1333 patients with acute abdominal pain. Scandinavian Journal of Gastroenterology 1994; 21: 534–540.
9. Dixon JM, Elton RA, Rainey JB. Rectal examination in patients with pain in the right lower quadrant of the abdomen. British Medical Journal 1991; 302: 386–389.
10. Wagner JM, McKinney WP, Carpenter JL. Does this patient have appendicitis? Journal of American Medical Association 1996; 276: 1589–1594.
11. Liddington MI, Thomson WH. Rebound tenderness test. British Journal of Surgery 1991; 78: 795–796.
12. Kalinski M., Guss DA. Hemorrhagic shock from a ruptured ectopic pregnancy in a patient with a negative urine pregnancy test result. Annals of Emergency Medicine 2002; 40: 102–105.
13. Scott JH 3rd, Amin M, Harty JI. Abnormal urinalaysis in appendicitis. Journal of Urology 1983; 129: 1015.
14. Acheson AG, Graham AN, Weir C, et al. Prospective study on factors delaying surgery in ruptured abdominal aortic aneurysms. Journal of the Royal College of Surgeons of Edinburgh 1998; 43: 182–184.
15. Parker JS, Vukov LF, Wollan PC. Abdominal pain in the elderly: use of temperature and laboratory testing to screen for surgical disease. Family Medicine 1996; 28: 193–197.
16. Chi CH, Shiesh SC, Chen KW. C-reactive protein for evaluation of acute abdominal pain. American Journal of Emergency Medicine 1996; 14: 254–256.
17. Badgett RG, Hansen CJ, Rogers CS, et al. Clinical usage of the leukocyte count in emergency room decision making. Journal of General Internal Medicine 1990; 5: 198–202.
18. Chase CW, Barker DE, Russell WL, et al. 1996 Serum amylase and lipase in the evaluation of acute abdominal pain. American Surgery 62: 1028–1033.
19. Hallen S, Asberg A. The accuracy of C-reactive protein in acute appendicitis – a meta-analysis. Scandinavian Journal of Clinical and Laboratory Investigation 1997; 57: 373–380.
20. Albu E, Miller EM, Choi Y, et al. Diagnostic value of C-reactive protein. Diseases of the Colon and Rectum 1994; 37: 49–51.
21. Nagurney JT, Brown DF, Chang T, et al. Use of diagnostic testing in the emergency department for patients presenting with non-traumatic abdominal pain. Journal of Emergency Medicine 2003; 25: 363–371.
22. Gore RM, Miller FH, Pereles FS, et al. Helical CT in the evaluation of the acute abdomen. American Journal of Roentgenology 2000; 174: 901–913.
23. Esses D, Birnbaum A, Bijur P, et al. Ability of CT to alter decision making in elderly patients with acute abdominal pain. American Journal of Emergency Medicine 2004; 22: 270.

24. Miller LA, Shanmuganathan K. Multi-detector CT evaluation of abdominal trauma. Radiologic Clinics of North America 2005; 43: 1079–1095.
25. deDombal FT. Acute abdominal pain in the elderly. Journal of Clinical Gastroenterology. 1994; 19: 331–335.
26. deDombal FT. The OMGE acute abdominal pain survey. Progress report. Scandinavian Journal of Gastroenterology 1998; 144: 35–42.
27. Simmens HP, Decurtins M, Rotzer A, et al. Emergency room patients with abdominal pain unrelated to trauma: Analysis in a surgical university hospital. Hepatogastroenterology 1991; 38: 279–282.
28. Bugliosi TF, Meloy TD, Vukov LF. Acute abdominal pain in the elderly. Annals of Emergency Medicine 1990; 19: 1383–1386.
29. Graff L, Radford MJ, Werne C. Probability of appendicitis before and after observation. Annals of Emergency Medicine 1991; 20: 503–507.
30. Singer AJ. Brandt LJ. Pathophysiology of the gastrointestinal tract during pregnancy. American Journal of Gastroenterology 1991; 86: 1695–1712.
31. Markle GB. 4th A simple test for intraperitoneal inflammation. American Journal of Surgery 1973; 125: 721–22.
32. Bennett DH, Tambeur Luc JMT, Campbell WB. Use of coughing test to diagnose peritonitis. British Medical Journal 1994; 308: 136.
33. Jeddy TA, Vowles RH, Southam JA. 'Cough sign: A reliable sign in the diagnosis of intra-abdominal inflammation. British Journal of Surgery 1994; 81: 278.

7.3 Bowel obstruction

Kim Yates

ESSENTIALS

1 Small bowel obstruction is most often caused by adhesions. Large bowel obstruction more commonly results from neoplasms.

2 The common clinical features of bowel obstruction are colicky, poorly localized abdominal pain, constipation/obstipation, abdominal distension and hyperactive or high-pitched bowel sounds. Examination for hernias is essential.

3 The presence of dilated loops of bowel with multiple air–fluid levels on abdominal X-ray is diagnostic of bowel obstruction.

4 Initial treatment consists of correction of dehydration and electrolyte abnormalities, decompression, analgesia and assessment particularly to identify strangulating bowel obstruction.

5 Strangulating bowel obstruction is an indication for urgent surgery.

Introduction

Bowel obstruction is the interruption of the normal peristaltic progression of intestinal contents. Mechanical bowel obstruction can be caused by lesions outside or within the bowel wall, or within the lumen itself. It may be partial or complete, strangulating or non-strangulating. Paralytic ileus may mimic obstruction but there is no mechanical cause; rather, it is associated with abnormal propulsive motility. Pseudo-obstruction is also associated with abnormal neuromuscular activity but is more chronic.

Aetiology and pathophysiology

Common causes of small bowel obstruction (SBO) include adhesions, hernias, and neoplasms. Less common causes include inflammatory bowel disease, gallstones, foreign bodies, strictures, radiation, diverticulitis, endometriosis and abscesses. Common causes of large bowel obstruction (LBO) include neoplasm, diverticulitis, and volvulus. Faecal impaction, inflammatory bowel disease, strictures and extraintestinal tumours are less common causes.

Paralytic ileus can be caused by a wide range of conditions. Metabolic causes include hypokalaemia (most common), hyponatraemia, hypomagnesaemia, and hypoalbuminaemia. Drugs such as tricyclic antidepressants, opiates, antihistamines, β-adrenergic agonists and quinidine have also been implicated.

The pathophysiology of mechanical bowel obstruction relates to rising intraluminal pressure, mucosal injury, bacterial overgrowth and inflammatory response. Bowel proximal to the obstruction distends with gas, fluid and electrolytes, then hypersecretion escalates, bowel absorptive ability decreases, and progressive systemic volume losses occur. As obstruction persists and intraluminal pressure rises, local vascular compromise can occur, especially venous stasis. Vomiting may ensue, worsening dehydration and electrolyte disturbances. As pressures rise and/or blood flow diminishes, strangulation, haemorrhagic necrosis and/or gangrene may follow, with consequent perforation and sepsis. A closed-loop obstruction implies both proximal and distal obstruction (e.g. strangulating hernia or volvulus), leading to vascular compromise more quickly, hence a higher risk of strangulation, necrosis and perforation.

Clinical features

History

In early bowel obstruction abdominal pain is poorly localized and colicky, but later may become more constant and, if severe, suggests ischaemia or peritonitis. Pain from SBO tends to be more severe earlier, and cramps tend to be more frequent, compared to LBO where dull, lower abdominal cramps are more common. Vomiting is more common in SBO and is a late symptom in LBO. Faeculent vomiting or distension suggests a more distal SBO. Obstipation was thought typical, but the passage of flatus and stool may continue.

The gastrointestinal and surgical history helps differentiate causes of mechanical obstruction, and drug history and systems enquiry may identify potential causes of non-mechanical obstruction.

Examination

Fever, tachycardia, abdominal tenderness or mass, guarding or peritonism suggest strangulating obstruction, but vascular compromise can occur in their absence. Signs of dehydration are often present. Abdominal distension is more commonly present in LBO or distal SBO. On auscultation rushes or high-pitched tinkles may be heard, but are not absolute indicators of obstruction. Surgical scars suggest adhesions as a cause of obstruction, and examination for hernias is essential. Rectal examination may be normal in SBO, but the presence of faecal impaction, blood or a mass may assist with diagnosis of cause. Pelvic examination may be useful if abscesses or inflammation are suspected.

A focused medical examination should also be performed to exclude causes of ileus and pseudo-obstruction, and to assess anaesthetic risk.

Investigations

Laboratory tests

Laboratory tests are of limited value for diagnosing bowel obstruction but help in assessment of severity and guiding resuscitation. Of all laboratory tests, only lactate and interleukin (IL)-6 levels appear to have significant predictive value for strangulating obstruction. If both are raised, the positive predictive value is 95% and the negative predictive value 97%. Haematocrit may be raised if dehydration is present. Electrolyte abnormalities, such as hyponatraemia, hypokalaemia and impaired renal function, are common. Serum amylase may be mildly raised in SBO. Arterial blood gases may show metabolic alkalosis if vomiting is severe, metabolic acidosis if shock, dehydration or ketosis is present, or hypoxaemia/hypercapnia if distension impairs breathing. A blood or urine pregnancy test, where appropriate, and urine microscopy are important in excluding other causes of abdominal pain.

Radiology

The presence of dilated loops of bowel with multiple air–fluid levels on abdominal X-ray (supine and erect or decubitus films) is diagnostic for bowel obstruction, but the accuracy of plain films is low. The dilated bowel loops may indicate the level of the obstruction, for example, dilated colon, identified by haustral sacculation, suggests LBO. The dilated single loop of colon ('bent inner tube') in the left abdomen suggests sigmoid volvulus or, in the midabdomen or epigastrium, caecal volvulus. Dilated small bowel, identified by valvulae conniventes that extend across the bowel, may be present in either SBO or LBO. Absence of bowel gas distal to the obstruction may be seen. Abdominal X-rays are rarely helpful in distinguishing strangulating from non-strangulating bowel obstruction. An erect chest X-ray or left lateral decubitus film should be checked, looking for free gas indicating perforation.

Abdominal computed tomography (CT) is used increasingly for determining the level and cause of obstruction, and for detecting closed-loop SBO or LBO. It is 91–95% accurate in detecting high-grade or complete SBO, and can show ischaemia, but is less accurate for low-grade SBO. Multidetector CT is most useful for diagnosing ischaemia. CT enteroclysis, where contrast is infused into the duodenum by catheter, is an emerging investigation for SBO. Magnetic resonance imaging (MRI) and ultrasound are used useful in evaluating bowel obstruction.

Oral water-soluble contrast (Gastrografin) progressing to the colon in serial abdominal X-rays within 24 hours predicts resolution of adhesive SBO.

Endoscopy

Careful sigmoidoscopy is safe in LBO and therapeutic in sigmoid volvulus when used to place a rectal tube. In some centres, endoscopy is performed acutely to decompress LBO by inserting drainage tubes or self-expanding metal stents.

Management

Resuscitation and general measures

Most patients with bowel obstruction are dehydrated, so treatment with i.v. crystalloid fluid therapy is usual, and electrolyte disturbances should be corrected. Urinary catheterization and monitoring of urine output, vital signs and electrolytes should guide ongoing fluid and electrolyte therapy.

Nasogastric decompression is customary, but evidence of benefit in patients without significant vomiting is weak. Analgesia is often required, with titrated i.v. increments of opiates the most appropriate option. Antibiotics are prescribed by some to counter bacterial translocation, but evidence of their effectiveness is sparse.

Conservative therapy

Ongoing intravenous fluid therapy and decompression are indicated in partial bowel obstruction and in those awaiting surgery. Long nasointestinal tubes have been trialled in SBO, but no benefit over standard nasogastric tubes is apparent. Monitoring of vital signs, urine output and clinical state should continue, and deterioration or failure to improve are indications for surgical therapy. Where malignant bowel obstruction is inoperable, octreotide appears superior to hyoscine butylbromide in relieving symptoms, and although corticosteroids are commonly advocated, evidence for their effectiveness is less clear. In patients with acute colonic pseudo-obstruction unresponsive to conservative therapy, i.v. neostigmine 2 mg has initiated rapid colonic decompression. A non-strangulating sigmoid volvulus can be temporarily decompressed by a rectal tube inserted via sigmoidoscope.

Endoscopic placement of self-expanding metallic stents can relieve malignant LBO, either prior to elective surgical resection or as definitive palliative therapy if the malignancy is inoperable. Reported complications of metallic stents include perforation, stent migration and reobstruction.

Surgical therapy

Bowel obstruction due to hernias and complete SBO usually requires surgery. Strangulating bowel obstruction is an indication for urgent surgery and is suspected in the presence of severe pain, localized tenderness, mass, fever, acidosis, marked leukocytosis, hernia, shock, sepsis or confirmatory CT findings. It can, however, occur without these features. Raised lactate and/or IL-6 levels may be more useful in diagnosis. Broad-spectrum parenteral antibiotics are indicated preoperatively and if sepsis is suspected.

In strangulating bowel obstruction or perforation mortality escalates dramatically the

DIGESTIVE

longer surgery is delayed (~30% compared to 3–5% in non-strangulating bowel obstruction), so prompt surgery is vital. The surgical approach adopted will depend on the suspected pathology and operative findings. Some centres use laparoscopy to treat SBO, with variable success rates (33–87%), better success being apparent in those with a history of appendicectomy only, or with band adhesions. In LBO, decompressive stomas followed by a definitive operation at a later date are sometimes useful in very sick patients; however, right-sided lesions can often be resected at laparotomy with a primary anastomosis, thereby avoiding a stoma completely. Single-stage resection/anastomosis is possible with left-sided lesions, but there is a higher risk of contamination in unprepared bowel and higher mortality rates.

Disposition

Patients with bowel obstruction associated with haemodynamic compromise, shock or sepsis require combined ongoing management by surgical and intensive-care teams. Patients with suspected strangulating bowel obstruction or perforation should have urgent surgery. Stable patients and those with partial bowel obstruction can be started on conservative therapy and monitored closely as surgical inpatients for signs of deterioration.

Controversies

- Diagnosis of strangulating bowel obstruction. Clinical features and plain radiography may not be helpful. Of all blood tests, lactate and IL-6 levels appear most predictive. CT findings are helpful, and multidetector CT may be most useful.

- Tube decompression therapy in SBO. Both short nasogastric and long nasointestinal tubes have been used in adhesive SBO, but long tubes have not shown a definite advantage.

- Non-operative therapy. Some surgeons prefer early surgery because of the difficulty of diagnosing strangulating bowel obstruction. In adhesive partial SBO, without signs of strangulation, a 48-hour trial of non-operative therapy with frequent reassessment appears safe. With inoperable malignant obstruction octreotide may be more effective than corticosteroids in relieving symptoms.

Further reading

Abbas S, Bissett IP, Parry BR. Oral water soluble contrast for the management of adhesive small bowel obstruction. Cochrane Database of Systemic Reviews (4): CD004651, 2004.

Czechowski J. Conventional radiography and ultrasonography in the diagnosis of small bowel obstruction and strangulation. Acta Radiologica 1996; 37: 86–218.

Ellis H. The clinical significance of adhesions: focus on intestinal obstruction. European Journal of Surgery 1997; 577: 5–9.

Evers BM. Small intestine. In: Townsend CM, Beauchamp RD, Evers BM, Mattox KL, eds. Sabiston textbook of surgery: the biological basis of modern surgical practice, 17th edn. Philadelphia: WB Saunders 2004; 1278–1331.

Fischer JE, Nussbaum MS, Chance NT, et al. Manifestations of gastrointestinal disease. In: Schwartz SI, ed. Principles of surgery, 7th edn. New York: McGraw-Hill, 1999; 2653–2673.

Levard H, Boudet MJ, Msika S, et al. Laparoscopic treatment of acute small bowel obstruction: a multicentre retrospective study. Australia and New Zealand Journal of Surgery 2001; 71: 641–646.

Maglinte DD, Kelvin FM, Sandrasegaran K, et al. Radiology of small bowel obstruction: contemporary approach and controversies. Abdominal Imaging 2005. 30: 160–178.

Mallo RD, Salem L, Lalani T, et al. Computed tomography diagnosis of ischemia and complete obstruction in small bowel obstruction: a systematic review. Journal of Gastrointestinal Surgery 2005; 9: 690–695.

Marincek B. Nontraumatic abdominal emergencies: acute abdominal pain: diagnostic strategies. European Radiology 2002; 12: 2136–2150.

Mercadante S, Casuccio A, Mangione S. Medical treatment for inoperable malignant bowel obstruction: a qualitative systematic review. Journal of Pain and Symptom Management 2007; 33: 217–223.

Nicholson DA, Driscoll PA. ABC of emergency radiology. London: BMJ Publishing, 1995.

Ponec RJ, Saunders MD, Kimmey MB. Neostigmine for the treatment of acute colonic pseudo-obstruction. New England Journal of Medicine 1999; 341: 137–141.

Suri S, Gupta S, Sudhakar PJ, et al. Comparative evaluation of plain films, ultrasound and CT in the diagnosis of intestinal obstruction. Acta Radiologica 1999; 40: 422–428.

Turnage RH, Heldman M, Cole P. Intestinal obstruction and ileus. In: Feldman M, Friedman LS, Friedman LJ, Brandt LJ, eds. Sleisinger and Fordtran's gastrointestinal and liver disease: pathophysiology, diagnosis, management. Philadelphia: WB Saunders, 2006; 1033–1061.

Yamamoto T, Umegae S, Kitagawa T. The value of plasma cytokine measurement for the detection of strangulation in patients with bowel obstruction: a prospective, pilot study. Diseases of the Colon and Rectum 2005; 48: 1451–1459.

7.4 Hernia

Andrew Dent • Neil Goldie

ESSENTIALS

1 A diagnosis of symptomatic hernia mandates early surgical repair to avoid life-threatening complications.

2 Hernia may present as a reducible lump, or may incarcerate, strangulate and/or present as bowel obstruction.

3 Femoral herniae are often misdiagnosed and are associated with high morbidity when complicated.

4 All herniae presenting with a complication should undergo surgical repair promptly.

Introduction

A hernia is defined as a protrusion of a viscus or part of a viscus through a weakness in the wall of the containing cavity. It has an aperture, coverings (usually peritoneum and abdominal wall layers) and contents, which may be any intra-abdominal organ but are usually omentum or small bowel. Surgical treatment requires reduction of the contents and closure of the aperture, with reinforcement to prevent recurrence.

There are a number of described sites for herniae. This chapter will focus on the more common, but the principles of assessment and treatment apply in general to herniae at other sites as well.

Inguinal hernia

Inguinal herniae are extremely common, with a lifetime risk of occurrence of 27% for men and 3% for women, and an annual incidence of 130 per 100 000 population. Up to 9% of hernia repairs are performed urgently. Emergency repairs are more common in the elderly and carry greater morbidity than elective repair.[1]

As their name implies, direct inguinal herniae bulge directly through the posterior wall of the inguinal canal. They are caused by weak abdominal musculature, are common in the elderly, and frequently bilateral. They have a large neck and hence seldom become irreducible or strangulate until they are of considerable size.

For indirect inguinal herniae, the hernial sac comes through the internal inguinal ring, travels the length of the inguinal canal and emerges from the external inguinal ring. Thus it usually lies above and medial to the symphysis pubis. Later the internal inguinal ring may stretch and the hernial sac and its contents may descend to and fill the scrotum, occasionally becoming very large. As the internal inguinal ring is usually narrow, irreducibility is common. Indirect inguinal herniae occur throughout life.

Direct and indirect inguinal herniae may be distinguishable by simple clinical tests. When an indirect hernia is reduced, finger pressure over the site of the internal ring may hold it reduced; however, a direct inguinal hernia will flop out again unless several fingers or the side of the hand props up the entire length of the inguinal canal.

Femoral hernia

Femoral herniae appear lateral and inferior to the symphysis pubis. They are formed by the peritoneal sac and contents, which occupy the potential space of the femoral canal, medial to the femoral vein. They are proportionately more common in women and rarely large. Symptoms usually occur early and complications are common.

The femoral canals should be closely examined in any patient presenting with abdominal pain or signs of bowel obstruction, as femoral herniae are frequently overlooked, especially in patients who are elderly and obese.[2] Diagnosis of a femoral hernia mandates early surgery. Morbidity from emergency femoral hernia repair increases with the presence of small bowel obstruction, and mortality with emergency surgery can be as high as 5%.[3]

Umbilical hernia

Umbilical and periumbilical herniae protrude through and around the umbilicus. They are very common in the newborn, but most resolve by 4 years of age. As they have a broad neck, emergency complications are uncommon. They can be difficult to diagnose in very obese people. If complicated, they can present resembling abdominal wall cellulitis.

Epigastric hernia

Epigastric herniae appear in the midline above the umbilicus. A small extraperitoneal piece of fat may be stuck in this hernia, causing pain.

Other herniae

Obturator hernia

Rarely, viscera may pass through a defect in the obturator foramen and present as a small bowel obstruction. This occurs most commonly in elderly emaciated women with chronic disease.[4] Diagnosis of this internal hernia, and the hernia of the foramen of Winslow, is seldom made preoperatively.

Spigelian hernia

These are rare and are due to a defect in the anterolateral abdominal wall musculature. They usually present as a reducible lump in the elderly male, lateral to the rectus muscle in the lower half of the abdomen.[5] Complications are rare.

Incisional hernia

These may occur at the site of any previous abdominal wound, such as appendicectomy or laparotomy. The wound area becomes weak, allowing the protrusion of a viscus or part of a viscus.

Sportsman's (athlete's) hernia

This is a term used for those who present with the painful symptoms of a hernia in the groin following exertion.[6] It is defined as an occult hernia caused by weakness or tear of the posterior inguinal wall without a clinically recognizable hernia.[7] Generally, by the time of diagnosis non-operative treatment options have failed and surgery often results in a return to sport.[8] Ultrasound can be a useful diagnostic medium to detect herniae which are intermittently symptomatic but without clinical signs.

Complications

In the early stages herniae are usually reducible, producing only intermittent pain in the groin, but reducible herniae may become irreducible (incarcerated). Incarcerated herniae may lead to a bowel obstruction. Strangulation and interruption of the blood supply to the contents of the hernia (usually small bowel) may supervene. In this case there will be increasing local pain and tenderness, warmth and overlying erythema accompanied by signs of bowel obstruction, accompanied by leukocytosis.

Rarely only part of the bowel wall is caught in a hernial constricting ring. Bowel wall necrosis ensues that is not circumferential; this is termed a Richter's hernia. In this case, there may be signs of strangulation without signs of obstruction.

Very rarely, neglected herniae can fistulate, with bowel contents appearing at the abdominal wall or through the hernial orifices.

Treatment

Reduction

It may be possible to reduce a hernia that initially appears irreducible in the emergency department (ED), but caution must be exercised. If the skin over the hernia is already inflamed and pain is severe, the contents may be compromised and urgent surgical exploration is required. Reduction of the contents in this circumstance can be dangerous, as false reassurance can occur followed by the later development of peritonitis due to intra-abdominal perforation of the hernia contents.

As a general rule, if the hernia has been irreducible for less than 4 hours, vital signs are normal and there are no symptoms of bowel obstruction, reduction of an incarcerated hernia may be attempted. This is achieved by giving adequate analgesia to relax the patient and applying gentle pressure manipulating the hernia site for several minutes. Elevating the foot of the bed may be helpful. Successful reduction relieves pain, may prevent strangulation and reduces the urgency for surgical intervention. Notwithstanding, all herniae that have undergone a complication require surgical consultation at the time of presentation.

Surgical repair

Inguinal hernia repair is a very common operation in general surgery. Rates of repair range from 10 per 10 000 population in the UK to 28 per 10 000 in the USA.[9]

Timely repair of herniae reduces the incidence of complications and avoids the greater risk associated with emergency surgery.[10] Until the introduction of synthetic mesh, inguinal hernia repair had changed little for over 100 years. The mesh can be placed by an open method or laparoscopically. Laparoscopic transabdominal preperitoneal hernia repair takes longer than open surgery and has a more serious complication rate with regard to visceral injuries, but is being increasingly performed as it reduces postoperative pain and significantly reduces time off work.[11] It is also much more operator dependent, is more difficult to learn and has higher overall hospital costs.[12]

Patients requiring emergency surgery for bowel obstruction or strangulation should be prepared with adequate fluid resuscitation and analgesia.

Controversies

- The diagnosis and management of 'sportsman's hernia'.

- The role of laparoscopy in hernia repair.

References

1. Brittenden J, Heys SD, Eremerin O. Femoral hernia: mortality and morbidity following elective and emergency repair. Journal of the Royal College of Surgeons of Edinburgh 1991; 36: 86–88.
2. Camary VL. Femoral hernia: intestinal obstruction is an unrecognized source of morbidity and mortality. British Journal of Surgery 1993; 80: 230–232.
3. Chung L, O'Dwyer PJ. Treatment of asymptomatic inguinal hernias. Surgeon 2007; 5: 95–100; quiz 100, 121.
4. Devsine M, Grimson R, Soroff HS. Benefits of a clinic for the treatment of external abdominal wall hernias. American Journal of Surgery 1987; 153: 387–391.
5. Farber AJ, Wilckens JH. Sports hernia: diagnosis and therapeutic approach. Journal of the American Academy of Orthopedic Surgery 2007; 15: 507–514.
6. Fredberg U, Kissmeyer-Nielsen P. The Sportsman's hernia – fact or fiction? Scandinavian Journal of Medicine and Science in Sports 1996; 6: 201–204.
7. Lo CY, Lorentz TG, Lau PW. Obturator hernia presenting as small bowel obstruction. American Journal of Surgery 1994; 167: 396–398.
8. Spangen L. Spigelian hernia. World Journal of Surgery 1989; 13: 573–580.
9. McCormack K, Scott NW, Go PM, et al. Laparoscopic techniques versus open techniques for inguinal hernia repair. Cochrane Database Systematic Review (1): CD001785, 2003.
10. Primatesta P, Goldacre MJ. Inguinal hernia repair: incidence of elective and emergency surgery, readmission and mortality. International Journal of Epidemiology 1996; 25: 835–839.
11. Reuben B, Neumayer L. Surgical management of inguinal hernia. Advances in Surgery 2006; 40: 299–317.
12. Swan KG, Wolcott M. The athletic hernia: A systematic review. Clinical Orthopaedics and Related Research 2007; 455: 78–87.

7.5 Gastroenteritis

Corinne Ginifer • Simon Young • Gerard O'Reilly

ESSENTIALS

1 Gastroenteritis is usually a benign, self-limiting disease that can be diagnosed clinically, warrants no specific investigation, and settles spontaneously with symptomatic treatment and oral fluid therapy.

2 The cardinal clinical feature of gastroenteritis is diarrhoea, which may be accompanied by varying degrees of nausea and vomiting, abdominal cramping and pain, lethargy and fever.

3 The clinical examination is directed at confirming the diagnosis of gastroenteritis, excluding alternative diagnoses and determining the degree of dehydration.

4 A wide variety of viruses, bacteria and protozoa may cause gastroenteritis. In developed countries common viral agents include rotavirus and Norwalk virus. Common bacteria include *Campylobacter jejuni*, *Staphylococcus aureus*, *Escherichia coli*, *Shigella dysenteriae* and *Salmonella enteriditis*. Common protozoa include *Giardia lamblia*.

5 The principles of treatment of gastroenteritis are to replace the fluid losses orally or intravenously, minimize the patient's symptoms by the use of antiemetic therapy, and in some circumstances administer specific antimicrobial agents.

Introduction

Gastroenteritis is a common clinical syndrome. It poses one of the world's major clinical and public health problems, and in developing countries with poor-quality drinking water and low levels of sanitation it is a major cause of morbidity and mortality, especially among children and the elderly.

Gastroenteritis is caused by infection of the gastrointestinal tract by various viruses, bacteria and protozoa, which have most commonly been transmitted by the faecal–oral route. The syndrome consists of diarrhoea, abdominal cramping or pain, nausea and vomiting, lethargy, malaise and fever. Each of these features may be present to a varying degree, and may last from 1 day to more than 3 weeks.

In developed countries, even though serious morbidity and mortality are low, gastroenteritis may be an extremely painful and unpleasant event causing disruption to daily life and significant loss of working and school days. Patients often seek emergency medical care because of the acuteness of onset or the frequency of the diarrhoea, the severity of abdominal pain and cramps, and because of concerns regarding dehydration.

Gastroenteritis may occur in many settings. It may be a sporadic isolated event, a small outbreak either within a family or other close living group such as in a geriatric residential facility, or part of a larger community epidemic. The latter can place extreme strain upon emergency department (ED) resources. It may occur in a traveller, either while still overseas or on their return home. It is important to be aware of the circumstances and context in which the illness occurs, as these will often dictate the course of investigation or management.

Pathophysiology and microbiology

Micro-organisms of all descriptions are constantly entering the gastrointestinal tract through the mouth. Extremely few of these progress to cause clinical illness. The natural defences of the gastrointestinal tract against infection include gastric acid secretion, normal bowel flora, bile salt production, bowel motility, mucosal lymphoid tissue and secreted immunoglobulin A. People with disturbances in any of these defences are more prone to a clinical infection. For example, patients with achlorhydria, bowel stasis or blind loops, immunodeficiency states or recent antibiotic therapy that has disturbed bowel flora are prone to gastroenteritis. Some organisms such as rotavirus occur principally in children, as previous infection confers immunity.

A wide variety of viruses, bacteria and protozoa may cause gastroenteritis, and the list is continually growing. Viral agents include rotavirus, enteric adenovirus, astrovirus, calicivirus, Norwalk virus, coronavirus and cytomegalovirus. Bacteria include *Campylobacter jejuni*, *Staphylococcus aureus*, *Bacillus cereus*, *Escherichia coli*, *Vibrio cholerae*, *Shigella dysenteriae*, *Salmonella enteriditis*, *Yersinia enterocolitica*, *Clostridium perfringens* and *C. difficile*. Protozoa include *Giardia lamblia*, *Cryptosporidium parvum* and *Entamoeba histolytica*.

Micro-organisms cause gastroenteritis by a number of mechanisms. They may release preformed toxins prior to ingestion, multiply and produce toxins within the gastrointestinal lumen, directly invade the bowel wall, or use a combination of toxins and invasion. *Staphylococcus aureus* and *Bacillus cereus* produce a variety of toxins in stored food that are subsequently ingested. These toxins are absorbed and within hours act on the central nervous system to produce an illness characterized predominantly by vomiting and mild diarrhoea.

Invasive bacteria are characterized by *Salmonella*, which invades the mucosa, primarily of the distal ileum, producing cell damage and excessive secretion. *Shigella* likewise invades the mucosa but also produces toxins that have cytotoxic, neurotoxic and enterotoxic effects.

The many strains of *E. coli* have been divided into five groups, depending on the pathology of the diseases they cause. These are enteropathogenic, enterotoxigenic, enteroinvasive, enteroaggregative and enterohaemorrhagic. Enterohaemorrhagic *E. coli* is associated with haemorrhagic colitis and the haemolytic–uraemic syndrome, whereas enterotoxigenic *E. coli* is associated with traveller's diarrhoea. The protozoan *Giardia lamblia* adheres to the jejunum and upper ileum, causing mucosal inflammation, inhibition of disaccharidase activity and overgrowth of luminal bacteria.

Clinical presentation

The clinical history and examination are directed at confirming the diagnosis of gastroenteritis, excluding other diagnoses, and determining the degree of dehydration.

The principal clinical manifestation of gastroenteritis is diarrhoea. The World Health Organization syndromic definition of gastroenteritis is 'three or more abnormally loose or fluid stools over 24 hours'. The diarrhoea of gastroenteritis is often watery and profuse in the early stages of the illness, and may last for up to 3 weeks. It is important to determine as far as possible the frequency, volume and characteristics of the stool. Some organisms, such as enterohaemorrhagic *E. coli*, *Shigella*, *Salmonella*, *Campylobacter* and *Entamoeba*

histolytica, may cause acute and bloody diarrhoea, whereas others such as *Giardia* may cause loose, pale, greasy stools.

Abdominal pain is common and is most often described as a diffuse intermittent colicky pain situated centrally in the abdomen. It may occur just prior to, and be partially relieved by, a bowel action. Severe pain is often caused by *Campylobacter*, *Yersinia* and *E. coli*. Abdominal pain is also the hallmark of many other forms of intra- and extra-abdominal pathology. Diagnoses other than gastroenteritis should be seriously considered if the pain is well localized, constant and severe, or radiates to the back or shoulder.

Vomiting may be present, particularly early in the illness, and can be variable in severity and persistence. The amount of vomiting and the ability to keep down clear fluids should be determined, as this will dictate the management of dehydration. Severe vomiting often occurs with organisms that produce preformed toxin, although it does not usually persist for longer than 24 hours. Anorexia, nausea and lethargy are common. Fever and systemic symptoms such as headache are prominent with organisms that invade the bowel wall and enter the systemic circulation, such as *Yersinia*. Lethargy may be related to the dehydration or merely the strain of constant and persistent diarrhoea from any aetiology.

Specific inquiry regarding fluid status is essential. The aim should be to determine the amount of fluids that have been taken orally and kept down over the course of the illness, along with the estimated urine output. It is also important to ascertain pre-existing or intercurrent illness, such as diabetes or immunosuppression, which may alter management.

Clinical examination

Suitable infection control procedures should be instituted prior to the examination to prevent spread to the examining doctor and hence to other patients. The patient should be in an isolated cubicle. Hand hygiene procedures before and after the consultation, the use of gloves and prompt disposal of soiled clothing and linen are important.

A careful clinical examination should be performed, concentrating on the abdomen and the circulatory state of the patient. The vital signs, temperature and urinalysis should be obtained.

In mild to moderate gastroenteritis the clinical examination is often unremarkable. There may be some general abdominal tenderness, active bowel sounds and facial pallor, but little else. In more severe disease the abdominal tenderness may be pronounced and signs of dehydration present. Of note, uncomplicated gastroenteritis is extremely unlikely if the abdominal examination reveals localized tenderness or signs of peritoneal irritation.

Fluid losses through diarrhoea, vomiting and fever, together with poor oral fluid intake, can lead to clinically apparent dehydration. This may be manifest as tachycardia, tachypnoea, reduced tissue turgor, delayed capillary return, reduced urine output and, in its more severe stages, hypotension, impaired conscious state and death.

Extra-abdominal signs of a primary gastroenteritis can occur. *Campylobacter* has been associated with reactive arthritis and Guillain–Barré syndrome. The clinical features, course and complications for various causative agents are summarized in Table 7.5.1.

Diarrhoea in certain circumstances

Traveller's diarrhoea
Millions of travellers each year are affected by diarrhoea. Southeast Asia, the Middle East, the Mediterranean basin, Central and South America are areas of frequent occurrence. The incidence of diarrhoea in travellers to these areas is as high as 30–50%.[1] Bacteria are the most common cause of traveller's diarrhoea. Pathogens include enterotoxigenic *E. coli* (ETEC), enteroaggregative *E. coli* (EAEC), *Salmonella*, *Shigella* and *Campylobacter*. Protozoans such as *Giardia*, *Cryptosporidium* and *Entamoeba histolytica* account for 10% of cases. Rotavirus and norovirus are the principal viral pathogens, but account for less than 10% of traveller's diarrhoea.[2] Many cases do not become symptomatic until after return home. A history of recent travel to one of these areas should be sought.

Antibiotic prophylaxis for traveller's diarrhoea, although effective, is not usually recommended as in most instances the illness will be self-limiting.

The immunocompromised patient
Patients with impaired immunity (AIDS, IgA deficiency, immunosuppressive therapy following organ transplantation and long-term corticosteroid usage) are not only more susceptible to the common causes of gastroenteritis, but are also vulnerable to the less common organisms such as *Cryptosporidium*, *Microsporidium*, *Isospora* and *Cytomegalovirus*. Infections are often more severe, have a higher incidence of complications, and may be more resistant to conventional therapy. Isolation of the causative organism and determination of antibiotic sensitivity are essential to guide management.

Hospital-acquired diarrhoea
Antibiotic-associated diarrhoea as a result of *Clostridium difficile* infection is the most common cause of acute diarrhoea in hospitalized patients.[1,3] It may range from a mild disease to life-threatening pseudomembranous colitis and can follow treatment with almost any antibiotic, but particularly cephalosporins and clindamycin. Methods of laboratory detection include tissue culture cytotoxicity, ELISA tests, and PCR.[3] Patients should be treated with oral metronidazole or oral vancomycin.

Differential diagnosis

Many pathological conditions, especially early in their course, may present with a clinical picture similar to that of gastroenteritis. Appendicitis, mesenteric adenitis, small bowel ischaemia and inflammatory bowel disease can all present in a similar fashion. Conversely, *Campylobacter* may cause severe abdominal pain with little diarrhoea, and may be misdiagnosed as appendicitis or inflammatory bowel disease. Medical conditions such as toxic ingestions, diabetic ketoacidosis, hepatitis and pancreatitis can present with vomiting, abdominal pain, tenderness and 'loose' stools.

Although a thorough history and examination, combined with judicious use of investigations, should be able to differentiate many of these at the time of presentation, careful observation over a period of time looking for a change in signs and symptoms may be necessary.

Investigations

In most circumstances no investigations are necessary in order to make the diagnosis of gastroenteritis or to manage the patient effectively.

Identification of the infective agent may be useful when there is an outbreak of gastroenteritis to ensure that adequate public health measures are instituted, in an attempt to limit spread of the disease. Additionally, in a patient who has a persistent illness or clinical features of a specific illness, such as *Campylobacter*, *Giardia* or *Salmonella*, identification of the organism may be helpful in directing antimicrobial therapy or identifying a carrier state. Although the history and examination may give clues as to the aetiological agent, they are unreliable as many similarities exist between the clinical syndromes produced by each organism. Laboratory identification is the only accurate method.

The infective agent may be identified by microscopy and culture of faeces, looking specifically for pathogenic bacteria, cysts, ova or parasites. A fresh specimen of faeces will assist in detection. Occasionally multiple specimens are required, especially for organisms which may shed into the faeces only sporadically. Once collected, the specimen must be kept cool (4°C) and transported promptly to the laboratory.

Rotavirus infection is detected by looking for rotavirus antigen in the stool by electron microscopy, PCR, ELISA or latex agglutination.

If a patient is dehydrated or systemically unwell, a full blood examination, serum electrolyte determination and serum glucose are warranted. In rare cases, where there are signs suggestive of septicaemia or severe systemic illness, blood cultures and liver function tests may be indicated.

Abdominal X-rays are only useful if it is necessary to exclude a bowel obstruction or free intra-abdominal gas.

Table 7.5.1 Pathogen-specific syndromes

Causative agent	Incubation period	Duration of illness	Predominant symptoms	Foods commonly implicated
Bacteria				
Campylobacter jejuni	1–10 days (usually 2–5 days)	2–5 days occasionally >10 days	Sudden onset of diarrhoea, abdominal pain, nausea, vomiting	Raw or undercooked poultry, raw milk, raw or undercooked meat, untreated water
E. coli enterohaemorrhagic (STEC, VTEC)	2–10 days	5–10 days	Severe colic, mild to profuse bloody diarrhoea can lead to haemolytic uraemic syndrome	Many raw foods (especially minced beef), unpasteurised milk, contaminated water
E. coli enteropathogenic enterotoxigenic enteroinvasive	12–72 hrs (enterotoxigenic)	3–14 days	Severe colic, watery to profuse diarrhoea, sometimes bloody	Many raw foods, food contaminated by faecal matter, contaminated water
Salmonella serovars (non-typhoid)	6–72 hrs	3–5 days	Abdominal pain, diarrhoea, chills, fever, malaise	Raw or undercooked meat and chicken, raw or undercooked eggs and egg products
Shigella spp.	12–96 hrs	4–7 days	Malaise, fever, vomiting, diarrhoea (blood & mucus)	Foods contaminated by infected food handlers and untreated water contaminated by human faeces
Yersinia enterocolitica	3–7 days	1–21 days	Acute diarrhoea sometimes bloody, fever, vomiting	Raw meat especially pork, raw or undercooked poultry, milk and milk products
Vibrio cholerae	A few hours to 5 days	3–4 days	Asymptomatic to profuse painless watery diarrhoea, dehydration	Raw seafood, contaminated water
Vibrio parahaemolyticus	4–30 hours (usually 12–24 hrs)	1–7 days	Abdominal pain, diarrhoea, vomiting and sometimes fever. Illness of moderate severity	Raw and lightly cooked fish, shellfish, other seafoods
Viruses				
Norovirus (and other viral gastroenteritis)	24–48 hrs	12–60 hrs	Severe vomiting, diarrhoea	Oysters, clams, foods contaminated by infected food handlers and untreated water contaminated by human faeces
Rotaviruses	24–72 hrs	Up to 7 days	Malaise, headache, fever, vomiting, diarrhoea	Foods contaminated by infected food handlers and untreated water contaminated by human faeces
Parasites				
Cryptosporidium	1–12 days	4–21 days	Profuse watery diarrhoea, abdominal pain	Foods contaminated by infected food handlers and untreated water contaminated by human faeces
Giardia lamblia	1–3 weeks	1–2 weeks to months	Loose pale greasy stools, abdominal pain	Foods contaminated by infected food handlers and untreated water contaminated by human faeces
Entamoeba histolytica	2–4 weeks	Weeks to months	Colic, mucous or bloody diarrhoea	Foods contaminated by infected food handlers and untreated water contaminated by human faeces
Toxin producing bacteria				
B. cereus (toxin in food)	1–6 hrs (vomiting) or 6–24 hrs (diarrhoea)	<24 hrs	Two known toxins causing nausea and vomiting or diarrhoea and cramps	Cereals, rice, meat products, soups, vegetables
C. perfringens (toxin in gut)	6–24 hrs	24 hrs	Sudden onset colic, diarrhoea	Meats, poultry, stews, gravies, (often inadequately reheated or held warm)
Staphylococcus aureus (toxin in food)	30 min–8 hrs	24 hrs	Acute vomiting, and cramps, may lead to collapse	Cold foods (much handled during preparation) milk products, salted meats

Adapted from Guidelines for the Control of Infectious Diseases – The Blue Book. Communicable Diseases Section, Public Health Group, Victorian Government Department of Human Services, 2005. (Reproduced with the kind permission of the Communicable Diseases Section, Public Health Group, Victorian Government Department of Human Services).

Treatment

The principles of treatment for gastroenteritis are to replace fluid and electrolyte losses, minimize symptoms if possible, and in selected cases administer specific antimicrobial therapy. Clear fluids for 24 hours are often recommended, with the rationale that keeping the stomach empty will minimize vomiting. If the patient wishes to eat it is allowed. Strictly withholding feeding, especially from children, is not necessary.

Replacement of fluid losses may be achieved enterally, either by mouth or via a nasogastric tube, or intravenously. The method selected will depend on the cooperation of the patient, the degree of dehydration, the rate at which rehydration is desired, and the presence of other diseases such as diabetes.

Specific oral rehydration solutions are the most appropriate for oral or nasogastric use. There are a number of commercial preparations available through pharmacies without prescription. These consist of a balanced formula of glucose, sodium and potassium salts, and in worldwide trials have been shown to be extremely effective and safe, even when used in the most primitive of conditions.[4] Although many commonly available fluids may be used and will probably be effective in mild disease, fluids that contain large amounts of glucose, such as degassed lemonade or undiluted fruit juice, should not be encouraged in adults and are contraindicated in children. These fluids are hyperosmolar and deficient in electrolytes, thus promoting further fluid losses. Glucose-containing electrolyte solutions use the gut's co-transport system for glucose and sodium, thereby facilitating the absorption of water as well. Milk and other lactose-containing products should be avoided during the acute phase of the illness, as viral or bacterial enteropathogens often result in transient lactose malabsorption. Caffeine-containing products should also be avoided.[1] Caffeine increases cyclic AMP levels, thereby promoting the secretion of fluid and worsening diarrhoea.

Intravenous rehydration is necessary in patients who are shocked or who are

DIGESTIVE

Table 7.5.2 Antibiotic treatment regimens

Giardia lamblia

Tinidazole 2 g (child: 50 mg/kg up to 2 g) orally, as a single dose. OR
Metronidazole 2 g (child: 30 mg/kg up to 2 g) orally, daily for 3 days.

Amoebiasis

Tinidazole 2 g (child: 50 mg/kg up to 2 g) orally, daily for 3 days. OR
Metronidazole 600 mg (child: 15 mg/kg up to 600 mg) orally, 8 hourly for 7–10 days. PLUS
Paromycin 500 mg (child: 10 mg/kg up to 500 mg) orally 8 hourly for 7 days (to prevent relapse).

Shigellosis

Norfloxacin 400 mg (child: 10 mg/kg up to 400 mg) orally, 12 hourly for 5 days. OR
Ampicillin 1 g (child: 25 mg/kg up to 1g) orally, 6 hourly for 5 days. OR
Co-trimoxazole 160/800 mg (child: 4/20 mg/kg up to 160/800 mg) orally, 12 hourly for 5 days.

Campylobacter

Erythromycin 500 mg (child: 10 mg/kg up to 500 mg) orally, 6 hourly for 5–7 days.

Traveller's diarrhoea

Norfloxacin 800 mg (child: 20 mg/kg up to 800 mg) orally, as a single dose. OR
Azithromycin 1 g (child: 20 mg/kg up to 1 g) orally, as a single dose.

Clostridium difficile

Metronidazole 400 mg (child: 10 mg/kg up to 400 mg) orally, 8 hourly for 7–10 days.
If unresponsive or severe disease: Vancomycin 125 mg (child: 3 mg/kg up to 125 mg) orally 6 hourly for 7–10 days.

Reference: Therapeutic Guidelines: Antibiotic. Version 13, 2006. Therapeutic Guidelines Limited. Antibiotic Expert Committee, Melbourne.

becoming progressively more dehydrated despite oral or nasogastric fluids. Resuscitation should be commenced with normal saline at a rate which accounts for ongoing losses, as well as replacing the estimated fluid deficit. In severely dehydrated patients one or two 20 mL/kg boluses of normal saline may be necessary. Patients should also be encouraged to take oral fluids, unless vomiting is prohibitive. As soon as an adequate intake is achieved the intravenous fluids can be scaled back and ceased.

Close monitoring of the serum electrolytes is necessary during intravenous rehydration. In particular it is important to monitor serum sodium, as the exclusive use of normal saline for rehydration can lead to hypernatraemia. Potassium should be added to the fluid as determined by the serum potassium, remembering that a low serum potassium in this circumstance is indicative of a low total body potassium.

In adults, parenterally administered antiemetic drugs such as metoclopramide, prochlorperazine, or ondansetron may be useful in the management of severe vomiting. In children, an unacceptably high incidence of dystonic reactions precludes their use. Antimotility agents such as loperamide may be used, and have been shown to reduce the number of diarrhoeal stools and the duration of the illness.[5] Antimotility agents have significant side effects and should only be used if it is essential.

Even though many bacteria that cause gastroenteritis respond to antibiotics they are rarely indicated. Recent antibiotic guidelines suggest that most infections with *Campylobacter*, *Salmonella*, *Shigella*, *Yersinia* and *E. coli* do not need antibiotics. In the majority of these cases the illness will be short-lived and mild. Because of the previous widespread use of antibiotics to treat gastroenteritis from any cause, and the current use of antibiotics in animals bred for food, many isolates of *Campylobacter jejuni*, *Shigella* and *Salmonella* are resistant to many antibiotics.[1] Choice of antibiotics should be based on antibiotic sensitivity patterns. Antibiotics may be indicated in *Giardia* infections, *Shigella* causing severe disease, *Salmonella* in infants, the immunosuppressed or the elderly, *Campylobacter* in food handlers, and in traveller's diarrhoea. Antibiotics are contraindicated in uncomplicated *Salmonella* infections as they may prolong the carrier state. Recommended antibiotic regimens are summarized in Table 7.5.2.

Controversies

- The role of faecal microscopy and culture.

- The public health role of emergency departments in monitoring and reporting the prevalence of gastroenteritis in the community.

- When is it appropriate to prescribe antiemetic or antidiarrhoeal therapy, given that this is most commonly a benign and self-limiting disease?

- The reliability of clinical examination in determining the degree of dehydration.

- The circumstances in which the empirical use of antibiotics may be appropriate.

References

1. Aranda-Michel J, Giannella RA. Acute diarrhea: a practical review. American Journal of Medicine 1999; 106: 670–676.
2. Centers for Disease Control and Prevention. Health information for international travel. Atlanta: CDC, 2005.
3. Riley TV. Nosocomial diarrhoea due to *Clostridium difficile*. Current Opinion in Infectious Disease 2004; 17: 323–327.
4. Guerrant RL, Van Gilder T, Steiner S, et al. Practice guidelines for the management of infectious diarrhea. Clinical Infectious Diseases 2001; 32: 331–350.
5. Cheng AC, McDonald JR, Thielman NM. Infectious diarrhea in developed and developing countries. Journal of Clinical Gastroenterology 2005; 39: 1–17.

7.6 Haematemesis and melaena

Colin Graham

ESSENTIALS

1 Resuscitation is the priority, with particular attention to restoring perfusion of vital organs by replacing intravascular volume.

2 Upper gastrointestinal endoscopy is the key investigation and frequently allows definitive therapy. It should be performed at the earliest opportunity.

Introduction

Upper gastrointestinal bleeding (UGIB) is a common medical emergency with significant morbidity and mortality. Over the last two decades there have been advances in drug therapy for peptic ulcer disease and varices, improvements in endoscopic techniques, interventional radiology and surgical management, in addition to advances in resuscitation and supportive care. Despite these advances, mortality for patients presenting with UGIB remains around 6–11%, with approximately 6–8% requiring emergency surgery. Patients with UGIB are increasingly elderly and have more comorbidity than in the past, which helps to explain the lack of apparent improvement in mortality. Patients now rarely die of exsanguination, but more commonly of multiple organ failure secondary to pre-existing comorbidities.[1–6]

Epidemiology, aetiology and differential dignosis

Peptic ulceration remains the most common cause of UGIB despite the recognition and treatment of *Helicobacter pylori* infection as a primary cause of peptic ulcer disease, accounting for between 35% and 50% of all cases. This represents a significant reduction compared to around 66% two decades ago. The pathogenesis of peptic ulcer disease is complex but is closely related to a variety of risk factors, including *Helicobacter pylori* infection, use of non-steroidal anti-inflammatory drugs (NSAIDs), smoking and alcohol use (see Chapter 7.7).

Gastroduodenal erosions and oesophagitis make up a further 15% of cases.

Oesophagogastric varices, resulting from portal hypertension, are the source of up to 10% of episodes of UGIB. Mallory–Weiss tears, the result of repeated vomiting, account for 5–15% of cases of UGIB and usually do not require specific treatment. The remaining causes (all <1%) include vascular lesions such as angiodysplasia, Dieulafoy's lesion and aortoenteric fistula.

Prevention

The development of peptic ulcer disease is closely related to management of the risk factors. The effective identification and eradication of *H. pylori* has led to a significant reduction in the incidence of peptic ulcer disease as the cause of UGIB.

There is little doubt that restricting the prescription of NSAIDs in the elderly (the highest risk group for development of UGIB from NSAIDs, and the age group with the highest risk of mortality from UGIB) would prevent a significant number of episodes of UGIB. This is particularly relevant to emergency medicine practice, where NSAIDs are frequently prescribed as analgesia for musculoskeletal conditions. Care should be taken to prescribe the safest drugs (ibuprofen has the lowest risk profile) for the shortest possible time at the lowest effective dose.

Definitions

Upper gastrointestinal bleeding is defined as any bleeding within the gastrointestinal (GI) tract proximal to the ligament of Treitz. Any bleeding arising distal to that is a lower GI bleed. Haematemesis is the vomiting of bright red blood. 'Coffee-ground vomiting' is the vomiting of digested blood clot, whereas melaena is the passage of black, tarry stools as a result of bacterial degradation of haemoglobin within the gut. Melaena usually represents a source of UGIB, but it can rarely occur due to a lower gastrointestinal source of bleeding. Haematochezia is the passage of bright red blood per rectum, and in the context of UGIB represents a briskly bleeding source of haemorrhage. Melaena of itself is not associated with poorer outcomes in UGIB, but haematochezia is associated with a three times higher risk of death.[3]

Clinical features

It is usually necessary to determine whether the blood loss is from a gastrointestinal source. Blood from the nose or oropharynx can be swallowed, resulting in haematemesis and/or melaena. If bleeding is thought to be from the upper GI tract, then a number of diagnoses need to be considered (see below).

Some historical clues and caveats must be considered:

- A history of epigastric pain or dyspepsia suggests peptic ulcer disease. However, peptic ulcer disease may be painless, particularly in the elderly, and particularly in those taking NSAIDs and steroids.
- A positive history of gastric or duodenal ulcer disease or reflux oesophagitis is associated with an approximately 50% chance of finding the same diagnosis at endoscopy.
- The risk of UGIB in patients taking NSAIDs is double that of patients not taking NSAIDs.
- The classic history of nausea and repeated vomiting prior to bleeding occurs in approximately one-third of cases of Mallory–Weiss tear.
- UGIB with a history of alcohol abuse and the stigmata of portal hypertension is suggestive of varices. However, up to 40% of patients with cirrhosis who

present with GI bleeding are bleeding from causes other than varices (commonly from gastric erosions).

- Conditions associated with stress ulcers include burns, major trauma, head injury, sepsis and hypotension.
- Patients with chronic renal failure have a high incidence of angiodysplasia, peptic ulcer disease and oesophagitis.
- A history of aortic surgery and gastrointestinal bleeding should alert the clinician to the possibility of an aortoenteric fistula, even if the initial bleeding episode is not significant (the first bleed is often the so-called 'herald bleed').
- Clinical evidence of a coagulopathy should be sought, as this will influence subsequent investigation, treatment and prognosis.
- A rectal examination is essential. As previously described, stool colour has prognostic significance. Testing for occult blood further increases the sensitivity of this examination, as kits such as the Hematest are able to detect as little as 6 mg of haemoglobin per gram of stool. A positive test is dependent on the time of onset of bleeding in relation to gastrointestinal transit time. False positives may be produced by certain bacterial and vegetable peroxidases, such as bananas and horseradish. False negatives may result from ferrous salts.

Clues to the speed or acuity of blood loss include:

- The most likely diagnosis: Varices produce large amounts of dark (venous) blood; aortoenteric fistulae produce massive bright red haematemesis and haematochezia, with profound circulatory collapse.
- Signs of haemodynamic instability and response to initial resuscitation: If there is a poor response there is likely to be significant haemorrhage.
- The character of the vomitus: Ongoing haematemesis is associated with large blood loss; 'coffee-ground' altered vomiting or clear fluid is often associated with a slower rate of bleeding.
- The colour of the stool (see previous discussion).
- The nasogastric aspirate if a tube is already in the stomach (commonly

retirement home residents receiving enteral nutrition). Note that the practice of inserting a nasogastric tube in the emergency department (ED) to assess the aspirate is no longer recommended.

The key message is that if there is haemodynamic instability or other evidence of significant ongoing UGIB, fluid resuscitation should continue but arrangements should be made to expedite emergency upper gastrointestinal endoscopy. The accuracy of diagnosis is not important at this stage, but the identification of major ongoing bleeding is.

Clinical investigation

Blood tests

At the time of insertion of two wide-bore (>16 G) intravenous cannulae, blood should be drawn for full blood count, coagulation studies (INR/PT, APTT and fibrinogen), electrolytes, urea, creatinine, glucose level, liver function tests and urgent cross-matching. The initial haemoglobin is of limited value, as 24–48 hours are required for the intravascular volume to equilibrate. Thrombocytopenia and leukocytosis are associated with increasing morbidity and mortality. UGIB may also result in an elevation of the urea level (relative to the creatinine), as there is a combination of an increased protein load in the gut and intravascular hypovolaemia. Blood should be taken for blood gas analysis to assess acid–base balance in those with significant bleeds. Similarly, a serum lactate level can help to identify those with clinically occult hypoperfusion who are at high risk of significant haemorrhage.

Imaging

A chest X-ray may be indicated where aspiration is suspected, in the elderly, or in patients with cardiopulmonary comorbidities. It should also be performed if perforation is suspected; however, perforation associated with significant UGIB is very rare.

Endoscopy

Although clinical and historical features can point towards the most likely diagnosis, they are not specific. There is no empirical therapy that effectively treats all causes of UGIB.

As a result, a specific endoscopic diagnosis needs to be made. Exceptions may include those with a classic history suggestive of a Mallory–Weiss tear with no ongoing UGIB symptoms and stable haemoglobin and haemodynamic status, and the very elderly with major comorbidity and poor health status.

Most centres rely on endoscopy to:

- provide information on the source of bleeding with a high degree of specificity (90–95%);
- allow prediction of the likelihood of rebleeding and mortality, according to the nature and location of the lesion and stigmata of recent haemorrhage. These factors help in deciding the level of patient monitoring or whether they may be treated as an outpatient;
- provide therapy. Endoscopy facilitates haemostasis through sclerotherapy, coagulation techniques and banding of varices, and allows histological or microbiological diagnosis. In high-risk peptic ulcers, endoscopic therapy has been shown to decrease rebleeding by 75% and mortality by 40%;
- diagnose with safety (morbidity < 0.01%). Safety is further maximized if endoscopy is delayed until the patient is haemodynamically stable and the airway patent and protected.

The sensitivity of endoscopy is optimized if performed within 12–24 hours of presentation. Urgent endoscopy should be performed in patients with active or recurrent bleeding, bright red blood on haematemesis, large bleeds (>2 units of blood required), and when variceal bleeding is suspected. Endoscopic visualization of the mucosa is enhanced by giving a single bolus of 250 mg intravenous erythromycin to promote gastric emptying 30–90 minutes before endoscopy – this should be given in the ED if an early endoscopy is warranted.[7,8]

Early endoscopy facilitates management and results in earlier discharge.

Treatment

Oxygen should be administered to all patients. Massive ongoing bleeding may compromise the airway to the extent that endotracheal intubation may be required to secure and protect the airway. Intubation in these circumstances can be both difficult and hazardous, and high-volume effective suction is essential. The extent of bleeding is often underestimated, and under these conditions doses of induction agents should be dramatically reduced from normal levels.

The intravascular volume should then be optimized. The presence of shock (in most studies this was defined as a systolic blood pressure <100 mmHg) places the patient at high risk for rebleeding, requirement for surgery and death. Note that in the elderly, patients with autonomic neuropathies (frequently found in diabetics) and those taking β-blockers or calcium channel antagonists, vital signs, including postural hypotension, may not be a reliable indicator of the degree of blood loss. Propranolol is a commonly used (and effective) prophylaxis for the prevention of variceal bleeding in cirrhotic patients, and this may blunt the haemodynamic responses of patients with acute massive variceal bleeding.

Intravascular volume should initially be replaced with isotonic crystalloid (saline or Hartmann's) or colloid. There is no evidence of superiority for either class of intravenous fluid in UGIB at this time. Blood should be given promptly if there is persistent haemodynamic instability despite 2 L of crystalloid or colloid, if the initial haemoglobin level is <8 mg/dL, if there is a significant risk of rebleeding, and in those patients with comorbidities making them unable to tolerate periods of anaemia (e.g. chronic obstructive pulmonary disease). Aggressive resuscitation with early blood transfusion is indicated in the elderly. However, overhydration of patients with suspected varices should be avoided, as raising the portal venous pressure will cause further bleeding.

Monitoring

Continuous ECG monitoring, non-invasive blood pressure monitoring and pulse oximetry should be instituted, with frequent clinical reassessment. Urine output should also be measured. Invasive arterial and central venous pressure monitoring may be necessary in massive bleeds, intubated patients and those with comorbidities.

Coagulation

Those needing blood often require infusions of fresh frozen plasma and platelets, and these blood products should be requested early.

Fresh frozen plasma should be given when the prothrombin time is 3 seconds greater than the control, or when large transfusions are required. In all patients requiring massive transfusion, attempts should be made to avoid hypothermia by using blood warmers, heating blankets and overhead heaters.

Endoscopy

Although endoscopy is diagnostic for UGIB, it can also be therapeutic in the majority of cases and should be performed within 24 hours of admission in all cases. It must be available 24 hours per day and should be carried out without delay when patients remain unstable despite initial fluid and blood product resuscitation. Although many guidelines stress the need for 'haemodynamic stability' prior to endoscopy, in cases where this is difficult to achieve, consideration must be given to achieving haemostasis by endoscopic means as part of the ongoing resuscitation process.

Specific therapy

Peptic ulcer disease

Bleeding ceases spontaneously in 80% of cases and the mortality rate is approximately 5–6%, significantly less than with variceal bleeding.

Drug therapy

Haemostasis is known to be a pH dependent process, so it was hypothesized that medications which inhibit acid secretion will also reduce the rates of rebleeding, need for surgery and mortality. The two main drug classes are the histamine (H_2) antagonists and the proton pump inhibitors (PPIs).

H_2 antagonists Most data relating to the benefit of H_2 antagonists in acute upper GI bleeds are unconvincing. A large meta-analysis in 2002 reported that H_2 antagonists had only modest effects on bleeding gastric ulcers, reducing rebleeding by 7.2%, surgery by 6.7% and death by 3.2%.[9,10] There were no effects on bleeding duodenal ulcers. H_2 antagonists are not recommended in the contemporary management of UGIB.

Proton pump inhibitors The PPIs are the most commonly used class of drugs used for peptic disease based on their profound and persistent acid suppression. A recent Cochrane Systematic Review suggested an overall reduction in rebleeding and surgery compared to placebo or H_2-antagonist therapy in UGIB secondary to peptic ulcer.[11] However, there has been no demonstrable effect on all-cause mortality. In summary, the available data suggest that:

- The beneficial effects of PPIs may be more pronounced in Asian patients owing to differences in drug metabolism and longer-term effectiveness in terms of raising intragastric pH to around 6.
- There are no high-quality data to support the different modes of administration of PPIs (oral versus intravenous), doses or duration of treatment, or timing of initiation of treatment (before or after UGI endoscopy).

For patients with peptic ulcer disease the aim should be to eliminate reversible risk factors such as *H. pylori* and NSAIDs, and aim for long-term healing. As PPIs have been shown to provide better rates of ulcer healing, they are therefore the drugs of first choice. It is reasonable to initiate oral therapy when oral intake is allowed or intravenous therapy when feeding is delayed. Oral doses of PPIs should be at least double the standard clinical dose.

Somatostatin/octreotide Studies have found conflicting results in the use of somatostatin and octreotide in peptic ulcer disease. The only meta-analysis on this topic[12] suggested that there may be a reduction in rebleeding and the need for surgery in patients with bleeding ulcers. There was no effect on mortality. Somatostatin and octreotide may have a role in reducing these complications in high-risk patients, or may be considered if there are going to be unavoidable delays in performing emergency UGI endoscopy.

Endoscopy

Endoscopic therapy has been shown to achieve haemostasis in approximately 90% of cases, reduce rebleeding by 62%, reduce emergency surgery by 64% and reduce mortality by 45%. The incidence of bleeding and perforation associated with endoscopic therapy was 0.38% and 0.61%, respectively.[13] The ongoing development of new endoscopic techniques for haemostasis means that endoscopy is continuing to supplant surgery as definitive therapy. Combination therapy using submucosal adrenaline injections combined with thermal coaptive therapy appears to be the best option for ulcers requiring endoscopic treatment.[3]

Surgery

Surgery is required in approximately 6–8% of patients. It is indicated for continuous or recurrent active bleeding, especially in patients aged over 60, in whom early elective surgery produces significant benefits in terms of mortality. Other indications include blood transfusion exceeding 5 units, refractory shock, and failure to respond to endoscopic therapy. Early elective surgery in selected cases is preferable to emergency surgery because of the significant mortality associated with the latter.

Surgical consultation should be considered early in patients aged over 60, those with significant comorbidities, those with evidence of active bleeding (active bright red haematemesis, haematochezia), when there is a significant risk of rebleeding, or when there is haemodynamic instability at any stage.

Embolization

This evolving technique appears to offer selected patients with bleeding that is not manageable by conventional endoscopic means a good alternative to open surgery. Success rates of up to 69% have been reported, which is comparable to the results of open surgery.[14,15]

Gastro-oesophageal varices

Although haemorrhage from gastro-oesophageal varices accounts for 2–15% of all UGIB, it represents a significant therapeutic challenge. Bleeding ceases spontaneously in only 20–30%, yet as bleeding is often more severe and recurrent, mortality approaches 25–40% for each episode of variceal haemorrhage. Factors influencing mortality include the stage and rate of deterioration of the underlying liver disease, the presence of comorbidities, variceal size, and specific endoscopic criteria. Patients with

known severe varices should be considered for early transfer to a specialist hepatology centre with expertise in dealing with acute massive variceal bleeding.

Drug therapy

Drugs should be used when endoscopic expertise is not available, if massive bleeding prevents immediate sclerotherapy, or as an adjunct to further treatment if continued variceal haemorrhage is suspected. However, sclerotherapy or other surgical procedures are still required after drug therapy.

Somatostatin/octreotide This therapy produces dramatic reductions in splanchnic arterial blood flow and portal venous pressure, while preserving cardiac output and systemic blood pressure. It is the pharmacological method of choice as it is comparable to injection sclerotherapy, vasopressin and balloon tamponade in terms of bleeding control and survival, with the advantage of fewer side effects. Treatment results in the control of bleeding in 74–92% of cases, with endoscopic evidence of cessation of bleeding in 68% of patients within 15 minutes. The suggested rate of administration of somatostatin is 250 mg/h after an initial bolus of 250 mg. Octreotide is administered at 50 mg/h after an initial bolus of 50 mg. There may be additional benefits from daily boluses.

Vasopressin This drug increases peripheral vascular resistance and mean arterial pressure, with reduced cardiac output and coronary blood flow. It is contraindicated in patients with coronary artery disease, and is associated with complications necessitating withdrawal of treatment in up to 25% of patients. This makes vasopressin a second choice for drug therapy. However, combination with i.v. nitroglycerin (if tolerated) reduces the incidence of complications with no deterioration in efficacy. Vasopressin results in the control of bleeding in 50–75% of cases. The recommended infusion rate is 0.2–0.4 U/min to a maximum of 0.8 U/min with nitroglycerin if tolerated (40 mg/min, increasing to 400 mg/min, titrated to blood pressure).

Terlipressin Terlipressin is a synthetic analogue of vasopressin. It can be given by bolus i.v. injection and has been shown

to have a 34% relative risk reduction in mortality from acute variceal haemorrhage and a much lower incidence of side effects than vasopressin. A systematic review showed no difference between terlipressin and somatostatin treatment or between terlipressin and endoscopic therapy.[16] Terlipressin (in an initial dose of 2 mg i.v. bolus) is therefore recommended for patients with known or highly suspected oesophagogastric varices with UGIB.

Endoscopic techniques

Sclerotherapy Endoscopy is essential to confirm the diagnosis of variceal haemorrhage, as in up to 81% of patients with known varices an alternative bleeding site is found. Endoscopy may also have therapeutic benefits, as sclerotherapy (EST) can be performed at the time of the initial endoscopy. Control of bleeding can be achieved subsequently in up to 95% of cases,[12] with a reduction in the risk of rebleeding. Therefore, EST is considered first-line therapy in the control of bleeding from oesophageal varices.

However, complications occur in up to 41% of patients. These include perforation, aspiration, pyrexia, chest pain, tachycardia, oesophageal ulcers and strictures. Because recurrence rates are 20–30%, patients need repeated treatments.

EST is not recommended for gastric varices owing to a high complication rate and poor efficacy. Two possible alternative therapeutic strategies of benefit are tissue adhesives or thrombin.

Endoscopic variceal ligation Although technically more difficult, endoscopic variceal ligation (EVL) has been shown to be as effective as EST in the control of variceal haemorrhage, with significantly fewer complications, less rebleeding and lower mortality. It also requires fewer treatment sessions. Additional benefits (more effective control of variceal bleeding) may be gained by combining sclerotherapy with octreotide or terlipressin.

Balloon tamponade

Compression of fundal and distal oesophageal varices by balloon tamponade results in control of bleeding in 70–90% of cases. Balloon tamponade may be used as a temporary means of controlling bleeding which is refractory to medical or endoscopic treatment, or when it is too massive for endoscopy to be performed successfully.

Because of the problems of pooling of secretions in the oesophagus (thereby increasing the risk of pulmonary aspiration), the standard Sengstaken–Blakemore tube has been modified to the form of the Minnesota tube to incorporate an oesophageal aspiration port. Further modifications have been made with the Linton–Nachlas tube, which incorporates a single large (600 mL) gastric balloon for the tamponade of gastric varices. Balloon tamponade may be used as a bridge to facilitate transfer to a specialist hepatology or endoscopy centre for ongoing care.

There are number of problems with balloon tamponade:

- It can only be used for a maximum of 48–72 hours. As up to 50% of patients rebleed when the tube is deflated, further definitive procedures (EVL, EST, surgery) need to be performed.
- There is a significant (25–30%) risk of complications, particularly pulmonary aspiration and oesophageal perforation.
- Balloon tamponade requires skilled staff and monitoring in an intensive-care setting for the initial insertion and maintenance of balloon position and function.
- Owing to the risks of pulmonary aspiration, endotracheal intubation should be considered in all patients requiring balloon tamponade.

Transjugular intrahepatic portosystemic stent

Transjugular intrahepatic portosystemic stent-shunt (TIPS) involves the insertion of a stent under radiological guidance via the jugular vein, forming a portosystemic shunt between the hepatic and portal veins. This technique is effective, achieving control of bleeding in up to 90% of patients, and is less invasive and faster to perform (range 30 minutes to 3 hours) than other surgical shunt procedures. However, it requires an experienced operator and often results in complications similar to those seen after other portosystemic shunts, particularly encephalopathy and deteriorating liver function.

The main role of TIPS, therefore, appears to be in patients who continue to bleed in spite of sclerotherapy or ligation therapy, and who do not have hepatic encephalopathy, pre-terminal liver failure, portal vein thrombosis, intrahepatic sepsis or significant cardiac disease. TIPS then acts as a bridging procedure until other definitive surgical procedures can be performed (such as liver transplantation, shunt surgery or oesophageal transection).

Surgery

Since the advent of EST, the role of surgery in the control of acute variceal bleeding has decreased and it is now largely confined to patients who continue to bleed despite endoscopic intervention. Shunt surgery and oesophageal transection have been shown to reduce bleeding. However, these techniques have not been shown to improve survival, and provide no cost advantage over EST.

Other issues

The primary decision in most cases is whether the patient is to be admitted to the general ward or to an intensive care (ICU) or high-dependency unit (HDU). Ideally, patients with UGIB should be admitted under the joint care of a physician and a surgeon in a specific gastrointestinal bleeding unit.

The main indications for ICU/HDU admission include:

- Known or suspected variceal bleeding.
- Haemodynamic instability.
- Significant comorbidities, including cardiac, renal, pulmonary or hepatic dysfunction.
- Endoscopic features suggesting recent haemorrhage (arterial bleeding, adherent clot or visible vessel).

It is been suggested that the threshold for ICU/HDU admission be lowered in patients over 60 years of age, owing to the high incidence of comorbidities and poor physiological compensatory reserve. Lower-risk patients may be admitted to the general ward. The usual length of stay is 2–3 days, as the major risk of rebleeding is during the first 24–48 hours.

The guidelines for outpatient management of upper GI bleeding are less clear. Most UGIB ceases spontaneously and most patients compensate well, not requiring transfusion or surgery. Some authors have suggested outpatient management for selected patients. To minimize the risk of adverse events if the patient is managed as an outpatient, early endoscopy has been advocated. Early discharge is then suggested for those who are found to have clean-based ulcers or non-bleeding Mallory–Weiss tears. In this group, with no stigmata of recent haemorrhage, the risks of rebleeding and the need for emergency surgery are between 0 and 5% and death is rare.[17] The pressure on acute hospital resources is such that it would be useful to develop clinical scoring systems that could facilitate early safe discharge with or without endoscopy. Current scoring systems have not yet been evaluated sufficiently rigorously to allow their routine use in clinical practice.

Likely developments over the next 5–10 years

- There is likely to be a continuing increase in the incidence or UGIB as the population ages, and particularly variceal bleeding as the incidence of liver disease rises in most developed countries.
- Further studies on doses, route of administration, and duration of therapy for PPIs after UGIB will help to clarify the optimum treatment for UGIB patients.
- Improvements in delivery of critical care may help to improve survival in patients with UGIB.
- Clinical risk evaluation tools allowing outpatient management will be validated and come into clinical practice.

Controversies

- The optimum dose, route of administration, and duration of therapy for PPIs after UGIB has not been clarified and requires further study.
- Despite improvements in rebleeding rates and a reduction in the

requirement for surgical intervention, mortality rates have not improved.

- Increasing comorbidities and the increasingly elderly population may require more intensive critical care to improve survival, rather than further improvements in endoscopic haemostasis.

- The pressure to manage more patients in the outpatient setting means that there is a need to validate and refine scoring systems to evaluate risk or adverse outcomes in UGIB, both with and without early endoscopy.

References

1. American Society for Gastrointestinal Endoscopy. ASGE guideline: the role of endoscopy in acute non-variceal upper-GI hemorrhage. Gastrointestinal Endoscopy 2004; 60: 497–504.

2. Barkun A, Bardou M, Marshall JK. Consensus recommendations for managing patients with nonvariceal upper gastrointestinal bleeding. Annals of Internal Medicine 2003; 139: 843–857.
3. British Society of Gastroenterology Endoscopy Committee. Non-variceal upper gastrointestinal haemorrhage: guidelines. Gut 2005; 51: iv1–iv6.
4. Chen IC, Hung MS, Chiu TF, et al. Risk scoring systems to predict need for clinical intervention for patients with nonvariceal upper gastrointestinal tract bleeding. American Journal of Emergency Medicine 2007; 25: 774–779.
5. Coffin B, Pocard M, Panis Y, et al. Erythromycin improves the quality of EGD in patients with acute upper GI bleeding: a randomized controlled study. Gastrointestinal Endoscopy 2002; 56: 174–179.
6. Cook DJ, Guyatt GH, Salena BJ. Endoscopic therapy for acute nonvariceal upper gastrointestinal hemorrhage: a meta-analysis. Gastroenterology 1992; 102: 139–148.
7. Ferguson JW, Tripathi D, Hayes PC. Review article: the management of acute variceal bleeding. Alimentary Pharmacology and Therapeutics 2003; 18: 253–262.
8. Frossard JL, Spahr L, Queneau PE, et al. Erythromycin intravenous bolus infusion in acute upper gastrointestinal bleeding: a randomized, controlled, double-blind trial. Gastroenterology 2002; 123: 17–23.
9. Imperale TF, Birgisson S. Somatostatin or octreotide compares with H_2-antagonists and placebo in the management of acute non-variceal upper gastrointestinal haemorrhage: a meta-analysis. Annals of Internal Medicine 1997; 127: 1062–1071.

10. Ioannou GN, Doust J, Rockey DC. Systematic review: terlipressin in acute oesophageal variceal haemorrhage. Alimentary Pharmacology and Therapeutics 2003; 17: 53–64.
11. Kwan V, Norton ID. Endoscopic management of non-variceal upper gastrointestinal haemorrhage. Australia and New Zealand Journal of Surgery 2007; 77: 222–230.
12. Levine JE, Leontiadis GI, Sharma VK, et al. Meta-analysis: the efficacy of intravenous H_2-receptor antagonists in bleeding peptic ulcer. Alimentary and Pharmacologic Therapy 2002; 16: 1137–1142.
13. Leontiadis GI, Sharma VK, Howden CW. Proton pump inhibitor treatment for acute peptic ulcer bleeding. Cochrane Database of Systematic Reviews (1): CD002094. DOI: 10.1002/14651858.CD002094.pub3, 2006.
14. Longstreth GF, Feitelberg SP. Outpatient care of selected patients with acute non-variceal upper gastrointestinal haemorrhage. Lancet 1995; 345: 108–111.
15. Palmer K. Management of haematemesis and melaena. Postgraduate Medical Journal 2004; 80: 399–404.
16. Ripoll C, Banares R, Beceiro I, et al. Comparison of transcatheter arterial embolization and surgery for treatment of bleeding peptic ulcer after endoscopic treatment failure. Journal of Vascular and Interventional Radiology 2004; 15: 447–450.
17. Schenker MP, Duszak R Jr, Soulen MC, et al. Upper gastrointestinal hemorrhage and transcatheter embolotherapy: clinical and technical factors impacting success and survival. Journal of Vascular and Interventional Radiology 2001; 12: 1263–1271.

7.7 Peptic ulcer disease and gastritis

Shirley Ooi • Stuart Dilley

ESSENTIALS

1 *Helicobacter pylori* is responsible for 70–90% of peptic ulcers, with non-steroidal anti-inflammatory drugs accounting for most of the remainder.

2 Emergency presentations of peptic ulcer disease vary from mild indigestion to severe life-threatening complications.

3 Endoscopy is the investigation of choice for definitive diagnosis.

4 Most patients can be managed medically with a combination of anti-secretory drugs and antibiotics as indicated.

5 Surgical treatment may be indicated for complications such as haemorrhage, perforation and obstruction.

6 A 'negative' erect chest X-ray does not exclude ulcer perforation.

Introduction

In recent years the discovery of the organism *Helicobacter pylori* has resulted in a dramatic change in our understanding of the aetiology and pathophysiology of peptic ulcer disease. What was once a chronic disease prone to relapse and recurrence has now become eminently treatable and curable.

Patients presenting to emergency departments may do so with 'classic' ulcer symptoms, undifferentiated abdominal or chest pain, or more dramatically with life-threatening complications such as perforation or haemorrhage.

Pathophysiology

Definitions

Peptic ulcers are defects in the gastrointestinal mucosa that extend through the muscularis mucosa. The term gastritis is used to denote inflammation associated with mucosal injury. Gastropathy is defined as epithelial cell damage and regeneration without associated inflammation.

Pathophysiology

Peptic ulcer disease is associated with two major factors: *Helicobacter pylori* (*H. pylori*) infection and the consumption of non-steroidal anti-inflammatory drugs (NSAIDs). Although the vast majority of patients harbouring *H. pylori* are asymptomatic, it is now accepted that *H. pylori* is the major cause of peptic ulceration, or at least a major cofactor in the development of peptic ulcer disease. *H. pylori* has been isolated from 20–50% of patients with dyspeptic symptoms. More importantly, 90–95% of patients with duodenal ulcers and 70% of those with gastric ulcers are infected with the organism. Eradication of *H. pylori* has been shown to markedly reduce the recurrence rate for ulceration. NSAIDs, including low-dose aspirin, are the second most common cause of peptic ulceration and account for most ulcers not due to *H. pylori*. NSAIDs cause ulcers by inhibiting the production of prostaglandins in the stomach and duodenum (a vital part of the stomach's mucosal defence mechanisms), and hence may also cause ulceration when given by non-oral routes. NSAIDs are more commonly associated with gastric ulceration. At least 50% of patients taking NSAIDs will have endoscopic evidence of erythema, erosions or ulcers, even if asymptomatic.

There are several risk factors that influence gastrointestinal toxicity due to NSAIDs, the most important being a prior history of clinical ulcer disease or ulcer complications. Other risk factors are the dose, duration of action and duration of therapy with NSAIDs, age of the patient (greater risk above 75 years) and comorbidity, especially with cardiovascular disease. Combined therapy of NSAIDs with corticosteroids, anticoagulants, other NSAIDs or low-dose aspirin dramatically increases the risk of ulcer complications. In a study of high-risk patients with a prior history of GI bleeding, the antiplatelet agent clopidogrel was associated with a 12-month rebleeding rate of 8.6%, compared to 0.7% for aspirin combined with a proton pump inhibitor. Thus, clopidogrel is contraindicated in high-risk patients used either alone or in combination with NSAIDs.

Some NSAIDS are more likely to produce ulcers than others. In general, shorter-acting agents such as ibuprofen and diclofenac are less likely to lead to ulcers than longer-acting agents. Controlled trials with COX-2 selective inhibitors (coxibs) have demonstrated a reduction in the risk of peptic ulcers and their complications. Importantly, valdecoxib and refecoxib were removed from the market by the US Food and Drug Administration because of data indicating an increased risk of thrombotic cardiovascular disease. Although there are concerns about the cardiovascular risks of celecoxib, especially at higher doses, it remains available at present. There is no evidence that coxibs have advantages over other NSAIDs for patients with unhealed ulcers. Coxibs appear to inhibit healing of peptic ulcers. Thus, they are not an attractive alternative for patients with active peptic ulcer disease.

Acid is an important ingredient in the pathogenesis of both NSAID- and *H. pylori*-induced ulceration. The interaction between NSAIDs and *H. pylori* is controversial and complex, but evidence from two controlled trials and a meta-analysis of observational studies identified synergism between *H. pylori* and NSAIDs in producing peptic ulcer and ulcer bleeding. Traditional risk factors such as smoking, alcohol and stress may increase the risk of ulceration and delay healing, but their relative importance as aetiological agents has fallen considerably with the discovery of *H. pylori*. Other causes of peptic ulceration, such as Zollinger–Ellison syndrome, are rare.

Gastritis is usually due to infectious agents (such as *H. pylori*) and autoimmune and hypersensitivity reactions. In contrast, gastropathy is usually caused by irritants such as drugs (e.g. NSAIDs and alcohol), bile reflux, hypovolaemia and chronic congestion.

Clinical features

History

Peptic ulcers may present with a wide variety of symptoms, or may be completely asymptomatic until complications such as haemorrhage or perforation occur. 'Indigestion' is the most common symptom in patients found to have peptic ulcer disease. Patients describe a burning or gnawing pain in the epigastrium that may radiate into the chest or straight through to the back. Food may either exacerbate or relieve the pain. The pain is classically both fluctuating and periodic, with bouts of discomfort of variable severity interspersed with symptom-free periods.

The symptoms 'indigestion' or 'dyspepsia', however, have relatively poor sensitivity and specificity for diagnosing the various peptic syndromes. Less than 25% of patients with dyspepsia have peptic ulcer disease proven by gastroscopy, and between 20% and 60% of patients presenting with complications of ulcer disease report no antecedent symptoms.

Some patients may present with the classic symptom complex. Others present with chest or abdominal pains that need to be differentiated from conditions such as myocardial ischaemia, biliary tract disease, pancreatitis and other abdominal emergencies.

Patients also present with the two most common complications of ulcer disease, namely acute gastrointestinal haemorrhage or acute perforation. The former gives symptoms of melaena with or without haematemesis, and the latter presents with sudden, severe abdominal pain.

Examination

In uncomplicated peptic ulcer disease abdominal findings may be limited to epigastric tenderness without peritoneal signs. If perforation has occurred, patients are in severe pain and look unwell. Abdominal findings include generalized tenderness, widespread peritonism and so-called 'board-like' rigidity. Those with gastrointestinal bleeding will usually have melaena on PR examination.

Investigations

The extent of investigations depends greatly on the patient's presentation and the degree of severity of symptoms.

Haematology and biochemistry

There are no established blood tests that can reliably predict the presence of peptic ulcer disease. Pathology investigations are aimed primarily at eliminating alternative diagnoses or identifying the complications of peptic ulceration.

Full blood examination

Anaemia is most likely to represent chronic rather than acute blood loss, unless bleeding is particularly heavy and hence clinically obvious. A microcytic, hypochromic anaemia suggests chronic blood loss with iron deficiency, and can be confirmed with iron studies. Unexplained anaemia warrants a detailed evaluation and may raise concern for an underlying malignancy.

Blood cross-match

Patients with active bleeding may need replacement with blood products. Several units of blood may be required.

Clotting studies

These are indicated in patients taking warfarin and those with massive bleeding and/or a history of liver disease or alcoholism.

Liver function tests/amylase/lipase

Biliary tract disease and pancreatitis are common differential diagnoses in patients presenting with non-specific epigastric or upper abdominal pain. Pancreatitis may also be the consequence of ulcer penetration through the posterior wall of the stomach.

Radiology

Radiological imaging has a very limited place in the diagnosis of uncomplicated peptic ulcer disease. However, an erect chest X-ray (CXR) is an important investigation when perforation is being considered. Gas is usually visible under the diaphragm, but its absence does not rule out perforation. Several studies have reported the sensitivity of erect CXR for detection of pneumoperitoneum as ranging from 70% to 80%. Lateral decubitus abdominal X-rays may be needed to demonstrate free gas in those unable to sit erect. CT scans of the abdomen may be more sensitive in detecting small pneumoperitoneums.

Contrast studies are no longer considered first-line investigations in the assessment of patients with dyspeptic symptoms. Abdominal X-ray and ultrasound studies are useful to exclude alternative diagnoses, as indicated.

Endoscopy

Endoscopy is the investigation of choice for patients with dyspeptic symptoms, allowing direct visualization of the mucosa of the oesophagus, stomach and proximal duodenum. It provides a definitive diagnosis, which forms the basis of drug therapy and allows biopsies to be taken to exclude malignant disease and to isolate H. pylori. Endoscopy may also be therapeutic in some cases of upper gastrointestinal haemorrhage. Patient selection for referral for endoscopy is described below.

H. pylori status

The discovery of H. pylori was quickly followed by the development of tests to identify its presence. Currently there are a number of tests available, both invasive and non-invasive, though their exact role in the emergency department (ED) setting has not been defined. It should be remembered that the majority of patients infected with H. pylori do not in fact have peptic ulcer disease, and that the identification of H. pylori infection often bears little relation to presenting symptoms. In particular, neither of the non-invasive tests can make a diagnosis of peptic ulcer disease, only of H. pylori infection. However, a negative test in a patient not taking NSAIDs makes the likelihood of peptic ulcer low.

The invasive tests for H. pylori include haematoxylin and eosin staining of mucosal biopsies and rapid urease tests (e.g. CLOtest). The non-invasive tests include urease breath tests and IgG serology. Urease breath tests are highly sensitive and specific for the presence of H. pylori. They are most useful in assessing H. pylori eradication without the need for further gastroscopy.

A number of IgG serology tests are available with varying specificities and sensitivities. They are inexpensive, non-invasive and well suited to primary care, and potentially emergency medicine, practice. Large studies have found uniformly high sensitivity (90–100%), but variable specificity (76–96%); the accuracy has ranged from 83% to 98%.

Management

Traditional management of patients with dyspeptic symptoms requires the exclusion of other diseases, the removal of known precipitants such as NSAIDs, alcohol and cigarettes, the institution of simple treatment measures aimed at symptomatic relief, and referral for further investigation and management. This remains a reasonable option. Alternatively, cost-effectiveness analysis and consensus statements support the treatment of H. pylori-positive dyspeptic patients with antimicrobial and anti-secretory therapy, followed by endoscopic study only in those with persistent symptoms, so it would also be reasonable to begin symptomatic

therapy, order serological testing for H. pylori, and refer for early follow-up with a primary care provider for initiation of antibacterial therapy if the test results are positive. The choice of approach is open to debate. Early treatment prior to endoscopy may cure some patients without the need for expensive invasive procedures. However, this plan of action may hinder subsequent H. pylori isolation and delay definitive diagnosis, including the diagnosis of malignant disease.

It should be noted that the prevalence of H. pylori is lower in patients with complicated duodenal ulcers (those complicated by bleeding or perforation) than in those with uncomplicated disease. Patients with H. pylori-negative ulcers appear to have a significantly worse outcome, especially if treated empirically for infection. Thus, documenting infection is an appropriate caution prior to initiating antimicrobial therapy.

For patients with mild symptoms of recent onset, empirical treatment with antacids and/or histamine receptor antagonists aimed at symptomatic relief is reasonable.

Given the poor correlation between dyspeptic symptoms and gastro-oesophageal disease, gastroscopy should be considered, particularly if symptoms are not controlled or promptly recur.

A recent review of the literature concluded that for patients with non-ulcer dyspepsia, H_2-receptor blockers were significantly more effective than placebo at reducing symptoms, whereas proton pump inhibitors and bismuth salts were only marginally so. Antacids and sucralfate were not statistically superior to placebo.

Antacids

'Antacids', containing combinations of calcium, magnesium, local anaesthetics and alginates, are useful in providing symptomatic relief for patients with relatively mild symptoms. In many instances patients have already tried these agents prior to presentation.

Histamine-receptor antagonists

The H_2-receptor antagonists such as cimetidine, ranitidine, famotidine and nizatidine all have similar efficacies with regard to ulcer healing. All are well absorbed orally, but their absorption may be reduced when used with antacids but not by food. Eighty to 90% of duodenal ulcers will be healed in 4–8 weeks, and 70% of gastric ulcers within 8 weeks. Relapse rates of 80% over the course of 1 year are to be expected if *H. pylori* eradication is not also undertaken. H_2 antagonists are also useful in the treatment of gastro-oesophageal reflux disease and management of dyspepsia. Due to renal excretion, dosage adjustments must be made in patients with renal failure.

Proton pump inhibitors (PPIs)

The PPIs omeprazole, lansoprazole, rabeprazole, pantoprazole and esomeprazole effectively block acid secretion by irreversibly binding to and inhibiting the $H^+/K^+ATPase$ pump of the gastric parietal cells, thereby inhibiting the cells' proton pump. Acidic compartments within the stimulated parietal cell are essential for activation of a PPI. Thus PPIs work poorly in fasting patients or those with simultaneous dosing with other antisecretory agents (H_2-receptor antagonists, anticholinergic agents or somatostatin). PPIs are most effective when taken with or shortly before meals. Compared to H_2-receptor antagonists, these agents result in more rapid ulcer healing and pain relief over 2–4 weeks, although differences at 8 weeks are not significant. Again, relapse rates are high, particularly if *H. pylori* is present and eradication therapy is not used.

Cytoprotectants

Cytoprotective agents include colloidal bismuth subcitrate (De-Nol) and sucralfate. Both act by binding to or chelating with proteins in the base of the ulcer. Bismuth compounds also suppress *H. pylori*. A 6–8-week course is recommended, and relapse rates are still high. Bismuth compounds lead to the formation of black stools that may be confused with melaena. The primary concern with bismuth is bismuth intoxication. Sucralfate should not be taken with antacids as it requires an acid environment to achieve its optimal effects. Sucralfate has minimal adverse effects other than possible aluminium toxicity.

Prostaglandin analogues

Misoprostol, a synthetic analogue of PGE_1, interferes with histamine-dependent gastric acid secretion as well as being cytoprotective. It is particularly useful in the prevention of NSAID-induced ulcers, although it is probably no better than the other agents in actually treating such ulcers.

H. pylori eradication

All patients with duodenal ulcers associated with *H. pylori* infection should undergo therapy to eradicate the organism. This recommendation is based on overwhelming data showing that cure of *H. pylori* infection reduces ulcer recurrence and complications such as bleeding. A number of eradication therapies have been postulated, all with very high eradication (>80%) and low relapse rates (<5%). The development of resistance to metronidazole has resulted in amoxicillin and clarithromycin being recommended as the antibiotics of choice. These are usually combined with a proton pump inhibitor or colloidal bismuth subcitrate for 1 week. Several single-prescription packages are now available. It is generally accepted that acid suppression therapy be continued for 4–8 weeks after cessation of antibiotic therapy.

H. pylori eradication therapy in patients with non-ulcer dyspepsia may have a small yet statistically significant effect on symptoms.

Misoprostol significantly reduces the risk of endoscopic ulcers. Standard doses of H_2-blockers were effective at reducing the risk of duodenal but not gastric ulcers. Double-dose H_2-blockers and proton pump inhibitors were effective at reducing the risk of both duodenal and gastric ulcers, and were better tolerated than misoprostol.

Treatment of NSAID-induced ulcers

NSAIDs, including aspirin, should be ceased if at all possible. Treatment should consist of a 4–8-week course of an H_2-receptor antagonist or proton pump inhibitor.

Surgical management

With the success of medical treatment for peptic ulcer disease, surgical intervention has been restricted to the management of complications rather than of the primary disease.

Complications

There are four major complications of peptic ulcer:

- Haemorrhage
- Perforation
- Penetration
- Obstruction.

Haemorrhage

Peptic ulceration is a common cause of upper GI bleeding, occurring in 10–20% of ulcer patients and accounting for approximately 50% of all upper GI bleeds. Urgent endoscopy is usually indicated, and surgical intervention may be required in a small proportion of patients. A recent meta-analysis concluded that the use of acid-reducing agents was associated with a statistically significant decrease in rebleeding, but not mortality. Assessment and management of these patients is discussed in detail in Chapter 7.6.

Perforation

Perforation occurs in approximately 5% of ulcers, with duodenal, antral and gastric body ulcers accounting for respectively 60%, 20% and 20% of perforations. One-third to one-half of perforated ulcers are associated with NSAID use; these usually occur in elderly patients. Chemical peritonitis develops suddenly, with acute severe generalized abdominal pain. Examination reveals a sick patient with a rigid, quiet abdomen and rebound tenderness. Delay in presentation and treatment, which may occur in the elderly and debilitated, sees the rapid development of bacterial peritonitis and subsequent sepsis and shock. The overall mortality rate is about 5%.

Rapid diagnosis is essential as the prognosis is excellent if treated within the first 6 hours, but deteriorates to probable death after more than a 12-hour delay. Diagnosis should be confirmed with an erect chest X-ray, bearing in mind a sensitivity of 70–80%. If free air is found, no other diagnostic studies are necessary. If there is diagnostic uncertainty, CT or ultrasound can be useful to detect small amounts of free air or fluid.

Vigorous fluid resuscitation should be instituted and renal function (via urine output) should be closely monitored. Ampicillin, gentamicin and metronidazole should be given, along with adequate analgesia. Cardiac and respiratory support may be needed in some cases.

The majority of patients with perforation should undergo surgery for decontamination and repair. Non-operative management, including intravenous fluids, nasogastric suction, antibiotics and anti-secretory drugs, may be successful in some patients in whom the leak seals quickly in response to medical management. There is some evidence that an initial period of non-operative treatment with careful observation is safe in younger patients (under 70 years), but this is not yet regarded as standard practice.

Penetration

Posterior ulcers may perforate the gastric or duodenal wall and continue to erode into adjacent structures, most commonly the pancreas, without free perforation and leakage of luminal contents into the peritoneal cavity. Surgical series suggest that penetration occurs in 20% of ulcers, but only a small proportion of penetrating ulcers become clinically evident. Patients may describe their pain as becoming more severe and constant, radiating to the back, and no longer eased by antacids and food. There is also loss of cyclicity of pain with meals. The serum amylase level may be mildly raised. Endoscopy may reveal ulceration, but 'penetration' is difficult to confirm.

Gastric outlet obstruction

This is the least frequent ulcer complication and may occur in up to 2% of patients with ulcer disease. It may arise acutely secondary to inflammation and oedema of the pylorus or duodenal bulb, or more commonly as a consequence of scarring due to chronic disease.

Disposition

Indications for admission

- Bleeding: haemetemesis or melaena or both.
- Perforation.
- Obstruction: difficult to diagnose in the ED, but patients present with vomiting or signs of intestinal obstruction.
- Severe symptoms not responsive to treatment.
- Abdominal pain with fever and jaundice.
- Inability to rule out serious differential diagnoses.

Indications for referral for early gastroenterology review as an outpatient

- Recent onset of new symptoms in patient >40 years old.
- Presence of concerning features such as weight loss, loss of appetite, early satiety, haemetemesis, melaena, unexplained anaemia, dysphagia, palpable abdominal mass.
- Persistence of symptoms despite a trial of empirical treatment (H_2-antagonists or PPIs).

A single episode of abdominal pain/discomfort (without any alarm features) does not need to be referred for further work-up, as this complaint is very common and is usually self-limiting and non-specific.

Discharge advice

Patients should be asked to return to the ED immediately should they develop fever, lower abdominal pain, persistent diarrhoea or vomiting. This is because upper abdominal pain may be an early symptom of other pathologies, e.g. acute appendicitis.

Controversies

- Should specific H_2-blockers, proton pump inhibitors or *H. pylori* eradication therapy be instituted prior to formal diagnosis via gastroscopy?
- Conservative versus surgical management of perforated ulcer.

Further reading

Chan F, Ching J, Hung L, et al. Clopidogrel versus aspirin and esomeprazole to prevent recurrent ulcer bleeding. New England Journal of Medicine 2005; 352: 238.

Cutler A. Testing for *Helicobacter pylori* in clinical practice. American Journal of Medicine 1996; 100: 35S–41S.

Huang J, Sridhar S, Hunt R. Role of *Helicobacter pylori* infection and NSAIDs in peptic ulcer disease: a meta-analysis. Lancet 2002; 359: 14.

Hooper L, Brown TJ, Elliott R, et al. The effectiveness of five strategies for the prevention of gastrointestinal toxicity induced by NSAIDs: systematic review. British Medical Journal 2004; 329: 948.

Laine L, Hopkins RJ, Girardi LS, et al. Has the impact of *H. pylori* therapy on ulcer recurrence in the United States been overstated? A metaanalysis of rigorously designed trials. American Journal of Gastroenterology 1998; 93: 1409.

Malfertheiner P, Megraud F, O'Morain C, et al. Current concepts in the management of *H. pylori* infection – The Maastricht 2-2000 consensus report. Alimentary Pharmacology and Therapeutics 2002; 16: 167.

Ofman JJ, Etchason J, Fullerton S, et al. Management strategies for H. pylori seropositive patients with dyspepsia: Clinical and economic consequences. Annals of Internal Medicine 1997; 126: 280.

Perini RF, Ma L, Wallace JL. Mucosal repair and COX-2 inhibition. Current Pharmaceutical Design 2003; 9: 2207.

Peterson WL, Fendrick AM, Cave DR, et al. H. pylori-related disease: guidelines for testing and treatment. Archives of Internal Medicine 2000; 160: 1285.

Soll AH. Medical treatment of peptic ulcer disease: Practice guidelines. Journal of the American Medical Association 1996; 275: 622.

Sonnenberg A, Olson CA, Zhang J. The effect of antibiotic therapy on bleeding from duodenal ulcer. American Journal of Gastroenterology 1999; 94: 950.

Svanes C, Salvesen H, Bjerke Larssen T, et al. Trends in and value and consequences of radiologic imaging of perforated gastroduodenal ulcer. Scandinavian Journal of Gastroenterology 1990; 25: 257–262.

Woodring J, Heiser M. Detection of pneumoperitoneum on chest radiographs: Comparison of upright lateral and posteroanterior projections. American Journal of Roentgenology 1995; 165: 45–47.

7.8 Biliary tract disease

Andrew Walby • Michael Bryant

ESSENTIALS

1 More than 95% of biliary tract disease is attributable to gallstones.

2 Most patients with gallbladder disease present with abdominal pain.

3 Investigations are directed to confirming the diagnosis and detecting the presence of complications.

4 The management of acute biliary pain is supportive, and discharge is often possible.

5 The management of cholecystitis and other complications of gallbladder disease is both supportive and surgical.

6 Acalculous cholecystitis occurs in the absence of gallstones.

7 Antibiotics are indicated for the treatment of cholecystitis and ascending cholangitis.

8 Ultrasound is the imaging test of choice for most biliary tract disease.

Introduction

The most frequent cause of gallbladder disease is gallstones (95%). It is more common in women than men, and the incidence increases with age. Recurring episodes of symptoms are characteristic. Gallbladder disease is diagnosed by a combination of clinical features, laboratory investigations and organ imaging. Patients present with biliary pain caused by obstruction of biliary flow, leading to dilatation of the biliary system. Cholecystitis and ascending cholangitis develop when secondary infection occurs. Calculous disease is the most frequent cause of pancreatitis. Acalculous cholecystitis occurs in the absence of gallstones and may complicate major illness.

Gallstones

Clinical features

History

Patients usually present with abdominal pain which may be midline and visceral or somatic and right upper quadrant. Visceral pain may be referred around the right costal margin or to the right shoulder area. Despite the use of the term biliary colic, the pain is usually constant and may be severe. Nausea and vomiting are often present. Complaints of fevers and chills may be indicative of either cholecystitis or ascending cholangitis. Rigors are suggestive of cholangitis.

Examination

Right upper quadrant tenderness is the most common examination finding. Fever and tachycardia are usually present in acute cholecystitis, although at presentation they may be absent in 59–90% of cases. Local peritonism and Murphy's sign also suggest acute cholecystitis. Jaundice is usually absent in biliary colic and acute cholecystitis. The presence of pain, jaundice, high fever and shaking chills (Charcot's triad) is indicative of ascending cholangitis.

Differential diagnosis

The differential diagnosis of right upper quadrant pain includes:

- Peptic ulcer disease, including perforation.
- Acute pancreatitis.
- Coronary ischaemia, especially involving the inferior myocardial surface.
- Appendicitis, especially retrocaecal or in pregnancy.
- Renal disease, including renal colic and pyelonephritis.
- Colonic conditions.
- Hepatic pathology, especially hepatitis.
- Right lower lobe pneumonia.

Investigations

Investigation of biliary pain are aimed at confirming the diagnosis, establishing the presence of gallstones and the detection of complications.

Imaging

Ultrasound is the investigation of choice to confirm the diagnosis and measure the thickness of the gallbladder wall and the diameter of the common bile duct (CBD). It can also detect the presence of calculi in the CBD and the presence of any local fluid collection. It has high sensitivity and specificity, is non-invasive, and requires little preparation of the patient. It does, however, require experience in technique and interpretation.

In the majority of cases plain radiographs are not helpful in the diagnosis of gallbladder disease, but on occasion they may be useful to rule out other potential diagnoses. Rare X-ray findings include radio-opaque calculi (only 10–15% of biliary calculi are radio-opaque), the presence of gas in the biliary tree indicating a biliary–gastrointestinal fistula, gas or an air–fluid level in emphysematous cholecystitis, or a localized ileus in the right upper quadrant.

Blood tests

Blood tests are relatively non-specific. Bilirubin and alkaline phosphatase levels are mildly elevated in uncomplicated biliary colic and cholecystitis. Amylase and lipase are elevated if pancreatitis is also present. Full blood examination shows a leukocytosis and left shift in the majority of cases of cholecystitis and cholangitis; however, 32–40% do not have a leukocytosis.

Complications

Complications of biliary disease include:

- Cholecystitis
- Obstructive jaundice
- Ascending cholangitis and Gram-negative septicaemia
- Gallstone ileus
- Perforation: the elderly and diabetics are at particular risk of rapid necrosis and perforation
- Pancreatitis.

Management

The management of biliary pain depends on the presence or absence of complications. In the emergency department (ED) phase patients should receive analgesia in the form of titrated intravenous opioids, and intravenous fluids. In selected patients, parenteral non-steroidal anti-inflammatory drugs (NSAIDs) may be effective. There is some evidence that a short course of NSAIDs may prevent progression to cholecystitis in some patients with biliary colic. In the absence of cholecystitis or complications such as biliary obstruction, ascending cholangitis or pancreatitis patients may be discharged for outpatient surgical follow-up if the pain settles.

Antibiotics are indicated for the treatment of cholecystitis or ascending cholangitis. The appropriate antibiotics for cholecystitis in which Gram-negative organisms are most frequently implicated are ampicillin and gentamicin, or cefotaxime if the patient is penicillin allergic. Ascending cholangitis should be treated with cefotaxime or ceftriaxone.

Endoscopic retrograde cholangiopancreatography (ERCP) is indicated for the treatment of biliary obstruction. Surgical removal of gallstones is indicated for all patients who are fit for the procedure. The timing of surgery is a matter of surgeon preference and theatre availability.

Disposition

Many patients with biliary colic can be discharged. Most patients with complications such as acute cholecystitis, ascending cholangitis or pancreatitis require hospital admission. Admission may also be indicated in some cases because of recurrent severe pain.

Cholelithiasis

Epidemiology

The most common abdominal pathology leading to hospital admission in developed countries is cholelithiasis. Gallstones are present in 10–20% of the adult population in developed countries, but more than 80% are 'silent'. In developed countries, the majority of gallstones are formed predominantly from cholesterol (up to 80%). Increased age is associated with lithogenic bile and an increased rate of gallstones. In young adults, more females are affected than males, but the disparity narrows with age. The lifetime risk of cholesterol gallstones is 35% in women, compared to 20% in men. This is likely to be due to endogenous sex hormones that enhance cholesterol secretion and increase bile cholesterol saturation. In addition, progesterone may contribute by relaxing smooth muscle and thereby impairing gallbladder emptying. Other than older age and female gender, predisposing factors include obesity, a high-calorie diet, total parenteral nutrition, weight loss (especially if rapid), drugs (including clofibrate, oral contraceptives and other exogenous oestrogens and ceftriaxone), genetic predisposition, diseases of the terminal ileum and abnormal lipid profile. Pregnancy is also a predisposing condition. Gallstone precipitation is common, especially in late pregnancy, but most remain asymptomatic, at least until delivery. Symptomatic cholelithiasis can complicate the puerperium and each first postnatal year. Forceful gallbladder contraction postpartum increases the potential for cystic or common bile duct obstruction.

Clinical features and investigation

Many gallstones are present for decades before symptoms develop and 70–80% remain asymptomatic throughout life. Asymptomatic patients convert to symptomatic at a rate of 1–4% per year (the risk decreases with time). The most common presentations are biliary colic, cholecystitis, obstructive pancreatitis (5% of all patients) and ascending cholangitis. Less common presentations are empyema, perforation, fistula formation, gallstone ileus, hydrops or mucocoele of the gallbladder and carcinoma of the gallbladder.

The investigation of choice is ultrasound, which has a sensitivity of 84–97% and a specificity of 95–100%.

Treatment

Cholecystectomy is the definitive treatment of choice for symptomatic cholelithiasis. It provides symptomatic relief in up to 99% of patients. Laparoscopic cholecystectomy is the technique of choice. Dissolution methods and lithotripsy are of limited utility owing to restricted indications for their use and gallstone recurrence at 5 years in approximately 50% of cases. Prophylactic cholecystectomy is not recommended in asymptomatic patients as the risks of the procedure outweigh the potential benefits.

Acute cholecystitis

Epidemiology

Distribution parallels that of cholelithiasis. Acute cholecystitis develops in 1–3% of patients with symptomatic stones.

Pathology

Cholelithiasis is present in most acute cases, a single large calculus being the most common finding. A small group of patients develop biliary sludge, which is a mixture of particulate matter and bile. More than 90% of cases result from cystic duct obstruction. Bacteria are present in approximately 20–50% of cases, but bacterial infection is not thought to cause acute cholecystitis: rather, it results from chemical irritation and inflammation of the obstructed gallbladder due to obstruction of the cystic or common bile duct. Secondary bacterial infection is usually caused by aerobic bowel flora (such as *Escherichia coli*, *Klebsiella* species and, less commonly, *Enterococcus faecalis*). Anaerobes are found infrequently, usually in the presence of obstruction.

Clinical features

Right upper quadrant pain and fever are the most common features. Usually patients have experienced previous episodes of biliary pain.

Nausea and vomiting are commonly present. A distended, tender gallbladder is not usually evident: the right upper quadrant mass palpated in approximately 20% of patients represents omentum overlying the inflamed gallbladder. Only approximately 20% of patients are jaundiced. The presence of hyperbilirubinaemia suggests common bile duct obstruction. Neutrophilia may be present.

Imaging

Ultrasound

Findings on ultrasound are often diagnostic, showing cholelithiasis, an increase in transverse gallbladder diameter >4–5 cm in up to 87% of cases, gallbladder wall thickening >5 mm and pericholecystic fluid. A positive Murphy's sign on ultrasound is a sensitive indicator of cholecystitis.

Plain abdominal X-rays

Abdominal X-rays are rarely helpful, but in 10% of cases may show radio-opaque gallstones. In emphysematous cholecystitis, gas may be seen within the gallbladder wall.

Complications

Complications include bacterial superinfection leading to ascending cholangitis or sepsis, gallbladder perforation leading to local abscess formation or diffuse peritonitis, biliary enteric (cholecystenteric) fistula, with a risk of gallstone-induced intestinal obstruction (gallstone ileus), and deterioration in pre-existing medical illness.

Treatment

Treatment is with antibiotics, hospital admission and cholecystectomy. (Amoxy)ampicillin 1 g i.v. 6-hourly, plus gentamicin at 4–6 mg/kg i.v. daily is recommended (the latter should be adjusted for decreased renal function). If these are contraindicated the alternatives are ceftriaxone 1 g i.v. daily or cefotaxime 1 g i.v. 8-hourly. It is important to note that cephalosporins are not active against enterococci. In the presence of biliary obstruction, metronidazole should be added to treat anaerobes. Most patients will respond to conservative management, with the gallstone disimpacting and falling back into the gallbladder, thereby allowing the cystic duct to drain. If the gallstone does not disimpact, gangrenous cholecystitis (2–30% of cases), empyema of the gallbladder or gallbladder perforation (10% of cases) may occur. Cholecystectomy is required to prevent recurrence or other complications. Approximately 20% of patients require emergency surgery, usually via a laparoscopic approach. If performed within 72–96 hours of the onset of symptoms, the surgery is easier and complication rates are lower. The timing of cholecystectomy for the remaining 80% will be determined by the treating surgical unit.

Acalculous cholecystitis

Acute acalculous cholecystitis is acute inflammation of the gallbladder in the absence of gallstones, generally in the severely ill patient, and accounts for 10% of cases of acute cholecystitis. Predisposing factors include postoperative state after major, non-biliary surgery, severe trauma or burns, multisystem organ failure, sepsis, prolonged intravenous hyperalimentation, and the postpartum state. It is thought to be ischaemic in pathogenesis, with more than 70% of patients having underlying atherosclerotic disease. Contributing factors include dehydration, multiple blood transfusions, gallbladder stasis, accumulation of biliary sludge, viscous bile and gallbladder mucus, and bacterial contamination. Compared with acute calculous cholecystitis, there is a much higher incidence of empyema, gangrene and perforation of the gallbladder, and consequently an increased mortality rate (up to 50%).

Choledocholithiasis

Features

Gallstones are present within the biliary tree, almost all derived from the gallbladder. Approximately 10% of patients with cholelithiasis have choledocholithiasis, which may be asymptomatic, intermittently or permanently obstructive. Choledocholithiasis is the second most common cause of CBD obstruction after neoplasms.

Symptomatic cases present due to obstruction (resulting in jaundice), pancreatitis, cholangitis, hepatic abscess, secondary biliary cirrhosis or acute acalculous cholecystitis.

Imaging and treatment

Ultrasound is less reliable in choledocholithiasis. CBD measurement may yield false positive or false negative results, but is more accurate in jaundiced patients, approaching 80% accuracy. In addition, the precise level and cause of obstruction is sometimes difficult to identify, especially if it lies near the pancreatic head. ERCP is more accurate and often therapeutic. Interval cholecystectomy to prevent recurrence is recommended. The management of asymptomatic duct calculi is controversial. Options include laparoscopic cholecystectomy with endoscopic sphincterotomy and stone extraction, or laparoscopic exploration of the common bile duct.

Cholangitis

Aetiology

Cholangitis is a purulent bacterial infection of the biliary tree, including the intrahepatic ducts related to obstruction to bile flow (e.g. choledocholithiasis, stents, tumours, acute pancreatitis and strictures). Parasitic infections are a rare cause in developed countries but are common in developing countries. Bacteria are usually Gram-negatives such as *E. coli*, *Klebsiella*, *Clostridium* spp., *Bacteroides* and *Enterobacter* or group D streptococci. They are thought to enter the biliary tree via the sphincter of Oddi.

Charcot's biliary triad (fluctuating jaundice, recurrent right upper quadrant abdominal pain and intermittent high fever with rigors) is present in 70% of patients.

Treatment

The principles of treatment are broad-spectrum antibiotics and prompt drainage of the obstruction. For the latter, the method will depend on the underlying cause, surgical preference and availability, and the state of the patient. The recommended antibiotics are (amoxy)ampicillin 2 g i.v. 6-hourly, plus gentamicin 4–6 mg/kg i.v. daily. Metronidazole 500 mg i.v. 12-hourly should be added in patients with a history of previous biliary tract surgery or known biliary obstruction. If these are contraindicated the alternatives are ceftriaxone 1 g i.v. daily or cefotaxime 1 g i.v. 8-hourly. Delay in management may lead to septicaemia and hepatic abscess formation, which are associated with a high mortality.

Controversies

- The role of NSAIDs in management of biliary colic.

- The optimal management of asymptomatic duct calculi.

Further reading

Beckingham IJ. ABC of diseases of liver, pancreas, and biliary system: gallstone disease. British Medical Journal 2001; 322: 91–94.

Beckingham IJ, Ryder SD. ABC of diseases of liver, pancreas, and biliary system: investigation of liver and biliary disease. British Medical Journal 2001; 322: 33–36.

Cotran RS, Kumar V, Collins T. Robbins pathologic basis of disease, 6th edn. Philadelphia: WB Saunders, 1999.

Epstein FB. Acute abdominal pain in pregnancy. Emergency Medical Clinics of North America 1994; 12: 151–165.

Feldman M, et al. Sleisenger and Fordtran's gastrointestinal and liver disease, 6th edn. Philadelphia: WB Saunders, 1998.

Gruber PJ, Silverman RA, Gottesfeld S, et al. Presence of fever and leukocytosis in acute cholecystitis. Annals of Emergency Medicine 1996; 28: 273–277.

Hudson PA, Promes SB. Abdominal ultrasonography. Emergency Medical Clinics of North America 1997; 15: 825–848.

Indar AA, Beckingham IJ. Acute cholecystitis. British Medical Journal 2002; 325: 639–643.

Johnson CD. ABC of the upper gastrointestinal tract: upper abdominal pain – gall bladder. British Medical Journal 2001; 323: 1170–1173.

Kumar A, Deed JS, Bhasin B, et al. Comparison of the effect of diclofenac with hyoscine-N-butylbromide in the symptomatic treatment of acute biliary colic. American New Zealand Journals of Surgery 2004; 74: 573–576.

Moscati RM. Cholelithiasis, cholecystitis and pancreatitis. Emergency Medical Clinics of North America 1996; 14: 719–737.

Singer AJ, McCracken G, Henry MC. Correlation among clinical, laboratory and hepatobiliary scanning findings with acute cholecystitis. Annals of Emergency Medicine 1996; 28: 267–272.

Therapeutic Guidelines (Australia): Antibiotic. Version 11. Therapeutic Guidelines Limited, 2007. Accessed at http://etg.hcn.net.au/ December 2007.

7.9 Pancreatitis

Kenneth Heng • Eillyne Seow

ESSENTIALS

1 The majority of acute pancreatitis is mild and self-limiting, However, 20% develop severe pancreatitis with a mortality of 20%.[1]

2 When clinical presentation or biochemical tests are equivocal, contrast-enhanced CT is the investigation of choice.

3 Contrast-enhanced CT establishes the diagnosis, excludes the alternative diagnoses, anatomically scores severity and detects local complications.

4 At presentation the focus should be on identification of severe pancreatitis, as these patients require aggressive management to reverse organ failure in an intensive care setting.[2]

Acute pancreatitis

The twin challenges of acute pancreatitis are to establishi the diagnosis and stratify severity. The difficulty in diagnosing pancreatitis lies in its non-specific symptomatology, which is shared by a number of other gastrointestinal diseases. Patient outcome may be dependent on prompt recognition of severe pancreatitis. These patients require aggressive treatment to reverse organ failure and admission to intensive care or a high-dependency area for ongoing management. The hunt for the aetiology is the next priority, but this may be deferred to the inpatient team.

Pathogenesis and aetiology

The pathogenesis of acute pancreatitis relates to inappropriate activation of trypsinogen to trypsin, which in turn releases digestive enzymes causing pancreatic injury. In 20% of cases, when pancreatic necrosis occurs it is coupled with infection from translocation of gut bacteria. An inflammatory response ensues, resulting in systemic inflammatory response syndrome, multiorgan dysfunction syndrome and, in some cases, death.

The commonest risk factor for pancreatitis in males is excessive alcohol use, and in females gallstone disease. The other aetiological factors are listed in Table 7.9.1.

Epidemiology

The incidence of pancreatitis is rising, reflecting an increase in alcohol consumption and gallstone disease. However, despite advances in care, overall mortality remains unaltered at 2–10%.

Clinical features

Gallstone pancreatitis typically presents with a sudden onset of severe, constant epigastric pain radiating to the back. In

Table 7.9.1 Aetiologies of acute pancreatitis

Common

Gallstone (including microlithiasis)
Alcohol
Idiopathic
Dyslipidaemia
Hypercalcaemia (hyperparathyroidism, metastatic bone disease, sarcoidosis)
Sphincter of Oddi dysfunction
Drugs (azathioprine, valproate, pentamidine, didanosine, co-trimoxazole)
Toxins
Post ERCP
Traumatic
Post operative

Uncommon

Structural (cancer of the pancreas/periampullary, pancreas divisum)
Vasculitis

Rare

Infective (Coxsackie, mumps, HIV, parasitic, ascariasis)
Autoimmune (systemic lupus erythematosus, Sjögren's syndrome)
α_1-Antitrypsin deficiency

contrast, pain in pancreatitis from other causes (e.g. alcohol) has a more insidious onset and may be poorly localized. This is often accompanied by nausea and vomiting. Abdominal wall ecchymosis around the umbilicus (Cullen's sign), flanks (Grey Turner's sign) and inguinal ligament (Fox's sign –an uncommon finding) does not occur till 36–72 hours after the onset of pain.

Differential diagnosis

The most important differential diagnoses to exclude are perforated viscus, ischaemic colitis, leaking abdominal aortic aneurysm and myocardial ischaemia.

Clinical investigations

Amylase rises in 2–12 hours and normalizes in about a week. In 10% of cases of pancreatitis, amylase is falsely negative due to depleted acinar cell mass. False positives may occur with salivary gland disease, macroamylasaemia and some cancers.

Lipase rises in 4–8 hours and normalizes in 1–2 weeks. It has superior sensitivity and specificity compared to amylase, as it is only produced in the pancreas. Amylase or lipase levels more than three times the upper limit of normal are diagnostic of acute pancreatitis. Lesser elevations must be interpreted against the timing of the test from symptom onset. The peak amylase and/or lipase level does not correlate with the severity of the disease.

When clinical signs and biochemical tests are equivocal, a contrast-enhanced CT scan of the abdomen is the radiological investigation of choice as it can establish the diagnosis, exclude most of the differential diagnoses listed above, stage the disease (see below) and detect complications. The use of ultrasound is not as helpful as the pancreas is poorly seen in 25–50% of patients, though it may show gallstones and/or a dilated common bile duct, giving a clue to its aetiology.

Plain radiography of the chest and abdomen has poor sensitivity for the diagnosis. Chest X-ray may show a pleural effusion or features of acute respiratory distress syndrome, and abdominal films may show gallstones, a sentinel bowel loop or peripancreatic retroperitoneal gas, the latter signifying infection of the pancreas.

Other tests to aid severity scoring and identification of aetiology include full blood count with haematocrit, urea, electrolytes, lactate dehydrogenase, alanine aminotransferase, blood gas analysis, calcium and lipid profile.

Severity scoring

Biochemical

Severe pancreatitis is identified either using a predictive scoring system or when a patient presents in frank organ failure (e.g. respiratory, renal or cardiovascular). Of the three predictive severity scoring systems in use, only the APACHE II allows scoring at presentation.[3,4] A score $\geq$8 indicates severe pancreatitis with a mortality of 11–18%. The Ransom[5] and Glasgow[6] scores (Table 7.9.2) can only be completed at 48 hours, which limits their usefulness in the ED. Likewise, an elevated C-reactive protein (CRP) >150 mg/dL 24 or 48 hours after presentation also reliably predicts severe pancreatitis.[3]

Radiological

Once severe pancreatitis is identified, contrast-enhanced CT is used to anatomically score the severity using the system described by Balthazar (Table 7.9.3).[7]

In summary, severe pancreatitis should be considered at presentation if the following risk factors are present: age>65 years, body mass index >30 kg/m^2, presence of pleural effusion on chest X-ray, contrast-enhanced CT shows >30% necrosis, APACHE II score $\geq$8, symptoms and signs of organ failure (e.g. poor urine output, progressive tachycardia, tachypnoea, hypoxaemia, agitation, confusion, rising haematocrit level).[1,8]

Emergency department treatment

The treatment for acute pancreatitis is supportive, with emphasis on fluid replacement and prevention of hypoxia.

- Supplemental oxygen. Hypoxia may indicate ARDS or significant pleural effusions. Mechanical ventilation may be required in patients with respiratory distress. Uncorrected, gut hypoxia promotes translocation of Gram-negative bacteria.

- Fluid resuscitation. Significant third-space losses may occur. Fluid replacement should be titrated to blood pressure and urine output. A worsening haematocrit indicates insufficient replacement. Central venous monitoring should be considered in severe cases.

- Analgesia. Opioid analgesia is often required. Morphine, administered intravenously, is the agent of choice and dose should be titrated against response. On occasion, large doses are required for pain control. There are no human studies to support the belief that morphine causes spasm of the sphincter of Oddi.[1]

- Disposition. Patients with pancreatitis require admission for treatment and observation of disease progression. Mild pancreatitis can be managed in the general ward, but severe pancreatitis should be managed in intensive care or a high-dependency unit.[2]

Prognosis

The majority of patients with acute pancreatitis experience a mild, self limiting course. Twenty per cent of patients develop severe pancreatitis, with a mortality of 20%;[1] 50% of deaths occur in the first week from multiorgan dysfunction syndrome, whereas death after 1 week is usually due to infective complications. If organ failure is reversed within 48 hours, the prognosis is good.

Complications

Local complications include pancreatic pseudocyst, abscess, splenic vein thrombosis, duodenal obstruction and progression to chronic pancreatitis. Systemic complications include hypocalcaemia, pleural effusion, ARDS and multiorgan dysfunction syndrome.

Likely developments over the next 5–10 years

New early markers of severe pancreatitis are being developed, such as urinary trypsinogen-activating peptide, the level of which correlates with severity. Other markers being investigated include interleukin 6 and 8, polymorphonuclear elastase and phospholipase A2.[1]

Table 7.9.2 Biochemical severity scoring systems

Ranson's score (1 point for each positive factor. Score ≥3 indicates severe pancreatitis)

At presentation	
Age	> 55 yr
Blood glucose	> 10 mmol/L
White cell count	> 16 000/mm^3
Lactate dehydrogenase	> 350 IU/L
Alanine aminotransferase	> 250 IU/L
Within 48 h after presentation	
Haematocrit	> 10% decrease
Calcium	< 2 mmol/L
Base deficit	> 4 mEq/L
Urea	> 1.8 mmol/L increase since admission
Fluid sequestration	> 6 L
Partial pressure of arterial oxygen	< 60 mmHg

Glasgow scoring system for prediction of severity in acute pancreatitis (1 point for each positive factor. Score ≥3 indicates severe pancreatitis)

Partial pressure of arterial oxygen	< 60 mmHg
Albumin	< 32 g/L
Calcium	< 2 mmol/L
White cell count	> 15 000/mm^3
Aspartate aminotransferase	> 200 IU/L
Lactate dehydrogenase	> 600 IU/L
Blood glucose	> 10 mmol/L
Urea	> 16 mmol/L

Table 7.9.3 CT severity index [6] (Score = sum of CT grade and necrosis. Score >6 indicates severe pancreatitis)

	CT grade		Necrosis score
Normal pancreas	0	No necrosis	0
Focal or diffuse enlargement	1	Necrosis of 1/3 of pancreas	2
Intrinsic change, fat stranding	2	Necrosis of 1/2 of pancreas	4
Single, fluid collection	3	Necrosis of >1/2 of pancreas	6
Multiple fluid/gas collection	4		

Chronic pancreatitis

Patients with chronic pancreatitis may present with recurrent abdominal pain radiating to the back. This may be associated with weight loss because of fear of eating due to postprandial exacerbations of pain. There may be signs of pancreatic exocrine insufficiency (steatorrhoea) or endocrine insufficiency (diabetes mellitus). Physical examination may reveal a mass in the epigastrium, suggesting a pseudocyst, and the patient may assume a characteristic pain-relieving posture of lying on the side with the knees drawn up to the chest.

The aetiology of chronic pancreatitis is usually metabolic in nature, with excessive alcohol consumption accounting for 60–90% of cases.[9] The primary process is chronic irreversible inflammation, fibrosis and calcification of the pancreas, affecting its exocrine and endocrine functions.

In chronic pancreatitis, serum amylase and lipase levels are not as elevated as in acute pancreatitis. Occasionally enzyme levels may be normal due to atrophy of the gland. ERCP is the gold standard for diagnosis of chronic pancreatitis.[10] Contrast-enhanced CT and magnetic resonance cholangiopancreatography are non-invasive and provide information about the pancreatic parenchyma as well.

Management

The key issues in the management of chronic pancreatitis are as follows:

- Continued alcohol intake is associated with increased risk of painful relapses and hastening of pancreatic dysfunction. Alcohol cessation may require a team approach incorporating counsellors and psychiatrists for cognitive therapy and behavioural modification.
- Providing adequate analgesia in chronic pancreatitis is a challenge, with many patients going on to develop chronic pain syndrome, and opioid dependency is a risk. Analgesia should not be withheld during acute episodes. Early referral to a pain management specialist may attenuate/manage opioid dependence. CT-guided coeliac ganglion blockade provides only temporary relief.[11]
- Malabsorption is treated by a low-fat diet and restoration of pancreatic exocrine function with supplementation of pancreatic enzymes, fat soluble vitamins and vitamin B_{12}. Diabetes mellitus results from endocrine dysfunction and requires insulin therapy.
- Relief of mechanical obstruction is achieved by endoscopy or surgical resection or drainage.[12]

Controversies

- The role of antibiotics. Although prophylactic antibiotics are not indicated in mild pancreatitis, empirical imipenem has been shown to reduce sepsis in severe pancreatitis with >30% necrosis on contrast-enhanced CT.[1] Antibiotic therapy should be aided by cultures obtained by CT-guided fine needle aspiration.

- Nutritional support. In severe pancreatitis, current evidence supports early nasojejunal tube feeding[1] over total parenteral nutrition, as it is more physiological, prevents gut mucosal atrophy and eliminates the risk of TPN-associated line sepsis. In mild pancreatitis, a low-fat and low-calorie diet may be started once the pain subsides.

- Gallstone eradication. In mild gallstone pancreatitis, cholecystectomy and bile duct clearance should occur prior to discharge[1] to prevent a potentially severe and fatal recurrence. In severe gallstone pancreatitis, especially where there is suspicion of cholangitis, current evidence supports endoscopic retrograde cholangiopancreatography with sphincterotomy within the first 24 hours.[8]

- Debridement of infected necrotic pancreatic tissue is required, although current opinion is that it should be delayed for 2 weeks as early surgery is associated with a high mortality.[7]

- Octreotide, aprotinin and glucagon have not been shown to improve outcome.[2]

References

1. Toouli J, Brooke-Smith M, Bassi C, et al. Working Party Report – Guidelines for the management of acute pancreatitis. Journal of Gastroenterology and Hepatology 2002; (Supplement 17): 515–539.
2. UK Working Party on Acute Pancreatitis. UK guidelines for the management of acute pancreatitis. Gut 2005; 54 (Supplement III): iii1–iii9.
3. Papachristou GI, Whitcomb DC. Predictors of severity and necrosis in acute pancreatitis. Gastroenterology Clinics of North America 2004; 33: 871–890.
4. Banks P, Freeman M, and the Practice Parameters Committee. Practice guidelines in acute pancreatitis. American Journals of Gastroenterology 2006; 101: 2379–2400.
5. Ransom JH. Etiological and prognostic factors in human acute pancreatitis: a review. American Journal of Gastroenterology 1982; 77: 633–638.
6. Blamey SL, Imrie CW, O'Neill J, et al. Prognostic factors in acute pancreatitis. Gut 1984; 25: 1340–1346.
7. Balthazer EJ. Acute pancreatitis. Assessment of severity with clinical and CT evaluation. Radiology 2002; 223: 603–613.
8. Whitcomb DC. Acute pancreatitis. New England Journal of Medicine 2006; 354: 2142–2150.
9. Dufour MC, Adamson MD. The epidemiology of alcohol-induced pancreatitis. Pancreas 2003; 27: 286–290.
10. Neiderau C, Grendell JH. Diagnosis of chronic pancreatitis. Gastroenterology 1985; 88: 1973.
11. AGA Technical Review. Treatment of pain in chronic pancreatitis. Gastroenterology 1998; 115: 765–776.
12. Cahen DL, Gouma DJ, Nio Y, et al. Endoscopic versus surgical drainage of the pancreatic duct in chronic pancreatitis. New England Journal of Medicine 2007; 356: 676–684.

7.10 Acute appendicitis

Ashis Banerjee

ESSENTIALS

1 Appendicitis is the most common cause of acute abdominal pain requiring surgical treatment.

2 The diagnosis is primarily clinical, but can often be difficult to confirm in the absence of a pathognomonic sign or conclusive first-line diagnostic test.

3 Diagnostic delay is the primary cause for morbidity and mortality, and is a major reason for litigation related to medical negligence in emergency departments.

4 Specialized imaging techniques may enhance diagnostic accuracy and help reduce the negative laparotomy rate for suspected appendicitis.

5 Surgical management is indicated once the diagnosis is confirmed or strongly suspected.

Introduction

Appendicitis remains the commonest cause of acute abdominal pain requiring surgical intervention, even though there has been a steady decline in incidence in industrialized countries, as measured by appendicectomy rates. The peak incidence is in the second and third decades of life. There is a male preponderance (male: female ratio of 1.4:1), with an overall incidence of around 1.9 per 1000 persons per year. Diagnostic delay is more common in children, women of childbearing age and the elderly. Early diagnosis is essential to avoid the risk of appendiceal perforation leading to intra-abdominal sepsis, abscess formation and/or generalized peritonitis.

Presentation

Appendicitis is a clinical diagnosis, but the clinical presentation may be atypical or equivocal, requiring a period of active observation or recourse to specialized imaging to confirm the suspicion. When evaluating any patient with acute abdominal pain in the emergency department (ED), one of the focused questions that has to be asked is whether the presentation could be due to appendicitis.

History

The classic presentation of acute appendicitis is with upper midline or periumbilical pain (70%), which represents visceral midgut pain due to appendiceal distension. This progresses over a period of 12–24 hours to right lower quadrant pain (50%), which represents somatic pain caused by localized irritation of the parietal peritoneum. The migratory pattern of the pain is the most characteristic symptom of appendicitis.

Pain is associated with nausea, anorexia (often a prominent feature) and vomiting. Low-grade fever – typically 37.5–38.0°C – may be present. Once pain localizes in the right lower quadrant, it becomes persistent, is aggravated by movement, deep inspiration and coughing, and tends to progress in severity. Pelvic appendicitis may present with irritative urinary symptoms (frequency of urination and dysuria) or with diarrhoea.

Localization of pain may, however, occur in atypical locations, such as the right upper quadrant or right flank with a retrocaecal appendix (the most common atypical location), or the left lower quadrant with a pelvic appendix or in the presence of situs inversus. Right upper quadrant pain may also be seen in the uncommon event that acute appendicitis complicates pregnancy (on an average one per every 1000 pregnancies).

Symptoms continuing longer than 72 hours make the diagnosis of appendicitis unlikely unless a mass has developed.

Examination

Examination findings vary according to the stage of evolution. Vital signs may be normal, but a mild tachycardia is usual along with low-grade fever. There may be some facial flushing, fetor oris and a dry, coated tongue.

Typically, there is localized tenderness in the right lower quadrant, classically maximal at McBurney's point (two-thirds of the way from the umbilicus to the anterior superior iliac spine). This is accompanied by reduction in respiratory movement and by involuntary muscle rigidity (guarding). Rigidity may be difficult to elicit in the obese, the elderly, children, and in the presence of atypical locations. Attempted demonstration of rebound tenderness is unkind. The same information can be obtained by noting aggravation of pain by deep inspiration or forced expiration (drawing in or blowing out the abdominal wall), with coughing, or by percussion of the anterior abdominal wall. Right lower quadrant pain may be provoked by pressure on the left lower quadrant (Rovsing's sign), and there may be accompanying hyperaesthesia of the overlying skin (Sherren's sign).

Unfortunately, the classic constellation of symptoms and signs is seen in only 50–70% of patients with acute appendicitis. Ancillary clinical signs may be of value in arriving at a diagnosis in patients with atypical symptoms, usually related to atypical locations of the tip.

Psoas muscle irritation, caused by a retrocaecal appendix, may be associated with a flexion deformity of the right hip. A positive psoas sign refers to pain with, and resistance to, passive extension of the right hip with the patient in the left lateral position. This has a high specificity but a low sensitivity. Irritation of the obturator internus muscle, caused by a pelvic appendix, may be associated with a positive obturator sign (pain on passive internal rotation of the flexed right hip). An abdominal mass may be palpable in 10–15% of cases. This represents inflamed omentum and adherent bowel loops in the presence of appendiceal perforation.

In most cases, rectal examination in patients with suspected appendicitis is of little value and does not alter management. It may be helpful when the diagnosis is in doubt, particularly in the elderly, when tenderness may be elicited in the right lateral wall of the rectum. Rectal examination may also help diagnose a pelvic abscess in the presence of a ruptured pelvic appendix.

Perforation of the appendix should be suspected in the presence of symptoms of over 24 hours' duration, a temperature higher than 38°C, and possibly a white cell count > 15 000 cells/mm^3.

Differential diagnosis

Appendicitis can mimic most acute abdominal conditions and should be considered in any patient with acute symptoms referable to the abdomen. There are a wide range of conditions that may resemble appendicitis (Table 7.10.1). On occasion the diagnosis of appendicitis may only be confirmed at surgery or laparoscopy; however, there is a 10–20% negative laparotomy rate associated with a preoperative diagnosis of appendicitis. Diagnostic delay can be associated with perforation, progression to abscess formation or to generalized peritonitis. These complications can contribute to wound infection, septicaemia and death.

Table 7.10.1 Differential diagnosis
Non-specific abdominal pain
Female genital tract: pelvic inflammatory disease; ruptured tubal gestation; ovarian cyst accident; ovarian follicle rupture
Small intestine: Meckel's diverticulitis; Crohn's disease; ileitis
Colon: caecal carcinoma; caecal diverticulitis; ileocaecal tuberculosis; *Campylobacter* colitis
Renal tract: acute pyelonephritis; ureteric colic
Lymph nodes: mesenteric lymphadenitis
Referred testicular pain

Investigation

Urinalysis

A urine dipstick examination should be performed in all patients to exclude urinary tract infection, but pyuria and microscopic haematuria can coexist with appendicitis. Qualitative β-hCG testing should be performed in all women of childbearing age in order to exclude pregnancy and the possibility of ectopic gestation.

Blood tests

The white cell count (WCC) lacks sufficient sensitivity and specificity for the diagnosis of appendicitis. A raised white cell count can also be seen with other causes of an acute surgical abdomen. A raised white cell count is a poor prognostic predictor, lacking correlation with gangrene and perforation. Undue reliance on the white cell count may lead to delays in definitive treatment and a higher perforation rate.

CRP measurement is of no diagnostic value in excluding the diagnosis of appendicitis. It would, however, appear that raised white cell count and CRP add weight to an already highly likely diagnosis of appendicitis, and some data suggest that appendicitis is unlikely if both investigations are normal.

Imaging

Plain abdominal radiography rarely provides helpful information in the work-up of clinical appendicitis and is not currently indicated, having a low sensitivity and specificity, as well as being frequently misleading. If an X-ray has been inadvertently obtained, the presence of a faecolith in the right lower quadrant may favour a diagnosis of appendicitis.

The normal appendix is usually not seen on ultrasonography but, if seen, has a diameter of < 6 mm when compressed with the examining probe. Ultrasound signs of acute appendicitis include a non-compressible appendix > 6 mm in diameter (measured outer wall to outer wall) and visualization of an appendicolith. With perforation, a loculated pericaecal fluid collection, a discontinuous wall of the appendix and prominent pericaecal fat are seen. Graded compression ultrasonography may be particularly useful in the presence of atypical presentations. In one study it had pooled sensitivity and specificity of 88% and 94%, respectively, for the diagnosis of appendicitis in children. It can also potentially identify other pathologies, especially in female patients. Ultrasound is, however, highly operator dependent, relying on skill and experience. Focused bedside ultrasound for evaluation of the appendix is an evolving option, with one study reporting sensitivity of 67%, specificity of 92% and overall accuracy of 80% for the diagnosis of acute appendicitis.

The precise role of limited helical computed tomography (CT) in the diagnosis of acute appendicitis awaits clarification, but it appears to be primarily of benefit in equivocal cases. CT signs of appendicitis include distension >6 mm, circumferential thickening of the wall, and periappendiceal inflammation and oedema. Contrast enhancement can be achieved by the intravenous, oral or rectal routes. Improved diagnostic accuracy with intravenous contrast material has reported. Sensitivity and specificity of 98% have been reported. The cost of CT scanning can be offset against the cost savings accruing from reduced rates of hospital admission and of negative laparotomy. Compared to ultrasonography, CT has been reported to have superior accuracy for appendicitis in all reported studies. This must be weighed against radiation exposure, availability and the diagnoses under consideration when selecting the preferred test for an individual patient.

A role has more recently been shown for magnetic resonance imaging (MRI) scanning in the diagnosis of acute appendicitis in the pregnant woman, with one study of 51 patients reporting sensitivity of 100% and specificity of 93.6%. The main MRI sign of acute appendicitis is an enlarged fluid-filled appendix >7 mm in diameter.

Clinical decision tools

Several tools have been described to assist clinical diagnosis. The best known of these is the 10-point Alvarado score for acute appendicitis, also known as the MANTRELS criteria (Table 7.10.2). These criteria were derived from a retrospective study of hospitalized patients with possible acute appendicitis, but have been applied to ED practice. The score was developed as a guide to determine the need for further investigation and to help decide on the need for laparotomy. Diagnostic accuracy may be improved by combining the score with ultrasonography.

Ultimately, improving diagnostic accuracy for appendicitis remains a challenge. A large population-based study concluded that the introduction of CT, ultrasonography and laparoscopy had not led to improved diagnostic accuracy.

Table 7.10.2 Alvarado score (MANTRELS criteria)	
Criterion	Point(s)
Symptoms	
M migration of pain to RLQ	1
A anorexia	1
N nausea and vomiting	1
Signs	
T tenderness in RLQ	2
R rebound pain	1
E elevated temperature	1
Laboratory findings	
L leukocytosis	2
S shift of WBCs to left	1
Total score (out of)	10
Interpretation	
1–4	Appendicitis unlikely
5–6	Appendicitis possible
7–8	Probable appendicitis
9–10	Surgery indicated

Treatment

Analgesia, usually small doses of intravenous opioids titrated to the patient's response, should be given as required, even before the diagnosis is confirmed. There is no evidence that the provision of adequate analgesia is associated with delayed diagnosis, as positive abdominal signs related to peritoneal irritation are not eliminated. Intravenous hydration should also be initiated.

The definitive treatment for appendicitis remains appendicectomy, which may be open or laparoscopic. Laparoscopy is being increasingly preferred, as it allows for combined diagnosis and treatment, as well as the recognition and potential treatment of alternative diagnostic conditions. There is an increase in operative time, but a reduction in postoperative analgesia requirements and length of inpatient stay, as well as earlier return to work. Broad-spectrum antimicrobial agents, when given preoperatively or intraoperatively, reduce the incidence of postoperative wound infection and intra-abdominal abscess.

Conservative management (intravenous hydration and broad-spectrum antimicrobial therapy) may be preferred in the presence of an appendix mass (a surgical decision), or in difficult circumstances when surgical help is not readily available, such as remote locations or while at sea.

Although a negative laparotomy rate of around 15–20% has been accepted in the past, it must be remembered that a negative laparotomy is associated with a more prolonged stay, higher complication rate and measurable mortality. Reducing this remains a major surgical challenge.

Acute appendicitis in Pregnancy

Acute appendicitis is the commonest non-obstetric reason for laparotomy in the pregnant woman, occurring in about 1 in 1000 pregnancies. Symptoms of appendicitis are similar to those in the non-pregnant state, but in late pregnancy the site of tenderness tends to be higher and more lateral. The incidence of perforation is higher. Fetal loss as a result of appendicitis and laparotomy may be as high as 20%.

Likely developments over the next 5–10 years

- Improved clinical decision support tools.
- Portable bedside ultrasound as part of the emergency department repertoire.

- A focus on a diagnostic strategy that rules out appendicitis while simultaneously ruling in other potential diagnoses.
- Reduction in the negative laparotomy rate to 5% or less.

Controversies

- An enhanced role for cross-sectional imaging, including ultrasound, CT and MRI, in confirming the diagnosis in equivocal cases.
- The threshold of acceptability for negative laparotomy.
- The role of laparoscopy in diagnosis and treatment.

Further reading

Cardall T, Glasser J, Guss DA. Clinical value of the total white blood cell count and temperature in the evaluation of patients with suspected appendicitis. Academic Emergency Medicine 2004; 11: 1021–1027.
Donnelly NJ, Semmens JB, Fletcher DR, et al. Appendicectomy in Western Australia: profile and trends, 1981–1997. Medical Journal of Australia 2001; 175: 15–18;
Doria AS, Moineddin R, Kellenberger CJ, et al. US or CT for diagnosis of appendicitis in children and adults? A meta-analysis. Radiology 2006; 241: 83–94.
Douglas CD, MacPherson NE, Davidson PM, et al. Randomized controlled trial of ultrasonography in diagnosis of acute appendicitis, incorporating the Alvarado score. British Medical Journal 2000; 321: 919–992.
Flum DR, Koepsell T. The clinical and economic correlates of misdiagnosed appendicitis: nationwide analysis. Archives of Surgery 2002; 137: 799–804.
Fox JC, Solley M, Zlidenny A, Anderson C. Bedside ultrasound for appendicitis. Academic Emergency Medicine 2005; 12: 76.
Frei SP, Bond WF, Bazuro RK, et al. Is early analgesia use associated with delayed diagnosis of appendicitis? Academic Emergency Medicine 2005; 12: 18.
Guttman R, Goldman RR, Koren G. Appendicitis during pregnancy. Canadian Family Physician 2004; 50: 355–357.
Pedrosa I, Levine AD, Eyvazzadeh B, et al. MR imaging evaluation of acute appendicitis in pregnancy. Radiology 2006; 238: 891–899.

7.11 Inflammatory bowel disease

Kim Yates

ESSENTIALS

1 The two major forms of inflammatory bowel disease (IBD) are Crohn's disease and ulcerative colitis. The principal clinical features are diarrhoea and/or abdominal pain.

2 IBD is chronic and relapsing. Patients may present with increased disease activity or with complications of the disease process or treatment.

3 Gastrointestinal complications may include dehydration, bleeding, strictures, obstruction, fistulae, sepsis, perforation, neoplasia and toxic megacolon.

4 Acute arthropathy is a common extraintestinal manifestation in IBD, but thromboembolic, ocular and hepatobiliary complications are potentially more serious.

5 Patients with moderate or severe IBD require admission to hospital. Most patients are managed initially with medical therapy such as aminosalicylates and corticosteroids, but those with intra-abdominal sepsis, perforation, obstruction or toxic megacolon are likely to require emergency surgery.

Introduction

Inflammatory bowel disease (IBD) classically refers to Crohn's disease and ulcerative colitis (UC). Both are chronic inflammatory diseases of the gastrointestinal (GI) tract of uncertain aetiology.[1]

Aetiology, genetics, pathogenesis and pathology

Although aetiologies are unknown, the consensus is that IBD is a response to environmental triggers (infection, drugs or other agents) in genetically susceptible people.[1] Whatever the initiator, an immune response against gut constituents – predominantly cell-mediated in Crohn's disease and humoral and cell-mediated in UC – appears critical to pathogenesis, and production of inflammatory mediators such as cytokines are crucial.[1-4] The genetics and immunology of IBD are reviewed in detail elsewhere.[2-5]

Pathologically the two forms differ. Crohn's disease is a focal intestinal inflammation characterized by aphthous ulcers, transmural lesions, granulomas, fat wrapping and skip lesions. It is associated with fistulas, abscesses, strictures and obstruction.[2] Any part of the GI tract can be affected, ileocolonic disease being the most common.[2] In contrast, UC is a continuous, symmetrical, colonic mucosal inflammation, often associated with bleeding.[3] Around 45% of UC patients have disease limited to the rectosigmoid, and only 20% have pancolitis.[3]

Epidemiology

IBD is more common in cooler latitudes and can occur at any age, but is most commonly diagnosed in late adolescence or early adulthood.[6] Crohn's disease is more common in women and smokers; UC more common in men and non-/ex-smokers.[6]

Clinical Features

Clinical features vary depending on the form and anatomic distribution of the disease. In acute presentations, assessing disease activity and identifying potentially serious complications of the disease and its treatments are equally important. To determine severity, the Truelove and Witts criteria for UC use stool frequency, rectal bleeding, fever, tachycardia, anaemia, and raised ESR.[3] The Crohn's Disease Activity Index uses abdominal pain, general well-being and opiate use, stool frequency, presence of complications, abdominal masses, anaemia and weight loss.[2]

GI complications may include fulminant colitis, toxic megacolon, bleeding, obstruction, abscesses, perforation, fistulas, strictures, and neoplasia.[1-3,7] Acute arthropathy and rashes are common extraintestinal manifestations of IBD, but thromboembolic, ocular and hepatobiliary complications can be more serious and require specific therapy.[2,3,7]

History

Diarrhoea is a frequent complaint, and the duration, number and type of motions per day are useful in assessing the activity and form of IBD.[2,3]

In UC more than six motions per day suggests severe disease, and fewer than four mild disease.[3] Bloody diarrhoea, mucus, tenesmus and rectal complaints are more common in UC.[1,3,8] In Crohn's disease abdominal pain and anal complaints including fissures, along with diarrhoea without rectal bleeding, are more common.[1,2,8]

Abdominal pain in Crohn's disease is commonly right-sided, and worse with eating.[8] In UC, pain is less frequent and usually crampy, lower abdominal, and relieved by passing a motion.[3,8] If pain is more severe, other GI complications should be considered. Fever is a marker of disease severity in IBD.[1,2] Weight loss is more common in Crohn's disease than in UC.[1,2]

Enquiry for extraintestinal manifestations and past surgical procedures is helpful. A careful drug history is essential, as treatments such as steroids and immunosuppressants can cause complications.

Examination

Anaemia, fever >37.5°C, pulse more than 90/min and abdominal tenderness are markers of more severe disease, particularly in UC.[1,2] The presence of fever, dehydration, orthostatic hypotension, abdominal tenderness, distension and hypoactive bowel sounds suggests fulminant colitis.[7] An abdominal mass is more common in Crohn's disease and is associated with increased disease severity.[2] Abdominal distension raises the question of fulminant colitis, toxic megacolon or obstruction.[1,2,7] Toxic megacolon (colonic dilatation with severe colitis, fever, abdominal distension and tachycardia) is potentially lethal but uncommon.[7] Rectal examination may show anal fissures, abscesses or fistulae (more common in Crohn's disease).[2] In patients taking immunosuppressants, signs of sepsis should be sought. A survey of joints, eyes, skin and vasculature can identify extraintestinal complications.

Clinical investigation

Laboratory tests

A full blood count to quantify anaemia[2,3] and determine the need for transfusion is helpful. Leukocytosis may be present in acute disease, but leukopenia may be seen if the patient is on immunosuppressants.[1,8] The ESR is usually > 30 mm/h in severe UC.[3] Electrolytes and renal function may be abnormal in dehydration.[3] Iron, folate and vitamin B_{12} deficiencies, and hypoalbuminaemia are common in IBD.[1-3] Disturbed liver function tests suggest hepatobiliary complications or drug toxicity.[1,3,9] Faecal cultures may be helpful to rule out infective diarrhoea as a cause of symptoms.[8]

Radiology

On acute presentation, particularly with abdominal pain, abdominal and chest X-rays looking for free gas with perforation, dilated bowel loops and air–fluid levels with obstruction, or dilated transverse colon (>6 cm) with toxic megacolon may be helpful, depending on clinical features.[2,3,7,10] If the transverse colon is dilated more than 12 cm, perforation is imminent.[10] Computed tomography (CT) is indicated when fistulas, intra-abdominal or retroperitoneal abscesses are suspected.[2,3,7] Barium studies will diagnose and differentiate between Crohn's disease and UC, but are contraindicated in acutely unwell patients because of the risks of perforation or obstruction.[11] MRI and ultrasound are used acutely in some centres.[2,3,12]

Endoscopy

Endoscopy is useful for diagnosing IBD, for staging activity, and in screening for strictures or cancer.[1-3,11] Cautious sigmoidoscopy is safe in the acutely unwell patient, but colonoscopy carries a risk of perforation.[1-3,11] The role of wireless video capsule endoscopy is unclear.[1,12]

Management

General measures

Initial assessment should focus on the detection and treatment of life-threatening conditions such as septic or hypovolaemic shock, severe anaemia or dehydration.

Thereafter, assessment focuses on disease activity/severity and the presence of complications. Intravenous fluid therapy, correction of electrolytes and/or transfusion may be necessary. For abdominal pain, appropriate analgesia should be provided. Opiates should be used with caution in severe colitis as it has been suggested that toxic megacolon may be precipitated.[1,7] Non-selective non-steroidal anti-inflammatory drugs (NSAIDs) appear to exacerbate IBD.[13] Selective NSAIDs such as celecoxib may not exacerbate IBD but carry other risks.[13] If toxic megacolon is suspected, nasogastric drainage, intravenous steroids and other medical therapy as discussed below should be commenced.[7] Complications requiring surgery, such as bowel obstruction, intra-abdominal sepsis or perforation, should be ruled out early.

Treatment for IBD is usually a stepwise approach depending on severity and response, with aminosalicylates and antibiotics first, then corticosteroids and immunomodulators, progressing to biologic agents and surgery.[14]

Medical therapy

Aminosalicylates (sulfasalazine, 5ASA/mesalamine) are used to treat mild to moderate IBD, but are more commonly effective in maintaining remission in UC.[1–3,14] Metronidazole and/or ciprofloxacin is effective in treating perianal fistulas in Crohn's disease.[1,2,14] In UC, antibiotics are used preoperatively or to treat pouchitis, but otherwise are not of proven benefit, although some studies show that rifaximin, a poorly absorbed antibiotic, may be effective.[1,3,7]

Corticosteroids induce remission of IBD but are not useful as maintenance therapy.[1–3] Rectal steroids are used in mild to moderate distal UC, and prednisone 40–60 mg/day or equivalent is used for moderate or more proximal IBD.[1–3,14] High-dose parenteral steroids (48–60 mg methylprednisolone/day) are reserved for fulminant disease.[7] Budesonide, which has low bioavailability but high potency, appears effective both topically and orally in IBD, with fewer systemic side effects.[1–3]

Immunomodulators such as azathioprine and 6-mercaptopurine are used as steroid-sparing agents or in steroid-resistant disease, but bone marrow suppression, pancreatitis and hepatotoxicity can be problems.[1–3] Methotrexate may be useful in Crohn's disease, and ciclosporin may be useful in severe UC.[1,15] Infliximab (anti-tumour necrosis factor (TNF) antibody) has been shown to be effective for severe or refractory Crohn's disease, although active sepsis is an absolute contraindication.[1,2] Infliximab also appears effective for refractory UC.[3,16] Other immunosuppressants have been trialled.

Nutritional support, such as elemental diets or parenteral nutrition, is more helpful in Crohn's disease than in UC.[1–3,15] Vitamin and trace element supplements are more important in Crohn's disease than UC, and in those on steroids.[2,3] Antidiarrhoeals may be useful for symptom control in mild disease.[3]

Surgical therapy

Indications for surgery in IBD include fulminant colitis, toxic megacolon, perforation, severe GI haemorrhage, intractable disease, stricture with obstruction, abscesses, fistulas or cancer.[1–3,7] In patients with fulminant colitis or toxic megacolon who do not respond to medical therapy, or deteriorate, subtotal colectomy is indicated.[1,3,7] Intra-abdominal abscesses, more common in Crohn's disease, can be drained percutaneously under CT or ultrasound guidance, but may require laparotomy.[2,7]

In UC, proctocolectomy is curative; however, subtotal procedures and anastomoses are often performed when disease is limited or when patients wish to avoid a stoma.[3] As Crohn's disease has a high recurrence rate after segmental resection, surgery is conservative to preserve bowel length and function.[1,2,15]

Disposition

Patients with moderate or severe IBD require admission, usually for a trial of medical therapy. Surgical admission is indicated for perforation, obstruction, intra-abdominal sepsis or toxic megacolon. Patients with mild IBD and no complications can be managed as outpatients, with gastroenterology follow-up.

Controversies

- Causes of IBD.[1–3,5,6,15] Numerous triggers for IBD in the genetically susceptible have been postulated. Although the mechanism is unknown, smoking and appendicectomy appear protective for UC, but are risk factors for Crohn's disease. Many infectious agent triggers have been proposed, including *Mycobacteria*, paramyxovirus (measles), *Listeria*, *Pseudomonas* and *Chlamydia*, but there is no definitive evidence to date. Non-infectious triggers under investigation include NSAIDs, diet, food additives, oral contraceptive agents and changes in gut flora.

- Medical therapies. Methotrexate is effective for inducing remission or reducing relapse in Crohn's disease, but owing to toxicity concerns (pneumonitis or hepatotoxicity) is reserved for refractory disease or where azathioprine or 6-mercaptopurine are not tolerated.[1,14,15] Ciclosporin is effective as salvage therapy in refractory colitis or to prevent proctocolectomy, but is controversial due to toxicity (renal impairment, infections, neurotoxicity) and long-term failure rate.[1,14,15] The place of nicotine therapy in UC is unclear.[3] Other biological therapies being investigated include adulimamab, certolizumab, interleukin-10, anti-interleukins, and natalizumab.[2,3,15] Immunomodulators such as tacrolimus, mycophenolate, and thalidomide show promise, as do heparin, porcine whipworm, granulocyte colony-stimulating factor and probiotics.[2,3,15]

- Cancer and IBD. Patients with UC are more at risk of colorectal cancer, particularly with increasing duration and extent of disease. Colonoscopic surveillance programmes for dysplasia have been developed for patients opting out of colectomy, but their effectiveness is controversial.[1,3]

DIGESTIVE

7

References

1. Carter MJ, Lobo AJ, Travis SPL. Guidelines for the management of IBD in adults. Gut 2004; 53: v1–v16.
2. Sands BE. Crohn's disease. In: Feldman M, Friedman LS, Friedman LJ, Brandt LJ, eds. Sleisinger and Fordtran's gastrointestinal and liver disease: pathophysiology, diagnosis, management. Philadelphia: WB Saunders, 2006; 2460–2490.
3. Su C, Lichtenstein GR. Ulcerative colitis. In: Feldman M, Friedman LS, Friedman LJ, Brandt LJ, eds. Sleisinger and Fordtran's gastrointestinal and liver disease: pathophysiology, diagnosis, management. Philadelphia: WB Saunders, 2006; 2499–2583.
4. Podolsky DK. IBD. New England Journal of Medicine 2002; 347: 417–429.
5. Thoreson R, Cullen JJ. Pathophysiology of IBD: an overview. Surgical Clinics of North America 2007; 87: 575–585.
6. Loftus EV. Clinical epidemiology of IBD: incidence, prevalence and environmental influences. Gastroenterology 2004; 126: 1504–1517.
7. Cheung O, Regueiro MD. IBD emergencies. Gastroenterology Clinics of North America 2003; 32: 1269–1288.
8. Sands BE. From symptom to diagnosis: clinical distinctions among various forms of intestinal inflammation. Gastroenterology 2004; 126: 1518–1532.
9. Ahmad J, Slivka A. Hepatobiliary disease in IBD. Gastroenterology Clinics of North America 2002; 31: 329–345.
10. Marincek B. Nontraumatic abdominal emergencies: acute abdominal pain: diagnostic strategies. European Radiology 2002; 12: 2136–2150.
11. Scotiniotis I, Rubesin SE, Geinsberg GG. Imaging modalities in IBD. Gastroenterology Clinics of North America 1999; 28: 391–421.
12. MacKalski BA, Bernstein CN. New diagnostic imaging tools for IBD. Gut 2006; 55: 733–741.
13. Korzenik JR, Podolsky DK. Selective use of selective nosteroidal anti-inflammatory drugs in IBD. Clinics in Gastroenterology and Hepatology 2006; 4: 157–159.
14. Katz JA. Management of IBD in adults. Journal of Digestive Diseases 2007; 8: 65–71.
15. Sands BE. IBD: past, present, and future. Journal of Gastroenterology 2007; 42: 16–25.
16. Lawson MM, Thomas AG, Akobeng AK. Tumour necrosis factor alpha blocking agents for induction of remission in ulcerative colitis. Cochrane Database Systematic Review 3: CD005112, 2006.

7.12 Acute liver failure

Abel Wakai • John M Ryan

ESSENTIALS

1 The diagnosis of acute liver failure is based on the presence of increasing coagulopathy, hepatic encephalopathy and deepening jaundice.

2 The aetiology is varied and related to a number of geographical and social factors. Viral hepatitis remains the commonest cause worldwide, but paracetamol toxicity is an increasingly common cause in the western world.

3 Early diagnosis is important because of the therapeutic option of using antidotes in the presence of a reversible cause.

4 Patients should be transferred to an intensive care unit or a specialized liver unit once the diagnosis of acute liver failure has been made.

5 Management involves optimizing the patient's haemodynamic, renal, pulmonary and cerebral status, in addition to preventing bacterial and fungal infections.

6 Orthotopic liver transplantation is the only definitive therapy for patients with acute liver failure unable to achieve regeneration of sufficient hepatocyte mass to sustain life.

7 Bridging devices are available to provide adequate liver function and maintain the patient well enough until the native liver recovers or until a graft is found.

Introduction

Acute liver failure (ALF) remains one of the most challenging medical emergencies. It is a rare condition in which rapid deterioration of liver function results in altered mentation and coagulopathy in previously normal individuals. United States estimates are placed at approximately 2000 cases per year. The most prominent causes include drug-induced liver injury, viral hepatitis, autoimmune liver disease and shock or hypoperfusion; many cases (≈20%) have no discernible cause. Acute liver failure often affects young persons and carries a high morbidity and mortality. Prior to transplantation, most series suggested less than 15% survival. Currently, overall short-term survival with transplantation is greater than 65%. Because of its rarity, ALF has been difficult to study in depth and very few controlled therapeutic trials have been performed. As a result, standards of intensive care for this condition have not been established.

Aetiology, pathogenesis and pathology

ALF occurs when the rate of hepatocyte death exceeds the rate of hepatocyte regeneration as a result of various insults that lead to a combination of apoptosis or necrosis. Apoptosis is associated with nuclear shrinkage, but without cell membrane rupture. Therefore, there is no release of intracellular content and no subsequent secondary inflammation. In contrast, necrosis is associated with ATP depletion, resulting in a swollen cell that eventually lyses, with the release of intracellular content associated with secondary inflammation. Most causes of ALF result in either apoptosis or necrosis; for example, paracetamol toxicity results in apoptosis, and ischaemia results in necrosis. The clinical result of the cellular damage is a catastrophic illness that can lead rapidly to coma and death caused by multiorgan failure.

Epidemiology

There is significant worldwide variation in the cause of ALF. It is relatively uncommon in the UK, causing fewer than 500 deaths and being responsible for less than 15% of liver transplantations per annum (fewer than 100 transplants per year).[5] Meanwhile, in the USA ALF affects approximately 2000 people per year. Although it accounts for fewer than 10% of all liver transplantations in the United States, it accounts for more than two-thirds of transplantations in the Far East.[5]

Paracetamol poisoning is the commonest cause of ALF in the UK and USA, causing up to 70% of cases in the United Kingdom and 51% of cases in the United States. Up to 10% of patients with paracetamol self-poisoning develop severe liver damage, but less than 2% go on to develop ALF, the worst outcomes being in patients with concurrent alcohol use.

Other major causes of ALF in the United States include idiosyncratic drug reactions (13%), secondary to hepatitis B (HBV; 8%) and secondary to hepatitis C (HCV; 4%). Seventeen per cent of ALF cases in the United States are of indeterminate cause. A small number of cases in the United States result from miscellaneous causes such as Wilson's disease, cardiogenic, pregnancy related, autoimmune disease and Budd–Chiari syndrome.

In the United Kingdom, approximately 5% of cases are caused by non-paracetamol drugs such as anti-tuberculous therapy, anticonvulsants, steroids, NSAIDs, herbal remedies and recreational drugs (for example Ecstasy and cocaine). Less than 0.05% of cases of acute hepatitis A and B lead to ALF, with these viruses contributing less than 5% of all ALF cases. Seronegative (non-A–E) hepatitis, a diagnosis of exclusion, is the commonest presumed viral cause in the United Kingdom and other western countries, but contributes less than 10% of all ALF cases. In the UK, unusual viral causes include herpes simplex, Epstein–Barr, cytomegalovirus, and varicella zoster. Small numbers of ALF cases in the United Kingdom result from miscellaneous causes such as pregnancy, Wilson's disease, Budd–Chiari syndrome, autoimmune hepatitis, ischaemic hepatitis and malignant infiltration.

Although ALF is most commonly drug-induced in the west, in the developing world and the Far East it is most often caused by viral hepatitis. Particularly common causes are exacerbations of chronic HBV, which is endemic in many countries, including Hong Kong, and hepatitis E in India. Flares of chronic HBV may be spontaneous, represent a secondary response to increased levels of replicating wild-type or mutant virus, occur after immunosuppressive and cytotoxic therapy, or occur

following superinfection with other hepatotropic viruses such as hepatitis D and HCV.

Prevention

Primary prevention of ALF in the west mainly involves strategies to combat increasing rates of paracetamol-induced ALF, including legislation to reduce the over-the-counter availability of paracetamol, printing specific warnings about overdose in the packets, use of paracetamol/methionine combination analgesics and the promotion of alternatives.

Secondary prevention involves immunization strategies. Hepatitis A and B vaccination is safe and immunogenic in patients with mild to moderate chronic liver disease (CLD), albeit less effective in those with decompensated liver cirrhosis or after liver transplantation.

Clinical features

History should include a careful review of possible exposures to viral infection and drugs or other toxins. If severe encephalopathy is present, a collateral history may be all that is available, or a history may be unavailable. In this setting information is limited, particularly regarding possible toxin/drug ingestions.

Physical examination must include careful assessment and documentation of mental status and a search for stigmata of CLD. Jaundice is often (but not invariably) seen at presentation. Right upper quadrant tenderness is variably present. Inability to palpate the liver or even to percuss a significant area of dullness over the liver can be indicative of reduced liver volume due to massive hepatocyte loss. Hepatomegaly may be seen early in viral hepatitis or with malignant infiltration, congestive heart failure or acute Budd–Chiari syndrome. History or signs of cirrhosis should be absent, as such features suggest underlying CLD, which may have different management implications.

Differential diagnosis

Common causes of ALF are hepatitis viruses or drugs (Table 7.12.1). In western countries, drug-induced ALF predominates,

comprising 19–75% of all cases. In India 91–100% of cases are due to viruses, with drug-induced cases responsible for 0–7.4%.

Idiosyncratic drug reactions account for 13% of cases of ALF in the United States and 5% of cases in the UK. Examples of causative drugs include antibiotics (amoxicillin–clavulanic acid, ciprofloxacin, doxycycline, erythromycin, isoniazid, nitrofurantoin, tetracycline, sulphonamides), antivirals (fialuridine), antidepressants (amitriptyline, nortriptyline), oral hypoglycaemic drugs (troglitazone, metformin), anticonvulsants (phenytoin, valproic acid), anaesthetics (halothane, isoflurane), statins (atorvastatin, lovastatin, simvastatin), immunosuppressants (cyclophosphamide, methotrexate, gold), NSAIDs, salicylates (Reye's syndrome), anti-thyroid drugs (propylthiouracil), anti-arrhythmics (amiodarone) disulfiram and flutamide.

Infectious diseases such as falciparum malaria, typhoid fever, leptospirosis and dengue fever may mimic ALF at presentation. They can present with fever, jaundice and features of encephalopathy, and should be considered in all patients presenting with ALF, particularly in the tropics, or in patients who have recently travelled in the tropics. Baseline routine clinical and laboratory investigations will provide supportive evidence of an infective cause. After reaching a definitive diagnosis, specific therapy for the infectious disease in addition to supportive therapy for ALF reduces mortality.

Clinical investigations

Initial laboratory investigation in the emergency department (ED) is aimed at evaluating both the aetiology and severity of ALF (Table 7.12.2). Other urgent investigations, mainly aimed at evaluating the aetiology of ALF following hospital admission, include viral hepatitis serologies (anti-HAV IgM, HBSAg, anti-HBc IgM, anti-HEV IgM, anti-HCV IgM), autoimmune markers (antinuclear, anti-smooth muscle antibodies, immunoglobulin levels) and ceruloplasmin level. Plasma ammonia, preferably arterial, may also be helpful. A liver biopsy, most often done via the transjugular route because of coagulopathy, may be indicated when certain conditions such as autoimmune

Table 7.12.1 Differential diagnosis of ALF

Viruses	Hepatitis A and B viruses(typical viruses causing viral hepatitis)
	Hepatitis C virus (rare)
	Hepatitis D virus
	Hepatitis E virus (often in pregnant women in endemic areas)
	Cytomegalovirus
	Haemorrhagic fever viruses
	Herpes simplex virus
	Paramyxovirus
	Epstein–Barr virus
Drugs	Paracetamol hepatotoxicity
	Idiosyncratic hypersensitivity reactions (e.g. isoniazid, statins, halothane)
	Illicit drugs (e.g. ecstasy, cocaine)
	Alternative medicines (e.g. chaparral and *Teucrium polium*)
Toxins	Mushroom poisoning (usually *Amanita phalloides*)
	Bacillus cereus toxin
	Cyanobacteria toxin
	Organic solvents (e.g. carbon tetrachloride)
	Yellow phosphorus
Vasculopathy	Ischaemic hepatitis
	Hepatic vein thrombosis (Budd–Chiari syndrome)
	Hepatic veno-occlusive disease
	Portal vein thrombosis
	Hepatic arterial thrombosis
Metabolic	Acute fatty liver of pregnancy/HELLP (haemolysis, elevated liver enzymes, low platelets) syndrome
	α_1-Antitrypsin deficiency
	Fructose intolerance
	Galactosaemia
	Lecithin–cholesterol acyltransferase deficiency
	Reye's syndrome
	Tyrosinaemia
	Wilson's disease
Autoimmune	Autoimmune hepatitis
Malignancy	Primary liver malignancy (hepatocellular carcinoma or cholangiocarcinoma)
	Secondary (e.g. extensive hepatic metastases or infiltration of adenocarcinoma)
Miscellaneous	Adult-onset Still's disease
	Heatstroke
	Primary graft non-function (in liver transplant recipients)
	Indeterminate aetiology (≈20% of ALF cases)

Table 7.12.3 Grades of hepatic encephalopathy

Grade 1	Drowsy but coherent, mood change
Grade 2	Drowsy, confused at times, inappropriate behaviour
Grade 3	Very drowsy and stuporose but rousable; alternatively restless, screaming
Grade 4	Comatose, barely rousable

autoimmune hepatitis may be included in spite of the possibility of cirrhosis if their disease has only been recognized for less than 26 weeks.

A number of other terms have been used, including fulminant hepatic failure and fulminant hepatitis or necrosis. It is intuitively logical that acute liver failure is a better overall term that should encompass all durations up to 26 weeks. Terms that signifying duration of illness, such as hyperacute (<7 days), acute (7–21 days) and subacute (>21 days and <26weeks), are not particularly helpful as they do not have prognostic significance distinct from the cause of the illness.

Treatment

The most important step in the treatment of ALF is to identify the cause, as the prognosis depends on this. Death in ALF is predominantly related to sepsis, multiorgan failure and intracranial hypertension. The circulatory disturbances in ALF, which contribute to the often-associated renal failure, are characterized by a generalized vasodilatation that results in increased cardiac output and reduced systemic vascular resistance and mean arterial pressure.

Emergency liver transplantation is the only proven therapeutic intervention for ALF. Whereas treatments for specific aetiologies are also initiated, emergency management requires intensive care support because deterioration can be rapid. Careful attention must be paid to fluid management, haemodynamics and metabolic parameters, as well as surveillance for and treatment of infection. Maintenance of nutrition and prompt recognition and resuscitation of gastrointestinal bleeding are crucial as well. Coagulation parameters,

Table 7.12.2 Emergency department investigations for ALF

Haematology	Full blood count
	Prothrombin time/INR
	Blood type and screen
Biochemistry	Liver function tests
	Urea & electrolytes
	Arterial blood gas
	Arterial lactate
	Arterial ammonia
	Glucose
	Calcium
	Magnesium
	Phosphate
	Amylase
Toxicology	Paracetamol level
	Toxicology screen
Urinalysis	hCG (females)
Imaging studies	Chest radiography
	Liver ultrasonography
Miscellaneous	Electrocardiogram

hepatitis, metastatic liver disease, lymphoma, or herpes simplex hepatitis are suspected.

Other investigations may be required as clinically indicated, for example determination of HIV status in patients who are candidates for liver transplantation.

Criteria for diagnosis

The most widely accepted definition of ALF includes impairment of liver function with evidence of coagulation abnormality (usually an international standardized ratio of prothrombin (INR) ≥1.5) and any degree of mental alteration (encephalopathy; Table 7.12.3) in a patient without existing cirrhosis and with an illness of less than 26 weeks' duration.[7] Patients with Wilson's disease, vertically acquired HBV, or complete blood counts, metabolic panels (including glucose) and arterial blood gas should be checked frequently. Liver function tests (LFTs) are generally measured daily to follow the course of the condition; however, changes in aminotransferase levels correlate poorly with prognosis.

General measures

Fundamental to the management of patients with ALF is the provision of good intensive care support. Aggressive monitoring is required to detect respiratory and haemodynamic complications, neurological changes, infections and gastrointestinal haemorrhage. Airway protection and endotracheal intubation may be required, because as patients become comatose their ability to protect their airway from aspiration is reduced. Central venous access and invasive and non-invasive arterial blood pressure monitoring are useful for monitoring vascular status. Swan–Ganz pulmonary artery pressure monitoring may provide helpful information about cardiac output. All patients should have a urinary catheter placed to monitor output. Volume resuscitation should ideally be with colloids and titrated to a pulmonary wedge pressure of 12–14 mmHg. Intravenous dopamine may be required to encourage renal perfusion, and noradrenaline (norepinephrine) may be required for systemic hypotension. Metabolic derangements such as hypoglycaemia should be sought and treated aggressively. Hypokalaemia is common and should be managed with intravenous supplements. Intravenous phosphate and magnesium supplements may also be required. Platelets may be required if the count falls below 20 000/mL. H_2-receptor blockers are given for prophylaxis against gastrointestinal bleeding. Nasogastric tube insertion for stomach decompression may be required in comatose patients. Dialysis may be required for deteriorating renal function and worsening acidosis.

Maintaining adequate cerebral perfusion is paramount, and the patient should be nursed in a quiet environment with 10° head-up tilt. Intracranial pressure monitoring may be helpful in some patients for directing therapy to prevent brainstem herniation.

Withdrawal of dietary protein is commonly recommended to treat acute hepatic encephalopathy, although the traditional use of lactulose for enteral decontamination is now more controversial. Instead, other agents such as metronidazole and neomycin have been recommended to treat acute hepatic encephalopathy. Systemic antimicrobial therapy with or without enteral decontamination reduces the infection rate in patients with acute liver failure.[11]

Specific measures

N-acetylcysteine (NAC)

Several clinical trials support the use of NAC in ALF.[5] In late-presenting paracetamol overdose, mortality and progression to grade III–IV encephalopathy is reduced in those receiving NAC.

Penicillin G and silibinin

Penicillin G and silibinin (silymarin or milk thistle) are accepted antidotes for mushroom poisoning (usually *Amanita phalloides*), despite no controlled trials proving their efficacy.[12] Although some reports have not found penicillin G to be helpful, enough efficacy has been reported to warrant consideration of the drug (given intravenously in doses of 300 000–1 million units/kg/day) in patients with known or suspected mushroom poisoning. Silibinin has generally been reported to be more successful than penicillin G, although the latter has been used more frequently. Silibinin/silymarin is not available as a licensed drug in the United States, although it is widely available in Europe and South America. When used for the treatment of mushroom poisoning, silymarin has been given in average doses of 30–40 mg/kg/day either intravenously or orally, for an average of 3–4 days.

Drug-induced hepatotoxicity

There are no specific antidotes for idiosyncratic drug reactions; corticosteroids are not indicated unless a drug hypersensitivity reaction is suspected. Current recommendations are: (1) obtain details (including onset of ingestion, amount and timing of last dose) concerning all prescription and non-prescription drugs, herbs and dietary supplement taken over the past year; (2) determine the ingredients of non-prescription medications whenever possible; (3) in the setting of ALF due to possible drug hepatotoxicity, discontinue all but essential medications.

Lamivudine and nucleoside analogues

ALF due to reactivation of hepatitis B may occur in the setting of chemotherapy or immunosuppression. The nucleoside analogue lamivudine (and possibly adefovir), used widely in the treatment of chronic hepatitis B, may be considered in patients with acute hepatitis B, although these dugs have not been subjected to controlled trials in acute disease. It is currently recommended that nucleoside analogues be given prior to and continued for 6 months after completion of chemotherapy in patients with hepatitis B surface antigen positivity to prevent reactivation/acute flare of disease.

Aciclovir

Although herpes virus infection rarely causes ALF, immunosuppressed patients or pregnant women (usually in the third trimester) are at increased risk. In addition, the occurrence of herpes virus ALF has been reported in previously healthy individuals. Meanwhile, other viruses such as varicella zoster have occasionally been implicated in causing hepatic failure. Patients with known or suspected herpes virus or varicella zoster as the cause of ALF should be treated with aciclovir.

Corticosteroids

Patients with autoimmune hepatitis may have unrecognized pre-existing chronic disease and yet still be considered as having ALF, if their illness is of less than 26 weeks' duration. Such patients represent the most severe form of the disease, and would generally fall into the category of patients recommended for corticosteroid therapy (prednisone, 40–60 mg/day). Initiation of steroid therapy may constitute a therapeutic trial for some patients, and placement on the transplant list is indicated as although some patients with ALF due to autoimmune hepatitis respond to steroid therapy, others require transplantation.

Cardiovascular support

In patients with evidence of ischaemic injury cardiovascular support is the treatment of choice. In such patients the ability to manage heart failure or other causes of ischaemia (for example, significant hypovolaemia) will determine outcome.

Liver transplantation

Orthotopic liver transplantation (OLT) remains the only definitive therapy for patients who are unable to achieve regeneration of sufficient hepatocyte mass to sustain life. Urgent liver transplantation is indicated where prognostic indicators suggest a high likelihood of death. Post-transplant survival rates for ALF have been reported to be as high as 80–90%, but accurate long-term outcome data are not yet available.

Patients with ALF secondary to the following causes should be listed for transplantation: mushroom poisoning, Wilson's disease, autoimmune hepatitis and hepatic vein thrombosis (provided underlying malignancy is excluded). In such patients, initial laboratory investigations should include determination of their HIV status, because this has implications for potential liver transplantation. Early liaison with a liver transplantation unit is mandatory, and any contraindications to transplantation should be identified with collateral histories through the family, friends and primary care physicians, if necessary. Planning for transfer to a transplant centre should begin in patients with grade I or II encephalopathy (see Table 7.12.3) because they may worsen rapidly. Early transfer is important as the risks involved with patient transport may increase or even preclude transfer once stage III and IV encephalopathy develops.

'Bridging options'

The aim of bridging devices is to provide adequate liver function and maintain the patient well enough until native liver function recovers or until a graft is found. In one study, only 29% of patients listed for transplantation received a liver graft, and 10% of the overall group (one-quarter of patients listed for transplantation) died on the waiting list. Other series have reported death rates as high as 40% of those listed for liver transplantation, despite most organ donor allocation systems prioritizing ALF.

The many and diverse function of the liver (metabolic, immunological and physiological) make the task of developing bridging devices a major challenge: the effects of the 'toxic liver' itself also require consideration. Bridging devices can be classified into four categories: (1) auxiliary transplant; (2) liver support devices (biological and non-biological); (3) hepatocyte transplantation; (4) innovative/experimental techniques (Table 7.12.4).

The current data regarding the efficacy, cost effectiveness and safety of liver support devices, both biological and non-biological (artificial) are conflicting and less promising in ALF. Currently available liver support systems are therefore not recommended outside clinical trials; their future in the management of ALF remains unclear.

Prognosis

The prognosis of ALF is variable and depends on the cause. Outcomes are much better for patients who have ALF associated with paracetamol, pregnancy or hepatitis A than those who have seronegative hepatitis, non-A non-B viral hepatitis, idiosyncratic drug reactions or Wilson's disease. Hepatitis B has an intermediate outcome. The age of the patient and the rate of disease progression also determine outcome. Generally, patients with slow disease progression tend to do worse than those with a rapid downhill course to encephalopathy. Other factors associated with a poor prognosis include the presence of a metabolic acidosis and, in cases of paracetamol toxicity, a continuing rise in the prothrombin time at days 3–4, which may rise to 180 seconds.

Given that the only proven beneficial therapeutic intervention in advanced ALF is transplantation, the timing of transplantation and selection of patients is crucial.

Although scoring systems have been proposed, the variety of causes of ALF tends to limit their accuracy. Validating selection criteria is difficult because of poor methodology in several reported series. Furthermore, ALF is rare; therefore, most case series involve small numbers and span long periods of time, during which important supportive medical therapies may have evolved that could affect prognosis.

Two main prognostic scoring systems are currently in use: the Clichy and the King's College (London) criteria. Both include different demographic, clinical and biochemical variables to identify a group most likely to require transplantation. Other prognostic criteria have been proposed, including severity of SIRS, α-fetoprotein (AFP) levels, ratios of factor VIII and factor V, liver histology, CT scanning of the liver, cytokine levels, serum phosphate levels and adrenal insufficiency. The Model for Endstage Liver Disease (MELD) score, now widely used to predict mortality among patients with chronic liver disease who are under consideration for liver transplantation, has been reported by some studies to have similar or better predictive value than the more established scores.

Table 7.12.4 'Bridging options' for ALF	
Auxiliary transplant	Heterotopic auxiliary liver transplantation (HALT)
	Auxiliary partial orthotopic liver transplantation (APOLT)
Liver support devices	Bioartificial liver (BAL) devices
	Demetriou's Hepatassist BAL
	Amsterdam Medical Centre BAL
	Extracorporeal liver assist device (MELS)
	Bioartificial liver support system (BLSS)
	Non-biological liver devices
	Molecular adsorbents
	Recirculating system (MARS)
	Prometheus system
	Plasmapheresis and high-volume plasmapheresis
Hepatocyte transplantation	Cryopreserved human hepatocytes via: intraportal hepatocyte infusions
	Splenic artery infusion
Innovative/experimental techniques	Total emergency hepatectomy
	Portal vein arterialization
	Auxiliary liver organ formation by implantation of spleen-encapsulated hepatocytes

Likely developments over the next 5–10 years

- Evidence base for NAC in non-paracetamol ALF.
- Mild hypothermia to prevent and treat brain oedema in ALF.
- Optimal biocomponent for liver support devices in ALF.
- Hepatocyte progenitor cells (including fetal liver cells, multipotent hepatic cells and bone marrow-derived stem cells) as genuine functional hepatocytes for use in hepatocyte transplantation.
- Auxiliary partial liver transplantation as a bridge to transplantation or spontaneous recovery in ALF.

Controversies

- Efficacy of penicillin G and silibinin (silymarin or milk thistle) as antidotes for mushroom poisoning .
- Selection of patients for transplantation.
- Role, selection and efficacy of bridging options for patients awaiting transplantation.

Further reading

Broussard CN, Aggarwal A, Lacey SR, et al. Mushroom poisoning – from diarrhea to liver transplantation. American Journal of Gastroenterology 2001; 96: 3195.

Brunetto MR, Giarin MM, Oliveri F, et al. Wild-type and e antigen-minus hepatitis B viruses and course of chronic hepatitis. Proceedings of the National Academy of the Sciences USA 1991; 88: 4186–4190.

Clavien PA. Acute liver failure: Where are the challenges? Journal of Hepatology 2007; 46: 553–554.

Ellis A, Rhodes A, Jackson N, et al. Acute liver failure (ALF) in a specialist intensive care unit; a 7 year experience. Critical Care 1998; 2: 150.

Jalan R. Acute liver failure: current management and future prospects. Journal of Hepatology 2005; 42: S115–123.

Khan SA, Shah N, Williams R. Acute liver failure: a review. Clinics in Liver Disease 2006; 10: 239–258.

Larson AM, Polson J, Fontana RJ, et al. Acetaminophen-induced acute liver failure: results of a United States multicenter, prospective study. Hepatology 2005; 42: 1364–1372.

Lee WM. Acute liver failure in the United States. Seminars in Liver Disease 2003; 23: 217–226.

O'Grady J. Modern management of acute liver failure. Clinics in Liver Disease 2007; 11: 291–303.

Ostapowicz GA, Fontana RJ, Schiodt FV, et al. Results of a prospective study of acute liver failure at 17 tertiary care centers in the United States. Annals of Internal Medicine 2002; 137: 947–954.

Polson J, William ML. AASLD Position Paper: The management of acute liver failure. Hepatology 2005; 42: 1179–1197.

Rolando N, Grimson A, Wade J, et al. Prospective study comparing prophylactic parenteral antimicrobials, with or without enteral decontamination, in patients with acute liver failure. Hepatology 1993; 17: 196–201.

Singhal A, Neuberger J. Acute liver failure: bridging to transplant or recovery – are we there yet? Journal of Hepatology 2007; 46: 557–564.

Trey C, Davidson CS. The management of fulminant hepatic failure. In: Popper H, Schaffner F, eds. Progress in liver disease. New York: Grune & Stratton, 1970.

Weisner R, Edwards E, Freeman R, et al. Model for end-stage liver disease (MELD) and allocation of donor livers. Gastroenterology 2003; 124: 91–96.

7.13 Rectal bleeding

Andrew Walby • Suresh David

ESSENTIALS

1 Rectal bleeding is a common presentation in patients aged over 50 years and can result in shock due to large volume loss.

2 Elderly patients with rectal bleeding should have complete investigation of their large bowel, regardless of the presence of anorectal disease.

3 Most cases of lower gastrointestinal haemorrhage resolve spontaneously.

4 Colonoscopy is the investigation of choice, but is unreliable in the unprepared bowel.

5 Despite improved diagnostic imaging, no source of bleeding will be identified in up to 10–20% of patients.

6 Treatment options consist of colonoscopic, angiographic and surgical techniques.

7 Emergency surgery is necessary in approximately 10% of patients, and the morbidity is reduced by prior haemodynamic stabilization.

Introduction

Rectal bleeding or haematochezia is the passage of bright red, bloody stools from the rectum, and is to be distinguished from melaena, which is stool with blood that has been altered by the gut flora and appears black and 'tarry'. Commonly associated with lower gastrointestinal bleeding, rectal bleeding affects 20% of western society at some stage in their lives. Patients may present with minor self-limiting episodes, evidence of occult blood loss with anaemia, or more severe bleeding with haemodynamic instability. Acute lower gastrointestinal haemorrhage accounts for approximately 20% of all cases of gastrointestinal haemorrhage.

Rectal blood loss usually originates distal to the ligament of Treitz (the duodenal suspensory ligament at the junction of the duodenum and the jejunum) in the distal duodenum. However, in a small group of cases the cause may be more proximal – in the duodenum, stomach or distal oesophagus.

Appropriate investigation and management is dictated by the severity of blood loss. Those with minor bleeds can often be investigated and managed as outpatients. Moderate bleeding may require inpatient investigation. Severe or continuous bleeding or significant re-bleeding within 1 week warrants in-hospital management. Massive lower gastrointestinal haemorrhage is characterized by haemodynamic instability and transfusion of at least two units of packed red blood cells.

Mortality from acute lower gastrointestinal bleeding is approximately 5–10%, and the risk increases with age (particularly in those over 60), concomitant medical problems, difficulty in locating a bleeding source, transfusion requirement of more than 5 units of blood, and surgery in the unstable patient.

Aetiology

The aetiology of rectal bleeding varies with age. In patients under 50 years, haemorrhoids are by far the most common cause, followed by anal fissures, benign polyps and inflammatory bowel disease. Diverticulosis and angiodysplasia are the most common causes in patients aged over 50, followed by carcinoma, polyps, colitis and rare malignancies such as anorectal melanoma. In this age group, the risk of colonic neoplasms increases with every year of age.

Diverticulosis

Colonic diverticula are acquired defects in the bowel wall occurring at the point of entry of nutrient vessels. They are present in more than 50% of people over 60 years of age, and the incidence increases with age. Diverticula are common in the distal colon and are the source of lower gastrointestinal bleeding in up to 60% of cases in adults. The bleeding is arterial and usually from a single diverticulum. It is acute, painless, and can be alarming in its volume. However, in most patients the blood loss stops spontaneously.

Angiodysplasia

Angiodysplastic lesions are acquired submucosal vascular ectasia and account for up to 12% of cases of lower gastrointestinal bleeding in adults. Rare vascular anomalies include arteriovenous malformation, haemangioma, and syndromes such as hereditary haemorrhagic telangiectasia. Blood loss is usually chronic, although a minority can present with acute haemorrhage. Although most cases tend to resolve spontaneously, they often re-bleed.

Neoplasia

Neoplasms of the bowel present as painless bleeding and may have associated symptoms of weight loss, altered bowel habit, abdominal pain or intestinal obstruction.

Inflammatory bowel disease (see Chapter 7.11)

Small to moderate amounts of bright blood mixed in with the stool occur in patients with ulcerative colitis and Crohn's disease. These patients are usually young (25–30 years) with widespread disease.

Colitis

Colitis can be due to parasitic and bacterial infections, ischaemic bowel and post-radiation therapy. Haemorrhagic radiation proctitis is a potential complication of prostate brachytherapy.

Anorectal disorders (see chapter 7.14)

Haemorrhoids are the most common cause of rectal bleeding, usually causing intermittent painless bleeding associated with defecation. Rectal varices may occur in association with portal hypertension. It is prudent to remember that benign anorectal disease on examination does not exclude the possibility of a more proximal source of bleeding or pathology.

Aortoenteric fistula

This complication occurs as a rare sequela of endovascular abdominal aortic aneurysm repairs and is probably due to inflammation and prosthetic leak. There may be a 'herald bleed' prior to catastrophic exsanguinating haemorrhage. High levels of suspicion should be maintained for all patients with gastrointestinal bleeding and previous abdominal aortic aneurysm repair.

Miscellaneous

Rectal ulcers may result from local trauma due to insertion of foreign bodies and aberrant sexual practices. Non-steroidal anti-inflammatory drugs (NSAIDs), inherited or acquired bleeding disorders, and rarely, infection in association with HIV, need to be considered.

History

Patients' estimates of blood loss are unreliable. However, the number and frequency of bowel movements, their colour and composition (e.g. mixed with stool, presence of clots), associated symptoms (e.g. abdominal pain, weight loss) and symptoms of volume depletion (syncope, dizziness, dyspnoea) are helpful. The diagnosis of neoplasia may be suggested by a history of altered bowel habit or abdominal pain, and constitutional symptoms such as weight loss and lethargy. Pain is unusual with bleeding from diverticular disease or angiodysplasia.

A history of haematemesis is useful in directing initial investigation to the upper tract (see Chapter 7.6). Enquiry should include past medical history (especially of cardiorespiratory disease), antithrombotic and antiplatelet therapy, NSAID use and alcohol intake.

Examination

Initial evaluation should focus on the assessment of haemodynamic stability. Respiratory rate is an important early indicator of shock. Orthostatic hypotension indicates a significant blood volume loss, although it can also be caused by drugs and autonomic dysfunction. Examination should look for abdominal signs, evidence of chronic liver disease and coagulopathy. Digital rectal examination is essential to confirm rectal bleeding and detect local pathology.

Investigations

Blood tests

A full blood examination (principally for anaemia) and serum electrolyte analysis (for renal function) is indicated in all but the young patient with mild bleeding and obvious anorectal disease. Other tests will be guided by the clinical presentation.

Endoscopy

Proctoscopy is particularly useful for the diagnosis of anorectal disease, offering the highest detection rate for haemorrhoids and anal fissures. Rigid or flexible sigmoidoscopy enables inspection of the mucosa of the rectum, sigmoid colon and distal descending colon. Colonoscopy offers the added ability to establish tissue diagnosis by biopsy and perform therapeutic interventions. It is the investigation of choice in the stable patient with adequate bowel preparation.

Imaging

Angiography

Selective mesenteric angiography has for many years been the investigation of choice for localization of bleeding, by injection of contrast into the superior mesenteric artery, inferior mesenteric artery and coeliac trunk, in sequential order. Sensitivity varies widely, but it is reported to detect bleeding at a rate of more than 0.5 mL/min. Angiography also offers a therapeutic option, through either selective vasopressin infusion or embolization. Unlike colonoscopy and scintigraphy, angiography does not require any special preparation.

CT

CT colonography, also known as virtual colonoscopy, is a relatively new technique that is becoming increasingly popular. This three-dimensional CT imaging is a sensitive diagnostic tool for the detection of colorectal polyps in cases with adequate bowel preparation. Magnetic resonance imaging (MRI) is another useful modality for rectal cancer and provides good visualization of important local prognostic factors. Endoscopic ultrasound is the modality of choice for small, superficial tumours. Given its current promise of offering high sensitivity, specificity and accuracy, the indications for positron emission tomography (PET) may well expand in the future, but its final role is yet to be confirmed.

Double-contrast barium enema

Barium studies have no place in the acute setting, largely because of practical difficulties and an inadequately prepared bowel. In addition, it hampers subsequent diagnostic investigations, including angiography and colonoscopy. It lacks sensitivity in detecting smaller dysplastic lesions, and cannot provide a tissue diagnosis. Barium studies may complement colonoscopy if a source is not found, or may be used in conjunction with sigmoidoscopy in the younger patient.

Technetium-labelled red blood cell (^{99m}Tc RBC) scans

The role of nuclear scintigraphic imaging is controversial. It has high sensitivity (up to 85%) and can detect bleeding at a rate as slow as 0.1 mL/min. However, its specificity is low (around 50%), and localization of the bleeding source is often imprecise. Serial scans can be obtained up to 36 hours after injection of the tracer, which may be useful in intermittent bleeding. It is reported to be 10 times more sensitive than mesenteric angiography in detecting ongoing bleeding.

Other investigations

If investigation of the colon has failed to identify a cause of bleeding, evaluation of the upper gastrointestinal tract (e.g. by gastroscopy) may be the most appropriate next step. Helical CT scanning of the abdomen and pelvis may occasionally be helpful. However, despite a range of modalities of investigation, no demonstrable bleeding source is identified in up to 10–20% of patients.

Treatment

The approach to the patient with rectal bleeding will differ depending on the severity of bleeding. The priorities are haemodynamic stabilization, localization of the bleeding site, and the formulation of an interventional plan.

Minor intermittent bleeding

Proctoscopy and rigid sigmoidoscopy can potentially be performed in the ED, although performer experience and adequate bowel preparation need to be considered. After initial assessment, many patients with mild bleeding or bleeding that has ceased can be investigated on an outpatient basis. Those discharged home should have adequate arrangements for outpatient follow-up with either a surgical or a gastroenterology service. The presence of anorectal pathology requires proximal evaluation of the colon in those aged over 50. The extent of further investigation in the younger age group is dependent on the clinician as well as predisposing factors for malignancy.

Major and/or persistent rectal bleeding

Immediate assessment should follow the standard ABC approach, with care to ensure adequate fluid resuscitation, followed by blood products if necessary. A haemodynamically stable, resuscitated patient has less morbidity and improved tolerance of further procedures. Most severe bleeding will cease spontaneously, and further investigation can proceed when the bowel has been properly prepared. In some cases, bleeding continues and active management is required on an emergency basis. Early colonoscopy preceded by bowel preparation with saline/polyethylene glycol results in improved diagnostic and treatment rates. Technetium-labelled red blood cell scanning and angiography are valuable adjuncts.

Treatment

Vasopressin may give temporary control of bleeding, with significant reported success. Colonoscopic control of bleeding is achieved in most cases. Risks include re-bleeding and perforation. In addition to proven efficacy, emergency colonoscopy may be the most cost-effective management approach. Other treatment modalities include electrocoagulation, laser and polypectomy. Most success has been achieved in cases of angiodysplasia, and occasionally with diverticulosis. Transcatheter embolization of angiodysplastic lesions has been reported, but has a significant risk of intestinal ischaemia and infarction. If the bleeding source is unknown, an upper gastrointestinal endoscopy should be considered prior to surgical exploration.

Surgery is most useful as an interval procedure in a resuscitated stable patient for definitive treatment of an established diagnosis. Emergency surgery has a high morbidity and mortality, as patients are usually elderly and haemodynamically unstable. Laparotomy is indicated if the patient continues to bleed and if non-operative management is unsuccessful.

Conclusion

Rectal bleeding is a common problem but rarely acutely life-threatening. Large-volume rectal bleeding can cause shock. Resuscitation should include active intravascular volume replacement with appropriate fluids and blood products. Surgical colleagues should be involved early so that plans can be made regarding appropriate investigation and intervention.

Further reading

Blachar A, Sosna J. CT colonography (virtual colonoscopy): technique, indications and performance. Digestion 2007; 76: 34–41.

Burling D, East JE, Taylor SA. Investigating rectal bleeding. British Medical Journal 2007; 335: 1260–1262.

Cagir B, Cirincione E. Lower gastrointestinal bleeding: surgical perspective. www.emedicine.com/med/topic2818.htm. Accessed December 2007.

Demarkles MP, Murphy JR. Acute lower gastrointestinal bleeding. Medical Clinics of North America 1993; 77: 1085–1099.

Douek M, Wickramasinghe M, Clifton MA. Does isolated rectal bleeding suggest colorectal cancer? Lancet 1999; 354: 393.

Ellis DJ, Reinus JF. Lower intestinal haemorrhage. Critical Care Clinics 1995; 11: 369–387.

Fleischer DE, Goldberg S, Browning T et al. Detection and surveillance of colorectal cancer. Journal of the American Medical Association 1992; 61: 580–585.

Gane EJ, Lane MR. Colonoscopy in unexplained lower gastrointestinal bleeding. New Zealand Medical Journal 1992; 105: 31–33.

Helfaud M, Marton KI, Zimmer-Gembeck MK. et al. History of visible rectal bleeding in a primary care population. Initial assessment and 10 year follow-up. Journal of the American Medical Association 1997; 1277: 44–48.

Jenson DM, Machicado GA. Diagnosis and treatment of severe hematochezia: the role of urgent colonoscopy after purge. Gastroenterology 1988; 95: 1569–1574.

Katkov WN. Case records of the Massachusetts General Hospital. Case 14–1992. New England Journal of Medicine 1992; 326: 936.

Korkis AM, McDougall CJ. Rectal bleeding in patients less than 50 years of age. Digestive Disease Sciences 1995; 40: 1520–1523.

Lichtiger S, Kornbluth A, Saloman P, et al. Lower gastrointestinal bleeding. In: Taylor MB, Gollan JL, Peppercorn MA et al., eds, Gastrointestinal emergencies. Baltimore: Williams & Wilkins, 1992.

Machicado GA, Jensen DM. Acute and chronic management of lower GI bleeding: Cost effective approaches. Gastroenterologist 1997; 5: 189–201.

Mehanna D, Platell C. Investigating chronic, bright red, rectal bleeding. Australia and New Zealand Journal of Surgery 2001; 71: 699–700.

Rana A. 2004 Gastrointestinal bleeding, lower. www.emedicine.com/radio/topic301.htm Accessed December 2007.

Richter JM, Christensen MR, Kaplan LM, et al. Effectiveness of current technology in the diagnosis and management of lower gastrointestinal haemorrhage. Gastrointestinal Endoscopy 1995; 41: 93–98.

Santos JC Jr, Aprilli F, Guimaraes AS, et al. Angiodysplasia of the colon: endoscopic diagnosis and treatment. British Journal of Surgery 1998; 75: 256–258.

Zuckerman DA, Bocchini TP, Birnbaum EH. Massive haemorrhage in the lower gastrointestinal tract in adults: diagnostic imaging and intervention. American Journal of Roentgenology 1993; 161: 703–711.

7.14 Perianal conditions

Andrew Dent • Michael Augello

ESSENTIALS

1 Perianal and pilonidal abscesses require incision and drainage. In some cases this can be done safely in the emergency department, but some surgeons prefer that all anorectal abscesses be drained in theatre.

2 Incision and drainage of cutaneous abscesses is not associated with bacteraemia in immunocompetent, afebrile adults, so routine antibiotic cover is not required.

3 Supralevator, intersphincteric and ischiorectal abscesses require formal surgical exploration and drainage in theatre.

4 Irreducible haemorrhoids require urgent reduction and surgery.

Pilonidal disease

Pilonidal disease is an acquired recurrent disease of young adults, affecting men twice as often as women. The natural history of the disease is for spontaneous regression in the fourth decade of life.[1] The pathological basis of the condition is the migration of loose hair ends into the natal cleft, where they become embedded and cause irritation. A pilonidal sinus or abscess may then form around these loose hairs. Patients who present usually describe a painful lump in the sacrococcygeal area, with or without seropurulent discharge, sometimes after a preceding period of prolonged sitting or physical exercise. Systemic symptoms are uncommon. Examination reveals an abscess in the presacral area about 5 cm cephalad to the anus, with one or more midline draining pits or sinuses. Occasionally hair is seen protruding from a pit.

The optimal treatment strategy is controversial. Initial treatment for a pilonidal abscess should be a cruciate incision, just off the midline or over the area where the abscess is pointing, with drainage and evacuation of pus and hair. This may take place under local or general anaesthesia, and in up to 58% of patients no further treatment is required. Healing may take up to 10 weeks, so additional surgery should not be considered early.[2,3] Prevention of recurrence by careful attention to hair control with natal cleft shaving and improved perineal hygiene is recommended.[4] More aggressive complex procedures, including various forms of open and closed excision and marsupialization, should probably be reserved for disease that fails more simple procedures, as they produce similar results at greater cost and more loss of working days.[3,5]

Anorectal abscesses

Anorectal abscesses are two to three times more common in men than in women. In most cases no specific aetiological cause can be found, but specific factors may include inflammatory bowel disease, infection, trauma, surgery, malignancy, radiation and immunosuppression. Clinically they tend to present with perianal pain, swelling, and sometimes fever. Examination reveals a tender, erythematous and fluctuant mass. Complex and recurrent anorectal abscesses may be well delineated by intrarectal ultrasound.[6] One classification is according to the four potential anorectal spaces they may occupy.

Perianal abscess

Perianal abscess presents as a painful lump around the anal verge, usually lateral and posterior to the anus. It may result from an infected anal gland or, more rarely, is a presentation of Crohn's disease. Systemic symptoms are uncommon. On examination most will be pointing, with an indurated red area which may be fluctuant.

Such abscesses can be drained under local anaesthesia, with the assistance of sedation or inhalation analgesia. Incision should be stab-like, circumferential to the anal ring, but long enough to allow complete evacuation of pus.

Ischiorectal abscess

Ischiorectal abscesses usually tend to be larger, yet may present with less dramatic cutaneous findings because of the compressibility of ischiorectal fat. Patients may be febrile and look toxic, with systemic symptoms. The area of induration is likely to be large and more lateral than a simple perianal abscesses. Pointing may not occur until late, and may seem more like buttock cellulitis. Treatment should be exploration and drainage under general anaesthesia, usually with proctosigmoidoscopy and possibly biopsy at the same time.

Supralevator abscess

This abscess arises from above the levator ani. In reality, it is a pelvic abscess and is often secondary to an intra-abdominal condition such as diverticular disease or Crohn's disease. Fever is common, and it may present as a pyrexia of unknown origin. The patient may present with pain on defaecation and altered bowel habit. Inspection of the perineum may be normal, but rectal examination will reveal a firm, spongy, tender mass. Treatment is

exploration and drainage under general anaesthesia by a surgeon with colorectal experience.

Intersphincteric or submucous abscess

These abscesses may be associated with severe pain and with urinary symptoms. They are within the anal canal, so no external swelling may be visible. They point within the anal canal and may rupture spontaneously. Treatment is exploration and drainage under general anaesthesia by a surgeon with colorectal experience.

Treatment

The treatment of all anorectal abscesses is incision and drainage. Depending on local practice, some small superficial abscesses may be able to be treated in the emergency department (ED) if anaesthesia to achieve adequate drainage can be achieved. Larger and more complicated abscesses are best treated under general anaesthesia by a surgeon with colorectal experience. The drained wound should be kept open long enough for the abscess to heal from below. This can be achieved by excising an ellipse of skin, or a cruciate incision with the skin edges excised, or by packing with a gauze wick. Aggressive probing of the cavity should be avoided as it can lead to iatrogenic fistulas. Regular review and dressing change should continue until healing is confirmed. The concern for the emergency physician is to identify those that can be safely drained in the ED without harming continence, causing seeding infection, or missing another diagnosis. Antibiotics are ineffective, and are only indicated in patients with valvular or rheumatic heart disease, diabetes, immunosuppression, extensive cellulitis or a prosthetic device.

Traditionally, in acute perianal abscesses the search for a fistulous internal opening followed by fistulotomy has been the standard treatment. Although fistulas are often present, immediate management of associated fistula tracts may result in higher rates of further fistulas, incontinence, and unnecessary treatment of fistulas that will resolve spontaneously and not require treatment.[7] Simple drainage is thus advocated for acute abscesses, as in most cases

this will be the only treatment required. The risk of recurrence is low.[8]

Anal fistula

Anal fistula rarely presents as an emergency de novo, but rather as recurrent perianal suppuration. A fistula is a connection between two epithelial surfaces, in this setting between rectal lumen and perianal skin. Fistula formation and recurrence following the first presentation of an anorectal abscess occurs in up to 50% of cases, and is more common with bowel-derived organisms such as *Escherichia coli* and *Bacterioides fragilis*.[9] Other causes include Crohn's disease, diverticular disease and, rarely, carcinoma. Diagnosis is suspected on a history of recurrent perianal suppuration and is confirmed by the delineation of fistulous tracks during surgery under anaesthesia. Fistula surgery can be difficult and complex, and recurrence is common.

Haemorrhoids

Haemorrhoidal tissue is a normal anatomic structure located in the anal canal that plays a role in differentiating between liquids, solids and gas, and maintaining anal continence. Haemorrhoids are composed of cushions of submucosal vascular tissue, usually located in the 3, 7 and 11 o'clock positions as viewed through a proctoscope with the patient in the lithotomy position. Haemorrhoidal disease occurs when there are symptoms such as bleeding, prolapse, pain, thrombosis, a mass, discharge or pruritus. Straining, inadequate fibre intake, prolonged sitting on the toilet, constipation, diarrhoea, pregnancy and other conditions with elevated intra-abdominal pressure have been suspected to contribute to the development of the disease.

The dentate line divides haemorrhoidal tissue into internal and external. Internal haemorrhoids are classically divided into four categories, depending on the degree of any prolapse. First-degree haemorrhoids do not prolapse, but cause symptoms by bleeding. Second-degree haemorrhoids prolapse, usually after straining at stool, but spontaneously reduce. Third-degree haemorrhoids prolapse and require digital replacement. Fourth-degree haemorrhoids are permanently prolapsed and cannot be reduced.

Bleeding is the most common symptom, and is typically painless and bright red. It is often described as a splash in the pan or streaks on toilet paper. Bleeding between bowel actions or blood mixed with the stool should raise suspicion of other pathologies, such as diverticular disease or carcinoma, and requires further investigation.

Examination involves observing the perineum with the patient straining. Redundant skin tags may be present. Grape-like structures may be seen to bulge around the classic 3, 7 and 11 o'clock positions. Proctosigmoidoscopy may reveal one or more haemorrhoids.

Differential diagnoses to consider include colorectal malignancy, inflammatory bowel disease, anal warts and other anorectal conditions. Some patients with haemorrhoidal symptoms should be evaluated further with colonoscopy to exclude more serious disease. These include patients with any suspicious findings on history or examination, iron-deficiency anaemia, positive faecal occult blood tests, those aged over 40 with a positive family history of neoplasia, and those aged over 50 with no recent colonoscopy.[10]

Treatment is directed at relieving symptoms. Conservative treatment is often successful, especially in lesser-grade disease. This includes increasing dietary fibre and using stool softeners to reduce straining and constipation, as well as anal hygiene such as Sitz baths. Increased dietary fibre reduces bleeding and overall symptoms.[11] There are many popular over-the-counter medications available, but despite their popularity there is limited high-level evidence for most topical medications. However, a recent randomized controlled trial of 0.2% glyceryl trinitrate paste (Rectogesic) applied topically showed a reduction in overall haemorrhoidal symptoms as well as bleeding.[12] Other over-the-counter products available include suppositories, creams, ointments, and pads that may contain ingredients such as local anaesthetics, corticosteroids, vasoconstrictors, antiseptics, keratolytics, protectants (such as mineral oils, cocoa butter), and astringents. There is no evidence that spicy food worsens haemorrhoidal symptoms.[13]

Procedural techniques used for more severe grades of disease that have failed conservative measures include rubber band ligation or sclerosant injection, progressing to more invasive surgical procedures including haemorrhoidectomy and stapled haemorrhoidopexy. All surgical techniques may be associated with a significant amount of postoperative pain and bleeding.

Prolapsed irreducible haemorrhoids

Prolapsed and oedematous irreducible haemorrhoids may become gangrenous and usually cause severe pain. Reduction can sometimes be achieved by the use of adequate analgesia, a foot-up tilted trolley, ice, local anaesthetic and firm slow pressure applied digitally. If successful, the requirement for surgery may change from emergency to urgent elective.

Thrombosed external haemorrhoids

This usually presents as a painful tender mass in the anus, frequently following an episode of constipation or diarrhoea. Examination reveals a bluish, exquisitely tender skin-covered lump sited lateral to the anus.

Surgical excision results in less pain on day 4, as well as reduced rates of recurrence at 1 year compared to incision alone or conservative treatment.[14,15] After the instillation of local anaesthetic, an elliptical piece of overlying skin and the associated thrombus are removed, leaving the skin open.[10] Incision and evacuation of the clot alone (without excision) is also widely practised, but has a higher rate of pain, bleeding and recurrence, and is less recommended than in the past. Conservative treatment will also ultimately result in resolution of symptoms but averaged 24 days in one study.[15]

Anal fissure

Anal fissure is a painful linear ulcer situated in the anal canal and extends from just below the dentate line to the margin of the anus. It has a similar incidence in both males and females, and is classically found in the posterior midline. Occasionally it is found in the anterior midline in women. The most widely accepted theory of its pathogenesis is that it results from the mechanical forces imposed on the anal canal during the passage of stool. Hard stool is most commonly implicated, although diarrhoea may also be associated. Most acute anal fissures heal spontaneously or with conservative treatment. Some go on to become chronic and develop secondary changes forming a fibrous skin tag, often referred to as a sentinel pile, as well as hypertrophied anal papillae and relative anal stenosis due to scarring. Anal hypertonicity and decreased blood flow to the anoderm, as well as constipation, is thought to contribute to the pathogenesis.

The history is often strongly suggestive of the condition. Typically, patients describe severe, knifelike, intense anal pain initiated during the passage of stool, described as being 'split open'. The pain may persist for hours, with a tight throbbing quality, and is usually accompanied by a small amount of bright red rectal blood, often as a smear on the toilet paper.

Inspection of the perineum may reveal tightening of the corrugator cutis ani, an almost diagnostic sign of anospasm that is usually secondary to a fissure. If a small midline 'sentinel' pile is seen, the diagnosis is confirmed. Gentle retraction of the perianal skin usually allows one to visualize the fissure directly. Rectal examination and proctosigmoidoscopy should be deferred until the acute pain has subsided. Anal fissure is sometimes complicated by abscess formation in the sentinel pile. This is suggested by a very swollen oedematous tag and requires surgical drainage.

Medical treatment is likely to be effective in acute fissures. Acute relief of pain and spasm around the acute fissure can be achieved by the use of local anaesthetic gel. Avoidance of constipation is probably the single most important non-operative treatment. Stool softeners, bulk-forming laxatives and high-fibre food are the mainstay of medical treatment. Warm baths may also help relieve sphincter spasm. Recurrence of symptoms after initial success with conservative treatment is not uncommon, but conservative treatment still has a good success rate on recurrent episodes.[16] Pharmacological agents that reduce internal sphincter tone and improve ano-dermal blood flow have also been used. Application of 0.2% glyceryl trinitrate ointment to the fissure two to three times daily may be successful in up to 88% of cases, but headache is a side effect and recurrence is common.[16,17] Injection with botulinum toxin is reported to be effective, but its optimal dose is unclear.[18,19] Topically applied calcium channel blockers (unavailable in Australia) have also been trialled, with initial good results but high rates of disease recurrence.[10]

Although most acute fissures can be dealt with conservatively as described, failure of medical treatment warrants surgical referral for consideration of sphincterotomy. Lateral internal sphincterotomy heals and relieves the symptoms of chronic anal fissure in more than 98% of patients.[10]

Pruritus ani

Pruritus ani is a dermatological condition characterized as an unpleasant itchy or burning sensation in the perianal region. Although it may be due to a definable perianal dermatological condition, including psoriasis, eczema and lichen sclerosis, most cases are idiopathic. Fungal, bacterial or parasitic infections such as pinworm and pediculosis are rare causes (except in children). Contributing factors may include excessive attempts at hygiene causing local irritation, loose stools, prolapsing haemorrhoids, and the frequent use of anorectal creams and ointments which may lead to perianal wetness with maceration of the skin and contact dermatitis. An itch and scratch cycle is then set up which can be very difficult to break. It is important to note that neoplasms such as Bowen's disease, lymphoma and Kaposi's sarcoma may cause pruritus.

Persistent itchiness in the anal region can be a difficult condition to treat. Potential identified causes should be treated appropriately. Idiopathic cases may benefit from reassurance, discontinuation of previously tried anorectal medications, and avoidance of irritants such as bar soap and vigorous scrubbing. Avoiding foods identified as exacerbating symptoms may be tried, as well as air-drying the area. A short course of topical hydrocortisone or sorbolene cream may provide relief and a break in the itch–scratch cycle.

Proctalgia fugax

Proctalgia fugax is the sudden and unpredictable onset of shearing or knife-like pain in the anus and rectum. It is usually of very short duration and is most common in males. It is thought to be due to dysfunction of the internal anal sphincter.[20] Apart from reassurance, no specific therapy is usually required. Salbutamol inhalation may shorten attacks of severe pain, but the mechanism of action is uncertain.[21]

Injuries to the perianal region

History is paramount and abuse needs to be excluded. Examination should focus on the function of the sphincter and be alert to the possibility of intra-abdominal extension of penetrating injuries. Where there is a history of foreign body insertion, plain films will determine position of the object and the presence or absence of free intra-abdominal gas.

Other anorectal conditions

Other important local conditions not covered in this chapter, but to be considered in the differential diagnosis of most anorectal conditions, include condylomata acuminata (warts associated with human papilloma virus), condylomata lata (flat white lesions associated with secondary syphilis), rectal prolapse and carcinoma. A complete anorectal examination reduces the risk of such conditions being missed or misdiagnosed.

Controversies

- Optimal treatment strategy for pilonidal abscesses.

- Role of drainage in ED of selected abscesses under local anaesthesia.

- Optimal surgical approach for treatment of high-grade haemorrhoidal disease.

- Optimal treatment for thrombosed external haemorrhoids.

- The relative efficacy of glyceryl trinitrate ointment, botulinum toxin and topical calcium channel blockers in treatment of acute anal fissure.

References

1. Clothier PR, Haywood IR. The natural history of the post anal (pilonidal) sinus. Annals of Royal College of Surgeons of England 1984; 66: 201–203.
2. Jensen SL, Harling H. prognosis after simple incision and drainage for a first episode acute pilonidal abscess. British Journal of Surgery 1988; 75: 60–61.
3. Hull T. Pilonidal disease. Surgical Clinics of North America 2002; 82: 1169–1185.
4. Armstrong JH, Barcia PJ. Pilonidal sinus disease. The conservative approach. Archives of Surgery 1994; 129: 914–919.
5. Aydede H, Erhan Y, Sukharya A, Kumkumoglu Y. Comparison of three methods in surgical treatment of pilonidal disease. Australia and New Zealand of Journal of Surgery 2001; 71: 362–364.
6. Cataldo PA, Senagore A, Luchtefeld MA. Intrarectal ultrasound in the evaluation of perirectal abscesses. Diseases of the Colon and Rectum 1993; 36: 554–558.
7. Rickard M. Anal abscesses and fistulas. Australia and New Zealand of Journal of Surgery 2005; 75: 64–72.
8. Tang CL, Chew SP, Seow-Choen F. Prospective randomized trial of drainage alone vs. drainage and fistulotomy for acute perianal abscesses with proven internal opening. Diseases of the Colon and Rectum 1996; 139: 1415–1417.
9. Janicke DM, Pundt MR. Anorectal disorders. Emergency Medicine Clinics of North America 1996; 14: 757–788.
10. Billingham RP, Isler JT, Kimmins MH. The diagnosis and management of common anorectal disorders. Current Problems in Surgery 2004; 41: 586–645.
11. Alonso-Coello P, Guyatt G, Heels-Ansdell D. Laxatives for the treatment of hemorrhoids. Cochrane Database Systematic Review (4): CD004649, 2005.
12. Tjandra JJ, Tan Y, Lim JF. Rectogesic® (glyceryl trinitrate 0.2%) ointment relieves symptoms of haemorrhoids associated with high resting anal canal pressures. Colorectal Diseases 2007; 9: 457–463.
13. Altomare DF, Rinaldi M, La Tore F, et al. Red Hot Chili Pepper and hemorrhoids: the explosion of a myth: results of a prospective, randomized, placebo-controlled, crossover trial. Diseases of the Colon and Rectum 2006; 49: 1018–1023.
14. Cavcic J, Turcic J, Martinac P, et al. Comparison of topically applied 0.2% glyceryl trinitrate ointment, incision and excision in the treatment of perianal thrombosis. Digestive and Liver Diseases 2001; 33: 335–340.
15. Greenspon, J, Williams SB, Young HA, et al. Thrombosed external hemorrhoids: Outcome after conservative or surgical management. Diseases of the Colon and Rectum 2004; 47: 1493–1498.
16. Lund JN, Armitage NC, Schofield JH. Use of glyceryl trinitrate ointment in the treatment of anal fissure. British Journal of Surgery 1996; 83: 776–777.
17. Beart R. Anorectal Surgery. Surgical Clinics of North America. 2002; 82: 1115–1297.
18. Watson J, Kamm MA, Nicholls RJ, et al. Topical glyceryl trinitrate in the treatment of chronic anal fissure. British Journal of Surgery 1996; 83: 771–775.
19. Hananel N, Gordon PH. Re-examination of clinical manifestations and response to therapy of fissure in ano. Diseases of the Colon and Rectum 1997; 40: 229–233.
20. Babb RR. Proctalgia fugax, would you recognise it? Postgraduate Medicine 1996; 99: 263–264.
21. Eckardt VF. Treatment of proctalgia fugax with salbutamol inhalation. American Journal of Gastroenterology 1996; 91: 686–689.

8.1 Headache

Anne-Maree Kelly

ESSENTIALS

1 The pathophysiological basis of headache is traction or inflammation of extracranial structures, the basal dura or the large intracranial arteries and veins; or dilatation/distension of cranial vascular structures.

2 Severity of headache is not a reliable indicator of the underlying pathology.

3 History is of paramount importance in the assessment of headache.

4 A normal physical examination does not rule out serious pathology.

5 Sudden, severe headache or chronic, unremitting headache is more likely to have a serious cause and should be investigated accordingly.

6 NSAIDs are the most effective treatment for tension headache.

7 As most patients have tried oral medications prior to attending the emergency department, parenterally administered agents are usually indicated for treatment of migraine.

8 Based on current evidence, the most effective agents for treating migraine are phenothiazines and triptans. Pethidine is not indicated because it is less effective than other agents, has a high rebound headache rate, and carries the potential for the development of dependence.

9 Carbamazepine is the agent of choice for treatment of trigeminal neuralgia.

Introduction

Headache is a common ailment that is often due to a combination of physical and psychological factors. The vast majority are benign and self-limiting and are managed by patients in the community.

Only a very small proportion of patients experiencing headache attend emergency departments (ED) for treatment. The challenges are to distinguish potentially life-threatening causes from the more benign, and to effectively manage the pain of headache.

Pathophysiology

The structures in the head capable of producing headache are limited. They include:

- Extracranial structures, including skin and mucosae, blood vessels, nerves, muscles and fascial planes.
- The main arteries at the base of the skull (as arteries branch they progressively lose the ability to produce painful stimuli).
- The great venous sinuses and their branches.
- The basal dura and dural arteries, but to a lesser extent than the other structures.

The bulk of the intracranial contents, including the parenchyma of the brain, the subarachnoid and pia mater and most of the dura mater, are incapable of producing painful stimuli.

The pathological processes that may cause headache are:

- Tension. This usually refers to contraction of muscles of the head and/or neck, and is thought to be the major factor in the so-called 'tension headache'.
- Traction. Traction is caused by stretching of intracranial structures due to a mass effect, as with a tumour. Pain caused by this mechanism is characteristically constant, but may vary in severity.

Table 8.1.1 A pathophysiological classification of headache

	Extracranial	Intracranial
Tension/traction	Muscular headache 'Tension headache'	Intracranial tumour Cerebral abscess Intracranial haematoma
Vascular	Migraine	Severe hypertension
Inflammatory	Temporal arteritis Sinusitis Otitis media Mastoiditis Tooth abscess Neuralgia	Meningitis Subarachnoid haemorrhage

- Vascular processes. These include dilatation or distension of vascular structures, and usually result in pain that is throbbing in nature.
- Inflammation. This may involve the dura at the base of the skull or the nerves or soft tissues of the head and neck. This mechanism is responsible for the initial pain of subarachnoid haemorrhage and meningitis, and for sinusitis.

The pathophysiological causes of headache are summarized in Table 8.1.1.

Assessment

In the assessment of a patient with headache, history is of prime importance. Specific information should be sought about the timing of the headache (in terms of both overall duration and speed of onset), the site and quality of the pain, relieving factors, the presence of associated features such as nausea and vomiting, photophobia and alteration in mental state, medical and occupational history and drug use.

Intensity of the pain is important from the viewpoint of management but is not a reliable indicator of the nature of underlying pathology. This said, sudden, severe headache and chronic, unremitting or progressive headache are more likely to have a serious cause.

Physical examination should include temperature, pulse rate and blood pressure measurements, assessment of conscious state and neck stiffness and neurological examination, including funduscopy (where indicated). Abnormal physical signs are uncommon, but the presence of neurological findings makes a serious cause probable. In addition, a search should be made for sinus, ear, mouth and neck pathology and muscular or superficial temporal artery tenderness.

Headache patterns

Some headaches have 'classic' clinical features: these are listed in Table 8.1.2. It must be remembered that, as with all diseases, there is a spectrum of presenting features and the absence of the classic features does not rule out a particular diagnosis. Every patient must be assessed on their merits and, if symptoms persist without reasonable explanation, further investigation should be undertaken.

Investigation

For the vast majority of patients with headache no investigation is required. The investigation of suspected subarachnoid haemorrhage and meningitis is discussed elsewhere in this book. If tumour is suspected, the investigations of choice are magnetic resonance imaging (MRI) or a contrast-enhanced computed tomography (CT) scan. An elevated ESR may be supporting evidence for a diagnosis of temporal arteritis. With respect to sinusitis, facial X-rays are of very limited value.

Table 8.1.2 Classic clinical complexes and cause of headache

Clinical complex	Cause
Preceded by an aura Throbbing unilateral headache, nausea Family history	Migraine
Sudden onset Severe occipital headache; 'like a blow' Worst headache ever	Subarachnoid haemorrhage
Throbbing/constant frontal headache Worse with cough, leaning forward Recent URTI Pain on percussion of sinuses	Sinusitis
Paroxysmal, fleeting pain Distribution of a nerve Trigger manoeuvres cause pain Hyperalgesia of nerve distribution	Neuralgia
Unilateral with superimposed stabbing Claudication on chewing Associated malaise, myalgia Tender artery with reduced pulsation	Temporal arteritis
Persistent, deep-seated headache Increasing duration and intensity Worse in morning Aching in character	Tumour: primary or secondary
Acute, generalized headache Fever, nausea and vomiting Altered level of consciousness Neck stiffness +/- rash	Meningitis
Unilateral, aching, related to eye Nausea and vomiting Raised intraocular pressure	Glaucoma
Aching, facial region Worse at night Tooth sensitive to heat, pressure	Dental cause

Tension headache

The pathological basis of tension headaches remains unclear, but increased tension of the neck or cranial muscles is a prominent feature. A family history of headaches is common, and there is an association with an injury in childhood or adolescence. The most common precipitants are stress and alteration in sleep patterns.

Aspirin, non-steroidal anti-inflammatory agents (NSAIDs) and paracetamol have all been shown to be effective in the treatment of tension headaches, with success rates between 50% and 70%. Ibruprofen 400 mg or ketoprofen 25–50 mg appear to be the most effective, followed by aspirin 600–1000 mg and paracetamol 1000 mg.

Migraine

Migraine can be a disabling condition for the sufferer. Most migraine headaches are successfully managed by the patient and their general practitioner, but a small number fail to respond or become 'fixed', and sufferers may present for treatment at EDs. As most patients (up to 80% in some studies) have tried oral medications prior to presenting, parenterally administered agents are usually indicated for ED treatment.

Migraine is a clinical diagnosis, and in the ED setting a diagnosis of exclusion. Other causes of severe headache, such as subarachnoid haemorrhage and meningitis, must be ruled out before this diagnosis is made. In particular, the response of the headache to anti-migraine therapy should not be used to assume that the cause was migraine. There have been reports that the headaches associated with subarachnoid haemorrhage and meningitis have, on occasion, responded to these agents.

Pathophysiology

The pathophysiology of migraine is complex and not completely understood. It is probably the result of interaction between the brain and the cranial circulation in susceptible individuals.

The phenomenon of 'cortical spreading depression' is probably the event underlying the occurrence of an aura in migraine.

This is a short-lasting depolarization wave that moves across the cerebral cortex. A brief phase of excitation is followed by prolonged depression of nerve cells. At the same time there is failure of brain ion homoeostasis, an efflux of excitatory amino acids from nerve cells, and increased energy metabolism. This phenomenon appears to be dependent on the activation of an N-methyl-D-aspartate receptor, which is a subtype of the glutamate receptor.

The headache pain of migraine seems to result from the activation of the trigeminovascular system. The trigeminal nerve transmits headache pain from both the dura and the pia mater. The triggers for the development of migraine headache are probably chemical and are thought to originate in the brain, the blood vessel walls and the blood itself. These triggers stimulate trigeminovascular axons, causing pain and the release of vasoactive neuropeptides, including calcium G-related peptide (CGRP) from perivascular axons. These neuropeptides act on mast cells, endothelial cells and platelets, resulting in increased extracellular levels of arachidonate metabolites, amines, peptides and ions. These mediators and the resultant tissue injury lead to a prolongation of pain and hyperalgesia.

Serotonin has also been specifically implicated in migraine. By activation of afferents, it causes a retrograde release of substance P. This in turn increases capillary permeability and oedema.

Classification and clinical features

Migraine is defined as an idiopathic recurring headache disorder with attacks that last 4–72 hours. Typical characteristics are unilateral location, pulsating quality, moderate or severe intensity, and aggravation by routine physical activity. There is also usually nausea, photophobia and phonophobia.

In some patients migraine is preceded by an 'aura' of neurological symptoms localizable to the cerebral cortex or brain stem, such as visual disturbance, paraesthesia, diplopia or limb weakness. These develop gradually over 5–20 minutes and last less than 60 minutes. Headache, nausea and/or photophobia usually follow after an interval of less than an hour.

Several variant forms of migraine have been defined, including ophthalmoplegic, abdominal, hemiplegic and retinal migraine, but all are uncommon. In ophthalmoplegic migraine the headache is associated with paralysis of one or more of the nerves supplying the ocular muscles. Horner's syndrome may also occur. Abdominal migraine manifests as recurrent episodes of abdominal pain for which no other cause is found. Retinal migraine, which is fortunately very rare, involves recurrent attacks of retinal ischaemia which may lead to bilateral optic atrophy. Hemiplegic migraine is a stroke mimic.

Treatment

The complexity of the mechanisms involved in the genesis of migraine suggests that there are a number of ways to interrupt the processes to provide effective relief from symptoms.

A wide variety of pharmacological agents and combinations of agents have been tried for the treatment of migraine, with varying results. Interpreting the evidence is challenging, as the majority of the studies have small sample sizes, compare different agents or combinations of agents, are conducted in settings other than EDs, and the outcome measure(s) tested varies widely. Because the ED migraine population appears to be different from the general outpatient population, the data presented here are based on studies in EDs.

The effectiveness of commonly used agents is summarized in Table 8.1.3. Dosing and administration are summarized in Table 8.1.4. At present the most effective agents seem to be the phenothiazines (chlorpromazine, prochlorperazine, droperidol and possibly haloperidol) and the triptans, each of which has achieved > 70% efficacy in a number of studies. Note that triptans are contraindicated in patients with a history of ischaemic heart disease, uncontrolled hypertension or with the concomitant use of ergot preparations.

Pethidine is not indicated for the treatment of migraine. Its reported effectiveness is only 56%, it has a high rate of rebound headache and it carries a risk of dependence. In two small RCTs haloperidol administered as 5 mg in 500 mL normal saline

Table 8.1.3   Pooled effectiveness data from ED studies of the treatment of migraine. (Clinical studies, defined 'success' endpoint, minimum of 50 patients studied in aggregate, NNT calculated assuming placebo effectiveness rate of 25%)

Agent	No. of studies	Total patients	Clinical success rate (%)	NNT: Clinical success
Chlorpromazine i.v.	6	171	85	1.67
Droperidol i.m.	3	233	83	1.72
Prochlorperazine (i.m. or i.v.)	4	113	79	1.85
Sumatriptan (s.c.)	5	659	69	2.27
Metoclopramide (i.v.)	5	169	67	2.38
Ketorolac (i.m. or i.v.)	6	155	66	2.44
Tramadol (i.m.)	2	174	59	2.94

Table 8.1.4   Drug dosing and administration

Agent	Drug dosing/administration
Chlorpromazine i.m.	12.5 mg intravenously, repeated every 20 minutes as needed to a maximum dose of 37.5 mg, accompanied by 1 L normal saline over 1 hour to avoid hypotension OR 25 mg in 1 L normal saline over 1 hour, repeated if necessary
Droperidol (i.m. or i.v.)	2.5 mg
Prochlorperazine (i.m. or i.v.)	10 mg/12.5 mg (depending on packaging)
Sumatriptan (s.c., i.n.)	6 mg SC, 20 mg i.n.
Metoclopramide (i.v.)	10–20 mg
Ketorolac (i.m. or i.v.)	30 mg i.v.; 60 mg i.m.
Tramadol (i.m.)	100 mg

was reported to give significant pain relief in more than 80% of patients. Lignocaine (lidocaine) has been shown to be no more effective than placebo. The data on dihydroergotamine are difficult to interpret because it is often used in combination with other agents, e.g. metoclopramide; however, it has also been shown to be less effective than chlorpromazine and sumatriptan in acute treatment, and to have a high rate of unpleasant side effects. There are insufficient data to assess the effectiveness of CGRP receptor antagonists. Sodium valproate has also shown moderate effectiveness in small studies, but there are insufficient data to draw a valid conclusion. The efficacy of intravenous magnesium sulphate (1 or 2 mg) remains unclear. It was shown in a small placebo-controlled trial to be effective, but in another study the combination of magnesium with metoclopramide was less effective than metoclopramide and placebo.

There is some preliminary evidence that oral or i.v. dexamethasone, in addition to standard migraine therapy for selected patients, may reduce the proportion of patients who experience early recurrence (so-called rebound headache). Unfortunately, different studies have identified different groups who might benefit. There are insufficient data to recommend this as standard therapy.

Trigeminal neuralgia

Trigeminal neuralgia is a debilitating condition in which patients describe 'lightning'- or a 'hot poker'-like pain that is severe and follows the distribution of the trigeminal nerve. Individual episodes of pain last only seconds, but may recur repeatedly within a short period and can be triggered by minor stimuli such as light touch, eating or drinking, shaving or passing gusts of wind. It is most common in middle or older age.

Pathophysiology

Evidence suggests that the pathological basis of trigeminal neuralgia is demyelination of sensory fibres of the trigeminal nerve in the proximal (CNS) portion of the nerve root or rarely in the brain stem, most commonly due to compression of the nerve root by an overlying artery or vein.

Treatment

The mainstay of therapy for trigeminal neuralgia is carbamazepine. The usual starting dose is 200–400 mg/day in divided doses, increased by 200 mg/day until relief up to a maximum of 1200 mg/day. The average dose required is 800 mg/day. There is preliminary evidence that baclofen alone and the addition of lamotrigene to carbamazepine or phenytoin may be effective. Case series suggest that in acute crises of trigeminal neuralgia subcutaneous sumatriptan or intravenous infusions of lidocaine, phenytoin or fosphenytoin may be helpful. Early reports also suggest that for second-division trigeminal neuralgia, lignocaine administered intranasally by metered-dose inhaler provides acute but temporary relief.

A significant proportion of patients fail to obtain adequate relief from medical therapy. In these cases interventions such as microvascular decompression or partial destruction of the trigeminal nerve (for example by glycerol injections, radiofrequency thermal ablation or stereotactic gamma knife radiosurgery) may be indicated.

Controversies

- Choice of drug therapy for migraine.

- Role and timing of investigations in atypical migraine. CT or MRI may be indicated acutely to rule out other intracranial pathology.

- The role of corticosteroids in prevention of recurrent/ rebound migraine.

- Role and timing of investigations, in particular neuroimaging, for persistent or atypical headache.

- Second-line treatment for trigeminal neuralgia.

Further reading

Australian and New Zealand College of Anaesthetists and Faculty of Pain Medicine. Acute pain management: scientific evidence, 2nd edn. Canberra: National Health and Medical Council (Australia) 2005.

Friedman BW, Greenwald P, Bania TC, et al. Randomized trial of IV dexamethasone for acute migraine in the emergency department. Neurology 2007 (Epub ahead of print).

Kelly AM. Specific pain syndromes: Headache. In: Mace S, Ducharme J, Murphy M, eds. Pain management and procedural sedation in the emergency department. New York: McGraw-Hill, 2006.

Kelly AM, Kerr D, Clooney M. Impact of oral dexamethasone versus placebo after ED treatment of migraine with phenothiazines on the rate of recurrent headache: a randomized controlled trial. Emergency Medicine Journal 2008; 25:26–29.

8.2 Stroke and transient ischaemic attacks

Philip Aplin

ESSENTIALS

1 Ischaemic strokes and transient ischaemic attacks (TIAs) are most commonly due to atherosclerotic thromboembolism of the cerebral vasculature or emboli from the heart. Other causes should be considered in younger patients, those presenting with atypical features, or when evaluation is negative for the more common aetiologies.

2 Haemorrhagic and ischaemic strokes cannot be reliably differentiated on clinical grounds alone, therefore further imaging, most commonly CT scanning, is required prior to the commencement of anticoagulant or thrombolytic therapy.

3 The risk of a completed stroke following a TIA is much higher than was previously appreciated (up to 30% in the first week). Clinical scoring systems such as the ABCD score have been proposed as an assessment tool for a stroke risk following TIA. This may help guide the urgency of investigations to detect a cause for a TIA, the treatment of which may prevent a subsequent major stroke.

4 Differentiating strokes from other acute neurological presentations may be difficult in the emergency department. This issue has implications for the use of high-risk therapies such as thrombolysis.

5 The early phase of stroke management concentrates on airway and breathing, rapid neurological assessment of conscious level, pupil size and lateralizing signs, and blood sugar measurements. Hyperglycaemia may worsen neurological outcome in stroke, and so glucose should not be given in likely stroke patients unless a low blood sugar level is objectively demonstrated.

6 Outcomes in stroke patients are improved when they are admitted to a dedicated stroke unit. This involves a multidisciplinary approach to all aspects of stroke management.

7 Treating doctors should be fully aware of the risks/benefits and indications/contraindications of thrombolytic therapy in treating acute strokes. Currently tPA is approved for use in selected acute ischaemic strokes when administered within 3 hours of symptom onset, but remains controversial.

Introduction

Cerebrovascular disease is the third highest cause of death in developed countries, after heart disease and cancer. A stroke is an acute neurological injury secondary to cerebrovascular disease, either by infarction (80%) or by haemorrhage (20%). The incidence of stroke is steady, and although mortality is decreasing, it is still a leading cause of long-term disability. Transient ischaemic attacks (TIAs) have traditionally been defined as a focal loss of brain function attributed to cerebral ischaemia that lasts less than 24 hours, although most last considerably less time than this. Causes are similar to those of ischaemic stroke, particularly atherosclerotic thromboembolism related to the cerebral circulation and cardioembolism. Diagnosis of the cause of TIAs with appropriate management is important in order to prevent a potentially devastating stroke.

Pathophysiology

Brain tissue is very sensitive to the effects of oxygen deprivation. Following cerebral vascular occlusion a series of metabolic consequences may ensue, depending on the extent, duration and vessels involved, which can lead to cell death. Reperfusion of occluded vessels may also occur, either spontaneously or via therapeutic intervention, with a potential for reperfusion injury. An area of threatened but possibly salvageable brain may surround an area of infarction. The identification of this so-called ischaemic penumbra, and therapeutic efforts to ameliorate the extent of irreversible neuronal damage, have been the subject of ongoing research efforts.

Large anterior circulation ischaemic strokes can be associated with increasing mass effect and intracranial pressure in the hours to days following onset. Secondary haemorrhage into an infarct may also occur, either spontaneously or related to therapy. Clinical deterioration often follows.

Ischaemic strokes

These are the results of several pathological processes (Table 8.2.1):

Table 8.2.1 Causes of stroke

Ischaemic stroke

Arterial thromboembolism
    Carotid and vertebral artery atheroma
    Intracranial vessel atheroma
    Small vessel disease – lacunar infarction
    Haematological disorders – hypercoagulable
    states
Cardioembolism
    Aortic and mitral valve disease
    Atrial fibrillation
    Mural thrombus
    Atrial myxoma
    Paradoxical emboli
Hypoperfusion
    Severe vascular stenosis or a combination of
    these factors]
    Hypotension]
    Vasoconstriction – drug induced, post SAH,
    pre-eclampsia
Other vascular disorders
    Arterial dissection
    Gas embolism syndromes
    Moyamoya disease
    Arteritis

Intracerebral haemorrhage

Hypertensive vascular disease –
Lipohyalinosis and microaneurysms
Aneurysms
    Saccular
    Mycotic
Arteriovenous malformations
Amyloid angiopathy
Bleeding diathesis
    Anticoagulation
    Thrombolytics
    Thrombocytopenia/disseminated
    intravascular coagulation
    Haemophilia
Secondary haemorrhage into a lesion – tumour
or infarction

- Ischaemic strokes are most commonly due to thromboembolism originating from the cerebral vasculature, the heart, or occasionally the aorta. Thrombosis usually occurs at the site of an atherosclerotic plaque secondary to a combination of shear-induced injury of the vessel wall, turbulence and flow obstruction. Vessel wall lesions may also be the site of emboli that dislodge and subsequently occlude more distal parts of the cerebral circulation. Atherosclerotic plaque develops at the sites of vessel bifurcation. Lesions affecting the origin of the internal carotid artery (ICA) are the most important source of thromboembolic events. The more distal intracerebral branches of the ICA, the aorta and the vertebrobasilar system are also significant sites. Acute plaque change is likely to be the precipitant of symptomatic cerebrovascular disease, particularly in patients with carotid stenosis. Hence the most effective therapies will probably not only target the consequences of acute plaque change, such as thrombosis and embolism, but also aim for plaque stabilization using such agents as antiplatelet drugs, statins and antihypertensive drugs along the lines used in the management of acute coronary syndromes.

- Approximately 20% of cerebrovascular events are due to emboli originating from the heart. Rarely emboli may arise from the peripheral venous circulation, the embolus being carried to the cerebral circulation via a patent foramen ovale.

- Lipohyalinosis of small arteries is a degenerative process associated with diabetes and hypertension that mainly affects the penetrating vessels that supply areas such as the subcortical white matter, and is the postulated cause of lacunar infarcts.

- Dissection of the carotid or vertebral arteries may cause TIAs and stroke. This may occur spontaneously or following trauma to the head and neck region, particularly in young people not thought to be at risk of stroke. Distal embolization from the area of vascular injury is the main pathological process involved.

- Haemodynamic reduction in cerebral flow may occur as a result of systemic hypotension or severe carotid stenosis. In these cases cerebral infarction typically occurs in a vascular watershed area.

- The cerebral vasoconstriction that may occur in association with subarachnoid haemorrhage (SAH), migraine and pre-eclampsia, and with drugs such as sympathomimetics and cocaine, may precipitate stroke.

- Less common vascular disorders such as arteritis, venous sinus thrombosis, sickle cell disease and moyamoya disease may be causes of stroke.

- Venous sinus thrombosis may occur spontaneously or in relation to an underlying risk factor such as an acquired or congenital prothrombotic disorder, dehydration or meningitis. The consequences depend on the extent and localization of the thrombosis. Stroke secondary to venous thrombosis is due to venous stasis, increased hydrostatic pressures and associated haemorrhage.

Haemorrhagic stroke

Haemorrhagic stroke is the result of vessel rupture into the surrounding intracerebral tissue or subarachnoid space. Subarachnoid haemorrhage is the subject of a separate chapter in this book (see Chapter 8.3). The neurological defect associated with an intracerebral haemorrhage is the consequence of direct brain injury, secondary occlusion of nearby vessels, reduced cerebral perfusion caused by associated raised intracranial pressure, and cerebral herniation. The causes of intracerebral haemorrhage (ICH) include:

- Aneurysmal vessel dilatation. Vascular dilatation occurs at a site of weakness in the arterial wall, resulting in an aneurysm that expands until it ruptures into the subarachnoid space, and in some cases the brain tissue as well.

- Arteriovenous malformation (AVM). A collection of weakened vessels exists as a result of abnormal development of the arteriovenous connections. AVMs may rupture to cause haemorrhagic stroke, or more rarely cause cerebral ischaemia from a 'steal' phenomenon.

- Hypertensive vascular disease. Lipohyalinosis, mentioned above as a cause of microatheromatous infarcts, is also responsible for rupture of small penetrating vessels causing haemorrhage in characteristic locations, typically the putamen, thalamus, upper brain stem and cerebellum.

- Amyloid angiopathy. Postmortem pathological examination has found these changes, particularly in elderly patients with lobar haemorrhages.

- Haemorrhage into an underlying lesion, e.g. tumour or infarction.

- Drug toxicity from sympathomimetics and cocaine.

- Anticoagulation and bleeding diatheses.

Prevention

This particularly applies to ischaemic strokes. Non-modifiable risk factors for stroke include:

- Increasing age: the stroke rate more than doubles for each 10 years above age 55.
- Gender: slightly more common in males than females.
- Family history.

Primary prevention

Hypertension is the most important modifiable risk factor. The benefit of antihypertensive treatment in stroke prevention has been well shown. The other major risk factors for atherosclerosis and its complications – diabetes, smoking and hypercholesterolaemia – often contribute to increased stroke risk. These should be managed according to standard guidelines. The most important cardiac risk factor for TIA and stroke is atrial fibrillation, both chronic and paroxysmal. Warfarin is recommended to prevent cardioembolism, except in unsuitable patients. Those with contraindications to warfarin should initially receive aspirin. Other major cardiac risk factors include endocarditis, mitral stenosis, prosthetic heart valves, recent myocardial infarction and left ventricular aneurysm. Less common risk factors include atrial myxoma, a patent foramen ovale and cardiomyopathies.

A carotid bruit or carotid stenosis found in an otherwise asymptomatic patient is associated with an increased stroke risk. However, the role of carotid endarterectomy in these patients is controversial. In a highly selected patient group, the asymptomatic carotid atherosclerosis study (ACAS)[1] showed a small but significant benefit in reduction of stroke or death at 5 years following surgery for angiographically proven stenosis >60% compared to medical therapy. The benefit was much lower than that achieved in symptomatic carotid stenosis shown in the North American Symptomatic Carotid Endarterectomy Study (NASCET 2),[2] and can only be achieved with low perioperative mortality and stroke rates.

Secondary prevention

This relates principally to the prevention of a disabling stroke following a TIA or minor stroke, and will be covered under Investigation and Management of TIAs.

Ischaemic stroke syndromes

The symptoms and signs of stroke or TIA correspond to the area of the brain affected by ischaemia or haemorrhage (Table 8.2.2).

In ischaemic brain injury the history and pattern of physical signs may correspond to a characteristic clinical syndrome according

Table 8.2.2 Location of TIA			
		Arterial territory	
Symptom	Carotid	Either	Vertebrobasilar
Dysphasia	+		
Monocular visual loss	+		
Unilateral weakness*		+	
Unilateral sensory disturbance*		+	
Dysarthria**		+	
Homonymous hemianopia		+	
Dysphagia**		+	
Diplopia**			+
Vertigo**			+
Bilateral simultaneous visual loss			+
Bilateral simultaneous weakness			+
Bilateral simultaneous sensory disturbance			+
Crossed sensory/motor loss			+

*Usually regarded as carotid distribution
**Not necessarily a transient ischaemic attack if an isolated symptom.
(Reproduced with permission from Hankey GJ. Management of first time transient ischaemic attack. Emergency Medicine 2001; 13: 70–81)

to the underlying cause and the vessel occluded. This has a bearing on the direction of further investigation and treatment decisions. Differentiating between anterior and posterior circulation ischaemia/infarction is important in this respect, but is not always possible on clinical grounds alone.

Determining the cause of the event is the next step. Once again, clues may be present on clinical evaluation. For accurate delineation of the site of the lesion, exclusion of haemorrhage and assessment of the underlying cause, it is usually necessary to undertake imaging studies.

Anterior circulation ischaemia

The anterior circulation supplies blood to 80% of the brain and consists of the ICA and its branches, principally the ophthalmic, middle cerebral and anterior cerebral arteries. Hence this system supplies the optic nerve, retina, frontoparietal and most of the temporal lobes. Ischaemic injury involving the anterior cerebral circulation commonly has its origins in atherothrombotic disease of the ICA. Atherosclerosis of this artery usually affects the proximal 2 cm, just distal to the division of the

common carotid artery. Advanced lesions may be the source of embolism to other parts of the anterior circulation, or cause severe stenosis with resultant hypoperfusion distally if there is inadequate collateral supply via the Circle of Willis. This is usually manifest by signs and symptoms in the middle cerebral artery (MCA) territory (Table 8.2.3). Less commonly, lesions of the intracranial ICA and MCA may cause similar clinical features.

Embolism to the ophthalmic artery or its branches causes monocular visual symptoms of blurring, loss of vision and field defects. When transient, this is referred to

Table 8.2.3 Signs of middle cerebral artery (MCA) occlusion
Homonymous hemianopia
Contralateral hemiplegia affecting face and arm more than leg
Contralateral hemisensory loss
Dysphasias with dominant hemispheric involvement (usually left)
Spatial neglect and dressing apraxia with non-dominant hemispheric involvement.

as amaurosis fugax, or transient monocular blindness.

The anterior cerebral artery territory is the least commonly affected by ischaemia because of the collateral supply via the anterior communicating artery. If occlusion occurs distally or the collateral supply is inadequate, then ischaemia may occur. This manifests as sensory/motor changes in the leg – more so than in the arm. More subtle changes of personality may occur with frontal lobe lesions, as may disturbances of micturition and conjugate gaze.

Major alterations of consciousness, with Glasgow Coma Scores <8, imply bilateral hemispheric or brainstem dysfunction. The brain stem may be primarily involved by a brainstem stroke or secondarily affected by an ischaemic or haemorrhagic lesion elsewhere in the brain, owing to a mass effect and/or increased intracranial pressure.

Posterior circulation ischaemia

Ischaemic injury in the posterior circulation involves the vertebrobasilar arteries and their major branches which supply the cerebellum, brain stem, thalamus, medial temporal and occipital lobes. Posterior cerebral artery occlusion is manifested by visual changes of homonymous hemianopia (typically with macular sparing if the MCA supplies this part of the occipital cortex). Cortical blindness, of which the patient may be unaware, occurs with bilateral posterior cerebral artery infarction.

Brainstem and cerebellar involvement manifests as a combination of motor and sensory abnormalities, which may be uni- or bilateral; cerebellar features of vertigo nystagmus and ataxia; and cranial nerve signs of ophthalmoplegia, diplopia, facial weakness and dysarthria.

Specific brainstem syndromes include:

- Lateral medullary syndrome: Clinical features include sudden onset of vertigo, nystagmus, ataxia, ipsilateral loss of facial pain and temperature sensation with contralateral loss of pain and temperature sensation of the limbs, ipsilateral Horner's syndrome and dysarthria and dysphagia.
- 'Locked-in' syndrome: This is caused by bilateral infarction of a ventral pons, with or without medullary involvement. The patient is conscious due to an intact

brainstem articular formation, but cannot speak and is paralysed. Patients can move their eyes due to sparing of the third and fourth cranial nerves in the midbrain.

Lacunar infarcts

Lacunar infarcts are associated primarily with hypertension and diabetes. They occur in the small penetrating arteries supplying the internal capsule, thalamus and upper brain stem. Isolated motor or sensory deficits are most commonly seen.

Pre-hospital care

The pre-hospital care of the possible stroke patient involves the usual attention to the ABCs of resuscitation and early blood sugar measurement; however, it is unusual for interventions to be required.

Of potentially greater significance is the development of stroke systems (along the lines of trauma systems) in which the sudden onset of neurological signs and symptoms, identified in the pre-hospital evaluation as being consistent with acute stroke, is then used to direct patients to stroke centres with the facilities and expertise to manage them, particularly with regard to the delivery of thrombolytic agents. Closer hospitals without these capabilities may be bypassed. Studies of stroke centres have shown an increase in the use of thrombolytic agents and admission to stroke units. The effect on outcomes continues to be evaluated.

A pre-hospital evaluation tool that has been developed and validated is the Cincinatti Prehospital Stroke Scale or FAST: F –facial movements, A –arm movements, S – speech, and T – test.[3] Pre-hospital personnel who identify patients with acute onset of neurological deficits identified using this simple scale can then notify the ED in order to mobilize appropriate staff and forewarn Radiology, so as to expedite assessment and imaging, particularly if thrombolysis is being considered.

Clinical evaluation in the ED

History

This includes the circumstances, time of onset, associated symptoms such as

headache, and any resolution/progression of signs and symptoms. It may be necessary to take a history from a relative or friend, particularly in the presence of dysphasia or reduced conscious state. The history of a stroke is usually of acute onset of a neurological deficit over minutes, but occasionally there may be a more gradual or stuttering nature to a presentation over a period of hours. A past history of similar events suggestive of a TIA should be carefully sought. The presence of a severe headache with the onset of symptoms may indicate ICH. However, headache may also occur with ischaemic strokes.

A declining level of consciousness may indicate increasing intracranial pressure due to an ICH or a large anterior circulation infarct – so-called malignant MCA infarction. It may also be caused by pressure on the brain stem by an infratentorial lesion such as a cerebellar haemorrhage.

The possibility of trauma or drug abuse should be remembered along with the past medical and medication history, particularly anticoagulant/antiplatelet therapy. Risk factors for vascular disease, cardiac embolism, venous embolism and increased bleeding should be sought.

In young patients with an acute neurological deficit, dissection of the carotid or vertebral artery should be considered. This is often associated with neck pain and headaches/facial pain with or without a history of neck trauma, which may be minor, as in a twisting or hyperextension/flexion injury sustained in a motor vehicle accident, playing sports or neck manipulation.

Cardioembolism tends to produce ischaemic injury in different parts of the brain, resulting in non-stereotypical recurrent TIAs, whereas atherothrombotic disease of the cerebral vessels tends to cause recurrent TIAs of a similar nature, particularly in stenosing lesions of the internal carotid or vertebrobasilar arteries.

Examination

Central nervous system

This includes assessing the level of consciousness, pupil size and reactivity, extent of neurological deficit, presence of neck stiffness and funduscopy for signs of papilloedema and retinal haemorrhage. Quantifying the neurological deficit using a stroke scale such as the 42-point National Institute of Health Stroke Scale (NIHSS)[4] is useful in the initial assessment, and also for monitoring progress in a more objective way than clinical description alone. Strokes with a NIHSS score >22 are classified as severe.

In the case of TIA all clinical signs may have resolved. The average TIA lasts less than 15 minutes.

Cardiovascular

This includes carotid auscultation and is directed towards findings associated with a cardioembolic source. A carotid bruit in a symptomatic patient is likely to predict a moderate to severe carotid stenosis. Conversely, the absence of a carotid bruit does not exclude significant carotid artery disease as a cause of a TIA or stroke. Major risk factors for cardioembolism that can be identified in the ED include atrial fibrillation, mitral stenosis, prosthetic heart valves, infective endocarditis, recent myocardial infarction, left ventricular aneurysm and cardiomyopathies. Obviously an ECG is an important part of this assessment.

Differential diagnosis
(Table 8.2.4)

The acute onset of stroke and TIA is characteristic; however, misdiagnoses can occur, even by experienced clinicians. The most common are seizures (particularly when there is associated Todd's paresis), systemic infection, brain tumour and toxic metabolic disorders. Others include subdural haematoma, hypertensive encephalopathy, encephalitis, multiple sclerosis, migraine and conversion disorder. This has implications when considering more aggressive stroke interventions, such as thrombolysis.

Complications of stroke

CNS complications include:

- Cerebral oedema and raised intracranial pressure (ICP). This is an uncommon problem in the first 24 hours following ischaemic stroke, but it may occur with large anterior circulation infarcts. It is more commonly seen with ICH, where acutely raised ICP may lead to herniation

Table 8.2.4 Differential diagnosis of stroke
Intracranial space-occupying lesion
Subdural haematoma
Brain tumour
Brain abscess
Postictal neurological deficit – Todd's paresis
Head injury
Encephalitis
Metabolic or drug-induced encephalopathy
Hypoglycaemia, hyponatraemia etc.
Wernicke–Korsakoff syndrome
Drug toxicity
Hypertensive encephalopathy
Multiple sclerosis
Migraine
Peripheral nerve lesions
Functional

and brainstem compression in the first few hours.

- Haemorrhagic transformation of ischaemic strokes may occur either spontaneously or associated with treatment.
- Seizures can also occur and should be treated in the standard way. Seizure prophylaxis is not generally recommended.
- Non-CNS complications include aspiration pneumonia, hypoventilation, DVT and pulmonary embolism, urinary tract infections and pressure ulcers. In the ED it is particularly important to be aware of the risk of aspiration.

Investigations

The investigations of TIA and stroke often overlap, but the priorities and implications for management may differ significantly.

General

Standard investigations that may identify contributing factors to stroke/TIA or guide therapy include: a complete blood picture, blood glucose, coagulation profile, electrolytes, liver function tests and CRP (in selected cases). Arterial blood gases performed if the adequacy of ventilation is in doubt. An ECG should be performed to identify arrhythmias and signs of pre-existing cardiac disease. Holter monitoring can be considered to identify paroxysmal arrhythmias, but has a low yield. A prothrombotic screen may be indicated, particularly in younger patients. Further investigations depend on the nature of the neurological deficit and other risk factors for stroke that are identified on evaluation, but usually involve a combination of brain, vascular and cardiac imaging.

TIAs and non-disabling strokes should be evaluated similarly in order to promptly diagnose and manage a potentially treatable process that might lead to a subsequent major stroke. The risk of a stroke following a TIA is now appreciated to be much higher than previously thought, and may be as high as 30% in the first week. The ABCD stroke risk score from TIA has been developed and validated to evaluate the risk of a stroke in the first 7 days following a TIA.[5] This has the potential to guide the urgency of investigations, such as carotid ultrasound, required to determine the underlying causes of the TIA. The scoring system is outlined in Table 8.2.5. In patients with an ABCD score <4 there is minimal short-term risk of stroke. With scores of 4, 5 and 6 the risk is 2.2%, 16.5% and 35%, respectively. Other patient groups are at increased risk of stroke independent of the ABCD scoring system. These include patients with diabetes, multiple TIAs within a short period, and patients with a probable or proven cardioembolic source. Diabetes has been incorporated in the recently published ABCD2 scoring system (see Further Reading).

Brain imaging

A head CT or MRI scan is indicated in most patients with TIA to exclude lesions that occasionally mimic TIA, such as subdural haematomas and brain tumours. CT, and more particularly MRI, may show areas of infarction which match the symptoms of an ischaemic event that, on clinical grounds, has completely resolved. CT is less sensitive than MRI in detecting posterior territory ischaemic lesions, particularly in the brain stem. In TIAs due to atrial fibrillation or another known cardiac source, brain imaging to exclude ICH is necessary prior to commencing anticoagulation. The exception is in cases of emboli from endocarditis

Table 8.2.5 The ABCD TIA Risk Score (From Rothwell PM, Giles MF, Flassmann E, et al. A simple score (ABCD) to identify individuals at high risk of stroke after transient ischaemic attack. Lancet 2005; 366: 29–36)

ABCD	Risk factor	Score
Age	Below 60	0
	Above 60	1
Blood pressure	BP > systolic 140 mmHg, and/or diastolic 90 mmHg	1
Clinical	Unilateral weakness of face, arm, hand or leg	2
	Speech disturbance without weakness	1
Duration	Symptoms lasted >60 min	2
	Symptoms lasted 10–60 min	1
	Symptoms lasted < 10 min	0

in which anticoagulation is contraindicated owing to the increased risk of secondary ICH.

Imaging vessels

- Ultrasound: If the aetiology of a TIA is likely to be carotid disease, such that there is a history of amaurosis fugax or hemispheric TIAs, with or without a carotid bruit, then a carotid ultrasound is the initial investigation of choice to investigate the presence and degree of a carotid stenosis.
- Magnetic resonance imaging (MRI) and magnetic resonance angiography (MRA): This provides non-invasive imaging of the brain and major cerebral vasculature. MRA can show lesions suggestive of a vascular aetiology for TIAs, such as a stenosis due to atheromatous disease and dissection. MRI/MRA is not routine in TIA work-up, but may be indicated in more prolonged TIAs, in patients in whom an uncommon cause is suspected, or in younger patients.
- Angiography: Formal angiography may be indicated in selected cases to confirm high-grade carotid stenosis and to confirm/exclude complete carotid occlusions shown on ultrasound. Angiography and MRI/MRA may be performed to investigate for intracranial cerebrovascular disease.

Cardiac imaging

If the clinical evaluation indicates that a cardioembolic source is the most likely cause of a TIA, such as a patient with atrial fibrillation or a recent myocardial infarction, then echocardiography is a priority. However, if there is no evidence of cardiac disease on clinical evaluation and the ECG is normal, then the yield of echocardiography is relatively low. A transthoracic echocardiogram (TTE) is the first line of investigation in cardiac imaging. A transoesophageal echocardiogram (TOE) is more sensitive than TTE in detecting potential cardiac sources of emboli, such as mitral valve vegetations, atrial/mural thrombi and atrial myxoma. It should be considered in patients with inconclusive or normal TTE with ongoing clinical concern for a cardioembolic source or patent foramen ovale. This particularly applies to younger patients with unexplained TIA/non-disabling stroke.

Imaging in stroke

Brain imaging

- CT: In the setting of completed stroke the usual first-line investigation is a non-contrast CT scan. The main value of CT is its sensitivity in the detection of ICH and its ready availability. However, CT scans are often normal in the first hours following ischaemic stroke. In only about half of cases will there be changes detected at 24 hours after the onset of symptoms. The earliest sign of ischaemic stroke is loss of the cortical grey/white matter distinction in the affected arterial distribution. Early signs of cerebral oedema, such as effacement of the cortical sulci or compression of the ventricular system, are indicative of large infarcts. Occasionally a hyperdense clot sign will be seen in the region of the MCA.
- A CT scan should be performed as soon as possible following stroke onset, and certainly within 24 hours. Urgent CT scanning is indicated in patients with a reduced level of consciousness, deteriorating clinical state, symptoms suggestive of ICH, associated seizures, prior to thrombolytic therapy, in younger patients, in patients who are on warfarin, and in cases of diagnostic doubt. A CT scan should also be performed to exclude haemorrhage prior to the commencement of antiplatelet therapies. It should, however, be noted that ICH may be subtle and difficult to diagnose, even for radiologists.
- CT angiography is replacing formal angiography in the evaluation of primary ICH to identify the underlying cause, such as an aneurysm or AVM. It may also show the site of major vessel occlusion in ischaemic stroke. CT perfusion imaging is being evaluated as a technique for the detection of areas of hypoperfused brain at risk of infarction.
- MRI: There are many magnetic resonance modalities available for imaging the brain in acute stroke. Even standard MRI is superior to CT in showing early signs of infarction, with 90% showing changes at 24 hours on T_2-weighted images. Multimodal MRI typically involves additional modes such as gradient recalled echo (GRE) for the detection of acute and chronic haemorrhage, and diffusion-weighted imaging (DWI) for the detection of early ischaemia or infarction. MR diffusion-weighted images show areas of reduced water diffusion in the parts of the brain that are ischaemic and likely to be irreversibly injured. This occurs rapidly after vessel occlusion (less than an hour after stroke onset) and manifests as an area of abnormal high signal in the area of core ischaemia. Hence it is much more sensitive in detecting early ischaemia/infarction than standard T_2-weighted MRI modalities or CT. Perfusion-weighted MR scans (PWI) reveal areas of reduced or delayed cerebral blood flow. This area of the brain is likely to become infarcted if flow is not restored. The DWI and PWI lesions can then be compared. A PWI lesion significantly larger than a DWI lesion is a marker of potentially salvageable brain: the ischaemic penumbra. It is postulated that acute ischaemic stroke patients with this

pattern are most likely to benefit from vessel opening strategies such as thrombolysis. Large areas of diffusion abnormality may also be a marker for increased risk of ICH with thrombolysis. An MRA can be performed at the same time to identify a major vessel occlusion.

Recent studies have suggested that MRI is as accurate as CT in diagnosing acute ICH.[6] This is significant, as it means that, where facilities are immediately available, CT may be bypassed in acute stroke and MRI can be used to both to exclude ICH and to scan for ischaemia/infarction with DWI. As already mentioned, other modalities such PWI and MRA/MRV may also give important diagnostic information and influence treatment decisions. However, MRI may not be feasible in a significant number of stroke patients, due either to standard contraindications to MRI or other factors such as haemodynamic instability, impaired consciousness or vomiting and agitation. In one study the proportion of patients intolerant of MRI was 1:10.

MRI is indicated in strokes involving the brain stem and posterior fossa where CT has poor accuracy. MRA/MRV is particularly useful in the evaluation of unusual causes of stroke such as arterial dissection, venous sinus thrombosis and arteritis. Basilar artery thrombosis causes a brain-stem stroke with an associated high mortality. If the diagnosis is suspected, urgent neurology consultation should be obtained. If MRA or CTA confirms the diagnosis, aggressive therapies such as thrombolysis may improve outcome.

Other investigations may be indicated, particularly in young people, in whom the cause of strokes/TIA may be obscure. These include tests to detect prothrombotic states and uncommon vascular disorders. A list of tests is potentially long and includes a thrombophilia screen, vasculitic and luetic screens, echocardiography and angiography.

Treatment

The treatment of cerebrovascular events must be individualized as determined by the nature and site of the neurological lesion and its underlying cause. The benefits and risks of any treatment strategy can then be considered and informed decisions made by the patient or their surrogate. This is particularly the case with the use of more aggressive therapies such as anticoagulation, thrombolysis and surgery.

General

The ED management of a TIA and stroke requires reassessment of the ABCDs and repeated blood glucose testing. Airway intervention may be necessary in the setting of a severely depressed level of consciousness, neurological deterioration, or signs of raised intracranial pressure and cerebral herniation. This is particularly the case with ICH, with its associated high mortality and morbidity rates. Hypotension is very uncommon in stroke patients, except in the terminal phase of brainstem failure. Hypertension is much more likely to be associated with stroke because of the associated pain, vomiting and raised intracranial pressure and/or pre-existing hypertension, but rarely requires treatment. It may be a physiological response to maintain cerebral perfusion pressure in the face of cerebral hypoxia and raised intracranial pressure. The use of antihypertensives in this situation may aggravate the neurological deficit. There is a paucity of scientific data to support the pharmacological lowering of blood pressure in the ischaemic stroke patient. Stroke guidelines recommend cautious and controlled lowering of a persistently raised blood pressure >220/140 mmHg or a mean arterial pressure greater than 130, using rapidly titratable intravenous drugs such as sodium nitroprusside, esmolol or glycerine trinitrate at low initial doses, and with continuous haemodynamic monitoring in a critical care setting. The aim is for a 10–15% reduction. Oral or sublingual nifedipine is contraindicated as it may cause a rapid uncontrolled fall in blood pressure that may aggravate cerebral ischaemia. Analgesia is appropriate if pain is thought to be contributory, and urinary retention should be excluded.

An elevated temperature can occur in stroke and should be controlled. It should also raise the suspicion of other possible causes for the neurological findings or an associated infective focus.

TIAs

As already stated, the main aim of therapy in TIA and minor strokes is to prevent a major subsequent cerebrovascular event.

- Antiplatelet therapy: Following CT scanning that excludes ICH, aspirin can be commenced at a dose of 300 mg and maintained at 75–150 mg/day in patients with TIAs or minor ischaemic strokes, and has been shown to be effective in preventing further ischaemic events. The ESPRIT trial[7] showed a modest additional benefit from a combination of dipyridamole with aspirin, over aspirin alone. There was no increased risk of bleeding complications, but there was a significantly increased rate of withdrawal of patients from the combination arm because of side effects of dipyridamole, principally headache. Clopidogrel may be substituted for aspirin if the patient is intolerant of aspirin or aspirin is contraindicated. There is some evidence that clopidogrel is more effective than aspirin in the prevention of vascular events, but at greater expense.[8] The combination of aspirin and clopidogrel at this stage is not recommended as it does not appear to give any greater therapeutic benefits and there is increased bleeding risk. Anticoagulation with heparin and warfarin has not been shown to be superior to aspirin, except in cases of TIA/minor stroke due to cardioembolism (excluding endocarditis).
- Anticoagulant therapy: Patients with a cardioembolic source of TIA should be considered for full anticoagulation following neurological consultation and normal brain imaging, with the exception of those with endocarditis, in whom the risk of haemorrhagic complications is increased.
- Surgery: Trials have demonstrated a beneficial outcome of urgent surgery for symptomatic carotid stenosis in patients with anterior circulation TIAs and minor stroke with a demonstrated carotid stenosis of between 70% and 99%.[2] The benefit of surgery may extend to lesser grades of stenosis down to 50% in selected patients. The patient's baseline neurological state, comorbidities and

operative mortality and morbidity rate also need to be assessed when considering surgery.

- Other medical therapies: Risk factors for stroke and TIAs should be identified and treated. Statins should be considered regardless of cholesterol levels. The benefit of lowering LDL cholesterol levels using atorvastatin in preventing further cerebro- and cardiovascular events following an initial episode of cerebral ischaemia was demonstrated in the recent SPARCL study.[9]

Ischaemic stroke

A more active approach to the acute management of ischaemic stroke is seen as having the potential to improve neurological outcomes. The ED is the place where these important treatment decisions will largely be made. Most patients with a stroke will require hospital admission for further evaluation and treatment, as well as for observation and possible rehabilitation. Studies of stroke units show that patients benefit from being under the care of physicians with expertise in stroke and a multidisciplinary team that can manage all aspects of their care.[10]

- Aspirin: In two large trials, aspirin, when administered within 48 hours of the onset of stroke, was found to improve the outcomes of early death or recurrent stroke compared to placebo.[11,12] A CT scan should be performed to exclude ICH prior to commencing aspirin. The combination of low-dose aspirin and dipyridamole may confer some additional benefit.
- Thrombolysis: Thrombolytic agents are seen as having an important place in the management of acute ischaemic stroke, although their use is still controversial.[13] In Australia, the United Kingdom and the United States tPA has been approved for use in acute stroke patients when administered within 3 hours of onset. It is recommended that the inclusion and exclusion criteria that were used in the NINDS study[14] should be strictly adhered to when deciding to administer tPA. For inclusion, treatment must be commenced within 3 hours of a known stroke onset and patients must have a CT scan excluding ICH. In the NINDS study,

thrombolysis resulted in improved neurological outcomes in patients receiving tPA compared to placebo, with a 13% absolute increase in the number of patients having good neurological outcomes (numbers needed to treat = 8). In the thrombolysis group, there was a significant increase in intracerebral haemorrhage rate (6.4% versus 0.6% in the placebo group), of which half were fatal, although there was no overall excess mortality. Factors that may be associated with increased haemorrhage risk include increased age (especially > 80 years), increased severity of stroke and early CT changes of a large ischaemic stroke. Studies of acute stroke patients given tPA outside controlled trials have yielded conflicting results.[15–17] They suggest that when tPA is used by specialists in well-equipped stroke centres in accordance with strict guidelines, the complication rate for acute stroke patients can be similar to that achieved in the NINDS trial. However, protocol violations are associated with an increased risk of poor outcomes. Trials of thrombolysis are ongoing, with the aim of identifying patients most likely to benefit from reperfusion therapy, reducing the risk of ICH, and extending the time window for treatment, particularly through the use of advanced imaging modalities such as diffusion/perfusion MRI.

- Anticoagulation: Anticoagulation should only be considered in stroke patients with a proven cardioembolic source. The risk of commencing anticoagulation soon after a vascular stroke is of inducing haemorrhagic transformation, which may result in clinical deterioration. A CT scan to exclude ICH and a neurological consultation should be obtained prior to considering anticoagulation in any patient with a stroke of likely cardio-embolic origin.
- Neuroprotection: A range of neuroprotective agents have been trialled in the setting of acute stroke in the hope that modulation of the ischaemic cascade of metabolic changes that follows vascular occlusion may result in improved neurological outcomes. At this stage, however, none of these

therapies is recommended for the treatment of acute stroke.

- Surgery: As for TIAs, patients with non-disabling stroke should be considered for investigation with carotid ultrasound to detect a significant stenosis that may be appropriate for urgent carotid endarterectomy. The use of endovascular stents in carotid surgery is also being developed and studied.

Large anterior circulation infarcts have a significant risk of developing cerebral oedema and raised ICP with associated clinical deterioration, particularly manifest by a declining conscious state with or without progression of other signs. Along with standard measures for managing raised ICP, there may be a place for decompressive craniotomy in selected cases. Intensive care and neurosurgical consultation should be considered.

Intracerebral haemorrhage (ICH)

Primary ICH is most commonly caused by long-standing hypertension induced small vessel disease. The site of hypertensive haemorrhage tends to occur in characteristic locations such as the basal ganglia, thalamus and cerebellum. Berry aneurysms most commonly arise around the Circle of Willis, hence ICH due to aneurysmal rupture is often located around this area. Secondary ICH may occur into an underlying lesion such as a tumour or infarct, and clinical deterioration may result – so-called symptomatic ICH (SICH) – but this is not always the case.

The clinical presentation of primary ICH is typically of sudden onset of a neurologic deficit with associated headache, collapse/transient loss of consciousness, hypertension and vomiting. However, clinical features alone are unable to differentiate ICH from infarction, hence the requirement for brain imaging to confirm the diagnosis. Both CT and MRI (using gradient echo sequences) are equivalent in the detection of ICH.

Medical management

Primary ICH is a medical emergency with a high mortality of between 35% and 50%, with half of these deaths occurring in the first 2 days. There is also a very high risk of dependency. Haematomas can expand rapidly, and there is a significant risk of early neurological deterioration and increasing intracranial pressure (ICP). Treatment of raised ICP in a setting of ICH involves a range of modalities similar to those used in head trauma. These include elevation of the head of the bed, analgesia, sedation, an osmotic diuretic such as mannitol and hypertonic saline, hyperventilation, drainage of CSF via ventricular catheter, and neuromuscular paralysis.

There is no good evidence regarding the management of hypertension in the setting of ICH sufficient to make firm recommendations. Guidelines have been published, but treatment should be individualized and take place in consultation with neurology/neurosurgery/intensive care specialists.[18] Sudden falls in blood pressure and hypotension should be avoided, as they may aggravate cerebral ischaemia in the setting of raised ICP, which is often associated with ICH.

Early studies of the use of recombinant factor VIIa have shown promise when administered within 3 hours of stroke onset, showing a significant reduction in haematoma expansion and improved mortality.[19] Steroids are not indicated in ICH. Anticonvulsant prophylaxis is common practice.

Management of ICH associated with anticoagulation or thrombolysis is a matter of urgency and should be done in consultation with a haematologist and a neurosurgeon. Agents such as protamine sulphate, vitamin K, prothrombin complex concentrate and FFP may be indicated. Factor VIIa normalizes the INR very rapidly, but with a greater potential for thromboembolism.

Surgical management

Surgical management of ICH depends on the location, cause, neurological deficit and overall clinical state. Early neurosurgical consultation should be obtained. High-level evidence for improved outcomes following drainage of supratentorial haematomas by craniotomy is lacking, but the procedure may be indicated in selected patients, particularly in those with lobar clots within 1 cm of the surface. In patients presenting in coma with deep haemorrhages, craniotomy is not recommended

and may worsen outcomes. The presence of a cerebellar haematoma is a particular indication for surgery, with a potential for a good neurological recovery. A variety of other techniques, such as minimally invasive haematoma evacuation, are under investigation.

Controversies

- Thrombolysis is a high-risk therapy which may improve neurological outcome in patients with ischaemic stroke when given within 3 hours of onset. Only one of a number of studies has so far demonstrated improved neurological outcomes without excess overall mortality. Problematic issues for thrombolytic therapy in stroke include the small number of patients who currently present within the time window for treatment; delays in ED assessment and obtaining an expertly reported CT, particularly after hours; identification in the ED of subgroups with higher risk of haemorrhagic complications or lesser treatment benefit; the significant rate of stroke misdiagnosis, with subsequent potential for unnecessary exposure to a high-risk therapy; and the large number of contraindications to thrombolysis, as well as the potential for protocol violations which increases the risk of a poor outcome.

- Advances in neuroimaging, particularly diffusion/perfusion MRI, and perfusion CTA, show promise for improved selection of patients likely to benefit from thrombolytic therapy. The optimal imaging strategy remains unclear.

- Selection of the most appropriate antiplatelet agent for the treatment of TIAs has become clearer. Aspirin, despite being cost-effective, is probably inferior to the combination of aspirin and dipyridamole. Clopidogrel is an effective single agent but usually reserved for patients with intolerance or contraindications to aspirin. A combination of clopidogrel and aspirin is not recommended.

- Treatment of hypertension associated with stroke. Antihypertensive therapy is rarely necessary. An elevated blood pressure may be a physiological response to maintain cerebral perfusion pressure. Rapid uncontrolled blood pressure reduction can occur with some antihypertensive agents, thereby aggravating cerebral ischaemia.

- Patients with so-called malignant MCA occlusion – that is, a large MCA infarct associated with decreased or deteriorating conscious state suggesting increased intracranial pressure – should be managed in an intensive care setting and appropriate measures to reduce intracranial pressure should be considered. Recent evidence suggests that the use of decompressive craniotomy in selected patients in this group can improve mortality and may improve neurological outcomes.[20]

- Aspects of the management of primary ICH remain controversial, particularly the use of recombinant factor VIIa and the role of surgery. New therapies such as minimally invasive clot evacuation continue to be evaluated.

- Neuroprotective therapies continue to be evaluated, but at this stage cannot be recommended outside a clinical trial.

References

1. Executive Committee of the Asymptomatic Carotid Atherosclerosis Study. Endarterectomy for asymptomatic carotid artery stenosis. Journal of the American Medical Association 1995; 273: 1421–1428.
2. North American Symptomatic Carotid Endarterectomy Trial Collaborators (NASCET). Beneficial effects of carotid endarterectomy in symptomatic patients with high grade carotid stenosis. New England Journal of Medicine 1991; 325: 445–453.
3. Kouthari RU, Panciolli A, Liu T, et al. Cincinatti Pre Hospital Stroke Scale: reproducibility and validity. Annals of Emergency Medicine 1999; 33: 373–378.
4. Goldstein LB, Samsa GP. Reliability of the National Institute of Health Stroke Scale: extension to non-neurologists in the context of a clinical trial. Stroke 1997; 28: 307–310.
5. Rothwell PM, Giles MF, Flassmann E, et al. A simple score (ABCD) to identify individuals at high risk of stroke after transient ischaemic attack. Lancet 2005; 366: 29–36.

6. Kidwell, CS, Chalela JA, Saver JL, et al. Comparison of MRI and CT for detection of acute intracerebral hemorrhage. Journal of the American Medical Association 2004; 292: 1823–1834.

7. The ESPRIT Study Group. Aspirin plus dipyridamole versus aspirin alone after cerebral ischaemia of arterial origin (ESPRIT). Lancet 2006; 367: 1665–1673.

8. CAPRIE Steering Committee. A randomized, blinded, control trial of clopidogrel versus aspirin in patients at risk of ischaemic events (CAPRIE). Lancet 1996: 348: 1329–1339.

9. The Stroke Prevention by Aggressive Reduction in Cholesterol levels (SPARCL) Investigators. High dose atorvastatin after stroke or transient ischaemic attack. New England Journal of Medicine 2006: 355: 549–559.

10. Duffy BK, Phillips PA, Davis SM, et al. Evidence based care and outcomes of acute stroke managed in hospital specialty units. Medical Journal Australia 2003; 178: 318–323.

11. International Stroke Trial Collaborative Group. The International Stroke Trial (IST): a randomised trial of aspirin, subcutaneous heparin, both, or neither among. 19435 patients with acute ischaemic stroke. Lancet 1997; 349: 1569–1581.

12. CAST (Chinese Acute Stroke Trial) Collaborative Group. CAST: randomised placebo controlled trial of early aspirin use in. 20000 patients with acute ischaemic stroke. Lancet 1997; 349: 1641–1649.

13. Hoffman J. Tissue plasminogen activator (tPA) for acute ischaemic stroke: why has so much been made of so little? Medical Journal Australia 2003; 179: 333–334.

14. National Institute of Neurological Disorders and Stroke rt-PA Stroke Study Group (NINDS). Tissue plasminogen activator for acute ischaemic stroke. New England Journal of Medicine 1995; 333: 1581–1587.

15. Albers GW. Intravenous tissue-type plasminogen activator for treatment of acute stroke: the Standard Treatment with Alteplase to Reverse Stroke (STARS) study. Journal of the American Medical Association 2000; 83: 1145–1150.

16. Katzan IL, Furlan AJ, Lloyd LE, et al. Use of tissue type plasminogen activator for acute ischaemic stroke: the Cleveland Area Experience. Journal of the American Medical Association 2000; 283: 1511–1518.

17. Wahlgren N, Ahmed N, Davalos A, et al. Thrombolysis with alteplase for acute ischaemic stroke in the Safe Implementation of Thrombolysis in Stroke (SITS-MOST): an observational study. Lancet 2007; 369: 275–282.

18. Broderick, JP, Connolly S, Feldman E, et al. AHA/ASA Guidelines for the management of spontaneous intracerebral hemorrhage in adults. ICH. Stroke 2007; 38: 2001.

19. Mayer S, Brun MC, Begtiup K, et al. Recombinant Factor 7a for acute ICH. New England Journal of Medicine 2005; 352: 777–785.

20. Vahedi K, Hofmijer J, Juettler E, et al. Early decompressive surgery in malignant infarction of the middle cerebral artery: a pooled analysis of three randomised controlled trials. Lancet Neurology 2007; 6: 215–222.

Further reading

Rothwell PM. Atherothrombosis and ischaemic stroke. British Medical Journal 2007; 334: 379–381.

Alberts MJ, Latchaw RE, Selman WR, et al. Brain Attack Coalition. Recommendations for comprehensive stroke centres: a consensus statement of the Brain Attack Coalition. Stroke 2005; 36: 1597–1616.

Libman RB, Wirkowski E, Alvir J. Conditions that mimic stroke in the emergency department. Archives of Neurology 1995; 52: 1119–1122.

Schriger DL, Kalafut M, Starkman S, et al. Cranial computed tomography interpretation in acute stroke. Physician accuracy in determining eligibility for thrombolytic therapy. Journal of the American Medical Association 1998; 279: 1293–1297.

Adams HP Jr, Zoppo G, Alberts MJ, et al. AHA/ASA Guidelines for the early management of adults with ischaemic stroke. Stroke 2007; 38: 1655.

Diener H, Bogousslavsky J, Brass LM, et al. on behalf of the MATCH Investigators. Acetylsalicilic acid on a background of clopidogrel in high risk patients randomized after recent stroke or transient ischaemic attack: The Match trial results. Lancet 2004; 364: 331–337.

Sacco RL, Adams R, Albers G, et al. AHA/ASA Guidelines for the prevention of stroke with ischaemic stroke or transient ischaemic attack. Stroke 2006; 37: 577.

Johnston SC, Rothwell PM, Nguyen-Huynh MN, et al. Validation and refinement of a score to predict very early stroke risk after transient ischaemic attack. Lancet 2007; 369:283–292.

8.3 Subarachnoid haemorrhage

Pamela Rosengarten

ESSENTIALS

1 The diagnosis of subarachnoid haemorrhage (SAH) demands a high index of suspicion for the condition.

2 Up to 50% of patients with SAH experience a warning leak – the sentinel haemorrhage – in the hours to days prior to the major bleed.

3 Severe sudden headache is the primary clinical feature.

4 Brain CT scan without contrast is the initial investigation of choice.

5 A negative CT scan for SAH must be followed by lumbar puncture and examination of the cerebrospinal fluid.

6 The patient with SAH requires urgent neurosurgical referral and management.

7 Early definitive isolation and occlusion of the aneurysm reduces early complications and improves outcome.

8 Endovascular treatment is the treatment of choice in most cases.

Introduction

Patients with headache account for approximately 1% of all emergency department (ED) visits, and of these 1–4% have been demonstrated to have subarachnoid haemorrhage. Early accurate diagnosis of aneurysmal subarachnoid haemorrhage is imperative, as early occlusion of the aneurysm has been shown to reduce early complications of re-bleeding and vasospasm and improve outcome.

Pathology and epidemiology

SAH is the presence of extravasated blood within the subarachnoid space. The incidence is 5–7 per 100 000 patient-years, but is significantly higher (around 20 per 100 000) in Japan and Finland, for reasons that are unclear. Although incidence increases with age, about half of those affected are under 55, the condition being most common in the 40–60 age group. Excluding head trauma, which remains the most common cause, non-traumatic or spontaneous SAH results from rupture of a cerebral aneurysm in approximately 85% of cases, non-aneurysmal perimesencephalic haemorrhage in 10%, and the remaining 5% from other rare causes including rupture of mycotic aneurysms, intracranial arterial dissection, aterio-venous malformations, vasculities, central venous thrombosis, bleeding diatheses, tumours and drugs such as cocaine, amphetamines and anticoagulants.

Aneurysms

Intracranial aneurysms are not congenital. Rather, they develop during the course of life. An estimate of the frequency for an adult without risk factors is 2.3%, with the proportion increasing with age. Most aneurysms will never rupture, but the risk increases with size. Paradoxically, as the vast majority of aneurysms are small, most aneurysms that rupture are small. An aneurysm of the posterior circulation is more likely to rupture than one of comparable size in the anterior circulation.

Risk factors can be considered as those that are modifiable and those that are not. Modifiable risk factors include cigarette smoking, hypertension, cocaine use and excessive alcohol intake. Non-modifiable factors include a family history of first-degree relatives with SAH, heritable connective tissue disorders (particularly polycystic kidney disease and neurofibromatosis), sickle cell disease and α_1-antitrypsin deficiency.

Non-aneurysmal perimesencephalic haemorrhage

This type of SAH is defined by the characteristic distribution of blood in the cisterns around the midbrain in combination with normal angiographic studies. It usually carries a relatively benign prognosis. A small proportion of patients with this distribution of blood may have a ruptured aneurysm of a vertebral or basilar artery.

Clinical features

History

The history is critical to the diagnosis of SAH:

- Headache is the principal presenting symptom, being present in up to 95% of patients with SAH and being the solitary symptom in up to 40% of patients. It is typically of sudden onset (75% within a few seconds) and severe, often being the worst headache ever experienced by the patient. It may be the only symptom in up to one-third of patients. Approximately one in four patients presenting with sudden severe headache will have SAH. Other causes include

benign thunderclap headache (40%), migraine, cluster headache, headache associated with sexual exertion, vascular headaches of stroke, intracranial haemorrhage, venous thrombosis, and arterial dissection, meningitis, encephalitis, acute hydrocephalus, intracranial tumour, and intracranial hypotension.

- Up to 50% of patients experience a warning leak (sentinel haemorrhage) in the hours to days before the major bleed. This headache may be mild, generalized or localized, resolve spontaneously within minutes to hours, or respond to analgesic therapy. It does, however, tend to develop abruptly and differ in quality from other headaches that the patient may have previously experienced. Hence a patient's worst or first headache is suggestive of SAH.
- Upper neck pain is common.
- One-third of patients will develop SAH during strenuous exercise, e.g. bending or lifting, whereas in the remaining two-thirds it will occur during sleep or routine daily activities.
- Nausea and vomiting are present in 75% of patients.
- Brief or permanent loss of consciousness occurs in the majority of patients. Severe headache is usually experienced when the patient regains consciousness, although a brief episode of excruciating headache may occur prior to losing consciousness.
- Seizures occur in 15% of patients and when associated with a typical headache are a strong indicator of SAH, even if the patient is neurologically normal when assessed.
- Prodromal symptoms particularly third cranial nerve with pupillary dilatation and sixth cranial nerve palsies are uncommon, but may suggest the presence and location of a progressively enlarging unruptured aneurysm.
- No clinical feature can reliably identify SAH.

Examination

There is a wide spectrum of clinical presentations, the level of consciousness and clinical signs being dependent on the site and extent of the haemorrhage:

- On ED presentation, two-thirds of patients have impaired level of

consciousness – 50% of these have coma. Consciousness may improve or deteriorate. An acute confusional state can occur which may be mistaken for a psychological problem.
- Signs of meningism, including fever, photophobia and neck stiffness, are present in 75% of patients, but may take several hours to develop and may be absent in the deeply unconscious. Absence of neck stiffness does not exclude SAH.
- Focal neurological signs may be present in up to 25% of patients and are secondary to associated intracranial haemorrhage, cerebral vasospasm, local compression of a cranial nerve by the aneurysm (e.g. oculomotor nerve palsy by posterior communicating aneurysm) or raised intracranial pressure (sixth-nerve palsy) or bilateral lower limb weakness (anterior communicating aneurysm).
- Ophthalmological examination may reveal unilateral or bilateral subhyaloid haemorrhages or papilloedema.
- Systemic features associated with SAH include severe hypertension, hypoxia and acute ECG changes that may mimic acute myocardial infarction.
- A small proportion of patients present in cardiac arrest. Resuscitation attempts are vital, as half of survivors regain independent function.

Patients are categorized into clinical grades from I to V, according to their conscious state and neurological deficit. Two grading schemes, that of Hunt and Hess and that of the World Federation of Neurosurgeons, which is preferred, are depicted in Table 8.3.1. The higher the score, the worse the prognosis.

Investigations

Imaging

A brain CT scan without contrast is the initial investigation of choice. In the first 24 hours after haemorrhage it can demonstrate the presence of subarachnoid blood in more than 95% of cases. (Fig. 8.3.1). The sensitivity, however, decreases with time owing to the rapid clearance of blood, with only 80% of scans positive at 3 days and 50% positive at 1 week. CT will also demonstrate the site and extent of the

Table 8.3.1	Clinical grading schemes for patients with SAH		
		Grading scheme of WFNS	
Grade	Grading scheme of Hunt and Hess	GCS	Motor deficit
1	No symptons or minimal headache, slight nuchal rigidity	15	No
2	Moderate to severe headache, no neurological deficit other than cranial nerve palsy	13–14	No
3	Drowsy, confused, mild focal deficit	13–14	Yes
4	Stupor, moderate to severe hemiparesis, vegetative posturing	7–12	Yes or No
5	Deep coma, decerebration, moribund	3–6	Yes or no

WFNS = World Federation of Neurosurgeons, GCS = Glasgow Coma Score.
(Reproduced with permission from Sawin PD, Loftus CM 1997 Diagnosis of spontaneous subarachnoid hemorrhage. American Family Physician 55(1): 145–156.)

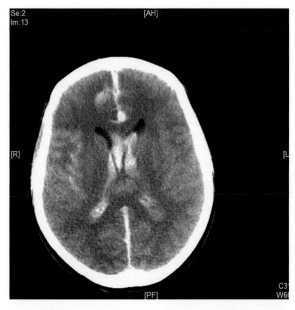

Fig. 8.3.1 Non-contrast head CT scan demonstrating widespread subarachnoid and intraventricular blood.

haemorrhage, indicate the possible location of the aneurysm, and demonstrate the presence of hydrocephalus and other pathological changes.

Magnetic resonance imaging (MRI) with FLAIR (fluid attenuated inversion recovery) is reliable in demonstrating early SAH and is superior to CT in detecting extravasated blood in the days (up to 40 days) following haemorrhage. Availability and logistical considerations make MRI impractical for use in the initial diagnostic work-up of SAH, but it may be considered in patients who present late.

CT angiography (CTA) is the preferred angiographic technique once SAH has been identified. Compared to catheter angiography it has a sensitivity of 95%, is readily available, and has a lower complication rate than catheter angiography. It should be performed as soon as the diagnosis is made. Where diagnosis has been made by CT, CTA should preferably be performed while the patient is still in the scanner. CTA is usually of sufficient quality to allow planning of endovascular or neurosurgical interventions.

Four-vessel cerebral angiography is the gold standard for confirming the presence of an aneurysm, its location and the presence of vasospasm, and was previously the preferred angiographic test. It is not, however, without risk. Neurological complications occur in ~1.8% of cases, with re-rupture of an aneurysm reported in 2–3%. It is also less available than CTA. These factors have seen it become less favoured and used in selected cases only.

MR angiography is currently useful as a screening tool for the diagnosis of intracranial aneurysms in patients at increased risk.

In patients where SAH is present and no cause is found, then the distribution of extravasated blood on the CT scan should be reviewed. If this conforms to the perimesencephalic distribution of non-aneurysmal haemorrhage, then no repeat investigations are warranted. If, however, an aneurysmal pattern of haemorrhage is present, then a second CTA is recommended as occasionally an aneurysm may have gone undetected on the original test.

Lumbar puncture

Lumbar puncture is necessary when there is clinical suspicion of SAH, the CT scan is negative, equivocal or technically inadequate, and no mass lesion or signs of raised intracranial pressure are found. In about 3% of patients with SAH the CT scan will be normal.

The diagnosis of SAH, then, is dependent on the finding of red blood cells not due to traumatic tap, or red blood cell breakdown products within the CSF. Lumbar puncture should be delayed for at least 6 and preferably 12 hours after symptom onset to allow bilirubin to be formed from cell breakdown in SAH. Detection of bilirubin and xanthochromia is the only reliable method of distinguishing SAH from a traumatic tap. Proceeding to angiographic studies in every patient with bloodstained CSF would be expected to identify an incidental finding of a small unruptured aneurysm in about 2%.

It is important to measure the opening pressure when performing a lumbar puncture, as CSF pressure may be elevated in SAH or in other conditions such as intracranial venous thrombosis or pseudotumour cerebri, or low in spontaneous intracranial hypotension.

Xanthochromia, the yellow discolouration of CSF caused by the haemoglobin breakdown products oxyhaemoglobin and bilirubin due to lysis of red blood cells, is generally agreed to be the primary criterion for diagnosis of SAH and differentiates between SAH and traumatic tap. It is usually present within 6 hours of SAH and has been demonstrated in all patients with SAH between 12 hours and 2 weeks following the haemorrhage. Xanthochromia is not reliably detected by visual examination of centrifuged CSF. Spectrophotometric analysis of CSF for bilirubin is considered the most sensitive means of detecting xanthochromia. Owing to the time taken for haemoglobin to degrade into bilirubin and oxyhaemoglobin, xanthochromia may take up to 12 hours to develop. Hence controversy exists as to the optimal timing of lumbar puncture. Early lumbar puncture within 12 hours may have negative or equivocal CSF findings, whereas delayed lumbar puncture may result in an increased risk of early re-bleeding as well as having practical implications for the ED. In general, at least 6–12 hours should have elapsed between the onset of headache and lumbar puncture. Although detection of xanthochromia is indicative of SAH, it does not entirely rule out traumatic lumbar puncture and can occur in extremely bloody taps (>12 000 RBC/mL) or where the lumbar puncture has been repeated after an initial traumatic tap.

Other studies of the CSF, such as three tube cell counts, D-dimer assay and detection of erythrophages, have been found to be inconsistent in differentiating SAH from traumatic tap.

General investigations

General investigations to be performed include full blood examination, erythrocyte sedimentation rate, urea, electrolytes including magnesium, blood glucose, coagulation screen, chest X-ray and 12-lead ECG. ECG changes are frequently present and include ST and T-wave changes which may mimic ischaemia, QRS and QT prolongation and arrhythmias.

Complications

Early complications

- Rebleeding: Up to 15% within hours of the initial haemorrhage, and overall 40% of patients re-bleed within the first 4 weeks without intervention. Re-bleeding is associated with a 60% mortality, and half of the survivors remain disabled.
- Subdural haematoma or large intracerebral haematoma can be life-threatening and require immediate drainage. Similarly, a large intracerebral haematoma may be contributing to the poor clinical condition and warrant drainage simultaneously with treatment of the aneurysm.
- Global cerebral ischaemia: Irreversible brain damage resulting from haemorrhage at the time of aneurysm rupture. This is probably secondary to a marked rise in incranial pressure resulting in inadequate cerebral perfusion.
- Cerebral vasospasm: Clinically significant vasospasm occurs in approximately 20% of patients with SAH and is a major cause of death and morbidity. It tends to occur between days 3 and 15 after SAH, with a peak incidence at days 6–8. Vasospasm causes ischaemia or infarction and should be suspected in any patient who suffers a deterioration in their neurological status or develops neurological deficits. The best predictor of vasospasm is the amount of blood seen on the initial CT scan.
- Hydrocephalus occurs in approximately 15% of patients with SAH. It can occur within 24 hours of haemorrhage and should be suspected in any patient who suffers a deterioration in mentation or conscious state, particularly if associated with slowed pupillary responses.
- Seizures.
- Fluid and electrolyte disturbances: Patients with SAH may develop hyponatraemia and hypovolaemia secondary to excessive natriuresis (cerebral salt wasting), or alternatively may develop a syndrome of inappropriate ADH (SIADH).
- Hyperglycaemia and hyperthermia, both of which are associated with a poor outcome.

- Medical complications include pulmonary oedema, cardiogenic or neurogenic (23%), cardiac arrythmias (35%), sepsis, venous thromboembolism and respiratory failure.

Late complications

- Late re-bleeding, from a new aneurysm or regrowth of the treated aneurysm, is estimated at ~1.3% in 4 years for coiling and ~2–3% in 10 years for surgical clipping.
- Anosmia: up to 30%.
- Epilepsy: 5–7%.
- Cognitive deficits and psychosocial dysfunction are common even in those who make a good recovery; 60% of patients report personality change.

Management

The management of SAH requires general supportive measures, particularly airway protection and blood pressure control, as well as specific management of the ruptured aneurysm and the complications of aneurysmal haemorrhage.

General measures

- Stabilization of the unconscious patient, with particular attention to the airway. Endotracheal intubation with oxygenation and ventilation will be required in patients with higher-grade (4–5) SAH.
- Close observation of GCS and vital signs.
- In all patients, maintain oxygenation and circulation ensuring adequate (euvolaemic) blood volume.
- Analgesia, using reversible narcotic analgesic agents, sedation and antiemetics as required. Ensure bed rest with minimal stimulation. Avoid aspirin and non-steroidal analgesic agents (NSAIDs).
- Blood pressure control: Blood pressure levels are often of the order of 150/90 immediately following SAH, and in most patients can be adequately controlled by sedation and analgesia. Normotensive levels extending to mild to moderately hypertensive levels, especially in patients with pre-existing hypertension, are acceptable. Antihypertensive therapy should be reserved for patients with

severe (mean arterial pressure >130 mmHg) hypertension, or where there is evidence of progressive end-organ dysfunction, and short-acting antihypertensive agents (e.g. esmolol or nitroprusside) and intensive haemodynamic monitoring should be employed.

- Seizures should be treated as they occur. The use of prophylactic phenytoin is controversial and has been linked with unfavourable functional and cognitive outcomes.
- Correct electrolyte imbalances. Hyponatraemia of excessive natriuresis must be differentiated from that of SIADH. Hypovolaemia is to be avoided.
- Venous thromboembolism prophylaxis, initially with compressive devices and later with subcutaneous heparin following treatment of the aneurysm.
- Treatment of hydrocephalus by ventricular drainage may be required.

Specific treatment

Prevention of re-bleeding

Early occlusion within 72 hours secures the aneurysm, prevents re-bleeding, removes the clot and reduces the incidence of early complications and improves outcomes.

Endovascular occlusion by placing detachable coils in aneurysms under radiological guidance (coiling) has largely replaced surgical occlusion as the method of choice for prevention of re-bleeding in suitable cases. Current evidence suggests that the relative risk reduction for poor outcome (death or severe disability) at 1 year with coiling versus surgical occlusion (clipping) is of the order of 24%, with an absolute risk reduction of 7%. Choice depends somewhat on antomical considerations, as aneurysms are not equally amenable to this option.

Surgical clipping is now a second-line option for most patients. Modern techniques provide an estimated absolute risk reduction for poor outcome of 10%, with a relative risk reduction of 19%. Clipping is usually done early – within 3 days, and preferably within 24 hours.

Antifibrinolytic agents, including ε-aminocaproic acid, which inhibit clot lysis, reduce the incidence of re-bleeding after initial aneurysmal rupture. Their use has, however, been associated with an increase in neurological deficits and failed to improve outcome. They are not advocated for routine use in SAH.

Prevention of delayed cerebral ischaemia

Cerebral ischaemia is often gradual in onset and involves the territory of more than one cerebral artery. Peak frequency is at 5–14 days after SAH. Calcium channel antagonists improve outcome in SAH, with a relative risk reduction of 18% and an absolute risk reduction of 5.1%. The current standard regimen is nimodipine 60 mg orally every 4 hours for 3 weeks. It should be commenced within 48 hours of haemorrhage.

Magnesium sulphate may also be useful as hypomagnesaemia is common and associated with the occurrence of delayed cerebral ischaemia and poor outcome. There is currently insufficient evidence to assess its effectiveness.

There are conflicting data about whether antiplatelet agents reduce the rate of cerebral ischaemia, and there is no evidence that they reduce the proportion of patients with poor outcome.

There are no proven treatments for delayed cerebral ischaemia, although induced hypertension, hypervolaemia and haemodilution are plausible. In vasospasm unresponsive to medical management, emergency cerebral angiography with intra-arterial vasodilator infusion or transluminal balloon angioplasty may be considered where focal vessel narrowing is demonstrated.

Prognosis

SAH has a 40–60% mortality rate from the initial haemorrhage, with up to one-third of survivors having a significant neurological deficit. The most important prognostic factor is the clinical condition at the time of presentation, with coma and major neurological deficits generally being associated with a poor prognosis. Survival rates have been reported at 70% for grade I, 60% for grade II, 50% for grade III, 40% for grade IV and 10% for grade V SAH.

It is worth noting, however, that survival without brain damage is possible even after respiratory arrest. Even patients who make a good recovery may suffer cognitive and psychosocial dysfunction.

Aneurysm screening in patients who have survived aneurysmal SAH is not advocated, as although these patients are at increased risk of new or recurrent aneurysmal bleeds, screening cannot be demonstrated to be cost effective or increase quality of life.

Incidental unruptured aneurysms

If an unruptured aneurysm is found incidentally, it raises the dilemma of the risk–benefit rationale between intervention and conservative management. Factors taken into account include age, aneurysm size and location, gender, country, comorbidity and family history. Such patients should be referred to a neurosurgical service for advice and counselling.

Conclusion

Clinical suspicion of the diagnosis of SAH gained from a history of sudden, severe or atypical headache demands a full investigation, including brain CT scan and, if necessary, lumbar puncture. Once SAH has been diagnosed, urgent neurosurgical referral and management are required.

Controversies

- The timing of lumbar puncture following a negative CT scan for SAH.
- Vascular imaging for patients with a negative CT scan and negative CSF is indicated in those with ambiguous test results, those at high risk for SAH and patients presenting after more than 2 weeks.
- Prophylactic anticonvulsant therapy for patients with SAH.
- Follow-up for patients after coiling.
- Role of magnesium sulphate for prevention of cerebral oedema.

Further reading

Al-Shahi R, White PM, Davenport RJ, et al. Subarachnoid haemorrhage. British Medical Journal 2006; 333: 235–240.

de Gans K, Nieuwkamp DJ, Rinkel GJ, et al. Timing of aneurysmal surgery in subarachnoid hemorrhage: a systematic review of the literature. Neurosurgery 2002; 50: 336–340.

Dorhout Mees SM, Rinkel GJE, Vermeulen M, van Gijn J. Calcium antagonists for aneurysmal subarachnoid haemorrhage. Cochrane Database of Systematic Reviews, (4): CD000277. DOI: 10.1002/14651858.CD000277. pub3, 1999.

Dorhout Mees SM, van den Bergh WM, et al. Antiplatelet therapy for aneurysmal subarachnoid haemorrhage. Cochrane Database of Systematic Reviews (4): CD006184. DOI: 10.1002/14651858.CD006184.pub2, 2007.

Edlow JA, Caplan LR. Primary care: Avoiding pitfalls in the diagnosis of subarachnoid hemorrhage. New England Journal of Medicine 2000; 342: 29–36.

Naval NS, Stevens RD, Mirski MA. Controversies in the management of subarachnoid haemorrhage. Critical Care Medicine 2006; 34: 511–524.

Roos YBWEM, Rinkel GJE, Vermeulen M, et al. Antifibrinolytic therapy for aneurysmal subarachnoid haemorrhage. Cochrane Database of Systematic Reviews (4): CD001245. DOI: 10.1002/14651858.CD001245, 1998.

Sawin PD, Loftus CM. Diagnosis of spontaneous subarachnoid hemorrhage. American Family Physician 1997; 55: 145–156.

Suarez JI, Tarr RW, Selman WR. Current concepts: Aneurysmal subarachnoid haemorrhage. New England Medical Journal 2006; 354: 387–398.

van Gijn J, Kerr RS, Rinkel GJE. Subarachoid haemorrhage. Lancet 2007; 369: 306–318.

8.4 Altered conscious state

Ruth Hew

ESSENTIALS

1 For clinical purposes, the ability of the individual to respond appropriately to environmental stimuli provides a quantifiable definition of consciousness. The Glasgow Coma Score is used to quantify conscious state and monitor progress.

2 The causes of altered conscious state can be divided pathophysiologically into structural and metabolic insults.

3 A thorough history and examination is the key to guiding investigation choices and identifying the cause of the primary insult, whereas management is directed towards resuscitation, specific correction of the primary pathology and minimization of secondary injury.

4 Bedside blood glucose measurement is essential and may be life-saving.

Introduction

Consciousness can be defined as a state of awareness of self and the environment. This presumes subjectivity, unity and intentionality, implying that each individual's perception is unique, consisting of a moulding of various sensory modalities over time and interpreted within the full range of that individual's experiences.

It is clear even from this limited description that the definition of consciousness is metaphysical and difficult to quantify. It would also include what is clinically described as mental state, but psychiatric disease and its differentiation from medical pathology is excluded from this discussion as it is discussed elsewhere.

For clinical purposes, the ability of the individual to respond appropriately to environmental stimuli provides a quantifiable definition of consciousness. Pragmatically, consciousness equals responsiveness.

Pathophysiology

The level of consciousness describes the rousability of the individual, whereas the content of consciousness may be assessed in terms of the appropriateness of the individual's response. Broadly speaking, the first is a brainstem function and the second is an attribute of the forebrain.

The physical portions of the brain involved in consciousness consist of the ascending arousal system that begins with monoaminergic cell groups in the brain stem and culminates in extensive diffuse cortical projections throughout the cerebrum. En route there is input and modulation from both thalamic and hypothalamic nuclei, as well as basal forebrain cell groups.

The integration of the brain stem and the forebrain is illustrated by individuals who have an isolated pontine injury. They remain awake, but the intact forebrain is unable to interact with the external world, hence the aptly named 'locked-in syndrome'. At the other end of the spectrum are individuals in a persistent vegetative state who, in spite of extensive forebrain impairment, appear awake but totally lack the content of consciousness. These clinical extremes emphasize the important role of the brain stem in modulating motor and sensory systems through its descending pathways and regulating the wakefulness of the forebrain through its ascending pathways.

Impairment of conscious state implies dysfunction of the ascending arousal system in the paramedian portion of the upper pons and midbrain, its targets in the thalamus or hypothalamus, or both cerebral hemispheres. The resultant changes in the conscious state range from awakeness through lethargy and stupor to coma with a progressively depressed response to various stimuli.

Numerous scales have been proposed to define consciousness but the one that has found universal acceptance is the Glasgow Coma (or Responsiveness) Scale (GCS) (Table 8.4.1). Initially described in 1974 for the assessment of traumatic head injuries, 25 years of experience have shown that the scale can also be used in non-traumatic situations to provide a structured assessment of an individual's conscious state at various points in time, and also to monitor progress. Trends

Table 8.4.1	The Glasgow Coma Scale

The GCS is scored between 3 and 15, 3 being the worst and 15 the best. It is composed of three parameters: Best Eye Response, Best Verbal Response, Best Motor Response, as given below.

Best eye response (score out of 4)
1 – No eye opening
2 – Eye opening to pain
3 – Eye opening to verbal command
4 – Eyes open spontaneously

Best verbal response (score out of 5)
1 – No verbal response
2 – Incomprehensible sounds
3 – Inappropriate words
4 – Confused
5 – Orientated

Best motor response (score out of 6)
1 – No motor response
2 – Extension to pain
3 – Flexion to pain
4 – Withdrawal from pain
5 – Localizing pain
6 – Obeys commands

Table 8.4.2	Mnemonics for causes of altered conscious state

T	Trauma
I	Infection
P	Psychogenic
(P)	(Porphyria)
S	Seizure
	Syncope
	Space-occupying lesion
A	Alcohol and other toxins
E	Endocrinopathy
	Encephalopathy
	Electrolyte disturbances
I	Insulin – Diabetes
O	Oxygen: Hypoxia of any cause
	Opiates
U	Uraemia including Hypertension
C	erebral
O	verdose
M	etabolic
A	sphyxia and other **A** ssociations

Table 8.4.3	Causes of alteration in conscious state

STRUCTURAL INSULTS

Supratentorial
Haematoma
- epidural
- subdural
Cerebral tumour
Cerebral aneurysm
Haemorrhagic CVA

Infratentorial
Cerebellar AVM
Pontine haemorrhage
Brainstem tumour

METABOLIC INSULTS

Loss of substrate
Hypoxia
Hypoglycaemia
Global ischaemia
Shock
- hypovolaemia
- cardiogenic
Focal ischaemia
- TIA/CVA
- vasculitis

Derangement of normal physiology
Hypo- or hypernatraemia
Hyperglycaemia/hyperosmolarity
Hypercalcaemia
Hypermagnesaemia
Addisonian crisis
Seizures
- status epilepticus
- post-ictal
Post-concussive
Hypo- or hyperthyroidism
Cofactor deficiency
Metastatic malignancy
Psychiatric illness
Dementia

Toxins
Drugs
- alcohol
- illicit
- prescription
Endotoxins
- subarachnoid blood
- liver failure
- renal failure
Sepsis
- systemic
Focal
- meningitis
- encephalitis
Environmental
- hypothermia/heat exhaustion
- altitude illness/decompression
- envenomations

provided by repeated measurements of the GCS give clinicians an objective measure to monitor a patient's deterioration or improvement in response to therapy. In quantifying and standardizing the various responses, the GCS has enabled clinicians worldwide to compare data and therapies. In the spectrum from full awareness to unrousable, coma or unconsciousness is arbitrarily defined as a GCS ≤ 8.

Differential diagnoses

As the main diagnostic challenge in a patient with an altered conscious state is to identify the cause, it is reasonable to approach the assessment of the patient armed with a knowledge of the possible differential diagnoses.

There are several well known mnemonics to assist in remembering the rather diverse list. Some are listed in Table 8.4.2. However, the long list of apparently disparate causes can be divided pathophysiologically into structural insults and metabolic insults.

Structural insults are usually focal intracranial lesions that exert direct or indirect pressure on the brain stem and the more caudal portions of the ascending arousal system. They tend to produce lateralizing neurological signs that can assist in pinpointing the level of the lesion. As there is little space in and around the brain stem, any extrinsic or intrinsic compression will rapidly progress through coma to death, unless the pressure on the brain stem is relieved surgically or pharmacologically.

Metabolic insults are usually due to systemic pathology that affects primarily the forebrain, although direct depression of the brain stem may also occur. There are seldom lateralizing signs. The solution to the problem is the correction of the underlying metabolic impairment. Naturally, as in all clinical practice, there are no absolute distinctions. Uncorrected, any of the metabolic causes can eventually cause cerebral oedema and herniation, leading thence to brainstem compression with lateralizing signs and death. Table 8.4.3 lists the more common and important causes of an altered conscious state.

Clinical assessment

As in all life-threatening conditions, assessment and management must proceed concurrently. There are two primary considerations, which are not mutually exclusive: identify and correct the primary insult while preventing or minimizing secondary injury, e.g. hypoxia, acidosis, raised intracranial pressure. As in other time-critical situations, the primary and secondary survey approach often proves useful.

Primary survey

This focuses on attention to the airway, breathing and circulation. It begins the identification of life-threatening problems and allows immediate therapeutic measures such as airway support to be implemented. Supplemental oxygen is indicated, as is frequent monitoring of vital signs and GCS. Endotracheal intubation is required at this stage if the patient is unable to maintain a safe airway or adequate ventilation. This usually corresponds with a GCS of 8 or less. Mild hyperventilation to a PCO_2 of 30–35 mmHg will help correct underlying acidosis and reduce intracranial pressure. Cervical spine precautions are imperative if trauma is suspected, until clearance of the spine can be obtained.

A bedside glucose determination may identify clinical or biochemical hypoglycaemia, which should be treated with glucose. There is no evidence that 50 mL of intravenous 50% dextrose will cause harm even in an already hyperglycaemic patient, and a case could be made for routinely administering glucose to any patient with an altered conscious state if a bedside glucose estimation is not readily available.

A history of opiate use combined with the clinical signs of pinpoint pupils and hypoventilation may make the administration of naloxone both diagnostic and therapeutic. Parenterally, 0.2–0.4 mg aliquots can be given, to a maximum of 10 mg. The likelihood of serious adverse reactions such as pulmonary oedema is very low. However, in combination overdoses, the negation of the opiate effect may unmask the effects of other toxins, including those with proconvulsant or proarrhythmic tendencies. Parenteral administration in uncontrolled situations with a flailing patient is not without its risks to both patient and staff. In particular, there is a risk to staff from needle-stick injuries and bloodborne infections. Intranasal administration of naloxone via an atomizer has entered mainstream pre-hospital practice and eliminates this risk.

The administration of 100 mg thiamine is advocated in patients suspected of having hepatic encephalopathy, but its effect is rarely immediate and a delay in its use will not change the course of the initial resuscitation. The old dogma that thiamine should be withheld until hypoglycaemia is corrected to avoid precipitating Wernicke's encephalopathy is unfounded, as the absorption of thiamine is so much slower than that of glucose as to render the timing irrelevant.

The routine use of the 'coma cocktail' consisting of intravenous 50% dextrose, naloxone and thiamine is no longer advocated.

Secondary survey

After initial resuscitation, it is important to complete the assessment by obtaining a full history, conducting a full examination and performing any adjunctive investigations. This will assist in identifying the cause of the condition and planning further management.

History

Obtaining a full history can be difficult as the patient may be confused or obtunded. Details have to be garnered from supplemental sources such as ambulance or police officers, relatives or carers, and primary care physicians. Medical records, when obtainable, may provide clues, and patients will occasionally carry cards or wear bracelets with alerts for particular conditions.

It is crucial to establish the events leading up to the presentation with specific questioning about prodromal events, ingestions, i.v. drug usage, trauma, underlying illness, medications, allergies, and associated seizures and abnormal movements. For example, the presence or absence of a headache and its onset and duration might aid in the clinical diagnosis of a subarachnoid haemorrhage, and a history of head injury with loss of consciousness would increase the likelihood of an extra-axial intracranial collection. Patients who are taking anticoagulants also have an increased risk of intracranial haemorrhage with minimal trauma.

In the elderly, dementia, itself a progressive illness, may be exacerbated by delirium caused by an acute illness, and often only a careful, corroborated history from all care providers and the passage of time will allow the two to be distinguished. In these patients it is important to remember that dementia as a cause of altered conscious state is a diagnosis of exclusion.

Examination

A general physical examination, bearing in mind the various differential diagnoses, is the next step. Vital signs may suggest sepsis or other causes of shock. A keen sense of smell might detect fetor hepaticus or the sweet breath of ketosis. A bitter almond scent is pathognomonic of cyanide poisoning. Of note, alteration of consciousness can be attributed to alcoholic intoxication only by the process of exclusion. Thus the characteristic odour of alcoholic liquor is indicative but cannot be presumed to be diagnostic. A bedside blood glucose determination is mandatory, as deficits are easily correctable.

Neurological examination clearly must be as comprehensive as possible. There are several obstacles to this. Initial resuscitation measures such as endotracheal intubation will reduce the ability of the patient to cooperate with the examination, and language difficulties will be accentuated as the neurological examination is strongly language oriented. Thus patients who do not share a common language and those with dysphasia may be disadvantaged. Also, sensory modalities are difficult to assess in patients with impaired mentation, although these deficits are often paralleled by deficits in the motor system.

The aim of the neurological examination is, primarily, to differentiate structural and nonstructural causes; secondly, to identify groups of signs that may indicate specific diagnoses such as meningitis; and finally, to pinpoint the precise location of a structural lesion. Therefore, emphasis needs to be placed on signs of trauma, tone, reflexes, papillary findings and eye signs, as well as serial estimations of GCS. Circumstances permitting, some or all of the neurological examination should be attempted before the patient receives neuromuscular paralyzing agents.

Signs of trauma need to be documented and spinal precautions taken as indicated. Palpation of the soft tissues and bones of the skull may detect deformity or bruising, and a haemotympanum may herald a fracture of the base of the skull.

Hypotonia is common in acute neurological deficits. Specific examination of anal sphincter tone will uncover spinal cord compromise and is crucial in trauma patients with a depressed level of consciousness. An upgoing Babinski response is indicative of pyramidal pathology, and asymmetry of the peripheral limb reflexes may help to 'side' a lesion. Conversely, heightened tone in the neck muscles (neck stiffness) may indicate meningitis or subarachnoid haemorrhage.

Pupillary findings and eye signs may also be useful to differentiate metabolic and structural insults, and more importantly to detect incipient uncal herniation. Intact oculocephalic reflexes and preservation of the 'doll's eyes' response indicates an intact medial longitudinal fasciculus and by default an intact brain stem, suggesting a metabolic cause for coma (Table 8.4.4). There are four pairs of nuclei governing ocular movements, and they are spread between the superior and inferior midbrain and the pons. The pattern of ocular movement dysfunction can be used to pinpoint the site of a brainstem lesion (Table 8.4.4). Likewise, specific testing of the oculovestibular reflex and the cranial nerve examination can be used to precisely locate a

Table 8.4.4 Ocular responses to cold caloric testing of the oculovestibular reflex

Response	Cerebrum	Medial longitudinal fasciculus	Brain stem
Bilateral nystagmus	Intact	Intact	Intact
Bilateral conjugate deviation towards the stimulus	Metabolic dysfunction	Intact	Intact
No response			Structural or metabolic dysfunction
Ipsilateral dysconjugate deviation			Structural dysfunction

Table 8.4.5 Patterns of dysfunction in various parameters determined by the site of the structural or metabolic insult

	Respirations	Motor response	Pupillary light response	Eye movements
Forebrain	Cheyne–Stokes - waxing & waning	Localizing to pain	Symmetrical, small, reactive Pretectal - symmetrical, large, fixed	
Midbrain	Hyperventilation	Decorticate	Fixed	Upper midbrain - CN III palsy Lower midbrain - CN IV deficit - loss of ipsilateral adduction
Pons	Apneusis - halts briefly in full inspiration	Decerebrate	Symmetrical, pinpoint, reactive. Uncal – ipsilateral, fixed, dilated	CN VI deficit - loss of ipsilateral abduction
Medulla	Ataxic irregular rate & uneven depth Apnoeic Bilateral ventrolateral medulla lesions			

brainstem lesion but is of limited use in the emergency setting except as a predictor of herniation (Table 8.4.5).

More generally, skin examination may reveal needle tracks suggestive of drug use or a meningococcal rash. Mucosal changes such as cyanosis or the cherry-red glow of carbon monoxide poisoning can be diagnostic. Cardiac monitoring and cardiovascular examination should identify rhythm disturbances, the murmurs of endocarditis and valvular disease, or evidence of shock from myocardial ischaemia or infarction. Respiratory patterns may aid in identifying the site of the lesion (Table 8.4.5). Abdominal examination may detect organomegaly, ascites, bruits or pulsatile masses.

Investigations

Specific laboratory and radiological investigations must be guided by the history and examination, and their timing determined by the priorities of resuscitation.

Haematology

A full blood examination may reveal anaemia, immunocompromise, thrombocytopenia, inflammation or infection, but is rarely specific. CRP and ESR are non-specific acute-phase reactants and single determinants are not initially useful, although they may later be followed to monitor resolution of the illness or response to therapy. Coagulation profiles are particularly useful in haematological and liver disease, or if patients are taking anticoagulants such as warfarin.

Biochemistry

Serum electrolyte levels aid in the differentiation of the various hypo- and hyperelemental causes of coma. Electrolyte imbalances may also be secondary to the causative insult and may not need specific correction.

In hypotensive patients, a high to normal sodium and a low potassium suggests primary or secondary addisonian crisis.

Liver, renal and thyroid function tests may confirm focal organ dysfunction. The last may not always be readily available, but hypothyroidism should be considered in the hypothermic patient and hyperthyroidism in the presence of tremor and tachyarrhythmias.

A serum glucose provides confirmation of bedside testing. Serum lactate determinations may reveal a metabolic acidosis and reflect the degree of tissue hypoxia, which again may be primary or secondary. Creatinine kinase and myoglobinuria are useful to determine the presence and extent of rhabdomyolysis and to predict the likelihood of requiring dialysis. Serum and urine osmolarity may be useful in toxic ingestions such as ethylene glycol.

Blood gas analysis may give important information regarding acid–base balance, and along with the anion gap and the serum electrolytes can help distinguish between the various types and causes of acidosis and alkalosis. Knowledge of the partial pressures of oxygen and carbon dioxide is vital to resuscitative efforts.

Microbiology

Sepsis is a major metabolic cause of conscious state alteration and may present with no localizing symptoms or signs, especially in the elderly. In this case, blood cultures – preferably multiple sets obtained before antibiotic therapy – may be the only means of isolating the causative organism. Naturally, system-specific specimens such as sputum, urine and cerebrospinal fluid should be collected when clinically indicated. Although as a rule specimens should be obtained prior to therapy, in suspected meningitis or encephalitis the administration of antibiotics or antiviral agents should not be delayed while a lumbar puncture/CT scan is performed.

Specific laboratory testing

Based on information from the history and examination, specific drug assays and urine screens may be indicated. These may include prescribed medications such as lithium or theophylline, or drugs of addiction such as amphetamine or opiates. Routine urine drug screens are of very limited value.

Venom detection kits can be used in specific clinical situations, and evidence of systemic envenomation can be screened for with other tests, such as coagulation profiles and creatinine kinase.

Imaging

A chest X-ray may reveal primary infection or malignancy. In a patient with an altered conscious state and any suspicion of head trauma, a full cervical spine series is mandatory. Inadequate plain films should be supplemented by CT imaging of the cervical spine, as allowed by resuscitation imperatives while spinal immobilization is maintained. Imaging of the rest of the spine and the pelvis should be guided by clinical assessment.

Intracranial imaging is best achieved with a plain CT of the head which, if normal and concern regarding intracranial pathology persists, may be followed by a contrast-enhanced scan or MRI. The latter has a higher sensitivity for encephalitis and cerebral vasculitis, although it may not always be easily accessible from the ED. Also, the technical constraints of MRI require a stable patient. Emergency CT angiography has a role in the delineation of cerebral aneurysms, and interventional angiography can provide therapeutic options, particularly in a patient who is progressing towards herniation.

Other tests

The 12-lead ECG can highlight rate and rhythm disturbances. Specific changes, such as the U wave of hypokalaemia, the J wave of hypothermia and focal infarction and ischaemic patterns, serve to confirm and offer pointers to the cause of the coma. It is worth noting that intracranial bleeding such as subarachnoid haemorrhage can be associated with an ischaemic-looking ECG. Care is required in cases of depressed level of consciousness with ECG changes, as the use of thrombolysis or anticoagulation based on the ECG in the presence of intracranial bleeding may well be fatal.

It is clear from the previous discussion that a good history and thorough examination are key to the appropriate choice of investigations.

Management

Assessment and management are also inextricably linked and must take place concurrently. The clinical findings on assessment guide management, and the response to treatment may further aid assessment and diagnosis.

The algorithm in Figure 8.4.1 is aimed at correcting immediate life-threatening pathology and then identifying and treating reversible structural and metabolic causes.

Following initial resuscitation, it is important to identify patients in whom trauma is known or suspected. These have a higher risk of skull fractures and focal intracranial pathology, and are more likely to have increased intracranial pressure requiring urgent imaging and subsequent neurosurgical consultation and definitive management. The same pathway is required for patients who have a non-traumatic cause for coma but who have lateralizing signs suggesting a focal intracranial lesion. Evidence of brainstem herniation is a neurosurgical emergency. A CT scan is helpful in

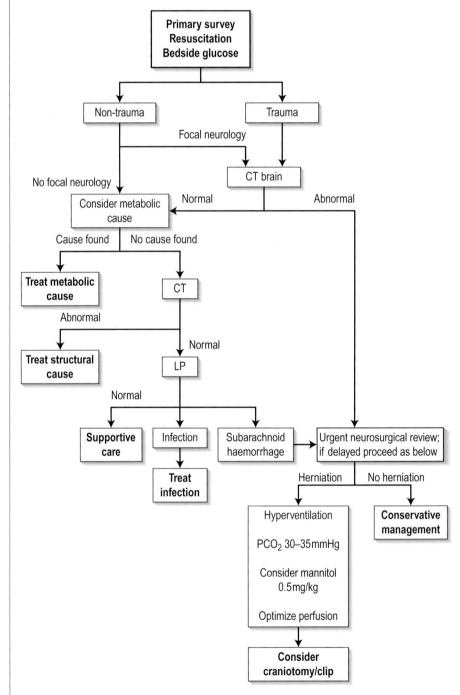

Fig. 8.4.1 Altered conscious state: management algorithm.

diagnosing the cause of cerebral herniation and should be obtained expeditiously. Neurosurgical consultation can be arranged concurrently so as not to impede smooth transit to theatre for those requiring urgent craniotomy. Cerebral resuscitation is continued concurrently, with relative hyperventilation to maintain a PCO_2 of 30–35 mmHg. The role of mannitol is still controversial, but it may be used in consultation with the neurosurgical team. The diuretic effect may, however, add to haemodynamic compromise and secondary neurological embarrassment.

Should there be no lateralizing signs, then a metabolic cause needs to be sought. A metabolic screen and, if indicated, a toxicological screen, is performed. If a cause is found, it is further specifically investigated and definitively managed. If no cause is identified or suggested on initial or other first-line specific investigation, a brain CT scan is performed. Thereafter, patients with identified causes are stabilized and referred for appropriate continuing care. Depending on the pathology, prophylactic anticonvulsants and corticosteroids may be considered.

A normal CT scan does not completely exclude treatable intracranial infection or subarachnoid haemorrhage. Therefore, depending upon the patient's conscious state and the level of clinical suspicion, a lumbar puncture may further assist with diagnosis. However, it must be emphasized that, in suspected intracranial infection, an obtunded patient should be treated empirically with appropriate antiviral agents and antibiotics, and the lumbar puncture deferred till the risk of herniation is minimized. In the absence of any identifiable cause, supportive care is provided until specific investigation or the natural evolution of the disease process points to the diagnosis.

Self-limiting causes for altered conscious states, such as seizures and vasovagal syncope, have not been addressed here as they are covered elsewhere.

Disposition

Patients with continuing altered consciousness should be admitted to a hospital with the range of services and clinical disciplines to manage the primary diagnosis. The level of care required will depend on the state of the patient on presentation and their subsequent response to treatment. Patient wishes, premorbid status and prognosis may also temper treatment choices and pathways.

Prognosis

Discussion of prognosis is difficult, as it depends on the cause and patient-specific factors. Effective cerebral resuscitation with optimal oxygenation and minimization of intracerebral hypercarbia and acidosis will promote the best recovery potential while addressing the underlying disease process. Prognosis is naturally dependent on the degree of irreversible cellular damage and the ability to correct the primary insult while minimizing secondary brain injury.

Controversies

- The timing of the lumbar puncture in an obtunded patient suspected of a central nervous system infection.

- The role of hyperventilation and mannitol in the management of acute elevation in intracranial pressure.

- Patient management that acknowledges the interplay between patient and family wishes, premorbid status, diagnosis and prognosis.

Further reading

Hasbun R, Abrahams J, Jekel J, Quagliarello VJ. Computed tomography of the head before lumbar puncture in adults with suspected meningitis. New England Journal of Medicine 2001; 345: 24: 1727–1732.

Hoffman JR, Schriger DL, Luo JS. The empiric use of naloxone in patients with altered mental status: A reappraisal. Annals of Emergency Medicine 1991; 20: 246–252.

Hoffman JR, Schriger DL, Votey SR, et al. The empiric use of hypertonic glucose in patients with altered mental status: A reappraisal. Annals of Emergency Medicine 1992; 21: 20–24.

Hoffman DS, Goldfrank LR. The poisoned patient with altered consciousness: Controversies in the use of a 'coma cocktail'. Journal of the American Medical Association 1995; 274: 562–569.

Kelly AM, Kerr D, Dietze P, et al. A randomised trial of intranasal versus intramuscular naloxone in prehospital treatment for suspected opioid overdose. Medical Journal Association 2005; 182: 24–27.

Teasdale G, Jennett B. Assessment of coma and impaired consciousness: A practical scale. Lancet 1974; 2: 81–84.

Teasdale G, Jennett B. Aspects of coma after head injury. Lancet 1977; 1: 878–881.

8.5 Seizures

Garry J. Wilkes

ESSENTIALS

1 Up to 10% of the population will have at least one seizure in their lifetime, but only 1–3% will develop epilepsy.

2 The management of an acute episode is directed at rapid control of seizures, identification of precipitating factors, and prevention/correction of complications.

3 Investigation of first seizures should be directed by history and clinical findings. Routine laboratory and radiological investigations are not warranted for uncomplicated first seizures with full recovery.

4 Persistent confusion should not be assumed to be due to a post-ictal state until other causes are excluded.

5 Benzodiazepines and phenytoin are the principal anticonvulsant agents for acute seizures.

6 Status epilepticus and eclampsia are severe life threats. Management plans for these conditions should be developed in advance.

7 Pseudoseizures are important to distinguish from neurogenic seizures in order to prevent inadvertent harm to patients and allow appropriate psychotherapeutic treatment.

8 Management of drug-related seizures (including those related to alcohol) includes measures to reduce drug absorption and enhance elimination. Specific therapy is available for only a few agents. Phenytoin is usually ineffective in the management of alcohol and drug-related seizures.

9 Severe head injuries are associated with an increased incidence of post-traumatic epilepsy, more than half of which will be manifest in the first year. Phenytoin is effective as prophylaxis for the first week only.

10 Patients with epilepsy should be encouraged to have ongoing care.

Introduction

The terms 'seizure', 'convulsion' and 'fit' are often used both interchangeably and incorrectly. A seizure is an episode of abnormal neurological function caused by an abnormal electrical discharge of brain neurons. The seizure is also referred to as an ictus or ictal period. A convulsion is an episode of excessive and abnormal motor activity. Seizures can occur without convulsions, and convulsions can be caused by other conditions. The term 'fit' is best avoided in medical terminology, but is a useful term for non-medical personnel.

Seizures are common. It has been estimated that up to 10% of the population will have at least one seizure in their lifetime, and 1–3% of the population will develop epilepsy.[1] A single seizure may be a reaction to an underlying disorder, part of an established epileptic disorder, or an isolated event with no associated pathology. The challenge is to rapidly identify and treat life-threatening conditions as well as to identify benign conditions that require no further investigation or treatment.

The manifestations of epileptic disorders are extremely varied. Two international classifications have been developed: the International Classification of Epileptic Seizures, and the International Classification of Epilepsy and Epileptic Syndromes.[2,3] The former divides epileptic seizures into two major categories: partial and generalized. Partial epileptic seizures are further classified according to the impairment or the preservation of consciousness into simple partial and complex partial seizures. Either condition may secondarily generalize into tonic–clonic seizures. Generalized seizures can be divided into convulsive and non-convulsive types.

Convulsive seizures are generalized tonic–clonic seizures or grand mal seizures. Non-convulsive generalized seizures include absence seizures (previously termed petit mal seizures), myoclonic, tonic and atonic seizures. Under the International Classification, epilepsy and epileptic syndromes are initially classified according to their corresponding types of seizure into localization related and generalized disorders. Each disorder can be further classified according to its relationship to aetiological or predisposing factors into symptomatic, cryptogenic or idiopathic types.[3] Different seizure types are associated with differing aetiological and prognostic factors. The details of the classification systems are not as important in emergency medicine as the concept of recognizing the different seizure types and being aware of the accepted terminology when discussing and referring cases.

Given the high frequency of this condition in emergency departments (ED) it is important to have a management strategy formulated in advance. One such approach has been developed by the American College of Emergency Physicians.[4] The four main management concepts are as follows:

- Altered mental state should be thoroughly assessed and not assumed to be due to a post-ictal state.
- Patients with known epilepsy who have recovered completely from a typical seizure require little further investigation. If they remain obtunded or have atypical features they must be fully evaluated, e.g. biochemical analysis, CT scan, etc.
- Patients with epilepsy should be encouraged to seek continuing care.
- Patients at risk of recurrent seizures should be advised about situations of

increased personal risk, such as driving, operating power machinery or swimming alone.

First seizures

A generalized convulsion is a dramatic event. Patients and those accompanying them will often be frightened, anxious and concerned, not only for the acute event but for what it may signify. A diagnosis of epilepsy carries important implications. The patient's occupation, social activities, ability to drive a car and long-term health implications may all be profoundly influenced. It is therefore vital that the diagnosis is correct and explained fully to the patient and relatives.

The majority of patients will have completed the seizure before arrival in the ED. Patients still seizing are treated immediately according to the guidelines below for status epilepticus.

The first and most important task is to determine whether a seizure has occurred. As the majority of patients will have returned to normal by the time they are reviewed in the ED, the diagnosis is made primarily on history. Patients will not remember seizures other than simple partial seizures, and the reports of witnesses may be unreliable or inconsistent. With the exception of partial seizures, generalized seizures are not accompanied by an aura. Most seizures last less than 2 minutes, are associated with impaired consciousness, loss of memory for the event, purposeless movements, and a period of post-ictal confusion. Although witnesses may grossly overestimate the duration, prolonged seizures, those occurring in association with a strong emotional event and those with full recall of events, should be regarded with suspicion. Similarly, motor activity that is coordinated and not bilateral, such as side-to-side head movements, pelvic thrusting, directed violence and movement that changes in response to external cues, are less likely to be true seizures.

Conditions such as syncope may be accompanied by myoclonic activity and are important to distinguish from true seizures. Migraine, transient ischaemic attacks, hyperventilation episodes and vertigo are all important conditions to consider in the differential diagnosis. Pseudoseizures will be discussed below.

The history, examination and investigation process is aimed at identifying associated conditions and treatable causes of seizures. The aetiology of seizures can be classified into five groups on this basis:

- Acute symptomatic: Occurring during an acute illness with a known central nervous system insult. Causes of this large, important group are listed in Table 8.5.1.
- Remote symptomatic: Occurring without provocation in a patient with a prior central nervous system insult known to be associated with an increased risk of seizures, e.g. encephalopathy, meningitis, head trauma or stroke.
- Progressive encephalopathy: Occurring in association with a progressive neurological disease, e.g. neuro-degenerative diseases, neurocutaneous syndromes and malignancies not in remission.
- Febrile: Patients whose sole provocation is fever. This is almost exclusively confined to children, and as such is beyond the scope of this book.
- Idiopathic: Patients who present de novo, or during the course of their illness, in the absence of an acute precipitating central nervous system insult. This is probably the most common group; however, this classification is by exclusion of the other causes.

Table 8.5.1 Acute symptomatic causes of seizures (Reproduced with permission from Brown AF, Wilkes GJ. Emergency department management of status epilepticus. Emergency Medicine 1994; 6: 49–61)

Hypoxia
Hypoglycaemia
Head trauma
Meningitis and encephalitis, including HIV disease
Metabolic, including hyponatraemia, hypocalcaemia, hyperthyroidism, uraemia and eclampsia
Drug overdose, including alcohol, tricyclics, theophylline, cocaine, amphetamine and isoniazid
Drug withdrawal, including alcohol, benzodiazepines, narcotics, cocaine and anticonvulsants
Cerebral tumour or stroke

A careful history is needed to decide whether this is part of an ongoing process or an isolated event. Patients may not recall previous events, may not recognize their significance, or may even avoid reporting previous episodes for fear of being labelled 'epileptic', with the associated consequences. Particular attention should be paid to any history of unexplained injuries, especially when they occur during blackouts or during sleep. Any history of childhood seizures, isolated myoclonic jerks and a positive family history increases the likelihood of epilepsy.

A complete physical and neurological examination is mandatory. Evidence of alcohol and drug ingestion and head trauma is particularly important. A comprehensive medication history may include agents known to reduce the seizure threshold in susceptible individuals, e.g. tramadol, selective serotonin reuptake inhibitors.[5] A careful mental state examination in seemingly alert patients may reveal evidence of a resolving post-ictal state or of underlying encephalopathy. All patients not fully alert should not be assumed to simply be in a post-ictal state until other causes are excluded. Of particular importance is any evidence of underlying illness, such as fever, nuchal rigidity (meningitis) or cardiac murmurs (endocarditis). Needle tracks, evidence of chronic liver disease, dysmorphic features and marks such as café-au-lait spots (neurofibromatosis) are important aetiological clues. Complications such as tongue biting, broken teeth and peripheral injuries are not uncommon in generalized seizures. Stress fractures can occur, particularly in the elderly, and posterior dislocation of the shoulder is an uncommon but significant and easily overlooked finding.

The investigations necessary following an uncomplicated seizure are minimal. Although it is common practice to order a variety of tests, such as electrolytes, blood sugar level and full blood count, these are rarely of benefit in the fully recovered patient. Elevated neutrophil counts in blood and CSF may be seen as a result of a generalized seizure in the absence of an infectious disorder. Although electrolyte abnormalities may cause seizures they are unlikely to be the cause if the patient has recovered. A serum prolactin level at 20 and 60 minutes post seizure may be helpful if the diagnosis is in doubt. Patients with an abnormal physical or neurological examination should be managed according to clinical findings and the results of laboratory and radiological investigations. Findings suggestive of meningitis, encephalitis or subarachnoid haemorrhage are indications for cranial CT scan and lumbar puncture.

There are no clear guidelines to the routine need for or urgency of neuroimaging following a single uncomplicated seizure. Patients with focal neurological signs, those who do not recover to a normal examination, and those with a history of head trauma or intracranial pathology should all undergo cranial CT as soon as possible. The dilemma arises in patients with complete recovery and no focal signs. The incidence of abnormalities on CT in this group of patients is less than 1%.[6] The decision as to whether and when to scan patients in this group will be determined largely by local factors. Generally, a contrast CT (more sensitive for subtle lesions) is performed on an outpatient basis prior to review. MRI is more sensitive than CT for infarcts, tumours, inflammatory lesions and vascular lesions, but cost and availability limit its use as a primary investigative modality.

Electroencephalography (EEG) at the time of a seizure will make a definitive diagnosis. It is not usually performed in the acute setting except when non-convulsive activity is suspected. Typically, an EEG is obtained electively on an outpatient basis, when it may still indicate an underlying focus of activity and may be able to detect specific conditions.

Once a diagnosis of first seizure is made and intercurrent conditions are excluded or treated, the patient may be discharged home. In most cases no treatment is needed. It must be stressed to the patient that a diagnosis of epilepsy has not been made but is being considered. When the suspicion is reasonable the patient should be given the same precautionary advice as epileptic patients with regard to driving and other activities that may place them or others at risk.

The planning of investigation and follow-up for patients suspected of having a first seizure is best done in conjunction with a neurology service. Planning and consultation will ensure that appropriate investigations are completed in a timely fashion. Generally, an inter-ictal EEG and contrast CT are completed prior to review.

Status epilepticus

Status epilepticus (SE) may be defined as 'two or more seizures without full recovery of consciousness between seizures, or recurrent epileptic seizures for more than 30 minutes'.[7]

Status epilepticus has been reported to account for 1–8% of all hospital admissions for epilepsy, 3.5% of admissions to neurological intensive care, and 0.13% of all visits to a university hospital ED. It is more common at the extremes of age, with over 50% of all cases occurring in children and a disproportionately high incidence in those over 60 years of age. SE is also more frequent in the mentally handicapped and in those with structural cerebral pathology, especially of the frontal lobes. Four to 16% of adults and 10–25% of children with known epilepsy will have at least one episode of SE. However, SE occurs most commonly in patients with no previous history of epilepsy.[8]

Many compensatory physiological changes accompany seizures. As the duration is increased these mechanisms begin to fail, with an increased risk of permanent damage. Brain damage resulting from prolonged SE is believed to be caused by excitatory amino acid neurotransmitters such as glutamate and aspartate. These lead to an influx of calcium into neuronal cytoplasm and an osmotolysis with cell destruction. Continuing seizure activity itself contributes substantially to neuronal damage, which is further exacerbated by hypoxia, hypoglycaemia, lactic acidosis and hyperpyrexia. When seizures continue for over 60 minutes, the risk of neuronal injury increases despite optimal delivery of oxygen and glucose. The longer an episode of SE continues, the more refractory to treatment it becomes, and the more likely it is to result in permanent neuronal damage. Mortality increases from 2.7% with seizure duration under 1 hour, to 32% with duration beyond this.[8] Generalized convulsive SE is therefore a medical emergency.

Treatment of SE is along the same lines as the resuscitation of all seriously ill patients. Management is in a resuscitation area with attention to four specific factors:

- Rapid stabilization of airway, breathing and circulation.
- Termination of seizure activity (clinical and electrical).
- Identification and treatment of precipitating and perpetuating factors.
- Identification and treatment of complications.

Each stage of resuscitation is made more difficult by the presence of active convulsions. No attempt should be made to prise clenched teeth apart to insert an oral airway: a soft nasal airway will suffice. Oxygen should be given by tight-fitting mask and the patient positioned in the left lateral position to minimize the risk of aspiration. Intravenous access is important for drug treatment and fluid resuscitation, but may be difficult in actively seizing patients. Although SE cannot be diagnosed until seizures have persisted for 30 minutes, patients still seizing on arrival at the ED should be treated with anticonvulsants immediately.

The principal pharmacological agents used are benzodiazepines and phenytoin. The benzodiazepines used vary between countries, with little clinical evidence to support any particular one. In Australasian centres midazolam is preferred, in increments of 1–2 mg i.v. If i.v. access cannot be rapidly secured, midazolam i.m. at a dose of 0.2 mg/kg will terminate most seizures.[9] Alternatives to midazolam are diazepam and clonazepam. Diazepam can be administered rectally if necessary, and this technique can be taught to parents with high-risk children. However, onset of action by this route in adults is slow and unpredictable. All benzodiazepines share the disadvantages of respiratory depression, hypotension, and a short duration of clinical effect.

Phenytoin is usually used as a second-line agent in a dose of 15–20 mg/kg at a rate of no more than 50 mg/min. Rapid administration is associated with bradyarrhythmias and hypotension. The common practice of administering 1 g is inadequate for most adults. The effect of phenytoin does not commence until 40% of the dose has been administered; for this reason it should be commenced at the same time that i.v. benzodiazepines are given. Most people on anticonvulsants who present in SE have negligible drug levels, and the side effects from a full loading dose on top of a therapeutic level are minimal. The full loading dose should therefore be given even when the patient is known to be on therapy.[10]

The most common causes of failure to control seizures are:

- Inadequate antiepileptic drug therapy.
- Failure to initiate maintenance antiepileptic drug therapy.
- Hypoxia, hypotension, cardiorespiratory failure, metabolic disturbance, e.g. hypoglycaemia.
- Failure to identify an underlying cause.
- Failure to recognize medical complications, e.g. hyperpyrexia, hypoglycaemia.
- Misdiagnosis of pseudoseizures.

Causes of failure to regain consciousness following treatment of seizures include the medical consequences of SE (hypoxia, hypoglycaemia, cerebral oedema, hypotension, hyperpyrexia), sedation from antiepileptic medication, progression of the underlying disease process, non-convulsive SE and subtle generalized SE.

When benzodiazepines and phenytoin are ineffective, expert advice should be sought. Drugs that may be used in the control of SE are summarized in Table 8.5.2. Inhalational or barbiturate anaesthesia can also be used. Both require expert airway control, and in some cases inotropic support. Management in an intensive care unit is mandatory.

For all patients with SE, early consultation with intensive care and neurology services is essential in planning definitive management and disposition.

Non-convulsive seizures

Not all seizures are associated with convulsive activity. Convulsive seizures are generally easy to recognize, whereas non-convulsive seizures are more subtle and often require a high index of suspicion. These types of seizure are an important cause of alterations in behaviour and conscious level, and may precede or follow convulsive episodes. Seizures can involve any of the sensory modalities, vertiginous episodes, automatism, autonomic dysfunction or psychic disturbances, including *déjà vu* and *jamais vu* experiences. Non-convulsive seizures can easily be confused with migraine, cerebrovascular events or psychiatric conditions. The definitive diagnosis can only be made by EEG during the event.

Non-convulsive seizures may be partial (focal) or generalized. Complex partial seizures and focal seizures account for approximately one-third of all seizures, whereas primary generalized non-convulsive seizures (absence seizures) account for 6%.[11]

Non-convulsive status epilepticus (NCS) accounts for at least 25% of all cases of SE and is diagnosed more frequently when actively considered. Absence seizures rarely result in complete unresponsiveness, and patients may appear relatively normal to unfamiliar observers. NCS may precede or follow convulsive seizures and may easily create the perception of a cerebral vascular or psychiatric event. The longest reported episode of absence status is 60 days, and that of complex partial status 28 days.[12]

Treatment of non-convulsive seizures in the acute setting is the same as for convulsive seizures.[12] The event is terminated with benzodiazepines in most instances, and should be followed by a search for precipitating causes. An estimated 50% of patients with simple partial seizures have abnormal CT scans.[12] Long-term seizure control uses different agents from those used for convulsive seizures, highlighting the importance of involving a neurological service when planning follow-up.[12]

Pseudoseizures

Pseudoseizures or psychogenic seizures are events simulating neurogenic seizures but without the accompanying abnormal neuronal activity. Differentiation from neurogenic seizures may be extremely difficult, even for experienced neurologists. Neurogenic and psychogenic seizures may coexist, making the diagnostic dilemma even more complex. Differentiation will often require video-EEG monitoring, but this facility is not available in the ED and other methods must be used. It is important to recognize pseudoseizures so as to prevent the possible iatrogenic consequences of unnecessary treatment, while at the same time not withholding treatment from patients with neurogenic seizures.

Pseudoseizures are more common in women, less common after 35 years of age, and rare in patients over 50.[13] They may be associated with a conversion disorder, malingering, Munchausen syndrome or Munchausen syndrome by proxy. Patients with conversion disorder differ from malingerers by being unaware of the psychiatric cause of their actions.

Pseudoseizures typically last more than 5 minutes, compared to neurogenic seizures which usually terminate within 1–2 minutes. Multiple patterns of seizures tend to

Table 8.5.2 Doses of drugs used in refractory SE (Modified with permission from Brown AF, Wilkes GJ. Emergency department management of status epilepticus. Emergency Medicine 1994; 6: 49–61)		
Drug	*Bolus (i.v. unless stated otherwise)*	*Maintenance infusion*
Midazolam	0.02–0.1 mg/kg 0.15–0.3 mg/kg i.m.	0.05–0.4 mg/kg/h
Phenytoin	15–20 mg/kg at up to 50 mg/min, followed by further 5 mg/kg	N/A
Phenobarbitone	10–20 mg/kg at 60–100 mg/min	1–4 mg/kg/day
Thiopentone	5 mg/kg	1–3 mg/kg/h
Pentobarbitone (USA only)	5 mg/kg at 25 mg/min	0.5–3 mg/kg/h
Propofol	2 mg/kg	5–10 mg/kg/h
Lignocaine	2 mg/kg	3–6 mg/kg/h
Chlormethiazole	0.8% solution, 40–100 mL over 10 minute	0.8% solution 0.5–4 mL/min
Paraldehyde	0.15 mL/kg i.m. or 0.3–0.5 mL/kg rectally diluted 1:1 with vegetable oil	

occur in individual patients, and post-ictal periods are either very brief or absent. Patients with recall of events during what appears to be a generalized convulsive seizure are likely to have had a psychogenic seizure. Extremity movement out of phase from one side to the other and head turning from side to side typify pseudoseizures. Forward pelvic thrusting occurs in 44% of patients with pseudoseizures and is highly suggestive of the diagnosis.[14]

Several manoeuvres are useful in identifying pseudoseizures. Eye opening and arm drop tests are accompanied by avoidance, eyes turning away from the moving examiner, and termination of the event when the mouth and nostrils are occluded are characteristic. Simple verbal suggestion and reassurance are also frequently successful.

The most definitive means of differentiating pseudoseizures is by ictal EEG or video-EEG monitoring. Unfortunately, this is of little value in the ED. Blood gas determinations demonstrate a degree of acidaemia in neurogenic tonic–clonic seizures, but not in patients with pseudoseizures. Pulse oximetry will detect a fall in SaO_2 during neurogenic but not pseudoseizures. Serum prolactin levels rise and peak 15–20 minutes after generalized tonic–clonic seizures, and then fall with a half-life of 22 minutes. The levels do not consistently rise with partial seizures, and remain normal with pseudoseizures.[15]

Patients presenting with pseudoseizures are often treated with anticonvulsant medications, both acutely and for maintenance. Such patients usually demonstrate resistance to anticonvulsant medication, and many will therefore present with therapeutic or supratherapeutic levels. It is difficult to resist the temptation to immediately administer pharmacotherapy when confronted with a convulsing patient, but to do so will result in patients with pseudoseizures receiving unnecessary and potentially harmful treatment.

Careful examination of eye movements, pupil reactions, asynchronous limb movements, rapid head turning from side to side, forward pelvic thrust movements, testing for avoidance manoeuvres and monitoring pulse oximetry may enable the diagnosis to be made and drug therapy avoided. In doubtful cases, blood gas determinations are helpful and serum prolactin levels can be collected for later analysis. Doubtful cases should be discussed with a neurology service and arrangements made for emergency EEG.

Once the diagnosis is confirmed it must be presented in an open and non-threatening manner. Patients often have underlying personal and/or family problems that will need to be addressed. Psychotherapy is effective, but seizures often relapse at times of stress.

Alcohol-related seizures

Seizures represent 0.7% of ED visits, and alcohol contributes to approximately 50% of these.[16] The majority of alcohol-related seizures occur as part of the alcohol withdrawal syndrome.[17]

Although the precise pathophysiology of alcohol-related seizures has not been elucidated, it is clear that alcohol is a direct CNS toxin with direct epileptogenic effects. Acute toxicity and withdrawal are both associated with an increased incidence of seizures. Alcohol intoxication and chronic alcohol abuse are also associated with increased incidences of intercurrent disease such as trauma, coagulopathy, falls, assaults and other drug intoxication, all of which further increase the likelihood of seizures. The management of seizures presumed to be alcohol related must include a search for associated disease and other causes.

Benzodiazepines are the principal anticonvulsant agent for acute seizures. These agents are also valuable in the treatment of withdrawal. Phenytoin is ineffective in the control of acute seizures or as a preventative.

Drug-related seizures

Seizure activity in the setting of acute drug overdose is an ominous sign associated with greatly increased mortality and morbidity. The most commonly reported are in association with cyclic antidepressants (CA), antihistamines, theophylline, isoniazid, and drugs of addiction such as cocaine and amphetamines. The diagnosis and management of these toxic syndromes are discussed in the section on toxicology.

Some medications are also associated with lowering seizure threshold in susceptible individuals. Tramadol in particular has been increasingly prescribed for analgesia in recent times and associated with new-onset seizures at normal therapeutic doses.[5] A complete medication history is therefore essential.

Post-traumatic seizures

Post-traumatic epilepsy develops in 10–15% of serious head injury survivors.[18] More than half will have their first seizure within 1 year. Significant risk factors are central parietal injury, dural penetration, hemiplegia, missile wounds and intracerebral haematomas.[19] Early treatment with phenytoin for severe head injuries reduces the incidence of seizures in the first week only.[20]

Seizures developing after significant head trauma have a higher incidence of intracranial pathology. Contrast CT is the initial investigation of choice. MRI will demonstrate more abnormalities but has not been shown to affect outcome. Long-term treatment with anticonvulsants should be planned in conjunction with a neurosurgical service.

Seizures and pregnancy

Seizures can occur during pregnancy as part of an established epileptic process, as new seizures, or induced by pregnancy. The most significant situations are eclampsia and generalized convulsive status epilepticus. At all times the management is directed at both mother and baby, with the realization that the best treatment for the baby will relate to optimal maternal care.

In previously diagnosed epileptics there is an increased risk of seizures during pregnancy of 17%.[21] Anticonvulsant levels are influenced by reduced protein binding, increased drug binding and reduced absorption of varying degrees. The final effect on free drug levels is unpredictable and is most variable around the time of delivery.[22] Careful clinical monitoring is essential, and monitoring of free drug levels rather than total serum levels may be necessary in selected patients. Anticonvulsants also interfere with the metabolism of vitamins D, K and folic acid. Supplementation is advisable.

Isolated simple seizures place both mother and fetus at increased danger of injury, but are otherwise generally well tolerated. Generalized seizures during labour cause transient fetal hypoxia and bradycardia of uncertain significance. Generalized convulsive SE is life-threatening to both mother and fetus at any stage of pregnancy.

All of the anticonvulsants cross the placenta and are potentially teratogenic. The risk of malformation in children is increased from 3.4% in the general population to 3.7% in epileptic mothers.[23] In general, the types of malformation associated are not drug specific, apart from the increased risk of neural tube defects associated with valproate and carbamazepine. Prenatal screening for such defects is advised in patients who become pregnant while taking these agents. The risk from uncontrolled seizures greatly outweighs the risk from prophylactic medication in patients with good seizure control.[3,24]

The management of seizures in pregnant patients is along the same lines as for non-pregnant patients. After 20 weeks' gestation the patient should have a wedge placed under the right hip to prevent supine hypotension, and eclampsia must be considered. Investigation will include an assessment of fetal wellbeing by heart rate, ultrasound and/or tocography, as indicated. Management and disposition should be decided in consultation with neurology and obstetric services.

Eclampsia is the occurrence of seizures in patients with pregnancy-induced toxaemia occurring after the 20th week of pregnancy, and consists of a triad of hypertension, oedema and proteinuria. One in 300 women with pre-eclampsia progresses to eclampsia. Seizures are typically brief, self-terminating, usually preceded by headache and visual disturbances, and tend to occur without warning.[25] Treatment is directed at controlling the seizures and hypertension, and expedient delivery of the baby. Magnesium sulphate is effective in seizure control and is associated with a better outcome for both mother and baby than standard anticonvulsant and antihypertensive

therapy.[26-29] The mechanism of action is unclear.[25]

Management of SE in pregnancy includes consideration of eclampsia, positioning in the left lateral position, and assessment and monitoring of fetal wellbeing. Urgent control of seizures is essential for both mother and baby. Phenobarbital may reduce the incidence of intraventricular haemorrhage in premature infants, and should be considered in place of phenytoin in this circumstance.[30] Early involvement of obstetric and neurology services is essential.

Future directions

Non-invasive portable modalities allowing definitive precise diagnosis of seizures in the ED will reduce the need for subsequent investigations in the majority of patients who do not have true epilepsy, and permit early focused therapy. Advances in pharmacotherapy and neurosurgical techniques will also improve seizure control with minimal side effects, allowing patients to more effectively resume normal activities.

Controversies

- Investigation required for patients with first seizures.

- Place of lumbar puncture in the investigation of first seizures.

- Role of antipyretics in febrile seizures.

References

1. Engel J Jr, Starkman S. Overview of seizures. Emergency Medicine Clinics of North America 1994; 12(4): 895–923.
2. Mosewich RK, So EL. A clinical approach to the classification of seizures and epileptic syndromes [see Comments]. Mayo Clinic Proceedings 1996; 71(4): 405–414.
3. Cavasos JE et al. Seizures and Epilepsy: Overview and Classification 2005. http://www.eMedicine.com Accessed August 2007.
4. American College of Emergency Physicians. Clinical policy for the initial approach to patients presenting with a chief complaint of seizure, who are not in status epilepticus. Annals of Emergency Medicine 1993; 22(5): 875–883.
5. Labate A, Newton MR, et al. Tramadol and new-onset seizures. Med J Aust 2005; 182(1): 42–43.
6. Reinus WR, Wippold FJD, Erickson KK. Seizure patient selection for emergency computed tomography. Annals of Emergency Medicine 1993; 22(8): 1298–1303.
7. Treiman DM. Electroclinical features of status epilepticus. Journal of Clinical Neurophysiology 1995; 12(4): 343–362.
8. Brown AF, Wilkes GJ. Emergency department management of status epilepticus. Emergency Medicine 1994; 6: 49–61.
9. McDonagh TJ, Jelinek GA, Galvin GM. Intramuscular midazolam rapidly terminates seizures in children and adults. Emergency Medicine 1992; (4): 77–81.
10. Lowenstein DH, Alldredge BK. Status epilepticus. New England Journal of Medicine 1998; 338(14): 970–976.
11. Hauser WA, Annegers JF, Kurland LT. Incidence of epilepsy and unprovoked seizures in Rochester, Minnesota: 1935–1984. Epilepsia 1993; 34(3): 453–468.
12. Jagoda A. Nonconvulsive seizures. Emergency Medical Clinics of North America 1994; 12(4): 963–971.
13. Riggio S. Psychogenic seizures. Emergency Medicine Clinics of North America 1994; 12(4): 1001–1012.
14. Gates JR, Ramani V, Whalen S, et al. Ictal characteristics of pseudoseizures. Archives of Neurology 1985; 42(12): 1183–1187.
15. Dana-Haeri J, Trimble MR. Prolactin and gonadotrophin changes following partial seizures in epileptic patients with and without psychopathology. Biology Psychiatry 1984; 19(3): 329–336.
16. Morris JC, Victor M. Alcohol withdrawal seizures. Emergency Medicine Clinics of North America 1987; 5(4): 827–839.
17. Krumholz A, Grufferman S, Orr ST, et al. Seizures and seizure care in an emergency department. Epilepsia 1989; 30(2): 175–181.
18. Dugan EM, Howell JM. Posttraumatic seizures. Emergency Medicine Clinics of North America 1994; 12(4): 1081–1107.
19. Feeney DM, Walker AE. The prediction of posttraumatic epilepsy. A mathematical approach. Archives of Neurology 1979; 36(1): 8–12.
20. Temkin NR, Haglund MM, Winn HR. Causes, prevention, and treatment of post-traumatic epilepsy. New Horizons 1995; 3(3): 518–522.
21. Shuster EA. Seizures in pregnancy. Emergency Medicine Clinics of North America 1994; 12(4): 1013–1025.
22. Yerby MS, Friel PN, McCormick K. Antiepileptic drug disposition during pregnancy. Neurology 1992; 42(4 Suppl 5): 12–16.
23. Stanley FJ, Priscott PK, Johnston R, et al. Congenital malformations in infants of mothers with diabetes and epilepsy in Western Australia, 1980–1982. Medical Journal of Australia 1985; 143(10): 440–442.
24. Yerby MS. Risks of pregnancy in women with epilepsy. Epilepsia 1992; 33(Suppl 1): S23–26; discussion S26–27.
25. Sibai BM. Medical disorders in pregnancy, including hypertensive diseases. Current Opinion in Obstetrics and Gynaecology 1991; 3(1): 28–40.
26. The Eclampsia Trial Collaborative Group. Which anticonvulsant for women with eclampsia? Evidence from the Collaborative Eclampsia Trial [published erratum appears in Lancet 346(8969): 258]. Lancet 1995; 345(8963): 1455–1463.
27. Lucas MJ, Leveno KJ, Cunningham FG. A comparison of magnesium sulfate with phenytoin for the prevention of eclampsia [see Comments]. New England Journal of Medicine 1995; 333(4): 201–205.
28. Duggan K, Macdonald G. Comparative study of different anticonvulsants in eclampsia. Journal of Obstetric and Gynaecological Research 1997; 23(3): 289–293.
29. Jagoda A, Riggio S. Emergency department approach to managing seizures in pregnancy. Annals of Emergency Medicine 1991; 20(1): 80–85.
30. Morales WJ. Antenatal therapy to minimize neonatal intraventricular hemorrhage. Clinical Obstetrics and Gynecology 1991; 34(2): 328–335.

8.6 Syncope and vertigo

Rosslyn Hing

ESSENTIALS

1 It is important to distinguish between syncope and true vertigo.

2 The most common cause of syncope is neurally mediated syncope.

3 A detailed history and physical examination are more useful than extensive investigations.

4 It is essential to identify high-risk patients for the serious potential cardiac causes of syncope so that appropriate treatment can be given.

5 Determine whether a central or peripheral cause of vertigo is more likely.

6 Dynamic manoeuvres may be both diagnostic and therapeutic.

Introduction

Syncope and vertigo are relatively common symptoms. They are often described by patients using the term 'dizziness'; however, it is essential to differentiate between the two. Syncope and vertigo both represent a significant diagnostic challenge and it is important to risk-stratify patients accurately to distinguish between potentially life-threatening and benign causes.

Syncope

Syncope as a presenting symptom represents about 1–1.5% of all emergency department (ED) attendances.[1] It is a symptom, not a diagnosis. It is defined as a loss of consciousness induced by the temporarily insufficient flow of blood to the brain. Patients recover spontaneously, without therapeutic intervention or prolonged confusion.

There is no simple test to distinguish between the benign and the potentially life-threatening causes of syncope, but a careful history, examination and bedside investigations can help determine appropriate disposition.

The causes of syncope are summarized in Table 8.6.1. The most common cause in all age groups is neurally mediated syncope, also known as neurocardiogenic or vasovagal syncope.[2] Orthostatic hypotension and cardiac causes are the next most common.[3]

Clinical features

Patients with syncope are often completely asymptomatic by the time they arrive at hospital. A thorough history and physical examination is the key to finding the correct cause for the syncope. The history should focus on the patient's recollection of the preceding and subsequent events, including environmental conditions, physical activity, prodromal symptoms and any intercurrent medical problems. Accounts from eyewitnesses or first responders are also vital. Medications that may impair autonomic reflexes need to be scrutinized and a postural blood pressure measurement performed. Physical examination should concentrate on finding signs of structural heart disease, as well as assessing any subsequent injuries.

Neurally mediated syncope causes a typical prodrome: patients complain of feeling lightheaded and faint, and often describe a blurring or 'tunnelling' of their vision. This may be accompanied by other vagally mediated symptoms such as nausea or sweating. More pronounced vagal symptoms include an urge to open their bowels. If patients are unable or unwilling to follow their body's natural instincts to lie flat, they may collapse to the ground as they lose consciousness. This reflex brings the head level with the heart, resulting in an improvement in cerebral perfusion and a return to consciousness. During this time the patient may exhibit brief myoclonic movements, which can be mistaken for seizure activity, but in contrast to true epileptic seizures, there are no prolonged post-ictal symptoms. Fatigue is common following syncope.

Table 8.6.1 Aetiology of syncope	
Neurally mediated	**Cardiac**
Vasovagal/neurocardiogenic	Structural valvular disease such as aortic stenosis
Situational: cough, micturition, defaecation	Cardiomyopathy
Carotid sinus syndrome	Unstable angina
	Myocardial infarction
	Bradyarrhythmias such as sinus node disease, AV block
	Tachyarrhythmias such as VT, SVT and *torsades de pointes*
	Pacemaker/defibrillator dysfunction
	Pulmonary hypertension
	Pulmonary embolus
	Aortic dissection
Orthostatic hypotension	**Neurological**
Dehydration	Vertebrobasilar transient ischaemic attack
Vasodilatation	Subclavian steal
	Migraines
Medication	Psychiatric
Antihypertensives	
β-Blockers	
Cardiac glycosides	
Diuretics	
Antiarrhythmics	
Antiparkinsonian drugs	
Nitrates	
Alcohol	

NEUROLOGY

Orthostatic hypotension occurs when the patient moves from a lying position to a sitting or standing position. If the required autonomic changes fail to compensate adequately, even healthy individuals will experience lightheadedness or blurring of their vision, and possibly a loss of consciousness. The most vulnerable people are those with blunted or impaired autonomic reflexes, such as the elderly, those on certain medications (particularly vasodilators, antihypertensive agents and β-blockers) and those who are relatively volume depleted due to heat, excessive fluid losses or inadequate oral intake.

Cardiac syncope is more likely to present with an absent or brief prodrome. Sudden unexplained loss of consciousness should raise suspicion for a cardiac arrhythmia, particularly in the high-risk patient. Both tachycardia and bradycardia can be responsible. A syncopal event while supine is of particular concern, and a predictor for a cardiac cause.[4] Those that occur during exertion should prompt a search for structural heart disease, in particular aortic stenosis.

Risk stratification

Most of the published literature on assessment of patients presenting to EDs with syncope has focused on identifying risk factors for mortality or adverse cardiac outcome. Colivicchi et al.[5] developed the OESIL score, based on four high-risk factors identified in a multicentre Italian study aimed at predicting mortality at a year. These were age over 65 years, a history of cardiovascular disease (which encompasses ischaemic heart disease, congestive cardiac failure, cerebrovascular disease and peripheral vascular disease), an abnormal ECG (including signs of ischaemia, arrhythmias, prolonged QT interval, AV block or bundle branch block) and absence of the typical prodrome. Martin[6] derived a similar group of risk factors in a cohort of syncope patients and then validated these prospectively. More recently, Quinn et al.[7,8] devised and then validated the San Francisco Syncope Rule (SFSR), where five factors were used to predict serious short-term and longer-term outcomes. These factors are:

❶ History of congestive cardiac failure.
❷ Haematocrit < 30%.

❸ Abnormal ECG.
❹ Patient complaining of shortness of breath.
❺ Systolic blood pressure < 90 mmHg at triage.

Distilling these factors, patients with syncope can be divided into high- and low-risk groups as shown in Table 8.6.2. Low-risk patients can be safely discharged for outpatient follow-up, but controversy over high-risk patients remains. It is likely that there is a significant proportion of patients in the high-risk group who are actually intermediate risk, and given further evaluation in the ED or a short-stay unit could also be safely discharged; however, it is more difficult to identify this subset.

A number of projects have attempted to further define risk groups or assess risk stratification approaches. The Risk Stratification of Syncope in the Emergency department (ROSE pilot)[9] compared the performance of the OESIL score, SFSR and the Edinburgh Royal Infirmary ED Syncope Guidelines and found that although the SFSR showed the best sensitivity for detecting adverse events, this was at the expense of increased hospital admissions. Similarly, an Australian validation study found that the SFSR was fairly sensitive but that it would have increased admissions by 9% if all high risk patients were admitted.[10] The Syncope Evaluation in the Emergency Department Study (SEEDS)[11] randomized patients deemed to be intermediate risk to either conventional assessment or assessment in a specialized syncope unit.

Table 8.6.2 Risk stratification for an adverse outcome	
High risk	**Low risk**
Chest pain consistent with IHD	Age < 45 years
History of congestive cardiac failure	Otherwise healthy
History of ventricular arrhythmias	Normal ECG
Pacemaker/defibrillator dysfunction	Normal cardiovascular exam
Abnormal ECG (findings such as prolonged QTc interval, conduction abnormalities, acute ischaemia)	Prodrome (consistent with neurally mediated syncope or orthostatic hypotension)
Exertional syncope/valvular heart disease	
Age > 60 years	

It reported that a specialized unit increased the diagnostic yield and reduced the need for inpatient hospital admission.

Differential diagnosis

Seizures are commonly listed as a cause for syncope. Although they do cause a transient loss of consciousness, the pathophysiology is very different. Post-ictal confusion often helps to differentiate the two; however, urinary incontinence may also occur in syncope. True tonic–clonic activity needs to be distinguished from the brief myoclonic jerks occasionally seen in syncope.

Transient ischaemic attacks (TIAs) are often attributed as potential causes for syncope, but this is rare. Only vertebrobasilar territory TIAs can affect the reticular activating system of the brain to cause a loss of consciousness.

Clinical investigations

The only two mandatory investigations are a 12-lead ECG and blood glucose. These should add enough information to the clinical findings to stratify the patient as high or low risk for an adverse outcome. Research has found that a serum troponin taken at least 4 hours after a syncopal event is not a sensitive predictor of an adverse cardiac outcome.[12]

Syncope may also be the presenting symptom of a potentially life-threatening condition such as pulmonary embolus, subarachnoid haemorrhage, gastrointestinal bleed or aortic aneurysm. If these are suspected, appropriate investigations based on clinical suspicion should be initiated.

Treatment

Treatment depends on the presumptive diagnosis. Those with neurally mediated syncope require explanation and reassurance only. After ensuring that the vital signs have returned to baseline, their blood glucose and ECG are within normal limits, and that they have had something to eat and drink, these patients may be discharged without further investigations.

Patients with orthostatic hypotension often require intravenous fluids and an adequate oral intake to reverse their postural blood pressure changes. Any decision regarding potential changes to chronic medications should ideally include the patient's primary care/treating doctor.

Patients who are deemed high risk for a cardiac cause need continuous cardiac monitoring for at least 24 hours and admission for further evaluation. This may include echocardiography to identify structural heart problems and to quantify an ejection fraction, or electrophysiological studies.

Prognosis

Syncope in a patient with underlying heart disease implies a poor prognosis, with data suggesting that a third will die within a year of the episode.[13] Overall, those with syncope on a background of congestive cardiac failure are at the highest risk for an adverse outcome.[1] In the absence of underlying heart disease, syncope is not associated with excess mortality.[2]

Vertigo

Vertigo is defined as the disabling sensation in which the affected individual feels that he himself or his surroundings are in a state of constant movement. It has a reported 1-year incidence of 1.4%.[14] Like syncope, it is a symptom not a diagnosis, and has as many causes. The difficulty is that whereas many of the causes of vertigo are benign, it may be a symptom of serious neurological conditions such as vertebrobasilar stroke.

Aetiology

The causes of vertigo may be divided into peripheral and central (Table 8.6.3).

Clinical features

It is vital to establish whether the patient is suffering true vertigo, as opposed to pre-syncope, loss of consciousness or mild unsteadiness. It is also necessary to clarify whether they have a sense of continuous motion (vertigo) or whether they feel 'light-headed' or 'dizzy'.

If the patient feels they are moving in relation to their surroundings this is termed subjective vertigo; however, if the patient feels that the surroundings are spinning around them, this is termed objective vertigo.

As previously described, vertigo may be central or peripheral in origin. Peripheral vertigo tends to be more intense and associated with nausea, vomiting, diaphoresis and auditory symptoms such as tinnitus or hearing loss (although hearing loss can rarely occur with vascular insufficiency in the posterior cerebral circulation, as the auditory apparatus is supplied via the anterior inferior cerebellar artery or the posterior inferior cerebellar artery). There may also be a history of ear trauma, barotrauma, ear infection or generalized illness. The onset of the vertigo tends to be subacute, coming on over minutes to hours. Central vertigo tends to be less severe and associated with neurological symptoms and signs such as headache, weakness of the limbs, ataxia, incoordination and dysarthria. These symptoms may be the harbinger of more serious causes, such as cerebellar lesions or demyelinating diseases (Table 8.6.4).

Physical examination concentrates on any positional factors plus a detailed search for neurological signs, in particular nystagmus. This is the main objective sign of vertigo. Any spontaneous movement of the eyes needs to be noted, plus direction and persistence. Peripheral vertigo tends to produce unidirectional nystagmus with the slow phase towards the affected side. In addition, patients with vestibular nystagmus are often able to suppress it by fixating on a stationary object.

Cardiovascular examination should focus on the risk factors for central nervous system thromboembolic events, such as arrhythmias, murmurs and bruits.

Clinical investigations

Most patients who present with vertigo do not need laboratory tests, apart from a blood glucose level. If there is a history of trauma or a space-occupying lesion is suspected, then a CT or MRI scan of the brain is indicated. An ECG should also be performed to help rule out arrhythmias if syncope is the possible problem.

Dynamic manoeuvres can be both diagnostic and therapeutic. The Dix–Hallpike test[15] can diagnose benign paroxysmal positional vertigo (BPPV). It should not be performed on patients with carotid bruits, and patients must be warned that the test may provoke severe symptoms.

Initially, the patient should be seated upright, close enough to the head of the bed so that when they are supine the head will be able to extend back a further 30–45°. To test the right posterior semicircular canal, the head is initially rotated 30–45° to the right. Keeping the head in this position, the patient is quickly brought to the horizontal position with the head placed 30–45° below the level of the bed. A positive test is indicated by rotatory nystagmus

Table 8.6.3	Aetiology of vertigo
Peripheral	Central
Benign paroxysmal positional vertigo (BPPV)	Cerebellar haemorrhage and infarction
Vestibular neuritis	Vertebrobasilar insufficiency
Acute labyrinthitis	
Ménière's disease	Neoplasms
Ototoxicitiy	Multiple sclerosis
Eighth-nerve lesions such as acoustic neuromas	Wallenberg's syndrome (lateral medullary syndrome)
Cerebellopontine angle tumours	Migrainous vertigo
Post-traumatic vertigo	

Table 8.6.4	Clinical features of vertigo	
	Peripheral	Central
Onset	Acute	Gradual
Severity	Severe	Less intense
Duration, pattern	Paroxysmal, intermittent; minutes to days	Constant; usually weeks to months
Positional	Yes	No
Associated nausea	Frequent	Infrequent
Nystagmus	Rotatory – vertical, horizontal	Vertical
Fatigue of symptoms, signs	Yes	No
Hearing loss/tinnitus	May occur	Not usually
CNS symptoms, signs	No	Usually

towards the affected ear. The test is then repeated on the left side.

Treatment

Treatment depends on the cause. Benign paroxysmal positional vertigo (BPPV) has the classic history of position-induced vertigo lasting only seconds. If BPPV is suspected, the Dix–Hallpike test is performed to identify the affected ear. The Epley manoeuvre[15] or 'canalith repositioning manoeuvre' aims to move any unwanted particles out of the semicircular canals and thus ease the symptoms for which they are responsible. The steps of this manoeuvre are:

❶ The patient is seated as for the Dix–Hallpike test with the head turned 45° toward the affected ear.

❷ The patient is brought to the horizontal position with the head hyperextended 30–45° below the bed.

❸ The head is gently rotated 45° towards the midline.

❹ The head is then rotated a further 45° towards the unaffected ear.

❺ The patient rolls onto the shoulder of the unaffected side, at the same time rotating the head a further 45°.

❻ The patient is returned to the sitting position and the head returned to the midline.

These movements may induce nystagmus in the same direction as that seen during the Dix–Hallpike test. Be aware that nystagmus in the opposite direction indicates an unsuccessful test. The manoeuvre may need to be repeated a few times.

Vestibular neuritis is unilateral and thought to be caused by a viral infection or inflammation. Episodes are acute in onset and may be severe, lasting for days, usually associated with nausea and vomiting. The sense of perpetual movement is present even with the eyes closed, and is made worse by movement of the head. Symptomatic treatment, with medications such as antihistamines, antiemetics and benzodiazepines, is often all that is indicated. If nausea and vomiting are severe, intravenous fluid therapy may be needed. There are some reports of trials using steroids for vestibular neuritis, but this treatment remains unproven.[16]

Acute labyrinthitis may be viral or bacterial in origin. If it is viral, the course and treatment are similar to those of vestibular neuritis. Bacterial labyrinthitis may develop from an otitis media. The key feature here is severe vertigo with hearing loss. Patients are febrile and toxic and require admission for intravenous antibiotics.

Ménière's disease has the classic triad of vertigo, sensorineural hearing loss and tinnitus. Attacks last from minutes to hours, and may recur with increasing frequency as the disease progresses. It is caused by dilatation of the endolymphatic system due to excessive production or problems with reabsorption of the endolymph (endolymphatic hydrops). Medical management traditionally involves salt restriction and diuretics, although a Cochrane Review has questioned the efficacy of this.[17]

Vertebrobasilar insufficiency can produce vertigo, often accompanied by unsteadiness and visual changes. Symptoms may be provoked by head position and often include headache. Importantly, however, patients with cerebellar infarction occasionally present with vertigo without other symptoms or signs of neurological impairment.[18] Treatment involves addressing cardiovascular risk factors as well as antiplatelet therapy.

Migrainous vertigo is an increasingly recognized condition that is incompletely understood. In the acute setting it poses a diagnostic challenge that will often necessitate exclusion of other central causes for vertigo, such as cerebrovascular disease.

Controversies

- Identifying and determining disposition for syncope patients who do not fall into the high- or low-risk groups.

- Role of a dedicated syncope evaluation unit.

- The use of corticosteroids to treat vestibular neuritis.

References

1. American College of Emergency Physicians. Clinical Policy: Critical issues in the evaluation and management of adult patients presenting to the emergency department with syncope. Annals of Emergency Medicine 2007; 49: 431–444.
2. Strickberger SA, Benson DW, Biaggioni I, et al. AHA/ACCF Scientific Statement on the Evaluation of Syncope. Circulation 2006; 113: 316–327.
3. Linzer M, Yang EH, Estes M, et al. Diagnosing syncope Part 1: Value of history, physical examination and electrocardiography. Clinical Efficacy Assessment project of the American College of Physicians. Annals of Internal Medicine 1997; 126: 989–996.
4. Jhanjee R, van Dijk JG, Sakaguchi S, et al. Syncope in adults: terminology, classification and diagnostic strategy. Pacing and Clinical Electrophysiology 2006; 29: 1160–1169.
5. Colivicchi F, Ammirati F, Melina D, et al. Development and prospective validation of a risk stratification system for patients with syncope in the emergency department. European Heart Journal 2003; 24: 811–819.
6. Martin TP, Hanusa BH, Kapoor WN. Risk stratification of patients with syncope. Annals of Emergency Medicine 1997; 29: 459–466.
7. Quinn JV, Stiell IG, McDermott DA, et al. Derivation of the San Francisco Syncope Rule to predict patients with short-term serious outcomes. Annals of Emergency Medicine 2004; 43: 224–232.
8. Quinn JV, Stiell IG, McDermott DA, et al. Prospective validation of the San Francisco Syncope Rule to predict patients with short-term serious outcomes. Annals of Emergency Medicine 2006; 47: 448–454.
9. Reed MJ, Newby DE, Coull AJ, et al. Risk Stratification of Syncope in the Emergency Department (ROSE) pilot study: A comparison of existing Syncope guidelines. Emergency Medicine Journal 2007; 24: 270–275.
10. Cosgriff T, Kelly AM, Kerr D. External validation of the San Francisco Syncope Rule in the Australian context. Canadian Journal of Emergency Medicine 2007; 9: 157–161.
11. Shen WK, Decker WW, Smars PA, et al. Syncope evaluation in the Emergency Department (SEEDS). Circulation 2004; 110: 3636–3645.
12. Hing R, Harris R. Relative utility of serum troponin and the OESIL score in syncope. Emergency Medicine of Australasia 2005; 17: 31–38.
13. Crane SD. Risk stratification of patients with syncope in an accident and emergency department. Emergency Medicine Journal 2002; 19: 23–27.
14. Neuhauser HK, von Brevern M, Radtke A, et al. Epidemiology of vestibular vertigo: a neurotological study of the general population. Neurology 2005; 65: 898–904.
15. Tintinalli J, Kelen G, Stapczynski S (eds). Emergency medicine. A comprehensive study guide, 6th edn. American College of Emergency Physicians 2003; 1402–1405.
16. Strupp M, Zingler VC, Arbuso V, et al. Methylprednisolone, valaciclovir, or the combination for vestibular neuritis. New England Journal of Medicine 2004; 351: 354–361.
17. Seemungal BM. Neuro-otological emergencies. Current Opinion in Neurology 2007; 20: 32–39.
18. Lee H, Yi HA, Cho YW, et al. Nodulus infarction mimicking peripheral vestibulopathy. Neurology 2003; 60: 1700–1702.

9.1 Approach to undifferentiated fever in adults

Allen Yung • Jonathan Knott

ESSENTIALS

1 Over one-third of patients who have fever for more than 2–3 days with no localizing symptoms and signs are likely to have a bacterial infection; half of these will be in the respiratory or urinary tracts.

2 An unexplained fever in a person over the age of 50 should be regarded as due to a bacterial infection until proved otherwise.

3 An undifferentiated fever in an alcoholic patient, an intravenous drug user or an insulin-dependent diabetic is generally an indication for admission to hospital.

4 Any fever in a traveller returned from a malaria-endemic area should be regarded as due to malaria until proved otherwise.

5 Severe muscle pain, even in the absence of overt fever, may be an early symptom of meningococcaemia, staphylococcal or streptococcal bacteraemia.

6 An unexplained rash in a febrile patient should be regarded as meningococcaemia until proved otherwise.

7 The diagnosis of meningococcaemia should be considered in every patient with an undifferentiated fever.

8 There will always be a small number of febrile patients whose sepsis is not initially recognized because they do not appear toxic and their symptoms are non-specific. It is essential that all patients are encouraged to seek review if they have any clinical deterioration.

Introduction

Fever is a common presenting symptom to the emergency department (ED): about 5% of patients give fever as the reason for their visit. Most patients with fever have symptoms and signs that indicate the site or region of infection. A prospective study of patients aged 16 years or older who presented to an ED with fever $\geq 37.9°C$ found that 85% had localizing symptoms and signs that suggested or identified a source of fever, and 15% had unexplained fever after the history and examination.[1]

Fever with no localizing symptoms or signs at presentation is often seen in the first day or two of the illness. Many patients with such a problem will ultimately prove to have self-limiting viral infections, but others will have non-viral infections requiring treatment. Among this latter group are illnesses that may be serious and even rapidly fatal.

Over one-third of patients, who have fever for more than a few days with no localizing symptoms and signs are likely to have a bacterial infection.[1,2]

If no cause is found in an adult with fever present for over 3 days there is a good chance the patient will have a bacterial infection that needs treatment. Over half of these infections are likely to be in the respiratory or urinary tracts.[1]

The most important task in the ED for febrile patients without localizing features is not to miss early bacterial meningitis, bacteraemia such as meningococcaemia, and early staphylococcal and streptococcal toxic shock syndromes.

Approach

The management of febrile patients varies according to the severity, duration and tempo of the illness, the type of patient and the epidemiological setting. Although the steps in management of a febrile patient in the ED, listed below, may be set out in a sequential manner, in reality the mental processes involved occur simultaneously by the bedside.

- Step 1: Identify the very ill.
- Step 2: Find localizing symptoms and signs.
- Step 3: Look for 'at-risk' patients.

Step 1: Identify the seriously ill patient who requires urgent intervention

The first step in managing febrile patients is to identify those in need of immediate resuscitation, urgent investigations and empirical therapy. The presence of any of the following features justifies immediate intervention: shock, coma/stupor, cyanosis, profound dyspnoea, continuous seizures and severe dehydration.

Step 2: Identify those with localized infections or easily diagnosable diseases

Having excluded those who need urgent intervention, the doctor has more time to attempt a diagnosis. The history and physical examination are usually sufficient to localize the source of community-acquired fever in most cases, especially if the illness has been present for several days.

History

A precise history remains the key to diagnosis of a febrile illness. An inability to give a history and to think clearly is a sign of potential sepsis.

Illness

An abrupt onset of fever, particularly when accompanied by chills or rigors and generalized aches, is highly suggestive of an infective illness.

Localizing symptoms, their evolution and relative severity, helps to identify the site of infection; localized pain is particularly valuable in this way.

The severity and the course of the illness can be assessed by the patient's ability to work, to be up and about, to eat and sleep, and the amount of analgesics taken.

Previous state of health

Underlying diseases predispose patients to infection at certain sites or caused by certain specific organisms. Knowledge of any defects in the immune system is similarly helpful. For example, asplenic patients are more prone to overwhelming pneumococcal septicaemia, and renal transplant patients to *Listeria* meningitis.

A past history of infectious diseases, particularly if properly documented, may be useful in excluding infections such as measles and hepatitis.

Predisposing events

Recent operations, accidents and injuries and medications taken may be the direct cause of the illness (e.g. drug fever, or rash from co-trimoxazole, ampicillin) or may affect the resistance of the patient, predisposing to certain infections. Concurrent menstruation raises the possibility of toxic shock syndrome.

Epidemiology

Information on occupation, exposure to animals, hobbies, risk factors for blood-borne viruses, and travel overseas or to rural areas may suggest certain specific infections, e.g. leptospirosis, acute HIV infection, hepatitis C, malaria etc.

Contact with similar diseases and known infectious diseases

This information is useful in the diagnosis of problems such as meningococcal infection, viral exanthema, respiratory infection, diarrhoea, and zoonoses.

Examination

Physical examination in the febrile patient serves two purposes: to assess the severity of the illness and to find a site of infection.

Bedside assessment of severity and 'toxicity' based on intuitive judgement is frequently wrong, and many patients with severe bacterial infections do not appear obviously ill or toxic.

Physical examination may yield a diagnosis in a febrile patient who has not complained of any localizing symptoms. A checklist of special areas to be examined is useful.

- Eyes: Conjunctival haemorrhages are seen in staphylococcal endocarditis, and scleral jaundice may be present before cutaneous jaundice is obvious.
- Skin: Rashes of any sort, especially petechial rash; cellulitis in the lower legs may present with fever and constitutional symptoms before pain in the leg develops. Evidence of intravenous drug use should be sought at the common injection sites.
- Heart: Murmurs and pericardial rubs.
- Lungs: Subtle crackles may be heard in pneumonic patients without respiratory symptoms.
- Abdominal organs: Tenderness and enlargement without subjective pain may be the only clue to infections in these organs.
- Lymph nodes: Especially the posterior cervical glands. Tenderness of the jugulodigastric glands is a good sign of bacterial tonsillitis.
- Sore throat may be absent in the first few hours of streptococcal tonsillitis. Examination of the throat may give the diagnosis. Oedema of the uvula is also a useful sign of bacterial infection in that region.
- Marked muscle tenderness is a frequent sign of sepsis.
- Neck stiffness may be a clue to meningitis in a confused patient who cannot give a history.
- Any area that is covered, e.g. under plasters or bandages, for evidence of sepsis.

There are two caveats when assessing local symptoms and signs.

- Localizing features may not be present or obvious early in the course of a focal infection, e.g. the absence of cough in bacterial pneumonia, sore throat in tonsillitis or diarrhoea in gastrointestinal infections in the first 12–36 hours of the illness.

- Localizing features may occasionally be misleading. For example, diarrhoea, which suggests infection of the gastrointestinal tract, may be a manifestation of more generalized infection, such as Gram-negative septicaemia, and crepitations at the lung base may indicate a subdiaphragmatic condition rather than a chest infection.

Step 3: Look for the 'at-risk' patient

If no diagnosis is forthcoming after the first two steps, the next task is to identify the 'at-risk' patient who may not appear overtly ill but who nonetheless requires medical intervention. This applies particularly to those with treatable diseases that can progress rapidly, such as bacterial meningitis, bacteraemia and toxic shock syndromes.

Four sets of pointers are helpful in identifying these 'at-risk' patients: the type of patient (host characteristics), exposure history, the nature of the non-specific symptoms, and how rapidly the illness evolves.

Clinical pointers: type of patient

Clinical manifestations of infections are often subtle or non-specific in young children, the elderly and the immunocompromised. The threshold for intervention in these patients should be lowered. The issue of fever in children is not addressed in this chapter.

Elderly patients Elderly patients with infections often do not mount much of a febrile response, and fever may be absent in 20–30% of these patients.[3]

Infectious diseases in the elderly, as in the very young, often present with non-specific or atypical symptoms and signs, and may progress rapidly.[4]

In adult patients with unexplained fever up to one-third may have bacteraemia or focal bacterial infection. This proportion is even higher in those over the age of 50.[1] In the elderly a fever $> 38°C$ indicates a possible serious infection[5] and is associated with increasing risk of death.[6]

The urinary tract is the most frequent site of infection and source of bacteraemia; symptoms of urinary tract infection are frequently absent in the elderly. The

respiratory tract is the next most common site of infection; fever and malaise may be the only clues of pneumonia in the elderly. Urinalysis and chest X-ray will identify about half of occult infections.[1]

An unexplained fever in a person over the age of 50 should be regarded as being caused by a bacterial infection until proved otherwise, and is generally an indication for admission to hospital.

Alcoholic patients Alcoholic patients present with multiple problems, many of which cause fever. Most are caused by infections, the commonest of which is pneumonia. Multiple infections may occur at the same time.[7]

Non-infectious causes of fever frequently coexist with infections, and conditions such as subarachnoid haemorrhage, alcoholic withdrawal and alcoholic hepatitis require admission.

The initial history and physical examination in the alcoholic may be unreliable and diagnosis may be difficult.

Alcoholic patients with fever for which no obvious cause is found should be admitted to hospital for investigations and observation.

Injecting drug users The risk of injecting drug users acquiring serious or unusual infections is high through repeated self-injection with non-sterile illicit substances, the use of contaminated needles and syringes, and poor attention to skin cleansing prior to injections.[8]

Most intravenous drug users presenting with fever have a serious infection. Some have obvious focal infections such as cellulitis and pneumonia. Others present simply with fever, and the presence of bacteraemia and endocarditis must be suspected.

Clinical assessment cannot differentiate trivial from potentially serious conditions in these patients.[8] A history of chills, rigors and sweats strongly suggest the presence of a transient or ongoing bacteraemia. Back pain may be a subtle symptom of endocarditis or vertebral osteomyelitis.

It is difficult to distinguish the patient with endocarditis from other drug users with fever due to another cause. Hospitalization of febrile injecting drug users would be prudent if 24-hour follow-up is not possible. Intravenous drug use in the previous

5 days is a predictor of occult major infection, and is an indication for admission to hospital.[9]

Patients with diabetes mellitus Diabetic patients are more prone to developing certain bacterial infections.[1] A diabetic patient with an unexplained fever is more likely to have an occult bacterial infection than a non-diabetic patient. In general an insulin-dependent diabetic patient, especially if aged over 50, with fever and no obvious source of infection, should be investigated and preferably admitted.

Febrile neutropenic patients Febrile neutropenic patients (absolute neutrophil count $<500/\mu L$, or $<1000/\mu L$ and falling rapidly) must be hospitalized for intravenous antibiotics regardless of their clinical appearance. Infections may become fulminant within hours in these patients, and the clinical manifestations of their infective illnesses are frequently modified by the underlying disease, therapy received and coexisting problems.

Splenectomized patients Splenectomized patients with fever must be very carefully assessed because of their increased risk of overwhelming bacterial infection. If the fever cannot be readily explained, admission for intravenous antibiotics is usually indicated.

Other immunocompromised patients Fever in transplant patients (renal, hepatic or cardiac) and those with HIV infection is not an absolute indication for admission, but the threshold of intervention should be considerably lowered and they are best assessed by their usual treating doctors.

Patients recently discharged from hospital may have hospital-acquired infections or infections caused by multi-resistant organisms. Recent operations or procedures may be a clue to the site of infection.

Clinical pointers: exposure history

Overseas travellers or visitors Returned travellers or overseas visitors may have diseases such as malaria and typhoid fever that need early diagnosis and treatment. Any fever in a traveller returned from a malaria-endemic area should be regarded as due to malaria until proved otherwise.

Influenza in febrile returned travellers is a concern to EDs worldwide. Outbreaks of avian influenza occur periodically in bird populations throughout Asia. Although the virus does not typically infect humans, direct bird-to-human transmission of H5N1 influenza has been documented. The virus is highly pathogenic, and the mortality of the disease is high. Travellers acquiring influenza overseas may also introduce this infection. Most cases occur within 2–4 days after exposure, but incubation is as long as 8 days. Suspected influenza infection requires isolation and respiratory precautions. The peak season is generally during the winter months, but can vary, especially in the tropics.[10]

Although rare, viral haemorrhagic fever in returned travellers represents a true medical emergency and a serious public health threat. Viral haemorrhagic fevers are caused by several distinct families of virus, including Ebola and Marburg, Lassa fever, the New World arenaviruses (Guanarito, Machupo, Junin, and Sabia), and Rift Valley fever and Crimean Congo haemorrhagic fever viruses. Most exist in Africa, the Middle East or South America. Although some types cause relatively mild illnesses, many can cause severe, life-threatening disease. Viral haemorrhagic fever should be considered in any febrile patient who has returned from an area in which viral haemorrhagic fever was endemic, especially if they have come into contact with blood or other body fluids from a person or animal infected with viral haemorrhagic fever, or worked in a laboratory or animal facility handling viral haemorrhagic fever specimens. All these infections have incubation periods of up to 2–3 weeks, so it may be possible to exclude viral haemorrhagic fever on epidemiological grounds alone. Isolation measures should be instituted immediately in these persons.[11]

Contact with animals A contact history with animals, either at work or at home, is frequently the clue to a zoonosis, particularly if the illness is a perplexing fever of several days' duration. The occurrence of multiple cases at work or at home should also make one suspect these infections early.

Contact with meningococcal and *Haemophilus* meningitis Close contacts of patients with these infections have a high risk of acquiring the same infections.

Early symptoms may be subtle and a high index of suspicion must be maintained.

Clinical pointers: non-specific clinical features (Table 9.1.1)

There are several non-specific clinical features whose presence should suggest the possibility of sepsis. These warrant careful scrutiny even when the patient does not appear toxic. They are by no means specific indicators of serious problems and there will be many false positives. However, ignoring them is frequently the cause of missed or delayed diagnosis of sepsis.

Severe pain in muscles, neck or back Severe muscle pain, even in the absence of overt fever, may be an early symptom of meningococcaemia, staphylococcal or streptococcal bacteraemia. It is also a feature of myositis and necrotizing fasciitis.

Impairment of conscious state A change in conscious state may be the sole presenting manifestation of sepsis, especially in the elderly.

Vomiting Unexplained vomiting, especially in association with headache or abdominal pain, should raise concern. Vomiting without diarrhoea should not be attributed to a gastrointestinal infection. It is a common symptom of CNS infections and occult sepsis.

Severe headache in the presence of a normal CSF This is especially important in a person who seldom gets headaches. Severe headache in a febrile patient with

Table 9.1.1 Clinical pointers: non-specific clinical features ('alarm bells')

Severe pain in muscles, neck or back
Impairment of conscious state
Vomiting especially in association with headache or abdominal pain
Severe headache in the presence of a normal CSF
Unexplained rash
Jaundice
Severe sore throat or dysphagia with a normal looking throat
Repeated rigors

normal CSF should not be diagnosed as a viral infection; many focal infections, e.g. pneumonia and bacterial enteritis may also present in this manner. CSF may be normal in cerebral abscess and in the prodromal phase of bacterial meningitis.

Unexplained rash An unexplained rash in a febrile patient should be regarded as meningococcaemia until proved otherwise, even in the absence of headache or CSF pleocytosis.

Jaundice Jaundice in the febrile patient is associated with a greatly increased risk of death, admission to ICU and prolonged hospital stay.[6] Jaundice in a febrile patient is unlikely to be due to viral hepatitis, but occurs in serious in bacterial infections such as bacteraemia, cholangitis, pyogenic liver abscess and malaria.

Sore throat or dysphagia Severe sore throat or dysphagia with a normal-looking throat is frequently the presenting symptoms of *Haemophilus influenzae* epiglottitis in adults.

Repeated rigors Although repeated rigors may occur in some viral infections they should generally be regarded as indicators of sepsis, in particular abscesses, bacteraemia, endocarditis, cholangitis and pyelonephritis.

Clinical pointers: evolution of illness (Table 9.1.2)

How rapidly the illness evolves is often an indication of its severity. Previously healthy individuals do not seek medical attention unless they are worried. Notice should be taken of any person seeking help within 24 hours of the onset of illness, or a person whose illness appears to have progressed rapidly within 24–48 hours (e.g. from being up and about to being bedridden). Similarly, the patient who presents to the ED

Table 9.1.2 Clinical pointers: evolution of illness

Those present early (< 24 hours)
Those presenting with rapidly evolving symptoms
Patients presenting to ED on > 1 occasion over a 24–48-hour period

on more than one occasion over a 24–48-hour period warrants a careful work-up.

Step 4: A final caveat

A major concern in the management of undifferentiated fever in adult is missing the diagnosis of meningococcal bacteraemia when the patient does not appear ill on presentation.

There are a number of infections that must be treated rapidly to minimize morbidity and mortality (Table 9.1.3). With the exception of meningococcal bacteraemia, there are usually some clues in the history or physical examination.

Meningococcal infection is peculiar in its wide spectrum of severity and variable rate of progression in different individuals (Table 9.1.4). It may be fulminant and cause death within 12 hours, or it may assume a chronic form that goes on for weeks.

When the patient presents with fever and a petechial rash, meningococcaemia can easily be suspected if one remembers the golden rule of medicine that 'fever plus a petechial rash is meningococcaemia (or staphylococcal bacteraemia) until proved otherwise'. However, only 40% of meningococcal diseases present with a petechial rash.

It is less well known that the early meningococcaemic rash may be macular, i.e. one that blanches with pressure. This is the basis of another golden rule in infectious disease: early meningococcal rash may resemble a non-specific viral rash.

Table 9.1.4 Presentations of meningococcal disease

Acute bacterial meningitis ± petechial rash
Localized infection other than meningitis
Fever + petechial rash
Fever + macular rash
Fever + alarm bells
Fever + contact history
Fever alone

Rarely, meningococcal disease presents with symptoms and signs of a localized infection other than meningitis, e.g. pneumonia, pericarditis or urethritis. These presentations should not pose any management problems.

The risk of missing the diagnosis increases markedly when the patient with meningococcal disease presents with fever and non-specific symptoms without a rash. Abrupt onset of fever and generalized aches may be due to influenza, but it could be due to meningococcaemia.

It is prudent to single out meningococcal disease and ask oneself, Could this patient have meningococcaemia? If in doubt, the safest course is to take cultures, give antibiotics and admit.

Clinical investigation

Most febrile patients seen in the ED justify a fever work-up.

Full blood examination is of limited use. White cell count ($> 15 \times 10^9$/L), marked left shift, neutropenia or thrombocytopenia are pointers to a possible bacteraemia or occult bacterial infections, but they may also be seen in viral infections.[12] Similarly, non-specific markers of inflammation such as C-reactive protein and erythrocyte sedimentation rate have not been shown to be useful in predicting outcomes for febrile patients in the ED.[13]

Urinalysis and urine culture should be done in febrile adults over the age of 50 unless the pathology clearly lies in another body system. However, if the history does not suggest urinary sepsis and the dipstick urinalysis is normal, then urine cultures are usually negative.[14]

A chest X-ray is usually indicated unless a definite diagnosis has been made, e.g. chickenpox, tonsillitis.

Blood cultures should be done in anyone suspected of having bacteraemia, endocarditis or meningitis, in compromised patients with a fever, all febrile patients over the age of 50, and possibly in anyone with an unexplained high fever. It should be noted that only 5% of blood cultures in this setting will be positive, and less than 2% will alter clinical management.[15] In general, a patient considered 'sick enough' to warrant blood cultures should be admitted to hospital or followed up within 24 hours.

Disposition

Patients who have any of the following features are in need of resuscitation, followed by work-up and admission: shock, coma/stupor, cyanosis, profound dyspnoea, continuous seizures and severe dehydration.

With few exceptions the following groups of febrile adults should be investigated and admitted:

- Those over 50 years of age.
- Patients with diabetes mellitus.
- Alcoholic patients.
- Injecting drug users.
- Immunologically compromised patients.
- Overseas travellers or visitors.
- Those with 'alarm bells' as described in Step 3.

In general there should be close liaison with the admitting unit, and the issue of

Table 9.1.3 Infections requiring urgent treatment

Disease	Clues
Meningococcaemia	Myalgia, rash. May be none
Falciparum malaria	Travel history, blood film
Bacterial meningitis	Headache, change in conscious state, CSF findings
Post-splenectomy sepsis	Past history, abdominal scar
Toxic shock syndromes	Presence of shock and usually a rash
Infections in the febrile neutropenic	Past history, blood film
Infective endocarditis	Past history, murmur, petechiae
Necrotizing soft tissue infections	Pain, tenderness, erythema and swelling in skin/muscle, toxicity
Space-occupying infection of head and neck	Localizing symptoms and signs
Focal intracranial infections	Headache, change in conscious state, neurological signs, CT findings

empirical therapy for septic patients should be discussed. For the dangerously ill, e.g. those with septic shock or bacterial meningitis, antibiotics should be commenced almost immediately.

There is an increasing tendency to start antibiotics in the ED as soon as possible to reduce the length of hospital stay. Time to antibiotic therapy is used as a key performance indicator for the ED, e.g. for febrile neutropenic patients.

Patients who do not require intervention after the basic work-up in the ED are discharged home after a period of observation. Because of the time taken to interview the patient, perform investigations and wait for the results, the patient will usually have been observed for 1–2 hours, and progression or lack of progression may be a help in deciding what to do. During observation one must be aware that the apparent improvement of the patient may be the result of pain relief or a fall in temperature due to antipyretics.

Arrangement must be made for the patient to be reviewed by their general practitioner or at the hospital. This is an essential component of the care of a febrile patient seen in an ED.

There is no easy way of detecting occult bacterial sepsis. The infectious process is a dynamic one, and the doctor must maintain contact with the patient or family during the 24–72 hours following the initial visit.

Patients with fever > 39°C must be seen within 24 hours. Review by a doctor within 6–12 hours may be necessary in those who have had a lumbar puncture, and is advisable in those who have had blood cultures taken. A verified phone number should be clearly recorded in the medical history.

All febrile patients discharged from the ED should be encouraged to seek review if there is any adverse change to their condition. A patient re-presenting to the ED has provided an opportunity to ensure that

they are being managed appropriately and to rectify any errors.

Fever due to most common viral infections will resolve by about 4 days. Many other infections will be diagnosed when new symptoms or signs appear.

If fever persists beyond 4–5 days without any localizing symptoms or signs, a less common infection or non-infective cause should be suspected and the patient should be thoroughly investigated. In this situation the threshold of admission to hospital should be low.

The establishment of ED short-stay units allows fast-track treatment and observation, usually for 24–48 hours, for carefully selected febrile patients who are not suitable for immediate discharge home.

Future research directions

- The subject of undifferentiated fever of short duration in the adult has not been well studied. There are few data on the spectrum of diseases producing this clinical problem.

Controversies

- Whether empirical antibiotics should be given to adult patients with undifferentiated fever of short duration in order to minimize the risk of death from unrecognized sepsis or meningitis is a perennial question, and there are no algorithms capable of directing management of this problem.

- The safe and ideal course of action is to admit for observation all those patients who are ill enough to warrant a blood culture or a lumbar puncture. The limitation of hospital beds precludes this policy, and there

will be unnecessary admissions. The introduction of ED short-stay units provides an alternative for selected patients.

References

1. Mellors JW, Horowitz RI, Harvey MR, et al. A simple index to identify occult bacterial infection in adults with acute unexplained fever. Archives of Internal Medicine 1987; 147: 666–671.
2. Gallagher EJ, Brooks F, Gennis P. Identification of serious illness in febrile adults. American Journal of Emergency Medicine 1994; 12: 129–133.
3. Norman DC, Yoshikawa TT. Fever in the elderly. Infectious Disease Clinics of North America 1996; 10: 93–99.
4. Fontanarosa PB, Kaeberlein FJ, Gerson FW, et al. Difficulty in predicting bacteraemia in elderly emergency patients. Annals of Emergency Medicine 1992; 21: 842–848.
5. Marco CA, Schoenfeld CN, Hansen KN, et al. Fever in geriatric emergency patients: clinical features associated with serious illness. Annals of Emergency Medcine 1995; 26: 18–24.
6. Tan SL, Knott JC, Street AC, et al. Outcomes of febrile adults presenting to the emergency department. Emergency Medicine 2002; 14: A22.
7. Wrenn KD, Larson S. The febrile alcoholic in the emergency department. American Journal of Emergency Medicine 1991; 9: 57–60.
8. Marantz PR, Linzer M, Feiner CJ. Inability to predict diagnosis in febrile intravenous drug abusers. Annals of Internal Medicine 1987; 106: 823–826.
9. Samet JH, Shevitz A, Fowle J, et al. Hospitalisation decisions in febrile intravenous drug users. American Journal of Medicine 1990; 89: 53–57.
10. Beigel JH, Farrar J, Han AM, et al. Avian influenza A (H5N1) infection in humans. New England Journal of Medicine 2005; 353: 1374–1385.
11. Ufberg JW, Karras DJ. Commentary (viral haemorrhagic fever). Annals of Emergency Medicine 2005; 45: 324–326.
12. Wasserman MR, Keller EL. Fever, white blood cell count, and culture and sensitivity: their value in the evaluation of the emergency patient. Top Emergency Medicine 1989; 10: 81–88.
13. Van Laar PJ, Cohen J. A prospective study of fever in the accident and emergency department. Clinical Microbiology and Infection 2003; 9: 878–880.
14. Sultana RV, Zalstein S, Cameron PA, et al. Dipstick urinalysis and the accuracy of the clinical diagnosis of urinary tract infection. Journal of Emergency Medicine 2001; 20: 13–19.
15. Kelly A. Clinical impact of blood cultures in the emergency department. Journal of Academic Emergency Medicine 1998; 15: 254–256.

Further reading

Talan DA. Infectious disease issues in the emergency department. Clinical Infectious Diseases 1996; 23: 1–14.

9.2 Meningitis

Andrew Singer

ESSENTIALS

1 Bacterial meningitis can be a rapidly progressive and fatal illness. A high level of suspicion is necessary, as well as rapid diagnosis and treatment.

2 Eighty-five per cent of cases have headache, fever, meningism and mental obtundation, but these are often absent or diminished in very young or old patients, those partially treated with oral antibiotics, and those with some form of immunocompromise.

3 Treatment should not be delayed if lumbar puncture cannot be performed within 20 minutes of arrival in the emergency department. Blood cultures should be taken prior to the first dose of antibiotics, if at all possible.

4 The combination of a third-generation cephalosporin and benzylpenicillin will treat most cases of suspected bacterial meningitis, and should be given as soon as the diagnosis is suspected (benzyl penicillin is sufficient in the pre-hospital setting).

5 Steroids are of benefit to both adults and children with bacterial meningitis, and should be given either before or with the first dose of antibiotic.

Introduction

Definition

Meningitis is an inflammation of the leptomeninges, the membranes that line the central nervous system, as well as the cerebrospinal fluid (CSF) in the subarachnoid space. It is usually the result of an infection, but can be due to an inflammatory response to a localized or systemic insult.

Classification

Meningitis is usually classified according to the aetiology or location as bacterial, aseptic (viral, tuberculous, fungal, or chemical) or spinal (where the infection specifically affects the spinal meninges).

Aetiology

Bacterial

Bacterial meningitis is a serious cause of morbidity and mortality in all age groups. The causes vary according to age, as shown in Table 9.2.1. *Neisseria meningitidis* serogroups A and C tend to cause endemic cases of meningitis, especially in Aboriginal

populations, whereas serogroup B is more commonly associated with epidemics.[1] There has been an increase in the incidence of penicillin-resistant *Streptococcus pneumoniae*, especially in children.[2]

Aseptic

Aseptic meningitis may be either due to an immune response to a systemic infection (usually viral), or to a chemical insult.

Viral

Enteroviruses are the most common cause of meningitis, often in clusters of cases. Herpes viruses often cause meningitis as part of a more generalized infection of the brain (meningoencephalitis), or as part of an immune response to a systemic infection. A generalized viraemia may also cause aseptic meningitis, owing to an immune reaction without direct infection.

Fungal

Fungal causes of meningitis, especially that due to *Cryptococcus neoformans*, tend to occur in immunocompromised patients, such as those with HIV/AIDS, or those on immunosuppressant medication or cancer chemotherapy. It can occur in

immunocompetent individuals as well, particularly the elderly.

Tuberculous

Tuberculous meningitis is rare in industrialized countries, but can occur in all age groups. It tends to follow an insidious course, with a lack of classic signs and symptoms. Diagnosis is often difficult, owing to the low yield from CSF staining, and the 4-week time frame required to culture the organism. Suspicion should be high in patients with immunocompromise or chronic illness. It tends to have a high mortality.

Spinal

Spinal meningitis is usually bacterial and due to direct spread from a localized infection in the spine.

Epidemiology

The epidemiology of meningitis is different for groups according to age, as well as immunocompetence:

- Neonates: Table 9.2.1 shows the main causes of bacterial meningitis in neonates. There is an overall incidence of 0.17–0.32 cases per 1000 live births. There is 26% mortality, which is even higher in premature infants.[3]
- Children: Until the introduction of Haemophilus influenzae type b (Hib) immunization in the early 1990s, this organism was the major cause of bacterial meningitis in children under 5 years (until 1990, the incidence of childhood Hib meningitis was 26.3 per 100 000 (152 per 100 000 in Aboriginal children)).[4] Between 1990 and 1996 there was a 94% reduction in the incidence of Hib disease. *N. meningitidis* and *S. pneumoniae* remain common causes of both meningitis and generalized sepsis.[5]
- Adults: N. meningitidis and *S. pneumoniae* are common causes in all age groups, with *N. meningitidis*

Table 9.2.1 Causes of meningitis

Viral	Bacterial	Other
Echovirus 6, 9,11, 30 Coxsackie viruses A9, A16, B1, B5, B6 Enterovirus 71H Herpes simplex 1 & 2 Cytomegalovirus Varicella zoster Epstein–Barr virus	**Neonates** (<3 months old): Group B streptococcus *Escherichia coli* *Listeria monocytogenes* Coagulase-negative *Staphylococcus aureus* *Pseudomonas aeruginosa* **Children** (<6 years old): *Haemophilus influenzae* type b *Neisseria meningitidis* *Streptococcus pneumoniae* **Adults** *Neisseria meningitidis* (especially in young adults) *Streptococcus pneumoniae* *Listeria monocytogenes* (especially in adults over 45) *Klebsiella pneumoniae* *Staphylococcus aureus* *Escherichia coli* (in the immunocompromised)	*Mycobacterium tuberculosis* *Cryptococcus neoformans* (especially in immunocompromised) Aseptic

predominating in adults under 24 years. *Listeria monocytogenes* is more common in adults over 45 years. The overall incidence in adults is 3.8 per 100 000 population.[6] More unusual organisms occur in patients following neurosurgery or chronic illness, such as alcoholism, hepatic cirrhosis, chronic renal failure, and connective tissue disease[7] (GNRs, coagulase-negative *Staphylococcus aureus*, *Mycobacterium tuberculosis*, *Klebsiella pneumoniae*).

- Patients with HIV/AIDS: *Cryptococcus neoformans* is relatively common, with an incidence of 5 per million of population, or 10% of HIV-infected patients. Tuberculosis, *Listeria*, *Klebsiella* and syphilis are also causes of meningitis in this group, as well as viral causes of meningoencephalitis.[8]
- Tuberculous meningitis occurs in around 2% of patients with TB, and around 10% of HIV-infected patients with TB. It has a poor prognosis, with 20% mortality.

Pathogenesis

Initially, there is colonization of the infectious agent, commonly in the nasopharynx in the case of the enteroviruses and bacteria such as meningococcus and Hib. Other infections may spread from already established foci such as otitis media, or sinusitis (e.g. pneumococcus). There is either haematogenous or local spread to the meninges and subarachnoid space, with inflammation of this area and the production of a purulent exudate approximately 2 hours after invasion of the area. The inflammatory response is initiated by bacterial subcapsular components, such as lipoteichoic acid in *S. pneumoniae*, a lipo-oligosaccharide in *H. influenzae*, and other Gram-negative endotoxins. These substances stimulate the release of cytokines such as interleukin-1 and -6, tumour necrosis factor (TNF) and arachidonic acid metabolites, as well as the complement cascade. There is a subsequent increase in neutrophil and platelet activity, with increased permeability of the blood–brain barrier. This response is often worse after the initial destruction of bacteria by antibiotics. If left untreated, fibrosis of the meninges may occur. In viral and aseptic meningitis there is a more limited inflammatory response, with mild-to-moderate infiltration of lymphocytes. In the more chronic causes, such as fungi or tuberculosis, the exudate is fibrinous, the main cells being a mixture of lymphocytes, monocytes/macrophages, and plasma cells. The base of the brain is most commonly affected.

Presentation

History

There are some differences in the history with different causes of meningitis, which may allow an early differential diagnosis to be made. There are no pathognomonic single symptoms or signs for meningitis, so a high index of suspicion is necessary.

The combination of fever, headache, meningism and mental obtundation is found in approximately 85% of cases of bacterial meningitis.[9] It is also a common pattern in viral or aseptic meningitis, where obtundation is less of a feature. In fungal or tuberculous meningitis these symptoms are much less common (less than 40% of cases of cryptococcal meningitis). Elderly patients or those who have had recent neurosurgery may present with subtle or mild symptoms, and lack a fever.[10]

The headache is usually severe and unrelenting. It may be either global, or located in a specific area. The main symptoms of meningism are nuchal rigidity (neck stiffness), and photophobia. The nuchal rigidity is something more than merely pain on movement of the neck. It is clinically important when the patient complains of a painful restriction of movement in the sagittal plane (i.e. forwards and backwards only). Up to 35% of cases have associated nausea and vomiting.

As a general rule, the height of the fever is a poor indication of the possible cause, though the fever may often only be mild in tuberculous or fungal meningitis, or in bacterial meningitis that has been partially treated by antibiotics. The spectrum of mental obtundation can range from mild confusion, to bizarre behaviour, delirium or coma. The severity of obtundation is a good indication of the severity of the illness.

Focal neurological signs occur in around 10–20% of cases of bacterial meningitis, but are also associated with cerebral mass lesions, such as toxoplasmosis or brain abscess. They are also a feature of tuberculous meningitis. Seizures are relatively uncommon (13–30%), but may occasionally be the only sign of meningitis if the patient has been partially treated with oral antibiotics.

There may also be associated systemic symptoms. Myalgias and arthralgias are often associated with viral causes, but may also be the sole presenting symptom in meningococcal meningitis. HIV/AIDS patients may show stigmata associated with that disease.

The course of the illness may also indicate the cause. Meningococcal or pneumococcal meningitis is often characterized by a rapid, fulminating course, often going from initial symptoms to death over an interval of hours. Viral causes tend to be a slower course over days. Fungal or tuberculous meningitis shows a more chronic course over days to weeks, with milder symptoms.

Risk factors for meningitis include the extremes of age, pre-existing sinusitis or otitis media, recent neurosurgery, CSF shunts, splenectomy, immunological compromise, and chronic diseases such as alcoholism, cancer, connective tissue disorders, chronic renal failure and hepatic cirrhosis.

Examination

The physical examination will often reflect symptoms elicited in the history, with fever, physical evidence of meningism, stigmata of AIDS, etc.

As stated above, neck stiffness is only clinically significant when it occurs in the sagittal plane. There will be a restriction of both passive and active movement. Other tests to elicit meningism include Kernig's sign and Brudzinski's sign, though these are only present in 50% of adult cases of bacterial meningitis. Kernig's sign is elicited by attempting extend the knee of a leg that has been flexed at the hip with the patient lying supine and the other leg flat on the bed. The sign is positive if the knee cannot be fully extended due to spasm in the hamstrings. The test can be falsely positive in patients with shortening of the hamstrings, or other problems involving the legs or lumbar spine. In Brudzinski's sign, flexing the head causes the thighs and knees to also flex. It can also be tested in children by the inability to touch the nose with the flexed hips and knees in the sitting position. These are both late signs.

Focal neurological signs should be a cause for concern, as they can indicate a poor prognosis.

Papilloedema is rare and late, as is a bulging fontanelle in infants, and should alert one to alternative diagnoses.

A rash, often starting as a macular or petechial rash on the limbs, is seen in sepsis due to *N. meningitidis* and *S. pneumoniae*. A petechial rash is a particularly serious sign, and is an indication to start antibiotics immediately. A maculopapular rash is also a feature of viral causes.

Investigations

Lumbar puncture

A CSF sample via a lumbar puncture (LP) is an important source of information for making the diagnosis and determining the likely aetiology and treatment. As the procedure may be time-consuming, treatment should not be delayed if there will be more than a 20-minute delay before the lumbar puncture and there is a reasonable clinical suspicion that a bacterial cause is present. Blood cultures should be taken prior to the administration of antibiotics.

Indications

- Symptoms suggestive of meningitis, especially the combination of fever, headache, neck stiffness and photophobia.
- Any patient with fever and an altered level of consciousness.
- Fever associated with seizures, especially in a neonate, older child or adult.
- Seizures in any patient who has been on oral antibiotics.

Precautions

- Deep coma: A patient with a Glasgow Coma Score (GCS) of 8 or less should have the lumbar puncture delayed until they are more awake. A normal brain CT does not exclude the risk of herniation in this group.
- Focal neurological signs: The patient should have CT first, to exclude a space-occupying lesion, which may increase the risk of cerebral herniation following the lumbar puncture.
- Surgery to the lumbar spine.
- Local skin infection around the lumbar spine.

The main features to note during lumbar puncture are the opening pressure and the physical appearance of the CSF. The sample should be sent for Gram staining, culture, sensitivities, a cell count, and protein and glucose levels. If fungal meningitis is suspected, an India-ink stain and cryptococcal antigen screen should be requested. If tuberculous meningitis is suspected, multiple 5 mL samples of CSF will be required to increase the likelihood of a positive result. If there has been prior administration of antibiotics, a bacterial antigen screen should also be requested.

Turbid CSF is indicative of a significant number of pus cells, and is an indication for immediate administration of antibiotics. The patient should usually rest supine for a few hours after the procedure to prevent a worsening of the headache. This has been known to occur up to 24 hours following the procedure. The evidence for the benefits of enforced rest after lumbar puncture is equivocal.

The pattern of cell counts and glucose and protein levels is shown in Table 9.2.2. This can act as a guide only, and the

Table 9.2.2 Expected CSF values in meningitis				
Parameter	Normal range	Bacterial	Viral	Fungal or TB
Pressure (cmH$_2$O)	5–20	>30	Normal or mildly raised	
Protein (g/L)	0.18–0.45	>1.0–5.0	<1.0	0.1–0.5
Glucose (mmol/L)	2.5–3.5	<2.2	normal	1.6–2.5
Glucose ratio -CSF/serum	0.6 (0.8 in infants)	<0.4 (allow 2–4 h equilibration)	0.6	<0.4
White cell count/μL	<3, usually lymphocytes (if the tap is traumatic, allow 1 WBC for every 1000 RBC)	>500 (90% PMN)	<1000, predominantly monocytes (10% are >90% PMN, 30–40% >50% PMN)	100–500
Gram stain	No organisms	60–90% positive	No organisms	

clinician needs to be guided by the complete clinical picture.

A leukocyte count (WCC) of more than 1000/μL with a predominantly neutrophilic pleocytosis is considered positive for bacterial meningitis. Ten per cent of cases, especially early in the course of the illness, may have a predominance of lymphocytes. As a general rule, bacterial meningitis is characterized by a raised CSF protein and a low CSF glucose level. The ratio of CSF to serum glucose levels is also lowered. The combination of CSF glucose <1.9 mmol/L, CSF to serum glucose ratio <0.23, CSF protein >2.2 g/L, and either a total WCC >2000/μL or a neutrophil count of >1180/μL has been shown to have a 99% certainty of diagnosing bacterial meningitis.[11] Aseptic meningitis will often have cell counts near the normal range. This does not exclude infection with less common agents, such as herpes viruses, or *L. monocytogenes*.

CT scan

CT scanning of the brain is indicated as a prelude to lumbar puncture in the presence of focal neurological signs, mental obtundation or abnormal posturing. It must be noted, though, that a normal CT does not exclude the risk of cerebral herniation in bacterial meningitis,[12] and therefore those with the above signs should have lumbar puncture delayed until they are conscious and stable.

Microbiology

Apart from microscopy and culture of CSF, there are a number of other methods that may allow the causative organism to be identified.

Skin lesion aspirate

In cases where a petechial rash is present, Gram staining or culture from some of the skin lesions may yield the causative organism. This has a reported sensitivity of 30–70%.

Throat swab

Throat swabs are useful in identifying a bacterial cause spread by nasopharyngeal carriage, and should be performed in a case of suspected bacterial meningitis.

Polymerase chain reaction

This potentially allows identification of the causative organism, and even the serotype for organisms such as meningococcus. The test can be performed on CSF or EDTA blood samples, and may remain positive for up to 72 hours after the commencement of antibiotics. In CSF the reported sensitivity is 89% with a specificity of 100%, and in blood a sensitivity of 81% with a specificity of 97%.[13]

Serology

Tests to detect IgM to specific organisms are available for meningococcus and some viruses. For meningococcus, the test has a sensitivity and specificity of 97% and 95%, but is only reliable in adults and children over 4 years old, and takes 5–7 days after onset of the illness to reach diagnostic levels.

Antigenic studies

Latex agglutination, immunoelectrophoresis or radioimmunoassay techniques can be used to screen for antigens from *S. pneumoniae*, Hib, group B streptococcus (*S. agalactiae*), *Escherichia coli* K1, *N. meningitidis* and *C. neoformans*. The tests can be performed on serum, CSF or urine. Serum or urine samples tend to allow greater sensitivities (around 96–99%) than CSF (82–99%). The test is no more sensitive in untreated cases than either a positive Gram-stain or the presence of CSF pleocytosis.[14] The main purpose of antigenic studies is in allowing rapid identification of the causative organism in cases confirmed by the CSF findings, or in cases where partial treatment with antibiotics renders the CSF sterile on culture. In many laboratories, these tests have been superseded by PCR methods.

General investigations

FBC, UEC, blood cultures, ESR and a throat swab can assist in building an overall picture.

Blood cultures should be taken prior to parenteral antibiotics, especially in patients where lumbar puncture has been delayed. One study found that blood cultures grew the causative organism in 86% of proven cases of bacterial meningitis, and that the combination of blood culture, CSF Gram staining and antigen testing identified the cause in 92% of cases.[15]

Differential diagnosis

- Generalized viral infections, with meningism as a component.
- Encephalitis: This is a more generalized viral infection of the brain. Clinically, there may be no difference.
- Brain abscess: This tends to produce focal signs due to local pressure at the site of the abscess.
- Focal cerebral infections, such as those due to *Toxoplasma gondii* in HIV/AIDS patients.
- Subarachnoid haemorrhage: This will often produce identical symptoms of meningism, but generally without any other evidence of infection, such as fever.
- Migraine and other vascular headaches: Again, meningism is a similar feature. The patient will often have a known history of the illness.
- Severe pharyngitis with cervical lymphadenopathy causing neck stiffness.

Management

Management depends on the likely causative agents, as well as the severity of the illness.

General

Patients should rest in bed, particularly following a lumbar puncture. A quiet, darkened room will be beneficial to those with headache or photophobia. Simple analgesics may be used to treat the headache, with or without codeine. Opiates may be required in severe headache.

Sedation may be necessary if the patient is very agitated or delirious. Suitable drugs are diazepam 5–10 mg i.v. or midazolam 2–10 mg i.v. or i.m., with or without the addition of a antipsychotic such as haloperidol 5–20 mg i.v. or i.m., or chlorpromazine 12.5–50 mg i.v. or i.m.

Seizures should be treated appropriately, initially with a benzodiazepine, then maintenance with phenytoin or phenobarbitone. Meningitis can occasionally be associated with status epilepticus, which should be treated in the standard way.

Patients with raised intracranial pressure may need pressure monitoring, and measures to reduce the pressure, such as nursing the patient 30° head up, and the administration of hyperosmotic agents such as mannitol. Hyperventilation is controversial, as it may reduce intracerebral pressure at the expense of reduced cerebral perfusion.

Obstructive hydrocephalus requires appropriate neurosurgical treatment with CSF shunting.

If septic shock has intervened, it should be treated in the usual way, with i.v. fluids and inotropes.

Antimicrobials

The choice of antimicrobial agent will be determined by the likely causative organism, and is therefore determined primarily by age and immune status. It is important that antibiotic therapy is not delayed by investigations such as lumbar puncture or CT, and should be administered as soon as the diagnosis is made. Table 9.2.3 shows the recommended choice of antimicrobial for different situations and organisms. Table 9.2.4 shows the recommended dosage of each. As a general rule, the combination of a third-generation cephalosporin and benzylpenicillin will cover most organisms in all age groups. It is important to note that there is emerging resistance to penicillins in *S. pneumoniae* (currently 7.6% of isolates in Australia). If Gram-positive diplococci are found or *S. pneumoniae* is identified on antigen or PCR testing, vancomycin should be added to the therapy.

Steroids

Steroids have been shown to improve the prognosis of bacterial meningitis in both adults and children. There is a reduction in both mortality and longer-term complications, such as sensorineural deafness, and neurological deficits. Steroids are usually administered as dexamethasone 0.15 mg/kg i.v. q6h (up to 10 mg), started before or with

the first dose of antibiotics, and continued for 4 days. The main adverse effect is gastrointestinal bleeding, which may be reduced by limiting treatment to 2 days.[16]

Disposition

All cases of bacterial meningitis require admission for i.v. antibiotics, as well as supportive therapy. They often require intensive therapy, especially if septic shock has supervened. Viral meningitis will usually require supportive therapy only, but this may require admission. Mild cases of viral or aseptic meningitis, with a clear diagnosis, can be safely sent home.

Prognosis

Over the last 20 years the mortality of bacterial meningitis has ranged from 6% to 20%, and is higher in the very young or the very old. Meningitis in immunocompromised individuals carries a high mortality of up to 50%. Bacterial meningitis in children can lead to a number of long-term sequelae, such as sensorineural hearing loss, learning difficulties, motor problems, speech delay, hyperactivity, blindness, obstructive hydrocephalus and recurrent seizures. These sequelae are less common in adults.

Prevention

Prophylaxis should be offered in cases of *H. influenzae* type b, or *Meningococcus* infection to:

- The index case.
- All household or childcare contacts who have either stayed overnight in the same house or have been in the same room as

Table 9.2.4 Antibiotic doses in treating meningitis[1]

Antibiotic	Daily dose mg/kg/day	Max daily dose	Route	Divided doses
Cefotaxime	200	12 g	i.v.	50 mg/kg q6h
Ceftriaxone	100	4 g	i.v.	100 mg/kg once or twice daily
Benzylpenicillin	1080	12 g	i.v.	60 mg/kg q4h
Ampicillin	360	12 g	i.v.	50 mg/kg q4h
Chloramphenicol	80–100	4 g	i.v.	20–25 mg/kg q6h
Aciclovir	30	1500 mg/m²/day in children 2–12 years	i.v.	10 mg/kg q8h
Amphotericin B	0.5–0.7		i.v.	0.5–0.7 mg/kg daily
Flucytosine	100–150		po	100–150 mg/kg daily
Vancomycin	50	2 g	i.v.	12.5 mg/kg q6h

Table 9.2.3 Choice of antimicrobial in meningitis

Organism	First-line drug	Second-line drug	Duration
Pre-hospital	Benzylpenicillin		
Organism unknown	Cefotaxime or ceftriaxone PLUS benzylpenicillin	Ampicillin instead of benzylpenicillin and gentamicin instead of a 3rd gen. cephalosporin in neonates	7–10 days
H. influenzae type b	Cefotaxime or ceftriaxone	Ampicillin or chloramphenicol	7–10 days
N. meningitidis	Benzylpenicillin or cefotaxime or ceftriaxone		5–7 days
S. pneumoniae	Benzylpenicillin	Cefotaxime or ceftriaxone or vancomycin	10 days
L. monocytogenes	Benzylpenicillin	Ampicillin	3–6 weeks
C. neoformans	Amphotericin PLUS flucytosine	Fluconazole	4–6 weeks
Herpes simplex	Aciclovir		14 days

the index case for any period of 4 hours or more in the preceding 7 days (in Hib, if less than 24 months old, or less than 4 years and incompletely immunized against Hib).

- Passengers adjacent to the index case on a trip of 8 hours' or longer duration.
- Any person who has potentially shared saliva (such as eating utensils or drink bottles) with the index case.
- Healthcare workers who have given mouth-to-mouth resuscitation to an index case.
- Appropriate regimens are:
  - For meningococcus:
    - Ciprofloxacin 500 mg orally as a single dose – preferred for females on oral contraceptives
    - Ceftriaxone 250 mg (125 mg in children <12 years) i.m. in 1% lidocaine – preferred in pregnant women
    - Rifampicin 600 mg orally 12-hourly for 2 days (5 mg/kg in neonates <1 month, 10 mg/kg in children).
  - For Hib:
    - Rifampicin 600 mg orally daily for 4 days (10 mg/kg in neonates <1 month, 20 mg/kg in children)
    - Ceftriaxone 1 g i.m. daily for 2 days (50 mg/kg in children)
    - If the index case is <24 months old, Hib vaccination should be given as a full course as soon as possible after recovery. Unvaccinated contacts under 5 years of age should be immunized as soon as possible.

Casual, neighbourhood or hospital contacts are not required to receive prophylaxis.

Meningococcal vaccine should be considered in populations where cases are clustered. The vaccine is currently only available for serogroup C.

Controversies

- Whether all patients should have a CT scan before lumbar puncture. In general it is safe without CT in those with a clear history consistent with meningitis and normal sensorium. Comatose patients should have lumbar puncture delayed until they are conscious.

- The use of steroids. Steroids have only been shown to improve outcome in adults and children, but are known to cause adverse outcomes in patients with generalized sepsis.

References

1. Munro R, Kociuba K, Jelfs J, et al. Meningococcal disease in urban south western Sydney, 1990–1994. Australia and New Zealand Journal of Medicine 1996; 26: 526–532.
2. Collignon PJ, Bell JM. Drug-resistant *Streptococcus pneumoniae*: the beginning of the end for many antibiotics? Australian Group on Antimicrobial Resistance. Medical Journal of Australia 1996; 164: 64–67.
3. Francis BM, Gilbert GL. Survey of neonatal meningitis in Australia: 1987–1989. Medical Journal of Australia 1992; 156: 240–243.
4. Bower C, Payne J, Condon R, et al. Sequelae of *Haemophilus influenzae* type b meningitis in aboriginal and non-aboriginal children under 5 years of age. Journal of Paediatric and Child Health 1994; 30: 393–397.
5. Herceg A. The decline of *Haemophilus influenzae* type b disease in Australia. Communicable Diseases Intelligence 1997; 21: 173–176.
6. Sigurdardottir B, Bjornsson OM, Jonsdottir KE. Acute bacterial meningitis in adults. A 20-year overview. Archives of Internal Medicine 1997; 157: 425–430.
7. Segreti J, Harris AA. Acute bacterial meningitis. Infectious Disease Clinics of North America 1996; 10: 797–809.
8. Jones PD, Beaman MH, Brew BJ. Managing HIV. Part 5: Treating secondary outcomes. 5.5 HIV and opportunistic neurological infections. Medical Journal of Australia 1996; 164: 418–421.
9. Tunkel AR, Scheld WM. Acute bacterial meningitis. Lancet 1995; 346: 1675–1680.
10. Miller LG, Choi C. Meningitis in older patients: how to diagnose and treat a deadly infection. Geriatrics 1997; 52: 43–44.
11. Spanos A, Harrell FE Jr, Durack DT. Differential diagnosis of acute meningitis: an analysis of the predictive value of initial observation. Journal of the American Medical Association 1989; 262: 2700–2707.
12. Rennick G, Shann F, de Campo J. Cerebral herniation during bacterial meningitis in children. British Medical Journal 1993; 306: 953–955.
13. Communicable Diseases Network Australia, Australian Government Department of Health and Ageing. Guidelines for the early clinical and public health management of Meningococcal Disease in Australia. The 2007 revision of the document is available at: http://www.health.gov.au/internet/main/publishing.nsf/Content/cda-pubs-other-mening-2007.htm
14. Feuerborn SA, Capps WI, Jones JC. Use of latex agglutination testing in diagnosing pediatric meningitis. Journal of Family Practice 1992; 34: 176–179.
15. Coant PN, Kornberg AE, Duffy LC, et al. Blood culture results as determinants in the organism identification of bacterial meningitis. Pediatric Emergency Care 1992; 8: 200–205.
16. van de Beek D, de Gans J, McIntyre P, Prasad K. Corticosteroids for acute bacterial meningitis. The Cochrane Database of Systematic Reviews Volume 3, 2007.

9.3 Septic arthritis

Trevor Jackson

ESSENTIALS

1 Delayed or inadequate treatment can lead to irreversible joint damage.

2 Diagnosis is usually straightforward, based on clinical features and synovial fluid examination; imaging techniques have a role in difficult cases.

3 *Staphylococcus aureus* and *Neisseria gonorrhoeae* are the most frequent pathogens.

4 Successful treatment hinges on rapid and complete joint drainage, and high-dose parenteral antibiotics guided by culture results.

5 Outcomes are good in paediatric and gonococcal subgroups, but the presence of chronic arthritis or polyarticular involvement is associated with up to 15% mortality and 50% chronic joint morbidity.

Introduction

Septic arthritis is defined as infection of the synovial lining and fluid of a joint. Bacteria are the usual pathogens by haematogenous seeding of the joint. Direct spread from adjacent infection or via trauma are less common routes of infection. Once established, phagocytic and neutrophil responses to the bacteria lead to proteolytic enzyme release and cytokine production, resulting in synovial abscess formation and cartilage necrosis.[1]

Comorbidity or deficient host defences are risk factors for infection[2] and can be associated with more rapid and severe disease (Table 9.3.1).

The majority of cases are community acquired and occur in children and young adults.[3] Prosthetic joint surgery and invasive management of chronic arthritis are factors in the increased prevalence observed in older age groups.

Presentation

History

This will usually reveal the recent onset of a painful, hot and swollen joint, most commonly the hip or knee, although any joint may be affected. Systemic features of fever or rigors should be sought, plus the presence of any risk factors.

Examination

Typical findings include a hot, tender joint with marked limitation of passive or active movement owing to pain. An effusion will be evident in most cases. A polyarticular presentation is more common in gonococcal infection or in the setting of chronic arthritis. In general, fever is low grade and few patients will appear 'toxic' and unwell. The elderly and immunosuppressed may present non-specifically with anorexia, vomiting, lethargy or fever.

Investigation

Synovial fluid examination and culture

Aspiration should be performed promptly with local anaesthetic and a large-bore needle to confirm the diagnosis and obtain a culture specimen. Typical findings in septic arthritis and its differential diagnoses are shown in Table 9.3.2[4]

A Gram stain and culture should be performed immediately after aspiration to focus antibiotic therapy and maximize the yield of positive cultures. Most infections are acute and bacterial (Table 9.3.3),[4] although fungal and mycobacterial pathogens have been recognized in chronic infections.

Other laboratory investigations

Blood cultures should always be taken, and may be positive in up to 50%. Inflammatory markers (ESR and C-reactive protein) are elevated, with typically a neutrophil-predominant leukocytosis. These are non-diagnostic, but aid in monitoring response to therapy.

Imaging studies

Plain radiographs should be performed in all cases: they may reveal effusions or local oedema, and help to exclude alternative

Table 9.3.1 Risk factors for septic arthritis	
Risk factors	**Examples**
Direct penetration	Trauma Medical (surgery, arthrocentesis) i.v. drug use
Joint disease	Chronic arthritis
Host immune deficit	Glucocorticoid, or immunosuppressive therapy HIV infection Chronic illness Cancer

Table 9.3.2 Synovial fluid characteristics			
Characteristic	**Septic arthritis**	**Non-septic arthritis**	**Non-inflammatory effusion**
Colour	Yellow/Green	Yellow	Colourless
Turbidity	Purulent, turbid	Turbid	Clear
Leukocytes/µL	10–100 000	5–10 000	<1000
Predominant cell	PMN*	PMN*	Monocyte

*PMN, Polymorphonuclear leukocyte.

Table 9.3.3 Bacterial causes of septic arthritis

Age group	Typical bacteria
Children	Staphylococcus aureus Group A streptococci (B in neonates) Haemophilus influenzae
Young adults	Neisseria gonorrhoeae Staphylococcus aureus
Older adults	Staphylococcus aureus Gram-negative species* Group A streptococci

*Pseudomonas sp. and Enterobacteriaceae

conditions. Ultrasound is very sensitive in detecting effusions, and excellent for facilitating needle aspiration.

Fluoroscopy may also be used. Nuclear medical studies are very sensitive early, but not specific for sepsis. Computed tomography (CT) and magnetic resonance imaging (MRI) have a small role in difficult joints (e.g. hip, sacroiliac).

Differential diagnosis

Non-septic arthritis or synovitis may be differentiated on clinical features and joint fluid analysis. Fractures will generally be evident on joint radiographs, but detection of osteomyelitis may require more advanced imaging techniques such as nuclear or CT scanning. Rheumatic fever and brucellosis are rare causes.

Management

Joint drainage and empiric parenteral antibiotic therapy must take place without delay. Surgical drainage is usually employed in children, with needle drainage more commonly first line in adults. Newer arthroscopic techniques are increasingly being used.[1,5–7] Repeated drainage procedures will often be necessary to ensure complete resolution of the infection.

Antibiotic therapy is initiated after culture specimens have been obtained, with clinical presentation and Gram stain guiding the choice of agents. All regimens must include an antistaphylococcal agent, with Gram-negative cover as indicated by the clinical setting.

Suggested initial empiric regimen[8]

Di(Flu)cloxacillin: 2 g (25–50 mg/kg up to 2 g) intravenously, 6-hourly. If Gram-negative bacteria are suspected, add ceftriaxone 2 g (25–50 mg/kg up to 2 g) intravenously daily. If methicillin resistance is suspected, add vancomycin 1 g (25 mg/kg) intravenously 12-hourly.

Definitive therapy will be tailored to later laboratory identification of the organism and its sensitivities.

The duration and route of therapy remain controversial, but in uncomplicated acute cases parenteral antibiotics will be required for at least 3 days in children and 2 weeks in adults, with a total treatment duration of 3–6 weeks.[7,9] Specific organisms such as Neisseria sp. will respond more rapidly, whereas chronic infections and comorbidity will necessitate aggressive and more prolonged therapy.

General care, with initial joint rest, appropriate analgesia and physical therapy, is important.

Disposition

All patients require admission until their joint sepsis is controlled. Thereafter, ongoing therapy may be monitored as an outpatient or via domiciliary hospital services.

Prognosis

This depends upon the organism, patient comorbidity, and the adequacy and rapidity of treatment. Gonococcal and paediatric infections have a generally good response, with low rates of ensuing joint morbidity. Polyarticular sepsis in rheumatoid arthritis has been associated with mortality rates of up to 15%, and major morbidity in up to 50% of survivors.[1,4,9]

Prevention

Safe sexual practice can reduce gonorrhoeal infections. Strict aseptic technique, good patient selection and prophylactic antibiotics help prevent cases associated with invasive joint procedures. The overall incidence of infection after arthroplasty ranges from 0.5 to 2%.[1]

Controversies

- The total duration of therapy has gradually been reduced, but optimum duration is unclear, as is the balance between parenteral and oral routes.[10]

- Consensus has not been reached on the best method of joint drainage. Surgical arthrotomy is usually employed for the hip and in children, but arthroscopic techniques are also available. Most centres still use repeated needle aspiration as first line for most joints.

- Difficulties still exist with the differentiation of septic arthritis from new-onset non-septic arthritis, especially when polyarticular. Joint fluid analysis and medical imaging are used, but nuclear and CT scanning techniques may have difficulty in distinguishing infective from non-infective inflammation.

References

1. Goldenberg DL. Bacterial arthritis. In: Kelley WN, Harris ED, Ruddy S, Sledge CB, eds. Textbook of rheumatology, 4th edn. Philadelphia: WB Saunders, 1993; 1449–1466.
2. Goldenberg DL. Septic arthritis. Lancet 1998; 351: 197–202.
3. Sonnen GM, Henry N. Paediatric bone and joint infections. Paediatric Clinics of North America 1996; 4: 933–947.
4. Brooks GF, Pons VG. Septic arthritis. In: Hoeprich PD, Jordan MC, Ronald AR, eds. Infectious diseases, 5th edn. Philadelphia: JB Lippincott, 1994; 1382–1389.
5. Stanitski CL, Harwell JC, Fu FH. Arthroscopy in acute septic knees. Clinical Orthopaedics 1989; 241: 209.
6. Broy SB, Schmid FR. A comparison of medical drainage (needle aspiration) and surgical drainage (arthrotomy or arthroscopy) in the initial treatment of infected joints. Clinics in Rheumatological Disease 1986; 12: 501–522.
7. Manadan AM, Block JA. Daily needle aspiration versus surgical lavage for the treatment of bacterial septic arthritis in adults. American Journal of Therapeutics 2004; 11: 412–415.
8. Skin, muscle and bone infections. In: Therapeutic Guidelines. Antibiotic, 13th edn. Therapeutic Guidelines Ltd. 2006. Available at http://www.tg.com.au. qelibresources.health.wa.gov.au/index.php
9. Youssef PP, York JR. Septic arthritis: a second decade of experience. Australia and New Zealand Journal of Medicine 1994; 24: 307–311.
10. Syrogiannopoulos GA, Nelson JD. Duration of antimicrobial therapy for acute suppurative osteoarticular infections. Lancet 1988; 1: 37–40.

9.4 Osteomyelitis

Trevor Jackson

ESSENTIALS

1 *Staphylococcus aureus* is the most frequent pathogen in all age groups.

2 Surgery, trauma and diabetes predispose to chronic adult infections.

3 Diagnosis may be difficult, relying on the triad of clinical features, imaging studies and microbiological culture.

4 Successful treatment requires appropriate parenteral antibiotics and complete surgical clearance of necrotic bone.

Introduction

Infection of bone is an infrequent but important emergency department (ED) presentation. Most cases occur in children and the aged, with the former occurring via haematogenous spread and the latter associated with comorbidity such as trauma, surgery, vascular insufficiency and diabetes. Bacteria enter bone via the blood vessels, by direct spread from contiguous infection, or by direct inoculation during trauma or surgery. Initially metaphyseal, infection usually extends to the subperiosteal space, forming an abscess and stimulating new bone deposition known as an involucrum. Necrosis of cortical bone follows, whereby bone fragments or sequestra are formed that harbour bacteria.[1] Successful treatment requires eradication of the bacteria and complete removal of necrotic tissue.

Presentation

History

New onset of localized bone pain and fever is typical. Inadequate vascular supply, diabetes, and prior surgery such as arthroplasty or compound fracture are all important risk factors. Chronic infections are commonly indolent, with few or no symptoms.

Intravenous drug use has been associated with infections in unusual sites such as the spine and clavicle.

Examination

Most patients will not appear toxic or unwell. Typical findings include mild fever with warmth, tenderness and swelling at the site of pain. Joint movements may be restricted if osteomyelitis is periarticular or has involved the joint space. Chronic infections may present with overlying scars, ulcers or draining sinuses.

Investigations

General laboratory tests

Inflammatory markers (erythrocyte sedimentation rate and C-reactive protein) will be significantly elevated in acute infections and are useful for monitoring the response to treatment. The white cell count is an unreliable guide to severity, typically showing low-grade neutrophil-predominant leukocytosis.

Imaging studies[2]

Plain radiographs may reveal early soft tissue oedema and periosteal elevation, particularly in children. However, in adults, radiographs typically remain normal for at least 10–14 days; thereafter the findings reflect bony destruction. Cortical rarefaction, involucrum formation and sequestra may all be seen. In subacute infection a bone abscess known as Brodie's abscess may appear as a lucent lesion at the metaphysis.

Nuclear medical scans with three-phase ^{99m}TC MDP are sensitive early and well tolerated by children, but may lack specificity.[3] They are most useful when combined with clinical features and plain radiography. Computed tomography (CT) and magnetic resonance imaging (MRI) scans are excellent for displaying the extent of established infection and soft tissue involvement, and for investigation of difficult sites (e.g. the spine).

Microbiology

Culture of infected bone obtained by needle aspiration or surgery[4] provides definitive evidence in up to 80% of cases. Blood cultures will be positive for a single bacterium in over 50% of infections, especially if established via haematogenous spread. Common bacterial pathogens are listed in Table 9.4.1. Polymicrobial infection will be encountered in the setting of chronic infection or a compromised host (e.g. diabetic foot ulcers). Non-bacterial pathogens occur rarely.

Differential diagnosis

Tumours such as Ewing's sarcoma or osteoid osteoma, traumatic injuries and septic arthritis are the most important. The latter may coexist with osteomyelitis in joints such as the hip and shoulder.

Table 9.4.1 Bacterial causes of osteomyelitis

Age group	Typical bacteria
Children <2 years	Staphylococcus aureus Streptococcus spp.
Older children	Staphylococcus aureus
Adults	Staphylococcus aureus Streptococcus spp. Gram-negative species*

*Pseudomonas sp. and enterobacteriaceae

Management

After appropriate microbiological specimens have been obtained, treatment requires prolonged parenteral and oral antibiotics guided by the results of Gram stain and culture. All initial antibiotic regimens should include an anti-staphylococcal agent, with vancomycin added if methicillin resistance is suspected. The duration and routes of therapy must be adjusted individually, but at least 4 weeks are necessary for acute uncomplicated cases.[5,6,8]

The relative duration, or balance of parenteral and oral antibiotic use, remains controversial. Newer treatments for chronic infections, including antibiotic-impregnated beads and hyperbaric oxygen therapy, are emerging, but are not yet in widespread use.

Suggested initial empiric regimen[6]

Di(flu)cloxacillin: 2 g (25–50 mg/kg up to 2 g) intravenously, 6-hourly; if Gram-negative bacteria are suspected, add ceftriaxone 2 g (25–50 mg/kg up to 2 g) intravenously daily; if methicillin resistance is suspected, add vancomycin 1g (25 mg/kg) intravenously 12-hourly.

In all cases, orthopaedic management will be essential to obtain culture specimens and ensure complete removal of necrotic bone at the site. This may be unnecessary in acute haematogenous cases in children, or complex in chronic postoperative cases with prosthetic implants involving major revision. Some of these latter infections may be managed with long-term suppressive antibiotic therapy.

Disposition

Confirmed acute cases require admission. Unless the patient is toxic or immunosuppressed, antibiotic treatment should commence after a definitive diagnosis has been established. After inpatient investigation and stabilization, patients may be able to complete antibiotic treatment at home.

Prognosis

Acute haematogenous osteomyelitis can be expected to resolve with few sequelae if prompt and adequate therapy is instituted. If epiphyses are involved, ongoing orthopaedic review will be necessary as bone growth may be impaired. Chronic osteomyelitis and sinus tracts will only be controlled with antibiotic therapy alone: surgery is necessary for eradication. Squamous cell carcinoma in the tract is a rare, long-term complication.

Prevention

Thorough debridement, careful wound management and antibiotic therapy are essential in the setting of open skeletal trauma. Careful patient selection, meticulous technique and antibiotic prophylaxis may all help to prevent infection following joint prosthetic surgery.

Controversies

- The optimum duration for parenteral antibiotics, and the balance between parenteral and oral routes, are still to be determined in both simple and complicated cases.[5,7,8]

References

1. Brooks GF, Pons VG. Septic arthritis. In: Hoeprich PD, Jordan MC, Ronald AR, eds. Infectious diseases, 5th edn. Philadelphia: Lippincott, 1994; 1382–1389.
2. Sonnen GM, Henry NK. Paediatric bone and joint infections. Paediatric Clinics of North America 1996; 43: 933–947.
3. Boutin RD, Brossmann J, Sartoris DJ, et al. Update on imaging of orthopaedic infections. Orthopaedic Clinics of North America 1998; 29: 41–66.
4. Weinstein SL, Buckwalter JA (eds) Turek's orthopaedics, 6th edn. Philadelphia: Lippincott, Williams & Wilkins, 2005; 127–150.
5. Syrogiannopoulos GA, Nelson JD. Duration of antimicrobial therapy for acute suppurative osteoarticular infections. Lancet 1998; 1: 37–40.
6. Skin, muscle and bone infections. 2006 in: Therapeutic guidelines. Antibiotic, 13th edn. Therapeutic guidelines Ltd. Available at http://www.tg.com.au. qelibresources.health.wa.gov.au/index.php
7. Lazzarini L, Lipsky BA, Mader JT. Antibiotic treatment of osteomyelitis: what have we learned from 30 years of clinical trials? International Journal of Infectious Diseases 2005; 9: 127–138.
8. Davis JS. Management of bone and joint infections due to *Staphylococcus aureus*. Internal Medicine Journal 2005; 35: s79–96.

INFECTIOUS DISEASES

9.5 Urinary tract infection

Salomon Zalstein

ESSENTIALS

1 Urinary tract infection (UTI) is the most common bacterial infection.

2 Between 20% and 30% of women will have a UTI at some time in their lives.

3 Most UTIs are caused by *Escherichia coli*, but *Staphylococcus saprophyticus* is responsible for up to 15% of infections in young, sexually active women.

4 There is a genetic predisposition in some women to recurrent UTI.

5 There are specific bacterial virulence factors determining uropathogenic strains of bacteria.

6 The clinical differentiation of lower from upper urinary tract infection is inaccurate. Up to 50% of patients presenting with typical lower tract symptoms will have concurrent upper tract involvement.

7 Up to half of women presenting with dysuria and frequency will have $<10^5$ organisms/mL of urine, but about half of these do have bacterial UTI.

8 For the majority of outpatients with typical symptoms urine culture is not necessary.

9 In institutionalized elderly patients, non-specific symptoms or a decline in function correlate poorly with UTI despite the presence of pyuria and bacteriuria. Non-UTI causes must be sought.

Introduction

Urinary tract infections are the most common bacterial infections, and the major cause of Gram-negative sepsis in hospitalized patients.[1,2]

Definitions

Urinary tract infection

Contrary to the commonly held view that the term 'urinary tract infection' (UTI) represents a group of specific diagnoses with clear-cut clinical syndromes, the term is non-specific and may refer to a variety of clinical conditions, including asymptomatic bacteriuria, urethritis, cystitis, female urethral syndrome, and acute and chronic pyelonephritis. The most common clinical presentations are cystitis and acute pyelonephritis, although the clinical distinction between these diagnoses may not be as straightforward as the terms imply, with up to 50% of patients having unrecognized pyelonephritis.

UTI is considered in two main groups: simple (or uncomplicated) and complicated. Simple UTIs occur in an otherwise healthy person with a normal urinary tract, most commonly young, non-pregnant women. A complicated UTI is one associated with anatomical abnormality, urinary obstruction or incomplete bladder emptying due to any cause: instrumentation or catheterization, pregnancy, or significant underlying disease such as immunosuppression or diabetes mellitus.

Significant bacteriuria

Significant bacteriuria most commonly refers to more than 10^5 bacteria/mL of urine, reported as colony forming units per mL (cfu/mL). This usually represents infection as opposed to contamination (see Quantitative culture), although there are significant exceptions to this generalization (see Urethral syndrome). Asymptomatic bacteriuria (ASB) refers to significant bacteriuria in the absence of symptoms of infection.

Epidemiology

In Australia, approximately 250 000 adults per year are diagnosed with urinary tract infection.[3] UTIs occur most commonly in women, in whom age, degree of sexual activity and the form of contraception used are all factors that affect the incidence and prevalence of infection.[4–6] At least 20% and up to 40–50% of women will have a UTI at some time in their life.[7,8] The overall rate of infection is difficult to estimate, as UTI is not a reportable disease, but in non-pregnant women aged 18–40 years has been stated to be between 0.5–0.7 per person per year.[6] Infection rates are much higher in pregnancy. Stated another way, based on USA statistics, a woman presenting with one or more symptoms of UTI has a probability of infection of approximately 50%.[9]

In males the prevalence of bacteriuria beyond infancy is 0.1% or less. Between the ages of 21 and 50, infection rates may be as low as 0.6–0.8/1000.[10] With increasing prostatic disease the frequency of bacteriuria may rise to 3.5% in healthy men, and to more than 15% in hospitalized men by age 70.[11,12] Homosexual men are at increased risk of UTI.

In the presence of chronic disease and institutionalization in the elderly, the incidence of bacteriuria may be as high as 50%.[11,13–15]

Aetiology

The aetiology of uncomplicated UTI has remained consistent for over 20 years, although increased antibiotic resistance in the bacteria responsible has been well documented. More than 95% of all UTIs are caused by the Enterobacteriaceae and *S. faecalis*. Of these, *E. coli* accounts for about 90% of acute infections in outpatients and some 50% in inpatients. Which bacteria are isolated is influenced by factors such as whether the infection is initial or recurrent; the presence of obstruction, instrumentation or anatomical abnormalities; and whether the patient is an inpatient or an outpatient. In simple acute cystitis, the most common presentation of UTI, a single organism is usually isolated. On the other hand, non-*E. coli* organisms are more commonly seen in complicated UTI. In the presence of structural abnormalities it is more common to isolate multiple organisms, and antibiotic resistance is frequently found. Perhaps surprisingly, the common skin commensal *Staphylococcus saprophyticus* has been identified as a cause of infection in young, sexually active females and is responsible for 5–15% of acute cystitis.[7,16–19]

Pathogenesis

In healthy individuals the perineum, vagina, vaginal introitus and urethra and periurethral areas each have their respective flora and are normally colonized by bacteria different from those commonly associated with UTI. The periurethral area may become colonized by such UTI-causing (uropathogenic) bacteria, which then ascend via the urethra into the bladder, and thence may ascend further to the kidney, causing pyelonephritis. The reservoir for these bacteria is the gastrointestinal tract.[7] Both host and bacterial mechanisms are involved in determining whether a UTI will occur.

Host mechanisms

Anatomical considerations (men) and prostatic secretions

In males the length of the urethra, its separation from the anus and the presence of prostatic secretions all contribute to the prevention of colonization and subsequent UTI.

Secretor/non-secretor status

Blood group antigens are secreted in the body fluids by some women. The urethral and periurethral mucosae in women who do not secrete these antigens (non-secretors) in their body fluids have a higher affinity for bacterial adhesins (see below) than the mucosae of women who do. These non-secretors are more susceptible to recurrent infections.[7,20]

Sexual activity, contraceptive practices, use of diaphragm/spermicides

Sexual activity is a risk factor for acute cystitis, with recent or frequent sexual activity increasing that risk. The use of a diaphragm with a spermicide (an inhibitor of normal vaginal flora) promotes vaginal colonization with uropathogenic bacteria, and has also been shown to increase the risk of UTI.[5,6,21]

Entry of bacteria into the bladder

Instrumentation of the bladder (see below) is a well recognized mechanism by which bacteria are introduced into the bladder. Other factors have been considered but have not been conclusively demonstrated. These include frequency and timing of voiding, hormonal changes, and personal hygiene habits.[4,5,22]

Bladder defence mechanisms

The healthy bladder can normally clear itself of bacteria. There are three factors involved: voiding; urinary bacteriostatic substances such as organic acids, high urea concentrations and immunoglobulins; and active resistance by the bladder mucosa to bacterial adherence.

Obstruction

This may be extrarenal (congenital anomalies such as urethral valves, calculi, benign prostatic hypertrophy) or intrarenal (nephrocalcinosis, polycystic kidney disease, analgesic nephropathy). Complete obstruction of the urinary tract predisposes to infection by haematogenous spread. In the absence of such obstruction, haematogenous seeding of bacteria to the kidneys accounts for about 3% of infections. Partial obstruction does not have this effect.

Vesicoureteric reflux

Incompetence of the vesicoureteric valve is a congenital problem that is five times more common in boys than in girls, but tends not to be a significant factor in adults. It allows infected urine to ascend to the kidney, and is the most common factor predisposing to chronic pyelonephritic scarring.

Instrumentation

Although any instrumentation of the urinary tract predisposes to infection, catheterization is the most common. A single catheterization will result in UTI in 1% of ambulatory patients, but in hospitalized patients 10% of women and 5% of men will develop a UTI after one catheterization. Once in place, catheters produce infection in up to 10% of patients per day, and nearly all catheterized patients will be bacteriuric by 1 month.[23] All chronically catheterized patients are bacteriuric.

Pregnancy

Changes to the urinary tract occur normally during pregnancy as a result of both anatomical alterations and hormonal effects: dilatation of the ureters and renal pelves, reduced peristalsis in the ureters and reduced bladder tone. These changes begin before the end of the second month. The prevalence of bacteriuria rises with age and parity. A large proportion of asymptomatic, bacteriuric women develop symptomatic pyelonephritis later in the pregnancy, with significant increases in toxaemia and prematurity.[24]

Diabetes mellitus

The relationship between diabetes mellitus on the one hand and asymptomatic bacteriuria and UTI on the other has been debated. Current evidence indicates that asymptomatic bacteriuria is more common in diabetic women than in non-diabetic women. The evidence in men is less clear cut. Good evidence from prospective studies for an increased incidence of symptomatic urinary tract infection in diabetics is lacking, but other studies indicate that this is true. What appears to be quite unequivocal is that diabetes is a significant and independent risk factor for pyelonephritis, complicated UTI, urosepsis, hospitalization and other, often rare, complications (such as emphysematous pyelonephritis, papillary necrosis and candidal infections). The precise pathogenetic mechanism is unclear, but involves many factors not necessarily related to glycaemic control.[25–28]

Ageing

Asymptomatic bacteriuria is highly prevalent in residents of long-term care facilities, with up to 30% of men and 50% of women showing bacteriuria, with a correlation between degree of functional impairment and likelihood of bacteriuria. UTI is the most frequent bacterial infection in residents of such facilities. Several factors may be involved: chronic degenerative neurological diseases may impair bladder function as well as bladder and bowel continence; prostatic enlargement in men and oestrogen deficiency in women can both lead to incomplete bladder emptying; the use of devices such as indwelling catheters or condom drainage predisposes to bacteriuria.[12–15,29]

Bacterial factors

A number of studies[30–32] have shown that the strains of *E. coli* (and a number of other Gram-negative bacteria) that cause UTI are not just the most prevalent in the bowel of the patient at the time of the infection, but have specific characteristics, termed virulence factors, that give them certain capabilities: increased intestinal carriage, persistence in the vagina, and the ability to ascend and invade the normal urinary tract. Thus there are clearly uropathogenic strains of these bacteria. In cases of complicated UTI (e.g. those associated with reflux, obstruction or foreign body) these virulence factors are not significantly involved. The two most important virulence factors are resistance to phagocytosis – which is a function of O and K antigens on the bacterial surface – and adherence to uroepithelium, which is a function of adhesins, molecular components expressed on the tips of the pili of the bacteria, and receptors on the uroepithelium.

Presentation

History

A careful history should be taken in any patient presenting with symptoms of apparent UTI, looking for risk factors for complicated or recurrent infection (such as previous UTIs and their treatment, the presence of known anatomical abnormalities and investigations or instrumentation, the possibility of pregnancy, and history of diabetes mellitus), as well as seeking to identify those patients with urethritis and vaginitis. In men, the most common cause of recurrent lower tract UTI is prostatitis, so evidence of prostatitis, such as chills, dysuria and prostatic tenderness, should be sought.

Lower tract infections typically present with irritative micturition symptoms such as dysuria and frequency, suprapubic discomfort, and sometimes macroscopic haematuria. There is usually no fever. The classic symptom complex of loin pain, fever and urinary symptoms is usually associated with pyelonephritis, but is not always present. It is important to note that the symptoms of pyelonephritis can be quite variable, and even absent. Studies have shown that, of patients presenting with typical lower tract symptoms and who have significant bacteriuria, 30–50% will have upper tract involvement in the infective process.[1,33,34] This has significant implications for treatment, particularly if short-course treatment is considered (see Treatment). Severe pain should raise the suspicion of a ureteric calculus, which, combined with infection, poses a greater risk of sepsis and of permanent injury to the kidney.

Patients with chronic indwelling catheters usually have no lower tract symptoms at all, but may develop loin pain and fever.

In elderly patients, particularly in long-term care facilities, the long-held view that symptoms of increased confusion and reduced mobility in the absence of fever are due to urinary tract infection has been cast into doubt (see Treatment of specific groups: Elderly patients).[13,15,35]

Examination

The clinical signs of lower UTI are few and non-specific; however, patients should be examined to exclude other causes for their symptoms, particularly vaginitis in women and prostatitis in men. The presence of fever and renal angle tenderness both suggest pyelonephritis but, as previously indicated, their absence does not rule it out.

Investigations

The key step in the diagnosis of UTI is examination of the urine, most commonly a midstream specimen. Catheterization is appropriate in patients with altered mental state or who cannot void for neurological or urological reasons. Suprapubic aspiration is commonly used in paediatric practice, but can be used in adults if other techniques have failed or are unable to be used.

The next step is to look for the presence of pyuria, and subsequently the specimen may be sent for quantitative culture. Testing for haematuria, proteinuria and nitrites may be of supportive value but is not diagnostic.

Reagent test strips

When considering the use of reagent strips in the diagnosis of UTI it should be noted that variations in published sensitivity and specificity exist and are due to 1) the use of different brands of reagent strips, 2) the use of different 'gold standards' against which comparison is made (e.g. counting chamber or cells/HPF counts, 'cut off' criterion of the test used), 3) the nature of the study (blinded, unblended), 4) the reader of the test (laboratory worker, doctor, nurse), and most importantly, 5) the clinical setting or target population (e.g. symptomatic ED patients rather than an asymptomatic population in a clinic or office environment) – in other words, the pretest probability.[36]

A reagent strip test for leukocyte esterase is now the most common screening test for pyuria (see below). Taken alone, this has a sensitivity of 48–86% and a specificity of 17–93%% for detecting $>10/mm^3$ of urine in various published studies. A positive predictive value (in symptomatic individuals) of 50% and a negative predictive value of 92% make it a valuable test for screening the ED population. Most studies indicate that when the combination of leukocyte esterase and nitrite is considered, the sensitivity of the test is 68–88%, and a negative test excludes the presence of infection.[36] Recent work by Sultana and others[37] has shown that reagent strips significantly improve the clinician's accuracy in diagnosing UTI in symptomatic ED patients. The clinical probability of UTI must be considered when using such screening tests. In the patient with typical urinary tract symptoms it may provide an adequate screen. It should, however, be used with great caution in the presence of fever of unknown cause in the elderly, the patient with an indwelling catheter or the patient with an impaired mental state, as pyuria and the implied bacteriuria may not be the cause of the problem.

Pyuria

Pyuria indicates inflammation in the urinary tract, and as an indicator of infection is second only to bacteriuria determined by quantitative culture (see below). The 'gold standard' definition of pyuria is based on early work involving the measurement of the rate of excretion of polymorphs in the urine. This work showed that excretion of 400 000 polymorphs per hour was always associated with infection, and was also found to be represented by 10 polymorphs/mm^3 in a single (unspun) midstream specimen of urine.[38] Thus 'significant pyuria' was defined as 10 000 polymorphs per mL of urine. It was subsequently shown that > 96% of symptomatic patients defined as having significant bacteriuria had significant pyuria, and conversely <1% of asymptomatic people without bacteriuria have this degree of pyuria. Other definitions of pyuria, such as >5 leukocytes/high-power field are based on examination of either the urinary sediment or of centrifuged urine, and are inherently inaccurate because they cannot be standardized, but are nevertheless often used.[39] 'Sterile' pyuria indicates the presence of significant pyuria without the presence of bacterial growth in standard culture (Table 9.5.1).

Nitrites

This reagent strip-based test is dependent on the bacterial reduction of urinary nitrate to nitrite, a function of coliform bacteria but not of *Enterococcus* spp. nor *S. Saprophyticus*. The test has a low sensitivity (45–60%), better specificity (85–98%) but a high false negative rate (about 45% in many studies).[7,40] False negative results are likely if the infecting organism is Gram positive or *Pseudomonas*, if the diet lacks nitrate, or if there is diuresis or extreme frequency, as a period of bladder incubation is necessary to form nitrites.[41]

Haematuria

Despite being a frequent accompaniment of UTI, this finding is non-specific as there are many other causes of haematuria.

Proteinuria

Most commonly with UTI, protein excretion is < 2g/24 h. It is another common but non-specific finding.

Table 9.5.1 Common causes of sterile pyuria[73]
Non-specific urethritis in males
Prostatitis
Renal tract neoplasm
Renal calculi
Catheterization
Renal TB
Previous antibiotic treatment

Quantitative culture

Urine culture is not essential in the management of the premenopausal sexually active woman with an uncomplicated UTI. However, culture should be performed in patients with recurrent infection, potentially complicated UTI, males, the elderly, or in cases where the cause of infection is not clinically evident. In symptomatic patients a single specimen with a bacterial count $>10^5$/mL has a 95% probability of representing infection, but in asymptomatic women one specimen with $>10^5$ bacteria/mL has only an 80% probability of indicating UTI, with the probability rising to 95% with two specimens showing the same organism in this concentration.[42] However, about one-third of young females with symptoms will have bacterial counts $<10^5$/mL (see Urethral syndrome).[43,44] In men, counts as low as 10^3/mL suggest infection.[45]

Urethral syndrome or UTI with low numbers of bacteria (Fig. 9.5.1)

Up to half of women with typical lower tract symptoms will have fewer than 10^5 bacteria/mL. Of these, about half have bacterial UTI, with low numbers of bacteria. Of the rest, one group has urethritis due to *Chlamydia trachomatis* or *Neisseria gonorrhoeae*, and the other has negative cultures and may have *Ureaplasma urealyticum* urethritis. All except this last group have pyuria.[44,46]

Blood cultures

Current evidence indicates that blood cultures do not alter management and are therefore unnecessary in the majority of cases of uncomplicated pyelonephritis.[47–50] Blood cultures may be of value in the following circumstances:

- Recent instrumentation.
- Known anatomic abnormality.
- Failure of empiric treatment.
- Immunosuppression.
- Significant comorbidity, such as diabetes mellitus.
- Major sepsis.
- Fever of unclear cause.

Imaging

Imaging is not required in cases of uncomplicated cystitis. In pyelonephritis, imaging should be performed in the following circumstances:

- Pain suggestive of renal colic or obstruction.
- Failure to defervesce within 72 hours.
- Rapid relapse on cessation of antibiotic treatment, or within 2 weeks.
- Infection with an unusual organism.

These circumstances have been shown to be associated with stones or renal scarring.[7,51–54] Helical CT is the preferred

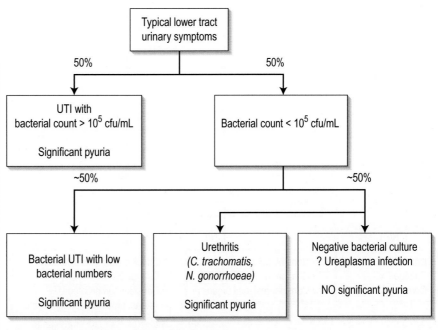

Fig. 9.5.1 UTI symptoms with low bacterial counts.

modality, as this has greater sensitivity for demonstrating not only stones and obstruction, but also rare gas-forming infections, haemorrhage and inflammatory masses.[55,56]

Management

Ideally, treatment of UTI should rapidly relieve symptoms, prevent short-term complications such as progression from cystitis to pyelonephritis and subsequent sepsis, or long-term sequelae such as renal scarring, and prevent recurrences by eliminating uropathogenic bacteria from vaginal and perineal reservoirs. Treatment should be cost-effective and have few or no side effects. There is no evidence that non-specific treatments such as pushing fluids or attempting to alter urinary pH improve the outcome of normal antibiotic treatment.

Antibiotic treatment

Serum levels of antibiotics are largely irrelevant in the elimination of bacteriuria.

Reduction in urinary bacterial numbers correlates with the sensitivity of the organism to the urinary concentration of the antibiotic. Inhibitory concentrations are usually achieved in the urine after oral doses of the commonly used antibiotics. On the other hand, blood levels are vitally important in the treatment of bacteraemic or septic patients, or those with renal parenchymal infections. The choice of antibiotic is based on the clinical presentation and the bacteria likely to be involved (Table 9.5.2).

Management of specific groups (Fig 9.5.2)

Frequency dysuria syndrome: presumed simple cystitis

A non-pregnant, non-diabetic woman first presenting with typical lower urinary symptoms should have vulvovaginitis excluded and an MSU taken and examined or tested by dipstick for pyuria. If pyuria is confirmed, culture of the urine specimen is not necessary and treatment should be commenced empirically.

There is now good evidence that in this group of patients a short course of treatment is effective in both treating the infection and eradicating uropathogenic strains of bacteria from reservoirs. Three-day treatment is superior to a single dose in eradicating the reservoirs of uropathogenic organisms, thereby reducing the incidence of recurrence. Longer courses have an increased incidence of side effects but not higher cure rates. The antibiotics of choice for 3-day treatment are trimethoprim or a fluoroquinolone; however, in order to postpone the emergence of bacterial resistance, the latter should only be used if an organism resistant to other agents is proven.[53,57–59] It is noteworthy that despite such recommendations, the emergence of trimethoprim-resistant uropathogens has been well documented in some communities, with local experts recommending the use of fluoroquinolones as first-line agents in these communities in Europe and the USA.[17,19,60–62] There is also worrying evidence of emerging resistance to extended-spectrum β-lactamases (such as third-generation cephalosporins), and to ciprofloxacin.[63,64] Awareness of local antibiotic resistance patterns is thus an important factor in choosing the most appropriate antibiotic.

Amoxicillin/clavulanic acid, nitrofurantoin and cephalexin are suitable for 5-day therapy, but amoxicillin alone should not be used as there is a high incidence (25%–30%) of resistant *E. coli* in community-acquired UTI. If there is no clinical response, MSU should be sent for culture and, in sexually active women, treatment for *C. trachomatis* commenced (doxycycline 100mg bd). In non-sexually active women, further treatment is guided by the results of sensitivity testing. Short-course treatment is inappropriate in women who are at risk of upper UTI (despite lower tract symptoms), which includes those with a history of previous infections due to resistant organisms, with symptoms for more than 1 week, or those with diabetes mellitus.

Males must have urine culture initially and should have at least 14 days of treatment with any of the agents used for treatment of young women with simple cystitis (Table 9.5.2). In men over 50 there is a high probability of invasion of prostatic tissue, and treatment may need to be continued for 4–6 weeks.

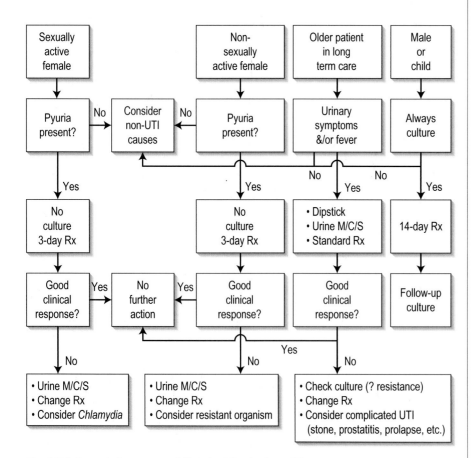

Fig. 9.5.2 Suggested management flow chart for simple cystitis.

Table 9.5.2 Choice of treatment depending on bacteria involved (see text) (Adapted from Stamm W, Hooton T. Management of urinary tract infections in adults. New England Journal of Medicine 1993; 329: 1328–1334)

Condition	Bacteria involved	Suggested treatment
Acute simple cystitis	E. coli, E.faecalis, S.saprophyticus, enterococci, Proteus spp., Klebsiella spp., Pseudomonas spp., staphylococci, Corynebacterium spp.	Trimethoprim 300 mg daily for 3 days OR cephalexin 500 mg 12-hourly for 5 days OR amoxicillin/clavulanate 500/125 mg 8-hourly for 5 days OR nitrofurantoin 50mg 6-hourly for 5 days Males or patients with recurrent infection should be treated for up to 14 days Norfloxacin 400mg 12-hourly for 3 days in resistant infection only
UTI with structural abnormalities (complicated) and inpatients	Increased frequency of Proteus spp., Pseudomonas spp., Klebsiella spp., enterococci, staphylococci, Corynebacterium spp.	Mild infection: trimethoprim or a fluoroquinolone Severe infection: aminoglycosides plus amoxicillin or imipenem/cilastatin Treatment may need to be continued (orally) for 4–6 weeks
Dysuria with low bacterial numbers (urethral syndrome)	Ureaplasma urealyticum*	Doxycycline in young women
Acute uncomplicated pyelonephritis	E. coli, Proteus spp., Klebsiella spp., S.saprophyticus	Mild infection: oral treatment with trimethoprim 300 mg/day, OR amoxicillin/clavulanate 500/125 mg 8-hourly, OR cephalexin 500 mg 6-hourly Severe infection: parenteral treatment initially then oral, use aminoglycoside, plus (ampicillin or) amoxicillin or a third-generation cephalosporin Consider piperacillin or fluoroquinolones. Treatment must be continued for 14 days in all patients
Malignancy causing obstruction/infection	Anaerobes	Add metronidazole or clindamycin
Pregnancy- associated cystitis	E. coli, E. faecalis, S.saprophyticus, Proteus spp., Klebsiella spp.	Nitrofurantoin 50 mg 6-hourly, amoxicillin/clavulanate 500/125 mg 8-hourly, orcephalexin 500 mg 6-hourly Follow closely. Treat for 10–14 days
Catheter-associated	E. coli, Proteus spp., Klebsiella spp., Pseudomonas spp., enterococci, staphylococci	Treat only if symptomatic Change catheter Treat as for 'complicated UTI'

*May have chlamydial or gonococcal urethritis.

Recurrent UTI

Recurrent UTI is defined as a symptomatic UTI which follows the resolution of a previous UTI. These may be re-infections (with the same organism or another) or relapses (regrowth of the same organism within 2 weeks of treatment). Re-infections are more common than relapses, but the two may be indistinguishable.[65] It is important to consider the risk factors specific to the age and gender of the patient, e.g. sexual activity and use of spermicides in the young premenopausal woman, or the higher rate of asymptomatic bacteriuria in the older patient. A careful search for causes and reversible factors (e.g. of complicated UTI due to stone or obstruction, previously undiagnosed diabetes mellitus) should be made, together with urine culture and sensitivity testing. Treatment with an appropriate antibiotic guided by the results of sensitivity tests for at least 10–14 days is required. The patient may benefit from post-intercourse or maintenance prophylaxis, e.g. with nitrofurantoin or trimethoprim for several months (see Host factors).

Acute pyelonephritis

Patients presenting with the typical symptoms of pyelonephritis are at risk of bacteraemia or sepsis syndrome and therefore must rapidly have adequate concentrations of appropriate antibiotics delivered to both the blood and the urine. In order to meet this requirement, particularly in patients who are vomiting, parenteral (intravenous) treatment is usually required initially, but seldom for longer than 24–48 hours, by which time the patient is usually afebrile and not vomiting.

The choice of antibiotics is necessarily empirical at this stage. In cases of mild-to-moderate infection, 10–14-day treatment with one of the antimicrobials used for simple cystitis is appropriate (with ciprofloxacin replacing norfloxacin for resistant organisms). For severe infections, parenteral ampicillin or amoxicillin together with gentamicin, both in high dose, are appropriate, with a third-generation cephalosporin as an alternative to gentamicin when the use of aminoglycosides is inappropriate.

Parenteral fluoroquinolone, and ureidopenicillins (e.g. piperacillin) may be appropriate for seriously ill patients with community-acquired infections. In patients with hospital-acquired infections and suspected Gram-negative sepsis, broader-spectrum agents such as ceftazidime, ticarcillin/clavulanic acid and imipenem, perhaps in combination with aminoglycosides, may be required.

Parenteral treatment is followed by oral therapy for 2 weeks.[58,66]

As part of the drive to more efficient use of hospital resources, the use of short-stay observation units is now a standard part of the practice of emergency medicine.[67,68] The safety and efficacy of treatment of pyelonephritis in such units with intravenous antibiotics and fluid administration, followed by oral therapy, is widely accepted.[69] Many hospitals also have active 'hospital in the home (HITH)' or 'outpatient antibiotic treatment (OPAT)' programmes, allowing close supervision of these patients by hospital-based staff and once- or twice-daily intravenous antibiotic administration at home.[70] This is an appropriate alternative to observation unit treatment suitable for milder cases, but requires careful patient selection to exclude those at risk of complicated infections. Appropriate follow-up is essential, although repeat urine cultures are not recommended in asymptomatic patients following simple pyelonephritis.

Pregnancy

UTIs in pregnancy are associated with an increased incidence of premature delivery and low-birthweight infants. This has also been demonstrated to occur with asymptomatic bacteriuria, although up to 40% of asymptomatic women develop acute pyelonephritis later in pregnancy. Therefore, screening for bacteriuria and treatment of pregnant women is essential, and urine must be sent for culture and antibiotic sensitivity testing. Three-day courses of treatment are not widely recommended, although it may be reasonable to use them with close follow-up in an effort to reduce antibiotic usage. Ten-day treatment courses are, however, the norm. Nitrofurantoin, amoxicillin/clavulanate or cephalexin are appropriate for use in pregnancy, sulphas and trimethoprim being contraindicated.[66]

Complicated UTI

As there is a greater range of organisms causing infection in these circumstances, and a higher probability of antibiotic resistance, urine culture is essential and initial empiric treatment must cover the broader spectrum of organisms potentially involved. Trimethoprim or a quinolone is appropriate for mild infections. More serious infections may need combinations of agents, such as aminoglycosides with amoxicillin or imipenem/cilastatin.

Catheter-associated UTI

Catheter-associated UTIs are the most common nosocomial infections.[71,72] In patients with short-term catheters who develop infection, the catheter must be changed and treatment instituted as for complicated UTI. For those with chronic indwelling catheters (such as patients with spinal injuries), bacteriuria is universal and treatment is only indicated in the presence of symptoms, such as fever, chills or loin pain. Antibiotic selection should again be based on culture.

Elderly patients

As previously stated, asymptomatic bacteriuria and UTI are very common in older patients, and more so with increasing functional impairment. There is good evidence that treatment of asymptomatic patients is of no benefit and may paradoxically be associated with increased morbidity. Conversely, symptomatic infection is a significant cause of morbidity and mortality, as this age group also has a higher incidence of bacteraemia associated with pyelonephritis, and septic shock commonly follows. Given the high rate of asymptomatic bacteriuria, the diagnosis of UTI in such individuals is difficult. The traditional view that non-specific symptoms such as increased confusion (without fever), falling or deteriorating mobility are due to UTI has been called into question, and it is currently held that UTI should only be considered in patients with fever or specific genitourinary symptoms, or both. In patients with non-specific symptoms non-infective causes should be sought, and in the case of fever alone, other potential sources of infection must be considered.[13,15,35]

Antibiotic treatment of symptomatic UTI in the elderly patient is no different initially from that of younger patients, but it should be borne in mind that a greater variety of organisms may be cultured in this age group, and urine for culture should be obtained at the outset whenever possible.

Disposition

Patients with simple UTI should have follow-up to confirm clinical cure. Failure of symptomatic improvement in 48 hours may indicate antibiotic resistance, which requires urine culture to elucidate. Recurrence of symptoms within 1–2 weeks may indicate occult renal infection, and necessitates urine culture and at least 7 days' treatment.

Prognosis

In adults with a normal urinary tract UTI does not cause long-term sequelae. In the presence of urinary tract abnormalities, infection may be a factor in producing renal damage or altering its rate of onset. Imaging of adults as part of their follow-up should detect this group of patients. In the elderly, bacteriuria may be a marker of functional deterioration. Opinion has been divided on whether or not asymptomatic bacteriuria leads to reduced survival in this age group. Treatment of asymptomatic bacteriuria in the elderly is not currently recommended, as there is no evidence of any benefit and some indication of increased morbidity due to antibiotic-related complications and the emergence of resistant organisms.

Controversies

- The level of bacteriuria representing infection – traditionally 10^5cfu/mL, or lower counts such as 10^2cfu/mL.

- Best first-line treatment of uncomplicated cystitis in the face of emerging resistance of uropathogens to common antibiotics such as trimethoprim.

- The role of blood cultures as part of the investigation of pyelonephritis. Although traditionally used, they add little to the diagnosis and management.

- Management of asymptomatic bacteriuria in the elderly – active treatment or observation?

References

1. Bergeron M. Treatment of pyelonephritis in adults. Medical Clinics of North America 1995; 79: 33, 619–649.
2. Kreger B, Craven DE, Carling PC, et al. Gram-negative bacteremia III. Reassessment of etiology, epidemiology and ecology in 612 patients. American Journal of Medicine 1980; 68: 332–343.
3. Anonymous. Urinary Tract Infections. Better Health Channel Website. Department of Human Services, State Government of Victoria. 2007.
4. Kelsey M, Mead MG, Gruneberg RN, et al. Relationships between sexual intercourse and urinary tract infection in women attending a clinic for sexually transmitted diseases. Journal of Medical Microbiology 1979; 12: 511–512.
5. Foxman B, Frerichs R. Epidemiology of urinary tract infection: I. Diaphragm use and sexual intercourse. American Journal of Public Health 1985; 75: 1308–1313.
6. Hooton TM, Scholes D, Hughes JP. A prospective study of risk factors for symptomatic urinary tract infection in young women. New England Journal of Medicine 1996; 335: 468.
7. Kunin C. Urinary tract infections in females. Clinical Infectious Diseases 1994; 18: 1–12.
8. Ronald A, Pattullo A. The natural history of urinary infection in adults. Medical Clinics of North America 1991; 75: 299–312.
9. Bent S, Nallamothu BK, Simel DL, et al. Does this woman have an acute uncomplicated urinary tract infection? Journal of the American Medical Association 2002; 287: 2701–2710.
10. Vorland L, Carlson K, Aalen O. An epidemiological survey of urinary tract infections among outpatients in

Northern Norway. Scandinavian Journal of Infectious Diseases 1985; 17: 277.

11. Dontas A, Kasviki-Charvati P, Papanayitotou PC, et al. Bacteriuria and survival in old age. New England Journal of Medicine 1981; 304: 939–943.

12. Nicolle L, Bjornson J, Harding GKM, et al. Bacteriuria in elderly institutionalized men. New England Journal of Medicine 1983; 309: 1421–1425.

13. Nicolle L. Urinary tract infection in geriatric and institutionalized patients. Current Opinion in Urology 2002; 12: 51–55.

14. Nicolle L. Asymptomatic bacteriuria in the elderly. Infectious Disease Clinics of North America 1997; 11: 647.

15. Nicolle L. Urinary tract infection in long-term-care facility residents. Clinical Infectious Diseases 2000; 31: 757–761.

16. Ronald A. The etiology of urinary tract infection: traditional and emerging pathogens. Disease A Month 2003; 49: 71–82.

17. Gupta K, Hooton T, Stamm W, et al. Increasing antimicrobial resistance and the managment of uncomplicated community-acquired urinary tract infections. Annals of Internal Medicine 2001; 135: 41–50.

18. Jordan P, Irvani A, Richard GA, et al. Urinary tract infection caused by Staphylococcus saprophyticus. Journal of Infectious Diseases 1980; 42: 510–515.

19. David RD, DeBlieux PM, Press R. Rational antibiotic treatment of outpatient genitourinary infections in a changing environment. American Journal of Medicine 2005; 118:7–13.

20. Kinane D, Blackwell CC, Brettle RP, et al. ABO blood group, secretor state and susceptibility to recurrent urinary tract infection in women. British Medical Journal 1982; 285: 7–9.

21. Scholes D, Hooton TM, Roberts PL, et al. Risk factors for recurrent urinary tract infection in young women. Journal of Infectious Diseases 2000; 182: 1177–1182.

22. Bran J, Levinson M, Kaye D. Entrance of bacteria into the female urinary bladder. New England Journal of Medicine 1972; 286: 626–629.

23. Turck M, Goffe B, Petersdorf R. The urethral catheter and urinary tract infection. Journal of Urology 1962; 88: 834–837.

24. Kincaid-Smith P, Bullen M. Bacteriuria in pregnancy. Lancet 1965; 1: 1312–1314.

25. O'Sullivan D, Fitzgerald MG, Meyness MJ, et al. Urinary tract infection, a comparative study in the diabetic and general population. British Medical Journal 1961; 1: 786–788.

26. Ronald A, Ludwig E. Urinary tract infection in adults with diabetes. International Journal of Antimicrobial Agents 2001; 17: 287–292.

27. Stapleton A. Urinary tract infections in patients with diabetes. Excerpta Medica 2002; 113: 80S–84S.

28. Karunajeewa H, McGechie D, Stuccio G, et al. Asymptomatic bacteriuria as a predictor of subsequent hospitalization with urinary tract infection in diabetic adults: The Fremantle Diabetes Study. Diabetologia 2005; 48: 1288–1291.

29. Pfisterer MH, Griffiths DJ, Schaefer W, et al. The effect of age on lower urinary tract function: a study in women. Journal of the American Geriatrics Society 2006; 54: 405–412.

30. Mabeck C, Orskov R, Orskov I. Escherichia coli serotypes and renal involvement in urinary tract infection. Lancet 1971; 1: 1312–1314.

31. Hagberg L, Hull R, Hull S, et al. Contribution of adhesion to bacterial persistence in the mouse urinary tract. Infection and Immunity 1983; 40: 265–272.

32. Svanborg-Eden C, Hausson S, Jodal Y, et al. Host–parasite interactions in the urinary tract. Journal of Infectious Diseases 1988; 157: 421–426.

33. Sandford J. Urinary tract symptoms and infections. Annual Review of Medicine 1976; 26: 485–499.

34. Rubin R, Cotran R, Tolkoff-Rubin N. Urinary tract infection, pyelonephritis, and reflux nephropathy. In:

Brenner B ed. The kidney.: Philadelphia: WB Saunders, 1991; 1597–1654.

35. Bentley D, Bradley S, High K, et al. Practice guidelines for evaluation of fever and infection in long-term care facilities. Clinical Infectious Diseases 2000; 31: 640–653.

36. Deville WL, Yzermans JC, van Duijn NP, et al. The urine dipstick test useful to rule out infections. A meta-analysis of its accuracy. Bio Med Central Urology 2004; 4: 2.

37. Sultana R, Zalstein S, Cameron P, et al. Dipstick urinalysis and the accuracy of the clinical diagnosis of urinary tract infection. Journal of Emergency Medicine 2001; 20: 13–19.

38. Brumfitt W. Urinary cell counts and their value. Journal of Clinical Pathology 1965; 18: 550.

39. Stamm W. Measurement of pyuria and its relation to bacteriuria. American Journal of Medicine 1983; 75: 53–58.

40. Pappas P. Laboratory in the diagnosis and management of urinary tract infections. Medical Clinics of North America 1991; 75: 313–325.

41. Morgan M, McKenzie H. Controversies in the laboratory diagnosis of community-acquired urinary tract infection. European Journal of Clinical Microbiology and Infectious Diseases 1993; 12: 491–504.

42. Kass E. Bacteriuria and the diagnosis of infection of the urinary tract. Archives of Internal Medicine 1957; 100: 709.

43. Stamm WE, Counts GW, Running KR, et al. Diagnosis of coliform infection in acutely dysuric women. New England Journal of Medicine 1982; 307: 463.

44. Stamm W, Wagner KJ, Amsel R, et al. Causes of the acute urethral syndrome in women. New England Journal of Medicine 1980; 303: 409–415.

45. Lipsky B. UTI in men: epidemiology, pathophysiology, diagnosis and treatment. Annals of Internal Medicine 1989; 110: 138–150.

46. Stamm W, Running K, McKevitt M, et al. Treatment of the acute urethral syndrome. New England Journal of Medicine 1981; 304: 956–958.

47. McMurray B, Wrenn K, Wright S. Usefulness of blood cultures in pyelonephritis. American Journal of Emergency Medicine 1997; 15: 137–140.

48. Velasco M, Martinez JA, Moreno-Martinez A, et al. Blood cultures for women with uncomplicated pyelonephritis: are they necessary? Clinical Infectious Diseases 2003; 37: 1127–1130.

49. Thanassi M. Utility of urine and blood cultures in pyelonephritis. Academic Emergency Medicine 1997; 4: 797–800.

50. Wing DA, Park AS, DeBuque L, et al. Limited clinical utility of blood and urine cultures in the treatment of acute pyelonephritis during pregnancy. American Journal of Obstetrics and Gynecology 2000; 182: 1437–1440.

51. Kanel K, Kroboth JF, Schwentker FN, et al. The intravenous pyelogram in acute pyelonephritis. Archives of Internal Medicine 1988; 148: 2144–2148.

52. Sandberg T, Stokland E, Brolin I, et al. Selective use of excretory urography in women with acute pyelonephritis. Journal of Urology 1989; 141: 1290–1294.

53. Stamm W, Hooton T. Management of urinary tract infections in adults. New England Journal of Medicine 1993; 329: 1328–1334.

54. Hooton T, Stamm W. Diagnosis and treatment of uncomplicated urinary tract infection. Infectious Disease Clinics of North America 1997; 11: 551.

55. Meyrier A, Condamin MC, Fernet M, et al. Frequency of development of early cortical scarring in acute primary pyelonephritis. Kidney International 1989; 35: 696–703.

56. Tsugaya M, Hirao N, Skagami H, et al. Computerized tomography in acute pyelonephritis: the clinical correlations. Journal of Urology 1990; 144: 611–613.

57. Anonymous. Urinary Tract Infections. In: eTG complete (Internet). Therapeutic Guidleines Limited. 2007.

58. Warren J, Abrutyn E, Hebel JR, et al. Guidelines for antimicrobial treatment of uncomplicated acute bacterial cystitis and acute pyelonephritis in women. Clinical Infectious Diseases 1999; 29: 745–758.

59. Vogel T, Verrault R, Gourdean M, et al. Optimal duration of antibiotic therapy for uncomplicated urinary tract infection in older women: a double-blind randomized controlled trial. [see comment]. Canadian Medical Association Journal 2004; 170: 469–473.

60. Raz R, Chazan B, Kennes Y, et al. Empiric use of trimethoprim-sulfamethoxazole (TMP-SMX) in the treatment of women with uncomplicated urinary tract infections, in a geographical area with high prevalence of TMP-SMX-resistant uropathogens. Clinical Infectious Diseases 2002; 34: 1165–1169.

61. Alos JI, Serrano MG, Gomez-Garces JL, et al. Antibiotic resistance of Escherichia coli from community-acquired urinary tract infections in relation to demographic and clinical data. Clinical Microbiology and Infection 2005; 11: 199–203.

62. Zahar JR, Lecuit M, Carbonelle E, et al. Is it time to reconsider initial antibiotic treatment strategies for severe urinary tract infections in Europe? Clinical Microbiology and Infection 2007; 13: 2. 19–21.

63. Paterson DL. Resistance in gram-negative bacteria: enterobacteriaceae. American Journal of Medicine 2006; 1: 19.

64. Gagliotti C, Nobilio L, Moro ML, et al. Emergence of ciprofloxacin resistance in Escherichia coli isolates from outpatient urine samples. Clinical Microbiology and Infection 2007; 13: 328–331.

65. Franco A. Recurrent urinary tract infections. Best Practice and Research in Clinical Obstetrics and Gynaecology 2005; 19: 861–873.

66. Anonymous. Urinary Tract Infections. In: eTG complete (Internet). Melbourne Therapeutic Guidleines Limited. 2006.

67. Williams A, Jelinek GA, Rogers IR, et al. The effect on hospital admission profiles of establishing an emergency department observation ward. Medical Journal of Australia 2000; 173: 411–414.

68. Jelinek G, Galvin G. Observation wards in Australian hospitals. Medical Journal of Australia 1989; 151: 80–83.

69. Ward G, Jorden R, Severance H. Treatment of pyelonephritis in an observation unit. Annals of Emergency Medicine 1991; 20: 258–261.

70. Montalto M, Dunt D. Home and hospital intravenous therapy for two acute infections: an early study. Australia and New Zealand Journal of Medicine 1997; 27: 19–23.

71. Haley R, Culver DH, White JW, et al. The nationwide nosocomial infection rate. A new need for vital statistics. American Journal of Epidemiology 1985; 121: 159–167.

72. Tambyah P, Maki D. Catheter-associated urinary tract infection is rarely symptomatic. Archives of Internal Medicine 2000; 160: 678–682.

73. Graham J, Galloway A. The laboratory diagnosis of urinary tract infection. Journal of Clinical Pathology 2001; 54: 911–919.

Further reading

Rubin RH, Cotran RS, Tolkoff-Rubin NE. Urinary tract infection, pyelonephritis, and reflux nephropathy. In: Brenner BM, ed. The kidney, 5th edn. Philadelphia: WB Saunders, 1991; 1597–1654.

Sobel JD, Kaye D. Urinary tract infections. In: Mandell GL, Bennett JE, Dolin R eds. Principles and practice of infectious diseases, 4th edn. New York: Churchill Livingstone, 1995; 662–690.

9.6 Skin and soft-tissue infections

Rabind Charles

ESSENTIALS

1 The time-honoured principles of wound management, together with the judicious evidence-based use of antibiotics remain the basis for preventing and treating skin and soft-tissue infections.

2 All wounds, no matter how trivial, should be assumed to be tetanus prone and treated accordingly.

3 Skin and soft-tissue infections are common and range from mild to life-threatening; they occasionally require surgical intervention, and usually respond to narrow-spectrum antibiotics.

4 Deep soft-tissue infections have high morbidity and mortality and, unless treated aggressively, can rapidly result in loss of limb or death of the patient.

5 Infections due to unusual organisms, including organisms not usually considered to be pathogenic, frequently cause serious infections in the immunocompromised, diabetics and patients with hepatic disease.

Introduction

Infectious disease is one of the most common reasons for patients to present to the emergency department (ED), and skin and soft tissue infections (SSTIs) make up an important subset of these. Bacteria cause the majority of SSTIs encountered in the ED. The pathogenesis of these infections usually involves direct inoculation of bacteria as a result of violation of the skin or its defences, although there may also be spread of infection from a distant source via the haematogenous or lymphatic systems, The severity of infections encountered may range from mild to life-threatening. Most recommendations for the diagnosis and treatment of SSTIs are based on tradition or consensus, as there are a few randomized clinical trials on the subject. Some of the challenges to the emergency physician include:

- Early and accurate diagnosis of the type of infection, based on clinical grounds and limited use of laboratory and radiological investigations.
- Early identification of potentially high-risk situations, when the initial presentation is seemingly innocuous, by looking at patient factors (e.g. diabetes, immunosuppression) and local factors (bite wounds, site of infection, e.g. orbital cellulitis).
- Role of antibiotics: (a) appropriate antibiotics for use, where indicated, taking into account the emergence of new infections and changing bacterial resistance patterns; (b) optimal route by which the antibiotic is delivered, i.e. topical versus oral versus initial i.v. or i.m. bolus, followed by oral antibiotics versus intravenous therapy; (c) duration of the antibiotic treatment.
- Need for surgical intervention, e.g. drainage of abscess, early debridement in necrotizing fasciitis.
- Disposition issues: whether the patient can be discharged with outpatient follow-up or will need hospitalization for management.

Aetiology

The majority of SSTIs are caused by aerobic Gram-positive bacteria, commonly *Staphylococcus aureus* and group A streptococcus. Deeper complicated infections, commonly seen in the immunocompromised host, are usually caused by Gram-negative, anaerobic or mixed organisms (Table 9.6.1).

Examination

History

When taking a history, it is important to elicit the following:

- The presence of trauma leading to a breach in skin integrity triggering the infection, e.g. human or animal bite, 'clenched fist' injury. This is important because it will help in determining the likely pathogen and choice of antibiotics, as well as the need to rule out any potential foreign body that may be embedded in the wound.
- The speed with which the infection has progressed will serve as a guide as to how aggressive the infection is, and the urgency of treatment needed.
- Patient factors that may complicate the treatment of the infection:
  - History of immunosuppression, e.g. diabetes, steroid use, chronic liver disease, alcoholism, HIV, oncology patients on chemotherapy, nephrotic syndrome
  - Recent use of antibiotics, i.e. failed treatment
  - History of prosthetic heart valves, mitral valve prolapse with regurgitation, previous history of endocarditis
  - Chronic venous stasis or lymphoedema in limbs
  - Intravenous drug use (IVDU).
- Tetanus status.
- Contamination with soil or water, which would suggest unusual pathogens as the cause of the infection.

Physical examination

- Identification of severe sepsis: unstable vital signs, hyperpyrexia, 'toxic'-looking patient.
- Specific features of the infection to help narrow down the diagnosis, e.g. raised erythematous margins in erysipelas; presence of bullae and crepitus or tenderness out of proportion to physical signs, suggestive of necrotizing fasciitis; fetid odour suggesting anaerobic

Table 9.6.1

Risk factor/setting	Expected pathogen
Simple cutaneous infection	*Staphylococcus aureus*. Also *Staph. epidermidis*, *Staph. hominis*, *Streptococcus viridans*
Perianal, genital, buttocks, ungual and cervical areas	*Bacteroides fragilis*, *Escherichia coli*, *Klebsiella* and *Proteus*
Immunocompromised host	*Cryptococcccus neoformans*, *Coccidioides*, *Aspergillus*, *Mycobacterium kansasii*, *M. tuberculosis* and *Yersinia enterocolitica*.
Human bite	*Eikenella corrodens*, *Fusobacterium*, *Prevotella*, *Streptococci*
Dog bite	*Pasteuralla multocida*, *Capnocytophaga canimorsus*
Cat bite	*P. multocida*
Injection drug abuse	*S. aureus*, *Clostridium* sp, *E. corrodens*, *S. pyogenes*
Body piercing	*S. aureus*, *S. pyogenes*, *P. aeruginosa*, *C. tetani*
Hot tub/wading pool	*Ps. aeruginosa*
Fresh water injury	*A. hydrophila*
Salt water injury	*V. vulnificus*
Fish tank exposure	*Mycobacterium marinum*

infection, or green exudates typical of *Pseudomonas* spp.

- The extent of the infection, e.g. mapping areas of erythema to track progress.
- Location of the infection, as involvement of certain critical areas (e.g. head, face, perineum) may require more intensive inpatient management and specialist consultation.
- Complicating factors that might impair successful treatment, e.g. needle tracks in i.v. drug users, the presence of prosthetic heart valves.

Investigations

SSTIs are usually diagnosed from their clinical presentation. Laboratory and radiological investigations play a secondary and limited role in routine evaluation but may be useful in the ED management of immunocompromised patients or those with signs and symptoms of severe sepsis. In such situations the following parameters should be considered:[1]

- Full blood examination with differential: Presence of marked leukocytosis,

leukopenia or an extreme left shift in the white cell differential; new-onset anaemia or thrombocytopenia may suggest sepsis syndrome.
- Urea/creatinine: Elevated levels suggest intravascular volume depletion or renal failure.
- Creatine kinase: Elevated levels may indicate myonecrosis caused by necrotizing fasciitis.
- Blood culture and drug susceptibility tests: The yield from these may be less than 10% and may be compounded by false positive results.[2] In addition, emergency physicians do not have the luxury of time to await blood culture results before initiating the appropriate antibiotic treatment.
- Other investigations: It is prudent to test for diabetes mellitus in patients presenting with an abscess because of the strong association of the two. Patients with a chronic, recurrent or unusual infection should have their immune status checked, including serology for HIV. Soft tissue radiographs may demonstrate a foreign body or gas in deep tissues. Computed tomography

(CT) or magnetic resonance imaging (MRI) may be needed to define the depth and extent of the infective process when entertaining the diagnoses of fasciitis or myonecrosis. Ultrasonography in the ED may be a useful adjunct in evaluating soft tissue infections for the presence of subcutaneous abscesses.

Management

Key points in the management of SSTIs include:

- Analgesia
- Appropriate use of antibiotics
- Appropriate surgical intervention
- Tetanus and other prophylaxis
- Disposition plans and options.

Analgesia

Oral or parenteral analgesia should be prescribed, as most patients with SSTIs will present with pain. Simple measures such as immobilization, elevation, heat or moist warm packs should not be overlooked as they may help to alleviate pain in cellulitis. Abscess pain is best resolved by timely incision and drainage.

It is important to have a high index of suspicion for necrotizing fasciitis in any patient who has cellulitis with an inordinate amount of pain, or exquisite muscle tenderness where there is no history of musculoskeletal trauma.

Antibiotic therapy

Antibiotics are recommended for patients with signs of systemic toxicity, high fever, tachycardia, who are flushed and who look unwell, who are immunocompromised, who have abscesses in high-risk areas (hands, perineal region or face) and where deep necrotizing infection is suspected.[2]

It is important for the emergency physician to recognize patients with serious skin and soft-tissue infections and to initiate appropriate care. The choice of antibiotic is often empiric and thus must be guided by the patient's history, where they have been recently institutionalized and knowledge of the typical range of pathogens associated with each type of infection and their resistance patterns. The antibiotic of choice is the one that has proven efficacy against the range of expected pathogens;

is associated with minimal toxicity; and is cost-effective. Where possible, narrow-spectrum antibiotics should be used in preference to broad-spectrum ones.[3]

Surgical intervention

Certain SSTIs are best treated surgically. Effective treatment of abscesses and carbuncles and large furuncles entails incision, drainage of pus and breaking up of loculations, followed by regular dressings. Necrotizing fasciitis requires *early* aggressive surgical debridement together with broad-spectrum antibiotics, in order to achieve best morbidity and mortality outcomes.[4]

Tetanus and other prophylaxis

All wounds should be considered to be tetanus prone and treated accordingly. The patient's immunization status should be checked and, where appropriate, tetanus toxoid plus tetanus immunoglobulin should be administered. Deep and penetrating wounds and wounds that have significant tissue devitalization or where there is heavy contamination (e.g. soil, dust, manure, wood splinters) are best treated with prophylactic antibiotic cover. The antibiotic of choice is penicillin; patients who are allergic to penicillin should receive cephalexin. If there is a history of severe penicillin allergy, use erythromycin or vancomycin.

Rabies prophylaxis should be considered for all feral and wild animal bites, and in geographical areas where there is a high prevalence of rabies.

In cases involving human bites, consideration should also be given to screening for bloodborne pathogens such as hepatitis B virus, hepatitis C virus, HIV and syphilis.

Disposition

SSTIs are among the most frequently encountered conditions in the emergency observation setting. Good candidates for the observation/short-stay unit include patients likely to respond to empirical therapy, with a low likelihood of infection with unusual and/or resistant organisms.

Patients who have systemic toxicity (fever, tachycardia, rigors, altered mentation, severe pain), involvement of vital structures (fingers, hand, face and neck, genitourinary, scrotal and anal regions),

those unable to take oral medication, who have failed outpatient therapy or who are immunocompromised (HIV positive, cancer, diabetes mellitus, hepatic or renal failure) are highly likely to require admission. Other prognostic factors include low serum bicarbonate, elevated creatinine, elevated creatine kinase, and marked left shift polymorphonuclear neutrophils. The emergency physician must also be alert to scenarios requiring not just inpatient care but also urgent subspecialty consultation, e.g. necrotizing fasciitis.

Superficial skin infections

Clinical presentation

Patients usually present with a complaint of localized pain, redness and swelling. They may have been self-treating or have had previous treatment with oral antibiotics without success. Frequently an abscess is fluctuant and indurated, with surrounding erythema. The patient may also have associated lymphadenitis, regional lymphadenopathy and cellulitis. If the patient is febrile or there is systemic involvement, their immune status needs to be examined.

The possibility of a foreign body associated with an abscess needs to be considered. A careful history needs to be taken to determine whether this is possible, and radiography may be necessary. Ultrasound can be useful in identifying the presence of a foreign body. The patient should also be questioned in relation to use of immunosuppressive agents.

Impetigo

This is a localized purulent skin infection, usually caused by group A streptococcus (*Strep. pyogenes*) and is seen more in warm humid climates. Topical therapy with mucipirocin often suffices, but oral antibiotics (first-generation cephalosporin or erythromycin) may be needed in cases with extensive lesions or perioral lesions.

Folliculitis

A superficial infection characterized by reddened papules or pustules of the hair follicles. Most cases are caused by *Staphylococcus aureus*. *Pseudomonas aeruginosa* may be the cause following swimming pool or hot tub (spa) exposure. Treatment may only require

the use of an antibacterial soap or solution. Removal of the hair in limited infections usually results in rapid resolution.

Furuncle and carbuncle

A furuncle arises secondarily to an infected hair follicle, where an abscess forms in the subcutaneous tissue. Furuncles most commonly occur on the back, axilla or lower extremities. *Staphylococcus* species are the most common associated organism. When the infection extends to involve several adjacent follicles, resulting in a coalescent inflammatory mass, the lesion is termed a carbuncle. Small furuncles are best treated with moist heat. Larger furuncles and all carbuncles require incision and drainage. The most common site is the back of the neck, and diabetics are particularly prone to this. Systemic antibiotics are usually unnecessary unless there is extensive surrounding cellulitis or fever, or if the patient has diabetes or is immunocompromised, in which case di(flu)cloxacillin (500 mg q6h oral), cephalexin (500 mg q6h) or clindamycin (450 mg q8h oral) can be used.

Erysipelas

Erysipelas is a rapidly progressive, erythematous, indurated, painful, sharply demarcated superficial skin infection caused by *Strep. pyogenes* (other causes are non-group A streptococci, *Haemophilus influenzae*, *Staph. aureus* and *Strep. pneumoniae*). The classic description is of a butterfly facial distribution, but recent evidence suggests that erysipelas is commonly found on the lower limbs. There is a clear line of demarcation between involved and uninvolved skin. It is common in young children and the elderly. Systemic symptoms (fever, chills, rigors and diaphoresis) are common, and 5% will have bacteraemia. Erysipelas may rapidly progress to cellulitis (i.e. involvement beyond the upper dermis), abscess formation and occasionally fasciitis. Treatment consists of the use of antibacterial soap and oral penicillin (di(flu)cloxacillin 500 mg q6h oral).

Herpetic whitlow

Herpetic whitlow is a superficial infection with herpes simplex virus and is an occupational hazard of jobs having contact with oral mucosa, e.g. dentistry and anaesthesiology.

Incision and drainage is contraindicated and may in fact spread the viral infection.

Cellulitis

Cellulitis is an acute spreading infection of the skin involving the deeper dermis and subcutaneous fat. In patients with a normal immune system who are otherwise healthy, the infection is caused by bacteria that normally colonize skin, principally *Staph. aureus* and group A β-haemolytic streptococci. Predisposing factors include conditions leading to a disrupted cutaneous barrier and/or impaired local host defences such as trauma and inflammatory dermatoses, e.g. eczema, oedema from venous insufficiency or lymphatic obstruction.

Despite the common occurrence of cellulitis, there is a paucity of published research on issues such as criteria for antibiotics and admission, and severity assessment.

Treatment consists of elevation of the affected part and administration of an anti-staphylococcal penicillin such as di(flu)cloxacillin (2 g q6h i.v.) or a first-generation cephalosporin such as cephazolin (2 g q12h i.v.).

Therapy may need to be escalated in special settings such as diabetes, or particular anatomical areas. Anaerobes or Gram-negative organisms have been identified in 95% of affected diabetic foot ulcers, with *Staph. aureus* found in approximately 33%. Broad-spectrum antibiotic treatment e.g. metronidazole (400 mg q12h orally) plus cephazolin (2g q12h i.v.) is recommended.

Infections that originate from wounds involving the feet may be due to *Pseudomonas aeruginosa*; this organism is also associated with osteomyelitis of the foot. Antibiotic treatment should consist of an antipseudomonal β-lactam such as carbenacillin, or a third-generation cephalosporin such as ceftriaxone and an aminoglycoside.

Cellulitis is a well-known complication in women who have undergone axillary lymph node dissection and surgery for breast cancer. The major mechanism is thought to be an altered lymphatic and/or venous circulation related to the surgical procedure and to radiation therapy. Empiric antibiotic therapy is targeted at *Staph. aureus* and β-haemolytic streptococci, and choices include cephalexin or cefazolin. If the patient has received recent chemotherapy and is neutropenic, then the antibiotic regimen must be broadened to include coverage for aerobic Gram-negative bacilli, including *Pseudomonas aeruginosa*.

Facial cellulitis, including periorbital and orbital cellulitis is a serious infection occurring in adults and children.[5] The causal organisms include *Staph. aureus*, *H. influenzae* type b and *Staph. pneumoniae*. This type of cellulitis may arise from an infected sinus. Broad-spectrum antibiotic therapy is required, the agent of choice being dicloxacillin 1 g i.v. 6-hourly. Radiological evaluation, including CT scanning, may be necessary to identify underlying sinusitis.

Abscesses

Pilonidal abscess

Pilonidal abscesses occur in the superior gluteal fold and arise from the disruption of the epithelium, causing the formation of a pit lined with epithelial cells that may become plugged with hair and keratin, leading to an abscess. Treatment involves incision and drainage, usually in the operating theatre, although smaller abscesses can be drained in the ED under local anaesthetic. They are usually associated with mixed organisms, both aerobic and anaerobic.

Hidradenitis suppurativa

This is a chronic suppurative abscess of the upper apocrine sweat glands in the groin and axilla. It is much more common in females, in obesity, and in patients who have poor hygiene or who shave the region. Organisms include *Staph. aureus*, *Strep. viridans* and *Proteus* spp. Treatment is incision and drainage, usually in the operating theatre. Definitive treatment may require removal of the apocrine sweat glands from the region.

Bartholin's abscess

This occurs as a result of the obstruction of a Bartholin's duct and is usually composed of mixed vaginal flora. *Neisseria gonorrhoeae* and *Chlamydia trachomatis* may also be involved. Treatment is incision, drainage and marsupialization of the cyst in the operating theatre.

Paronychia

This is a superficial abscess of the lateral aspect of the nail, commonly associated with patients whose hands are frequently wet. Common organisms involved are *Staph. aureus*, *Candida* and anaerobes. Some cases may require incision and drainage, with advice to keep the hands dry.

Perianal abscess

These are thought to originate in the anal crypts and extend into the ischiorectal space. Patients frequently complain of pain on defecation and sitting. Perianal abscesses may be associated with inflammatory bowel disease and fistula formation. Treatment should be incision and drainage in the operating theatre under general anaesthesia. When the abscess is superficial and 'pointing', drainage in the ED is possible.

Infected sebaceous cyst

Sebaceous cysts become infected when the duct is obstructed. They can occur anywhere on the body, but tend to favour the head and neck region. Treatment is incision and drainage, recurrence is not uncommon.

Treatment

Incision and drainage of cutaneous abscesses is the key to treatment. Some patients require oral antibiotic therapy. Patients who are immunosuppressed or who have diabetes mellitus should be treated with appropriate antibiotic therapy based on a knowledge of the probable pathogen. Patients at risk of developing bacterial endocarditis require prophylactic antibiotics prior to incision and drainage. The treatment of superficial skin abscesses has in recent years been complicated by the emergence of MRSA. Proponents of the practice of 'routine culture' of abscess fluid say that surveillance of antimicrobial susceptibility allows therapeutic adjustment. Detractors point out that for simple abscesses, incision and drainage without antibiotics is usually sufficient, and thus if antibiotics are not considered clinically useful it is unlikely that culture results will alter the management.

Deep soft-tissue infections

Necrotizing fasciitis

Necrotizing fasciitis is a rare, rapidly progressing, life-threatening infectious process involving primarily the superficial fascia (i.e. all the tissue between the skin and

429

INFECTIOUS DISEASES

9

underlying muscles – the subcutaneous tissue). Patients usually present with the triad of exquisite pain – often out of proportion to initial physical findings – swelling and fever. Early diagnosis is sometimes thwarted by the paucity of cutaneous findings early in the course of the disease. The clinician should have a high index of suspicion based on the clinical presentation as well as the patient's underlying comorbidities (diabetes, chronic alcoholism, and immunosuppression).

Numbness of the involved area is characteristic of advanced necrotizing fasciitis – this is a result of infarction of the cutaneous nerve. Eighty per cent of cases show clear origins for an accompanying skin lesion (insect bite minor abrasion, furuncle, IVDU injection site) but in the remaining 20% no skin lesion can be found.[6,7]

Patients appear extremely toxic with a high fever, tachycardia and malaise. Pathognomonic features include extensive undermining of the skin and subcutaneous tissues, with separation of the tissue planes. The subcutaneous tissues may have a hard, wooden feel. Bullous lesions and skin ecchymoses may also be evident. Crepitation may be clinically evident and gas may be visualized on X-ray in some 80% of patients. The gas is typically layered along fascial planes. CT or MRI may aid in confirming the clinical suspicion.

Bacteria involved in this infection are usually mixed: *Staph.aureus*, haemolytic streptococci, Gram-negative rods and anaerobes. Sometimes only group A streptococci, either alone or in combination with *Staph.aureus*, are found. Aggressive therapy is essential, as mortality approaches 50%. Immediate surgical intervention to extensively open and debride the wound is required, as myonecrosis may be present.[8] Appropriate antimicrobial therapy should be commenced immediately: meropenam (1 g q8h i.v.) plus clindamycin (600 mg q8h i.v.) or lincomycin (600 mg q8h i.v.). Hyperbaric oxygen therapy should be considered.

Fournier's gangrene is a form of necrotizing fasciitis which involves the scrotum, penis or vulva and is usually seen in diabetics. It usually originates from perianal or urinary tract infections (which extend into the periurethral glands) and can progress explosively. The management is early recognition and surgical debridement and i.v. antibiotics.

Gas gangrene

Gas gangrene is an acute life-and-limb threatening deep-tissue infection, also known as clostridial myonecrosis. Aetiological agents include *Clostridium perfringens*, *Cl. histolyticum*, *Cl. septicum* and *Cl. novyi*. *Cl. perfringens* is the most common cause in traumatic gas gangrene, whereas spontaneous gangrene is principally associated with *Cl. septicum*. This infection is characterized by the rapid development (often within hours) of intense pain in the region of a wound, followed by local swelling and a haemoserous exudate. A characteristic foul smell is also a good indication of the diagnosis. The area becomes tense and may develop a bluish and bronze or dusky discoloration. The presence of gas is typical, although it may be a late finding. It is frequently found on X-ray, where it has a feathered pattern as gas develops within the muscle itself. Aggressive treatment is required, as the patient may present in an advanced stage with tachycardia, altered mental status, shock, and haemolytic anaemia.

Classically the gas gangrene occurs in extensive and or deep wounds with predisposing factors, including vascular ischaemia, diabetes and presence of foreign bodies. Gram stain frequently reveals relatively few white blood cells and large numbers of club shaped Gram-positive rods.

Early surgical intervention is essential, including wide debridement of necrotic muscle and other tissues, administration of high-dose penicillin G (benzylpenicillin 2.4 g q4h i.v.), an aminoglycoside and hyperbaric oxygen therapy. Early hyperbaric oxygen therapy has been demonstrated to result in improved outcome.[3,7–10]

One should note that the presence of gas certainly raises the suspicion of a deep-tissue infection, including gas gangrene, but that it may also be present because of previous wound manipulation, self-injection of air, localized gas abscess or other gas-producing organisms, including anaerobes, *E. coli*, streptococci and staphylococci.

Pyomyositis

Pyomyositis is the presence of pus within individual muscle groups, and the usual culprit is *Staph. aureus*. A positive blood culture yield is found in only 5–30% of cases. Typical presenting symptoms included localized pain in a single muscle group, usually in an extremity, and fever. Ultrasonography or CT may be warranted to differentiate the condition from a suspected deep vein thrombosis.

Toxic complications of wound infections

A number of bacteria produce toxins that result in systemic symptoms.

Tetanus

Tetanus, albeit rare in developing countries, still occurs despite the fact that immunization is completely effective in preventing it. All wounds should be treated as tetanus prone. Tetanus may occur with trivial wounds that may not even be apparent. The incubation period is variable, ranging from 3 days to several weeks after inoculation; the disease is more severe at the extremes of age. Difficulty in swallowing and a fever with progression to stiffness and trismus is pathognomonic. Tetanus is also associated with autonomic nervous system dysfunction. Occasionally localized tetanus may occur with muscle spasm in the area adjacent to the wound. This is sometimes associated with cranial nerve dysfunction. Treatment is largely supportive, often requiring deep sedation, paralysis, and ventilation for prolonged periods. Antibiotic therapy with high-dose penicillin should also be given in addition to tetanus immunization and tetanus immunoglobulin (Table 9.6.2).

Toxic shock syndrome

Toxic shock syndrome (TSS) is a life-threatening multisystem disease caused by inflammatory immune responses to toxogenic strains of *Staph. aureus*. TSS has been classically associated with the use of tampons, although 10–40% of cases are non-menstrual related. Onset of menstrual TSS symptoms occurs within 3 days of the menstrual cycle and usually has no preceding clinically apparent infection. Non-menstrual cases occur after childbirth, abortions, in bone and skin infections including postoperative wound infections, burns, mastitis and varicella-related cellulitis. The wound

INFECTIOUS DISEASES

Table 9.6.2 Tetanus prophylaxis (Reproduced with permission from Antibiotic Expert Group. Therapeutic guidelines: antibiotic. Version 13. Melbourne: Therapeutic Guidelines Limited; 2006. p.269.[20])

Time since vaccination	Type of wound	Tetanus toxoid	Tetanus immunoglobulin
History of 3 or more doses of tetanus toxoid			
< 5 yrs	All wounds	-	-
5–10 yrs	Clean minor wounds	-	-
	All other wounds	yes	-
>10 yrs	All wounds	yes	-
Uncertain vaccination history or <3 doses of tetanus toxoid			
	Clean minor wounds	yes	-
	All other wounds	yes	yes

itself may look insignificant. There is a rapid onset of fever, usually ≥38.9°C, hypotension, and an initial diffuse and later desquamating erythematous rash. Multiorgan involvement may include muscular (myalgia), neurological (headache, altered sensorium) and gastrointestinal (nausea, diarrhoea) symptoms. Occasionally *Staph. aureus* can be cultured locally, although blood cultures are rarely positive. Antibiotics do not affect the course of TSS but may lower the recurrence rate by 59–73%.[11] An antistaphylococcal agent should be given with an aminoglycoside. Patients are frequently haemodynamically compromised, requiring aggressive fluid resuscitation and inotropic support. Debridement of necrotic wounds, if present, and elimination of the source of infections – e.g. removal of the tampon – should be carried out urgently. A similar syndrome can develop due to infection with group A β-haemolytic streptococci. This is known as 'wound' or 'surgical' scarlet fever. Treatment is the same as for TSS.

Special infections

Human bites

Human bite wounds may occur as a result of an accidental injury, deliberate biting or closed fist injuries. The bacteriology reflects the normal oral flora of the biter: streptococci in 80% of wounds, staphylococci, *Eikenella corrodens* and anaerobic organisms. Therapy consists of irrigation and topical wound cleansing, and prophylactic antibiotics should be initiated as early as possible in all patients, regardless of the appearance of the wound.

Clenched fist injuries over the metacarpophalangeal joint warrant hospitalization for formal washout and i.v. antibiotics.

Appropriate antibiotic choices include amoxicillin–clavulanate (875 + 125 mg q12h oral), metronidazole (400 mg q12h oral) plus either ceftriaxone (1 g daily i.v.) or cefotaxime (1 g daily i.v.). In cases of β-lactam allergy, metronidazole plus doxycycline, ciprofloxacin or trimethoprim–sulfamethoxazole may be used.

Animal bites

Most bites are from dogs (80%) or cats, but bites from exotic pets and feral animals also occur. *Pasteurella* species are the most common bacterial isolate, and *Capnocytophaga canimorsus* can cause bacteraemia and fatal sepsis, especially in patients with underlying liver disease or asplenia. Wounds should be cleansed with sterile normal saline, and infected wounds should not be closed. Cat bite wounds have less crush injury and wound trauma than dog bites, but have a higher proportion of osteomyelitis and septic arthritis. The oral agent of choice for both dog and cat bites is amoxicillin–clavulanate, with doxycycline as an alternative. Intravenous options include second-generation cephalosporins, piperacillin–tazobactam and carbapenams. Cellulitis and abscesses usually respond to 5–10 days of therapy. Rabies prophylaxis should be considered for all feral and wild animal bites, and in geographical areas where there is a high prevalence of rabies.

Water-related infections

Water-related infections may be caused by unusual organisms. *Vibrio vulnificus, V. alginolyticus* and other non-cholera vibrios are found in salt and brackish water and can result in serious and life-threatening infections, especially in patients with hepatic disease. Aggressive infection can progress rapidly over 2–4 hours. It is associated with saltwater exposure or the ingestion of raw shellfish. Infections can mimic gas gangrene, with rapid progression and tissue destruction; septicaemia may occur, and can be fatal. If parenteral therapy is required, a third-generation cephalosporin can be combined with an aminoglycoside and/or doxycycline.

Exposure to fresh or brackish water (rivers, mud and caving) can result in infection with the Gram-negative bacillus *Aeromonas hydrophila*.[12] *Aeromonas* infections can result in superficial skin infections, myositis and septicaemia. Treatment consists of administration of cefotaxime 1 g i.v. 8-hourly or ceftriaxone 1 g i.v. daily. If oral therapy is possible, consider ciprofloxacin 500 mg orally 12-hourly.

Mycobacterium marinum, M. ulcerans, M. chelonei, M. gordanae. and *M. fortuitum*, are found in fish tanks and can result in 'fish fancier's finger'. After 2–6 weeks of incubation, an ulcerating granuloma develops. Treatment options include clarithromycin, trimethoprim–sulfamethoxazole or a combination of ethambutol and rifampicin.

Saltwater fish handlers may develop infections due to *Erysipelothrix rhusiopathiae*; this causes erysipeloid, a type of cellulitis. It also causes infections in people handling fish, poultry, meat and hides. Coral cuts are often infected with *Streptococcus pyogenes*; other marine pathogens may be involved (including *Vibrio* species). Treatment should consist of phenoxymethylpenicillin 500 mg 6-hourly.

Mastitis

Infections of the breast can occur in both sexes and in all ages; however, breast infections are most common in nursing mothers, and the prevalence of lactational mastitis in Australia is estimated at 20%.[13] *Staphylococcus aureus* is the most common pathogen in infective mastitis.

Treatment consists of regular emptying of the breast. If breastfeeding needs to be stopped because of the severity of the infection or the risk to the neonate, a pump or manual expression methods should be employed (at least temporarily). If symptoms are not resolving within 12–24 hours of effective milk removal and analgesia, antibiotic treatment should be commenced to prevent abscess formation. Eleven per cent of patients who are not treated appropriately with antibiotics will develop an abscess. Options include di(flu)cloxacillin (500 mg q6h oral) or a first-generation cephalosporin such as cephalexin (500 mg q6h oral) or erythromycin (250 500 mg q6h oral). Severe infections may require parenteral or more prolonged therapy. Local care to the region is also important, including warm compresses, breast support, analgesia and the application of a moisturizing cream to the nipple and areolar region. Patients who develop an abscess will require percutaneous aspiration or open drainage.[14]

Decubitus ulcers

Decubitus ulcers are cutaneous ulcerations caused by prolonged pressure that results in ischaemic necrosis of the skin and underlying soft tissue. They are most commonly found in patients who are bedbound, particularly elderly nursing home patients and patients with sensory deficits such as paraplegia and quadriplegia. Immobility, compounded by vascular insufficiency and neuropathy, results in ulcer formation, and unless treated aggressively, serious complications can follow.[15] Complications include cellulitis and deep soft tissue necrosis, osteomyelitis, septic thrombophlebitis, bacteraemia and sepsis. Culture of the ulcer invariably reveals a mixed bacterial flora of both aerobes and anaerobes, which do not distinguish between colonization and tissue infection. The most common organisms found are staphylococci, streptococci, coliforms and a variety of anaerobes. Systemic antibiotics are required for patients with clinical signs of sepsis or osteomyelitis.

Varicose ulcers

Varicose ulcers are cutaneous ulcers caused by oedema and poor tissue drainage as a result of dysfunction of the venous system, including varicose veins. These are more common in the elderly and obese. They may be chronic, and healing is often difficult. Complications include cellulitis and occasionally bacteraemia. Culture of the ulcer variably reveals a mixed bacterial flora of both aerobes and anaerobes that cannot distinguish between colonization and tissue infections. The most common organisms found are staphylococci, streptococci, coliforms and a variety of anaerobes.

Treatment consists of debridement of necrotic tissue, pressure area and general nursing care, as well as treatment of infection, if present. Antibiotic treatment is only indicated where there is systemic evidence of infection or where there is a complicating infection such as osteomyelitis or bacteraemia. Surgical debridement is frequently as important, if not more important, than antibiotic therapy, particularly where the bacterial infection is localized.

Diabetic foot infections

Foot infections are a common complication of diabetes, and require both local (foot) treatment and systemic (metabolic) optimization, which is best undertaken by a multidisciplinary team including surgeons, podiatry services and the endocrinologist or physician.

The peripheral neuropathy associated with diabetes results in the loss of protective pain sensation and results in repetitive injuries, followed by the development of ulcers that become infected. Vascular insufficiency and impaired immune function contribute to the increased risk of acute and chronic infection. Infections in foot ulcers are often polymicrobial, and both the number of bacterial groups and bacterial density are thought to affect healing.[16] Aerobes include *Staph. aureus*, coagulase-negative staphylococci and streptococci. Enterobacteriaceae and *Corynebacterium* are not uncommon. Anaerobes which have been isolated from up to 48% of patients include *Bacteroides*, and *Clostridium* spp. The presence of anaerobes is associated with a high frequency of fever, foul-smelling lesions, and the presence of an ulcer. Cultures obtained using curettage following debridement should be used in preference to wound swabs to identify causative organisms and sensitivities.

Local signs and symptoms predominate, and include those secondary to infection, vasculopathy and neuropathy. Pain and tenderness is often minimal due to the neuropathy, and pulses are frequently reduced or absent. Wound infections must be diagnosed clinically on the basis of local (and occasionally systemic) signs and symptoms of inflammation. Laboratory (including microbiological) investigations are of limited use for diagnosing infection, except in cases of osteomyelitis radiography, and/or a bone scan may be warranted to exclude osteomyelitis.

A recent systemic review[16] reported that there is no strong evidence for any particular antimicrobial agent in the prevention of amputation, resolution of infection, or ulcer healing. For mild to moderate infections with no evidence of osteomyelitis or septic arthritis, consider amoxicillin–clavulanate (875 + 125 mg q12h oral) for at least 5 days. Alternatives include ciprofloxacin 500 mg q12h with clindamycin 600 mg q8h. For severe limb- or life-threatening infections, intravenous piperacillin–tazobactam 4–0.5 g q8h or ticarcillin–clavulanate 3 + 0.1 g q6h or meropenem 500 mg q8h are all acceptable empiric therapy. Prolonged use of appropriate bactericidal antibiotics may be required, especially in the setting of osteomyelitis or septic arthritis.

Surgical site/postoperative wound infection

Surgical site infections are the most commonly occurring adverse events in patients who have undergone surgery, accounting for as much as 38% of nosocomial infections in postoperative patients. Surgical site infections are usually diagnosed by the usual features of inflammation: wound pain, redness, swelling and purulent discharge. These external signs of inflammation may manifest late in morbidly obese patients or those with deep, multilayer wounds. Most bacterial wound infections present with fever only after 48 hours. Earlier symptoms may be seen in *Strep. pyogenes* and clostridial infections.

The mainstay of treatment for surgical site infections is early opening of the incision, coupled with evacuation of any infected material and sending off of wound cultures. This should be done after consultation with the surgeon involved, where possible. There has been a paucity of evidence regarding the use of antibiotics combined with drainage,[17] but expert consensus generally advocates the use of empirical antibiotics for patients with temperature > 38.5°C and/or pulse rate > 100 in the presence of obvious wound infection.[4]

Post-traumatic wound infection

The goals of wound care are to avoid infection and to achieve a functional and cosmetically acceptable scar. Adequate wound management requires a thorough history, with particular attention directed at factors adversely affecting healing. Factors such as the extremes of age, diabetes, chronic renal failure, malnutrition, alcoholism, obesity, and patients on immunosuppressive agents cause an increased risk of infections and impaired wound healing. Wounds located in highly vascular areas such as the scalp or face are less likely to become infected than wounds in less vascular areas.

In order to reduce the incidence and severity of infections, wounds need to be thoroughly cleansed and irrigated. Devitalized tissue should be removed, injuries to associated structures need to be excluded and the wound closed appropriately. The method of closure depends on the location of the wound, the level of contamination and whether it is an 'old' wound (over 6 hours old). Wounds that should not be closed because of a high risk of infection, such as heavily contaminated wounds, should be treated by delayed primary closure 3–5 days after initial management. Where primary closure is possible the wound should be closed and a protective non-adherent dressing applied for a minimum of 24–48 hours, with both the wound and the dressing kept dry.[18]

The use of prophylactic antibiotics is not recommended except where there is significant bacterial contamination, foreign bodies, the patient is immunosuppressed, or the wound is the result of a bite (human or animal) or associated with an open fracture. Most wounds can be treated with amoxicillin–clavulanate (875 + 125 mg q12h oral), or metronidazole (400 mg q12h oral) plus di (flu)cloxacillin (500 mg q6h oral). Broad-spectrum antibiotics should be limited to heavily contaminated and bite wounds, and immunosuppressed patients (see Table 9.6.2).

Intravenous drug users

Intravenous drug users frequently develop unusual infections because the needles and the drug paraphernalia used are contaminated. They also have alterations to their skin and flora and frequently have poor nutrition and immune function.[19] Many are hepatitis B, C and HIV positive.

Intravenous drug users frequently have mixed organisms, particularly anaerobes, including: *Klebsiella*, *Enterobacter*, *Serratia* and *Proteus*. They have mixed Gram-positive and Gram-negative infections. Some develop fungal infections, including candidaemia. Subacute bacterial endocarditis and endocarditis need to be considered in i.v. drug users. If endocarditis is not suspected, treatment should consist of flucloxacillin 2 g i.v. 6-hourly and gentamicin 5–7 mg/kg/day as a single daily dose.

Controversies

- The timing and method of closure of contaminated or 'old' (more than 6 hours since injury) wounds.

- The prophylactic use of antibiotics in patients with 'clean' wounds.

- Which antibiotics to use in treating skin and soft tissue infections: narrow-spectrum, first-generation cephalosporin or broad-spectrum third-generation cephalosporin? Do you use antibiotics to cover Gram-negative, Gram-positive organisms, anaerobes and aerobes?

- Can more patients be treated wholly as outpatients using parenteral therapy, or after early discharge once the acute toxic phase is over?

- Management of cutaneous abscesses: are antibiotics necessary after incision and drainage? Are cultures of the abscess fluid needed?

References

1. Simonart T, Simonart JM, Derdelinckx I, et al. Value of standard laboratory tests for the early recognition of group A beta-hemolytic streptococcal necrotizing fasciitis. Clinical Infectious Diseases 2001; 32: E9–12.

2. Perl B, Gottehrer NP, Raveh D, et al. Cost-effectiveness of blood cultures for adult patients with cellulitis. Clinical Infectious Diseases 1999; 29: 1483–1488.
3. Antibiotic Expert Group. Therapeutic guidelines: antibiotics. Version 13. Melbourne: Therapeutic Guidelines Limited. 2006.
4. Stevens DL, Bisno AL, Chambers HF, et al. Infectious Diseases Society of America. Practice guidelines for the diagnosis and management of skin and soft-tissue infections. Clinical Infectious Diseases 2005; 41: 1373–1406.
5. Leong WC, Lipman J, Hon H. Severe soft-tissue infections–a diagnostic challenge. The need for early recognition and aggressive therapy. South African Medical Journal 1997; 87: 648–652, 654.
6. Gabillot-Carre M, Roujeau JC. Acute bacterial skin infections and cellulitis. Current Opinion on Infectious Diseases 2007; 20: 118–123.
7. Wong CH, Chang HC, Pasupathy S. Necrotizing fasciitis: clinical presentation, microbiology, and determinants of mortality. Journal of Bone and Joint Surgery 2003; 85A: 1454–1460.
8. Bosshardt TL, Henderson VJ, Organ CH Jr. Necrotizing soft-tissue infections. Archives of Surgery 1996; 131: 846–852.
9. Lille ST, Sato TT, Engrav LH, et al. Necrotizing soft tissue infections: obstacles in diagnosis. Journal of the American College of Surgeons 1996; 182: 7–11.
10. Ben-Aharon U, Borenstein A, Eisenkraft S, et al. Extensive necrotizing soft tissue infection of the perineum. Israel Journal of Medical Sciences 1996; 32: 745–749.
11. Nakase JY. Update on emerging infections from the centers for disease control and prevention. Annals of Emergency Medicine 2000; 36: 268–269.
12. Weber CA, Wertheimer SJ, Ognjan A. *Aeromonas hydrophila* – its implications in freshwater injuries. Journal of Foot and Ankle Surgery 1995;34: 442–446.
13. Amir LH, Forster DA, Lumley J, et al. A descriptive study of mastitis in Australian breastfeeding women: incidence and determinants. BMC Public Health 2007; 25: 62.
14. File TM Jr, Tan JS. Treatment of skin and soft-tissue infections. American Journal of Surgery 1995; 169: 27S–33S.
15. Lertzman BH, Gaspari AA. Drug treatment of skin and soft tissue infections in elderly long-term care residents. Drugs and Aging 1996; 9: 109–121.
16. Nelson EA, O'Meara S, Golder S, et al. DASIDU Steering Group. Systematic review of antimicrobial treatments for diabetic foot ulcers. Diabetic Medicine 2006; 23: 348–359.
17. Huizinga WK, Kritzinger NA, Bhamjee A. The value of adjuvant systemic antibiotic therapy in localised wound infections among hospital patients: a comparative study. Journal of Infectious Diseases 1986; 13: 11–16.
18. Singer AJ, Hollander JE, Quinn JV. Evaluation and management of traumatic lacerations. New England Journal of Medicine 1997; 337: 1142–1148.
19. Henriksen BM, Albrektsen SB, Simper LB, et al. Soft tissue infections from drug abuse. A clinical and microbiological review of 145 cases. Acta Orthopaedica Scandinavica 1994; 65: 625–628.
20. Table 2- Tetanus prophylaxis [revised 2006 June]. In: eTG complete [Internet]. Melbourne: Therapeutic Guidelines Limited; 2006Jan. Accessed 2007 Aug 1 http://etg.hcn.net.au/tgc/about/5a57c76.htm.

9.7 Hepatitis

Helen E. Stergiou

ESSENTIALS

1 Acute and chronic viral hepatitis are of global public health importance.

2 Owing to the non-specific symptomatology in the early phases of acute viral hepatitis, definitive diagnosis may be delayed in the emergency setting.

3 Supportive care is fundamental in the management of hepatitis.

4 Prevention of viral hepatitis is possible via the introduction of public health programmes which include appropriate education regarding high-risk practices.

Introduction

Hepatitis is a non-specific clinicopathological term that encompasses all disorders characterized by hepatocellular injury and by histological evidence of a necroinflammatory response.[1] Prolific research has resulted in the identification of specific hepatotrophic viruses. An important distinction is that between acute and chronic viral hepatitis. Acute viral hepatitis refers to a process of self-limited liver injury of less than 6 months' duration.[1] Chronic viral hepatitis is diagnosed on pathological criteria and is characterized by a duration of more than 6 months.[1]

Clinical presentations of viral hepatitis

An appropriate clinical pattern of illness and specific laboratory confirmation are necessary for the diagnosis of acute viral hepatitis. Patients with acute viral hepatitis may present quite variably: they may be asymptomatic with only mildly deranged liver function tests (LFTs), they may be symptomatic with or without jaundice, or they may present with fulminant disease (severe liver failure which develops within eight weeks of symptom onset).[2]

Various clinical phases characterize acute viral hepatitis.[1-4] The incubation phase is the time between the original infection and the initial symptoms, and is the time of viral replication and laboratory evidence of hepatitis. During the pre-icteric phase non-specific symptoms evolve, such as malaise, fatigue, anorexia, nausea, vomiting, myalgias,

arthralgias, abdominal discomfort. If fever is present it is generally low grade. Cough, coryza, pharyngitis and a distaste for alcohol and tobacco smoke may be evident. Rarely meningoencephalitis may occur.

The icteric phase features a variable degree of jaundice, dark urine (bilirubinuria), pale stools (absence of bile pigment in the stool), pruritus, hepatomegaly and splenomegaly. During the convalescent phase symptoms resolve, as do liver enzyme abnormalities. In patients presenting to the emergency department (ED) during the pre-icteric phase the diagnosis may be challenging, given their non-specific symptomatology. If the patients present during the icteric phase, focused history-taking, examination and the appropriate investigations should result in a definitive diagnosis.

Laboratory investigations

Blood test abnormalities are a prominent aspect of acute viral hepatitis. Serum transaminases are typically elevated at $>500 \mu/L$ and often $>1000 \mu/L$.[5] Alanine aminotransferase (ALT) may be characteristically higher than aspartate aminotransferase (AST).[5] Alkaline phosphatase may be normal or mildly elevated. Serum bilirubin is variably elevated and is usually divided between conjugated and unconjugated fractions. Albumin and the prothrombin time should be normal unless hepatic synthetic function is significantly impaired. Neutropenia and lymphopenia may be evident transiently. Severe acute hepatitis may cause hypoglycaemia. Further specific laboratory tests for viral hepatitis will be presented subsequently.

Management

In cases of acute viral hepatitis the fundamental management is supportive care. Many of these patients can be managed on an outpatient basis. Patients require hospitalization when they have intractable vomiting with inadequate oral intake, and when they demonstrate clinical features of liver failure. Bed rest is recommended during the symptomatic phase. A well-balanced diet is beneficial. It is recommended that alcohol be avoided during the acute phase, but there is no definitive evidence that alcohol consumption post recovery causes either relapses or progression to chronic disease.[2] Given that the liver is involved in the metabolism of a plethora of drugs, all medications must be carefully prescribed to patients with acute hepatitis.

Interferon-α (IFNα) may prevent progression from acute HBV infection to the chronic phase.[2] This glycoprotein has both direct antiviral effects and it may also enhance the body's immune response.[3,5] The limiting factor in the use of IFNα is the side-effect profile, which includes an influenza-like illness, gastrointestinal symptoms, psychological sequelae (particularly depression), bone marrow suppression, thyroid dysfunction and possible birth defects.[5] Agents such as ribavirin may be used synergistically with IFNα.[5]

In managing fulminant hepatic failure it is imperative that potential patients be identified as early as possible. In the emergency setting intubation and the concomitant critical care are necessary for patients with progressive encephalopathy. Early referral to an appropriate intensive care unit (ICU) is mandatory.

Prevention and immunization

Prevention of viral hepatitis is possible via the introduction of public health programmes, improved sanitation and vaccination programmes. Post-exposure prophylaxis regimens are particularly relevant to healthcare workers.

Hepatitis A virus

As the most common cause of viral hepatitis, HAV contributes significantly to the global burden of disease. Multiple genotypes exist, and infection with one genotype confers immunity against others.[6] See Table 9.7.1 for virology.

Epidemiology

HAV is highly endemic in developing countries and can often be traced to contaminated water or food.

Natural history

Virus is excreted in the stool of the infected person for 1–2 weeks prior to and for 1 week after the onset of symptoms. A non-specific prodrome may be followed by jaundice and tender hepatomegaly. The clinical severity of the illness increases with age, with more than 80% of children being asymptomatic.[1] HAV has been associated with extrahepatic features such as cutaneous vasculitis, renal failure, pancreatitis, bradycardia and rarely convulsions, transverse myelitis and aplastic anaemia.[7] Relapsing hepatitis has been described in 20% of those with HAV infection.[2] Relapses are generally benign and may occur 4–15 weeks after the original illness. Complete recovery is the typical outcome. Fulminant hepatic failure occurs in less than 1% of cases. Chronic infection never ensues.

Laboratory investigations

Serum antibody is present from the onset of HAV disease in both IgM and IgG forms. After approximately 3–12 months anti-HAV IgM disappears and anti-HAV IgG persists, thereby conferring lifelong immunity against re-infection.

Management

Supportive management is of primary importance. Bed rest is indicated until any jaundice settles. Potentially hepatotoxic medications must be ceased. Alcohol must not be consumed during acute episodes because of the direct nephrotoxic effects.

Prevention and immunization

General measures are imperative – safe water supplies, proper sewage disposal and careful handwashing. HAV vaccines can prevent HAV infection and, importantly, they have excellent safety profiles. Persons who have been exposed to HAV and who have not been previously vaccinated should receive the vaccine within 2 weeks of exposure. Travellers to endemic areas require inactivated hepatitis vaccine, which confers long-term immunity to more than 90% of persons.

Hepatitis B virus

Of the viral causes of hepatitis few are of greater global importance than HBV. HBV infection is endemic in certain parts of the world – Southeast Asia, China and sub-Saharan Africa. It is estimated that there are 350 million carriers worldwide.[8] See Table 9.7.1 for virology.

Epidemiology

Transmission occurs by percutaneous and mucosal exposure to infected blood products and bodily fluids, hence unprotected sexual contact with infected individuals, the use of contaminated paraphernalia during intravenous drug use and vertical transmission from mother to infant are commonly implicated.

Natural history

Many acute HBV infections are asymptomatic, particularly in younger patients. The non-specific symptoms of the acute episode may be preceded by a serum-sickness syndrome with fevers, urticaria and arthralgias.[5]

Approximately 90% of patients completely recover from an acute episode of HBV infection. Fulminant hepatic failure may develop in 1% of patients and has a mortality rate of up to 80%.

Progression to chronic HBV infection occurs in 5–10% of cases, with 90% of these experiencing an asymptomatic carrier state and the remaining 10% proceeding to cirrhosis and hepatocelluar carcinoma. The risk of developing chronic disease is related to the age at which HBV is first contracted – there is a greater than 90% risk of developing chronic HBV in neonates and a less than 5% risk in immunocompetent adults.[1,2] Although chronic HBV infection is generally a lifelong condition, a small percentage of infected individuals will experience complete viral eradication.

Laboratory investigations

HBsAg indicates acute hepatitis or a carrier state if it persists beyond 6 months. Anti-HBc IgM indicates acute HBV and high infectivity. Anti-HBc IgG indicates previous infection. HBeAg indicates ongoing viral replication, high infectivity or chronic hepatitis.

Management

Supportive care is the primary aim of management. Household contacts require adequate education. In cases of chronic HBV infection the aims are to suppress HBV replication and to reduce liver injury.

Prevention and immunization

The pre-exposure administration of HBV vaccine is fundamental to immunoprophylaxis. The vaccine is protective in over 90% of individuals.[1] Current recommendations include all infants at birth and individuals with high exposure risk, such as healthcare personnel, injecting drug users and high-risk

Table 9.7.1 Characteristics of the main hepatitis viruses					
	HAV	**HBV**	**HCV**	**HDV**	**HEV**
Family	Picornavirus	Hepadnavirus	Flavivirus	Incomplete	Calicivirus
Nucleic Acid	RNA	DNA	RNA	RNA	RNA
Diameter	27 nm	42 nm	32 nm	36 nm	34 nm
Incubation Period (weeks)	2–6	6–24	2–26	6–9	2–10
Spread Faeces	Yes	No	No	No	Yes
Blood	Uncommon	Yes	Yes	Yes	No
Sexual	Uncommon	Yes	Uncommon	Yes	?
Vertical	No	Yes	Uncommon	Yes	No
Chronic Infection	No	Yes	Yes	Yes	No
Vaccine	Available	Available	Nil	Nil	Nil

sexual workers. Antibody titres may decrease with time, but the protective effects persist. The risk of HBV infection in the occupational setting is related primarily to the degree of contact with blood and to the HBeAg status of the donor. In needle-stick injuries the risk of developing clinical hepatitis if the blood is both HBsAg- and HBeAg-positive has been estimated to be up to 30%. Post-exposure prophylaxis involves the administration of hepatitis B immunoglobulin in addition to the recombinant vaccine series.

Hepatitis C virus

International studies estimate that up to 3% of the world's population is infected with HCV.[2,9] See Table 9.7.1 for virology. The identification of six major genotypes of the HCV has important clinical implications in that such genomic sequence variation makes vaccine development extremely difficult.

Epidemiology

Parenteral exposure leads to HCV infection, the use of contaminated needles and syringes being a predominant factor. Sexual and perinatal transmission of HCV is negligible. Transfusion-related HCV transmission has essentially been eradicated via donor screening. Up to 10% of HCV cases do not have an identifiable source of infection.

Natural history

A pre-icteric phase featuring non-specific symptoms develops in 15–20% of patients. When the icteric phase develops it typically lasts for 1–2 weeks. Fulminant hepatic failure rarely results from acute HCV infection.

Following an acute episode, 75–85% of adults and 55% of children will enter a chronic phase.[9] There is a high proportion of subclinical chronic HCV infection, hence patients may not manifest any pathology until incidental blood tests or end-stage liver disease many years after the initial infection. Approximately 20–30% of chronic HCV patients develop cirrhosis, with subsequent hepatocellular carcinoma occurring in up to 20% of the latter group.[1,5]

Laboratory investigations

A fluctuating titre of HCV RNA is detectable within days to weeks of the initial HCV infection. The rate at which HCV antibodies develop is variable. Notably, HCV

antibodies are neither neutralizing nor protective. It may not be possible to distinguish between acute and chronic HCV infection, given that the same laboratory markers can be present in both conditions. Further specific laboratory tests for viral hepatitis are presented in Table 9.7.2.

Management

Supportive management is fundamental in addressing HCV infection. Relevant education and counselling regarding high-risk behaviours and referrals to appropriate support networks are necessary. Avoidance of alcohol is advisable as some studies indicate that alcohol may promote the progression of HCV infection.[10,11] Interferon therapy is offered to some chronic HCV patients.

Prevention and immunization

Currently there is no effective vaccination available against HCV infection, nor is there any specific post-exposure prophylaxis

regimen. Vaccination against HAV and HBV is advisable. HCV is not transmitted efficiently through occupational exposures to blood. The average incidence of anti-HCV seroconversion after accidental exposure from an HCV-positive source is <2%.[12]

Hepatitis D virus

As a defective virus, HDV requires the presence of HBV for virion assembly and for viral replication.[1,2] See Table 9.7.1 for virology.

Epidemiology

Only patients with acute or chronic HBV infection are susceptible to infection with HDV. An estimated 5% of HBV carriers are infected with HDV worldwide.[1,2,5] Parenteral exposure is the primary transmission mode. HDV can occur as a co-infection with acute HBV (acquired at the same time) or as a superinfection in chronic HBV carriers.

Table 9.7.2 Laboratory tests in viral hepatitis (Modified from Talley N, Martin C. Clinical gastroenterology: A practical problem-based approach, 2nd edn. Edinburgh: Churchill Livingstone, 2006.)		
Test	Interpretation of positive test	Clinical significance
Tests for HAV		
Anti-HAV IgM	Recently acquired HAV	Acute hepatic illness
Anti-HAV IgG	Previous infection/vaccination	Immunity
Tests for HBV		
HBsAg (surface Ag)	Current/chronic infection	Structural viral component
Anti-HBsAg (surface Ab)	Previous infection/vaccination	Immunity
Anti-HBcIgM (core Ab)	Recently acquired HBV	Test for acute HBV
HBeAg	Marker of viral replication	High infectivity
Anti-HBeAg	No viral replication	Low infectivity
HBV DNA	Complete virus present	High infectivity
Tests for HCV		
Anti-HCV	HCV exposure	Variable infectivity
HCV RNA	Virus present	
Tests for HDV		
Anti-HDV IgG/IgM	HDV exposure	Acute or chronic HDV
Delta Ag	HDV present	Acute or chronic HDV
Tests for HEV		
Anti-HEV IgM	Recently acquired HEV	Acute hepatic illness
Anti-HEV IgG	Previous exposure	

Natural history

In cases of HDV and HBV coinfection, acute HDV infection generally presents as a benign acute hepatitis with subsequent resolution in up to 80–95% of patients. Chronic HDV/HBV infection may occur in 5–10% of patients.[2] HDV superinfection results in progression to chronic HDV/HBV in 70–80% of cases.[5] Chronic HDV/HBV infection manifests as a chronic healthy carrier state or severe liver disease. HDV superinfection may result in fulminant hepatitis in 2–20% of cases.[5]

Laboratory investigations

HBsAg must be detected to diagnose acute HDV-HBV coinfection. Anti-HDV IgM is transiently present in acute infections. Anti-HDV IgG appears late in acute infections.

Management

There is no specific treatment for HDV infection other than suppressing HBV replication.

Prevention and immunization

Currently there is no vaccine for preventing HDV infection. HBV immunization has been shown to provide protection against the development of HDV.

Hepatitis E virus

Refer to Table 9.7.1 for virology.

Epidemiology

HEV is endemic in developing countries such as Southeast and Central Asia and the Indian subcontinent. The primary transmission mode is the faecal–oral route, with contaminated drinking water and food supplies being primary sources of infection. Young adults are often predominantly affected.

Natural history

The clinical course is similar to that of acute HAV infection. Full recovery from the acute HEV infection is the norm. There have not been any recorded cases of chronic HEV infection.

For reasons which remain unclear, fulminant hepatic failure with a subsequent high mortality rate occurs in 25% of women with HEV infection during the third trimester of pregnancy.

Laboratory investigations

Anti-HEV IgM occurs between 1 week and 6 months after the illness onset. Anti-HEV IgG is evident during the convalescent phase or post exposure.

Management

Supportive management is the key.

Prevention and immunization

Disease control depends on good personal hygiene and improved environmental sanitation. There is no effective vaccine.

Hepatitis G virus

The clinical significance of the parenterally transmitted HGV infection is yet to be clarified. To date there is no substantial evidence to suggest that the HGV causes serious liver disease at any age.

Non-hepatotrophic viruses

Several non-ABCDE viruses cause viral hepatitis. The cytomegalovirus (CMV) and Epstein–Barr virus (EBV) commonly contribute to abnormal LFTs, and icteric hepatitis may also occasionally be noted. In immunocompromised patients herpes simplex may lead to a hepatitic picture. Progression to chronic hepatitis has not been demonstrated with any of these viruses.

Non-viral hepatitis

Of the causes of non-viral hepatitis the following are important in the emergency setting: alcoholic hepatitis, non-alcoholic steatohepatitis (NASH), drug-induced hepatitis and autoimmune hepatitis.

Alcoholic hepatitis

Alcoholic hepatitis is an important clinical syndrome which is variably characterized by anorexia, nausea, jaundice, hepatomegaly and features of portal hypertension such as ascites and encephalopathy. Cirrhosis and death are possible sequelae if the patients do not cease their alcohol consumption.

Non-alcoholic steatohepatitis

Defects in the processing of fatty acids through the liver may cause steatosis-induced inflammation (steatohepatitis). Ten to 50% of patients with NASH are at risk of developing cirrhosis.[11]

Drug-induced hepatitis

Toxic exposure to certain medications, vitamins, herbal remedies and food supplements may result in a drug-induced hepatitis. Drug-induced hepatitis may occur as an expected consequence of a drug's toxicity profile or as an idiosyncratic reaction to a standard dose. Hepatotoxic agents result in variable clinicopathological patterns of liver injury via toxic and immune mechanisms.[13] Commonly, the formation of reactive hepatotoxic metabolites is the primary underlying mechanism.[14] Extensive lists of hepatotoxic drugs can be found in the literature. Acute liver injury may be necroinflammatory (e.g. paracetamol), cholestatic (e.g. chlorpromazine) or of a mixed type. Table 9.7.3 lists drugs which may induce hepatitis and which are encountered in the emergency setting.[13,14]

Autoimmune hepatitis

Autoimmune hepatitis is a self-perpetuating hepatocellular inflammation of unknown cause which is associated with hypergammaglobulinaemia and serum antibodies.[11] Fatigue, anorexia and jaundice may progress to liver failure. Corticosteroids are the basis of treatment.

Table 9.7.3 Hepatitis-inducing drugs[13,14]	
Drug	Pathology
Allopurinol	Hepatic granulomas
Cloxacillin	Lobular hepatitis
Chlorpromazine	Cholestatic hepatitis
Dantrolene	Cytolytic hepatitis
Erythromycin	Cholestasis with hepatitis
Flucloxacillin	Cholestatic hepatitis
Halothane	Hepatocellular injury
Isoniazid	Cytolytic hepatitis
Non-steroidals	Primarily cholestasis
Paracetamol	Cytolytic hepatitis
Phenothiazines	Cholestatic hepatitis
Phenytoin	Non-caseating granulomas
Sulphonamides	Cytolytic hepatitis

Future directions

- Global emphasis on adequate public health schemes, including vaccination programmes, to control the transmission of viral hepatitis.
- Emphasis on public education regarding high-risk practices.
- Surveillance of the long-term immunity conferred by the hepatitis A and B vaccinations.
- Development of a vaccine for hepatitis C.
- Optimization of the management algorithms for chronic viral hepatitis.

References

1. Yamada T, Hasler W, Inadomi J, et al. Handbook of gastroenterology, 2nd edn. Baltimore: Lippincott Williams & Wilkins, 2005.
2. Mandell G, Bennett J, Dolin R. Principles and practice of infectious diseases 6th edn. Edinburgh: Churchill Livingstone, 2005.
3. Talley N, Martin C. Clinical gastroenterology: A practical problem-based approach, 2nd edn. Edinburgh: Churchill Livingstone, 2006.
4. Boon N, Colledge N, Walker B, et al. Davidson's principles and practice of medicine, 20th edn. Edinburgh: Churchill Livingstone, 2006.
5. Friedman S, McQuaid K, Grendell J. Current diagnosis and treatment in gastroenterology, 2nd edn. McGraw-Hill, 2003.
6. Lemon S, Jansen RW, Brown EA, et al. Genetic, antigenic and biological differences between strains of hepatitis A virus. Vaccine 1992; 10: S40–S44.
7. Schiff E. Atypical clinical manifestations of hepatitis A. Vaccine 1992; 10: S18–S20.
8. Kane M, Clements J, Hu D. Disease control priorities in developing countries. In: Jamison D, Mosley W, Measham A, Bobadilla J, eds. Disease control priorities in developing countries. New York: Oxford University Press, 1993; 330.
9. Lavanchy D. Public health measures in the control of viral hepatitis: A World Health Organization perspective for the next millennium. Journal of Gastroenterology and Hepatology 2002; 17: S452–S459.
10. Thomas D, Astemborski J, Rai R. The natural history of hepatitis C virus infection. Journal of the American Medical Association 2000; 284: 450.
11. FriedmanL, Keeffe E, Schiff E. Handbook of liver disease, 2nd edn. Edinburgh: Churchill Livingstone, 2004.
12. Mitsui T, Iwano K, Masuko K. Hepatitis C virus infection in medical personnel after needlestick accident. Hepatology 1992; 16: 1109–1114.
13. Farrell G. Drug-induced liver injury. New York: Churchill Livingstone, 1994.
14. Bircher J, Benhamou J-P, McIntyre N, et al. Oxford textbook of clinical hepatology, 2nd edn. Oxford: Oxford University Press, 1999.

9.8 HIV/AIDS

Alan C. Street

ESSENTIALS

1 Globally, heterosexual transmission accounts for most HIV infections, but in Australia HIV infection remains predominantly a disease of homosexual and bisexual men.

2 Patients with previously undiagnosed HIV infection may present to the emergency department at any time during the course of infection, from early (acute seroconversion illness) to late (opportunistic infection) stages.

3 Most serious HIV-related complications occur when the CD4 T-lymphocyte count is $< 0.2 \times 10^9$/L (bacterial pneumonia and tuberculosis are exceptions).

4 The emergency physician should be able to provide expert HIV pre- and post-test counselling in a sensitive and non-judgemental fashion.

5 Combination antiretroviral therapy has dramatically reduced HIV mortality and morbidity; well-tolerated and potent once daily regimens are now the standard of care as initial therapy, and new agents that target additional steps in the viral life cycle provide new treatment options for patients who have failed antiretroviral therapy with currently available agents.

6 Close liaison between emergency department staff and the patient's hospital or local doctor is vital for optimal management of HIV-infected patients.

- The natural history and clinical manifestations of HIV infection.
- The principles of HIV diagnosis, including the ability to engage patients in discussions about HIV testing and test results.
- The principles of management of patients with common HIV-related disease syndromes.
- Familiarity with antiretroviral agents in current use, including toxicity and drug interactions.

The first cases of AIDS were recognized in the USA in 1981 and in Australia in 1982. The causative agent, human immunodeficiency virus (HIV), was discovered in 1984 and a diagnostic blood test developed soon thereafter. In 1986 the first effective antiviral drug (AZT, later renamed zidovudine) became available. Since the late 1990s the use of combination antiretroviral therapy has led to dramatic reductions in HIV-associated morbidity and mortality in resource-rich countries. Antiretroviral use is rapidly increasing in poor countries, but the global HIV situation remains serious; in 2006, the World Health Organization (WHO) estimated that there were 4.3 million new HIV infections, 2.9 million deaths, and 39.5 million people living with HIV, 24.7 million in sub-Saharan Africa and 8.5 million in Asia.[1] A major challenge

Introduction

HIV medicine is a complex and specialized field and emergency physicians are not the usual primary care providers for people with HIV infection. However, the emergency department (ED) is often the first point of contact for patients presenting with acute HIV-related complications, whether or not they have already been diagnosed with HIV.

Emergency medicine physicians do not need to be HIV experts, but they should develop knowledge and skills in the following areas:

in the coming years will be to develop an effective HIV vaccine.[2]

Epidemiology

Globally, the great majority of HIV infections arise as a result of heterosexual transmission. In developed countries, injecting drug use and sex between men account for a greater proportion of HIV infections, although the contribution of specific behaviours to overall transmission varies greatly between countries and over time.

In Australia up to December 2005 more than 22 000 people had been diagnosed with HIV infection, of whom 9872 have progressed to AIDS and 6668 have died. Eighty-one per cent of people infected with HIV report male-to-male sex, 12% have become infected through heterosexual transmission, 4% of cases have occurred in injecting drug users, and 2% in recipients of contaminated blood or blood products. Women account for 8% of HIV-infected people and children for less than 1%.[3] A worrying recent development has been an increase in the number of new HIV notifications for each of the past few years, from 757 in 2000 to 954 in 2005; this increase predominantly involves gay men. Compared to some other countries, the prevalence of HIV infection in injecting drug users has remained low, of the order of 1–2%.

Pathogenesis

Once HIV infection becomes established, one billion or more HIV virus particles are produced per day, chiefly in lymph nodes and other lymphoid tissue, accompanied by the daily turnover of up to 1 billion CD4 T lymphocytes. The number of CD4 cells falls secondary to mechanisms such as immune activation and direct infection of CD4 cells, resulting in reduced helper function for cell-mediated and humoral immunity.[4]

HIV replication occurs at a relatively constant rate, producing a stable level of HIV in the blood, and this can be measured with quantitative HIV RNA detection tests. The HIV viral load is used as a prognostic marker (because it is associated with the rate at which CD4 T lymphocytes are lost) and to monitor the efficacy of antiretroviral therapy.

The peripheral blood CD4 T-lymphocyte count is an accurate indicator of the degree of immunosuppression. The normal count is $0.5–1.5 \times 10^9/L$; susceptibility to opportunistic infection, and to most other serious HIV-related complications, is greatest when the CD4 cell count is less than $0.2 \times 10^9/L$. In untreated patients, the average rate of CD4 cell decline is $0.05–0.1 \times 10^9 L/year$.

Classification and natural history (Fig. 9.8.1)

HIV infection can be conveniently divided into four stages on the basis of time after infection, CD4 T-lymphocyte count and the presence of complications:[5]

- Primary infection: a febrile illness that occurs soon after infection (discussed in more detail below)
- Early infection: CD4 cell count $>0.5 \times 10^9/L$ – generally asymptomatic period
- Intermediate infection: CD4 cell count $0.2–0.5 \times 10^9/L$ – asymptomatic or less serious complications
- Late infection: CD4 cell count $<0.2 \times 10^9/L$ – susceptibility to AIDS-defining opportunistic infections and malignancies.

Patients are categorized as having AIDS when they develop a defined opportunistic infection, an HIV-related malignancy, a wasting syndrome or AIDS dementia complex.

Presentation

Patients with underlying HIV infection who present to the ED fall into three distinct groups. First, they may present with a manifestation of previously unrecognized HIV infection. To identify these patients, the physician must know who is potentially at risk of HIV infection (see Epidemiology above) and be aware of the many different ways in which previously undiagnosed HIV infection may present. Prompt consideration of the possibility of HIV infection is important because the differential diagnosis of the presenting problem will broaden to encompass a variety of other conditions, some of which may be life-threatening.

The second group includes those who are already known to be HIV infected. These patients usually present with one of a limited number of clinical syndromes, such as diarrhoea, fever or shortness of breath and cough, or with a complication of antiretroviral therapy. The initial diagnostic and treatment approach is based on knowledge of the differential diagnosis for each of these syndromes.

Finally, there will be patients whose ED presentation is not related to an HIV complication at all but who are at risk of HIV

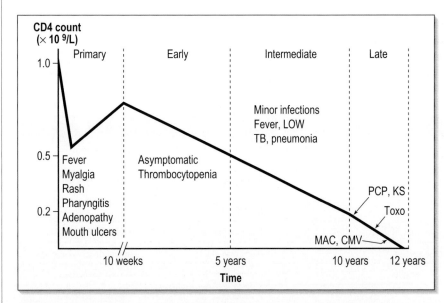

Fig. 9.8.1 Natural history of untreated HIV infection. 'Time' represents time after infection.
(Modified with permission from Stewart G (ed) Managing HIV. Sydney: Australasian Medical Publishing Co, 1997.)

infection. Patients with a sexually transmitted infection belong to this category and are readily identifiable; otherwise, a brief history, including a sexual history, is required to elicit HIV risk factors. Presentation of these patients to the ED offers an important opportunity to discuss the benefits of earlier HIV diagnosis and the desirability of HIV testing.

Previously undiagnosed HIV infection[6]

Primary HIV infection (acute seroconversion illness) (Table 9.8.1)

Up to 50% of patients will develop a glandular fever-like illness of varying severity 2–3 weeks after acquiring HIV. The most common features are fever, myalgia, headache, erythematous maculopapular rash, diarrhoea, lymphadenopathy and mouth ulcers. Complications include aseptic meningitis, encephalitis and Guillain–Barré syndrome. The diagnosis is often missed at this stage, as patients may be considered to have infectious mononucleosis, or a 'viral illness', or the possibility of HIV infection is not considered in a patient with (for example) encephalitis.

Early infection (CD4 cell count >0.5 × 10⁹/L)

People are generally healthy during this phase. Thrombocytopenia may occur, and so HIV infection should be considered in appropriate patients with idiopathic thrombocytopenia.

Intermediate HIV infection (CD4 cell count 0.2–0.5 × 10⁹/L)

This is a phase when previously undiagnosed HIV-infected patients often present with HIV-related conditions, but the clues may not be recognized and the diagnosis is missed. Manifestations include:

- Minor infections: shingles, recurrent orolabial or genital herpes, oral thrush.
- Skin conditions: extensive seborrhoeic dermatitis, worsening psoriasis.
- Constitutional symptoms: fever, weight loss, diarrhoea.
- Generalized lymphadenopathy.
- More serious complications: bacterial pneumonia, tuberculosis and, rarely, Kaposi's sarcoma or non-Hodgkin's lymphoma.

Late HIV infection (CD4 cell count 0.2 × 10⁹/L)

It is often not appreciated that patients may remain completely well during the early and intermediate stages of HIV infection, and only present when they develop a serious opportunistic infection; the ED is a common point of initial care for such patients. If the history reveals risk factors for HIV infection, HIV testing can be performed and initial investigations directed at specific HIV-related complications. However, if the patient does not volunteer this information, is not specifically asked about HIV risk factors, or does not belong to a 'conventional' HIV risk group, diagnosis of the presenting illness and the underlying HIV infection is often delayed.

The following clinical situations should prompt consideration of the possibility of underlying HIV infection:

- Diffuse bilateral pulmonary infiltrates (as a manifestation of *Pneumocystis jiroveci* pneumonia, PCP) – this is the commonest serious opportunistic infection in patients with previously undiagnosed HIV infection; it is often misdiagnosed as atypical pneumonia, leading to incorrect initial treatment with a macrolide agent or doxycycline.
- Ring-enhancing space-occupying cerebral lesion – initially thought to be a bacterial brain abscess or tumour, and prompting brain biopsy; in the setting of HIV infection, cerebral toxoplasmosis is the most likely diagnosis and brain biopsy can be avoided.
- Tuberculosis – although the overlap between those at risk for HIV and tuberculosis is not as great in Australia as in other countries, all patients with tuberculosis should be encouraged to undergo HIV testing after appropriate counselling.
- Kaposi's sarcoma – well-developed lesions (purple, oval and nodular) are easy to recognize, but early lesions are often non-descript (brown or pink and flat) and biopsy may be required for diagnosis.
- Other presentations – conditions such as non-Hodgkin's lymphoma, cryptococcal meningitis, chronic cryptosporidial diarrhoea, AIDS dementia complex (manifesting as impaired cognition and motor performance) and unexplained cytopenias (including pancytopenia) are occasionally the first manifestation of previously unsuspected HIV infection.

Disease syndromes in those with known HIV infection[7]

Cough, shortness of breath, fever

Respiratory pathogens are listed in Table 9.8.2. The most important issue to decide is whether the patient has *Pneumocystis jiroveci* pneumonia (PCP) or not, because this complication is common and potentially serious. Tuberculosis must also be considered because of the need to place the patient in respiratory isolation.

Table 9.8.1 Manifestations of primary HIV infection		
Common (present in > 30% of patients)	Less common	Complications
Fever	Diarrhoea	Aseptic meningitis
Rash	Generalized lymphadenopathy	Guillain–Barré syndrome
Myalgia/arthralgia	Painful swallowing	Encephalitis
Headache	Abdominal pain	Interstitial pneumonitis
Pharyngitis	Cough	Rhabdomyolysis
Cervical lymphadenopathy	Photophobia	Haemophagocytic syndrome
Mouth ulcers	Tonsillitis	

Table 9.8.2 Respiratory complications in HIV-infected patients

Common	Uncommon
Pneumocystis jiroveci pneumonia (PCP)	Tuberculosis
Bacterial pneumonia:	Atypical mycobacteria
pneumococcus	*Aspergillus* pneumonia
Haemophilus influenzae	Other infections:
Bronchitis	*Rhodococcus equi*, CMV
	Non-infectious:
	Pulmonary Kaposi's sarcoma
	Lymphoma

- PCP (occurs in patients with $<0.2 \times 10^9$ CD4 cells/L): the presentation is subacute or chronic, with a non-productive cough, dyspnoea, fever and chest tightness. Physical examination reveals fever, tachypnoea and reduced chest expansion, but chest auscultation is often normal. PCP is very unlikely in patients taking regular co-trimoxazole because this drug is virtually 100% effective as PCP prophylaxis.
- Bacterial pneumonia (may occur when the CD4 cell count is $>0.2 \times 10^9$/L): patients usually present with a short history, a productive cough and sometimes pleuritic chest pain. Physical examination may be normal or reveal signs of consolidation, a pleural rub or pleural effusion.
- Tuberculosis: the clinical features vary according to the degree of immunosuppression. If the CD4 cell count is $>0.2 \times 10^9$/L, patients usually present with typical symptoms and signs of tuberculosis (chronic cough, haemoptysis, fever and weight loss), but in late-stage infection atypical manifestations such as disseminated disease are common and diagnosis is more difficult.

Focal neurological signs, convulsions or altered conscious state

These features generally indicate the presence of an intracerebral space-occupying lesion, the most common causes of which are:

- Cerebral toxoplasmosis: this infection occurs when the CD4 cell count is $<0.2 \times 10^9$/L. The specific focal features depend on the site of the usually multiple lesions, and may include hemiparesis, visual field defects, personality change or cerebellar signs.
- Primary intracerebral lymphoma: this complication occurs with advanced HIV infection (CD4 cell count usually $<0.05 \times 10^9$/L), develops in 2–3% of AIDS patients and is closely associated with Epstein–Barr virus (EBV) infection. Clinical presentation is indistinguishable from that of cerebral toxoplasmosis.
- Progressive multifocal leukoencephalopathy: caused by JC virus (a polyoma virus); patients present with cognitive decline or focal signs and seizures are relatively uncommon. Differentiation from cerebral toxoplasmosis and primary cerebral lymphoma requires computed tomography (CT) or magnetic resonance imaging (MRI) scanning (see below).

Diarrhoea, with or without abdominal pain or fever

A wide range of gastrointestinal pathogens cause diarrhoea in HIV-infected patients (Table 9.8.3). Patients should be asked about recent travel or antibiotic use. Bloody, small-volume diarrhoea with cramping lower abdominal pain is suggestive of a large bowel pathogen such as cytomegalovirus, *Entamoeba histolytica* or *Clostridium difficile*, whereas profuse watery diarrhoea suggests an infection of the small bowel, such as cryptosporidiosis. However, clinical features are often of limited diagnostic value and the specific diagnosis rests on identification of the pathogen in a faecal or biopsy specimen. Prominent anal pain or tenesmus suggest the possibility of proctitis due to a sexually acquired infection such as gonorrhoea, *Chlamydia* (including lymphogranuloma venereum) or herpes.

Table 9.8.3 Gastrointestinal pathogens in HIV-infected patients

Bacterial	Protozoal
Salmonella,	Cryptosporidiosis
Campylobacter	Giardiasis
Clostridium difficile	*Entamoeba histolytica*
Mycobacterium avium complex (MAC)	Microsporidiosis
Viral	**Non-infectious**
CMV	Lactose intolerance
	Gastrointestinal Kaposi's sarcoma and lymphoma

Fever without localizing features

This is chiefly a problem in those with a CD4 cell count $<0.2 \times 10^9$/L. The differential diagnosis is extensive, the major causes being:

- Disseminated opportunistic infections: disseminated *Mycobacterium avium* complex (MAC), disseminated tuberculosis, disseminated histoplasmosis (USA and South America), *Salmonella* bacteraemia, CMV.
- Focal opportunistic infections with non-focal presentation: PCP, cryptococcal meningitis, tuberculosis.
- Bacterial infections: sinusitis, bacterial pneumonia, primary bacteraemia (especially in patients with an indwelling long-term intravenous device, or neutropenia).
- Non-HIV specific infections: right-sided endocarditis, secondary syphilis.
- Non-infectious causes: non-Hodgkin's lymphoma, drug fever.

Difficult or painful swallowing

This is usually due to *Candida* oesophagitis, in which case oral candidiasis is often present. Other causes include idiopathic aphthous ulceration, CMV oesophagitis and herpes simplex oesophagitis.

Headache, fever, neck stiffness

Cryptococcal meningitis is the most common cause of this syndrome, although headache may be mild and signs of meningism subtle or absent. Less common causes include tuberculous meningitis, syphilitic meningitis, HIV itself and lymphomatous meningitis.

Complications of antiretroviral therapy

Antiretroviral drugs are discussed in more detail below, and drug side effects are outlined in Table 9.8.4. Examples of more serious side effects that may prompt presentation to the ED include:

- Pancreatitis – didanosine.
- Hepatitis – nevirapine.
- Drug rash – nevirapine, abacavir, fosamprenavir, efavirenz.
- Renal calculi – indinavir.
- Lactic acidosis – stavudine, zidovudine.
- Renal impairment – tenofovir.
- Anaemia – zidovudine.

Table 9.8.4 Side effects of antiretroviral agents

Agent	Side effect
Nucleoside/nucleotide reverse transcriptase inhibitors (NRTI) agents	
Class effects	Hyperlactataemia, lactic acidosis
Zidovudine	Nausea, headache, myalgia, anaemia, neutropenia
Didanosine	Pancreatitis, diarrhoea, nausea, peripheral neuropathy
Lamivudine	Abnormal liver function, neutropenia, pancreatitis (all uncommon)
Emtricitabine	Skin pigmentation
Stavudine	Peripheral neuropathy, pancreatitis
Abacavir	Hypersensitivity reaction (challenge contraindicated); associated with HLA *B57–01 (8% of Caucasian populations), perform HLA B locus typing pre-therapy
Tenofovir	Renal tubular dysfunction, renal impairment
Non-nucleoside reverse transcriptase inhibitors (NNRTI) agents	
Nevirapine	Rash, hepatitis, fever
Efavirenz	Neuropsychological (vivid dreams, insomnia, difficulty concentrating, light headedness), rash, abnormal liver function, teratogenic
Delavirdine	Rash, abnormal liver function
Protease inhibitors (PI)	
Class effects	Hyperglycaemia, hyperlipidaemia, redistribution of body fat, abnormal liver function
Nelfinavir	Diarrhoea
Indinavir	Renal calculi, back pain, nausea, hyperbilirubinaemia
Saquinavir	Diarrhoea, nausea
Lopinavir	Diarrhoea, nausea
Atazanavir	Hyperbilirubinaemia
Fosamprenavir	Rash, diarrhoea, nausea
Entry Inhibitors	
enfuvirtide	Injection site reactions, hypersensitivity

Other presentations

- Cutaneous manifestations: Kaposi's sarcoma, infections (e.g. secondary syphilis, zoster, warts, molluscum contagiosum, crusted scabies), eosinophilic folliculitis, drug rashes.
- Abdominal pain: pancreatitis due to antiretroviral therapy, HIV cholangiopathy, intra-abdominal lymphadenopathy secondary to MAC or lymphoma, lactic acidosis and hepatic steatosis associated with antiretroviral therapy.
- Neuropsychiatric manifestations: depression, mania, cognitive decline.
- Visual complaints: CMV retinitis (when CD4 cell count $<0.05 \times 10^9$/L), syphilitic uveitis or chorioretinitis, uveitis, rarely toxoplasma or cryptococcal chorioretinitis.

Clinically silent HIV infection with risk factors

Sexually transmitted infections

Perianal or rectal sexually transmitted infections (STIs) in men are obvious markers of HIV infection risk and should prompt testing for infection. However, STIs often 'hunt in packs', so any patient diagnosed with gonorrhoea, *Chlamydia*, syphilis, genital warts, genital herpes or another STI should also be investigated for HIV.

Other risk groups

After appropriate pre-test discussion (see below), other patients who present with a problem unrelated to HIV but who should be considered for opportunistic HIV testing include those with the following risk factors:

- Unprotected male-to-male intercourse.
- Sharing of injecting equipment.
- Being the sexual partner of an HIV-positive person.
- Being from a country with a high HIV prevalence.

Investigation

Requesting an HIV antibody test[8]

In Australia, doctors are obliged to provide patients with information about the medical, psychological and social consequences of a positive or negative HIV antibody test. Ideally, such discussions should take place in a private and quiet environment, but this is not always possible in an open-design, overcrowded and noisy ED! If the patient does not speak English well, an accredited interpreter (not a family member or friend) must be used.

Areas covered in the pre-test discussion should include the following:

- Asking the patient about risk factors for HIV infection.
- Providing information about the test itself, including its limitations (e.g. 'window period') and the meaning of a positive or negative test.
- Briefly discussing the transmission of HIV, the natural history of HIV infection, (including the difference between HIV and AIDS) and the improved outlook with modern antiretroviral therapy.
- Addressing any concerns about the confidentiality of results.
- Assessing whether additional testing for other sexually transmitted infections is required.
- Reinforcing preventive messages, such as safer sexual practices.
- Assessing the patient's preparedness to be tested.
- Obtaining informed consent from the patient (verbal is sufficient) and documenting this in the medical record.

The doctor who originally discusses HIV testing, obtains the patient's informed consent and requests the antibody test is responsible for notifying the patient of the result. This post-test discussion should be carried out in person (not over the telephone or by post) and applies equally to positive and negative results.

Primary HIV infection

- Full blood examination, heterophile antibody test.
- HIV antibody: the antibody test may be negative initially, in which case it is vital to repeat the test in 2, 4 and 6 weeks.
- p24 antigen: this viral protein can be detected in blood during primary infection and has a diagnostic role in those with an initially negative antibody test. HIV RNA (viral load) tests are not recommended for diagnosis of primary HIV infection because false positives may occur.

Patients with previously unrecognized infection

The HIV antibody test will be positive in all patients, and other tests are not needed for diagnosis. As indicated in the previous section, appropriate pre- and post-test discussion is vital.

Patients known to be HIV infected

Cough, shortness of breath, fever

If the CD4 cell count is $>0.2 \times 10^9/L$, most patients can be managed as if they did not have HIV infection. Investigations required for patients with suspected bacterial pneumonia or tuberculosis include a chest X-ray, full blood examination, sputum examination and blood cultures.

If the CD4 cell count is $<0.2 \times 10^9/L$ investigation is almost always indicated, the extent of which will be guided by the patient's condition and the likely diagnostic possibilities, and may include some or all of the following:

- Oxygen saturation
- Chest X-ray
- Blood cultures
- Sputum Gram stain, culture, and AFB smear and culture
- Induced sputum for detection (by microscopy or PCR) of PCP
- Bronchoscopy – usually during inpatient admission.

A high index of suspicion for tuberculosis must be maintained; the diagnosis is generally suggested by one or more suggestive epidemiological, clinical or radiological features.

Focal neurological signs, convulsions or altered conscious state

A brain CT scan (with contrast) should be done in all patients, often as a matter of some urgency, and should always precede a lumbar puncture. MRI will often provide additional important information. The commonest causes of focal lesions are cerebral toxoplasmosis and primary intracerebral lymphoma. An IgG test for *Toxoplasma gondii* will have usually been performed in those with previously diagnosed HIV infection: if positive, this indicates a predisposition to the development of cerebral toxoplasmosis; if negative, toxoplasmosis is much less likely. Diagnosis of cerebral lymphoma is primarily based on non-response to empiric treatment for cerebral toxoplasmosis; CSF cytology, detection of EBV DNA in CSF by polymerase chain reaction or occasionally brain biopsy are required for a specific diagnosis. Progressive multifocal leukoencephalopathy manifests as focal white matter lesions visible on T_2-weighted MRI scans.

Diarrhoea, with or without abdominal pain and fever

Faecal examination (preferably three fresh specimens collected on different days) for:

- Microscopy for ova, cysts and parasites.
- Cryptosporidium antigen test or stain, microsporidium stain.
- Culture for *Salmonella*, *Campylobacter* and *Shigella*.
- *Clostridium difficile* culture and toxin if recent antibiotic therapy.

Selected patients with undiagnosed diarrhoea may require colonoscopy or upper GI endoscopy if infections such as CMV, MAC or microsporidiosis are suspected. Swabs for gonorrhoea, *Chlamydia* and herpes should be taken from patients with symptoms of proctitis.

Fever without localizing features

If the CD4 cell count is $>0.2 \times 10^9/L$ serious HIV-related causes are uncommon, and so investigation will be guided by clinical features, severity of illness and so on. If the CD4 cell count is $<0.2 \times 10^9/L$ most patients will need investigation, beginning with the following basic work-up:

- Blood cultures, including mycobacterial blood cultures if CD4 cell count $<0.05 \times 10^9/L$.
- Chest X-ray.
- Serum cryptococcal antigen.

Additional tests for selected patients include faecal examination, sputum examination, abdominal ultrasonography or CT scanning, and occasionally bone marrow or liver biopsy.

Difficult or painful swallowing

Oesophagoscopy and biopsy are reserved for those who fail an empirical course of antifungal therapy (see below).

Headache, fever, neck stiffness

The serum cryptococcal antigen test is a useful screening test for cryptococcal meningitis because a negative result effectively excludes the diagnosis. A lumbar puncture should only be performed after a CT brain scan, and if the CT does not show a space-occupying lesion or evidence of increased intracranial pressure. CSF should be routinely sent for the following:

- Protein and glucose.
- Gram stain and culture (and AFB smear and culture if tuberculosis is suspected).
- India ink stain and cryptococcal antigen.
- Cytology.
- VDRL or RPR test – only indicated if serum syphilis serology is positive.

Management

Primary HIV infection

- Symptomatic treatment.
- Specific antiretroviral therapy – role not determined.

Specific HIV syndromes

ED physicians should consult doctors experienced in treating HIV-infected patients for advice about the management of specific syndromes and opportunistic infections. The following guidelines focus on initial and empiric therapy and provide examples of treatment options, but detailed information about indications for specific agents, toxicity and so on is omitted. For more comprehensive treatment recommendations, a specialized text should be consulted.[9,10]

Cough, fever, shortness of breath

Any person with suspected pulmonary tuberculosis must be placed in respiratory isolation until the diagnosis is excluded. On the basis of the initial diagnostic evaluation, patients can be categorized and management proceed as follows:

- Significant infection unlikely: no treatment.
- Possible PCP: empirical PCP therapy with co-trimoxazole, and corticosteroids if PaO_2 on room air <60 mmHg.
- Possible bacterial pneumonia:
  - Non-severe, outpatient – oral amoxicillin with or without either macrolide (e.g. roxithromycin) or doxicycline
  - Non-severe, inpatient – i.v. penicillin plus either oral macrolide (e.g. roxithromycin) or doxycycline
  - Severe – i.v. ceftriaxone plus i.v. azithromycin.

- Possible tuberculosis: admission, respiratory isolation; treatment with isoniazid, rifampicin, pyrazinamide and ethambutol if diagnosis confirmed; empirical therapy sometimes necessary depending on clinical circumstances (e.g. suspected tuberculous meningitis).

Focal neurological signs, convulsions, altered conscious state

Treatment is guided by the results of the brain CT scan. If a space-occupying lesion is found patients are treated empirically for cerebral toxoplasmosis with sulfadiazine and pyrimethamine. The CT scan is repeated after 2–3 weeks, and if no response is evident a brain biopsy might be considered in selected patients to diagnose cerebral lymphoma. If the CT scan is normal or non-diagnostic, MRI scanning is usually indicated, supplemented by lumbar puncture.

Diarrhoea, with or without abdominal pain and fever

Any infection identified on initial faecal examinations is treated on its merits. Symptomatic treatment with an antimotility agent such as loperamide is contraindicated if bloody diarrhoea and fever are present, but otherwise can be given safely to most patients. Endoscopy is generally reserved for those in whom no specific cause is identified on initial evaluation, and whose diarrhoea persists despite antimotility therapy.

Fever without localizing features

Empirical antibacterial therapy (with an anti-pseudomonal agent such as ceftazidime, with or without an aminoglycoside or vancomycin) is indicated for patients with an absolute neutrophil count $<0.5 \times 10^9$/L; otherwise the need for specific treatment is guided by the condition of the patient and the results of the diagnostic work-up. Any long-term i.v. access device should be removed if infection of the device is confirmed on clinical or microbiological grounds, or if diagnostic evaluation reveals no other focus of infection. Treatment for disseminated MAC (with clarithromycin and ethambutol, with or without rifabutin) is generally given only after the organism has been isolated, although occasional patients with debilitating fevers, weight loss and no other diagnosis may be treated empirically.

Difficult or painful swallowing

Empirical antifungal therapy is started with an azole agent, usually oral fluconazole. Some patients with *Candida* infections resistant to azoles need treatment with a short course of i.v. amphotericin B. Patients undergo endoscopy if they do not respond to antifungal treatment, and the results of histology and cultures determine subsequent treatment.

Headache, fever, neck stiffness

Patients with confirmed cryptococcal meningitis are treated with a combination of i.v. amphotericin B and oral 5-fluorocytosine for 1–2 weeks, then remain on suppressive therapy with oral fluconazole. If tuberculous meningitis is suspected empirical therapy should be started immediately, pending the results of CSF cultures.

Specific treatment of other infections

- CMV infections: i.v. ganciclovir or i.v. foscarnet.
- *Salmonella* infections: ciprofloxacin.

Antiretrovirals in the management of HIV infection

Combination antiretroviral therapy has transformed the lives of people living with HIV infection, by improving their quality of life and by reducing the incidence of HIV-related complications and deaths by 80% or more. More than 90% of patients starting treatment with one of the current recommended antiretroviral regimens will achieve a non-detectable plasma HIV viral load and a substantial CD4 cell count increase, and in the great majority of patients these benefits are sustained in the long term. Modern antiretroviral regimens are much more convenient, less toxic and more potent than earlier combination antiretroviral therapy, but antiretroviral therapy is not without its costs: difficulty in maintaining life-long adherence, short- and long-term toxicities of antiretroviral agents, and the potential development of antiretroviral resistance.[11]

New antiretroviral agents, including some with novel mechanisms of action, provide options for those patients failing therapy because of drug resistance or intolerance. Examples include 'new-generation' protease inhibitors (tipranavir and darunavir), inhibitors of HIV integrase and inhibitors of CCR5, the latter a host chemokine receptor involved in HIV cell entry.[12]

The emergency physician does not require a detailed knowledge of antiretroviral therapy, but should be aware of the agents in current use, their side effects, and the potential importance of drug–drug interactions. More detailed information can be referenced in regularly updated antiretroviral guidelines; examples are those produced by a panel of the US Department of Health and Human Services with an added Australian commentary, accessible at http://www.ashm.org.au/aust-guidelines/, and British HIV treatment guidelines, accessible at http://www.bhiva.org/.

Indications

- Symptomatic HIV infection.
- Asymptomatic HIV infection – CD4 cell count $<0.35 \times 10^9$/L.
- Pregnant women with HIV infection.[13]
- After significant HIV exposure sustained by healthcare worker (see Chapter 9.10).

Classes of drug

- Nucleoside/nucleotide reverse transcriptase inhibitors (NRTIs): zidovudine (ZDV or AZT), didanosine (ddI), lamivudine (3TC), stavudine (d4T), abacavir, tenofovir, emtricitabine (FTC).
- Protease inhibitors (PIs): nelfinavir, indinavir, saquinavir, fosamprenavir, lopinavir/ritonavir, atazanavir, tipranavir, darunavir.
- Non-nucleoside reverse transcriptase inhibitors (NNRTIs): nevirapine, efavirenz, delavirdine.
- Entry inhibitors: enfuvirtide (chemokine receptor inhibitors, e.g. maraviroc undergoing clinical evaluation).
- Integrase inhibitors (e.g. raltegravir): undergoing clinical evaluation.

Initial regimens – at least three drugs

- Two NRTIs – tenofovir + FTC (Truvada) OR abacavir + 3TC (Kivexa) or zidovudine + 3TC (Combivir) plus one NNRTI – nevirapine or efavirenz; OR
- Two NRTIs (as listed above) plus one PI (lopinavir OR fosamprenavir OR saquinavir OR atazanavir) boosted with low-dose ritonavir.

Side effects[14] (see Table 9.8.4)

If an antiretroviral drug is suspected or known to be the cause of a serious side effect, the patient's treating HIV doctor or a hospital HIV doctor should be consulted. In the interim, or unless advised otherwise by the treating or hospital doctor, all antiretroviral medications, and not just the incriminating drug, should be withheld to reduce the risk of development of resistance on a less than fully suppressive therapy.

Drug–drug interactions

Some commonly used drugs metabolized by hepatic cytochrome P450 oxidases are contraindicated with certain PIs or NNRTIs; in addition, many other drugs will require dose modification or closer monitoring. The following list of contraindicated drugs is not exhaustive, and physicians are urged to consult a pharmacist or HIV physician if there is any doubt about a potential antiretroviral drug interaction. A useful web site is www.hiv-druginteractions.org.

- Contraindicated with ritonavir-boosted PIs: astemizole, terfenadine, cisapride, rifampicin, midazolam, triazolam, simvastatin, ergotamine, dihydroergotamine, amiodarone (indinavir and tipranavir), flecainide, pimozide, St John's wort, proton pump inhibitors (atazanavir), inhaled fluticasone.
- Contraindicated with efavirenz: voriconazole plus as for ritonavir-boosted PIs, except rifampicin, simvastatin and amiodarone.
- Contraindicated with nevirapine: St John's wort, ketoconazole, rifampicin.

Disposition

Patients with newly diagnosed HIV infection should be referred to a specialized HIV clinic, or to a doctor with expertise in HIV medicine.

HIV medicine is a complex and rapidly changing field. For this reason, the management of patients with known HIV infection presenting to the ED should always involve consultation with a hospital doctor knowledgeable about HIV infection, such as an infectious diseases physician or immunologist. The patient's usual HIV doctor (a hospital specialist, sexual health physician or general practitioner with a high HIV caseload) can be contacted to obtain important details such as recent CD4 cell count and current antiretroviral agents in the event that such information is not otherwise immediately available. In general, patients with a suspected or confirmed serious opportunistic infection will need to be admitted for investigation and management. Patients in the final stages of AIDS, or those with less serious complications, can often be managed in the community, in which case liaison with the local doctor, home-care nurses or community-care agencies is vital.

Prognosis

Prior to the widespread use of opportunistic infection prophylaxis and effective antiretroviral therapy, 50% of patients developed AIDS 10 years after becoming HIV infected, and 75% of patients after 13 years. Following an AIDS-defining illness, the median survival was 12–24 months. Long-term non-progressors, who have a normal CD4 count and no HIV-related complications without antiretroviral therapy after 10 or more years of HIV infection, comprise less than 5% of patient cohorts.

Most AIDS-defining infections, such as PCP, now have low mortality and high 1-year survival rates if the infection is treated appropriately and patients are started on combination antiretroviral therapy, but survival rates following diagnosis of disseminated MAC and CMV end-organ disease are lower because these two opportunistic infections usually occur at a very advanced stage of HIV infection. Combination antiretroviral therapy has reduced the mortality and incidence of opportunistic infections by over 80%.

The ultimate prognosis of patients on long-term antiretroviral therapy is unknown, but emerging data suggest that life expectancy will be shorter than average. Surprisingly, this seems to be accounted for by an excess of deaths due to chronic conditions not typically associated with HIV infection, such as cardiovascular disease, malignancy and liver disease, rather than to expected complications such as opportunistic infections.

Prevention

Prevention of HIV transmission
- Public health and educational efforts to encourage the adoption of safer sex practices.
- HIV screening of blood, blood products and tissue donors.
- Non-sharing and use of clean needles and syringes by injecting drug users.
- Observance of standard precautions by workers in healthcare settings.
- Use of antiretroviral therapy and avoidance of breastfeeding to prevent transmission from an HIV-infected mother to her baby.
- Use of antiretroviral prophylaxis after significant occupational exposures to HIV-infected blood (see Chapter 9.10). (Similar use after sexual exposure may be considered but is of unproven benefit.)
- Male circumcision – shown to reduce the acquisition of HIV infection by 60% in studies in sub-Saharan Africa.[15,16]

Prevention of HIV-related complications[17]

Infection	Preventive measure
Pneumococcal pneumonia	Pneumococcal vaccination
Latent tuberculous infection	Isoniazid
PCP	Co-trimoxazole
Toxoplasmosis	Co-trimoxazole
MAC	Azithromycin or rifabutin

Controversies

- Why has there been a recent increase in HIV diagnoses among gay men in Australia and some other developed countries, and how can this be reversed?

- Can a vaginal microbicide be developed that will reduce the risk of HIV transmission to females in developing countries?

- Should a large-scale programme of male circumcision be undertaken in developing countries in sub-Saharan Africa, and what are the barriers to implementation of such a programme?

- With the availability of more potent, more convenient and better-tolerated antiretroviral drugs, should therapy be started at a higher CD4 cell count than is currently recommended?

- Is long-term HIV infection associated with a broader range of chronic medical conditions than previously thought?

- Can an effective HIV vaccine be developed?

References

1. UNAIDS 2006. AIDS epidemic update. Special report on HIV/AIDS: December2006. UNAIDS, Geneva.
2. Simon V, Ho DD, Abdool Karim Q. HIV/AIDS epidemiology, pathogenesis, prevention, and treatment. Lancet 2006;368:489–504.
3. National Centre in HIV Epidemiology and Clinical Research 2006. HIV/AIDS, viral hepatitis and sexually transmitted infections in Australia Annual Surveillance Report 2006. National Centre in HIV Epidemiology and Clinical Research, The University of New South Wales, Sydney, NSW.
4. Kelly M 2003. HIV immunopathology. In Hoy J, Lewin S (eds). HIV management in Australasia: a guide for clinical care. Australasian Society for HIV Medicine, Sydney, 23–40.
5. Stewart G (ed.) 1994. Could it be HIV? Australasian Medical Publishing Company Ltd, Sydney
6. Workman C 2003. Clinical manifestations and the natural history of HIV. In Hoy J, Lewin S (eds). HIV management in Australasia: a guide for clinical care. Australasian Society for HIV Medicine, Sydney, 123–130.
7. Post JJ, Workman C, Kelly M, Clezy K 2003. Key opportunistic infections. In Hoy J, Lewin S (eds). HIV management in Australasia: a guide for clinical care. Australasian Society for HIV Medicine, Sydney, 131–162
8. Ministerial Advisory Committee on AIDS, Sexual Health and Hepatitis 2006. National HIV testing policy 2006. Department of Health and Ageing, Canberra.
9. Hoy J, Lewin S (eds) 2003. HIV management in Australia: a guide for clinical care. Australasian Society for HIV Medicine, Sydney.
10. Crowe S, Hoy J, Mills J (eds) 2001. Medical Management of the HIV-infected Patient, 2nd edn. Martin Dunitz, Cambridge
11. Chen LF, Hoy J, Lewin SR. Ten years of highly active antiretroviral therapy for HIV infection. Med J Aust 2007;186:146–51.
12. Hirschel B, Perneger T. No patient left behind—better treatments for resistant HIV infection. Lancet 2007;370:3–5.
13. Perinatal HIV Guidelines Working Group 2006. Public Health Service Task Force Recommendations for Use of Antiretroviral Drugs in Pregnant HIV-1 Infected Women for Maternal Health and Interventions to Reduce Perinatal HIV-1 Transmission in the United States. October 12, 2006 1–65. Available at http://aidsinfo.nih.gov/ContentFiles/PerinatalGL.pdf. Accessed 21/08/07.
14. Calmy A, Hirschel B, Cooper DA, Carr A. Clinical update: adverse effects of antiretroviral therapy. Lancet 2007;370:12–14.
15. Gray RH, Kigozi G, Serwadda D, Makumbi F, et al. Male circumcision for HIV prevention in men in Rakai, Uganda: a randomised trial. Lancet 2007;369:657–666.
16. Bailey RC, Moses S, Parker CB, et al. Male circumcision for HIV prevention in young men in Kisumu, Kenya: a randomised controlled trial. Lancet 2007;369:643–656.
17. Centers for Disease Control and Prevention 2002. Guidelines for preventing opportunistic infections among HIV-infected persons – 2002: recommendations of USPHS and IDSA. Morbidity and Mortality Weekly Report 51(No.RR-8): 1–27.

9.9 Antibiotics in the emergency department

John Vinen

ESSENTIALS

1 Infectious disease presentations are common in emergency departments.

2 There are changing patterns of infectious disease, largely due to immunosuppression from chemotherapy, HIV, and new and emerging infections.

3 Many bacteria are becoming increasingly resistant to available antimicrobials, with some resistant to multiple agents.

4 The growing world trade in wildlife, factory farming, increasing air travel and increased population density increases the risk of infectious disease transmission.

5 There are relatively few new antimicrobials to counter these changing patterns of resistance.

6 Antimicrobial prescribing should follow evidence-based guidelines.

7 Some patients with infection can be treated wholly as outpatients using parenteral therapy, or after early discharge once the acute toxic phase is over.

8 Early administration of appropriate antibiotics combined with supportive therapy is the key to a good outcome.

9 The increasing incidence of terrorism may result in patients presenting with novel, unusual or clusters of infections caused by biological agents.

Principles of antimicrobial therapy

The first decision to be made regarding antimicrobial therapy is whether the administration of these agents is truly indicated. In many cases antibiotics are administered without clear need. This practice is potentially dangerous, as some agents can cause serious toxicity, diagnoses may be masked if appropriate cultures are not taken prior to therapy, and micro-organism resistance may emerge. The choice of an appropriate antimicrobial agent requires consideration of the following factors.

The micro-organism

The identity of the infecting organism must be known or suspected. In the emergency department (ED) setting almost all antimicrobial decisions will be made without the benefit of cultures, and the physician applies knowledge of the organisms most likely to cause infection in a given clinical setting.[1] However, certain 'rapid methods' of microbial identification may be employed. These include Gram-stain preparations (bacterial, some fungal and leukocyte identification) and immunological methods for antigen detection (enzyme-linked immunoabsorbent assay, latex agglutination, polymerase chain reactions).

Micro-organism susceptibility

The emergency physician is unlikely to have this information, and therapeutic decisions will generally be based on a knowledge of likely susceptibilities.[1] For example, group A streptococci remain susceptible to the penicillins and cephalosporins, and virtually all anaerobes (except *Bacteroides* spp.) are susceptible to penicillin G. However, when the identity or susceptibility of the infecting organism is sufficiently in doubt, the patient's clinical condition is atypical, serious or potentially serious, or where antimicrobial resistance is suspected, it is good practice to obtain appropriate specimens for culture and susceptibility testing prior to empirical antimicrobial therapy (Table 9.9.1).

Host factors

An adequate history of drug allergies must be obtained in order to prevent the administration of an agent that may have serious or fatal consequences. The age of the patient may have clinically significant effects on drug absorption (e.g. penicillin absorption is increased in the young and the elderly),[2] metabolism (e.g. reduced chloramphenicol metabolism in the neonate)[2] and excretion (e.g. declining renal function with age[3] may reduce the excretion of penicillins, cephalosporins and aminoglycosides). Furthermore, tetracyclines bind and discolour the developing bone and tooth structures in children aged 8 years or less.[2] Pregnant women and nursing mothers may pose certain problems in the selection of appropriate antimicrobial agents, as all of these agents cross the placenta to varying degrees. The administration of antibiotics to pregnant patients must be based on guidelines.[4] The administration of antibiotics to patients on the oral contraceptive pill can reduce the effectiveness of the pill and

result in unwanted pregnancy. Other host factors that may require consideration include the patient's renal and hepatic function, their genetic (e.g. liver acetylation rate) or metabolic abnormalities (e.g. diabetes mellitus), and the site of the infection.[5]

Route of administration

In general, the oral route is chosen for infections that are mild and can be managed on an outpatient basis. In this situation, consideration needs to be given to compliance with treatment, the variability of absorption with food in the stomach, and interaction of the agent with concomitant medications.[5] The parenteral route is used for agents that are inefficiently absorbed from the gastrointestinal tract, and for the treatment of patients with serious infections in whom high concentrations of antimicrobial agents are required.[5] Intramuscular administration will provide adequate serum concentrations for most infections, and may be appropriate where antimicrobial depots are desirable, e.g. procaine penicillin injections where patient compliance with oral medication is doubtful. Intravenous administration allows large doses of drugs to be given with a minimal amount of discomfort to the patient, e.g. infection prophylaxis in compound fractures, life-threatening infections and shock. For intravenous administration large veins should be used followed by saline flushing of the veins to help to minimize the incidence of venous irritation and phlebitis.

Supportive care

Supportive care in association with antimicrobial therapy is essential in many infections, fluid resuscitation and vasopressors being essential for a good outcome in sepsis.[6]

Antibiotic resistance

Bacteria can be resistant to an antimicrobial agent because the drug fails to reach the target or is inactivated, or because the target is altered.[7–9] Bacteria may produce enzymes that inactivate the drug, or have cell membranes impermeable to the drug. Having gained entry into the micro-organism, the drug must exert a deleterious effect. Natural variation, or acquired changes at the target

site that prevent drug binding or action, can lead to resistance.

Resistance is most commonly acquired by horizontal transfer of resistance determinants from a donor cell, often of another bacterial species, by transformation, transduction or conjugation. Resistance may also be acquired by mutation, and passed vertically by selection to daughter cells. Antimicrobial agents can affect the emergence of resistance by exerting strong selective pressures on bacterial populations favouring those organisms capable of resisting them.[10]

The increasing emergence of antibiotic resistance is a very serious development that threatens the end of the antibiotic era. Penicillin-resistant strains of pneumococci account for 50% or more of isolates in some European countries. The worldwide emergence of *Haemophilus* and gonococci that produce β-lactamase is a major therapeutic problem.[11] Methicillin-resistant strains of *Staphylococcus aureus* are widely distributed among hospitals and are increasingly being isolated from community-acquired infections.[12] There are now strains of enterococci (VRE), *Pseudomonas* and enterobacters that are resistant to all known drugs.[13] Epidemics of multiply drug-resistant strains of *Mycobacterium tuberculosis* have been reported.[13]

A more responsible approach to the use of antimicrobial agents is essential to slow the development of multidrug-resistant organisms. Their use should be avoided in viral infections, and rational policies for their use in prophylaxis and in established bacterial infections must be developed and followed.[1] The use of narrow-spectrum antimicrobial agents to which the organism is susceptible is encouraged, and in certain circumstances the use of combinations of agents may prevent the emergence of resistant mutants during therapy.

Prophylactic use of antibiotics

Antimicrobial prophylaxis is the use of antimicrobial agents before infection takes place. It is indicated in many circumstances, including the prevention of recurrent rheumatic fever, endocarditis, meningitis, tuberculosis, and urinary-tract and surgical infections.[1] Antimicrobial prophylaxis in

Table 9.9.1 Antimicrobial agents of choice in selected infections

Micro-organism	Diseases	First choice	Second choice
Gram-positive cocci			
Staphylococcus aureus*	Abscesses penicillinase-negative: Osteomyelitis	benzylpenicillin (penicillin G), phenoxymethyl penicillin (penicillin V)	cephalosporin (G1), clindamycin
	Bacteraemia penicillinase-positive: Endocarditis	nafcillin, oxacillin	cephalosporin (G1) vancomycin, clindamycin
	Pneumonia methicillin-resistant: Cellulitis	vancomycin ± rifampicin	co-trimoxazole + rifampicin ciprofloxacin + rifampicin
Streptococcus (A, B, C, G and bovis)	Pharyngitis, scarlet fever, otitis media, cellulitis, erysipelas, pneumonia, bacteraemia, endocarditis, meningitis	benzylpenicillin (penicillin G), phenoxymethylpenicillin (penicillin V), ampicillin	erythromycin, cephalosporin (G1) vancomycin
Streptococcus pneumoniae*	Pneumonia, arthritis, sinusitis, otitis media, meningitis, endocarditis	benzylpenicillin (penicillin G), phenoxymethylpenicillin (penicillin V), ampicillin, penicillin G	erythromycin, cephalosporin (G1–3) vancomycin + rifampicin, ceftriaxone
Streptococcus viridans*	Bacteraemia, endocarditis	benzylpenicillin (penicillin G) ± gentamicin	ceftriaxone, vancomycin ± gentamicin
Enterococcus	Bacteraemia, endocarditis, urinary tract infection	ampicillin + gentamicin, benzylpenicillin (penicillin G) + gentamicin	vancomycin + gentamicin, nitrofurantoin, fluoroquinolone, ampicillin + clavulanic acid
Gram-negative cocci			
Moraxella catarrhalis	Otitis, sinusitis, pneumonia	co-trimoxazole amoxicillin + clavulanic acid	cephalosporin (G2,3), erythromycin, tetracycline
Neisseria gonorrhoeae	Gonorrhoea, disseminated disease	ceftriaxone, ampicillin + probenecid	ciprofloxacin, doxycycline spectinomycin
Neisseria meningitidis	Meningitis, carrier state	benzylpenicillin (penicillin G) rifampicin	cephalosporin (G3), chloramphenicol
Gram-positive bacilli			
Clostridium perfringens*	Gas gangrene Tetanus	benzylpenicillin (penicillin G)	clindamycin, metronidazole, cephalosporin
Clostridium tetani	Tetanus	benzylpenicillin (penicillin G), vancomycin	doxycycline, clindamycin
Clostridium difficile	Antimicrobial-associated colitis	metronidazole (oral)	vancomycin (oral)
Corynebacterium diphtheriae	Pharyngitis, tracheitis, pneumonia	erythromycin	benzylpenicillin (penicillin G), clindamycin
Listeria monocytogenes	Meningitis, bacteraemia	ampicillin ± gentamicin	co-trimoxazole, erythromycin
Gram-negative bacilli			
Brucella	Brucellosis	doxycycline + gentamicin	co-trimoxazole + gentamicin/rifampicin
Campylobacter jejuni*	Enteritis	fluoroquinolone	erythromycin, azithromycin
Escherichia coli*	Urinary tract infection, bacteraemia	ampicillin, co-trimoxazole cephalosporin (G1)	ampicillin + gentamicin, fluoroquinolone, nitrofurantoin
Enterobacter species	Urinary tract and other infections	fluoroquinolone imipenem	gentamicin + broad-spectrum penicillin, co-trimoxazole
Haemophilus influenzae*	Otitis, sinusitis, pneumonia	co-trimoxazole, ampicillin, amoxicillin	amoxicillin + clavulanic acid, azithromycin cefuroxime
	Epiglottitis, meningitis	cephalosporin (G3)	chloramphenicol
Klebsiella pneumoniae*	Urinary tract infection, pneumonia	cephalosporin ± gentamicin	co-trimoxazole, fluoroquinolone
Legionella pneumophila	Legionnaires' disease	erythromycin ± rifampicin	ciprofloxacin, azithromycin, co-trimoxazole
Pasteurella multocida	Animal bite infections, abscesses, bacteraemia, meningitis	benzylpenicillin (penicillin G), amoxicillin + clavulanic acid	doxycycline, cephalosporin
Proteus mirabilis*	Urinary tract and other infections	ampicillin, amoxicillin	cephalosporin, co-trimoxazole, gentamicin
Proteus (other species)*	Urinary tract and other infections	cephalosporin (G3), gentamicin	co-trimoxazole, fluoroquinolone
Pseudomonas aeruginosa*	Urinary tract infection, pneumonia, bacteraemia	broad-spectrum penicillin ± gentamicin	ceftazidime ± gentamicin fluoroquinolone ± gentamicin
Salmonella species*	Typhoid fever, paratyphoid fever, bacteraemia, gastroenteritis	fluoroquinolone, ceftriaxone	ampicillin, co-trimoxazole, chloramphenicol
Shigella*	Acute gastroenteritis	fluoroquinolone	ampicillin, co-trimoxazole
Vibrio cholerae	Cholera	doxycycline, fluoroquinolone	co-trimoxazole
Miscellaneous agents			
Chlamydia species	Pneumonia, trachoma, urethritis, cervicitis	doxycycline	azithromycin, erythromycin
Mycoplasma pneumoniae	Atypical pneumonia	erythromycin, doxycycline	azithromycin
Pneumocystis carinii	Pneumonia in impaired host	co-trimoxazole	trimethoprim + dapsone, pentamidine
Rickettsia	Typhus fever, Q fever, Rocky Mountain spotted fever	doxycycline	chloramphenicol
Treponema pallidum	Syphilis	benzylpenicillin (penicillin G)	ceftriaxone, doxycycline

*All strains should be examined in vitro for sensitivity to various antimicrobial agents.
G1, first-generation cephalosporin; G2, second-generation cephalosporin; G3, third-generation cephalosporin.

the emergency department is usually indicated to prevent trauma-related infection following contamination of soft tissue, crush injuries, bites, clenched fist injuries, and compound fractures. Other risk factors for wound infection include 'old' wounds (>6 hours), penetrating injuries, contaminated wounds, comorbid illness, shock, colon injury and massive haemorrhage.[14]

Antimicrobial prophylaxis should be considered where there is a significant risk of infection, but cannot be relied upon to overcome excessive soiling, damage to tissues, inadequate debridement or poor surgical technique. Adequate wound care, with splinting and elevation of the affected area as indicated, will remain important factors in trauma-related infection prophylaxis.

Antimicrobial prophylaxis should be directed against the likely causative organism(s). However, an effective regimen need not necessarily include antimicrobials that are active against every potential pathogen. Regimens that only reduce the total number of organisms may assist host defences and prevent infection.[1] The type, dose, duration and route of administration of antimicrobial therapy will vary according to the nature, site and aetiology of the injury, as well as host factors, and should be based on established guidelines. In all cases of open traumatic injury, no matter how trivial, tetanus prophylaxis must be considered.

Penicillins

Chemistry and mechanism of action

The penicillins constitute one of the most important groups of antimicrobial agents and remain the drugs of choice for a large number of infectious diseases. The basic structure of the penicillins consists of a thiazolidine ring connected to a β-lactam ring, and a side chain. The penicillin nucleus is the chief structural requirement for biological activity, whereas the side chain determines many of the antibacterial and pharmacological characteristics of the particular type of penicillin.

Peptidoglycan is an essential component of the bacterial cell wall, and provides mechanical stability by virtue of its highly cross-linked latticework structure. Penicillin is thought to acetylate and inhibit a transpeptidase enzyme responsible for the final cross-linking of peptidoglycan layers. Penicillin also binds to penicillin-binding proteins (PBPs), causing further interference with cell wall synthesis and cell morphology. The lysis of bacteria is ultimately dependent on the activity of cell wall autolytic enzymes – autolysins and murein hydrolases. Although the relationship between the inhibition of PBP activity and the activation of autolysins is unclear, the interference with peptidoglycan assembly in the face of ongoing autolysis activity might well lead to cell lysis and death.

Bacterial resistance to penicillins

Micro-organisms may be intrinsically resistant to the penicillins because of structural differences in PBPs. Resistance may be acquired by the development of high molecular weight PBPs that have reduced affinity for the antibiotic.[9] Bacterial resistance can also be caused by the inability of the agent to penetrate to its site of action.[15] Unlike Gram-positive bacteria, Gram-negative bacteria have an outer membrane of lipopolysaccharide which functions as an impenetrable barrier to some antibiotics. However, some broader-spectrum penicillins, such as ampicillin and amoxicillin, can diffuse through aqueous channels (porins) of this outer membrane to reach their sites of action.

Bacteria can destroy penicillins enzymatically. Different bacteria elaborate a number of different β-lactamases, and individual penicillins vary in their susceptibility to these enzymes. In general, Gram-positive bacteria produce a large amount of β-lactamase, which is secreted extracellularly. Most of these enzymes are penicillinases which disrupt the β-lactam ring and inactivate the drug. In Gram-negative bacteria, β-lactamases are found in relatively small amounts strategically located between the inner and outer bacterial membranes for maximal protection.

Classification of penicillins

Benzylpenicillin (penicillin G) and phenoxymethyl penicillin (penicillin V)

These drugs are the so-called 'natural penicillins'. The antimicrobial spectra of benzyl penicillin (penicillin G) and phenoxymethyl penicillin (penicillin V) are very similar for aerobic Gram-positive microorganisms. Benzyl penicillin is the drug of choice against many Gram-positive cocci (streptococci, penicillin-sensitive staphylococci), Gram-negative cocci (Neisseria meningitidis and N. gonorrhoeae), Gram-postive bacilli (Bacillus anthracis, Cl. diphtheria), anaerobes (peptostreptococcus, Actinomyces israeli, Clostridium and some Bacteroides), Pasteurella multocida and Treponema pallidum. Phenoxymethyl penicillin is an acceptable alternative for Streptococcus pneumoniae, Strep. pyogenes (A) and Actinomyces israeli.

The sole virtue of benzylpenicillin compared to phenoxymethyl penicillin is that it is more stable in an acid medium and therefore much better absorbed from the gastrointestinal tract. Benzylpenicillin is administered parenterally but has a half-life of only 30 minutes. Accordingly, repository preparations (penicillin G procaine, penicillin G benzathine) are often used, and probenecid may be administered concurrently to block the renal tubular secretion of the drug. Once absorbed, both penicillins are distributed widely throughout the body. Significant amounts appear in the liver, bile, kidney, semen, joint fluid, lymph and intestine. Importantly, penicillin does not readily enter the CSF when the meninges are normal. However, when the meninges are acutely inflamed penicillin penetrates into the CSF more easily. Under normal circumstances, penicillin is eliminated unchanged by the kidney, mainly by tubular secretion.

The penicillinase-resistant penicillins

These drugs remain the agents of choice for most staphylococcal disease. Methicillin is a penicillin resistant to staphylococcal β-lactamase, although the increasing incidence of isolates of methicillin-resistant micro-organisms is cause for concern. Methicillin-resistant Staph. aureus (MRSA) contain a high molecular weight PBP with a very low affinity for β-lactam antibiotics.[9] From 40% to 60% of strains of Staph. epidermidis are also resistant to penicillinase-resistant penicillins by the same mechanism. As bacterial sensitivies are usually not known in the emergency department, methicillin is rarely administered in this setting.

The isoxazolyl penicillins (oxacillin, cloxacillin, dicloxacillin and flucloxacillin) are congeneric semisynthetic penicillins which are pharmacologically similar. All are relatively stable in an acid medium and are adequately absorbed after oral administration. These penicillins undergo some metabolism but are excreted primarily by the kidney with some biliary excretion. All are remarkably resistant to cleavage by penicillinase, and inhibit both penicillin-sensitive and some penicillin-resistant staphylococci. Methicillin-resistant staphylococci are resistant to these penicillins. Isoxazolyl penicillins inhibit streptococci and pneumococci but are virtually inactive against Gram-negative bacilli.

The aminopenicillins

Ampicillin is the prototypical agent in this group. It is stable in acid medium and, although well absorbed orally, is often administered parenterally. Amoxicillin is a close chemical and pharmacological relative of ampicillin. The drug is stable in acid and was designed for oral use. It is more rapidly and completely absorbed from the gastrointestinal tract than is ampicillin. The antimicrobial spectra of these agents are essentially identical, with the important exception that amoxicillin appears to be less effective for shigellosis. Ampicillin is the penicillin of choice for many Gram-negative bacilli (H. influenzae, Escherichia coli, Proteus mirabilis, Salmonella typhi and Salmonella spp.), some Gram-positive bacilli (Listeria monocytogenes) and some Gram-positive cocci (Enterococcus faecalis). It also has activity against Pneumococcus spp., Neisseria spp., Peptostreptococcus, Fusobacterium, Clostridium and Erysipelothrix.

Bacterial resistance to these drugs is becoming an increasing problem. Many pneumococcal isolates have varying levels of resistance to ampicillin. H. influenzae and the viridans group of streptococci are usually inhibited by very low concentrations of ampicillin. However, strains of H. influenzae (type b) that are highly resistant to ampicillin have been recovered from children with meningitis. It is estimated that 30% or more cases of H. influenzae meningitis are now caused by ampicillin-resistant strains. Similarly, ampicillin-resistant strains of H. influenzae have been increasingly isolated from cases of acute

otitis media. An increasing percentage of N. gonorrhoeae, E. coli, P. mirabilis, Salmonella and Shigella are now resistant to ampicillin, and practically all species of Enterobacter are now insensitive.

β-Lactamase inhibitors have been introduced to combat many penicillin-resistant microorganisms. These molecules bind to β-lactamases and inactivate them, thereby preventing the destruction of β-lactamase antibiotics. Clavulanic acid binds to the β-lactamases produced by a wide range of Gram-positive and Gram-negative microorganisms. It is well absorbed orally and can also be given parenterally. It has been combined with amoxicillin as an oral preparation (Augmentin) and with ticarcillin as a parenteral preparation (Timentin). Augmentin is effective for β-lactamase-producing strains of staphylococci, H. influenzae, gonococci and E. coli. Sulbactam is another β-lactamase inhibitor which also can be administered orally or parenterally. In combination with ampicillin (Unasyn), good coverage is provided for Gram-positive cocci (including β-lactamase-producing strains of Staph. aureus), Gram-negative anaerobes (but not Pseudomonas) and anaerobes.

Adverse reactions to penicillin

Hypersensitivity reactions are the major adverse effects of penicillins. Penicillins are capable of acting as haptens to combine with proteins contaminating the solution, or with human protein after the penicillin has been administered. Penicilloyl and penicillanic derivatives are the major determinants of penicillin allergy. All acute hypersensitivity reactions to penicillin are mediated by the IgE antibody, and range in severity from rash to anaphylaxis. Anaphylactic reactions are uncommon, occurring in only 0.2% of 1000 courses of treatment, with 0.001% out of 100 000 courses resulting in death.[16] Morbilliform eruptions that develop after penicillin therapy are likely to be mediated by IgM antibodies, and the uncommon serum sickness is likely to be mediated by IgG antibodies. All forms of penicillin are best avoided in patients with a history of penicillin allergy.

Otherwise, the penicillins are generally well tolerated. CNS toxicity, in the form of myoclonic seizures, can follow the administration of massive doses of benzylpenicillin

(penicillin G), ampicillin or methicillin. Massive doses have also been associated with hypokalaemia. Haematological toxicity – usually neutropenia – and nephrotoxicity have also been reported. Gastrointestinal disturbances have followed the use of all oral penicillins, but have been most pronounced with ampicillin. Enterocolitis due to the overgrowth of Cl. difficile is well documented and abnormalities in liver function have been reported, especially with flucloxacillin.

Cephalosporins

The antimicrobial activity of cephalosporins, like that of other β-lactam antibiotics, results at least in part from their ability to interfere with the synthesis of the peptidoglycan component of the bacterial cell wall. However, the exact bactericidal and lytic effects of cephalosporins are not completely understood.

Classification and uses

The first-generation compounds (cephalothin, cefazolin, cefalexin) have a relatively narrow spectrum of activity focused primarily on the Gram-positive cocci, especially penicillin-sensitive streptococci and methicillin-sensitive Staph. aureus. These compounds have modest activity against Gram-negative organisms, including E. coli and Klebsiella spp. Cefaclor has extended Gram-negative activity and is active against H. influenzae and M. catarrhalis.

The second generation of cephalosporins (cefuroxime, cefamandole) are more stable against Gram-negative β-lactamases. They have variable activity against Gram-positive cocci, but have increased activity against Gram-negative bacteria (E. coli, Proteus, Klebsiella). In spite of relatively increased potency against Gram-negative aerobic and anaerobic bacilli (Bacteroides fragilis), the cephamycins (cefoxitin, cefotetan) are included in this generation.

The third-generation cephalosporins (cefotaxime, ceftriaxone, ceftazidime, cefpirome) have very marked activity against Gram-negative bacteria. Most are useful against Ps. aeruginosa, Serratia and Neisseria species and some Enterobacteriaceae. Some of these compounds have limited activity against Gram-positive cocci, particularly methicillin-sensitive *Staph. aureus*. This generation of cephalosporins is particularly effective in meningitis because of their better penetration into the CSF and higher intrinsic activity. However, as these third-generation drugs are more expensive and have a wide antimicrobial spectrum, their use should be based on established guidelines.

Recently, several compounds have been considered as possibly meriting classification as a fourth generation. Cefepime has activity against Gram-positive cocci and a broad array of Gram-negative bacteria, including *Ps. aeruginosa* and many of the Enterobacteriaceae with inducible chromosomal β-lactamases.

Adverse reactions

Hypersensitivity reactions are the most common side effects of the cephalosporins and all compounds have been implicated. The reactions appear to be identical to those caused by the penicillins. Immediate reactions such as anaphylaxis, bronchospasm, angio-oedema and urticaria have been reported. More commonly a maculopapular rash develops, usually after several days of therapy. Because of the similarity in structure between the penicillins and the cephalosporins, patients allergic to one class of agents may manifest cross-reactivity when a member of the other class is administered. Studies indicate that about 0.5% of patients allergic to penicillin will demonstrate a clinically apparent reaction when a first-generation cephalosporin is administered (0% for second- and third-generation cephalosporins).[17] Patients with a mild or temporarily distant reaction to penicillin appear to be at low risk of rash or other allergic reaction following the administration of a cephalosporin. However, subjects with a recent history of an immediate reaction to penicillin should not be given a cephalosporin. Other reactions to cephalosporins are uncommon and include diarrhoea, nephrotoxicity, intolerance of alcohol and bleeding disorders.

Bacterial resistance

The most prevalent mechanism for resistance to cephalosporins is their destruction by β-lactamase hydrolysis. The cephalosporins have variable susceptibility to β-lactamase, with the later-generation compounds being more resistant to the β-lactamases produced by Gram-negative bacteria. However, third-generation cephalosporins are susceptible to hydrolysis by inducible, chromosomally encoded (type 1) β-lactamases. The induction of type 1 β-lactamases by treatment of infections due to many aerobic Gram-negative bacilli with second- or third-generation cephalosporins may result in resistance to all third-generation cephalosporins.

Macrolides

Erythromycin was originally isolated from soil bacteria and contains a many-membered lactone ring to which are attached one or more deoxy sugars. Clarithromycin, azithromycin and roxithromycin are new semi-synthetic derivatives of erythromycin. Clarithromycin differs only by methylation of a hydroxyl group and azithromycin contains a methyl-substituted nitrogen atom in the lactone ring. Roxithromycin is a good alternative to oral erythromycin and has good oral bioavailability, but is more expensive. The macrolides are usually bacteriostatic and inhibit protein synthesis by binding reversibly to 50S ribosomal subunits of sensitive micro-organisms. They are thought to inhibit the translocation step wherein a newly synthesized peptidyl tRNA molecule moves from the acceptor site on the ribosome to the peptidyl (donor) site.

Clinical uses

Erythromycin is most effective against aerobic Gram-positive cocci and bacilli. It is active against *Strep. pyogenes, Strep. pneumoniae, Cl. perfringens, Cl. diphtheriae, L. monocytogenes* and some staphylococci. Useful activity has also been seen with *P. multocida, Borrelia* spp., *B. pertussis, Campylobacter jejuni, L. pneumophila, M. pneumoniae, C. trachomatis* and some atypical mycobacteria. It has modest activity in vitro against some Gram-negative organisms, including *H. influenzae* and *N. meningitidis*, and excellent activity against most strains of *N. gonorrhoeae*.

Clarithromycin is more potent against erythromycin-sensitive strains of streptococci and staphylococci, but has only modest activity against *H. influenzae* and *N.* *gonorrhoeae*. However, it has good activity against *M. catarrhalis, Chlamydia* spp., *L. pneumophila* and *M. pneumoniae*. Azithromycin is generally less active than erythromycin against the Gram-positive organisms and is more active than the other two macrolides against *H. influenzae* and *Campylobacter* spp. Azithromycin is very active against *M. catarrhalis, P. multocida, Chlamydia* spp., *M. pneumoniae, L. pneumophila* and *N. gonorrhoeae*.

Adverse reactions

Erythromycin is one of the safest antibiotics and causes serious adverse effects only rarely. Dose-related abdominal cramps, nausea, vomiting, diarrhoea and flatulence occur, but are uncommon in children and young adults. Allergic reactions observed include fever, eosinophilia and skin eruptions. Cholestatic hepatitis, transient hearing loss, polymorphic ventricular tachycardia, superinfection of the gastrointestinal tract and pseudomembranous colitis have been reported. Intravenous use of erythromycin is often associated with thrombophlebitis, but the incidence of this complication can be reduced with appropriate dilution of the dose. Adverse reactions to the other macrolides, at the usual dose, are rare and usually confined to the gastrointestinal tract. For this reason roxithromycin is often prescribed instead of erythromycin.

Erythromycin and, to a lesser extent, the other macrolides, has been reported to cause clinically significant drug interactions.[18] Erythromycin has been reported to potentiate astemizole, terfenadine, carbamazepine, corticosteroids, digoxin, theophylline, valproate and warfarin, probably by interfering with cytochrome P450-mediated drug metabolism. Care should be used in the concurrent administration of the macrolides with these drugs.

Bacterial resistance

Resistance to erythromycin may be the result of reduced permeability through the cell envelope. This form of resistance is exhibited by the Enterobacteriaceae and *Pseudomonas* spp. Alteration of ribosomal proteins, especially the 50S protein, often affects binding of the drug and has led to the emergence of resistant strains of *B.*

subtilis, Strep. pyogenes and Strep. pneumoniae, Campylobacter spp., E. coli, Staph. aureus, Cl. perfringens, Listeria spp. and Legionella spp. Finally, enzymatic degradation of the drug has conferred high-level resistance among strains of Enterobacteriaceae.

Tetracycline

Tetracyclines are generally bacteriostatic and are thought to inhibit bacterial protein synthesis by binding to the 30S bacterial ribosome and preventing access of aminoacyl tRNA to its acceptor site.

Clinical uses

The antimicrobial spectra of all the tetracyclines are almost identical. They possess a wide range of antimicrobial activity against aerobic and anaerobic Gram-positive and Gram-negative bacteria. Clinically, the tetracyclines are useful against Strep. pneumoniae, H. influenzae, Neisseria spp., E. coli, Brucella spp., H. ducreyi, Vibrio cholera, Campylobacter spp., and some Shigella and Mycobacterium spp. Many pathogenic spirochaetes are susceptible, including Borrelia burgdorferi. They are also effective against some micro-organisms that are resistant to cell-wall active antimicrobial agents, such as Rickettsia, Coxiella burnetti, Mycoplasma pneumonia, Chlamydia spp., Legionella spp. and Plasmodium spp.

Adverse reactions

The tetracyclines all produce gastrointestinal irritation in some individuals, although doxycycline is usually well tolerated. Epigastric discomfort, nausea, vomiting and diarrhoea are commonly reported. Renal and liver toxicity, and photosensitivity may occur. Tetracyclines are deposited in the skeleton and teeth during gestation and childhood, and can cause abnormalities of bone growth and discolouration of the teeth. It is therefore prudent not to administer these agents to pregnant women or children under 8 years of age. Hypersensitivity reactions, including skin reactions, burning of the eyes, pruritus ani, vaginitis, angio-oedema and anaphylaxis, are rarely seen.

Bacterial resistance

Bacteria develop resistance to the tetracyclines mainly by preventing the accumulation of the drug within the cell. This is accomplished by reducing the influx or increasing the ability of the cell to export the antibiotic. Rarely, the tetracyclines are inactivated biologically or inhibited in their ribosomal attachment.[18] Resistance to one tetracycline usually means resistance to all. Clinically, most strains of enterococci are now resistant to tetracycline; group B streptococci are 50% susceptible, and only 65% of Staph. aureus remain susceptible. Resistant pneumococci are now found in many geographical areas, and many strains of Neisseria spp. are now resistant.

Aminoglycosides

Each aminoglycoside demonstrates concentration-dependent bactericidal activity against susceptible micro-organisms. Gentamicin is the most commonly administered aminoglycoside in the ED and is a mixture of three closely related constituents. It binds to a specific area on the interface between the smaller (30S) and the larger (50S) bacterial ribosomal subunits, causing an increase in misreading of messenger RNA and a measurable decrease in protein synthesis. However, these effects do not provide a complete explanation for the rapidly lethal effect of gentamicin on bacteria.

Clinical uses

The antibacterial activity of gentamicin is directed primarily against aerobic and facultative Gram-negative bacilli. It has little activity against anaerobic micro-organisms and facultative bacteria under anaerobic conditions, and its activity against most Gram-positive bacteria is very limited. Gentamicin is clinically effective against Pseudomonas aeruginosa, Proteus mirabilis, Klebsiella pneumoniae, E. coli, Enterobacter spp. and Serratia spp. It is particularly effective when used in combination with cell-wall active antimicrobial agents, e.g. penicillin, cephalosporin. Interactions between these agents result in synergistic effects on bacterial death and may be useful against enterococci, Strep. pyogenes, some staphylococci, Enterobacteriaceae and Pseudomonas aeruginosa.

Adverse reactions

Like most other aminoglycosides, gentamicin has the potential to cause injury to the renal proximal convoluted tubules, damage to the cochlear and/or vestibular apparatus, and neuromuscular blockade. As the drug is eliminated almost entirely by glomerular filtration, gentamicin dosing in renal failure must be undertaken with care and drug-level monitoring is recommended. Gentamicin has little allergenic potential. Anaphylaxis, rash and other hypersensitivity reactions are unusual.

Bacterial resistance

Bacteria defend themselves against the aminoglycosides by a combination of alteration of uptake, synthesis of modifying enzymes, and a change of ribosomal binding sites.

In several centres a significant percentage of clinical isolates are highly resistant to all aminoglycosides.[19] At present, other widespread bacterial resistance to the aminoglycosides remains limited. However, there are reports of resistance emerging among some strains of Ps. aeruginosa, Enterobacteriaceae, E. coli, Serratia spp. and Staph. aureus.

Metronidazole

The toxicity of metronidazole is due to short-lived intermediate compounds or free radicals that produce damage by interaction with DNA and possibly other macromolecules.

Clinical uses

Metronidazole is active against a wide variety of anaerobic protozoal parasites. It is directly trichomonicidal. Sensitive strains of Trichomonas vaginalis are killed by very low concentrations of the drug under anaerobic conditions. The drug also has potent amoebicidal activity against E. histolytica, even in mixed culture, and substantial activity against the trophozoites of Giardia lamblia. Metronidazole manifests antibacterial activity against all anaerobic cocci and both anaerobic Gram-negative bacilli and anaerobic spore-forming Gram-positive bacilli. Bacteroides, Clostridium, Helicobacter, Fusobacterium, Peptococcus and Peptostreptococcus spp. are all susceptible.

Adverse reactions

In general, metronidazole is well tolerated. The most common side effects are headache, nausea, dry mouth and a metallic taste. Vomiting, diarrhoea and abdominal distress are occasionally experienced.[20] Furry tongue, glossitis and stomatitis may occur during therapy and are associated with a sudden intensification of moniliasis. Of clinical importance is metronidazole's well-documented disulfiram-like effect (Antabuse). Some patients experience abdominal distress, vomiting, flushing or headache if they drink alcohol during therapy with this drug.

Bacterial resistance

Fortunately, very few strains of *Bacteroides* spp. have demonstrated resistance. Some resistant strains of *T. vaginalis* have been isolated from patients with refractory cases of trichomoniasis, but these patients have usually responded to higher doses of metronidazole and prolonged courses of therapy.[21]

Co-trimoxazole

Co-trimoxazole is a combination of sulphamethoxazole, a sulphonamide antibiotic, and trimethoprim, a diaminopyrimidine. The antimicrobial activity of this combination results from actions on two steps of the enzymatic pathway for the synthesis of tetrahydrofolic acid. Sulfamethoxazole inhibits the incorporation of PABA into folic acid, and trimethoprim prevents the reduction of dihydrofolate to tetrahydrofolate. The latter is the form of folate essential to bacteria for one-carbon transfer reactions. Mammalian cells utilize preformed folate from the diet and do not synthesize this compound. This combination has been associated with serious sulphonamide-induced side effects. It has been recommended that the combination product be restricted to the few situations where combined use is the treatment of choice.[1]

Clinical uses

Trimethoprim is effective in the treatment of most urinary tract infections and should be used alone for this indication. However, co-trimoxazole is active against a wide range of Gram-positive and Gram-negative micro-organisms. *Cl. diphtheriae* and *N. meningitidis* are susceptible, as are most strains of *Strep. pneumoniae*. From 50% to 95% of strains of *H. influenzae*, *Staph. aureus* and *epidermidis*, *Strep. pyogenes* and *viridans*, *E. coli*, *Proteus mirabilis*, *Enterobacter* spp., *Salmonella*, *Shigella* and *Serratia* are inhibited. Also sensitive are *Klebsiella* spp., *Brucella abortis*, *Pasteurella haemolytica* and *Yersinia* spp. Co-trimoxazole has an important place in the treatment and prophylaxis of *P. carinii* infection, and the treatment of *L. monocytogenes* and *Nocardia* infection.

Adverse reactions

In routine use the combination appears to produce little toxicity. About 75% of adverse reactions involve the skin. These reactions are typical of those produced by sulphonamides and include a wide variety of rashes, erythema nodosum, erythema multiforme of the Stevens–Johnson type, exfoliative dermatitis and photosensitivity. Severe reactions tend to be more common among the elderly and HIV-infected patients. Gastrointestinal reactions include nausea and vomiting, but rarely diarrhoea. Glossitis and stomatitis are relatively common. Central nervous system reactions (headache, depression and hallucinations) and haematological disorders (anaemias, coagulation disorders and granulocytopenia) have been reported.

Bacterial resistance

The frequency of development of bacterial resistance to co-trimoxazole is lower than it is to either of the constituent compounds alone. Resistance to sulfamethoxazole is presumed to originate by random mutation and selection, or by transfer of resistance by plasmids. Such resistance is usually persistent and irreversible. Resistance to all sulphonamides is now becoming widespread in both community and nosocomial strains of bacteria, including streptococci, staphylococci, Enterobacteriaceae, *Neisseria* spp. and *Pseudomonas* spp. Trimethoprim-resistant microorganisms may arise by mutation, but resistance in Gram-negative bacteria is often associated with the acquisition of a plasmid that codes for an altered dihydrofolate reductase. Increasing incidences of resistance have been found in Enterobacteriaceae, *Ps. aeruginosa*, *Staph. aureus*, *E. coli*, *Salmonella* and *Shigella*.

Quinolones

The 4-quinolones, including nalidixic acid, are a family of compounds that contain a carboxylic acid moiety attached to a basic ring structure. The newer fluoroquinolones also contain a fluorine substituent, e.g. ciprofloxacin, ofloxacin. Some may also contain a piperazine moiety. Bacterial DNA gyrase is an essential enzyme involved in DNA function. The quinolones inhibit the enzymatic activities of DNA gyrase and promote the cleavage of DNA within the enzyme–DNA complex.

Clinical uses

The early quinolones are most active against aerobic Gram-negative bacilli, particularly Enterobacteriaceae and *Haemophilus* spp., and against Gram-negative cocci such as *Neisseria* spp. and *M. catarrhalis*. The fluoroquinolones are significantly more potent and have a much broader spectrum of antimicrobial activity. Relative to nalidixic acid, the fluoroquinolones also have additional activity against *Ps. aeruginosa* and some staphylococci. Ciprofloxacin remains the most potent fluoroquinolone against Gram-negative bacteria. Several intracellular bacteria are inhibited by the fluoroquinolones, including *Chlamydia*, *Mycoplasma*, *Legionella*, *Brucella* and some mycobacteria. Recently a new drug, moxifloxacin, has been released that is useful for sinusitis, community-acquired pneumonia and acute bronchitis.

Adverse reactions

Generally, these drugs are well tolerated. Gastrointestinal symptoms of anorexia, nausea, vomiting, diarrhoea and abdominal discomfort are commonly seen, particularly with the older quinolones. Headache, dizziness, insomnia and alteration in mood are the next most commonly reported symptoms. Allergic and skin reactions, including phototoxicity, may occur. Rarely, arthralgias and joint swelling, leukopenia, eosinophilia, thrombocytopenia and haemolysis are reported.

Bacterial resistance

Resistance patterns over time have indicated that resistance increased following the introduction of fluoroquinolones, and occurred most often with *Pseudomonas* spp. and staphylococci, and in soft-tissue infections and in infections associated with foreign bodies. Possibly reflecting the pressures of extensive use, increasing fluoroquinolone resistance has been reported among strains of *Cl. jejuni* and *E. coli*. Focused quinolone use should be considered to avoid compromising the utility of the fluoroquinolones.

Nitrofurantoin

The mechanism of action is poorly understood, but activity in many cases appears to require enzymatic reduction within the bacterial cell.[22] The reduced derivatives are thought to bind to and damage intracellular proteins, including DNA, and inhibit bacterial respiration, pyruvate metabolism and the synthesis of inducible enzymes.

Clinical uses

Nitrofurantoin is active against over 90% of clinical strains of *E. coli*, *Citrobacter* spp., *Staph. saprophyticus* and *E. faecalis*. However, most species of *Proteus*, *Pseudomonas*, *Serratia*, *Providencia*, *Morganella* and many *Enterobacter* and *Klebsiella* spp. are resistant. Given its spectrum of activity and concentration in the urine, nitrofurantoin is usually administered for the treatment of urinary-tract infections or for urinary antisepsis. However, it may have activity against bacteria not usually associated with urinary tract infections, including *Salmonella*, *Shigella*, *Staph. aureus*, *Strep. pneumoniae* and *pyogenes*, and *Bacteroides*. Fortunately, bacteria that are susceptible to nitrofurantoin rarely become resistant during therapy.

Adverse reactions

Gastrointestinal upsets, particularly nausea, vomiting and diarrhoea, are the commonest side effects of nitrofurantoin. The frequency of these symptoms may be reduced if the macrocrystalline formulation is administered. Rashes, presumably allergic in nature, have been seen quite commonly. Cholestatic jaundice, acute and chronic hepatitis, pulmonary and haematological reactions, and peripheral neuropathies have all been reported.

Antiviral drugs

Several antiviral drugs are available, although famciclovir, aciclovir and valaciclovir (prodrug of aciclovir that requires a lower dosage frequency) are the most frequently prescribed. Their mechanism of action is similar. Each drug targets virus-infected cells and inhibits viral DNA polymerase. Consequently, viral DNA synthesis and therefore viral replication are inhibited.

Clinical uses

These drugs are primarily used for the management of herpes zoster (within 72 hours of rash onset), treatment and suppression of genital herpes, and the management of patients with advanced symptomatic HIV disease. Famciclovir is well absorbed in the gut and has the advantage of three times daily dosage compared to five times daily for aciclovir.

Adverse reactions

These drugs are generally well tolerated. However, headache, gastrointestinal disturbance, dizziness and fatigue have been reported. Adverse effects are generally mild.

Antiretroviral drugs

Emergency physicians are unlikely to initiate these drugs as they form the basis of HIV treatment. However, an appreciation of their uses and side effects is useful. Furthermore, the management of patients with HIV disease can be difficult, and advice from an appropriate specialist source is recommended.

Clinical uses

The antiretrovirals are used in the treatment of established HIV infection. This includes patients with HIV-associated illnesses (e.g. CNS disease, malignancies, opportunistic diseases) and asymptomatic patients with low CD4 cell counts and/or high HIV viral loads. The drugs are also of use in the prevention of maternofetal transmission and as post-exposure prophylaxis for significant exposure from a known HIV-infected source.[23]

Three major classes of antiretroviral are available. For initial therapy, three drugs are generally used in combination. The recommended regimen is:

- Two nucleoside reverse transcriptase inhibitors (NRTI) e.g. zidovudine, lamivudine, didanosine
- PLUS EITHER
- One protease inhibitor (PI) e.g. indinavir OR
- One non-nucleoside reverse transcriptase inhibitor (NNRTI) e.g. nevirapine.[1]

Adverse reactions

The toxicity associated with the different regimens stems from the component drugs. As classes, the NRTIs are associated with lactic acidosis and hepatic steatosis; the NNRTIs with rash, abnormal liver function tests and fever; and the PIs with lipodystrophy, hyperglycaemia, hyperlipidaemia and abnormal liver function tests.

Importantly, the PIs and NNRTIs are metabolized by cytochrome P450 enzymes and interact with many other drugs. These drugs should not be prescribed with cisapride, dihydroergotamine, ergotamine, benzodiazepines and rifampicin. There are many other potential drug interactions with the antiretroviral agents, and new prescriptions should be made with care.

Outpatient parenteral antibiotic therapy

Outpatient parenteral antibiotic therapy (OPAT) has been widely used for the treatment of moderate to serious infections, either as an alternative to hospitalization or following initial hospitalization and early discharge once the patient is over the toxic phase of the infection. A wide range of infections are suitable for OPAT therapy (Table 9.9.2).

Significant savings both in terms of direct and indirect costs are possible utilizing OPAT. Appropriate patient selection is essential for safe and effective outpatient parenteral therapy. (Tables 9.9.3 and 9.9.4). Patients should be clinically stable, willing to participate and physically and mentally capable of being treated at home (Table 9.9.4).

Some patients require initial hospitalization (Table 9.9.5), following which they may be suitable for early discharge to continue treatment at home.

Table 9.9.2 Conditions that can be treated on an outpatient basis with parenteral antibiotic therapy

AIDS	Soft-tissue infections
Associated Infections	Cellulitis
	Wound infections/abscesses
Cardiac	**Bone and joint infections**
Endocarditis	Osteomyelitis
Prosthetic-valve infections	Septic arthritis
	Prosthetic infections
	Neurological infections
	Meningitis
Genitourinary	**Other infections**
Pyelonephritis	Bacteraemia
Complicated urinary-tract infections	Mastoiditis
Prostatitis	
Pelvic inflammatory disease	
Respiratory	
Pneumonia	
Lung abscess	

Table 9.9.3 Patient selection process

Condition suitable for outpatient therapy
Patient does not fulfil need to admit criteria (Table 9.9.5)
OR
Patient meets discharge criteria (Table 9.9.6)
Home environment suitable
Patient/family consent

Table 9.9.4 Patient selection criteria

Able to give consent
Adequate social support at home
The antibiotic(s) chosen is/are appropriate for OPAT use
Patient's condition is stable
Concurrent illness does not require hospital care
Adequate venous access can be maintained
Patient is mobile
The infection is amenable to outpatient parenteral therapy
Adequate monitoring by the treating medical team is possible

Table 9.9.5 Criteria for admission to hospital

Confused
Persistent high fever
Systolic blood pressure <100 mmHg
Respiratory rate >30/min
Pulse rate >100/min
Requires specialized nursing care assistance with activities of daily living
Hypoxic on room air (PaO$_2$ <80 mmHg)
Concurrent illness requiring inpatient care
Personal or social reasons
Pneumonic consolidation in more than one lobe.

Table 9.9.6 Discharge criteria

Medical
Afebrile
Clinical improvement
No specialized nursing care required
Stable
Bacterial pathogens identified
Response to inpatient therapy
Complications unlikely
Social
Parents interested and motivated
Parents capable
Home environment acceptable
Telephone and transport access

Once patients comply with predefined discharge criteria (Table 9.9.6) they may be able to be discharged into an outpatient parenteral therapy programme.

Close patient monitoring is essential, with daily reviews by a nurse either by telephone or face to face while patients are in the programme. Patients should be reviewed at least weekly by a physician.

The benefits of OPAT include a reduction in overall costs of patient care through avoidance or reduction in hospitalization, reduction of the costs associated with the hazards of hospitalization, and increased patient satisfaction.[24,25]

Other issues

The risks associated with bioterrorism need to be taken into account with each and every patient presenting with a febrile illness or signs and symptoms of infection.

Numerous bacterial agents and bacterial toxins have been identified as potential biological agents. Patients presenting in clusters or with unusual or uncommon infections, particularly those that can be used as biological agents, should be quarantined, with staff utilizing PPE and strict infection control procedures. It may be necessary to activate the hospital's Mass Casualty Incident Plan when biological agents are suspected.[26]

Likely developments over the next 5–10 years

The most important challenge regarding infectious disease in the future will be:

❶ The containment of and management of antimicrobial resistance patterns. In part, these patterns have emerged as a result of poor prescribing habits.[27]

❷ Fewer new antimicrobial drugs are being developed, with the result that with developing resistance patterns there will be very few effective antibiotics available for use against infection.

❸ The implementation of prescribing guidelines based on scientific evidence will form the basis of all antibiotic prescribing.

❹ Human behaviour, wildlife trade, factory farming, poor hygiene, global warming and increasing travel will increase the risk of pandemics, evolution and spread of new and old infections.[28–30]

Detailed descriptions of the drugs described above are available on the Internet by accessing MIMS Online[31] and Antibiotic Guidelines.[32]

References

1. Therapeutic Guidelines Limited 2000 Therapeutic Guidelines: Antibiotic, Version 11, Therapeutic Guidelines Limited (pub), Melbourne.
2. Weinstein L, Dalton AC. Host determinants of response to antimicrobial agents. New England Journal of Medicine 1968; 279: 467.
3. Moellering RC Jr. Factors influencing the clinical use of antimicrobial agents in elderly patients. Geriatrics 1978; 33: 83.
4. Philipson A. The use of antibiotics in pregnancy. Journal of Antimicrobiological Chemotherapy 1983; 12: 101.
5. Moellering RC Jr. Principles of anti-infective therapy. In: Mandell GL, Bennett JE, Dolin R, eds. Principles and practice of infectious diseases, 4th edn. New York: Churchill Livingstone, 1995; 199–212.
6. Schlichting D, McCollam JS. Recognising and managing severe sepsis: a common and deadly threat. Southern Medical Journal 2007; 100: 594–600.
7. Davies J. Inactivation of antibiotics and the dissemination of resistance genes. Science 1994; 264: 375–382.
8. Nikaido H. Prevention of drug access to bacterial targets: permeability barriers and active efflux. Science 1994; 264: 382–388.
9. Spratt BG. Resistance to antibiotics mediated by target alterations. Science 1994; 264: 388–393.
10. Kopecko D. Specialized genetic recombination systems in bacteria: their involvement in gene expression and evolution. Proceedings in Molecular and Subcellular Biology 1980; 7: 135–243.
11. Elwell LP, Roberts M, Mayer LW, et al. Plasmid-mediated beta-lactamase production in Neisseria gonorrhoeae.

Antimicrobiological Agents and Chemotherapy 1977; 11: 528–533.
12. Lyon BR, Skurray R. Antimicrobial resistance of Staphylococcus aureus: genetic basis. Microbiology Review 1987; 5: 88–134.
13. Chambers HF, Sande MA. Antimicrobial agents. In: Goodman and Gilman's The pharmacological basis of therapeutics, 9th edn. New York: McGraw-Hill, 1995; 1029–1032.
14. Stillwell M, Caplan ES. The septic multiple-trauma patient. Infectious Disease Clinics of North America 1989; 3: 155.
15. Kobayashi Y, Takahashi T, Nakae T. Diffusion of beta-lactam antibiotics through liposome membranes containing purified porins. Antimicrobiological Agents and Chemotherapy 1982; 2: 775–780.
16. Idsoe O, Gothe T, Wilcox RR, et al. Nature and extent of penicillin side reactions with particular reference to fatalities from anaphylactic shock. Bulletin of the WHO 1968; 38: 159.
17. Pichichero ME. A review of evidence supporting the American Academy of Pediatrics recommendation for prescribing cephalosporin antibiotics for penicillin-allergic patients. Pediatrics 2005; 115: 1048–1057.
18. Periti P, Mazzei T, Mini E, Novelli A. Pharmacokinetic drug interactions of macrolides. Clinical Pharmacokinetics 1992; 23: 106–131.
19. Spera RV Jr, Farber BF. Multiply-resistant Enterococcus faecium. The nosocomial pathogen of the 1990s. Journal of the American Medical Association 1992; 268: 2563–2564.
20. Lau AH, Lam NP, Piscitelli SC, et al. Clinical pharmacokinetics of metronidazole and other

nitroimidazole anti-infectives. Clinical Pharmacokinetics 1992; 2: 328–364.
21. Johnson PJ. Metronidazole and drug resistance. Parasitology Today 1993; 9: 183–186.
22. McCalla DR, Reuvers A, Kaiser C. Mode of action of nitrofurazone. Journal of Bacteriology 1970; 104: 1126–1134.
23. Speer BS, Shoemaker NB, Salyers AA. Bacterial resistance to tetracycline: mechanisms, transfer and clinical significance. Clinical Microbiology Review 1992; 5: 387–399.
24. Tice AD. Outpatient Parenteral Antibiotic Therapy (OPAT) in the United States: Delivery models and indications for use. Canadian Journal of Infectious Diseases 2000; 11A: 45A–48A.
25. Vinen JD. Intravenous antibiotic treatment outside the hospital: safety and health economic aspects Review of Contemporary Pharmacotherapy 1995; 6: 435–44, 525.
26. www.bt.cdc.gov/Agent/agentlist.asp, last accessed November 2007.
27. Gross EA, Stephens D. Multi-drug resistant bacteria: implications for the emergency physician. Emergency Medicine Reports 2007; 28.
28. WHO World Health Report. 2007: A Safer Future. www.who.com.
29. Singer JI, Williams M. Imported infections in pediatric travelers. Emergency Medicine Reports 2007; 28.
30. CDC. 2007 Travellers' Health: Yellow Book wwwn.cdc.gov/travel/contentYellowBook.aspx, last accessed November 2007.
31. MIMS Online. http://mims.hcn.net.au/, last accessed November 2007.
32. Therapeutic Guidelines – Antibiotic version 13, 2006 – www.tg.com.au

9.10 Needlestick injuries and related blood and body fluid exposures

Sean Arendse • Alan C. Street

ESSENTIALS

1 Avoiding blood and other body fluid exposure remains the primary means of preventing occupationally acquired bloodborne virus infections.

2 The risks of acquiring infection after occupational exposure to bloodborne viruses are: HIV 0.3%,[1] hepatitis B (HBV) 1–62%,[2] hepatitis C (HCV) 1.8%.[3,4]

3 HBV immunization is an integral part of workplace safety.

4 Effective post-exposure prophylaxis (PEP) is available for both HBV and HIV, but not HCV.

5 Significant emotional distress often complicates needlestick and related occupational injuries.

Introduction

Management of the healthcare worker who sustains an occupational exposure to blood or other potentially infectious body fluids (e.g. semen, vaginal secretions, CSF and fluids containing visible blood,) is an important issue for the emergency department (ED) doctor. An estimated 800 000 such injuries occur each year in the USA,[5] although this figure is a conservative estimate as many needlestick injuries go unreported. HBV, HCV and HIV are the most important occupationally acquired bloodborne pathogens, although many other organisms, including malaria, syphilis, cytomegalovirus, and possibly the prion diseases such as Creutzfeld–Jakob disease, may also be transmissible via this route.

Most exposures do not result in infection, and the risk of infection following significant exposure varies with factors such as:

- The pathogen involved (hepatitis B, hepatitis C or HIV).
- The fluid involved – blood is generally the most infectious body fluid.
- The type of exposure – percutaneous or mucous membrane/non-intact skin.
- The amount of blood or other infectious body fluid involved in the exposure.
- The amount of virus in the patient's blood at the time of exposure.

General issues

Prevention of needlestick injuries

The old adage 'prevention is better than cure' certainly rings true when considering needlestick injuries.

The potentially infectious nature of all blood and bodily fluids necessitates the implementation of infection control practices. The universal application of standard precautions should be the minimum level of infection control when treating patients to prevent bloodborne virus transmission. The important elements of standard precautions are:

- The use of gloves when contact with blood, body fluids or secretions is anticipated.
- The use of masks and protective eyewear during procedures that have the potential to generate splashes or sprays of blood or bodily fluids.
- The use of gowns to protect skin and clothing from soiling by blood and other bodily fluids.
- Correct handling and disposal of needles and other sharp instruments.
- Correct handling and disposal of needles and other sharp instruments.
  - Disposal of sharps directly from patient immediately into sharps bins
  - Locating sharps bins conveniently to reduce the unnecessary transportation of uncapped devices
  - Avoiding overfilling sharps containers
  - Never re-sheathing or re-capping needles
  - 100% attention when handling sharps.

More than 50 products with features designed to prevent needlestick injuries are currently available, and fall broadly into two categories: those providing 'passive' or automatic protection and those with a safety mechanism that the user must activate. These devices include i.v. connectors, needle guards, sheathed syringes, needle-recapping products, blood-drawing devices, i.v. catheters, and needleless injection devices. Pilot studies conducted at 10 hospitals in New York State in 1990 and 1991 found that needlestick injuries declined by 75–94% in the hospitals using these preventive devices.[6]

Hospital systems

Hospitals need to have appropriate policies and procedures to deal with occupational exposures to blood and body fluids; these are best implemented through a comprehensive and coordinated occupational exposure programme. Depending on the individual institution, such a programme is usually managed by infection control personnel, and also involves staff health, occupational health, laboratory services, the ED and the infectious diseases service.

Staff need to be aware of the appropriate steps to take in the event that they sustain an exposure, such as who to notify, incident reporting requirements, and where and how to seek medical evaluation. The programme should develop processes for consent and testing of the source individual (including situations where the individual refuses or is unable to give consent), prompt bloodborne virus testing, and communication of results to the exposed person. Clear written guidelines and clinical pathways should be accessible to medical staff involved in managing these exposures (including specific recommendations for exposures involving a bloodborne virus positive source, and antiretroviral post-exposure prophylaxis).

Initial management

Occupational exposure to blood or other potentially infectious body fluids should be considered a medical emergency to ensure timely management. Following exposure the exposed person should be removed from the area and general first aid measures applied:

- For skin exposures – wash the exposed area well with soap and water; if no water is available, use an alcohol-based antiseptic.
- For eye exposures – remove contact lenses if present, and irrigate eyes with copious amounts of water or saline.
- For oral mucous membrane exposures – spit out contaminating material and rinse the mouth with water several times.

Hepatitis B

Hepatitis B vaccination is recommended for all healthcare workers who are involved in direct patient care or who handle human blood or tissues,[7] and is an important infection control and occupational health strategy. Healthcare workers should be aware of their HBV immunization status and should undergo antibody testing 4–8 weeks after the last dose of the HBV vaccine to ascertain their immune status.

The risk of acquiring HBV from occupational blood/body fluid exposure to a patient positive for hepatitis B surface antigen (HBsAg) is well recognized and related primarily to the degree of contact with blood and the hepatitis B e antigen (HBeAg) status of the source. Following contact with a source positive for HBeAg, the risk of clinical hepatitis is 22–31% and serological evidence of HBV infection develops in 37–62% of exposed, non-immune individuals. In contrast, after exposure to HBeAg-negative blood, there is a 1–6% risk of clinical hepatitis and a 23–37% risk of serological evidence of HBV infection.[2] The average time from exposure to the development of symptoms is 10 weeks (range 4–26 weeks). Routine vaccination against HBV has been recommended for healthcare workers since the early 1980s,[8] with a consequent marked reduction in the incidence of infection in this population.

Post-exposure management following an occupational blood/body fluid exposure to HBV requires evaluation of the source's HBsAg status, and the HBV vaccination and vaccine response status of the exposed person.[9,10] HB immunoglobulin (HBIG) is indicated for people who are non-immune (either because of no prior vaccination, or because of vaccine non-responsiveness) and are exposed to blood or other infectious body fluids from a HBsAg-positive source. HBIG is prepared from human plasma (screened for bloodborne viruses) known to contain a high titre of antibody to HBsAg (antiHBs). The dose of HBIG is 400 IU, given i.m. Concomitantly, HBV vaccination should be injected at a separate site and a full course completed. Table 9.10.1 provides more detailed information about specific indications for HBIG and hepatitis B vaccination following occupational exposures.

Hepatitis C

The risk associated with occupational exposure to hepatitis C following a parenteral injury is estimated to range between 1.8% and 10%.[11]

Transmission to healthcare workers has never been documented from skin contamination and rarely from mucous membrane

INFECTIOUS DISEASES

Table 9.10.1 HBV prophylaxis following occupational exposure

Source	Unvaccinated healthcare worker	Vaccinated healthcare worker
HBs antigen positive	HBIG course of vaccination	1. if >10 mIU/ml – reassure 2. if<10 mIU/ml – HBIG & repeat course of vaccination 3. if result not available within 24 h, consider HBIG
HBs antigen negative	Course of vaccination	1. if >10 mIU/ml – reassure 2. if <10 mIU/ml – consider repeat vaccination
Unknown source	1. Consider HBIG 2. Commence course of vaccination	1. if >10 mIU/ml – reassure 2. if <10 mIU/ml – booster HBV vac ± HBIG

HBIG if indicated should preferably be given within 24 hours.
HBV vaccine should also be administered as soon as possible (preferably within 24 hours).
Exposed healthcare workers do not need to take any special precautions to prevent secondary transmission.[12]

exposure. In contrast to HBV, environmental contamination is not significant.[13]

Numerous studies and laboratory experiments have failed to demonstrate a role for either immunoglobulin[14] or antiviral agents (e.g. interferon-α and/or ribavirin)[15] in post-exposure prophylaxis. However, it is important to document infection because chronic hepatitis will develop in more than 50% of infected adults, and these patients may respond to treatment with interferon-α.

Recommendations for the management of occupational exposures to HCV are aimed at achieving early identification of infection. Recent data suggest that antiviral treatment of acute HCV infection increases rates of HCV clearance.[16,17] If the source's HCV antibody test is positive, then polymerase chain reaction (PCR) testing for HCV RNA should be performed. Transmission is much less likely to occur from a source who is PCR negative, and the exposed individual can be reassured that the transmission of HCV in this case is negligible. If the source is positive for HCV RNA, a baseline serum from the exposed person is tested for anti-HCV and

ALT with follow-up testing 3 and 6 months after the exposure (Table 9.10.2). HCV viraemia can be detected by PCR between 10 days and 6 weeks after infection[18] early diagnosis by PCR may reduce the already low potential risk of HCV transmission to patients from healthcare workers who perform exposure prone procedures.

Early recognition of acute HCV infection in healthcare workers may reduce the risk of staff-to-patient transmission, as recent data suggest that early antiviral treatment of acute HCV infection vastly increases viral clearance.[16]

Human immunodeficiency virus

The average risk of acquiring human immunodeficiency virus (HIV) infection from all types of reported percutaneous exposure to HIV-infected blood is 0.3%.[1] This is increased for exposures involving:

- A deep injury.
- Visible blood on the device causing the injury.

- A device previously placed in the source's artery or vein.
- A source with terminal AIDS who has died as a result of AIDS within 60 days of the exposure, and thus is presumed to have a high titre of HIV.[19]

These factors are also probably significant for mucous membrane and skin exposures to HIV-infected blood, where the average risk of HIV transmission is approximately 0.09% and <0.09% respectively.[20] Prolonged or extensive skin contact or visibly compromised skin integrity would also suggest a higher risk.

Healthcare workers potentially exposed to HIV need to be evaluated as soon as possible after the exposure, preferably within 2 hours. If the source is seronegative for HIV, baseline testing and further follow-up of the exposed person is normally not necessary. If the source HIV antibody test is positive or inconclusive, or the source is not available for testing, HIV antibody testing of the exposed person should be performed at 6 weeks, 12 weeks and (if antiretroviral post-exposure prophylaxis is given – see below) 6 months (Table 9.10.3). Extended HIV follow-up testing (12 months) is recommended for healthcare workers who become infected with HCV following exposure to a source coinfected with HIV/HCV.

Table 9.10.3 Recommended HIV post-exposure

Basic (2-drug) regimens	Expanded (3-drug) regimens
Zidovudine (ZDV) 300 mg and lamivudine (3TC) 150 mg one tablet bd or tenofovir (TDF) 300 mg and emtricitabine (FTC) 200 mg one tablet daily	Either basic regimen plus (lopinavir 200 mg/ritonavir 50 mg) two tablets bd.

Table 9.10.2 Serology testing for recipient

Source	At time of exposure	6 weeks	3 months	6 months	12 months
Low risk source and negative serology	Hep B surface antibody and store serum		HIV and Hep C antibody test may be offered		
High risk source and positive serology	Baseline HIV, Hep C and Hep B Surface antibody recommended	HIV and Hep C antibody test	HIV and Hep C antibody test recommended	HIV and Hep C antibody test recommended	HIV and Hep C antibody test recommended
Unknown source	Baseline HIV, Hep C and Hep B Surface antibody recommended		HIV and Hep C antibody test recommended	HIV and Hep C antibody test recommended	

Recommendations for post-exposure prophylaxis (PEP) with antiretroviral agents have been guided by a better understanding of the pathogenesis of primary HIV infection, which indicates that HIV infection does not become established immediately; this leaves a brief window of opportunity during which post-exposure antiretroviral intervention might modify or prevent viral replication. An early case–control study demonstrated that use of zidovudine decreased the risk of occupational HIV seroconversion by 81%,[21] and it is likely (but not proven) that combination antiretroviral therapy provides even greater protection. Animal data also support the use of antiretroviral prophylaxis after exposure to HIV, provided prophylaxis is administered promptly and for an adequate period. Failures of HIV PEP are well documented with both single drug and combination drug regimens.[22]

HIV PEP should be initiated promptly, preferably within 2 hours of the exposure, although it may still be effective for up to 72 hours. Recommendations for HIV PEP include a basic 4-week regimen of two drugs for most HIV exposures, and an expanded regimen that includes the addition of a third drug for HIV exposures that pose an increased risk of transmission (Table 9.10.2). Decisions about the need for HIV PEP and choice of antiretroviral agents should only be made in consultation with a physician who has expertise in this area, such as an infectious diseases physician. A 3–5-day supply of PEP antiretroviral agents (a 'starter pack') should be kept in the ED.

Most occupational exposures do not result in transmission of HIV, and the potential benefits of PEP need to be carefully weighed against the toxicity of the drugs involved. Nearly 50% of healthcare workers taking HIV PEP experience adverse symptoms (e.g. nausea, malaise, headache, diarrhoea and anorexia) and approximately 33% cease because of side effects.[23,24] The importance of completing the prescribed regimen needs to be stressed, and measures taken to minimize side effects.

The emotional effect of an occupational HIV exposure is substantial[25,26] and often underestimated. The exposed person may need time off work, short-term use of a night-time sedative, or even referral for formal psychological or psychiatric counselling. Patients should be advised of measures to prevent secondary transmission (e.g. safer sexual practices) during the follow-up period, especially the first 6–12 weeks.

Maintaining confidentiality for the staff member sustaining exposure is a priority, as it may have lasting implications both personally and professionally.

The circumstances surrounding the exposure should be reviewed as part of the hospital's occupational exposure policy, and appropriate preventive and educational measures taken if indicated.

Exposures that occur in the community

Blood or body fluid exposures may be sustained in the community, as well as in healthcare settings; examples include needlestick injuries from improperly discarded needles and syringes, or blood splashes to the eye or mouth in the course of an altercation. The exposed person may be a member of the public, or of an emergency service such as a policemen or ambulance officer. These exposures are usually managed in the ED.

Although the principles of management are broadly similar to those for occupational exposures, there are some important differences. First, the source is almost never available for testing. (If the source syringe has been retrieved by the exposed person, this should *not* be tested for bloodborne viruses because such testing is only validated on serum.) Second, needlestick exposures almost always involve old dried blood; this is much less infectious than fresh blood because the viral titre falls with time, and dried blood does not pass easily from the lumen of the needle into the exposed person's subcutaneous tissue. Third, these exposures often provoke a considerable degree of distress in the affected person, and there may be considerable pressure from the exposed person, a family member or a colleague to 'do something'. Some of these incidents even attract media attention.

In Australia, only 1–2% of injecting drug users are HIV infected, so the risk of HIV transmission from a discarded needlestick injury is negligible: 1:100 (risk source is HIV positive) × 1:300 (risk of HIV transmission after needlestick) × undefined factor to account for old dried blood (say 1:5), or approximately 1 in 150 000. Similar calculations show a potentially higher risk of hepatitis B and C transmission, but in reality documented instances of bloodborne virus infection resulting from these community exposures are extremely rare, and people should be reassured about this.

In Australia, antiretroviral prophylaxis is not recommended for these exposures unless there are particularly compelling epidemiological circumstances to indicate a high HIV risk in the source. People not previously vaccinated against HBV should be given HBIG and the first dose of a hepatitis B vaccination course. Despite the low risk of bloodborne virus transmission, many patients feel more reassured if they are offered baseline and follow-up testing. As with exposures in the hospital setting, the attending doctor needs to provide the affected person with information, support and a sympathetic ear!

Provision of antiretroviral prophylaxis following sexual exposures in the community is a highly specialized field and is outside the scope of this chapter; advice should be sought from a doctor with HIV expertise. Interested readers are referred to guidelines produced by the Australian Department of Health and Ageing, available at http://www.ashm.org.au/pep-guidelines/

Illustrative cases

Case 1

A 4-year-old child presents to the ED after stepping on a needle at the beach. The parents have the needle. The child has never been vaccinated against hepatitis B.

Management

- Reassurance: risk of transmission of HBV ~30%, HCV ~10%, HIV <0.3% where source is known to be infected with these viruses. With regard to HIV (usually the chief concern of parents), the needle is likely to have come from an injecting drug user but the risk of HIV transmission is miniscule (see calculation above). Therefore, PEP is not indicated (but note that it may be indicated in other countries if the risk of HIV in injecting drug users is higher).
- No benefit in testing needle.
- Obtain baseline serum specimen from child.

- Offer:
  - HBIG/HIV vaccination if not previously vaccinated
  - Tetanus prophylaxis and vaccination if indicated
  - Advise parents of symptoms of hepatitis
  - Serology for HIV at 6 weeks and 3 months, HCV at 3 months and 6 months, HBsAg at 6 months.

Case 2

A 23-year-old intern sustains a needlestick injury through a glove to the pulp of the left index finger after taking arterial blood gases from a newly diagnosed HIV patient with *Pneumocystis jiroveci* pneumonia who is not on antiretroviral therapy. The source patient is HBsAg and hepatitis C antibody negative.

Management

- Medical emergency – urgent medical assessment.
- Contact infectious diseases doctor (or nominated specialist, as per hospital policy).
- Risk assessment – percutaneous injury with needle previously in patient's artery (higher risk exposure), untreated HIV positive source (high-titre exposure), antiretroviral resistance unlikely.
- Obtain baseline serum from intern.
- Begin antiretroviral prophylaxis as quickly as possible – three-drug (expanded) regimen.
- Provide support – counselling, information about PEP drugs, advice about safe sex, contact telephone numbers (e.g. of infectious diseases physician).
- Organize specialist follow-up in next 48–72 hours as per hospital policy.
- Ensure that incident is reported through usual hospital incident reporting mechanism.

Case 3

A healthcare worker presents to the ED having had blood on her ungloved hands while caring for an HIV patient. She has no visible cuts or other skin defects on her hands. She received HBV vaccination some years previously and responded serologically. The source patient is known to be HBsAg and hepatitis C antibody negative.

Management

- Counselling regarding negligible risk of HIV transmission with intact skin exposures.
- Discuss with infectious disease physician or specialist nominated in hospital policy (chiefly to reassure staff member) – very low risk exposure and PEP not indicated.
- Despite low risk, anticipate psychological distress.
- Reinforce practice of standard precautions (e.g. wearing gloves).
- Follow-up serology not necessary, unless specifically requested by exposed person.

References

1. Bell DM. Occupational risk of human immunodeficiency virus infection in health-care workers: an overview. American Journal of Medicine 1997; 102: 9–15.
2. Werner BG, Grady GF. Accidental hepatitis-B-surface-antigen-positive inoculations: use of e antigen to estimate infectivity. Annals of Internal Medicine 1982; 97: 367–369.
3. Lanphear BP, Linnemann CC Jr, Cannon CG, et al. Hepatitis C virus infection in healthcare workers: risk of exposure and infection. Infection Control and Hospital Epidemiology 1994; 15: 745–570.
4. Mitsiu T, Iwano K, Masuko K, et al. Hepatitis C viral infection in medical personnel after needlestick accident. Hepatology 1992; 16: 1109–1114.
5. Jagger JI. Preventing HIV transmission in health care workers with safer needle devices. 6th International Conference on AIDS, San Francisco, California, 22 June 1990.
6. Chiarello LA, Nagin D, Laufer F March. Pilot study of needlestick prevention devices, Report to the legislature, New York State Department of Health, 1992; 16.
7. Australian Immunization Handbook 8th Edition. 2003 (National Health and Medical Research Council). http://www.immunise.health.gov.au.
8. CDC. Recommendation of the Immunization Practices Advisory Commitee (ACIP) inactivated hepatitis B virus vaccine. Morbidity and Mortality Weekly Report 1982; 31: 317–328.
9. Grady GF, Lee VA, Prince AM, et al. Hepatitis B immune globulin for accidental exposures among medical personnel; final report of a multicenter controlled trial. Journal of Infectious Diseases 1978; 138: 625–638.
10. Seeff LB, Zimmerman HJ, Wrught EC, et al. A randomized, double blind controlled trial of the efficacy of immune serum globulin for the prevention of post-transfusion hepatitis: a Veterans Administation cooperative study. Gastroenterology 1977; 72: 111–121.
11. HIV/Viral hepatitis – a guide for primary care, Australian society for HIV medicine inc. 2001.
12. CDC. Recommendations for the prevention and control of hepatitis C virus (HCV) infection and HCV-related chronic disease. Morbidity and Mortality Week Report 1998; 47(No. RR-19).
13. Polish LB, Tong MJ, Co RL, Risk factors for hepatitis C virus infection among health care personnel in a community hospital. American Journal of Infection Control 1993; 21: 196–200.
14. Alter MJ. Occupational exposure to hepatitis C virus: a dilemma. Infection Control and Hospital Epidemiology 1994; 15: 742–744.
15. Peters M, Davis GL, Dooley JS. The interferon system in acute and chronic viral hepatitis. Progress in Liver Disease 1986; 8: 453–467.
16. Jaeckel E, Cornberg M, Wedemeyer H, et al. Treatment of acute hepatitis C with interferon alpha-2b. New England Journal of Medicine 2001; 345: 1452–1457.
17. Gerberding JL. 2003 Clinical practice. Occupational exposure to HIV in health care settings. The New England Journal of Medicine 348: 826.
18. Zaaijer HL, Cuypers HT, Reesink HW, et al. Reliability of polymerase chain reaction for detection of hepatitis C virus Infection. Lancet 1993; 341: 722–724.
19. CDC. Case-control study of HIV seroconversion in health care workers after percutaneous exposure to HIV-infected blood -France, United Kingdom and United States, Jan. 1988-Aug. 1994. Morbidity and Mortality Weekly Report 1995; 44: 929–933.
20. Gerberding JL. Management of occupational exposure to blood borne viruses. New England Journal of Medicine 1995; 332: 444–551.
21. Cardo DM, Culver DH, Ciesielski CA, et al. A case-control study of HIV seroconversion in health care workers after percutaneous exposure. New England Journal of Medicine 1997 337: 1485–1490.
22. Jochimsen EM. Failures of zidovudine postexposure prophylaxis. American Journal of Medicine 1997 102 (suppl 5B): 52–55.
23. Wang SA, Panlilio AL, Doi PA, et al. Experience of healthcare workers taking postexposure prophylaxis after occupational HIV exposure: findings of the HIV postexposure prophylaxis registry. Infection Control and Hospital Epidemiology 2000; 21: 780–785.
24. Parkin JM, Murphy M, Anderson J, et al. Tolerability and side effects of post-exposure prophylaxis for HIV infection [Letter]. Lancet 2000; 335: 722–723.
25. Armstrong K, Gordon R, Santorella G. Occupational exposures of health care workers (HCWs) to human immunodeficiency virus (HIV): stress reactions and counselling interventions. Social Work and Health Care 1995; 21: 61–80.
26. Henry K, Campbell S, Jackson B, et al. Long-term follow-up of health care workers with work-site exposure to human immunodeficiency virus [Letter]. Journal of the American Medical Association 1990; 236: 1765.

Further reading

CDC guidelines 2001 (available at NH&MRC infection control guidelines (available at http://www.health.gov.au/internet/wcms/publishing.nsf/Content/Guidelines-2)

GENITOURINARY

Edited by **George Jelinek**

10.1 Acute kidney injury

Nicholas Adams • Linas Dziukas

ESSENTIALS

1 Acute renal dysfunction occurs when there is a rapid reduction in the glomerular filtration rate; serum creatinine (SCr) concentration increases rapidly.

2 Definitions of acute renal failure have focused on patients who have a marked increase in SCr or need renal replacement treatment. However, even small rises in SCr increase morbidity and mortality.

3 Acute kidney injury (AKI) includes the complete spectrum of acute renal dysfunction: prerenal azotaemia, and the RISK, INJURY and FAILURE stages of the RIFLE classification of acute renal dysfunction. The commonly used term 'acute renal failure' (ARF) corresponds to the FAILURE stage.

4 The early stages of AKI are usually asymptomatic, and the diagnosis is based on a decrease in urine output or elevated SCr. It may take 24 h or more for an initially normal SCr concentration to definitely increase, and up to 48 h to distinguish between early AKI and renal failure.

5 The basic processes causing AKI are renal hypoperfusion (prerenal causes), damage to glomeruli, tubules, interstitium or blood vessels (renal causes), or obstruction to urine flow (postrenal causes).

6 Prerenal factors are present in about 40% of persons with AKI. They are caused by hypovolaemia, hypotension, oedematous states with a reduced 'effective' circulating volume, renal hypoperfusion and drugs.

7 Bedside correction of hypovolaemia should be based on jugular venous pulse and urine output, and their response to intravenous fluid resuscitation. Assessment of the patient's volume state by measurement of the central venous pressure does not improve outcome.

8 Renal factors are present in about 50% of persons with AKI. Acute tubular necrosis (ATN) is the most common pathological process causing ARF, and is classified as ischaemic ATN or ATN due to damage by toxins (e.g. myoglobin) or drugs. No therapeutic intervention has hastened the recovery of renal function in established ATN.

9 Obstruction is present in about 10% of persons with AKI. Hydronephrosis can occur in the absence of obstruction, and some persons with obstruction do not have a dilated urinary collecting system.

10 Urine output usually decreases in AKI, and the patient may be oliguric (less than 400 mL per day) or anuric (less than 100 mL per day). Only a few conditions cause complete anuria: total obstruction, vascular lesions, severe ATN or rapidly progressive glomerulonephritis.

11 Intravenous mannitol and sodium bicarbonate to produce an alkaline diuresis as a means of preventing ATN in severe rhabdomyolysis has not been shown to be effective.

12 The evidence that sodium bicarbonate is effective in treating acute hyperkalaemia is equivocal.

13 There is no evidence that potassium-exchange resins are effective in the acute treatment of hyperkalaemia.

Introduction

The first recognition of illness caused by a sudden decline in renal function ('ischuria renalis') was by William Heberden in 1802.[1] In 1888 Delafield described a form of 'acute Bright's disease' that was caused by toxins, various infectious diseases and extensive injuries, and where there was degeneration or death of tubule cells.[2] Impaired renal function in injured soldiers was described in World War I ('war nephritis') and in World War II.[3,4] The term 'acute renal failure' (ARF) was first used in 1951.[5]

The basic process in ARF is a rapid (hours to days) reduction in the glomerular filtration rate (GFR) due to renal hypoperfusion (prerenal causes), damage to glomeruli, tubules, interstitium or blood vessels (renal causes), or obstruction to urine flow (postrenal causes). The GFR is inversely related to the serum creatinine (SCr) concentration. The diagnosis of ARF is made when there is an increase in the SCr concentration, with or without a decrease in the urine output. A simple definition of ARF is an acute and sustained (lasting for 48 h or more) increase in the SCr of 44 μmol/L if the baseline is less than 221 μmol/L, or an increase in the SCr of more than 20% if the baseline is more than 221 μmol/L.[6] A more comprehensive definition (the RIFLE system) is used to classify persons with acute impairment of renal function[7] (Table 10.1.1).

The term 'acute kidney injury' (AKI) includes the spectrum of functional and structural changes seen in renal failure. AKI includes prerenal azotaemia, and the RISK, INJURY and FAILURE stages of the RIFLE system. ARF is applied to the FAILURE stage of the RIFLE system.

Aetiology and pathogenesis

The causes of AKI are grouped according to the probable source of renal injury: prerenal, renal (parenchymal) and postrenal. More than one cause can be present in AKI.

Prerenal acute kidney injury

Prerenal AKI is an adaptive response to severe volume depletion and hypotension in structurally intact nephrons. Prerenal AKI that is prolonged or inadequately treated can be followed by parenchymal renal damage. Prerenal AKI is a potentially reversible cause of ARF.

Reductions in renal blood flow (RBF) and GFR occur in the setting(s) of hypovolaemia, hypotension (cardiogenic shock, anaphylaxis, sepsis), oedematous states with a reduced 'effective' circulating volume (cardiac failure, hepatic cirrhosis, nephrotic syndrome) or renal hypoperfusion (renal artery stenosis, hepatorenal syndrome). Drugs that interfere with autoregulation (e.g. prostaglandin inhibitors, angiotensin converting enzyme (ACE) inhibitors or angiotensin II receptor antagonists) also reduce glomerular perfusion. The physiological responses to volume depletion and hypotension, and the link to prerenal AKI, are shown in Figure 10.1.1.

In the early stages of hypovolaemia the serum urea concentration can increase before there is a rise in SCr concentration. An increase in the serum urea concentration or the blood urea nitrogen (BUN) concentration with a normal SCr concentration when renal perfusion is reduced is called prerenal azotaemia. If acute renal hypoperfusion is prolonged the serum urea concentration and the SCr concentration are both increased.

Renal (parenchymal) acute kidney injury

Ischaemic, cytotoxic or inflammatory processes damage the renal parenchyma. The causes of the damage are grouped according to the major structures that are damaged: vessels, glomeruli, renal tubules or renal interstitial tissue.

Vascular causes involving the larger vessels are acute thrombosis of the renal artery, embolism of the renal arteries, renal artery dissection and renal vein thrombosis. Damage to the renal microvasculature is caused by inflammatory damage (e.g. glomerulonephritis or vasculitis), malignant hypertension or thrombotic microangiopathy (TMA).

Glomerulonephritis causes proteinuria, haematuria, nephrotic syndrome, nephritic syndrome or chronic renal failure. Rapidly progressive glomerulonephritis (RPG) is a rare type of glomerulonephritis with extensive cellular crescents in the glomeruli. Patients with RPG can develop oliguric AKI that progress within weeks to end-stage renal failure.

Acute tubular necrosis (ATN) is the most common pathological process that causes ARF. While the terminology suggests that the main cause is tubular damage, the actual pathophysiology is more complex: impaired autoregulation and marked intrarenal vasoconstriction (the main mechanism for the greatly reduced GFR), tubular damage (with cytoskeleton breakdown), increased tubuloglomerular feedback, endothelial cell injury, fibrin deposition in the microcirculation, release of cytokines, activation of inflammation and activation of the immune system.[8,9]

ATN is classified as ischaemic ATN or cytotoxic ATN (due to damage by toxins); both processes are present in some patients. In ischaemic ATN there is a continuum between prerenal azotaemia, the RISK and INJURY stages of AKI, and the development of ATN. ATN caused by administration of intravenous or intra-arterial contrast agents is due to renal vasoconstriction, reduced

Table 10.1.1	RIFLE classification of acute renal failure	
Stage	Serum creatinine (SCr) concentration	Urine output
RISK	Increase of 1.5 times the baseline	<0.5 mL/kg/h for 6 h
INJURY	Increase of 2.0 times the baseline	<0.5 mL/kg/h for 12 h
FAILURE	Increase of 3.0 times the baseline or SCr is 355 μmol/L or more when there has been an acute rise of greater than 44 μmol/L for 24 h or anuria for 12 h	<0.3 mL/kg/h
LOSS	Persistent acute renal failure; complete loss of kidney function for longer than 4 weeks	
END-STAGE RENAL DISEASE	End-stage renal disease for longer than 3 months	

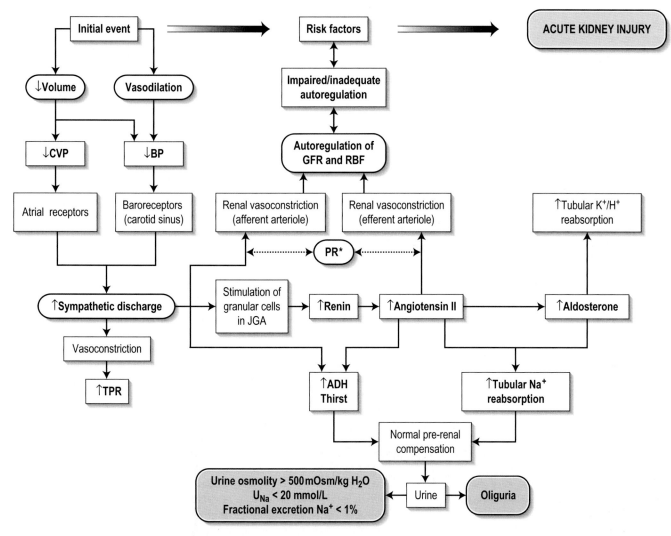

Fig. 10.1.1 Physiological response of the kidney to hypovolaemia or reduced perfusion. The normal response results in a reduced volume of concentrated urine. The presence of risk factors, impaired autoregulation or prolonged hypovolaemia can cause acute kidney injury. ADH, antidiuretic hormone; BP, blood pressure; CVP, central venous pressure; GFR, glomerular filtration rate; JGA, juxtaglomerular apparatus; PR*, renal prostaglandins; RBF, renal blood flow; TPR, total peripheral resistance.

medullary blood flow and tubular injury.[10] The main mechanisms of AKI or ATN caused by drugs are vasoconstriction, altered intra-glomerular haemodynamics, tubular cell tox-icity, interstitial nephritis, crystal deposition, thrombotic microangiopathy and osmotic nephrosis.[11]

Important causes of cytotoxic ATN are listed in Table 10.1.2. Non-steroidal anti-inflammatory drugs (NSAIDs), ACE inhibi-tors and angiotensin receptor blockers (ARBs) often cause a gradual and asymp-tomatic decrease in the GFR, but can cause AKI (including ATN). NSAIDs do not impair renal function in a healthy person, but can reduce the GFR in elderly persons with atherosclerotic cardiovascular disease, in persons with chronic renal failure, when

chronic prerenal hypoperfusion is present (e.g. cardiac failure, cirrhosis), or in persons using diuretics and calcium channel blockers.[12]

Renal damage is uncommon after admin-istration of intravenous or intra-arterial radiocontrast agents if renal function is normal, but the likelihood is increased by chronic renal impairment, diabetes, heart failure, hypertension, hypovolaemia, hyper-uricaemia, proteinuria or multiple mye-loma. Patients usually develop renal injury (with a rise in SCr concentration that returns to baseline within 3 to 5 days, and no reduction in the urine output) rather than ATN. Drugs that alter angiotensin levels (ACE inhibitors and ARBs) reduce renal perfusion by their antihypertensive

effects, or by impairing vasoconstriction of the efferent arteriole when renal perfusion is reduced by renal artery stenosis.

The haem pigments that damage the kidney are haemoglobin and myoglobin. The clinical spectrum of AKI due to rhabdo-myolysis ranges from a biochemical domi-nated presentation (elevated serum concentrations of muscle enzymes, a rapidly reversible increase in SCr concentration and no clinical features of muscle damage) to a presentation where the skeletal muscles are often swollen and painful, the muscle enzymes are very elevated and the patient rapidly develops ATN. The nephrotoxicity of haem pigments is enhanced by volume depletion, low urine flow rates and low urine pH.

Table 10.1.2 Causes of toxic acute tubular necrosis
Exogenous agents
Radiocontrast
Non-steroidal anti-inflammatory drugs
Antibiotics: aminoglycosides, amphotericin B
Antiviral drugs: aciclovir, foscarnet
Immunosuppressive drugs: ciclosporin
Organic solvents: ethylene glycol
Poisons: snake venom, paraquat, paracetamol
Chemotherapeutic drugs: cisplatin
Herbal remedies
Heavy metals
Endogenous agents
Haem pigments: haemoglobin, myoglobin
Uric acid
Myeloma proteins
Correct intravascular volume depletion
Maintain perfusion pressure
Choice of resuscitation fluid
Diuresis in rhabdomyolysis
Avoid nephrotoxins
Use derived GFR or creatinine clearance when calculating drug doses

Once ATN is established there is a persistent and marked reduction in RBF and in GFR that lasts for 1 to 2 weeks. During this time the patient is usually oliguric, and cannot excrete concentrated urine. Renal autoregulation is impaired, and renal perfusion depends directly on the systemic blood pressure. A fall in systemic blood pressure during the ATN phase causes more renal damage. Recovery from ATN is associated with increased renal blood flow (reperfusion), an increase in GFR and (often) a large volume urine output because the concentrating ability of the regenerating nephrons is impaired.

Abnormalities of renal interstitial structure and function are present in ATN. However, AKI and ATN can be caused by a primary abnormality of the interstitial tissues: acute tubulointerstitial nephritis (ATIN). The damage in ATIN is due to immunological mechanisms, the most important involving cell-mediated immunity. ATIN is usually due to a drug reaction, but can also be caused by infections (e.g. infection with hantavirus, a RNA virus that causes haemorrhagic fever with renal syndrome.[13] Drugs that cause ATIN include antibiotics (β-lactam antibiotics, sulphonamides, fluoroquinolones), NSAIDs, cyclooxygenase-2 inhibitors, proton pump inhibitors, diuretics, phenytoin, carbamazepine and allopurinol.

Postrenal (obstructive) acute kidney injury

Obstructive uropathy refers to the functional or structural processes in the urinary tract that impede the normal flow of urine, and obstructive nephropathy is the renal damage caused by the obstruction. Hydronephrosis is a dilatation of the ureter(s); it can occur in the absence of obstruction, and some persons with obstruction do not have a dilated urinary collecting system.[14-16]

Casts or crystals within the renal tubular lumen can cause intrarenal obstruction. Extrarenal obstruction can develop in the urethra, bladder, ureter or the pelvicureteric junction. Obstructive uropathy in adults is commonly caused by prostate disease or retroperitoneal neoplasm (cancer of the cervix, uterus, bladder, ovary or colon). Metastatic cancer, lymphomas or inflammatory processes in the retroperitoneum (appendicitis, diverticulitis, Crohn's disease) or a neurogenic bladder can also cause obstructive uropathy. Renal stones passing through the ureter(s) cause pain, haematuria and varying degrees of (usually unilateral) obstructive uropathy.

Obstructive nephropathy usually develops gradually and can cause chronic renal failure if the obstruction involves the urethra, the bladder or both ureters. Unilateral ureteric obstruction will cause ARF if it involves a single kidney, or if the obstructed kidney is the only functioning kidney.

Epidemiology

The annual incidence of ARF in European communities is between 209 and 620 cases per million per year, with an incidence of severe acute renal failure (SCr greater than 500 μmol/L) of 172 cases per million per year.[17-20] About 1% of patients in the USA have ARF on admission to hospital, and ARF develops in 5–7% of all hospitalized patients.[21-23] The frequency of ARF in hospitalized patients is about 19 per 1000 admissions.[24]

Studies of the pathogenesis of community acquired ARF have produced conflicting results. In one study the major processes were identified as prerenal in 70% of cases, renal in 11% of cases and postrenal in 17% of cases.[21] Other studies found a lower incidence of prerenal factors (present in 21–48% of cases) and a higher incidence of renal factors (present in 34–56% of cases, most commonly due to ATN).[19,25] Acute on chronic renal failure was present in 13% of persons in one study.[19] The basic processes in hospital acquired ARF are prerenal in 35–40% of cases, renal in 55–60% of cases and postrenal in 2–5% of cases.[6]

Using the RIFLE criteria the community incidence of AKI is 1811 per million of population, and AKI occurs in 18% of hospitalized patients (9% had changes in SCr concentration and urine output consistent with RISK, 5% had renal INJURY and 4% developed FAILURE).[26,27]

There are geographical differences in the causes of ATN. In Africa, India, Asia and Latin America ATN is usually caused by infections (e.g. diarrhoeal illnesses, malaria, leptospirosis), ingestion of plants or medicinal herbs, envenomation, intravascular haemolysis due to glucose-6-phosphate dehydrogenase deficiency or poisoning.[28] The incidence of ATN due to crushing injuries is increased in earthquake-prone areas.

Prevention

The processes involved in the prevention of AKI are shown in Table 10.1.3.

Maintaining intravascular volume and renal perfusion

The rate and volume of intravenous fluid given to hypovolaemic persons depends on the nature of the intravascular depletion, the blood pressure and heart rate, the (estimated) volume of fluid lost, cardiac function and ongoing circulatory losses. The response to treatment is evaluated by simple bedside measurements (heart rate, blood pressure, urine output). Fluid replacement that is predominately determined by formulas (e.g. in burns) often underestimates the magnitude of the fluid loss.

Acute haemorrhage causes prerenal azotaemia, but the incidence of ARF is low (1.5% in major gastrointestinal bleeding[29]) if the hypovolaemia is treated promptly

Table 10.1.3   Use derived GFR or creatinine clearance when calculating drug doses

Correct intravascular volume depletion
Maintain perfusion pressure
Choice of resuscitation fluid
Diuresis in rhabdomyolysis
Avoid nephrotoxins

and there are no other risk factors. In severe trauma the incidence of ARF needing dialysis is about 0.1%.[30] Severe progressive ARF after cardiopulmonary resuscitation is rare, and pre-existing and post resuscitation haemodynamics are more important risk factors for AKI than the degree of hypoperfusion during resuscitation.[31]

Choice of resuscitation fluid

Hypovolaemia is initially treated with crystalloid rather than colloid, with colloid being added in specific clinical settings (e.g. burns, anaphylaxis) or if there is no initial improvement in vital signs or urine output following crystalloid administration (e.g. in sepsis). The liberal use of crystalloid and colloid in high-output sepsis with AKI may increase the incidence of ARF or need for dialysis.[32]

Use of derived GFR in drug administration

Formulas are available to calculate the estimated creatinine clearance or estimated GFR from the measured SCr concentration.[33,34]

Rhabdomyolysis

Most studies on the prevention of ATN after rhabdomyolysis have been in persons with crush injury after earthquakes, where the incidence of AKI is about 50%. In this situation fluid resuscitation should, if possible, begin before the crush is relieved. These patients may require massive amounts of fluid because of fluid sequestration in the injured muscles. The goal of intravenous fluid treatment is to produce a urine output of 200–300 mL/h while myoglobinuria (discoloured urine) persists. There is no evidence to support this rate

of fluid replacement in persons who have rhabdomyolysis and AKI without crush injury, although a urine output of 100 mL/h would be reasonable while the urine is discoloured. The intravenous administration of mannitol and sodium bicarbonate to produce an alkaline diuresis as a means of preventing ATN in severe rhabdomyolysis has not been shown to be effective.[35]

Radiocontrast nephropathy

The incidence of radiocontrast nephropathy can be reduced by saline infusion to produce intravascular volume expansion, by using low osmolar contrast agents and by N-acetyl cysteine administration before and after radiocontrast administration.

Envenomation and poisoning

Specific antidotes, if available, should be used to treat persons who develop AKI after envenomation or poisoning.

Clinical features

The diagnosis of AKI should be considered when there is a decrease in urine output, an elevated SCr concentration or increases in SCr concentration. The clinical features depend on the pre-existing conditions that increase the risk of developing AKI, the initiating factor(s), and the effects of AKI (Fig. 10.1.2). The history should include a detailed drug history, enquiry about recent invasive vascular or radiological procedures, and any family history of renal disease. This is followed by clinical examination and evaluation of investigations. A number of key issues then need to be resolved (Table 10.1.4).

Evaluation of prerenal (intravascular volume) status

Imprecise or lazy terminology such as 'dry' or 'dehydrated' should be avoided. 'Dehydration' refers to situations where more water than electrolyte(s) has been lost, shrinking body cells and increasing the serum sodium concentration and osmolality.[36] In other words, 'dehydration' means water depletion. Hypovolaemia is a decrease in the intravascular volume due to loss of blood (haemorrhage, trauma) or loss of sodium and water (e.g. vomiting, diarrhoea, sequestration of fluid in the bowel, etc.).

The (bedside) assessment of the (extracellular) volume status determines the initial resuscitation strategy. This involves evaluation of heart rate and blood pressure, the state of the skin and mucous membranes, and the jugular venous pulse. The examination also includes auscultation of the lungs (for pulmonary crackles), abdominal examination (for ascites or masses) and examination of the legs (for peripheral oedema).

The 'typical' features of intravascular volume depletion (tachycardia or hypotension or both in the supine position, or postural hypotension) are not as consistent or reliable as implied by textbook descriptions. About one-third of persons with hypovolaemia due to trauma have bradycardia rather than tachycardia.[37,38] The presence of (supine) tachycardia has low sensitivity as a diagnostic feature of increasing acute blood loss in healthy persons.[39] An increase in the pulse rate of 30 beats per minute or more between the supine value and the standing values is a highly sensitive and highly specific sign of hypovolaemia after phlebotomy of large volumes (600–1100 mL) of blood, but the sensitivity is much less after phlebotomy of smaller volumes.[39] The inability to stand long enough for vital signs to be measured because of severe dizziness is a sensitive and specific feature of acute large blood loss.[39] The persistence of tachycardia after intravenous administration of fluids in clinical conditions causing hypovolaemia suggests that hypovolaemia is still present, but tachycardia due to other causes (pain, fever) will persist after correction of hypovolaemia.

A systolic blood pressure of 95 mmHg or less in the supine position has high specificity but low sensitivity after acute blood loss.[39] Postural hypotension is present in 10% of normovolaemic person younger than 65 years, and in up to 30% of normovolaemic person older than 65 years. Postural hypotension in persons who can stand without developing severe dizziness is of no diagnostic value after blood loss due to acute phlebotomy.[39]

The textbook descriptions of the signs of saline depletion in adults (dry mucous membranes, shrivelled tongue, sunken eyes, decreased skin turgor, weakness, confusion) are neither specific nor sensitive compared to laboratory tests for hypovolaemia. The

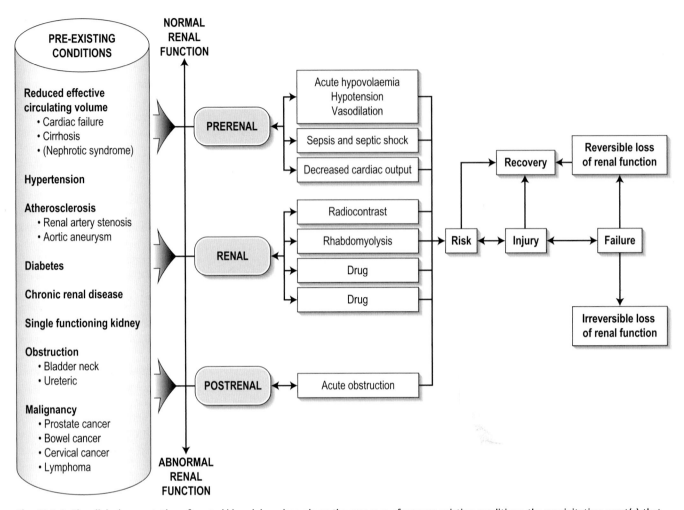

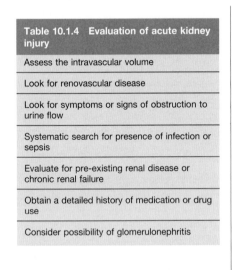

Fig. 10.1.2 The clinical presentation of acute kidney injury depends on the presence of any pre-existing conditions, the precipitating event(s) that caused the acute kidney injury and the severity of the acute kidney injury.

Table 10.1.4   Evaluation of acute kidney injury
Assess the intravascular volume
Look for renovascular disease
Look for symptoms or signs of obstruction to urine flow
Systematic search for presence of infection or sepsis
Evaluate for pre-existing renal disease or chronic renal failure
Obtain a detailed history of medication or drug use
Consider possibility of glomerulonephritis

presence of a dry axilla argues somewhat for the presence of saline depletion; the absence of tongue furrows and the presence of moist mucous membranes argue against the presence of saline depletion.[39]

The central venous pressure (CVP) is an indicator of the vena caval or right atrial pressure. A vertical distance greater than 3 cm between the top of the jugular venous pulsation (using the external jugular vein or internal jugular vein) and the sternal angle indicates that the CVP is elevated. An elevated venous pressure in persons with pulmonary crackles or peripheral oedema means that the intravascular volume is greater than normal. A markedly elevated CVP is the cardinal finding of cardiac tamponade and constrictive pericarditis.

The absence of visible venous pulsation in the neck veins when the patient is supine or in a head down position indicates significant intravascular volume depletion. The presence of visible venous pulsations in the neck at or below the level of the sternal angle that is seen only when the patient is supine indicates that the intravascular volume is below normal.

Evaluation of the renovascular state

Acute renal infarction is caused by dissection of the aorta or renal artery, embolism, renal artery thrombosis, renal vein thrombosis or renal artery aneurysm. Acute arterial occlusion is usually symptomatic, with the development of pain (loin, abdominal or back pain), haematuria, proteinuria, nausea or vomiting. Vascular occlusion of a single functioning kidney produces anuria.

Atherosclerosis can cause abdominal aortic aneurysms that may be palpable on abdominal examination. Inflammation of the adventitia of some abdominal aortic aneurysms can cause ureteric obstruction. There is an increased incidence of dissection of the thoracic aorta in persons with autosomal dominant polycystic kidney disease.

Atheromatous disease of the renal arteries is common in persons older than

50 years with widespread atherosclerosis. There is a 7% prevalence of renal artery stenosis in persons older than 65 years, and one-third of elderly persons with heart failure have renovascular disease.[40,41] Persons with stenosis or occlusion of one or both renal arteries can develop an elevation in SCr concentration after starting treatment with ACE or ARB drugs, or develop acute on chronic renal failure.

Exclusion of thrombotic microangiopathy

TMA is a syndrome of microangiopathic haemolytic anaemia, thrombocytopenia and varying degrees of organ injury caused by platelet thrombosis in the microcirculation. There are two clinically distinct entities: haemolytic uraemic syndrome (HUS) and thrombotic thrombocytopenic purpura (TTP). HUS affects young children and causes ARF with absent or minimal neurological abnormalities. TTP occurs in adults and causes severe neurological involvement in most cases, and variable degrees of renal damage.

Pre-existing renal disease or chronic renal failure

It can be difficult to distinguish between chronic and acute renal impairment. The following features suggest the presence of chronic renal failure: documented renal impairment in the past, family history of renal disease, polyuria or nocturia, uraemic pigmentation, normochromic and normocytic anaemia, or small kidneys on ultrasound or computed tomography (CT) scans. Renal size may be normal or increased in chronic renal failure associated with diabetes, polycystic kidney disease or amyloidosis.

Infection and sepsis[42]

Infection with virulent organisms or spread of organisms into the blood releases toxins and cytokines that produce a systemic inflammatory response. This causes systemic vasodilatation and increased permeability of capillaries. Compensatory physiological responses produce a secondary increase in the cardiac output, but this is not maximal because of the myocardial depressant effect of cytokines. Renal vasoconstriction occurs (even in the absence of hypotension), compensatory renal vasodilatation responses are impaired and the renal endothelium is injured. One half of all patients with septic shock develop ARF, and the combination of ARF and sepsis is associated with a greater than 80% mortality.

Exclusion of urinary obstruction

The symptoms and signs of urinary tract obstruction depend upon the site and cause, and the rapidity with which it develops. Pain is more common in acute obstruction and is felt in the lower back, flank or suprapubic region, depending on the level of the obstruction. Chronic obstruction is usually painless. Symptoms of prostatic obstruction include frequency, nocturia, hesitancy, post-void dribbling, poor urinary stream and incontinence. Bladder neck obstruction usually results in an enlarged (and palpable) bladder.

Recognition of rhabdomyolysis

Muscle necrosis releases intracellular contents into the circulation. This causes red-brown urine (that tests positive for haem in the absence of visible red cells on microscopy, or tests positive for myoglobin with specific tests), pigmented granular casts in the urine, elevated serum creatine kinase (CK) levels that are five times or more above the upper limit of normal and clear serum (serum is reddish in haemolysis). The severity of the rhabdomyolysis ranges from asymptomatic elevations of muscle enzymes in the serum to AKI and life-threatening electrolyte imbalances.

Urine dipstick findings may be normal because myoglobin is cleared from the serum more rapidly than CK, so serum CK levels can be elevated in the absence of myoglobinuria. Myoglobinuria may be absent in patients with renal failure or those who present later in the illness. Muscle pain is absent in about 50% of cases, and muscle swelling is an uncommon finding. Muscle weakness occurs in those with severe muscle damage. Fluid sequestration in muscles can cause hypovolaemia. Marked muscle swelling can cause a compartment syndrome.

Other blood test abnormalities include hyperkalaemia, AKI with rapid and marked elevation in SCr (e.g. 220 μmol/L per day), hypocalcaemia (which occurs early, and is usually asymptomatic), hyperuricaemia, hyperphosphataemia, metabolic acidosis and disseminated intravascular coagulopathy. About one-third of persons with ATN due to rhabdomyolysis develop hypercalcaemia during the recovery phase.

Acute kidney injury and acute renal failure

The early stages of AKI are usually asymptomatic, and the diagnosis is based on an elevated SCr concentration. It may take 24 h or more for an initially normal SCr concentration to show a definite increase, and up to 48 h after the event(s) that caused the AKI to distinguish between the early stages of AKI (risk and injury) and the development of renal failure.

The urine output usually decreases, and the patient may be oliguric (urine output less than 400 mL per day) or anuric (urine output less than 100 mL per day). Persons with AKI and oliguria have more severe kidney impairment than those without oliguria. Only a few conditions cause complete anuria: total obstruction, vascular lesions, severe ATN or rapidly progressive glomerulonephritis. The clinical features caused by ARF are shown in Table 10.1.5.

Differential diagnosis

The diagnosis of AKI requires synthesis of data from the patient's history, physical examination, laboratory studies and urine output. The category of AKI (RISK, INJURY or FAILURE) may be difficult to determine in the emergency department (ED) if the

Table 10.1.5 Clinical features of acute renal failure
1. Anorexia, fatigue, confusion, drowsiness, nausea and vomiting, and pruritus
2. Signs of salt and water retention in the intravascular and interstitial spaces: an elevated jugular venous pressure, peripheral oedema, pulmonary congestion, acute pulmonary oedema
3. Abnormal plasma electrolyte concentrations, particularly hyperkalaemia
4. Metabolic acidosis
5. Anaemia
6. Uraemic syndrome: ileus, asterixis, psychosis, myoclonus, seizures, pericardial disease (pericardial effusion, tamponade).

baseline SCr is unknown. The reversibility of the AKI may be inferred if there is a marked increase in urine output after correction of prerenal problems, but a reduction in SCr (due to an increase in GFR) may not be seen for 12–24 h.

Criteria for diagnosis

Serum biochemistry

The following are measured: serum concentration of electrolytes (sodium, potassium, bicarbonate, chloride, calcium, phosphate), serum urea and SCr concentrations, random blood glucose, liver function tests, coagulation tests and CK concentration.

AKI causes acute elevation in the SCr concentration or serum urea concentrations or both. In prerenal AKI the low urine flow rate favours urea reabsorption out of proportion to decreases in GFR, resulting in a disproportionate rise of serum urea concentration or BUN concentration relative to the SCr concentration. However, serum urea concentrations depend on nitrogen balance, liver function and renal function. Severe liver disease and protein malnutrition reduce urea production, resulting in a low serum urea concentration. Increased dietary protein, gastrointestinal haemorrhage, catabolic states (e.g. infection, trauma), and some medications (corticosteroids) increase urea production and increase serum urea concentration without any change in GFR.

The SCr concentration is the best available guide to the GFR. Acute reductions in GFR produce an increase in the SCr concentration. The changes in SCr concentration lag behind the change in GFR, and can be affected by the dilution effect of intravenous fluid. Correct interpretation of the SCr concentration extends beyond just knowing the normal values (Fig. 10.1.3). Creatinine is a metabolic product of creatine and phosphocreatine, which are found almost exclusively in skeletal muscle. The SCr concentration is affected by the muscle mass, meat intake, GFR, tubular secretion (which can vary in the same individual and increases as the GFR decreases) and breakdown of creatinine in the bowel (which increases in chronic renal failure). The GFR decreases by 1% per year after 40 years of age, yet the SCr concentration remains unchanged because the decrease in muscle mass with age reduces the production of

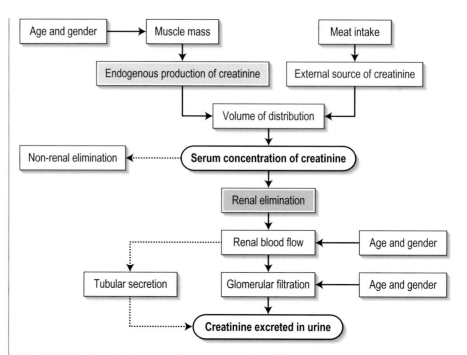

Fig. 10.1.3 Factors that determine the serum creatinine (SCr) concentration.

creatinine. The GFR (corrected for body surface area) is 10% greater in males than females, but men have a higher muscle mass per kilogram of body weight. The SCr concentration in men is thus greater than in women.

The creatinine clearance (CCr) or GFR are estimated indirectly using formulae (Cockcroft–Gault formula or the Modification of Diet in Renal Disease (MDRD) Study Equation) based on the SCr concentration[33,34] (Fig. 10.1.4). These equations assume a steady-state SCr concentration, and are inaccurate if the GFR is changing rapidly. They will also be less accurate in amputees, very small or very large persons, or persons with muscle-wasting diseases.

Knowledge of a patient's baseline SCr concentration is important in assessing the severity and progression of AKI. Small changes when the baseline SCr concentration is low are more important than larger changes when the baseline SCr concentration is high. Major decreases in GFR can occur in the normal range of SCr concentration. If the previous SCr concentration is not known, the MRDR equation can estimate the expected (normal) SCr concentration (using a value for the GFR at the lower range of normal).

Hyperkalaemia is a common complication, with the serum K^+ usually rising by 0.5 mmol/L/day in ARF. The serum Ca^{2+}

$$CCr = \frac{(140-age) \times weight}{0.814 \times SCr\ (\mu mol/L)} \quad \text{in males}$$

$$CCr = \frac{(140-age) \times weight \times 0.85}{0.814 \times SCr\ (\mu mol/L)} \quad \text{in females}$$

Cockcroft–Gault formula

$$\frac{GFR}{(mL/min/1.73m^2)} = 186 \times \left[\frac{SCr\ (\mu mol/L)}{88.4}\right]^{-1.154} \times age^{-0.203} \times \underset{\text{(if female)}}{0.742} \times \underset{\text{(if black)}}{1.210}$$

MDRD equation

Fig. 10.1.4 Formulae for calculating the creatinine clearance (CCr) or the glomerular filtration rate (GFR) from the serum creatinine concentration (SCr). MDRD, modified diet renal disease.

concentration may be normal or reduced in ARF. Both hypocalcaemia and hypercalcaemia may occur at different stages of ARF in rhabdomyolysis. Rhabdomyolysis is characterized by a very high blood CK concentration. Abnormal liver function tests invariably accompany hepatorenal syndrome and hepatic cirrhosis.

Full blood examination

Anaemia develops rapidly in ARF, but its presence or the degree of anaemia does not reliably distinguish between acute and chronic renal failure. Leukocytosis is usually seen if sepsis is the cause of ARF. Eosinophilia is often present in acute interstitial nephritis, polyarteritis nodosa and atheroembolic disease. Anaemia and rouleaux formation suggest a plasma cell dyscrasia. Disseminated intravascular coagulation can complicate ARF due to rhabdomyolysis. A microangiopathic blood film associated with ARF occurs in vasculitis or thrombotic thrombocytopenic purpura.

Serological tests

Tests for the detection of antinuclear antibody (ANA) or antineutrophil cytoplasmic antibody (ANCA) or measurement of complement concentration are indicated in suspected cases of vasculitis or glomerulonephritis.

Urine tests

The results of urine analysis may be normal. A positive test for leukocytes or nitrates or both is found in urinary tract infections. A positive test for blood or protein or both suggests a renal inflammatory process. The presence of red cell casts on microscopy is diagnostic of glomerulonephritis.

The measurement of the concentration of electrolytes in the urine, and the calculation of their fractional excretion, is of intellectual interest in understanding the pathophysiological responses of the nephron to different types of AKI. The calculations are cumbersome, the results are inconsistent, and the information obtained does not alter the patient's immediate treatment.[43]

Imaging

A chest X-ray is taken to assess the heart size and the presence of cardiac failure, infection, malignancy or other abnormalities.

An abdominal X-ray focusing on the kidneys, ureter and bladder may reveal radio-opaque calculi (calcium, cysteine or struvite stones).

Ultrasound can define renal size and demonstrate calyceal dilation and hydronephrosis, but the findings depend on the expertise of the operator. Obtaining adequate images is difficult in obese patients, in ascites or where there is a large quantity of gas within the bowel. Ultrasound also provides information about bladder size and can detect prostamegaly.

A normal ultrasound examination can occur in the very early stages of obstruction, or if ureteric obstruction is due to retroperitoneal fibrosis or to infiltration by tumour.[14-16] Hydronephrosis not due to obstruction occurs in pregnancy, vesicoureteric reflux or in diabetes insipidus.

Doppler scans are useful for detecting the presence and nature of renal blood flow in thromboembolism or renovascular disease. Because renal blood flow is reduced in prerenal or intrarenal AKI, test findings are of little use in the diagnosis of AKI. CT scans of the urinary tract evaluate renal size and renal position, renal masses, renal calculi, the collecting system and the bladder. Non-contrast CT is the examination of choice in persons with suspected renal calculi, and can be used to assess the urinary tract in persons at risk of radiocontrast AKI. Injection of intravenous contrast is used for CT urography, CT angiography and CT venography. Radionuclide is used to assess renal blood flow and tubular functions.

Renal biopsy

A renal biopsy provides a tissue diagnosis of the intrarenal cause of AKI and is indicated if the findings will identify a treatable condition. A renal biopsy is also valuable when renal function does not recover after several weeks of ARF and a prognosis is required for long-term management.

Treatment

The basis of emergency management is recognizing that AKI is present, correcting reversible factors, providing haemodynamic support, treating life-threatening complications and treating infection. This is followed by treatment (if available) of the specific cause of AKI and management of ARF by supportive measures and (if required) renal replacement treatment.

Correction of hypovolaemia

Hypovolaemia not only causes AKI but also worsens all forms of AKI. The clinical diagnosis of hypovolaemia can be difficult if the jugular venous pressure is not easily seen or if there is pre-existing cardiac failure. A 'normal' blood pressure reading does not exclude hypovolaemia. When there are definite signs of hypovolaemia the patient is resuscitated with rapid infusion of crystalloid. If hypovolaemia is a possibility, or if the person's urine output has decreased markedly, the patient should have 250–500 mL of crystalloid infused rapidly (fluid challenge) and the response (urine output, vital signs, jugular venous pressure) evaluated. An increase in urine output or an increase in blood pressure following a fluid challenge suggests that hypovolaemia was present.

Invasive measurement of volume status using central venous and pulmonary artery catheters can increase mortality, lengthen hospital stay and increase the cost of care. There is no evidence to justify the routine use of these invasive measures in patients with AKI. The main indications for central venous cannulation in AKI in the ED are difficulties obtaining intravascular access in the limbs or the need to give inotrope drugs.

Haemodynamic support

AKI impairs autoregulation of GFR and renal blood flow throughout all ranges of mean arterial pressure. Renal perfusion in ATN is linearly dependent on mean arterial pressure even in the normal range of blood pressure. Episodes of mild or severe decrease in blood pressure lead to recurrent ischaemic injury. Inotrope drugs (noradrenaline or adrenaline) should be commenced if hypotension persists after correction of hypovolaemia.

Monitoring and maintaining urine output

Urinary Catheter

Accurate measurement of urine output requires insertion of a urinary catheter, but this is not needed in the less severe forms of AKI if there is frequent spontaneous voiding. A catheter is required initially in persons with oliguria or (apparent) anuria, shock or obstruction to bladder outflow.

Diuretics

Furosemide is used to produce a diuresis in the treatment of AKI due to hypercalcaemia and in the treatment of severe rhabdomyolysis. A trial of high-dose furosemide (80–120 mg) can be used in persons with AKI who have acute pulmonary oedema. Persons with less severe forms of AKI (e.g. RISK or INJURY) who have a low urine output (less than 0.5 mL/kg/h) that does not increase after correction of hypovolaemia and an intravenous fluid challenge are given furosemide (e.g. 20–40 mg). An increase in urine is not necessarily associated with a decrease in the SCr concentration. There is no evidence that the use of diuretics to convert the less severe forms of AKI from a (presumed) oliguric to a non-oliguric stage affects outcome.

Electrolyte abnormalities

Potassium

The serum potassium concentration may be low, normal or high. AKI due to diarrhoea causes hypokalaemia and metabolic acidosis, while AKI due to vomiting or diuretics causes hypokalaemia with metabolic alkalosis. A serum $[K^+]$ less than 3.0 mmol/L is treated with oral or intravenous potassium. Diabetic ketoacidosis (DKA) causes renal loss of K^+, depleting the body of potassium. Persons with AKI due to DKA who have a normal or low serum $[K^+]$ need intravenous potassium during treatment with intravenous fluids and insulin.

Hyperkalaemia is due to an imbalance between potassium intake and renal potassium excretion, or follows redistribution of potassium from the intracellular to the extracellular space. Hyperkalaemia (often with metabolic acidosis) is a frequent finding in chronic obstruction.[44,45] Hyperkalaemia in AKI can be asymptomatic, produce electrocardiogram (ECG) changes or cause potentially fatal changes in cardiac rhythm.

The initial ECG changes in hyperkalaemia are shortening of the PR and QT interval, followed by peaked T waves that are most prominent in leads II, III and V2 through V4[46,47] (Fig. 10.1.5). Marked ST-T segment

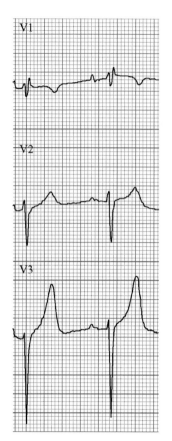

Fig. 10.1.5 The initial electrocardiograph changes in hyperkalaemia. The T waves in leads V3 to V5 are very tall and have a 'peaked' tip. The other findings (which may be unrelated to the hyperkalaemia) are the presence of a right bundle branch block pattern and a slightly prolonged PR interval.

elevation (pseudomyocardial infarction pattern) may occur.[48] Bradycardia with sinoatrial (SA) block or atrioventricular block (including complete heart block) can develop and progress to periods of cardiac standstill or asystole. More commonly the PR interval is prolonged and the QRS complex is widened, with the QRS complex having a left or right bundle branch block configuration (Fig. 10.1.6). At high serum $[K^+]$ (8–9 mmol/L) the sinoatrial (SA) node may stimulate the ventricles without ECG evidence of atrial activity (sinoventricular rhythm).[49] When the serum $[K^+]$ is 10 mmol/L or greater SA conduction no longer occurs and junctional rhythms are seen. The QRS complex width continues to increase and eventually the QRS complexes and the T wave blend, producing a sine wave ECG. At this stage ventricular fibrillation or asystole are imminent.

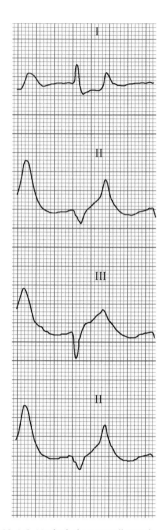

Fig. 10.1.6 Marked electrocardiograph changes in hyperkalaemia. The QRS complexes are widened, and have a right bundle branch block type configuration. Tall T waves are seen in the inferolateral leads. P waves are not visible, and a junctional rhythm is present.

The higher the serum $[K^+]$ concentration the more likely is the occurrence of ECG changes or life-threatening arrhythmias or both. However, nearly half of persons with a serum $[K^+]$ greater than 6.8 mmol/L do not have ECG changes of hyperkalaemia.[50,51] Physicians predict the presence of hyperkalaemia solely on the basis of ECG changes with a sensitivity of less than 45%.[52]

Drugs such as oral potassium tablets, ACE inhibitors and aldosterone antagonists should be ceased in AKI. Hyperkalaemia is treated when the serum $[K^+]$ is greater than 6.5 mmol/L (even if there are no ECG changes) or when there are ECG changes of hyperkalaemia. The emergency treatment of hyperkalaemia is covered in Chapter 12.2 Electrolyte disturbances.

Sodium

The sodium concentration in AKI may be normal, low (when water excess is present) or high (when water depletion is present). Hyponatraemia in ARF is usually asymptomatic and is treated by water restriction. Patients with ARF and symptomatic hyponatraemia should be treated with haemofiltration or dialysis. Hypernatraemia is treated by slow intravenous infusion of hypotonic saline or 5% dextrose.

Calcium, phosphate, uric acid and magnesium

The serum calcium concentration is normal or slightly reduced in the RISK and INJURY stages of AKI, and is moderately reduced in ARF. Hypocalcaemia does not require therapy unless tetany is present. Hyperphosphataemia is present in nearly all persons with ARF, but does not need treatment in the ED.

Hyperuricaemia is common in ARF, but also occurs in chronic renal failure and in persons without AKI. Episodes of acute gout are very uncommon in ARF, and the hyperuricaemia does not need treatment. Hypermagnesaemia is common in ARF, but is usually asymptomatic. Severe symptomatic hypermagnesaemia can occur if magnesium is administered to persons with ARF.

Acid base abnormalities

Increased loss of bicarbonate rich intestinal secretions (diarrhoea or an ileal conduit) can cause AKI with a normal anion gap metabolic acidosis. AKI accompanied by acid loss from the stomach (vomiting or nasogastric suction) or caused by diuretics can result in a hypochloraemic metabolic alkalosis. Persons with the RISK and INJURY stages of AKI often have a decrease in the serum bicarbonate concentration. ARF causes a mild-to-moderate metabolic acidosis with an increased anion gap. This acidosis does not usually require specific treatment. Severe acidosis occurs in rhabdomyolysis and in lactic acidosis. The presence of a very severe metabolic acidosis in ARF is an indication for dialysis.

Fluid overload

The management of AKI in patients with peripheral oedema or pulmonary congestion due to cardiac failure is challenging. The clinical diagnosis of hypovolaemia in these patients is difficult, and rapid intravenous administration of large volumes of fluid can worsen the pulmonary congestion or heart failure. Hypovolaemia is treated (or excluded) in these cases by assessing the response to small volume (200 mL) fluid challenges.

Patients with acute pulmonary oedema may have a raised SCr, which can be due to chronic renal failure, AKI or acute on chronic renal failure. These patients usually improve following treatment with vasodilators, continuous positive airway pressure (CPAP) ventilation and loop diuretics (40–80 mg furosemide intravenously). Patients with AKI and acute pulmonary oedema who do not respond to these measures need haemofiltration or haemodialysis or both.

Some persons with severe hypertension and chronic renal impairment who have recurrent episodes of acute pulmonary oedema ('flash' pulmonary oedema) have significant renovascular disease. Renal revascularization in these patients can reduce or abolish the episodes of pulmonary oedema.[53]

Hypertension

Persons with AKI may have an elevated blood pressure that predated the renal injury, or AKI may cause hypertension. A markedly elevated blood pressure reading (greater than 180/120 mmHg) in a person with AKI can be treated with glyceryl trinitrate applied as a skin patch (at a dose of 25–50 mg), sublingual nifedipine (5–10 mg) or oral hydralazine (20 mg). Intravenous drugs (glyceryl trinitrate or hydralazine) are used if AKI is associated with a hypertensive emergency such as acute pulmonary oedema, hypertensive retinopathy or hypertensive encephalopathy. Persons with AKI and acute aortic dissection should be treated with beta-adrenergic blocking drugs combined with an intravenous infusion of glyceryl trinitrate or sodium nitroprusside.

Specific causes of AKI

Obstruction

Obstruction is relieved by decompression or diversion of the urinary tract. The site of the obstruction determines the technique used: placement of a Foley catheter or insertion of a suprapubic catheter, ureteral catheters (stents) or nephrostomy tubes. Relief of obstruction is often followed by a post-obstructive diuresis. Fluid replacement after relief of obstruction is based on frequent measurements of urine volume and urinary electrolytes.

Other causes

Specific treatments include immunosuppressive agents (glomerulonephritis, vasculitis), plasma exchange (thrombotic microangiopathy), systemic anticoagulation or stents (renovascular disease).

Management of ATN

Reduction of damage/accelerating recovery

Despite much experimental laboratory work and numerous clinical trials, no therapeutic intervention has hastened the recovery of renal function in established ATN. Therapeutic trials of dopamine, atrial natriuretic peptide and various growth factors have been ineffective. The use of high-dose loop diuretics to convert oliguric ATN to non-oliguric ATN was based on the observation that patients with non-oliguric ATN had a lower mortality and better renal recovery rates than those with oliguric ATN. The use of high-dose loop diuretics does not affect the duration of ATN, the need for dialysis or the outcome.[54]

Supportive treatment

This includes monitoring fluid input and fluid output, measuring serum electrolyte values frequently, preventing sepsis by reducing the number of intravenous lines and removing urinary catheters, culturing periodically and using antibiotics when indicated clinically. The fluid intake is restricted to insensible water loss (about 500 mL per day in the absence of fever) plus all measured fluid losses (urine output, gastrointestinal losses, chest tube drainage). Nephrotoxic agents should be avoided and the dosage of renally excreted drugs reduced. Because the increase in SCr lags behind the decrease in GFR, drug doses should be calculated based on a GFR of less than 10 mL/min per 1.73 m^2 rather than on the SCr value.

Renal replacement treatment

Renal replacement treatment (RRT) is required in most patients with oliguric ARF, and one-third of patients with nonoliguric ARF. The indications for RRT are summarized in Table 10.1.6.

Table 10.1.6 Indications for renal replacement treatment in acute kidney injury*

Oliguria (urine output <200 mL/12 h) or anuria (urine output 0–50 mL/12 h)

Serum urea concentration >35 mmol/L

Serum creatinine concentration >400 μmol/L

Serum potassium concentration >6.5 mmol/L or rapidly rising

Serum sodium concentration <100 mmol/L or >160 mmol/L

Pulmonary oedema not responding to diuretics

Severe (uncompensated) metabolic acidosis with pH < 7.1

Uraemic syndrome (asterixis, psychosis, myoclonus, seizures, pericarditis)
Overdose with a toxin that is dialyzable

*Presence of two or more indications in a patient means that renal replacement will be needed.

Prognosis

The prognosis of ARF is largely dependent on the underlying cause and the presence of comorbidities. Mortality varies from about 40% in those with no comorbidity to more than 80% in those who have three or more failed organ systems.

References

1. Eknoyan G. Emergence of the concept of acute renal failure. American Journal of Nephrology 2002; 22: 225–230.
2. Delafield F. Acute Bright's disease. Med Rec1888; 33: 151–155.
3. Davies F, Weldon R. A contribution to the study of 'war nephritis'. Lancet 1917; II: 118–120.
4. Bywaters EG, Beall D. Crush injuries with impairment of renal function. British Medical Journal 1941; 1: 427–432.
5. Oliver J, Mac DM, Tracy A. The pathogenesis of acute renal failure associated with traumatic and toxic injury: renal ischemia, nephrotoxic damage and the ischemic episode. Journal of Clinical Investigation 1951; 30: 1307–1439.
6. Singri N, Ahya SN, Levin ML. Acute renal failure. Journal of the American Medical Association 2003; 289: 747–751.
7. Bellomo R, Ronco C, Kellum JA, et al. Acute renal failure—definition, outcome measures, animal models, fluid therapy and information technology needs: the Second International Consensus Conference of the Acute Dialysis Quality Initiative (ADQI) Group. Critical Care 2004; 8: R204–R212.
8. Esson ML, Schrier RW. Diagnosis and treatment of acute tubular necrosis. Annals of Internal Medicine 2002; 137: 744–752.
9. Gill N, Nally JV, Fatica RA. Renal failure secondary to acute tubular necrosis: epidemiology, diagnosis, and management. Chest 2005; 128: 2847–2863.
10. Tumlin J, Stacul F, Adam A, et al. on behalf of the CIN Consensus Working Panel. Pathophysiology of contrast-induced nephropathy. American Journal of Cardiology 2006; 98(suppl): 14K–20K.
11. Schetz M, Dasta J, Goldstein S, et al. Drug-induced acute kidney injury. Current Opinion in Critical Care 2005; 11(6): 555–565.
12. Huerta C, Castellsague J, Varas-Lorenzo C, et al. Nonsteroidal anti-inflammatory drugs and the risk of ARF in the general population. American Journal of Kidney Diseases 2005; 45(3): 531–539.
13. Settergren B, Ahlm C, Alexeyev O, et al. Pathogenetic and clinical aspects of the renal involvement in hemorrhagic fever with renal syndrome. Renal Failure 1997; 19(1): 1–14.
14. James B, Naidich JB, Rackson ME, et al. Nondilated obstructive uropathy: percutaneous nephrostomy performed to reverse renal failure. Radiology 1986; 160: 653–657.
15. Charasse C, Camus C, Darnault P, et al. Acute nondilated anuric obstructive nephropathy on echography: difficult diagnosis in the intensive care unit. Intensive Care Medicine 1991; 17: 387–391.
16. Leong W, Sells H, Moretti KL. Anuric, obstructive uropathy in the absence of obvious radiological evidence of obstruction. Australian and New Zealand Journal of Surgery 2004; 74 (7):611–613.
17. Khan IH, Catto GR, Edward N, et al. Acute renal failure: factors influencing nephrology referral and outcome. QJM 1997; 90(12): 781–785.
18. Stevens PE, Tamimi NA, Al-Hasani MK, et al. Non-specialist management of acute renal failure. QJM 2001; 94:533–540.
19. Liano F, Pascual J. Epidemiology of acute renal failure: a prospective, multicentre, community based study. Madrid Acute Renal Failure Study Group. Kidney International 1996; 50(3): 811–818.
20. Feest TG, Round A, Hamad S. Incidence of severe acute renal failure in adults: results of a community based study. British Medical Journal 1993; 306: 481–483.
21. Kaufman J, Dhakal M, Patel B, et al. Community acquired acute renal failure. American Journal of Kidney Disorder 1991; 17(12): 191–198.
22. Shusterman N, Strom BL, Murray TG, et al. Risk factors and outcomes of hospital acquired ARF: clinical epidemiologic study. American Journal of Medicine 1987; 83: 65–71.
23. Nash K, Hafeez A, Hou S. Hospital-acquired renal insufficiency. American Journal of Kidney Diseases 2002; 39(5): 930–936.
24. Liangos O, Wald R, O'Bell JW, et al. Epidemiology and outcomes of acute renal failure in hospitalized patients: a national survey. Clinical Journal of American Society of Nephrology 2006; 1(1): 43–51.
25. Sesso R, Roque A, Vicioso B, et al. Prognosis of ARF in hospitalized elderly patients. American Journal of Kidney Diseases 2004; 44(3): 410–419.
26. Ali T, Khan I, Simpson W, et al. Incidence and outcomes in acute kidney injury: a comprehensive population-based study. Journal of American Society of Nephrology 2007; 18: 1292–1298.
27. Uchino S, Bellomo R, Goldsmith D, et al. An assessment of the RIFLE criteria for acute renal failure in hospitalized patients. Critical Care Medicine 2006; 34(7): 1913–1917.
28. Uchino S. The epidemiology of acute renal failure in the world. Current Opinion in Critical Care 2006; 12: 538–543.
29. Anderson RJ, Schrier RW. Acute renal failure. In: Schrier RW, Gottschalk CW, eds. Diseases of the kidney. 6th edn, Chapter 41. Little Brown: Boston; 1997: 1069–1113.
30. Morris JA, Mucha P, Ross SE, et al. Acute post traumatic renal failure: a multicentre perspective. Journal of Trauma 1991; 31(12): 1584–1590.
31. Domanovits H, Schillinger M, Mullner M, et al. Acute renal failure after successful cardiopulmonary resuscitation. Intensive Care Medicine 2001; 27(7): 1194–1199.
32. Bagshaw SM, Bellomo R. Fluid resuscitation and the septic kidney. Current Opinion in Critical Care 2006; 12: 527–530.
33. Cockcroft DW, Gault MH. Prediction of creatinine clearance from serum creatinine. Nephron 1976; 16(1): 31–41.
34. Stevens LA, Coresh J, Greene T, et al. Assessing kidney function-measured and estimated glomerular filtration rate. New England Journal of Medicine 2006; 354: 2473–2483.
35. Brown CV, Rhee P, Chan L, et al. Preventing renal failure in patients with rhabdomyolysis: do bicarbonate and mannitol make a difference? Journal of Trauma 2004; 56(6): 1191–1196.
36. Mange K, Matsuura D, Cizman B, et al. Language guiding therapy: the case of dehydration versus volume depletion. Annals of Internal Medicine 1997; 127: 848–853.
37. Demetriades D, Chan LS, Bhasin P, et al. Relative bradycardia in patients with traumatic hypotension. Journal of Trauma 1998; 45(3): 534–539.
38. Victorino GP, Battistella FD, Wisner DH. Does tachycardia correlate with hypotension after trauma? Journal of American College of Surgeons 2003; 196: 679–684.
39. McGee S. Evidence based physical diagnosis. 2nd edn. St Louis: Saunders Elsevier; 2007: 94–96, 153–173.
40. MacDowall P, Kalra PA, O'Donoghue DJ, et al. Risk of morbidity from renovascular disease in elderly patients with congestive cardiac failure. Lancet 1998; 352: 13–16.
41. Hansen KJ, Edwards MS, Craven TE, et al. Prevalence of renovascular disease in the elderly: a population based study. Journal of Vascular Surgery 2002; 36(3): 43–51.
42. Schrier RW, Wang W. Acute renal failure and sepsis. New England Journal of Medicine 2004; 351: 159–169.
43. Bagshaw SM, Langenberg C, Bellomo R. Urinary biochemistry and microscopy in septic acute renal failure: a systematic review. American Journal of Kidney Diseases 2006; 48: 695–705.
44. Batlle DC, Arruda JA, Kurtzman NA. Hyperkalemic distal renal tubular acidosis associated with obstructed uropathy. New England Journal of Medicine 1981; 304 (7): 373–380.
45. Pelleya R, Oster JR, Perez GO. Hyporeninemic hypoaldosteronism, sodium wasting and mineralocorticoid-resistant hyperkalemia in two patients with obstructive uropathy. American Journal of Nephrology 1983; 13(4): 223–227.
46. Dittrich KL, Walls RM. Hyperkalemia: ECG manifestations and clinical considerations. Journal of Emergency Medicine 1986; 4(6): 449–455.
47. Quick G, Bastani B. Prolonged asystolic hyperkalemic cardiac arrest with no neurologic sequelae. Annals of Emergency Medicine 1994; 24: 305–311.
48. Simon BC. Pseudomyocardial infarction and hyperkalemia: a case report and subject review. Journal of Emergency Medicine 1988; 6(6): 511–515.
49. Cohen HC, Gozo EG Jr, Pick A. The nature and type of arrhythmias in acute experimental hyperkalemia in the intact dog. American Heart Journal 1971; 82(6): 777–785.
50. Acker CG, Johnson JP, Palevsky PM, et al. Hyperkalemia in hospitalized patients: causes, adequacy of treatment, and results of an attempt to improve physician compliance with published therapy guidelines. Archives of Internal Medicine 1998; 158(8): 917–924.
51. Martinez-Vea A, Bardaji A, Garcia C, et al. Severe hyperkalemia with minimal electrocardiographic manifestations: a report of seven cases. Journal of Electrocardiology 1999; 32(1): 45–49.
52. Wrenn KD, Slovis CM, Slovis BS. The ability of physicians to predict hyperkalemia from the ECG. Annals of Emergency Medicine 1991; 20(11): 1229–1232.
53. Bloch MJ, Trost DW, Pickering TG, et al. Prevention of recurrent pulmonary edema in patients with bilateral renovascular disease through renal artery stent placement. American Journal of Hypertension 1999; 12 (1): 1–7.
54. Ho KM, Sheridan DJ. Meta-analysis of frusemide to prevent or treat acute renal failure. British Medical Journal 2006. 333: 420–425.

10.2 The acute scrotum

Gino Toncich

ESSENTIALS

1 Torsion is the most time-critical diagnosis in acute scrotal pain.

2 Early surgery is mandatory if the diagnosis is strongly suspected. No investigation should delay surgery.

3 Colour Doppler ultrasound is of limited use and is best used when testicular ischaemia needs to be excluded in an inflammatory mass or in the older patient.

4 Torsion of an appendage can be diagnosed clinically by finding a small blue lump in the scrotal sac (with normal scrotum and testes) and can be managed non-operatively.

5 Epididymo-orchitis is rare in adolescence and torsion should be suspected. Colour Doppler ultrasound may be used to exclude torsion if suspicion remains.

6 Masses found on ultrasound should be followed up as traumatic injury can bring attention to an undiscovered tumour.

7 Ultrasound is unreliable in diagnosing testicular rupture.

8 Early surgery in scrotal trauma allows diagnosis and treatment of rupture, as well as early evacuation of other haematomas with shorter inpatient stays and less pain.

TORSION OF THE SPERMATIC CORD (TESTICLE)

Torsion is a twisting, not of the testicle (as is commonly described), but of the spermatic cord, which then interferes with the vascularity of the testicle, ultimately leading to infarction.

Aetiology

Torsion is due to a powerful contraction of the cremaster muscles in an abnormally attached testis. A normal testis is anchored posterolaterally to the scrotal sac and is, therefore, fixed in place. The main abnormality found in patients with torsion is an enlarged tunica vaginalis, which surrounds the whole of the testes and epididymis, preventing the testis from creating any attachment to the scrotal wall. The testis, therefore, floats freely like a clapper inside a bell. The contraction of the cremaster causes the testes and adnexa to be rotated, thereby twisting the cord.[1]

Pathology

The twisting of the cord causes obstruction of the lymphatic and venous outflows, but allows arterial inflow, leading to venous engorgement. Eventually the pressure rises to occlude the arterial inflow.

The extent and rapidity of the damage depends on the degree of torsion, that is the number of turns:

- An incomplete turn (<360°) may not completely occlude arterial flow.
- One turn (360°) causes necrosis in 12–24 h.
- Two or more turns (>720°) cause necrosis in less than 2 h because arterial flow is completely obstructed.[1,2]

Clinical presentation

There is a sudden onset of severe scrotal or abdominal pain. There are no irritative voiding symptoms. Between 29 and 50% of patients have had previous episodes of acute scrotal pain.[3,4]

The patient looks pale and may vomit. The testis is tender and riding high in the scrotum. Other signs are loss of cremasteric reflex, scrotal oedema testicular swelling and retraction. One study in which all children had mandatory exploration found these clinical signs had sensitivities of 60–91% and specificities of 27–68%.[5]

Systemic signs such as fever are classically absent. Urinalysis is normal.

Intermittent torsion of the testis

This is a syndrome of recurrent acute scrotal pain, usually lasting less than 2 h, which resolves spontaneously. Creagh and McDermott[4] describe a series of 27 patients who underwent elective orchidopexy for these symptoms. Three patients developed acute torsion while on the waiting list; of those coming to operation, one had an atrophic testis and four had evidence of torsion of the appendages of the testis. One patient subsequently had torsion after surgery because absorbable sutures were used.[4]

Differential diagnosis of acute testicular pain

Differential diagnoses to consider in acute testicular pain are listed in Table 10.2.1.

Table 10.2.1 Differential diagnosis of acute testicular pain
Epididymo-orchitis
Strangulated hernia
Haematocoele
Hydrocoele
Testicular tumour
Henoch Schonlein purpura in children
Idiopathic scrotal oedema.

Traps in the clinical diagnosis

There are many potential pitfalls in the clinical diagnosis of the acute scrotum:

- Age: The abnormality is present for life, so the torsion could potentially occur at any age. In those under 18 years of age an acutely painful scrotum should always be considered to be torsion.[3] Most of the literature concerns itself with the paediatric <18-year-old population. Less than 4% of torsions occur in patients over 30 years. It is most common in adolescence (12–18 years).[6] In teenagers there is an increasing amount of sexually transmitted disease, which may confuse the diagnosis. There is an old surgical aphorism: 'Question: When do you diagnose epididymo-orchitis in a teenager? Answer: After you have fixed the torsion.'
- Pain: In 25% of cases there is no sudden onset of pain, nor is it necessarily severe. Some patients with epididymo-orchitis (EDO) have severe pain.[1,3]
- Localization: Some patients may have no scrotal pain but may have all their pain referred to the lower abdomen or inguinal area. The scrotum must always be examined in males with lower abdominal pain.
- Abnormal position of testis: this is only seen if 360° or greater rotation occurs.[3]
- Previous repair: Torsion can occur in a testis that has previously been fixed, especially if absorbable sutures have been used.[4]
- Dysuria: Irritative voiding symptoms rarely occur with torsion and suggest infection.[3]
- Fever: Temperatures >102°F have been noted in up to 15% of torsion patients.[1]

Clinical findings remain misleading and none can reliably exclude the diagnosis of torsion.[7]

Investigations

Surgical exploration of the scrotum

This is the investigation of choice where the diagnosis of torsion is likely, and maximizes the chance of saving the testis.

Delaying the diagnosis is 'castration by neglect'.[3,7] Surgical exploration requires only a skin incision and has no major complications.[5,7]

Low rates of torsion diagnosed at operation have led to interest in other tests to predict torsion preoperatively.

Scintigraphic scanning

Classically radionucleotide scintinography was said to be more sensitive and specific than Doppler ultrasound. However, this test is rarely performed due to time constraints, lack of reporting expertise and its replacement with colour Doppler ultrasound or direct surgical exploration. It is for the time being consigned to the dustbin of medical imaging.

Colour Doppler imaging of the testis

This is the ultrasound examination of choice. It is useful in diagnosing torsion but also in elucidating other scrotal pathology. Comparison of blood flow to the asymptomatic side is crucial. If there is reduced flow to one side then some degree of torsion must be suspected. If the testis has untwisted, hyperaemic flow may be noted. The sensitivity of colour Doppler imaging (CDI) for torsion can be as low as 82%, missing one in five cases, and is affected by:

- lack of sensitivity in low flow states
- inappropriate settings
- inexperience of the operator
- incomplete torsion
- failure to compare low flow to the normal side
- spontaneous untorting, giving an increased flow to the affected side, not reduced or absent flow.[2]

Role of investigations in suspected testicular torsion

When the diagnosis of torsion remains probable then the only investigation is surgical exploration of the scrotum, and any investigations that delay theatre are unnecessary. If torsion is unlikely clinically, but needs to be excluded, then CDI can be used, provided it is available on an urgent basis.[1,3,7] It is important that there is early communication and discussion with the responsible surgeon so no unavoidable delays are instituted between the suspicion of torsion and any surgical intervention.[1–3]

Treatment

Manual untwisting

This manoeuvre is not universally recommended and should be done only as a temporizing measure or when surgical exploration cannot be performed. The spermatic cord is infiltrated with local anaesthetic and the testis is untwisted. Untwisting is done by turning the left testis anticlockwise (outward) and the right one clockwise, like opening the pages of a book.[8]

Surgery

The scrotum is opened and the testis is delivered, untwisted and inspected for return of colour and bleeding. An obviously infarcted testis is removed at the initial surgery. A viable testis is sutured into place on the scrotal wall. The tunica should be inverted and also sutured to the scrotal wall. It is vital that the normal side is also explored and fixed to the scrotal wall, as the abnormality is bilateral in most cases. Retorsion following orchidopexy has occurred when absorbable sutures have been used.[1,3–6]

Prognosis

Viability depends on the number of twists and the time taken to untwist the testis. There is 100% salvage if the testis is untwisted in less than 4 h. Up to 24 h the rate falls to 50%. Rare case reports of salvage after 30 h have been reported.

Testicular salvage (return of circulation at surgery) does not mean no injury to the testicle. Long-term follow-up of salvaged testes shows that 75% have a reduction in volume. Abnormalities are also seen in sperm volume, motility and morphology. These abnormalities are not seen in patients who have had an infarcted testis removed at the initial operation. This suggests some antispermatogenesis effect caused by the damaged testicle.[1,3,4]

Torsion of a testicular appendage

These are embryological remnants with no function. They are small (<5 mm) pedunculated structures that may twist on their pedicle. If the appendage can be isolated in the scrotum a small blue lump may be isolated: 'the blue dot sign'. These do not need surgery and can be treated with analgesia. Late presentations may have scrotal or testicular swelling, in which case they should be treated as torsion until proved otherwise.[1]

ACUTE EPIDIDYMO-ORCHITIS

Introduction

This is a clinical syndrome resulting from pain and swelling of the epididymis (and the testis) of less than 6 weeks' duration. Chronic epididymitis is a long-standing condition of epididymal or testicular pain, usually without swelling.[2]

Aetiology

A variety of organisms may be responsible for EDO (Table 10.2.2).

The most likely cause depends on the patient's demographic group. For heterosexual males under 35 years of age, the agent is usually gonococcus or chlamydia. These organisms are also responsible for infection in homosexual males under 35 years (where anal sex is practised), but coliforms and even haemophilus can cause

Table 10.2.2 Causative agents in EDO
Bacterial: *Neisseria gonorrhoeae*, *Escherichia coli*, *Pseudomonas aeruginosa*, coliforms, *Klebsiella*, *Mycobacterium tuberculosis*
Chlamydial: *C. trachomatis*
Viral: mumps
Drugs: amiodarone epididymitis
Fungal: cryptococcal
Parasitic: filariasis (usually chronic).

infection. In males older than 35 years, EDO is usually due to obstructive urological disease, so coliforms predominate. EDO may also be part of a systemic disease, for example brucellosis or cryptococcus.

EDO is usually thought to be an ascending infection from the urethra or prostate, but it can be part of a generalized systemic disease. The infection spreads from epididymis to testicle, and eventually they may become one large inflammatory mass. Isolated orchitis is rare and usually due to viral causes, which are spread via the bloodstream.[9–11]

Clinical presentation

The exact features depend on the underlying cause and whether both the epididymis and the testicle are involved. The pain may come on suddenly or slowly. There is scrotal swelling and tenderness that is relieved by elevating the testis. The spermatic cord is usually tender and swollen. Associated symptoms of urethritis are common. In younger males (under 35 years) a history of sexually transmitted disease may be elicited. In the older patient there is a history of instrumentation, intercurrent urinary tract infection (UTI) or prostatism. Pyuria is common.

Investigations

Urethral swabs

Urethral discharge may not be seen if the patient has just voided, so a urethral swab and smear should be examined for white blood cells (WBC). If there are more than five WBC per high-powered field, then urethritis is likely. The presence of intracellular diplococci confirms the diagnosis of gonorrhoea; their absence suggests chlamydia.[9]

Midstream urine

Look for the presence of WBC or Gram-negative organisms.

Differential diagnosis

In the acute non-traumatic setting the most important differential diagnosis is torsion of the testicle.[9] If the clinical features, urethral swabs or mid-stream urine do not

differentiate, then ultrasound or isotope scans may help. In young men, if these are not available and there is no evidence of UTI or urethritis, then surgical exploration may be necessary. Ultrasound can help differentiate other causes of the acute scrotum.

Treatment

Symptomatic treatment consists of bed rest, analgesia and scrotal supports.

If the cause is secondary to a sexually transmitted disease, then appropriate antibiotics should be chosen after urethral swabs have been taken, for instance a single dose of ceftriaxone (250 mg stat) for gonorrhoea and a 14-day course of doxycycline (100 mg) or roxithromycin (300 mg) for chlamydia. The patient's sexual partners should be investigated and treated. Tests for syphilis or HIV should be performed.

If the infection is secondary to UTIs then an appropriate antibiotic, such as amoxyl/clavulanic acid (500/125) b.d. or trimethoprim (300 mg daily) for 14 days, should be used. Antibiotic choice can be adjusted according to the urine culture results. Investigation for underlying urinary tract obstruction should be undertaken according to clinical features.

Complications

These include abscess formation, testicular infarction, chronic pain and infertility.

Blunt traumatic injury to the testicle

The mobility of the testicle, cremaster muscle contraction and the tough capsule usually protect the testicle from injury. However, a direct blow that drives the testicle against the symphysis pubis may result in contusion or rupture of the testicle. Typical mechanisms are a direct kick to the groin, or handlebar and straddle injuries.[12,13]

The types of injury include scrotal-wall haematomas, tunica vaginalis haematoma (haematocoele) or intratesticular (subcapsular) haematoma.

The most serious is testicular rupture, where the tunica is split, allowing blood and seminiferous tubules to extrude into the tunica vaginalis. This occurs in up to 50% of blunt trauma. Complete disruption of the testis may occur.[12-14]

Ultrasound examination is not 100% sensitive in detecting testicular rupture, so early surgical exploration is the investigation and treatment of choice.

Indications for exploratory surgery include:

- uncertainty in diagnosis after appropriate clinical and radiographic evaluations
- clinical findings consistent with testicular injury
- disruption of the tunica albuginea on ultrasound
- absence of blood flow on scrotal ultrasound images with Doppler studies
- clinical hematocoeles that are expanding or of considerable size (e.g. 5 cm or larger) should be explored
- smaller haematocoeles are often explored because it has been shown that such practice allows for more optimal pain control and shorter hospital stays.

It should be noted that 10–15% of testicular tumours present after an episode of trauma, and so any abnormalities on ultrasound examination should be followed to resolution if surgery is not performed.[15]

Early surgical exploration with evacuation of blood clots in the tunica vaginalis and repair of testicular rupture, if present, results in a shortened hospital stay, a greatly reduced period of disability and a faster return to normal activity compared to patients managed conservatively. Conservative management is complicated by secondary infection of the haematocoele, frank acute necrosis of the testis and delayed atrophy due to pressure effects of haematoma. The orchidectomy rate for early exploration is only 9%, compared to 45% for those managed non-operatively.[13]

Controversies and future directions

❶ Should all patients with suspected torsion should go straight to surgical exploration or is there is any role for investigations in older or low probability patients?

❷ Should all patients with scrotal and testicular injury have routine surgical exploration regardless of ultrasound findings?

❸ Should all attempts at testicular salvage be abandoned in favour of orchidectomy of the affected side in order to preserve the spermatogenesis of the other side?

References

1. Lutzker LG, Zuckier LS. Testicular scanning and other applications of radionuclide imaging of the genital tract. Seminars in Nuclear Medicine 1990; 20(2):159–188.
2. Herbener TE. Ultrasound in the assessment of the acute scrotum. Journal of Clinical Ultrasound 1996; 24: 405–421.
3. Cass AS. Torsion of the testis. Postgraduate Medicine 1990; 87: 69–74.
4. Creagh TA, McDermott TE, McLean PA, et al. Intermittent torsion of the testis. British Medical Journal 1988; 297: 525–526.
5. Van Glabeke E, Khairouni A, Larroquet M, et al. Acute scrotal pain in children: results of 543 surgical explorations. Pediatric Surgery International 1999; 15: 353–357.
6. Rajfer J. Testicular torsion. In: Walsh PC, Retik AB, Darracott VE, Wein AJ eds. Campbell's urology Vol. 2, 7th edn London: WB Saunders; 1997: 2184–2186.
7. Murphy FL, Fletcher L, Pease P. Early Scrotal exploration in all cases is the investigation and intervention of choice in the acute paediatric scrotum. Pediatric Surgery 2006; 22(5): 413.
8. Schneider RE. Testicular torsion. In: Tintinalli JE, Ruiz E, Krome RL, eds. Emergency medicine: a comprehensive study guide. 4th edn. New York: McGraw-Hill; 1996.
9. Berger R. Epididymitis. In: Walsh PC, Retik AB, Darracott VE, Wein AJ, eds. Campbell's urology Vol. 1, 7th edn. London: WB Saunders; 1997: 670–673.
10. Tintanalli JE, Ruiz E, Krome RL. Epididymitis. In: Tintinalli JE, Krome RL, eds. Emergency medicine: a comprehensive study guide. 4th edn. New York: McGraw-Hill; 1996.
11. Therapeutic Guidelines: Antibiotics. 10th edn. Melbourne: Therapeutic Guidelines Limited; March 2006.
12. Bertini JE, Corriere JN. The etiology and management of genital injuries. Journal of Trauma 1990; 28: 1278–1281.
13. Cass AS. Testicular trauma. Journal of Urology 1983; 129: 299–300.
14. Kukadia AN, Ercole CJ, Gleich P, et al. Testicular trauma: potential impact on reproductive function. Journal of Urology 1996; 156: 1643–1646.
15. Cass AS, Luxenberg M. Testicular injuries. Urology 1991; 38: 528–530.

10.3 Renal colic

Sean Arendse

ESSENTIALS

1 Renal colic affects 2–5% of the population, with 50% of patients having a recurrence within 5 years.

2 Management includes adequate analgesia and hydration.

3 Computerized tomography or intravenous pyelography establish the diagnosis and evaluate the severity of obstruction.

4 Most stones (90%) are passed spontaneously within 1 month.

5 Obstruction, infection and intractable pain necessitate admission to hospital.

6 Urology follow-up is essential to minimize further episodes.

Introduction

Nephrolithiasis is a common disorder affecting 2–5% of the population at some point in their lives.[1] It occurs most frequently between the ages of 20 and 50 years, with a male:female ratio of approximately 3:1. About 50% of patients have a single episode but the remaining 50% have recurrent episodes within 5 years.[2]

Most calculi are believed to originate in the collecting system (renal calyces and pelvis) before passing into the ureter. Supersaturation with stone-forming substances (calcium, phosphate, oxalate, cystine or urate) combined with a decrease in urine volume and lack of chemicals that inhibit stone formation (such as magnesium, citrate and pyrophosphate) result in production of a calculus. In addition, infection with urea-splitting organisms that produce an alkaline urinary pH frequently contributes to the growth of 'struvites' or triple phosphate (calcium, magnesium and ammonium phosphate) stones.

Less commonly, mixed stones occur via nucleation with sodium hydrogen, urate, uric acid and hydroxyapatite crystals providing a core to which calcium and oxalate ions adhere (heterogeneous nucleation).

Approximately 75% of all stones are calcium based, consisting of calcium oxalate, calcium phosphate or a mixture of the two. Ten per cent are uric acid based, 1% are cystine based and the remainder are primarily struvite.

Predisposing factors for stone formation include prolonged immobilization, strong family history of nephrolitiasis, hyperparathyroidism or peptic ulcer disease (hyperexcretion of calcium), small bowel disease, such as Crohn's disease or ulcerative colitis (hyperoxaluria), and gout (hyperuricaemia). Myeloproliferative disorders, malignancy, glycogen storage disorders, renal tubular acidosis and the use of certain medications (calcium supplements, acetazolamide, vitamins C and D, and antacids) may also be conducive to nephrolithiasis.[3]

Persistent obstruction of the ureter leads to hydronephrosis of the urinary tract and may precipitate renal failure.

Pathophysiology of pain

The mechanisms implicated in the production of the pain of renal colic are an increase in renal pelvic pressure, ureteric spasm, local inflammatory effects at the level of the calculus, and increased peristalsis and pressure proximal to the calculus.

Acute obstruction of the upper urinary tract from a calculus results in increased pressure in the renal pelvis, which, in turn, induces the synthesis and secretion of renal prostaglandins, in particular PGE2, which promotes a diuresis by causing dilatation of the afferent arteriole, further elevating the renal pelvic pressure.[4,5] The acute obstruction and renal capsular tension are believed to be the cause of the constant ache in the costovertebral angle.

In experiments with isolated ureteric smooth muscle, prostaglandins have also been shown to increase phasic and tonic contractile activity,[6] resulting in ureteric spasm and severe, colicky pain.

Presentation

The pain of renal colic has been described as the worst pain a person can endure. The classic textbook description is of severe, intermittent, flank pain of abrupt onset originating from the area of the costovertebral angle and radiating anteriorly to the lower abdominal and inguinal regions. Testicular or labial pain may be present and may suggest the location of the stone as a low ureteric position. Urinary frequency or urgency often develops as the stone nears the bladder, and nausea and vomiting frequently accompany the pain. One-third of patients complain of gross haematuria.[7]

Examination usually reveals an agitated, pacing patient unable to find a comfortable position. Pulse rate and blood pressure may be elevated secondary to the pain. Fever is unusual and suggests infection. The abdominal examination may only reveal signs of an early ileus with hypoactive bowel sounds and distended abdomen, but should not be omitted as it is extremely useful in excluding intra-abdominal or retroperitoneal causes of the pain (such as pancreatitis, cholecystitis, appendicitis, or leaking or rupture of the abdominal aorta).

Urinalysis usually shows red blood cells, although the absence of red cells in the urine in the setting of colicky flank loin to groin pain does not rule out nephrolithiasis, and between 10 and 30% of patients with documented nephrolithiasis do not have haematuria.[8] Nitrites, leukocytes or microorganisms in the urine suggest either the complication of infection or a diagnosis of acute pyelonephritis. Urine culture is indicated to rule out infection with urea-splitting organisms such as *Klebsiella* and

Proteus spp. Electrolyte studies may demonstrate obstruction or suggest an underlying metabolic abnormality such as hypercalcaemia, hyperuricaemia or hypokalaemia. A slightly elevated white blood cell count may occur with renal colic, but a count greater than 15 000/mm^3 suggests active infection.

A pregnancy test should be performed in all women of childbearing age, as a positive result needs further investigation to exclude ectopic pregnancy.

Many conditions may have a similar presentation to renal colic, and examination and investigations should be directed towards confirming the diagnosis of nephrolithiasis and excluding the other conditions in the differential diagnosis (Table 10.3.1).

Radiological examination

A variety of imaging modalities is used to evaluate renal colic. Their pros and cons are listed in Table 10.3.2.

Most stones (90%) are radio-opaque and theoretically should be visible on plain X-ray; if seen, they are irregularly shaped densities on abdominal radiography (KUB). However, a KUB alone is not usually sufficient to make the diagnosis of nephrolithiasis as it has poor sensitivity of between 58 and 62%.[9] Phlebitis in the pelvic veins and calcified mesenteric lymph nodes may add confusion, and many small stones may be obscured by the bony density of the sacrum. Thus, plain X-ray should only be used in conjunction with another imaging

Table 10.3.1 Differential diagnosis of renal colic

- Renal carcinoma producing blood clots temporarily occluding the ureter
- Ectopic pregnancy
- Ovarian torsion
- Abdominal aortic aneurysm
- Acute intestinal obstruction
- Pyelonephritis
- Appendicitis
- Diverticulitis
- Narcotic seekers and Munchausen's syndrome

Table 10.3.2 Pros and cons of imaging modalities in renal colic

	Pros	Cons
CT	High sensitivity (97%) High specificity (96%) Nearly all stones opaque Can accurately measure stone size Can detect obstruction Can diagnose other causes of flank pain Can avoid the use of contrast	Exposes patient to radiation Higher cost
Abdominal radiography (KUD)	Readily available Fast	Low sensitivity Exposes patient to radiation
Intravenous urography	Provides information regarding size and location of stone Measure of renal function	Potential for contrast reaction Exposes patient to radiation More time-consuming than CT Unable to exclude alternative diagnoses
MRI	Useful in pregnant patients Does not use ionizing radiation Does not use contrast	Not readily available Time consuming Accuracy may be less than IVU
Ultrasound	Non invasive No exposure to ionizing radiation Modality of choice in pregnant patients	Lower sensitivity than IVU Size of stone cannot be accurately measured May not be available 24 h Requires skilled operator

modality such as ultrasound in the setting of renal colic.

Computerized tomography (CT), with or without contrast, is the first-line test in many centres, and has become the adopted gold standard with high sensitivity (97%) and specificity (96%) for ureterolithiasis.[10] Nearly all stones are opaque on CT, and thus the size of the stone and its position can be accurately measured. Other positive findings include perinephric stranding, dilatation of the kidney (hydronephrosis) or ureter, and low density of the kidney, suggesting oedema. Non-contrast CT is equivalent to intravenous urography (IVU) in the diagnosis of obstruction and is more reliable in the detection of ureterolithiasis.[11] It is also useful in the exclusion or confirmation of the other intra-abdominal differential diagnoses such as appendicitis, abdominal aortic aneurysm or diverticulitis. As no contrast is used there is not the risk of contrast reaction that is associated with IVU. It is more rapid than IVU and does not depend on the technical expertise required by other imaging modalities such as ultrasound, but it does subject the patient to a larger dose of radiation than IVU.

The intravenous pyelogram had been the standard investigation for the evaluation of renal colic until the widespread adoption of CT. It establishes the diagnosis of calculus disease in 96% of cases and determines the severity of obstruction.[12] Classic findings of acute obstruction include a delay in the appearance of one kidney, a dilated ureter and a dilated renal pelvis.[13] IVU is useful in estimating the size of the stone, in identifying extravasation of dye and in evaluating renal function. Its main disadvantage is the use of ionizing radiation, although less than in CT, and the administration of intravenous iodinated contrast media with its risk of contrast reaction. Compared with CT it is time-consuming and unable to offer alternative diagnoses.

Ultrasonography is a useful, safe and a non-invasive alternative when renal function is impaired or contrast media contra-indicated. It can identify the stone, its location and demonstrate proximal obstruction such as hydroureter or a dilated pelvis, as well as the size and configuration of each kidney, but unfortunately not size of the stone. Ultrasound has significantly lower sensitivity than IVU and misses more than 30% of stones.[14].

Magnetic resonance imaging (MRI) can easily depict a dilated ureter and demonstrate the level of obstruction without using ionizing radiation or contrast. The accuracy of MRI for stones may be lower than IVU as its special resolution is not high enough to detect small stones, but when used in combination with ultrasound it may have a role in the evaluation of loin pain, especially in the pregnant patient. MRI is, however, expensive, time-consuming and usually not readily available to most emergency departments (EDs).

Management

As 90% of stones are passed spontaneously, the most urgent therapeutic step is relief of pain, providing adequate hydration and antiemetics. Opioid analgesics and non-steroidal anti-inflammatory drugs (NSAIDs) remain the mainstay of treatment.

Intravenous narcotics provide rapid analgesia, are titratable to effect and relieve anxiety in most cases. However, prolonged use may cause dependence and tolerance. Side effects are common and include nausea, vomiting, drowsiness, constipation and with larger doses precipitate respiratory depression and hypotension. The data are very variable with regards to the effect of opioids on ureteric tone. Results indicate an increase in ureteric tone or no effect at all.[15]

Codeine, a less potent opioid than morphine, is effective for relieving mild to moderate pain associated with renal colic. Constipation is a significant side effect and limits its long-term use. One hundred milligrams of tramadol, an opioid-like agents but with fewer side effects when used for treating renal colic, has been shown to be as effective as pethidine 50 mg in one study,[16] but more research is needed before adopting tramadol as an alternative to conventional opioids.

NSAIDs appear to be equally effective when compared with opioids.[17] A double-blind study comparing diclofenac and an opioid demonstrated a better effect with diclofenac and fewer side effects, but slower onset of action.[18] There are many NSAIDs available, differing in preparation and route of administration, the major differences between them being the incidence and nature of side effects, predominantly gastric irritation, ulceration and precipitation of renal failure. Ibuprofen has the fewest side effects and the lowest risk of gastrointestinal effects, but the weakest analgesic action. Naproxen and diclofenac provide stronger analgesia and a relatively low incidence of side effects. Oral diclofenac and oral/rectal indometacin have

both been shown to be effective in reducing the number of new renal colic episodes as well as further admission to hospital, but have no effect on spontaneous stone passage rates.[19,20] Thus, it has been suggested that one should give both a rapidly acting titratable opioid and a slower acting NSAID, which may result in earlier discharge from the ED.[21] Intravenous preparations of NSAIDs have limited availability in Australian EDs and have been reported to have a faster onset of action but a higher incidence of side effects, and therefore if available should be used with caution.

Buscopan, an antimuscarinic agent used for treating smooth muscle spasm, has been shown to decrease ureteric activity to some degree in 80% of the subjects studied.[22] However, one study comparing its use to a NSAID found that buscopan was less effective[23] and was associated with significant side effects, including dry mouth, photophobia, urgency, retention and constipation, significantly limiting its use in renal colic.

Recently the use of alpha-blockers in renal colic has been reported, with a number of studies showing that patients treated with alpha-blockers as well as standard therapy achieve stone clearance more often and take less time to do so than controls.[24]

Intravenous crystalloid should be administered to ensure a urine volume of 100–200 mL/h in those unable to tolerate oral fluids.

The size, shape and site of the stone at initial presentation are factors that determine whether a stone passes spontaneously or requires removal. Stones less than 5 mm in patients without associated infection or anatomic abnormality pass within 1 month in 90% of cases, stones 4–6 mm pass 50% of the time but only 5% of stones larger than 7 mm pass, and hence usually require elective surgical removal.[8] The overall passage rate for ureteral stones is:

- proximal ureteral stones 25%
- mid-ureteral stones 45%
- distal ureteral stones 70%.

Most patients with renal colic can be discharged with oral analgesia (codeine, paracetamol and NSAIDs), hydration

Table 10.3.3 Indications for hospital admission in renal colic
• Presence of infection
• Deteriorating renal function
• Persistent pain requiring parenteral narcotics
• Stone greater than 5 mm in diameter
• Extravasation of dye (uncommon)

and a referral for outpatient urology. Rectal administration of indometacin is particularly effective if tolerated by the patient.

Indications for admission to hospital are listed in Table 10.3.3.

Further intervention is required if obstruction with hydronephrosis is present, the stone is a large stag horn calculus or the patient continues to have pain and no stone is passed within 2–3 days. A percutaneous nephrostomy allows drainage of an obstructed kidney until the blockage can be removed, either by ureteroscopic procedures for low stones or by open surgery for large or infected stones. Extracorporeal shockwave lithotripsy is preferred for single or small (>2 cm) otherwise uncomplicated stones as it has minimal complications and morbidity.

Urology follow-up is essential for all patients, for elective removal of stones when complications have not ensued and for the prevention of recurrence. Indications for stone removal include stone diameter >7 mm, stone obstruction associated with infection, single kidneys with obstruction and bilateral obstruction.

Precautions

Renal colic, with its minimal findings on examination, is a commonly used presentation for those seeking narcotics or with Munchausen's syndrome, and treating physicians should be aware of this. However, it is essential to give analgesia to those patients suffering from renal colic and it is probably preferable to give patients analgesia unnecessarily than cause unnecessary suffering. Features suggesting narcotic seeking are discussed in Chapter 21.5.

Conclusion

Renal colic is an acutely distressing medical condition that requires a careful evaluation of symptoms and signs to ensure timely analgesia, recognition of other causes of acute abdominal pain and avoidance of inappropriate narcotic usage.

Controversies and future directions

❶ Controversies in the management of renal colic relate largely to analgesia. Traditionally, it has been taught that parenteral narcotics provide fast and effective pain relief, but with the advent of injectable NSAIDs some argue that these should be first-line of care.

References

1. Lingeman J. Calculous disease of the kidney and bladder. In: Harwood-Nuss A, ed. The clinical practice of emergency medicine. Philadelphia: JB Lippincott; 1991.

2. Trivedi BK. Nephrolithiasis. Postgraduate Medicine 1996; 100(6): 3–78.
3. Coe FL, Parks JH, Asplin JR. The pathogenesis and treatment of kidney stones. New England Journal of Medicine 1992; 327(16): 1141–1152.
4. Holmlund D. The pathophysiology of ureteric colic. Scandinavian Journal of Urology and Nephrology 1983; 75(suppl): 25–27.
5. Nishikawa K, Morrisin A, Needleman P. Exaggerated prostaglandin biosynthesis and its influence on renal resistance in the isolated hydronephrotic rabbit kidney. Journal of Clinical Investigation 1977; 59: 1143–1150.
6. Cole RS, Fry CH, Shuttleworth KED. The action of prostaglandins on isolated human ureteric smooth muscle. British Journal of Urology 1988; 61: 19–26.
7. Smith DR. General urology. 9th edn. Los Altos, California: Lange Medical Publishers; 1978.
8. Teichman JM. Acute renal colic from ureteral calculus. New England Journal of Medicine 2004; 350: 684.
9. Mutgi A, Willliams JW, Nettleman M. Renal colic. The utility of the plain abdominal roentgenogram. Archives of Internal Medicine 1991; 151: 1589–1592.
10. Kenney PJ. CT evaluation of urinary lithiasis. The Radiological Clinics of North America 2003; 41: 979–999.
11. Sourtzis S, Thibeau JF, Damry N, et al. Radiologic investigation of renal colic: unenhanced helical CT compared with excretory urography. American Journal of Roentgenology 1999; 172: 1491–1494.
12. Harrison JH, et al. (eds) Campbell's urology. Vol. 1, 4th edn. Philadelphia: WB Saunders; 1987.
13. Samm BJ, Dmochowski RR. Urologic emergencies. Postgraduate Medicine 1996; 100(4): 177–184.
14. Svedstorm E, Alanen A, Nurmi M. Radiologic diagnosis of renal colic: the role of plain films, excretory urography and sonography. European Journal of Radiology 1990; 11: 180–183.
15. Lennon GM, Bourke J, Ryan PC, et al. Pharmacological options for the treatment of acute ureteric colic. British Journal of Urology 1993; 71: 401–407.
16. Salehi M, Ghaserni H, Shiery H, et al. Intramuscular tramadol versus intramuscular pethidine for the treatment of acute renal colic. Journal of Endourology 2003; 17(suppl 1): A243.
17. Cordell WH, Larson TA, Lingerman JE, et al. Indomethacin suppositories versus intravenous titrated morphine for treatment of ureteric colic. Annals of Emergency Medicine 1994; 23: 262–269.
18. Lundstam SO, Leissner KH, Wahlandar LA, et al. Prostaglandin synthetase inhibition of diclofenac in the treatment of renal colic: comparison with use of a narcotic analgesic. Lancet 1982; 1096–1097.
19. Laerum E, Omundsen OE, Gronseth JE, et al. Oral diclofenac in the prophylactic treatment of recurrent renal colic. European Journal of Urology 1995; 28:108–111.
20. Grenabo L, Holmlund D. Indomethacin as prophylaxis against recurrent ureteral colic. Scandinavian Journal of Urology and Nephrology 1984; 18: 325–327.
21. Larkin GL, Peacock WF, Pearl SM, et al. Efficiency of ketorolac tromethamine verses meperidine in ED treatment of acute renal colic. American Journal of Emergency Medicine 1999; 17(1): 6–10.
22. Ross JA, Edmond P, Kirkland IS. The action of drugs on the intact human ureter. In: Behaviour of the human ureter in health and disease. Chapter 9. Churchill Livingstone; 1972: 118–129.
23. Al-waili NS, Saloom KY. Intravenous tenoxicam to treat acute renal colic: comparison with buscopan. Journal of the Pakistan Medical Association 1998; 48(12): 370–372.
24. De Sio M, Autorino R, Lorenzo GD, et al. Medical expulsive treatment of distal-ureteral stones using tamsulosin. Journal of Endourology 2006; 20(1): 12–16.

ENDOCRINE

Edited by **Anthony F. T. Brown**

11.1 Diabetes mellitus and hypoglycaemia: an overview

Anthony F. T. Brown

ESSENTIALS

1 Optimal blood sugar control aids in reducing the incidence of multisystem diabetic complications.

2 Hypoglycaemic coma requires immediate treatment with intravenous glucose. Intramuscular glucagon can be used if liver glycogen stores are adequate, and may be given pre-hospital.

DIABETES MELLITUS

Classification system and diagnostic criteria

The classification system and diagnostic criteria for diabetes were re-examined in 1996 by the American Diabetes Association and the World Health Organization.[1] The classification of type I and type II diabetes mellitus was retained, although the recommended criterion for the diagnosis of diabetes has become a fasting plasma glucose of 7 mmol/L or greater, or a random plasma glucose of over 11 mmol/L associated with polyuria, polydipsia and weight loss. The oral glucose tolerance test is no longer routinely recommended.

Aetiology

The exact aetiology of diabetes is unclear. Evidence regarding type I diabetes suggests genetic and environmental factors associated with certain human leukocyte antigen (HLA) types (90% of patients are HLA-DR3 or DR4 or both) and abnormal immune responses. Certain genes are also implicated as possible co-contributors, particularly sites on chromosomes 6, 7, 11, 14 and 18. Genetic factors are implied by familial aggregation of cases with type II diabetes, and environmental factors in the context of genetic susceptibility, as well as obesity and diet. For instance, the introduction of a high fat and high calorie 'Western' diet rather than traditional crop foods has seen countries such as India now record amongst the fastest growth rate of new diabetes anywhere.

Although type I diabetes occurs most frequently among Caucasians throughout the world, diabetes in Australia is more common in the Aboriginal community. Other groups with a high prevalence include Native Americans and Pacific Islanders.

Diabetes secondary to other conditions

Diabetes mellitus may be secondary to conditions including chronic pancreatitis, carcinoma of the pancreas and pancreatectomy, haemochromatosis, cystic fibrosis, pregnancy, Cushing's syndrome, acromegaly, phaeochromocytoma and glucagonoma.

Drug-induced diabetic state

Certain drugs can impair glucose tolerance or cause overt diabetes mellitus. These include glucocorticoids, the oral contraceptive pill, thiazide diuretics used at higher doses, tacrolimus and ciclosporin, and HIV protease inhibitors.

Emergency presentations of a high blood sugar

Diabetic ketoacidosis (DKA) and hyperosmolar hyperglycaemic non-ketotic state (HHNS) are both life-threatening acute complications of diabetes mellitus. Although important differences do exist, the pathophysiology and treatment are similar. DKA is usually seen in type I diabetes and HHNS in patients with type II, but both complications can occur in type I and type II diabetes. See Chapter 11.2 for the diagnosis and management of DKA and HHNS.

General management of diabetes mellitus

Aims of long-term blood sugar control

The aim of excellent long-term blood sugar control is an HbA1c (glycated haemoglobin) level of less than 7.5% without frequent disabling hypoglycaemia for the prevention of microvascular disease, and 6.5% in those at increased risk of arterial disease.[2] This should be represented by a pre-prandial blood glucose level of 4.0–7.0 mmol/L, and a post-prandial blood glucose level of less than 9.0 mmol/L.

Insulins

Insulin was first administered to humans in 1922. Animal insulins (bovine, porcine) have been used for many years, but in the 1980s human insulins became commercially available. Today, with the widespread availability of human insulins, animal insulins are of historical interest only.

Types of insulins

Table 11.1.1 illustrates the different types of insulins and the important parameters of each type. Mixtures of short- and intermediate-acting insulins are also available: 70/30 (70% NPH/30% regular) and 50/50 (50% NPH/50% regular).

Antidiabetic drugs

Two major groups of oral hypoglycaemic agents important in the management of type II diabetes are the sulphonylureas and the biguanides. The sulphonylurea group of drugs acts by stimulating the pancreatic secretion of insulin, and the biguanide metformin acts by suppressing hepatic glucose production and enhancing the peripheral use of glucose.

Two newer types of oral agents are available for the treatment of diabetes. The alpha-glucosidase inhibitor acarbose acts on the gastrointestinal tract to interfere with carbohydrate digestion. The other group is the thiazolidinediones, such as pioglitazone and rosiglitazone. The thiazolidinediones act primarily by reducing insulin resistance, thereby enhancing the effect of circulating insulin. However, roziglitazone increases the risk of myocardial infarction and cardiovascular deaths, and thus should be avoided in ischaemic heart disease.[3] In addition, all thiazolidinediones must be avoided in people with moderate or severe heart failure.

Other non-diabetic drugs

Statins are important in the strict treatment of dyslipidaemia in diabetic patients. Angiotensin converting enzyme inhibitors also delay the onset of diabetic nephropathy even in normotensive patients with diabetes.

DIABETIC HYPOGLYCAEMIA

Hypoglycaemia most commonly occurs in type I diabetes. The critical plasma level at which hypoglycaemia manifests varies between different individuals, but symptoms are likely below a plasma glucose of 3.5 mmol/L. Common precipitants include exercise, a late meal, inadequate carbohydrate intake, ethanol ingestion and errors of insulin dosage. Hypoglycaemia may also occur in the non-diabetic patient, precipitated by a variety of conditions (see Table 11.1.2).[4]

Table 11.1.2 Causes of hypoglycaemia
Diabetic patients
• Medication change or error, particularly with insulin or oral hypoglycaemic sulphonylurea (very rarely metformin)   • Inadequate dietary intake   • Excessive calorie use such as exercise
Any patient
• Deliberate self-harm with insulin, sulphonylurea, salicylates, β-blockers, quinine, chloroquine, valproic acid   • Ethanol   • Liver disease   • Sepsis   • Starvation, including anorexia nervosa   • Post-gastrointestinal surgery 'dumping syndrome'   • Adrenal insufficiency   • Hypopituitarism   • Islet cell tumour/extrapancreatic tumour   • Tumour-related, such as mesenchymal, epithelial or endothelial tumours   • Artefact 'Munchausen syndrome'

Clinical features

Hypoglycaemia produces neurological and mental dysfunction. Less commonly, it can present as hypothermia, depression and psychosis. In some instances hypoglycaemia is asymptomatic.

Management of hypoglycaemic coma

- The ABC approach is important in a patient with coma.
- Give 50 mL of 50% glucose i.v. initially after taking a blood sugar level. Further glucose administration is often necessary, including an infusion of 10% dextrose.
- Alternatively give 0.5–2 mg of glucagon i.m. when venous access to administer i.v. glucose has not been established. This is unhelpful in the patient with liver disease and depleted glycogen reserves.

Table 11.1.1 Pharmacokinetic characteristics of currently available human insulins			
Insulin	Onset of action	Peak of action	Duration of action
Lispro*	5–15 min	1–2 h	4–5 h
Regular	30–60 min	2–4 h	6–8 h
NPH	1–2 h	5–7 h	13–18 h
Lente	1–3 h	4–8 h	13–20 h
Ultralente	2–4 h	8–10 h	18–30 h

*Lispro insulin (Humalog®) is the first rapidly acting insulin analogue. It produces a peak blood insulin level 2–3 times higher than regular insulin.

Controversies

❶ Non-parenteral insulin delivery such as nasal, oral or intra-pulmonary.

❷ The risk–benefit profile of newer antidiabetic drugs, such as the thiazolidinediones.

References

1. Alberti KGMM, DeFronzo RA, Keen H, et al. International textbook of diabetes mellitus. Chichester: John Wiley & Sons Ltd; 1992: 31–98.
2. NICE Clinical Guideline 15. Type 1 diabetes: diagnosis and management of type 1 diabetes in children, young people and adults. July 2004. Available: http://www.nice.org.uk/nicemedia/pdf/CG015NICEguideline.pdf (accessed Dec 2007).
3. Nissen SE, Wolski K. Effect of rosiglitazone on the risk of myocardial infarction and death from cardiovascular causes. New England Journal of Medicine 2007; 356: 2457–2471.
4. eMedicine. Hypoglycaemia. Available: http://www.emedicine.com/emerg/topic272.htm (accessed Dec 2007).

11.2 Diabetic ketoacidosis and hyperosmolar, hyperglycaemic non-ketotic state

Richard D. Hardern

ESSENTIALS

1 Diabetic ketoacidosis (DKA) gives rise to hyperglycaemia, ketosis and a high anion gap metabolic acidosis.

2 DKA is often caused by insulin error or omission, intercurrent illness (especially infections) or a combination of these.

3 There are four key components to the management of DKA:

- Fluids (usually 0.9% normal saline) at 3 L in the first 8 h. This is preferred to faster rates of infusion, in the absence of shock.

- Insulin as an intravenous infusion of soluble insulin at 0.1 unit/kg/h to a maximum of 6 units/h. Avoid an insulin sliding scale, as regular review with recent biochemistry results should determine what adjustment to the insulin infusion rate is necessary. Do not commence the insulin until the serum potassium [K] has been confirmed as >3.4 mmol/L (risk of hypokalaemic cardiac arrest).

- Potassium replacement will be needed, providing the serum potassium is less than 6.0 mmol/L and there is no anuria (rare in DKA).

- Education. All patients treated with insulin need to know the 'sick day rules', plus be familiar with regular home testing for capillary blood sugar.

4 The treatment of DKA is not complicated, but meticulous monitoring and documentation are essential.

5 The mortality and morbidity of the hyperglycaemic, hyperosmolar non-ketotic state (HHNS) are greater than with DKA.

6 Treatment of HHNS is similar to that of DKA except:

- a lower infusion rate of insulin is often sufficient

- this insulin infusion rate is titrated against the serum osmolarity rather than to ketoacids

- half normal (0.45%) saline is often used

- low molecular weight heparin (LMWH) thromboprophylaxis indicated

- shock may have a cardiogenic component.

Introduction

Diabetic ketoacidosis (DKA) is potentially fatal and overall is a common presentation to the emergency department (ED) for insulin-dependent diabetics. Shortfalls in the quality of care for patients with DKA have been highlighted. Hyperglycaemic, hyperosmolar non-ketotic state (HHNS) is less common than DKA, but has a worse prognosis, with an increased mortality and greater morbidity, often related to underlying chronic medical disorders.

Aetiology, genetics, pathogenesis and pathology

DKA may be the presenting feature of diabetes mellitus, and is usually seen in patients with type I diabetes when there has been an insulin error and/or an intercurrent illness. A variant of type II diabetes is also ketosis prone. This is most often seen in racial groups with a high prevalence of inherited glucose-6-phosphate dehydrogenase (G6PD) deficiency.

DKA arises from a lack of insulin and an excess of counter regulatory hormones such as glucagon. Insulin absence leads to increased gluconeogenesis and therefore to hyperglycaemia. The less complete the lack of insulin, the greater the hyperosmolarity.

Lack of insulin and excess counter regulatory hormones increase lipolysis with subsequent ketone body formation and a reduced capacity to prevent ketoacid formation.

HHNS is at the other end of the spectrum from DKA. It occurs with a relative rather than an absolute deficiency of insulin, leading to greater hyperglycaemia, which may approach 100 mmol/L. The hyperosmolarity is therefore greater than that seen in DKA and the degree of dehydration is greater (typically 10–15% body weight), but significant ketosis does not occur. HHNS is more insidious in onset than DKA, and patients with HHNS are typically older patients with pre-existing type II diabetes.

Epidemiology

An annual incidence of DKA of approximately 1:170 patients with type I diabetes has been reported.[1]

Clinical features

Although there are no clinical features specific to DKA, often the diagnosis can be made from the end of the trolley. Malaise and fatigue on a background of polyuria, polydipsia and sometimes weight loss are common, but gastrointestinal symptoms such as nausea and abdominal pain may predominate. The lack of a history of diabetes does not rule out the diagnosis, as it may be the first presentation.

An increased rate and depth of respiration, known as Kussmaul breathing, is most noticeable, in association with dehydration causing a dry mouth and tongue. The breath may smell of pear drops but this is not always noticed. The conscious level may be reduced or the patient may present in coma.

Look carefully for signs of the underlying cause such as chest, urinary or skin infection, as many cases of DKA are secondary to a stressor such as this.

The urine output should be measured regularly, although this does not always require urinary catheterization.

Invasive haemodynamic monitoring should not be instituted as a 'routine' for patients for DKA, but should be reserved for those with reduced capacity to handle fluid overload.

DKA differential diagnosis

Other causes of high (greater than 16) anion gap metabolic acidosis:

- alcoholic or starvation ketoacidosis
- lactic acidosis
- renal failure
- ethanol, methanol, ethylene glycol, salicylate ingestion.

Other causes of hyperglycaemia:

- HHNS
- hyperglycaemia without DKA or HHNS.

Clinical investigations in DKA

Venous blood

The capillary blood glucose should be measured hourly and the venous pH measured until both are near to the normal range. Venous urea and electrolytes (U&Es) and glucose should also be measured hourly initially, then 2-hourly once the venous glucose and capillary glucose are in agreement.

A mild leukocytosis is often seen in DKA, but should not be interpreted as signifying infection. Likewise hyperamylasaemia is common and does not imply pancreatitis.

Urinalysis

This diagnosis is highly likely in an unwell patient in the presence of glycosuria and ketonuria.

Electrocardiograph (ECG)

T-wave changes may be the first indication of hyperkalaemia (tall and peaked) or hypokalaemia (flat or inverted), or a clinically silent myocardial infarction (MI) may precipitate DKA.

Point-of-care testing

Point-of-care testing for blood ketones such as beta-hydroxybutyrate can be helpful in triage and when monitoring the response to treatment.

Similar investigations are needed in HHNS, although monitoring the pH and ketone bodies is not needed.

Criteria for diagnosis

DKA

- Hyperglycaemia. This is rarely >40 mmol/L since in DKA presentation is usually within 24 h of onset.
- Metabolic acidosis with serum bicarbonate <15 mmol/L.
- Ketonaemia or heavy ketonuria, associated with a high anion gap.

HHNS

- Hyperglycaemia. Serum glucose >33.3 mmol/L.
- Hyperosmolarity with serum osmolarity >320 mOsm/kg.
- pH > 7.30, anion gap normal and bicarbonate >15 mmol/L.
- Minimal ketosis with no more than 1+ ketonuria on urinalysis.

Treatment of DKA

The treatment of DKA is not complicated, but requires careful monitoring of the patient both clinically and biochemically.

Ideally all observations and results should be recorded on a purpose-designed record sheet, such as an integrated care pathway that includes guidance and data recording.[2]

Resuscitation environment

Patients with DKA require an environment that provides nursing staff familiar with monitoring patients with DKA and familiar with infusion equipment, and medical staff used to managing DKA and who have access to senior advice and or a written guideline, and, importantly, access to timely laboratory facilities for frequent biochemistry testing.

Access in the ED to glucose strips and a blood gas analyser with the ability to measure electrolytes, anion gap and lactate is also useful.

Standard resuscitative measures should be provided for sicker patients, including oxygen, especially for patients who are shocked, with airway protection in comatose patients, and at least a nasogastric tube to prevent aspiration of gastric contents in patients who are not intubated, but whose airway reflexes are impaired.

Early aggressive volume resuscitation should be used in shocked patients, then slow i.v. fluids and insulin infusion once the shocked circulatory status has been restored to normal.

Fluids

Intravenous fluids should be started within 30 min of the patient's arrival in the ED. Shocked patients require rapid fluid resuscitation, although care is needed in patients with comorbidities to avoid fluid overload.

Give patients who are not shocked 0.9% normal saline at a rate of 500 mL/h for 4 h, then 250 mL/h for the next 4 h.[3] A suggested fluid regime is shown in Table 11.2.1.

Most intravenous fluid regimes suggest replacing the volume deficit (often 10% of body weight) over 24 h. However, in patients with significant comorbidites, it is prudent (although unproven) to aim to correct half the fluid deficit in the first 24 h, and the remainder in the next 24 h. There are no data from randomized controlled trials to support the choice of one crystalloid over another in the treatment of DKA.

Once serum [glucose] has fallen to <15 mmol/L, change the intravenous fluid to 5% dextrose rather than 0.9% saline, but

Table 11.2.1 Replacement fluid regime in patients with DKA who are not haemodynamically compromised or in shock	
Litre	Timing (hours from starting treatment)
First at 500 mL/h	0–2
Second at 500 mL/h	2–4
Third at 250 mL/h	4–8
Fourth at 100 mL/h	8–18
Fifth at 100 mL/h	18–28
Sixth at 100 mL/h	28–38
Seventh at 100 mL/h	38–48

continue the insulin infusion until the ketoacidosis has cleared.

Insulin

An intravenous insulin infusion should be started within 60 min of the patient's arrival in the ED.

Insulin infusion regime

The standard regime is a continuous intravenous infusion of soluble insulin, making up 50 units of insulin to a total of 50 mL with 0.9% saline to produce a solution containing 1 unit/mL. When prescribing insulin always write 'units' in full rather than as 'u', as the latter is too easily confused with a 0 (zero), and a 10-fold dose increase can be given in error.

Run the infusion at an initial rate of 0.1 units/kg/h (to a maximum of 6 units/h). Adjust the rate to reduce the serum [glucose] by not more than 5 mmol/L/h. Avoid using a sliding scale in this setting, as this may lead to a failure of medical staff to review patients regularly and frequently.

When the serum [glucose] is less than 15 mmol/L, halve the insulin infusion rate and then adjust it to maintain the serum [glucose] between 9 and 14 mmol/L.[2]

Do not start the insulin infusion until it has been checked that the serum [potassium] is not below the bottom of the reference range, i.e. it should be greater than 3.4 mmol/L. If it is lower than this, start an infusion of potassium with i.v. fluid first prior to commencing the insulin infusion.

Although there are few data on the benefits or harm of giving a bolus of insulin

before starting the infusion, the short half-life of insulin makes it unnecessary. Providing the insulin infusion is prepared and started with minimal delay, there is no justification for a bolus (despite a bolus appearing in many published guidelines).

Although switching from an insulin infusion to intermittent insulin is most likely to occur in the inpatient setting, ED staff must be aware that the insulin infusion is still needed even after the hyperglycaemia resolves, as the ketoacidosis may persist for longer. It may therefore be necessary to combine the insulin infusion with isotonic 5% or hypertonic 10% dextrose to prevent hypoglycaemia.

Stopping an insulin infusion

If ED staff do supervise cessation of the insulin infusion, they must ensure the first sub cut dose is given at least 1 h before the infusion is stopped, providing *all* the following criteria have been met before stopping the insulin infusion:

- serum [glucose] < 11 mmol/L
- serum bicarbonate > 18 mmol/L
- pH > 7.30
- patient eating and drinking normally, with normal conscious level.

Potassium replacement

Hyperkalaemia and then hypokalaemia are the most common life-threatening electrolyte problems seen in DKA. Therefore the serum [K] should be monitored closely, and treatment planned to treat either condition rapidly, particularly the risk of hypokalaemia. The typical total body deficit of potassium in DKA is 3–5 mmol/kg.[1]

Hyperkalaemia seen in the early phase of DKA may cause life-threatening dysrhythmias due to potassium movement out of the cells from the lack of insulin, prior to insulin and fluid management. Hyperkalaemia resolves soon after insulin treatment begins.

Add potassium to intravenous fluids once serum [K] is below the upper end of the reference range, i.e. <6.0 mmol/L. However, never add potassium to the first fluids infused rapidly for volume resuscitation.

Usually adding 20 mmol/h is sufficient, but this may need to be altered in the light of serum [K] measurements, with the aim of maintaining serum [K] in the range 4–5 mmol/L. Use an intravenous fluid pump or driver to avoid unregulated or inadvertently rapid potassium infusion.

Education

Arguably all episodes of DKA represent a failure of patient education, except for those patients in whom DKA is the first presentation of diabetes mellitus. All patients treated with insulin must understand 'sick day rules' to increase their normal insulin dose by 4 units or more when they have an intercurrent illness, even if they are not eating, as their insulin requirements will rise. Stopping insulin because a patient is 'not eating properly' is all too common and an entirely avoidable precipitant of DKA.

Treatment of HHNS

The treatment of HHNS is similar to that of DKA. Use 0.9% normal saline for volume resuscitation if there is hypovolaemic shock. Give insulin by intravenous infusion and potassium supplementation to maintain serum [K] between 4 and 5 mmol/L. A typical deficit of sodium in HHNS is 5–13 mmol/kg and of potassium is 4–6 mmol/kg, both generally greater than in DKA.

Important management differences

- The patient with HHNS may be more sensitive to insulin. Give an initial dose of 0.05 units/kg/h to a maximum of 3 units, titrated to a controlled fall in serum osmolarity. Aim for a rate of decline in serum osmolarity of less than 3 mOsm/kg/h, avoiding more rapid falls.
- Reduce the insulin infusion rate when the serum [glucose] drops to 18 mmol/L or less, to maintain serum [glucose] in the range 14–18 mmol/L until the serum osmolarity is less than 315 mOsm/kg.

- Shock may be partly or entirely cardiogenic rather than due to volume depletion. Thus invasive monitoring, central venous access and the use of vasoactive drugs rather than fluid alone will be required in this circumstance.
- LMWH is given for thromboprophylaxis although there are no trial outcome data to support this.
- Infuse 0.45% half-normal saline at 250 mL/h, unless the corrected serum [Na] is low (see below the correction of serum [Na] for an elevated glucose level). Aim for a rate of decline of serum [Na] not exceeding 1 mmol/L/h. If the corrected serum [Na] is low, use 0.9% normal saline.
- To correct serum [Na] for hyperglycaemia, adjust the serum [Na] up by 1 mmol/L for every 3 mmol/L elevation in serum glucose.

Prognosis

DKA has an overall mortality of less than 5%, which has not changed for many years, but this is higher at extremes of age and with significant comorbidity. The mortality is 25–33% in HHNS.

Miscellaneous issues

There are no data to support the use of phosphate in the treatment of DKA, despite there often being hypophosphataemia.

Heparin thromboprophylaxis is not used routinely in DKA, nor are antibiotics in the absence of a focus of infection or sepsis.

Sodium bicarbonate should never be used in DKA if the pH is greater than 7.0 and even below that level its value is unproven. Significant disadvantages of giving i.v. bicarbonate are a rapid fall in serum [K] and a worsened intracellular acidosis.

Controversies

- Choice and rate of intravenous fluid replacement, and whether this has any impact on the unexpected but devastating development of cerebral oedema (usually seen in children).

- Point-of-care measurement of beta-hydroxybutyrate may become more widespread, although the precise role in the care of patients with DKA has yet to be determined.[4]

- Titrating insulin use against beta-hydroxybutyrate rather than against serum glucose.

- Earlier recognition of ketosis by measuring beta-hydroxybutyrate to reduce incidence and severity of DKA.

- Use of ultrafast-acting insulin analogues subcutaneously in the treatment of DKA in children. Although they would not generally be used in adults with DKA, they may have a role when there is inadequate equipment for continuous intravenous insulin infusion.

References

1. American Diabetes Association. Clinical practice recommendations. Diabetes Care 2004; 27(Suppl 1): S94–102.
2. McGeoch SC, Hutcheon SD, Vaughan SM, et al. Practical Diabetes International 2007; 24(5): 257–261.
3. Adrogue HJ, Barrero J, Eknoyan G. Salutary effects of modest fluid replacement in the treatment of adults with diabetic ketoacidosis. Use in patients without extreme volume deficit. Journal of the American Medical Association 1989; 262(15): 2108–2113.
4. Wallace TM, Matthews TR. Recent advances in the monitoring and management of diabetic ketoacidosis. Quarterly Journal of Medicine 2004; 97: 773–780.

11.3 Thyroid and adrenal emergencies

Andrew Maclean • Pamela Rosengarten

ESSENTIALS

1 The thyroid and adrenal emergencies posing an acute threat to life are thyroid storm, myxoedema coma and acute adrenal insufficiency. Diagnosis of these conditions requires a high index of suspicion and treatment frequently must be initiated on clinical rather than laboratory diagnosis.

2 Common features of thyroid storm are fever, alteration in mental state, cardiovascular complications such as tachyarrhythmias and cardiac failure, and signs of hyperthyroidism. Treatment is with β-blockers, drugs that block thyroid hormone synthesis and release, and corticosteroids.

3 Common clinical features of myxoedema coma are an alteration in conscious state, hypothermia and features of hypothyroidism. Treatment is with intravenous tri-iodothyronine and corticosteroids.

4 The most important clinical feature of acute adrenal insufficiency is hypotension unresponsive to fluid therapy. Although hyponatraemia and hyperkalaemia are usual in acute adrenal insufficiency, serum electrolytes may be normal. Treatment is with intravenous corticosteroid replacement on suspicion of the diagnosis.

5 General supportive measures and the treatment of the precipitating event must parallel the specific treatment regimes in all of these conditions.

Table 11.3.1	Causes of thyrotoxicosis
Primary hyperthyroidism	Graves disease Toxic multinodular goitre Toxic adenoma
Thyroiditis	de Quervains Postpartum Radiation
Central hyperthyroidism	Pituitary adenoma Ectopic thyroid tissue Metastatic thyroid tissue
Drug induced	Lithium Iodine (including radiographic contrast) Amiodarone Excess thyroid hormone ingestion (factitious thyrotoxicosis)

Introduction

Four conditions are covered in this chapter: thyrotoxicosis, hypothyroidism, hypoadrenal states and hyperadrenal states. Patients with the first three present relatively infrequently to emergency departments (EDs), but all four conditions are potentially fatal if they go unrecognized and untreated. The most common cause of Cushing's syndrome is exogenous steroid administration. An inability to produce endogenous steroids in times of physiological stress and therefore the potential for adrenal insufficiency must be considered in such patients.

THYROTOXICOSIS

Aetiology, genetics, pathogenesis and pathology

Normal secretion of thyroid hormone relies on an intact feedback loop involving the hypothalamus, pituitary gland and thyroid gland. Thyrotropin-releasing hormone (TRH) released from the hypothalamus stimulates thyroid-stimulating hormone (TSH) production in the anterior pituitary, which stimulates thyroid hormone release from thyroid follicular cells. Thyroid hormones suppress TRH and TSH production. Thyroid hormones act at a cellular level, binding with nuclear receptors to enable gene expression and protein synthesis. Thyroid hormone may also have an effect on modulating cellular metabolism.

There are a number of pathological causes of thyrotoxicosis (see Table 11.3.1). Graves' disease is an autoimmune condition related to a combination of genetic and environmental factors, including iodine intake, stress and smoking. The thyrotoxicosis of Graves' disease is caused by autoantibodies, which stimulate the thyroid resulting in excess thyroid hormone production.

Thyroiditis may be acute (rare), subacute or chronic. Inflammation of the thyroid is associated with damage to follicles with release of thyroid hormone. Subacute thyroiditis (de Quervain's) is related to a viral infection.

Multinodular goitre occurs in areas of both iodine deficiency and sufficiency, indicating that a multiplicity of genetic and environmental factors are at play. Fibrosis, hypercellularity and colloid cysts are the main pathological findings.

Epidemiology

Graves' disease accounts for at least 80% of cases of thyrotoxicosis.[1] The prevalence increases in areas with high iodine intake. Graves' disease has a strong female predominance, affecting up to 2% of all women.[1,2] Thyrotoxicosis due to Graves' disease usually occurs in the second to fourth decades of life, whereas the prevalence of a toxic nodular goitre increases with age.

Clinical features

The signs and symptoms of hyperthyroidism are secondary to the effects of excess thyroid hormone in the circulation. The severity of the signs and symptoms is related to the duration of the illness, the magnitude of the hormone excess and the age of the patient. These symptoms and signs are summarized in Table 11.3.2, which illustrates the wide spectrum of possible clinical features.

Table 11.3.2 Clinical features of thyrotoxicosis
Nervousness, irritability
Heat intolerance and increased sweating
Tremor
Weight loss and alterations in appetite
Palpitations and tachycardia, in particular atrial fibrillation
Widened pulse pressure
Exertional intolerance and dyspnoea
Frequent bowel movements
Fatigue and muscle weakness
Thyroid enlargement (depending on cause)
Pretibial myxoedema (with Graves' disease)
Menstrual disturbance and impaired fertility
Mental disturbances
Sleep disturbances
Changes in vision, photophobia, eye irritation, diplopia, lid lag or exophthalmos
Dependent lower extremity oedema
Sudden paralysis, with or without hypokalaemia.

A comprehensive history and physical examination should be performed, with particular attention to weight, blood pressure, pulse rate and rhythm, looking specifically for cardiac failure, palpation and auscultation of the thyroid to determine thyroid size, nodularity and vascularity, neuromuscular examination, and an eye examination for evidence of exophthalmos or ophthalmoplegia.

Clinical investigation and criteria for diagnosis[1-3]

The TSH level is the single best screening test for hyperthyroidism. The recent development of sensitive TSH assays has greatly facilitated the diagnosis of hyperthyroidism. Hyperthyroidism of any cause (except excess TSH production from the anterior pituitary) results in a lower than normal TSH. The reference range is 0.4–5.0 mIU/L depending on the method.

Other laboratory and isotope tests may include:

- Free thyroxine (T4) or free tri-iodothyronine (T3) assay, when there is strong clinical suspicion of hyperthyroidism but the TSH is high or high normal.
- Thyroid autoantibodies, including TSH receptor antibody. These are not routine but may be helpful in selected cases.
- Radioactive iodine uptake and/or thyroid scan. These tests are helpful in establishing the cause of hyperthyroidism, but are not part of the ED assessment.

Treatment

Mild hyperthyroidism does not require any treatment in the ED and may simply be referred to an appropriate outpatient clinic. Any features of thyroid storm (see below) mandate admission, as does any significant intercurrent illness. Atrial arrhythmias should be controlled by the use of β-blockers, aiming to achieve a rate of less than 100 beats per minute.

Ensure that all bloods have been collected first if thyroid-blocking drugs are to be commenced in the ED. High doses of thyroid-blocking drugs are often required to gain an initial response, after which the dose can be tapered.

Give carbimazole 10–45 mg daily bd or tds, or propylthiouracil 200–600 mg daily bd or tds initially, using the larger doses for more severe cases.[4] It is preferable to discuss initiation of these agents with the physician who will be managing the patient after their discharge from the ED. Ninety per cent of patients will be controlled within weeks with these drugs.[5] Treatment for 12–18 months will result in a long-term remission in 40–60% of patients with Graves' disease.[2]

Thyroid storm

Aetiology

Thyroid storm occurs in about 1% of patients with hyperthyroidism. It usually occurs as an acute deterioration in a patient with poorly controlled or undiagnosed hyperthyroidism, precipitated by factors such as surgery, trauma, infection, radioiodine treatment, use of iodinated contrast, exogenous thyroxine ingestion or any other significant stressor.

The diagnosis is entirely clinical, as there is no test to differentiate a thyroid storm from thyrotoxicosis. The mortality rate if left untreated or if the diagnosis is missed is 90%, which with treatment is reduced to 10–15%. Death is usually due to cardiovascular collapse.

Clinical features

The symptoms and signs of thyrotoxicosis are present and significantly exaggerated, with the abrupt onset of a combination of the following features:

- fever >37.6°C up to 41°C
- cardiovascular complications:
  - tachycardia with pulse rates up to 200–300/min, including rapid atrial fibrillation
  - wide pulse pressure
  - high output cardiac failure
- alteration in mental state, varying from agitation and restlessness to delirium, coma and seizures
- abdominal pain with vomiting and diarrhoea.

Differential diagnosis

The following differential diagnoses need to be considered:

- sepsis
- heat stroke
- malignant hyperthermia
- neuroleptic syndrome
- sympathomimetic ingestion
- drug withdrawal (including alcohol)
- phaeochromocytoma crisis.

Treatment

The treatment of thyroid storm is directed to blocking thyroid hormone synthesis and release, the peripheral effects of the thyroid hormones, and corticosteroids.

β-blockers

β-blockade is the most important factor in decreasing morbidity and mortality. Many of the peripheral manifestations of hyperthyroidism, in particular the cardiovascular effects, are reduced by the use of propranolol. Propranolol inhibits the peripheral conversion of T4 to T3 as well as antagonizing the effects of thyroid hormones and the hypersensitivity to catecholamines.

Give intravenous increments of 0.5 mg initially up to 10 mg total with continuous cardiovascular monitoring. Subsequent doses of 40–120 mg 6-hourly can be given orally. β-blockers should treat the cardiac failure secondary to the tachyarrhythmia or high cardiac output, but may cause complications in patients with pre-existing heart disease or asthma.

In this situation the short-acting β-blocker esmolol should be used, as any adverse effects will be of brief duration. Give a 250–500 μg/kg bolus followed by an infusion starting at 50–100 μg/kg/min titrated to effect. Another option is to use a combination of a β-blocker and digoxin.

Thyroid-blocking drugs

Give propylthiouracil 900–1200 mg loading dose orally or via a nasogastric tube if necessary. This is followed by 200–300 mg 4–6-hourly. Propylthiouracil acts by preventing hormone synthesis by blocking the iodination of tyrosine, and also inhibits the peripheral conversion of T4 to T3.

Iodine in large doses inhibits the synthesis and release of thyroid hormones, and may be given either orally as Lugol's iodine, 30–60 drops daily in divided doses, or intravenously as sodium iodide 1 g 12-hourly. Lithium carbonate may be used in patients allergic to iodine or added when there is difficulty with control.[4]

Cholestyramine may also be considered, which acts by binding with thyroxine after biliary excretion and hence increasing elimination.

Corticosteroids

Corticosteroids are given to inhibit the peripheral conversion of T4 to T3 and as a relative deficiency may also be present. Hydrocortisone 100 mg i.v. 6-hourly or dexamethasone 2 mg i.v. 6-hourly are used.

General supportive measures

Dehydration and electrolyte disturbances need correction. Aggressive treatment of hyperthermia with paracetamol and cooling measures are necessary, but induction of shivering should be avoided. Salicylates are contraindicated as they displace T4

from binding proteins. In addition it is essential to look for and treat any precipitating cause, which will improve the prognosis.

Prognosis

Mortality rates are high, at 10–75% despite treatment.

Apathetic hyperthyroidism

Patients with this condition are generally older, although it has been recorded in all age groups. The clinical picture is of a depressed mental state with cardiac complications, in particular cardiac failure. Weight loss is usually not significant and eye signs are rare. Most of the usual hyperkinetic manifestations of hyperthyroidism are absent. Treatment is as for standard hyperthyroidism.

HYPOTHYROIDISM

Aetiology, genetics, pathogenesis and pathology

Hypothyroidism results from undersecretion of thyroid hormone from the thyroid gland. Causes of primary hypothyroidism include iodine deficiency, chronic autoimmune thyroiditis (Hashimoto's thyroiditis), congenital, surgical removal of the thyroid gland, post-radioactive iodine, thyroid gland ablation and external irradiation. A significant number of cases are idiopathic. Secondary causes of hypothyroidism include pituitary and hypothalamic disease.

Epidemiology

Iodine deficiency is the most common cause worldwide, whereas in areas of iodine sufficiency, autoimmune disease and hypothyoidism secondary to treatment of hyperthyroid disease are most common. The prevalence of hyperthyroidism in adults is of the order of 1.4% in women and <0.1% in men.[6] Congenital hypothyroidism is rare, occurring in about 1:4000 births.

Clinical features

The symptoms of hypothyroidism are related to the duration and severity of hypothyroidism, the rapidity with which hypothyroidism occurs and the psychological characteristics of the patient. These are summarized in Table 11.3.3.

A complete evaluation, including a comprehensive history, physical examination and appropriate laboratory evaluation, should be performed in every patient with a goitre. Patients with chronic thyroiditis have a higher incidence of other associated autoimmune diseases such as vitiligo, rheumatoid arthritis, Addison's disease, diabetes mellitus and pernicious anaemia.

Table 11.3.3 Clinical features of hypothyroidism
Dry skin and cold intolerance
Coarse facial features
Enlarged tongue
Coarse brittle hair or loss of hair, loss of outer third of eyebrows
Periorbital oedema
Fatigue
Constipation
Weight gain/obesity
Memory and mental impairment, decreased concentration
Depression, personality changes
Yellow skin
Swelling of ankles
Irregular or heavy menses and infertility
Hoarseness
Myalgias
Goitre
Hyperlipidaemia
Delayed relaxation phase of tendon reflexes, ataxia
Sinus bradycardia (atrioventricular block, rare)
Cardiac failure, pericardial effusion (rare)
Hypothermia (uncommon)

Clinical investigation and criteria for diagnosis

Laboratory evaluation

Perform a TSH assay as the primary test to establish the diagnosis of hypothyroidism. The reference range is 0.4–5.0 mIU/L depending on the method. Additional tests may include free thyroxine assay and thyroid autoantibodies. A combination of an elevated TSH and low free thyroxine is diagnostic.[3,4,6] A patient may be hypothyroid with a TSH greater than twice the reference interval, but with a free thyroxine within the normal range. Subnormal thyroxine with a normal TSH can occur in secondary hypothyroidism.

Thyroid autoantibodies are positive in 95% of patients with autoimmune thyroiditis (Hashimoto's thyroiditis). The high titres are of great value in making this specific diagnosis.

Other investigations

A thyroid scan and/or an ultrasound are useful if structural thyroid abnormalities are suspected.

Thyroid nodules are not uncommon with chronic thyroiditis and carry a small risk of thyroid cancer.

Treatment

Start thyroxine at 50–100 μg orally daily in adults under 60 years of age without evidence of ischaemic heart disease. Rapid commencement of full thyroid hormone replacement may cause myocardial ischaemia, from increased myocardial oxygen consumption without a corresponding increase in cardiac output. The initial daily replacement dose is therefore 25 μg thyroxine in the elderly and where there is suspicion of heart disease. This dose should remain unchanged for 3–4 weeks to allow a steady state to be reached. It is appropriate to start this in the ED, when a firm diagnosis has been made and appropriate follow-up arranged.

The dose of thyroxine is then increased in 25–50 μg increments until the optimum dose is reached, determined by clinical response and TSH level. Consider admission for any patient with coexistent unstable angina to monitor cardiac function. Any features of myxoedema coma (see below) also mandate admission.

Myxoedema coma

The clinical syndrome of altered mental state, features of hypothyroidism and hypothermia is referred to as myxoedema coma. There is usually a precipitating event such as infection, stroke, trauma, myocardial infarction or administration of drugs, particularly phenothiazines, phenytoin, amiodarone, propranolol or lithium that initiates this terminal decompensation phase of hypothyroidism.

The mortality for myxoedema coma remains up to 50% despite aggressive treatment.

Clinical features

- Altered mental state, usually coma due to cerebral oedema, hypoxia and hypercarbia.
- Seizures may precede coma in 25% patients.
- Hypothermia with temperature usually less that 32.2°C. Notably, patients do not shiver.
- Hypoventilation resulting in hypoxia and hypercarbia.
- Cardiovascular complications, including hypotension and bradycardia, with heart rate inappropriate for the hypotension. Pericardial effusion, rarely cardiac tamponade.
- Hypoglycaemia (common).
- Hyponatraemia.
- Paralytic ileus, megacolon, urinary retention.
- Usual clinical features of hypothyroidism.

Treatment

Treatment should commence on clinical suspicion.

Administration of thyroid hormones

Tri-iodothyronine There is no consensus as to whether T3 or T4 replacement is preferable.[7,8] Intravenous T3 may give a faster clinical response in myxoedema coma, as it is the active form of the hormone. Give T3 as an initial i.v. bolus of 25–50 μg followed by 10–20 μg 8-hourly to a maximum of 60 μg per day. Alternatively, commence an infusion with a lower total dose of 20 μg per day, as large initial doses appear unnecessary for recovery and may in fact be harmful. Oral or nasogastric replacement of T3 is not recommended in the initial phase of management because of unreliable gastrointestinal absorption.

Thyroxine The use of T4 is supported as the gradual delivery of T3 through the peripheral conversion of T4 is better tolerated and as the onset of action is more predictable. Give a 400–500 μg i.v. bolus (300 μg/m²), followed by 50 μg i.v. daily until oral therapy is tolerated. Combined approaches are now also described.

Corticosteroids These are given as there is impaired response to stress and the potential for coexistent adrenal insufficiency. Give hydrocortisone 100 mg i.v. 6-hourly.

General supportive measures This requires correction of ventilatory, circulatory, temperature and metabolic abnormalities, and includes the use of warm humidified oxygen. Look for and treat any precipitating cause. Finally avoid sedative drugs and take care to avoid water overload.

HYPOADRENAL STATES

Aetiology, genetics, pathogenesis and pathology

Glucocorticoids act to produce multiple effects on metabolism, including gluconeogenesis, mobilization of fatty acids and amino acids, inhibiting the effects of insulin and ketogenesis. Glucocorticoids have anti-inflammatory effects related to the inhibition of production, and reduction of the effects of cytokines, and reduction of cell-mediated immunity. They also maintain the normal response of the vascular system to vasoconstrictors. Glucocorticoids also affect the regulation of body water by increasing free water excretion. This occurs by an increase in the glomerular filtration rate as well as inhibition of migration of water into cells. Aldosterone acts primarily to cause the reabsorption of sodium and the excretion of potassium and hydrogen ions.

The adrenals normally respond within minutes by elevating corticosteroid levels in response to any physiological or pathological stress. When glucocorticoid insufficiency is present such stressors may result in hypotension, shock and ultimately death if left untreated.

Primary adrenal insufficiency

Primary adrenal insufficiency is due to inability of the adrenal cortex to produce adequate levels of adrenal hormones. Hyponatraemia, hyperkalaemia, acidosis and elevated serum creatinine mainly occur due to aldosterone deficiency in primary adrenal insufficiency. Hypoglycaemia is related to cortisol deficiency. Hypercalcaemia occurs as a result of reduction in glomerular filtration rate as well as increased proximal tubular reabsorption of calcium. There may also be some increased mobilization of calcium from bone in patients with adrenal insufficiency.

Secondary adrenal insufficiency

Secondary adrenal insufficiency is due to failure of adequate adrenocorticotrophic hormone (ACTH) from the pituitay gland (Table 11.3.4). Hyponatraemia still occurs in secondary adrenal insufficiency, but is due to cortisol deficiency.[9,10]

The majority of presentations of acute adrenal insufficiency occur as an exacerbation of a chronic disease process, where there is a malfunctioning adrenal system. Acute precipitating factors include sepsis, major trauma, surgery and a myocardial infarct.

Causes of primary or secondary adrenal insufficiency

The cause of 80% of primary adrenal insufficiency is autoimmune (Addison's disease). Other causes include primary or secondary malignancy, infection such as tuberculosis, adrenal infarction or haemorrhage (Waterhouse-Friedrichsen syndrome) seen in meningococcaemia or severe

Table 11.3.4	Causes of adrenal insufficiency
Primary	Addison's disease Surgical removal Infectious (TB, viral, fungal) Haemorrhage, including Waterhouse–Friedrichsen syndrome Congenital
Secondary	Exogenous steroid suppression (single most common cause of hypoadrenalism overall) Endogenous steroid (tumour) Pituitary failure

sepsis, and drugs. Primary adrenal insufficiency also occurs in up to 20% of patients with AIDS. Up to 60% of patients with sepsis have a low baseline cortisol level, although fewer meet criteria of insufficiency on suppression testing.[11,12]

The most common cause of secondary adrenal insufficiency is suppression of the adrenopituitary axis by long-term steroid therapy, although other causes include pituitary failure.

Clinical features

Suspect adrenocortical failure in any hypotensive patient when no apparent cause is found, particularly anyone who is unresponsive to fluid therapy. Orthostatic hypotension is almost always present. Other common features include abdominal pain, which may be severe, with vomiting.

Less obvious findings are weakness, anorexia, diarrhoea, postural syncope, mucocutaneous pigmentation/vitiligo (only with primary adrenal disease) and a dulled mental state.

Hypercalcaemia and/or hyperkalaemia may be the first sign of adrenal insufficiency in the critically ill patient.[10] The other features of adrenal insufficiency may be masked by coexisting illness, but the possibility of adrenal insufficiency should always be considered in such cases.

Differential diagnosis

The diagnosis of adrenal insufficiency in the early stages is difficult as weakness, lethargy and gastrointestinal symptoms are common and non-specific. Consider adrenal insufficiency in any patients presenting with these symptoms when more common causes have been excluded.

Clinical investigation

Laboratory findings

The classical laboratory findings are hyponatraemia (due to sodium depletion and the intracellular movement of sodium), hypochloraemia and hyperkalaemia (due to acidosis and aldosterone deficiency). Mild hypercalcaemia (in 10–20% of cases) and a non-anion gap metabolic acidosis may be present. Hypoglycaemia if present

is usually mild. However, all basic laboratory investigations may be within normal limits, even in the presence of an addisonian crisis.

Anti-adrenal antibodies are positive in 70% of patients with autoimmune adrenalitis.

Criteria for diagnosis 3

Baseline cortisol and ACTH levels should be taken prior to treatment. The normal reference range for cortisol is 200–650 nmol/L. ACTH levels should normally be <50 ng/L, although interpretation needs to take into account the time of day the sample is taken. ACTH should be high in primary adrenal disease and low in pituitary disease.

The Synacthen® stimulation test is the definitive test and may be required if the initial test results are not diagnostic, usually performed as an inpatient. Synacthen® 250 μg is administered intramuscularly and cortisol levels are taken at baseline, 30 min and 60 min. A baseline or post-Synacthen® cortisol level of >550 nmol/L is considered normal.

Treatment

Corticosteroid replacement

Do not delay treatment awaiting confirmatory results if acute adrenal insufficiency is suspected.

Give immediate corticosteroid replacement with either intravenous hydrocortisone or dexamethasone. Dexamethasone is recommended when the diagnosis has not been confirmed by laboratory investigations, as it does not interfere with the cortisol assay. Give 10 mg dexamethasone i.v. stat followed by 4 mg i.v. 8-hourly. Alternatively, give hydrocortisone in a dose of 250 mg stat followed by 100 mg i.v. 6-hourly.

Fluid replacement therapy

Give normal saline 1 L stat, then titrated to response, although the total volume deficit is rarely greater than 10% body weight. Intravenous dextrose should be given at the same time, either separately or as 5% dextrose in normal saline to avoid hypoglycaemia.

General supportive measures

General supportive measures include treatment of hypoglycaemia and other electrolyte replacement abnormalities, although most will be corrected with saline rehydration alone. Mineralocorticoid replacement is usually not necessary in the acute crisis if salt and water replacement is adequate.

Once the crisis has been successfully treated it is important to investigate and manage the cause and develop a maintenance regime.

Prognosis

The patient may die with acute adrenal insufficiency if the diagnosis is not made. When the diagnosis is suspected and treatment is early, the outcome is favourable depending on the nature of any precipitating illness.

Response to severe illness

The normal response to severe illness should see cortisol levels rising to at least 500 nmol/L. States of 'relative adrenal insufficiency' are described where glucocorticoid administration diminishes or even eliminates the requirements for vasopressor agents, even though measured cortisol levels are normal or close to normal.[11] There is no consensus on what constitutes 'normal' cortisol levels in severe illness.

Up to 60% of patients in sepsis may have some degree of adrenal insufficiency depending upon the threshold cortisol level used.[12] Moreover, it appears that it is the delta cortisol rather than the basal cortisol level that is associated with clinical outcome.[13] Repeat adrenal function testing is indicated in patients with severe illness who remain unstable or who fail to improve with aggressive supportive therapy.[14]

The use of hydrocortisone has been recommended in septic shock after a 250 μg Synacthen® stimulation test.[15–17] This should continue for a week if adrenal insufficiency is confirmed.

HYPERADRENAL STATES

Aetiology, pathogenesis and epidemiology

Cushing's disease usually refers to hyperadrenalism due to a pituitary adenoma.

Cushing's syndrome occurs as a result of hyperadrenalism from exposure to excess glucocorticoids over a prolonged period. Endogenous causes of Cushing's syndrome are related to primary adrenal disorders, such as adrenal adenoma, carcinoma or hyperplasia, or are secondary to ACTH or CRH stimulation, and ectopic ACTH production from bronchogenic carcinoma or carcinoid tumours in particular. However, by far the most common cause of Cushing's syndrome is from the exogenous (iatrogenic) administration of steroids.

The incidence of Cushing's syndrome ranges from 0.7 to 2.4 per million population per year, but the reported prevalence in obese patients with type II diabetes may be between 2 and 5%.[18]

Clinical features

The classical clinical features of Cushing's syndrome are increased body weight with central obesity, rounded face, hypertension, fatigue, weakness and proximal myopathy, hirsutism, striae, bruising, decreased libido, amenorrhoea, depression and or personality changes, osteopenia or fracture. Proximal weakness or myopathy is useful to differentiate simple obesity (strong limbs) from possible Cushing's syndrome (relative weakness for patient's size).

Clinical investigation and criteria for diagnosis

Laboratory tests
Full blood examination may reveal polycythaemia, neutrophilia and eosinophilia. Electrolytes may show hyperkalaemia, metabolic alkalosis and hyperglycaemia.

24-h urinary cortisol level
A measured 24-h urinary cortisol level with a value more than four times the upper normal range is rare except in Cushing's syndrome (normal range 100–300 nmol/24 h).

Overnight dexamethasone suppression test
This is an outpatient screening test for Cushing's syndrome:[3]

Day 1 0900 hours: 5 mL blood taken for baseline cortisol
Day 1 2300 hours: 1 mg dexamethasone taken orally
Day 2: 5 mL blood for cortisol

The baseline reference range for cortisol is 200–650 nmol/L. The day 2 cortisol level should drop to lower than 50% of the baseline level, indicating normal suppression and excluding Cushing's syndrome.

Long dexamathasone suppression test
The long dexamathasone suppression test is performed as an inpatient, using increasing doses of dexamethasone to determine at what level suppression occurs, with testing of both cortisol and ACTH levels. Cushing's disease will only suppress at high doses.

Other tests
A chest X-ray is important if bronchogenic carcinoma of the lung is suspected. Magnetic resonance imaging of the adrenals and/or head is used for the identification of tumours.

Treatment

Treatment will depend on the cause. When a pituitary or adrenal adenoma is identified, optimal treatment is removal of the tumour.[4,18] Glucocorticoid replacement is then required for up to 2 years following surgery to allow full recovery of the normal pituitary–adrenal axis.

Pharmacological blockade of adrenal corticosteroid production may be required in some circumstances. Ketaconazole, aminoglutethimide, metapyrone and mitotane may be used for this purpose.

Controversies

❶ What constitutes 'normal' cortisol levels in severe illness?

❷ Whether T3 or T4 replacement therapy is preferable in myxoedema coma.

❸ Differentiating simple obesity with hypertension from Cushing's syndrome.

References

1. Cooper DS. Hyperthyroidism. Lancet 2003; 362(9382): 459–468.
2. Pearce EN. Diagnosis and management of thyrotoxicosis. British Medical Journal 2006; 332: 1369–1372.
3. Royal College of Pathologists of Australasia. Manual Version 4.0. Surrey Hills: Royal College of Pathologists of Australasia; 2004.
4. Endocrinology Expert Group. Endocrinology. Guidelines. Melbourne: ©Therapeutic Guidelines Limited; 2004.
5. Cooper DS. Antithyroid drugs. New England Journal of Medicine 2005; 352: 905–917.
6 Lindsay RS, Toft AD. Hypothyroidism. Lancet 1997; 349: 413–417.
7. Jordan RM. Myxedema coma. Medical Clinics of North America 1995; 79: 185–194.
8. Vedig AE. Thyroid emergencies. In: Oh's intensive care manual. 5th edn. Edinburgh: Elsevier; 2004.
9. Oelkers W. Adrenal insufficiency. New England Journal of Medicine 1996; 335: 1206–1212.
10. Nair G, Simmons D. Adrenal insufficiency presenting as hypercalcemia. Hospital Physician 2003; 33–35.
11. de Herder W, van der Lely A. Addisonian crisis and relative adrenal failure. Reviews in Endocrine & Metabolic Disorders 2003; 4: 143–147.
12. Marik P, Zaloga G. Adrenal insufficiency during septic shock. Critical Care Medicine 2003; 31: 141–145.
13. Lipner Fredman D, Sprung C, et al. Adrenal function in sepsis: the retrospective Corticus cohort study. Critical Care Medicine 2007; 35: 1012–1018.
14. Marik P. Adrenal-exhaustion syndrome in patients with liver disease. Intensive Care Medicine 2006; 134: 275–280.
15. Cooper MS, Stewart PM. Current concepts: corticosteroid insufficiency in acutely ill patients. New England Journal of Medicine 2003; 348: 727–734.
16. Annane D. Glucocorticoids in the treatment of severe sepsis and septic shock. Current Opinion in Critical Care 2005; 11: 449–453.
17. Luce JM. Physicians should administer low-dose corticosteroid selectively to septic patients until an ongoing trial is completed. Annals of Internal Medicine 2004; 141: 70.
18. Newall-Price J, Bertagna X, Grossman AB, et al. Cushing's syndrome. Lancet 2006; 367: 1605–1617.

Further reading

Jameson L, Weetman AP. Disorders of the thyroid gland. In: Kaspar DL, et al, eds. Harrison's principles of internal medicine. 16th edn. New York: McGraw-Hill; 2005.

Maclean A, Dunn R. Endocrinology. In: The emergency medicine manual. 4th edn. Adelaide: Venom Publishing; 2006.

Vedig AE. Thyroid emergencies. In: Oh's intensive care manual. 5th edn. Edinburgh: Elsevier; 2004.

Vedig AE. Adrenocortical insufficiency. In: Oh's intensive care manual. 5th edn. Edinburgh: Elsevier; 2004.

Williams GH, Dluhy RG. Disorders of the adrenal cortex. In: Kaspar DL, et al, eds. Harrison's principles of internal medicine. 16th edn. New York: McGraw-Hill; 2005.

12.1 Acid–base disorders

Robert Dunn

ESSENTIALS

1 Acid–base homeostasis is maintained by buffering, respiratory and renal mechanisms.

2 Acidosis increases serum potassium concentration and may have protective effects on tissues.

3 Lactic acidosis is the most common cause of metabolic acidosis seen in emergency medicine practice.

4 Respiratory acidosis is caused by alveolar hypoventilation.

5 Treatment of acidosis is directed towards correction of the underlying cause.

6 Administration of $NaHCO_3$ is indicated in severe hyperkalaemia, sodium channel blocking agent, salicylate, ethylene glycol and methanol toxicity.

7 Metabolic alkalosis in the emergency department is usually secondary to prolonged vomiting, and its management is directed towards rehydration with normal saline and correction of the underlying cause.

8 Respiratory alkalosis commonly presents with features of hypocalcaemia with hypoxia, early sepsis, cerebral oedema and anxiety being important causes.

Introduction

Acid–base disorders are commonly encountered in the emergency department (ED), and their recognition is important for the diagnosis, assessment of severity and monitoring of many disease processes. Although these disorders are usually classified according to the major metabolic abnormality present (acidosis or alkalosis) and its origin (metabolic or respiratory), it is important to realize that acid–base disorders of a mixed type commonly occur and that the recognition and assessment of these are more complex.

Acid–base homeostasis

The acid–base status is one of the most tightly regulated systems in the body. Normal metabolic activity generates CO_2 and smaller amounts of lactate and other acids. The effects of these substances on plasma and intracellular pH are limited by buffering, respiratory and renal mechanisms. Buffering systems provide the most immediate mechanism. The most important intracellular buffers are HCO_3^- and plasma protein systems, whilst the most important extracellular buffers are intracellular proteins (especially haemoglobin in red blood cells) and phosphate. The production of CO_2 stimulates ventilation, with the result that respiratory excretion of CO_2 accounts for the vast majority of acid secretion from the body. The respiratory compensatory effects start to occur within minutes. Renal elimination of acid accounts for a smaller percentage of total acid elimination and usually takes hours to days to take effect.

Acidosis

Systemic acidosis is defined as the presence of an increased concentration of H^+ ions in the blood. The physiological effects of acidosis are a decrease in the affinity of haemoglobin for oxygen and an increase in serum K^+ of approximately 0.4–0.6 mmol/L for each decrease in pH of 0.1, although this does not appear to occur during anaesthesia.[1] It is commonly believed that acidosis decreases myocardial contractility, but this is usually of little clinical significance at a pH of more than 7.1. Although the presence of acidosis is often associated with a poor prognosis, the presence of acidosis per se usually has few clinically significant effects, and it is the nature and severity of the underlying illness that determines its outcome. There is also evidence that acidosis may have a protective effect in tissues by decreasing phospholipase activity and inhibiting the development of the mitochondrial permeability transition defect that leads to apoptosis. In certain situations, such as in pregnant women and the neonate, increased acid production may result in a greater change in serum pH (and possibly greater adverse physiological effects) than expected, owing to the decreased buffering capacity of the plasma. A decrease in measured serum HCO_3^- of up to 5 mmol/L has also been reported as a result of underfilling of vacuum-type specimen tubes.[2]

Metabolic acidosis

Metabolic acidosis is defined as an increase in the $[H^+]$ of the blood as a result of increased acid production or decreased acid elimination by routes other than the lungs. The cause is often multifactorial and can be further classified into 'anion-gap' and 'non-anion gap' (or hyperchloraemic) metabolic acidosis.

Anion-gap metabolic acidosis

As electroneutrality must exist in all solutions, the anion gap represents the concentration of anions that are not commonly measured. The most commonly used formula for the calculation of the anion gap is:

$$anion\ gap = ([Na] + [K]) - ([Cl] + [HCO_3^-])$$

The normal value for the anion gap depends on the type of biochemical analyser used and whilst the upper limit of normal has been commonly quoted as 18, the mean range with some modern analysers is only 5–12.[3] In the normal resting state the serum ionic proteins account for most of the anion gap, with a lesser contribution from other 'unmeasured' anions such as PO_4^- and SO_4^-. In pathological conditions where there is an increase in the concentration of unmeasured anions, an anion-gap metabolic acidosis results. The anions responsible for the increase in the anion gap depend on the cause of the acidosis. Lactic acid is the predominant anion in hypoxia and shock, PO_4^- and SO_4^- in renal failure, ketoacids in diabetic and alcoholic ketoacidosis, oxalic acid in ethylene glycol poisoning and formic acid in methanol poisoning.

Of the causes of an anion-gap metabolic acidosis, lactic acidosis is the most commonly encountered in the ED and is defined as a serum lactate of >2.5 mmol/L. The presence of lactic acidosis is determined by the balance between lactate production and metabolism. In the seriously ill patient, it is common for increased production and decreased metabolism to be present simultaneously. Tissue hypoxia of any cause decreases oxidative phosphorylation and results in the increased conversion of pyruvate to lactate. This commonly occurs in major haemorrhage and in the presence of severe cardiorespiratory disease. An alternative cause for increased lactate production may be the uncoupling of oxidative phosphorylation following exposure to toxins, such as cyanide, salicylates, metformin and iron. Severe thiamine deficiency may result in a marked increase in lactate production known as warm beriberi. A mild metabolic acidosis is common in acute ethanol intoxication and is associated with an elevated anion gap in 80% of cases; however, it is multifactorial in origin. Metabolism of lactic acid occurs in the liver and kidney, and is reduced when these organs are diseased or in the presence of alkalosis, hypothermia and diabetes mellitus.

It is important to realize that, in many conditions, a variety of factors may produce the acidosis, and that multiple anions may be involved in the production of an anion-gap acidosis. For example, in a patient with severe diabetic ketoacidosis, poor tissue perfusion, renal failure, increased lactic and ketoacid production, decreased SO_4^- and PO_4^- elimination and decreased lactic acid metabolism may all be present. Lactic acidosis is generally considered to be severe if serum lactate is >4 mmol/L.

Non-anion gap metabolic acidosis

Non-anion gap metabolic acidosis results from loss of HCO_3^- from the body, rather than increased acid production. To maintain electroneutrality, chloride is usually retained by the renal tubules when HCO_3^- is lost, and the hallmark of non-anion gap acidosis is an elevation of the serum chloride. The causes of non-anion gap metabolic acidosis are further classified according to the site of HCO_3^- loss. Gastrointestinal losses can occur with lower gastrointestinal tract (GIT) fluid losses that are rich in HCO_3^-, or with cholestyramine ingestion due to binding of HCO_3^- in the gut. Renal losses can occur with renal tubular acidosis, carbonic anhydrase inhibitor therapy or adrenocortical insufficiency. Acid is rarely ingested in sufficient quantity to cause systemic acidosis.

Renal tubular acidosis Renal tubular acidosis (RTA) is a group of conditions where there is an impaired ability to secrete H^+ in the distal convoluted tubule or absorb HCO_3^- in the proximal convoluted tubule. This may result in a chronic metabolic acidosis, with hypokalaemia, nephrocalcinosis, rickets or osteomalacia. There are many subtypes of RTA and many different causes. Those most commonly encountered in the ED are due to inherited renal tubular transportation disorders, chronic renal diseases, toluene toxicity, heavy metal toxicity or therapy with various drugs, including lithium. Chronic treatment of type I RTA with citrated HCO_3^- decreases the systemic acidosis and may prevent renal calculi formation, and progression of renal and secondary bone disease.

Treatment of metabolic acidosis

The treatment of acidosis should usually be directed primarily towards correction of the underlying cause. Intravenous HCO_3^- is of use in the presence of acidosis and severe hyperkalaemia, severe sodium channel (e.g. tricyclic antidepressant), salicylate, methanol or ethylene glycol toxicity. It should be used to attempt to normalize the pH before Factor VIIa therapy is administered. It may be of use in rhabdomyolysis and cardiac arrest in young children or pregnant women or cardiac arrest of more than 15 min duration. The use of HCO_3^- in patients with diabetic ketoacidosis and lactic acidosis associated with sepsis or severe cardiorespiratory disease does not appear to improve outcome.[4–6] The potential hazards of HCO_3^- therapy include a high solute load, hyperosmolarity, hypokalaemia, decreased ionized serum calcium, worsening of cerebrospinal fluid acidosis (which may precipitate hepatic encephalopathy in susceptible patients) and decreased metabolic degradation of citrate, lactate and ketone bodies in the liver. It also reduces oxygen off-loading by haemoglobin in the tissues and may inactivate calcium and adrenaline when administered through the same intravenous line.[7]

Respiratory acidosis

Respiratory acidosis is defined as an elevation of the arterial partial pressure of carbon dioxide (PCO_2) and is due to alveolar hypoventilation. The effects of mild-to-moderate hypercarbia are usually confined to its effect on decreasing the alveolar partial pressure of oxygen (see alveolar gas equation). With more significant elevations, sweating, tachycardia, confusion and mydriasis occur. When the PCO_2 is greater than 80 mmHg, the level of consciousness is usually depressed. There are many possible causes of alveolar hypoventilation. Central nervous system causes include severe hypotension, drugs with respiratory depressant effects (especially opioids and sedatives), cerebrovascular events, tumours, infections, neurotrauma and metabolic derangements. Ventilatory drive may also be reduced by high partial pressures of oxygen in patients with chronic obstructive airways disease (COAD) and chronic CO_2 retention. Lesions of the spinal cord, such as tumours, infections, trauma or demyelination, may also result in alveolar hypoventilation if the lesion is above the level of C4. Lower in the afferent limb of respiratory muscle innervation, lesions of peripheral nerves such as Guillain–Barré syndrome or trauma to both phrenic nerves may also be causative. Neuromuscular junction dysfunction following postsynaptic destruction of acetylcholine receptors in myaesthenia gravis, inactivation of cholinesterase in organophosphate poisoning or the effects of spider or snake venoms and muscle relaxant drugs may also cause ventilatory failure. Aminoglycoside antibiotics may also precipitate ventilatory failure in susceptible patients. Muscular dystrophy, myopathies and severe electrolyte disorders may cause muscular weakness, and lesions of the chest wall, such as flail chest, severe kyphoscoliosis or arthritis, may also impair effective ventilation.

Pleural abnormalities, such as tension pneumothorax, massive haemothorax/pleural effusion, pulmonary conditions, such as severe fibrosis, pulmonary oedema or pneumonia, and severe airway obstruction due to severe croup, asthma or the inhalation of a foreign body are additional causes. In the intubated patient, causes such as the improper connection of the anaesthetic circuit, mechanical ventilator failure and the use of inappropriate equipment in small children should be considered.

Treatment

The treatment of respiratory acidosis is directed towards reversal of the causative factors. Ventilatory assistance is usually indicated in the presence of severe hypoxia,

depressed level of consciousness or an acute elevation of PCO_2 of greater than 80 mmHg.

Alkalosis

Alkalosis is defined as a decrease in $[H^+]$ in the blood. Its physiological effects are the same as those of the administration of HCO_3 except that it does not cause hyperosmolarity. In very severe cases altered mental state, seizures and respiratory depression may also occur. The most common symptoms of metabolic alkalosis are related to a decrease in the concentration of ionized calcium, and are more commonly present in respiratory alkalosis due to anxiety, than from other causes. Reduced levels of ionized calcium may cause neurological symptoms such as light headedness, dizziness, chest tightness and difficulty swallowing. On examination, the respiratory rate is elevated, muscular tremor is often present and, if severe, carpopedal spasm may also be observed. Chovstek's and Trousseau's signs may also be present.

Metabolic alkalosis

This is caused by loss of acid from the GIT or kidney, or the addition of exogenous alkali. Upper GIT acid losses as a result of severe and prolonged vomiting are the most common cause encountered in the ED. Other causes, such as hyperaldosteronism, Bartter's and Gitelman's syndromes and severe hypokalaemia, result in the loss of H^+ in the urine due to increased H^+–K^+ exchange in the distal convoluted tubule. Diuretics may also induce alkalosis by the same mechanism; however, the pH is rarely raised to >7.5.

Alkali may be added to the body in the form of citrate by red cell transfusion, intravenous $NaHCO_3$ administration or as urinary alkalinizers. The milk alkali syndrome may occur as a result of the chronic ingestion of more than 2 g of calcium salts each day (commonly in conjunction with vitamin D).[8] The metabolic derangement known as post-hypercapnic alkalosis is caused by the decrease of a chronically elevated PCO_2 to normal levels, when relative hyperventilation occurs. In such patients the HCO_3^- is usually elevated as a result of chronic hypercarbia, and when the PCO_2 is acutely lowered to normal levels the appearance

on blood gas analysis is that of a metabolic alkalosis, rather than that of a relative respiratory alkalosis. The most common example of this in the ED occurs in a patient who has chronic CO_2 retention with an acute exacerbation of COAD. The ingestion of strong alkali is almost never a cause of systemic alkalosis.

The causes of metabolic alkalosis can be further classified according to their response to intravenous saline (which is also related to the urinary chloride concentration). If the urinary Cl is <10 mmol/L, this is considered to be saline responsive and is usually caused by GIT losses, diuretics or the acute correction of chronic hypercapnia. If the urinary Cl is >10 mmol/L, the metabolic alkalosis is considered to be saline resistant and is usually caused by mineralocorticoid excess, oedema states or renal failure.

The treatment of metabolic alkalosis should be directed primarily towards correction of the underlying cause. In the presence of upper gastrointestinal fluid losses, intravenous fluids with high chloride content (such as 0.9% saline) should be used initially for rehydration, and correction of hypokalaemia may also be required.

Respiratory alkalosis

This is the only acid–base disturbance in which compensation may be complete. In a fully compensated chronic respiratory alkalosis the pH returns to 7.4 in approximately 4 days, and the reduction in serum HCO_3^- that occurs results in an increase in the anion gap.

Common causes of respiratory alkalosis in the general population include exercise, altitude-elated hypoxia and stimulation of the medullary respiratory centre by progesterones during pregnancy. In the ED setting, causes such as hypoxia, early sepsis, cerebral oedema, hepatic cirrhosis, mechanical ventilation, anxiety and salicylate, theophylline and carbon monoxide toxicity should be considered.[9] Treatment is directed towards correction of the underlying cause and the treatment of hypokalaemia or hypocalcaemia as required. Hydrochloric acid can be administered to correct the metabolic abnormality, but it is rarely required. A dose of 1– 3 mmol/kg of hydrochloric acid can be given through a central venous line at a rate of no faster than 1 mEq/min.[10]

Controversies

Whilst it was previously thought that, due to levels decreasing rapidly following sampling, serum lactate needed to be measured by immediate assay of arterial blood, more recent evidence has challenged this assumption with one study failing to demonstrate any significant difference in lactate levels measured at 15 min after sampling.[11]

References

1. Natalini G, Seramondi V, Fassini P, et al. Acute respiratory acidosis does not increase plasma potassium in normokalaemic anaesthetized patients. A controlled randomized trial. European Journal of Anaesthesiology 2001; 18(6): 394–400.
2. Herr RD, Swanson T. Pseudometabolic acidosis caused by underfill of vacutainer tubes. Annals of Emergency Medicine 1992; 21(2): 177–180.
3. Paulson WD, Roberts WL, Lurie AA, et al. Wide variation in serum anion gap measurements by chemistry analyzers. American Journal of Clinical Pathology 1998; 110(6): 735–742.
4. Cooper DJ. Bicarbonate does not improve haemodynamics in critically ill patients who have lactic acidosis: a prospective controlled clinical study. Annals of International Medicine 1990; 112: 492–498.
5. Mathieu D, Neviere R, Billard V, et al. Effects of bicarbonate therapy on hemodynamics and tissue oxygenation in patients with lactic acidosis: a prospective, controlled clinical study. Critical Care Medicine 1991; 19(11): 1352–1356.
6. Okuda Y, Adrogue HJ, Field JB, et al. Counterproductive effects of sodium bicarbonate in diabetic ketoacidosis. Journal of Clinical Endocrinology and Metabolism 1996; 81(1): 314–320.
7. Australian Resuscitation Council, Medications in cardiac arrest. February 2006.
8. Whiting SJ, Kim K, Wood R. Calcium supplementation. Journal of the American Academy of Nurse Practitioners 1997; 9(4): 187–192.
9. Laffey JG, Kavanagh BP. Hypocapnia. New England Journal of Medicine 2002; 347(1): 43–53.
10. Adrogue HJ, Madias NE. Management of life-threatening acid base disorders. New England Journal of Medicine 1998; 338(2): 107–111.
11. Jones AE, Leonard MM, Hernandez-Nino J, et al. Determination of the effect of in vitro time, temperature, and tourniquet use on whole blood venous point-of-care lactate concentrations. Academic Emergency Medicine 2007; 14: 587–591.

12.2 Electrolyte disturbances

John Pasco

ESSENTIALS

1 Sodium disorders are relatively common in hospitalized patients and elderly people.

2 The brain is most at risk from hyponatraemia because the osmotically expanded intracellular volume may induce increased intracranial pressure (hyponatraemic encephalopathy).

3 Treatment of hyponatraemia needs to be carefully individualized because of the risk of osmotic myelinolysis.

4 Hypernatraemia has a high in-hospital mortality rate, which often reflects severe associated medical conditions.

5 Although usually benign, hypokalaemia may cause cardiac arrhythmias and rhabdomyolysis. Oral replacement is usually sufficient, except where there is severe myopathy or cardiac arrhythmias.

6 Electrocardiogram changes in the presence of hyperkalaemia require urgent potassium-lowering measures and myocardial protection with calcium.

7 Management of severe hypercalcaemia includes enhancement of renal excretion of calcium, inhibition of osteoclast activity and treatment of the underlying condition.

8 Acute symptomatic hypocalcaemia should be treated with i.v. calcium.

9 Hypomagnesaemia is difficult to diagnose because its symptoms are non-specific and the serum level often does not reflect the true magnesium status of the patient. It usually exists as a 'deficiency triad' with hypokalaemia and hypocalcaemia.

10 Hypermagnesaemia is often iatrogenic, particularly in elderly patients or patients with renal impairment and/or chronic bowel conditions receiving magnesium therapy.

HYPONATRAEMIA

Introduction

Hyponatraemia, defined as serum sodium concentration of less than 130 mmol/L, is a common condition. The prevalence is estimated at 2.5% in hospitalized patients, of which two-thirds develop the condition whilst in hospital.[1]

Pathophysiology

Hyponatraemia is almost always associated with extracellular hypotonicity, with an excess of total body water relative to sodium. The exceptions are:

- Normotonic hyponatraemia (pseudohyponatraemia): an artefactually low sodium measurement seen in hyperlipidaemia and hyperproteinaemia. It is rarely seen now because of the routine use of direct ion-selective electrodes to measure sodium.
- Hypertonic hyponatraemia: a dilutional lowering of the measured serum sodium concentration in the presence of osmotically active substances, most commonly glucose, but also mannitol, glycerol and sorbitol. In the presence of hyperglycaemia the true serum sodium

497

can be estimated by adjusting the measured serum sodium upwards by 1 mmol/L for each 3 mmol/L rise in glucose.

Hyponatraemia causes cellular swelling as water moves down an osmotic gradient into the intracellular fluid. Most of the symptomatology of hyponatraemia is produced in the central nervous system (CNS) by the swelling of brain cells within the rigid calvarium, causing raised intracranial pressure (hyponatraemic encephalopathy). As intracranial pressure rises, adaptive responses come into play. Initially there is a reduction of the cerebral blood and cerebrospinal fluid (CSF) pools. Later, neuronal intracellular osmolality is reduced by extrusion of potassium, followed within hours to days by organic solutes such as amino acids, phosphocreatine and myoinositol. These processes return brain volume towards normal and restore cellular function.

Patients become symptomatic when hyponatraemia develops rapidly and the adaptive responses have not had time to develop, or when the adaptive responses fail.

Aetiology and classification

Hypotonic hyponatraemia may be classified according to the volume status of the patient (hypovolaemic, euvolaemic or hypervolaemic).

Hypovolaemic hyponatraemia
These patients have deficits in both total body sodium and total body water, but the sodium deficit exceeds the water deficit. Causes include renal and extra-renal fluid losses, and are listed in Table 12.2.1. Determination of the urinary sodium concentration

Table 12.2.1 Causes of hypovolaemic hyponatraemia

Renal losses (urinary [Na] >20 mmol/L)
Diuretics
Mineralocorticoid deficiency—Addison's disease
Salt-losing nephropathy
Ketonuria
Osmotic diuresis—glucose, mannitol, urea
Bicarbonaturia with metabolic alkalosis

Extrarenal losses (urinary [Na] <20 mmol/L)
Vomiting—self-induced, gastroenteritis, pyloric obstruction
Diarrhoea
Excessive sweating
Blood loss
Third-space fluid loss—burns, pancreatitis, trauma

can differentiate these two groups. Extrarenal losses are associated with low urinary sodium concentrations (<20 mmol/L) and hyperosmolar urine. The exception is with severe vomiting and metabolic alkalosis, where bicarbonaturia obligates renal sodium loss and urinary sodium is high (>20 mmol/L), despite volume depletion. However, urinary chloride, a better indicator of extracellular fluid (ECF) volume, is low.

Euvolaemic hyponatraemia
Total body water is increased with only minimal change in total body sodium. Volume expansion is mild and usually not clinically detectable. Causes are listed in Table 12.2.2.

Hypervolaemic hyponatraemia
Total body water is increased in excess of total body sodium. Causes include congestive cardiac failure, hepatic cirrhosis with ascites, nephrotic syndrome and chronic renal failure.

Clinical features

In addition to the features of the underlying medical condition and alteration in extracellular volume, clinical manifestations of hyponatraemia per se usually develop when

Table 12.2.2 Causes of euvolaemic hyponatraemia

Psychogenic polydipsia

Iatrogenic water intoxication
  Absorption of hypotonic irrigation fluids during TURP
  Inappropriate intravenous fluid administration

Postoperative hyponatraemia (elevated ADH levels)

Non-osmotic ADH secretion
  Glucocorticoid deficiency
  Severe hypothyroidism
  Thiazide diuretics

Drugs (ADH analogues, potentiation of ADH release, unknown mechanisms)
  Psychoactive agents: phenothiazines, SSRIs, TCAs, MAOIs, 'ecstasy'
  Oxytocin
  Anticancer agents: cyclophosphamine, vincristine, vinblastine
  NSAIDs
  Carbamazepine
  Chlorpropamide

SIADH

TURP, transurethral resection of prostate; ADH, antidiuretic hormone; SSRI, selective serotonin reuptake inhibitor; TCA, tricyclic antidepressant; MAOI, monoamic oxidase inhibitor; SIAOH, syndrome of inappropriate antidiuretic hormone secretion.

serum sodium is less than 130 mmol/L. The severity of symptoms depends partly on the absolute serum sodium concentration and partly on its rate of fall. At sodium concentrations from 125 to 130 mmol/L the symptoms are principally gastrointestinal, whereas at concentrations below 125 mmol/L the symptoms are predominantly neuropsychiatric. The principal signs and symptoms of hyponatraemia are listed in Table 12.2.3.

Mild chronic 'asymptomatic' hyponatraemia in the elderly contributes to an increased rate of falls, probably due to impairment of attention, posture and gait mechanisms.[2]

Hyponatraemic encephalopathy carries a high mortality (50%) if left untreated.[3] Population groups prone to hyponatraemic encephalopathy have been identified (Table 12.2.4).[3–8]

Premenopausal women appear at risk of developing hyponatraemic encephalopathy because oestrogen and progesterone are

Table 12.2.3 Clinical manifestations of hyponatraemia

Anorexia

Nausea

Vomiting

Lethargy

Muscle cramps

Muscle weakness

Headache

Confusion/agitation

Altered conscious state

Seizures

Coma

Table 12.2.4 Patient groups at risk of hyponatraemia

Postoperative

Menstruating females

Elderly women on thiazide diuretics

Prepubescent children

Psychiatric polydipsic patients

Hypoxaemic patients

AIDS patients

Patients taking 'Ecstasy' (MDMA)

Endurance athletes

thought to inhibit the brain Na-K-ATPase and increase circulating levels of antidiuretic hormone (ADH).[5]

Psychogenic polydipsia refers to a condition in which kidney function is normal and dilute urine is produced, but free water intake overwhelms the kidney's capabilities and the serum sodium falls. It occurs primarily in patients which schizophrenia or bipolar disorder. These patients develop hyponatraemia with a far lower fluid intake than is usually necessary (over 20 L of water/day in a 60-kg man, in the absence of elevated levels of ADH)[4,5] and it may arise through a combination of factors: antipsychotics, increased thirst perception, enhanced renal response to ADH and a mild defect in osmoregulation.

Exercise-associated hyponatraemia occurs in endurance athletes and mainly relates to the consumption of excessive fluid although non-osmotic release of vasopression and other mechanisms may be implicated.[9,10]

Hyponatraemia in AIDS is common and associated with a high mortality. It may be secondary to syndrome of inappropriate ADH (SIADH), adrenal insufficiency or volume deficiency with hypotonic fluid replacement.[4]

The use of 'Ecstasy' at 'rave' parties has been associated with acute hyponatraemia.[6,7] This may be due to a combination of drug effect and drinking large quantities of water in an attempt to prevent dehydration.

Syndrome of inappropriate ADH secretion

This is a diagnosis of exclusion and is characterized by inappropriately concentrated urine in the setting of hypotonicity. It accounts for approximately 50% of all cases of hyponatraemia. These patients have elevated serum ADH levels without an obvious volume or osmotic stimulus. The diagnostic criteria for SIADH secretion are shown in Table 12.2.5 and conditions associated with the syndrome are listed in Table 12.2.6.

Clinical investigation

Measurement of serum and urine sodium concentrations and osmolalities, in addition to clinical assessment of volume status, are essential for the assessment of hyponatraemia (Fig. 12.2.1).

Table 12.2.5   Diagnostic criteria for SIADH
Hypotonic hyponatraemia
Urine osmolality >100 mmol/kg (i.e. inappropriately concentrated)
Urine sodium >20 mmol/mL while on a normal salt and water intake
Absence of extracellular volume depletion
Normal thyroid and adrenal function
Normal cardiac, hepatic and renal function
No diuretic use

Table 12.2.6   Conditions associated with SIADH
Neoplasms (ectopic ADH production)
Bronchogenic carcinoma
Pancreatic carcinoma
Lymphoma
Mesothelioma
Thymoma
Carcinoma of the bladder
Pulmonary disease
Pneumonia
Tuberculosis
Aspergillosis
Cystic fibrosis
Chronic obstructive airways disease
Positive-pressure ventilation
CNS disease
Encephalitis
Acute psychosis
Head trauma
Brain abscess
Meningitis
Hydrocephalus
Brain tumour
Delirium tremens
Guillain–Barré syndrome
Stroke
Subdural or subarachnoid belled
HIV infection
Pneumocystis carinii pneumonia

Treatment

There is ongoing controversy over the treatment of hyponatraemia because of the risk of osmotic demyelination, which is discussed below.

Treatment should be carefully individualized and depends on the presence of symptoms, the duration of the hyponatraemia and the absolute value of sodium. Ideally correction of the serum sodium should be of a sufficient pace and magnitude to reverse the manifestations of hypotonicity but not be so rapid and large as to pose a risk of the development of osmotic demyelination.[11] Treatment of the underlying cause is obviously essential and may

correct the hyponatraemia. For hypovolaemic hyponatraemia, adequate volume replacement is essential.

Acute symptomatic hyponatraemia

Symptomatic hyponatraemia developing within 48 h is a medical emergency requiring prompt and aggressive treatment. The risks of developing osmotic demyelination are clearly outweighed by those of the encephalopathy.[4] An immediate increase in serum sodium concentration by 8 mEq/L over 4–6 h is recommended.[12] This can be achieved by infusing hypertonic saline (3% NaCl) at a rate of 1–2 mL/kg/h, which should raise the serum sodium by 1–2 mmol/L/h. Where neurological symptoms are severe, hypertonic saline can be infused at 4–6 mL/kg/h. Indications for ceasing rapid correction of hyponatraemia are cessation of life-threatening manifestations, moderation of other symptoms or the achievement of a serum sodium of 125–130 mEq/L.[11] Other measures to reduce intracranial pressure, such as intubation and intermittent positive pressure ventilation (IPPV), may also be required.

Chronic symptomatic hyponatraemia

Hyponatraemia present for more than 48 h, or where the duration is unknown, presents the greatest dilemma. Care must be taken with correction of sodium as these patients are at the greatest risk of developing osmotic demyelination, yet the presence of encephalopathy mandates urgent treatment.[4,5,13] Hypertonic saline can be infused so that a correction rate of no more than 1–1.5 mmol/L/h is maintained. Therapy with hypertonic saline should be discontinued when (a) the patient becomes asymptomatic, (b) the serum sodium has risen by 20 mmol/L or (c) the serum sodium reaches 120–125 mmol/L. Thereafter, slower correction with water restriction should follow. The serum sodium should never be acutely elevated to hypernatraemic or normonatraemic levels, and should not be elevated by more than 25 mmol/L during the first 48 h of therapy.

Chronic asymptomatic hyponatraemia

In this situation saline infusion is usually not required, and patients can be managed by

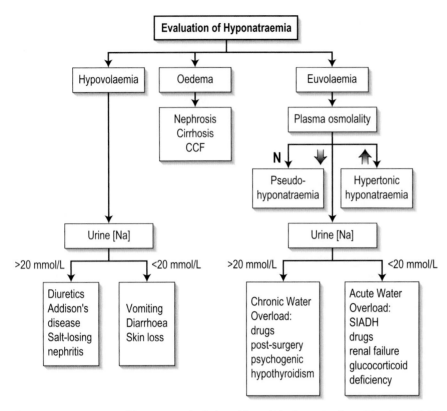

Fig. 12.2.1 Assessment of hyponatraemia. (Adapted from Walmsley R, Guerin M. Disorders of fluid and electrolyte balance. Bristol: John Wright & Sons; 1984.)

treating the underlying disorder, discontinuing diuretic therapy or restricting fluids. Fluid restriction is inexpensive and effective but is often limited by patient non-compliance. Other treatment options include pharmacological inhibition of ADH with demeclocycline, which is limited by its neuro- and nephrotoxic side effects, or increasing solute with the use of furosemide or urea.[4,14]

Osmotic myelinolysis

This is an iatrogenic disorder which develops progressively over 3–5 days following the correction of hyponatraemia. It classically produces symmetrical lesions centred on the midline of the pons and was originally described as 'central pontine myelinolysis'. However, about 10% of cases involve extrapontine lesions. It is reported as occurring in 25% of severely hyponatraemic patients following correction of serum sodium.[15] Clinically, the disorder is initially manifested by dysarthria, mutism, lethargy and affective changes, which may be mistaken for psychiatric illness. Classically, pseudo-bulbar palsy and spastic quadripar-

esis are observed. Recovery is usually gradual and incomplete although both fatalities and complete recovery are reported.[16] Demyelination in the central pons and extrapontine sites can be demonstrated on magnetic resonance imaging (MRI) scan or at autopsy.[17]

It appears that the risk of developing osmotic myelinolysis is associated with severity and chronicity of hyponatraemia. It rarely occurs if the serum sodium is >120 mmol/L or where hyponatraemia has been present for <48 h. Alcoholics, malnourished patients, hypokalaemic patients, burn victims and elderly patients on thiazides seem to be most at risk of developing osmotic demyelination.[3,4]

Both the rate and the magnitude of sodium correction appear important in the development of osmotic myelinolysis. Although there is as yet no agreed rate of correction that is regarded as completely safe, most authorities suggest that the serum sodium concentration should not rise by more than 10–14 mmol/L during any 24-h period.[4,5,13]

HYPERNATRAEMIA

Introduction

Hypernatraemia is much less common than hyponatraemia and may be defined as a serum sodium concentration greater than 150 mmol/L.

It is important to recognize hypernatraemia because it is usually associated with severe underlying medical illness. It is a condition of hospitalized patients, elderly and dependent people. The incidence of hypernatraemia in hospitalized patients ranges from 0.3 to 1%, with from 60 to 80% of these developing hypernatraemia after admission.[14] In-hospital mortality is high (40–55%) and may be due to a combination of hypernatraemia and the severity of the underlying disease.[14,18]

Pathophysiology

Hypernatraemia is a relative deficiency of total body water compared to total body sodium, thus rendering the body fluids hypertonic. The normal compensatory response includes stimulated thirst—the most important response—and renal water conservation through ADH secretion. In the absence of ADH, water intake can match urinary losses because of increased thirst, but where the thirst mechanism is absent or defective, patients become hypernatraemic even in the presence of maximal ADH stimulation. Therefore, hypernatraemia is usually seen where water intake is inadequate, i.e. in patients too young, too old or too sick to drink, with no access to water or with a defective thirst mechanism.

Extracellular hypertonicity causes a shift of water from the intracellular space until there is osmotic equilibrium. The resultant cellular contraction may explain some of the clinical features of hypernatraemia. The brain is especially at risk from shrinkage because of its vascular attachments to the calvarium. Haemorrhage may occur if these vascular attachments tear.

As with hyponatraemia, the rate and magnitude of the rise in sodium determine the severity of the symptoms, which is a reflection of the brain's capacity to adapt to the deranged osmotic conditions.[14]

Aetiology and classification

The clinical causes of hypernatraemia are listed in Table 12.2.7. Population groups at particular risk of developing hypernatraemia are listed in Table 12.2.8.[4,14]

Hypernatraemia is classified into these categories based on extracellular volume status: hypovolaemic, hypervolaemic and euvolaemic.[4,14,19]

Hypovolaemic hypernatraemia

This occurs where there is loss of both total body water and sodium, but with a greater loss of water. Renal causes include osmotic diuresis and diuretic excess. Urinary sodium is usually >20 mmol/L. Extrarenal losses include profuse diarrhoea, sweating, burns and fistulae. Urinary sodium is usually <20 mmol/L.

Table 12.2.7   Causes of hypernatraemia
Altered perception of thirst

Osmoreceptor damage/destruction
   Exogenous: trauma
   Endogenous: vasculitis, carcinoma,
     granuloma

Idiopathic: psychogenic, head injury
Drugs
Normal perception of thirst

Poor intake
   Confusion
   Coma
   Depression
   Dysphagia
   Odynophagia

Increased water loss and decreased intake
Diuresis Renal loss Diabetes insipidus Chronic renal failure Diuretic excess GIT loss: fistulae, diarrhoea
Exogenous increase in salt intake

Table 12.2.8   Groups at particular risk for hypernatraemia
Elderly or disabled, unable to obtain oral fluids independently
Infants

Inpatients receiving:
   hypertonic infusions
   tube feedings
   osmotic diuretics
   lactulose
     mechanical ventilation

Altered mental status
Uncontrolled diabetes mellitus
Underlying polyuric disorders

Euvolaemic hypernatraemia

This is the most common form of hypernatraemia. Patients have pure water losses, with intracellular dehydration as water shifts according to the osmotic gradient. Hypernatraemia in these patients occurs only when there is no accompanying water intake, i.e. restricted access to water or a defect in thirst sensation.

Extrarenal losses are usually seen in skin losses in burns patients and via the respiratory system in respiratory infections and at high altitude. Renal water loss is usually due to diabetes insipidus—a failure of ADH production or secretion (central diabetes insipidus), or a failure of the collecting duct of the kidney to respond to ADH (nephrogenic diabetes insipidus).

Hypervolaemic hypernatraemia

This is not very common. These patients are typically extracellular volume expanded but intracellular volume depleted. It is seen following resuscitation with sodium bicarbonate, with the use of hypertonic saline solutions, with excess salt intake, in primary hyperaldosteronism and in Cushing's syndrome.

Clinical features

In addition to the features of the underlying medical condition and alteration in extracellular volume, the clinical features of hypernatraemia per se are primarily CNS. Early symptoms are anorexia, nausea and vomiting; lethargy, hyperreflexia, confusion, seizures and coma occur later.

Treatment

The speed at which hypernatraemia is corrected should take into account the rate of development and severity of symptoms. Too rapid correction, especially in chronic hypernatraemia, can cause cerebral oedema or isotonic water intoxication. The rate of correction of chronic hypernatraemia should not exceed 0.5–0.7 mmol/L/h.

Treatment is based on clinical assessment of the patient's volume status.

Hypovolaemic hypernatraemia

These patients require restoration of the volume deficit with isotonic saline, colloid or blood in the first instance, to prevent peripheral vascular collapse, and treatment of the underlying cause. Following this, the water deficit is corrected with 0.45% saline, 5% dextrose or oral water.[4,14]

The water deficit is calculated as follows:

$$\text{water deficit} = \text{total body water} \times (1 - Na2/Na1)$$

where Na2 = desired sodium, Na1 = actual sodium and total body water is usually 60% of the body weight. The calculated normal daily maintenance fluids should be added to the above volumes.

Euvolaemic hypernatraemia

Calculate the water deficit as above and replace the deficit and ongoing losses with 5% dextrose, 0.45% saline or oral water.[4,14] To avoid cerebral oedema, particularly in chronic hypernatraemia, 50% of the water deficit should be replaced over the first 6–12 h and the rest given slowly over 1–2 days. Serum sodium estimations should be repeated at regular intervals.

Hypervolaemic hypernatraemia

Removal of sodium is required with the use of diuretics such as furosemide and discontinuation of causative agents. Furosemide causes excretion of more water than sodium, so a hypotonic fluid such as 5% dextrose may need to be infused. In severe cases, or in renal failure, dialysis may be required.

HYPOKALAEMIA

Introduction

Hypokalaemia may be defined as a serum potassium concentration of less than 3.5 mmol/L. It is usually considered to be severe when this is less than 2.4 mmol/L.

Pathophysiology

Hypokalaemia may develop as a consequence of potassium depletion or a shift of potassium into cells. In either case there is an increase in the ratio of intracellular to extracellular potassium concentrations. This in turn produces hyperpolarization across excitable membranes, and is responsible for the effects of hypokalaemia on striated muscle and the cardiac conducting system.

Aetiology

The causes of hypokalaemia are listed in Table 12.2.9.

Clinical presentation

Hypokalaemia commonly produces no symptoms in otherwise healthy subjects.

Clinical features may include weakness, constipation, ileus and ventilatory failure. Myopathy may develop, with weakness of the extremities which characteristically worsens with exercise. If the hypokalaemia is severe and untreated, rhabdomyolysis may occur. Polyuria and polydipsia may result from the effect of hypokalaemia on the distal renal tubule (nephrogenic diabetes insipidus of hypokalaemia). Cardiac effects include ventricular tachycardias and atrial tachycardias, with or without block. Characteristic electrocardiogram (ECG) changes include PR prolongation, T-wave flattening and inversion and prominent U waves.[20]

Table 12.2.9 Causes of hypokalaemia

Inadequate dietary intake

Abnormal losses
  Gastrointestinal
    Vomiting, nasogastric aspiration
    Diarrhoea, fistula loss
    Villous adenoma of the colon
    Laxative abuse
  Renal
    Mineralocorticoid excess
      Conn syndrome
      Bartter syndrome
      Ectopic ACTH syndrome
        Small cell carcinoma of the lung
        Pancreatic carcinoma
        Carcinoma of the thymus
    Renal tubular acidosis
    Magnesium deficiency

Drugs
  Diuretics
  Corticosteroids
  Gentamicin, amphotericin B
  Cisplatin

Compartmental shift
  Alkalosis
  Insulin
  Na-K-ATPase stimulation
  Sympathomimetic agents with β_2 effect
  Methylxanthines
  Barium poisoning
  Hypothermia
  Toluene intoxication
  Hypokalaemic periodic paralysis

Treatment

Oral replacement is safe for asymptomatic patients and 40–60 mmol of potassium every 1–4 h is usually well tolerated.

Intravenous administration of potassium is recommended when hypokalaemia is associated with cardiac arrhythmias, familiar periodic paralysis or severe myopathy. Usual infusion rates are 10–20 mmol/h. Rates greater than 40 mmol/h are not recommended. Potassium is a slerosant and should, therefore, be given via a large peripheral or central vein. Lignocaine, heparin and hydrocortisone can be used to ameliorate symptoms. Serum potassium estimations every 1–4 h and continuous cardiac monitoring are mandatory.

HYPERKALAEMIA

Introduction

Hyperkalaemia, defined as a serum potassium concentration greater than 5.5 mmol/L, is less common than hypokalaemia. Moderate (6.1–6.9 mmol/L) and severe (>7 mmol/L) hyperkalaemia can have grave consequences, particularly if acute.

Pathophysiology

Two homeostatic mechanisms are responsible for maintaining potassium balance. The renal system maintains external potassium balance by excreting 90–95% of the average daily potassium load (100 mmol/day); the gut excretes the remainder. This is a relatively slow process: only half the administered load of potassium will have been excreted in the urine after 3–6 h.[21,22] The extra-renal system involves hormonal and acid–base mechanisms that rapidly translocate potassium intracellularly. This system

is critical in the management of acute hyperkalaemia.

Aetiology

The causes of hyperkalaemia are listed in Table 12.2.10.

Clinical features

The clinical features of hyperkalaemia are often non-specific. Diagnosis depends on clinical suspicion, measurement of potassium concentration in the plasma and the characteristic changes on the ECG.

Generalized muscle weakness, flaccid paralysis and paraesthesiae of the hands and feet are common, but there is poor correlation between the degree of muscle weakness and serum potassium concentration.

The ECG changes (Table 12.2.11) are characteristic, but are an insensitive method of evaluating hyperkalaemia.

Table 12.2.10 Causes of hyperkalaemia

Pseudohyperkalaemia
  Delay in separating red cells
  Specimen haemolysis during or after venesection
  Severe leukocytosis/thrombocytosis
Excessive intake
  Exogenous: i.v. or oral KCl, massive blood transfusion
  Endogenous: tissue damage
  Burns
  Trauma
  Rhabdomyolysis
  Tumour lysis
Decrease in renal excretion
  Drugs
    Spironolactone, triamterene, amiloride
    Indometacin
    Captopril, enalapril
  Renal failure
  Addison's disease
  Hyporeninaemic hypoaldosteronism
Compartment shift
  Acidosis
  Insulin deficiency
  Digoxin overdose
  Succinylcholine
  Fluoride poisoning
  Hyperkalaemic periodic paralysis

Table 12.2.11 ECG changes of hyperkalaemia

Plasma potassium (mmol/L)	ECG characteristics
6–7	Tall peaked T waves (>5 mm)
7–8	QRS widening, small-amplitude P waves
8–9	Fusion of QRS complex with T wave producing sine wave
>9	AV dissociation, ventricular tachycardia, ventricular fibrillation

Serum biochemistry in almost all patients with hyperkalaemia shows some degree of renal impairment and metabolic acidosis. In dialysis patients, hyperkalaemia may develop without concomitant metabolic acidosis.

Treatment

Pseudohyperkalaemia is common and, if hyperkalaemia is an unexpected finding, the serum potassium should be remeasured.

Hyperkalaemia with ECG changes requires urgent management. The priorities are as follows:[20,23]

❶ Antagonize potassium cardiac toxicity:
- i.v. calcium chloride 10%, 5–10 mL or
- i.v. calcium gluconate 10%, 5–10 mL. The effects of calcium should be evident within minutes and last for 30–60 min. A calcium infusion may be required. Calcium antagonizes the myocardial membrane excitability induced by hyperkalaemia. It does not lower serum potassium levels.

❷ Shift potassium into cells:
- i.v. soluble insulin, 20 U with dextrose 50 g or
- salbutamol nebulized (10–20 mg) or i.v. (0.5 mg diluted in 100 mL over 10–15 min)[20,24] or
- i.v. sodium bicarbonate, 50–200 mmol.

❸ Enhance potassium excretion:
- oral and/or rectal resonium A 50 g. This is a cation exchange resin; as the resin passes through the gastrointestinal tract Na and K are exchanged and the cationically modified resin is then excreted in the faeces.
- furosemide diuresis
- haemodialysis. This is usually reserved for cases of acute renal failure or end-stage renal disease. It is the most effective treatment for acutely lowering serum potassium, but there is usually a time delay in instituting dialysis and the temporizing measures outlined above must be employed in the interim.

The use of insulin and glucose is well supported in the literature.[19,22] A response is usually seen within 20–30 min, with lowering of plasma potassium by up to 1 mmol/L and reversal of ECG changes. Transient hypoglycaemia may be observed within 15 min of insulin administration. In some patients, particularly those with end-stage renal failure, late hypoglycaemia may develop. For this reason, a 10% dextrose infusion at 50 mL/h is recommended and the blood glucose should be monitored closely. The exact mechanism by which insulin translocates potassium is not known; it is thought to be stimulation of Na-K-ATPase independent of cAMP.

β_2-Agonists significantly lower plasma potassium when given intravenously or via a nebulizer.[21,22] Potassium levels are reduced by up to 1.00 mmol/L within 30 min following 10–20 mg of nebulized salbutamol. The effect is sustained for up to 2 h. Adverse effects of salbutamol administration include tachyarrhythmias and precipitation of angina in patients with coronary artery disease. Patients on non-selected β-blockers may not respond. Some patients with end-stage renal disease are also resistant to this therapy. The reason for this is unknown. Greater decreases in potassium have been observed when salbutamol treatment is combined with insulin and glucose. The additive effect is thought to be due to stimulation of Na-K-ATPase via different pathways. Transient hyperglycaemia may occur with combined therapy, but delayed hypoglycaemia does not occur.

HYPOCALCAEMIA

Introduction

A reduction in serum calcium concentration manifests principally as abnormal neuromuscular function.

Pathophysiology

Calcium is involved in smooth and skeletal muscle contraction and relaxation, platelet aggregation, neurotransmission, hepatic and adipose glycogenolysis, thermogenesis and neutrophil function. In addition, most endocrine and exocrine gland function is calcium dependent.

Aetiology

Hypocalcaemia occurs when calcium is lost from the extracellular fluid at a rate greater than can be replaced by the intestine or bone. The major cause of severe hypocalcaemia is hypoparathyroidism, as a result of surgery for thyroid disease, autoimmune destruction or from developmental abnormalities of the parathyroid glands. Other causes are listed in Table 12.2.12.

Clinical features

Patients with acute hypocalcaemia are more likely to be symptomatic than those with chronic hypocalcaemia. Symptomatic hypocalcaemia is characterized by abnormal neuromuscular excitability and neurological sensations.[24] Early signs are perioral numbness and paraesthesia of distal extremities. Hyperreflexia, muscle cramps and carpopedal spasm follow. Chvostek's sign (ipsilateral contraction of the facial muscles elicited by tapping the facial nerve just anterior to the ear) and Trousseau's sign (carpopedal spasm with inflation of a blood pressure cuff for 3–5 min) are signs of neuromuscular irritability. If muscle contractions become uncontrollable tetany results, and this can prove fatal if laryngospasm occurs. Seizures may occur when there is CNS instability. Cardiovascular manifestations include hypotension, bradycardia, impaired cardiac contractility and arrhythmias. ECG evidence of hypocalcaemia includes prolonged QT interval, and possibly ST prolongation and T-wave abnormalities.

Table 12.2.12   Causes of hypocalcaemia
Factitious EDTA contamination
Hypoalbuminaemia
Decreased PTH activity Hypoparathyroidism Pseudohypoparathyroidism Hypomagnesaemia
Decreased vitamin D activity
Acute pancreatitis
Hyperphosphataemia Renal failure Phosphate supplements
'Hungry bone' syndrome
Drugs Mithramycin Diuretics: furosemide, ethacrynic acid

Treatment

Acute symptomatic hypocalcaemia

In the emergency situation where seizures, tetany, life-threatening hypotension or arrhythmias are present, i.v. calcium is the treatment of choice. Infusion of 15 mg/kg of elemental calcium over 4–6 h increases the total serum calcium by 0.5–0.75 mmol/L.[24]

Administration of 10–20 mL of 10% calcium gluconate (89 mg elemental calcium per 10 mL) i.v. over 5–10 min is recommended. This should be followed by a continuous infusion because the effects of a single i.v. dose last only about 2 h. The infusion rate should be adjusted according to serial calcium measurements obtained every 2–4 h. Over-rapid infusion may cause facial flushing, headache and arrhythmias.

Calcium chloride 10% may also be used. This contains more calcium per ampoule (272 mg in 10 mL), resulting in a more rapid rise in serum calcium, but is more irritant to veins and can cause thrombophlebitis with extravasation.

Where hypcalcaemia and metabolic acidosis are present (usually in sepsis or renal failure) correction of the acidosis with bicarbonate may result in a rapid fall in ionized calcium as the number of calcium-binding sites is increased. Therefore, hypocalcaemia must be corrected before the acidosis. Bicarbonate or phosphate should not be infused with calcium because of possible precipitation of calcium salts.

Cardiac monitoring is recommended during rapid calcium administration, especially if the patient is taking digoxin, when calcium administration may precipitate digitalis toxicity.

If coexisting magnesium deficiency is suspected, or when symptoms do not improve after calcium administration, $MgSO_4$ 1–5 mmol i.v. over 15 min may be given.

Chronic asymptomatic hypocalcaemia

These patients are usually managed with oral calcium supplements taken between meals. Calcitriol, the active hormonal form of vitamin D, 0.5–1.5 mg daily, can also be given.

HYPERCALCAEMIA

Introduction

The normal total serum calcium concentration is 2.15–2.55 mmol/L. Hypercalcaemia is a relatively common condition with a frequency estimated at 1:1000–1:10 000.[25] Although there are many causes, the most frequent are malignancy and hyperparathyroidism, with the former the most likely to cause hypercalcaemia requiring urgent attention.[25]

Pathophysiology

Total serum calcium is made up of protein-bound calcium (40%, mostly albumin and not filterable by the kidneys), ion-bound complexes (13%, bound to anions such as bicarbonate, lactate, citrate and phosphate), and the unbound, ionized fraction (47%). The ionized fraction is the biologically active component of calcium and is closely regulated by parathyroid hormone (PTH). Total serum calcium is affected by albumin and does not necessarily reflect the level of plasma ionized calcium. Normal ionized calcium levels are 1.14–1.30 mmol/L. Protein binding in turn is influenced by extracellular fluid pH and alterations in serum albumin. Acidaemia decreases protein binding and increases the level of ionized calcium.

To correct for pH:

ionized calcium rises 0.05 mmol/L for each 0.1 decrease in pH.

To correct for serum albumin:

$$corrected[Ca^+] = measured [Ca^+] + (40 - albumin\ g/L) \times 0.02\ mmol/L$$

Corrected calcium is used for all treatment decisions except where direct measurement of ionized calcium using an ion-specific electrode is available.

Three pathophysiological mechanisms may produce hypercalcaemia:[25]

- Accelerated osteoclastic bone resorption. This is the most common cause of severe hypercalcaemia. Osteoclasts are activated by PTH and various humoral tumour products, the most common being parathyroid hormone-related protein (PTHRP).
- Increased gastrointestinal absorption (rarely important).
- Decreased renal excretion of calcium. PTH and PTHRP stimulate renal tubular reabsorption of calcium. Hypercalcaemia per se causes polyuria by interfering with renal mechanisms for reabsorption of water and sodium. If there is inadequate fluid intake to compensate, extracellular volume depletion occurs, reducing glomerular filtration and exacerbating the hypercalcaemia.

Aetiology

The majority of cases of hypercalcaemia requiring urgent treatment are due to malignancy or, less commonly, primary hyperparathyroidism (parathyroid crisis). Malignant hypercalcaemia is most commonly seen with the solid tumours: lung and breast cancer, squamous cell carcinoma of the head and neck and cholangiocarcinoma and the haematological malignancies multiple myeloma and lymphoma.[24] Other causes of hypercalcaemia are uncommon (Table 12.2.13).

Table 12.2.13   Causes of hypercalcaemia

Factitious
  Haemoconcentration
  Postprandial

Malignancy
Primary hyperparathyroidism

Drugs
  Thiazides
  Vitamin D
  Lithium
  Vitamin A

Hormonal
  Thyrotoxicosis
  Acromegaly
  Hypoadrenalism
  Phaeochromocytoma

Granulomas
  Tuberculosis
  Sarcoidosis

Renal failure
Milk alkali syndrome
Immobilization

Clinical features

Hypercalcaemia causes disturbances of the gastrointestinal, cardiovascular, renal and central nervous systems.[24,26]

Gastrointestinal manifestations include anorexia, nausea, vomiting and constipation. Cardiovascular manifestations include hypertension and a shortened QT interval on the ECG. Renal manifestations include polyuria, polydipsia and nephrocalcinosis (rare). CNS symptoms include psychotic behaviour, seizures, apathy, cognitive difficulties, obtundation and coma. Renal elimination of digoxin is also impaired.

Moderately elevated total serum calcium (3.00–3.50 mmol/L) is usually associated with symptoms. Markedly elevated total serum calcium (>3.5 mmol/L) mandates urgent treatment regardless of symptoms.

Treatment

Irrespective of the cause, the management of hypercalcaemic crisis is the same. There are four primary treatment goals:[26–29]

❶ hydration of the patient
❷ enhancement of renal excretion of calcium
❸ inhibition of accelerated bone resorption
❹ treatment of the underlying problem.

Hydration and diuresis

Hydration expands intravascular volume, dilutes calcium and increases calcium clearance. Infusion rates of 200–300 mL/h of 0.9% saline, depending on the degree of hypovolaemia and the ability of the patient to tolerate fluid, may be required.

Frusemide 20–40 mg i.v. every 1–4 h, or by infusion, is usually added once the patient is adequately hydrated. This inhibits the function of the ascending loop of Henle and increases the excretion of calcium and sodium. This treatment, although effective, results in a relatively modest reduction in serum calcium, and patients with severe hypercalcaemia usually require additional treatment.

Enhancement of renal excretion

Haemodialysis is the treatment of choice to rapidly decrease serum calcium in patients with heart failure or renal insufficiency.[30]

Inhibition of bone resorption

Pharmacological inhibition of osteoclastic bone resorption is the most effective treatment for hypercalcaemia, particularly hypercalcaemia of malignancy. Bisphosphonates, analogues of pyrophosphate, are the principal agents used. They inhibit osteoclast function and hydroxyapatite crystal dissolution. Unfortunately, normalization of calcium levels may take 3–6 days, which is too slow in critically ill patients.

Etidronate given as a dose of 7.5 mg/kg daily over 4 h for 3–7 days produces normocalcaemia in most patients after a 7-day course. Adverse reactions include a transient elevation in serum creatinine, a metallic taste and transient hyperphosphataemia.

Disodium pamidronate is more potent and lowers serum calcium more rapidly and predictably than etidronate. It is currently the bisphosphonate of choice. The dose is 60 mg i.v. (in 500 mL 0.9% saline over 4 h) if serum calcium is <3.5 mmol/L, and 80 mg i.v. if serum calcium is >3.5 mmol/L. Calcium levels normalize in up to 80% of patients within 7 days, and this effect can persist for up to a month. Common adverse reactions include a mild transient elevation in temperature, local infusion site reactions, mild gastrointestinal symptoms and mild hypophosphataemia, hypokalaemia and hypomagnesaemia.

An alternative treatment to pamidronate is sodium clodronate 1500 mg in 500 mL 0.9% saline i.v. (4–6 mg/kg daily) over 4 h.

Glucocorticoids are the treatment of choice in selected patient populations where the production of 1.25-dihydroxy-vitamin D is the known mechanism for causing hypercalcaemia. Such conditions include vitamin D toxicity, sarcoidosis, other granulomatous diseases, and haematological malignancies such as multiple myeloma and lymphoma. The usual dose is 200–300 mg hydrocortisone i.v. for 3–5 days. However, the maximal calcium-lowering effect does not occur for several days, and glucocorticoids should only be regarded as adjunctive therapy in hypercalcaemic crises.

Treat the underlying disorder

The definitive treatment for hypercalcaemia is to treat the underlying disease: surgery for hyperparathyroidism and tumour-specific therapy for hypercalcaemia of malignancy.

HYPOMAGNESAEMIA

Introduction

The diagnosis of magnesium deficiency is difficult and often overlooked largely because the symptoms are non-specific and do not usually appear until the patient is severely deficient.

Serum magnesium concentration (normal range: 0.76–0.96 mmol/L) is not a sensitive indicator of magnesium deficiency as it may not truly reflect total body stores. However, it is commonly used in the absence of other reliable methods to estimate the 'true' magnesium status. A low serum magnesium concentration is usually present in symptomatic magnesium deficiency, but it is important to remember that it may be normal in the presence of significant intracellular depletion.

Pathophysiology

Magnesium plays a critical role in metabolism; as an enzyme co-factor, in the maintenance of cell membranes and in electrolyte balance. It is the fourth most common cation in the body and is predominantly an intracellular ion with the majority found in bone (>50%) and soft tissue. Only 0.3% of total body magnesium is located extracellularly, of which 33% is protein bound, 12% is complexed to anions such as citrate, bicarbonate and phosphate, and 55% is found in the free ionized form.

Hypokalaemia is present in 40–60% of cases of magnesium deficiency, due to renal wasting of potassium. The hypokalaemia is resistant to potassium replacement alone, as a result of a combination of factors, including impaired cellular cation pump activity and increased cellular permeability to potassium.

Hypocalcaemia is usually present at serum magnesium concentrations below 0.49 mmol/L. This may be due to impaired PTH synthesis or secretion, or to PTH resistance as a result of magnesium deficiency.

Aetiology

From an emergency medicine perspective, hypomagnesaemia is most frequently encountered in the context of acute and chronic diarrhoea, acute pancreatitis, diuretic use, in

Table 12.2.14 Causes of magnesium deficiency[31]
Gastrointestinal losses
Acute and chronic diarrhoea
Acute pancreatitis
Severe malnutrition
Intestinal fistulae
Extensive bowel resection
Prolonged nasogastric suction
Renal losses
Osmotic diuresis – diabetes, urea, mannitol
Hypercalcaemia and hypercalciuria
Volume expanded states
Chronic parenteral fluid therapy
Drugs
ACE inhibitors
Alcohol
Aminoglycosides
Amphotericin B
Cisplatin
Ciclosporin
Diuretics – thiazide or loop
Other
Phosphate depletion

Table 12.2.15 Clinical manifestations of severe magnesium deficiency[32]		
Cardiac effects	*Metabolic effects*	*Neurological effects*
Atrial fibrillation	Hypokalaemia	Grand mal seizures
Atrial flutter	Hypocalcaemia	Focal seizures
Supraventricular tachycardia	Hyponatraemia	Paraesthesias
Ventricular tachycardia	Hypophosphataemia	Dizziness
Torsades des pointes	Metabolic alkalosis	Vertigo
Coronary artery spasm	Hyperglycaemia	Ataxia
Hypertension	Hyperlipidaemia	Nystagmus
ECG changes		Tremor
Atherosclerosis		Myopathy
		Dysphagia
		Oesophageal spasm
		Delirium, personality changes
		Depression
		Coma

alcoholics and in diabetic ketoacidosis, secondary to glycosuria and osmotic diuresis. Table 12.2.14 details causes of magnesium deficiency.

Hypomagnesaemia has been found in 30% of alcoholics admitted to hospital and results from a combination of the direct effect of alcohol on the renal tubule, which increases magnesium excretion, and associated malnutrition, diarrhoea and metabolic acidosis.[31]

Clinical features

The clinical manifestations of severe magnesium deficiency include metabolic, neurological and cardiac effects (Table 12.2.15).

The presenting symptoms are non-specific and can be attributed to associated metabolic abnormalities such as hypocalcaemia, hypokalaemia and metabolic alkalosis. In particular, patients may present with symptoms of hypocalcaemia: neuromuscular hyperexcitability, carpo-pedal spasm and positive Chvostek's and Trousseau's signs.

Early ECG changes of magnesium deficiency include prolongation of the PR and QT intervals, with progressive QRS widening and U-wave appearance as severity progresses. Changes in cardiac automaticity and conduction, atrial and ventricular arrhythmias, including torsades des pointes, can occur. Administration of a magnesium bolus can abolish torsades des pointes, even in the presence of normal serum magnesium levels.[32] Magnesium is a co-factor in the Na-K-ATPase system and so magnesium deficiency enhances myocardial sensitivity to digitalis and may precipitate digitalis toxicity. Digitalis-toxic arrhythmias, in turn, can be terminated with intravenous magnesium.

Treatment

Oral replacement is the preferred option in asymptomatic patients, although this route takes longer.

Symptomatic moderate-to-severe magnesium deficiency should be treated with parenteral magnesium salts. The patient should be closely monitored and therapy discontinued if deep tendon reflexes disappear or serum magnesium exceeds 2.5 mmol/L.[32] Suggested dosing regimes are outlined in Table 12.2.16.

HYPERMAGNESAEMIA

Hypermagnesaemia (serum magnesium above 0.95 mmol/L) is rare and usually iatrogenic.

Table 12.2.16 Magnesium doses (in mmol magnesium)
Emergency – i.v. route
8–16 mmol statim
40 mmol over next 5 h
Severely ill – i.m. route
48 mmol on day 1
17–25 mmol on days 2–5
Asymptomatic – oral route
15 mmol/day

The elderly and patients with renal impairment or chronic bowel disorders are particularly at risk, especially when i.v. magnesium or magnesium-containing cathartics or antacids are used.

Clinical manifestations include mental obtundation progressing to coma, cardiac arrhythmias, loss of deep tendon reflexes, refractory hypotension and respiratory arrest, nausea and vomiting, muscle paralysis and flushing.

Magnesium administration should be immediately discontinued. Further management is largely supportive. Maintain urine output at greater than 60 mL/h with fluid administration to enhance renal excretion. Furosemide (40–80 mg i.v.) may also be given once the patient is adequately hydrated. Haemodialysis may be of benefit in severe cases, particularly if there is impaired renal function.

Controversies

❶ The safest and most effective ways of correcting hyponatraemia remain controversial because of the risk of inducing osmotic myelinolysis.

❷ The usefulness of bicarbonate for the acute therapy of hyperkalaemia has been questioned. A number of studies have shown that bicarbonate fails to lower potassium levels sufficiently in the acute, life-threatening situation to justify its use as first-line treatment.[21,22] It is still recommended, however, when hyperkalaemia is associated with severe metabolic acidosis (pH < 7.20).

References

1. Anderson RJ, Chung HM, Kluge R, Scrier RW. Hyponatremia: a prospective analysis of its epidemiology and the pathogenetic role of vasopressin. Annals of Internal Medicine 1985; 102: 164–168.

2. Decaux G. Is asymptomatic hyponatraemia really asymptomatic? American Journal of Medicine 2006; 119: S79–S82.

3. Berl T. Treating hyponatraemia: what is all the controversy about? Annals of Internal Medicine 1990; 113: 417–419.

4. Kumar S, Berl T. Sodium-electrolyte quintet. Lancet 1998; 352: 220–228.

5. Fraser C, Arieff A. Epidemiology, pathophysiology, and management of hyponatremic encephalopathy. American Journal of Medicine 1997; 102: 67–77.

6. Maxwell D, Polkey M, Henry J. Hyponatraemia and catatonic stupor after taking 'ecstasy'. British Medical Journal 1993; 307(6916): 1399.

7. Box SA, Prescott LF, Freestone S. Hyponatraemia at a rave. Postgraduate Medical Journal 1997; 73(855): 53–54.

8. Yeong-Hau HL, Shapiro JI. Hyponatremia: clinical diagnosis and management. American Journal of Medicine 2007; 120: 653–658.

9. Almod CS, Shin AY, Fortescure EB, et al. Hyponatremia among runners in the Boston Marathon. New England Journal of Medicine 2005; 352: 1550–1556.

10. Noakes TD, Sharwood K, Speedy D, et al. Three independent biological mechanisms cause exercise-associated hyponatraemia: evidence from 2,135 weighed competitive athletic performances. Proceedings of the National Academy of Science USA 2005; 102: 18550–18555.

11. Androgue HJ, Madias NE. Hyponatremia. New England Journal of Medicine 2000; 342: 1581–1589.

12. Kokko JP. Symptomatic hyponatraemia with hypoxia is a medical emergency. Kidney International 2006; 69: 1291–1293.

13. Cluitmans F, Meinders A. Management of severe hyponatraemia: rapid or slow correction? American Journal of Medicine 1990; 88: 161–166.

14. Fried L, Palevsky P. Myelinolysis after correction of hyponatraemia. Annals of Internal Medicine 1997; 3: 585–689.

15. Sterns RH, Cappuccio JD, Silver SM, et al. Neurologic sequelae after treatment of severe hyponatremia: a multicenter perspective. Journal of the American Society of Nephrology 1994; 4: 1522–1530.

16. Karp BI, Laureno R. Pontine and extrapontine myelinolysis: a neurological disorder following rapid correction of hyponatraemia. Medicine (Baltimore) 1993; 72: 359–373.

17. Laureno R, Karp BI. Myelinolysis after correction of hyponatraemia. Annals of Internal Medicine 1997; 126: 57–62.

18. Long C, Marin P, Byer A, et al. Hypernatraemia in an adult in-patient population. Postgraduate Medical Journal 1991; 67: 643–645.

19. DeVita M, Michelis M. Perturbations in sodium balance. Clinics in Laboratory Medicine 1993; 13(1): 135–148.

20. Mandel A. Hypokalemia and hyperkalemia. Medical Clinics of North America 1997; 81(3): 611–639.

21. Allon M. Treatment and prevention of hyperkalemia in end-stage renal disease. Kidney International 1993; 43: 1197–1209.

22. Salem MM, Rosa RM, Battle DC. Extrarenal potassium tolerance in chronic renal failure: implications for the treatment of acute hyperkalemia. American Journal of Kidney Disease 1991; 18: 421–440.

23. Halperin M, Kamel K. Potassium-electrolyte quintet. Lancet 1998; 352: 135–140.

24. Bourke E, Delaney V. Assessment of hypocalcemia and hypercalcemia. Clinics in Laboratory Medicine 1993; 13(1):157–177.

25. Deftos L. Hypercalcemia. Postgraduate Medicine 1996; 100(6):119–126.

26. Bushinskey D, Monk R. Calcium-electrolyte quintet. Lancet 1998; 352: 306–311.

27. Chisholm M, Mulloy A, Taylor T. Acute management of cancer-related hypercalcemia. Annals of Pharmacotherapy 1996; 30: 507–513.

28. Bilezikian J. Management of acute hypercalcemia. New England Journal of Medicine 1992; 326(18): 1196–1203.

29. Falk S, Fallon M. Emergencies—ABC of palliative care. British Medical Journal 1997; 315: 1525–1528.

30. Edelson GW, Kleerekoper M. Hypercalcemic crisis. Medical Clinics of North America 1995; 79: 79–92.

31. Weisinger JR, Bellorin-Font E. Magnesium and phosphorus-electrolyte quintet. Lancet 1998; 352: 391–396.

32. Fawcett WJ, Haxby EJ, Male DA. Magnesium: physiology and pharmacology. British Journal of Anaesthesia 1999; 83(2): 302–320.

13.1 Anaemia

Lindsay Murray

ESSENTIALS

1 Anaemia is a condition in which the absolute number of red cells in the circulation is abnormally low.

2 Anaemia is not a diagnosis: it is a finding, which should prompt the search for an underlying cause.

3 The anaemic patient is doing at least one of three things: not producing enough red cells, destroying them too quickly or bleeding.

4 Bleeding is the most common cause of severe anaemia encountered in the emergency department.

Introduction

Anaemia is a condition in which the absolute number of red cells in the circulation is abnormally low. The diagnosis is usually made on the basis of the full blood count (FBC). This, together with the blood film, offers qualitative as well as quantitative data on the blood components, and a set of normal values is shown in Table 13.1.1.

The average lifespan of a normal red blood cell in the circulation is from 100 to 120 days. Aged red cells are removed by the reticuloendothelial system, but under normal conditions are replaced by the marrow such that a dynamic equilibrium is maintained. Anaemia develops when red cell loss exceeds red cell production. It follows that the anaemic patient is doing at least one of three things: not producing enough red cells, destroying them too quickly or bleeding.

The overriding functional importance of the red cell resides in its ability to transport oxygen, bound to the haemoglobin molecule, from the lungs to the tissues. Functionally, anaemia may be regarded as an impairment in the supply of oxygen to the tissues and the adverse effects of anaemia, from whatever cause, are a consequence of the resultant tissue hypoxia. Anaemia is not a diagnosis: rather, it is a clinical or a laboratory finding that should prompt the search for an underlying cause (Table 13.1.2).

ANAEMIA SECONDARY TO HAEMORRHAGE

Aetiology

By far the most common cause of severe anaemia encountered in the emergency department (ED) is haemorrhage. Therefore, the assessment of the anaemic patient is often chiefly concerned with the search for a site of blood loss. The most common causes of haemorrhage are outlined in Table 13.1.3. However, the emergency physician must remain alert to the possibility that the patient is not bleeding but manifesting a rarer pathological condition.

Clinical features

While it may be obvious on history and examination that a patient is bleeding, occasionally the source of blood loss is occult and the extent of loss underestimated.

In the context of trauma the history often gives clear pointers to both sites and extent of blood loss. Consideration of the mechanism of injury may allow anticipation of occult pelvic, intraperitoneal or retroperitoneal bleeding. Intracranial bleeding is never an explanation for hypovolaemic shock in

Table 13.1.1 Full blood count: normal parameters

Haemoglobin (Hb)

Males	13.5–18 g/dL
Females	11.5–16.5 g/dL

Red blood cell count

Males	$4500–6500 \times 10^9$/L
Females	$3900–5600 \times 10^9$/L

Haematocrit

Males	42–54%
Females	37–47%
MCH	27–32 pg
MCHC	32–36 g/dL
MCV	76–98 fL
Reticulocytes	0.2–2%
White blood cells	$4–11 \times 10^9$/L
Neutrophils	$1.8–8 \times 10^9$/L
Eosinophils	$0–0.6 \times 10^9$/L
Basophils	$0–0.2 \times 10^9$/L
Lymphocytes	$1–5 \times 10^9$/L
Monocytes	$0–0.8 \times 10^9$/L
Platelets	$150–400 \times 10^9$/L

MCH, Hb divided by RBC; MCHC, Hb divided by HCT; MCV, HCT divided by RBC.
Most automated counting machines now give the red cell distribution width (RDW), a measure of degree of variation of cell size.

Table 13.1.2 Causes of anaemia

Haemorrhage

Traumatic
Non-traumatic
Acute or chronic

Production defect

Megaloblastic anaemia
Vitamin B12 deficiency
Folate deficiency
Aplastic anaemia
Pure red cell aplasia
Myelodysplastic syndromes
Invasive marrow diseases
Chronic renal failure

Decreased RBC survival (haemolytic anaemia)

Congenital
Spherocytosis
Elliptocytosis
Glucose-6-phosphate-dehydrogenase deficiency
Pyruvate kinase deficiency
Haemoglobinopathies: sickle cell diseases
Acquired autoimmune haemolytic anaemia, warm
Acquired autoimmune haemolytic anaemia, cold
Microangiopathic haemolytic anaemias
RBC mechanical trauma
Infections
Paroxysmal nocturnal haemoglobinuria

RBC, red blood cell.

Table 13.1.3 Common causes of haemorrhage in the emergency department

Trauma

Blunt trauma to mediastinum
Pulmonary contusions/haemopneumothorax
Intraperitoneal injury
Retroperitoneal injury
Pelvic disruption
Long bone injury
Open wounds: inadequate first aid

Non-trauma

Gastrointestinal haemorrhage
Oesophageal varices
Peptic ulcer
Gastritis/Mallory–Weiss
Colonic/rectal bleeding
Obstetric/gynaecological bleeding
Ruptured ectopic pregnancy
Menorrhagia
Threatened miscarriage
Antepartum haemorrhage
Postpartum haemorrhage
Other
Epistaxis
Postoperative
Secondary to bleeding diathesis

an adult. In the context of non-trauma it is essential to obtain an obstetric and gynaecological history in women of childbearing age. The remainder of the formal history may supply information essential in determining the aetiology of anaemia. The past medical history may point to a known haematological abnormality or to a chronic disease process. A drug and allergy history is always relevant. Many drugs cause marrow suppression, haemolytic anaemia and bleeding. The family history points to hereditary disease; the social history may alert the clinician to an unusual occupational exposure in the patient's past or, more likely, to recreational activities liable to exacerbate an ongoing disease process. The systems review is particularly relevant to the consultation with middle-aged or elderly male patients, who must be asked about symptoms of altered bowel habit and weight loss.

The symptomatology of anaemia proceeds from vague complaints of tiredness, lethargy and impaired performance through to more sharply defined entities such as shortness of breath on exertion, giddiness, restlessness, apprehension, confusion, and collapse. Comorbid conditions may be exacerbated (the dyspnoea of chronic obstructive airway disease) and occult pathologies unmasked (exertional angina in ischaemic heart disease).

Anaemia of insidious onset is generally better tolerated than that of rapid onset because of cardiovascular and other compensatory mechanisms. Acute loss of 40% of the blood volume may result in collapse, whereas in certain developing countries it is not rare for patients with haemoglobin concentrations 10% of normal to be ambulant. Trauma superimposed on an already established anaemia can lead to rapid decompensation.

The cardinal sign of anaemia is pallor. This can be seen in the skin, the lips, the mucous membranes and the conjunctival reflections. Yet not all anaemic patients are pallid, and not all patients with a pale complexion are anaemic. Patients who have suffered an acute haemorrhage may show evidence of hypovolaemia: tachycardia, hypotension, cold peripheries and sluggish capillary refill. The detection of postural hypotension is an important pointer towards occult blood loss. Conversely, patients with anaemia of insidious onset are not hypovolaemic and may manifest high-output cardiac failure as a physiological response to hypoxia.

Other features of the physical examination may provide clues to the aetiology of anaemia. The glossitis, angular stomatitis, koilonychia and oesophageal web of iron-deficiency anaemia are uncommon findings. Bone tenderness, lymphadenopathy, hepatomegaly and splenomegaly may point to an underlying haematological abnormality. The rectal and gynaecological examinations can sometimes be diagnostic.

Clinical investigations

The full blood count often reveals an anaemia that has not been clinically suspected and that must be interpreted in the light of the history and examination. If the anaemia is mild it may be a chance finding with little relevance to the patient's presenting complaint, but such a finding should never be ignored. At the very least a follow-up blood count should be arranged.

Anaemic patients have a low red cell count, a low haematocrit and a low haemoglobin, but some caveats need to be borne in mind:

- Patients who are bleeding acutely may initially have a normal FBC.
- Normal or high haematocrits may reflect haemoconcentration.
- Mixed pictures can be difficult to interpret, e.g. that of a polycythaemic patient who is bleeding.

Red cell morphology, particularly the mean corpuscular volume (MCV), can help elucidate the cause of anaemia. The finding of a pancytopenia suggests a problem in haematopoiesis, rather than haemolysis or blood loss. In women of childbearing age, assay of blood or urine β-HCG is important.

Treatment

The principles of management of haemorrhage are as follows:

- Maintain the circulation.
- Identify the site of bleeding.
- Control the bleeding.
- Identify the underlying pathological process.
- Arrange for definitive treatment.
- Restore the blood volume.

The indications for red cell transfusion are discussed in Chapter 13.5. The faster the onset of the anaemia, the greater the need for urgent replacement. Patients who are tolerating their anaemia may require no more than an appropriate diet with or without the addition of haematinics. Elderly patients with severe bleeding often need red cells urgently. Excessive administration of colloid and/or crystalloid precipitates left ventricular failure, and it can then be difficult to administer red cells.

Chronic haemorrhage

The finding of a hypochromic microcytic anaemia on blood film is usually indicative of iron deficiency and, in the absence of an overt history of bleeding, should prompt the search for occult blood loss. Iron-deficiency anaemia may be due to malnutrition, but inadequate dietary intake of iron is not usually the sole cause of anaemia in developed countries: much more commonly it is the result of chronic blood loss from the gastrointestinal (GI) tract, the uterus or the renal tract. More unusual causes are haemoptysis and recurrent epistaxes.

Patients present with insidious and rather vague symptoms. They may be unaware that they are bleeding and will probably show none of the trophic skin, nail and mucosal changes of iron deficiency. The automated cell count, in addition to

showing a hypochromic, microcytic picture, may also show a raised red cell distribution width, which reflects anisocytosis on the blood film.

Iron studies may confirm the diagnosis of iron deficiency without pointing to the underlying cause. Serum iron and ferritin are low and total iron-binding capacity is high.

Disposition

If the source of blood loss is obvious, for example heavy menstrual bleeding, then appropriate referral may be all that is indicated. If the source is not obvious, particularly in older patients, then sequential investigation of the GI tract and the renal tract may be indicated. Decisions to admit or discharge these patients depend on the red cell reserves, the patient's cardiorespiratory status, home circumstances and the likelihood of compliance with follow-up.

The anaemia itself can be corrected with oral iron supplements: 200 mg of ferrous sulphate three times daily is an appropriate regimen, although single daily doses are often more acceptable to the patient and have fewer GI side effects.

ANAEMIA SECONDARY TO DECREASED RED CELL PRODUCTION

Megaloblastic anaemia

The finding of a raised MCV is common in the presence or absence of anaemia. Alcohol abuse is a frequent underlying cause, and other causes are listed in Table 13.1.4. MCVs greater than 115 fL are usually due to megaloblastic anaemia, which in turn is usually due to either vitamin B12 or folate deficiency. Vitamin B12 and folate are essential to DNA synthesis in all cells. Deficiencies manifest principally in red cell production because of the sheer number of red cells that are produced. B12 deficiency is usually the result of a malabsorption syndrome, whereas folate deficiency is of dietary origin. Tetrahydrofolate is a co-factor in DNA synthesis and, in turn, the formation of tetrahydrofolate

Table 13.1.4 Some causes of a raised mass cell volume
Alcohol
Drugs
Hypothyroidism
Liver disease
Megaloblastic anaemias (B12 and folate deficiency)
Myelodysplasia
Pregnancy
Reticulocytosis

from its methylated precursor is B12-dependent. Unabated cytoplasmic production of RNA in the context of impaired DNA synthesis appears to produce the enlarged nucleus and abundant cytoplasm of the megaloblast. These cells, when released to the periphery, have poor function and poor survival.

B12 deficiency is an autoimmune disorder in which autoantibodies to gastric parietal cells and the B12 transport factor (intrinsic factor) interfere with B12 absorption in the terminal ileum. Patients have achlorhydria, mucosal atrophy (a painful smooth tongue) and sometimes evidence of other autoimmune disorders, such as vitiligo, thyroid disease and Addison's disease. This is so-called 'pernicious anaemia'.

A rare, but important, manifestation of this disease is 'subacute combined degeneration of the spinal cord'. Demyelination of the posterior and lateral columns of the spinal cord manifests as a peripheral neuropathy and an abnormal gait. The central nervous system abnormalities worsen and become irreversible in the absence of B12 supplementation. Treatment of B12 deficient patients with folate alone may accelerate the onset of this condition.

Undiagnosed untreated pernicious anaemia is not a common finding in the ED, but the laboratory finding of anaemia and megaloblastosis should prompt haematological consultation. The investigative workup, which includes B12 and red cell folate levels, autoantibodies to parietal cells and intrinsic factor, a marrow aspirate, and Schilling's test of B12 absorption, may well necessitate hospital admission.

The work-up for folate deficiency is similar to that for B12. Occasionally, patients require investigation for a mal-absorption syndrome (tropical sprue, coeliac disease), which includes jejunal biopsy. Folate deficiency is common in pregnancy because of the large folate requirements of the growing fetus. It can be difficult to diagnose because of the maternal physiological expansion of plasma volume and also of red cell mass, but diagnosis and treatment with oral folate supplements are important because of the risk of associated neural tube defects.

Both B12 and folate deficiency are usu-ally manifestations of chronic disease pro-cesses. Rarely, an acute megaloblastic anaemia and pancytopenia can develop over the course of days and nitrous oxide therapy has been identified as a principal cause of this condition.

Anaemia of chronic disorders
Patients with chronic infective, malignant or connective tissue disorders can develop a mild-to-moderate normochromic normo-cytic anaemia. Evidence of bleeding or haemolysis is absent, and there is no response to haematinic therapy. The path-ophysiology of this anaemia is complex and probably involves both decreased red cell production and survival. Possible underlying mechanisms include reticuloen-dothelial overactivity in chronic inflamma-tion, and defects in iron metabolism mediated by a variety of acute-phase reac-tants and cytokines such as interleukin-1, tumour necrosis factor and interferon γ, which impair renal erythropoietin produc-tion and function.

Anaemia of chronic disorders (ACD) is generally not so severe as to warrant emergency therapy. The importance of ACD in the ED lies in its recognition as a pointer towards an underlying chronic process. Difficulties can arise in distinguishing ACD from iron deficiency, and the two conditions may coexist – in rheumatoid arthritis, for example. Iron studies generally elucidate the nature of the anaemia. In iron deficiency, iron and ferritin are low and total iron binding is high, whereas in ACD iron and total iron binding are low and ferritin is normal or high.

Other causes of decreased red cell production

Bone marrow failure is rarely encountered in emergency medicine practice. The physi-cian must be alert to the unusual, insidious or sinister presentation, and be particularly attuned to the triad of decreased tissue oxygenation, immunocompromise and a bleeding diathesis that may herald a pancy-topenia. An FBC may dictate the need for haematological consultation, hospital admission and further investigation.

Among the entities to be considered are the aplastic anaemias, characterized by a pancytopenia secondary to failure of plurip-otent myeloid stem cells. Half of cases are idiopathic, but important aetiologies are infections (e.g. non-A, non-B hepatitis), inherited diseases (e.g. Fanconi's anaemia), irradiation, therapeutic or otherwise, and – most important in the emergency setting – drugs. Drugs that have been implicated in the development of aplastic anaemia include, in addition to antimetabolites and alkylating agents, chloramphenicol, chlorpromazine and streptomycin.

Characteristic of patients with a primary marrow failure is the absence of splenomeg-aly and the absence of a reticulocyte response. There is a correlation between prognosis and the severity of the pancytope-nia. Platelet counts less than $20 \times 10^9/L$ and neutrophil counts less than 500/mL equate to severe disease. Depending on the severity of the accompanying anaemia, patients may require red cell and sometimes platelet transfusion in the ED, as well as broad-spectrum antibiotic cover. It is imper-ative to stop all medications that might be causing the marrow failure. Other forms of marrow failure include pure red cell aplasia, where marrow red cell precursors are absent or diminished. This can be a complication of haemolytic states in which a viral insult leads to an aplastic crisis (see haemolytic anaemias).

The myelodysplastic syndromes are a group of disorders primarily affecting the elderly. In these states there is no reduction in marrow cellularity but the mature red cells, granulocytes and platelets generated from an abnormal clone of stem cells are disordered and dysfunctional. There is peripheral pancytopenia. These disorders

Table 13.1.5 Classification of the myelodysplastic syndromes
Refractory anaemia
Refractory anaemia with ringed sideroblasts
Refractory anaemia with excess of blasts
Chronic myelomonocytic leukaemia

are classified according to observed cellular morphology (Table 13.1.5). These condi-tions were once termed 'preleukaemia', and one-third of patients progress to acute myeloid leukaemia.

Two more causes of failure of erythropoi-esis might be mentioned. One is due to invasion of the marrow and disruption of its architecture by extraneous tissue, the commonest cause being metastatic cancer. Finally, but not at all uncommon, is the anaemia of chronic renal failure, where deficient erythropoiesis is attributed to decreased production of erythropoietin. Most patients with chronic renal failure on dialysis treatment tolerate a moderate degree of anaemia, but occasionally require either transfusion or treatment with eryth-ropoietin. Emergency physicians should recognize anaemia as a predictable entity in patients with chronic renal failure, usu-ally not requiring any action.

ANAEMIA SECONDARY TO DECREASED RED CELL SURVIVAL: THE HAEMOLYTIC ANAEMIAS

Patients whose main problem is haemolysis are encountered rarely in the ED. The most fulminant haemolytic emergency one could envisage is that following transfusion of ABO-incompatible blood (discussed in Ch. 13.5), a vanishingly rare event where proper procedures are followed. Haemolysis and haemolytic anaemia are occasionally encountered in decompensating patients with multisystem problems. Rarely, first presentations of unusual haematological conditions occur.

Some of the haemolytic anaemias are hereditary conditions in which the inherited disorder is an abnormality intrinsic to the red cell, its membrane, its metabolic path-ways or the structure of the haemoglobin contained in the cells. Such red cells are liable to be dysfunctional, and to have increased fragility and a shortened lifespan. Lysis in the circulation may lead to clinical jaundice as bilirubin is formed from the breakdown of haemoglobin. Lysis in the reticuloendothelial system generally does not cause jaundice but may produce splenomegaly. The anaemia tends to be normochromic normocytic; sometimes a mildly raised MCV is due to an appropriate reticulocyte response from a normally functioning marrow. Serum bilirubin may be raised even in the absence of jaundice. Urinary urobilinogen and faecal stercobilinogen are detectable and serum haptoglobin is depleted. The antiglobulin (Coombs') test is important in the elucidation of some haemolytic anaemias. In this test, red cells coated in vivo (direct test) or in vitro (indirect test) with IgG antibodies are washed to remove unbound antibodies, then incubated with an antihuman globulin reagent. The resultant agglutination is a positive test.

Any chronic haemolytic process may be complicated by an 'aplastic crisis'. This is a usually transient marrow suppression brought on by a viral infection which can result in a severe and life-threatening anaemia. Red cell transfusion in these circumstances may be life-saving.

Hereditary spherocytosis

A deficiency of the red cell wall protein, spectrin, leads to loss of deformability and increased red cell fragility. These cells are destroyed prematurely in the spleen. The condition may present at any age, with anaemia, intermittent jaundice and cholelithiasis. Patients are Coombs' negative and show normal red cell osmotic fragility. Splenectomy radically improves general health. Hereditary elliptocytosis is a similar disease, with usually a milder course.

Glucose-6-phosphate dehydrogenase deficiency

Glucose-6-phosphate dehydrogenase (G6PD) generates reduced glutathione, which protects the red cell from oxidant stress. G6PD deficiency is an X-linked disorder present in heterozygous males and homozygous females. The disorder is commonly seen in West Africa, southern Europe, the Middle East and South East Asia. Oxidant stress leads to severe haemolytic anaemia. Precipitants include fava beans, antimalarial and analgesic drugs, and infections. The enzyme deficiency can be demonstrated by direct assay, and treatment is supportive.

Sickle cell anaemia

Whereas in the thalassaemias there is a deficiency in a given globin chain within the haemoglobin (Hb) molecule, in the haemoglobinopathies a given globin chain is present but structurally abnormal. HbS differs from normal HbA by one amino acid residue: valine replaces glutamic acid at the sixth amino acid from the N-terminus of the β-globin chain. Red cells containing HbS tend to 'sickle' at states of low oxygen tension. The deformed sickle-shaped red cell has increased rigidity, which causes it to lodge in the microcirculation and sequester in the reticuloendothelial system – the cause of a haemolytic anaemia.

Sickle cell disease is encountered in Afro-Caribbean people. The higher incidence in tropical areas is attributed to the survival value of the β-S gene against falciparum malaria. Heterozygous individuals have 'sickle trait' and are usually asymptomatic. Homozygous (HbSS) individuals manifest the disease in varying degrees. The haemolytic anaemia is usually in the range of 60–100 g/L and can be well tolerated because HbS offloads oxygen to the tissues more efficiently than HbA.

A patient with sickle cell disease may occasionally develop a rapidly worsening anaemia. This may be due to:

- a production defect – reduced marrow erythropoiesis may be secondary to folate deficiency or to a parvovirus infection; this is an aplastic crisis
- a survival defect – increased haemolysis is usually secondary to infection
- splenic sequestration.

In any of these circumstances transfusion may be life-saving. However, these events are unusual and more commonly encountered is the vaso-occlusive crisis. A stressor – for example infection, dehydration, or cold – causes sickle cells to lodge in the microcirculation. Bone marrow infarction is one well-recognized complication of the phenomenon, but virtually any body system can be affected. Common presenting complaints include acute spinal pain, abdominal pain (the mesenteric occlusion of 'girdle sequestration'), chest pain (pulmonary vascular occlusion), joint pain, fever (secondary to tissue necrosis), neurological involvement (translent ischaemic attacks, strokes, seizures, obtundation, coma), respiratory embarrassment and hypoxia, priapism, 'hand-foot syndrome' (dactylitis of infancy), haematuria (nephrotic syndrome, papillary necrosis), skin ulcers of the lower limbs, retinopathies, glaucoma and gallstones.

Most patients presenting with a vaso-occlusive crisis know they have the disease but otherwise the differential diagnosis is difficult. Sickle cells may be seen on the blood film, and can also be induced by deoxygenating the sample. Hb electrophoresis can establish the type of Hb present. Other investigations are dictated by the presentation, and may include blood cultures, urinalysis and culture, chest X-ray, arterial blood gases and electrocardiograph.

Pain relief should commence early. A morphine infusion may be required for patients with severe ongoing pain. Other supportive measures are dictated by the presentation. Intravenous fluids are particularly important for patients with renal involvement. Aim to establish a urine output in excess of 100 mL/h in adults. Antibiotic cover may be required in the case of febrile patients with lung involvement. It may be impossible to differentiate between pulmonary vaso-occlusion and pneumonia. Many patients with sickle cell disease are effectively splenectomized owing to chronic splenic sequestration with infarction, and are prone to infection from encapsulated bacteria. The choice of antibiotic depends on the clinical presentation. Indications for exchange transfusion are shown in Table 13.1.6. The efficacy of exchange transfusion in painful crises remains unproven.

Table 13.1.6 Indications for exchange transfusion in sickle cell crisis
Neurological presentations: TIAs, stroke, seizures
Lung involvement (PaO$_2$ < 65 mmHg with FiO$_2$ 60%)
Sequestration syndromes
Priapism

TIA, transient ischaemic attack

Haemoglobin S-C disease

Sickle trait or Hb S-C disease occurs in up to 10% in the black population. The clinical presentation resembles that of sickle cell disease but is usually less severe.

Haemoglobin C disease

In HbC, lysine replaces glutamic acid in the sixth position from the N terminus of the β-chain. Red cells containing HbC tend to be abnormally rigid, but the cells do not sickle. Homozygotes manifest a normocytic anaemia but there is no specific treatment and transfusion is seldom required.

Thalassaemias

There is a high incidence of β-thalassaemia trait among people of Mediterranean origin, although in fact the region of high frequency extends in a broad band east to South East Asia.

Thalassaemias are disorders of haemoglobin synthesis. In the haemoglobin molecule, four haem molecules are attached to four long polypeptide globin chains. Four globin chain types (each with their own minor variations in amino acid order) are designated α, β, γ and δ. Haemoglobin A comprises two α and two β chains; 97% of adult haemoglobin is HbA. In thalassaemia there is diminished or absent production of either the α chain (α-thalassaemia) or the β chain (β-thalassaemia). Most patients are heterozygous and have a mild asymptomatic anaemia, although the red cells are small. In fact, the finding of a marked microcytosis in conjunction with a mild anaemia suggests the diagnosis.

There are four genes on paired chromosome 16 coding for α-globin and two genes on paired chromosomes 11 coding for β-globin. α-Thalassaemias are associated with patterns of gene deletion as follows: (-/-) is Hb-Barts hydrops syndrome, incompatible with life, and (-α/-) is HbH disease.

Patients who are heterozygous for β-thalassaemia have β-thalassaemia minor or thalassaemia trait. They are usually symptomless. Homozygous patients have β major.

Diagnosis of the major clinical syndromes is usually possible through consideration of the presenting features in conjunction with an FBC, blood film and Hb electrophoresis.

HbH disease patients present with moderate haemolytic anaemia and splenomegaly. The HbH molecule is detectable on electrophoresis and comprises unstable β tetramers. α Trait occurs with deletion of one or two genes. Hb, MCV and mean corpuscular haemoglobin (MCH) are low, but the patient is often asymptomatic.

β major becomes apparent in the first 6 months of life with the decline of fetal Hb. There is a severe haemolytic anaemia, ineffective erythropoiesis, hepatosplenomegaly and failure to thrive. With improved care many of these patients survive to adulthood, and may possibly present to the ED, where transfusion could be life-saving. Patients with β trait may be encountered in the ED relatively frequently. They are generally asymptomatic, with a mild hypochromic microcytic anaemia. It is important not to work these patients up continually for iron deficiency, and not to subject them to inappropriate haematinic therapy.

Acquired haemolytic anaemias

Many of the acquired haemolytic anaemias are autoimmune in nature, a manifestation of a type II (cytotoxic) hypersensitivity reaction. Here, normal red cells are attacked by aberrant autoantibodies targeting antigens on the red cell membrane. These reactions may occur more readily at 37°C (warm autoimmune haemolytic anaemia, or AIHA), or at 4°C (cold AIHA). Warm AIHA is more common. Red cells are coated with IgG, complement or both. The cells are destroyed in the reticuloendothelial system. Fifty per cent of cases are idiopathic, but other recognized causes include lymphoproliferative disorders, neoplasms, connective tissue disorders, infections and drugs (notably methyldopa and penicillin). Patients have haemolytic anaemia, splenomegaly and a positive Coombs' test. In the ED setting it is important to stop any potentially offending drugs and search for the underlying disease. The idiopathic group may respond to steroids, other immunosuppressive or cytotoxic drugs or splenectomy.

In cold AIHA, IgM attaches to the I red cell antigen in the cooler peripheries. Primary cold antibody AIHA is known as cold haemagglutinin disease. Other causes include lymphoproliferative disorders, infections such as mycoplasma, and paroxysmal cold haemoglobinuria. Patients sometimes manifest Reynaud's disease and other manifestations of circulatory obstruction. Symptoms worsen in winter. Red cell lysis leads to haemoglobinuria.

Microangiopathic haemolytic anaemia

In this important group of conditions intravascular haemolysis occurs in conjunction with a disorder of microcirculation. Important causes are shown in Table 13.1.7.

Haemolytic uraemic syndrome and thrombotic thrombocytopenic purpura

These are probably manifestations of the same pathological entity, with haemolytic uraemic syndrome occurring in children and thrombotic thrombocytopenic purpura most commonly in the fourth decade, especially in women. The primary lesion is likely to be in the vascular endothelium. Fibrin and platelet microthrombi are laid down in arterioles and capillaries, possibly as an autoimmune reaction. The clotting system is not activated. Haemolytic anaemia, thrombocytopenia and acute renal failure are sometimes accompanied by fever and neurological deficits.

Table 13.1.7 Causes of microangiopathic haemolytic anaemia
Disseminated intravascular coagulation
Haemolytic uraemic syndrome
HELLP
Malignancy
Malignant hypertension
Snake envenoming
Thrombotic thrombocytopenic purpura
Vasculitis

In adults, the presentation is usually one of a neurological disturbance (headache, confusion, obtundation, seizures or focal signs). The blood film reveals anaemia, thrombocytopenia, reticulocytosis and schistocytes. Coombs' test is negative.

Patients require hospital admission. Adults with this condition may require aggressive therapy with prednisone, antiplatelet therapy, further immunosuppressive therapy and plasma exchange transfusions.

HELLP syndrome

HELLP stands for haemolysis, elevated liver enzymes and a low platelet count, and is seen in pregnant women in the context of pre-eclampsia. Treatment is as for pre-eclampsia, early delivery of the baby being of paramount importance.

Disseminated intravascular coagulation

The introduction of procoagulants into the circulation resulting in the overwhelming of anticoagulant control systems may occur as a consequence of a substantial number of pathophysiological insults – obstetric, infective, malignant and traumatic. Disseminated intravascular coagulation has an intimate association with shock, from any cause. The widespread production of thrombin leads to deposition of microthrombi, bleeding secondary to thrombocytopenia and a consumption coagulopathy, and red cell damage within abnormal vasculature leading to a haemolytic anaemia.

Recognition of this condition prompts intensive care admission and aggressive therapy. Principles of treatment include definitive management of the underlying cause and, from the haematological point of view, replacement therapy that may involve transfusion of red cells, platelets, FFP, and cryoprecipitate. There may be a role for heparin and other anticoagulant treatments if specific tissue and organ survival is threatened by thrombus.

Paroxysmal noctural haemoglobinuria

This entity is unusual in that an intrinsic red cell defect is seen in the context of an acquired haemolytic anaemia. A somatic stem cell mutation results in a clonal disorder. A family of membrane proteins (CD55, CD59 and C8 binding protein) is deficient and renders cells prone to complement-mediated lysis. Because the same proteins are deficient in white cells and platelets, in addition to being anaemic patients are prone to infections and haemostatic abnormalities. They may go on to develop aplastic anaemia or leukaemia. Treatment is supportive. Marrow transplant can be curative.

Other causes of haemolysis

Haemolysis may be due to mechanical trauma, as in 'March haemoglobinuria'. Artificial heart valves can potentially traumatize red cells. Historically, ball-and-cage type valves have been most prone to cause haemolysis, whereas disc valves are more thrombogenic. Improvements in design have made cardiac haemolytic anaemia very rare. Haemolysis is sometimes seen in

Table 13.1.8   Infections associated with haemolysis
Babesiosis
Bartonella
Clostridia
Cytomegalovirus
Coxsackie virus
Epstein-Barr virus
Haemophilus
Herpes simplex
HIV
Malaria, especially *Plasmodium falciparum* (Blackwater fever)
Measles
Mycoplasma
Varicella

Table 13.1.9   Drugs and toxins associated with haemolysis
Antimalarials
Arsine (arsenic hydride)
Bites: bees, wasps, spiders, snakes
Copper toxicity
Dapsone
Lead (plumbism)
Local anaesthetics: lidocaine, benzocaine
Nitrates, nitrites
Sulfonamides

association with a number of infectious diseases, notably malaria. Other infections that have been implicated are listed in Table 13.1.8. Certain drugs and toxins are associated with haemolytic anaemia (Table 13.1.9). The haemolytic anaemia that is commonly seen in patients with severe burns is attributed to direct damage to the red cells by heat.

Further reading

Bain BJ. Morphology in the diagnosis of red cell disorders. Hematology 2005; 10S(1):178–181.

Bayless PA. Selected red cell disorders. Emergency Medicine Clinics of North America 1993; 11(2): 481–493.

Bojanowski C. Use of protocols for ED patients with sickle cell anaemia. Journal of Emergency Nursing 1989; 15: 83–87.

Brookoff D, Polomano R. Treating sickle cell pain like cancer pain. Annals of Internal Medicine 1992; 116(5): 364–368.

Carbrow MB, Wilkins JC. Haematologic emergencies. Management of transfusion reactions and crises in sickle cell disease. Postgraduate Medicine 1993; 93(5): 183–190.

Erslev A. Erythropoietin. New England Journal of Medicine 1991; 316: 101.

Evans TC, Jehle D. The red blood cell distribution width. Journal of Emergency Medicine 1991; 9(suppl 1): 71–74.

Friedman EW, Webber AB, Osborn HH, et al. Oral analgesia for painful crisis in sickle cell anaemia. Annals of Emergency Medicine 1986; 15: 787–791.

Gaillard HM, Hamilton GC. Hemoglobin/hematocrit and other erythrocyte parameters. Emergency Medicine Clinics of North America 1986; 4(1): 15–40.

Gregory SA, McKenna R, Sassetti RJ, et al. Hematologic emergencies. Medical Clinics of North America 1986; 70(5): 1129–1149.

Losek JD, Hellmich TR, Hoffman GM. Diagnostic value of anemia, red blood cell morphology, and reticulocyte count for sickle cell disease. Annals of Emergency Medicine 1992; 21(8): 915–918.

Pollack CV. Emergencies in sickle cell disease. Emergency Medicine Clinics of North America 1993; 11(2): 365–378.

Powers RD. Management protocol for sickle-cell disease patients with acute pain: impact of emergency department and narcotic use. American Journal of Emergency Medicine 1986; 4(3): 267–268.

Thomas C, Thomas L. Anemia of chronic disease: pathophysiology and laboratory diagnosis. Laboratory Hematology 2005; 11(1): 14–23.

13.2 Neutropenia

Simon Wood

ESSENTIALS

1 The risk of infection increases significantly as the absolute neutrophil count drops below 1.0×10^9/L.

2 Life-threatening neutropenia is most likely to be due to impaired haematopoiesis.

3 A detailed medication history is vital to the 'work-up' of neutropenia.

4 Fever in the presence of severe neutropenia constitutes a true emergency that mandates rapid assessment and aggressive management to prevent progression to overwhelming sepsis.

5 Strategies of early empiric broad-spectrum antibiotic administration have significantly reduced the overall mortality of febrile neutropenia.

Table 13.2.1 Important causes of neutropenia

Decreased production

Aplastic anaemia
Leukaemias
Lymphomas
Metastatic cancer
Drug-induced agranulocytosis
Megaloblastic anaemias
   Vitamin B12 deficiency
   Folate deficiency
CD8 and large granular lymphocytosis
Myelodysplastic syndromes

Decreased survival

Idiopathic immune related
Systemic lupus erythematosis
Felty syndrome
Drugs

Redistribution

Sequestration (hypersplenism)
Increased utilization (overwhelming sepsis)
Viraemia

Introduction

Neutropenia is defined as a decrease in the number of circulating neutrophils. The neutrophil count varies with age, sex and racial grouping. The severity of neutropenia is usually graded as follows:[1]

- Mild: neutrophil count $1.0–1.5 \times 10^9$/L
- Moderate: neutrophil count $0.5–1.0 \times 10^9$/L
- Severe: neutrophil count $<0.5 \times 10^9$/L

The risk of infection rises as the neutrophil count falls and becomes significant once the neutrophil count drops below 1.0×10^9/L. Febrile neutropenia is a term used to describe the clinical scenario where a patient has a neutrophil count less than 1.0×10^9/L in the presence of a temperature greater than or equal to 38°C or if the patient is systemically unwell with signs or symptoms of sepsis. Neutropenic patients are at greater risk of overwhelming infection if the onset of the neutropenia is acute rather than chronic and, in the case of patients receiving cancer chemotherapy, if the absolute neutrophil count is in the process of falling rather than rising.

Signs or symptoms of infection in the presence of severe neutropenia constitute a true emergency that mandates rapid assessment and aggressive management to prevent progression to overwhelming sepsis. In the emergency department (ED) setting this is most commonly encountered when a patient presents with fever in the context of chemotherapy for cancer.

Pathophysiology and aetiology

Polymorphonuclear neutrophils are formed in marrow from the myelogenous cell series. Pluripotent haematopoietic stem cells are committed to a particular cell lineage through the formation of colony-forming units, which further differentiate to form given white cell precursors. The mature neutrophil has a multilobed nucleus and granules in the cytoplasm. The cells are termed 'neutrophilic' because of the lilac colour of the granules caused by the uptake of both acidic and basic dyes.

The neutrophils leave the marrow and enter the circulation, where they have a lifespan of only 6–10 h before entering the tissues. Here they migrate by chemotaxis to sites of infection and injury, and then phagocytose and destroy foreign material. In health, about half of the available mature neutrophils are in the circulation. 'Marginal' cells are adherent to vascular endothelium or in the tissues and are not measured by the full blood count. Some individuals have fixed increased marginal neutrophil pools and decreased circulating pools; they are said to have benign idiopathic neutropenia.

For a previously normal individual to become neutropenic there must be decreased production of neutrophils in the marrow, decreased survival of mature neutrophils or a redistribution of neutrophils from the circulating pool. The important causes are shown in Table 13.2.1.

It is a defect in neutrophil production that is most likely to prove life threatening. Consumption of neutrophils in the periphery, as occurs early in infectious processes, is likely to be rapidly compensated for by a functioning marrow. Fortunately, most of the primary diseases of haematopoiesis are rare, and in practice many of the acquired neutropenias are drug induced. Processes interfering with haematopoiesis, often involving autoimmune mechanisms, may affect neutrophils both in the marrow and in the periphery. Some drugs cause neutropenia universally but many more reactions are idiosyncratic, be they dose-related or independent of dose. Some commonly implicated drugs are listed in Table 13.2.2. Cancer chemotherapy drugs are now recognized as the commonest cause of neutropenia.

515

Table 13.2.2 Drugs commonly associated with neutropenia

Antibiotics: chloramphenicol, sulfonamides, isoniazid, rifampicin, β-lactams, carbenicillin

Antidysrhythmic agents: quinidine, procainamide

Antiepileptics: phenytoin, carbamazepine

Antihypertensives: thiazides, ethacrynic acid, captopril, methyldopa, hydralazine

Antithyroid agents

Chemotherapeutic agents: especially methotrexate, cytosine arabinoside, 5-azacytidine, azothioprine, doxorubicin, daunorubicin, hydroxyurea, alkylating agents

Connective tissue disorder agents: phenylbutazone, penicillamine, gold

H_2-receptor antagonists

Phenothiazines, especially chlorpromazine

Miscellaneous: imipramine, allopurinol, clozapine, ticlopidine, tolbutamide

Clinical features

Neutropenia is frequently anticipated based on the clinical presentation, such as fever developing in the context of cancer chemotherapy, by far the most common scenario in which severe neutropenia is seen in the ED. Alternatively, it may be identified in the course of investigation for a likely infective illness, or it might be an incidental finding during investigation for an unrelated condition.

Chronic neutropenia may be asymptomatic unless secondary or recurrent infections develop. Acute severe neutropenia may present with fever, sore throat, and mucosal ulceration or inflammation.[2] Symptoms or signs of an associated disease process may also be present, such as pallor from anaemia, or bleeding from thrombocytopenia, as might occur in conditions causing pancytopenia.

The history of the mode of onset and duration of the illness is important. Systems enquiry may reveal cough, headache and photophobia, a diarrhoeal illness, or urinary symptoms. The past history may reveal a known haematological illness or previous evidence of immunosuppression, such as frequent and recurrent infections. A detailed drug history is vital. Most neutropenic drug reactions occur within the first 3 months of taking a drug.

In the ED, vital signs, including pulse, blood pressure, temperature, respiratory rate and pulse oximetry, should be performed at initial assessment and monitored regularly until disposition. Attention should be paid to identifying early signs of severe sepsis and the progression to septic shock.

Physical examination may reveal necrotizing mucosal lesions, pallor, petechial rashes, lymphadenopathy, bone tenderness, abnormal tonsillar or respiratory findings, spleno- or other organomegaly.[2] Careful examination of the skin of the back, the lower limbs and the perineum for evidence of infection is important. The presence of indwelling venous access devices should be noted and insertion sites inspected for evidence of inflammation or infection.

Clinical investigation

Investigation in the ED is firstly aimed at confirming and quantifying the severity of neutropenia, identifying the cause, and then at identifying the focus and severity of infection. An urgent full blood count and blood film should be ordered in any patient who is suspected of suffering febrile neutropenia. A coagulation profile and biochemistry, including electrolytes and creatinine, glucose and liver function tests may be indicated once severe neutropenia is confirmed. Anaemic patients may require a group-and-hold or cross-match.

Microbiological cultures aimed at isolating a causative organism should be taken but antibiotics should not be unreasonably delayed in the presence of fever and confirmed significant neutropenia. Blood cultures should be taken at the time of cannulation and if possible prior to the instigation of antibiotic therapy. Throat swab, swabs of skin lesions and indwelling venous access device sites, urinalysis and urine culture may be indicated depending on the clinical picture. Patients with apparent central nervous system infections might require a lumbar puncture, but this should be postponed or even cancelled in the presence of an uncorrected coagulopathy, signs of raised intracranial pressure, focal neurological signs, or haemodynamic instability. Antibiotics, if clinically indicated, should be commenced prior to lumbar puncture.

Treatment

Management of the patient with confirmed febrile neutropenia in the ED involves early recognition and treatment of bacterial infection, and institution of supportive care to prevent progression to overwhelming sepsis and shock. Evolving or established haemodynamic instability requires immediate, aggressive resuscitation.

Empiric broad-spectrum antibiotic therapy should be started in the ED after drawing blood for culture in any patient with fever and confirmed significant neutropenia. This strategy has played a pivotal role in reducing mortality rates in febrile neutropenia.[3] There is no clear consensus approach to which particular empiric antibiotic regime should be used. Practices vary widely amongst institutions and regions, and are influenced by local patterns of infection, prevalence and risk of inducing resistant organisms, and acquisition costs.[4] In general antibiotics should provide good cover for both Gram-positive and Gram-negative organisms. With increased use of indwelling venous access devices for cancer chemotherapy, there has been an increase in the incidence of sepsis due to Gram-positive organisms such as coagulase negative staphylococci, *S. aureus* and MRSA.[5] Although occurring infrequently, bacteraemia due to *Pseudomonas aeruginosa* is associated with a high morbidity and mortality and therefore should also be covered.[6] A reasonable initial regime might include ticarcillin/clavulanate plus either a cephalosporin, such as ceftazidime, or an aminoglycoside, such as gentamicin. The addition of vancomycin might be considered if the patient is in shock, is known to be colonized with MRSA or has clinical evidence of a catheter-related infection in a unit with a high incidence of MRSA. Empiric antifungal therapy is not generally required unless there is persistent fever in high-risk patients beyond 96 h of antibacterial therapy.[6]

Disposition

The presence of significant neutropenia with fever generally mandates admission to hospital. Patients with severe acute neutropenia without an established aetiology will also generally require admission regardless of the presence or absence of fever. Both the haematological abnormality and the likely presence of infection require investigation. Sometimes the aetiology of the neutropenia will be evident; on other occasions marrow aspiration and biopsy will be required.

There is emerging evidence that a subset of febrile neutropenic patients can be identified who are at low risk of life-threatening complications and in whom duration of hospitalization and intensity of treatment may be safely reduced.[7] Strategies that involve outpatient treatment of low-risk patients with oral antibiotics have also been evaluated.[3] Such regimens are reliant upon accurate prediction of risk, as well as the availability of structured programmes and resources, and are not yet in widespread use.

Prognosis

The prognosis of the neutropenic patient is largely dependent upon the underlying aetiology of the condition. Febrile neutropenia has in the past been associated with a significant mortality rate which varies depending on the organism causing the infection. Improvements in therapy, such as rapid treatment with empiric broad-spectrum antibiotics, have significantly reduced mortality rates from this condition. Overall mortality rates for patients with febrile neutropenia have reduced from more than 20% to less than 4% in recent data sets.[3,7]

Controversies

❶ The prophylactic use of granulocyte colony-stimulating factors, such as filgrastim and pegfilgrastim, to reduce the incidence of febrile neutropenia during cancer chemotherapy.[8]

❷ The indications for and efficacy of granulocyte transfusions in the management of febrile neutropenia.[9]

❸ The development and validation of clinical decision rules to stratify risk patients with febrile neutropenia and the use of these to determine suitability for oral antibiotic and/or outpatient therapy.[3]

References

1. Palmblad J, Papadaki HA, Eliopoulos G. Acute and chronic neutropenias. What's new? Journal of Internal Medicine 2001; 250: 476–491.
2. Dale DC. Neutropenia and neutrophilia. In: Lichtman MA, et al., eds. Williams haematology. 7th edn. New York: McGraw-Hill; 2006.
3. Viscoli C, Varnier O, Machetti M. Infections in patients with febrile neutropenia: epidemiology, microbiology, and risk stratification. Clinical Infectious Diseases 2005; 40: S240–S245.
4. Glasmacher A, von Lilienfeld-Toal M, Schulte S, et al. An evidence-based evaluation of important aspects of empirical antibiotic therapy in febrile neutropenic patients. Clinical Microbiology and Infection 2005; 11(suppl 5): 17–23.
5. Picazo JJ. Management of the febrile neutropenic patient: a consensus conference. Clinical Infectious Diseases 2004; 39: S1–S6.
6. Severe sepsis: empirical therapy (no obvious source of infection): febrile neutropenic patients. In: eTG, Therapeutic Guidelines Limited 2007.
7. Chisholm JC, Dommett R. The evolution towards ambulatory and day-case management of febrile neutropenia. British Journal of Haematology 2006; 135: 3–16.
8. Waladkhani AR. Pegfilgrastim 2004: a recent advance in the prophylaxis of chemotherapy-induced neutropenia. European Journal of Cancer Care 2004; 13: 371–379.
9. Bishton M, Chopra R. The role of granulocyte transfusions in neutropenic patients. British Journal of Haematology 2004; 127: 501–508.

13.3 Thrombocytopenia

Simon Wood

ESSENTIALS

1 A low platelet count detected on automated blood count should always be confirmed by examination of the blood film prior to further investigation or treatment.

2 The cause of isolated thrombocytopenia can often be determined by a careful history and physical examination in addition to assessment of the full blood count and blood film.

3 Platelet transfusion is unnecessary in the management of the thrombocytopenic patient unless the platelet count is extremely low or there is ongoing bleeding.

4 In the absence of other clotting disorders or abnormal platelet function, bleeding in the thrombocytopenic patient is often amenable to local measures of haemostasis.

Introduction

Thrombocytopenia is defined as a reduction in the number of circulating platelets, the normal circulating platelet count being $150–400 \times 10^9$/L. It is the most common cause of abnormal bleeding.[1] Like anaemia, thrombocytopenia itself is not a diagnosis, but rather a manifestation of another underlying disease process.

In the emergency department setting, thrombocytopenia may present as an incidental finding on a routine blood count or may be diagnosed in the context of abnormal bleeding. In most cases, the underlying aetiology can be determined by a careful history and physical examination combined with interpretation of the blood count.

Aetiology

The clinically important causes of thrombocytopenia are outlined in Table 13.3.1. Diagnoses are classified by pathological process. It should be noted that more than one pathological process may be present.

Artifactual thrombocytopenia

Artifactual thrombocytopenia results from an underestimation of the platelet count as

Table 13.3.1 Causes of thrombocytopenia

Pseudothrombocytopenia
Platelet clumping
Collection into anticoagulant (EDTA)
Platelet agglutinins
Giant platelets

Increased platelet destruction
Immune
   Primary
      Idiopathic thrombocytopenic purpura
      (ITP)
   Secondary
      Autoimmune thrombocytopenia
      associated with other disorders
         Graves' disease, Hashimoto's
         thyroiditis, systemic lupus
         erythematosus
      HIV-related thrombocytopenia
      Drug-induced thrombocytopenia
         Heparin, gold salts, quinine/
         quinidine, sulfonamides, rifampicin,
         H2-blockers, indometacin,
         carbamazepine, valproic acid,
         ticlopidine, clopidogrel, monoclonal
         antibodies (infliximab, efalizumab,
         rituximab)
      Post-transfusion purpura
Non-immune
   Thrombotic thrombocytopenic purpura –
   haemolytic uraemic syndrome
   Pregnancy
   Gestational benign thrombocytopenia
   Pre-eclampsia/HELLP
   Disseminated intravascular coagulation

Decreased platelet production
Congenital
   TAR (thrombocytopenia with absent
   radius), Wiskott–Aldrich syndrome,
   Fanconi anaemia
Acquired
   Viral infection
   Epstein-Barr virus, rubella, dengue
   fever
   Marrow aplasia
   Malignant bone marrow infiltrates
   Chemotherapeutic agents
   Radiation therapy
Abnormal distribution and dilution
   Splenic sequestration (hypersplenism)
   Splenic enlargement
   Hypothermia
   Massive blood transfusion

measured by an automated particle counter. The most common mechanism is platelet clumping. Clumping is most often due to the anticoagulant EDTA, but may also result from auto-antibodies such as cold agglutinins. The presence of giant platelets and platelet satellitism may also yield falsely low automated platelet counts.[2]

Artifactual thrombocytopenia should be suspected when the automated platelet count is low in the absence of symptoms or signs of abnormal bleeding or disorders associated with thrombocytopenia. It is best excluded by examination of the blood film by an experienced observer. Any case of thrombocytopenia found on an automated blood count should be confirmed by examination of the peripheral smear prior to further investigation or treatment.

Immune-related thrombocytopenia

Idiopathic thrombocytopenic purpura

Idiopathic thrombocytopenic purpura (ITP) is defined as an isolated thrombocytopenia (low platelet count with an otherwise normal complete blood count and peripheral blood smear) in a patient with no clinically apparent associated conditions that can cause thrombocytopenia.[3] It is a common cause of low platelet count and abnormal bleeding in both children and adults. ITP is thought to be caused by the development of auto-antibodies to platelet membrane antigens.

Treatment is aimed at modulating the immune response and reducing the rate of platelet destruction and is indicated in all patients who have counts less than 20×10^9/L, and those with counts less than 50×10^9/L accompanied by significant mucous membrane bleeding. First phase treatment includes parenteral glucocorticoids and intravenous IgG. Splenectomy is usually reserved for patients who do not respond to medical therapy and have ongoing bleeding symptoms.[3] Platelet transfusions may cause temporary increases in platelet count and may be used in cases of life-threatening haemorrhage but are otherwise not usually indicated.[4]

In addition to the primary idiopathic form, immune thrombocytopenic purpura may also accompany autoimmune disorders such as Graves' disease and systemic lupus erythematosus. It is the main mechanism of the thrombocytopenia related to HIV infection.

Drug-related thrombocytopenia

A large number of drugs have been reported to cause immune-related thrombocytopenia. By far the most commonly implicated are quinine, quinidine and heparin. Heparin is associated with a syndrome of thrombosis due to diffuse platelet activation accompanied by a consumptive thrombocytopenia. Some platelet inhibitors, particularly ticlopidine and less commonly clopidogrel, are associated with severe thrombocytopenia and other signs and symptoms of thrombotic thrombocytopenic purpura. Recently developed monoclonal antibodies, such as infliximab (anti-tumour necrosis factor-α antibody), efalizumab (anti-CD11α antibody) and rituximab (anti-CD20 antibody) are also associated with an acute, severe, but usually self-limited thrombocytopenia.[5]

In most cases of drug-related thrombocytopenia, recovery occurs rapidly after withdrawal of the offending agent. The exception is patients with gold sensitivity, who may remain thrombocytopenic for months due to the slow clearance of this drug.[6]

Post-transfusion purpura

Post-transfusion purpura is clinically distinct from thrombocytopenia due to dilution of platelets following massive transfusion. It is an acute, severe thrombocytopenia occurring about 1 week after blood transfusion and is associated with a high titre of platelet-specific alloantibodies. It is most commonly reported in multiparous women following their first blood transfusion. The mechanism for alloantibody formation is unclear. Spontaneous recovery occurs within weeks, although fatalities from severe haemorrhage have been reported.[6]

Non-immune platelet destruction

Thrombotic thrombocytopenic purpura

Thrombotic thrombocytopenic purpura (TTP) is considered to be the adult form of the haemolytic uraemic syndrome (HUS). Essentially, a thrombotic microangiopathy the classic pentad of clinical findings is: (1) fever, (2) thrombocytopenia, (3) microangiopathic haemolytic anaemia,

(4) neurological abnormalities and (5) renal involvement.

TTP can occur sporadically as an idiopathic disorder or may be associated with pregnancy, epidemics of verotoxin-producing *Escherichia coli* and *Shigella dysenteriae*, malignancy, chemotherapy, marrow transplantation, and drug-dependent antibodies. Treatment with plasma exchange has dramatically influenced the outcome of TTP. Mortality has fallen from more than 90% prior to introduction of plasma exchange to less than 20% with this treatment.[7]

Thrombocytopenia in pregnancy

Gestational thrombocytopenia develops during an otherwise normal pregnancy and is clinically distinct from autoimmune thrombocytopenias such as ITP. It is thought to be due to decreased platelet survival consequent to activation of the coagulation system. Thrombocytopenia is usually mild and there is no corresponding thrombocytopenia in the infant. The platelet count returns to normal after delivery, although thrombocytopenia may recur in subsequent pregnancies.[8]

Autoimmune thrombocytopenias, on the other hand, are often associated with more severe reductions in the platelet count. Antiplatelet antibodies are capable of crossing the placenta and may result in significant thrombocytopenia in the fetus and newborn. This can lead to complications, such as intracranial haemorrhage, during the delivery. Treatment of the mother with autoimmune thrombocytopenia is similar in principle to the treatment of non-pregnant cases.[8]

In the context of pregnancy, thrombocytopenia may also be seen as part of the HELLP (haemolysis, elevated liver enzymes, low platelets) and pre-eclampsia syndromes. The two syndromes are thought to be related. Common to both is a process of microvascular endothelial damage and intravascular platelet activation. This leads to release of thromboxane A and serotonin, which provoke vasospasm, platelet aggregation and further endothelial damage.[9] In both syndromes, the process is terminated by delivery.

Disseminated intravascular coagulation

Thrombocytopenia is one manifestation of the syndrome of disseminated intravascular coagulation (DIC). DIC is an acquired syndrome of diffuse intravascular coagulation up to the level of fibrin formation, accompanied by secondary fibrinolysis or inhibited fibrinolysis.[10] It occurs in the course of severe systemic diseases or may be provoked by toxins such as snake venoms.

Thrombocytopenia due to impaired platelet production

Congenital disorders of impaired platelet production usually present in childhood and will not be discussed.

Of the acquired disorders of impaired platelet production, the most commonly seen in the emergency setting is the incidental finding of reduced platelet count in patients suffering viral illness. Causative viruses include Epstein–Barr virus, rubella and dengue fever. Thrombocytopenia in these cases is reversible and requires no specific therapy other than monitoring of the platelet count to ensure normalization.

Disorders of bone marrow dysfunction, such as malignant infiltration and bone marrow suppression, cause thrombocytopenia accompanied by reductions in numbers of other blood components. Examination of the full blood count (FBC) and blood film usually distinguishes these from other causes of isolated thrombocytopenia. Further investigation is best referred to a haematologist.

Massive blood transfusion and thrombocytopenia

Massive blood transfusion is defined as the transfusion of a volume equivalent to the patient's normal blood volume within a 24-h period. Thrombocytopenia results from dilution of the patient's remaining platelets and, where whole blood is used, decreased survival of platelets in stored blood. It is possibly the most important factor contributing to the haemostatic abnormality seen in massively transfused patients. Platelet transfusion should be reserved for cases where the platelet count falls below 50×10^9/L.[4]

Hypersplenism

Hypersplenism refers to the thrombocytopenia due to pooling in patients with splenic enlargement. It is the primary cause of thrombocytopenia in hepatic cirrhosis, portal venous hypertension, and congestive splenomegaly. In these cases, thrombocytopenia is rarely severe and not usually of clinical importance.[2]

Transient thrombocytopenia has been described in patients suffering severe hypothermia and is due to splenic sequestration. Platelet counts usually return to normal within days of rewarming.[2]

Clinical features

Thrombocytopenia may be an incidental finding on the FBC or may be diagnosed in the context of abnormal bleeding. There are distinct differences in the patterns of abnormal bleeding associated with disorders of platelet deficiency and disorders of impaired coagulation.

Spontaneous bleeding related to thrombocytopenia typically manifests as cutaneous petechiae and/or purpura, most commonly in dependent areas such as the legs and buttocks.[1,3] Other spontaneous manifestations include multiple small retinal haemorrhages, epistaxis, gingival and gastrointestinal bleeding. Bleeding following trauma or surgery in thrombocytopenic patients is often immediate and may respond to local methods of haemostasis. In contradistinction to this the bleeding associated with coagulation disorders is most commonly in the form of large haematomata or haemarthroses that occur spontaneously or develop hours to days following trauma.[1]

In addition to the haemorrhagic manifestations of platelet insufficiency, patients with thrombocytopenia may present with the clinical features of the underlying causative disorder. Splenic enlargement may be present in cases where thrombocytopenia is due to hypersplenism but is not a feature of immune-related thrombocytopenia.

The level of platelets associated with clinically significant abnormal bleeding is not precisely defined. It varies depending on the platelets' functional integrity, and with the presence or absence of other risk factors, such as coagulation disorder, trauma, and surgery. There is evidence that platelet counts above 5×10^9/L are sufficient to prevent bleeding when the platelets are functionally normal and there are no other risk factors. Severe haemorrhage is uncommon at platelet counts above 20×10^9/L and in the setting of surgery the risk of abnormal haemorrhage is reduced at counts above 50×10^9/L.[4]

Clinical investigation

The FBC and examination of the blood film are diagnostic of thrombocytopenia. The pattern of deficiency should be considered. Isolated thrombocytopenia refers to a low platelet count in the presence of an otherwise normal FBC and blood film. In these cases, FBC combined with a careful clinical history and examination is often sufficient to lead to a final diagnosis.[3] Coexistent anaemia and/or leukopenia suggest bone marrow dysfunction as the primary aetiological process.

Other useful investigations may include coagulation studies and D-dimer (DIC, preeclampsia), electrolytes, urea and creatinine (TTP), liver function tests (HELLP, liver disease), and thyroid function tests (autoimmune thyroid disorders). Platelet antibody titres are indicated in the work-up of pregnancy-related thrombocytopenia, and bone marrow aspirate may be indicated in investigation of thrombocytopenia due to bone marrow dysfunction, but neither of these tests is useful in the emergency department setting.

Treatment

Treatment for specific causes of thrombocytopenia has already been discussed. Bleeding in the face of low platelet count may be responsive to local methods of haemostasis if the remaining platelets are functionally normal

and there is no other disorder of coagulation present. Individual case reports provide some support for the use of recombinant Factor VIIa as an enhancer of haemostasis in the treatment of bleeding in the context of severe thrombocytopenia, although evidence from randomized clinical trials is lacking.[11] Platelet transfusion may be helpful in cases of severe haemorrhage and is sometimes used prophylactically to prevent bleeding in patients with very low platelet counts.

Platelet transfusion is primarily indicated in patients in whom thrombocytopenia is due to impaired platelet production and who are bleeding or have very low counts. The threshold for prophylactic transfusion in these patients is controversial. It is indicated when the platelet count is below 5×10^9/L, but is probably not indicated above this level unless other risk factors for bleeding are present.[4]

Platelet transfusion is rarely indicated in immune-related thrombocytopenias as the transfused platelets are rapidly destroyed. Transfusion of platelets may aggravate TTP.[4] In DIC, platelet transfusion has not been proven to be effective but may be indicated in bleeding patients. There is little evidence to support the suggestion that blood component therapy aggravates DIC.[12] In cases of massive blood transfusion, platelets are not routinely indicated unless there is ongoing bleeding and the platelet count is below 50×10^9/L.[4]

Raising the platelet count to 20–50 $\times$ 10^9/L is sufficient to prevent serious bleeding. In patients undergoing surgery or other invasive procedures counts up to 60–100 $\times$ 10^9/L may be required. A useful rule of thumb is that in a 70 kg adult, transfusion of one unit of platelets will increase the platelet count by 11×10^9/L.[4]

At present, platelet preparations for transfusion are stored in liquid at 22°C. Problems include the continued risk of febrile non-haemolytic reactions, transmission of infectious agents and graft-versus-host disease. Alternatives to conventional liquid storage include frozen storage, cold liquid storage, photochemical treatment and lyophilized platelets. None of these methods is currently widely available. Several platelet substitutes have been developed but remain untested in the clinical setting. Some examples are red cells with

surface-bound fibrinogen, fibrinogen-coated albumin microcapsules and liposome-based haemostatic agents.[13]

Disposition

Disposition will depend on the presence and extent of abnormal bleeding, the degree of thrombocytopenia and the underlying aetiology. In general, patients who present with abnormal bleeding and a low platelet count should be admitted for further evaluation and treatment. In the absence of bleeding, patients who have isolated thrombocytopenia with counts above 20×10^9/L may be investigated on an outpatient basis.[3]

Controversies

❶ The platelet count at which prophylactic platelet transfusion is indicated.

❷ The development and clinical testing of alternative methods of platelet preparation and platelet substitutes.

❸ The role of recombinant Factor VIIa in the treatment of bleeding in the context of severe thrombocytopenia.

References

1. Rodgers GM, Bithell TC. The diagnostic approach to the bleeding disorders. In: Lee GR, Wintrobe MM, Lee GR, et al, eds. Wintrobe's clinical hematology. 10th edn. Maryland: Lippincott Williams & Wilkins; 1999: 1557–1578.
2. George JN. Thrombocytopenia: pseudothrombocytopenia, hypersplenism, and thrombocytopenia associated with massive transfusion. In: Beutler E, Beutler E, Williams WJ, eds. Williams Hematology. 5th edn. New York: McGraw-Hill; 1995: 1355–1360.
3. American Society of Hematology. ITP Practice Guideline Panel. Diagnosis and treatment of idiopathic thrombocytopenic purpura. American Family Physician 1996; 54(8): 2437–2447, 2451–2452.
4. Mollison PL, Engelfriet CP, Contreras M. Blood transfusions in clinical medicine. 10th edn. Oxford: Blackwell Science; 1997.
5. Aster RH, Bougie DW. Drug-induced immune thrombocytopenia. New England Journal of Medicine 2007; 357(6): 580–587.
6. George JN, El-Harake M, Aster RH. Thrombocytopenia due to enhanced platelet destruction by immunological mechanisms. In: Beutler E, et al, eds. Williams hematology. 5th edn. New York: McGraw-Hill; 1995: 1315–1354.
7. George JN, El-Harake M. Thrombocytopenia due to enhanced platelet destruction by nonimmunological mechanisms. In: Beutler E, et al, eds. Williams hematology. 5th edn. New York: McGraw-Hill; 1995; 1290–1314.

8. Schwartz KA. Gestational thrombocytopenia and immune thrombocytopenias in pregnancy. Hematology and Oncology Clinics of North America 2000; 14(5): 1101–1116.
9. Padden MO. HELLP syndrome: recognition and perinatal management. American Family Physician 1999; 60(3): 829–836.
10. Ten Cate H. Pathophysiology of disseminated intravascular coagulation in sepsis. Critical Care Medicine 2000; 28(9 suppl): S9–S11.
11. Goodnough LT, Lublin DM, Zhang L, et al. Transfusion medicine service policies for recombinant factor VIIa administration. Transfusion 2004; 44: 1325–1331.
12. Levi M, de Jonge E, van der Poll T. Novel approaches to the management of disseminated intravascular coagulation. Critical Care Medicine 2000; 28 (9 suppl): S20–S24.
13. Lee DH, Blajchman MA. Novel treatment modalities: new platelet preparations and substitutes. British Journal of Haematology 2001; 114: 496–505.

13.4 Haemophilia

Sean Arendse

ESSENTIALS

1 Haemophilia is a disorder which should be managed by the emergency physician in consultation with their nearest haemophilia centre.

2 Patients should carry their treatment regime cards with them. If not, they should be encouraged to do so.

Introduction

Haemophilia is a group of congenital disorders of blood coagulation that arise as a result of a deficiency of clotting factor proteins, which are essential to the normal intrinsic coagulation pathway. The classic form, haemophilia A, is attributable to deficiency of Factor VIII while haemophilia B (also known as Christmas disease) is attributable to deficiency of Factor IX. Both these diseases have a classic X-linked pattern of inheritance and thus affect males while female carriers may also have mild deficiency of the appropriate coagulation factor.

Haemophilia A is the commoner disease (80%), with an incidence of 1 in 8000–10 000 live male births, compared to an incidence of 1 in 25 000–30 000 for haemophilia B (20%).

Pathophysiology

The normal clotting system is activated in the presence of vascular injury to produce: (1) vascular spasm, (2) platelet plug formation, (3) coagulation: factor activation and the production of fibrin. Normal coagulation of blood is dependent on the generation of adequate thrombin via the clotting cascade. Deficiency of Factor VIII or IX reduces the amplification of the clotting cascade and causes haemophilia. The severity of the bleeding disorder is inversely related to the level of functional factor present and is categorized into mild, moderate and severe disease:

- Mild disease (6–30% of normal factor level) – manifests with persistent bleeding after surgery, dental extractions and trauma. Spontaneous bleeds do not occur in this group of patients.
- Moderate disease (1–5% of normal factor level) – manifests with bleeding into joints and muscles after minor trauma and excessive bleeding after surgery and dental extractions.
- Severe disease (<1% of normal factor level) – manifests with spontaneous joint and muscle bleeding, and excessive bleeding following minor trauma, surgery or dental extractions.

Clinical features

Haemophilia A and B are clinically indistinguishable and symptoms vary according to the severity of the inherited disorder. Mild disease may not present till adulthood, whereas moderate to severe disease usually presents in infancy or early childhood.

Bleeding in haemophilia tends to occur spontaneously or following minor trauma and is typically delayed and persistent. This is because although initial platelet 'plugging' function is normal, the subsequent coagulation 'cascade' response is abnormal. This delay is usually hours, occasionally days. Once bleeding occurs it may persist for days or even weeks. Patients who are severely affected may present with bleeding episodes on a weekly basis.

The most common manifestations of haemophilia are:

- bleeding into joints (knees, elbows, ankles, shoulders, hips, wrists in descending order of frequency)
- bleeding into soft tissues and muscles (the iliopsoas muscle around the hip, calf, forearm, upper arm, Achilles tendon, buttocks)
- bleeding in the mouth from a cut, bitten tongue or loss of a tooth
- haematuria
- superficial bruising
- haemarthroses – the bleeding is from synovial membrane apendicular structure, with inflammation of the synovium, and leads to degenerative arthritis, joint destruction and loss of joint mobility and function
- bleeding into tissue planes – tense flexor haematomas in limbs can cause compartment syndromes, and haemorrhage into muscles may lead to atrophy and contracture
- bleeding into the neck (may cause airway compromise)
- central nervous system bleeding
- retroperitoneal bleeding.

Patients may also present with a complication of therapy. Most haemophiliac patients treated before 1985 have been exposed to pathogenic viruses, of which the most important are hepatitis C, hepatitis B and HIV. Of those who received plasma prior to the mid-1980s, 90% are hepatitis B positive, 85–100% are hepatitis C positive, and 60–90% are HIV positive.

Clinical investigation

Investigations are tailored to the individual presentation. A full blood count, blood film and coagulation profiles are useful in the evaluation of first presentations, or major bleed, but unlikely to be helpful in patients with an established diagnosis. Plain radiography of affected joints and computerized tomography (CT) scanning of the head, chest, abdomen and pelvis may be essential to establish the presence or absence of bleeding complications.

The prothrombin time measures primarily Factors II, VII, V and X, thus patients with both haemophilia A and B have a normal prothrombin time, and a normal thrombin clotting time. The partial thromboplastin time measures activation of all factors other than Factor VIII and is prolonged in haemophilia (although it can be normal if factor activity exceeds 30%). Specific factor assays are required to distinguish between haemophilias A and B.

Treatment

Treatment of haemophilia has evolved dramatically in the past 40 years with the discovery in the 1960s that coagulation Factor VIII was concentrated in cryoprecipitate. More recently, highly purified concentrates of Factor VIII and Factor IX have been developed.

Products currently available for the treatment of haemophilia include:

❶ 'Recombinate' (recombinant Factor VIII)
❷ 'BeneFix' (recombinant Factor IX)
❸ 'Biostate' (plasma derived Factor VIII, includes von Willebrand factor)
❹ 'Monofix' (plasma derived Factor IX)
❺ DDAVP (desmopressin).

Treatment of acute bleeding episodes primarily involves administration of factor replacement therapy. Complications of bleeding may require specific intervention. Adjunctive therapies include pain relief, rest and immobilization. Specific treatment is influenced by:

• the type of haemophilia
• the severity of haemophilia
• the severity of the bleed.

Haemophilia patients presenting with suspected bleeds should be triaged as ATS 3 and receive prompt assessment by a senior doctor. For muscle and joint bleeds 'R.I.C.E.S' should be initiated on arrival to limit bleeding and reduce pain.

• R = rest (in position of comfort)
• I = ice (cold pack to reduce bleeding and pain)
• C = gentle compression bandage
• E = elevation
• S = splint (severe/recurrent bleeds).

Options for adequate analgesia include:

• paracetamol and/or codeine
• inhaled nitrous oxide
• tramadol
• I.V. morphine
• may require patient controlled analgesia (PCA)/opioid infusion.

In the context of pain relief, aspirin (or other platelet-modifying drugs) should be avoided and NSAIDs used with caution. Intramuscular injections should never be administered. In major bleeds there may be a requirement for red cell transfusion. Developing limb compartment syndromes may require surgical decompression and intracranial bleeds may require neurosurgical intervention. In all of these cases, factor replacement must commence as quickly as possible. Management of complex presentations requires a multidisciplinary approach, and early consultation with the relevant state haemophilia centre, especially if the presentation is a major bleed or the patient has inhibitors.

Intravenous cannulation is best performed by a skilled practitioner to help ensure vein preservation. Invasive procedures such as arterial puncture and lumbar puncture must only be performed after clotting factor replacement. Intramuscular injections should be avoided.

Some patients with Factor VIII levels higher than 10% may be successfully treated with 1-amino-8-D-arginine vasopressin (desmopressin, DDAVP). It acts by releasing von Willebrand Factor stored in the lining of the blood vessels. Von Willebrand Factor is a protein that transports Factor VIII in the bloodstream and as such plays an important role in blood clotting. Desmopressin appears to mobilize available Factor VIII stores and may raise Factor VIII activity by a factor of three. If the patient has previously had a documented good response to desmopressin, this can be used as first line therapy for minor bleeding such as haemarthroses.

Desmopressin can be administered intravenously, subcutaneously or by nasal spray. The intravenous dose is 0.3 mcg/kg in 100 mL saline over no less than 45 min. A response should be evident within the first hour. More rapid administration can be associated with blood pressure changes. Side effects, including facial flushing and headache, are usually well tolerated. Tachyphylaxis tends to develop after three or four doses. The antidiuretic properties of desmopressin (which can last up to 24 h after a dose) can produce fluid retention and hyponatraemia (leading to seizures), and the serum sodium levels should be measured before giving further doses. Desmopressin is useful in treating mild and very rarely moderate haemophilia A. It is not of value in severe haemophilia A or with any type of haemophilia B. In serious bleeds or major surgery, desmopressin alone will not control bleeding. In such a case, most patients should also receive Factor VIII concentrate, recombinant Factor VIII replacement and recombinant Factor IX replacement.

Most haemophiliac patients are usually well known to their state haemophilia centres, who often hold specialized treatment protocols for difficult or complex patients. Patients should have their treatment regime cards with them. If not they should be encouraged to do so.

One unit of Factor VIII concentrate provides the amount of Factor VIII activity in 1 mL of normal plasma. Given that a 70-kg adult has a plasma volume of 3500 mL, we can expect that an infusion of 3500 units of Factor VIII will produce 100% Factor VIII activity in a haemophiliac with negligible activity prior to treatment.

The half-life of Factor VIII is approximately 12 h. Accordingly, a further dose of 1750 units in 12 hours' time will again restore 100% activity.

It is not always necessary to provide 100% Factor VIII activity in order to ensure haemostasis: levels of 30–50% may be sufficient in the context of haemarthrosis or dental extraction. Larger infusions should be reserved for life-threatening situations.

Treatment of bleeding

Minor bleed (e.g. spontaneous haemarthrosis or muscle bleed):

- recombinate 20 units/kg single dose only
- BeneFIX 40 units/kg single dose only
- DDAVP (0.3 micrograms/kg in patients proven to be responsive).

Moderate bleed (e.g. epistaxsis, traumatic haemarthrosis, excluding hip):

- recombinate 30 units/kg for first dose then 20 units/kg at 12 and 24 h
- BeneFIX 60 units/kg for first dose then 30 units/kg at 24 h
- DDAVP.

Major bleed (e.g. intracerebral, hip, neck, throat, psoas muscle):

- recombinate 45 units/kg stat and urgent haematology consultation
- BeneFIX 90 units/kg stat and urgent haematology consultation.

Many patients can administer Factor VIII concentrate at home 'on demand'. Indeed, the availability of Factor VIII and the ease of administration have revolutionized the care of haemophiliac patients in the community. However, the following are indications for hospital admission:

- suspected intracranial haemorrhage
- a large bleed
- ongoing bleed
- suspected bleeding into the head, neck or throat
- need for ongoing therapy, especially infusions
- suspected compartment syndrome (especially of forearm and calf)
- bleeding into hip or inguinal area, suspected iliopsoas haemorrhage
- undiagnosed abdominal pain
- persistent haematuria

- ongoing analgesia requirements
- inadequate social circumstances.

Antifibrinolytic agents such as tranexamic acid (cyclokapron) and aminocaproic acid (amicar) have been used as adjunctive therapy in episodes of gastrointestinal and mucosal bleeding, for example following dental extraction. Fibrin tissue adhesives containing fibrinogen, thrombin and Factor XIII have also been successfully placed in tooth sockets and similar surgical sites.

Tranexamic acid and aminocaproic acid are useful in treating both haemophilia A and B. These drugs help to hold a clot in place once it has formed. They act by stopping the activity of plasmin, which dissolves blood clots. They do not help to actually form a clot which means they cannot be used instead of desmopressin or Factor VIII or IX concentrate, but can be used to hold a clot in place on mucous membranes, including in the oral cavity, nasal cavity, intestinal and uterine walls. Tranexamc acid and aminocaproic acid are associated with minor side effects including nausea, lethargy, vertigo, diarrhoea and abdominal pain.

Oral/dental bleeds

First line therapy should be topical tranexamic acid mouthwash (5%). Patients hold 10 mL of the solution in the mouth near the site of bleeding (without gargling) for 2 min repeated five times a day for a week.

Haematuria

Factor replacement and anti-fibrinolytic therapy is not usually recommended in these cases due to the risk of clot retention and renal tract obstruction.

Head injury

Haemophiliac patients with even apparently minor head trauma need hospital assessment and CT head scanning. Beware of subtle signs of a developing subdural haematoma. If an intracranial bleed is suspected, replacement therapy should be initiated prior to radiological investigation.

Antibodies to factor VIII

Some patients develop antibodies to Factor VIII, known as 'inhibitors'. Treatment has to be modified according to the titre of inhibitor present (measured by the Bethesda Inhibitor Assay). Patients are classified as 'high responders' if their baseline inhibitor titre exceeds 10 Bethesda Units (BU) or if the titre rises above 10 BU on exposure to Factor VIII. Different management strategies are employed according to the severity of the bleed. These include increasing the dose of Factor VIII or alternative therapies such as activated prothrombin complex, porcine Factor VIII or recombinant Factor VIIa.

Most patients who develop inhibitors do so early in life and are known to have severe hereditary haemophilia, but inhibitors can also arise in previously normal individuals to produce an acquired haemophilia. The incidence of this phenomenon is from 0.2 to 1/1 000 000/year. Patients tend to be elderly and some have autoimmune disease, but there is also an association with pregnancy as well as with some drugs, notably penicillin. Patients haemorrhage into muscle and soft tissues, and may present with haematemesis, or with unusual postoperative bleeding. In the laboratory the patient's blood shows a prolonged APPT that is not corrected by 'mixing', that is, by the addition of normal plasma. Factor VIII levels are low. Management is directed towards control of the bleeding episode, replacement therapy and the prevention of further reactions using a variety of immunosuppressive remedies.

Disposition

- Patients with 'minor' bleeds and no other complicating issues may be discharged after treatment in the emergency department but management should ideally be discussed first with the treating haemophilia unit and early review arranged.
- Patients with 'moderate' bleeds may need admission, preferably at the state treatment centre. These cases must be discussed with the treating unit before discharge from the emergency department.
- All patients with 'major' bleeds **must** be admitted and management discussed on an urgent basis with the treating haemophilia unit, prior to transferring care.

von Willebrand disease

Factor VIII has an intimate association with von Willebrand factor (vWF). This is an adhesive glycoprotein secreted by endothelium and megakaryocytes, which is required for the normal instigation of platelet plug formation and for stabilization and transport of Factor VIII within the circulation. Thus von Willebrand disease (vWD) is a result of dysfunction, reduction, or a complete lack of the vWF and is often associated with low Factor VIII activity. It is the most common inherited bleeding disorder, affecting 0.1–1% of the population, and affects males and females equally.

Three types of von Willebrand disease are recognized:

- type I (common): reduced levels of vWF – clinically associated with mild bleeding
- type II (uncommon): abnormally functioning vWF – clinically associated with a variable bleeding pattern
- type III (rare): a near absence of vWF – clinical presentation is similar to that of moderate-to-severe haemophilia

Common symptoms of vWD are:

- frequent nose bleeds
- easy bruising
- bleeding from gums following tooth extractions
- menorrhagia
- gastrointestinal bleeding.

Treatment

If the patient has previously had a documented good response to DDAVP, this can be used as first line in Type I vWD. It is occasionally also effective in Type II vWD, but never effective in Type III vWD. The dose is the same as used in haemophilia (0.3 μg/kg). Antifibrinolytic agents such as tranexamic acid are often helpful for mucosal bleeding, epistaxis and menorrhagia. 'Biostate' (plasma derived Factor VIII, includes von Willebrand factor) may be required in Type I vWD if bleeding is severe or unresponsive to DDAVP and it can also be used to treat bleeding in patients with Type II and Type III vWD.

Useful contacts

Websites

Australian Haemophilia Centre Directors' Organisation: www.ahcdo.org.au
Haemophilia Foundation Australia: www.haemophilia.org.au
Canadian Hemophilia Society: www.hemophilia.ca
Hemophilia Federation of America: www.hemophiliafed.org
Haemophilia Foundation Australia: www.haemophilia.org.au
Haemophilia Foundation of New Zealand: www.haemophilia.org.nz
Haemophilia Society (UK): www.haemophilia.org.uk
World Federation of Hemophilia: www.wfh.org

Contact numbers for advice/referrals

ACT

Canberra
The Canberra Hospital
Haemophilia Centre
Ward 14A Yamba Drive Garran ACT 2605
Telephone 02 6244 2188 / 2286
Emergency 02 6244 2222
Fax 02 6244 2271

NSW

Newcastle
Mater Misericordiae Hospital
Haemophilia Centre
Edith Street Waratah NSW 2298
Telephone 02 4921 1240
Emergency 02 4921 1211
Fax 02 4960 2136

Sydney
Royal Prince Alfred Hospital
Haemophilia Centre
Page Building, Level 9 Missenden Road Camperdown NSW 2050
Telephone 02 9515 7013
Emergency 02 9515 6111
Fax 02 9515 8946

The Children's Hospital
Cnr Hawkesbury Rd & Hainsworth St Westmead NSW 2145
Telephone 02 9845 0000 and page haematologist on call
Emergency 02 9845 0000 and page haematologist on call
Fax 02 9845 3082

NT

Darwin
Royal Darwin Hospital
Rocklands Drive, Tiwi NT 0812
Telephone 08 8920 6176
Emergency 08 8922 8888
Fax 08 8920 6183

QLD

Brisbane
Royal Brisbane & Women's Hospital
Queensland Haemophilia Centre
Level 4, West Block, Butterfield Street, Herston QLD 4029
Telephone 07 3636 5727 / 8760
Emergency 07 3636 8111
Fax 07 3636 4221

Royal Children's Hospital
Haemophilia Centre
Banksia Ward, Level 3 Woolworths Building, Herston Road, Herston QLD 4029
Telephone 07 3636 9030
Emergency 07 3636 7472
Fax 07 3636 1552

SA

Adelaide
Royal Adelaide Hospital
Haematology Day Centre
Level 7 East Wing, North Terrace, Adelaide 5000
Telephone 08 8222 4308 / 5632
Emergency 08 8222 4000
Fax 08 8222 4358

Women's and Children's Hospital
McGuiness-McDermott Foundation Children's Clinic
72 King William Roadd, North Adelaide SA 5006
Telephone 08 8161 7411
Emergency 08 8161 7000
Fax 08 8161 6567

TAS

Hobart
Royal Hobart Hospital
Paediatric Ambulatory Care Unit
Liverpool Street, Hobart TAS 7000
Telephone 03 6222 8045
Emergency 03 6222 8308
Fax 03 6222 8900

VIC

Melbourne
The Alfred
Ronald Sawers Haemophilia Centre
Commercial Road, Melbourne Vic 3004
Telephone 03 9076 2178
Emergency 03 9076 2000
Fax 03 9076 3021

Royal Children's Hospital
The Henry Ekert Haemophilia Treatment
   Centre
Flemington Road Parkville Vic 3052
Telephone 03 9345 5099
Emergency 03 9345 5522
Fax 03 9345 5099

WA

Perth

Royal Perth Hospital
Haemophilia Centre
Kirkman House, 10 Murray Street, Perth
   WA 6000
Telephone 08 9224 2937 / 2897

Emergency 08 9224 2244
Fax 08 9224 8475
Princess Margaret Hospital for Children
Oncology & Haematology Ward 3B
Roberts Road, Subiaco WA 6008
Telephone 08 9340 8682 / 8234
Emergency 08 9340 8222
Fax 08 9341 9842

Fremantle

Fremantle Hospital
Alma Street, Fremantle WA 6160
Telephone 08 9431 2210 / 2886
Emergency 08 9431 3333
Fax 08 9431 2881

Further reading

Bell BA, Birch K, Glazer S. Experience with recombinant factor VIIA in an infant with haemophilia with inhibitors to FVIII:C undergoing emergency central line placement. A case report. American Journal of Pediatrics, Hematology and Oncology 1993; 15(1): 77–79.

Bush MT, Roy N. Hemophilia emergencies. Journal of Emergency Nursing 1995; 21(6): 531–538.

De Behnke DJ, Angelos MG. Intracranial hemorrhage and hemophilia: case report and management guidelines. Journal of Emergency Medicine 1990; 8(4): 423–427.

Pfaff JA. Geninatti M. Hemophilia. Emergency Medicine Clinics of North America 1993; 11(2): 337–363.

Warrier I, Ewenstein BM, Koerper MA, et al. Factor IX inhibitors and anaphylaxis in hemophilia B. Journal of Pediatrics, Hematology and Oncology 1997; 19(1): 23–27.

13.5 Blood and blood products

Sean Arendse

ESSENTIALS

1 The decision to transfuse packed red cells should ultimately be based on the knowledge that the patient's own oxygen carrying capacity has dropped to an unacceptably low level.

2 The administration of blood products is not without risk. The emergency physician should always ensure that potential benefits outweigh potential risks, and communicate these risks and benefits in order to obtain informed consent where possible.

3 Meticulous documentation and vigilant monitoring minimize the risk of serious adverse reaction from administration of blood products.

Introduction

Blood is a living tissue composed of blood cells suspended in plasma; it transports nutrients and oxygen, and facilitates temperature control. An average 70-kg male has a blood volume of about 5 L. The cellular elements comprise red blood cells, white blood cells and platelets, and make up about 45% of the volume of whole blood. Plasma, which is 92% water, makes up the remaining 55%.

Early attempts at blood transfusion were thwarted by adverse reactions. In 1900 Karl Landsteiner demonstrated the ABO blood group system and explained many of the observed severe incompatibility reactions (Table 13.5.1). He won the Nobel prize for

medicine in 1930 and went on to discover the Rhesus factor in 1940. The next major advance in transfusion medicine occurred with the development of long-term anticoagulants such as sodium citrate, which allowed extended preservation of blood. Development of refrigeration procedures allowed

Table 13.5.1	The ABO group system	
ABO blood group	Antigens on red cells	Antibody in serum
O	None	Anti-A, Anti-B
A	A	Anti-B
B	B	Anti-A
AB	A, B	None

storage of anticoagulated blood. The addition of a citrate-glucose solution extended the viability of collected blood to several days. The ability to preserve blood for longer than a few hours paved the way for the establishment of the first blood bank in a Leningrad hospital in 1932.

Transfusion of blood and blood products is now routine and vital to the practice of emergency medicine. As with any prescribed treatment, these products are associated with potential hazards as well as advantages. The hazards are more likely to be encountered with blood products used during emergencies. The blood products available in most Australian emergency departments (EDs) are packed red blood cells, platelets, fresh frozen plasma (FFP), cryoprecipitate, activated Factor VII, prothrombin complex concentrates and other factor concentrates.

In the Australian urban hospital setting, 50% of packed red cells are used for the treatment of anaemia, 22% pre- or perioperatively and 13% for abnormal, excessive or continued bleeding.[1] Medical oncology uses 78% of all platelets.[2] Forty-one per cent of all FFP is used to correct coagulopathy associated with surgery, 27% to correct coagulopathy in bleeding, 16% to reverse haemostatic disorders in patients having massive blood transfusion, 11.5% for reversal of warfarin effect and the remaining 4.5% for a number of miscellaneous conditions, including liver disease and disseminated intravascular coagulation (DIC).

In the ED setting, blood products are most often administered to patients with acute rather than chronic blood loss. In most EDs, trauma patients are the major consumers of blood products and in this setting they need to be provided rapidly and infused often in large quantities. However, as short stay units are developed, non-time critical transfusions of blood products for other medical indications are increasingly the responsibility of ED staff.

Packed red blood cells

Packed red blood cells are produced from whole blood collections by removing most of the plasma by centrifugation and then resuspending the red cells in citrate-based anticoagulant-preservative solution to prolong storage time. Each unit of packed cells contains approximately 200 mL of red cells. Transfusion of one unit can be expected to raise the haematocrit by 3% and the haemoglobin by 10 g/L provided there is no ongoing blood loss.

Packed red cells are the blood product most commonly prescribed in the ED, the usual indication being the replacement of acute blood loss.[3] Transfusion of packed red cells is indicated where the patient's oxygen-carrying capacity is so impaired that control of bleeding alone, if indeed it can be readily achieved, is regarded as insufficient to take the patient out of danger. Occasionally it may be necessary

to transfuse a patient with a primary haematological condition, a failure of erythropoiesis or a haemolytic process. The indication for transfusion is the same as for haemorrhage: a severe reduction in oxygen-carrying capacity. Complex multisystem failure, such as DIC or septic shock, may result in simultaneous blood loss, circulatory collapse, haemolysis and a coagulopathy. Transfusion therapy may be life saving in this context (Table 13.5.2).

Fluid administration is the cornerstone of management during initial trauma reception and resuscitation, as hypovolaemia is one of the leading causes of death in trauma. Fluid resuscitation must be rapid and appropriate, and should be reassessed and adjusted at regular intervals. This has led to a significant decrease in morbidity and mortality from major trauma.[4]

The American College of Surgeons estimates fluid and blood loss by using six physiological parameters to grade patients into classes I–IV (Table 13.5.3). This allows more accurate characterization of a patient's immediate haemodynamic status than do laboratory parameters such as haemoglobin and haematocrit. It is recommended that patients in groups III and IV receive blood.

Transfusion is not indicated when alternative haematinic therapy is deemed safe and appropriate. A moderately anaemic patient who is asymptomatic and not bleeding, with some reserve oxygen-carrying capacity, does not require blood transfusion. A haemoglobin of 7 g/dL is sometimes taken as the failsafe point in the decision whether to transfuse, although of course the patient's unique circumstances need to be taken into account: treat the patient, not the number. The National Health and Medical Research Council together with the Australasian Society of Blood Transfusion have published transfusion guidelines for red blood cells and other products (Table 13.5.4).

Prior to transfusion, except in an extreme emergency, the patient's informed consent should be sought, obtained and documented. Rarely, patients may be encountered who refuse transfusion, either on religious grounds or for fear of adverse reactions, particularly with respect to the transfer of viral agents. This can pose problems if the patient appears incompetent to give or withhold informed consent. The situation of an exsanguinating minor whose parents refuse permission to transfuse is

Table 13.5.2 Potential indications for red cell transfusion

Haemorrhage
Dilutional anaemia following severe burns
Iron-deficiency anaemia
Megaloblastic anaemia
Anaemia of chronic disorders
Chronic renal failure
Failure of erythropoiesis
Sickle cell disease
Septic shock
Disseminated intravascular coagulopathy

Table 13.5.3 Estimated fluid and blood losses (for a 70-kg man)

	Blood loss (mL)	Blood loss (% blood volume)	Pulse rate (beats/min)	Blood pressure	Pulse pressure (mmHg)	Respiratory rate (breaths/min)	Urine output (mL/h)	CNS/mental status	Fluid replacement (3:1 rule)
Class I	Up to 750	Up to 15	<100	Normal	Normal or increased	14–20	>30	Slightly anxious	Crystalloid
Class II	750–1500	15–30	>100	Normal	Decreased	20–30	20–30	Mildly anxious	Crystalloid
Class III	1500–2000	30–40	>120	Decreased	Decreased	30–40	5–15	Anxious, Confused	Crystalloid and blood
Class IV	>2000	>40	>140	Decreased	Decreased	>35	Negligible	Confused, Lethargic	Crystalloid and blood

CNS, central nervous system.
Adapted from Advanced Trauma Life Support Students Course Manual (7th edn). American College of Surgeons 2007.

Table 13.5.4 Guidelines for transfusion of blood components

Indications	Considerations
Red blood cells	
Hb	
<70 g/L	Lower thresholds may be acceptable in patients without symptoms and/or where specific therapy is available
70–100 g/L	Likely to be appropriate during surgery associated with major blood loss or if there are signs or symptoms of impaired oxygen transport
>80 g/L	May be appropriate to control anaemia-related symptoms in a patient on a chronic transfusion regimen or during marrow suppressive therapy
>100 g/L	Not likely to be appropriate unless there are specific indications
Platelets	
Bone marrow failure	At a platelet count of $<10 \times 10^9$/L in the absence of risk factors and $<20 \times 10^9$ in the presence of risk factors (e.g. fever, antibiotics, evidence of systemic haemostatic failure)
Surgery/invasive procedure	To maintain platelet count at $>50 \times 10^9$/L. For surgical procedures with high risk of bleeding (e.g. ocular or neurosurgery) it may be appropriate to maintain at 100×10^9/L
Platelet function disorders	May be appropriate in inherited or acquired disorders, depending on clinical features and setting. In this situation, platelet count is not a reliable indicator
Bleeding	May be appropriate in any patient in whom thrombocytopenia is considered a major contributory factor
Massive haemorrhage/transfusion	Use should be confined to patients with thrombocytopenia and/or functional abnormalities who have significant bleeding from this cause. May be appropriate when the platelet count is $<50 \times 10^9$/L ($<100 \times 10^9$/L in the presence of diffuse microvascular bleeding)
Fresh frozen plasma	
Single factor deficiencies	Use specific factors if available
Warfarin effect	In the presence of life-threatening bleeding. Use in addition to vitamin-K-dependent concentrates
Acute DIC	Indicated where there is bleeding and abnormal coagulation. Not indicated for chronic DIC
TTP	Accepted treatment
Coagulation inhibitor deficiencies	May be appropriate in patients undergoing high-risk procedures. Use specific factors if available
Following massive transfusion or cardiac bypass	May be appropriate in the presence of bleeding and abnormal coagulation
Liver disease	May be appropriate in the presence of bleeding and abnormal coagulation
Cryoprecipitate	
Fibrinogen deficiency	May be appropriate where there is clinical bleeding, an invasive procedure, trauma or DIC

TTP, idiopathic thrombocytopenia purpura ;DIC, disseminated intravascular coagulation.
Adapted from the National Health and Medical Research Council and Australasian Society Clinical Practice Guidelines on appropriate use of blood components http://www.nhmrc.gov.au/publications/synopses/-files/cp82.pdf.

particularly difficult. Court orders can be obtained to treat minors without parental consent, and in such an extreme situation many doctors would feel justified in applying to obtain one, even retrospectively.

Effect of storage on red blood cells

Although it makes intuitive sense that blood loss should be replaced by blood products, there is evidence that the immediate observed benefit is from volume replacement rather than improved oxygen carriage.[5,6] Red blood cells may not be fully functional until 2–6 h after transfusion because storage affects the oxygen-carrying capacity of blood. This is probably due to decreased intracellular 2,3-diphosphoglycerate (2,3-DPG), loss of red cell viability, decreased red cell deformability, relative acidosis and potassium leakage.[7]

Storage reduces 2,3-DPG levels, leading to a leftward shift of the oxyhaemoglobin dissociation curve and increased affinity of oxygen binding. The transfused red cell does regenerate 2,3-DPG to normal levels but this can take 6–24 h post transfusion. With increasing age of stored red cells, levels of 2,3-DPG progressively fall such that by 5–6 weeks the level is 10% of normal. It is still uncertain whether this abnormality is physiologically important, even in critically ill patients.[8]

When red cells are transfused, some of the cells are removed from the circulation within a few hours, with the rest surviving normally; as the storage time increases to 42 days, more cells are removed immediately after transfusion. This loss of viability is highly dependent upon the anticoagulant-preservative solution used.[9]

Potassium gradually leaks out of stored red cells and this raises the plasma potassium by approximately 1 meq/L per day.[10]

Choice of red cell product

The choice of red cell product is determined by time and safety considerations. O-negative red cells, the universal donor group, are readily available in most major hospitals. Supplies of O-negative blood are limited and the product should be used with care. It is preferable that blood be collected prior to infusion of such cells so as to characterize the recipient's blood group serology. Premenopausal female patients should be given group O Rhesus negative, Kell negative blood in an emergency situation in order to avoid sensitization and possibility of haemolytic disease of newborn in subsequent pregnancies. Male patients, however, can be transfused either Rhesus positive or negative blood. The incidence of adverse reaction using this type of blood is approximately 3%. O-negative may be given immediately on arrival where the patient has not responded to adequate crystalloid given during transport, or the patients are in class III or IV shock.[11] By contrast, the provision of group-specific blood requires matching a blood sample to the major (ABO) and Rhesus D compatibility groups only. Group-specific blood can be available for transfusion within 35 min depending on the logistic support and staffing levels within the haematology laboratory. It has an incidence of adverse reaction similar to O-negative blood. As O-negative blood is usually in short supply it is preferable where possible to infuse group-specific blood. A more comprehensive cross match where there are no atypical antibodies identified in the initial screening can take 30 min or more and the incidence of adverse transfusion reaction is reduced to 0.01%. Due to the time required for sample collection and cross matching, it is generally not possible to provide fully cross-matched blood within the first 30 min of trauma reception.

Precautions when cross-matching and transfusing blood

Although most patients do not require transfusion in the ED, it is often appropriate to 'group and hold' or cross-match the patient while in the department. Many hospitals have written protocols detailing the anticipated requirements for a given surgical procedure. Documentation should be meticulous. It is preferable that the person drawing the blood for cross-matching should also fill in and sign the laboratory request form. Most severe incompatibility reactions to blood transfusion result not from exposure to unusual antigens but from an administrative error. Any systematic change in documentation protocols, for example the adoption of an electronic record, needs to be accompanied by an obsessive risk management strategy.

The checking of the compatibility details of blood to be transfused must be meticulous. Blood products should not be left lying around workbenches. Universal precautions must be observed by staff setting up transfusions. Rapid or large transfusions should be via a blood warmer. Blood is transfused intravenously through sterile giving sets containing 170 µm filters. Alternative routes (arterial, intraperitoneal or intraosseous) are only used in exceptional circumstances. Lines for transfusion should be dedicated lines; drugs and other additives should be administered at separate sites. Normal saline is compatible with all blood components.

Pulse, blood pressure and temperature are measured at regular intervals, and particular attention is paid to the patient during the first 25 min of the transfusion. The transfusion is started slowly. The rate at which it continues depends upon the clinical urgency. The usual regime is 500 mL over 1–2 h. As a general rule, the faster the anaemia has developed the more rapidly it needs to be corrected. Rapid infusion techniques may be indicated in patients who appear to be exsanguinating, but over-rapid infusion can precipitate cardiac failure in the elderly. Hypothermia may be a problem if a blood warmer is not used.

Adverse reactions to transfusion

The principal adverse reactions to blood transfusion are listed in Table 13.5.5. Serious adverse reactions are relatively rare (Table 13.5.6) although some are more likely to occur when blood is administered urgently.

Immunological transfusion reactions

Immunological transfusion reactions may be immediate or delayed in onset.

Immediate

Febrile non-haemolytic reactions   The most common transfusion reaction is a febrile, non-haemolytic transfusion reaction (FNHTR), which is defined as an increase in temperature of 1°C or more over baseline during a transfusion. It manifests as fever and occasionally shortness of breath 1–6 h after transfusion. FNHTRs are benign, but their presentation is very similar to acute haemolytic transfusion reaction and infection, which have a higher rate of mortality and morbidity, mandating early clinical review to exclude more serious complications.

Acute haemolytic reactions   Acute haemolytic transfusion reactions (ATHRs) result from the rapid destruction of donor red cells by preformed recipient antibodies and are a medical emergency. They are usually due to ABO incompatibility and most often the result of clerical or procedural error.[12] Some acquired allo-antibodies, such as anti-Rh or anti-Jka, are

Table 13.5.5 Adverse effects of blood transfusion	
Immunological transfusion reactions	*Transmission of infection*
Immediate	**Bacterial**
Febrile non-haemolytic reactions	Brucella
Acute haemolytic transfusion reactions	Pseudomonas
Allergic reactions and anaphylaxis	Salmonella
Transfusion-related acute lung injury	Treponema pallidum
Delayed	**Parasites**
Delayed haemolytic transfusion reactions	Babesia
Alloimmunization	Plasmodium
Transfusion-associated graft versus host disease	Toxoplasma
Hypothermia	Trypanosoma
Dilutional coagulopathy	**Viruses**
Volume overload	Cytomegalovirus
	Hepatitis B and delta agent
	Hepatitis A
	Hepatitis C
	Other hepatitis 'non-A, non-B'
	HIV-1 and HIV-2
	HTLV-1 and HTLV-2
	Parvovirus

HIV, human immunodeficiency virus; HTLV, human T-cell lymphotropic virus.

Table 13.5.6 Incidence of adverse transfusion reactions (per unit packed red cells transfused)		
Adverse transfusion reaction	*Incidence*	*Mortality*
Bacterial sepsis	1 in 40 000–500 000	1 in 4–8 million
Acute haemolytic reaction	1 in 12 000–38 000	1 in 600 000–1.5 million
Delayed haemolytic reaction	1 in 1000–12 000	1 in 2.5 million
Anaphylaxis	1 in 20 000–50 000	
Transfusion-related acute lung injury	1 in 5000–100 000	1 in 5 million
Fluid overload	1 in 100–700	
Transfusion-associated graft versus host disease	Rare	90% fatality

Adapted from Australian Red Cross website: http://www.transfusion.com.au/TRANSFUSIONPOCKETGUIDES/Pocket_RiskConsent.asp (accessed 25th February 2008).

occasionally implicated, but AHTRs more typically occur when a group O recipient is transfused with non-group O red cells. This may lead to DIC, shock and acute tubular necrosis precipitating acute renal failure. These reactions usually manifest with fever and rigors, lumbar pain, crushing chest pain, tachycardia, hypotension and haemoglobinaemia with subsequent haemoglobinuria. The symptoms usually develop within the first 30 min of transfusion.

Anaphylactoid transfusion reactions

Anaphylactoid reactions usually begin within 1–45 min of the start of transfusion of blood products but less severe reactions can be delayed up to 2–3 h. Generally, the shorter the time between commencement of the transfusion and onset of symptoms, the more severe the reaction. These reactions are manifested by rapid onset of shock, hypotension, angio-oedema and respiratory distress. They are almost always due to the presence of class-specific IgG, anti-IgA antibodies in patients who are IgA deficient. Selective IgA deficiency is not uncommon, occurring in about 1 in 300–500 people. The incidence of anaphylactic transfusion reactions can be reduced by the use of washed products (e.g. washed red cells) and by pre-medicating the patient with antipyretics and antihistamines.

Treatment of an anaphylactoid transfusion reaction consists of immediate cessation of transfusion and standard treatment of anaphylaxis including, oxygen fluids and adrenaline (see Ch. 28.7).

Transfusion-related acute lung injury

This complication is characterized by onset of acute respiratory distress, hypoxaemia, hypotension, tachycardia, fever and pulmonary oedema, initially without signs of left ventricular failure. The central venous pressure is normal, which helps distinguish the condition from transfusion-associated circulatory overload. Treatment is supportive. High-dose steroid therapy has been used but appears to be ineffective.[13] The blood bank needs to be notified and the donor identified.

Delayed

Delayed haemolytic transfusion reaction These reactions occur in patients who have developed antibodies from previous transfusions or pregnancy but, at the time of pre-transfusion testing, the antibody in question is too weak to be detected by standard procedures. Subsequent transfusion with red cells having the corresponding antigen results in an anamnestic antibody response and haemolysis of transfused red cells. These delayed reactions are seen generally within 2–10 days after transfusion. Haemolysis is usually extravascular, gradual and less severe than with acute reactions, but rapid haemolysis can occur. A falling haematocrit, slight fever, mild increase in serum unconjugated bilirubin and spherocytosis on the blood smear may be noted.

No treatment is required in the absence of brisk haemolysis. However, future transfusions containing the implicated red cell antigen need to be avoided.

Alloimmunization Transfused (non-leukocyte depleted) red cells and platelets contain leukocytes to which antibodies can be made. This may cause patients to become resistant to subsequent platelet transfusions. Approximately 50% of patients undergoing multiple blood transfusions become alloimmunized and are refractory to further platelet transfusions. Refractory patients require platelets matched to their specific platelet/human leukocyte antigen (HLA) type. Patients receiving leukocyte reduced blood products are at a much lower risk for refractoriness to platelet transfusion than are recipients of non-leukocyte reduced blood products.

Transfusion-associated graft versus host disease Transfusion-associated graft versus host disease results from transfusion of viable T lymphocytes which proliferate and damage the recipient's tissue, particularly skin, gastrointestinal tract, liver, spleen and bone marrow. This is a rare and almost always fatal complication of transfusion. Clinical manifestations typically develop 10–14 days following transfusion and consist of fever, erythematous skin rash, pancytopenia, diarrhoea and abnormal liver function. High-risk patients for this complication include bone marrow transplant recipients, patients receiving granulocyte transfusions, transfusions from a biologically related donor (directed donation), the fetus (intrauterine transfusion), exchange transfusion, patients with Hodgkin lymphoma, and patients with congenital cellular immune deficiency. Irradiation of products in this situation will reduce the risk and is recommended for the above patient groups.

Transmission of infection

In Australia, blood is tested for ABO and Rh (D) blood groups, red cell antibodies, and the following infections:

- human immunodeficiency virus 1 and 2
- hepatitis B and C
- human T-cell lymphotropic virus I and II
- syphilis.

In terms of viral safety Australia has one of the safest blood supplies in the world (Table 13.5.7).

Hypothermia

Red blood cells are stored at 4°C. Rapid infusion of large volumes of stored blood can contribute to hypothermia. Blood warmers should be used during massive blood transfusion. In addition, other intravenous fluids should be warmed and other measures instituted to maintain patient body temperature (see Ch. 28.2).

Table 13.5.7 Risks of transfusion transmitted infection (per unit tested blood transfused)

Infection	Residual risk
CMV	1 in 127 000
Hepatitis B	Approximately 1 in 660 000
Syphilis	Considerably less than 1 in a million
Hepatitis C	<1 in 10 million
HIV	<1 in 10 million
HTLV I and II	<1 in 10 million
Variant CJD	Possible and cannot be excluded

CMV, cytomegalovirus; HIV, human immunodeficiency virus; HTLV, human T-cell lymphotropic virus; CJD, Creutzfeldt–Jakob disease.
Adapted from Australian Red Cross website: http://www.transfusion.com.au/ TRANSFUSIONPOCKETGUIDES/ Pocket_RiskConsent.asp (accessed 25th February 2008).

Dilutional coagulopathies

Clinically significant depletion of coagulation proteins and platelets is a complication of massive transfusion, secondary to dilution and the consumptive coagulopathy of trauma. Stored red cells are deficient in platelets and clotting factors, and transfusion of large amounts can complicate bleeding when not accompanied by assessment and correction of coagulation disturbances. Coagulation parameters including the prothrobin time (PT), activated partial thromboplastin time (APTT), platelet count and fibrinogen level should be monitored and corrected if deficiencies occur in the presence of abnormal bleeding.

Volume overload

This complication occurs when excessive volume of fluid is administered. Pulmonary oedema is a particular risk in the elderly, in infants and in patients with chronic severe anaemia where the red cell mass is decreased but the blood volume is normal.

Management of transfusion reactions

The first action to be taken in the management of any suspected transfusion reaction is to stop the transfusion immediately and assess the patient. The bag containing the transfused cells, along with all attached labels, should not be discarded so as to allow repeat typing and cross-matching of this unit by the blood bank. Management then proceeds as follows:

- Maintain the patient's airway, blood pressure and heart rate.
- From the other arm, obtain a sample for a direct antiglobulin test, plasma-free haemoglobin, and repeat blood group and cross-match. Save a urine sample for haemoglobin testing.
- Culture the patient's blood.
- Commence broad-spectrum antibiotics to cover Gram-positive skin organisms and Gram-negative organisms.

The laboratory which tested and issued the blood should be alerted immediately, and a search for any clerical error instituted. Every hospital has a protocol for evaluating transfusion reactions, which should be rigorously followed. The haematology unit should notify the local blood bank, who have a haematologist on-call at all times and are responsible for the recall of any other implicated components from the same donor in the case of suspected infection or transfusion-related acute lung injury. If there is any suggestion (e.g. clerical mistake, hypotension, pink plasma or urine) that an AHTR is possible, oxygen should be applied to the patient and fluid resuscitation with saline to maintain a urine output of 2–3 mL/kg/h, in an attempt to prevent acute oliguric renal failure. A vasopressor such as adrenaline may be required. If massive intravascular haemolysis has already occurred, hyperkalemia is likely and cardiac monitoring and acute haemodialysis may be required.

Platelets

Platelets are one of the main cellular components of blood and are central to haemostasis. Platelet products commonly available for transfusion are obtained by apheresis from a single donor or from donated blood using buff-coat or platelet-rich plasma techniques. Modifications to reduce the risk of viral transmission and prevent graft-versus-host disease include leukocyte reduction, irradiation, plasma depletion and the use of platelet additive solutions.

Platelets are transfused to prevent or treat haemorrhage in patients with thrombocytopenia or defects in platelet function. Specific indications for platelet transfusion are shown in Table 13.5.4. Use of platelets is not generally considered appropriate in the treatment of immune-mediated platelet destruction, thrombotic thrombocytopenic purpura, haemolytic uraemic syndrome or drug-induced or cardiac bypass thrombocytopenia without haemorrhage.[3]

In general, one platelet unit will raise the platelet count about $5–10 \times 10^9$/L in an average adult. Depending on the method of manufacture the volume of each unit of platelets varies from 100–160 mL, with a storage life of about 5 days at 20–24°C.

Compatibility testing is not necessary in routine platelet transfusion, although platelet components should preferably be ABO and Rh type compatible with the recipient. ABO-incompatible platelets may be used if ABO compatible platelets are not available. The usual dose in an adult patient is four units, which is equivalent to one unit of apheresis platelets or one unit of pooled platelets.

Fresh frozen plasma

FFP is prepared from anti-coagulated blood by separating the plasma from the blood cells through centrifugation of whole blood or apheresis. It is stored frozen until used. It contains all coagulation factors including small amounts of Factor V and approximately 200 units of Factor VIII. Fresh frozen plasma can be stored at below −25°C for up to 12 months. Indications for use of FFP are shown in Table 13.5.2.

The appropriate dose depends on the clinical indication, patient size and results of laboratory tests. A general guide is 10–15 mL/kg per dose, but in some situations dosages greater than this may be required (e.g. dilutional coagulopathy in the context of massive transfusion). On average 1 mL of FFP/kg patient weight will raise most coagulation factors by 1%, therefore a dose of 10–15 mL/kg would be expected to increase levels by 10–15%.[3] Compatibility testing is not required; however, ABO compatible plasma should be used wherever possible. Group AB plasma can be used for all patients in an emergency.

Cryoprecipitate

Cryoprecipitate is prepared by thawing FFP to between 1 and 6°C and recovering the precipitable protein fraction. It contains most of the Factor VIII, fibrinogen, Factor XIII, von Willebrand factor and fibronectin from the FFP. It may be stored for up to 12 months at 25°C or below. Once thawed it must be used immediately or stored at 2–6°C for up to 24 h. Cryoprecipitate is indicated in fibrinogen deficiency with clinical bleeding or prior to an invasive procedure, and in DIC.[3] Cryoprecipitate is transfused to keep fibrinogen levels above 1.0 g/L in the acutely bleeding patient. Compatibility tests before transfusion are not necessary. It is preferable to use an ABO group compatible with the recipient's red cells; however, ABO incompatible can be used with caution. Up to 4 units/10 kg body weight may be required to raise the fibrinogen concentration by approximately 0.5 g/L in the absence of continued haemorrhage.

The use of cryoprecipitate is not generally considered appropriate in the treatment of haemophilia, von Willebrand's disease or deficiencies of Factor XIII or fibronectin, unless alternative therapies are unavailable.[3]

Massive transfusion

In the 1970s, massive transfusion was defined as more than 10 units of blood over a 24-h period. This is equivalent to approximately one patient blood volume in a person of average weight person.[14] Recent reviews in the literature have expanded this definition, with some reports using up to 50 units of blood in 24 or 48 h.[15]

There is wide institutional variation in massive or emergency transfusion protocols. Many recommend a ratio of red cells to clotting factors. One institution advocates for every 10 units of red blood cells one should consider transfusing 6 units of FFP, 5 units of platelets and 5 units of cryoprecipitate, and if the fibrinogen level is less than 1.0 g/L, then 10 units of cryoprecipitate. If laboratory parameters are available then one should consider treatment when platelets $<100 \times 10^9$/L, international normalized ratio (INR) >1.5, fibrinogen <1.0 g/L or when there is ongoing and uncontrollable ooze from damaged tissue. This should always be in close consultation with the transfusionist/haematologist as each individual shocked trauma patient should be assessed and transfusion decisions made on physiological and haematological parameters, as well as availability and access to appropriate transfusion products available at the time. As products such as FFP and cryoprecipitate require up to 25 min preparation time, and if one is anticipating a major transfusion situation (i.e. greater than 10 units of red cells)

then the laboratory should be notified of the potential need for cryoprecipitate and FFP, and the provision of pre-thawed AB plasma, O-negative cells.

Controversies

❶ While the changes observed during red cell storage affect overall red cell viability and function, there are no randomized controlled studies examining the effect of storage duration on recipient morbidity and mortality.[16]

❷ Significant coagulopathy is seen in up to 50% of cases of major trauma (ISS > 15), in particular where there is major head injury, hypothermia (temperature <34°), acidosis or massive transfusion.[17] There is no current reliable evidence defining the best practice for use of platelets, cryoprecipitate or FFP in the shocked trauma patient.

❸ Recently, there has been much interest in recombinant activated Factor VII (rFVIIa). Developed primarily for use in patients with haemophilia especially with inhibitors, this compound is a potent activator of the extrinsic clotting system when bound to exposed tissue factor. There has been increasing experience in the use of rFVIIa in normal patients with acquired coagulopathy after surgery or trauma and rFVIIa holds promise for further use. Randomized controlled clinical trials are required to assess the efficacy and safety of rFVIIa for haemorrhaging patients without a pre-existing coagulation disorder.[18–20]

❹ The potential for prions, thought to be the infective molecules in the variant form of Creutzfeldt–Jakob disease, to be transmitted by blood transfusion has become a subject for intense scrutiny for transfusion medicine.

References

1. Rubin GL, Schofield WN, Dean MG, et al. Appropriateness of red blood cell transfusions in major urban hospitals and effectiveness of an intervention. Medical Journal of Australia 2001; 175: 354–358.
2. Metz J, McGrath KM, Copperchini ML, et al. Appropriateness of transfusions of red cells, platelets and fresh frozen plasma. An audit in a tertiary care teaching hospital. Medical Journal of Australia 1995; 162: 572–577.
3. Practice Guidelines on the Use of Blood Components. National Health and Medical Research Council and Australasian Society of Blood Transfusion Clinical, 2001 http://www.nhmrc.gov.au/publications/synopses/_files/cp78.pdf (accessed 4 August 2008).
4. Champion H, Bellamy RF, Roberts CP, et al. A profile of combat injury. Journal of Trauma 2003; 54(suppl): s31–s19.
5. Dabrowski GP, Steinberg SM, Ferrara JJ, et al. A critical assessment of endpoints of shock resuscitation. Surgical Clinics of North America 2000; 80: 825–844.
6. Revell M, Greaves I, Porter K. Endpoints for fluid resuscitation in hemorrhagic shock. Journal of Trauma 2003; 54(suppl): s63–s67.
7. McKinley BA, Valdivia A, Moore FA. Goal orientated shock resuscitation for major torso trauma. Current Opinions in Critical Care 2003; 9: 292–299.
8. Walsh TS, McArdle F, McLellan SA, et al. Does the storage time of transfused red blood cells influence regional or global indexes of tissue oxygenation in anaemic critically ill patients? Critical Care Medicine 2004; 32: 364–371.
9. Council of Europe. Guide to the preparation, use and quality assurance of blood components. Recommendation R (95) 15, 11th edition. Strasbourg: Council of Europe Publishing; 2005: 1–266.
10. Simon GE, Bove JR. The potassium load from blood transfusion. Postgraduate Medicine 1971; 49: 61–64.
11. Advanced Trauma Life Support Students Course Manual 7th edn. Chicago: American College of Surgeons 2007.
12. Serious Hazards of Transfusion Annual Report 2004; http://www.shotuk.org/SHOTREPORT2004.pdf (accessed 4 August 2008).
13. Popovsky MA, Chaplin HC Jr, et al. Transfusion-related acute lung injury: a neglected, serious complication of hemotherapy. Transfusion 1992; 32: 589–592.
14. Wilson RF, Mammen E, Walt AJ. Eight years of experience with massive blood transfusions. Journal of Trauma 1971; 11: 275–285.
15. American Society of Anesthesiologists. Practice Guidelines for Blood Component Therapy. Baltimore: Williams & Wilkins; 2003.
16. Ho J, Sibbald WJ, Chin-Yee IH. Effects of storage on efficacy of red cell transfusion: when is it not safe?. Critical Care Medicine 2003; 31: S687–S697.
17. Reiss RF. Hemostatic defects in massive transfusion: rapid diagnosis and management. American Journal of Critical Care 2000; 9: 158–165.
18. Boffard KD, Riou B, Warren B, et al. NovoSeven Trauma Study Group. Recombinant factor VIIa as adjunctive therapy for bleeding control in severely injured trauma patients: two parallel randomized, placebo-controlled, double-blind clinical trials. Journal of Trauma-Injury Infection & Critical Care 2005; 59(1): 8–15.
19. Dutton RP, McCunn M, Hyder M, et al. Factor VIIa for correction of traumatic coagulopathy. Journal of Trauma-Injury Infection & Critical Care 2004; 57(4): 709–718.
20. Levi M, Peters M, Buller HR. Efficacy and safety of recombinant factor VIIa for treatment of severe bleeding: a systematic review. Critical Care Medicine 2005; 33: 883–890.

14.1 Rheumatological emergencies

Michael J. Gingold • Adam B. Bystrzycki • Flavia M. Cicuttini

ESSENTIALS

1 Emergencies in the rheumatological population are related to either the disease or toxicity from treatment.

2 Understanding the basics of inflammatory conditions helps diagnose emergencies early.

3 Infection must be diagnosed and promptly treated in patients on antirheumatic and immunosuppressive medication.

Introduction

Rheumatological conditions are common among the population and broadly encompass inflammatory/connective tissue diseases and mechanical/musculoskeletal conditions. Life-threatening emergencies are generally rare, and relate to either the underlying condition or its treatment. The challenge is in making the distinction between the two, as treatment is frequently diametrically opposed; for example, the difference between administering further immunosuppression and giving antibiotics.

The most common rheumatological emergency seen in the emergency department (ED) is acute monoarthritis (see Ch. 14.2). This chapter discusses the important emergencies associated with general rheumatological conditions. Many of these are multisystem diseases and emergencies may be related either to a primary joint problem or to an extra-articular manifestation of the disease. As many of these conditions are autoimmune, suppression of the immune system is usually central to their management. This can be complicated by infection, which can relate to usual pathogens but also opportunistic infection.

RHEUMATOID ARTHRITIS

Rheumatoid arthritis (RA) affects 1–2% of the population across most ethnic subgroups and is two to three times more common in females than males. RA is a systemic inflammatory condition of unknown aetiology characterized by widespread synovitis resulting in joint erosions and destruction. It may also produce extra-articular manifestations, including vasculitis and visceral involvement.

Management typically involves symptom relief with non-steroidal anti-inflammatory drugs (NSAIDs) and/or corticosteroids, and prevention of disease progression with disease modifying antirheumatic drugs (DMARDs). These include methotrexate, leflunomide, sulfasalazine and hydroxychloroquine. Newer, so-called biologic agents act by inhibiting tumour necrosis factor-α (TNF-α) (infliximab, etanercept, adalimumab) or interleukin-1 (anakinra) and are currently used for patients who fail traditional DMARD therapy. Rituximab is also recently available for those who fail the aforementioned medications – its mechanism of action is B-cell depletion. See Chapter 14.3 for further details on the clinical features of RA, its diagnosis, useful investigations and principles of management.

EMERGENCIES IN RA – ARTICULAR MANIFESTATIONS

Acute monoarthritis

The patient with established RA may present with an acutely painful, hot, swollen joint that may be a manifestation of the underlying condition. Alternatively, it may signal septic arthritis, a condition to which patients with RA are 2–3 times more susceptible than matched controls.[1] The possibility of septic arthritis should be considered in a patient with RA who has acute monoarthritis out of keeping with their disease activity. See Chapter 14.2 for the approach to acute monoarthritis.

Cervical spine involvement

Cervical spine involvement in RA is a common finding with a prevalence of up to 61%.[2] It is more common in those with long-standing, erosive disease and disease of greater severity and activity.[3] Cervical spine involvement is associated with increased mortality.[4] Involvement of the cervical spine may manifest as atlanto-axial subluxation (most commonly anterior movement on the axis) or subluxation of lower cervical vertebrae. Either of these can result in cervical myelopathy.

Cervical spine subluxation is frequently asymptomatic, up to 44% in one study.[3] The most common symptom of cervical spine involvement is neck pain that may radiate towards the occiput. Other suggestive symptoms include slowly progressive spastic quadriparesis, sensory loss in hands or feet and paraesthesiae or weakness in the distribution of cervical nerve roots.

Important 'red flag' features suggestive of cervical myelopathy are shown in Table 14.1.1.

Table 14.1.1 Symptoms and signs of cervical myelopathy
Symptoms
Pain
Weakness
Peripheral paraesthesiae
Gait disturbance
Sphincter dysfunction
Changes in consciousness
Respiratory dysfunction
Signs
Spasticity
Weakness
Hyperreflexia of deep tendon reflexes
Extensor plantar response
Gait ataxia
Respiratory irregularity

Investigations

Plain X-rays of the cervical spine (lateral view) may demonstrate an increase in separation between the odontoid and arch of C1. Prior to taking flexion-extension films, perform plain 'peg' X-rays through the open mouth to exclude odontoid fracture or severe atlanto-axial subluxation. Computerized tomography (CT) can occasionally provide additional useful information; however, if there is concern regarding myelopathy, magnetic resonance imaging (MRI) is the most sensitive imaging technique.

Management

The primary implication of RA of the cervical spine in the ED is when endotracheal intubation is required. Inappropriate manipulation of the rheumatoid cervical spine in preparation for intubation can result in significant morbidity and even mortality from atlanto-axial and subaxial subluxation. Where possible, patients with RA who are scheduled to undergo surgery should have imaging of their cervical spine performed prior to intubation. Anaesthetic consultation may be required.

Patients with subluxation and signs of spinal cord compression are a neurosurgical emergency and prompt referral is essential.

EMERGENCIES IN RA – EXTRA-ARTICULAR MANIFESTATIONS

Rheumatoid vasculitis

Vasculitis in RA can occur in both small- and medium-sized vessels. Patients typically have long-standing, aggressive joint disease.

Clinical features

Presentations with rheumatoid vasculitis are varied and non-specific. Patients frequently present with constitutional symptoms and fatigue. The most common manifestation is of cutaneous vasculitis with deep skin ulcers on the lower limbs,[5]

digital ischaemia and gangrene (medium vessels) or palpable purpura (small vessels). Mononeuritis multiplex is another common presentation and results from infarction of the vasa nervorum due to vasculitis. It typically has an acute onset.

Medium vessel rheumatoid vasculitis can also produce organ infarction and necrosis. Rheumatoid vasculitis may mimic polyarteritis nodosa (PAN) with involvement of the renal arteries, and less commonly the mesenteric circulation. Pericarditis may accompany rheumatoid vasculitis but coronary vasculitis is rare. Ocular manifestations include episcleritis and peripheral ulcerative keratitis. Central nervous system (CNS) involvement is rare.

Investigations

Rheumatoid factor titre is typically elevated in rheumatoid vasculitis, although this is a non-specific finding. Rheumatoid vasculitis in the absence of rheumatoid factor is rare. Erythrocyte sedimentation rate (ESR) and C-reactive protein (CRP) are also elevated. Check a mid-stream urine specimen for active urinary sediment and a full blood count, urea and electrolytes.

Further investigations are directed by the relevant organ system involved and usually require specialist consultation:

- skin biopsy
- nerve conduction studies/ electromyography (EMG)
- sural nerve biopsy
- kidney biopsy.

Angiography findings are non-specific and not always diagnostic.

Diagnosis

Suspect rheumatoid vasculitis in patients with a long-standing history of seropositive RA who presents with constitutional symptoms and one of the above clinical features, such as a typical rash, digital gangrene, red eye, neurological symptoms or active urinary sediment.

Management

Systemic rheumatoid vasculitis has a poor prognosis without immune-suppressive therapy. Urgent rheumatology consultation is required as treatment usually consists of high-dose corticosteroids as well as cyclophosphamide.

Summary of other extra-articular manifestations of RA

Lung disease

Lung disease may manifest as a pleural-based disease such as pleurisy or pleural effusions, or parenchymal lung disease such as interstitial lung disease (the most common manifestation), organizing pneumonia and rheumatoid nodules. Caplan's syndrome occurs when RA is associated with pneumo-coniosis. Important differential diagnoses include infection due to immune-suppression, treatment-related toxicity (e.g. methotrexate-induced pneumonitis) and other medical comorbidities such as chronic obstructive pulmonary disease.

Pleural disease often resolves without treatment, alternatively a NSAID may be used. Parenchymal disease as documented on chest X-ray or high-resolution CT requires specialist treatment.

Cardiac disease

Pericarditis occurs in 30% of RA patients based on echocardiography, but less than 10% have any clinical features. It generally occurs when there is active joint and other extra-articular disease. Management consists of NSAIDs or prednisolone.

Myocarditis is a rare manifestation of RA. It can be granulomatous and depending on its location may produce valvular (especially mitral) incompetence or conduction defects.

Sjogren's syndrome

Sjogren's syndrome may present in its primary form as a systemic disease, but can also occur secondary to RA and other connective tissue disorders. The classic symptoms are dry gritty eyes, dry mouth or both. Treatment is usually symptomatic in patients with no other features.

Felty's syndrome

Felty's syndrome is characterized by seropositive RA, splenomegaly and neutropenia. There may be other cytopenias, as well as leg ulcers.

Kidney disease

Renal involvement in RA is rare and includes vasculitis and glomerulonephritis. Secondary amyloidosis can occur in patients with long-standing active disease. However, many medications used in RA are nephrotoxic, in particular NSAIDs and ciclosporin.

Neurological disease

Vasculitis may produce mononeuritis multiplex, as mentioned previously, otherwise central nervous system involvement is rare.

Cardiovascular disease in RA and other connective tissue diseases

Patients with RA and other connective tissue diseases such as systemic lupus erythematosus (SLE) have an increased risk of ischaemic heart disease (IHD).[6] This occurs independently of traditional risk factors such as smoking or dyslipidaemia, and is more common in those with extra-articular disease.[7] The higher incidence of IHD could be related to disease factors such as widespread inflammation, or to medications used such as NSAIDs (including selective COX-2 inhibitors) and corticosteroids.

The emergency physician needs a low threshold for ruling out ischaemic causes of chest pain in the RA patient. Routine investigations are no different to those undertaken for non-RA patients. A patient with suggestive history but negative cardiac biomarkers and normal electrocardiograms should proceed to stress testing as per the recommendations for the general population. Management of acute coronary syndrome in RA is no different.

SYSTEMIC LUPUS ERYTHEMATOSUS

SLE is a multisystem, autoimmune disease. It is the prototype disease of immune complex deposition resulting in tissue damage across a variety of organ systems. It is one of the most common autoimmune conditions among women of childbearing age.

Clinical features

Common presenting features of SLE include general constitutional symptoms such as fatigue, malaise and weight loss. There are a variety of skin manifestations that can occur in SLE which are lupus-specific (malar rash, discoid lupus, subacute cutaneous lupus erythematosus) or non-specific (panniculitis, alopecia, oral ulceration). Arthralgias or an acute non-erosive arthritis are the most common presenting symptoms of SLE. Myositis may also occur. Another common manifestation is serositis producing pleurisy, pericarditis or peritonitis. SLE also causes renal and CNS disease (see below) and rarely can involve the lung (pneumonitis, pulmonary hypertension) and the heart (myocarditis, endocarditis).

Investigations

A full blood examination often reveals cytopenias which are a common feature of SLE. Biochemistry investigations may indicate renal involvement. Clotting abnormalities may include a prolonged activated partial thromboplastin time due to the lupus anticoagulant. ESR and CRP may be raised.

Serological abnormalities

Serological abnormalities may reveal decreased levels of complement components C3 and C4, as well as the presence of auto-antibodies. The antinuclear antibody (ANA) is present in 95% of patients with SLE, but may also occur in a variety of other connective tissue and inflammatory diseases. The anti-Smith (Sm) and anti-dsDNA (double-stranded DNA) antibodies are more specific for SLE but less sensitive. The anti-Sm is obtained as part of a panel of tests for extractable nuclear antigens (ENA).

Other tests are directed towards the organ system involved, for example midstream urine specimen looking for proteinuria or glomerular haematuria (>70% dysmorphic red blood cells or red-cell casts) or chest X-ray for the patient with serositis.

Assessing SLE disease activity

It is important in the ED to determine SLE disease activity. Useful symptoms of disease activity include mouth ulcers, alopecia and constitutional symptoms, as well as organ-specific symptoms such as arthralgia or pleuritic chest pain.

Investigations used to assess disease activity include complement levels (low in active SLE), CRP and ESR (elevated), as well as anti-dsDNA titre. These are not diagnostic and many people with quiescent SLE may remain hypocomplementaemic or display elevated anti-dsDNA titres.

A mid-stream urine for urinary sediment is an essential part of the assessment of the SLE patient, as a marker of renal involvement.

Management

Management of SLE is directed by the organ system involved, and includes topical therapies for cutaneous lupus and NSAIDs for arthralgias and mild serositis. Most patients with SLE will be on an anti-malarial such as hydroxychloroquine, which is helpful for skin and musculo-skeletal manifestations, as well as organ involvement. Many patients will also be on corticosteroids. Those with major organ involvement will also be taking other immunosuppressants such as methotrex-ate, cyclophosphamide or azathioprine. Mycophenolate mofetil is emerging as an alternative to cyclophosphamide for lupus nephritis.

Lupus nephritis

Early diagnosis of lupus nephritis is essential in instituting prompt management and preventing the progression of renal damage. Patients may be asymptomatic, or present with nocturia or 'frothy' urine. Other presentations include hypertension, the nephritic syndrome and the nephrotic syndrome.

Urinalysis is the most useful investigation in detecting lupus nephritis, and pro-teinuria is the most common abnormality detected. The fresh urine specimen should be sent for phase contrast microscopy in order to detect the presence of dysmorphic erythrocytes (>70 % indicates glomerular disease) or cellular casts.

Urinalysis can expedite the investigation and further management of this potentially organ-threatening condition. Prompt referral to a rheumatologist or renal physician for consideration of renal biopsy and further management is indicated.

Neuropsychiatric SLE

There are a myriad of neuropsychiatric manifestations of neuropsychiatric SLE. Neurological presentations include:

- stroke (due to vasculitis, emboli, atherosclerosis or antiphospholipid antibodies)
- seizure
- migraine
- aseptic meningitis.

Psychiatric presentations include:

- psychosis
- cognitive deficit
- dementia
- anxiety.

These presentations are non-specific and have a broad differential diagnosis which includes medication side effects, infection and tumour. Unfortunately, there is no spe-cific diagnostic test which helps differenti-ate SLE from other potential aetiologies. Thus, the diagnosis is made from a range of diagnostic tests and clinical features. The role of the emergency physician in this setting is to exclude common non-SLE pre-sentations such as meningitis or intracra-nial haemorrhage.

Imaging studies are necessary in addi-tion to tests for SLE activity (see above). CT brain scan may detect changes of acute infarction but is also useful in excluding other unrelated causes such as haemorrhage or tumour. MRI is more sen-sitive in detecting white matter abnormal-ities although these are frequently non-specific.

Cerebrospinal fluid (CSF) analysis is essential to exclude infection, but may be normal in SLE. Changes such as ele-vated protein, low glucose or even a posi-tive ANA are non-specific and do not always reflect active SLE. The electro-encephalogram is occasionally useful in cases of suspected non-convulsive status epilepticus with unexplained altered conscious level.

Giant cell (temporal) arteritis

Giant cell arteritis (GCA) is the most common vasculitis and almost exclusively affects Caucasians. It is a large and medium vessel vasculitis of unknown aetiology, which pre-dominantly affects the cranial branches of arteries originating from the aortic arch.

Polymyalgia rheumatica (PMR) is a syn-drome of inflammatory pain and stiffness in the shoulder and pelvic girdles that occurs alone or frequently in association with GCA.

Epidemiology

GCA and PMR rarely occur before the age of 50 years of age.[8] The mean age at diag-nosis is approximately 72 years, with an incidence of GCA of roughly 1 in 500 of people over the age of 50 years. The inci-dence and prevalence of PMR are less well studied.

Clinical features

The most common symptom of GCA is headache, usually localizing to the tempo-ral region, although it can be more diffuse. The area is often tender and worsened by brushing the hair. Most patients complain of constitutional symptoms such as malaise, fatigue, anorexia and weight loss. Jaw clau-dication (pain after a period of chewing) is the most specific symptom for GCA, although not sensitive, as it is only present in 34%.[8] On examination the temporal arteries may be thickened, 'ropey' and ten-der with an absent or reduced pulse.

The most significant complication of GCA is anterior ischaemic optic neuropathy resulting in sudden painless loss of vision. Less commonly, other branches of the aorta may be involved resulting in hemiparesis, arm claudication, aortic dissection or myo-cardial infarction.

Polymyalgia rheumatica

PMR usually affects the neck, shoulder and pelvic girdles resulting in stiffness and inflammatory pain, worse in the morning and after rest. The pain is often poorly localized and there may be muscle atrophy late in the disease. There can also be evidence of synovitis affecting the shoulders, knees, wrists and hands.

The relationship between onset of symptoms of GCA and PMR is highly variable. PMR symptoms may occur before, after or with GCA symptoms.

Differential diagnosis of PMR and GCA

The differential diagnosis of PMR includes late-onset RA, inflammatory myositis and other myopathies, fibromyalgia and hypothyroidism. GCA can mimic any of the other vasculitides. Non-arteritic anterior ischaemic optic neuropathy can also mimic GCA.

Investigations

The classic non-specific laboratory finding in GCA and/or PMR is a markedly elevated ESR (often >100 mm/h). CRP is also usually elevated, and full blood count often shows a mild normochromic normocytic anaemia.

A temporal artery biopsy confirms the diagnosis of GCA and is particularly useful when the diagnosis is doubtful or the presentation atypical. Unfortunately, there is a false negative rate of 10–30%, so a negative biopsy does not exclude GCA.

Criteria for diagnosis

The ACR classification criteria for GCA are helpful in differentiating GCA from other forms of vasculitis.[9] They include age at onset >50 years, a new headache, temporal artery tenderness or decreased pulsation and an ESR >50. An abnormal artery biopsy showing vasculitis with mononuclear infiltrate or granulomatous inflammation with multi-nucleated giant cells is also required to confirm the diagnosis.

Management

Corticosteroids are the treatment of choice and should not be withheld to perform a biopsy, if there is a strong clinical suspicion.

The initial dose for GCA is unclear, but prednisone 1 mg/kg/day is usually indicated[10] especially for ischaemic complications; however, lower doses such as prednisone 40–50 mg have been used.[11] The dose of prednisone for PMR alone is lower at 10–20 mg/day.[11] Most patients do not require hospital admission, provided a temporal artery biopsy can be organized within a few days. However, patients with visual loss at diagnosis require urgent treatment, often with pulsed parenteral corticosteroids, and inpatient admission. Patients with GCA should also be commenced on aspirin.

An approach to the systemic vasculitides

The systemic vasculitides are a group of disorders characterized by an inflammatory infiltrate in the walls of blood vessels resulting in damage to the vessel wall. The clinical manifestations depend upon the size of vessel and location in the vascular tree and may result in systemic or organ-specific manifestations. Table 14.1.2 classifies vasculitic syndromes according to vessel size (there is much overlap).

Clinical features

An underlying vasculitis should be considered in patients who present with one or more of the following:

Table 14.1.2 Classification of systemic vasculitis according to vessel size	
Vessel size	Vasculitis
Large	Takayasu's arteritis Giant cell arteritis
Medium	Polyarteritis nodosa Kawasaki disease
Small	Wegener's granulomatosis (ANCA+) Microscopic polyangiitis (ANCA+) Churg–Strauss syndrome Henoch–Schonlein purpura Cryoglobulinaemic vasculitis Leukocytoclastic cutaneous vasculitis

- unexplained systemic illness – fatigue, fevers, nightsweats, malaise
- unexplained ischaemia of an organ or limb
- rash of palpable purpura
- chronic inflammatory sinusitis and chronic discharge or bleeding from the nose or ears
- mononeuritis multiplex
- pulmonary infiltrates
- microscopic haematuria, especially if dysmorphic glomerular erythrocytes
- any of the above in the setting of atopy and peripheral blood eosinophilia.

Investigations and diagnosis

Baseline investigations should include FBE, U&E, LFTs and clotting studies as well as CRP and ESR. Blood cultures should be taken if the patient is systemically unwell.

A panel of auto-immune serological tests is carried out in suspected cases. This includes ANA, ENA, rheumatoid factor, dsDNA, anti-cyclic citrullinated peptides (anti-CCP), complement levels (C3, C4), antineutrophil cytoplasmic antibodies (ANCA) and cryoglobulins. PAN is associated with hepatitis B and cryoglobulinaemic vasculitis with hepatitis C infection.

Collection of a mid-stream urine specimen to look for glomerular haematuria is mandatory when vasculitis is suspected. Imaging is required such as chest X-ray, CT scan of the chest or sinuses or other areas depending on the suspected organ involved. The definitive diagnosis of vasculitis requires biopsy of affected tissue or angiography.

Differential diagnosis of systemic vasculitis

Other conditions which may mimic vasculitis include:

- infections such as infective endocarditis, meningococcaemia, gonococcaemia
- disorders of haemostasis and thrombosis such as thrombotic thrombocytopenic purpura, antiphospholipid syndrome
- malignancy such as lymphoma, myxoma
- sarcoidosis.

Management of systemic vasculitis

Treatment is usually with high-dose corticosteroids and, depending on the condition, additional immunosuppression such as cyclophosphamide. Urgent specialist referral is essential.

Emergencies associated with rheumatology therapy

The medications used most commonly in rheumatology include NSAIDs, corticosteroids and DMARDs. Over the past 5 to 10 years, the 'biologic' DMARDs have become available for the treatment of RA, psoriatic arthritis and ankylosing spondylitis. These medications are all associated with adverse effects which occasionally result in serious morbidity.

Non-steroidal anti-inflammatory drugs

NSAIDs are used for symptom relief in a variety of conditions, especially inflammatory joint pain. They are of equal efficacy, although those with shorter half lives appear to have less gastrointestinal toxicity.[12] NSAIDs should be used in the lowest possible dose for the shortest duration and combination of NSAIDs (not aspirin) should be avoided.[12]

The most common adverse effects of NSAIDs seen as an emergency include peptic ulcer disease and acute renal failure, both related to inhibition of prostaglandin synthesis. GI toxicity is more common in the elderly, those on anticoagulants and with high doses or prolonged duration of NSAIDs. Prescribe a proton pump inhibitor when there is concern about GI toxicity. The COX-2 selective inhibitors such as celecoxib have a reduced incidence of peptic ulcer disease, but a similar incidence of other adverse effects including hypertension, peripheral oedema and cardiac failure and in particular an increased risk of cardiovascular deaths with prolonged courses.

Corticosteroids

Corticosteroids are the mainstay of treatment for most inflammatory rheumatological conditions. At high doses they provide rapid control of inflammatory disease and are often required for long-term management at low doses. Long-term use is associated with numerous adverse effects such as diabetes, hypertension and osteoporosis. In addition, psychosis and mood disorders related to corticosteroid use as well as peptic ulcer disease may present as an emergency.

Immunosuppressants/disease modifying antirheumatic drugs

This heterogeneous group of medications is used to prevent joint destruction in the inflammatory arthritides and as steroid-sparing therapy in many connective tissue diseases. They include methotrexate, leflunomide, hydroxychloroquine, sulfasalazine, ciclosporin, azathioprine and cyclophosphamide. Each drug has its own range of adverse effects, but common adverse effects presenting at an ED include cytopenias, rashes including the Stevens–Johnson syndrome, abnormal liver function tests, GI toxicity and heightened susceptibility to infections (see Table 14.1.3).

Biologic disease modifying antirheumatic drugs

The so-called 'biologic' DMARDs are a newer and expanding collection of therapies directed against molecules that mediate joint destruction and help drive the inflammatory process. Principally, agents are directed against TNF-α such as adalimumab, etanercept and infliximab, and against interleukin-1 (IL-1) such as anakinra. More recently, rituximab has become available for those who fail the above therapies. Its main function is to deplete B lymphocytes from peripheral circulation. These therapies are being increasingly used for those who fail conventional DMARD therapy for RA.

Adverse effects of biologic DMARDs

Adverse effects associated with the use of TNF-α inhibitors include a heightened risk of all infections, particularly soft-tissue and joint infections, as well as re-activation of tuberculosis. Other opportunistic infections appear more common such as listeriosis. Patients may also develop local injection site reactions and infusion-related reactions, which may be delayed. Less common adverse effects include a form of drug-induced lupus and demyelination.

Presentations of treatment-related emergencies

Bone marrow suppression

Anaemia, leukopenia and thrombocytopenia all occur in patients taking DMARDs such as methotrexate, cyclophosphamide,

---

Table 14.1.3   Adverse effects of disease modifying antirheumatic drugs (DMARDs)

DMARD	Adverse effects
Methotrexate	Nausea and other GI upset, mouth ulcers, abnormal liver function (transaminases), bone marrow suppression, rash, alopecia, pneumonitis Teratogenic Increased bone marrow toxicity in renal impairment – withhold in acute renal failure
Leflunomide	Abnormal liver function (transaminases), diarrhoea, rash, alopecia, hypertension, peripheral neuropathy Teratogenic
Hydroxychloroquine	Nausea, rash, dizziness ('cinchonism'), retinal toxicity at higher doses (all uncommon)
Sulfasalazine	GI upset, uncommonly abnormal liver function and bone marrow suppression, rashes (rarely, Stevens–Johnson syndrome)
Ciclosporin	Renal impairment, hypertension, electrolyte disturbance, hyperuricaemia and gout, gingival hyperplasia, hirsutism
Cyclophosphamide	Bone marrow suppression especially neutropenia, GI upset, bladder toxicity, including haemorrhagic cystitis (acute) and bladder cancer (chronic), opportunistic infections Teratogenic
Azathioprine	GI upset, rash, systemic symptoms, abnormal liver function, bone marrow suppression, skin cancers, infections

GI, gastrointestinal.

sulfasalazine and azathioprine. The patient who presents with sepsis and leukopenia is a medical emergency and requires resuscitation, supportive care and broad-spectrum parenteral antibiotics.

Cytopenia in a patient taking methotrexate is uncommon but those at increased risk include the elderly and with renal impairment, related to the drug's mechanism of action as an inhibitor of dihydrofolate reductase. Management involves temporary cessation of treatment and administration of folinic acid.

The most common adverse effect of cyclophosphamide is myelosuppression, particularly leukopenia. The white cell nadir occurs at 2 weeks post infusion following intravenous therapy. Patients on oral therapy may experience a gradual decrease in white cell count.

Bone marrow suppression may also occur as a side effect of azathioprine treatment especially if given in combination with allopurinol, which inhibits its metabolism, thus potentiating bone marrow toxicity. Cytopenias are also more common in patients with deficient thiopurine methyltransferase enzyme. Sulfasalazine therapy is uncommonly complicated by bone marrow suppression.

Infections

Treatment of rheumatological conditions is directed at immunosuppression, thus infections are a common and expected adverse effect of corticosteroids, certain DMARDs and, in particular, anti-TNF-α therapy. Although studies have shown RA patients to have a de novo increased risk of infection, biologic DMARDs may further increase this risk.

Some studies have reported an increased risk of infection and serious infection in patients receiving anti-TNF therapy, although the largest study of infection risk in patients on anti-TNF agents showed that while there is an increased risk of skin and soft tissue injections, there was no significant difference in risk of serious infections.[13] Patients on anti-TNF therapy who develop infections are advised to temporarily cease their treatment and to commence antibiotics. If in doubt, they should be admitted to hospital to receive parenteral antibiotics. There is also an increased risk

of re-activation of tuberculosis and possibly of infections with other organisms such as Listeria and Salmonella.[13] Rigorous tuberculosis screening prior to commencement of anti-TNF therapy should now be universal.

DMARD-related pneumonitis

Methotrexate and leflunomide both result in lung toxicity. The incidence of methotrexate-induced lung toxicity is difficult to assess but uncommon. The most common type of toxicity is a hypersensitivity pneumonitis, but other forms of lung injury may also occur. Clinical features are non-specific and include constitutional symptoms, cough and progressive dyspnoea. Subacute presentations are more common, although acute and chronic presentations may also occur, with rapid progress to respiratory failure in more acute situations. Patients at higher risk for methotrexate-induced lung injury have prolonged duration of methotrexate treatment, pre-existing rheumatoid involvement of the lungs and pleura, increased extra-articular manifestations, diabetes mellitus, previous DMARD use and low serum albumin.[14] Age and smoking also appear to be important.

Imaging reveals interstitial opacities and patchy consolidation. High-resolution CT scanning typically shows a ground-glass appearance. The main differential diagnosis is of a respiratory infection which may be due to typical pathogens or opportunistic infections such as *Pneumocystis jirovecii*.

Management is supportive with empiric antibiotic therapy in case of infection. Corticosteroids are also used. Patients may become seriously ill and require intensive care, but mortality is still low (1%).

Leflunomide may also cause lung injury, typically in the first few months of therapy and usually when given in combination with methotrexate.

Allopurinol hypersensitivity syndrome

Minor hypersensitivity reactions to allopurinol occur in around 2% of patients and usually consist of a mild rash. Rarely, a severe hypersensitivity syndrome may present as an unwell patient with fever, erythematous rash, abnormalities of liver function, peripheral blood eosinophilia and acute renal failure due to interstitial nephritis.[15] It is more

common in those with renal impairment who do not have appropriate dose reduction. This presentation has a mortality rate of 25%. Treatment is supportive.

References

1. Margaretten ME, Kohlwes J, Moore D, et al. Does this adult patient have septic arthritis? Journal of American Medical Association 2007; 297: 1478–1488.
2. Collins DN, Barnes CL, Fitzrandolph RL. Cervical spine instability in rheumatoid patients having total hip or knee arthroplasty. Clinical Orthopaedics and Related Research 1991; 272: 127–135.
3. Neva MH, Hakkinen A, Makinen H, et al. High prevalence of asymptomatic cervical spine subluxation in patients with rheumatoid arthritis waiting for orthopaedic surgery. Annals of Rheumatic Diseases 2006; 65: 884–888.
4. Riise T, Jacobsen BK, Gran JT. High mortality in patients with rheumatoid arthritis and atlantoaxial subluxation. Journal of Rheumatoloy 2001; 28: 2425–2429.
5. Genta MS, Genta RM, Gabay C. Systemic rheumatoid vasculitis: a review. Seminars in Arthritis and Rheumatism 2006; 36: 88–98.
6. Turesson C, Jarenros A, Jacobsson L. Increased incidence of cardiovascular disease in patients with rheumatoid arthritis: results from a community based study. Annals of Rheumatic Diseases 2004; 63: 952–955.
7. Turesson C, Jarenros A, Jacobsson L. Severe extra-articular disease manifestations are associated with an increased risk of first ever cardiovascular events in patients with rheumatoid arthritis. Annals of Rheumatic Diseases 2007; 66(1): 70–75.
8. Smetana GW, Shmerling RH. Does this patient have temporal arteritis? Journal of American Medical Association 2002; 287: 92–101.
9. Hunder GG, Bloch DA, Michel BA, et al. The American College of Rheumatololgy 1990 criteria for the classification of giant cell arteritis. Arthrtitis Rheumatics 1990; 33: 1122–1128.
10. Spiera RF, Spiera H. Therapy for giant cell arteritis: can we do better? Arthritis Rheumatics 2006; 54: 3071–3074.
11. Kyle V, Hazleman BL. Treatment of polymyalgia and giant cell arteritis: 1. Steroid regimens in the first two months. Annals of Rheumatic Diseases 1989; 48: 658–661.
12. Therapeutic Guidelines: Rheumatology, Version 1. Melbourne: Therapeutics Guidelines Ltd; 2006.
13. Dixon WG, Watson K, Lunt M, et al. Rates of serious infection, including site-specific and bacterial intracellular infection in rheumatoid arthritis patients receiving anti-tumour necrosis factor therapy: results from the British Society of Rheumatology Biologics Register. 2006; 54: 2368–2376.
14. Alarcon GS, Kremer JM, Macaluso M, et al. Risk factors for methotrexate-induced lung injury in patients with rheumatoid arthritis: a multicentre, case control study. Annals of Internal Medicine 1997; 127: 356–364.
15. Guttierez-Macias A, Lizarralde-Palacios E, Martinez-Odriozola P, et al. Fatal allopurinol hypersensitivity syndrome after treatment of asymptomatic hyperuricaemia. British Medical Journal 2005; 331: 623–624.

Further reading

D'Cruz DP. Clinical review: systemic lupus erythematosus. British Medical Journal 2006; 332: 890–840.
Hochberg, M et al. (eds.) Rheumatology. 3rd edn. Edinburgh: Mosby; 2003.
Savage COS, et al. ABC of arterial and vascular disease: vasculitis. British Medical Journal 2000; 20:1325–1328.
Up To Date online: http://www.utdol.com/utd/content/search.do (accessed Jul 2008).

14.2 Monoarticular rheumatism

Michael J. Gingold • Adam B. Bystrzycki • Flavia M. Cicuttini

ESSENTIALS

1 Presenting features alone, including absence of fever, do not reliably exclude septic arthritis.

2 Synovial aspirate in appropriate pathology transport media may be diagnostic when performed prior to antibiotics in septic arthritis.

3 Acute monoarthritis affecting a prosthetic joint or the hip should *not* be aspirated in the emergency department. It requires urgent orthopaedic assessment.

Table 14.2.1 Most common presentations with acute monoarthritis to an emergency department[4]
Gout
Reactive arthritis such as post-viral, Reiters
Acute exacerbation of pre-existing inflammatory arthritis
Rheumatoid arthritis
Septic arthritis

Note: Orthopaedic-related joint problems such as trauma and/or haemarthrosis, plus osteoarthritis (OA) were not included in this series.

SEPTIC ARTHRITIS

The assessment of a patient with acute monoarthritis is focused on excluding a septic arthritis. Septic arthritis can cause rapid joint destruction, and mortality has been reported as high as up to 15%.[1]

Pathogenesis and pathology

Non-gonococcal bacterial arthritis occurs when bacteria enter the synovial lining of a joint via the haematogenous route, local spread from nearby soft tissue infections or following penetrating trauma or injury to a joint.

When the bacteria reach the synovium they trigger an inflammatory response, and bacteria and inflammatory cells enter the synovial fluid in the joint space, causing swelling and destruction of articular cartilage. These destructive changes may extend to subchondral bone and produce irreversible damage within days. The commonest causative organisms are staphylococci and streptococci.

Epidemiology and risk factors

The prevalence of septic arthritis among patients presenting to an emergency department with acute monoarthritis is up to 27%.[2]

Risk factors for septic arthritis include inflammatory arthritis (especially rheumatoid arthritis), diabetes mellitus and systemic factors such as age greater than 80 years, as well as local factors such as recent joint surgery, joint prosthesis and overlying skin infection. These individual risk factors increase the risk of septic arthritis by two- to three-fold.[3] Skin infection overlying a prosthetic joint increases the risk of infection by 15-fold.[3]

Clinical features

Septic arthritis presents with joint pain and swelling in over 80% of cases, which may or may not be associated with systemic symptoms such as sweats and rigors.[3] The hip and knee joints are the most commonly involved joints.

The patient may be febrile and the affected joint is usually swollen, warm, erythematous and tender. Classically, there is reduced ability to actively move the joint and marked pain on passive movement. Unfortunately, the symptoms and signs are non-specific and a patient with septic arthritis may present with all or only certain of these features. Thus, septic arthritis cannot be excluded with confidence on the history and examination alone.

Differential diagnosis

The differential diagnosis of acute monoarthritis is shown in Table 14.2.1. Ask the patient about a history of previous rheumatological disease such as rheumatoid arthritis, gout or other inflammatory arthritis, as well as risk factors for infection such as immunosuppression, including steroids and diabetes. Recent trauma or history of a bleeding diathesis or anticoagulant is also relevant. Finally, ask the patient about any recent sexually transmitted infection, including gonococcal infection or non-specific urethritis, and any systemic features, including uveitis and/or gastrointestinal infection, which may point towards a reactive arthritis.

Clinical investigations

Blood tests

Send blood for a full blood count, which may reveal an elevated peripheral white blood cell count, as well as C-reactive protein (CRP) and erythrocyte sedimentation rate (ESR). ESR and CRP are non-specific and not sensitive for septic arthritis, but may help in the differential diagnosis. Blood cultures are taken in the presence of fever. Finally, a serum urate may be elevated, but can be normal in acute gout.

X-rays

Imaging may be normal in septic arthritis, as it takes at least 1 week for destructive changes to appear on plain X-ray. Magnetic resonance imaging, if available, is non-specific but may be helpful to determine if the pathology is in the joint or juxta-articular bone.

Joint aspiration

The most useful investigation is synovial fluid aspiration and analysis. Send the aspirate in a sterile container for Gram stain and culture, as well as for polarizing light microscopy to look for the presence of urate (strongly negative birefringent) crystals or calcium pyrophosphate crystals (weakly positive birefringent crystals).

Place some of the aspirate in an EDTA tube for a cell count to be performed. The likelihood of septic arthritis increases from 2.9% with a synovial white cell count greater than 25 000/µL up to 28% with a synovial white cell count of greater than 100 000/µL. Synovial glucose and protein levels are unhelpful.

Criteria for diagnosis septic arthritis

There is no 'gold standard' test for the diagnosis of septic arthritis. Gram stain of synovial fluid has a sensitivity of only 50% maximum, while culture has a sensitivity of up to 85%.[3] However, combined with an appropriate clinical presentation, the presence of micro-organisms in synovial fluid on Gram stain and/or a positive synovial fluid culture with high synovial white cell count are diagnostic.

Treatment

Treatment of septic arthritis requires parenteral antibiotics, and urgent referral to orthopaedics for surgical drainage, with the patient admitted to hospital. Commence empirical antibiotic therapy with dicloxacillin or flucloxacillin 2 g i.v. 6-hourly, or cephalothin 2 g i.v. 6-hourly if patient is allergic to penicillin to cover against staphylococcus, until guided by microbiology results.

The patient with suspected hip sepsis or sepsis affecting a prosthetic joint must be referred to orthopaedics urgently without attempting joint aspiration.

GOUT

Gout is an intra-articular inflammatory response to monosodium urate crystal deposition usually related to hyperuricaemia. It is more common in males than females, but is extremely rare in the premenopausal female.

Aetiology and pathogenesis

Uric acid is derived from purine metabolism. Hyperuricaemia is the strongest predictor for gout and relates to either over-production or under-excretion of uric acid. Hyperuricaemia may also cause radiolucent renal calculi.

Over-production of uric acid is due to dietary factors such as beer, shellfish and other purine-rich foods, or endogenous factors associated with high cell turnover such as a haematological malignancy. Reduced excretion is related to chronic kidney disease, hypovolaemia, acidosis and medications such as diuretics, ciclosporin, pyrazinamide and ethambutol and low-dose aspirin. There is frequently a family history of gout.

Epidemiology

The peak incidence of acute gout occurs in men between the ages of 30 and 60 years and in women between 55 and 70 years. The presentation of gout in younger patients should prompt a search for a secondary cause (including lifestyle factors). Gout is more common in Maori and Polynesian populations.

Clinical features

The classic presentation is of acute onset of a hot, swollen and painful first metatarsophalangeal joint (75% of cases) known as podagra. Other commonly affected joints include other joints in the foot, the ankle, knee and small joints of the hand.

Common triggers of an acute attack include binges of alcohol or purine-rich foods, dehydration, severe illness such as sepsis, trauma and surgery. Sudden cessation or the introduction (especially in an acute attack) of hypo-uricaemic agents such as allopurinol or probenecid can also precipitate gouty arthritis, as can the introduction or a dose change of a diuretic.

Untreated, the symptoms will abate over the course of several days to 2 weeks. Occasionally, the patient may appear systemically unwell during an acute attack with malaise and septic symptoms. Examination reveals a tender, warm and erythematous joint with severely restricted range of movement. The patient may also be febrile. Presentations of acute gout may also be polyarticular.

Recurrent untreated acute gout and hyperuricaemia results in chronic tophaceous gout, where the patient is no longer pain-free between attacks. Examination will reveal joint deformity and tophus formation on the ears, fingers and around the elbows.

Investigations and diagnosis

Synovial fluid aspiration

Synovial fluid aspirate identifying monosodium urate crystals is diagnostic of acute gout. The crystals may be phagocytosed, and the synovial fluid will have a high white cell count. Send fluid for Gram stain and culture to rule out septic arthritis, which may rarely coexist with gout. Podagra in the typical clinical scenario has a sensitivity of 96% and specificity of 95% for acute gout.[5]

Blood tests

Hyperuricaemia on blood testing is not diagnostic of gout, and although up to 5% of adults may have a raised serum uric acid at some point, only one-fifth (1% overall) will ever have an attack of gout. Conversely, in about one-third of patients with gout the serum uric acid level is normal during an acute attack. Other blood tests such as FBE, ESR and CRP are sent, and may be abnormal including elevated inflammatory markers. Check the renal function with serum urea and creatinine, to both identify a potential aetiology and help guide treatment such as avoidance or reduced doses of non-steroidal anti-inflammatory drugs (NSAIDs).

Radiology

Plain X-ray is performed to exclude injury, but should be normal in the acute attack other than soft-tissue swelling. Periarticular punched-out erosions are seen in chronic gouty arthritis, which when associated with calcium deposition, deforming arthritis and soft-tissue swelling are quite characteristic of chronic tophaceous gout.

Management

The aim is to treat the acute pain and then prevent chronic relapse with hypo-uricaemic drugs.

Acute attack

Non-steroidal anti-inflammatory drugs

After excluding infection, give either colchicine and/or an NSAID in the absence of any contraindications. Give diclofenac 50 mg tds orally followed by 25 mg tds orally, or naproxen 500 mg followed by 250 mg tds orally until symptoms subside. A selective COX-2 inhibitor such as celecoxib 100 mg bd orally is preferred in patients with a history of peptic ulcer disease, although there is a similar risk of renal dysfunction in the elderly or with pre-existing renal disease.

Colchicine

When NSAIDs are contraindicated, colchicine is used. Doses of colchicine of 0.5 mg 6- or 8-hourly orally have equivalent efficacy and a lower rate of gastrointestinal toxicity compared to higher doses.[6] The higher doses such as colchicine 1.0 mg followed by 0.5 mg up to four times daily, with a maximum cumulative dose of 8 mg for an acute attack, are no longer recommended. All colchicine doses should be less with renal impairment, and may be restricted by the onset of nausea, vomiting and diarrhoea. Avoid prolonged colchicine use in patients with renal impairment as this may lead to a peripheral myoneuropathy.

Corticosteroids

Give patients with gout refractory to the above treatment or in whom both medications are contraindicated corticosteroids, such as prednisolone from 25 to 50 mg daily for 3 days then weaned over the course of 1 to 2 weeks.[7,8] An alternative approach is to give intra-articular corticosteroid for monoarticular gout provided sepsis has been excluded. Educate all patients to correct lifestyle factors where appropriate.

Recurrent attacks

Urate lowering therapy

A second attack of gout usually requires urate lowering therapy, although this is not usually commenced in the emergency setting, as treatment must be delayed until the acute flare up has settled. Allopurinol, a xanthine oxidase inhibitor, prevents the production of uric acid from xanthine. It is introduced at a low dose once the acute attack has settled and gradually titrated up to a maximum of 300 mg daily.[9] Typically, the patient will remain on a low-dose NSAID or colchicine (and/or prednisolone) as prophylaxis against precipitating further acute attacks. An alternative uricosuric agent to allopurinol is probenecid which should be avoided in renal impairment.

ACUTE PSEUDOGOUT

Acute pseudogout causes acute monoarthritis and is one of the several potential presentations of calcium pyrophosphate dihydrate (CPPD) deposition disease. It is more commonly seen in females and patients over 65 years old.

Aetiology and pathogenesis

Calcium pyrophosphate disease is characterized by deposition of CPPD crystals in cartilage causing chondrocalcinosis. When released, there may be uptake in other synovial structures and an inflammatory response producing acute synovitis, tenosynovitis or bursitis.

Advanced age is the strongest risk factor. Other associations are a family history, metabolic diseases such as haemochromatosis, Wilson's disease, hyperparathyroidism, hypophosphataemia or hypomagnesaemia and mechanical factors such as previous injury or osteoarthritis (OA).

Clinical features

CPPD deposition disease presents in a variety of ways. The two most common are acute pseudogout and chronic pyrophosphate arthropathy, which may mimic OA. CPPD deposition disease may also mimic rheumatoid arthritis or ankylosing spondylitis, as well as the neuropathic joint. Other presentations include tenosynovitis, bursitis or as an incidental radiographic finding of chondrocalcinosis.

Acute pseudogout typically presents in older patients, and the knee is the most commonly affected joint. Other common sites include the wrist, shoulder, elbow and ankle. Occasionally, there may be an oligoarticular presentation. Presentation is with a hot, red and swollen joint. There may be septic symptoms and the patient may be febrile. Triggers include trauma, surgery or illness, but most cases are spontaneous.

Investigations and clinical diagnosis

Joint aspiration

Diagnosis of pseudogout depends on the demonstration of CPPD crystals in synovial fluid, which is frequently blood stained. Polarizing light microscopy demonstrates weakly positive birefringent rhomboid-shaped crystals.

Plain X-rays

Plain X-rays of the joint may reveal chondrocalcinosis seen in fibrocartilage such as the knee menisci, triangular cartilage of the wrist and pubic symphysis. Other characteristic findings are of marked degenerative change in joints that are not usually affected by OA.

Younger patients presenting with polyarticular chondrocalcinosis should be screened for an underlying metabolic cause, checking serum calcium, magnesium, phosphate, alkaline phosphatase, parathyroid hormone, thyroid function and iron studies.

Management

Symptoms of acute pseudogout frequently improve once the joint has been aspirated. Intra-articular injection of corticosteroid is also appropriate for acute monoarthritis, once infection has been excluded. In addition, rest and splintage for 48–72 h is beneficial.

Give oral analgesics and NSAIDs similar to acute gout for polyarticular pseudogout, as performing multiple joint injections is also impractical and painful.

Take great care using NSAIDs in the elderly, and choose the smallest doses to avoid renal impairment and precipitating heart failure.

HAEMARTHROSIS

Haemarthrosis is bleeding into a joint which may be traumatic and related to intra-articular injury, or non-traumatic related to an underlying bleeding diathesis.

Aetiology

The causes of haemarthrosis are listed in Table 14.2.2.

Clinical features

A haemarthrosis causes a painful swollen joint with a reduced range of movement joint. The joint is often warm. Ask about a history of trauma, and if minimal or absent a bleeding disorder such as haemophilia should be considered. Also ask about troublesome bleeding during a previous operation, or following dental instrumentation, and about a family history.

Investigations and diagnosis

Perform plain radiography to exclude a fracture. Consider a computerized tomogrphy scan if there is a high index of clinical suspicion but normal plain imaging. Send a full blood count and a coagulation

---

Table 14.2.2 Causes of haemarthrosis

Traumatic
- Fracture
- Ligamentous (e.g. anterior cruciate or peripheral meniscal tear in the knee)

Non-traumatic
- Bleeding diathesis, e.g. haemophilia, von Willebrand's disease
- Anticoagulant use
- Neuropathic joint
- Acute pseudogout
- Septic arthritis
- Pigmented villonodular synovitis
- Vascular abnormalities such arteriovenous malformation, haemangioma

---

screen if there is no history of significant trauma. Haemarthrosis is diagnosed on aspiration of synovial fluid. An intra-articular fracture is indicated by observing fat globules floating on the surface of the blood.

Management

Management includes rest, immobilization, ice and compression as well as analgesia. Aspiration frequently provides some pain relief if performed within 24 h of onset. NSAIDs should be avoided in patients with a bleeding diathesis.

Haemophilia or other bleeding diathesis

Haemarthrosis due to haemophilia or other disorders of clotting factor deficiency requires immediate factor replacement therapy to a level of 40–50% of normal. This should be performed as soon as possible after the presentation, in consultation with a haematology specialist.

Often the patient will be able to advise on their normal treatment (and usually knows what factor they are deficient in, their usual basal levels and how much replacement is necessary in an acute bleed). Vitamin K and administration of fresh frozen plasma may be required in patients with elevated INR related to warfarin toxicity.

SERONEGATIVE SPONDYLO-ARTHROPATHIES

Monoarthritis is occasionally a presentation of a seronegative spondyloarthropathy such as reactive arthritis, psoriatic arthritis, inflammatory bowel disease-associated arthritis.

Clinical features suggesting reactive arthritis include a recent history of infective diarrhoea, or sexually transmitted infection, urethritis or uveitis. The patient may appear ill and be febrile with a tachycardia. The patient should be asked about a history of psoriasis or inflammatory bowel disease in the past.

Check for sites of enthesitis with inflammation at a tendon insertion points such as the Achilles tendon or plantar facia around the heel, or dactylitis causing 'sausage-shaped' digits.

Summary of the approach to the management of acute monoarthritis

The British Society for Rheumatology in conjunction with other medical associations published guidelines in 2006 regarding an approach to the hot swollen joint.[10] These guidelines are summarized below:

❶ The hot, swollen and tender joint should be considered as septic arthritis until proven otherwise. This may occur in the absence of fever.

❷ Synovial fluid must be obtained and sent for appropriate investigations prior to commencement of antibiotics. In situations of high clinical suspicion, a negative Gram stain or culture does not exclude septic arthritis.

❸ Other investigations should include blood cultures, CRP, ESR and full blood count.

❹ X-ray of the affected joint should be performed as a baseline.

❺ Septic joints require aspiration to dryness in addition to parenteral antibiotics.

❻ Prosthetic joints and suspected hip sepsis require an urgent orthopaedic opinion.

❼ The presentation of a hot and swollen first metatarso-phalangeal joint is almost always gout, and is diagnosed clinically.

References

1. Gupta MN, Sturrock RD, Field M, et al. Prospective comparative study of patients with culture proven and high suspicion of adult onset septic arthritis. Annals of Rheumatic Diseases 2003; 62: 327–331.
2. Jeng GW, Wang CR, Liu ST, et al. Measurement of synovial tumour necrosis factor-alpha in diagnosing emergency patients with bacterial arthritis. American Journal of Emergency Medicine 1997; 15: 626–629.
3. Margaretten ME, Kohlwes J, Moore D, et al. Does this adult patient have septic arthritis? Journal of American Medical Association 2007; 297: 1478–1488.

4. Sharma M, Leirisalo-Repo M. Arthritis patient as an emergency case at a university hospital. Scandinavian Journal of Rheumatology 1997; 26: 30–36.
5. Zhang W, Doherty M, Pascual E, et al. EULAR evidence based recommendations for gout. Part 1: Diagnosis. Annals of Rheumatic Diseases 2006; 65: 1301–1311.
6. Morris I, Varughese G, Mattingly P, et al. Colchicine in acute gout. British Medical Journal 2003; 327: 1275–1276.
7. Cronstein BN, Terkeltaub R, The inflammatory process of gout and its treatment. Arthritis Respiratory Therapy 2006; 8(suppl 1): S3.
8. Rheumatology Guidelines, Version 1. Therapeutic Guidelines Ltd., Melbourne; 2006.
9. Zhang W, Doherty M, Bardin T, et al. EULAR evidence based recommendations for gout. Part 1: Management. Annals of Rheumatic Diseases 2006; 65: 1312–1324.
10. Coakley G, Mathews C, Field M, et al. BSR and BHPR, BOA, RCGP and BSAC guidelines for management of the hot swollen joint in adults. Rheumatology 2006; 45: 1039–1041.

Further reading

Antibiotic Guidelines, Version 13. Melbourne: Therapeutic Guidelines Ltd; 2006.
Hochberg MC, et al. Rheumatology. 3rd edn. London: Elsevier; 2003.
Terkeltaub RA. Gout. New England Journal of Medicine 2003; 349: 1647–1655.
UpToDate online. http://www.utdol.com/utd/content/search.do (accessed August 2008).

14.3 Polyarticular rheumatism

Shom Bhattacharjee • Adam Bystrzycki • Flavia Cicuttini

ESSENTIALS

1 Polyarthritis is a common adult rheumatological presentation with a wide differential diagnosis.

2 Documenting articular and extra-articular involvement facilitates decision-making, particularly with regards to patient admission.

3 Joint aspiration is often useful for both diagnosis and excluding a septic arthritis. Other valuable tests include full blood examination, erythrocyte sedimentation rate and plain radiography.

4 Emergency management is with anti-inflammatory medication that may include systemic or intra-articular corticosteroids; early rheumatological consultation and/or admission, particularly in the presence of extra-articular features or sepsis; and organizing multidisciplinary follow-up on discharge from the emergency department.

Introduction

Polyarticular rheumatic disease is a frequent adult rheumatological presentation to the emergency department. This chapter focuses on the more common diseases encountered, the initial assessment and management, and most appropriate follow-up. These include rheumatoid arthritis (RA), the seronegative spondyloarthropathies, including psoriatic arthropathy, reactive arthritis with reference to arthritides occurring in association with enteric and urogenital infections, and infectious arthritis, including viral arthritis and rheumatic fever. Management principles include establishing the diagnosis, treating the acute problem and arranging appropriate follow-up.

ACUTE POLYARTHRITIS

Polyarthritis syndromes may be difficult to diagnose accurately due to the wide range of differential diagnoses, as shown in Table 14.3.1. Important measures are to rule out infection, quantify underlying inflammation and document extra-articular involvement.

Diagnosis and clinical features

History[2,3]

Take a focused history to include the following.

Table 14.3.1 Differential diagnosis of polyarthritis syndromes[1]

Inflammatory

Rheumatoid arthritis
Inflammatory osteoarthritis
Systemic connective tissue disease, including SLE, vasculitis, Behçet's disease, relapsing polychondritis
Seronegative spondyloarthropathies, commonly psoriatic arthropathy
Gout
Pseudogout (calcium pyrophosphate arthropathy)
Drug induced, including lupus syndromes
Infectious arthritis – bacterial including mycobacteria, endocarditis, protozoal, viral
Reactive or post-infectious arthritis including rheumatic fever

Non-inflammatory

Neoplastic/paraneoplastic disease including hypertrophic pulmonary osteoarthropathy
Sarcoidosis
Endocrine disease such as haemochromatosis, acromegaly
Haematological disease such as haemophilia, leukaemia

Mode of onset

- Acute (less than 6 weeks): gonococcal, viral including human immunodeficiency virus (HIV), reactive arthritis, rheumatic fever
- Chronic: RA, psoriatic arthropathy, systemic lupus erythematosus (SLE), scleroderma, dermatomyositis, other autoimmune diseases

Distribution

- Symmetric or asymmetric: large or small joint involvement

Course

- Progressive, intermittent or migratory

Constitutional symptoms

- Fever, night sweats, fatigue, significant weight loss >10%

Rheumatological systems review

- Symptoms including early morning stiffness, Raynaud's phenomenon, sclerodactyly, sicca syndrome, uveitis, scleritis, oral, digital or genital ulcers, rash, alopecia, urethritis, cervicitis, chronic bowel symptoms and serositis with pleuritis or pericarditis

Extra-articular organ involvement

Cough, dyspnoea, haematuria, hypertension, symptomatic peripheral neuropathy.

History of recent sore throat, febrile illness, new sexual contact, features of a sexually transmitted disease, diarrhoea, rash or uveitis.

Past medical history of gout, rheumatic fever, inflammatory bowel disease (IBD), malignancy and juvenile polyarthritis.

Family history of gout, psoriasis, IBD, uveitis or chronic back pain suggesting ankylosing spondylitis (AS) and other seronegative arthropathy.

Examination[4]

Perform a detailed physical examination and document:

- vital signs, painful joints with swollen soft tissue and their distribution
- cutaneous stigmata of underlying diseases such as psoriatic nails, rash and subcutaneous nodules, oral, genital or digital ulceration
- features of end-organ involvement such as a cardiac murmur, pleural or pericardial rub and pulmonary crackles
- lumbosacral spine and pelvis including sacroiliac joints.

Investigations[1,2]

Laboratory studies

Send blood for baseline haematology and biochemistry including full blood count (FBC), urea, electrolytes and liver function tests (ELFTs) and non-specific inflammatory markers, including erythrocyte sedimentation rate (ESR) and C-reactive protein (CRP).

Send serum antibody or antigen tests as indicated by the history including for infectious exposure such as hepatitis B serology, streptococcal antigen test and an autoantibody panel including antinuclear antibody (ANA), rheumatoid factor and antibodies against cyclic citrullinated peptide (anti-CCP). Antibody tests in particular should be interpreted with caution and interpreted in the context of each individual patient, due to their varying sensitivities and specificities.[5]

Joint aspiration

Joint aspiration and analysis of synovial fluid are of particular use in establishing the diagnosis of septic arthritis and crystal arthropathy (see Ch. 14.2).

Imaging studies

Imaging studies such as plain X-rays may demonstrate diagnostic features in erosive arthropathy, but these do not occur for some time after the acute onset.

RHEUMATOID ARTHRITIS

Rheumatoid arthritis (RA) is a chronic systemic inflammatory disorder of unknown aetiology characterized by symmetric synovitis, erosive polyarthritis and numerous extra-articular manifestations. It occurs in up to 2% of the general population and is two to three times more common in women.[6] Its onset is often indolent, and may lack the characteristic symmetry of joint involvement. Uncommonly it presents as an acute monoarthritis.

Diagnosis

The diagnosis in adults requires four or more of the American College of Rheumatology criteria:[7]

- Morning stiffness lasting at least 1 h.
- Arthritis of three or more joints.
- Swelling of proximal interphalangeal or metacarpophalangeal or wrist joints.
- Symmetrical involvement.
- Rheumatoid nodules.
- Abnormal level of serum rheumatoid factor.
- Radiological erosion or periarticular osteoporosis in hand or wrist joints.

Constitutional features such as malaise and fatigue are common.

Clinical features

Characteristic presentations in RA include the following.[8-10]

Upper limb

The wrist, metacarpophalangeal and proximal interphalangeal joints are typically affected, with sparing of the distal interphalangeal joints. Swan-necking and Boutonnière deformities are common, together with ulnar deviation at the metacarpophalangeal joints. Fixed flexion deformities may result in entrapment neuropathies, in particular carpal tunnel syndrome with median nerve involvement. Tenosynovitis may lead to tendon rupture, particularly of the extensor pollicis longus, or degenerative changes in the long extensors of the middle, ring and the little fingers with rupture of these tendons.

Lower limb

The hip and knee are frequently involved. Metatarsophalangeal joint subluxation may occur. Talonavicular joint inflammation causes pronation and eversion deformity, with overlying muscle spasm. A Baker's cyst due to posterior herniation of the joint capsule of the knee joint may occur, and require differentiation from a deep vein thrombosis by Doppler ultrasound. Entrapment of the posterior tibial nerve causes burning paraesthesiae on the sole of the foot.

Cervical spine

Cervical arthritis is common and may result in critical spinal problems from degeneration of the transverse ligament of the C1 vertebra that produces C1–2 instability in up to 5% of patients, and can result in cervical cord compression or vertebral artery insufficiency. In addition, decreased motion and myelopathy may result from longstanding joint involvement.

Extra-articular manifestations

The extra-articular manifestations of RA are protean, and may involve any organ system due to local inflammation causing functional or neurological deficits, rheumatoid vasculitis or distant inflammation. Patients may also present with the side effects of the treatment, including sepsis related to immunosuppression. Sepsis with encapsulated organisms is of particular concern in patients with Felty's syndrome of RA, neutropenia and splenomegaly.[11]

Investigations

Laboratory studies

Send blood for FBC and ELFTs and non-specific markers of inflammation such as ESR, and CRP, with assays for serum rheumatoid factor and anti-CCP.[12] Anti-CCP is less sensitive but more specific than rheumatoid factor for RA, and is more frequently positive early in the disease process. It is also thought to identify individuals at higher risk of erosive disease.[13] Send blood cultures as well as mid-stream urine for suspected sepsis.

Joint aspiration

Joint aspiration is essential to exclude co-existent or primary sepsis of any sudden hot, swollen joint.

Imaging

Initial plain imaging of affected joints at first presentation does not usually demonstrate erosive changes, but is useful in patients with longstanding disease. However, in any patient with any cervical or neurological features, always request plain X-rays of the cervical spine to look for an atlanto-dens interval of greater than 2.5 mm, which is diagnostic of instability.[14] Include a chest X-ray if there is a fever and/or any respiratory features. Request an ultrasound examination to differentiate deep vein thrombosis from a Baker's cyst.

Emergency management

The goals of emergency therapy are the relief of acute pain and reduction of joint inflammation. Longer term goals include restoration and maintenance of joint function, and the prevention of periarticular bony and cartilage destruction. Important principles include education, rest and exercise. Use non-steroidal anti-inflammatory drugs (NSAIDs), and the input of a multidisciplinary allied health team incorporating occupational therapy and physiotherapy.

Medication falls broadly under the categories of NSAIDs and disease-modifying anti-rheumatic drug (DMARD) therapy. Readers are referred to Chapter 14.1 for a brief overview of these medications and common adverse effects, as well as the references at the end of this chapter.[15-18]

Other long-term measures include orthopaedic and orthotic intervention. Surgery involving joint fusion, synovectomy, total joint arthroplasty and reconstruction may be required.

Early consultation with a rheumatologist is essential, particularly for patients with acute or first presentations. Exclusion of infection even for mild or moderate presentations is always imperative, and then to control symptoms with simple analgesics including NSAIDs and discharge for specialist follow-up. Admit patients if there is evidence of end-organ involvement, severe symptoms requiring nursing or allied health management, or if they are unable to tolerate oral therapies.

Prognosis[19,20]

The spontaneous remission rate in RA is less than 10%. High titres of rheumatoid factor, which is positive in up to 75% of cases or a high anti-CCP, the presence of nodules, and human leukocyte antigen (HLA)-DR4 haplotype are markers of severity. Overall, a patient's life expectancy is shortened by 10-15 years by infection, pulmonary and renal disease, and gastrointestinal bleeding.

SERONEGATIVE ARTHROPATHIES

The seronegative arthropathies are characterized by inflammation of the axial spine with sacroiliitis and spondylitis in particular, enthesopathy which is inflammation at the attachments of tendons and ligaments to bones, dactylitis, asymmetric polyarthritis, eye inflammation often of the lower limb and varied mucocutaneous features.[21] They are labelled 'seronegative' as serum rheumatoid factor is typically absent.

Epidemiology

The term 'seronegative arthropathies' covers conditions such as AS, reactive arthritis which occurs in the setting of viral or bacterial infection, psoriatic arthropathy and arthritis associated with IBD. The prevalence of the seronegative spondyloarthropathies varies widely, and is thought to parallel the prevalence of the HLA-B27 gene.

However, the exact role of HLA-B27 in the pathogenesis of the spondyloarthropathies has not been clearly defined. The proportion of HLA-B27 positive individuals who develop symptomatic arthropathy varies widely from 16% in patients with AS to 70% of patients with spondylitis in the setting of IBD.[22] HLA-B27 positive individuals may be less efficient at the intracellular removal of certain inciting bacteria, although this is controversial.[23]

Although diagnostic criteria exist for AS, they have yet to be validated for many of the other seronegative arthropathies. One of the problems is the late development of radiographic changes, particularly those of sacroiliitis. A useful set of criteria based on clinical findings, rather than on radiographic confirmation, has been developed by the European Spondyloarthropathy Study Group.[24]

Criteria for the classification of spondyloarthropathy[24]

Inflammatory spinal pain or synovitis (asymmetric, or predominantly lower limb), plus one or more of:

- positive family history
- psoriasis
- IBD
- alternate buttock pain
- enthesopathy
- sacroiliitis.

This discussion focuses on psoriatic arthropathy and reactive arthritis from among the conditions above.

RHEUMATOLOGY AND MUSCULOSKELETAL

PSORIATIC ARTHROPATHY

Psoriatic arthropathy is a heterogeneous disease with an identity distinct from other inflammatory arthritides. It occurs in 10% of patients with psoriasis, but may affect up to 40% of hospitalized psoriasis patients with widespread skin involvement.[25] It occurs between the ages of 30 years and 60 years, with an equal prevalence in males and females. It is thought to be inherited in a polygenic pattern that is significantly influenced by environmental factors including trauma and infectious agents. Multiple studies have confirmed the important role of class I HLA, particularly B13, B16 and B27 and certain C-subclasses.[26,27] The arthropathy pattern may be pauci-articular, but more than five peripheral joints are usually involved.

Diagnosis and clinical features

The diagnosis of psoriatic arthropathy is essentially clinical, requiring the demonstration of coexisting synovitis and psoriasis. A set of simple clinical diagnostic criteria (abbreviated to the CASPAR criteria) were recently proposed by a large international study group.[28]

The CASPAR diagnostic criteria for psoriatic arthropathy

Established inflammatory joint disease, and at least three points from the following features:

- current psoriasis (2 points)
- a history of psoriasis (in the absence of current psoriasis −1 point)
- a family history of psoriasis (in the absence of current or past history − 1 point)
- dactylitis (1 point)
- juxta-articular new bone formation (1 point)
- rheumatoid factor negativity (1 point)
- nail dystrophy (1 point).

Five clinical subtypes are recognized, including asymmetric oligoarthritis, symmetric small joint polyarthritis, predominant distal interphalangeal joint involvement, psoriatic spondyloarthropathy and arthritis mutilans.[29] Major extra-articular organ manifestations such as aortic insufficiency and pulmonary fibrosis occur rarely. However, up to 30% of patients have mild inflammation at the eye, most commonly conjunctivitis.

Asymmetric oligoarthritis

This occurs in 30–50% of patients.[30] It presents as an oligoarthritis involving a single large joint, in association with a 'sausage-shaped' or dactylitic digit or toe. Dactylitis occurs due to a combination of arthritis and tenosynovitis. Distal interphalangeal joint involvement is typical, and is almost invariably associated with psoriatic nail changes of pitting, ridging and onycholysis. Enthesopathy occurs most frequently with this form of the disease, and commonly manifests as plantar fasciitis or epicondylitis at the elbow.

Symmetric small joint polyarthritis

This occurs in 30% of patients, in a pattern strongly resembling RA, but with more frequent distal interphalangeal joint involvement.[30]

Psoriatic spondyloarthropathy

This occurs in 5% of patients.[30] It is often asymptomatic, but may present with inflammatory low back pain due to sacroiliitis in up to 30% of cases.

Arthritis mutilans

'Arthritis mutilans' is a rare (<5% of patients), but well-characterized feature of psoriatic arthritis, with severely deforming arthritis including telescoping of the fingers or toes from osteolysis of the metacarpal or metatarsal bones and phalanges.[30]

Dermatological features

Dermatological features include typical erythematous, scaling plaques on the extensor surfaces of the elbows and knees, scalp and ears, and nail changes. The nail changes include pitting with usually greater than 20 pits, ridging with transverse depressions, and onycholysis with separation of the nail from the underlying nail bed.[25] Nodules and vasculitic features such as digital ulcers do not occur.

Psoriatic arthritis can be difficult to distinguish from the other seronegative spondyloarthropathies in the absence of dermatological features or a positive family history.

Investigations

ESR and CRP are raised, but the rheumatoid factor and autoantibody screen are negative. Plain imaging studies of affected joints may reveal typical radiographic features, including soft tissue swelling, bone proliferation at the base of digital phalanges coupled with resorption of the distal tufts (the 'pencil-in-cup' deformity) and fluffy periostitis.[31] Chest radiographs are useful as a baseline when clinical examination suggests cardiac or pulmonary involvement.

Emergency and ongoing management

Emergency treatment involves the relief of pain and reduction of joint inflammation, with appropriate specialist follow-up. Education, rest and exercise, and referral to a multidisciplinary allied health team are the mainstay of ongoing management.

NSAIDs are useful for acute symptomatic relief, and intra- or peri-articular corticosteroids may be used for short-term relief of painful arthritis or enthesitis. Long-term therapy with disease modifying agents, such as sulphasalazine or methotrexate, is instituted at specialist review.[32] Oral corticosteroids are usually avoided, as their cessation often exacerbates the psoriasis. Therapy with tumour necrosis factor α antagonists[32] such as infliximab or etanercept has recently been approved to rheumatologists under strict access criteria for severe disease resistant to other DMARD therapy.

Emergency management of skin disease includes topical treatments such as emollients and keratolytic agents.[33] Phototherapy and photo-chemotherapy may be instituted on early dermatological consultation. Admit patients if their symptoms are severe enough to preclude oral therapy or safe discharge pending outpatient specialist follow-up.

Prognosis

Psoriatic arthropathy generally runs a more benign course than RA, but patients nonetheless suffer from considerable morbidity. Adverse prognostic factors include onset before 20 years of age, erosive disease and extensive skin involvement.[30]

REACTIVE ARTHRITIS

Reactive arthritis is aseptic peripheral arthritis following certain infections, which include bacterial infections of the urogenital tract usually by *Chlamydia trachomatis*, or of the gastrointestinal tract with organisms such as *Shigella*, *Salmonella* and *Campylobacter*. It may also follow viral infections such as HIV, although in the case of HIV, coinfection with sexually transmitted organisms rather than the virus itself is thought to cause the symptoms.[34] The seroconversion illness of HIV with its own constellation of articular symptoms is considered to be a separate entity.

Epidemiology

The prevalence of reactive arthritis has been difficult to define owing to diagnostic uncertainty particularly in the setting of asymptomatic sexually transmitted infection. The male preponderance is up to 9:1 following sexually transmitted infection, but males and females are equally affected following gastrointestinal tract infection.[35] The peak incidence is around the age of 35 years, and up to 75% of patients are HLA-B27 positive.[35] An important exception is with the reactive peripheral arthritis that occurs in 20% of patients with idiopathic IBD, a condition that may mimic gastrointestinal tract infection, but where patients are usually HLA-B27 negative.

Diagnosis and clinical features

The diagnosis of reactive arthritis is clinical. It typically manifests within a month of gastrointestinal or genitourinary infection, although the latter is frequently asymptomatic.[36] Musculoskeletal manifestations include myalgias and asymmetric polyarthritis affecting the knees, ankles and small joints of the feet in particular, although peripheral upper limb involvement is seen. Affected joints demonstrate marked inflammatory features with erythema, swelling, warmth and exquisite pain on active or passive movement. Fever and malaise are common.

Arthropathy and extra-articular manifestations

Symptomatic spondylitis and sacroiliitis cause low back and buttock pain and occur frequently. Dactylitis and enthesopathy are characteristic features of this disease with heel pain from plantar fasciitis or Achilles tendonitis.[36]

Extra-articular features associated with reactive arthritis include keratoderma blennorrhagicum; the scattered, thickened, hyperkeratotic skin lesions with pustules and crusts seen in Reiter syndrome, and circinate balanitis. An inflammatory aortitis occurs in 1% of patients and may result in aortic valvular incompetence, and/or heart block. Keratoderma blennorhagicum on the soles or palms may coalesce to form plaques virtually indistinguishable from those of psoriasis.[37] Circinate balanitis causes shallow meatal ulcers that are moist in uncircumcised men or hyperkeratotic and plaque-like in circumcised men.[37]

The peripheral arthritis associated with IBD is migratory and occurs in a similar distribution. Common features include large joint effusions, particularly involving the knee, and sacroiliitis or spondylitis.[38] Unlike peripheral arthritis following genitourinary infection, the spondylitis of IBD-associated arthropathy does not tend to settle with treatment of the bowel inflammation. Cutaneous features associated with this form of arthropathy occur mainly on the lower limbs, and include erythema nodosum and pyoderma gangrenosum.[38]

Investigations

Blood testing

An active inflammatory response is seen in the acute phase with a neutrophil leukocytosis and thrombocytosis, and raised ESR and CRP. The presence of a mild normochromic, normocytic anaemia suggests chronic disease. Send blood for HLA-B27.

Document the preceding genitourinary or gastrointestinal organism by stool culture or cervical/urethral swabs.[39] Rheumatoid factor and ANA are negative.

Joint aspiration

Joint aspiration may be necessary to exclude intra-articular sepsis (see Ch. 14.2). The synovial fluid may be turbid, viscous and with a neutrophil leukocytosis up to 50 000/mm^3, but Gram stain and bacterial culture are negative, and unlike true septic arthritis, the synovial glucose level is not significantly reduced compared to serum levels.[39] Macrophages with intracytoplasmic vacuoles containing ingested neutrophils are occasionally seen.

Radiography

Radiographic abnormalities are unusual with an acute arthritis, but are seen after several months. As with psoriatic arthropathy, a common finding is a 'fluffy' periosteal reaction, particularly at the calcaneus, and evidence of sacroiliitis or spondylitis with bridging syndesmophytes in longstanding disease.

Emergency and ongoing management

Exclude infection by synovial aspiration and culture for a markedly inflamed joint and early consultation with a rheumatologist, particularly in patients with a first presentation. Provide symptom relief with NSAIDs as the mainstay of emergency treatment. Corticosteroids may be given after rheumatological consultation, either systemic or topically for the skin manifestations. Disease modifying therapy with sulfasalazine may be initiated at specialist follow-up if NSAID therapy fails to control symptoms.

Give antibiotics such as doxycycline 100 mg orally bd for 7 days or azithromycin 1 g orally once for documented urethritis or cervicitis, and remember partner contact tracing and treatment. An infectious diseases opinion is useful in these cases.[39]

Admit patients with suspected septic arthritis until it is excluded, or if they are unable to tolerate simple oral therapies. Request a cardiology opinion for major cardiac involvement with valvular disease or a conduction abnormality, and a gastroenterology opinion when IBD is suspected, although the role of treatment and the effect on the arthropathy is unclear. Multidisciplinary physical therapy is essential on an outpatient basis.

Prognosis

Signs and symptoms usually remit within 6 months. However, up to 50% of patients suffer from recurrent arthritis, and up to 30% develop chronic arthropathy.[40] Post-dysenteric cases have a better prognosis than post-chlamydial cases. Poor prognostic signs include early onset under the age of 16 years, hip involvement and the presence of dactilytis.

POLYARTICULAR CRYSTAL ARTHROPATHY

Crystal-induced arthropathies result from the deposition of crystal in joint spaces, such as in gout or pseudogout. Both diseases cause debilitating joint inflammation resulting from the lysis of neutrophil polymorphs that have ingested monosodium urate in the case of gout or calcium pyrophosphate crystals in pseudogout. Although usually monoarticular, polyarticular involvement can occur in up to 5% of cases. See Chapter 14.2 for a detailed discussion of these diseases.

INFECTIOUS POLYARTHRITIS

Septic bacterial arthritis is most often monoarticular. However, it can present with polyarticular involvement. Infectious polyarthritis may occur as aseptic manifestation of certain viral infections, and following streptococcal infection as acute rheumatic fever (ARF).

Viral arthritis

Arthralgia affecting several joints is common in numerous viral infections, but few viruses cause frank polyarthritis. In general, these are self-limiting and managed symptomatically. Those viruses involved include alphaviruses such as the Ross River virus

(RRV), parvovirus B19 and hepatitis B and hepatitis C virus.

Alphaviruses

Alphaviruses are a mosquito-borne genus of the Togaviridae family. They are responsible for epidemics of febrile polyarthritis, including Ross River, Barmah Forest and Sindbis viruses in Australia, West Nile virus that has recently been documented in the USA, Chikungunya virus in East Africa, South and South-East Asia, O'nyong-nyong virus in East Africa and Mayaro virus in South America.[41]

Ross River virus

RRV is endemic to Australia, New Zealand and South Pacific islands, and is the most common arboviral disease in Australia. RRV is transmitted by the *Ochlerotatus* (formerly *Aedes*) *vigilex* mosquito via a marsupial reservoir.[42] Epidemics of acute febrile polyarthritis are most common between January and May, but can occur after periods of heavy rains.

Diagnosis and clinical features of Ross River virus

A detailed travel history is essential. There is usually low grade fever and other constitutional symptoms. A rash varying in distribution, character and duration occurs up to 2 weeks before, during or after the other symptoms. Polyarticular symptoms are present in most patients with a symmetric arthritis or arthralgia primarily affecting the wrist, knee, ankle and small joints of the extremities. Cervical lymphadenopathy occurs frequently, and paraesthesiae and tenderness of the palms and soles in a small percentage of cases.[43]

The diagnosis is predominantly clinical, particularly in endemic areas in the event of a local outbreak, and confirmed by serology.

Investigations

Serology for Ross River virus Serology testing distinguishes RRV from other causes of febrile polyarthritis such as Barmah Forest virus. A significant rise in IgM antibody titre to RRV indicates acute infection, or the virus itself may be isolated from the serum of acutely unwell patients. Radiographs are

unremarkable and uneconomic as the disease is largely self-limiting.[44]

Emergency and ongoing management

Patients with RRV require symptomatic treatment with simple analgesics or NSAIDs. Occasionally, a brief course of low-dose prednisolone may be used. RRV is a notifiable disease.[42] Conventional personal preventative measures such as protective clothing, effective mosquito repellent and avoidance of mosquito-prone areas should be recommended, as no vaccine currently exists. Refer to a rheumatologist if symptoms are severe or refractory to simple treatment measures.

Prognosis of Ross River virus infection

The illness is usually self-limiting, but prolonged symptoms may occur, and there may be relapses of decreasing intensity, separated by remissions, for up to a year or more.

Parvovirus B19

Human parvovirus B19 infection is caused by a small, single-stranded DNA virus that has a predilection for erythroid precursor cells and is transmitted by respiratory secretions. It causes the self-limiting illness *Erythema infectiosum* or 'slapped cheek disease' or 'fifth disease' in children. In adults, however, parvovirus B19 manifests with severe flu-like symptoms, and as many as 75% develop joint symptoms. It may be responsible for up to 12% of adult patients presenting with acute polyarthritis, most notably in those who have frequent exposure to children.[45]

Diagnosis and clinical features

The characteristic rash is usually absent in adults. An acute polyarthritis improves over 2 weeks, with symmetric involvement of peripheral small joints, including the hands (proximal interphalangeal and metacarpophalangeal joints in particular), wrists, knees and ankle joints. Morning stiffness is a prominent feature. These features are similar to those seen in patients with RA, and in fact up to 50% of affected patients meet the ACR diagnostic criteria for RA.[46] Uncommon but important extra-articular features of parvovirus B19 infection are detailed below.[47]

Extra-articular features of parvovirus

- Development of an aplastic crisis in patients with chronic haemolytic anaemia.
- Bone marrow suppression in immunocompromised patients.
- *Hydrops foetalis* in women infected during pregnancy.
- Henoch–Schönlein purpura.
- Thrombotic thrombocytopenic purpura.
- Wegener's granulomatosis or polyarteritis nodosa (rare).

Investigations

Always send an FBC, particularly given the potential for an aplastic crisis and bone marrow suppression. Non-specific markers of inflammation are likely to be elevated. Specific serological diagnosis is made by demonstrating high IgM antibody titres specific to the virus, and by isolation of the viral DNA by polymerase chain reaction (PCR). IgG antibodies to parvovirus B19 indicate past infection and are common in the adult population.[48]

Transient, moderate elevations of rheumatoid factor, anti-DNA, antilymphocyte or anticardiolipin antibodies sometimes occur.[48] Radiographs of the affected joints are normal.

Emergency and ongoing management

Rest and NSAIDs are the mainstay of emergency treatment, except in pregnant women, as NSAIDs are contraindicated in the third trimester.[49] A short course of prednisolone may be required. Significant extra-articular manifestations may require admission and consultation with the appropriate specialist. Blood transfusion or intravenous immunoglobulin infusions may be necessary.

Prognosis

Joint symptoms are self-limited in the majority of adult patients, but up to 10% may have prolonged relapsing and remitting symptoms lasting up to 9 years.[50]

Hepatitis B and Hepatitis C Viruses

The common hepatitis viruses A, B and C all cause viral polyarthritis. Hepatitis B virus (HBV) is responsible for 20–25%, and hepatitis A (HAV) up to 14% of causes in patients with viral polyarthritis.[51] The polyarthritis of HAV tends to occur during the infectious phase, and is self-limiting. The polyarthritis of HBV occurs in early infection during a period of significant viraemia, and is thought to be due to immune complexes.

Diagnosis and clinical features

HBV polyarthritis is acute and severe, and manifests in a symmetric, migratory or additive fashion most commonly involving the hand and knee joints.[52] Other large axial joints may be involved, and significant early morning stiffness is often present. The arthritis may precede the development of jaundice, and persist for several weeks after jaundice has developed.

Hepatitis C virus (HCV) polyarthritis is rapidly progressive and symmetrical, involving the hands, wrists, shoulders, knees and hips.[53] Carpal tunnel syndrome and tenosynovitis may occur. It is unusual for polyarthritis to be the first manifestation of the underlying disease in either HBV or HCV. Nonetheless, ask about exposure risk factors for these viruses such as intravenous drug abuse, unprotected sexual intercourse, past blood transfusions, tattoos, as well as about previous jaundice. Both hepatitis B and hepatitis C disease are associated with a number of important extra-articular, extra-hepatic manifestations.

Extra-articular, extra-hepatic manifestations

- HBV: polyarteritis nodosa, systemic necrotizing vasculitis, membranous glomerulonephritis.[54]
- HCV: mixed cryoglobulinaemia causing palpable purpura, arthritis and serum cryoglobulinaemia with cutaneous phenomena such as Raynaud's syndrome and digital ulcers, and membranous glomerulonephritis.[53,55]

Investigations

Blood testing

Send blood for ELFTs for evidence of raised transaminases with elevated bilirubin, hepatitis B surface antigen; antihepatitis B surface antigen IgM to indicate acute infection and/or viral DNA quantification by PCR. Check also for anti-HCV IgM and for viral DNA quantification by PCR.

Also check FBC and for ESR, CRP, cryogobulins and rheumatoid factor in the presence of a rash, ulcers or other vasculitic phenomena. Radiographs are normal other than showing soft tissue swelling.

Emergency and ongoing management

Commence symptomatic treatment of the polyarthritis with NSAIDs in the emergency department. Refer refractory HBV- or HCV-associated polyarthritis to a rheumatology specialist and/or combined hepatology clinic. Disease modifying agents such as prednisolone and sulphasalazine may be used cautiously with careful monitoring of the liver function tests and for increasing viraemia.[56]

Prognosis

The prognosis varies depending on the treatment of the underlying disease and on the presence of vasculitic phenomena. The polyarthritis of HBV is usually limited to the pre-icteric phase, but patients with chronic active hepatitis or chronic HBV viraemia may have recurrent arthritis.

RHEUMATIC FEVER

Acute rheumatic fever (ARF) refers to a constellation of non-infectious symptoms occurring after a pharyngeal infection with group A streptococci (GAS). Anecdotal evidence suggests that it may also occur in high-risk populations following skin infections with GAS.[57]

Epidemiology

ARF is characterized by inflammation of connective tissue including the joints, subcutaneous tissue, heart and blood vessels. Its prevalence has declined over time in developed countries, but it remains a major public health problem in developing countries, and in the more socially isolated parts of Australasia. The highest documented rates in the world occur in the Aboriginal Australian population and Torres Strait Islander populations of New Zealand and the Pacific Islands.[58]

ARF is primarily a disease of children aged 5–14 years. The annual incidence may reach 350 per 100 000 in Aboriginal children.[59] However, the polyarthritis of ARF is most commonly seen in adolescents and young adults.

Diagnosis and clinical features

The diagnosis of ARF worldwide is made on the 1944 Jones or more recently World Health Organization major and minor criteria. However, these criteria appear too restrictive for diagnosing ARF in Australian indigenous populations. Therefore, new criteria for use in high- and low-risk populations in Australia have been proposed (see Table 14.3.2).[60]

The polyarthritis of ARF is usually the earliest symptom of the disease, and is classically described as migratory affecting several joints in quick succession for a short time, commencing with the large joints of the lower limb then the large joints of the upper limb.[61] Affected joints are painful but objective signs of inflammation such as erythema and swelling are not prominent.

Fever and constitutional symptoms are common. Other important extra-articular major criteria (with polyarthritis) of the disease include the following.[61]

Major criteria (with polyarthritis) of acute rheumatic fever

- Carditis: symptomatic pericarditis with pain and/or congestive cardiac failure with breathlessness, new murmurs, cardiomegaly, electrocardiographic evidence of heart block.
- Sydenham's chorea (St Vitus' dance): choreiform movements particularly of the face and upper limbs, emotional lability, rarely transient psychosis.
- Subcutaneous Aschoff nodules: firm, painless, mobile nodules near bony prominences on the extensor surfaces of wrists, elbows and knees.
- Rash (*Erythema marginatum*): occurs in around 5% of ARF. It consists of

blanching ring-like pink macules with a serpiginous edge and central clear portion occurring on the trunk and inner surfaces of the arms and legs, which are not itchy and can come and go for months. They may be slightly raised, but spare the face. The rash may change from hour to hour and may seem to appear, disappear or move rapidly in front of you. It is exacerbated by heat and fades when the patient is cool.

Investigations

Measure antistreptolysin O and antideoxyribonuclease B (anti-DNase B) titres.[61] As these titres can take 6 weeks after infection to peak, interpretation in the acute phase should be cautious, and serial tests should be performed. Note that anti-streptococcal antibody titres are useful in low-risk populations, but are difficult to interpret in high-risk populations due to pre-existing high background titres.[62] Send a throat swab, although this is positive in less than 10% of high-risk populations. Other important tests include:

- ESR and CRP, which are almost invariably elevated
- FBC, which may demonstrate a leukocytosis and less commonly, a normochromic, normocytic anaemia
- electrocardiography to document the P-R interval
- chest X-ray to look for cardiomegaly or symptomatic cardiac failure.

Synovial fluid aspirate is usually inflammatory with an elevated white cell count, and sterile on microscopy and culture. Radiographs of affected joints generally demonstrate soft tissue swelling only.

Emergency and ongoing management

Emergency management of ARF depends on making the diagnosis, and treating the manifestations. Patients are severely symptomatic, and often require admission for initial observation and management. Request

Table 14.3.2	2005 Australian guidelines for the diagnosis of acute rheumatic fever	
	High-risk groups	*All other groups*
Initial episode of ARF	Two major **or** one major and two minor manifestations plus evidence of a preceding GAS infection	Two major **or** one major and two minor manifestations plus evidence of a preceding GAS infection
Recurrent attack of ARF in a patient with known past ARF or RHD	Two major **or** one major and two minor **or** three minor manifestations plus evidence of a preceding GAS infection	Two major **or** one major and two minor **or** three minor manifestations plus evidence of a preceding GAS infection
Major manifestations	• Carditis, including subclinical evidence of rheumatic valve disease on echocardiogram • Polyarthritis **or** aseptic monoarthritis **or** polyarthralgia • Chorea • *Erythema marginatum* • Subcutaneous nodules	• Carditis, excluding subclinical evidence of rheumatic valve disease on echocardiogram • Polyarthritis • Chorea • *Erythema marginatum* • Subcutaneous nodules

ARF, acute rheumatic fever; GAS, group A streptococci; RHD, rheumatic heart disease.

rheumatology and infectious diseases opinions and a neurology opinion if chorea is troublesome. The presence of heart block or, more importantly, frank cardiac failure or acute valvular regurgitation mandate cardiac admission.

The polyarthritis of rheumatic fever is exquisitely responsive to NSAID therapy, particularly aspirin, so much so that failure of NSAID therapy to rapidly relieve symptoms should prompt consideration of an alternative diagnosis.[63] Give aspirin at doses of 80–100 mg/kg/day in 4–5 divided doses in adults, usually for 1 to 2 weeks.[64]

Commence antibiotic therapy with phenoxymethylpenicillin 10 mg/kg up to 500 mg orally 12-hourly for 10 days to eradicate streptococcal pharyngitis as soon as possible, after obtaining appropriate diagnostic investigations as detailed above. Commence prophylaxis following resolution of the acute episode in high-risk indigenous communities. Ongoing rheumatology and infectious diseases specialist follow-up is recommended. Note that penicillin reduces the frequency and severity of post-streptococcal rheumatic fever, but has little effect on the course of immune-complex mediated post-streptococcal glomerulonephritis.

Prognosis

Recurrence of ARF commonly occurs within 2 years of the initial attack, despite prophylactic therapy. Most affected connective tissues do not sustain long-lasting damage, with the exception of the heart, which is prone to additive subclinical damage resulting in rheumatic heart disease.[65]

Controversies

❶ Role of DMARD therapy in the various causes of acute polyarthropathy.

❷ The exact role of HLA-B27 in the pathogenesis of the spondyloarthropathies.

❸ Pathogenetic mechanisms leading to reactive arthropathy.

References

1. Klinkhoff A. Rheumatology: 5. Diagnosis and management of inflammatory polyarthritis. Canadian Medical Association Journal 2000; 162: 1833–1838.
2. Pinals RS. Polyarthritis and fever. New England Journal of Medicine 1994; 330: 769.
3. Richie A, Francis M. Diagnostic approach to polyarticular joint pain. American Family Physcian 2003; 68(6): 1075–1088.
4. Talley NJ, O'Connor S. The rheumatological system. In: Talley NJ, O'Connor S, eds. Clinical examination: a systematic guide to physical diagnosis. 5th edn. Sydney: Churchill Livingstone.
5. Woolf SH, Kamerow DB. Testing for uncommon conditions. The heroic search for positive test results. Archives of Internal Medicine 1990; 150: 2451–2058.
6. Rindfleisch JA, Muller D. Diagnosis and management of rheumatoid arthritis. American Family Physician 2005; 72(6): 1037–1047.
7. Arnett FC, Edworthy SM, Bloch DA, et al. The American Rheumatism Association 1987 revised criteria for the classification of rheumatoid arthritis. Arthritis and Rheumatism 1988; 31: 315–324.
8. Rindfleisch JA, Muller D. Diagnosis and management of rheumatoid arthritis. American Family Physician 2005; 72(6): 1037–1047.
9. Scott DL. Rheumatoid arthritis: acute presentations and urgent complications. British Journal of Hospital Medicine 2006; 67(5): 235–239.
10. Tutuncu Z, Kavanaugh A. Rheumatic disease in the elderly: rheumatoid arthritis. Rheumatic Diseases Clinics of North America 2007; 33(1): 57–70.
11. Balint GP, Balint PV. Felty's syndrome. Best Practices and Research Clinics Rheumatology 2004; 18(5): 631–645.
12. Westwood OM, Nelson PN, Hay FC. Rheumatoid factors: what's new? Rheumatology 2006; 45: 379–385.
13. American College of Rheumatology. The use of anti-cyclic citrullinated peptide (anti-CCP) antibodies in RA. 2003. http://www.rheumatology.org/publications/hotline/1003anticcp.asp (accessed August 2008).
14. Macarthur A, Kleiman S. Rheumatoid cervical joint disease – a challenge to the anaesthetist. Canadian Journal of Anaesthesia 1993; 40(2): 154–159.
15. Emery P. Treatment of rheumatoid arthritis. British Medical Journal 2006; 332(7534): 152–155.
16. O'Dell JR. Therapeutic strategies for rheumatoid arthritis. New England Journal of Medicine 2004; 350 (25): 2591–2602.
17. Strand V, Hochberg MC. The risk of cardiovascular thrombotic events with selective cyclooxygenase-2 inhibitors. Arthritis and Rheumatism 2002; 47: 349–355.
18. Olsen NJ, Stein CM. New drugs for rheumatoid arthritis. New England Journal of Medicine 2004; 350: 2167–2179.
19. Alarcon GS. Predictive factors in rheumatoid arthritis. American Journal of Medicine 1997; 103(6A): 19S–24S.
20. Wagner U, Kaltenhauser S, Sauer H, et al. HLA markers and prediction of clinical course and outcome in rheumatoid arthritis. Arthritis and Rheumatism 1997; 40(2): 341–351.
21. Young JL, Smith L, Matyszak MK. HLA-B27 Expression does not modulate intracellular Chlamydia trachomatis infection of cell lines. Infection and Immunity 2001; 69 (11): 6670–6675.
22. Dougados M, van der Linden S, Juhlin R, et al. The European Spondylarthropathy Study Group preliminary criteria for the classification of spondylarthropathy. Arthritis and Rheumatism 1991; 34(10): 1218–1227.
25. Myers WA, Gottlieb AB, Mease P. Psoriasis and psoriatic arthritis: clinical features and disease mechanisms. Clinics in Dermatology 2006; 24(5): 438–447.
26. Eastmond CJ. Psoriatic arthritis. Genetics and HLA antigens. Baillières Clinical Rheumatology 1994; 8(2): 263–276.
27. Espinoza LR, van Solingen R, Cuellar ML, et al. Insights into the pathogenesis of psoriasis and psoriatic arthritis. American Journal of Medical Science 1998; 316(4): 271–276.
28. Taylor W, Gladman D, Helliwell P. Classification criteria for psoriatic arthritis: development of new criteria from a large international study. Arthritis and Rheumatism 2006; 54(8): 2665–2673.
29. Cuellar ML, Silveira LH, Espinoza LR. Recent developments in psoriatic arthritis. Current Opinion of Rheumatology 1994; 6(4): 378–384.
30. Mease P, Goff BS. Diagnosis and treatment of psoriatic arthropathy. Journal of the American Academy of Dermatology 2005; 52(1): 1–19.
31. Ory PA, Gladman DD, Mease PJ. Psoriatic arthritis and imaging. Annals of Rheumatic Diseases 2005; 2(64 suppl): ii55–ii57.
32. Mease P. Management of psoriatic arthritis: the therapeutic interface between rheumatology and dermatology. Current Rheumatology Reports 2006; 8(5): 348–354.
33. Menter A, Griffiths CE. Current and future management of psoriasis. Lancet 2007; 370(9583): 272–284.
34. Hamdulay SS, Glynne SJ, Keat A. When is arthritis reactive? Postgraduates in Medicine Journal 2006; 82(969): 446–453.
35. Toivanen A, Toivanen P. Reactive arthritis. Best practice and research. Clinical Rheumatology 2004; 18(5): 689–703.
36. Amor B. Reiter's syndrome. Diagnosis and clinical features. Rheumatic Diseases Clinics of North America 1998; 24(4): 677–695.
37. Angulo J, Espinoza LR. The spectrum of skin, mucosa and other extra-articular manifestations. Baillières Clinical Rheumatology 1998; 12(4): 649–664.
38. Holden W, Orchard T, Wordsworth P. Enteropathic arthritis. Rheumatic Diseases Clinics of North America 2003; 29(3): 513–530, viii.
39. Petersel DL, Sigal LH. Reactive arthritis. Infectious Disease Clinics of North America 2005; 19(4): 863–883.
40. Colmegna I, Espinoza LR. Recent advances in reactive arthritis. Current Rheumatological Reports 2005; 7(3): 201–207.
41. Suhrbier A, La Linn M. Clinical and pathologic aspects of arthritis due to Ross River virus and other alphaviruses. Current Opinion in Rheumatology 2004; 16(4): 374–379.
42. Ross River virus infection Factsheet. Australian Government Department of Health and Ageing, May 2004. http://www.health.gov.au/ (accessed August 2008).
43. Mylonas AD, Brown AM, Carthew TL, et al. Natural history of Ross River virus-induced epidemic polyarthritis. Medical Journal of Australia 2002; 177(7): 356–360.
44. Cheong IR. Ross River virus: are we wasting money doing tests ? Medical Journal of Australia 2003; 178(3): 143.
45. Servey JT, Reamy BV, Hodge J. Clinical presentations of parvovirus B19 infection. American Family Physician 2007; 75(3): 373–376.
46. Naides SJ, Scharosch LL, Foto F, et al. Rheumatologic manifestations of human parvovirus B19 infection in adults. Initial 2-year clinical experience. Arthritis and Rheumatism 1990; 31: 1297–1309.
47. Calabrese LH, Naides SJ. Viral arthritis. Infectious Disease Clinics of North America 2005; 19(4): 963–980, x.
48. Moore TL. Parvovirus-associated arthritis. Current Opinion in Rheumatology 2000; 12(4): 289–294.
49. Jacqz-Aigrain E, Koren G. Effects of drugs on the fetus. Seminars in Fetal and Neonatal Medicine 2005; 10(2): 139–147. Epub 2005 Jan 25.
50. Broliden K, Tolfvenstam T, Norbeck O. Clinical aspects of parvovirus B19 infection. Journal of Internal Medicine 2006; 260(4): 285–304.
51. Franssila R, Hedman K. Infection and musculoskeletal conditions: viral causes of arthritis. Best Practices and Research Clinics of Rheumatology 2006; 20(6): 1139–1157.
52. Chi ZC, Ma SZ. Rheumatologic manifestations of hepatic diseases. Hepatobiliary and Pancreat Diseases International 2003; 2(1): 32–37.
53. Sanzone AM, Bégué RE. Hepatitis C and arthritis: an update. Infectious Disease Clinics of North America 2006; 20(4): 877–889, vii.
54. Farrell GC, Teoh NC. Management of chronic hepatitis B virus infection: a new era of disease control. International Medicine Journal 2006; 36(2): 100–113.

55. Hoofnagle JH. Course and outcome of hepatitis C. Hepatology 2002; 36(5 Suppl 1): S21–S29.
56. Ramos-Casals M, Trejo O, García-Carrasco M. Therapeutic management of extrahepatic manifestations in patients with chronic hepatitis C virus infection. Rheumatology (Oxford) 2003; 42(7): 818–828. Epub 2003 Apr 16.
57. McDonald M, Currie B, Carapetis J. Acute rheumatic fever: a chink in the chain that links the heart to the throat? Lancet Infectious Diseases 2004; 4: 240–245.
58. Carapetis JR, et al. The global burden of group A streptococcal diseases. Lancet Infectious Diseases 2005; 5: 685–694.

59. Australian Institute of Health and Welfare. Rheumatic heart disease in Australia – all but forgotten except in Aboriginal and Torres Strait Islander peoples. Canberra: AIHW; 2004.
60. National Heart Foundation of Australia (RF/RHD guideline development working group) and the Cardiac Society of Australia and New Zealand. Diagnosis and management of acute rheumatic fever and rheumatic heart disease in Australia – an evidence based review. National Heart Foundation of Australia; 2006: 6–24. http://www.heartfoundation.org.au/Professional_Information/Clinical_Practice/ARF_RHD.html (accessed August 2008).

61. Carapetis JR, McDonald M, Wilson NJ. Acute rheumatic fever. Lancet 2005; 366(9480): 155–168.
62. Nimmo GR, Tinniswood RD, Nuttall N, et al. Group A streptococcal infection in an Aboriginal community. Medical Journal of Australia 1992; 156: 537–540.
63. Cilliers AM. Rheumatic fever and its management. British Medical Journal 2006; 333(7579): 1153–1156.
64. Thatai D, Turi DG. Current guidelines for the treatment of acute rheumatic fever. Drugs 1999; 57: 545–555.
65. Figueroa FE, Fernández MS, Valdés P. Prospective comparison of clinical and echocardiographic diagnosis of rheumatic carditis: long term follow-up of patients with subclinical disease. Heart 2001; 85(4): 407–410.

14.4 Musculoskeletal and soft tissue emergencies

Anthony Tzannes • Anthony F. T. Brown

ESSENTIALS

1 Soft tissue injuries may be as debilitating and painful, and take longer to heal, than fractures in the same area.

2 The mechanism of injury and biomechanics predict the soft tissue damage caused.

3 The so-called 'minor injury' can be associated with significant and prolonged morbidity that could be permanent if managed incorrectly. Adopting a careful, consistent approach that considers potential pitfalls is important to patient outcome.

4 Exclude potentially serious causes of back pain 'red flags' prior to discharging any patient with this presentation.

Common causes of soft tissue injuries

One way of classifying soft tissue injuries is to consider the mechanism of the trauma, with certain types of trauma noted due to specific management concerns.

Trauma

- Penetrating:
  - puncture
  - incised.
- Blunt (direct tissue injury from overload of anatomic structures):
  - acute:
    - disruption designated by tissue type e.g. fracture in bony injury

  - crush injury
  - shear (degloving):
    - open
    - closed
- chronic:
  - designated and graded by the tissue involved and the extent.

Many of the types of trauma above are covered in other chapters.

General evaluation of a soft tissue injury

Assessment

History

Obtain a history of:

- the nature of the injury, and when, where and how it was sustained with specific attention to the forces involved
- the possibility of a foreign body, wound contamination and damage to deeper structures
- patient function following the injury
- pain associated with the injury, including time course, nature and aggravating factors/actions
- any crush or shear injury
- current medical conditions and drug therapy
- allergies and tetanus immunization status.

Examination

Examine nerves and tendons for evidence of damage, *before* infiltrating with local anaesthetic.

Send the patient for X-rays if a radio-opaque foreign body such as metal or glass is suspected, *before* exploring a wound. Inform the radiographer the nature of the foreign body.

Specific issues with a possible chronic overload injury

- Change in activity/equipment or sudden change in load.
- At what point of activity the pain is felt (before, during, after or a combination).
- History of prior similar injury.

Puncture injuries

Clinical evaluation

This type of injury is caused by stepping on a nail or pin, penetration by a sewing machine needle, or industrial equipment such as a nail gun, high pressure hose or gun. Needlestick and sharps incidents are covered in Chapter 9.10.

Management

Refer all high-pressure gun injuries such as from paint or oil immediately to the appropriate surgical team, even if no apparent damage is seen initially. They will require extensive wound debridement and tissue plane cleaning, however innocuous they seem.

Otherwise, clean the wound with antiseptic and evaluate the need for tetanus prophylaxis and antibiotics. Treat a rusty nail injury to the foot by soaking in iodine in alcohol for 30 min and give amoxicillin 500 mg and clavulanic acid 125 mg one tablet orally tds for 5 days. Instruct the patient to return immediately if signs of infection or gross oedema supervene.

Pretibial lacerations

These are most common in elderly patients, often from trivial trauma tearing a flap of skin, particularly if taking steroids. Ask about general mobility and safety issues at home.

Management

Clean the wound, remove blood clots, trim obviously necrotic tissue and unfurl the rolled edges of the wound to determine actual skin loss. Refer the patient immediately to the orthopaedic or plastic surgery team for consideration of early skin grafting if there is significant skin loss or marked skin retraction preventing alignment of the skin edges.

Otherwise, lay the flap back over the wound and hold in place with adhesive skin-closure strips (Steristrips™). Cover the wound with a single layer of paraffin-impregnated gauze and a cotton-wool and gauze combine pad. Then apply a firm crêpe bandage and instruct the patient to keep the leg elevated whenever possible. Enquire about tetanus immunization status.

Arrange for review and dressing change within 5 days, or earlier if blood or serum has seeped through the wound dressing known as 'strike-through', as there is now an increased risk of secondary infection.

Expect the wound edges to heal by granulation tissue and new epidermal tissue laid down at the rate of approximately 1 mm per week. Refer the patient to the orthopaedic or plastic surgery team at this point, if healing is clearly not occurring. Otherwise, arrange follow-up with the GP, plus community nurse input as necessary.

Acute mechanical overload injuries

These include fractures, ligament sprains, muscle strains or tears and tendon ruptures. Many are covered in Section 4.

Classification of ligament sprains/muscle strains

Grade I Small number of fibres injured, with pain on stressing, but no laxity or loss of strength.

Grade II Significant number of fibres injured with laxity and or weakness and pain on stressing.

Grade III Complete tear with gross laxity and no strength.

Management

General principles

The initial management principles are the same for both and include rest, ice, compression and elevation (RICE) and analgesia, usually with a combination of paracetamol 1 g orally qid, plus a non-steroidal anti-inflammatory drug (NSAID) such as ibuprofen 400 mg orally tds (in the absence of significant asthma, peptic ulcer disease and renal impairment).

Ligament sprains

Ligament sprains that are grade I or II are managed with a protective brace or strapping and reduction of, but not cessation of physical activity. Consider grade III sprains for immobilization with a splint or plaster of Paris (POP) cast and/or operative repair if there is gross instability, and warn the patient that they may take up to 3 months or longer to heal. This is of particular relevance to the manual labourer and high-level athlete, although the latter usually has excellent access to physiotherapy and a formulated rehabilitation plan.

Muscle strains

Muscle strains require initial minimization of bruising and haematoma formation by RICE followed by graded return to activity. Physiotherapy may help improve return of function and prevent re-injury, although research is surprisingly limited. Consider complete muscle tears, especially in active individuals, for operative repair, and refer to an orthopaedic specialist. Assess the functional limitations imposed by these injuries, particularly in patients who live alone and or who are elderly and infirm, as loss of independence is likely. Consider the need for community services, respite care or admission until they are able to look after themselves again.

Tendon ruptures

Evaluation Acute rupture of the supraspinatus tendon, long head of biceps and Achilles tendon are the most common injuries. The extent of the rupture may be complete or partial. Injury may be secondary to an acute event or chronic overload that is often asymptomatic until a tear occurs.

Management Request an ultrasound to confirm the diagnosis, although magnetic resonance imaging (MRI) is equally or more sensitive and specific depending on which tendons are being imaged, although clearly much less readily available.

Treatment is aimed at the earliest return to normal function, with least likelihood of recurrence. Refer complete tears, particularly in active people, for orthopaedic surgery repair. Manage partial tears conservatively, but they too may have a better outcome if repaired surgically, depending on surgical availability and local hospital guidelines.

Degloving injuries

Evaluation

Degloving injuries are caused by either a shearing or traction force on skin, causing it to be torn from its capillary blood supply. When the skin tears and actually peels off it leaves an obvious exposed open injury.

Closed degloving injuries are harder to diagnose and may only lead to the skin feeling slightly less tethered than prior to injury, a failure to blanch with pressure, poor capillary return and most importantly altered cutaneous sensation. This is most easily and accurately assessed by 2-point discrimination. If 2-point discrimination is normal, a significant degloving injury has not occurred. Pain may or may not be prominent, and/or may relate to an underlying bony injury.

Management

Arrange specialist assessment and admission for all degloving injuries by the appropriate surgical team, usually orthopaedic and or plastic surgery. Keep any degloved skin available, as it may be used as a skin graft.

Do *not* be tempted to simply replace the skin into its original position and hold it there with sutures or adhesive skin-closure strips (Steristrips™) as this is inadequate. Degloving injuries are also considered as a high-risk wound for tetanus.

Chronic overload (overuse) injuries

Few of these injuries require emergency treatment. However, a general knowledge of these conditions is worthwhile. They develop wherever tissue microtrauma occurs at a rate that exceeds the body's ability to heal.

Classification

Bony overuse injuries follow a continuum from pain on activity only, through local tenderness, to pain at rest, and loss of function. Many will have led to a stress fracture by the time of presentation to an emergency department (ED).

Other overuse injuries are classified by tissue type and the extent of injury, and are often best diagnosed by the timing of the pain in relation to physical activity. They are further classified by the presence or absence of inflammation.

Classification of chronic overuse syndromes
Grade I   Pain after activity
Grade II Pain early on and after activity; activity not limited
Grade III Pain throughout activity, which is limited
Grade IV Pain at rest.

Management

Most chronic overuse injuries are managed with a decrease in activity and NSAIDs. Arrange referral to a physiotherapist or specialty physician as appropriate. Tendon-related injuries sometimes require a steroid injection, which should only be performed by doctors trained in the technique such as orthopaedic specialists, rheumatologists or sports physicians. Specific examples of chronic overuse syndromes with their management follow.

Stress fractures that require active specialist management
- Pars interarticularis causing low-back pain in adolescent athletes
- Femoral neck
- Mid-tibia
- Foot or ankle
  - talus
  - calcaneus
  - navicular
  - metatarsal base second or fifth toe
  - sesamoid bone of hallux.

Pars interarticularis

Diagnosis
The defect with a pars interarticularis stress injury represents a fatigue fracture caused by repetitive loading and unloading of this region of the vertebrae from physical activity, with progression through spondylolysis to spondylolisthesis, particularly in adolescents. Unilateral low-back pain occurs, worse on extension.

Those most at risk perform repeated hyperextension and or twisting movements such as female gymnasts in particular, ballet dancers and fast bowlers.

Management
The diagnosis is best made on MRI or computerized tomography (CT), but changes will be seen on plain X-ray and be confirmed by a bone scan. Treatment is primarily by understanding the mechanism, avoiding unnecessary movements and the use of a brace worn for 6–12 weeks to prevent hyperextension. The patient will then require core stability re-training under the guidance of a sports physiotherapist to minimize the risk of re-injury or chronic back pain.

Femoral neck

Diagnosis and management
Femoral neck stress fracture causes vague thigh or groin pain of insidious onset, worse on weight bearing, particularly with an increase in activity or loading, for instance in distance runners or athletes that do repeated jumping.

X-ray is often normal, so diagnosis usually requires a bone scan or MRI. Fractures that are greater than 50% of the femoral neck diameter are referred for operative fixation, otherwise a decrease in physical activity for at least 6 weeks is recommended to allow healing.

Anterior cortex of mid-tibia

Diagnosis and management
Stress fracture of the anterior cortex of the mid-tibial region causes progressive anterior leg pain – which is worse with and immediately following activity – most often in distance runners and ballet dancers.

A plain X-ray may show a line through the anterior cortex, often with cortical thickening as an early sign. Initial management is to decrease activity, and to refer patients for a bone scan as an outpatient. This is in part to determine if non-union has occurred, as these injuries often fail to heal or may progress to a complete fracture, which requires an intramedullary nail.

Talus

Diagnosis and management
Stress fracture of the talus is most common in pole vaulters, or in a person with a fall from a height, particularly if they have excessive foot pronation. It presents as foot or ankle pain that is worse with weight bearing and shock loading. On examination there may be tenderness over the mid-talus or localized swelling from a joint effusion.

X-ray is usually normal, but the diagnosis may be made on a bone scan, CT scan or MRI. Arrange for a non-weight bearing POP cast for 6 weeks, with referral to an orthopaedic specialist.

Calcaneus

Diagnosis and management

Stress fracture of the calcaneus causes the insidious onset heel pain, which is worse with weight bearing and is tender on lateral compression of the heel. It is most common in distance runners or in the military related to marching. X-ray is occasionally abnormal, but otherwise the diagnosis is made on a bone scan, CT scan or MRI. Arrange for a non-weight bearing POP cast for 6 weeks and referral to an orthopaedic specialist.

Navicular

Diagnosis and classification

Stress fracture of the navicular presents as vague mid-foot pain that radiates to the medial arch, with point tenderness over the navicular. This bone is best found by following the tendon of tibialis anterior during dorsiflexion.

Classification is grade I with a dorsal cortical break only, grade II with a fracture that propagates to the body and grade III with a fracture that extends to another cortex. Grade I and II stress fractures of the navicular usually have a normal X-ray, and require a bone scan, CT or MRI to confirm the diagnosis.

Management

Arrange for a non-weight bearing POP cast for 6–8 weeks, with referral to an orthopaedic specialist for follow-up with a repeat bone scan to assess the degree of healing.

Metatarsal

Diagnosis

Stress fracture of a metatarsal is most common in ballet dancers. Two fractures in particular require aggressive management. These are at the base of second metatarsal, which presents as forefoot pain on exercise, and the transverse fracture at the base of the fifth metatarsal, known as Jones fracture. This presents as mid-foot pain with activity. Both are diagnosed with X-ray and/or with a bone scan.

Management

A stress fracture at the base of second metatarsal requires non-weight bearing on crutches for 4–6 weeks. The Jones fracture of the base of the fifth metatarsal is managed with a non-weight bearing plaster of Paris cast (POP) for 6 weeks, or directly with open reduction and internal fixation particularly in the athlete, as non-union is common.

Sesamoid bone of the hallux

Diagnosis

A stress fracture of the sesamoid bone of the hallux leads to forefoot pain on weight bearing, with the patient deliberately walking on the outside (lateral) aspect of the foot. There is marked tenderness and swelling over the sesamoid at the base of the hallux on examination. X-rays are often difficult to interpret as the sesamoid bone may be multiple or bifid, so may require a bone scan to confirm the diagnosis.

Management

Arrange for 6 weeks of non-weight bearing with crutches and then an orthotic splint to correct faulty biomechanics, once the patient resumes weight bearing, to prevent a recurrence.

Non-articular rheumatism

General management of non-articular rheumatism

Joint pain, swelling and tenderness mimicking arthritis may be due to inflammation of periarticular structures. Most patients are treated with NSAIDs such as ibuprofen 200–400 mg orally tds or naproxen 250 mg orally tds, and/or with paracetamol in combination with codeine, usually as paracetamol 500 mg plus codeine 8 mg.

Avoid higher doses of codeine such as 30 mg per tablet, as there is no good evidence for an increase in analgesic effect, but the side effects including nausea, vomiting, disorientation and constipation are markedly increased with regular use. Refer the patient to outpatients or back to their GP.

Do *not* perform joint aspiration and steroid injection in the emergency department, as complications such as septic arthritis and joint destruction do occur. This is best left to the specialist who undertakes long-term care.

Aetiology

- Torticollis (wry neck)
- Frozen shoulder
- Rotator cuff tear (usually supraspinatus rupture)
- Supraspinatus tendonitis
- Subacromial bursitis
- Tennis and golfer's elbow
- Olecranon bursitis
- Prepatellar bursitis (housemaid's knee)
- de Quervain's stenosing tenosynovitis
- Plantar fasciitis
- Carpal tunnel syndrome.

Torticollis ('wry neck')

Diagnosis

Torticollis is abnormal unilateral neck muscle spasm, resulting in the head being held in a bent or twisted position. The aim of the history and examination is to exclude serious underlying causes such as local sepsis from a quinsy or submandibular abscess, recent trauma, cervical disc prolapse, acute drug dystonia from metoclopramide, or even a carotid artery dissection.

Management

Benign 'wry neck' occurs most commonly on waking after sleeping in an awkward position, or follows unaccustomed activity or minor trauma. Arrange for a cervical spine X-ray if there is a history of potential bony trauma or cervical pathology. Give benztropine 1–2 mg i.v. when drug-induced dystonia is suspected.

Once the serious causes have been excluded, use NSAIDs or paracetamol in combination with codeine 8 mg. Recommend gentle manipulation or muscle energy techniques to slowly work loose the muscles in spasm. Discharge the patient back to their GP with further analgesia and ongoing exercises/stretches to maintain neck alignment.

Frozen shoulder (adhesive capsulitis)

Diagnosis

Frozen shoulder (adhesive capsulitis) has a natural history over 1–5 years, with an average duration of 2.5 years. It begins with an acutely painful period of 3–9 months, with progressively decreasing range of motion at the glenohumeral joint over 4–12 months that starts soon after the pain. The decreased range of motion of about 15–45 degrees of movement usually entirely resolves but takes from

1 to 4 years to do so. The pain tends to be worse at night or when lying flat.

A frozen shoulder may occur spontaneously, but more commonly follows local trauma that can be trivial, immobilization, cerebrovascular accident or shingles. There is an increased risk in diabetic patients, where the condition may present bilaterally, and in smokers, and with hyperlipidaemia and treatment with protease inhibitors. There is a peak incidence at age 55 years and it is more common in females, and in the non-dominant arm. The most sensitive sign on examination is the loss of external rotation at the glenohumeral joint. Test for this by first immobilizing the scapula by placing a hand over top of shoulder, to exclude scapulothoracic movement.

Management

The only treatments with evidence of efficacy are high-dose intra-articular steroid injection that reduces early pain but without effect on the range of motion, and physical disruption of the joint capsule, for instance by arthroscopic capsule release. There is no evidence that NSAIDs or physiotherapy alone have any effect on outcome, and NSAIDs in particular have an increased risk of causing renal impairment, heart failure and gastrointestinal bleeding in the elderly (see Ch. 22.1).

Rotator cuff tear (usually rupture of supraspinatus)

Diagnosis

Sudden traction on the arm may tear the muscles that make up the rotator cuff. The onset of pain may be insidious, but a traumatic incident may complete a tear, causing sudden severe pain and reduced shoulder function. Evaluate the full range of active and passive movement at the glenohumeral joint. Typically, there is reduction of active shoulder motion with inability to initiate abduction and weakness of external rotation of the shoulder in particular.

Tenderness is localized over the greater tuberosity and the subacromial bursa, particularly with supraspinatus rupture. Other muscles forming the rotator cuff may also tear but are difficult to differentiate clinically in the acute stage.

Radiography

Shoulder X-ray may show a decrease in the space between the head of the humerus and the acromion, but ultrasound is used to best characterize the extent of a full-thickness rotator cuff tear and a biceps tendon dislocation. It is less sensitive for partial-thickness tears. MRI is highly sensitive and specific for delineating the degree, location and characteristics of rotator cuff pathology, when available.

Management

Refer a young patient with an acute tear to the orthopaedic specialist for consideration of operative repair, as this may ensure an optimal return to a full range of movement and function. Otherwise, conservative management consists of analgesics, an immobilizing sling and referral to the physiotherapy department for a physical therapy rehabilitation programme.

Supraspinatus tendonitis

Diagnosis and management

Supraspinatus tendonitis is one of the causes of the 'painful arc' between 60 and 120 degrees of shoulder abduction. Perform a shoulder X-ray, which may reveal calcification in the supraspinatus tendon, and/or arrange for an ultrasound both for diagnosis and to facilitate aspiration and local steroid injection.

Give an anti-inflammatory analgesic, and consider referral to the orthopaedic or rheumatology clinic for aspiration and local steroid injection, or via ultrasound by an interventional radiologist.

Subacromial bursitis

Diagnosis and management

Subacromial bursitis may follow rupture of calcific material into the subacromial bursa, again causing a 'painful arc' on attempted shoulder abduction, or a constant severe pain in the shoulder. Manage as for supraspinatus tendonitis above.

Tennis and Golfer's Elbow

Diagnosis and management

Tennis elbow (lateral epicondylitis) causes pain over the lateral epicondyle of the humerus from a partial tear of the extensor origin of the forearm muscles involved in repetitive movements such as using a screwdriver or playing tennis. Advise the patient to avoid the activity causing the pain, and to rest the arm.

Give an anti-inflammatory analgesic and refer for physiotherapy. Local steroid injection may reduce short-term pain and improve movement in the first 6 weeks, but has no effect on the medium or longer term outcome.

Golfer's elbow (medial epicondylitis) is a similar condition affecting the medial epicondyle and the flexor origin. Management is the same, and just as disappointing.

Olecranon bursitis

Diagnosis and management

Painful swelling of the olecranon bursa is due to trauma, gout or infection, usually with *Staphylococcus aureus*. Aspirate under sterile conditions and send fluid for Gram stain and microscopy and culture, plus polarizing light microscopy for crystals, if the latter two conditions are considered likely from the presence of severe pain and/or systemic features of sepsis.

Refer the patient for drainage of the bursa under anaesthesia if significant bacterial infection is confirmed, or if a septic arthritis itself is suspected by markedly reduced movement at the elbow (see Ch. 14.2). Otherwise, give an antistaphylococcal antibiotic such as di- or flucloxacillin 500 mg orally qid for 7 to 10 days, and/or a non-steroidal anti-inflammatory analgesic, and refer back to the GP.

Prepatellar bursitis (Housemaid's knee)

Diagnosis and management

This is a prepatellar bursitis secondary to friction or occasionally infection.

Treat by giving an anti-inflammatory analgesic, avoiding further trauma and, if necessary, by aspiration and steroid injection by an orthopaedic or rheumatology specialist, or by arrangement with the patient's GP. When infection is suspected, start an anti-staphylococcal antibiotic such as di- or flucloxacillin 500 mg orally qid for 7 to 10 days, and again refer back to the GP.

Refer the patient to the orthopaedic specialist for intravenous antibiotics and/or local drainage if systemic infection is suspected.

De Quervain's stenosing tenosynovitis

Diagnosis and management

This causes tenderness over the radial styloid, a palpable nodule from thickening of the fibrous sheaths of the abductor pollicis longus and extensor pollicis brevis tendons, and pain on moving the thumb. Treat by resting the thumb in a splint and by using an anti-inflammatory analgesic.

Refer to a rheumatology specialist for consideration of local steroid injection, although it may require surgical release of the tendon sheaths if local injection of steroid fails.

Plantar fasciitis

Diagnosis and management

Plantar fasciitis presents as a painful mid-foot, especially in the sole or arch, that is worse on first weight bearing and improves after 10–15 min of walking, recurring again during load bearing for an extended period. It is one of the most common causes of recurrent foot pain, and may be one manifestation of the spondyloarthropathy seen in Reiter syndrome, ankylosing spondylitis and psoriatic arthritis (see Ch. 14.3). On examination, there is tenderness of the plantar fascia especially at the calcaneal attachment.

X-ray may reveal a bony spur extending along the plantar fascia, but this has no bearing on the initial management. Symptomatic relief may be obtained by a soft heel pad. Longer term management and prevention is best achieved by a properly fitted orthotic splint.

Carpal tunnel syndrome

Diagnosis and management

This is a compressive neuropathy of the median nerve at the wrist, most commonly affecting middle-aged females. Secondary causes include rheumatoid arthritis, post-trauma such as a Colles' fracture, pregnancy and rarely myxoedema, acromegaly and amyloidosis. Most cases though are idiopathic or related to minor trauma.

Patients complain of pain and paraesthesiae in the distribution of the median nerve in the hand, primarily the thumb, index, middle and lateral aspect of the ring finger.

It is typically worse at night or following repetitive strain such as computer work.

Test for reduced sensation over the palmar aspect of the affected digits and weakness of thumb abduction, associated with thenar muscle wasting in chronic cases. Perform Phalen's test by reproducing paraesthesiae in the distribution of the median nerve following 60 s of wrist hyperflexion, or look for Tinel's sign eliciting median nerve paraesthesiae by tapping on the volar aspect of the wrist over the median nerve.

Treat with an anti-inflammatory analgesic, and immobilize the wrist in a volar splint in the neutral position, particularly at night. Refer resistant cases to an orthopaedic specialist for consideration of carpal tunnel decompression.

Back pain

This is a common problem that may be considered under four major groups that include back pain following direct major trauma, or minor indirect mechanical trauma; and severe or atypical non-traumatic back pain, or mild to moderate non-traumatic back pain. Direct major thoracic and lumbosacral spine trauma is covered in Chapter 3.3.

Indirect mechanical back trauma

Clinical features

History Bending, lifting, straining, coughing or sneezing may precipitate acute, severe low back pain, causing intense muscle spasm, or even complete immobility. The normal lumbar lordosis is lost, with the development of a scoliosis.

Examination Assess for a reduced straight-leg raise (SLR), but if a patient is able to sit up in bed with the legs out straight, this is equivalent to an SLR of 90 ° on both sides. Examine for signs of nerve-root irritation or compression from an acute lumbar disc prolapse. See Chapter 3.3 for a description of the myotomes, dermatomes and nerve roots in the leg.

Look for motor loss occurring in the following myotomes:

- L1, L2: hip flexion by iliopsoas
- S1: hip extension by gluteus maximus

- L5: knee flexion by the hamstring muscles
- L3, L4: knee extension by the quadriceps
- L5: ankle dorsiflexion by extensor hallucis longus
- S1: ankle plantar flexion by the calf muscles.

Assess for any reflex loss, with the knee jerk (L3, L4) and the ankle jerk (L5, S1).

Check for sensory loss occurring in the following dermatomes:

- L3 over medial lower thigh and knee
- L4 over the medial side of calf
- L5 over the lateral side of calf
- S1 over the lateral border of the foot and sole.

Finally, in *every* patient, examine for signs of a central disc prolapse causing a cauda equina compression with difficulty emptying the bladder or bowels, lax anal sphincter tone on rectal examination, saddle area anaesthesia over dermatomes S2, S3, S4 and S5 and bilateral leg weakness.

Management

Refer any patient with a suspected central disc prolapse causing cauda equina compression immediately to the orthopaedic or neurosurgical specialist, and arrange an MRI scan to best confirm the exact position and extent of the lesion.

Arrange a CT scan of the spine in other patients with new or recent exacerbation of low-back pain who present with focal pain or abnormal neurology down one leg. Arrange admission, usually under the orthopaedic specialist, for any patient completely unable to move despite a trial of adequate analgesia in the ED, for debilitating symptoms or signs of nerve-root compression with an abnormal CT scan, or if the patient is elderly and fails a trial of mobilization within the ED.

Discharge other patients with moderate pain and without nerve-root signs with a non-steroidal anti-inflammatory analgesic such as diclofenac 50 mg orally tds, or indometacin 100 mg pr twice-daily, or 25 mg orally tds. Encourage early return to ordinary activities within the limits of the pain, and make sure bed rest is kept to a minimum. Arrange review and follow-up by the GP for back care education, including posture, exercise and lifting.

Non-traumatic severe or atypical back pain

Clinical features

Consider the more likely causes according to the patient's age.

Under 30 years:

- ankylosing spondylitis
- rheumatoid arthritis
- osteomyelitis
- discitis
- extradural abscess.

Over 30 years:

- bony metastases
- myeloma
- lymphoma
- renal or pancreatic disease
- aortic aneurysm.

Over 60 years: as above plus:

- osteoporosis
- Paget's disease
- osteoarthritis
- spinal stenosis.

Enquire about previous back trouble, joint trouble, unremitting symptoms especially night-time pain, fever, weight loss, associated abdominal symptoms and/or urinary tract symptoms. These 'red flag' features should alert the clinician to a serious underlying cause for the pain that must be sought.

Record the vital signs and perform a full physical examination, including an abdominal, rectal, neurological and breast examination, and request a urinalysis.

Laboratory investigations

Send blood for a full blood count to look for anaemia or leukocytosis, an erythrocyte sedimentation rate and C-reactive protein as non-specific inflammatory markers, U&E and LFTs for signs of renal or hepatic dysfunction and an MSU.

Radiology

Request a chest X-ray, and thoracic and lumbosacral spine X-ray as appropriate. Consider a bone scan or CT scan if the diagnosis is still in doubt.

Management

Refer the patient to the appropriate specialist team according to the suspected aetiology. *Never* send home a patient with abnormal vital signs or an abnormal physical examination, or one who has failed an analgesia regime. Always consider the possibility of a serious cause and avoid diagnosing *'musculoskeletal pain ? cause'.* See Chapters 14.1, 14.2 and 14.3 for the management of associated rheumatological conditions.

Non-traumatic mild-to-moderate back pain

Diagnosis and management

This is a nebulous group of patients with none of the red flag features of a possible serious underlying cause, with no abnormal physical signs, who are apyrexial with a normal urinalysis. They should be discharged.

Prescribe a non-steroidal anti-inflammatory analgesic such as diclofenac 50 mg orally tds or ibuprofen 400 mg orally tds, and give the patient a letter for his or her GP to follow them up, to arrange physiotherapy, an exercise regime and behaviour modification as appropriate.

Also give a medical certificate for a suitable time off work, based on a clear proactive management plan.

Controversies

❶ Surgical versus conservative management for soft tissue or chronic overuse injuries, particularly for elite athletes who tend to get early surgery as it reduces the time to return to sport. The long-term outcomes have little research data.

❷ Timing of rotator cuff repair.

❸ Acute management of lateral and medial epicondylitis, and the impact on medium- to long-term outcome.

❹ Who should perform intra-articular or intralesional steroid injections, and how often is safe?

Further reading

Bolin D, Kemper A. Current Concepts in the Evaluation and Management of Stress Fractures. Current Sports Medicine Reports 2005; 4(6): 295–300.

Booth C. High pressure paint gun injuries. British Medical Journal 1977; 2: 1333–1335.

Brown AFT, Cadogan MD. Emergency medicine. Emergency and acute medicine: diagnosis and management. 5th edn. London: Hodder Arnold; 2006.

Brukner P, Khan K. Clinical Review of Sports Medicine. 2nd edn, 2001. Sydney McGraw-Hill.

Mehallo C, Drezner J, Bytomski J. Practical Management. NSAID use in athletic injuries. Clinical Journal of Sport Medicine 2006; 16(2): 170–174.

NHMRC Acute Pain Management: Scientific Evidence. 2nd ed, 2005. ANZCA and Faculty of Pain Medicine. Available at www.nhmrc.gov.au/publications/synopses/cp104syn.htm/ (Accessed Nov 2008).

NHMRC Evidence-Based Management of Acute Musculoskeletal Pain: A Guide for Clinicians. Australian Acute Musculoskeletal Pain Guidelines Group 2004. Available at www.nhmrc.gov.au/publications/synopses/cp94syn.htm/ (Accessed Nov 2008).

Tatso J, Elias D. Adhesive Capsulitis. Sports Medicine and Arthroscopy Review 2007; 15(4): 216–221.

UpToDate online version 15.2. http://www.utdol.com/utd/content/search.do (accessed August 2008).

DERMATOLOGY

Edited by **Anthony F. T. Brown**

15.1 Emergency dermatology

Edward Upjohn • George Varigos • Vanessa Morgan

ESSENTIALS

1 Emergency dermatology presentations may be divided into three major groups: acute-on-chronic, new localized and new generalized.

2 Acute-on-chronic complications can be due to non-compliance or a complication of the specific skin disease. A careful history usually differentiates.

3 A new acute rash may have a pattern that is localized, sharply defined or grouped. Look for the following lesion forms: papules, purpura, nodules, pustules, vesicles or blisters.

4 A generalized new acute rash is differentiated according to its duration and morphology such as targetoid lesions, associated pustules, purpura, scaling, weeping or blisters.

Introduction

The pattern and form of acute dermatological conditions that present to the emergency department (ED) are confusing in that the clinical features such as vasodilatation, exfoliation, blistering or necrosis are the common endpoint of many different inflammatory processes in the skin. The pathological response involves cytokines or chemokines, and their effects create the visible response(s). The important clinical differences seen in these acute reactions should be recognized by the trained observer (see Tables 15.1.1 and 15.1.2). This chapter aims to provide a clinical pathway from taking an appropriate history to having knowledge of the distinguishing clinical features of the likely differential diagnoses. The emergency presentations discussed are limited to specific dermatological conditions that may be

seen in an ED as a true urgency. The presentation of skin infections (Ch. 9.6) and anaphylaxis (Ch. 28.7) are covered elsewhere. It is important to use other resources with this book, such as a dermatology atlas or specialized texts, to provide greater detail on the conditions mentioned.

POTENTIALLY LIFE-THREATENING DERMATOSES

Toxic epidermal necrolysis and Stevens–Johnson syndrome

Toxic epidermal necrolysis (TEN) and Stevens–Johnson syndrome (SJS) are disorders of mucosal ulceration at two or more sites

with cutaneous blisters. Confusion exists between these two diagnoses and erythema multiforme (EM), although some consider SJS a severe form of EM major, and TEN a severe form of SJS. This distinction is not important in the emergency setting, but rather it is the recognition of a potentially serious dermatosis that is important.

The difference between TEN and SJS is defined by the extent of skin involvement. TEN affects more than 30% of the body surface area, whereas SJS affects 10% or less (see Fig. 15.1.1). TEN/SJS overlap refers to patients where there is between 10 and 30% body surface area involvement. Again this distinction is academic, as the rash may evolve over hours or days to become true TEN.

The key to making the diagnosis is recognizing mucosal involvement, which may include conjunctival, oral mucosal, genital and sometimes perianal erosions, as well as an often severe haemorrhagic cheilitis. Nikolsky sign is positive, that is dislodgement of the epidermis by lateral finger pressure in the vicinity of a lesion causes an erosion, or pressure on a bulla leads to lateral extension of the blister.

TEN is almost always due to drug ingestion, which can include in rare instances illicit drug ingestion. Therefore ask about prescribed and over the counter drugs such as NSAIDs, sulphonamides, and anticonvulsants such as sodium valproate and lamotrigine, as well as illicit drug use.

Table 15.1.1	Definition of macroscopic skin pathological lesions
Papule	Circumscribed firm raised elevation, less than 0.5 cm in diameter
Nodule	A solid or firm mass more than 0.5 cm in the skin which can be observed as an elevation or can be palpated
Purpura	Discolouration of skin or mucous membranes due to extravasation of red blood cells
Pustule	A visible accumulation of fluid, usually yellow, in the form of a vesicle or papule containing the fluid It may be centred around a pore such as a hair follicle or sweat glands, and sometimes appears in normal skin, not uncommonly palmar/plantar
Vesicle	A visible accumulation of fluid in a papule of <5 mm The fluid is clear, serous-like and is located within or beneath the epidermis
Blister or bulla	Large fluid containing lesion of more than 5 mm
Plaque	An area or sheet of skin elevated and with a distinct edge, of any shape and usually wider than 1 cm

With permission: Rook AJ, Burton JL, Champion RH, Ebling FJG 1992 Diagnosis of skin disease. In: Textbook of Dermatology, Bolognia J, Jorizzo J, Rapini R (eds). Blackwell Scientific, Oxford.

Table 15.1.2	Definitions of patterns in skin disorders
Annular	Ring-like or part of a circle
Linear	Line-like
Arcuate	Arch-like
Grouped	Local collection of similar lesions
Unilateral	One side
Symmetrical	Both sides

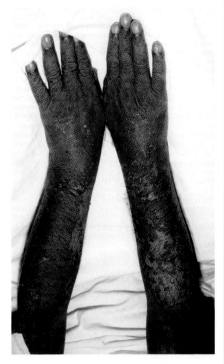

Fig. 15.1.1 Toxic epidermal necrolysis.

Investigations

Request a full blood count, urea and electrolytes, liver function tests (LFT), and a blood glucose level. These may also be used to calculate the prognostic SCORTEN (see below). Send blood for HIV testing also, after appropriate counselling, as the risk of developing TEN is increased in patients with HIV and AIDS. If a biopsy is taken, clearly state on the request slip that the differential diagnosis is of toxic epidermal necrolysis. Epidermal (keratinocyte) necrosis is the histological hallmark of this condition.

Management

Cease the triggering drug or agent immediately, and involve the intensive care unit and/or the burns unit. Arrange assessment and treatment by the ophthalmology and ear, nose and throat teams for ocular and oral/pharyngeal involvement, respectively.

TEN may continue to evolve and extend over days, unlike a burn, where the initial insult occurs at a defined time. The SCORTEN severity scoring system for TEN (see Table 15.1.3) is similar in concept to the Ranson's score for pancreatitis. Calculate the SCORTEN severity score within 24 h of admission and again on day 3 to aid the prediction of possible death (see Table 15.1.4).

Table 15.1.3 SCORTEN severity score for toxic epidermal necrolysis (TEN)
• Age >40 years
• Heart rate >120/min
• Presence of cancer or haematological malignancy
• Epidermal detachment involving body surface area >10% on day 1
• Blood urea nitrogen >10 mmol/L (28 mg/dL)
• Glucose >14 mmol/L (252 mg/dL)
• Bicarbonate <20 mEq/L
(One point is given for each variable.)

Table 15.1.4 SCORTEN mortality prediction*	
Score	Mortality
0–1	3.2%
2	12.1%
3	35.3%
4	58.3%
5 or greater	90.0%

*Guegan S, Bastuji-Garin S, Poszepczynska-Guigne E, et al 2006. Performance of the SCORTEN during the first five days of hospitalization to predict the prognosis of epidermal necrolysis. Journal of Investigative Dermatology 126: 272–76.

Erythema multiforme

EM presents with malaise, target lesions, blistering and sometimes pain or pruritus, but with only one mucous membrane involved (EM major) or none (EM minor).

Most cases of EM are due to drug ingestion, *Herpes simplex* or *Mycoplasma* infection, although in up to half no cause is identified (see Fig. 15.1.2). It is acceptable to treat erythema multiforme with a systemic steroid such as predinosolone (0.5–1 mg/kg/day).

Sweet's syndrome may resemble severe EM in the acute oedematous phase, presenting with fever, arthralgia, neutrophilia and sterile, non-infective but painful pustules, plaques or nodules over the head, trunk and arms. It may recur, and can be associated with a haematological malignancy such as myeloid leukaemia, pregnancy or infection such as *Yersinia* or Streptococcal (see Fig. 15.1.3). Sweet's syndrome is very responsive to systemic steroids; however, a sinister underlying cause such as leukaemia must be sought for and excluded by appropriate investigations.

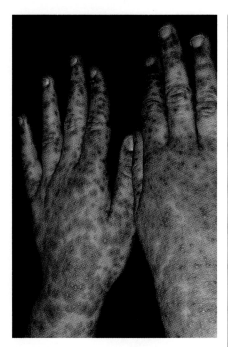

Fig. 15.1.2 Erythema multiforme.

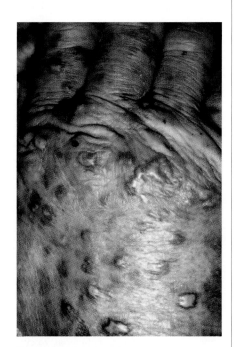

Fig. 15.1.3 Sweet syndrome.

Erythroderma

The causes of erythroderma include eczema (40%), psoriasis (22%), drugs (15%), lymphoma (Sezary syndrome) (10%) and idiopathic (8%).

Complications of erythroderma

These include:

- high output cardiac failure
- dehydration, which may result in renal failure
- protein loss with oedema that occurs often and contributes to the fluid loss with renal failure
- hypothermia/temperature dysregulation
- thrombophlebilitis/deep vein thrombosis (DVT)
- infection both cutaneous and respiratory, with pneumonia being a major cause of death
- side effects of treatment – obtain any history of previous skin disease, recent medications or recent changes to skin management, assess hydration and cardiac status, check for oedema, respiratory infection, DVT and arrange to admit the patient.

Investigations

Send a full blood count (FBC) with film and differential, UE&C, LFTs and blood cultures if the temperature is greater than 38 °C, or if the patient appears unwell with rigors (even if the temperature is normal, as the patient may have become poikilothermic but still be septic). Send skin swabs for microscopy and culture and request a chest X-ray. Arrange biopsy of the skin if the cause of the erythroderma is uncertain.

Management

Treatment is general and supportive, and includes:

- attention to temperature control, avoiding hypothermia
- i.v. fluid replacement with careful charting of the fluid balance chart, monitoring urine output in particular
- referral to dietitian for high protein diet in the first 24 h
- chest physiotherapy
- DVT prophylaxis.

Specific treatment includes:

- bath oil daily in bath or shower
- 50% soft and liquid paraffin all-over strictly every 6 h
- antibiotics for proven infection.

Arrange admission and supervision under the direction of the dermatology team. Intensive care may be necessary.

Other bullous and vesicular conditions

There are many causes of blistering skin rashes that range from common and harmless (but still distressing) to uncommon and potentially life-threatening, such as TEN and SJS. Always ask about recent drug ingestion, and also about drug allergy in the event a bacterial skin infection is diagnosed and antibiotics are required. See Table 15.1.5 for the differential diagnosis of a vesicobullous rash.

Table 15.1.5   Causes of a vesicular or bullous skin rash

Most common	Less common	Rare
Viral: • herpes zoster • herpes simplex Impetigo Scabies Insect bites and papular urticaria Bullous eczema and pompholyx Drugs – sulphonamides, penicillin, barbiturates	Erythema multiforme major ('target lesions' rash, plus one mucous membrane involved) or erythema multiforme minor (1–2 cm 'target lesions' only): • mycoplasma pneumonia • herpes simplex • drugs such as sulphur, penicillins • idiopathic (50%) SJS and TEN with epidermal detachment and mucosal erosions: • drugs such as anticonvulsants, sulphonamides, NSAIDs and penicillins Staphylococcal scalded-skin syndrome (children) Dermatitis herpetiformis (gluten sensitivity) Pemphigus and pemphigoid	Porphyria cutanea tarda Epidermolysis bullosa

Pemphigus vulgaris

Pemphigus vulgaris is characterized by flaccid bullae and erosions together with oral ulceration. The bullae often break down readily to form erosions as the split is epidermal. The Nikolsky sign is positive with dislodgement of the epidermis by lateral finger pressure in the vicinity of a lesion, causing an erosion, or pressure on a bulla leading to lateral extension of the blister. Vegetating lesions, particularly in flexures such as the axillae or on the scalp, may occur as 'pemphigus vegetans'.

Investigations

Send blood for FBC, U&E, LFTs and glucose as a baseline, and for thiopurine methyltransferase (TPMT) levels as adjuvant immunosuppression with azathioprine may be required. Also, send a serum autoantibody profile for anti-skin antibodies directed against a 130-kDa glycoprotein designated desmoglein 3 and located in desmosomes. Arrange biopsy of lesional skin for histology, and perilesional skin, which should be sent fresh and not in formalin, for direct immunofluorescence. An alternative medium is Michel's if fresh transport is not possible.

Management

Start high-dose prednisolone initially at a dose of 1–2 mg/kg/day to achieve remission. Prior to the introduction of systemic steroids this disease was uniformly fatal. Admit the patient under the care of an experienced dermatologist for consideration of other therapies such as immunosuppression with azothioprine, methotrextae or cyclophosphamide. Plasmapharesis and intravenous gamma-globulin may have an additive drug-sparing effect.

Bullous pemphigoid

The usual presentation is an elderly patient with tense skin bullae that may occur on an urticarial base, particularly in the axillae, medial thigh, groin, forearm and abdomen. Itch is a common accompaniment (see Fig. 15.1.4).

Investigations

Send for FBC, electrolytes, LFTs and glucose level as a baseline, plus serum for indirect immunofluorescence for autoantibodies. Also send a TPMT level, as adjuvant immunosuppression with azathioprine may be required. Arrange biopsy of an urticated or bullous lesion for histology, and perilesional skin for direct immunofluorescence. If this is not possible, blister fluid may be sent for indirect immunofluorescence.

Management

Start prednisolone at a moderate dose such as 1 mg/kg daily. An alternative approach is to apply super-potent topical steroids. Admit patients for supportive care.

PETECHIAL AND PURPURIC RASHES

Petechiae, bruising and ecchymoses

Consider and exclude potentially life-threatening causes such as thrombocytopenia and vasculitis, platelet abnormalities such as those associated with thrombasthenia or uraemia, or over-anticoagulation (see Table 15.1.6 for causes of a petechial or purpuric rash). Take a full drug history and ask about systemic symptoms, bleeding tendency, travel history, alcohol abuse and known HIV disease. Check also about anticoagulant medications.

'Senile purpura' are usually due to sun damage with subsequent loss of dermal support for blood vessels which then bleed into the skin. They are sometimes dramatic but always benign and resolve. Finally, if simple trauma is considered, remember non-accidental injury in all cases where the history is suspicious, 'hollow' or changes over time.

Cutaneous vasculitis

There are many potential causes of cutaneous vasculitis, such as viral and bacterial infection, autoimmune and connective tissue diseases, including systemic lupus erythematosus and rheumatoid arthritis, systemic vasculitis, such as Wegener's granulomatosis, polyarteritis nodosa and other causes, which include inflammatory bowel diseases (see Fig. 15.1.5). Rarely, malignant tumours and leukaemia may present with vasculitis.

However, 50% of all cases of cutaneous small vessel vasculitis remain of undetermined aetiology or 'idiopathic' after extensive investigation and are presumed to be of post-infectious origin. Cutaneous vasculitis is clinically best diagnosed when lesions are palpable and on the lower limbs, although they may spread to the buttocks and arms. Sharp edges with stellate or irregular shapes indicate full thickness ischaemia and are seen in septic embolic lesions or meningococcal infections, and in thrombotic occlusion states such as calciphilaxis.

Pyoderma gangrenosum is frequently a differential diagnosis of cutaneous vasculitis. It may begin as a discrete painful haemorrhagic pustule or grouped lesions that rapidly ulcerate, usually on the lower leg, causing larger lesions with neutrophilic inflammation with abscesses and necrosis, but not vasculitis on biopsy. It may be associated with inflammatory bowel disease, rheumatoid arthritis, blood dyscrasias, Behçet's syndrome and malignancy such as myeloma and leukaemia (see Fig. 15.1.6).

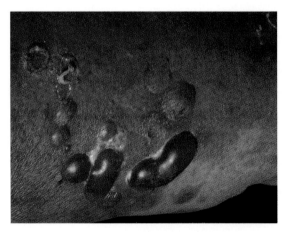

Fig. 15.1.4 Bullous pemphigoid.

Table 15.1.6 Causes of petechiae or purpura

Non-palpable purpura					Palpable purpura (vasculitis)
Non-thrombocytopenic	Thrombocytopenic disorders				
	With splenomegaly		Without splenomegaly		
	Normal marrow	Abnormal marrow	Normal marrow	Abnormal marrow	

Cutaneous disorders:
• trauma, sun
• steroids, old age
Systemic disorders:
• uraemia
• von Willebrand's disease
• scurvy, amyloid
	Liver disease with portal hypertension
	Myeloproliferative disorders
	Lymphoproliferative disorders
	Hypersplenism
		Leukaemia
		Lymphoma
		Myeloid metaplasia
			Immune: idiopathic thrombocytopenic purpura, drugs, infections including HIV
			Non-immune: vasculitis, sepsis, disseminated intravascular coagulation, haemolytic-uraemic syndrome, thrombotic thrombocytopenic purpura
				Cytotoxics
				Aplasia, fibrosis or infiltration
				Alcohol, thiazides
					Polyarteritis nodosa (PAN)
					Leukocytoclastic (allergic)
					Henoch-Schönlein purpura
					Infective:
					• meningococcaemia
					• gonococcaemia
					• other infections:
					  • staphylococcus
					  • rickettsia (Rocky Mountain spotted fever)
					  • enteroviruses
					Embolic

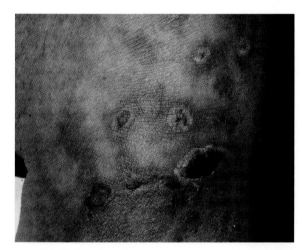

Fig. 15.1.5 Palpable purpura due to vasculitis.

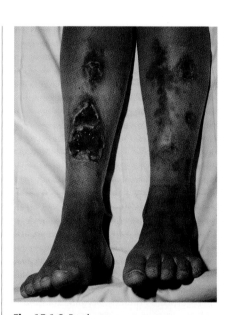

Fig. 15.1.6 Pyoderma gangrenosum.

Investigations

Send blood for a vasculitis screen, including FBC, erythrocyte sedimentation rate, C-reactive protein, U&E, LFTs, hepatitis B and C serology, anti-nuclear antibodies, rheumatoid factor, anti-nuclear cytoplasmic antibodies, antistreptolysin O titre, cryoglobulin screen, anticardiolipin and antiphospholipid screen, serum protein electrophoresis and C3 and C4 complement levels.

Send two sets of blood cultures prior to any immediate antibiotic therapy such as ceftriaxone 2 g i.v. if meningococcal infection is possible. Send a fresh urine specimen for microscopy and culture, looking specifically for glomerular infection and glomerular red cells and casts that indicate renal involvement (over 70% dysmorphic red cells or the presence of red cell casts indicate glomerular disease).

Arrange biopsy, although this is usually performed after admission or dermatology referral to clinic. Send a fresh specimen for both immunofluorescence (Henoch–Schönlein purpura suspected) and culture (infection suspected), as well as a specimen in formalin for histology.

Management

Potential triggers (see above) should be carefully sought and treated appropriately. General measures include rest and elevation of the legs, supportive stockings and topical steroids. If systemic treatment is required then non-steroidal anti-inflammatory drugs (NSAIDs) may be trialled before prednisolone. Antibiotics, steroids and cytotoxic immunosuppression are indicated based on the aetiology and severity of the disease, in consultation with a dermatologist.

PRURITIC (ITCHY) DERMATOSES

Itch can be localized or generalized and may present with or without rash. Whilst not an urgent problem, itch must be recognized as being distressing to the patient. The causes are many and the

Table 15.1.7 Causes of pruritus with, and without, skin disease	
With skin disease	*Without skin disease*
Drugs Scabies, pediculosis, insect bites, parasites (roundworm) Eczema Contact dermatitis Urticaria Lichen planus Pityriasis rosea ('Herald' patch) Dermatitis herpetiformis (with gluten sensitivity)	Hepatobiliary - jaundice, including primary biliary cirrhosis Chronic renal failure Haematological: • lymphoma • polycythaemia rubra vera Endocrine: • myxoedema • thyrotoxicosis Carcinoma: • lung • stomach Drugs

prevalence of chronic itch (like chronic pain) increases with age. See Table 15.1.7 for causes of pruritus with or without skin disease.

Urticaria may occur alone and be acute, relapsing or chronic (see Fig. 15.1.7). It may also be a warning of impending anaphylaxis that necessitates immediate assessment for upper airway swelling, wheeze and or hypotension (see Anaphylaxis, Ch. 28.7).

Scabies

Scabies must be excluded in the elderly patient, particularly nursing home residents. This involves careful examination of web spaces, flexural wrist and the instep of the foot for scabies burrows, and the penis and scrotum for nodules. Crusted 'Norwegian' scabies is predisposed to by glucocorticoid therapy, organ transplant and HIV infection, and in the elderly. It is usually not particularly itchy, but affected patients, who are infested with countless mites, are often the source of large-scale outbreaks in nursing homes and hospitals (see Fig. 15.1.8). Tinea incognito refers to tinea corporis, which has been suppressed and modified in appearance due to the inappropriate use of topical steroids. The topical steroid suppresses the erythema and allows for excessive growth of the causative fungus.

Investigations for pruritis
Send blood for the following tests:

• FBC for eosinophilia (a non-specific finding seen in atopy, scabies and parasitic infections) and to look for iron deficiency anaemia
• iron studies and ferritin level if there is a hypochromic, microcytic blood picture
• random glucose level to screen for diabetes
• urea, electrolytes and creatinine to exclude renal failure

• liver function tests to exclude hepatic impairment with jaundice, including from primary biliary cirrhosis
• serum protein electrophoresis to look for a monoclonal gammopathy, particularly in patients over 70 years
• thyroid stimulating hormone to exclude hypothyroidism or hyperthyroidism.

Take skin scrapes from any suspicious areas for fungal culture and microscopy. In suspected scabies, send material to look for scabies mites, eggs or faeces on microscopy.

Management
General measures include avoiding triggers, in particular overheating, and rehydrating the skin with an emollient such as aqueous cream combined with an anti-itch preparation (0.5% menthol) and an antihistamine in aqueous cream as an anti-itch emollient, and an antihistamine for short-term use, particularly if sleep is impaired, such as promethazine 10 mg

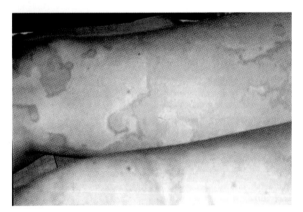

Fig. 15.1.7 Urticaria.

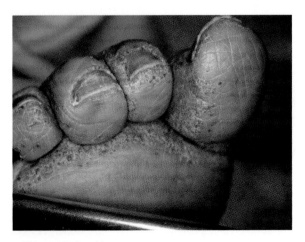

Fig. 15.1.8 Crusted 'Norwegian' scabies.

8-hourly or chlorpheniramine 4 mg 6-hourly, with a warning to avoid alcohol and not to drive or operate machinery. An attempt should be made to identify a cause in every case. Avoid giving prednisolone for an itchy dermatosis when a cause has not been identified. Arrange appropriate investigations and refer the patient for dermatologic follow-up, to avoid missing a treatable but otherwise chronic condition, such as dermatitis herpetiformis from gluten sensitivity.

ECZEMA AND PSORIASIS

Eczema

Atopic eczema is a common skin complaint often affecting the flexures (see Fig. 15.1.9). It may present in a number of ways as an emergency. See Table 15.1.8 for an overview of aetiology, clinical features and management principles.

Erythroderma

Eczema is one of the most common causes of erythroderma (40%), along with psoriasis (22%), drugs (15%), lymphoma (Sezary syndrome) (10%) and idiopathic (8%). See earlier for management principles, which should always involve a dermatologist and may require intensive care unit admission.

Discoid Eczema

Discoid eczema presents as discrete coin-like or 'nummular' erythematous plaques that may develop significant exudate and

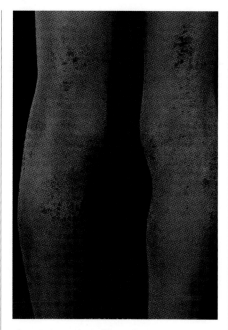

Fig. 15.1.9 Atopic flexural eczema.

crusting. 'Satellite' lesions are common and skin involvement is often progressive, as one area of involvement 'drives' other areas of skin to become eczematous.

Investigation
Take swabs to exclude staphylococcal super-infection.

Management
Prescribe a potent topical steroid such as mometasone 0.1% or betamethasone 0.1% cream or ointment. It is important to advise the patient that more than 1 week of daily or twice daily application may be required, and that lesions will tend to recur

at the same site. Relapses should be treated in the same manner. As a steroid alternative, topical coal tar preparations may be used such as 5–10% coal tar in either white soft paraffin or aqueous cream. Preparations are also available as a shampoo.

Allergic contact dermatitis

Allergy to plants typically presents in a 'streaky' or linear pattern. A severe facial flare of eczema may suggest an airborne allergen as a trigger. The use of hair dyes following a 'henna tattoo' (which may have been applied months or years before) can result in severe scalp and facial dermatitis. Henna used on hair is adulterated with paraphenylene diamine in high concentrations and the patient becomes sensitized to this compound, which is found in most hair dyes.

Some allergens require activation by the ultra-violet (UV) in sunlight to become active allergens. Nickel sensitivity is a common cause of reactions to jewellery, particularly costume jewellery, and occasionally to the clasp of a bra. The cause may or may not be obvious to the patient, so take a carefully focused history.

Irritant contact dermatitis

The hands are commonly involved and may become secondarily infected. Patients may be severely incapacitated if both hands are affected and may therefore need admission. Patients commonly have an atopic background, especially atopic eczema. Ask the patient how many times they wash their hands each day, as irritant contact dermatitis is often one of the first clinically detected signs of an obsessive–compulsive disorder.

Table 15.1.8	Atopic eczema: acute attacks and complications					
	Infective eczema		**Erythroderma**		**Acute eczema**	
	Eczema herpeticum	Impetiginized eczema	Unstable eczema	Psychological	Contact
Cause	Infection with herpes simplex, Varicella, which can rapidly disseminate over the skin	Staphylococcal	Due to many factors Systemic or external	Stressors	Allergen?
Examination	Grouped locally or generally Pinhead-sized papules or vesicles Clear or closed pustules Excoriated sharply defined circular erosions	Discharge and weeping Yellow and crusted blisters or erosions	Total body redness Scale or weeping pruritus Hypothermia Fever, sepsis	Severe Red Pruritus Disturbed sleep	Sharp edges Localized
Management	Antivirals if severe, early, and eyes at risk	Oral antibiotics Antiseptic (triclosan) soaks and wet dressings	Admission Oral steroids Ciclosporin	Admission topicals Oral steroids Paraffin, etc.	Oral steroids Admission

Psoriasis

Psoriasis may present acutely in the following patterns:

- Erythroderma: This is an unstable state that may be caused by systemic or external factors, including treatment. Clinically it is indistinguishable from the other causes of erythroderma, as there is total body redness with no typical features of psoriasis. At presentation, hypothermia and sepsis and high output cardiac failure must be considered.
- Pustular psoriasis: This is triggered by systemic or external factors, including pregnancy, topical treatments, medication and oral steroids. Examination reveals yellow sterile pustules on plaques, diffuse generalized or localized red areas, beginning around the paronychium of the digits or pulp (see Fig. 15.1.10). Arthritis may be present. Consider Reiter's syndrome or hypocalcaemia if the pustular psoriasis is generalized.

- Immune activated psoriasis flares: These are caused by bacterial or viral infective foci in respiratory, bowel, gallbladder or urinary bladder sites. Typically there are new guttate lesions or flares in old psoriatic plaques. Often there have been similarly triggered attacks in the past. Streptococcal pharyngitis is a common precipitant.
- Flare or rebound psoriasis following cessation or poor compliance with therapy: This may be seen in particular with the newer immunomodulatory monoclonal antibody or 'biologic' agents such as efaluzimab. Compliance with some of these drugs is complicated by the need for refrigerated transportation and storage.
- Palmar plantar psoriasis: This may be pustular or may show a keratoderma (thickened skin) which can be difficult to distinguish from eczema, or even inflammatory tinea pedis. Patients may be debilitated and unable to walk or care for themselves and therefore can require admission.

Investigation of acute presentations of psoriasis

Send blood for FBC, U&E and LFTs, including a serum calcium (which may be low with pustular psoriasis). Send further investigations for systemic complications such as infection including a skin swab and/or blood cultures, as well as monitoring for the side effects of therapy. A skin biopsy is usually performed in the ward or clinic if the diagnosis is in doubt.

Management

Treatments include UV therapy, methotrexate, ciclosporin, acitretin or anti-tumour necrosis factor (TNF) therapy such as etanercept or infliximab. These all require a dermatology consultation and careful review of past treatment. Older treatments such as Ingram's or Goerkerman's regimens use the combination of dithranol or coal tar, respectively, and UV phototherapy. They can be particularly effective, have low toxicity and may therefore be

considered as one option for patients. There is benefit in rotating therapies in psoriasis, and a past history of treatment failure does not necessarily indicate that the treatment will always be ineffective. Admission is required if the patient has extensive areas involved, is systemically unwell or unable to manage at home.

OTHER DERMATOSES

Skin cancer

Patients may present to an ED with lesions they, or a concerned family member or partner, are worried about. Important differential diagnoses not to miss include melanoma and non-melanoma skin cancer, including squamous cell and basal cell carcinoma. Refer the patient for prompt assessment by a dermatologist if the lesion looks suspicious, which will usually include a biopsy.

Herpes zoster

This can be a challenge unless the dermatomal distribution of the eruption is appreciated. The rash may also be preceded by pain or dysaesthesia, which may cause a diagnostic quandary itself. Take swabs for bacteriology and viral polymerase chain reaction to confirm the diagnosis. Prompt treatment with antiviral medication such as aciclovir 800 mg orally five times a day or famciclovir 250 mg orally tds, when seen within 72 h of vesicle eruption, may prevent post-herpetic neuralgia.

Non-accidental injury and neglect

Suspect this in the young and elderly with multiple purpura of different ages, particularly if hand- or finger-shaped, and associated with other injuries of differing ages. Burns without splashing suggest deliberate hot water immersion in children, and neglected ulcers and pressure sores in an elderly patient should prompt consideration of neglect.

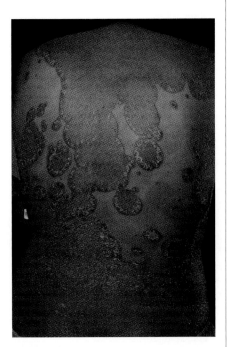

Fig. 15.1.10 Generalized psoriasis.

Controversies

- The treatment of TEN is controversial, with prednisolone, intravenous gamma globulin and ciclosporin all at one time or another being advocated and then discredited. The advent of the biologic therapies (in particular the TNF antagonists) may add to the controversy. Ideally, all patients with this rare disease should be included in a prospective register of patients.

- The use of immunomodifying agents and immunosuppressants, with the potential for unusual side effects or severe rebound of cutaneous disease following cessation or poor compliance.

- The take up of tele-dermatology may make it easier to obtain a second opinion in isolated areas, or to better triage patients for dermatological review. The effect on clinical outcome is unknown.

Further reading

Bolognia JL, Jorizzo JL, Rapini RP. Textbook of dermatology. London: Mosby; 2003.

Burns T, Breathnach S, Cox N, et al. Rook's textbook of dermatology. 7th edn. Oxford: Blackwell; 2004.

Du Vivier A. Atlas of clinical dermatology. 3rd edn. London: Churchill Livingstone; 2002.

eMedicine: Allergy and immunology: dermatology. http://www.emedicine.com/emerg/index.shtml (accessed Dec 2007).

Wolff K, Johnson RA, Suurmond D. Fitzpatrick's color atlas & synopsis of clinical dermatology. 5th edn. New York: McGraw-Hill; 2005.

16.1 Ocular emergencies

David V. Kaufman • James K. Galbraith • Mark J. Walland

ESSENTIALS

Injuries

1 Always assess and record vision.

2 Gentle examination with magnification is essential.

3 X-ray/computerized tomography where bony or penetration injury is suspected.

4 The principal first-aid measure for caustic burns is free irrigation with water, with subsequent removal of any particulate matter.

Painful loss of vision

1 Bacterial keratitis requires intensive, specific, topical antibiotic therapy.

2 Acute primary angle closure produces a rock-hard, inflamed eye with a fixed, mid-dilated pupil.

Painless loss of vision

1 It is imperative to test the pupils for a relative afferent pupillary defect, which is an objective sign of neuroretinal dysfunction.

2 Central retinal artery occlusion requires attempts to lower intraocular pressure acutely and immediate referral to an ophthalmologist is required.

3 Elderly patients with acute visual failure have giant cell arteritis until proven otherwise, and need oral steroid cover until the diagnosis is excluded.

4 Recent onset of distorted vision requires ophthalmic review within 1–2 days to exclude exudative age-related macular degeneration.

5 New onset of floaters, particularly in association with flashes, requires early ophthalmic review to exclude retinal detachment.

6 Local ocular pathology does not cause a visual field defect respecting a vertical midline.

Introduction

Ocular emergencies are common. A relatively trivial traumatic presentation may mask a more serious underlying injury. Similarly, a relatively transient episode of visual loss with no abnormality found on examination may indicate potentially life-threatening cerebrovascular disease. Therefore, all eye presentations in an emergency department (ED) should be carefully evaluated with the necessary equipment.

Basic sight testing equipment should include a Snellen 6-m chart and a black occlusive paddle with multiple pinhole perforations. A slit-lamp biomicroscope is needed for examination of the anterior segment and the removal of foreign bodies.

Emergency eye trolley setup

Examining equipment
- Torch
- Magnifying loupe
- Desmarres lid retractors/lid speculum
- Sterile dressing packs
- Normal saline for irrigation
- Fluorescein strips (sterile)
- Topical anaesthetic (e.g. tetracaine 1%).

Treating
- Mydriatics (dilating): tropicamide 1%, homatropine 2%
- Miotic (constricting): pilocarpine 2%
- Pressure control: acetazolamide 250 mg tablets; ampoules 500 mg (Diamox®)
- Eye pads, plastic shields, tape

- Cotton-tipped applicators (sterile)
- 25G, 23G disposable hypodermic needles (foreign body removal).

A portable slit lamp for examining reclining patients is valuable. A pressure-measuring device, such as a Tono-pen®, which is portable, accurate and easily used, is desirable.

OCULAR TRAUMA

History

Ocular injuries, however trivial, are a frightening experience for the patient, who may have a deep-rooted fear of blindness. The incidence of injuries varies with the environment and protective measures taken. The major injuries result from blunt trauma or penetrating injuries to the globe, with or without the retention of a foreign body. Mechanical interference with eye movement may result from orbital injury, either haematoma or interference with muscle function. Similarly, neurotrauma may disturb the visual pathways or ocular motor nerves.

It is necessary to elicit a history of the patient's prior visual status, including the wearing of glasses or contact lenses and ocular medication.

Examination

Visual acuity

After an eye toilet to remove any debris from the eyelids, vision is tested by a distance Snellen chart, if necessary using a pinhole device as a rough focusing aid. Vision less than 6/60 Snellen may be graded by the patient's ability to count fingers at a measured distance, discern hand movements or to project the direction of a light from various angles. The eye not being tested must be completely shielded by an opaque occluder.

It is essential to assess early whether the patient has sustained a relatively minor superficial injury or a severe injury which may be either blunt or penetrating. Reassurance and extreme gentleness in examining the eye, using topical anaesthetic, will allow a more definite assessment to be made in the ED. With penetrating trauma, any external pressure on the eye may result

in ocular structures being squeezed out of the wound, drastically worsening the prognosis.

To open lids that are adherent due to blood or discharge, gently bathe with sterile saline. Wipe the eyelid skin dry and apply gentle distractive pressure to skin below the brow and below the lower lid, i.e. over bony orbital rim to open the lids. Note that no pressure should be applied to the globe.

Investigation

All patients in whom a penetrating injury is suspected require X-ray or computerized tomography (CT) scanning to exclude a radio-opaque intraocular foreign body (IOFB). If there is any possibility of metallic IOFB, magnetic resonance imaging (MRI) scans are contraindicated. When an adequate examination cannot be made, or where occult perforation is suspected, examination under anaesthesia is mandatory.

Management of specific injuries

Superficial injury

Corneal abrasion

The corneal epithelium is easily dislodged by a glancing blow from fingers, twigs, stones or a paper edge. The trauma produces an acute sensation of a foreign body, with light sensitivity and excessive tearing.

After fluorescein staining, the size of the epithelial defect is recorded. Antibiotic ointment (chloramphenicol) is instilled and an eye pad applied if local anaesthetic is used. The condition heals spontaneously within 24–48 h. Large abrasions produce reflex ciliary spasm, which may require short-acting mydriatics such as homatropine 2% in addition to oral analgesia to relieve the pain.

Corneal foreign body

Small ferrous particles rapidly oxidize when adherent to the corneal epithelium, producing a surrounding rust ring within hours. The rusted particle requires removal under adequate topical anaesthesia using a slit-lamp microscope. An adherent rust ring may be loosened by the application of

antibiotic ointment and padding for 24 h, after which it is easily shelled out with the edge of a fine hypodermic needle. Mechanical dental burrs may cause large areas of epithelial removal and delay return to work. Wooden splinters are particularly dangerous as they may easily penetrate the eye and cause violent suppuration. In all suspected foreign body injury, the upper and lower lids should be everted and examined with suitable lighting and magnification. The conjunctival fornices may be swept gently with a moist cotton bud under topical anaesthesia.

Penetrating injury

A careful history is important in assessing penetrating injury, including prior visual status and the use of contact lenses or spectacles. Occupational trauma may be due to high-speed penetrating metal fragments. Agricultural trauma often involves heavily contaminated implements.

Examination of the eye involves the instillation of sterile topical anaesthetic drops, followed by a gentle eye toilet removing debris, clot and glass from the face and lids. The lids should be opened without pressure (Fig. 16.1.1). The penetration may be evidenced by an obvious laceration or presence of prolapsed tissue with collapse of the globe. Conjunctival oedema (chemosis) and low intraocular pressure (IOP) may indicate an occult perforation or bursting injury.

When a penetrating injury is either suspected or established, the patient must be

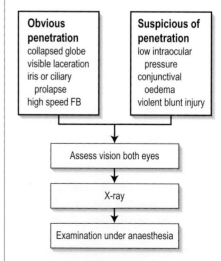

Fig. 16.1.1 Emergency department diagnosis of penetrating injury. FB, foreign body.

transferred without delay to a centre where appropriate surgical facilities are available. During transport, the eye should be covered with a sterile pad and a plastic cone. Vomiting should be prevented with antiemetics, and the fasted patient given intravenous fluids as necessary.

Penetrating trauma involving the cornea has the best prognosis. Lens involvement requires removal of the traumatized lens and usually a staged implantation of an intraocular lens. Posterior segment trauma involving tears or perforation of the choroid and retina requires staged vitreo–retinal surgery and has a guarded prognosis. Uncommonly, penetrating trauma excites an autoimmune reaction resulting in a destructive inflammation involving the uninjured fellow eye – sympathetic ophthalmitis. Long-term follow-up of all penetrating ocular trauma is mandatory.

Blunt trauma

Concussion of the globe may cause tearing of the iris root, resulting in blood in the anterior chamber. A hyphema greater than one-third of the anterior chamber usually indicates some damage to the drainage angle, and may also be associated with concussive lens damage. Uninterrupted absorption of the hyphema is essential, and is aided by sedation and an admission to hospital. The affected eye is padded and the patient nursed semirecumbent to encourage sedimentation of the blood in the anterior chamber to clear as much of the angle as possible. A hyphema may cause considerable pain due to raised IOP. To lower the pressure, oral or intravenous acetazolamide 500 mg initially is required.

Pain is relieved by paracetamol or narcotics, with antiemetics if necessary. Aspirin in any form should be avoided as it increases the risk of secondary haemorrhage. The patient should remain in bed until the blood has completely cleared from the anterior chamber. Bleeding recurs in up to 10% of patients, usually due to early mobilization in those with extensive iris damage. Total hyphema has a poor prognosis because of secondary glaucoma, field loss and corneal opacification. When angle damage occurs, long-term follow-up after hyphema is required to determine whether the IOP is raised. The fundus requires careful examination after the hyphema has

cleared completely, to exclude a traumatic retinal tear, which may be heralded by sudden onset of flashes and floaters.

Chemical burns

Chemical trauma requires priority assessment on arrival at an emergency centre.

Alcohol and solvent burns occur from splashes while painting and cleaning. Although the epithelium is frequently burnt, it regenerates rapidly. The condition is very painful initially, but heals with topical antibiotic and patching for 48 h.

Alkali and acid burns are potentially more serious because of the ability of the burning agent to alter the pH in the anterior chamber of the eye and inflict chemical damage on the iris and lens. Caustic soda, lime and plaster, commonly used in industry, may inflict painful, deep and destructive ocular burns. Splashes of acids, such as sulphuric and hydrochloric, if concentrated, will cause equally destructive injury.

The first principle of management at the injury site is copious irrigation of the eyes for at least 10 min with running water. Assessment of the ocular burn should be done using topical anaesthetic drops and fluorescein staining to determine the area of surface injury. The eyelids should be everted and the fornices carefully examined and swept gently with a cotton bud to ensure there is no particulate caustic agent remaining.

Chemical burns where the epithelium is intact or minimally disturbed can usually wait 24 h before review by an ophthalmologist. Burns involving more than one-third of the epithelium and the corneal edge, with any clouding of the cornea, are potentially more serious as subsequent melting of the cornea by collagenase action may ensue. These burns should all be further irrigated in the ED with a buffered sterile solution such as lactated Ringer's (Hartmann's). The irrigation should continue until the tears are neutral to litmus testing.

More serious caustic injuries have shown a significant improvement in outcome with the introduction of 10% citrate and ascorbate drops, commencing 2-hourly for 48 h and reducing over the week, in combination with 1 g oral ascorbic acid daily. This regimen has an inhibitory effect on corneal melting. Topical antibiotic (chloramphenicol) and soluble steroids such as

prednisolone phosphate 0.5% decrease inflammation.

Initial treatment of caustic injury:

- Immediate flooding of the eye with fresh water for 10 min.
- Transfer to medical centre.
- Assess visual acuity in both eyes.
- Ascertain chemical agent and time of injury.
- Sterile topical anaesthetic, e.g. tetracaine (amethocaine).
- Stain with fluorescein.
- Examine the cornea and conjunctiva.
- Evert lids and sweep tarsal plate with cotton bud.
- Reirrigate.

A minor injury is defined as less than one-third epithelial loss and a clear cornea. A major injury is a large epithelial defect, a conjunctival burn and a hazy media.

For major injury commence ascorbic acid 1 g daily and 10% topical ascorbate hourly.

Prevention

Children are constantly exposed to domestic hazards, particularly household utensils with sharp points and caustic substances in spray cans, which need to be kept out of reach. The well-known workshop injuries caused by iron fragments created while hammering or chipping, exploding car batteries and carbonated drinks bottles cause significant trauma. Protective glasses – preferably polycarbonate – may provide protection in racquet sports. Contact lenses do not protect.

Australian seatbelt legislation has markedly reduced the incidence of penetrating eye injuries in road trauma, but eye problems still occur from violent head and facial trauma in addition to the neurological complications of head injury.[1,2]

ACUTE INFLAMMATORY CONDITIONS

Acute primary angle-closure (glaucoma)

Acute primary angle-closure (APAC) is characterized by an acute impairment of the outflow of aqueous from the anterior chamber in an anatomically predisposed eye.

This results in a rapid and severe elevation in IOP. Normal IOP lies between 10 and 21 mmHg, but in cases of APAC can rise to >60 mmHg. This is manifested as severe pain, blurring of vision and redness. The pain may be severe enough to cause nausea and vomiting, and may be poorly localized to the eye. Visual disturbance can be preceded by halos around lights, and in established cases is due to corneal oedema. Relative hypoxia of the pupillary sphincter due to elevated pressure results in a pupil unresponsive to light stimulation. The pupil is classically fixed and mid-dilated. The associated inflammation induces congestion of conjunctival and episcleral vessels. The term 'acute angle-closure glaucoma' is no longer regarded as appropriate, as there may be no optic nerve head cupping or visual field loss – the features that define glaucoma – at the acute presentation.

Treatment of APAC is aimed at lowering the IOP and allowing the flow of aqueous from the posterior to the anterior chamber. Acetazolamide 500 mg i.v. and/or topical apraclonidine or brimonidine may be effective in acutely lowering the pressure and thereby reducing pain. If ineffective, subsequent constriction of the pupil with 2% pilocarpine, a parasympathomimetic, may alleviate the forward bowing of the iris, relieve the pupil block and re-establish aqueous flow and angle drainage. One drop is initially instilled every 5 min for 15 min, and then half-hourly. If the pressure is very high, however, the ischaemia induced will render the pupillary sphincter unresponsive to the pilocarpine. In these cases it may be necessary to move to early laser treatment.

A peripheral iridotomy (PI) is performed using the yttrium:aluminium:garnet (YAG) laser to allow aqueous permanently to bypass the pupil and remove the risk of further episodes of APAC. This may be done acutely or electively. The anatomical predisposition to APAC is usually bilateral, and a PI is also performed in the other eye as an elective procedure. Until this is done, miotics are instilled (G. pilocarpine 2% qid) in the unaffected eye to avoid the risk of APAC.

Early YAG laser PI in the affected eye may be hampered by corneal oedema. Argon laser peripheral iridoplasty may be used in the acute phase for resistant attacks, or where corneal oedema precludes YAG laser PI.[3,4]

Acute iritis

Acute iritis (AI) is an inflammatory response in the ciliary body and the iris. As part of this response there is an increase in vascular dilatation and permeability, with release of inflammatory mediators and cells that can damage intraocular structures.

Acute iritis (AI) is usually an idiopathic condition with no systemic cause or association. Less commonly, associated conditions may include HLA B27-related disease, sarcoidosis, inflammatory bowel disease, including ulcerative colitis and Crohn's disease, connective tissue disorders such as ankylosing spondylitis and ocular infection, including herpetic disease or toxoplasmosis. A complete history will often give clues to these associations.

Acute anterior iritis is generally unilateral, although bilateral involvement is seen. It is characterized by pain, redness and visual disturbance. The pain is constant and exacerbated by light owing to movement of the inflamed iris. Dilatation of the conjunctival and episcleral vessels is apparent, particularly in the vessels adjacent to the corneal limbus, often referred to as limbal flush. Visual acuity can be reduced by varying degrees depending on the severity of inflammation. The pupil is constricted due to irritation.

Examination of the anterior segment with the slit lamp will reveal evidence of increased vascular permeability, seen as fibrin clumps, flare and inflammatory cells in the aqueous released from the vessels. In some cases small collections of neutrophils can be seen aggregating on the posterior surface of the cornea as keratic precipitates (KP). In cases of severe inflammation, cells can accumulate in the inferior anterior chamber and a sediment level can be seen as a hypopyon. The IOP may be raised.

Treatment of AI is directed towards resolution of the inflammatory response and limiting the ocular effects of this response. The mainstay of treatment is intensive, topical steroid eye drops (prednisolone acetate 1%, up to hourly in severe cases). In severe cases, orbital steroid injections or oral steroids may be necessary. Mydriatic eye drops (G. homatropine 2% qid) are used to break

any lens–iris adhesions and to limit the extent of permanent adhesions. In 'splinting' the iris these drops also provide pain relief by limiting pupil movement.

As the degree of inflammation decreases on slit-lamp examination, the topical treatment is decreased in frequency. The long-term use of topical steroid drops is not without risk, and can be associated with the development of glaucoma, cataract and concurrent ocular surface infection, such as herpes simplex keratitis.

Acute infectious keratitis

The surface of the eye is protected by several mechanisms from penetration by infectious agents, both bacterial and viral. The flow of tears over the surface washes debris away and contains antibodies and lysozymes. The smooth surface of the corneal epithelium hinders the adherence of infectious agents, and the rapid repair of any defect in the epithelium limits the likelihood of penetration by such agents. If these defenses are impaired in any way there is the possibility of penetration into the corneal stroma, and active infection may occur.

Bacterial keratitis is characterized by a focus of infection with an associated inflammatory response. Patients complain of pain, redness, watering and a decrease in visual acuity. Fluorescein staining shows an area of ulceration over the infection, which appears as an opacity or area of whiteness within the cornea. Marked conjunctival and episcleral injection results in a unilateral red eye. Evidence of intraocular inflammation is usually present, with cells and flare being seen in the anterior chamber on slit-lamp examination. In severe cases, a collection of inflammatory cells can be seen in the inferior part of the anterior chamber as sediment, called a hypopyon.

The most important aspect of management is to identify the infectious agent and to commence appropriate antibiotic treatment. A specimen is taken via a scraping for microbiological assessment, including Gram staining and culture. Under topical anaesthetic, using a preservative-free single-use dispenser of benoxinate or tetracaine (amethocaine), a sterile 23G needle is used to gather a small specimen. This is transferred directly to glass slides and also plated on to HB and chocolate agar plates for culture. Fungal cultures may be indicated. Antibiotic therapy is not delayed until the results are available, but is commenced on a broad-spectrum basis, such as the intensive use of a fluoroquinolone eye drop (e.g. G. ciprofloxacin) on an hourly basis. Daily monitoring with slit-lamp examination is mandatory and severe infections require hospital admission. This regimen can be modified when culture and sensitivity results are available. It is sometimes necessary to add a topical steroid when the active infection is under control, to limit the amount of inflammation and vascularization – and hence damage – to the cornea.

Herpes simplex infection of the cornea usually presents initially as an infection of the epithelial cell layer, although with recurrent episodes stromal involvement may be seen. It is most often a unilateral infection. As with other herpetic infections it is not possible to eradicate the virus, but limitation of inflammatory-mediated damage is important. Patients complain of foreign body sensation, redness, watering and a variable decrease in visual acuity. On examination the areas of infected epithelium can be seen as a branching irregularity or *dendrite* on the surface of the eye. Multiple dendrites may be scattered over the surface, particularly in immunocompromised patients. These are best seen when the cornea is stained with fluorescein or Rose Bengal stains and viewed under the slit lamp.

Treatment is directed to clearing the virus from the cornea to promote epithelial healing and limit stromal involvement and damaging corneal inflammation. An antiviral ointment, aciclovir, is instilled five times daily until there is resolution of the epithelial lesions, and then ceased as long-term usage may be toxic to the unaffected corneal epithelium. Steroid eye drops are contraindicated except under the strict supervision of an ophthalmologist.

ACUTE VISUAL FAILURE

Introduction

Acute visual failure is any acute change in visual acuity, visual field or colour vision. Effective emergency management depends upon rapid recognition of those conditions for which acute therapy is available (Table 16.1.1). Some conditions have no effective therapy, or are more appropriately managed on an outpatient basis.

Clinical assessment

History

Particular attention should be paid to the rapidity of onset, degree and location in space of visual loss, previous episodes and associated symptoms. Most of the sinister causes of acute visual failure are painless (Table 16.1.2).

One should distinguish on history between acute onset and acute discovery of visual loss, as a patient may discover decreased vision from, for example, cataract, or retinal venous occlusion, by

inadvertently covering one eye for the first time.

Examination

Testing of the visual acuity and visual field will clarify uni- or binocular involvement.

Examination of the pupils is mandatory before pharmacological dilation. Test for a relative afferent pupillary defect (RAPD), one of the few objective signs. When required, pupils will dilate in 10–15 min with tropicamide 1.0% drops, which last 1–2 h.

Bilateral vision loss

Bilateral visual field loss usually implicates a retrochiasmal – and, therefore, non-ocular – cause. This visual field defect will, however, respect a vertical midline. In contrast, the retinal nerve fibre layer and retinal vascular elements within the eye are distributed around a horizontal midline, and may thus involve a superior or inferior (i.e. horizontal) hemifield. Localized ocular pathology does not cause a visual field defect respecting a vertical midline.

Bilateral acute, complete, visual failure is uncommon. Bilateral occipital infarction may present with bilateral blindness, but pupil responses would be expected to be intact. Rapidly progressive bilateral sequential visual loss from temporal arteritis is occasionally encountered. Other prechiasmal causes of bilateral, simultaneous, ocular involvement include toxic causes, such as poisoning with either quinine or methanol, where the patient presents with bilateral blindness and fixed, widely dilated pupils. Visual recovery in these cases is variable, and the efficacy of a range of therapeutic interventions is controversial.[5–7]

Central retinal artery occlusion

The history is typically of sudden, painless loss of vision in the affected eye over seconds. This may have been preceded by episodes of transient loss of vision (amaurosis fugax) in the previous days or weeks. Mean age of presentation is in the 60s. Men are more frequently affected, and the history may include evidence of previous cardiac or cerebrovascular disease. Systemic arterial hypertension and diabetes mellitus are often coexistent. Carotid disease is

Table 16.1.1 Acute visual failure for which acute therapy is available	
Condition	*Therapy*
Central (or branch) retinal artery occlusion	Acetazolamide Pulsed ocular compression Anterior chamber paracentesis
Anterior ischaemic optic neuropathy	Steroids
Exudative age-related macula degeneration	anti-VEGF injections Laser Verteporfin
Retinal detachment	Surgery

Table 16.1.2 Symptoms significant for cause in acute visual failure

Symptom	Condition
Floaters (if recent onset)	Posterior vitreous detachment Vitreous haemorrhage Retinal detachment
Flashes (especially temporal)	Retinal detachment Migraine aura
Shadow (billowing curtain/cloud)	Retinal detachment Vitreous haemorrhage
Distortion	Exudative macula disease
Amaurosis fugax	Retinal artery occlusion Anterior ischaemic optic neuropathy
Pain on eye movement	Optic neuritis
Visual field loss Horizontal hemifield	Anterior ischaemic optic neuropathy Branch retinal vein occlusion Branch retinal artery occlusion
Vertical hemifield (bilateral)	Retrochiasmal CVA/compression
Whole-field (unilateral)	Vitreous haemorrhage Central retinal artery occlusion Anterior ischaemic optic neuropathy Central retinal vein occlusion
Bilateral total loss of vision	Bilateral occipital infarction Toxic (methanol/quinine)

frequently implicated, with emboli often being the cause of the obstruction, but their absence does not preclude the diagnosis, as the obstruction may lie behind the lamina cribrosa.

The visual acuity is drastically reduced, often to the level of light perception, with a RAPD present on the affected side. Fundus examination shows creamy-white retinal oedema (cloudy swelling) with a central red fovea – the 'cherry-red spot' – caused by the absence of oedema in the thinner retina at the fovea. The arterioles may be attenuated, with segmentation ('cattle-trucking') of the blood column. An embolus may be seen at any point along the retinal arterioles, from the disc to the periphery.

Acute treatment proceeds on the assumption that the cause is embolic. The principles of therapy are, therefore, to vasodilate the retinal arterial circulation in order to promote dislodgement of the embolus from a proximal position and encourage its movement downstream to a less strategic site. All the measures currently used are directed to lowering the IOP, thereby relieving the compressive effect on the intraocular vasculature.

Intravenous or oral acetazolamide 500 mg will lower IOP within 15–30 min; pulsed ocular compression ('ocular massage') involves cyclical sustained compression of the globe for 10–15 s before sudden release of this compression, continuing for 5–10 min. The release of pressure may result in a momentary marked increase in the perfusion pressure gradient and dislodge an embolus. Definitive reduction of IOP is achieved with anterior chamber paracentesis by the removal of aqueous from the eye (see section on Anterior chamber paracentesis). Visual outcomes are generally poor in central retinal artery occlusion (CRAO), but occasional successes justify aggressive intervention if the patient presents within 12 h.

Intra-arterial fibrinolytic therapy is a promising technique that is not widely available at present and requires the services of an experienced interventional neuroradiology team.[8–11] The place of hyperbaric therapy is uncertain at this time.[12] The use of carbogen gas (95% oxygen/5% carbon dioxide) is now largely historical.

Non-acute management must include attempts to define the embolic source. Investigations may include Doppler and cardiac ultrasound, and perhaps angiography (including aortic arch studies), as well as assessment of cardiac and cerebrovascular risk factors. An erythrocyte sedimentation rate (ESR) and C-reactive protein (CRP) should exclude temporal arteritis – which causes 5% of cases of CRAO – as a non-embolic cause.

Anterior chamber paracentesis

The eye is anaesthetized with topical, unpreserved drops from single-use dispensers – tetracaine 1%. The fornices and globe are prepared with a drop of 10% povidone-iodine. An assistant is useful to steady the patient's head at the slit lamp. With toothed forceps to provide counterpressure opposite the site of entry into the anterior chamber, a 27 G needle on an insulin syringe with the plunger removed is inserted parallel to the iris plane: if the eye is phakic (i.e. natural lens present), then the needle course must be only over the iris, below the margin of the pupil, to avoid contact with the lens. Aqueous will drain along the barrel of the syringe and should be allowed to continue until the cornea starts to wrinkle. The needle is then withdrawn, taking great care not to allow the needle point to tip backwards against the lens in the softened eye. The entry wound is self-sealing. Antibiotic drops such as chloramphenicol should be commenced and used four times a day for 4 days. Vision will be worse immediately after the procedure.

Central (branch) retinal vein occlusion

Central or branch retinal vein occlusion may present as a painless blurring of vision that is not sudden. Patients are usually in the older age group, often with systemic hypertension, diabetes mellitus and glaucoma. Visual acuity varies with severity, as does the presence of an RAPD. The characteristic fundus appearance is of extensive intraretinal haemorrhage with a variable number of cotton wool spots. There may be disc oedema, with venous tortuosity and a generally congested appearance.

There is no emergency management specific to the vein occlusion that will positively influence the visual outcome, and the patient should therefore be referred to the next ophthalmic outpatient clinic. Systemic hypertension and raised IOP rarely require acute control.

Anterior ischaemic optic neuropathy

Arteritic anterior ischaemic optic neuropathy (AION) is the feared visual loss of giant cell (temporal) arteritis (GCA). The patient is commonly mid-70s or older, and more often female. Presentation is with profound vision loss in one eye. This may have been preceded by premonitory visual obscurations or double vision, to which the patient may not have ascribed significance. Systematic questioning may reveal specific features such as jaw claudication, headache, scalp tenderness, anorexia, malaise, weight loss or night sweats, and there may be a history of polymyalgia rheumatica in up to 50% of cases. Giant cell arteritis is a systemic illness with the potential for devastating visual loss, as well as long-term life-threatening non-ophthalmic complications.

Vision may be reduced at presentation to the level of perception of light only. An RAPD will be present. Total field loss in the affected eye is usual. Fundus examination will almost invariably show disc oedema, but the fundus may be otherwise normal. Evidence of decreased acuity, colour vision deficits and disc oedema should also be sought in the other eye. Palpation of the temporal arteries will often be abnormal, with the pulses perhaps absent or the arteries thickened and tender.

Clinical suspicion requires blood to be drawn for ESR and CRP. Treatment should then be started on an urgent basis and must not be delayed or deferred until after temporal artery biopsy. The biopsy will remain positive for at least several days despite steroids. Elevation of both ESR and CRP is highly specific for a diagnosis of GCA, but does not avoid the need for biopsy.[13] Urgent referral to an ophthalmologist is required.

Prednisolone 1 mg/kg daily is an accepted dose, although recent experience has suggested that 'pulse' methylprednisolone 500 mg i.v. daily or twice daily over 1–2 h is safe and more efficacious in suppressing the inflammation, and this has become standard therapy in a number of centres. This is generally used for 3 days, and oral prednisolone is then substituted.[14–16] Treatment will be prolonged (at least 6 months) and should be undertaken in cooperation with a physician. Attention should also be directed to the avoidance of steroid complications in this aged patient group.

Non-arteritic AION is classically seen in males in the late 50s and 60s, who have a history of cardiac or vascular disease, hypertension, diabetes or smoking. The presentation may be similar to that seen with GCA – although the visual acuity and field loss may not be as profound and the specific systemic symptoms are absent – so that management must be as for arteritic AION until GCA is excluded.

Retinal detachment

Retinal detachment is usually a result of retinal hole formation, with seepage of fluid into the subretinal space and lifting of the retina. This may occur as a result of trauma, but is more often seen in an older age group as a result of vitreous traction in spontaneous posterior vitreous detachment (PVD), and is predisposed to by high myopia (short-sightedness). Exudative retinal detachment is less common and is associated with underlying pathology.

Posterior vitreous detachment
Shrinkage and detachment of the vitreous is common in the older population, and produces a new onset of floaters – wispy spots, threads or 'spider webs' in the vision. As part of this process, vitreous traction on the retina may produce flashes of light (photopsia) seen particularly in the temporal periphery of vision in that eye. These flashes can usually be distinguished from the visual aura of migraine. While PVD is usually not serious in its own right, early elective ophthalmic review is required as it is not possible to exclude related changes predisposing to retinal detachment without dilated examination of the retinal periphery.

Retinal detachment
With a history of flashes and floaters, the presence of pigmented cells ('tobacco dust') in the anterior vitreous should alert one to the possibility of a retinal hole and subsequent retinal detachment. A detached retina shows a visual field defect, which will be described as a shadow or curtain, corresponding to the area of detachment, i.e. inferior field defect equals superior retinal detachment. Vision loss is painless. There may be an RAPD, depending on the amount of retina involved. Treatment will usually require surgery. If the visual acuity is normal, the macula is likely to be still attached and referral to an ophthalmologist specializing in vitreo-retinal surgery is urgent.

Vitreous haemorrhage

The most common causes are proliferative diabetic retinopathy, chronic branch retinal vein occlusion, posterior vitreous detachment or trauma. Patients with an acute vitreous haemorrhage may have symptoms varying from a few floaters causing blurred vision to a total loss of vision to a level of light perception, depending on the density of the haemorrhage. Any loss of vision is painless. The red reflex may be poor and the view of the retina may be similarly impaired. Media opacities do not affect pupil light reflexes, so there should be no RAPD, unless the underlying retina is damaged or detached.

The patient should be referred for early ophthalmic assessment – urgent if an RAPD is present – which may include B scan ultrasonography to exclude retinal detachment if the retinal view is inadequate. Aspirin should be avoided.

Age-related macular degeneration

In 10–20% of cases of age-related macular degeneration (AMD), an exudative-type disease is seen, and in its most sinister form this will involve subretinal neovascularization (SRNV). These patients may present with painless distortion of vision, particularly metamorphopsia – a complaint that objects that they know to be straight appear curved. Visual acuity is reduced, depending on the stage of the disease; an RAPD is rarely seen owing to the relatively small area of retina involved, which manifests as a central scotoma on field testing. Macular drusen (yellow spots), retinal thickening and haemorrhage may be seen, with at least drusen usually also seen in the fellow eye.

Acute symptoms must not be dismissed. With appropriate treatment, central vision may be preserved in a proportion of these patients. Rapid ophthalmic review is therefore appropriate. Treatment will be undertaken following fundus fluorescein angiography to delineate the subretinal vascular lesion. Laser photocoagulation has been the traditional therapy, but the emergence of verteporfin, and more recently anti-vascular endothelial growth factor (VEGF) agents such as ranibizumab (Lucentis) have revolutionized the treatment options and prognosis. Clinical trials with the anti-VEGF agents are ongoing.[17,18]

Optic neuritis

Optic neuritis classically presents in young females, and may be the first presentation of a demyelinating illness. Visual symptoms are not usually sudden, and presentation is thus seldom acute. The vision declines gradually over days, perhaps to the level of 6/36–6/60, with loss of colour vision being prominent. The common visual field defect is a central scotoma, but many variations are possible, and an RAPD should always be present. If disc oedema is not seen the diagnosis may be retrobulbar neuritis. There may be pain on medial or superior eye movement.

Good spontaneous recovery has made the value of treating optic neuritis controversial: the results of the Optic Neuritis Treatment Trial[19] would suggest that there is no place for oral prednisolone alone in management. The benefit of 'pulse' intrave-

nous methylprednisolone seems restricted to shortening the acute episode, without influencing the possibility of progression to multiple sclerosis or the final visual outcome.[20] However, there is usually no role for acute intervention, and referral within a day or two to a neurologist or an ophthalmologist is satisfactory.

Controversies

❶ What are the roles of hyperbaric oxygen and intra-arterial fibrinolytic therapy in central retinal artery occlusion?

❷ What is the appropriate therapy for acute optic neuritis: oral steroid, intravenous steroid or no treatment?

❸ What are the long-term results with anti-VEGF treatments for exudative age-related macula degeneration?

References

1. McCarty CA, Fu CLH, Taylor HR. Epidemiology of ocular trauma in Australia. Ophthalmology 1999; 106: 1847–1852.
2. Colby K. Management of open globe injuries. International Opthalmologic Clinic 1999; 39: 59–69.
3. Lai JSM, Tham CCY, Chua JK, et al. Laser peripheral iridoplasty as initial treatment of acute attack of primary angle-closure: A long-term follow-up study. Journal of Glaucoma 2002; 11: 484–487.
4. Lam DSC, Lai JSM, Tham CCY, et al. Argon laser peripheral iridoplasty versus conventional systemic medical therapy as first line treatment of acute angle closure: a prospective, randomised controlled trial. Ophthalmology 2002; 109: 1591–1596.
5. Canning CR, Hague S. Ocular quinine toxicity. British Journal of Ophthalmology 1988; 72: 23–26.
6. Bacon P, Spalton DJ, Smith SE. Blindness from quinine toxicity. British Journal of Ophthalmology 1988; 72: 219–224.
7. Stelmach MZ, O'Day J. Partly reversible visual failure with methanol toxicity. Australia and New Zealand Journal of Ophthalmology 1992; 20: 57–64.
8. Watson PG. The treatment of acute retinal arterial occlusion. In: Cant JS, ed. The ocular circulation in health and disease. St Louis: Mosby Year Book; 1969: 243–245.
9. Schmidt D, Schumacher M, Wakhloo AK. Microcatheter urokinase infusion in central retinal artery occlusion. American Journal of Ophthalmology 1992; 113: 429–434.
10. Weber J, Remonda L, Mattle HP, et al. Selective intra-arterial fibrinolysis of acute central retinal artery occlusion. Stroke 1998; 29: 2076–2079.
11. Beatty S, Au Eong KG. Local intra-arterial fibrinolysis for acute occlusion of the central retinal artery: a meta-analysis of the published data. British Journal of Ophthalmology 2000; 84: 914–916.
12. Beirna I, Reissman P, Scharf J, et al. Hyperbaric oxygenation combined with nifedipine treatment for recent-onset retinal arterial occlusion. European Journal of Ophthalmology 1993; 3: 89–84.
13. Hayreh SS, Podhajsky PA, Raman R, et al. Giant cell arteritis: validity and reliability of various diagnostic criteria. American Journal of Ophthalmology 1997; 123: 285–296.
14. Hayreh SS. Anterior ischaemic optic neuropathy. Differentiation of arteritic from non-arteritic type and its management. Eye 1990; 4: 25–41.
15. Liu GT, Glaser JS, Schatz NJ, et al. Visual morbidity in giant cell arteritis. Clinical characteristics and prognosis for vision. Ophthalmology 1994; 101: 1779–1785.
16. Cornblath WT, Eggenberger ER. Progressive visual loss from giant cell arteritis despite high-dose intravenous methylprednisolone. Ophthalmology 1997; 104: 854–858.
17. Rosenfeld PJ, Brown DM, Heier JS, et al. Ranibizumab for neovascular age-related macular degeneration. New England Journal of Medicine 2006; 355: 1419–1431.
18. Brown DM, Kaiser PK, Michels M, et al. Ranibizumab versus verteporfin for neovascular age-related macular degeneration. New England Journal of Medicine 2006; 355: 1432–1444.
19. Beck RW, Cleary PA, Anderson MA, et al. A randomized controlled trial of corticosteroids in the treatment of acute optic neuritis. New England Journal of Medicine 1992; 326: 581–588.
20. Kapoor R, Miller DH, Jones SJ, et al. Effects of intravenous methylprednisolone on outcome in MRI-based prognostic subgroups in acute optic neuritis. Neurology 1998; 50: 230–237.

Further reading

Kanski J. Clinical Ophthalmology, A systematic approach. 6th edn (rev). Oxford: Butterworth-Heinemann Ltd; 2007.
The Wills eye manual: Office and emergency room diagnosis and treatment of eye disease. 4th edn (rev). Philadelphia: Lippincott Williams and Wilkins; 2004.
Riordan-Eva P. Vaughan and Asbury's general ophthalmology, 16th edn. New York: McGraw-Hill Medical; 2003.

17.1 Dental emergencies

Sashi Kumar

ESSENTIALS

1 An avulsed tooth reimplanted within 30 min has a 90% survival rate.

2 Dental caries are the most common cause of dental emergency attendance.

3 Dental caries require analgesia in the emergency department and referral to a dentist for definitive care. Antibiotics are not required unless complicated by abscess.

Anatomy

The tooth consists of the crown, which is exposed, and the root, which lies within the socket covered by the gum and serves to anchor the tooth. The gingival pulp carries the neurovascular structures via the root canal and is covered by dentine, which in turn is covered by enamel, the hardest substance in the body (Fig. 17.1.1).

The deciduous teeth are 20 in number and erupt between the ages of 6 months and 2 years. The permanent dentition begins to erupt at around age 6 and in the adult consists of 32 teeth.

Dental caries

The most common cause of toothache or odontalgia is caries. Dental caries-related emergencies account for up to 52% of first contact with a dentist for children below the age of 3 years.[1] Dental caries is the cause of emergency visits to a dentist in 73% of paediatric patients.[2] Pain associated with dental caries is of a dull, throbbing nature, localized to a specific area and aggravated by changes in temperature in the oral cavity (hypersensitivity to hot and cold food or fluids).

Examination reveals tenderness of the offending tooth when tapped with a tongue depressor or a mirror. Management includes symptomatic pain relief using analgesics such as paracetamol with or without codeine non-steroidal anti-inflammatory drugs (NSAIDs) and urgent referral to the dentist.

Periodontal emergencies

Pain is the most common cause of self-referral to the emergency department for dental problems. The common conditions causing dental pain are acute apical periodontitis and reversible and irreversible pulpitis resulting from dental caries.[3] Symptoms include painful swollen gums with or without halitosis. On occasions frank pus or bleeding from the gums may be the presenting symptom. At all stages varying degrees of pain associated with inflammation are invariably present.[4]

Management includes diagnosis of the periodontal disease and the offending

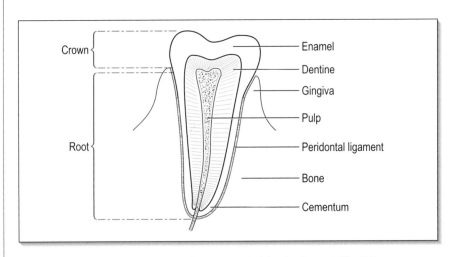

Fig. 17.1.1 The anatomy of the tooth. (From an original drawing by Ian Miller RN.)

Crown — Enamel, Dentine, Gingiva, Pulp

Root — Peridontal ligament, Bone, Cementum

tooth. Symptomatic pain relief can be achieved with analgesics, non-steroidal anti-inflammatory agents and warm saline rinses. Routine antibiotic therapy is not required unless there is evidence of gross infection locally, regional lymphadenopathy or fever. In all cases urgent review by the dentist is mandatory.

Alveolar osteitis (dry socket)

Dry socket occurs between 2 and 5 days following dental extraction. The dull throbbing pain is due to the collection of necrotic clot and debris in the socket. The condition is diagnosed on the history and examination, which confirms the acutely tender extraction site.

Treatment consists of irrigation of the extraction site to remove the necrotic material and packing the socket with sterile gauze soaked in local anaesthetic such as cophenylcaine, followed by urgent dental review.[5]

Postdental extraction bleeding

Bleeding from the socket post extraction within 48 h is due to reactionary haemorrhage due to opening up of the small divided blood vessels. Bleeding after 5 days is secondary haemorrhage due to infection that destroys the organizing blood clot.

General causes such as hypertension and warfarin therapy need to be addressed to control the bleeding.

Management is essentially reassurance, careful suction to clear the debris and clot in the socket, followed by packing with gauze soaked in lignocaine with adrenaline or cophenylcaine and pressure. Occasionally, the gingival flaps may need to be sutured under local anaesthetic.

Traumatic dental emergencies

Tooth avulsion is probably the most serious tooth injury. An avulsed tooth, if reimplanted in the socket within 30 min, has a 90% survival rate.[6] The mechanism of injury in such cases is usually either accidental sports-related facial injuries or assault.

Management

If the patient makes telephone contact with the emergency department the patient is advised to locate the tooth because, even if the crown is broken, the root may be intact. The tooth should not be handled by the root to avoid damage to the periodontal ligament fibres; it is washed in running cold water and replaced in the socket. If this is not possible, place the tooth in the cheek or under the tongue and proceed immediately to the dentist. Do not scrub the tooth.[7,8]

The best transportation medium for an avulsed tooth is saliva. Cold milk or iced salt water are suitable alternatives.

If the patient arrives in the emergency department with the tooth, clean it by holding it by the crown in cold running water; any foreign debris should be removed with forceps. The tooth should not be allowed to dry. Following irrigation the tooth should be placed in the socket as near the original position as possible, and the patient referred to a dentist for stabilization with an archbar or orthodontic bands.

If the reimplanted tooth remains mobile after 2 weeks it should be extracted. The complications of reimplantation are ankylosis and loss of viability.

Dentoalveolar trauma in children

Concussion and subluxation

Concussion is an injury to the tooth without displacement or mobility. Subluxation is when the tooth is mobile but not displaced.

Management
Periapical X-rays as base line, soft diet for a week and local dentist follow-up.

Intrusive luxation

Most common injury to upper primary incisors after a fall.

Management
If the crown is visible leave the tooth to re-erupt. If the whole tooth is intruded, extraction is required as it might affect the permanent dentition underneath.

Extrusive and lateral subluxation

If there is excessive mobility or displacement extraction is recommended.

Avulsion

Avulsed primary teeth should not be replanted. Unless there is extensive soft-tissue damage, antibiotics are not required.

Dental fractures

The incidence of fractured teeth is reported to be 5 and 4.4 per 100 adults per year for all teeth and posterior teeth respectively.[9] Based on the above statistics, it can be deduced that the likelihood of experiencing a fractured frontal/anterior tooth is about 1 in 20 in a given year in adults and in 1 in 23 for posterior teeth.

Traumatic injuries to the teeth have been classified as follows:[10]

Class I: Simple fracture of the enamel of the crown.
Class II: Extensive fracture of the crown involving dentine.
Class III: Extensive fracture of the crown involving dentine and dental pulp.
Class IV: Extensive involvement and exposure of the entire pulp.
Class V: Totally avulsed or luxated teeth.
Class VI: Fracture of the root with or without loss of crown structure.
Class VII: Displacement of tooth without fracture of crown or root.
Class VIII: Fracture of the crown in its entirety (Fig. 17.1.2).

Management

Emergency management includes reassurance, adequate analgesia, replacement of an avulsed tooth in the socket and

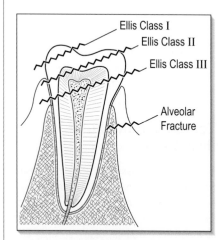

Fig. 17.1.2 Ellis classification. (From an original drawing by Ian Miller RN.)

immediate referral to a dentist for further evaluation and appropriate management.

Specific treatment depends on the type of fracture:[11]

- Class I: Treated by smoothing the enamel margins and applying topical fluoride to the fracture site.
- Class II A: Calcium hydroxide dressing is applied as a bandage to provide a stable form of temporary restoration, which will be replaced by a more aesthetic restoration as soon as the vitality of the pulp is assured.
- Class III: If seen within 6 h of the accident, calcium hydroxide direct pulp capping. If more than 6 h but less than 24 h, pulpotomy. If more than 24 h since the accident, total pulpectomy.
- Class IV: Conventional filling for permanent teeth and total pulpectomy for a primary tooth.
- Class V: Managed as for an avulsed tooth.
- Class VI: If the pulp is necrotic, pulpectomy and root canal therapy.
- Class VII: If the tooth is intruded it should be extracted. If driven through the labial plate of bone, extraction, and, if not, it should be left alone to re-erupt. If the tooth is extruded, slowly move it back to its original position using finger pressure. Primary teeth, if mobile after 2 weeks after the injury, should be extracted. Parents should be warned about possible damage to the developing permanent tooth.
- Class VIII: In a permanent tooth, pulpotomy or pulpectomy. Primary teeth with this amount of destruction should be extracted.
- When a tooth is missing following facial trauma, a thorough intraoral examination is followed by appropriate radiographs to avoid missing an intruded tooth. When full intrusion of a tooth is suspected, a facial computerized tomography (CT) scan may aid definite diagnosis.[12]

Temporomandibular dislocation

Temporomandibular dislocation can result from congenital weakness of ligaments, iatrogenic causes (traumatic extractions, prolonged dental procedures and direct laryngoscopy), trauma, drugs, epilepsy and even simple yawning. The dislocation may be unilateral but is more commonly bilateral.

The condyle is most frequently dislocated anterior to the articular eminence.

The patient presents with an open bite and malocclusion. If unilateral, the mandible deviates to the unaffected side. The patient complains of severe pain in the ear and is unable to fully open or close the mouth. Management includes diagnosis and reduction. The patient is seated, with posterior head support, and the muscle spasm is overcome by using intravenous benzodiazepines, such as midazolam, and narcotic analgesia such as fentanyl.

The mandible is held by the clinician by both hands, with the gloved thumbs intraorally just lateral to the lower molars. The mandibular condyle is then manipulated in a downward and backward direction below the articular eminence. In bilateral dislocation it may be easier to reduce one side at a time using a lateral rocking motion.

Following the procedure a postreduction radiograph is taken to confirm enlocation. The patient is discharged with a supportive bandage to the mandible and a soft diet advised for the next few days. Follow-up by the maxillofacial surgeon is essential, as temporomandibular dysfunction due to damage to the fibrous cartilage can lead to ongoing symptoms or recurrent dislocations.

Dental infection and abscess (odontogenic infection)

Dentofacial infections usually arise from necrotic pulps, periodontal pockets or pericoronitis.

The symptoms are pain and swelling of the adjacent gingival tissue with facial swelling and fever.

Examination reveals erythema and tender swelling of the gingival and in severe cases frank pus with halitosis. The offending tooth is tender on percussion.

Gingival probing, X-rays and orthopontomogram (OPG) confirm the diagnosis.

Management

Periapical abscess requires root canal (endodontic) treatment and extraction in severe cases.

Periodontal abscess requires scaling and root planing (periodontal) treatment and extraction in severe cases.

Complications include spread of infection into the submental, submandibular, parapharyngeal spaces of the neck and Ludwig's angina (cellulites of the floor of the mouth), which requires intravenous antibiotic therapy and drainage if a collection is diagnosed on the CT scan.

Controversies

❶ Dental services are generally not part of acute health service funding, therefore low-income patients may have to wait for medical complications of poor dental hygiene before being able to access appropriate care.

❷ Oil of cloves originated from India and was traditionally used topically for relief of dental pain such as dry socket prior to the availability of safe approved topical anaesthetic agents. However, it is highly toxic to human cells even at relatively low concentrations.

❸ 0.03% (v/v) and even small amounts can be life threatening if ingested.

References

1. Sheller B, Williams BJ, Lombardi SSM. Diagnosis and treatment of dental caries related emergencies in a children's hospital. American Academy of Pediatric Dentistry 1997; 19(8): 470–475.
2. Wilson S, Smith GA, Preisch J, Casamassimo PS. Non traumatic dental emergencies in a pediatric emergency department. Clinical Pediatrics 1997; 36(6): 333–337.
3. Matthews RW, Peak JD, Skully C. The efficacy of management of acute dental pain. British Dental Journal 1994; 176: 413–416.
4. Ahl DR, Hidgeman JL, Snyder JD. Periodontal emergencies. Dental Clinics of North America 1986; 30: 459–472.
5. Laskin DM, Steinberg B. Diagnosis and treatment of common dental emergencies. Medicine of Dentistry 1984; 77: 41–52.
6. Gaedeve Norris MK. Emergency treatment for tooth avulsion. Nursing – Springhouse INTERNATIONAL EDITION 1992; 92: 33–35.
7. Scheer B. Emergency treatment of avulsed incisor teeth. British Medical Journal 1990; 301: 4.
8. Rice RT, Bulford OG Jr. Clinical notebook. Emergency treatment of injured teeth. Journal of Emergency Nursing 1988; 14(1): 32–33.
9. Bader JD, Martin JA, Shugars DA. Preliminary estimates of the incidence and consequences of tooth fracture. Journal of the American Dental Association 1995; 126: 1650–1654.
10. Ellis RG, Davey KW. The classification and treatment of injuries to the teeth of children. 5th edn. Chicago: Yearbook Medical Publishers; 1970.
11. Braham RL, Roberts MW, Morris ME. Management of dental trauma in children and adolescents. Journal of Trauma 1977; 17(11): 857–865.
12. Tung-Chain T, Yu-Ray C, Chien-Tzung C, Chia-Jung L. Full intrusion of a tooth after facial trauma. Journal of Trauma 1977; 2: 357–359.

ENT

Edited by **Peter Cameron**

18.1 Ears, nose and throat

Sashi Kumar

ESSENTIALS

1 Removal of foreign bodies from the ear requires good lighting, a cooperative or fully restrained patient and a patient/gentle approach by the clinician.

2 Haematoma of the auricle requires urgent release by aseptic incision and immediate application of a firm mastoid bandage.

3 It is important to exclude septal haematoma in patients with a fractured nose. In general X-rays are not warranted.

4 Patients presenting with odynophagia but no dysphagia following ingestion of a fish bone, and negative physical examination and radiology, can be safely discharged for review within 48 h.

5 Sudden sensory neural hearing loss constitutes an ENT emergency, which requires urgent ENT consultation and audiometry.

THE EAR

Introduction

Emergency presentations for ear, nose and throat (ENT) problems are common and all emergency physicians need to be familiar with the basic skills required for assessment and management of these problems.

Foreign body

Foreign bodies in the ear are most common in children under the age of 5 and in mentally handicapped adults. Animate objects such as insects in the ear can affect all ages, especially adults who enjoy the outdoors, particularly at dusk.

Accidental foreign bodies, such as the end of a cotton bud or a matchstick, occur in people obsessed with cleaning their ears with such objects.

Management

Two simple rules in managing foreign bodies in the ear are:

- Do not attempt to remove a foreign body that is not there! (Identify the foreign body prior to attempts at removal.)
- Unless the object is alive, there is no emergency to remove it if it can be done safely at a later time under better conditions.

Removal of a live foreign body

This is a true ENT emergency. The insect should be killed as a matter of urgency, as considerable damage is being done to the sensitive skin of the bony meatus and the tympanic membrane by the flapping wings and appendages of the desperate insect trying to escape.

The movement of the insect also causes intense pain and tinnitus, thereby creating further anxiety and distress.

Any liquid used to kill the insect should be carefully chosen so as to avoid damage to the sensitive skin and tympanic membrane: strong corrosive agents, knockdown spray or alcohol should be avoided. The common agents of choice are lignocaine 2%, olive oil, water for injection or normal saline.

One of the preferred methods is to instil some water for injection from a 10 mL plastic ampoule and leave an examination light on the pinna. The insect swims up to surface towards the light and can be helped to safety by holding the tip of the ampoule.[1]

Removal of a foreign body in a child or a mentally handicapped adult may be done in one of two ways. The patient is either cooperative and unrestrained or fully restrained. It is vital not to attempt any procedure with partial restraint, as any movement of the patient during the attempt could cause trauma to the ear canal and the tympanic membrane.

There are two techniques used to remove a foreign body. The dry method is by using a Jobson Horne probe for solid objects such as beads or alligator forceps for an insect or a cotton bud. The wet method is by syringing the ear canal with tepid water. The water should be close to body temperature to avoid a caloric effect, which produces nystagmus and vertigo.

The key to success is good lighting, preferably through a head lamp, a cooperative or fully restrained patient, and a patient, gentle approach by the clinician, who knows when to stop if unsuccessful.

Trauma

Trauma to the ear canal requires the ear to be kept dry for about a week with antibiotic ear drops for 4–5 days in severe cases to avoid progressing into otitis externa.

Penetrating trauma can cause perforation of the eardrum and occasionally disruption of the ossicular chain. Dislocation of the footplate of the stapes following such an injury can cause permanent sensorineural hearing loss. Referral to an ENT specialist is essential in all cases of traumatic perforation with suspected ossicular chain disruption.

Blunt trauma

Boxing and other contact sports can lead to blunt trauma to the pinna. Accumulation of blood under the perichondrium, if not treated properly, may progress to cartilage necrosis and the end result is a 'cauliflower ear'.

A slap on the ear can also produce a ruptured tympanic membrane with or without ossicular chain disruption.

Assessment

Assessment of the injury includes a clinical assessment of the hearing loss. A ruptured eardrum without ossicular chain disruption does not usually cause a significant hearing loss. Any evidence of nystagmus or tinnitus suggests damage to the inner ear.

Management

A simple traumatic perforation of the eardrum is managed by simple analgesics and keeping the ear dry. On no account should any drops or water be allowed into the ear, as this may precipitate otitis media.

If ossicular chain disruption or inner ear trauma is suspected, an urgent ENT opinion is required to assess the need for urgent tympanotomy and repair.

Haematoma of the pinna requires urgent release of the accumulated blood by aseptic incision and drainage and the immediate application of a firm mastoid bandage to prevent reaccumulation and this should be left in place for up to a week. The patient should be placed on broad-spectrum antibiotics to prevent infection.

Infection

Otitis externa

Infection of the external ear is common and affects between 3 and 10% of the patient population.[2] It can be localized (furuncle) or diffuse. The symptoms are pain, itching and tenderness to palpation, followed by aural fullness, hearing loss and discharge. The common pathogens responsible are *Pseudomonas aeruginosa*, *Proteus* spp. and *Staphylococcus aureus*.[3]

The diagnosis is usually self-evident, but the diagnostic signs of otitis externa are tragal tenderness or pain on pulling the pinna. This is a disease of the cartilaginous ear canal, with swelling and discharge causing occlusion of the meatus. It may be extremely painful to pass the ear speculum and often the tympanic membrane is not able to be visualized.

Management

The most important step in the treatment is thorough and atraumatic cleansing of the ear canal.[4] Tolerance and cooperation between the patient and the clinician is vital. Pope Otowick (Xomed)® is very useful in the management of this condition. This is a semirigid foam wick that, when inserted into the ear canal, swells, absorbing moisture to increase the size of the ear canal. Topical otic drops, such as Sofradex® (Roussel), are used three to four times a day and the patient is reviewed on a daily basis to change the wick and continue the ear toilet. Occasionally oral antibiotics such as ciprofloxacin or flucloxacillin may be required,[5] particularly if there is evidence of cellulitis. The patient is advised to keep the ear clear of any water. Strong analgesics are usually required.

Fungal otitis externa (otomycosis) tends to be not that painful and is treated with ear toilet as described and topical antifungal ear drops such as Loco corten vioform.

Otitis media

Acute otitis media is a common infection and is due to blocking of the eustachian tube (eustachian catarrh), and negative pressure in the middle ear cavity. Although viral in origin, secondary bacterial infection often supervenes. The most frequently isolated pathogens are *Streptococcus pneumoniae*, *Haemophilus influenzae* and *Moraxella catarrhalis*.[6] The symptoms are earache, fullness, hearing loss and fever, with ear discharge if the drum has perforated. The development of discharge usually marks an improvement in the pain and fever.

The clinical findings vary from a retracted dull eardrum to a congested bulging drum or a white eardrum with pus behind, and a perforated tympanic membrane with discharge in the ear canal. A perforated eardrum without much pain is usually a sign of chronic otitis media.

Management

Treatment is almost always empiric and amoxicillin is a good first-line therapy. Cephalosporins and trimethoprim/sulpha are also used with considerable success. The newer macrolides, such as azithromycin and clarithromycin, are rational alternatives.[6]

In otitis media with a perforated eardrum, the mainstay of treatment should be toilet by dry mopping followed by antibiotic drops such as Sofradex®. The ear should be kept dry and regular follow-up arranged until the perforation has healed.

Labyrinthitis

Acute labyrinthitis usually has cochlear symptoms such as hearing loss and tinnitus, which should be referred for audiometry and urgent ENT evaluation. If the symptoms are limited to vertigo and nystagmus, it is more likely to be due to acute vestibular neuronitis.

Management

The management of labyrinthitis includes bed rest, antiemetics, e.g. prochlorperazine, benzodiazepine, e.g. diazepam, and admission if severely debilitating. In the presence of hearing loss a course of oral steroids or intra-tympanic dexamethasone may be started after discussions with the ENT surgeon.

Otitis media with effusion (glue ear)

This is most common in children in developed countries. The symptoms are fullness and hearing loss, and occasionally pain. Management includes the diagnosis based on history and examination, which reveals a dull, retracted drum or fluid behind the drum without redness. The most reliable sign of a glue ear is an immobile eardrum on valsalva manoeuvre or pneumatic otoscopy. Repeated attacks of glue ear are an indication for the insertion of tympanostomy tubes.

Mastoiditis

Acute mastoiditis is a complication of acute or chronic otitis media. It is a rare condition in the developed world, although still quite prevalent in the developing world and the aboriginal population of Australia. Otitis externa with a painful and tender postauricular lymph node is usually mistaken for acute mastoiditis due to the postauricular tenderness. Extension of infection can cause meningitis or cerebral abscess, with life-threatening complications if untreated.

Examination reveals infection in the middle ear cavity by way of an injected drum or a perforated drum with discharge. The cardinal sign of acute mastoiditis is tenderness at the base of the mastoid on digital pressure. The diagnosis is confirmed by CT scan.

Management

Admission, intravenous antibiotics and surgical intervention to drain the abscess.

THE NOSE

Foreign body

A foreign body in the nose is common in preschool children and adults with mental retardation. The most common types of foreign body are beads, buttons and pieces of paper.

The diagnostic sign of a neglected nasal foreign body is a unilateral foul-smelling nasal discharge. The patient or the parent usually provides the history as to the type of foreign body and for how long present.

Management

The removal of the foreign body follows the same rules as for a foreign body in the ear.

An additional method is to blow forcefully through the patient's mouth while occluding the unaffected nostril. This could be done by the parent with instruction.

The suggested method of removal is to pass the ring end of a Jobson–Horne probe above and behind the foreign body and to roll it along the floor of the nose. This patient should be cooperative and unrestrained, or fully restrained. At the first sign of trauma or bleeding removal should be organized under general anaesthesia as soon as practically possible.

Trauma

Fractured nose

This is a common presentation in the emergency department. The history is often quite clear and the findings include pain and tenderness over the nasal bones with or without crepitus, and swelling at the bridge of the nose with or without epistaxis.

Careful examination will usually rule out CSF rhinorrhoea due to cribriform plate fracture and any external deformity. Active bleeding from the nostril should be controlled by direct pressure by pinching the nostril; if it does not settle it may require nasal packing.

Radiographs are not indicated for nasal bone fracture as this is a clinical diagnosis. It is often difficult to visualize the fracture line on the X-rays and radiographs do not help in the management. If associated facial fractures are suspected, X-ray facial views or CT scan should be taken.

Management

Acute intervention is required in the following circumstances:

- Continuing epistaxis should be managed along the lines described later.
- Obvious external deformity of the nose needs cosmetic correction, either by immediate reduction under local anaesthetic or by referral to an ENT surgeon for review and reduction in 7–10 days time. A formal rhinoplasty may be required in severe cases. The acute management of a fractured nose is reassurance, analgesia and ice packs, followed by a review by the general practitioner or an ENT surgeon in 7–10

days. The patient is advised to avoid any form of contact sport for a week.
- CSF rhinorrhoea requires a CT scan and neurosurgical referral.
- A septal haematoma, which is clinically apparent as a widened and bulging septum, can become infected, causing a septal abscess that could result in the collapse of the external nose. The diagnosis is made by visualizing the boggy swelling on one or both sides of the septum, and management requires admission, drainage under local or general anaesthesia, followed by nasal packing.

Sinusitis

Approximately 90% of upper respiratory infections have associated sinus cavity disease.[7] Viral rhinosinusitis is the most common cause and is associated with the common cold. Approximately 0.5–2% of these cases progress to bacterial sinusitis.

Clinical features

Symptoms of viral sinusitis are rhinorrhoea, nasal obstruction and sneezing, and facial pressure with or without headache. With bacterial superinfection a purulent or coloured nasal discharge and fever of 38°C or higher develop. Significant facial pain and maxillary toothache with no obvious dental cause also occurs. The common organisms involved are *Streptococcus pneumoniae* and *H. influenzae*. Patients with allergic sinusitis typically have sneezing and itching, with watery eyes, as a leading symptom.

Radiographs of the sinus are not very helpful unless they demonstrate a distinct air-fluid level, as this increases with the likelihood of bacterial sinusitis. CT can indicate the presence of sinus abnormalities and evidence of infection. A raised white cell count is neither sensitive nor specific in the diagnosis of bacterial sinusitis.

Management of viral rhinosinusitis is symptomatic and it is generally self-limiting. Bacterial sinusitis must be treated with antibiotics: amoxicillin, augmentin or keflex could be used as first-line drugs. Although of unproven value, an oral decongestant or antihistamine is commonly used. Complications of sinus disease include meningitis, orbital extension and brain abscess.

Diagnosis is by CT scan and treatment is intravenous antibiotics with surgical intervention by an otolaryngologist.

Epistaxis

Nose bleeding is the most common ENT emergency: a Scottish study reported an incidence of 30/100 000 people[8] in which the cause could only be found in 15%.[9] The common identified causes are trauma, blood dyscrasias, anticoagulation therapy and occasionally hereditary haemorrhagic telangiectasia.[10] Although hypertension has been traditionally labelled as a cause of epistaxis, studies have shown that blood pressure in these patients is no higher than in the control population.[11,12]

The history is vital and all patients should be asked where the blood appeared first – anteriorly in the nose or in the back of the throat. Anterior epistaxis can usually be controlled in the emergency department and the patient safely discharged home without a nasal pack after cautery.

Management

The control of epistaxis due to a general cause such as uncontrolled warfarin therapy or a bleeding disorder is to reverse the cause. Local measures can still be used to stem the flow.

Idiopathic epistaxis, or that due to a local cause such as trauma, can be dealt with using local measures. The most common cause of anterior epistaxis is bleeding from Kiesselbach's plexus of the septum[13] (Fig. 18.1.1), which can easily be controlled by simple measures in the emergency department. Careful examination of a seated patient applying direct pressure to the bleeding vessel by pinching the anterior nares with the thumb and forefinger for up to 10 min will usually slow or cease the bleeding. At this point it is essential to remove all the blood clots from the nasal cavity and the postnasal space using a suction.

Following this, the application of cotton pledgets soaked in 5% cocaine or lignocaine with adrenaline or cophenylcaine (phenylephrine and lignocaine) will provide analgesia and vasoconstriction to the septum and the anterior part of the lateral wall.

Examination may reveal the bleeding vessel on the septum, which can be cauterized under direct vision using silver nitrate sticks. Following this the patient is observed for a short time and can be discharged from the emergency department. The patient is advised not to pick, rub or blow the nose for 10 days and is advised to keep the cauterized area moist by applying chloromycetin eye ointment or Vaseline twice a day.

If the bleeding cannot be controlled by the above measures, or the bleeding point is posteriorly placed, the nasal cavity should be packed. There are several ways to pack the nose, the most traditional being to use ribbon gauze to fill the entire nasal cavity in layers (Fig.18.1.2). A Foley urinary catheter can be used to control the posterior bleed, but it can be better controlled with a specifically designed epistaxis catheter such as a Brighton's epistaxis catheter, which has a double balloon for anterior

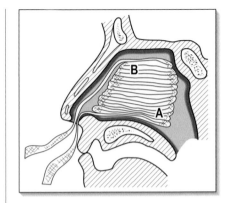

Fig. 18.1.2 Insertion of anterior nasal pack (begin at A and finish at B). (From an original drawing by Ian Miller RN.)

and posterior tamponade, or a Merocel® nasal pack (Xomed) or Rapid Rhino, which can be used as a nasal tampon, both of which are quite useful. Almost all patients with nasal packing need admission and observation. When the above measures are unsuccessful, further invasive procedures such as postnasal packing, examination under anaesthesia and septal surgery or arterial ligation may be required under general anaesthesia.

Summary

Patients with anterior nasal bleeds can usually be managed by chemical cautery with silver nitrate and then be discharged. Posterior bleeding or failure to control by simple measures may require nasal packing and admission for further invasive procedures.

THE THROAT

Foreign body

Coins are a common oesophageal foreign body in children. In adults the foreign body is usually a fish, chicken or meat bone, and occasionally objects such as partial dentures, safety pins, etc.

The common lodgement sites include the cricopharynx, the oesophagus at the level of the aortic arch, and the gastro-oesophageal junction. Fish bones can lodge in the tonsil, the posterior third of the tongue or the vallecula prior to entering the oesophagus.

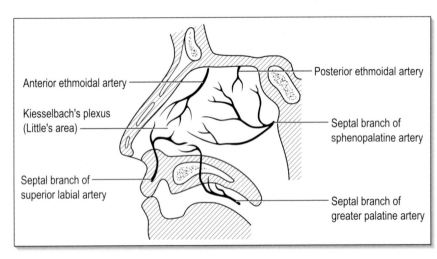

Fig. 18.1.1 Arterial supply to the nasal septum. (From an original drawing by Ian Miller RN.)

Anterior ethmoidal artery

Kiesselbach's plexus (Little's area)

Septal branch of superior labial artery

Posterior ethmoidal artery

Septal branch of sphenopalatine artery

Septal branch of greater palatine artery

Management

Careful examination of the oropharynx initially, especially if the patient localizes the foreign body above the level of the hyoid and to one side. If the foreign body is found it should be removed under direct vision.

A foreign body at or below the cricopharynx requires general anaesthesia and endoscopy.

Lateral X-ray of the neck is useful in identifying and localizing radio-opaque foreign bodies, such as coins and bones, including large fish bones.

Patients presenting with odynophagia but no dysphagia following the ingestion of a fish bone, and a negative physical examination, can be discharged safely for review in 48 h. Symptoms of increasing odynophagia, fever, haematemesis or dysphagia warrant admission for endoscopy. Patients with a confirmed foreign body should be admitted for endoscopy and removal.

A food bolus not containing bone causing obstruction should have a trial of i.v. glucagon 1 mg, i.v. buscopan 20–40 mg and sips of a fizzy drink before arranging for an endoscopy, as one of these may dislodge the obstruction, thereby avoiding an urgent endoscopy. Recurrent food bolus obstructions require an endoscopy to rule out stricture or malignancy.

Button batteries

Button battery lodged in the oesophagus can cause liquefaction necrosis and perforation so urgent endoscopy and removal is recommended.[14]

If the battery is lodged past the oesophagus in the stomach most, if not all, will pass in the next 48–72 h and the patient can be safely discharged following reassurance.[15]

Infection

Tonsillitis

Patients with acute tonsillitis present to the general practitioner and occasionally to the emergency department. The emergency department patients usually have severe symptoms or are not responding to oral antibiotics. They are often dehydrated, toxic, with a high temperature and unable to take adequate oral fluids. Treatment includes intravenous penicillin in high doses (e.g. 2 g 4 hourly), intravenous fluids and adequate analgesia.

Infectious mononucleosis (Glandular fever)

The symptoms are similar to severe tonsillitis with odynophagia, fever and a hot potato voice. The tonsils are quite swollen but have a smooth diffuse swelling with not much exudate on the fossa. The cervical lymph nodes are enlarged and tender and there may also be axillary and inguinal lymphadenopathy with or without hepatosplenomegaly.

The diagnosis is made by abnormal lymphocytes in the blood film and monospot test.

Treatment is symptomatic. Amoxicillin should not be used as it produces a rash.

Quinsy

Peritonsillar abscess or quinsy is a condition in which the infection in the tonsil has breached the capsule and caused cellulitis in the adjacent soft palate (peritonsillitis), and eventually a collection of pus (quinsy).

Examination reveals a congested tonsil being pushed medially and downwards by a diffuse swelling of the soft palate. The opposite tonsil may look injected. There are often unilateral or bilateral enlarged and tender jugulodigastric lymph nodes in the neck. The patient is usually febrile, toxic and dehydrated. There is marked trismus due to masseteric spasm and referred otalgia.

Management includes admission to hospital for intravenous fluids, penicillin or cephalosporin, and adequate analgesia. Aspiration of the pus using a large-bore needle or incision and drainage of the quinsy can be done in the emergency department under local anaesthesia in a conscious patient sitting up. Sometimes this needs general anaesthesia. Intubation of such patients should be performed by a skilled anaesthetist preferably by awake fibre optic technique and every effort must be made to avoid rupturing the abscess to avoid aspiration of pus.

Retropharyngeal abscess

This is predominantly a disease of young children, as the retropharyngeal lymph nodes atrophy after the age of 5. In older patients it could be secondary to trauma or lodgement of a foreign body, such as a fish bone. Diagnosis is made on symptoms of fever, swelling of the neck due to cervical lymphadenopathy and, especially in young children, stridor. Clinical suspicion leads to imaging procedures such as CT, which is diagnostic.

Management includes admission to hospital, intravenous antibiotics and urgent ENT consultation. Treatment is incision and drainage of the abscess under general anaesthesia.

Epiglottitis

Childhood epiglottitis is rare these days due to a highly successive immunization programme against *Haemophilus influenza*. Adults with epiglottitis are still occasionally seen in emergency departments. The classical symptoms are acutely painful throat, drooling, odynophagia and increased pain to speech with enlarged tender bilateral cervical lymph nodes.

A quick bedside test is to ask the patient to poke his or her tongue out and wiggle it from side to side as this will increase the pain substantially.

Management is mainly intravenous antibiotics and analgesia. If the patient is showing signs of imminent upper airway obstruction, an attempt should be made to intubate by the most skilled emergency doctor available with the surgical airway kit readily available in case of failure.

All other patients should be taken to the operating theatre for a gaseous induction by a skilled anaesthetist with an ENT surgeon standing by for immediate surgical airway if unable to intubate.

Post-tonsillectomy bleed

Haemorrhage from the tonsillar fossa that occurs 24 h after tonsillectomy is termed 'secondary haemorrhage'. This differs from primary, which happens during surgery, and reactionary haemorrhage, which occurs within 24 h of surgery whilst the patient is still in the hospital. The cause of secondary haemorrhage is usually infection and this occurs classically 10 days postoperatively. This incidence is about 1% and is usually not very severe. The management is intravenous antibiotics, usually penicillin. The patient should be admitted and bloods taken for estimation of haemoglobin and cross-matching. Application of a swab soaked in 1 in 1000 adrenaline (epinephrine) to the tonsillar fossa after removal of the clot may help to stop the bleeding. Rarely the patient may need to have a general anaesthetic to cauterize/ligate the bleeder.[16]

Controversies

❶ Timing of nasal fracture reduction. This may be performed either immediately or after 7–10 days.

❷ The method used for control of epistaxis. There is no clear advantage in using one method over another.

References

1. Kumar S. An interesting method of removal of live foreign body from the ear. Emerg. Med. 1998; 10: 278
2. Bojrab DI, Bruderly T, Razzak YA. Otitis externa. Otolaryngology Clinics of North America 1996; 29(5): 761–782.
3. Briggs RJ. Otitis externa: presentation and management. Australian Family Physician 1995; 24(10): 1859–1864.
4. Ali Raza S, Denholm SW, Wong JCH. An audit of the management of acute otitis externa in an ENT casualty clinic. Journal of Laryngology and Otology 1995; 109: 130–133.
5. Mirza N. Otitis externa - management in the primary care office. Postgraduate Medicine 1996; 99(5): 153–158.
6. Block SL. Causative pathogens, antibiotic resistance and therapeutic considerations in acute otitis media. Paediatric Infectious Diseases Journal 1997; 16(4): 449–456.
7. Bukata R. Sinusitis, a ubiquitous, yet enigmatic disease. Emergency Medicine and Acute Care Essays 1997; 21(3): 1–4.
8. Kotecha B, Fowler S, Harkness P, et al. Management of epistaxis: a national survey. Annals of the Royal College of Surgeons of England 1996; 78: 444–446.
9. Small M, Maran AGD. Epistaxis and arterial ligation. Journal of Laryngology and Otology 1984; 98: 281–284.
10. Juselius H. Epistaxis. Journal of Laryngology and Otology 1974; 88: 317–327.
11. Shaheen OH. Studies of nasal vasculature and problems of arterial ligation for epistaxis. Annals of the Royal College of Surgeons of England 1970; 47: 30–44.
12. Weiss NS. The relation of high blood pressure to headache and epistaxis and selected other symptoms. New England Journal of Medicine 1972; 287: 631–633.
13. Darry KW, Barlow F, Deleyiannis WB, Pinczower EF. Effectiveness of surgical management of epistaxis at a tertiary care center. Laryngoscope 1997; 107: 21–24.
14. Gordon AC, Gough MH. Oesophageal perforation after button battery ingestion. Ann Coll Surg Engl 1993; 75: 362–364.
15. Kumar S. Management of foreign bodies in the ear, nose and throat. Emergency Medicine 2004; 16: 17–20.
16. Evans JNG, ed. Scott Brown's Otolaryngology. 5th edn. Butterworth, London; 1987: 96

OBSTETRICS AND GYNAECOLOGY

Edited by **Anthony F. T. Brown**

19.1 Emergency delivery

Stephen Priestley

ESSENTIALS

1 Perform a rapid assessment of pregnant patients arriving in labour at the emergency department in order to decide on the most appropriate site for management.

2 Equipment, drugs and protocols must be placed within emergency departments so that unexpected deliveries can be managed safely.

3 Establish and maintain lines of communication with regional obstetric services so that decisions regarding management of labour and transfer of mothers and babies are optimum.

4 Emergency department staff must be prepared to provide newborn resuscitation following an emergency delivery. Preparedness for newborn resuscitation requires preparation of a suitable, warmed area, special equipment and trained personnel, and a structured approach to assessment and intervention.

Introduction

Occasionally doctors working in emergency departments (EDs) are faced with caring for a patient in labour and are required to manage a spontaneous vaginal delivery. This situation is generally accompanied by much anxiety on the part of the ED medical and nursing staff, but it is important that a calm, systematic approach is taken to minimize the risk of an adverse fetal or maternal outcome. This chapter describes the management of a normal delivery in the ED.

The setting

There are a number of settings where childbirth may need to occur in an ED. Pregnant patients at different gestational ages may present to the ED in varying stages of labour. Immediate management will depend on the availability of obstetric services, the gestational age and on both the stage of labour and its anticipated speed of progression.

Safe transfer to a delivery suite when there is adequate time is always preferable to delivery in the ED. If there is no delivery suite available and/or there is no time for transfer to an appropriate facility, or the patient arrives with full cervical dilatation and the fetal presenting part is on the perineal verge, then arrangements need to be rapidly made to perform the delivery in the ED.

Precipitate labour

Patients who have precipitate labour – an extremely rapid labour lasting less than 4 h (more common in the multiparous) – may have to stop in the ED even when *en route* to the delivery suite, or another hospital, because of the rapidity of the labour.

Concealed or unrecognized pregnancy

The diagnosis of a concealed or unrecognized pregnancy may also be made in the ED. Concealed pregnancies occur most commonly in teenage girls who do not tell anyone that they are pregnant and receive no antenatal care, whilst unrecognized pregnancies occur most commonly in obese females who may present to the ED complaining of abdominal pains or a vaginal discharge and are found to be pregnant and/or in labour. Women with intellectual impairment or mental illness are another group that may present with an unrecognized pregnancy.

'Born before arrival'

The term 'precipitous birth' or 'born before arrival' (BBA) is commonly associated with precipitate labour and refers to women who deliver their baby prior to arrival at a hospital, usually without the assistance of a trained person. Both the mother and the baby require assessment and may need resuscitation and completion of the third stage of labour on arrival in the ED. The incidence of BBA is low and in one series was found to occur 1 in 695 births (0.14%), whilst the incidence of precipitate labour is 17% in the total hospital population.[1]

History

Assessment of the patient in labour in the ED includes obtaining information regarding gestational age, antenatal care, progression of the pregnancy, past obstetric and a medical history. Always enquire if the patient has a copy of her antenatal care record with her. Then perform a physical and obstetric examination to confirm the progression of labour, the number of babies and the presence or absence of any complications related to the pregnancy and labour.

In hospitals where there is a delivery suite, a member of that unit should be called to attend the ED to either assist with immediate transfer to the delivery suite if possible, or with the assessment and conduct of the labour within the ED. Delivery in hospitals where there is no delivery suite should include immediate contact by telephone with the nearest or most appropriate obstetric unit to obtain advice and to organize transfer of the mother and newborn.

Gestational age

The gestational age may be determined from the last normal menstrual period (LNMP) if this is known. Naegle's rule is the most common method of pregnancy dating. The estimated date of delivery (EDD) is calculated by counting back three months from the last menstrual period and adding seven days. As an example, if the last menstrual period is December 20, then the EDD will be September 27. This method assumes the patient has a 28-day menstrual cycle with fertilization occurring on day 14. Inaccuracy occurs because many women do not have regular 28-day cycles, or do not conceive on day 14, and many others are not certain of the date of their last period.

Gestational age estimation

Antenatal ultrasound is useful in estimating the estimated date of confinement (EDC) where dates are uncertain, remembering that scans performed later in the pregnancy are less accurate in dating the gestational age of the baby than those performed early in the pregnancy. Additionally, a rough estimation of the gestational age of the baby can be made by abdominal examination. Between 20 and 35 weeks there is a rough correlation between gestational age and the height of the uterine fundus measured in centimeters from the pubic symphysis.

Past obstetric history

The past obstetric history should include the duration and description of previous labours, the types of deliveries and the sizes of previous babies in addition to a history of a previous caesarean section, the use of forceps or vacuum extraction, a neonatal death and history of abnormal presentations, shoulder dystocia, prolonged delivery of the placenta or a post-partum haemorrhage.

Maternal medical conditions

Maternal conditions such as cardiac and respiratory disease, diabetes, bleeding diatheses, hepatitis B and herpes simplex should be documented. Note all drugs whether prescribed, over-the-counter or illicit that the patient is taking. The presence of any bleeding or other complications during the pregnancy should also be noted. Obtain the results of antenatal investigations, including a full blood count, blood group, hepatitis-B status, HIV and syphilis serology.

Take a careful history regarding the onset and timing of contractions and the presence and nature of fetal movements, in addition to a history of vaginal bleeding or discharge, which may represent the rupture of membranes.

Examination

General examination

Carry out a general examination with particular emphasis on vital signs, and the abdominal and pelvic examination. Examine the breast, nipples, heart and chest and perform a urinalysis looking for evidence of infection, glucose or proteinuria, which may be associated with preeclampsia (see Ch. 19.7).

Abdominal examination

Perform an abdominal examination to ascertain the height of the fundus, the lie and presentation of the baby and to make an assessment of the engagement of the presenting part. The presence of scars and extrauterine masses should be noted. Assess the frequency, regularity, duration and intensity of uterine contractions.

Fetal heart rate

Count the fetal heart for 1 min using an ordinary stethoscope, Pinard or a Doppler stethoscope, which should normally be between 110 and 160 beats/min. Count the fetal heart for at least 30 s following a contraction. If bradycardia is detected, give the mother oxygen and position her in the left lateral position to ensure that uterine blood flow and fetal oxygenation is optimized.

If post-contraction bradycardias persist despite these measures then give an intravenous fluid bolus and seek specialist obstetric advice. Note any vaginal bleeding or discharge and record the amount remembering haemorrhage may also be concealed. Assess the colour and character of any amniotic fluid, looking for evidence of meconium staining.

Vaginal examination

Perform an aseptic vaginal examination with the patient in the dorsal lithotomy position to assess the effacement, consistency and dilatation of the cervix, the nature and position of the presenting part (i.e. vertex or breech) and to exclude a cord prolapse. If unsure of the nature of the presenting part, a portable ultrasound can aid in diagnosis.

The exception to performing a vaginal examination is the gravid patient with active vaginal bleeding who should be evaluated with an ultrasound to exclude placenta praevia, *before* performing any pelvic examination.

If the membranes are intact, there is no indication to rupture them if the labour is progressing satisfactorily, as there is a risk of cord prolapse when the presenting part is not engaged in the pelvis.[2] After the vaginal examination, apply a sterile perineal pad and allow the mother to assume whichever position gives her the most comfort, whilst avoiding the completely supine position with the potential for inferior vena cava (IVC) compression by the gravid uterus.

Considerations on transferring the patient

After this assessment the decision whether to transfer the patient to a delivery suite either within the hospital, or at a distant hospital, must be made. Cervical dilatation greater than 6 cm in a multiparous patient and 7–8 cm in the primiparous makes transfer to a distant hospital a hazardous procedure because of the risk of rapid progression to full cervical dilatation and imminent delivery of the baby. The availability and type of transport and personnel, and the distance to be travelled must be carefully considered. Consult with the obstetric unit regarding the safety of transfer and make arrangements for reception of the patient.

Management

Preparation for delivery

Ongoing assessment of maternal temperature, blood pressure, heart rate and contractions should be performed and recorded. Fetal heart rate should be counted every 15–30 min up to full cervical dilatation and every 5 min thereafter. The fetal heart rate is best measured with a Doppler device, commencing towards the end of a contraction and continuing for at least 30 s after the contraction has finished.

Unless there is a clear indication for an intravenous line such as a history of postpartum haemorrhage or antepartum haemorrhage, bleeding tendency, evidence of pre-eclampsia or history of a previous caesarean section, then placement for the normal delivery is unnecessary. Perform simple venepuncture for a haemoglobin and blood group, and put some blood aside for cross-matching.

Equipment and drugs

Obtain a delivery pack, sterile surgical instruments and oxytocic drugs and place close by (see Table 19.1.1). Resuscitation equipment and drugs should be available. Assemble personnel with clear task delegation, remembering that reassurance and emotional support for the mother and the mother's partner is crucial during the entire labour. A specific member of staff may be delegated to provide this.

If a midwife or doctor experienced in delivery is available then they should assume control of the procedure and continue the assessment of the progression of labour and conduct the delivery of both the baby and the placenta. A doctor or nurse with some experience in neonatal or paediatric resuscitation should perform a rapid assessment of the newborn immediately after the delivery of the baby, to ascertain the need for resuscitation.

Conduct of labour

Labour is divided into three stages: The first stage is from the onset of regular contractions to full (10 cm) dilatation of the cervix. The second stage is from full dilatation of the cervix to delivery of the baby and the third stage is from the birth of the baby until delivery of the placenta. A full description of the detailed management of the three stages of labour is beyond the scope of this chapter, but a brief summary of the management of a normal vertex delivery is described.

First stage

Examine the patient abdominally and vaginally as necessary to follow the progress of the labour. As mentioned earlier, perform measurement and recording of maternal vital signs and fetal heart rate. Gently wash the perineum with a non-irritating soap solution such as 0.1% chlorhexidine, particularly when operative vaginal delivery by forceps or vacuum extraction is anticipated. Neither shaving, urinary catheterization nor enema administration is required.

Table 19.1.1 Equipment and drugs required for emergency delivery	
Equipment	**Drugs**
Three clamps – straight or curved (e.g. Pean)	Adrenaline 1:10 000
Episiotomy scissors	Oxytocin 10 units
Scissors	Ergometrine 250 µg
Suture repair set	Vitamin K 1 mg
Absorbable suture material	Lignocaine 1%
Neonatal resuscitation equipment (ETT, laryngoscope etc)	Naloxone 400 µg/1 mL
Blanket	
Warmer	
Sterile drapes	
Huck towels	
Sterile gloves	
Soap solution	
Sterile bowls	
Umbilical vein catheters	

ETT, endotracheal tube.

Analgesia Analgesics are helpful for the patient with significant discomfort and are not injurious to the fetus. The timing and dose of analgesia must be decided with due regard to the stage and rate of progression of labour. Intramuscular opiates such as pethidine 1–1.5 mg/kg are commonly used and provide some relief from pain with varying degrees of sedation. The provision of other forms of analgesia such as epidural anaesthesia is more commonly employed in a delivery suite rather than in the ED delivery. Do not give sedatives and analgesic drugs immediately before anticipated delivery because of potential depressive effects on the baby.

The average duration of the first stage of labour in primiparous patients is 14 h, and in subsequent pregnancies is 6–8 h.

Second stage

Spontaneous delivery of the fetus presenting by vertex is divided into three phases: delivery of the head, delivery of the shoulders and delivery of the body and legs. The second stage of labour begins when the cervix is fully dilated and delivery will occur when the presenting part reaches the pelvic floor.

The normal duration of this stage in the absence of regional anaesthesia ranges from 20 to 60 min in the primiparous, down to 10–30 min in the multiparous patient. Prolongation of the second stage may be defined as 2 h or more in the primiparous patient, and 1 h or more in the multiparous patient. Preparations for delivery, including cleansing, are made as described earlier. Drape the patient in such a manner that there is a clear view of the perineum.

Maternal position Either a dorsal lithotomy or lateral Sims' position may be used for the actual delivery. The dorsal lithotomy position is recommended for inexperienced operators, as it is easier to visualize and manually control the delivery process, and perform an episiotomy. In the dorsal lithotomy position the mother should be tilted slightly over to the left side using a pillow or soft wedge, to avoid compression of the inferior vena cava by the gravid uterus and possible maternal hypotension and fetal hypoxia.

Episiotomy When the presenting part distends the perineum delivery is imminent.

Consider an episiotomy at this time, but one should *not* be performed routinely. Episiotomy refers to a surgical incision of the female perineum performed by the accoucheur at the time of parturition. The primary reason to perform an episiotomy is to prevent a large spontaneous, irregular laceration of the perineum. It is usually performed with scissors when the perineum is stretched and distended, just prior to crowning of the fetal head, following infiltration of a posterior area of the peritoneum with 5–10 mL of 1% lignocaine (lidocaine) between contractions.

Commonly a mediolateral perineal incision is made beginning at the fourchette and is extended towards the ischiorectal fossa. A midline episiotomy is no longer recommended due to an increased risk of tears extending through to the rectum. The patient should be encouraged to bear down during contractions and to rest in between.

Delivery of the head Delivery of the head must be controlled by the accoucheur so that it extends slowly after crowning, and does not 'pop out' of the vagina. Placing the palm of one hand over the head to control its extension most easily achieves this. At this point the patient should cease actively pushing and may need to be instructed to pant or breathe through her nose, in order to overcome her desire to push. The accoucheur's second hand covered with a sterile gauze pad or towel may be used to gently lift the baby's chin, which can be felt in the space between the anus and the coccyx.

As the occiput descends under the symphysis pubis, extension of the head occurs and progressively the forehead, nose, mouth and finally chin emerge. If there is evidence of meconium staining of the liquor, gently suction the baby's nose and mouth, although there is no evidence that this intervention reduces the risk of meconium aspiration or improves perinatal outcome.[3]

In 25–30% of patients the umbilical cord is looped around the neck, which should be checked for. Generally it is only loosely looped and can be drawn over the head. If there is tension, place two clamps on the cord 2–3 cm apart and cut the cord in between them. Release of additional loops is now straightforward by unwinding the clamped ends around the neck. The baby's head, having been delivered face down in the most common occipito-anterior position, is allowed to 'restitute' (or correct) to one or the other lateral position.

Restitution and delivery of the shoulders Once the head has restituted, the shoulders will lie in an antero-posterior plane within the pelvis, and delivery of the shoulders is now effected taking great care not to allow the perineum to tear. Usually the anterior shoulder slips under the symphysis pubis with the next contraction by exerting gentle downward and backward traction on the head to facilitate this. Do not use excessive force as this may result in a brachial plexus injury.

On delivery of the anterior shoulder, lifting the baby up will result in delivery of the posterior shoulder followed by the body and lower limbs. Grasp the baby firmly with one hand, securing the infant behind the neck and the other encircling both ankles and place on the mother's abdomen. The baby is slippery as a result of being covered with vernix and should never be held with one hand alone. Dry the baby and wrap in a warm, dry blanket to minimize heat loss, and record the time of birth.

Clamping the cord and Apgar score There is no need to immediately cut the cord if the baby is breathing spontaneously and is close to term. There appears to be a benefit in delaying cord clamping in preterm and possibly term infants, as more blood is transferred from the placenta to the infant when clamping is delayed.[4,5] Perform an assessment of the baby with Apgar scoring to determine the need for resuscitation.

If the baby is preterm or requires resuscitation, quickly clamp the cord following delivery and transfer the baby for further assessment and resuscitation to a resuscitation trolley that has a radiant heat source. Apply an umbilical clamp 1–2 cm from the baby's abdomen to cut the umbilical cord and trim the cord approximately 0.5 cm above the plastic clamp.

Use of oxytocics Following the birth of the baby, palpate the woman's abdomen to exclude the possibility of a second fetus, where no antenatal ultrasound result is available, and if none, administer an oxytocic agent. The commonest is oxytocin at a dose of 10 units given intramuscularly, or 5 units intravenously as a slow bolus. An alternative is ergometrine in a dose of 250 μg intramuscularly, or slowly intravenously, but as this agent is associated with nausea, vomiting and hypertension it is unsuitable for use in pre-eclampsia, eclampsia or hypertension. Ergometrine is also associated with an increased risk of retained placenta.

Third stage

After administration of the oxytocic agent, look for signs of separation of the placenta from the uterine wall. The three classic signs of placental separation are: (1) lengthening of the umbilical cord, (2) a gush of blood from the vagina signifying separation of the placenta from the uterine wall and (3) change in the shape of the uterine fundus from discoid to globular, with elevation of the fundal height. Following separation, and once the uterus is firmly contracted, apply traction on the cord in a backward and downward direction with one hand, whilst the other is placed suprapubically to support the uterus. Cease traction if the cord feels as though it is tearing.

Placental inspection As the placenta appears at the introitus, traction is then applied in an upward direction and the placenta is grasped and gently rotated to ensure that the membranes are delivered without tearing. Inspect the placenta and membranes to look for any missing segments or cotyledons, or evidence of a missing succenturiate lobe, which may prevent the uterus from contracting properly if they remain within the uterus.

Procedure post delivery

Uterine tone

Rub over the uterus to facilitate contraction and expulsion of clots. A common cause of post-partum haemorrhage is incomplete uterine contraction, as a result of clots or tissue remaining within the cavity, which may be expelled by massaging the fundus or by manual removal under anaesthesia. Further oxytocics may be necessary.

Bleeding may also occur from other sites so always perform a careful examination of the cervix, vagina, episiotomy wound and perineum following delivery. Full examination of the cervix for ongoing bleeding will require anaesthesia. The episiotomy wound and any other lacerations may be repaired with a synthetic absorbable suture.

Vitamin K

Keep the baby warm and dry and measure and record both mother and baby's vital signs. Also make regular observations of the maternal fundal height, uterine tone and vaginal loss. If vitamin K is available, administer it to the baby as a deep intramuscular 1 mg injection.

Disposition

Disposition of mother and baby to an obstetric unit either within the hospital or at a distant hospital should then be made when both are stable. The important information that must be provided includes the time of birth, drugs given to either mother or baby and the Apgar scores of the baby. Include the results of any blood tests and a copy of the observations. If either mother or baby is unstable then early consultation with the appropriate referral service is mandatory regarding the optimum timing and nature of the transfer.

Complications of delivery

Breech delivery

Breech presentation occurs in 3–4% of all deliveries, reducing in incidence with advancing gestation. Most breech presentations are delivered by caesarean section. Neonatal morbidity and mortality are worse in breech deliveries than in those fetuses delivering by cephalic presentation.[2] The object is safe delivery of the fetus.

Management of the breech delivery

Minimal interference is best. Perform an episiotomy as the fetal anus is climbing the perineum. Allow maternal effort to deliver the baby spontaneously to the umbilicus, delivering the legs with knee flexion. A loop of umbilical cord may be pulled down and allowed to hang. The mother is encouraged to bear down until the trunk becomes visible up to the scapula. Then rotate the trunk until the anterior shoulder delivers. Subsequent rotation of the trunk in the opposite direction results in delivery of the posterior shoulder.

Once the shoulders are delivered the accoucheur delivers the head either with the application of forceps, or by placing the middle finger in the baby's throat, and flexing the head with the other hand resulting in delivery (Mauriceau Smellie Veit manoeuvre).

Shoulder dystocia

Shoulder dystocia is one of the most frightening complications of vaginal delivery and is frequently unexpected. The rate is approx 1:300 deliveries. The important steps in management are recognizing the at-risk patient, getting assistance early and understanding the manoeuvres to deliver the fetus. The at-risk patient may have a large baby, gestational diabetes or have had a previous shoulder dystocia. In many cases of shoulder dystocia, however, there are no predisposing factors at all.

Recognizing shoulder dystocia

The problem encountered in shoulder dystocia is following delivery of the fetal head as the anterior shoulder does not deliver spontaneously, or with gentle traction by the accoucheur. The anterior shoulder becomes caught immediately above the symphysis. The first sign of shoulder dystocia is retraction of the fetal chin into the perineum, following the delivery of the head. Delivery in under 5 min is essential to prevent asphyxia.

Morbidity with shoulder dystocia

Fetal mortality and morbidity rates are significant. The effects of prolonged asphyxia include neuropsychiatric dysfunction. Brachial plexus injuries result from lateral traction on the fetal head during delivery. The Erb's palsy arises from damage to the C5 and C6 nerve roots, with paralysis of the deltoid and short muscles of the shoulder, and of brachialis and biceps, which flex and supinate the elbow. The arm hangs limply by the side with the forearm pronated and the palm facing backwards ('waiter's tip position'). About 90% of these lesions recover fully or almost fully.

Treatment of shoulder dystocia:

- McRoberts manoeuvre: exaggerated flexion of maternal legs resulting in widening of the pelvic diameter.
- Suprapubic pressure (these two usually result in delivery of the fetus).
- Woods corkscrew manoeuvre: the shoulders are rotated to a transverse position freeing the obstruction.
- Delivery of the posterior shoulder (may result in clavicular or humeral fracture).
- Zavanelli's procedure: replacing the head in the uterus and performing a caesarean section.

Post-partum haemorrhage

The average blood loss at vaginal delivery is generally estimated to be 500 mL. A post-partum haemorrhage (PPH) is best defined and diagnosed clinically as excessive bleeding that makes the patient symptomatic with lightheadedness, vertigo and syncope and/or results in signs of maternal hypovolaemia with hypotension, tachycardia or oliguria. It is also commonly defined as blood loss of 500 mL or greater after delivery of the fetus.

The causes of PPH may be broadly classified as those relating to retained products, uterine hypotonia or atony, trauma or coagulation abnormalities. Effective management relies on an accurate assessment and identification of the cause.

Causes of PPH

- Retained placenta or products of conception
- Uterine atony
- Soft-tissue laceration
- Coagulopathy
- Uterine rupture
- Uterine inversion

Risk factors for PPH

- Retained placenta
- Grand multiparity (reduced muscular tissue in uterus)
- Antepartum haemorrhage
- Over distension of the uterus from polyhydramnios, macrosomia or multiple pregnancy
- Large placental site associated with multiple pregnancy
- Past history of PPH or haemorrhagic disorders

- Fibroid uterus
- Precipitate labour
- Induced labour
- Prolonged labour
- Chorioamnionitis
- Tocolytic agents, inhalational anaesthetics.

No risk factors are found in up to 20% of cases.

Management of PPH

Prevention is the mainstay of treatment by identifying the at-risk patient, and the aggressive use of oxytocin, along with active management of the third stage of labour. These measures reduce the incidence of PPH by 40%. Resuscitate the patient with intravenous fluids and cross-match blood. Remember to rub up the fundus and deliver the placenta if undelivered. Examine the lower genital tract for tears.

Uterine rupture Suspect uterine rupture in patients with severe abdominal pain. If a coagulation or platelet defect is present then correct with either fresh frozen plasma (FFP) or platelets. Manage uterine atony by the initial administration of oxytocics such as oxytocin 5 units i.v., which may be followed by an infusion of 20–40 units of oxytocin in 1 L of 0.9% saline. Use an initial rate of 250 mL/h with the infusion rate slowed as uterine contraction occurs. Other agents that are effective in the management of uterine atony include misoprostol 800–1000 µg per rectum (PR) and/or ergometrine 250 µg by the intravenous or intramuscular route.

Further medical treatment of PPH Further medical treatment includes intra-myometrial PG F_2a 250–500 µg in aliquots up to a maximum of 2 mg. It is successful in 60–85% cases of refractory uterine atony. Side effects include nausea, vomiting, diarrhoea, pyrexia, hypertension and bronchoconstriction. Its use is therefore contraindicated in women with asthma and hypertension.

Should uterine atony persist, further measures may be required. Exploration of the uterine cavity may be required to identify and remove retained products and bimanual uterine compression may be employed as a temporizing measure.

Surgical management of PPH Surgical management of continuing PPH will require laparotomy.

- Uterine tamponade. The Bakri tamponade balloon was specifically designed for uterine tamponade to control post-partum bleeding. It is a silicone balloon with a capacity of 500 mL of saline, and strength to withstand a maximum internal and external pressure of 300 mmHg. A Sengstaken–Blakemore tube can be used to tamponade the uterus if the Bakri device is not available.
- Uterine artery ligation has minimal complications and reduces the pulse pressure by 60–70% to allow endogenous haemostatic mechanisms to control bleeding. Failing this, internal iliac artery ligation may be performed usually bilaterally.
- Uterine compression sutures. Uterine compression sutures are an effective method for reducing PPH and avoiding hysterectomy. The B-Lynch suture (or its modifications) envelops and compresses the uterus, similar to the result achieved with manual uterine compression.
- Hysterectomy is the operation of last resort. It may be necessary in uterine atony or rupture, as well as in placenta praevia, or be the procedure of choice in women of high parity.

Resuscitation of the neonate

Approximately 5% of infants require some resuscitation at birth such as stimulation to breathe, and between 1 and 10% of those born in hospital are reported to require assisted ventilation. Most newborn infants do not need any assistance establishing effective respiration at birth. Of those who do, the majority only need minimal help to start breathing. Few require intubation and ventilation, and the need for external cardiac massage with chest compressions is most unusual.[6]

Neonates who may need resuscitation

The need for resuscitation in the newborn should be anticipated in some groups such as the preterm birth, absent or minimal antenatal care, maternal illness, complicated or prolonged delivery, antepartum haemorrhage, multiple births and a previous neonatal death. Additionally there are occasions when the requirement for newborn resuscitation is unexpected, thus EDs must make available a suitable place, appropriate equipment and trained personnel to perform newborn resuscitation at short notice following an emergency delivery.

A structured and sequential approach to assessment and intervention in the newborn is required. This includes the initial steps in stabilization, including airway clearance, positioning and stimulation, ventilation, chest compressions and administration of drugs or i.v. volume expansion.[6] The initial assessment addresses the key elements of response to stimulation, breathing, heart rate, tone and colour. Ongoing assessment is focused on the breathing, heart rate, colour and tone.

The Australian Resuscitation Council has published a Neonatal Resuscitation Flowchart illustrating the assessment and resuscitation of a newborn baby (Fig. 19.1.1).

Positive pressure ventilation and chest compressions

Positive pressure ventilation alone is generally effective in raising the heart rate >100/min and establishing spontaneous respirations. Chest compressions are indicated if the newborn's heart rate fails to rise above 60/min following ventilation. These are achieved by using an encircling thumbs technique at the lower half of the sternum, or by a two-finger technique, if only one healthcare worker is available. Inflations and chest compressions should be synchronized with a 3:1 ratio of 90 compressions and 30 inflations to achieve approximately 120 'events' per minute.[7]

Use of adrenaline

Adrenaline is recommended if the heart rate remains <60 beats/min, after 1 min of effective ventilation and chest compressions. The recommended intravenous dose is 10–30 µg/kg or 0.1–0.3 mL/kg of a 1:10 000 adrenaline solution by a quick push followed by a small saline flush. This dose of adrenaline is repeated if the heart rate remains below 60 beats/min despite effective ventilation and cardiac compressions. Higher doses of adrenaline are not recommended.

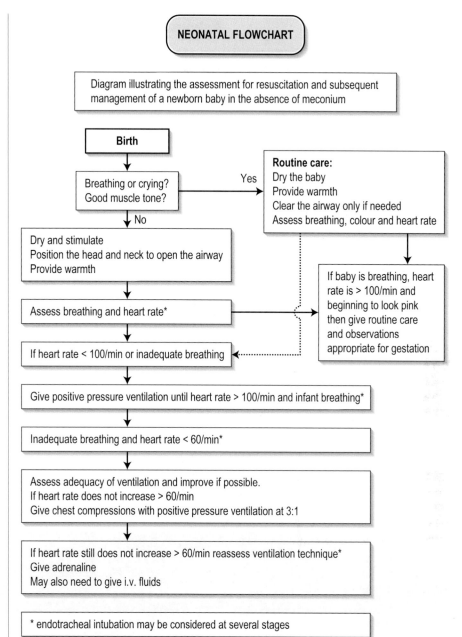

NEONATAL FLOWCHART

Diagram illustrating the assessment for resuscitation and subsequent management of a newborn baby in the absence of meconium

Birth

Breathing or crying? Good muscle tone? — Yes →

Routine care:
Dry the baby
Provide warmth
Clear the airway only if needed
Assess breathing, colour and heart rate

No ↓

Dry and stimulate
Position the head and neck to open the airway
Provide warmth

Assess breathing and heart rate*

If baby is breathing, heart rate is > 100/min and beginning to look pink then give routine care and observations appropriate for gestation

If heart rate < 100/min or inadequate breathing

Give positive pressure ventilation until heart rate > 100/min and infant breathing*

Inadequate breathing and heart rate < 60/min*

Assess adequacy of ventilation and improve if possible.
If heart rate does not increase > 60/min
Give chest compressions with positive pressure ventilation at 3:1

If heart rate still does not increase > 60/min reassess ventilation technique*
Give adrenaline
May also need to give i.v. fluids

* endotracheal intubation may be considered at several stages

Fig. 19.1.1 Neonatal Resuscitation Flowchart. Reproduced with permission from the Australian Resuscitation Council.

Route of administration of adrenaline

The preferred route of administration of adrenaline is via the umbilical vein. Other routes include those through an intraosseous catheter or peripheral vein catheter, although these are more technically challenging. Adrenaline can also be administered via the endotracheal tube, but there is insufficient evidence to support its routine use via this route. If the endotracheal route is used doses of 30–100 µg/kg are

recommended, although again the efficacy and safety of these higher doses has not been studied.[8]

Use of intravenous fluids

Consider intravenous fluids when there is suspected blood loss and/or the infant appears shocked, i.e. pale, with poor perfusion and a weak pulse, and has not responded adequately to the other resuscitative measures above. In the absence of suitable blood for neonatal transfusion, use isotonic crystalloid normal saline at an initial intravenous dose of 10 mL/kg given by bolus push. This dose may be repeated after observing the response.[8]

Use of naloxone

Naloxone should not be used routinely as part of the initial resuscitation of newborns with respiratory depression in the delivery room. It may be considered in situations of continuing respiratory depression following restoration of heart rate and colour by standard resuscitation methods as outlined above. The currently recommended naloxone dose is 0.1 mg/kg intravenously, or intramuscularly, though evidence to support this recommendation is lacking.[8]

Neonatal transfer

Neonates requiring resuscitation following emergency delivery will need to be referred to a regional or tertiary neonatal unit for ongoing care. Transfer of these babies requires careful communication and coordination between the two centres, and transport is usually undertaken by a specialized neonatal transport team.

Acknowledgements

The author wishes to acknowledge the assistance of Dr Ian Barabash, Senior Obstetric Registrar at Sunshine Hospital, Melbourne, and Dr Michael Gregora, Director of Obstetrics and Gynaecology, Sunshine Coast and Cooloola Health Service District, Queensland.

References

1. Weir PE, Beischer NA. Birth before arrival in hospital. Medical Journal of Australia 1980; 2: 31–33.
2. Brenner WE. Breech presentation. Clinical Obstetrics and Gynecology 1978; 21: 511–531.
3. Vain NE, Szyld EG, Prudent LM, et al. Oropharyngeal and nasopharyngeal suctioning of meconium-stained neonates before delivery of their shoulders: multicentre, randomised controlled trial. Lancet 2004; 364: 597–602.
4. Rabe H, Reynolds G, Diaz-Rossello J. Early versus delayed umbilical cord clamping in preterm infants. Cochrane Database of Systematic Reviews 2004; 4: CD003248.
5. Ceriani Cernadas JM, Carroli G, Pellegrini L, et al. The effect of timing of cord clamping on neonatal venous hematocrit values and clinical outcome at term: a randomized, controlled trial. Pediatrics 2006; 117(4): e779–786. Epub 2006 Mar 27.
6. Australian Resuscitation Council Guideline 13.1 February 2006. Introduction to resuscitation of the newborn infant. http://www.resus.org.au (accessed Jan 2008).
7. Australian Resuscitation Council Guideline 13.6 February 2006. Chest compression during resuscitation of the newborn infant http://www.resus.org.au (accessed Jan 2008).
8. Australian Resuscitation Council Guideline 13.7 February 2006. Medication or fluids for the resuscitation of the newborn infant. http://www.resus.org.au (accessed Jan 2008).

Further reading

Advanced Life Support Group. Advanced paediatric life support: the practical approach. 4th edn. Oxford: Blackwell British Medical Journal Books; 2005.
Beischer NA, Mackay EV, Colditz P (eds). Obstetrics and the newborn: an illustrated textbook. 3rd edn. Philadelphia, PA: W B Saunders; 1997.
Bobak IM, Jensen MD, eds. Essentials of maternity nursing. 3rd edn. St Louis: Mosby; 1991.
DeCherney AH, Nathan L, eds. Current obstetric and gynaecologic diagnosis and treatment. 9th edn. New Jersey: Lange, McGraw Hill Professional; 2002.
Funai EF, Norwitz ER. Management of normal labor and delivery. In: Rose BD, ed. Up to date. ; Waltham, MA. 2007.
Gianopoulos JG. Emergency complications of labour and delivery. Emergency Medical Clinics of North America 1994; 12(1): 201–217.
International Liaison Committee on Resuscitation. International consensus on cardiopulmonary resuscitation and emergency cardiovascular care science with treatment recommendations. Part 7: Neonatal Resuscitation. Resuscitation 2005; 67: 293–303.
James DK, Steer PJ, Weiner CP, et al. High risk pregnancy: management options. 3rd edn. Philadelphia, PA: WB Saunders; 2006.
Oates JK, Abraham S. Llewellyn-Jones fundamentals of obstetrics and gynaecology. 8th edn. St Louis: Mosby; 2004.
Tintinalli JE, Kelen GD, Stapczynski S. Emergency medicine: a comprehensive study guide. 6th edn. New York: McGraw-Hill Inc; 2003.

19.2 Ectopic pregnancy and bleeding in early pregnancy

Sheila Bryan

ESSENTIALS

1 Approximately 25% of all clinically diagnosed pregnancies are associated with bleeding in the first 12 weeks, of which approximately 50% of cases will be due to a failed pregnancy.

2 Ectopic pregnancy occurs at a rate of about 11:1000 diagnosed pregnancies.

3 The management of ectopic pregnancy and failed pregnancy may be surgical, medical or conservative.

Introduction

Bleeding in early pregnancy is a common problem affecting approximately 25% of all clinically diagnosed pregnancies, and of these approximately 50% will have bleeding due to a failed pregnancy.[1] Other causes of bleeding include incidental or physiological, which have no bearing on the outcome of the pregnancy, molar pregnancy and ectopic pregnancy.

Failed pregnancy

Failed pregnancies are defined on ultrasound criteria. Embryonic death is defined as an embryo greater than 6 mm with no cardiac activity. Fetal death is a fetus greater than 8 weeks with no cardiac activity. An anembryonic pregnancy ('blighted ovum') is a gestational sac equal to or greater than 20 mm with no embryo.

A failed pregnancy may then remain in the uterus (previously termed as a missed abortion), or may progress to either an incomplete or complete miscarriage, as defined by the presence or absence of pregnancy-related tissue in the uterus.

Ectopic pregnancy

An ectopic pregnancy is a pregnancy that is implanted outside of the normal uterine cavity. The most common location of an ectopic pregnancy is in the fallopian tube. Other sites include cervix (~1%), ovary (1–3%), interstitial (1–3%), abdomen (1%) and rarely in a uterine scar.

The natural history of an ectopic pregnancy may be one of resorption, spontaneous miscarriage (vaginal or tubal) or it may continue to grow and disrupt the surrounding structures (rupture).

History

History should include the date of the last normal menstrual period and a complete obstetric and gynaecological history including the use of assisted reproductive techniques. Risk factors for ectopic pregnancy include a past history of tubal damage, a previous ectopic pregnancy, pelvic infection, tubal surgery, assisted reproductive techniques, increased age, smoking and progesterone-only contraception. Intrauterine contraceptive devices (IUD) not only decrease the chance of intrauterine pregnancies, but also increase the likelihood of an ectopic pregnancy.[2]

When estimating the amount of vaginal bleeding it is useful to quantify the blood loss compared to the woman's normal menstrual loss. Ectopic pregnancy is rarely associated with heavy bleeding. Heavy bleeding and the passage of clots are more common with failed intrauterine pregnancy. However, the history of passage of fetal products should not be used as the basis for a diagnosis. Blood clots or a decidual cast may be misinterpreted as the products of conception. In addition, the correct identification of the products of conception does not exclude the possibility of a live twin or of a coexistent ectopic pregnancy (heterotopic pregnancy).

Examination

Determination of the patient's haemodynamic status and the rate of ongoing bleeding are a priority. Hypotension, tachycardia and signs of peritoneal irritation suggest a ruptured ectopic pregnancy or bleeding from a corpus luteal cyst.

Bimanual examination can localize tenderness and identify adnexal masses and can also give an estimate of the size of the uterus. However, bimanual examination lacks sensitivity and specificity in identification of small, unruptured ectopic pregnancies[3] and gives no information about the viability of the pregnancy. Speculum examination allows visualization of the vaginal walls and the cervix, and allows identification of the source of bleeding.

A complete physical examination should be performed including an assessment of the woman's mental state, as pregnancy loss may have a profound psychological impact on some women.

Investigations

Biochemistry

Beta subunit of human chorionic gonadotrophin

The beta subunit of human chorionic gonadotrophin (β-hCG) is produced by the outer layer of cells of the gestational sac (the syncytiotrophoblast) and may be detected as early as 9 days after fertilization.[4] The β-hCG level increases by approximately 1.66 times every 48 h, then plateaus, before falling at around 12 weeks to a lower level. At any stage of the pregnancy there is always a large range of normal values.

The half life of β-hCG is approximately 48 h, which results in the β-hCG level remaining elevated for a number of weeks post-termination or miscarriage. A positive pregnancy test or a single β-hCG level is therefore unreliable to confirm ongoing pregnancy, and cannot be used to identify retained products of conception. High levels of β-hCG may be associated with multiple or molar pregnancies.

Urine pregnancy test

Urine pregnancy tests are sensitive to a β-hCG level of 25–60 IU/L. Thus false negatives may occur in the setting of early pregnancy or dilute urine.

Haematology

A full blood count and cross-match should be arranged for haemodynamically unstable patients. Blood group and Rhesus factor should be determined on all patients.

Ultrasound

Ultrasound should be performed in every patient to identify the anatomical location of the pregnancy, and to look for a fetal heart beat. The introduction of emergency department (ED) ultrasound provides a cost-effective method for the assessment of patients presenting with bleeding in early pregnancy.[5]

Transvaginal ultrasound

A gestational sac can be identified as early as 31 days gestation using transvaginal ultrasound. The differential diagnosis of an early gestational sac is a pseudo-sac or an endometrial cyst. A pseudo-sac is a small collection of fluid seen in the uterine cavity, often in association with an ectopic pregnancy. A yolk sac can be identified within the gestational sac at 5–6 weeks when the β-hCG is around 1500 IU/L (except in the case of anembryonic pregnancies). Embryonic cardiac activity should be identified by approximately 39 days (5.5 weeks) gestation, at which stage the crown rump length of the embryo is approximately 5 mm.[6]

Transabdominal ultrasound

A developing pregnancy may be expected to be reliably identified by about 6 weeks using transabdominal ultrasound, when the β-hCG is approximately 6500 IU/L.

An ultrasound is still valuable when the β-hCG level is less then 1000 IU/L, while not expecting to identify an intrauterine gestational sac.[7] Ultrasound can assist in the diagnosis of a ruptured ectopic, if free fluid is identified in the pouch of Douglas and no pregnancy is identified in the uterus.

Heterotopic pregnancy

The identification of an interuterine pregnancy does not exclude an ectopic pregnancy. Ectopic pregnancy may coexist with an intrauterine pregnancy, which is known as a heterotopic pregnancy. The incidence of heterotopic pregnancy in the general population is around 1:3889, but in patients who have undergone assisted reproduction it increases significantly to up to 1:100–1:500.[8]

Management

Rh(D) immunoglobulin

All patients should have their blood group and Rhesus (Rh) factor determined. As little as 0.1 mL of Rh(D) positive fetal blood will cause maternal Rh iso-immunization. A dose of 250 IU of Rh(D) immunoglobulin should be given in early pregnancy bleeding with a singleton pregnancy to an Rh-negative woman as soon as possible, certainly within 72 h of onset of the bleeding. This dose will prevent immunization from a feto–maternal haemorrhage of up to 2.5 mL of fetal cells. Further doses may be required in the case of repeat or prolonged bleeding.[9]

A dose of 625 IU of Rh(D) is recommended in multiple pregnancies or with a gestation of greater than 13 weeks. The Kleihauer test is used in later pregnancy to quantify the amount of fetal cells in the maternal circulation, but is unreliable in early pregnancy.

Ectopic pregnancy

Haemodynamically unstable patients

Haemodynamically unstable patients with suspected ectopic pregnancy should be resuscitated and transferred to theatre for surgical intervention as soon as possible. A ruptured corpus luteal cyst may rarely cause similar haemodynamic compromise and is often diagnosed laparoscopically.

Haemodynamically stable patients

The management options for haemodynamically stable patients with an ectopic pregnancy include observation, medical treatment or surgical intervention.

Factors considered in reaching a management choice include the location of the ectopic pregnancy, the β-hCG level, the size of the ectopic pregnancy, the presence of fetal cardiac activity and patient factors.

Observation is sometimes considered in stable patients with a low β-hCG (<1000 IU/L), which is falling. Medical management using intramuscular methotrexate is an option in some patients.[10] Selection criteria include non-tubal ectopic pregnancy, or a small tubal ectopic pregnancy (<3 cm) with no cardiac activity, and a β-hCG level less than 5000 IU/L.

Failed pregnancy (miscarriage)

Haemodynamically unstable patients

Patients with heavy bleeding, hypotension and bradycardia should have a speculum examination. Occasionally the products of conception cause dilatation of the cervix, which leads to neurocardiogenic shock, or cervical shock. Removal of the clot and products of conception from the cervix usually results in reversal of the shock.

Haemodynamic compromise may also be secondary to significant blood loss related to the miscarriage. Fluid resuscitation should be instituted simultaneously with attempts to control the bleeding, by removal of blood clot and the products of conception from the cervix and vagina. Uterine contraction may be induced by administering ergometrine 200 μg i.m., if removal of clot and tissue fail to control the bleeding, while emergency surgical evacuation of the uterus is being arranged.

Haemodynamically stable patients

Haemodynamically stable patients have traditionally been treated by surgical evacuation of uterine contents known as evacuation of retained products of conception (ERPC), following the diagnosis of a failed pregnancy (miscarriage).

Other options for emptying the uterus include waiting for spontaneous expulsion (conservative management), or using agents such as misoprostol to induce uterine contraction and miscarriage (medical management). Currently there is insufficient evidence to support the superiority of any of these three treatment options. A number of studies have assessed the time to achieve complete miscarriage and the frequency of complications. These studies have varied with respect to inclusion criteria and duration of conservative management.

The success of conservative treatment is variable but in one study, 78.6% of women studied had an empty uterus at 8 weeks.[11]

Conservative management is generally associated with slightly longer duration of bleeding and pain, and in some studies the need for transfusion. The incidence of infection was similar in some studies, but higher in the surgical group in others. Complications of surgery such as cervical trauma, uterine perforation and intrauterine adhesions were uncommon. The current view is that a woman's preference should be a major consideration in recommending treatment options.[12]

Prognosis

Approximately 50% of patients with bleeding in early pregnancy will proceed to term. Only 60% of women with an ectopic pregnancy will conceive again naturally, and they will have an ectopic rate of 25–30% in subsequent pregnancies.

Disposition

There is an 85–90% chance of the pregnancy progressing to term in a patient with early pregnancy bleeding and an ultrasound confirming a live intrauterine gestation. Poor prognostic indicators include advanced maternal age, the ultrasound findings of an enlarged yolk sac and fetal bradycardia after 7 weeks' gestation. Patients may be reassured and discharged for review by the treating obstetrician or antenatal clinic in the absence of the above findings. They should be advised to avoid sexual intercourse and not to use tampons until after the bleeding has settled. There is no evidence to support improved pregnancy outcomes from prescribing bed rest.[13]

The patient with an ultrasound finding of a gestational sac <20 mm with no yolk sac should be followed up with either serial β-hCG levels or repeat ultrasound to ensure the exclusion of a pseudo-sac. Patients with a failed pregnancy or an ectopic pregnancy should be referred to a gynaecology service for ongoing management.

Referral for counselling or psychological support may be indicated in some women.

Investigation for an underlying cause is generally not indicated until after the third consecutive miscarriage due to the high frequency of first trimester miscarriage.

Controversies

❶ The role of emergency physician ultrasound within the ED.

❷ The indications for anti-D immunoglobulin.

❸ The management of patients with no intrauterine pregnancy identified on ultrasound.

❹ The best practice for emptying the uterus following a failed pregnancy.

❺ The best practice for managing an ectopic pregnancy.

References

1. Beischer NA, MacKay EV, Colditz PB. Obstetrics and the newborn. 3rd edn. Pennsylvania: WB Saunders: 2000: 176.
2. Tay JI, Moore J, Walker JJ. Ectopic pregnancy. British Medical Journal 2000; 320: 916–919.
3. Dart R, Kaplan B, Varakis K. Predictive value of history and physical examination in patients with suspected ectopic pregnancy. Annals of Emergency Medicine 1999; 33(3): 283–290.
4. Guyton AC, Hall JE. Textbook of medical physiology. 9th edn. Pennsylvania: WB Saunders; 1996: 1037–1039.
5. Durston W, Carl M, Guerra W, et al. Ultrasound availability in the evaluation of ectopic pregnancy in the ED: comparison of quality and cost effectiveness with different approaches. American Journal of Emergency Medicine 2000; 18(4): 408–417.
6. Cacciatore B, Titinen A, Stenman U-H, et al. Normal early pregnancy: Serum hCG levels and vaginal ultrasonography findings. British Journal of Obstetrics and Gynaecology 1990; 97: 899–903.
7. Dart RG, Kaplan B, Cox C. Transvaginal ultrasound in patients with low beta-human chorionic gonadotrophin values: how often is the study diagnostic. Annals of Emergency Medicine 1997; 30(2): 135–140.
8. Society for Assisted Reproductive Technology (SART)/ The American Fertility Society. In vitro fertilization-embryo transfer (IVF-ET) in the Unites States. 1990 results from the IVF-ET registry of the Medical Research International and Society for Assisted Reproductive Technology (SART)/The American Fertility Society. Fertility and Sterility 1992; 57: 15–24.
9. NHMRC. Guidelines on the prophylactic use of Rh D immunoglobulin (Anti-D) in obstetrics. NHMRC 1999. www.nhmrc.gov.au/index.htm/(Accessed Nov. 2007).
10. Hajenius PJ, Mol F, Mol BWJ, et al. Interventions for tubal ectopic pregnancy. Cochrane Database of Systematic Reviews 2007. CD000324.
11. Shelly JM, Healy D, Grover S. A randomised trial of surgical, medical and expectant management of first trimester spontaneous miscarriage. Australian New Zealand Journals of Obstetrics and Gynaecology 2005; 45: 122–127.
12. Nanda K, Peloggia A, Grimes D, et al. Expectant care versus surgical treatment for miscarriage 2006. Cochrane Database of Systemic Reviews 2006; 2: CD003518.DOI:10.1002/14651858.CD003518.pub2.
13. Aleman A, Althabe F, Belizan J, et al. Bed rest during pregnancy for preventing miscarriage 2005. Cochrane Database of Systemic Reviews 2005; 2: CD003576. DOI:10.1002/14651858.CD003576.pub2.

OBSTETRICS AND GYNAECOLOGY

19.3 Bleeding after the first trimester of pregnancy

Jenny Dowd • Sheila Bryan

ESSENTIALS

1 Up to 4% of pregnant women will have significant bleeding after 20 weeks' gestation.

2 Resuscitation of the mother followed by ultrasound localization of the placenta are the priorities of management for patients with heavy vaginal bleeding after 20 weeks' gestation.

3 Secondary post-partum haemorrhage is commonly caused by endometritis or retained products of conception.

Introduction

Vaginal bleeding after the first trimester may be due to a number of causes. The most common is classified as 'incidental', where the bleeding is not directly related to pregnancy.

Antepartum haemorrhage

Obstetric causes of bleeding include placenta praevia, accidental haemorrhage or abruption and vasa praevia. Bleeding that occurs after 20 weeks' gestation is classified as an antepartum haemorrhage (APH).

Post-partum haemorrhage

Primary post-partum haemorrhage (PPH) is defined as heavy (>600 mL) vaginal bleeding within 24 h of delivery and is discussed in Chapter 19.1 on emergency delivery.

Secondary post-partum haemorrhage

Secondary PPH is most commonly due to infection and/or retained tissue, and may cause significant bleeding up to 6 weeks post partum.

ANTEPARTUM HAEMORRHAGE

Differential diagnosis

Incidental causes

These include bleeding from the lower genital tract, most commonly from physiological cervical erosion or ectropion, which may be either spontaneous or post-traumatic such as post coital. Other causes that need to be excluded include bleeding from cervical polyps, cervical malignancy and cervical or vaginal infections.

Bleeding from haemorrhoids or vulval varices may also mistakenly be reported as vaginal bleeding.

Placenta praevia

Placenta praevia occurs when the placenta is situated in the lower part of the uterus and therefore is in front of the presenting part of the fetus. It occurs in 0.5% of pregnancies.[1] Bleeding in this situation is usually painless, unless associated with labour contractions, and often presents with several small, 'warning' bleeds.

Accidental haemorrhage (marginal bleed or placental abruption)

This is bleeding from a normally situated placenta. This may be from the edge of the placenta known as a marginal bleed, or from behind the placenta associated with placental separation (abruption). Vaginal bleeding may not always be present with a placental abruption, but it is usually associated with pain. A placental abruption that causes significant detachment of the placenta may cause fetal compromise and fetal death in up to 30% of cases.[2]

The retroplacental clot consists of maternal blood and up to 2–4 L may be concealed behind the placenta without vaginal loss. A placental abruption may follow relatively minor blunt trauma, such as a fall onto the abdomen, or a shearing force such as that applied in a motor vehicle deceleration crash. Placental abruption may also occur spontaneously associated with hypertension, inherited disorders of coagulation or with cocaine use.[3]

Vasa praevia

This is the presence of fetal vessels running in the amniotic membranes distant from the placental mass and across the cervical os. These vessels occasionally rupture, often in association with rupture of the amniotic membranes. When this happens the bleeding is from the fetus, which may quickly lead to fetal compromise. The first indication of this may be fetal bradycardia or other abnormalities of the fetal heart rate seen on cardiotocographic (CTG) tracing.

Physiological

Vaginal blood mixed with mucus is called a 'show' and is due to the mucus plug or operculum within the endocervical canal dislodging, as the cervix begins to dilate. This usually occurs at the time of, or within a few days of, the onset of labour, and is not significant unless the pregnancy is pre-term or associated with rupture of the membranes. As a general guide, when a woman needs to wear a pad to soak up blood, she should be assessed as having an APH.

History

The history should specifically include details of recent abdominal trauma or drug use suggesting a diagnosis of placental abruption. A history of recent coitus is commonly identified in bleeding from a cervical ectropion. The history should also include details regarding the presence and quality of fetal movements.

Constant pain over the uterus or sometimes in the lower back from separation of a posteriorly situated placenta is suggestive of placental abruption. Intermittent pains in the lower abdomen or back may represent uterine contractions. Women may describe this as 'period pains' or tightenings and may notice a general hardening over the whole uterus in association with the pain. Painless bleeding is suggestive of either an incidental cause or of placenta praevia.

An increase in pelvic pressure associated with a mucous vaginal fluid loss and spotting or mild bleeding suggests cervical incompetence. This usually presents between 14 and 22 weeks gestation. Prior cervical damage secondary to either a cone biopsy or a cervical tear is a risk factor for cervical incompetence.

Examination

Assessment of the mother is the priority. A relatively low blood pressure with a systolic of 90 mmHg and a resting tachycardia of up to 100 bpm is normal in pregnancy.

Examination after 30 weeks' gestation should be performed with the right hip elevated by a pillow to give a 15° tilt of the pelvis to the left. This avoids the problem of vena caval compression (supine hypotension syndrome) from pressure of the gravid uterus reducing inferior vena caval venous return.

Speculum or digital vaginal examination should *never* be performed until the site of the placenta is determined by ultrasound, to avoid disrupting a low-lying placenta and precipitating torrential haemorrhage.

Once an ultrasound scan has excluded a low-lying placenta, an experienced operator may proceed to a speculum examination to look for liquor in the vagina, in suspected rupture of the membranes, or to assess the cervix to localize the site of bleeding and to look for cervical dilation.

A sterile speculum examination is indicated, again by an experienced operator, if preterm pre-labour rupture of the membranes is possible, in order to decrease the risk of introducing infection. Digital vaginal examination should be performed to assess the cervix for dilation if labour is suspected.

Ideally, a CTG should be applied to assess the status of the fetus beyond 24 weeks' gestation. Auscultation of the fetal heart for several minutes should be attempted if this is not available. The baseline rate and variations related to contractions are important. The normal range of the fetal heart rate is 120–160 bpm, but a healthy term or post-term fetus may have a heart rate of between 100 and 120 bpm. Decelerations of the fetal heart rate may indicate fetal distress.

Investigations

Laboratory blood tests

Blood should be taken for a baseline haemoglobin, coagulation screen, Kleihauer test, blood group, Rhesus factor, Rhesus antibodies and a cross match.

A pre-eclampsia screen should be ordered if the patient is hypertensive, including liver function tests, a uric acid and platelet count.

Ultrasound

Ultrasound is used to assess fetal gestation, presentation, liquor volume and placental position. Many 'low-lying' placentas at 18 weeks are no longer classified as placenta praevia by 30–32 weeks, owing to the differential growth of the lower uterine segment as pregnancy progresses.

As only 50% of placental abruptions will be seen on ultrasound, it is not a reliable test for excluding this problem and the diagnosis is usually made on clinical grounds alone. Transvaginal ultrasound with an empty bladder is best to visualize the cervix to look for shortening, or 'beaking' of the amniotic sac into the internal os, which are signs of early cervical incompetence.

Management

Incidental causes of bleeding usually require no specific therapy apart from explanation and reassurance. Cervical polyps are rarely removed during pregnancy due to the risk of heavy bleeding.

Minor amounts of bleeding due to placenta praevia distant from term are managed by close observation, either as an inpatient or an outpatient.

Small placental abruptions may also be managed conservatively with serial ultrasound scans to monitor fetal growth and regular CTG assessments. Delivery is usually advised round 37 weeks to pre-empt a massive placental abruption developing. Sometimes a small retroplacental clot will cause weakening of the amniotic membranes and subsequent rupture of the amniotic sac 1–2 weeks after the initial bleed.

Massive antepartum haemorrhage, often with fetal demise when associated with placental separation, requires urgent delivery, possibly by caesarean section.

Hypovolaemia and coagulopathies are treated as per usual guidelines.

Prognosis

A decision needs to be made about when to transfer a patient to an obstetric unit, in a hospital where there are no obstetric or neonatal facilities. Corticosteroids should be administered to the mother if the fetus is between 23 and 34 weeks, and delivery can be delayed for 24 h. Two intramuscular doses of betamethasone or dexamethasone given over 24 h decrease the baby's risk of developing respiratory distress syndrome, necrotizing enterocolitis and intraventricular haemorrhages.[4]

The current survival rate of babies admitted to a neonatal intensive care unit (NICU) is 40, 50, 60 and 70% at 24, 25, 26 and 27 weeks, respectively.[4]

Disposition

Discharge home may be appropriate if the diagnosis of a benign physiological cause for bleeding can be made with certainty.

SECONDARY POST-PARTUM HAEMORRHAGE

Introduction

Secondary PPH is defined as excessive or prolonged bleeding from 24 h to 6 weeks post partum. Normal lochia is moderately heavy and red vaginal loss for some days, but settles to light bleeding or spotting by 2–4 weeks. Some women have a persistent brownish vaginal discharge for up to 8 weeks.[5]

Differential diagnosis

Common causes of secondary PPH

Common causes of secondary PPH include retained products of conception and endometritis. The bleeding is usually prolonged, moderate blood loss or a recurrence of blood loss after an initial decline.

Less common causes of secondary PPH

Less common causes include trophoblastic disease, uterine arterio-venous malformation (AVM) and any of the incidental causes outlined in the previous section. Reactivation of bleeding from an episiotomy or vaginal laceration is less common. Annoying spotting may occur for several weeks in women using progestogen-only contraception, especially when concurrently breastfeeding, in the setting of an oestrogen-deficient endometrium.

History

Distinguishing endometritis from retained products may be difficult clinically and the two conditions often coexist. Endometritis may follow any type of delivery, but is more commonly seen in women with a history of prolonged rupture of the membranes, and multiple vaginal examinations during labour.

Examination

Abdominal examination may show sub-involution of the uterus with retained tissue, while offensive lochia, uterine tenderness and systemic signs of infection support the diagnosis of endometritis.

An AVM presents with heavy vaginal bleeding and, occasionally, haemodynamic compromise.

Investigations

Full blood examination and blood cultures are indicated if the woman is clinically septic. Send cervical swabs for microscopy and culture, and *Chlamydia trachomatis* detection to help guide the management of endometritis.

Ultrasound is necessary to quantify the amount of retained products of conception and to confirm a diagnosis of an AVM.

Treatment

Empirical treatment with amoxicillin/clavulanic acid 875 mg/125 mg bd for 5–7 days as an outpatient is appropriate, if endometritis is suspected but the woman is systemically well. Erythromycin may be substituted in penicillin sensitive patients.

Admit women who are clinically septic for intravenous antibiotics.

Perform an ultrasound examination if bleeding persists to look for retained products of conception. Patients with small amounts of retained products of conception may be treated conservatively. Uterine curettage in the post-partum period is associated with the risks of uterine perforation or Asherman syndrome due to intrauterine adhesions.

Controversies

❶ The timing of delivery in patients with mild APH due to placental abruption.

❷ Suppression of labour in patients with APH.

❸ The timing and interpretation of ultrasound investigation in patients with secondary PPH.

References

1. Cotton D, Ead J, Paul R, et al. The conservative aggressive management of placenta praevia. American Journal of Obstetrics and Gynecology 1980; 17: 687–689.
2. Saftlas A, Olsen D, Atras H, et al. National trends in the incidence of abruptio placenta. Obstetrics and Gynecology 1991; 78: 1081–1086.
3. Paterson M. The aetiology and outcome of abruptio placentae in Sweden. Obstetrics and Gynecology 1986; 67: 523–528.
4. Koh THHG. Simplified way of counselling parents about outcomes of extremely premature babies. Lancet 1996; 348: 963.
5. Bonnar J. Massive obstetric haemorrhage. Best Practice & Research in Clinical Obstetrics and Gynaecology 2000; 14(1): 1–18.

19.4 Abnormal vaginal bleeding in the non-pregnant patient

Anthony F. T. Brown • Sheila Bryan

ESSENTIALS

1 Start the assessment of any patient with vaginal bleeding by excluding pregnancy.

2 Locate the anatomical site of bleeding and assess the severity.

3 Consider coagulopathy as a cause of heavy uterine bleeding in all patients, especially adolescents.

Introduction

Vaginal bleeding may be divided into two major categories, that which occurs in a pregnant patient and that in the non-pregnant patient. Therefore, the first step in a patient presenting with vaginal bleeding is to exclude pregnancy. See Chapter 19.2 if the woman is pregnant.

This chapter deals exclusively with bleeding in non-pregnant women. Bleeding may be from the external genitalia, vaginal walls, cervix or uterus. The pathological basis for bleeding from the vulva, vagina and cervix includes infection, trauma, atrophy or malignancy. Uterine bleeding may be physiological or pathological.

Physiological uterine bleeding

Physiological uterine bleeding occurs associated with ovulatory menstrual cycles, which occur at regular intervals every 21–35 days, and last for 3–7 days. The average volume of blood loss is 30–40 mL with >80 mL being defined as menorrhagia.

The menstrual cycle is controlled by the hypothalamic–pituitary–ovarian (HPO) axis. During the first 14 days oestrogen is produced by the developing follicle, leading to proliferation of the endometrium, which reaches a thickness of 3–5 mm. Oestrogen acts on the pituitary gland to cause the release of follicle stimulating hormone (FSH) and luteinizing hormone (LH) which result in ovulation. The corpus luteum then releases progesterone in excess of oestrogen.

Progesterone causes stabilization of the endometrium during the secretory phase of the menstrual cycle. In the absence of fertilization there is involution of the corpus luteum and a fall in oestrogen and progesterone levels. This results in vasoconstriction within the endometrium, which consequently becomes ischaemic and is shed as normal menstrual bleeding.

Pathological uterine bleeding

Pathological causes include infection, structural abnormalities such as polyps, fibroids, arteriovenous malformations (AVM) or malignancy, coagulopathy and thyroid endocrinopathy. Other causes also include abnormal uterine bleeding with ovulatory menstrual cycles and abnormal uterine bleeding with anovulatory menstrual cycles.

Abnormal uterine bleeding with ovulatory menstrual cycles

The most common cause of abnormal uterine bleeding is menorrhagia occurring in ovulatory menstrual cycles. This presents as regular heavy bleeding and may result in anaemia. In these women the menstrual blood has been shown to have increased fibrinolytic activity and/or increased prostaglandins.

Abnormal uterine bleeding with anovulatory menstrual cycles

Abnormal uterine bleeding due to anovulatory menstrual cycles, previously referred to as dysfunctional uterine bleeding (DUB), presents as irregular bleeding of variable volume. In anovulatory menstrual cycles and other high oestrogen states, there is a relative lack of progesterone to oppose the oestrogenic stimulation of the endometrium. This results in excessive proliferation and occasionally hyperplasia/metaplasia of the endometrium. The endometrium also becomes 'unstable' and prone to erratic sloughing.

Clinically this presents as irregular, often heavy, menstrual bleeding. Anovulatory cycles are due to immaturity or disturbance of the normal HPO axis. This is seen in the first decade after menarche, in premenopausal women and during periods of either physical or emotional stress.

Causes of abnormal vaginal bleeding

It is essential to initially review all possible causes of vaginal bleeding which may be considered by pathophysiology and/or pathological location (see Table 19.4.1).

History

A careful menstrual history helps determine the cause of the vaginal bleeding. A history of vaginal trauma may indicate vulval or vaginal wall bleeding. The vaginal trauma may be associated with either consensual or non-consensual intercourse, or a vaginal foreign body. Exposure in utero to diethyl stilboestrol (DES) should raise suspicion of vaginal malignancy.

Postcoital or intermenstrual bleeding may be symptomatic of cervical or uterine pathology. A history of an abnormal PAP smear, cervical polyp or cervical surgery may indicate cervical bleeding. Vaginal, cervical and/or uterine infection should also be considered in women at risk of a

Table 19.4.1   Differential diagnosis of menorrhagia (see reference 2)
• Ovulatory bleeding
• Anovulatory bleeding: previously known as dysfunctional uterine bleeding (DUB)

• Uterine and ovarian pathology:
  – uterine fibroids (pelvic pain, dysmenorrhoea)
  – endometriosis; adenomyosis (dysmenorrhoea, dyspareunia, pelvic pain, infertility)
  – pelvic inflammatory disease and pelvic infection (fever, vaginal discharge, pelvic pain, intermenstrual and postcoital bleeding)
  – endometrial polyps (intermenstrual bleeding)
  – endometrial hyperplasia; endometrial carcinoma (pelvic pain, abnormal bleeding, postcoital bleeding)
  – polycystic ovary syndrome (irregular bleeding and anovulatory menorrhagia)

• Systemic disease
  – coagulation disorder; bleeding diathesis (von Willebrand disease)
  – liver or renal disease
  – hypothyroidism (fatigue, constipation, coarse features, alopecia, pretibial myxoedema)

• Iatrogenic cause
  – anticoagulation
  – intrauterine device
  – chemotherapy
  – sex steroids

sexually transmitted infection, or following childbirth or instrumentation of the uterus.

Postmenopausal bleeding may be related to vulval or vaginal pathology such as infection, atrophy, trauma or malignancy. It may also be a symptom of uterine pathology with important common causes being a polyp or endometrial carcinoma.

A diagnosis of anovulatory bleeding is classically made from the history of irregular menses with periods of amenorrhoea followed by heavy bleeding, in the absence of features suggesting a structural or a histological uterine abnormality.[1] A menstrual cycle of less than 21 days or more than 35 days, even if regular, is usually anovulatory.

The patient's estimate of the amount of vaginal bleeding is often inaccurate and has limited use in diagnosis, other than the presence of clots, which is abnormal and suggests heavy bleeding.[2] Ask about additional information including known gynaecological cancer, a known bleeding disorder or a family history of a bleeding diathesis and exogenous sex steroid use.

Physical examination

First determine the haemodynamic stability of the patient. Physiological menorrhagia alone is rarely a cause of shock and other diagnoses such as cervical malignancy or endometrial AVMs should be considered. Examine also for evidence of anaemia, petechiae and thyroid endocrinopathy.

Abdominal and pelvic examination

Palpate the abdomen to assess for uterine enlargement. Inspect the vulva for local causes of bleeding including trauma and infection. The vaginal speculum examination should include assessment of the vaginal walls and the cervix, ideally with a clear plastic speculum for viewing the vaginal wall. Speculum examination will allow an assessment of the site and amount of bleeding. Bimanual examination is indicated to assess for local tenderness, uterine size and/or masses and adnexal masses or cervical motion tenderness.

Investigations

These are based around laboratory tests and ultrasound scanning.

Laboratory investigations

• Serum or urinary β-hCG pregnancy test. Perform this immediately on all women of childbearing age, even in the face of assurances from the patient that pregnancy could not be possible. Urine pregnancy tests are highly sensitive, detecting β-hCG levels as low as 25 IU/L.
• Full blood count. Perform this in all patients to identify anaemia. Add iron studies if the blood count shows a hypochromic, microcytic picture.
• Thyroid function tests. These are only indicated in women with menorrhagia and anovulatory bleeding, or if clear

evidence of thyroid endocrinopathy. Do *not* send routinely.
• A coagulation profile. Perform on all adolescents and any women with unusually heavy uterine bleeding.

Radiology

• Ultrasound is requested to assess the pelvic organs. Pay particular attention to the myometrium looking for fibroids or adenomyosis, the endometrial thickness and the endometrial cavity for polyps or retained products of conception.
• Ultrasound may also identify an AVM, which may be congenital or acquired either post partum or more commonly, post instrumentation of the uterus.

Management

Management may be considered as general supportive measures, and then specific treatment measures targeted at structural lesions or vaginal and endometrial infections, heavy uterine bleeding associated with either ovulatory or anovulatory uterine bleeding and at bleeding secondary to an excess of progesterone.

General supportive measures

Resuscitation should proceed in the usual manner with initial therapy determined by the degree of haemodynamic instability, or severity of anaemia.

Specific treatment measures for structural lesions

Vaginal wall bleeding

Vaginal wall bleeding secondary to trauma generally settles spontaneously. Examination under anaesthesia (EUA) is indicated for vaginal trauma if the laceration extends beyond the mucosa, or if examination is too uncomfortable for the woman.

Cervical bleeding

Cervical bleeding rarely requires immediate therapy. However, cervical bleeding from malignancy may occasionally be difficult to control because lesions tend to be friable. Attempt cautery with silver nitrate, and if this fails to control bleeding, pack the vagina with a vaginal pack. Refer the patient immediately to the gynaecology team.

Specific treatment for vaginal and endometrial infections

Vaginal and endometrial infections should be dealt with as outlined in Chapter 19.5. Arrange for the partner(s) to have contact tracing and simultaneous treatment as necessary.

Specific treatment for heavy uterine bleeding associated with ovulatory cycles

Tranexamic acid

The usual dose is 1 g three times a day for 3–4 days. Side effects include nausea and leg cramps but it is generally well tolerated. Tranexamic acid is a plasminogen activator inhibitor that promotes local haemostasis. Long-term studies have not shown any increase in thrombo-embolic events; however, active thrombo-embolic disease is considered a contraindication to its use.

Mefenamic acid, naproxen or ibuprofen

The usual dose of mefenamic acid is 500 mg three times a day, naproxen 250 mg three times a day and of ibuprofen 400 mg three times a day. These non-steroidal anti-inflammatory drugs (NSAIDs) block prostaglandin PGE_2, which is a vasodilator found in excess in patients with menorrhagia.[3] NSAIDs are especially helpful if there is associated dysmenorrhoea.

Specific treatment measures for heavy uterine bleeding associated with anovulatory uterine bleeding

Many different regimes are recommended, and emergency department (ED) physicians should select a range of agents with which to become familiar.[1,2,4] The underlying pathology is a relative lack of progesterone and so treatment should include progestin therapy to stabilize the endometrium. This may be combined with tranexamic acid and/or an NSAID, which decrease the amount of blood loss. If anovulatory cycles are expected to continue, then the progestin therapy may need to be long term.

Heavy uterine bleeding secondary to anovulation

Progestin therapy Give norethisterone 5–10 mg up to three times a day, tapering to 5–10 mg a day over 2–3 weeks, or medroxyprogesterone acetate 10–30 mg orally daily reducing to 10 mg daily over 2–3 weeks. Side effects include bloating, headache, acne and breast tenderness.

Tranexamic acid and NSAIDs These can be added to progestin therapy for heavy anovulatory bleeding.

Combined oral contraceptive pill Combined oral contraceptive pill (COCP) may be used to decrease blood loss in ovulatory cycles, and to regulate anovulatory cycles. It also provides contraception. Start a monophasic COCP that includes at least 30 µg of ethinyloestradiol and a progestin. Consider histological assessment of the endometrium in patients over 35 years of age, prior to commencing hormone therapy.

Specific treatment for bleeding secondary to an excess of progesterone

Patients who are exposed to exogenous progesterone such as for contraception or endometriosis may have abnormal bleeding requiring oestrogen therapy. Discuss this with their gynaecologist. Thin, young girls may also have a relative oestrogen deficiency and should be managed in conjunction with a paediatric gynaecologist.

Other treatments not usually commenced in the ED

Surgical procedures

Dilation and curettage is a method of endometrial sampling and *not* a treatment for menorrhagia or irregular menstrual cycles. It is often used in combination with hysteroscopy, which allows visual assessment of the uterine cavity and biopsy if indicated.

Other drug treatments

Other treatments that are not usually commenced in the ED include the levonorgestrel-releasing intrauterine system such as Mirena[R], or long-acting progestogens such as medroxyprogesterone acetate (Depo-Provera[R]), which may prove successful if oral agents fail.

Gonadotrophin-releasing hormone (GnRH) analogues should only be commenced by a gynaecologist when other medical and surgical treatments are contraindicated, or prior to proposed surgery.

Disposition

Admit patients with haemodynamic instability or profound anaemia. Consult the gynaecology team if a significant underlying cause for the abnormal bleeding is likely. However, most patients may be discharged and followed up in an outpatient clinic.

Conclusions

A systematic approach to abnormal vaginal bleeding must first exclude pregnancy and then include a search for the site of the bleeding. Investigations should be targeted to the presumed underlying pathology and most can be performed as an outpatient. Treatment is targeted at the likely underlying pathophysiology.

Controversies

❶ A precise regimen for progestins in the management of anovulatory bleeding.

❷ The indications for endometrial sampling, especially in postmenopausal women.

❸ The optimal form of endometrial sampling.

❹ The role of surgical versus medical therapy in the long-term management of menorrhagia.

References

1. National Institute for Health and Clinical Excellence. Heavy menstrual bleeding. NICE clinical guideline 44, Jan 2007. http://www.nice.org.uk/nicemedia/pdf/word/CG44NICEGuideline.doc (accessed Dec 2007).
2. National Health Service. Menorrhagia (heavy menstrual bleeding). Clinical knowledge summaries, Sept 2007. http://www.cks.library.nhs.uk/menorrhagia/view_whole_topic_review (accessed Dec 2007).
3. Duckitt K, Collins S. Menorrhagia. *Clinical evidence*, British Medical Journal Publications. http://clinicalevidence.bmj.com/ceweb/conditions/woh/0805/0805.jsp (accessed Dec 2007).
4. Smith SK, Abel MH, Kelly RW, et al. A role for prostacyclin (PGI 2) in excessive menstrual bleeding. Lancet 1981; 1: 522–524.

19.5 Pelvic inflammatory disease

Sheila Bryan

ESSENTIALS

1 Pelvic inflammatory disease (PID) is an infection and/or inflammation of the upper genital tract.

2 The clinical features cover a spectrum of presentations, which depend on the extent of infection and/or inflammation, the anatomical structures involved and the specific micro-organisms.

3 *Chlamydia trachomatis* is the most common pathogen identified in sexually transmitted PID. Other pathogens include *Neisseria gonorrhoeae* and mixed anaerobes.

4 The sequelae of PID include infertility, chronic pelvic pain and ectopic pregnancy.

5 Screening high-risk patients for sexually transmitted infections reduces the incidence of PID.

Introduction

Pelvic inflammatory disease (PID) refers to a clinical syndrome resulting from infection or inflammation involving the usually sterile upper genital tract.

The diagnosis encompasses endometritis, salpingitis, tubo-ovarian abscess and/or pelvic peritonitis.

Most cases of PID are caused by the ascent of micro-organisms from the vagina and endocervix into the upper genital tract.[1] The passage of organisms through the cervix is facilitated by mechanical disruption of the cervical barrier e.g. from dilation and curettage, childbirth or by sexually transmitted infections (STIs) such as *Chlamydia trachomatis* and *Neisseria gonorrhoeae*.

N. gonorrhoeae and *C. trachomatis* colonize the endometrium in sexually transmitted PID, causing asymptomatic endometritis, or may involve other structures resulting in symptomatic PID. The mechanism of tubular damage with *N. gonorrhoeae* is by direct cellular toxicity, and that by *C. trachomatis* is via a host immune response.[2,3]

Epidemiology

The exact incidence of PID is unknown as there are no standardized clinical criteria for diagnosis. The clinical significance of asymptomatic disease is thus unclear.

However, there are an estimated 59 000 patient encounters annually to Australian general practitioners, of which only 0.3% are referred to hospitals.[4]

Risk factors

Risk factors for PID include STIs and procedures or conditions that involve disruption of the normal cervical barrier. The presence of an intrauterine contraceptive device (IUCD) increases the risk of PID in the first 3 weeks following insertion.[5] There is also an increased risk of PID during or shortly after the menses.[6] Chlamydial infection is now the most common cause of sexually transmitted PID in Australia.

Presentation

Laparoscopy was considered the gold standard for investigation of presumed PID in the 1960s and 1970s.[7] At that time there was limited access to ultrasound scans, no reliable, simple tests for pregnancy or for *C. trachomatis*, and *N. gonorrhoeae* was the main causative organism.

A number of combinations of clinical and laboratory features have been proposed as criteria for initiating treatment, in an attempt to optimize the sensitivity and specificity of the clinical diagnosis of PID.[8] However, increasing the specificity by combining diagnostic criteria decreases the sensitivity. In view of the significant sequelae of untreated PID, the current recommendation is to consider treatment for PID in an at risk woman with adnexal tenderness, if no other cause for the local signs can be found.[9]

History

The history should assess the recognized risk factors for STIs such as young age at first sexual intercourse, younger age, multiple sexual partners, high frequency of sexual intercourse and non-barrier methods of contraception. History should also seek non-sexually transmitted causes such as recent instrumentation or other causes of disruption of the cervical barrier.

Abdominal pain of less than 3 weeks' duration is the most sensitive symptom of PID. Other symptoms may include new or changed vaginal discharge, dyspareunia, and abnormal vaginal bleeding.

Examination

Adnexal tenderness alone is the single most sensitive examination finding (95%), but has just a 3.8% specificity.[9] Other findings with a high sensitivity of over 90% include lower abdominal tenderness, uterine tenderness and cervical motion tenderness. However, as isolated findings, they again all lack sensitivity. Fever is less frequently found, but if present increases the specificity of the diagnosis.

Fitz-Hugh-Curtis syndrome (FHCS) peri-hepatitis

The presence of right upper quadrant pain in the absence of biliary tract disease in a patient with PID raises the possibility of the Fitz-Hugh–Curtis syndrome (FHCS). This is a peri-hepatitis with focal peritonitis resulting from the transcoelomic spread of inflammatory peritoneal fluid to the subphrenic and sub-diaphragmatic spaces. FHCS is usually an incidental finding in patients with PID, but occasionally is the presenting symptom.[10]

Perform a thorough examination to look for alternative causes of the presenting symptoms and to assess the severity of the infection. This should include upper abdominal ultrasound to exclude gall stones, as well as a pelvic examination and pelvic ultrasound (see later).

Investigations

Haematological tests

White cell count, erythrocyte sedimentation rate and C-reactive protein are all raised as non-specific markers of inflammation that alone lack sensitivity and specificity for the diagnosis.

Biochemical tests

A beta subunit of human chorionic gonadotrophin pregnancy test must be performed on all women of child-bearing age. PID in pregnancy, although rare, has significant implications. Pelvic pain secondary to a complication of pregnancy is an important differential diagnosis.

Microbiology

Collect endocervical swabs for microscopy and culture, and polymerase chain reaction (PCR) for *N. gonorrhoeae* and for *C. trachomatis*. A positive result retrospectively supports the diagnosis of PID, defines antibiotic sensitivities and identifies the need to treat sexual partners.

The presence of either mucopus or white blood cells (WBCs) in the vaginal discharge is a sensitive marker for PID. The diagnosis of PID is therefore unlikely if the cervical discharge appears normal and there are no WBCs in the wet slide preparation.[11]

Histological diagnosis

The identification of inflammatory cells on endometrial biopsy has been used to confirm the diagnosis of endometritis. The significance of different histological findings is yet to be defined.

Ultrasound

Ultrasound is valuable in the assessment of patients with moderate to severe PID and for identifying tubo-ovarian abscess, and in excluding other causes of pelvic pain. It lacks sensitivity in the diagnosis of mild to moderate PID.

Laparoscopy

Laparoscopy is valuable in diagnosing salpingitis and for identifying other causes of pelvic pain, but lacks sensitivity in identifying mild disease. It is usually reserved for patients with pelvic pain in whom a definitive diagnosis is unclear.

Differential diagnosis

Important differential diagnoses include ectopic pregnancy, endometriosis, complications of ovarian cysts and ovarian tumours, appendicitis and diverticulitis.

Management

Most patients with the clinical diagnosis of PID may be treated as outpatients. There is no evidence of improved outcomes between inpatient and outpatient treatment with respect to fertility, chronic pelvic pain or recurrence of PID.[12] Consider inpatient treatment for severe PID with clinical septicaemia, inability to tolerate oral antibiotics due to vomiting and when surgical emergencies cannot be excluded.

Antibiotic therapy

Sexually acquired PID[13]
- Mild-to-moderate infection
  Azithromycin 1 g orally as a single dose, plus doxycycline* 100 mg orally 12-hourly for 14 days, plus metronidazole 400 mg orally 12-hourly for 14 days.
  When gonorrhoea is suspected, add ceftriaxone 250 mg i.m. or i.v. as a single dose.
- Severe infection
  *Doxycycline 100 mg orally or i.v. 12-hourly, plus metronidazole 500 mg i.v. 12-hourly, plus either ceftriaxone 1 g i.v. once daily, or cefotaxime 1 g i.v. 8-hourly.
- Treat sexual partners in all proven cases of *N. gonorrhoeae* and *C. trachomatis*.

Non-sexually acquired PID:[13]
- Mild-to-moderate infection
  Amoxicillin plus clavulanate 875/125 mg orally 12-hourly for 14 days, plus doxycycline* 100 mg orally 12-hourly for 14 days.
- Severe infection
  Amoxicillin or ampicillin 2 g i.v. 6-hourly, plus gentamicin 4–6 mg/kg i.v. once daily (adjusted for renal function), plus metronidazole 500 mg i.v. 12-hourly.

Continue parenteral therapy until there is substantial improvement. Thereafter continue treatment as per mild-to-moderate infection guidelines to complete 14 days of treatment.

*Substitute roxithromycin 300 mg orally once daily for 14 days if the patient is pregnant or breast feeding, or when doxycycline is contraindicated (category B1).

Disposition

Review all patients discharged on oral medication within 24–48 h to assess the response to therapy.

Prognosis

Women with PID are at increased risk of chronic pelvic pain, ectopic pregnancy and infertility.

Controversies

❶ The clinical significance of asymptomatic PID.

❷ Clinical criteria to initiate treatment in PID.

❸ The indications for laparoscopy in PID.

References

1. Cunningham FG, Hauth JC, Gilstrap LC. The bacterial pathogenesis of acute pelvic inflammatory disease. Obstetrics and Gynecology 1978; 52(2): 161–164.
2. Melly MA, Gregg CR, McGee ZA. Studies on the toxicity of *Neisseria gonorrhoeae* for human fallopian tube mucosa. Journal of Infectious Diseases 1981; 143: 432–441.
3. Paton DL, Kuo CC, Wang SP, et al. Distal obstruction induced by repeated *Chlamydia trachomatis* salpingeal infection in pig-tailed macaques. Journal of Infectious Diseases 1987; 155: 1292–1299.
4. Chen M, Pan Y, Britt H, et al. Trends in clinical encounters for pelvic inflammatory disease and epididymitis in a national sample of Australian general

practices. International Journal of STD & AIDS 2006; 17: 384–386.

5. Farley TM, Rosenberg MJ, Rowe PJ. Intrauterine devices and pelvic inflammatory disease: an international perspective. Lancet 1992; 339: 785–788.

6 Nowicki S, Tassell AH, Nowiki B. Susceptibility to gonococcal infection during the menstrual cycle. Journal of the American Medical Association 2000; 283 (10): 1291–1292.

7 Jacobson L, Westrom L. Objectivized diagnosis of acute pelvic inflammatory disease. Diagnostic and prognostic value of routine laparoscopy. American Journal of Gynecology 1969; 105:1088–1098.

8. Centers for Disease Control and Prevention. Sexually transmitted diseases treatment guidelines. Morbidity and Mortality Weekly Reports 2006; 55(No. RR-11): 56–61.

9. Peipert JF, Ness RB, Blume J, et al. Clinical predictors of endometritis in women with symptoms and signs of pelvic inflammatory disease. American Journal of Obstetrics and Gynecology 2001; 184(5): 856–863.

10. Lopez-Zeno JA, Keith LG, Berger. The Fitz-Hugh–Curtis syndrome revisited. Changing perspectives after half a century. Journal of Reproductive Medicine 1985; 30: 567–582.

11. Peipert JF, Boardman J, Hogan JW. Laboratory evaluation of acute upper genital tract infection. Obstetrics and Gynecology 1996; 87(5): 730–736.

12. Ness R, Soper D, Holley R, et al. Effectiveness of inpatient and outpatient treatment strategies for women with pelvic inflammatory disease: results from the pelvic inflammatory disease evaluation and clinical health (PEACH) randomized trial. American Journal of Obstetrics and Gynecology 2002; 186: 929–937.

13. Pelvic inflammatory disease, version 13 2006. In: eTG complete. Melbourne: Therapeutic Guidelines Limited. http://www.tg.com.au/ip/complete/ (accessed July 2007).

19.6 Pelvic pain

Michael Cadogan • Anusch Yazdani • James Taylor

ESSENTIALS

1 Consider the possibility of pregnancy in *all* patients of reproductive age with abdominal or pelvic pain.

2 Give effective analgesia by the regular administration of non-steroidal anti-inflammatory drugs.

3 A negative pelvic examination should not preclude a gynaecological referral, even in the absence of other findings.

4 'Psychogenic pain' is a diagnosis of exclusion.

Introduction

Pelvic and lower abdominal pain in female patients is a complex and challenging complaint. It is the second most common gynaecological symptom after vaginal bleeding. The large differential diagnosis for female pelvic pain makes a definite diagnosis in the emergency department (ED) difficult, therefore a systematic approach is essential.

The emergency physician should aim to identify and stabilize the critically ill patient, identify those conditions that require early surgical intervention, and to expedite the investigation and further management of the female patient with pelvic pain, following adequate analgesia.

Classification

Conditions causing pelvic pain may be life threatening or mild, acute or chronic, gynaecological, non-gynaecological or non-organic, and cyclical or acyclic. They are often complex, requiring ongoing care and management by other specialties. This chapter outlines the initial investigation and management of the most common gynaecological conditions associated with acute and chronic pelvic pain.

History

A thorough history is essential to determine the potential cause(s) of the pain. Parietal pelvic pain may be well localized and occurs secondary to peritoneal irritation such as in appendicitis and Mittelschmerz. More generalized and diffuse abdominal pain is associated with intraperitoneal blood or pus resulting from the rupture of an ectopic pregnancy, or tubo-ovarian abscess.

Pain of sudden onset is associated with ovarian cyst rupture or adnexal torsion. Gradually worsening pain is suggestive of a long-term process, such as endometriosis or chronic pelvic inflammatory disease (PID). Pain with sexual intercourse (dyspareunia) may be associated with adnexal pathology and endometriosis.

Evaluating the patient's sexual and menstrual history indicates the potential for pregnancy-related problems or sexually transmitted diseases (STD), and defines chronic pain as cyclic or acyclic. This should include possible physical and sexual abuse, menarche, menopause, contraception, last menstrual period (LMP), previous STD, gravida, parity, tubal surgery and previous ectopic pregnancy.

The radiation of the pain may provide a clue to the underlying origin, such as pain referred via the hypogastric nerve plexus to the lower abdomen from the uterine fundus, adnexae and bladder dome. The S2–4 sacral nerve roots transmit pain from the lower uterine segment, cervix, bladder trigone and rectum to the lower back, buttocks, perineum and legs. It is also important to ask about associated urological, gastrointestinal and musculoskeletal symptoms.

Finally, consider psychosocial factors particularly in the evaluation of chronic pelvic pain. The symptoms of fatigue, loss of energy and depressed mood are commonly associated with chronic pelvic pain, thus a screen for anxiety, depressive and somatoform disorders is essential. Enquire about marital distress: the partner's understanding and response to the pain and the family's response to how the patient is handling the pain are all important.

Examination

Record the vital signs, provide early analgesia and establish rapport with the patient who may be reticent, frightened or embarrassed. Note the pulse, blood pressure and temperature to evaluate for potential life-threatening haemorrhage such as an ectopic pregnancy, or overwhelming sepsis associated with tubo-ovarian abscess.

Commence the abdominal examination with inspection for distension associated with obstruction, ascites or abdominal masses. Palpation and percussion delineate areas of generalized or localized tenderness and aim to replicate the patient's pain. Check for hernias, inguinal nodes and other non-gynaecological causes for the patient's symptoms at the same time (see Table 19.6.1).

Pelvic examination

A pelvic examination is essential in the sexually active patient. Perform this only in the presence of a chaperone, after providing adequate explanation for the procedure and gaining verbal consent. The pelvic examination includes:

- visual examination of the vulva and urethral meatus to identify varicosities, infection or abnormal lesions
- speculum examination to directly visualize the cervix, cervical os and the vaginal vault. Note vaginal discharge, take endocervical and vaginal swabs and perform a PAP smear, if follow-up of the result can be guaranteed.
- bimanual (vagino–abdominal) examination to examine the cervix, uterus and adnexae.

The uterus is normally mobile, but conditions such as endometriosis or adhesions may cause fixation. An enlarged uterus is associated with pregnancy, fibroids and adenomyosis. The uterine axis is dependent on a number of other local pelvic factors, such as the content of the bladder or bowel. A retroverted uterus is usually normal, but a fixed retroverted uterus is classically associated with pouch of Douglas pathology such as endometriosis.

Uterine tenderness occurs with any pelvic peritonism, adenomyosis or fibroid degeneration. An open cervical os may be associated with the passage of intrauterine pathology such as a failed pregnancy or clots. Cervical excitation pain on moving the cervix is non-specific and associated with conditions producing pelvic peritonism such as blood or other irritants in the peritoneal cavity. Palpable adnexal masses are associated with more gross pathology, such as ovarian cysts and endometriomata, again associated with adnexal tenderness.

A normal pelvic examination does not accurately exclude pelvic pathology. It still provides valuable information and helps in the selection of further definitive investigations, such as ultrasound scan (USS) and laparoscopy.

Rectal examination

The rectal examination completes the pelvic examination, taking note of stool consistency, faecal occult blood and the presence of mass lesions. A rectovaginal examination allows palpation of the posterior cul-de-sac for ovarian masses, the posterior wall of the uterus, and the uterosacral ligaments for nodularity and tenderness in association with endometriosis. This should only be performed once, preferably by the doctor with ongoing clinical care.

Laboratory investigations

Laboratory studies depend on the history and physical examination and are tailored to the individual patient. They include the following tests.

Blood tests

Beta subunit of human chorionic gonadotrophin testing
Screening for pregnancy is essential in a patient of reproductive age and a serum (or urine) pregnancy test should be performed. The beta subunit of human chorionic gonadotrophin (β-hCG) is produced by the outer layer of cells of the gestational sac (the syncytiotrophoblast) and may be detected as early as 9 days after fertilization (see Ch. 19.2). False-positive and false-negative serum and urine tests do occur, but are rare.

Full blood count, ESR and C-reactive protein
A full blood count may be helpful in identifying the presence and type of anaemia, but cannot determine the cause. A leukocytosis may indicate underlying infection or inflammation. An elevated ESR or C-reactive protein may indicate inflammation and acute pathology, and are included in the clinical diagnosis of PID in some centres.

Table 19.6.1 Causes of acute pelvic pain			
Gynaecological	Non-gynaecological		
	Intestinal	Urological	Other
Complication of pregnancy: ectopic, miscarriage	Appendicitis	Cystitis	Hernia
Complication of ovarian and adnexal cysts and masses	Diverticulitis	Acute urinary retention	Porphyria
Pelvic inflammatory disease	Inflammatory bowel disease	Urolithiasis	Pelvic vein thrombophlebitis
Adnexal torsion	Gastroenteritis	Pyelonephritis	
Leiomyoma complication	Bowel obstruction Constipation		

Tumour markers

Tumour markers have a limited role in the evaluation of pelvic pain in the ED. Markers such as the CA 125 have a role in the evaluation of an adnexal mass or when endometriosis is suspected. Serial levels improve the sensitivity and specificity of such markers, usually on an outpatient basis.

Urinalysis

Urinary β-hCG is fast, cheap and accurate. Perform this in all sexually active patients. The presence of leukocytes in the urine may indicate infection with a sensitivity of around 70–75%, but may also be associated with inflammation of adjacent pelvic organs. The presence of red cells and casts may indicate urolithiasis.

Send the urine for microscopy, culture and sensitivity if urinary tract pathology is suspected. The urine may also be sent for chlamydial PCR in suspected PID (see Ch. 19.5).

Microbiological swabs

Take endocervical swabs for chlamydia, gonorrhoea and ureaplasma during the speculum examination, and a swab of the introitus for agents associated with vulvar vestibulitis, one cause of dyspareunia.

Taking a PAP smear test is of little benefit in the patient with acute pelvic pain, and any inability to guarantee adequate follow-up of the result must preclude its performance.

Imaging

Ultrasound scan

Ultrasound is now regarded as a non-invasive extension of the physical examination, particularly in the female patient. It is the single most useful test in diagnosing acute gynaecological presentations within the ED.

Ultrasound may determine the uterine size, presence of fibroids, and the thickness and characteristics of the endometrium and myometrium. It may delineate adnexal pathology such as ovarian cysts, endometriomata, hydro/pyosalpinx, tubo-ovarian abscess and tumours.

USS is more accurate at predicting abnormal pelvic pathology, as confirmed by laparoscopy, than pelvic examination

alone. However, studies using laparoscopy as the 'gold standard' still found that half of the patients with either a normal pelvic examination or USS had abnormal laparoscopic findings.

Computerized tomography scan

Computerized tomography (CT) scan is helpful to delineate pelvic masses such as malignancy further or complex abscess formation. A CT scan may also help identify a urinary calculus, a Spigelian hernia, abdominal tuberculosis and appendicitis. The radiation risk must be considered, particularly if a repeat scan is requested.

Magnetic resonance imaging

Magnetic resonance imaging (MRI) may define adenomyosis and obstructive uterine anomalies associated with endometriosis, but is rarely ever available from the ED.

Differential diagnosis

Patients attending the ED may present with:

- acute pelvic pain
- an acute presentation of chronic pelvic pain (acute-on-chronic)
- chronic pelvic pain

Acute pelvic pain

Table 19.6.1 lists conditions that present to the ED with acute pelvic pain. The causes may be broken down into the following.

Pregnancy-related

Pregnancy should be excluded in all women of reproductive age and, if diagnosed, ectopic pregnancy must then be excluded. See Chapter 19.2.

Pelvic inflammatory disease

See Chapter 19.5 on the evaluation of pelvic inflammatory disease (PID).

Adnexal mass or cyst

Ovarian mass or cyst

- 'Functional' ovarian cysts are either follicular ovarian cysts that develop during the first 14 days of the menstrual cycle prior to ovulation, or corpus luteum cysts

that develop during the last 14 days following ovulation. 'Functional' cysts are usually asymptomatic unless complications occur. As these cysts are related to normal ovarian activity, ovarian cysts in the postmenopausal woman should never be considered 'functional'.
- Neoplastic masses may be either benign or malignant. Features that increase the risk of malignancy include being postmenopausal, the presence of ascites and increasing size or complexity.
- Infective masses usually arise as part of a tubo-ovarian mass in association with PID.
- Endometriomata are deposits of endometriosis in association with the ovary, forming a collection of altered blood and cellular debris, hence the term 'chocolate cyst'.

Non-ovarian adnexal mass or cyst

- Para-ovarian and paratubal cysts are related to either the ovary or, more commonly, the fallopian tube.
- Hydrosalpinx arises in the blocked fallopian tube.

Any of these structures may present acutely due to rupture, haemorrhage or torsion.

Rupture of ovarian cyst Follicular cyst rupture at ovulation may be accompanied by ovarian bleeding and peritoneal irritation during the mid-cycle known as Mittelschmerz. The rupture of a corpus luteum cyst usually occurs between days 20 and 26 of the menstrual cycle and is associated with intra-peritoneal bleeding. This bleeding may be catastrophic depending on the size of the torn ovarian blood vessel. USS helps differentiate a ruptured ectopic pregnancy from a bleeding corpus luteum cyst, although they may coexist.

Intra-ovarian haemorrhage Haemorrhage may occur into a cyst or tumour. The sudden onset of sharp unilateral pain with increasing intensity results from ovarian capsule distension. There may be localized or generalized peritonism dependent on the degree of peritoneal irritation and haemorrhage extravasation. Pelvic examination may reveal a focal expanding adnexal mass, which is confirmed by USS.

Haemorrhagic ovarian cysts may be managed conservatively. Indications for intervention include failure to obtain adequate analgesia, failure of rapid symptom resolution and haemodynamic instability.

Torsion of adnexae The adnexae include the ovary and fallopian tube. Torsion occurs when these structures twist on their supportive appendages causing compromise of their vascular supply. This most commonly occurs in the third decade of life and accounts for 3–5% of emergency gynaecological surgery. Over 90% of cases of adnexal torsion are associated with cystic tumours or simple cysts of the ovary. Torsion of the fallopian tube is less common and is associated with a hydrosalpinx, tubal ligation and pelvic adhesions. Both adnexal torsion and torsion of the fallopian tube are associated with an enlarging adnexal mass, secondary to venous obstruction and secondary oedema.

Pain associated with adnexal torsion is commonly sudden in onset, sharp, unilateral and increasingly severe on a background of a dull pelvic ache. It is associated with nausea, vomiting, low-grade pyrexia and with urinary symptoms secondary to bladder irritation. Late presentations may be associated with ovarian necrosis, frank peritonitis and shock.

Pelvic examination reveals cervical motion tenderness, adnexal tenderness and a discrete adnexal mass in the majority of patients. USS usually confirms the underlying pathology and defines the adnexal mass. Definitive diagnosis and treatment can be laparoscopic or via laparotomy.

Ovarian infection This may occur rarely as a primary event with mumps or tuberculosis, but usually occurs in the setting of PID with the formation of a tubo-ovarian abscess. See Chapter 19.5.

Acute-on-chronic pelvic pain and chronic pelvic pain

Chronic pelvic pain is defined as pain lasting more than 6 months, localized to the anatomic pelvis causing functional disability requiring medical or surgical treatment. It affects many millions of women worldwide, and accounts for 10% of gynaecology outpatient attendances. The commonest diagnoses associated with chronic pelvic pain are endometriosis and pelvic adhesions. However, up to 60% of patients have no visible pathology at laparoscopy and 25% of patients remain without a definitive diagnosis.

Patients usually present to the ED with an acute exacerbation of their chronic condition (acute-on-chronic pelvic pain), an acute unrelated cause of pelvic pain or an inability to cope with their debilitating condition.

Cyclic pelvic pain

Cyclic pelvic pain (see Table 19.6.2) occurs in 30–50% of women of reproductive age and interferes with normal daily activities in up to 12% of cases. It is usually related to ovulation or menstruation. Many conditions that cause cyclic pain may ultimately cause acyclic pain, such as endometriosis.

Mittelschmerz Mittelschmerz is defined as a transient mid-cycle pain occurring at or after ovulation. Increasing ovarian capsular pressure is associated with poorly localized pain, which becomes localized following follicular rupture and the release of fluid and/or blood causing peritoneal irritation.

There are usually minimal findings on physical examination, but thorough evaluation is essential to rule out other pelvic pathology. A slightly enlarged ovary may be palpated on the affected side.

Mittelschmerz is a clinical diagnosis, although USS may reveal the presence of a recently ruptured follicle. Provide regular NSAID tablets and reassurance as the mainstay of treatment. Although the pain on presentation may be severe, it usually resolves spontaneously.

Endometriosis Endometriosis occurs when ectopic endometrial glands and stroma occur outside the uterine cavity. Initially the pain is cyclic and associated with menses, but as pelvic adhesions develop the pain often becomes continuous and acyclic.

Endometriosis affects women aged 20–45 years and is the second most common cause of cyclic pain in reproductive age females. Over 70% of sufferers are nulliparous and up to 60% of patients investigated for infertility are found to have endometriosis.

Typically, the pain commences a few days prior to the menses and extends variably into or beyond this period. Persistent, unilateral mid-cycle pain is suggestive of an endometrioma. Patients may also commonly present with dysmenorrhoea (75%), dyspareunia (20%), following the finding of an adnexal mass (endometrioma) or with tenesmus.

Table 19.6.2 Causes of cyclic and acyclic pelvic pain	
Cyclic	**Acyclic**
Mittelschmerz	Chronic PID
Endometriosis*	Pelvic adhesions
Adenomyosis	Uterine prolapse
Cervical stenosis*	Chronic urethritis
Intra-uterine device	Diverticulitis
Leiomyoma (fibroid)	Irritable bowel syndrome
Primary and secondary dysmenorrhoea	Levator syndrome of the perirectal area
Pelvic congestion*	Detrusor instability
	Interstitial cystitis
	Abdominal hernias
	Abdominal wall myofascial pain
	Abuse syndromes: physical and sexual
	Depression

*This may become 'acyclic'. PID, pelvic inflammatory disease.

The physical examination is completely normal in the majority of women with endometriosis. Suggestive findings include adnexal tenderness during menses and a fixed retroverted uterus with posterior tenderness. In addition, uterosacral ligament and posterior uterus nodularity with tenderness on rectovaginal examination is characteristic of endometriosis, but may not always be present.

USS may reveal endometriomata, or focal endometriotic lesions. The definitive diagnosis is made on histology at laparoscopy. Excision is both diagnostic and therapeutic.

Adenomyosis Adenomyosis is a benign condition characterized by the ingrowth of the endometrial glands and stroma into the myometrium. The majority (>80%) of cases involve multiparous women in the fourth and fifth decade of life. Patients usually present with menorrhagia and dysmenorrhoea.

Pelvic examination reveals a symmetrically enlarged, slightly tender uterus with a diffusely boggy consistency. Rarely, a large mass (adenomyoma) may be palpated.

USS may reveal generalized uterine enlargement with indistinct myo-endometrial margins. MRI will clearly demonstrate the pathology, but is rarely necessary or available.

Hysteroscopy and endometrial biopsy may demonstrate adenomyosis, but definitive diagnosis is usually made at hysterectomy.

Leiomyomata (fibroids) Leiomyomata or fibroids are benign tumours of myometrial origin. They are the most common pelvic tumour and occur in 25% of Caucasian women and 50% of Negro women. Their aetiology is unknown but they enlarge in pregnancy and recede in the climacteric.

Symptoms are usually associated with chronic cyclic pelvic pain with or without bleeding. Acute pain occurs with torsion or degeneration. Torsion usually involves pedunculated subserosal lesions. Degeneration is usually associated with pregnancy and results from the rapidly expanding lesion restricting its own blood supply.

Fibroids may be palpated on bimanual pelvic examination. The lesions are usually painless unless associated with acute degeneration when uterine tenderness, pyrexia and leukocytosis are seen.

Treatment of chronic leiomyomata is usually conservative unless associated with anaemia. The patient with acute torsion or degeneration of a fibroid requires opiate analgesia and urgent gynaecological review for definitive management.

Primary or secondary dysmenorrhoea
Primary dysmenorrhoea This is painful menstruation in the absence of pelvic pathology and is a diagnosis of exclusion. Primary dysmenorrhoea is associated with the release of prostaglandins, principally PGF2α from the endometrium during menstruation. This causes abnormal uterine contractions, arteriolar vasoconstriction and uterine ischaemia, with the most intense pain occurring as the menstrual flow is subsiding. Primary dysmenorrhoea usually coincides with the onset of ovulatory cycles 4–12 months after menarche, and affects up to 10% of young nulliparous women.

Primary dysmenorrhoea is associated with spasmodic, crampy lower abdominal pain radiating to the lower back and upper thighs, and usually lasts 24–48 h. Associated symptoms include headache, nausea and vomiting. Symptoms may be alleviated by the regular administration of NSAID drugs or by suppressing ovulation with the oral contraceptive pill.

Secondary dysmenorrhoea This is painful menstruation associated with pelvic pathology including cervical stenosis, adenomyosis, leiomyomata, pelvic congestion syndrome and the intra-uterine contraceptive device. It usually affects women later in life and symptoms often start earlier in the menstrual cycle and can precede menstruation.

Acyclic pelvic pain
Chronic PID.
See Chapter 19.5.

Pelvic adhesions Adhesions occur when anatomical structures are abnormally bound to one another by bands of fibrous tissue. They are believed to account for the pain suffered by up to 33% of patients with chronic pelvic pain, although their exact role is uncertain. They are associated with PID, endometriosis, abdominal surgery,

perforated appendix and inflammatory bowel disease.

Adhesions contain their own nerve fibres and the pain perceived by patients is thought to originate within the fibrous tissue when it is under tension. The pain is often consistent in location and aggravated by sudden movements, intercourse or physical activity. Laparoscopy is the gold standard for diagnosis and treatment.

Pelvic congestion syndrome Pelvic congestion syndrome is characterized by dilation, congestion and venous stasis of the pelvic veins. This syndrome is associated with multiparity, polycystic ovarian syndrome, tubal ligation and lower limb varicosities. Patients commonly present with a chronic, dull ache localized to the pelvis and lower back with exacerbations of sharp stabbing pain. Other symptoms include dyspareunia (75%), dysfunctional uterine bleeding (54%) and mucoid vaginal discharge (47%).

Deep abdominal palpation, particularly over the adnexae, usually reproduces the pain. On external examination superficial vulval varices are seen and speculum examination may reveal a bluish tinge to the engorged cervix.

Pelvic venography can establish the size of varicosities and the site of incompetence. Ultrasound may demonstrate uterine enlargement and venous incompetence.

Psychological There is an association between chronic pelvic pain and somatization disorders. In addition, many women with chronic pelvic pain have suffered physical, sexual and emotional abuse, and psychiatric disease is often related.

Conclusion

Female pelvic pain presents a complex and challenging problem in the ED. A systematic evaluation may find a diagnosis in acute pelvic pain, but chronic conditions require review and follow-up by a specialist unit.

The resuscitation of the acutely unwell patient, exclusion of pregnancy-related problems, provision of adequate analgesia, prompt initiation of appropriate investigations and specialist referral for ongoing evaluation are fundamental to the management of gynaecological pelvic pain.

Controversies

❶ Accuracy of emergency physician focused pelvic ultrasound scan to evaluate pelvic pain.

❷ Diagnosis and management of acute-on-chronic and chronic pelvic pain syndromes.

Further Reading

Berchuk A, Boente MP, Bast RB. The use of tumour markers in the management of patients with gynaecological carcinomas. Clinical Obstetrics of Gynaecology 1992; 35(1): 45–54.

Carter JE. A systematic history for the patient with pelvic pain. Journal of the Society of Laparoendoscopic Surgeons 1993; 3: 245–252.

Howard FM. The role of laparoscopy in chronic pelvic pain: promise and pitfalls. Obstetrics and Gynaecological Surgery 1993; 48: 357–387.

Howard FM, Perry CP, Carter JE eds. Pelvic pain: diagnosis and management. New York: Lippincott; 2000.

Muse KN. Cyclic pelvic pain. Obstetrics and Gynecology Clinics of North America 1990; 17: 427.

Scialli AR, Barbieri RL, Glasser MH, et al. Chronic pelvic pain: An integrated approach. Medical Education Collaborative. Association of Professors of Gynaecology and Obstetrics 2000; 3–9.

19.7 Pre-eclampsia and eclampsia

Marian Lee

ESSENTIALS

1 Pre-eclampsia and eclampsia are part of the continuum of 'hypertensive disorders of pregnancy'.

2 Pre-eclampsia is a multi-system condition.

3 Oedema is no longer part of the definition of pre-eclampsia.

4 The pathogenesis of pre-eclampsia (and of eclampsia) remains incompletely deciphered.

5 Anti-angiogenic factors are associated with the pathogenesis of pre-eclampsia (and eclampsia).

6 The clinical manifestations of pre-eclampsia are an extension of the abnormalities in the utero–placental circulation.

7 Early recognition is essential as mortality and morbidity are high for the mother and the fetus.

8 Pre-eclampsia is a life-long disease with implications for future pregnancies and the subsequent cardiovascular health of the mother.

Introduction

Pre-eclampsia is a hypertensive emergency unique to pregnancy. It is part of the spectrum of hypertensive disorders of pregnancy (see Table 19.7.1), and is characterized by the presence of hypertension, proteinuria or other evidence of end-organ dysfunction.[1,2]

Definition of pre-eclampsia

Hypertension is defined by the International Society for the Study of Hypertension in Pregnancy as a diastolic blood pressure (dBP) of 90 mmHg on two consecutive occasions, or a single measurement of 110 mmHg. Proteinuria is defined by 1+ on dipstick urinalysis which correlates with >300 mg proteinuria per 24 h. Oedema is *no longer* a defining feature of pre-eclampsia.[3]

Definition of severe pre-eclampsia

Severe pre-eclampsia is defined when at least one of the following is present: evident target organ dysfunction (besides proteinuria), severe proteinuria with greater than 5 g/24 h, systolic blood pressure (sBP) greater than 160 mmHg, dBP greater than 110 mmHg and fetal growth retardation.

The *typical* period of onset of pre-eclampsia is between 20 weeks of gestation and 48 h post partum. The associated abnormalities resolve within 10 post-partum days.

Aetiology, genetics and pathogenesis of pre-eclampsia

The aetiology and pathogenesis of pre-eclampsia are incompletely understood.

Aetiology

Increasing evidence since 2001 has supported the importance of anti-angiogenic factors in the pathogenesis of this multi-system condition.[4] Two such factors produced by the placenta are soluble fms-like tyrosine kinase 1 (sFlt1) and endoglin.[3–6] Soluble fms-like tyrosine kinase 1 acts by binding the angiogenic factors vascular endothelial growth factor and placental growth factor. Endoglin, however, inhibits nitric oxide mediated vasodilatation. High levels of both in vitro lead to the changes found in pre-eclampsia. High levels of sFlt1 alone are found in early onset pre-eclampsia, i.e. before 32 weeks' gestation. This may be relevant to the early detection of pre-eclampsia in the future.[7]

Table 19.7.1 Spectrum of hypertensive disorders of pregnancy

Gestational hypertension	Hypertension in pregnancy without proteinuria or end-organ dysfunction
Pre-eclampsia	Hypertension in pregnancy with associated proteinuria and/or evidence of organ dysfunction.
Eclampsia	Seizure or coma complicating pre-eclampsia
Chronic hypertension	Hypertension pre-dating pregnancy

Pathogenesis

As the pathogenesis is currently incompletely deciphered, the abnormalities are best illustrated by comparing it with the changes in a normal pregnancy.

Normal pregnancy changes to blood pressure

The renin–angiotensin–aldosterone system (RAAS) is activated in normal pregnancy. Its promotion of vasoconstriction is countered by a reduced sensitivity of small vessels to vasopressors, and the release of systemic and renal vasodilatory mediators.[1,4] Consequently, the blood pressure (BP) falls after conception with a nadir at 24 weeks, before returning to pre-pregnancy level by the third trimester. A second fall occurs after delivery and again returns to pre-pregnancy range by the fifth postpartum day. These changes to the BP are accompanied by a 50% rise in the plasma volume.

Pre-eclamptic pregnancy

Two major aspects of difference in the pre-eclamptic pregnancy are abnormal placental vascularization, and an increased vasomotor tone in the maternal and utero–placental circulations.

Placental vascularization The placental vascularization in the pre-eclamptic pregnancy is both incomplete and abnormal. In normal pregnancy, trophoblasts invade through all layers of the uterine wall leading to the formation of sinusoids. This results in a highly vascular structure with high capacitance vessels. In a pregnancy destined for pre-eclampsia, the above changes do not occur, resulting in an utero–placental circulation at risk of hypoperfusion. Additionally, placental anti-angiogenic factors are released into the maternal circulation and contribute to the eventual maternal clinical manifestations.[7]

Maternal circulation The maternal circulation also suffers a number of abnormalities.[5,6] The RAAS is not activated as in normal pregnancy. Additionally, there is increased synthesis of endothelin and thromboxane, both vasopressors that lead to increased vasomotor tone, and the synthesis of the vasodilatory mediators prostacyclin and nitric oxide is reduced. These abnormalities all result in a maternal circulation that is volume-depleted with high vasomotor tone culminating in hypoperfusion of multiple target organs additional to the placenta.

Eclampsia[8]

The seizures in pre-eclampsia (that is, eclampsia itself) are thought to be secondary to cerebral ischaemia. Vasospasm has been demonstrated in the subcortical white matter and adjacent grey matter of the parietal and occipital lobes. The pathological findings of infarction, micro haemorrhages and oedema are similar to those found in hypertensive encephalopathy.

Epidemiology

The prevalence and risk factors for pre-eclampsia and eclampsia are as follows.

Prevalence[2,6,9]

In Australia, 10% of pregnancies are associated with a hypertensive disorder of pregnancy, including pre-eclampsia occurring in 1–4% of all pregnancies. The worldwide prevalence for comparison is 2–8% of pregnancies.

Risk factors[3,5,6,8,10,11]

Maternal

- Gestational hypertension: up to 25% will develop pre-eclampsia
- Primiparity: 2.4 × risk

- Past history or a family history of pre-eclampsia
- Increased BMI
- No prenatal care
- Renal disease
- Diabetes mellitus
- Hypercoagulable states: acquired (antiphospholipid syndrome with anticardiolipin antibodies, lupus anticoagulant or both) or inherited (Factor V Leiden deficiency)
- Collagen vascular disease.

Fetal factors

- Large placenta: multiple gestation, molar pregnancy, fetal hydrops.

Note that age alone is not a risk factor for pre-eclampsia. However, chronic hypertension is more prevalent in older women.

Prevention

Prevention of pre-eclampsia and eclampsia is as follows.

Pre-eclampsia[5,6]

The prevention of pre-eclampsia is hampered by incomplete knowledge of its pathogenesis. Aspirin, calcium and starting antihypertensives for mild-to-moderate hypertension have been investigated, but there is no clear evidence to support their use.

Eclampsia[8]

Magnesium sulphate ($MgSO_4$) is used to prevent eclampsia in women hospitalized with severe pre-eclampsia. In symptomatic patients with signs of imminent seizure such as headache and blurred vision, the number needed to treat (NNT) is 16. The benefit for asymptomatic patients is less impressive, with the NNT being 185.

Clinical features of pre-eclampsia and eclampsia

The clinical features of pre-eclampsia reflect its far reaching effects on the maternal circulation. Multiple body systems are affected as a result of the generalized increased vasomotor tone and volume depletion. The clinical manifestations are best described according to the target organ system involved. Discussion of atypical presentations highlights the need for vigilance by emergency physicians.

Magnitude of blood pressure[5]

The diastolic component of the BP rises disproportionately to the sBP, although as the sBP is usually less than 160 mmHg, an sBP greater than 200 mmHg suggests chronic hypertension.

Neurological manifestations

Typical features are headache, blurring of vision, hyperreflexia and an altered level of consciousness ranging from drowsiness to coma. The distinguishing feature from an acute stroke is reversibility of the above by lowering of the BP. Intracerebral haemorrhage is one of the most devastating complications, although fortunately uncommon.[12]

Eclampsia includes typically a generalized tonic–clonic seizure. Over 90% of seizures occur beyond 29 weeks of gestation, and approximately half (44%) take place in the post-partum period. Note that the risk period for pre-eclampsia and eclampsia includes the period from delivery to 4 weeks post partum.

Acute pulmonary oedema

Pulmonary oedema occurs as a consequence of pulmonary capillary leakage rather than of direct myocardial origin.[5]

Hepatic syndrome

The spectrum of hepatic injury ranges from mild elevation of liver enzymes to subcapsular bleeding, liver capsular rupture and the haemolysis, elevated liver enzymes (hepatic enzymosis) and low platelets (thrombocytopenia) (HELLP) syndrome.

HELLP syndrome

The HELLP syndrome refers to haemolysis, elevated liver enzymes (hepatic enzymosis) and low platelets (thrombocytopenia). This syndrome defines severe pre-eclampsia and is accompanied by severe hypertension, renal failure and disseminated intravascular coagulation (DIC).[5] It is associated with a significant morbidity and mortality for the patient.

Renal dysfunction[5,13]

Proteinuria is one hallmark of pre-eclampsia. However, renal involvement also includes between a 10 and 40% fall in the glomerular filtration rate (GFR) resulting in a rise in the serum creatinine, uric acid and calcium. Usually in a normal pregnancy, the serum creatinine is lowered as a result of a rise in the GFR with the normal level being less than 0.70 mmol/L.

Serum uric acid level is used as a marker for pre-eclampsia, as abnormally raised levels predate clinical manifestation of pre-eclampsia.

Atypical presentations

Hypertension is not present in 16% of pre-eclamptic patients who otherwise have typical features.[8]

Suspect underlying renal disease or undiagnosed chronic hypertension in patients with features of pre-eclampsia prior to 20 weeks' gestation.

Up to 10% of eclamptic patients less than 32 weeks' gestation at presentation may not have the distinguishing features of hypertension or proteinuria. However, over 70% of those who present after this period have severe hypertension.

Pre-eclampsia and eclampsia may occur up to 4 weeks' post partum. Hence, they must be considered in the differential diagnosis of blurred vision, headache and seizures presenting during this time frame.

Differential diagnosis

There are several differential diagnoses for pre-eclampsia, HELLP and eclampsia.

Pre-eclampsia and HELLP syndrome

Rare differential diagnoses include:[14]

- acute fatty liver of pregnancy
- thrombotic thrombocytopenic purpura (TTP)
- haemolytic uraemic syndrome
- systemic lupus erythematosus.

Eclampsia[8]

Consider the following differential diagnoses, particularly in those presenting with seizures prior to 20 weeks' gestation or if focal neurological deficits persist (both unusual in eclampsia):

- stroke
- primary seizure disorder
- space-occupying lesion
- metabolic causes such as hypoglycaemia, hypocalcaemia, uraemia
- haematological abnormalities: thrombophilia and TTP.

Clinical investigation

No single set of investigations predicts or confirms the diagnosis of pre-eclampsia. The following all contribute to the diagnosis or point to a potential complication.

Laboratory investigations

See Table 19.7.2.

Imaging

Similar to the above, no single imaging test confirms the diagnosis of pre-eclampsia or eclampsia. Imaging is necessary to confirm a differential diagnosis or complication. In particular, a cerebral CT scan is recommended under the following circumstances:

- prolonged coma
- persistent neurological deficit(s)
- seizure or altered mental status in a patient presenting at less than 20 weeks' gestation, or greater than 48 h post partum
- seizures which are refractory to treatment.

Other investigations

Urinalysis

Urinalysis for proteinuria contributes to the diagnosis. It may need to be followed by a

Table 19.7.2 Laboratory investigations for pre-eclampsia	
Investigation	Potential abnormality sought
Full blood count	Thrombocytopenia Haemoconcentration (volume depleted state)
Blood film	Haemolysis (microangiopathic haemolysis)
Coagulation profile (indicated if platelet count is $<100 \times 10^9$/L)	Disseminated intravascular coagulation
Serum creatinine	0.08–0.13 mmol/L (high for a normal pregnancy) Normal pregnancy (upper limit 0.07 mmol/L)[5]
LFT	Elevated transaminases
Serum uric acid	>354 µmol/L (abnormal)

24-h urinary collection to evaluate the extent of the proteinuria.

Lumbar puncture

A lumbar puncture may be indicated to exclude other differential diagnoses in eclampsia, although it is *essential* to check a full blood count for platelet numbers prior to spinal needle insertion, and if low, a clotting profile.

There are no pathognomonic EEG findings in eclampsia.

Treatment

The objectives in managing the pre-eclamptic patient in the ED are to treat the hypertension to prevent complications, in particular an intracerebral haemorrhage, to prevent maternal hypoxaemia and hypotension and to prevent or treat eclampsia. However, treatment of the hypertension per se in pre-eclampsia and eclampsia slows, but does not stop, the disease process.[3]

Anti-hypertensive medications

Some disagreement and misunderstanding exist about the choice and endpoint of anti-hypertensive medication in pre-eclampsia.

Initiation of medication

There is no consensus evidence on which to base recommendations for the initiation of anti-hypertensive medications.[5,12] However, the following guide is suggested:

sBP > 170 mmHg or dBP > 110 mmHg mandates treatment
sBP range of 155–160 mmHg to prevent a stroke.

Target range for the BP

There is also no consensus as to the target range for the BP once the decision to treat has been made. Various recommendations are commonly available including the following:

- sBP 140–160 mmHg[2]
- dBP 90–110 mmHg[2]
- mean arterial pressure reduction to <125 mmHg.[11]

The above are used only as a guide, as the maternal and fetal response to treatment are the final arbiter of the degree of BP reduction required.

Iatrogenic hypoperfusion

Overzealous treatment may cause iatrogenic hypoperfusion as there is no maternal cerebral auto-regulation, as well as a volume-depleted maternal circulation and no autoregulation of the utero–placental circulation. Thus, it is important to maintain vigilant maternal and fetal monitoring during treatment of the hypertension. The endpoint is titrated to the clinical status, rather than to the magnitude of the BP reduction.

Drug choice in treatment of hypertension in pre-eclampsia

Hydralazine is the traditional first line parenteral agent in Australia, whereas in New Zealand and other countries labetalol may be preferred parenterally, as it has fewer adverse effects (it is not available intravenously in Australia). Labetalol may also be used orally in pre-eclampsia.

Although a number of other intravenous antihypertensive agents are available, they are not often used for a variety of reasons (see Table 19.7.3). Hydralazine remains the drug of choice amongst Australian emergency physicians. Its profile is provided below.

Hydralazine[1,3,12,15]

Mechanism of action Hydralazine is a peripheral arteriolar vasodilator that improves uterine blood flow.

Adverse effects: maternal Well-recognized maternal adverse effects of hydralazine include headaches, palpitations with

Table 19.7.3 Antihypertensive drug side effects in pre-eclampsia

Drug	Disadvantages of use in pre-eclampsia
Nitroprusside	Fetal cyanide toxicity
Beta-blocker	Fetal bradycardia and hypotension
Diazoxide	Rapid vasodilatory effect leading to severe hypotension Also inhibits labour
Diuretics	Maternal circulation is already volume-depleted in pre-eclampsia

tachycardia from reflex sympathetic stimulation, epigastric pain and vomiting and sodium and water retention. Hydralazine has also been associated with placental abruption, and an increased need for delivery via caesarean section.

Be wary of reducing the intervals between administration and excessive dosing, as in the pre-existing volume-depleted maternal circulation, iatrogenic hypotension must be anticipated.

Adverse effects: fetal Potential fetal adverse effects of hydralazine used in the third trimester are thrombocytopenia, and a lupus-like syndrome in the neonate. Hydralazine has also been associated with fetal distress, and a low Apgar score. No congenital adverse effects have been evident.

Contraindications Coronary artery disease.

Onset of action Hydralazine must be metabolized to its active form, thus the onset of action is 10–20 min. Base the dosing interval on this.

Administration Give a fluid bolus first to offset the reflex tachycardia. Administer hydralazine as 2.5–5.0 mg boluses at 15–20 min intervals. The maximal bolus dose is 10 mg.

Treatment of eclampsia

The immediate objectives in treating eclampsia are to stop the seizure, prevent maternal complications and to prevent further seizures.

Magnesium sulphate

Magnesium sulphate is used as both a prophylactic agent and treatment for severe pre-eclampsia.[15–18] It is more effective at preventing a subsequent seizure than phenytoin, with the rate of eclampsia reduced by 58% when compared with placebo. It is also more effective than diazepam for treating seizures in eclampsia. Failure of magnesium sulphate in this context is 0.8%.

Mechanism of action of magnesium sulphate The mechanism of action of magnesium in eclampsia is unclear. Magnesium lowers BP through systemic vasodilatation, with a duration of action up to 6 h.

Dose of magnesium sulphate Give the magnesium intravenously at an initial dose of 6 g (24 mmol or 12 mL of 49.3% solution) over 15 min, followed by a maintenance dose of 2 g/h (8 mmol or 4 mL of 49.3% solution/h). Give a further bolus of 2 g (8 mmol or 4 mL of 49.3% solution) magnesium over 5 min in the event of seizure recurrence.

Side effects of magnesium sulphate
Adverse effects of magnesium are dose-related and include flushing (20%), nausea, weakness, drowsiness and respiratory depression at highest doses (1%). A useful indicator of a potential toxic level is the loss of tendon reflexes. Routine monitoring of the serum magnesium level is not useful, as there is no 'therapeutic range' established for its use in eclampsia, so the clinical assessment of respiratory status and motor reflexes is important. Check the magnesium level in patients with renal dysfunction, or in those who lose their motor reflexes.

Delivery of the fetus and placenta
The decision to deliver the fetus is made by the treating obstetric team, so early referral is crucial. Immediate delivery is considered essential, regardless of the gestation, in eclampsia and pre-eclampsia complicated by the HELLP syndrome.

Prognosis of pre-eclampsia and eclampsia

The morbidity and mortality of both the mother and fetus are considered.

Maternal morbidity and mortality[1,4,8]

Pre-eclampsia and eclampsia increase the maternal morbidity and mortality by 400 times compared to a normal pregnancy.

Maternal mortality is up to 1.8% for developed countries, but as high as 14% for developing countries. The major cause of mortality is haemorrhagic stroke.

Maternal morbidity is more likely with antepartum eclampsia. The major causes are cardiorespiratory arrest, non-cardiogenic pulmonary oedema, aspiration pneumonia, DIC and placental abruption.

Fetal morbidity and mortality[6]

The fetal mortality is 2% in a pre-eclamptic pregnancy, but increases in eclampsia to the range of 5.6–11.8%, caused by prematurity at delivery and placental abruption. Fetal growth retardation occurs in 25% of pre-eclamptic pregnancies.

Recurrence of pre-eclampsia[6]

Pre-eclampsia recurs in 25% of subsequent pregnancies for early onset (<32 weeks), and in 5–8% of subsequent pregnancies for late onset pre-eclampsia.

Maternal implications of pre-eclampsia[6]

Pre-eclampsia is a life-long disease, and has an impact on maternal cardiovascular health. There is a risk of hypertension in later life, and an eight-fold increase in risk of death from stroke for those with pre-eclampsia prior to 37 weeks' gestation.

Likely developments in the next 5–10 years

Although much progress has been made towards elucidating the pathogenesis of pre-eclampsia, it is likely that within the next 5–10 years the cause(s) will be found.

References

1. Vidaeff AC, Carroll MA, Ramin SM. Acute hypertensive emergencies in pregnancy. Critical Care Medicine 2005; 33(10): 307–312.
2. Abalos E, Duley L, Steyn DW, et al. Antihypertensive drug therapy for mild to moderate hypertension during pregnancy [reviews]. The Cochrane Collaboration 2007; 2.
3. Frishman WH, Schlocker SJ, Awad K, et al. Pathophysiology and medical management of systemic hypertension in pregnancy. Cardiology in Review 2005; 3(6): 274–284.
4. Lindheimer MD, Umans JG. Explaining and predicting preeclampsia. New England Journal of Medicine 2006; 355(10): 1056–1058.
5. Krane NK, Hamrahian M. Pregnancy: kidney diseases and hypertension. American Journal of Kidney Disorder 2007; 49(2): 336–345.
6. Wikström A, Larsson A, Nash P, et al. Placental growth factor and soluble FMS-like tyrosine kinase-1 in early-onset and late-onset preeclampsia. American College of Obstetrics and Gynaecology 2007; 109(6): 1368–1374.
7. Brown MA. Pre-eclampsia: a lifelong disorder. Medical Journal Association 2003; 179(4): 182–184.
8. Sibai BM. Diagnosis, prevention and management of eclampsia. American College of Obstetrics and Gynecology 2005; 105(2): 402–410.
9. Roberts CL, Algert CS, Morris JM, et al. Hypertensive disorders in pregnancy: a population-based study. Medical Journal of America 2005; 182(7): 332–335.
10. Luo Z-C, Na A, Xu H-R, et al. The effects and mechanisms of primiparity on the risk of pre-eclampsia: a systematic review. Paediatric and Perinatal Epidemiology 2007; 21: 36–45.
11. James PR, Nelson-Piercy C. Management of hypertension, before, during and after pregnancy. Heart 2004; 90: 1499–1504.
12. Martin JN, Thigpen BD, Moore RC, et al. Stroke and severe preeclampsia and eclampsia: a paradigm shift focusing on systolic blood pressure. American College of Obstetrics and Gynecology 2005; 105(2): 245–254.
13. Yankowitz J. Pharmacologic treatment of hypertensive disorders during pregnancy. Journal of Perinatal and Neonatal Nursing 2004; 18(3): 230–240.
14. Sibai BM. Imitators of severe preeclampsia. American College of Obstetrics and Gynecology 2007; 109(4): 956–966.
15. Magee LA, Cham C, Waterman EJ, et al. Hydralazine for treatment of severe hypertension in pregnancy: meta-analysis. British Medical Journal 2003; 327: 955–965.
16. Frias AE Jr, Belfort MA. Post Magpie: how should we be managing severe pre-eclampsia? Current Opinion in Obstetrics and Gynecology 2003; 15(6): 489–495.
17. Montan S. Drugs used in hypertensive diseases in pregnancy. Current Opinion in Obstetrics and Gynecology 2004; 16(2): 111–115.
18. Belfort MA, Clark S, Sibai B. Cerebral haemodynamics in preeclampsia: Cerebral perfusion and the rationale for an alternative to magnesium sulphate. Obstetrical and Gynaecological Survey 2006; 61(10): 655–665.

PSYCHIATRIC EMERGENCIES

Edited by **George Jelinek**

20.1 Mental state assessment

Sylvia Andrew-Starkey

ESSENTIALS

1 Prevalence of mental health disorders appears to be increasing in Western society.

2 Regardless of diagnosis and presentation, three brief risk assessments must be performed within the first few minutes of an individual's arrival in the emergency department (ED).[1,2,3] These are:

- suicide risk assessment
- violence risk assessment
- absconding risk assessment.

3 The role of organic illness masquerading as a behavioural disorder should not be forgotten.

4 Substance use/misuse resulting in presentations to EDs also appears to be increasing in the general population.

Epidemiology

Recent estimates place mental health disorders as one of the three leading causes of total burden of disease and injury in Australia, alongside cancer and cardiovascular disease.[4,5,6] In middle age, it is the leading cause of non-fatal disease burden in the Australian population. There is no doubt that mental health disorders have a high prevalence, are disabling and are high cost in both human and socioeconomic terms.[4,5]

In terms of disability, it has been estimated that having moderate to severe depression is the equivalent of having congestive cardiac failure,[6] chronic severe asthma or chronic hepatitis B.[5] Severe post traumatic stress syndrome was comparable to the disability from paraplegia and severe schizophrenia was comparable to quadriplegia, in terms of disability.[5] Over the last 10 years emergency department (ED) presentations have risen 8% in the USA, whereas mental health presentations for the same time period have risen 38%, contributing significantly to ED overcrowding.[7] This trend has been mirrored in Australia.

Contributing to this may be:

- lack of private health insurance
- lack of social supports
- lack of alternatives to care
- 24-h accessibility of the ED.[7]

The Australian Institute of Health and Welfare report into Mental Health Services in 2007 estimated that there were over 190 000 occasions of service to Australian EDs where the primary problem was thought to be due to a mental health disorder. This was estimated to be approximately 3.2% of total presentations to public hospital EDs.[4] This correlates well with other studies and US figures, which estimate 2–6 % of emergency medicine presentations are primarily due to mental health disorders.[1,7,8,9]

Two-thirds of these people are between the ages of 15 and 44 years (compared to 42% for the general population presenting to a suburban ED. 29% have anxiety and neurotic disorders, 21% mental and behavioural disorders due to psychoactive substance abuse, 19% mood disorders and 17% schizophrenia or delusional disorders.[7]

This, of course, is a gross underestimate of the prevalence of mental health disease in the ED as many patients remain undiagnosed, and many have active medical conditions and a mental health diagnosis may be secondary.[8]

It is estimated that 17.7% of adult Australians admitted to hospital report a mental health issue in the previous 12 months. An estimated 0.4–0.7% of the adult population suffer from a psychotic episode in any one year.[5] Mental health issues are highly prevalent and relevant.

Introduction to the mental state examination

The mainstreaming of mental health patients into general EDs has brought problems and anxieties for staff. Staff often feel a lack of confidence because they are dealing with a population of patients unfamiliar to them. They also feel inadequate due to poor assessment skills.[9,10]

Mental health patients are often seen as 'low yield', unrewarding and there is often a negative attitude expressed toward them.[9,10] A high proportion have drug and alcohol intoxication. This confounds the evaluation and treatment, lengthens the stay of these patients within the ED and delays their disposition. Mental health patients are sometimes perceived as 'frequent flyers' – victims of chronic disease that can never be cured – and can be seen as burdensome and unrewarding.

These negative attitudes have resulted in mental health patients being assigned lower triage categories and longer waits to be seen by staff than mainstream patients. They have a higher chance of leaving before assessment has begun or is complete and the overall increase in length of assessment time has the potential to increase violence in the ED.[9,10]

With this in mind, there has been much work over the last 10 years on the assessment of mental health patients in a general ED.

Bias and discrimination

It is important for health professionals assessing the mentally ill to be aware of their own potential biases. An interviewer's past history and personal beliefs can influence a mental state assessment and the interviewer should be aware of this. These beliefs may stem from past personal or professional experience (Table 20.1.1).

ABC of the MSE

A mental state examination (MSE) is analogous to the management of severe trauma. There is an initial risk assessment looking for immediately life-threatening risks to the patient or staff. The triage nurse and the treating doctor should then obtain a brief collateral history from the emergency services or carers, and initial management is based on this assessment. Regardless of threat, all assessments should balance the safety of both patient and staff with privacy and dignity.[9]

Assessment should be based on:[2]

- appearance and affect
- behaviour
- conversation
- drug and/or alcohol intoxication.

If the situation is relatively controlled, the formal mental health assessment should then take place. Further information is gathered from the community. A provisional assessment and management plan is developed in conjunction with the mental health team, and appropriate disposition is arranged (Fig. 20.1.1).

Triage

The Mental Health Triage Scale (Table 20.1.2) has been developed and modified to be included into the Australian Triage Scale (ATS).[3,9,11] It is very broad and asks the triage nurse to make four assessments: risk of suicide/self harm, risk of

Table 20.1.1   Factors which may influence an objective MSE
• Religious beliefs • Race/ethnicity/cultural beliefs and practices • Political opinion • Philosophical beliefs • Sexual preference or orientation (provided not criminal) • Promiscuity or immorality • Intellectual disability • Intoxication

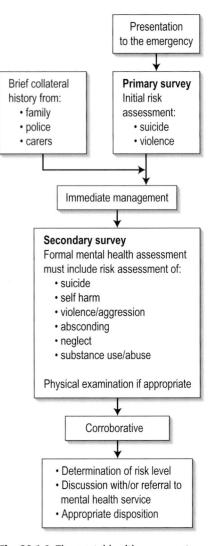

Fig. 20.1.1 The mental health assessment process.

aggression/harm to others, risk of absconding and whether the patient is intoxicated. From this, the triage nurse determines the ATS and urgency of initial treatment. It is also helpful to determine if the patient is known to a mental health service.

Many centres have developed a triage risk assessment proforma. For ease of use, many of these have included 'tick box' areas. A compilation of multiple assessment tools used throughout Australia is shown in Tables 20.1.3, 20.1.4 and 20.1.5.[1,2,3,5,11,12]

It is recommended that any patient who scores 'high risk' in any one area or 'medium risk' in two areas is treated as a 'high risk' patient. Ensuing management of 'high risk' patients depends on: local protocols, levels

Table 20.1.2	The Mental Health Triage Scale
ATS 2	Patient is violent, aggressive or suicidal, or is a danger to self or others Requires police escort/restraint
ATS 3	Very distressed or acutely psychotic Likely to become aggressive May be a danger to self or others
ATS 4	Long-standing or semi-urgent mental health problem and/or has supporting agency/escort present
ATS 5	Patient has a long-standing non-acute mental health disorder but has no support agency Many require referral to an appropriate community resource

Table 20.1.3	Brief screening suicide risk template
Mental state	☑ Active disease ☑ Depression ☑ Psychosis ☑ Hopelessness/despair/guilt/shame ☑ Anger/agitation ☑ Impulsivity
Suicide attempts/ thoughts	☑ Continual/specific thoughts ☑ Formulated plan ☑ Intent ☑ Past history of attempt with high lethality ☑ Means ☑ Suicide note ☑ Risk of being found ☑ Organizing personal affairs
Substance abuse	☑ Current misuse
Supports	☑ Lack of or hostile relationships
Loss	☑ Recent major loss (even perceived): significant relationship, job, housing, financial difficulties, independence ☑ Recent/new diagnosis of major illness or chronic illness
Patients then stratified into high, medium or low risk	

Table 20.1.4	Aggression risk tool
☑ Alert on chart ☑ Previous history of violence/threatening behaviour: verbal or physical ☑ Aggressive behaviour/thoughts ☑ Homicidal ideation ☑ Use of weapons previously ☑ Access to weapons ☑ Intoxicated ☑ Middle aged male	
Patient then stratified into high, medium or low risk	

Table 20.1.5	Risk of absconding
Mode of arrival ☑ Police ☑ Handcuffed ☑ Family/carer coercion ☑ Voluntary	
☑ Past history of absconding behaviour ☑ Alert on chart ☑ Verbalising intent to leave ☑ Lack of insight into illness ☑ Poor/non-compliance with medication	
Patients then stratified into high, medium or low risk	

and presence of security, police intervention, restraint and sedation guidelines and guidelines for the urgent assessment by ED and/or by mental health services.

Aims of mental health assessment

The aims of the formal mental health assessment are to determine the following:

- Does the patient have a mental illness?
- Is there a question of safety for the patient or for others?
- Does the patient have insight into their illness?
- Will the patient comply with suggested treatment?
- Can the patient be managed in the community or is hospitalization required?

Only if all of the above are answered, can management and appropriate disposition be considered.

The formal psychiatric interview

Introduction

The environment in which the mental state assessment is conducted is important. Behaviourally disturbed people are unable to tolerate noise and have short concentration spans. The interview room should be quiet, private, make the patient feel safe and the interviewer should avoid all interruptions. These prerequisites are increasingly difficult to attain in current access-blocked environments.

The interviewer should sit at the same level as the patient and impart empathy. The voice should be quiet and calming. The interviewer should use non-judgemental language and open-ended questions.[3,13] It is important that the interviewer also feels safe and secure. If any risk is felt, the interviewer should have security or police present in the room or just outside. Depending on state legislation and hospital policy, the interviewer may request to have the patient searched. The interviewer should also note the nearest duress alarm and/or choose to wear a personal alarm. The interviewer should sit within easy access of an exit and should never be boxed into a corner. If an interviewer begins to feel uncomfortable, there is always the option of leaving and returning to complete the assessment at a later stage. All threats, attempts and gestures suggestive of violence should be treated seriously.

First part of the interview: direct questioning

Basic demographic information

The formal interview has become less diagnosis focused and more problem based. Management is centred around the alleviation of symptoms and return to function. Thus the psychiatric interview has become somewhat less structured.

It is wise to establish rapport with the patient by introducing yourself and explaining the purpose of the interview. The interviewer can begin by asking a series of non-threatening questions such as demographics. This information is often required as many mental health services rely on an appropriate post code to determine follow-up management.

These questions assist by building a profile of lifestyle, relationships and thought processes. Likelihood of success or failure of particular treatment modalities may be assisted by knowledge of previous hospital admissions (both general hospital and mental health) (Table 20.1.6).

The process of obtaining a mental health assessment is different to that of a general medical assessment. In a general medical history, a series of questions is asked and the response is written. In a mental health assessment, responses are also interpreted. The interviewer is asked to form an opinion as to how thoughts are processed, based on observations. The interviewer is asked to interpret the patient's thought patterns by what and how the patient tells the interviewer.

Presenting complaint

The patient is asked to recall the sequence of events prior to presentation to the ED. The interviewer should explore the circumstances of the behaviour, reasons for it, degree of planning or impulsivity, and its context. Were drugs and alcohol involved? Was there a recent precipitating event? It is often useful to get the patient to recall the previous 48–72 h leading up to the event.

This usually leads to questioning regarding current difficulties. The interviewer should explore the nature of current problems. They may be financial or legal problems, isolation, bereavement, impending or actual loss, or diagnosis of major illness. Have there been any recent changes and who are their usual support people/person? An exploration of significant relationships is important along with the depth and duration of these relationships. It is useful to explore the patient's usual coping methods when under stress.

Mood and affect

There should be formal questioning regarding the patient's mood (internal feelings) and whether it is in keeping with affect (external expression). The mood may be incongruent with affect, swing wildly between extremes (labile) or be completely inappropriate.

Usually mood is assessed by asking about the patient's ability to cope with activities of daily living such as eating, weight loss or gain, sleep disturbance (early morning wakening or trouble getting to sleep) and general hygiene. The patient's ability to concentrate may also diminish with increasing mood disturbance, reflected by the ability to perform normal work duties.

This may lead to direct questioning regarding mood and thoughts of suicide. It is important to be direct in asking the patient about suicide and whether they have a formulated plan. A well thought out plan with clear means of carrying out threats is of great concern.

Delusions and hallucinations

Delusions and hallucinations are often personal and the patient may not want to disclose intimate thoughts and beliefs to the interviewer. Hallucinations may be auditory, visual, tactile, olfactory, somatic or gustatory. The context in which they occur should be explored. Hypnagogic (occurring just before sleep) and hypnopompic (occurring on wakening) hallucinations are more benign than others. Common themes for all types of hallucinations include suicide, persecution, religion, control, reference, grandeur or somatization.

Insight and judgement

Insight is the degree of understanding of what is happening and why. This may be:

- complete denial of illness
- slight awareness of being sick and needing help but denying it at the same time
- awareness of being sick but blaming it on external factors
- awareness that illness is due to something unknown within the patient
- intellectual insight: admission that the patient is ill and that symptoms are due to irrational feelings, but inability to apply this to the future
- true insight: being aware of motives and feelings and being aware of what can lead to changes in behaviour.

It is important to determine the patient's level of insight. This determines appropriate treatment and management, level of supervision required and the likelihood of compliance with treatment.

Second part of interview: observation

Key elements

The second part of the MSE can be more difficult to conceptualize. It relies on the interviewer actively observing the patient's behaviour and conversation, and interpreting their thoughts. A summary is given in Table 20.1.7.

This second part of the interview can be difficult to remember and different services have developed a multitude of acronyms for remembering the various elements of the remaining mental health assessment. Listed below are two.

ABC of Mental Health Assessment[2]
- Appearance
- Affect
- Behaviour
- Conversation and mood

GFCMA – 'Got Four Clients on Monday Afternoon'[3]
- General appearance
- Form of thought
- Content of thought
- Mood and affect
- Attitude

Table 20.1.6 Demographic information required
Age/date of birth
Address
Accommodation history
Other persons in household
Occupation
Occupational history
Social resources: • family, friends, partners • social history
Past medical history
Previous hospital admissions
Previous mental health admissions: • length of stay • type of treatment: medication/ECT • medications on discharge • follow-up arrangements
Forensic history: • trouble with police • jail terms/convictions
Alcohol
Drug use
Tobacco use

Table 20.1.7 Overview of mental state examination

General description:
- appearance
- behaviour
- attitudes

Mood and affect:
- mood
- affect
- appropriateness

Motivation/energy

Appetite

Sleep

Speech:
- perception

Thought process:
- form
- content

Cognition:
- consciousness
- orientation
- memory
- intelligence

Insight and judgement

Impulse control

Table 20.1.8 Appearance, attitude and behaviour

General:
- clothes
- application
- appropriate for climate?

Cleanliness:
- general grooming (hair, nails)
- tattoos, track marks on arms

Eye contact:
- avoids direct gaze
- decreases with increasing anxiety

Facial expression:
- variation in facial expression, voice, use of hands, and body movements

Reaction to interviewer:
- aggressive, submissive, cooperative, guarded, evasive, passive or hostile

Motor:
- restless
- repetitive behaviour, e.g. rocking, hand wringing
- tremor
- posturing
- tics
- tardive dyskinesia

Speech:
- rate, volume and rhythm
- mute
- poverty of speech (slow, monosyllabic responses)
- pressure of speech (extremely rapid, loud speech)
- normal inflection or flat and monotonous

somaticism (the extremes of which are nihilistic delusions – the belief that part of the self does not exist, is dead or decaying), or they may be grandiose in nature.

Perception

A patient may be actively hallucinating despite denying this on questioning. It is important to note if the patient's eyes suddenly switch direction for no apparent reason, or they appear to be listening to a voice. These movements are often quite subtle and easily missed if observation is not active.

Cognitive assessment and physical examination

A formal examination of cognitive function and a thorough physical examination complete the full psychiatric assessment. The interviewer should ensure that the patient does not have an acute confusional state secondary to a physical condition that may account for a behavioural problem.

A number of tools are available to assess cognitive functioning. These comprise assessments in orientation, concentration, memory, language, abstraction and judgement. An assessment of a patient's cognitive functioning and intelligence may assist in deciding the best way to deal with problems.

Approximately 20% of mental health patients have a concurrent active medical disorder requiring treatment and possibly contributing to the acute behavioural disturbance.[8] Investigations depend on physical findings but may include creatine kinase, urine drug screen, electroencephalogram, computerized tomography and lumbar

Appearance, attitude and behaviour

This determines the patient's ability to self care. Table 20.1.8 lists features that may require particular attention. Attitude is important as it may indicate whether a patient is compliant with management and treatment. Abnormal posturing or repetitive behaviours should be noted. These may indicate increasing thought disturbance. With increasing aggression and agitation, there may be motor restlessness, pacing and hand wringing. Tension may escalate rapidly, and steps should be taken early to diffuse the situation.

The interviewer should note the rate, volume and rhythmicity of speech. This can range from completely mute, through monosyllabic answers, to rapid, loud speech indicative of pressure of speech. The tone, inflection content and structure of speech should also be noted. The interviewer should determine if the speech is fluent, if the thoughts behind it are logical and whether it flows appropriately for the situation.

Thought disorder

This is speech that does not reach its goal, is not fluent and is interrupted often with

many pauses and/or changes in direction. A list with explanations is given in Table 20.1.9.

Thought content

There are often recurrent themes in the speech of an acutely disturbed patient. These may revolve around suicide, persecution, control, reference, religion or

Table 20.1.9 Thought disorders

Circumstantiality	Delays in reaching goals by long-winded explanations, but eventually gets there
Distractible speech	Changes topic according to what is happening around the patient
Loosening of associations	Logical thought progression does not occur and ideas shift from one subject to another with little or no association between them
Flight of ideas	Fragmented, rapid thoughts that the patient cannot express fully as they are occurring at such a rapid rate
Tangentiality	Responses that superficially appear appropriate, but which are completely irrelevant or oblique
Clanging	Speech where words are chosen because they rhyme and do not make sense
Neologisms	Creation of new words with no meaning except to the patient
Thought blocking	Interruption to thought process where thoughts are absent for a few seconds and are unable to be retrieved

puncture. Only after this can an emergency medicine practitioner plan the most appropriate management for the patient.

Conclusion

Although time-consuming and seemingly unrewarding, a good mental health assessment is vital for the appropriate management and disposition of what is an increasingly large group of patients in the ED. If able to formulate an opinion on the risk assessments regarding suicide, violence and flight risk and the aims of the MSE, the emergency medical officer will be able to present to mental health services a comprehensive picture of the patient.

Only then will the mental health professional be able to administer mental health first aid,[5] the principles of which are:

- Assess the risk of suicide/harm to others.
- Listen non-judgementally.
- Give reassurance and information.
- Encourage getting professional help.
- Encourage self-help strategies.

Controversies

❶ Whereas most general hospitals have integrated the assessment of mental health patients within the ED, there is now a growing trend towards the development of stand-alone psychiatric emergency centres – a separate area attached to the ED where mental health patients are assessed after initial triage. This is staffed by dedicated mental health professionals and has the potential to deskill emergency medicine personnel, both nursing and medical. It is uncertain as to whether this model or mainstreaming is more effective in the management of mental health patients.

❷ Despite an overall improvement in assessments, mainstreaming of mental health patients has exposed them to the increasing levels of access block within general hospitals and increasing overcrowding in EDs. This has resulted in mental health patients spending prolonged periods of time in the ED whilst waiting for inpatient beds to become available. This has the potential for increased violence, unnecessary use of sedation and increased morbidity and mortality of mental health patients whilst placing other patients, their carers and staff members at unnecessary risk.

References

1. Crowe M, Carlyle D. Deconstructing risk assessment and management in mental health nursing. Journal of Advanced Nursing 2003; 43(1): 19–27.
2. McSherry B. Risk July 2004 Assessment by Mental Health Professionals and the Prevention of Future Violent Behaviour. Australian Government. Australian Institute of Criminology.
3. NSW Department of Health. Framework for suicide risk assessment and management. Emergency Department; 2004. Online. Available www.health.nsw.gov.au
4. The Australian Institute of Health and Welfare. Mental health services in Australia 2004-5. (Mental Health Series No 9). Canberra: Australian Institute of Health and Welfare; 2007.
5. Kitchener B, Jorm A. Mental health first aid manual. Melbourne: Orygen Research Centre; 2002.
6. Clinical Practice Guidelines Team for Depression, Royal Australian and New Zealand College of Psychiatrists. Australian and New Zealand clinical practices. Practice guidelines for the treatment of depression. Australian and New Zealand Journal of Psychiatry 2004; 38: 389–407.
7. Larkin GL, Classen CA, et al. Trends in US Emergency Departments. Visits for mental health conditions, 1992-2001. Psychiatric Services June 2005; 56(6): 671–677.
8. ACEP Clinical Policies Subcommittee. Clinical policy: critical issues in the diagnosis and management of the adult psychiatric patient in the emergency department. Annals of Emergency Medicine 2006; 47(1): 79–99.
9. Smart D, Pollard C, Walpole B. Mental health triage in emergency medicine. Australian and New Zealand Journal of Psychiatry 1999; 33: 57–66.
10. Happell B, Summers M, Pinikahana J. Measuring the effectiveness of the national Mental Health Triage Scale in an emergency department. International Journal of Mental Health Nursing 2003; 12: 288–292.
11. Department of Health and Ageing. Emergency triage education kit. Australian Government; 2007: 37–48.
12. Department of Human Services, Victorian Emergency Department. Mental health triage tool. Online. Available: www.health.vic.gov.au/emergency/mhtriagetool.pdf
13. Meyers J, Stein, S. The psychiatric interview in the emergency department. Emergency Medicine Clinics of North America 2000; 18: 173–183.

20.2 Distinguishing medical from psychiatric causes of mental disorder presentations

David Spain

ESSENTIALS

1 Morbidity and health costs are reduced by correct distinction of medical from psychiatric causes of mental disorder in presentations to emergency departments.

2 Does any medical conditions exist in addition to the psychiatric complaints? This question will identify most medical causes of mental disorder.

3 Missed medical diagnosis is most commonly associated with failure to undertake an adequate medical history, mental state examination and physical examination.

4 Substance-related disorders are most easily identified on direct or collateral history.

5 The presence of delirium or other significant cognitive defects makes an organic or substance-related illness almost certain.

6 The diagnosis of delirium may require repeated assessments over time.

Introduction

Emergency physicians are facing a significantly increased volume and complexity of mental disorder presentations. Increased numbers relate to increased community care for chronic mental illness, the ageing population and frequent substance abuse. Intoxicated patients, with and without mental disorder, are increasingly being presented to emergency departments (EDs) for assessment due to concerns about patient or community safety. These patients frequently display impulsive, suicidal or violent behaviour and are often difficult to manage. A thorough understanding of the assessment and appropriate disposition of mental disorder presentations is essential for all emergency physicians.

The concept of differentiating an organic from a psychiatric basis for a mental disorder is becoming increasingly blurred as research shows the biological and genetic basis of many traditional psychiatric illnesses. The accepted terminology for classification of mental disorder is also rapidly changing. One accepted Western standard is the *Diagnostic and Statistical Manual of Mental Disorders*, 4th edition (DSM-IV).[1] To emphasize the biological basis of many traditional psychiatric illnesses, DSM-IV no longer uses the term 'organic mental disorder'. Despite this change, current clinical management and disposition still revolve around the traditional distinction of organic (medical) from psychiatric problems.

In practice emergency physicians need a simple classification defining the principal diagnosis of the presenting mental disorder consistent with current DSM-IV terminology. This should assist diagnostic, management and disposition accuracy. Table 20.2.1 is such a suggested classification. A more simplistic grouping into psychiatric, medical, substance-related or antisocial behaviour may even suffice. Correct assignment by the emergency physician to the appropriate classification, and hence appropriate disposition, reduces medical costs and morbidity.[2]

General approach

Patients with abnormal behaviour labelled as psychiatric after routine medical and psychiatric assessment frequently have a final diagnosis of a medical cause or precipitant for the mental disorder. The incidence of missed medical diagnosis ranges between 8 and 46%.[2–4] A prospective study of ED patients in the USA showed a medical diagnosis in 63% of patients with first psychiatric presentations.[5] Deciding whether a particular presentation of mental disorder is medical or psychiatric is often difficult, as there are very few absolutes that distinguish medical from psychiatric illness. Careful collection and weighing of appropriate information commonly leads to an accurate differential diagnosis.

Some diagnoses and dispositions can be determined quickly after a medical and psychiatric history, with the addition of a mental state and full physical examination. This may sometimes take place without expensive diagnostic procedures.[6] Other presentations are difficult and require extensive and intensive evaluation, repeat evaluation, observation in hospital and significant investigations before the diagnosis is clear.

Many initial assessments in EDs are difficult and inaccurate owing to the presence of intoxicating substances or difficult patient factors. The latter may include poor communication ability, poor cooperation with examination, antisocial behaviour, intentional obscuring of information or denial of problems. Intoxicated patients may have other complex and distracting issues, such as threats of violence or self-harm, possible head injury, possible unknown substance overdose, and poor cooperation with necessary history, examination and investigations. A non-judgemental

Table 20.2.1 A simple classification of principal diagnosis of mental disorder for emergency physicians

DSM-IV terminology	Broad traditional clinical grouping	Likely principal management and disposition
Axis 1		
Clinical disorder due to a general medical disorder	Organic	Medical
Delirium, dementia and amnestic and other cognitive disorders	Organic	Medical
Substance-related disorder – intoxication or withdrawal disorder	Organic	Medical
Substance-related disorder – substance induced persistent disorder	Organic	Psychiatric
Clinical disorder (not identified to above or axis II principal diagnosis)	Psychiatric	Psychiatric

Table 20.2.2 Triage safety questions[10]

Is the patient a danger to him or herself?

Is the patient at risk of leaving before assessment?

Is the patient a danger to others?

Is the area safe?

Table 20.2.3 High-yield indicators of organic illness

First presentation of mental disorder

Delirium
  Abrupt onset change in mental state
    Hours to days
    Fluctuates
  Change in cognition
    Disorientation
    Memory deficit
    Language disturbance.
  Disturbance of consciousness
    Fluctuating or decreased
    Poor attention
  Perceptual disturbance
    Hallucinations (especially visual)
    Illusions
    Misinterpretations

Drug use
  Recreational/illicit
  Overdose
  Prescribed or over-the-counter

Recent or new medical problems

Neurological signs or symptoms

Abnormal vital signs

approach with prudent intervention based on known or likely risks, close monitoring in a safe environment, and repeated reassessment of physical and mental state over time are necessary to obtain an accurate diagnosis and optimal outcome.

Studies on medical clearance by ED staff, primary-care physicians and psychiatrists have repeatedly shown a poor ability to discover medical conditions. This failure is commonly due to one or more of the following factors: inadequate history, failure to seek alternative information from relatives, carers and old records, poor attention to physical examination, including vital signs, absence of a reasonable mental state examination, uncritical acceptance of medical clearance by receiving psychiatric staff and failure to re-evaluate over time.[7] A recent study noted that medical conditions were most easily identified in the ED by the triage nurse or medical officer asking whether any medical conditions existed in addition to the patient's psychiatric complaints.[8]

Conversely, studies have shown that many patients admitted with a medical diagnosis frequently have a physical presentation of a classic psychiatric disorder. In addition, patients who frequently present to EDs with physical problems commonly have abnormal illness behaviour. Inability to recognize this leads to inappropriate diagnosis and management, with subsequent treatment failure.

Psychiatric patients also have a higher incidence of physical illness than the general population. The comorbid illness may not have been diagnosed previously in this socially disadvantaged population.

Evaluation requires a thorough approach and a commitment of time and effort. Special skills are required for medical clearance and psychiatric interview. A coordinated and focused medical and psychiatric assessment has the highest yield of correct diagnoses.[2] Proformas may improve compliance and documentation of important details.

Triage

Triage is vital, as many patients presenting with apparent psychiatric problems have medical conditions. The patient previously labelled psychiatric must be carefully triaged to avoid any new medical problems being overlooked. Psychiatric patients have been found to express their physical illnesses in different ways from those without mental illness. They may be suffering from severe or life-threatening illness, but fail to communicate this to their medical carers. Correct identification at the point of entry by nursing staff facilitates correct management and reduces morbidity and mortality.[9] Many patients with psychiatric illness are also a significant risk to themselves or others, and require urgent intervention. Questions regarding safety should always be raised[10] (Table 20.2.2).

Nursing staff should use a triage checklist to identify likely organic presentations (Table 20.2.3). These are indications for urgent medical assessment. If these are absent and a psychiatric diagnosis is likely, then an appropriate urgency rating by Australasian Triage Scale for psychiatric presentations should be applied. This triage categorization for psychiatric presentations has been developed and verified, and allows reasonable waiting time standards for urgency to be applied (Table 20.2.4).[11]

Triage should consider patient privacy issues if the history obtained is to be accurate. Collateral information from the carers with the patient should always be diligently obtained, carefully considered and documented. Integration of all this information should allow the patient to be placed in an appropriate and safe environment where continuing visual and nursing observations can occur while further assessment is awaited. An emerging trend is to use nursing triage to immediately refer likely psychiatric presentations to mental health clinicians without formal 'medical

Table 20.2.4   Guidelines for Australasian Triage Scale coding for psychiatric presentations[11]

Emergency: Category 2

Patient is violent, aggressive or suicidal, or is a danger to self or others, or requires police escort.

Urgent: Category 3

Very distressed or acutely psychotic, likely to become aggressive, may be a danger to self or others. Experiencing a situation crisis.

Semiurgent: Category 4

Long-standing or semi-urgent mental health disorder and/or has a supporting agency/escort present (e.g. community psychiatric nurse*)

Non-urgent: Category 5

Long-standing or non-acute mental disorder or problem, but the patient has no supportive agency or escort. Many require a referral to an appropriate community resource.

*It is considered advantageous to 'up triage' mental health patients with carers present because carers' assistance facilitates more rapid assessment.

clearance'. This method appears effective and efficient for both patient and clinicians. Most triage referral systems have built-in medical safety nets and have been operating now for some years without obvious increase in adverse outcomes. They are yet to be validated by scientific studies.

The interview environment

A climate of trust is very important, as many details of the psychiatric interview are quite intimate. The psychiatric interview should take place in as quiet and private an environment as possible. The choice of the interview site may be limited in emergencies to ensure safety for both patient and staff.

History

A careful traditional medical history is the most common identifier of medical illness as a cause of a mental disorder presentation. Substance-related disorders are also most easily identified on history. A careful drug history, including prescribed, recreational and over-the-counter medications, should always be included. A slow onset and a previous psychiatric history are more commonly associated with psychiatric illness. Conversely, rapid onset, no premorbid decline and no past psychiatric history favour a medical cause.

Poor recall of recent events may indicate delirium.

Family history is often a key indicator of psychiatric or medical cause. For example, a depressed 30-year-old man with a family history of Huntington's disease or porphyria is more likely to have a physical cause. Conversely, an 18-year-old man with a hypomanic presentation and a strong family history of bipolar disorder more likely has a psychiatric cause. Suicidal and homicidal risk should be assessed routinely to ensure safety. Escalating immediate risk can often be recognized by combining patient perceived lethality and inquiry about any transition from thoughts, to actual plans and finally to actions. For patients with previous psychiatric illness the system review is a useful screen for organic illness.

HIV is an increasingly important area as HIV-related illness becomes the new great mimic of modern psychiatry and medicine. Practices likely to have put the patient at risk should be explored. These may have been in the distant past. Known positive HIV status always warrants assessment for an organic cause of any new behavioural disturbance. Clinically, these problems often initially present with symptoms of mild anxiety or depression. Many treatable medical causes are only evident after significant investigations.[12]

Delirium, a highly specific but not absolute indicator of medical or substance-induced disorders, should always be sought. By definition this requires a history of recent onset and of fluctuation over the course of the day. Classically there will be subtle changes in level of consciousness or the sleep–wake cycle. Patients may not be able to attend sufficiently to give this history if delirious. The psychiatric history, including life profile, may give evidence of the presence or absence of premorbid decline. An abrupt onset of abnormal behaviour with no premorbid decline is more suggestive of an organic cause.

Collateral history

Collateral history is important as the patient is not always capable of or willing to give full information. This history often crystallizes a diagnosis that would otherwise be uncertain or completely missed. Previous discharge summaries may provide relevant information regarding alcohol and drug use, previous behaviour and diagnosis. The family should be asked to bring in all medications, including over-the-counter items. Family, friends and caregivers may give more rapid access to collateral history than waiting for past admission details. Family and friends may be the only source for obtaining a history of a patient's fluctuating mental status suggesting delirium, even when the patient appears quite lucid in the ED.

Examination

Lack of attention to important details of the examination is a frequently identified cause of missed medical illness. Areas that commonly yield positive findings, but which are frequently omitted, are the neurological examination, a search for general or specific appearances of endocrine disease, the toxidromes, examination for signs of malignancy, drugs or alcohol abuse, and vital sign examination.

Vital signs

Abnormal vital signs are frequently the only abnormality found on examination of patients with serious underlying medical disease. They must always be acknowledged and explained. Pulse oximetry should be included to rapidly exclude hypoxia. A bedside blood sugar level should be routine for patients with abnormal behaviour.

Mental state examination

This is an account of objective findings of mental state signs made at the time of interview. It is the psychiatric equivalent of the medical examination, and specifically details the current status.[13] Observations made by other staff in the department, such as hallucinations, may be very significant and can be included with the source identified. Careful consideration of the mental status frequently clearly distinguishes medical from psychiatric illness, and guides further investigation and management. For example, the presence of delirium or other significant cognitive defects make an organic illness almost certain. Delirium can be very subtle. Sometimes, owing to the fluctuating nature, the patient may appear normal on a single interview. Other less obvious features, such as lability of mood, variability of motor activity or lapses in patient concentration making the interview more difficult, can be the only clues and can be easily overlooked. The importance of formulation using collateral history and repeated mental state examination is stressed. Documentation is important so that mental status changes with time during assessment can be appreciated.

Examination tools

Cognitive defects may be rapidly and reliably identified in the ED during mental status examination by the use of Folstein's Mini Mental State Examination (MMSE)[14] (Table 20.2.5). A score of less than 20 suggests an organic aetiology. A fall of two or more points on serial MMSE is highly suggestive of delirium.[15] Elderly patients with delirium or cognitive defects are frequently not recognized by emergency physicians.[16] These patients are at high risk of morbidity and mortality.[17] Simple assessment methods such as the confusion assessment method (CAM) are rapid, reliable methods of identifying delirium in older patients, suitable for ED use.[18] Use of such simple methods should be encouraged to reduce inappropriate disposition.

Table 20.2.5 Mini-mental state examination[14,15]

Date of assessment *Cognition*			**Points**
Orientation 1. What is the date?			1
What is the day?			1
What is the month?			1
What is the year?			1
What is the season?			1
2. What is the name of this building?			1
What floor of the building are we on?			1
What city are we in?			1
What state are we in?			1
What country are we in?			1
Registration			
3. I am going to name three objects. After I have said them I want you to repeat them. Remember what they are because I am going to ask you to name them in a few minutes. APPLE TABLE PENNY		APPLE	1
		TABLE	1
		PENNY	1
Code first attempt and then repeat the answers until the patient learns all three.			
Attention and calculation 4. Can you subtract 7 from 100, and then subtract 7 from the answer you get and keep subtracting until I tell you to stop?		93	1
		86	1
		79	1
		72	1
		65	1
OR			
5. I am going to spell a word forwards and I want you to spell it backwards. The word is 'WORLD'. Now you spell it backwards. Repeat if necessary.		D	1
		L	1
		R	1
		O	1
		W	1
Recall 6. Now what are the three objects I asked you to remember?		APPLE	1
		TABLE	1
		PENNY	1
Language 7. Interviewer: Show wristwatch What is it called? Interviewer: Show pencil What is it called?			2
8. I'd like you to repeat a phrase after me. 'NO IFS ANDS OR BUTS'			1
9. Read the words on the bottom of this table and do what it says.			1
10. Interviewer: Read the full statement below before handing the respondent a piece of paper. 'Do not repeat or coach.' I am going to give you a piece of paper. What I want you to do is take the paper in your right hand, fold it in half and put the paper on your lap.		Takes with right hand	1
		Folds in half	1
		Puts on lap	1
11. Write a complete sentence on this piece of paper. Sentence should have subject, verb and make sense. Spelling and grammatical errors are okay.			1
12. Here is a drawing. Please copy the drawing on the same paper. Hand drawing to respondent. Correct if two convex five-sided figures and intersection makes a four-sided figure.			1
TOTAL SCORE..			
(Score best of question 4 or 5 to give a total out of 30) A score of 20 or less indicates cognitive impairment. CLOSE YOUR EYES			

The tests above are suitable screening tools for EDs but are not intended to replace formal neuropsychological assessment. Proformas of medical history, mental state examination and physical examination may improve thoroughness of assessment and documentation.

Investigations

Investigations should always be guided by clinical findings and must be tailored to each individual presentation. First presentations and suspicion of a medical cause that needs to be confirmed or excluded are the major indications. Baseline blood tests, such as full blood profile, blood sugar level, electrolytes, liver function tests, calcium and thyroid function tests, may at times detect clinically unsuspected problems. Examination and culture of urine and cerebrospinal fluid should be undertaken if occult infection is considered a possible cause. A urine drug screen may on occasion be the only way to confirm clinical suspicions of drug-related illness. Time delays for results, low specificity from cross-reactivity and uncertainty caused by drugs with long half-lives limit their usefulness. Newer drug-screening stat tests at the bedside may improve their usefulness in the ED. Mandatory brain computerized tomography (CT) is not indicated,[19–21] but the threshold for imaging in first presentations of altered mental state without obvious cause should be low. HIV and syphilis testing should be done on all patients with significant risk profile. Newer modalities such as magnetic resonance imaging, magnetic resonance spectroscopy, positron emission tomography and single-photon emission CT continue as research tools but may have a role in the future. Electroencephalogram examination is rarely a current ED test for psychiatric patients.

Diagnostic formulation

Emergency physicians should suspect organic disease until proved otherwise. In particular, reversible medical causes of abnormal mental state should be sought. Proformas improve documentation and summation.[22] Consideration of the factors in Table 20.2.6 may help to determine

Table 20.2.6 Factors influencing the likelihood of medical or psychiatric illness as the principal diagnosis	
Organic	**Psychiatric**
Abnormal vital signs	Family history of psychiatry disorder
Age >40 with first psychosis	Past psychiatric illness
Delirium	Fully orientated
Conscious level fluctuates	Clear sensorium
Inability to attend	
Memory impaired	
Impaired cognitive abilities	Intact cognition
Neurological signs, e.g. dysarthria	
Abnormal physical signs	
Abrupt onset	Slow onset
Dramatic change in general status (hours to days)	Premorbid slow deterioration in employment/family/ socially
Recent medical problem	Recent significant life event
Medication, drugs/alcohol/withdrawal	Non-compliance psychiatric medication
Marked new personality changes	
Visual, tactile or olfactory hallucinations more common Agitation/irritability HIV/AIDS Failed psychiatric treatment	Auditory hallucinations more common especially: Voices arguing Voices commentary Two voices discussing Audible thoughts
Disorganized delusions	Structured delusions
Movement disorders	Somatic passivity experiences.
Perseveration	
Confabulation	
Illusions or misinterpretations	
Circumstantiality	
Concretism	Thought withdrawal, insertion or broadcasting
FH degenerative brain disease	
FH heritable metabolic	

FH, family history.

doubtful cases. There are few absolutes that distinguish organic from psychiatric patients. Use of the five-axis DSM-IV system improves the ability to look at the patient's presentation in the context of total functioning.[1] It also allows emergency physicians to communicate with psychiatric peers in the recognized language.

Some patients require periods of observation, re-examination and further investigations before a definitive answer is obtained. Intoxicated patients frequently are not assessable till sober. Interim care and disposition varies depending on presentation, prior history and facilities available.

A common expectation of emergency physicians for patients referred to psychiatrists is to document that the patient is 'medically cleared'. The assessment is known to be imprecise and difficult.[2–5,8–10,22] Better documentation is to state that the ED assessment has revealed no evidence of an emergent medical problem.

Conclusion

A thorough medical history, psychiatric history, collateral history, physical examination, mental state examination and judicious specific investigation will identify most patients likely to have an underlying physical cause for a mental disorder presentation. Omission of any of these steps may lead to missed medical diagnosis and incorrect disposition.

Controversies and future directions

❶ Where and when should assessment of mental disorder occur? Urgent assessment in the traditional hospital-based general ED with strict 'medical clearance' is ideal and safest for rapid and new onset illness.

Increased demands and resource restraints are forcing alternative models for entry to care. Many EDs are triaging patients in crisis as likely medical, emergent psychiatric or non-emergent psychiatric. Depending on local service availability, early streaming based on this triage allows many psychiatric clients (some emergent and most non-emergent) to be directed away from the ED to appropriate community mental health services. Additionally, community-based psychiatric services are increasingly managing acute episodes of behaviour disorder in the community without the need for hospitalization or emergency department involvement. Hard outcome studies are yet to be undertaken on these new models.

❷ Should all mental disorder patients receive medical clearance by a doctor or can early referral to an acute care psychiatric team occur after triage? Many believe that this has produced significant benefits to patients, with shorter waiting times and better psychiatric assessments by psychiatric-trained nurses and psychologists when compared to junior medical staff. Initial experience to date indicates they need ready access to safety net medical systems and consultant psychiatric supervision to operate effectively and safely.

❸ How do we deal with increased numbers of drug and alcohol affected clients?

Providing adequate resources and a safe physical environment for assessment, management and disposition of the rapidly escalating number of patients with substance-related disorder is a major emergency department challenge. Assessments during intoxication are typically unhelpful. Intoxication may last hours to days and require medical therapy. New initiatives are exploring clinical pathways and memorandums of understanding with local police services to care for selected high-risk clients until sober.

References

1. American Psychiatric Association. Diagnostic and statistical manual of mental disorders. 4th edn. Washington, DC: American Psychiatric Association; 1994.
2. Hoffman RS. Diagnostic errors in the evaluation of behavioural disorders. Journal of the American Medical Association 1982; 248: 964–967.
3. Koranyi EK. Morbidity and rate of undiagnosed physical illnesses in a psychiatric clinic population. Archives of General Psychiatry 1979; 36: 414–419.
4. Hall RC, Popkin MK, Devaul RA, et al. Physical illness presenting as psychiatric disease. Archives of General Psychiatry 1978; 35: 1315–1320.
5. Henneman PL, Mendoza R, Lewis RJ. Prospective evaluation of emergency department medical clearance. Annals of Emergency Medicine 1994; 24: 672–677.
6. Allen MH, Faumann MA, Morin FX. Emergency psychiatric evaluation of 'organic' mental disorders. New Directions for Mental Health Services 1995; 67: 45–55.
7. Tintinalli JE, Peacock FW, Wright MA. Emergency medical evaluation of psychiatric patients. Annals of Emergency Medicine 1994; 23: 859–862.
8. Olshaker JS, Browne B, Jerrard DA, et al. Medical clearance and screening of psychiatric patients in the emergency department. Academic Emergency Medicine 1997; 4: 124–128.
9. Ferrera PC, Chan L. Initial management of the patient with altered mental status. American Family Physician 1997; 55: 1773–1780.
10. Pollard C. Psychiatry reference book – nursing staff. Hobart: Department of Emergency Medicine Royal Hobart Hospital; 1994.
11. Smart D, Pollard C, Walpole B. Mental health triage in emergency medicine. Australian and New Zealand Journal of Psychiatry 1999; 33: 57–66.
12. Sternberg DE. Testing for physical illness in psychiatric patients. Journal of Clinical Psychiatry 1986; 47 (suppl 1): 3–9.
13. Dakis J, Singh B. Making sense of the psychiatric patient. Foundations of clinical psychiatry. Melbourne: Melbourne University Press; 1994: 79.
14. Folstein MF, Folstein SE, McHugh PR. 'Mini Mental State': A practical method for grading the cognitive state of patients for the clinician. Journal of Psychiatric Research 1975; 12: 189–198.
15. O'Keefe ST, Mulkerrin EC, Nayeem K, et al. Use of serial Mini-Mental State Examinations to diagnose and monitor delirium in elderly hospital patients. Journal of American Geriatrics Society 2005; 53(5): 867–870.
16. Hustey FM, Meldon SW. The prevalence and documentation of impaired mental status in elderly emergency department patients. Annals of Emergency Medicine 2002; 39(3): 248–253.
17. Trzepacz P, McIntyre, Charles SC, et al. Practice guideline for the treatment of patients with delirium. American Journal of Psychiatry 1999; 156 (5 suppl): 1–20.
18. Inouye SK, van Dyck CH, Alessi CA, et al. Clarifying confusion. The confusion assessment method. A new method for detection of delirium. Annals of Internal Medicine 1990; 113: 941–948.
19. Weinberger DR. Brain disease and psychiatric illness: when should a psychiatrist order a CAT scan? American Journal of Psychiatry 1984; 41: 1521–1527.
20. Sata LS. Diagnosing organic psychosis. Maryland State Medical Journal 1970; 19(2): 61–64.
21. Ananth J, Gamal R, Miller M, et al. Is routine CT head scan justified for psychiatric patients? A prospective study. Journal of Psychiatry and Neuroscience 1993; 18: 69–73.
22. Riba M, Mahlon H. Medical clearance: fact or fiction in the hospital emergency room. Psychosomatics 1990; 31: 400–404.

20.3 Deliberate self-harm/suicide

Antonio Celenza

ESSENTIALS

1 Deliberate self-harm is a frequent presentation to emergency departments and is a symptom of diverse underlying problems, including suicidality, attention-seeking, psychosis and anxiety.

2 Patients with deliberate self-harm form a heterogeneous group, most of whom have an excellent prognosis and do not have ongoing suicidal behaviour.

3 Assessment of suicide risk following deliberate self-harm is difficult. It involves assessment of background demographic, psychiatric, medical and social factors as well as the suicidal behaviour itself and the acute psychosocial situation. Patients can then be stratified into risk groups and managed accordingly.

4 Risk assessment needs to be individualised based on local data, since suicide profiles vary considerably between countries, regions and cultures.

5 The most consistent factors predicting fatal and non-fatal repetition following deliberate self-harm are psychiatric illness, personality disorder, substance abuse, multiple previous attempts, and current suicidality and hopelessness.

6 Management requires emergency staff, observation wards, medical teams, mental health nurses, social workers and psychiatrists.

7 A planned strategy to deal with these patients should address triage, restraint and observation, medical and suicidality assessment, treatment and disposition.

8 Discharge following crisis intervention or brief problem-solving treatments can be helpful to many low-risk patients, but short-stay or overnight admission and repeat assessment should be encouraged for all patients. This may improve accuracy of psychiatric assessment and provide opportunity for early management.

Introduction

Suicide is a deliberate act of intentional self-inflicted death. It is the most extreme expression of suicidality, which also comprises suicidal thoughts, threats, planning and attempted suicide through deliberate self-harm (DSH). Although suicide is uncommon, 10% of people who commit suicide are seen in an emergency department (ED) in the month prior to death, with a substantial proportion not having psychosocial assessment, thus providing an opportunity for intervention.[1,2] The major ED impact, however, is in the assessment of large numbers of potentially suicidal patients, accurate risk stratification, and initial control and management of these patients.

DSH is a maladaptive response to stress and a manifestation of suicidality, but can also occur without any intent to die with other psychiatric and personality disorders.[3] Deliberate self-harm is a common ED presentation (approximately 0.5% of all ED visits[4]) and the goals of management include treatment of the physical sequelae, assessment of risk of non-fatal or fatal repetition, and diagnosing and commencing treatment of potentially reversible psychosocial causes.[5]

Incidence

In Australia there were approx 2100 deaths per year from suicide in 2004 and 2005, with age-standardized rates of approximately 16.4 per 100 000 in males and 4.3 in females.[6] Suicide accounts for 1.6% of deaths in Australia and is in the top 10 causes of death despite a reduction of approximately 30% in suicide rates from 1997 to 2004.[7] Suicide rates are similar in the UK, New Zealand, Canada and the USA, suicide accounting for 1–2% of all deaths in these countries.[6,8–11] The national rates of suicide vary: Japan, Scandinavian and Eastern European countries have population suicide rates as high as 25:100 000, whereas some southern European and Middle Eastern countries have rates less than 5:100 000.[11,12]

Hospital presentations for DSH are at least 10 times higher than suicide rates.[6,9] In the 1997 Australian National Survey of Mental Health, 0.3% of males and 0.4% of females reported they had made a suicide attempt in the previous 12 months. Most of these are not reported or are reported as accidents. Hence unrecognized DSH is at least as frequent as that recognized. The same survey reported 2.7% of males and 4.5% of females experienced suicidal thoughts within 12 months.[13] This rate may be as high as 25% in certain populations and age groups.[14,15]

Aetiology

No specific psychological or personality structure is associated with suicide, and patients who commit suicide or DSH do so for many unrelated reasons. The precipitant may be a personal crisis or life change amplified by poor social support, substance abuse or psychiatric disorder. Intoxication may decrease inhibitions enough to allow an act to proceed.

The most frequent methods of suicide in Australia are hanging (approximately 50% of male and 40% of female suicide deaths) and deliberate self-poisoning (approximately 30% of males and 40% of females). Firearms accounted for 7% of suicide deaths in Australia in 2005, a rate which has declined from 20% a decade prior, possibly due to firearm restriction legislation.[6] Proportions due to each method vary according to region, residence, age and sex.[1,16] In the USA, firearms accounted for 57% of male and 32% of female suicide

625

deaths. In many developing countries, organophosphate or antimalarial poisoning is the most common method of suicide.[17,18]

One-third of patients with DSH express a wish to die, but most seek attention or want to communicate distress. Other reasons include release of tension, escape from a stressful situation, blotting out distressing thoughts, eliciting guilt, manipulating others, expressing anger or grief, or escaping from custody. Many patients threaten suicide or exaggerate suicidality to increase the likelihood of admission to hospital. These patients are more likely to be substance dependent, antisocial, homeless, unmarried and in legal difficulty. However, these instances of secondary gain should not be assumed to be the cause of the suicidality and the behaviour should be taken seriously.

Most cases of medically serious DSH are due to self-poisoning, with 90% associated with alcohol intoxication. The most common drugs are non-prescription analgesics and psychotropic drugs. Many overdoses are related to recreational drug use and may be accidental rather than deliberate, although this distinction is often difficult. Self-injury usually involves cutting of the wrist or forearm. Some people self-inflict cigarette burns, excoriate their skin or hit themselves. More violent forms of self-injury are less common and suggest serious suicidal intent. Bizarre self-mutilation may occur in psychotic patients who may not necessarily have an intention to die. Self-immolation, suicide bombing and hunger striking as forms of protest are special concerns.

Patient characteristics

Demographic factors

Age

Suicide and DSH are rare in children under 12 years of age. Australian data suggest similar rates of suicide from the age of 20 to 50, with a peak at 30–34 years in males and 35–39 in females.[6,19] There is another peak in the elderly, with suicide rates increasing with age from 65 years. This bimodal distribution is also evident from USA and New Zealand data, with males aged over 80 years having the highest age specific rates of suicide.

The incidence of DSH increases throughout puberty, reaching a peak at 15–24 years of age and decreasing thereafter. The ratio of rates of DSH to suicide decreases markedly with age. DSH is uncommon in the elderly, who have a high ratio of successful to unsuccessful attempts.[20]

Gender

The overall rate for male suicide is approximately four times that for females. This is a consistent pattern internationally except for China, where the female suicide rate is higher than the male. The rate for male DSH has been increasing in Western countries recently with the male to female ratio approximately 1:2. Females choose methods that are less likely to be fatal, and may be more likely to present to hospital following DSH.

Employment

Unemployment increases the risk of DSH by 10–15 times, with the risk increasing with duration of unemployment. This may not be a cause or effect, but may be due to some underlying factor such as a psychiatric condition, personality disorder or substance abuse.

Social and cultural factors

Suicide rates are higher in those who live alone or are in a lower social group, especially in urban areas characterized by social deprivation and overcrowding. Marriage reinforced by children decreases the risk of suicidal behaviour. Being single, separated, divorced or widowed increases the risk of suicide two- to threefold.

Recent data in Australian Aboriginal people report substantially higher suicide rates that commence at a lower age than in the non-Aboriginal population.[6,19] This has also been reported in New Zealand Maoris, Native Americans and Inuit in Canada.[9,10,21] Suicide rates of migrants initially reflect rates in the country of origin and converge toward the Australian rate over time.

Some higher social status groups such as doctors, dentists, musicians, lawyers and law-enforcement officers are more prone to suicide.[22] Most adults (75%) with DSH have relationship problems with their partners, and teenagers with their parents. A major argument or separation often precedes the act on a background of ongoing social difficulties and substance use.

Medical factors

There is an increased rate of medical illness in patients who commit suicide, especially epilepsy, chronic ill-health, terminal illness or chronic pain. The majority of such patients have sought medical advice in the 6 months before suicide. Most patients with DSH have good health.

Psychiatric factors

There is a pre-existing psychiatric disorder in 90–100% of cases of suicide, of which depression accounts for 66–80%, but this rate may be based on retrospective psychological analysis.[23,24] The rate of suicide among psychiatric inpatients is 3–12 times higher than in the general population and involves more violent methods, such as jumping from buildings, hanging or jumping in front of vehicles. One-third of these episodes occur after self-discharge from hospital, with another third occurring during approved leave. The high-risk time is the first week of admission and during the first 3 months after discharge.[25] Psychiatric disorders are present in up to 60% of patients who commit DSH, but may be transient and secondary to acute psychosocial difficulties.

Affective disorders

The psychiatric diagnosis that carries the greatest risk of suicide is mood disorder, particularly major depression if associated with borderline personality disorder, anxiety or agitation.[26] Fifteen per cent of these high-risk patients commit suicide over a lifetime. Depression correlates well with the occurrence of suicidal desire and ideation, but may not be as strong a predictor of planning and preparation (intense thoughts, plans, courage and capability) and, therefore, suicide completion.[24] Hopelessness is the most important factor associated with suicide completion and may be of greater importance than suicidal ideation or depression itself.[24] Depressed patients should, therefore, have their attitudes towards the future carefully assessed.

Substance abuse

Fifteen per cent of alcohol-dependent persons eventually commit suicide. The majority of these are also depressed. The risk is higher if associated with social isolation, poor physical health, unemployment and previous suicidal behaviour. The increased risk may be more pronounced in males aged below 35 years.[27] There is an increased risk of suicide in patients who use recreational drugs. Young male heroin addicts may have 20 times the risk of the general population. Chronic alcohol dependence is uncommon in DSH, but alcohol intoxication is involved in 50–90% of suicide attempts.

Schizophrenia

Up to 10% of schizophrenics die by suicide. Young adult males are at high risk, especially if there is associated depression, previous suicidal behaviour, unemployment or social isolation. Most suicides occur during a relatively chronic or non-psychotic phase of the illness associated with some degree of insight into possible mental deterioration or with feelings of hopelessness.

Personality disorders

Patients with antisocial and borderline personality disorders are at high risk of DSH and suicide, especially if associated with labile mood, impulsivity, alienation from peers and associated substance abuse. This may be due to precipitation of undesirable life events, predisposition to psychiatric and substance-abuse disorders, and social isolation. Adjustment disorders are associated with 25% of adolescent suicide.[23]

Neuroses

Frequent attenders to EDs are also at high risk. This group has seven times the risk of the general population and rates of suicide similar to clinical psychiatric populations. This risk is particularly pronounced in patients who present with panic attacks, especially if associated with depressive symptoms.

Assessment

A person who expresses suicidal ideation or commits an act of DSH is sending a distress signal that emergency physicians must recognize and assess for further risk. Suicidality

should also be assessed in patients with symptoms or signs of depression, unusual behavioural changes, substance abuse, psychiatric disorders, complainants of sexual violence,[28] and those who present with injuries of questionable or inconsistent mechanism, such as self-inflicted lacerations and gunshot wounds or motor vehicle accidents involving one victim.

Assessment requires a systematic, multidisciplinary approach involving prior staff education, appropriate triage, observation and restraint procedures, and a planned strategy for assessment followed by treatment and disposition. The priorities are to define the physical sequelae of the act, risk of further suicidal behaviour, psychiatric diagnoses and acute psychosocial stressors. These aspects are those that can then be targeted for short-term interventions.

Triage

In a patient who has attempted DSH, initial management involves resuscitation, treatment of immediate life threats and preventing complications. The patient should be triaged according to the physical problem as well as current suicidality, aggressiveness and mental state. The mental health triage scale can be used for this purpose.[29] A triage score of 2 or 3 should be applied if patients are violent to themselves or others, actively suicidal, psychotic or distressed, or at risk of leaving before full assessment. Constant observation is required at this point and nursing staff, orderlies, security or police may be needed.

Medical assessment

The patient should be prevented from doing further harm by limiting availability of drugs, removing sharp implements, removing car keys, ropes, belts or sheets, and securing nearby windows. Other concurrent and concealed methods of self-harm should be sought. Assessment of the patient may be difficult either due to an organic cause or being unsettled from the precipitant of the act or from genuinely not wanting to be in hospital or allow medical intervention. This may necessitate the physical or chemical restraint of the patient if at high risk or unable to be fully assessed and wanting to self-discharge.

Emotional support of patient, friends and relatives is required during this phase.

Suicide risk assessment

Initially, this needs to be done in the ED so as to determine patient disposition, but full psychiatric assessment may need to wait until drug effects wear off. Other sources of information need to be accessed since patient history can be unreliable or incomplete. Friends, family, local doctor, ambulance officers, helping agencies already involved and previous presentations documented in the medical record can all add useful information in order to complete an assessment. A therapeutic relationship should be formed and the clinician should be non-judgemental, non-threatening and clearly willing to help. A negative attitude is common among emergency personnel, especially with repeat attenders. This may intensify the patient's already low self-esteem, increasing future suicide potential and making a therapeutic relationship difficult to establish.[30] When managing a patient who may be suicidal, the suicidal ideation should be discussed openly. This does not increase the likelihood of attempted suicide and may make the patient realize there are other options.

Assessment of suicide risk involves assessing background demographic, psychiatric, medical and social factors, as well as the current circumstances and suicidal behaviour itself, as outlined in Table 20.3.1. There are epidemiological differences between people who attempt suicide and those who complete suicide. Although the groups are different, there is an important overlap. The more an individual's characteristics resemble the profile of a suicide completer, the higher the risk of future suicide or suicide attempts. Despite this, in long-term follow-up studies very few of these factors have been shown to be good independent predictors of suicide following DSH. The most consistent factors are psychiatric illness, personality disorder, substance abuse, multiple previous attempts, and current suicidality and hopelessness. Guidelines are available to assist in suicide-risk stratification and describe characteristics associated with suicide-risk levels and the appropriate further assessment and disposition for each group.[31]

Table 20.3.1 Factors associated with suicide[30]

Variable	High risk	Low risk
Background factors		
Gender	Male	Female
Marital status	Separated, divorced, widowed	Married
Employment	Unemployed or retired	Employed
Medical factors	Chronic illness, chronic pain, epilepsy	Good health
Psychiatric factors	Depression, bipolar, schizophrenia, panic disorder, previous psychiatric inpatient, substance abuse	No psychiatric history, normally robust personality
Social background	Unresponsive family, socially isolated or chaotic, indigenous background	Supportive family, socially stable and integrated
Current factors		
Suicidal ideation	Frequent, prolonged, pervasive	Infrequent, transient
Attempts	Multiple	First attempt
Lethality	Violent, lethal and available method, aware of medical dangerousness	Low lethality, poor availability
Planning	Planned, active preparation, extensive premeditation	Impulsive, no realistic plan, telling others prior to act
Rescue	Act performed in isolation, event timed to avoid intervention, precautions taken to avoid discovery	Rescue inevitable, obtained help afterwards
Final acts	Wills, insurance, giving away property	
Coping skills	Unwilling to seek help, feels unable to cope with present difficulties	Can easily turn to others for help, can plan to overcome present difficulties, willing to become involved in aftercare
Current ideation	Admitting act was intended to cause death, no remorse, continued wish to die, hopelessness or helplessness	Primary wish to change, pleased to recover, suicidal ideation resolved by act, optimism
Precipitant	Similar circumstances can recur, acute precipitant not resolved	Stressful but transient life event, acute precipitant addressed

Use of scales

Many screens have been devised to identify high-risk groups within those presenting with DSH. PATHOS,[32] the Suicidal Intent Scale,[33] the Sad Persons Scale[34] and other scoring systems have been devised to complement medical assessment of suicide risk. The modified Sad Persons Scale (Table 20.3.2) incorporates some high-risk characteristics to predict suicide risk in patients with suicidal ideation or behaviour. However, many of these scales use outdated risk factors and patient populations unrepresentative of EDs. Scales need to be sensitive, but this misclassifies a large number of individuals as potentially suicidal. These deficiencies need to be considered when applying suicide risk scales in the ED and these scales should not be used as an absolute assessment of suicide risk or of the need for psychiatric admission.[35,36] The problems associated with suicide-risk assessment are summarized in Table 20.3.3.

Definitive treatment and disposition

Following necessary medical treatment and suicide-risk stratification, disposition may involve involuntary or voluntary admission to a psychiatric or medical ward, short-term or overnight observation, or discharge with appropriate follow-up. Restraint and involuntary admission may be necessary for the high-risk patient who wishes to self-discharge. Approximately 30% of DSH patients are admitted for psychiatric inpatient care but the factors involved in the decision for psychiatric hospitalization following DSH are not well understood and involve a complex evaluation of risk, potential for treatment and social supports.[37]

Overnight observation allows drug intoxication to resolve so that proper psychiatric assessment can take place. An overnight stay in hospital can also help resolution of many acute areas of conflict and make psychiatric evaluation more accurate. ED short-stay wards are appropriate for these admissions, especially if a multi-disciplinary team is available to review the patient and institute management and follow-up.

Important elements of management involve neutralizing the precipitating problem, treatment of psychiatric illness and environmental interventions such as family counselling, encouraging a support network, and developing coping and problem-solving skills.[38] Open discussion about suicide should be undertaken and a firm stance should be maintained that suicide is an ineffective solution. Alternative, non-suicide solutions should be reinforced.

Other factors that should be addressed whilst patients are in hospital include problems with relationships, employment, finances, housing, legal problems, social isolation, alcohol and drug abuse, and bereavement. In this regard, medical social workers or mental health nurses are invaluable.[39] For greatest effect, these should be available after hours and on weekends since the majority of DSH presents after hours.[40] For repeat attenders or manipulative patients who are often socially isolated, hospitalization should not be a substitute for social services, substance-abuse treatment and legal assistance, although admission may be necessary while appropriate supports are put in place.[41]

Discharge is appropriate for the low-risk patient who is cooperative, no longer suicidal, not intoxicated, has no underlying psychiatric or substance abuse disorder, and has strong social support with the precipitating problem having resolved due to the act or subsequent assessment and intervention in hospital. Discharged patients should make a commitment to seek help if they reach a crisis point, and the physician should be available to help. This can be part of a commitment to a non-suicidal behavioural plan between the patient and clinician. This contract should

Table 20.3.2 Modified Sad Persons Scale[34]

Variable	Score
Gender: male	1
Age: <19 or >45 years	1
Depression: hopelessness, despair, especially if associated with physiological shift symptoms	2
Psychiatric care: previous DSH, psychiatric care or severe personality disorder	1
Excessive drug use	1
Rational thinking loss: severe depression with psychotic features, organic brain syndrome, delusions	2
Single, separated, divorced, widowed	1
Organized attempt: planned, premeditated, lethal and available method	2
No life supports: social isolation, homeless, unemployed	1
States future intent: continued suicidal ideation	2

Table 20.3.3 Problems in assessing suicide risk

Suicide is rare, even in high-risk groups, so it cannot be predicted without a high rate of false-negative or false-positive errors
Suicidality presents in heterogeneous ways that may not be recognized
Suicidality is transient and affected by intoxication, stress and being in hospital
The patient may be reluctant, oppositional or manipulative
The patient may present in an atypical fashion, especially the elderly with physical complaints
Suicide risk factors identify high-risk subgroups but not individuals
The demographic factors associated with suicide have changed recently, thus changing the make-up of risk groups
Risk factors are based on studies of long-term follow-up and, therefore, long-term risk
Subtle changes in mental status and behaviour may be missed if not assessed by the usual doctor
Unexplained improvement in psychological status may be the result of increased motivation to die
Patients may deny their true intentions due to embarrassment, fear of being stopped in carrying out their own wishes, fear of being institutionalized or fear of the confidentiality of the interview
Patients may say life is not worth living or that they feel they would be better off dead, but not necessarily have an increased risk of suicide, unless they have made suicidal plans or attempts, or if they have pervasive hopelessness
Correlation between medical danger and suicidal intent is low unless the patient can accurately assess the probable outcome of their attempts if treatment had not been received

be with the clinician who will arrange definitive care. Contracts may delay the patient's suicidal impulses so that other treatment strategies can be implemented. If discharged, there should be liaison with the patient's general practitioner and therapist, and follow-up should be confirmed where possible within 1–2 days.

Pharmacotherapy involves the treatment of the underlying psychiatric disorder.

Antidepressants decrease the risk of attempting suicide, although the lethality of suicide attempts is increased if tricyclic antidepressants are taken in overdose. Selective serotonin reuptake inhibitors may have a more selective effect in decreasing suicidal behaviour and are less toxic in overdose. These factors make this class of drugs an attractive choice for depressed patients who are suicidal, but

any long-term therapeutic drug should, ideally, be prescribed by the doctor who will provide definitive follow-up.[42]

Consequences

Risk of suicide

An episode of DSH is probably the best predictor of future suicide. Approximately 1–2% of patients commit suicide during the year following an attempt and in approximately 40% of suicides there is a history of a previous attempt. A systematic review of fatal and non-fatal repetition of self-harm reported a suicide rate of 2% at 1 year and 7% after 9 years.[43] In a prospective Finnish 14-year follow-up study, and a UK 18-year follow-up study, the rate of suicide after an episode of DSH was 6.7%.[44,45] A 10-year follow-up study in New Zealand documented a suicide rate of 4.6% in patients admitted for DSH.[46] Hospitalization and aftercare decrease short-term risk of suicide, but have little impact on long-term risk of suicide. However, this may be due to under-treatment of psychiatric illness.[23,47,48]

Exposure to suicide in adolescents tends not to cause an increased risk of suicide among friends but may cause an increased incidence of depression anxiety, and post-traumatic stress disorder.[49]

Repeated episodes of DSH

DSH usually invokes help from friends, family and the medical profession so that the patient's social situation and psychological wellbeing tends to improve.[50] This cathartic effect is prominent in younger patients but may not occur in patients aged over 60 years.[51] The risk of repetition is 12–16% in the following year, with 10% of these occurring in the first week.[43,49] This is more likely in females who are unemployed, have cluster B personality traits or have substance-abuse problems.

Patients with DSH who leave the ED prior to a psychosocial assessment may have a higher risk for repeat DSH, probably associated with lack of specialist follow-up and treatment of reversible factors.[52,53]

Some patients have chronic suicidal ideation and multiple repetitions of DSH. They often suffer from personality disorders, psychotic disorders, chronic medical conditions, alcohol or drug use, a history of childhood sexual abuse[54,55] and violent behaviour. They use DSH as a means of fighting off anxiety, hopelessness, loneliness or boredom, or for manipulation of family, friends or health carers. These patients place a heavy burden on hospital resources, are difficult to treat and have a high rate of eventual suicide. Reversible potentiating factors should be addressed where possible.

Increased all cause mortality

A suicide attempt is associated with a severe risk of premature death with the increased mortality rate not entirely due to suicide.[56] There is a higher than expected rate of accidents, homicides and death from other medical conditions. This may indicate social disadvantage, a disengagement with the health system, underlying chronic illnesses or lifestyle factors.

Prevention

Comprehensive strategies for prevention of suicide have been or are being developed in Finland, Norway, Sweden, Australia and New Zealand.[12] Suicide prevention focuses on psychiatric, social and medical aspects, and usually involves public education, media restrictions on reporting of suicide, school-based programmes with teacher education, training of doctors in detection and treatment of depression and other psychiatric disorders, alcohol and drug-abuse information, enhanced access to the mental health system and supportive counselling after episodes of DSH. Decreasing the availability of lethal methods may involve legislative changes such as more stringent gun control, restricting access to well-known jumping sites or changes to availability or packaging of tablets.[57] Overall, studies into the effectiveness of suicide-prevention strategies have shown inconsistent reductions in suicide rates following interventions.[58] Approaches to reduce DSH repetition have also shown disappointing results.[59] Improved recognition and treatment of mental illness, improved social services, and drug- and alcohol-support services may be of greater benefit than specific suicide-prevention strategies.

Conclusion

Assessment of suicide risk is an important skill in emergency medicine since many patients present to EDs with suicidal thinking or behaviour. Although the risk of suicide for an individual patient is remote and cannot be predicted, emergency physicians can provide a system for assessment and identification of risk groups. Acute interventions can attempt to prevent short-term completion of suicide or repetition of DSH, since emergency physicians are predominantly involved in the care of these patients, often using short-stay wards. A team approach involving psychiatry and social work is necessary in most cases, with many minor problems resolved by a short-term hospital admission, brief crisis intervention and intense short-term follow-up.

Controversies

❶ Although in most cultures suicide has been considered morally wrong since ancient times, there are arguments that it may be rational, especially if active voluntary euthanasia is considered a suicidal act.

❷ The legal position is clear in not assisting suicide, and we have a duty of care for people who are suicidal. However, the question of how long doctors should have the power to keep suicidal people alive against their will remains controversial.

❸ Part of the role of EDs is in the epidemiological monitoring and further research of patient risk factors.

❹ Clinical trials of ED assessment and brief intervention strategies, including short-stay admissions, need to occur since more patients are managed entirely in EDs.

❺ Currently available guidelines need to be validated and refined, and current, local risk stratification scales produced.

References

1. Salter A, Pielage P. Emergency departments have a role in the prevention of suicide. Emergency Medicine 2000; 12: 198–203.
2. Gairin I, House A, Owens D. Attendance at the accident and emergency department in the year before suicide: retrospective study. British Journal of Psychiatry 2003; 183: 28–33.
3. Mitchell AJ, Dennis M. Self harm and attempted suicide in adults: 10 practical questions and answers for emergency department staff. Emergency Medicine Journal 2006; 23: 251–255.
4. Doshi A, Boudreaux ED, Wand N, et al. National study of US emergency department visits for attempted suicide and self-inflicted injury, 1997–2001. Annals of Emergency Medicine 2005; 46: 369–375.
5. Boyce P, Carter G, Penrose-Wall J, et al. Summary Australian and New Zealand clinical practice guideline for the management of adult deliberate self-harm. Australasian Psychiatry 2003; 11: 150–155.
6. Australian Bureau of Statistics. 3309.0 Suicides, Australia, 2005 [Internet homepage] [updated 2007, Mar 14; cited 2007, Nov 22]. Available: www.abs.gov.au/AUSSTATS/abs@.nsf/Lookup/3309.0Main+Features12005?.
7. Australian Bureau of Statistics. 3303.0 Causes of Death, Australia, 2005 [Internet homepage] [updated 2007, Apr 16; cited 2007, Nov 22]. Available: www.abs.gov.au/AUSSTATS/abs@.nsf/mf/3303.0/.
8. Office for National Statistics. Death rates from suicide [Internet homepage] [updated 2007, Feb 22; cited 2007, Nov 22]. Available: www.statistics.gov.uk/statbase/Product.asp?vlnk=13618.
9. New Zealand Health Information Service. Suicide facts: provisional 2003 all-ages statistics [Internet homepage] [updated 2006, Feb; cited 2007, Nov 22]. Available: www.nzhis.govt.nz/stats/suicidefacts2003.pdf.
10. American Association of Suicidology. USA Suicide: 2004 official final data [Internet homepage] [updated 2006, Dec 15; cited 2007, Nov 22]. Available: www.suicidology.org/associations/1045/files/2004datapgu1.pdf.
11. World Health Organisation. Suicide rates [Internet homepage] [updated 2003, May; cited 2007, Nov 22]. Available: www.who.int/mental_health/prevention/suicide/suiciderates/en/.
12. Taylor SJ, Kingdom D, Jenkins R. How are nations trying to prevent suicide? An analysis of national suicide prevention strategies. Acta Psychiatrica Scandinavia 1997; 95: 457–463.
13. Pirkis J, Burgess P, Dunt D. Suicidal ideation and suicide attempts among Australian adults. Crisis 2000; 21: 16–25.
14. McKelvey RS, Pfaff JJ, Acres JG. The relationship between chief complaints, psychological distress, and suicidal ideation in 15–24 year-old patients presenting to general practitioners. Medical Journal of Australia 2001; 175: 550–552.
15. Bertolote JM, Fleischmann A, De Leo D, et al. Suicide attempts, plans, and ideation in culturally diverse sites: the WHO SUPRE–MISS community survey. Psychological Medicine 2005; 35: 1457–1465.
16. Dudley MJ, Kelk NJ, Florio TM. Suicide among young Australians, 1964–1993: an interstate comparison of metropolitan and rural trends. Medical Journal of Australia 1998; 169: 77–80.
17. Arun M, Menezes RG, Babu YPR. Autopsy study of fatal deliberate self harm. Medicine, Science & the Law 2007; 47: 69–73.
18. Eddleston, M. Patterns and problems of deliberate self-poisoning in the developing world. Quarterly Journal of Medicine 2000; 93: 715–731.
19. Baume P. Suicide in Australia: do we really have a problem? Australian Journal of Education & Developmental Psychology 1996; 13: 3–39.
20. Hawton K, Harriss L. Deliberate self-harm in people aged 60 years and over: characteristics and outcome of a 20-year cohort. International Journal of Geriatric Psychiatry 2006; 21: 572–581.

21. Isaacs S, Keogh S, Menard C, et al. Suicide in the Northwest Territories: a descriptive review. Chronic Diseases in Canada [serial online]. 2000; 19 [cited 2007, Nov 22]. Available: www.phac-aspc.gc.ca/publicat/cdic-mcc/19-4/c_e.html.

22. Kaplan HI, Sadock BJ, Grebb JA. Kaplan and Sadock's synopsis of psychiatry. 7th edn. Baltimore: Williams & Wilkins; 1994: 803–809.

23. Lönnqvist JK, Henriksson MM, Isometsä ET, et al. Mental disorders and suicide prevention. Psychiatry and Clinical Neurosciences 1995; 49: S111–S116.

24. Hawton K. Assessment of suicide risk. British Journal of Psychiatry 1987; 150: 145–153.

25. Shah AK, Ganesvaran T. Inpatient suicides in an Australian mental hospital. Australia and New Zealand Journal of Psychiatry 1997; 31: 291–298.

26. Gilbody S, House A, Owens D. The early repetition of deliberate self harm. Journal of Royal College Physicians London 1997; 31: 171–172.

27. Cooper J, Kapur N, Webb R, et al. Suicide after deliberate self-harm: a 4-year cohort study. American Journal of Psychiatry 2005; 162: 297–303.

28. Campbell L, Keegan A, Cybulska B. Prevalence of mental health problems and deliberate self-harm in complainants of sexual violence. Journal of Forensic Legal Medicine 2007; 14: 75–78.

29. Smart D, Pollard C, Walpole B. Mental health triage in emergency medicine. Australian and New Zealand Journal of Psychiatry 1999; 33: 57–66.

30. Rund DA, Hutzler JC. Behavioral disorders: emergency assessment and stabilization. In: Tintinalli JE, Kelen GD, Stapczynski JS. (eds) Emergency medicine: a comprehensive study guide. 6th edn. New York: American College of Emergency Physicians, McGraw-Hill; 2004: 1812–1816.

31. Australasian College for Emergency Medicine and the Royal Australian and New Zealand College of Psychiatrists. Guidelines for the management of deliberate self harm in young people. Victoria: ACEM and RANZCP; 2000.

32. Kingsbury S. PATHOS: a screening instrument for adolescent overdose: a research note. Journal of Child Psychology and Psychiatry and Allied Disciplines 1996; 37(5): 609–611.

33. Beck AT, Schuyler D, Herman J. Development of suicidal intent scales. In: Beck AT, Resruk HLP, Lettieri DJ (eds).

The prediction of suicide. Maryland: Charles Press; 1974.

34. Hockberger RS, Rothstein RJ. Assessment of suicide potential by nonpsychiatrists using the SAD PERSONS score. Journal of Emergency Medicine 1988; 6: 99–107.

35. Cochrane-Brink KA, Lofchy JS, Sakinofsky I. Clinical rating scales in suicide risk assessment. General Hospital Psychiatry 2000; 22: 445–451.

36. Harriss L, Hawton K. Suicidal intent in deliberate self-harm and the risk of suicide: the predictive power of the Suicide Intent Scale. Journal of Affective Disorders 2005; 86: 225–233.

37. Carter GL, Safranko I, Lewin TJ, et al. Psychiatric hospitalisation after deliberate self-poisoning. Suicide and Life-Threatening Behavior 2006; 36(2): 213–222.

38. Brent DA. The aftercare of adolescents with deliberate self harm. Journal of Child Psychology and Psychiatry and Allied Disciplines 1997; 38(3): 277–286.

39. Brakoulis V, Ryan C, Byth K. Patients seen with deliberate self-harm seen by a consultation–liaison service. Australasian Psychiatry 2006; 14: 192–197.

40. Bergen H, Hawton K. Variations in time of hospital presentation for deliberate self-harm and their implications for clinical services. Journal of Affective Disorders 2007; 98(3): 227–237.

41. Lambert MT, Bonner J. Characteristics and six-month outcome of patients who use suicide threats to seek hospital admission. Psychiatric Services 1996; 47: 871–873.

42. Kasper S, Schindler S, Neumeister A. Risk of suicide in depression and its implication for psychopharmacological treatment. International Journal of Psychopharmacology 1996; 11(2): 71–79.

43. Owens D, Horrocks J, House A. Fatal and non-fatal repetition of self-harm. British Journal of Psychiatry 2002; 181: 193–199.

44. Suokas J, Suominen K, Isometsa E, et al. Long-term risk factors for suicide mortality after attempted suicide – findings of a 14-year follow-up study. Acta Psychiatrica Scandinavia 2001; 104: 117–121.

45. De Moore GM, Robertson AR. Suicide in the 18 years after deliberate self harm. British Journal of Psychiatry 1996; 169: 489–494.

46. Gibb SJ, Beautrais AL, Fergusson DM. Mortality and further suicidal behaviour after an index suicide attempt: a 10-year study. Australian and New Zealand Journal of Psychiatry 2005; 39: 95–100.

47. Kurz A, Moller HJ. Attempted suicide: efficacy of treatment programs. Psychiatry and Clinical Neurosciences 1995; 49: S99–S103.

48. McNeil DE, Binder RL. The impact of hospitalization on clinical assessments of suicide risk. Psychiatric Services 1997; 48: 204–208.

49. Brent DA, Moritz G, Bridge J. Long-term impact of exposure to suicide: a three-year controlled follow-up. Journal of the American Academy of Child and Adolescent Psychiatry 1996; 35: 646–653.

50. Sarfati Y, Bouchaud B, Hardy-Bayle M-C. Cathartic effect of suicide attempts not limited to depression: a short-term prospective study after deliberate self-poisoning. Crisis 2003; 24: 73–78.

51. Matsuishi K, Kitamura N, Sato M, et al. Change of suicidal ideation induced by suicide attempt. Psychiatry and Clinical Neurosciences 2005; 59: 599–604.

52. Hickey L, Hawton K, Fagg J, et al. Deliberate self-harm patients who leave the accident and emergency department without a psychiatric assessment: a neglected population at risk of suicide. Journal of Psychosomatic Research 2001; 50: 87–93.

53. Kapur N, Cooper J, Hiroeh U. Emergency department management and outcome for self-poisoning: a cohort study. General Hospital Psychiatry 2004; 26: 36–41.

54. Soderberg S, Kullgren G, Salander Renberg E. Childhood sexual abuse predicts poor outcome seven years after parasuicide. Social Psychiatry and Psychiatric Epidemiology 2004; 39: 916–920.

55. Vajda J, Steinbeck K. Factors associated with repeat suicide attempts among adolescents. Australian and New Zealand Journal of Psychiatry 2000; 34: 437–445.

56. Ostamo A, Lonnqvist J. Excess mortality of suicide attempters. Social Psychiatry and Psychiatric Epidemiology 2001; 36: 29–35.

57. Cantor CH, Baume PJM. Access to methods of suicide: what impact? Australian and New Zealand Journal of Psychiatry 1998; 2: 8–14.

58. Gunnell D, Frankel S. Prevention of suicide: aspirations and evidence. British Medical Journal 1994; 308: 1227–1233.

59. Burns J, Dudley M, Hazel P. Clinical management of deliberate self-harm in young people: the need for evidence-based approaches to reduce repetition. Australian and New Zealand Journal of Psychiatry 2005; 39: 121–128.

20.4 Depression

Simon Byrne

ESSENTIALS

1 Clinical depression is common, affecting 2–5% of the population at any time.

2 Depressive symptoms can be accurately assessed through a systematic interview.

3 The diagnosis of depressive syndrome depends on the severity, pervasiveness and persistence of the symptoms.

4 Management decisions include inpatient admission and referral to appropriate community outpatient services.

Introduction

The need to determine the presence and severity of a depressive syndrome is a very frequent task in the emergency department (ED). Assessment of depression is necessary in relation to a variety of patient presentations. The classic ED situation is the overdose, or other attempted suicide or self-harm, where the assessment of depression forms part of further evaluation after the patient has been medically stabilized.

It is also becoming more common for patients to present to the ED complaining of depression (often on the advice of family, friends or crisis helplines) without having harmed themselves. Patients with a variety of medical conditions, especially conditions which are chronic or disabling, also often develop a depressive syndrome that can form a major part of the reason behind an ED attendance. Some patients who present to EDs with personal crisis or self-harm may have been identified as suffering from a personality disorder, but nevertheless need assessment for comorbid depression. The evaluation of depressive symptoms is also an important aspect of the assessment of patients seen in the ED with alcohol and drug abuse problems.

In these assessments it is very important to have a clear concept of the syndrome of 'clinical depression'. This syndrome is called 'depressive episode' in The International Classification of Disease – 10th edition[1] (ICD-10) and 'major depression' in the Diagnostic and Statistical Manual of Mental Disorders – 4th edition[2] (DSM-IV). The importance of diagnosing a depressive episode lies principally in determining the presence of a clinical syndrome which is in need of treatment, is likely to respond to treatment and is likely to persist without treatment. The clear delineation of a depressive episode is also an essential basis for differential diagnosis from other medical and psychiatric conditions, and for distinguishing between the clinical syndrome of depression and the day-to-day fluctuations of mood and states of dejection, pessimism, frustration and disappointment which are the lot of all human beings.

The diagnosis of a depressive episode depends on the pervasive presence of a sufficient number of a specific list of symptoms. The list of symptoms contributing to the depressive episode syndrome in ICD-10 is shown in Table 20.4.1. The DSM-IV syndrome of major depression has the same list of symptoms, with the exception of 'loss of confidence or self-esteem'. An adequate number of these symptoms must be present for at least 2 weeks before the diagnosis of depressive episode can be made. The pervasiveness of the symptoms is defined principally by the specifications that they must be present 'most of the day' and for 'nearly every day'.

Table 20.4.1 Symptoms contributing to the diagnosis of a depressive episode in ICD-10[1]

1. Depressed mood, most of the day, nearly every day, largely uninfluenced by circumstances
2. Markedly diminished interest or pleasure in all, or almost all, activities, most of the day, nearly all day
3. Loss of energy or fatigue, nearly every day
4. Loss of confidence or self-esteem
5. Unreasonable feelings of self-reproach, or excessive or inappropriate guilt, nearly every day
6. Recurrent thoughts of death or suicide, or any suicidal behaviour
7. Diminished ability to think or concentrate, or indecisiveness, nearly every day
8. Psychomotor agitation or retardation, nearly every day
9. Insomnia or hypersomnia, nearly every day
10. Change in appetite (decrease or increase with corresponding weight change)

ICD-10 further classifies depressive episodes into mild, moderate and severe, according to the total number of symptoms present (mild = 4/10 symptoms, moderate = 6/10 symptoms and severe = 8/10 symptoms). However, it is important to note that both the mild and moderate categories require the presence of at least two of the first three symptoms, that is the patient must have two of depressed mood, loss of interest or loss of energy, most of the day, nearly every day, for at least 2 weeks. The diagnosis of severe depressive episode requires the presence of all three of the first three symptoms.

The diagnosis of a depressive episode does not in any way depend on the presence or absence of a precipitating life event or situation. The ICD-10 also has a category of brief depressive reaction (one of the 'adjustment disorders'), which forms part of the differential diagnosis of a depressive episode. This syndrome is defined by the presence of a precipitating life event and depressive symptoms. However, if the depressive symptoms are of sufficient number, pervasiveness and duration as to qualify for the description of a depressive episode, then this diagnosis should be made regardless of the presence of a precipitant. The notion that 'this patient's depression is understandable given the circumstances' should never detract from a proper evaluation of the severity and duration of the symptoms.

It is an ICD-10 requirement that depressive syndromes which form part of a bipolar disorder, or are secondary to alcohol or other drug abuse or to a medical condition, should be given a different diagnostic category ('bipolar affective episode, current episode mild, moderate or severe depression', 'mood disorder due to psychoactive substance use' or 'organic mood disorder'). The distinction is important because the treatment implications may be significant.

Epidemiology

Clinical depression, defined as 'major depression' or an ICD-10 'depressive episode', is a very common condition. Extensive epidemiological community surveys in many populations around the world have established that the 6-month prevalence rate of major depression is in the range of 2–5% in any population.[3] The epidemiological research has also shown that only a minority of persons with current depressive syndromes are receiving active treatment.[3]

The age onset of the first depressive episode is typically in the third decade, but can be at any age. The male to female ratio is 1:2. A person who has had one episode of clinical depression has an 80% chance of recurrence, and patients with recurrent depression have an average of four episodes in their lifetime.[4]

Incomplete recovery is common. Studies of hospitalized patients have shown that, while at least 50% of patients recover from an index episode within 6 months, 30% remain symptomatic for more than a year and 12% for more than 5 years.[5]

There is some evidence for an increase in the prevalence of major depression, and a younger age of onset, over the last 40 years.[6]

Aetiology

The aetiology of depression is complex, involving both genetic and environmental factors. Important environmental factors include childhood experiences of adversity or neglect, and stresses in adult life.

The effect of genetic factors may be mediated in part through inherited predispositions to excessive worry and anxiety.[3]

Precipitating life events, especially those involving loss, are known to play a part in triggering individual episodes of depression.[7] This effect is greatest for the first episode of depression. Second and subsequent episodes are more likely to occur without identifiable precipitating events,[8] suggesting that the first episode has a neurobiological priming effect.[9]

Neurobiological changes in depression are also complex. Based in part on the supposed mechanism of action of antidepressant medication, early work focused on evidence of depletion of amine neurotransmitters in the central nervous system.[10] More recent research has suggested depression may involve alterations in neural cell populations, especially in the hippocampus.[11]

Prevention

Depression is a major public health problem. The World Health Organization has determined that in 1990 depression was the fourth leading cause of disease burden in the world and that by 2020 it would be the second leading cause of disease burden.[12] Public health measures have included campaigns to raise awareness of depression both in the general public and in healthcare providers. ED staff can play a very significant role in case identification and in ensuring referral for effective treatment.

Clinical features

The syndrome described as a 'depressive episode' (or 'major depression') is defined principally by its symptoms and, to a lesser extent, signs. As the severity of the depressive episode is also dependent on specific characteristics of the individual symptoms and signs (as well as the total number of symptoms) it is also important to understand the varieties of their manifestations.

Symptoms

It is useful to start the history with an exploration of the problem which has brought the person to the ED. This problem may be an overdose or other attempted suicide or self-harm, a personal or relationship crisis, a period of alcohol or other drug abuse, an exacerbation of a chronic medical condition or chronic pain, or some other complaint. It is also important during the clinical assessment to begin to form some picture of who the patient is, including whether he or she lives alone or with others, the nature and quality of his or her personal relationships, and his or her daily occupation, interests and activities. These inquiries assist in building rapport through demonstrating an interest in the patient, but also elicit information that is necessary for understanding the patient's symptoms in context.

At some point, the patient can be told that the interviewer would now like to explore the symptoms of depression in more detail. It may be helpful to group the symptoms of depressive episode (Table 20.4.1) into various domains of the patient's experience. The first group ('depressed mood', 'markedly diminished interest', and 'loss of energy') refers to the pervasive mood state and the quality of the patient's spirits or enthusiasm for life. The second group ('loss of self-esteem', 'unreasonable self-reproach or guilt', and 'recurrent thoughts of death or suicide') refers to the cognitive contents of the patient's thoughts. The third group ('diminished concentration' and 'psychomotor agitation or retardation') refers to the degree of agitation or lethargy associated with the patient's thought processes and physical activity. The final group ('insomnia or hypersomnia' and 'change in appetite') refers to physiological changes.

Both the pervasiveness and duration of these symptoms should be assessed. Pervasiveness is important because most of the symptoms can only be rated as present for the specific diagnosis of a depressive episode if they are present 'nearly every day'. The syndrome is, by definition, one in which the symptoms have become persistent and inescapable, not the occasional or sporadic experience of these symptoms which nearly everybody endures sometimes. Duration is important because the syndrome must be present for at least 2 weeks before the diagnosis can be made.

The timing of onset of a depressive episode can be difficult to establish because the onset is often very gradual and insidious (although it can be relatively rapid). The patient may have experienced previous episodes which become confused with the present one, and patients often confuse long-term feelings of low self-esteem with the current episode. Hence the question 'How long have you been feeling like this?' is often unproductive. It is more useful to ask the patient to describe the presence and pervasiveness of each of the symptoms 'during the last 2 or 3 weeks or so' and in particular to try to identify some recent time at which there has been a change in the clinical state or function of the patient.

The pervasiveness and duration criteria taken together imply a diminished ability to carry out normal activities and meet responsibilities. Although many depressed patients push themselves to keep going, careful enquiry reveals that this has become more arduous. Difficulty in attending to tasks may range from diminished effectiveness at work, child care or study to, eventually, neglect of self-care and nutrition. Thus impairment in function is another indicator of the severity of the episode.

'Depressed mood, most of the day, nearly every day' is perhaps the most difficult of the symptoms to characterize. 'Mood' refers to a person's underlying emotional state, the emotional baseline that permeates each day. It is useful to ask not only 'Do you feel depressed?' but also 'What is that like for you?'. Some patients describe feeling much more unhappy than usual or sad all the time or unexpectedly tearful; others report feeling more irritable with others or more inclined to worry. The severity of the mood change may be shown in a loss of mood reactivity, which can be elicited by asking 'Can you cheer yourself up, take your mind off your worries?' and 'Do you find that the things which normally make you happy don't seem to cheer you up as much as usual?'.

'Markedly diminished interest or pleasure in all, or almost all, activities, most of the day, nearly every day' is somewhat easier to assess, especially if the interviewer takes the time to build up a picture of the patient's usual day. With careful inquiry a nuanced picture can be built up of the extent of the patient's withdrawal from his or her usual activities. Included within this criterion is a lack of pleasure or interest in sexual activity, which in more severe cases can be experienced as a profound loss of sexual feelings.

'Loss of energy or fatigue, nearly every day' is an important symptom which is sometimes overlooked. The emphasis should be on the loss of energy, that is whether the patient is aware of having much less energy or drive than usual. In severe cases, the patient may describe feeling the body is heavy or thoughts sluggish, at which point this symptom overlaps with 'psychomotor retardation'. Loss of energy is an important symptom in differential diagnosis, which may point to such conditions as anaemia, hypothyroidism, diabetes or other undiagnosed medical condition.

The diagnosis of depressive episode requires the enduring presence of at least two of these mood-related symptoms, that is depressed mood, diminished interest and loss of energy. The most important part of the assessment is therefore the systematic exploration of these three symptoms.

The cognitive symptoms of depression ('loss of self-esteem', 'unreasonable self-reproach or guilt' and 'recurrent thoughts of death or suicide') can to some extent be observed in listening to the patient's spontaneous comments, and as such form a part of the mental state examination. However, patients who are more introspective have some awareness of a change in thought processes and are able to describe the ways in which their thoughts have become more gloomy than usual. This insight is lost when depression becomes more severe and the patient tends to regard the self-reproach or thoughts of suicide as entirely justified.

In assessing 'loss of confidence or self-esteem', the emphasis should be on the loss or change in the person's self-concept. It can be helpful to approach the issue with suggestive questions, such as 'Tell me about a time when you felt better about yourself', 'Did you used to feel more confident at work?' or 'Was there a time when you felt more adequate as a parent?'.

'Unreasonable feelings of self-reproach, or excessive or inappropriate guilt, nearly every day' is probably one of the most consistently reliable symptoms pointing to a diagnosis of depressive episode. Sometimes a very conscientious person may habitually find fault with him- or herself without being clinically depressed. However, a person who is not depressed will usually be able to consider other points of view, to debate the sense of culpability internally and to consider whether the sense of guilt may be 'excessive', 'inappropriate' or 'unreasonable'. This capacity to rationalize about thought processes becomes progressively more impaired as the patient becomes more severely depressed, until the patient's guilt appears unquestionable.

In psychotic forms of depression the sense of guilt may take on bizarre dimensions in which the patient can feel responsible for all the evil in the world or for distant events. A not uncommon experience is for the patient to see a report on the television of a calamity such as an earthquake and to feel responsible for the event.

'Recurrent thoughts of death or suicide' can arise in a depressive episode in a variety of ways. Not uncommonly, the thoughts may simply come in to the patient's mind: the patient reports having thoughts of being dead, wanting to be dead or thoughts of suicide that are uncharacteristic, unbidden and apparently inexplicable. Sometimes the suicidal thoughts are directly linked to excessive or delusional guilt, in which the patient feels his or her death to be necessary and inevitable: here the risk of suicidal action is very high.

In other cases, the suicidal thoughts are a logical consequence of a sense of hopelessness, a lack of faith in the future. This last type of suicidal ideation is less specific for the diagnosis of depressive episode, as it may also reflect an apparently realistic appraisal of life circumstances, an attitude of philosophical pessimism or poor coping skills in a person with impaired personality function. These distinctions are important because the suicidal ideation which is a part of a depressive episode may be expected to resolve with treatment of the depression, whereas the other forms may not.

'Diminished ability to think or concentrate, or indecisiveness, nearly every day' is a relatively straightforward symptom to assess and is useful as an indicator of the severity of the depressive episode. It can be assessed by asking about ability to focus on work or a recreational activity such as watching television or reading a book. Some patients report that their mind is easily distracted or restlessly inattentive. Many report the intrusion of negative ruminations (concerning lack of worth, sense of failure or guilt, thoughts of suicide or other worries) which go round and round in their minds. Progressive impairment in the capacity to concentrate will demonstrate increasing severity of depression: a severely depressed patient may not even be able to focus on one newspaper story and take in the contents.

'Psychomotor agitation or retardation, nearly every day' refers to abnormalities of movement, facial expression, speech and thought processes which are directly assessed in the mental state examination and are discussed more fully below. However, this can also to some extent be assessed through the history from the family. 'Psychomotor agitation' includes restless, fidgety behaviour, inability to sit still or attend to a task, and anxious, repetitive speech or even perseveration. 'Psychomotor retardation' includes lack of spontaneous bodily movement, lack of facial expression, lack of verbal communication and slowness of response. Retardation is the more common, and the patient or family may report progressive withdrawal and decrease in activity to the point where the patient sits for long hours apparently doing nothing. The presence of significant psychomotor agitation or retardation is usually indicative of a severe depressive episode.

Changes in sleep pattern ('insomnia or hypersomnia, nearly every day') are very common in depression, even in mild episodes. It is worth enquiring in detail about the specific changes in sleep pattern, as these relate to the severity of the depressive episode. Initial insomnia, or delay in the onset of sleep, is not specifically associated with depression, as it can be strongly associated with anxiety or primary insomnia. Middle insomnia (waking after 2 or 3 h of sleep) and early morning waking are more specific to depression. The extent of difficulty the patient has in going back to sleep, and the mood and thought content when awake during the night are also relevant.

Change in appetite may involve an increase or decrease with corresponding weight change. Severe loss of appetite with marked loss of weight, in the absence of medical illness or deliberate dieting, is associated with severe depression.

Signs

The most important signs are:

- signs of psychomotor agitation or retardation
- the affective state of the patient
- the thought content
- the degree of insight.

The patient with psychomotor agitation demonstrates, in milder forms, fidgety or repetitive behaviours such as hand wringing or sighing. This can progress to an inability to sit still and, eventually, continuous pacing. The patient may say little while looking very apprehensive and preoccupied, or may importune all the staff with repetitive, anxious questions, apparently seeking reassurance which is never achieved. In severe cases, speech becomes perseverative.

By contrast, the psychomotor-retarded patient maintains a relative immobility, lying in bed or sitting in a chair for long periods, with infrequent changes in posture. The face may be relatively expressionless, look sad or show an anxious dread. Both the facial expression and the body language show diminished reactivity during interview. There is little spontaneous speech and, if responses to questions can be elicited, the responses lack richness, depth or elaboration. Slowness of thought processes is shown especially by a marked increase (sometimes as long as several minutes) in the time taken to supply an answer to a question. In severe cases the patient may be mute.

The affective state of the depressed patient during the interview is most often sad, but sometimes anxious or even hostile. As the depression becomes more severe, the patient tends to show a diminished range of affects and have an impaired affective reactivity (for example, the patient does not smile in response to social cues).

During the interview it is important to observe the themes evident in the patient's spontaneous conversation. Themes of despair, failure, guilt and death are typical of a depressive episode. The degree of insight may be a marker of the severity of the depressive episode.

Variants

Melancholic (somatic) depression

Some severe depressive episodes can be distinguished which have severe mood symptoms, marked changes in physiological function and significant psychomotor agitation or retardation.

This form of the depressive syndrome is designated 'major depression with melancholia' in DSM-IV and 'depressive episode with somatic syndrome' in ICD-10. The ICD-10 criteria for the 'somatic syndrome' are shown in Table 20.4.2. At least four of the eight symptoms must be present to make the diagnosis. Most 'depressive episodes with somatic syndrome' are also likely to meet the criteria for 'severe depressive episode'.

The clinical significance of making the diagnosis of melancholic depression is that this form of depression is likely to require intensive biological treatment.

Most of the symptoms contributing to the diagnosis of the 'somatic syndrome' are more severe and more specific forms of the symptoms of a 'depressive episode'. It is not just any sleep disturbance, but marked early morning waking which is important. Similarly, it is not just a change in appetite, but a significant loss of weight which is important. The presence and severity of the psychomotor agitation or retardation is the most important sign, since these phenomena can be objectively and systematically observed and rated.[13]

Psychotic depression

This is discussed in Chapter 20.5. The patient with a psychotic depression will usually meet the criteria for a severe depressive episode, often with the 'somatic syndrome'.

Mild and moderate depressive episodes

In clinical practice it is usually not difficult to recognize a 'severe' depressive episode, as the patient manifests eight out of 10 specified symptoms, including all three of the first three symptoms, and these symptoms must have been persistently present ('nearly every day') for at least 2 weeks.

Greater uncertainty may be associated with making the diagnosis of 'mild' or 'moderate' depressive episode, especially in patients who have a long-term history of poor self-esteem, or are temperamentally inclined to worrying, moodiness or irritability. Some research evidence[14] suggests that these temperamental factors can affect the presentation of the depressive syndrome. Thus a person who is a habitual worrier who develops a depressive episode is likely to worry more, and perhaps to withdraw from social contact, or abuse alcohol or anxiolytic drugs. A person who tends to be moody or irritable is likely to become more so in a depressive episode, and may appear demanding, complaining and unreasonable.

Nevertheless the essential and salient characteristic of even a mild or moderate depressive episode is that the patient has a persistent mood change, manifested by at least two of persistent depressed mood, persistent loss of interest and persistent loss of energy, which have been present for at least 2 weeks. These are the symptoms which the interviewer needs to explore in greatest detail because it is their enduring presence which makes the diagnosis clear. Of the additional symptoms contributing to the diagnosis of depressive episode, probably the most common are difficulty with sleep and diminished ability to think and concentrate.

A patient with persistent depressed mood and impaired concentration almost certainly has some functional impairment. A useful approach to this question is to ask the patient about normal daily activities and then assess the extent to which these activities are disrupted by the symptoms. Can the patient do household chores? Does this require unusual effort? Can the

---

Table 20.4.2 ICD-10 criteria for the 'somatic syndrome' (melancholia)[1]

1. Marked loss of interest in activities that are normally pleasurable

2. Lack of emotional reactions to events or activities that normally produce an emotional response

3. Waking in the morning 2 h or more before the usual time

4. Depression worse in the morning

5. Objective evidence of marked psychomotor retardation or agitation

6. Marked loss of appetite

7. Marked loss of libido

patient go to work? Is the patient functional at work? Are even simple leisure activities like watching television disrupted by the patient's mood state? It is this evidence of change in function which permits the identification of a mild or moderate depressive episode, regardless of pre-existing temperamental vulnerabilities.

Depression in the elderly

The symptoms of depression in older people are generally very similar to those in younger age groups and should be assessed in a similar way.[15] Symptoms such as loss of energy, insomnia or change in appetite may also be influenced by comorbid medical illness, but a persistent mood change or loss of interest should prompt consideration of a depressive episode. Older people may tend to minimize their feelings of depression and in these cases a collateral history of loss of interest in usual activities may be found. Not uncommonly older people are seen in the ED following an overdose that may appear medically trivial. These patients should always be carefully assessed for the presence of a depressive syndrome.

'Pseudo-dementia' is a term used to describe patients with a depressive syndrome who present with an apparent change in cognitive function. The patient with depressive pseudo-dementia is likely to have a relatively recent and relatively abrupt change in concentration and memory. In contrast to the patient with dementia, the patient with pseudo-dementia usually shows a great awareness of having memory difficulties and will tend to demonstrate the impairment to the interviewer with considerable anxiety. In addition, the patient with depressive pseudo-dementia manifests other symptoms of a depressive episode.

Differential diagnosis

The differential diagnosis of the depressive syndrome is important because there are several other clinical disorders involving depressed mood or other symptoms of depression which have a different prognosis and treatment.

Brief depressive reaction

A brief depressive reaction (also called 'adjustment disorder with depressed mood'

in DSM-IV) can be diagnosed when a person experiences some depressive symptoms without meeting the full criteria for a depressive episode, following stressful life events. Typically the person describes a depressed mood which is not persistent, that is there are good days and bad days, and the depressed mood can be relieved by distraction or pleasant activities. Common stressful life events include relationship crises or other interpersonal conflicts.

This is often the diagnosis in patients who are seen in the ED following overdose, although care should be taken to inquire about symptoms of a depressive episode. Treatment involves brief psychotherapy aimed at helping the person achieve some resolution of the personal crisis. If the hospital has a crisis counselling service, the patient can be referred to that service for brief therapy. Alternatively the patient can be referred to their GP or other community counselling service. Social work staff in the ED often have good knowledge of local crisis counselling services.

Grief

The symptoms of acute grief can be mood disturbance, guilt, impaired concentration, sleep and appetite disturbance, impaired function in daily activities, and preoccupation with memories of the deceased.[16] There is a considerable overlap with the symptoms of a depressive episode. However, it is customary to respect the feelings of the bereaved and to recognize that it is usually beneficial for the person to be supported through the natural process of grief, preferably by family, friends or other familiar persons such as the family GP.

However, if the symptoms become more severe or more prolonged (such as beyond 6 months) it is appropriate to consider the diagnosis of a depressive episode. Symptoms suggestive of the development of a depressive episode include persistent and progressive lowering of self-esteem, persistent thoughts of death and suicide, markedly impaired concentration and psychomotor retardation.

Bipolar depression

ICD-10 specifies that in a person who has a history of bipolar disorder, a diagnosis of 'depressive episode' should not be made even if the patient meets the criteria for a

depressive episode. Instead the diagnosis of 'bipolar affective episode, current episode mild, moderate or severe depression' should be made. The distinction is important because of the treatment and prognosis. In particular, antidepressant medication should be used very cautiously in the person with bipolar disorder because of the risk of provoking a switch to mania.

The symptoms of a bipolar depressive episode are in themselves not different from the symptoms of any other episode of depression. The distinction therefore rests on a previous history of treatment for bipolar disorder or a history of a manic episode that may not have been treated.

A manic episode, as defined in ICD-10,[1] involves an elevated or irritable mood sustained for at least a week, and at least three (or at least four if the mood is only irritable) of the signs shown in Table 20.4.3. Mania is discussed in more detail in Chapter 20.5.

The depressed patient seen in ED who is suspected of having a bipolar disorder should usually be referred to a psychiatrist for assessment and treatment. Bipolar disorder is a life-long condition, with a high rate of recurrent episodes, which requires specialized pharmacological and psychological management.

Organic mood disorder

Many medical conditions (Table 20.4.4) are especially associated with a typical depressive syndrome. Because the medical

Table 20.4.3 Signs contributing to the diagnosis of a manic episode in ICD-10[1]

1. Increased activity or physical restlessness

2. Increased talkativeness ('pressure of speech')

3. Flight of ideas or subjective experience of thoughts racing

4. Loss of normal inhibitions, resulting in behaviour that is inappropriate to the circumstances

5. Decreased need for sleep

6. Inflated self-esteem or grandiosity

7. Distractibility or constantly changing activity or plans

8. Behaviour that is foolhardy or reckless

9. Marked sexual energy or sexual indiscretions

Table 20.4.4 Medical conditions associated with depressive syndrome
Hyperthyroidism
Hypercalcaemia
Pernicious anaemia
Pancreatic cancer
Lung cancer
Stroke
Alzheimer's dementia
Vascular dementia
Parkinson's disease
Huntington's disease
AIDS
Central nervous system tumour
Multiple sclerosis
Neurosyphillis
Brucellosis

condition is considered likely to have a pathophysiological significance in the development of the depressive syndrome, these conditions are termed 'organic mood disorders'.

Occasionally the depressive syndrome may be the first presentation of a previously undiagnosed medical illness. Clinical or laboratory evidence of hypothyroidism was found in 5% of patients with a depressive syndrome in one series.[17] Hypercalcaemia due to unsuspected hyperparathyroidism very occasionally presents with depressed mood, lethargy or cognitive change as the presenting symptoms.[18] The first presentation of pancreatic cancer with a depressive syndrome is well recognized.[19] A depressive syndrome may be the first presentation of Huntington's disease, before the onset of the movement disorder, and the diagnosis will only be suggested by the family history.[20] Some patients with HIV infection have been found to present with a mood disorder before manifesting other symptoms of AIDS.[21] Because many medical conditions associated with depressive symptoms involve central nervous system disease, any neurological signs should prompt investigation for, for example, unsuspected cerebral tumour.

However, more commonly the depressive syndrome presents in a patient with an already recognized medical illness. In these cases it is important to evaluate carefully the severity and persistence of the depressive symptoms and not dismiss them as an understandable reaction to the illness. Symptoms such as loss of energy, sleep disturbance and anorexia may be difficult to evaluate, as they may be related to other pathophysiological change, but the patient with persistent depressed mood, loss of pleasure in activities, marked loss of self-esteem and feelings of guilt or hopelessness is likely to be experiencing a depressive episode. If such a depressive episode is diagnosed and treated, the patient will experience relief of suffering and a greater ability to deal effectively with other medical problems.

Many drugs have been associated with depressive symptoms, often based on only a few case reports.[22] Medications with a particularly strong association with depression include interferon, isotretinoin, methyldopa, benzodiazepines, digitalis, β-blockers, oral contraceptives and corticosteroids. A useful approach is to consider drugs which have recently been introduced in relation to the time course of the depressive symptoms.

Mood disorder due to psychoactive substance use

Chronic alcohol misuse is frequently associated with depressed mood, low self-esteem and feelings of guilt and hopelessness. Severe sleep disturbance can also be precipitated by rebound wakefulness as blood alcohol levels fall during the night. The person who regularly abuses alcohol is also likely to experience fatigue, impaired concentration, appetite disturbance and loss of sex drive. These symptoms may mimic those due to a depressive episode, such that it is not possible to make a differential diagnosis of a depressive episode while the patient continues to drink, nor is it likely that the depressive symptoms will remit without abstinence. Patients with alcohol-induced mood disorders should be encouraged to attend alcohol detoxification and rehabilitation programmes. There is some evidence that anti-depressant medication may help to reduce both depressive symptoms and alcohol consumption.[23]

Amphetamine withdrawal is often associated with a markedly depressed mood, which usually improves within a few days if the patient remains abstinent.

The abuse of alcohol and other drugs is sometimes an attempt to self-medicate for a pre-existing depressive syndrome. This history should be especially sought in the patient whose abuse of alcohol or other drugs is of recent onset or follows important life-change such as bereavement or divorce. Even if a pre-existing depressive syndrome is identified, however, the patient should be informed that abstinence is necessary for recovery.

Depressive stupor, catatonia and hysterical stupor

Sometimes a patient with profound psychomotor retardation presents with 'depressive stupor', that is the patient is mute but alert, and lacking spontaneous bodily movement. This presentation can give rise to a diagnostic uncertainty in the ED. Neurological conditions, such as pontine haemorrhage causing a 'locked-in syndrome', may have to be considered. Collateral history, if available, generally reveals that the patient with depressive stupor has a preceding history of the gradual onset of a depressive syndrome. Occasionally the condition of depressive stupor may be confused with the catatonic form of schizophrenia. However, in catatonia the patient is likely to display 'waxy flexibility' (maintenance of an uncomfortable posture such as an arm held up for a prolonged period against gravity), echopraxia (imitation of movements) and bizarre posturing and grimacing. These specific motor abnormalities are not usually associated with depressive stupor. Furthermore, the catatonic form of schizophrenia is now quite rare, especially as a first presentation. A final differential diagnosis of depressive stupor is hysterical stupor: in this condition the collateral history shows that the patient was well preceding the abrupt onset of apparent paralysis and mutism. There will usually be a history of a markedly stressful event.

Dysthymia

Dysthymia refers to a chronic form of depression in which the patient experiences symptoms such as lack of enjoyment in life and a gloomy or pessimistic outlook, without meeting the full criteria for a depressive episode. The depressed outlook tends to become interwoven with the personality of the patient, who tends to be somber, self-critical and lacking in confidence and motivation. Dysthymia often has onset in early adult life and can persist for many years. The disorder has been well characterized,[24] and found to be relatively common (about 3% of the general population) in epidemiological studies.[25]

Sometimes patients with a dysthymic disorder develop further symptoms indicating a super-imposed depressive episode, which can be termed a 'double depression'.

Patients with dysthymia may present to EDs as a consequence of suicidal ideation or behaviour. The condition should be regarded as serious because of its chronicity. The patient should be referred to a psychiatrist or mental health service as the treatment can be difficult.[26]

Anxiety

Anxiety disorders include panic disorder (recurrent panic attacks), generalized anxiety disorder (persistent worrying associated with muscular tension and autonomic symptoms), obsessive–compulsive disorder and phobic disorders such as agoraphobia or social phobia. The symptoms of each of these anxiety disorders may occur as a part of the symptoms of a depressive episode. However, primary anxiety disorders are also common. In these cases the patient gives a history of typical anxiety symptoms usually extending over many months or even years. Many patients with primary anxiety disorder go on to also develop a depressive syndrome.

Because of both the overlap in symptoms and the frequent comorbidity, it may be difficult to distinguish primary anxiety disorders from primary depressive disorders in the emergency setting. Probably the most important symptoms are persistent depressed mood and suicidal ideation, which may require inpatient treatment. Patients who do not have persistent depressed mood and suicidal ideation but who have a mixture of other depressive symptoms and anxiety symptoms can be safely directed to their GP or to an outpatient mental health service for further evaluation.

Personality disorder

The concept of personality disorder refers to enduring patterns of behaviour, including especially interpersonal behaviours, which are well outside the usually sanctioned range of behaviours in a particular culture and which are associated with substantial subjective distress or conflict with others. The diagnosis of personality disorder should only be made if the behaviour patterns are persistent, relatively inflexible and have been present since a young age, often beginning in childhood or adolescence.

Although a variety of specific personality disorders have been described, the two most common forms in the ED are antisocial personality disorder and borderline personality disorder.

Persons with antisocial personality have a long-term history of disregard for social rules, usually resulting in a chequered employment history, broken relationships and often violent or criminal behaviour. As a result of personal crisis precipitated by these behaviours, persons with antisocial personality not infrequently present to ED with acute brief depressive reactions, helplessness and suicidal ideation or behaviour. Assessment should be especially directed at clarifying if a superimposed persistent depressive episode is present and the severity of this episode. Inpatient psychiatric treatment is problematic because the patient often has difficulty adhering to ward rules and expectations.

If the depressive symptoms are not severe and seem to be reactive to recent stressors, it is preferable to try to engage the patient in a realistic discussion of the current problems and, if possible, make a referral to crisis counselling. In some cases, however, when the depressive symptoms are more severe and the risk of suicidal behaviour is high, it may be necessary to arrange inpatient admission.

The person with borderline personality disorder displays persistent severely immature interpersonal behaviour, as well as considerable impulsivity and recklessness. The interpersonal behaviours include a strong tendency to see others in 'all good' or 'all bad' terms, and to blame others for the patient's own feelings and behaviours. Reckless and impulsive behaviours include abrupt breaches in relationships, alcohol and other drug abuse, and self-damaging acts such as cutting. Persons with borderline personality often describe chronic feelings of emptiness and loneliness, often associated with suicidal ideation. These features are sometimes misdiagnosed as depression when they may actually represent the patient's usual way of feeling rather than a discrete depressive episode. Because borderline personality disorder is a long-term condition, intervention with the patient who presents in the ED in crisis should if possible be directed towards facilitating or enhancing the patient's engagement with outpatient treatment services.

As many as 50% of patients with borderline personality may also meet the criteria for a depressive episode at any one time.[27] Although a diagnosis of borderline personality may have been made on the basis of the longitudinal history, it is therefore also important to try to assess the severity, persistence and duration of current depressive symptoms. If the patient is already engaged with an outpatient mental health clinician, it is useful to liaise with the therapist regarding recent symptoms and function.

Assessment

The assessment of the patient for depression should cover:

- the current social circumstances of the patient
- recent stressors or precipitating events
- thorough evaluation of the symptoms of the syndrome of clinical depression and their severity
- consideration of previous depressive or manic episodes
- mental state examination
- risk assessment
- consideration of possible medical illness as cause of symptoms
- detailed evaluation of alcohol and other drug use
- identification of treatment services already available to patient.

It is generally a good idea to start the interview with some basic social information. Does the patient live alone? How is he or she occupied or employed? Is there a supportive relationship or other family? This information assists in understanding the context of the symptoms and helps with treatment planning.

Exploration of precipitating events is important partly because these worries are likely to be occupying the mind of the patient and discussion of these issues helps to build rapport in the interview.

Identification of the presence and severity of the depressive symptoms is the most important part of the assessment. Unfortunately, it is often not done systematically and the 'diagnosis' of depression is made only on the basis of a patient's statement about 'being depressed' and one or two other symptoms such as sleep and appetite disturbance. Systematic evaluation requires detailed exploration of the symptoms described above. Particular attention should be paid to the persistence, pervasiveness and duration of the symptoms. If this systematic approach is taken it is possible to determine:

- if the syndrome of clinical depression is present or not
- the severity of the syndrome.

The proper diagnosis of a depressive syndrome and the assessment of the severity of the syndrome are of major importance in treatment planning.

There may be insufficient time in an emergency interview to explore fully the previous psychiatric history. However, it is useful to ask if the patient has been depressed before, whether or not any previous episodes were treated and what was the response to previous treatment. It is also important to identify any previous episodes of mania in case the depressive episode may be a presentation of bipolar disorder.

Mental state examination focuses on the signs described above. Persistently sad affect and noticeable psychomotor agitation or retardation are indicators of more severe depression. Similarly, if the patient's conversation is very preoccupied with themes of failure, despair, guilt or death the depression is likely to be more severe. Inquiry about these matters should be extended to look for delusional beliefs. Useful questions may include 'Do you feel responsible for bad things happening?', 'Do you feel there is something drastically wrong with you?' or 'Do you believe you deserve punishment?'. Understanding the patient's level of insight into his or her condition is also important to treatment planning, particularly if

involuntary treatment should become necessary due to the risk of suicide.

Risk assessment is multi-faceted. If the patient has attempted suicide through overdose or other means, inquiry should be made about the circumstances of this attempt, the patient's understanding of the lethality of the attempt and whether or not the patient sought help afterwards or made an effort to conceal the attempt. The patient's current thoughts about suicide and his or her attitude to suicide are also relevant. Many patients admit to having thoughts of suicide but indicate that they would be deterred from suicidal action by, for example, having responsibility for dependent children. The disappearance of these 'protective factors' from a patient's considerations is an indicator of worsening risk. Patients with psychotic depression may be at higher risk because they lack such 'emotional' constraints on suicidal behaviour. Other factors associated with increased suicide risk include lack of supportive relationship, living alone, being unemployed and current alcohol abuse.

A primary medical condition causing depressive symptoms is likely to be suggested by other symptoms and signs, or be pre-existing. There are no mandatory investigations for the assessment of a depressive episode, although checking thyroid biochemistry is sensible.

Inquiry should be made about alcohol and other drug-use patterns, and especially recent changes in pattern use. A person with long-standing alcohol or other drug

abuse is likely to have a substance-induced mood disorder, and needs to address this as the major focus of treatment. A recent marked increase in alcohol or other drug use may indicate an attempt to self-medicate for a depressive syndrome.

It is always useful to ask the patient if she or he is currently seeing a psychiatrist, psychologist or other mental health therapist, or has a good relationship with a trusted GP. These existing healthcare professionals can often be the natural starting point in planning treatment interventions.

Treatment

Treatment for a depressive episode involves the prescription of specific antidepressant medication or a specific course of psychotherapy or both.

Medications

Commonly used first-line antidepressant medications are shown in Table 20.4.5. Because no one of these medications has been shown consistently to have superior efficacy, choice of medication is based on the acceptability of the side effect profile and previous treatment response.

The selective serotonin re-uptake inhibitors (SSRIs) are usually well tolerated and are a good first choice. Some patients experience agitation, nausea or gastrointestinal hypermotility when they start SSRI medications. These symptoms usually settle in a week or two. The most troublesome

Table 20.4.5	Commonly used antidepressant medications		
Drug	Class	Usual daily oral dose range (mg)	Half life (hours)
Fluoxetine	SSRI	20–60	24–144
Citalopram	SSRI	20–40	23–45
Escitalopram	SSRI	10–20	27–32
Fluvoxamine	SSRI	100–300	9–28
Paroxetine	SSRI	10–40	3–65
Sertraline	SSRI	50–200	22–36
Venlafaxine	SNRI	75–225	3–7
Moclobemide	RIMA	450–600	1–3
Mirtazapine	–	30–60	20–40
Reboxitene	–	8–10	12–13

SSRI, selective serotonin re-uptake inhibitor; SNRI, serotonin and noradrenaline re-uptake inhibitor; RIMA, reversible monoamine oxidase inhibitor.

long-term side effect of SSRIs is sexual dysfunction (especially delayed ejaculation or anorgasmia). These side effects sometimes require a change of medication. The side effects of venlafaxine are similar to SSRIs, with the addition of excessive sweating and itch at high doses.

Mirtazapine has useful sedating properties and can be very helpful in a patient with marked insomnia or agitation. Because it stimulates appetite, its use is limited in patients with a weight problem. Mirtazapine, reboxitine and moclobemide are useful alternatives for patients who experience sexual dysfunction with SSRIs or venlafaxine.

Tricyclic antidepressants (e.g. imipramine, amitriptyline and dothiepin) and irreversible monoamine oxidase inhibitors (MAOIs; phenelzine and tranylcypromine) continue to be prescribed for some patients, but they tend not to be first-line drugs. The use of tricyclics has decreased because of side effects (especially anticholinergic) and because of their cardiac toxicity in overdose. Irreversible MAOIs are generally inconvenient to take because of the need for dietary restrictions.

Psychotherapy

The psychotherapies commonly used for depression include supportive psychotherapy, cognitive behavioural therapy (CBT) and interpersonal psychotherapy (IPT). Most psychiatrists and clinical psychologists have appropriate training and skills to offer one or more of these therapies. It is also increasingly common for GPs and other health professionals such as social workers and occupational therapists to have received training in these therapies.

Supportive psychotherapy is the least well defined of the psychotherapeutic treatments. The core of the treatment is a supportive relationship, education about the nature of depression and practical advice. CBT is a structured psychotherapy, usually involving 10–20 sessions. The behavioural techniques include reversing social isolation, scheduling relaxing or pleasurable activities and working with family members to provide incentives for helpful behaviours. The main part of the therapy involves 'cognitive restructuring', a systematic exploration of the patient's unhelpful thought patterns, followed by collaborative work to help the patient substitute more positive responses.[28]

IPT is also a structured psychotherapy, typically of about 16 sessions. The therapy focuses on helping the patient to make changes in his or her interpersonal relationships which may be contributing to the depressive syndrome.[29]

Evidence

All currently available antidepressants have been shown to achieve better symptom reduction than placebo, with no one antidepressant consistently demonstrating superior efficacy.[30] In drug trials, up to 40% of patients in the placebo arm show improvement, which may include the non-specific effects of supportive interventions, as well as spontaneous remissions.[31] As the natural history of depression in a community sample (which includes relatively minor, untreated cases) shows a median episode duration of 12 weeks, spontaneous remission appears to be not uncommon.[32] Patients with psychotic depression respond better to the combination of an antidepressant and an antipsychotic medication than to an antidepressant medication alone.[33]

Both CBT and IPT have been shown to be effective in achieving symptom reduction compared to pill placebo control.[34,35] CBT and IPT have been shown to be as effective as medication for mild-to-moderate depression.[35] For a severe depressive episode, psychotherapy alone is not as effective as medication alone or a medication-psychotherapy combination.[36]

There are no systematic data regarding supportive psychotherapy (as it is not a standardized treatment) but substantial clinical experience attests to its efficacy.

Mild-to-moderate depressive episodes

As long as the suicide risk is containable, the great majority of these patients can be treated as outpatients. The most important part of treatment planning in ED is therefore to identify an appropriate referral pathway. If the patient is already in contact with a mental health professional or has a trusted GP, it is preferable to refer the patient back to these persons and, if possible, make phone contact with that doctor or therapist with advice regarding the emergency presentation. If the patient does not have their own doctor or mental health professional, it is appropriate to refer the patient to an outpatient mental health service.

Patients with mild-to-moderate depressive episodes can improve with either medication or psychotherapy, and can be advised to discuss these treatment options with the follow-up doctor. It is not essential to start the antidepressant medication in the ED; it is probably more appropriate to leave this to the follow-up doctor who can monitor for efficacy and side effects.

Some patients may only have mild-to-moderate symptoms but nevertheless be at significant suicidal risk, associated with recent suicidal behaviour and persistent suicidal ideation. The risk is increased if the patient lives alone. Such patients require admission to a psychiatry ward, where the options for medication and psychotherapy can be further explored.

Severe depressive episodes

Most patients with severe depressive episodes will be admitted because of significant suicide risk or substantial functional impairment. The evidence suggests that these patients require treatment with antidepressant medication and are often initially too symptomatic to engage in psychotherapy. Classical indications for electroconvulsive therapy are psychotic depression and severe retarded depression (especially if the patient has inadequate oral intake).

Controversies and future directions

❶ Population-based studies indicate that clinical depression is very common, possibly increasing in prevalence, and significantly under-treated.

❷ A major challenge for all health services is to improve the rate of case identification.

❸ Equally important will be the further development of effective referral pathways to appropriate treatment.

References

1. World Health Organization. The ICD-10 classification of mental and behavioural disorders. Geneva: WHO; 1993.
2. American Psychiatric Association. Diagnostic and statistical manual of mental disorders. 4th edn. American Psychiatric Association: Washington DC; 1994.
3. Joyce P. Epidemiology of mood disorders. In: Gelder M, Lopez-Ibor J, Andreasen N, eds. New Oxford textbook of psychiatry. Oxford: Oxford University Press; 2000: 695–701.
4. Judd J. The clinical course of unipolar major depressive disorders. Archives of General Psychiatry 1997; 54: 989–991.
5. Katz M, Secunda S, Hirschfeld R, et al. NIMH clinical research branch collaborative program on the psychobiology of depression. Archives of General Psychiatry 1979; 36: 765–771.
6. Cross National Collaborative Group. The changing rate of major depression. Cross national comparisons. Journal of American Medical Association 1992; 268: 3098–3105.
7. Tennant C. Life events, stress and depression: a review of recent findings. Australian and New Zealand Journal of Psychiatry 2002; 36: 173–182.
8. Frank E, Anderson B, Reynolds C. Life events and research diagnostic criteria endogenous subtype. Archives of General Psychiatry 1994; 51: 519–524.
9. Kendler K, Thornton L, Gardner C. Stressful life events and previous episodes in the etiology of major depression in women: an evaluation of the 'kindling' hypothesis. American Journal of Psychiatry 2000; 157: 1243–1251.
10. Schildkraut J. The catecholamine hypothesis of affective disorders: a review of supporting evidence. American Journal of Psychiatry 1965; 122: 509–522.
11. Jacobs B, Praag H, Gage F. Adult brain neurogenesis and psychiatry: a novel theory of depression. Molecular Psychiatry 2000; 5: 262–269.
12. Murray C, Lopez A. The global burden of disease and global health statistics. Boston: Harvard University Press; 1996.
13. Parker G, Hadzi-Pavlovic D. Melancholia: a disorder of movement and mood. Cambridge: Cambridge University Press; 1996.
14. Parker G, Hadzi-Pavlovic D, Roussos J, et al. Non-melancholic depression: the contribution of personality, anxiety and life-events to subclassification. Psychological Medicine 1998; 28: 1209–1219.
15. Musetti L, Perugi G, Soriani A, et al. Depression before and after age 65: a re-examination. British Journal of Psychiatry 1989; 155: 330–336.
16. Lindemann E. The symptomatology and management of acute grief. American Journal of Psychiatry 1944; 101: 141.
17. Gold M, Pottash A, Extein I. Hypothyroidism and depression. Journal of the American Medical Association 1981; 245: 1919–1922.
18. Watson L. Clinical aspects of hyperparathyroidism. Proceedings of the Royal Society of Medicine 1968; 61: 1123.
19. Joffe R, Rubinow D, Denicoff K, et al. Depression and carcinoma of the pancreas. General Hospital of Psychiatry 1986; 8: 241–245.
20. Folstein S, Abbott M, Chase G, et al. The association of affective disorder with Huntington's disease in a case series and in families. Psychological Medicine 1983; 13: 537–542.
21. Atkinson J, Grant I, Kennedy C et al. Prevalence of psychiatric disorders among men infected with human immunodeficiency virus. Archives of General Psychiatry 1988; 45: 859–864.
22. Hales R, Yudofsky S. The American psychiatric publishing textbook of clinical psychiatry. 4th edn. Washington: American Psychiatric Publishing; 2003: 462–463.
23. Cornelius J, Salloun I, Ehler J, et al. Fluoxetine reduced depressive symptoms and alcohol consumption in patients with co-morbid major depression and alcohol dependence. Archives of General Psychiatry 1997; 54: 700–705.
24. Akiskal H, Cassano G, eds. Dysthymia and the spectrum of chronic depressions. New York: Guildford Press; 1997.
25. Waintraub L, Guelfi J. Nosological validity of dysthymia. Part 1, historical, epidemiological and clinical data. European Psychiatry 1998; 13: 173–180.
26. Haykal R, Akiskal H. The long-term outcome of dysthymia in private practice. Clinical features, temperament and the art of management. Journal of Clinical Psychiatry 1999; 60: 508–518.
27. Gunderson J. Borderline personality disorder: a clinical guide. Washington: American Psychiatric Publishing; 2001.
28. Seligman M. Learned optimism. New York: Random House; 1991.
29. Weissman M, Markowitz J, Klerman G. Comprehensive guide to interpersonal psychotherapy. New York: Basic Books; 2000.
30. Nemeroff C, Schatzberg A. Pharmacological treatment of unipolar depression. In: Nathan P, Gorman J, eds. A guide to treatments that work. New York: Oxford University Press; 1998: 212–215.
31. Paykel E, Scott J. Treatment of mood disorders. In: Gelder M, Lopez-Ibor J, Andreasen, N, eds. New Oxford textbook of psychiatry. Oxford: Oxford University Press; 2000: 724–736.
32. Eaton W, Anthony J, Gallo G, et al. Natural history of diagnostic interview schedule/DSM-IV major depression: the Baltimore epidemiologic catchment area follow-up. Archives of General Psychiatry 1997; 54: 993–999.
33. Schatzberg A, Rothschild A. Psychotic (delusional) major depression: should it be included as a distinct syndrome in DSM-IV? American Journal of Psychiatry 1992; 149: 733–745.
34. Dobson K. A meta-analysis of the efficacy of cognitive therapy for depression. Journal of Consulting and Clinical Psychology 1988; 57: 414–419.
35. Elkin I, Shea M, Watkins J, et al. National Institute of Mental Health treatment of depression collaborative treatment programme. Archives of General Psychiatry 1992; 46: 971–982.
36. Thase M, Greenhouse J, Frank E, et al. Treatment of major depression with psychotherapy or psychotherapy-pharmacotherapy combinations. Archives of General Psychiatry 1997; 54: 1009–1015.

20.5 PSYCHOSIS

Simon Byrne

ESSENTIALS

1 In the age of community mental health treatment, emergency departments have become major sites for the assessment of patients with psychosis.

2 It is important to distinguish psychiatric causes of psychosis from psychosis due to medical conditions or to drug abuse.

3 Attention must be given to the proper management of the patient with psychosis in the emergency department environment.

4 Disposition decisions, including community referral or hospitalization, depend on the collection of information about treatment history, community supports and risk assessment, as well as assessment of the mental state of the patient.

Introduction

Psychotic illness is a frequent cause of presentation to the emergency department (ED), accounting for 0.5–1.0% of all visits and 10–20% of all mental health presentations.[1,2] Because these patients are usually severely mentally unwell, they also account for a significant share of the workload of EDs.

The tasks of the ED staff in relation to patients with psychotic illness are complex and varied. Initially there is usually a need for containment and stabilization of an aroused and frightened patient with impaired reality testing. The patient is often in the hospital unwillingly and frequently following a major crisis in the community or at home. There is often a need to manage behavioural disturbance, potentially involving risk of harm to the patient, staff or others, while the patient remains in the ED for often lengthy periods of assessment and for the implementation of disposition plans. It is also important to exclude medical causes for the psychotic symptoms and to consider the presence of comorbid medical conditions. In determining disposition, consideration must be given to the need for voluntary or involuntary admission, or alternatively referral to an array of community-based treatment services. Finally, it is often useful to involve families and other carers in both the assessment phase and in treatment planning. These tasks are summarized in Table 20.5.1.

Classification

Traditionally psychotic illnesses were classified into 'functional' (i.e. non-organic) psychoses and 'organic' psychoses. Developments in psychiatric nosology have expanded this classification and the ICD-10 Classification of Mental and Behavioural Disorders[3] now contains at least 16 different diagnoses, many with several sub-types, which could be used to describe patients with psychotic symptoms.

In emergency practice, however, the differentiation of the specific psychiatric syndrome is not always possible. The pragmatic classification shown in Table 20.5.2 is based on:

Table 20.5.1 Tasks of ED in relation to the patient with psychosis
1. Stabilization of the aroused or frightened patient
2. Management of behavioural disturbance in the ED
3. Exclusion of medical causes for the psychiatric presentation
4. Assessing the presence of comorbid medical illness
5. Determining the need for voluntary or involuntary admission
6. Arranging referral to community services
7. Liaison with family and other carers

ED, emergency department.

Table 20.5.2 Pragmatic classification of patients with psychotic symptoms

1. Psychotic symptoms due to general medical condition
  1.1. Delirium
  1.2. Dementia
  1.3. Psychosis in clear consciousness without cognitive impairment
  1.4. Psychosis caused by medications

2. Acute and chronic schizophrenia
3. Mania with psychosis
4. Depression with psychosis
5. Substance-induced psychosis
6. Psychotic-like reactive states

- excluding medical causes for the psychotic presentation
- considering the role of alcohol and other drugs of abuse
- making a provisional psychiatric diagnosis as a guide to initial management and
- considering the possibility that the symptoms may be related primarily to psychological stress.

A description of each of these categories is given in the section on clinical features.

Epidemiology and prognosis

The two principal 'non-organic' conditions which involve psychotic presentations are schizophrenia and bipolar affective disorder.

The prevalence of schizophrenia is 0.2–0.5% of the population. It is not a rare disorder. The male:female ratio is 1:1. Onset can be at any age, but mostly before the age of 30.[4]

Schizophrenia is usually a chronic condition, but with a variable course. In the long term, about 20% of cases have a good recovery, 20% have recurrent episodes with good recovery between episodes, 40% have recurrent episodes with incomplete remission and 20% have a severe chronic course.[5] The 20-year suicide rate may be as high as 14–22%.[5]

The prevalence of bipolar disorder (which by definition means that the patient has had at least one manic episode) is about 1.0% of the population. The male:female ratio is 1:1. The onset is often in late adolescence and 95% of cases have onset before the age of 26.[6]

A patient who has had one episode of mania has about an 80% chance of a recurrence within 5 years. Although there is usually a good recovery between episodes, there is a very high rate of recurrence, with an average of one episode of mania or depression every 2 years, although the frequency of episodes in the individual case varies greatly.[7] The 22-year suicide rate is 13%.[7]

Aetiology and prevention

The aetiology of schizophrenia and bipolar disorder is not well understood, despite intensive research. Both disorders involve genetic and environmental factors. A person who has one parent with schizophrenia has about a 10% chance of developing the disorder; this is similar for bipolar disorder. There is insufficient knowledge about the aetiology of either disorder to suggest effective strategies for primary prevention.

There is considerable scope for secondary prevention, that is early diagnosis and prompt treatment, especially in relation to recurrent episodes. Strategies include education of patients and families, the identification of early warning signs of relapse and the use of maintenance and prophylactic medication.[8] ED staff can make a major contribution to this preventative work by emphasizing the importance of continuing treatment and facilitating engagement with generalist and specialist mental health services.

Clinical features

Psychiatric symptoms due to a general medical condition

Delirium

Delirious patients often manifest psychiatric symptoms. Visual illusions (misperception of real objects, such as mistaking an innocuous object for a malevolent figure or animal) and delusions of persecution (such as the patient believing he is being poisoned by the doctors and nurses) are particularly common. Other symptoms including auditory hallucinations, affective lability, apparent formal thought disorder, and grandiose or religious delusions.

The pathognomonic features of delirium are disorientation (especially for time and place) and a fluctuating conscious state. Not uncommonly the patient plucks at the air or the bedclothes in apparent response to visual illusions or hallucinations. The abnormalities of mental state can fluctuate widely over the course of a day from relative lucidity to marked disturbance.

The delirious patient usually has a history or symptoms of a medical disorder and manifests abnormalities of vital signs or other abnormalities on physical examination or laboratory investigation.

The differentiation of medical and psychiatric causes of altered mental state is discussed in detail in Chapter 20.2.

Dementia

Psychotic symptoms in dementia can include auditory and visual hallucinations, delusions (often persecutory) and delusional misidentification (e.g. the delusion that a person closely related to the patient has been replaced by a double). These psychotic symptoms are common in dementias of all types, including Alzheimer's and vascular dementias. A mean prevalence of 44% has been found across several cross-sectional samples.[9] The diagnosis of dementia depends on the presence of multiple cognitive deficits, and will usually be evident from other features of the history and presentation. A change in the mental state of a patient with dementia should prompt consideration of superimposed delirium.

Psychosis in clear consciousness without cognitive impairment

Occasionally patients present with psychotic symptoms of organic cause, without features of delirium or dementia. The variety of medical conditions associated with psychotic presentations is shown in Table 20.5.3. Although these disorders are relatively rare as the cause of psychiatric presentation, they should be especially considered in relation to a patient with new-onset psychosis over the age of 40 (i.e. older than the usual age of onset of the much more common schizophrenia and bipolar disorder).

In emergency practice, the psychoses associated with epilepsy are probably those most likely to be associated with uncertainty in management. These psychoses are of two types. Some patients with established epilepsy develop chronic inter-ictal psychosis, that is a psychosis without specific

Table 20.5.3 Medical causes of psychotic presentations
Epilepsy
Hypo- or hyper-thyroidism
Huntington's disease
Wilson's disease
Porphyria
B12 deficiency
Cerebral neoplasm
Stroke
Viral encephalitis
Neurosyphilis
AIDS

temporal relationship to seizure activity. The clinical picture is often like schizophrenia and the disorder should be treated in its own right with anti-psychotic medication.[10] The second presentation is of a post-ictal psychosis, usually following a cluster of seizures and sometimes with a lucid interval of 1 or 2 days. The patient can present with both schizophrenia-like and mood symptoms. The mental state spontaneously returns to normal within a few days, as in the more common post-ictal delirium.[11]

Psychoses caused by prescribed medications

A long list of medications, many based on sporadic case reports, can sometimes be associated with psychotic symptoms.[12] The two most common are corticosteroids and dopamine agonists.

Steroid psychosis usually presents a manic-like picture and can show florid psychosis. It is most often associated with doses greater than 40 mg equivalents of prednisolone per day.[13]

Dopamine agonists used in the treatment of Parkinson's disease like levodopa and bromocriptine are associated with auditory and visual hallucinations, persecutory delusions and hypomania. The psychotic symptoms are dose-related but dose reductions may be associated with severe exacerbation of Parkinsonian symptoms.[14]

Acute and chronic schizophrenia

The symptoms of schizophrenia include the 'positive' symptoms of acute psychosis and the 'negative' symptoms such as apathy and social withdrawal.

Positive symptoms involve delusions hallucinations and formal thought disorder. The content of delusions may include beliefs that the patient is an important person (grandiose), that the patient has special communication with deities or spirits (religiose) or that there is something awry with the patient's body or the world (hypochondriacal and nihilistic). The most common delusions are beliefs that other persons or the TV or radio are making special reference to the person (delusions of reference) and beliefs that certain persons or agencies are engaged in conspiracies to harm the patient (delusions of persecution).

Hallucinations are usually auditory but can be in any sensory modality. The specific types of auditory hallucinations first described by Schneider,[15] although not specific to schizophrenia, are strongly supportive of the diagnosis. These include a voice making a running commentary on the patient's actions, two or more voices discussing or arguing about the patient and a voice repeating the patient's thoughts aloud.

Sometimes the most obvious positive symptom of psychosis is formal thought disorder. This usually takes the form of loosening of associations (lack of logical connection between statements) and tangential (off the point) replies to questions. The effect of these symptoms is to make it difficult or impossible to take a sequential history. In more severe cases the language itself becomes incoherent as grammatical conventions are abandoned and invented words ('neologisms') are used. In the emergency setting, the less severe forms of formal thought disorder may also be shown by highly anxious, delirious or intoxicated patients.

The negative symptoms include blunting of affect (lack of emotional response), apathy (loss of volition), poverty of speech (severely diminished verbal communication) and autistic withdrawal from social interaction. These symptoms can be difficult to distinguish in the acute setting from the effects of co-morbid depression or from the bradykinesia caused by anti-psychotic medications.

In emergency practice the three most common types of presentation of schizophrenia are the first psychotic episode, acute psychotic relapse of an established illness and a social crisis in a patient with chronic schizophrenia. It is useful to distinguish these types of presentation because of the management implications.

The patient with a first episode of psychosis is typically a young adult who has been brought to the ED by family or police often following months of concern about deterioration in the patient's mental state or behaviour. Sometimes there will have been an acute episode of bizarre, suicidal or aggressive behaviour. Exclusion of medical causes of psychosis is important in the first episode, especially in the older patient. It may be difficult to be certain whether the syndrome is one of mania (see below) or schizophrenia, but this distinction is not crucial in emergency assessment. More important is the fact that the patient is likely to be frightened and confused, as is also the family. The patient may require involuntary hospitalization.

The acute relapse of an established illness can also involve considerable distress to the patient and family. In these cases it is useful to look for changes in medication, problems in compliance, changes in the treatment system such as absence of the treating doctor, alcohol and other drug abuse, and recent stressful events. It may be possible to avoid hospitalization.

Patients with chronic schizophrenia are now treated most frequently through community mental health services. They may present with an exacerbation of the psychosis for the reasons outlined above. However, the presentation is often related to social problems, such as conflict with family or difficulties with accommodation or finances. In these cases it can be very useful to communicate with the community mental health services to clarify the patient's baseline level of function and current problems. Some patients with chronic illness are effectively homeless and have poor engagement with community services, irregular medication use and ongoing drug abuse. Although it is difficult in a busy ED, these patients ideally need some work towards establishment of continuity of care and long-term treatment plans.

The term 'schizo-affective disorder' has been used to describe an illness in which patients show typical symptoms of schizophrenia as well as having definite manic or depressive episodes. In practice in the ED such patients can be assessed and managed in a similar way to patients with schizophrenia.

Mania with psychotic symptoms

The manic syndrome is one form of presentation of bipolar disorder, the others being a depressive episode and mixed affective psychosis.

The typical manic syndrome is very distinctive. The patient presents with euphoric or irritable affect, pressure of speech (rapid, continuous speech which is difficult to interrupt), distractibility, and disinhibited or over-familiar behaviour. If delusions are present, they are grandiose (that the patient has an important mission) or persecutory (e.g. that other persons are engaged in a conspiracy to prevent the patient fulfilling his or her destiny). Collateral history will usually show that the patient has been well until the last few days, when the patient has become overactive and disorganized with a markedly decreased need for sleep.

In mixed affective psychosis, the patient often shows typically manic arousal and irritability, but may have a depressive theme evident in the content of speech. Depressive psychosis is discussed below.

Sometimes a delirious patient with affective lability, irritability, disinhibition and distractibility may be misdiagnosed as manic. The diagnosis should be considered in the older patient without previous history of bipolar disorder. The distinction can be made on the basis of the impairment of cognitive function (disorientation, fluctuating conscious state and memory impairment) in delirium, and clinical or laboratory evidence of medical illness.

It may be difficult to distinguish acute mania from acute schizophrenia in the emergency setting, especially in first episode cases. Being certain of the diagnosis is not crucial, as the short-term management is similar (see below).

Major depression with psychotic features

Patients who exhibit psychotic features during a depressive syndrome are severely depressed. The content of delusions and hallucinations relates to the patient's feelings of worthlessness or guilt, and may include the conviction that the patient should die. Because the patient is unable to rationally evaluate these beliefs, the risk of suicidal actions is high and these patients should be closely supervised.

The patient with a depressive psychosis will show the other typical features of a depressive syndrome. Most often, the mental state assessment will show a patient who lacks spontaneity and is withdrawn and sad. Occasionally, however, the patient may be agitated and irritable.

The differential diagnosis and management of depressive syndromes are discussed in Chapter 20.4.

Substance-induced psychosis

Drugs of abuse are associated with psychotic presentations in several ways: psychosis as a manifestation of acute intoxication, psychosis during withdrawal reactions, chronic psychosis following prolonged use and the exacerbation of pre-existing psychotic illness due to drug abuse. Drugs of abuse which may contribute to psychosis are listed in Table 20.5.4.

The psychosis associated with intoxication may include auditory and visual hallucinations, and persecutory or grandiose delusions. The patient is usually agitated, highly anxious and incoherent, and often shows autonomic signs such as dilated pupils. Some drugs, such as phencyclidine, are particularly associated with disinhibited rage. Management is focused on ensuring safety and maintaining vital functions in the expectation that the psychosis will clear when the intoxication resolves.

Table 20.5.4 Drugs of abuse associated with psychosis
Amphetamine and methamphetamine
Methylenedioxymethamphetamine (MMDA, Ecstasy)
Cocaine
Phencyclidine
Ketamine
LSD
Cannabis
Alcohol
Benzodiazepines

Alcohol and benzodiazepines can lead to psychotic symptoms (most commonly visual hallucinations) in the context of withdrawal delirium. The psychotic symptoms resolve through management of the withdrawal with benzodiazepines.

Amphetamine (and amphetamine derivatives), phencyclidine and lysergic acid diethylamide (LSD) have all been associated with chronic psychosis which can persist for weeks or months after cessation of drug use.[16–18] Whether or not the patients who develop these chronic psychoses may have been predisposed to psychotic illness is controversial, but nevertheless the psychosis should not be regarded purely as an intoxication effect but treated in its own right. Amphetamine dugs are most frequently associated with this chronic psychosis, usually following prolonged heavy amphetamine abuse. The clinical picture can be quite distinctive, including beliefs that the patient is being watched or followed or that thoughts may be monitored with an implanted device. 'Running commentary' auditory hallucinations may occur as well as tactile hallucinations, which may lead the patient to excoriate the skin in pursuit of a supposed infestation with insects.

The role of cannabis as a cause of chronic schizophrenia-like psychosis is uncertain, although cannabis frequently exacerbates psychotic symptoms in patients with an existing illness.[19]

Alcoholic hallucinosis is a relatively uncommon condition found in some patients with long-term alcohol abuse histories. The patient experiences auditory hallucinations of a derogatory or 'running commentary' type in clear consciousness, without being in a withdrawal state. This disorder may persist for weeks or months and the symptoms may respond to antipsychotic medications.

Because alcohol and drug abuse can exacerbate psychosis in patients with an established schizophrenic or bipolar disorder, inquiry should be made into their use with every patient.

Psychotic-like reactive states

Patients with histories of severe personality disorder, post-traumatic stress disorder and dissociative disorder sometimes present with quasi-psychotic states.[20,21] These episodes usually follow acute stress, such as a relationship or other social crisis, or events which trigger recall of traumatic experiences. The patient is usually extremely anxious and may have impaired verbal communication, further complicating assessment. Psychotic-like experiences can include intense subjective experiences of a derogatory internal monologue, which can seem like auditory hallucinations, or intense fears of being harmed which mimic persecutory delusions. Some patients' recall of traumatic experiences is so persistent and vivid that it seems as if it is actually happening again.

When such patients are seen in emergency settings, they often need containment and assessment in a similar manner to patients with true psychoses. Benzodiazepines and sedative anti-psychotic medications (see below) are often useful in reducing the high level of arousal.

Assessment

Objectives and sources of information

The assessment of the psychotic patient in ED has several objectives. The basic questions are:

- Is the altered mental state primarily due to a medical condition?
- To what extent are drugs or alcohol contributory?
- Can a primary psychiatric diagnosis be made?
- Can the patient be treated at home or is hospitalization necessary?
- Should the patient be detained under the mental health act?

These questions cannot be answered by considering only the clinical state of the patient. Decisions about risk assessment and disposition depend on a careful consideration of the social circumstances of the patient, recent events which have led to the emergency presentation and past and current engagement with community mental health treatment services. Diagnostic clarification is often greatly assisted by previous treatment records, which can usually be fairly quickly accessed.

Information should be sought from family and community mental health teams about recent function, symptoms, dangerous behaviours and alcohol and other drug use. The police who sometimes bring patients with psychosis to ED can often give important information about the circumstances which led to the presentation.

The assessment process is not a single one-off review of the patient's mental state, nor is it a linear process in which the various objectives of assessment can be serially addressed. It tends rather to be a back and forth process as multiple lines of inquiry are simultaneously pursued and the clinical data re-evaluated in the light of new information.

At the end of the assessment process it should be possible to record a summary of the various parameters of assessment as outlined in Table 20.5.5, which can then form the basis for management planning.

Initial stabilization of the patient

In order that conditions can be created for an adequate assessment, there is an immediate need to stabilize the patient. The acutely psychotic patient has distorted understanding and may be an unwilling participant in the process. It is preferable to try and engage the patient in a calm manner with straightforward and clear expectation of the need for assessment. The patient's own concerns and perceptions of the problem are worth listening to without initially trying to seek answers to specific questions. This attention is reassuring to the patient and provides an opportunity

Table 20.5.5 The psychotic patient – brief assessment schedule
1. Circumstances of referral
2. Presenting problem
3. Social circumstances
4. Previous treatment
5. Current mental health services
6. Current medication
7. Alcohol and other drug use
8. Mental state examination
9. Medical assessment and investigations
10. Provisional diagnosis
11. Risk assessment
12. Treatment and disposition plan

for observation of the mental state, even if the patient's account lacks coherence.

Patients who are aroused and agitated, intoxicated or have persecutory delusions may pose a risk of violent or aggressive behaviour. In these cases it is important to monitor safety by having security staff present, by not assessing the patient in a confined space and by remaining out of striking distance and not turning one's back on the patient. Sometimes the patient may have to be sedated before much assessment can be made. Sedating the aroused patient is discussed in Chapter 20.7.

Moderate use of benzodiazepines need not significantly complicate the mental state assessment, although these drugs may exacerbate delirium. High doses of benzodiazepines (especially diazepam which has active metabolites with long half lives) can produce a prolonged delirium, which will delay the assessment process.

Mental state assessment

Especially in the aroused patient, it is often difficult to carry out a formal mental state examination. Nevertheless it is possible to collect a lot of information by simple observation. The general appearance can give clues to the patient's level of self care. The rate and mode of speech can suggest the presence of formal thought disorder. Hostile or euphoric affects may suggest a manic syndrome or intoxication. Patients may spontaneously reveal delusional ideas or auditory hallucinations, or may admit to these on specific questioning. Orientation to time and place and recent events should always be assessed because of the strong association of disorientation with delirium. Although detailed cognitive assessment is usually not possible, an attempt should be made to assess short-term memory function, and attention and concentration.

As with all aspects of assessment, the assessment of mental state should not be based on a single evaluation but on serial assessments by medical staff and the observations of the nursing staff throughout the time the patient is in the ED.

Risk assessment

It is important to inquire directly about suicidal and homicidal ideation and to record the patient's statements. However, risk assessment depends on an objective evaluation of the whole situation. A patient with persistent persecutory beliefs may be at significant risk of behaving aggressively towards perceived persecutors, even though he or she may deny hostile intent. Conversely, a patient's expression of suicidal ideation may reflect long-standing frustration and dissatisfaction (which may be alleviated by receiving help) rather than intent to act in a suicidal manner. The degree to which the patient can exercise judgement is also important. A floridly psychotic or grossly disorganized patient is at greater risk than a patient with chronic symptoms who presents with a social crisis. The home situation and the views of family should also be considered and taken very seriously. Inquiry should be also made into the provision of care for dependent children.

Decisions about hospital admission and involuntary detention usually focus appropriately on danger to self and others. Uncertainty may sometimes arise regarding the use of mental health act detention powers in relation to manic (and some schizophrenic) patients who clearly deny any intent to harm themselves or others, but who are clearly in need of treatment, lack insight and are very unlikely to receive treatment unless compulsorily detained. Most jurisdictions, however, make some provision in their mental health legislation for such patients to be detained in the interests of their health or to prevent other 'harms' such as harm to reputation. The decision to detain involves balancing the patient's right to autonomy against the probable risks of not receiving treatment. In general, such a patient has only been brought to ED because family, friends or other carers have been concerned about the behaviour or mental state of the patient, and it is therefore wise to consult with these concerned others if there is doubt about the decision to detain.

Medical evaluation and investigation

Medical evaluation has three goals: excluding delirium (or dementia), considering other organic causes of psychosis and assessing for the presence of comorbid medical illness.

The practice of 'medical clearance' prior to psychiatric evaluation may detract from a comprehensive evaluation of the patient. A more satisfactory process is to compile an adequate history of the presenting illness, assess the mental state, review the medications and alcohol and other drug use, consider previous medical history, check vital signs and carry out as comprehensive a physical examination as possible, with particular attention to signs of injury, poisoning or intoxication.[22] In services where both emergency physicians and psychiatrists are available, direct discussion about cases of uncertain diagnosis is useful.

Medical causes for an altered mental state will usually be suggested by the history, mental state assessment, abnormal vital signs and physical examination. As noted above, particular consideration should be given to medical causes in a first presentation of psychosis, especially in an older patient.

Investigations should be driven by history and examination findings, such as neurological signs or signs of infection. Nevertheless, because of the difficulties in compiling comprehensive medical histories, it is often appropriate to do a number of 'screening' investigations as indicators of unsuspected medical illness. The range of suggested tests varies, but usually includes urea and electrolytes, full blood count, liver function tests, random blood sugar, blood alcohol level, thyroid function tests and B12 and folate levels.[23]

The availability of computerized tomography (CT) scanning in more centres has facilitated the use of neuroimaging as an aid to diagnosis. This investigation is likely to be indicated in patients where stroke, neoplasm, haemorrhage or central nervous system infection may be suspected. It is also appropriate to consider a CT scan of the brain in first episode psychosis cases to further assess the possibility of neurological disease presenting with only psychotic or affective symptoms. However, the yield of positive results with this investigation is low,[24] especially in the younger patient,[25] and neuroimaging is therefore generally not required as an emergency investigation if the patient is otherwise medically well.

It is well established that patients with chronic psychotic illness tend to have poorer physical health than the general population.[26] Common conditions include obesity, late onset diabetes, hypertension, arterio-sclerotic disorders, smoking-related disorders, and alcohol and other drug-related disorders. The prevalence of these problems can be related to lifestyle factors, the side effects of medication and difficulties in making effective use of primary medical care. It is worth considering the possible presence of these common conditions as they sometimes need acute treatment or contribute to an exacerbation of the mental state.

Treatment

Management in the ED

Once medical causes have been excluded, the primary psychiatric diagnosis is likely to fall into one of the following groups:

- Drug-induced psychosis
- acute schizophrenia
- mania
- chronic schizophrenia
- psychosis-like reactive state
- depressive psychosis.

Patients with psychotic illness often stay in ED for prolonged periods. Sometimes this is due to delays in the assessment process, but it is also significantly a result of access block, that is the lack of ready availability of beds in psychiatric wards. In some hospitals, these circumstances have resulted in the establishment of specific psychiatric 'holding beds', within or closely related to the ED, where patients may be observed and treated for up to 48 h while further management and disposition plans are being made.[27,28] The availability of such specialized psychiatric observation units is likely to reduce the need for reliance on sedative medications to manage behavioural disturbance. The patient can move around more freely, preferably with access to an outside secure area, and specialized mental health staff can provide assessment, supervision, explanation and reality orientation.

In the more conventional ED setting, behavioural management is more difficult as a balance must be achieved between imposing restrictions on the patient and maintaining the safety of all patients and staff. Psychotic patients should be in areas which can be easily observed and often one-to-one supervision will be necessary, preferably with trained mental health nurses. If possible, this should be in a quiet area without too much coming and going. Engagement of the patient in reality-based conversation (explanation of what is happening, attention to personal concerns) is often useful. It may be possible to enlist the help of family members in providing reassurance and comfort.

The use of specific medications will depend in part on the diagnostic picture. Patients with drug-induced psychosis are usually quite aroused and require significant levels of sedation. Benzodiazepines such as midazolam and diazepam are usually preferred as they are less likely to lead to medical complications (especially arrhythmias) in a person who has already taken other drugs and has a high sympathetic drive. The period of sedation may become prolonged for several hours (or even days if high doses of diazepam are used). The mental state needs to be reassessed for the presence of persistent psychosis when the sedation abates.

Patients with acute schizophrenia, mania or persistent psychosis following drug use all have similar management in the short term. These patients tend to be aroused and agitated and to have considerable difficulty in coping with the restrictions and the stimulation of the ED environment. If the patient will take oral medications, sedative antipsychotics (such as olanzapine) or benzodiazepines (such as lorazepam) can be used. These are better prescribed as regular doses (e.g. olanzapine 5 mg tds or 7.5 mg qid or lorazepam 1 mg qid or 2 mg qid) than on a pro re nata (PRN) basis to ensure consistency in dosing. Repeated divided doses to maintain a more constant level of sedation are preferable to infrequent large doses. Estimates of the probable appropriate dose can be made on the basis of the size of the patient and degree of arousal, and then titrated upward or downward on the basis of response in the first 24 h.

If the patient refuses oral medication, lorazepam (if available) or clonazepam can be used intramuscularly or intravenously. Olanzapine can also be used effectively intramuscularly. Patients who are likely to stay in the ED for more than 24 h can be given zuclopenthixol acetate 50–150 mg i.m. (dose dependent on the size of the patient). This is a medium acting depot antipsychotic preparation which will last for 3–4 days. However, the onset of action is delayed for 6–8 h, and this medication should be avoided in neurolept-naïve patients because of the risk of prolonged dystonia.

The patient who presents with acute schizophrenia who is not aroused may benefit from explanation and only small doses of medication, such as olanzapine 5 mg at night. Similarly the patient with chronic schizophrenia should be maintained on usual medications, possibly with the addition of a PRN benzodiazepine if very anxious.

Patients with psychotic depression can be quite agitated, but also may be quiet and withdrawn. They should be considered at high risk of suicidal behaviour and need close supervision. Their mental anguish may be helped in the short term with the use of benzodiazepines or sedative antipsychotics (olanzapine or quetiapine). Regular doses are better than PRN, although smaller doses are needed than in the treatment of the acutely schizophrenic or manic patient. It is not essential to commence an antidepressant medication during the time the patient is in the ED.

The patient with severe personality disorder or a history of severe trauma who presents with a psychosis-like reactive state often requires similar treatment to a patient with acute schizophrenia. The patient may require containment in a place of safety and will benefit from explanation and reassurance. Benzodiazepines and sedative anti-psychotics can be very useful in lowering arousal.

Admission to inpatient care

The decision to admit the patient for inpatient psychiatric care depends on the acuity of the presentation, the supports available at home, the degree of risk and the availability of community mental health services.

Patients with an acute episode of schizophrenia, especially a first episode, often require admission because they are often very disorganized, lack insight and are likely to be non-compliant with medication and may be at risk of suicide or aggressive behaviour. However, the increasing availability of mobile crisis teams (community mental health teams with the capacity for rapid and intensive follow-up in the home) has made it more possible to treat even these acutely unwell patients at home. This is usually preferred by the patient and sometimes by the family, especially where the patient is an adolescent or young adult still living in the family. In these cases, careful assessment of potential risks to the patient or others, and frank discussion of these issues with the family, is advisable.

The acutely manic patient who has been brought to the ED almost certainly requires admission. Once established, the manic syndrome is likely to persist for several weeks if untreated. In some cases, especially those involving recurrence of a previous bipolar disorder, the patient presents relatively early in the relapse and with sufficient insight to accept advice about increasing or changing medications. If such a patient is discharged to outpatient care, specific arrangements should be made with the family and the community mental health services for monitoring and follow-up.

The patient with an acute psychotic depression almost always requires admission because of the high risk of suicidal behaviour.

On the other hand, patients with chronic schizophrenia who present with a mild exacerbation of symptoms or family or social crisis should generally be managed in the community if possible. These are chronic conditions analogous to diabetes or asthma, and quality of life can be enhanced if the patient can be helped to engage with community treatment services, achieve stability of accommodation and daytime activity and learn to self-manage the condition.[29]

For patients with reactive psychoses in the context of personality disorder or trauma history, the individual circumstances vary widely and the decision to admit depends on careful assessment of the risk factors. Every effort should be made to return the patient as quickly as possible to reality-based perceptions of the world, and to restore a sense of autonomy and personal responsibility. It is sometimes not possible to achieve this during the course of an ED stay and a brief crisis admission to a psychiatric unit may be necessary.

Criteria for involuntary treatment

When inpatient admission is considered desirable but refused by the patient,

consideration should be given to the use of mental health act powers for referral and detention. Contemporary mental health legislation requires the person considering this option (which may be a doctor or other authorized mental health practitioner) to review options for less restrictive treatment before making this decision.

Mental health acts generally stipulate that persons can only be referred under the act if they suffer from a 'mental disorder' and are also at some 'risk'. Risks involving danger to self through suicidal intent or behaviour, and danger to others as a result of aggression or persecutory delusions, are usually straightforward grounds for referral and detention. The decision may be more difficult in relation to the mildly manic patient or the schizophrenic patient with partial insight. The need for detention involves weighing up the potential consequences of not receiving treatment, the possibility of access to community services and the availability of family or other social supports.

Where mental health specialists are not readily available to the ED, ED doctors may appropriately refer a patient under the mental health act so that assessment by a psychiatrist can take place at another location. Especially in cases where the need for involuntary treatment is uncertain, it is good practice for the ED doctor to make this referral to ensure that the decision to detain or release can be made by a psychiatrist, who is in a clearer position to take medico-legal responsibility.

Community referral

The range of potential community treatment options is now wide. Patients may receive outpatient treatment through GPs, private psychiatrists and psychologists, community mental health clinics, public and private drug and alcohol services, relationship counselling agencies, and various other specialized services (e.g. non-government community support services, services for indigenous persons and services for victims of trauma). In planning outpatient care, a good approach is to determine initially what service providers may be already involved in helping the patient and the strength of the patient's relationship with those services. Direct communication between the ED staff and the community

service providers is very desirable, especially if the patient is a new referral to those services.

Some of the more effective psychiatric emergency services work in close liaison with mobile crisis teams or acute care teams, who actively and intensively follow up discharged patients in their own homes or in crisis accommodation.[28,30]

Controversies and future directions

❶ As a result of the contemporary mental health community focus, EDs will continue to have a major role in the assessment and stabilization of patients with psychosis.

❷ Should this assessment occur within traditional EDs or should EDs should facilitate the development of co-located psychiatric emergency services?

❸ The models of care which will achieve the best integration of emergency mental health assessments with community services require better definition.

References

1. Gregory LL, Claassen CA, Edmond JA, et al. Trends in US emergency department visits for mental health conditions, 1992 to 2001. Psychiatric Services 2005; 56: 671–677.
2. Kalucy R, Thomas L, King D. Changing demand for mental health services in the emergency department of a public hospital. Australia and New Zealand Journal of Psychiatry 2005; 39: 74–80.
3. World Health Organization. The ICD-10 classification of mental and behavioural disorders. Geneva: WHO; 1993.
4. Jablensky A. Epidemiology of schizophrenia. In: Gelder MG, Lopez-Ibor JJ, Andreasen NC, eds. New Oxford textbook of psychiatry. London: New Oxford Press; 2000.
5. Jablensky A. Course and outcome of schizophrenia and their prediction. In: Gelder MG, Lopez-Ibor JJ, Andreasen NC, eds. New Oxford textbook of psychiatry. London: New Oxford Press; 2000.
6. Joyce PR. Epidemiology of mood disorders. In: Gelder MG, Lopez-Ibor JJ, Andreasen NC, eds. New Oxford textbook of psychiatry. London: New Oxford Press; 2000.
7. Angst J. Course and prognosis of mood disorders. In: Gelder MG, Lopez-Ibor JJ, Andreasen NC, eds. New Oxford textbook of psychiatry. London: New Oxford Press; 2000.
8. McGorry PD. The concept of recovery and secondary prevention in psychiatric disorders. Australia and New Zealand Journal of Psychiatry 1992; 26: 3–17.
9. Douglas S, Ballard C. Psychotic symptoms in dementia. In: Hassett A, Ames D, Chiu E, eds. Psychosis in the elderly. London: Taylor Francis; 2005.
10. Bredkjoer SR, Mortensen PB, Parnas J. Epilepsy and non-organic non-affective psychosis: national epidemiologic study. British Journal of Psychiatry 1998; 172: 235–238.

11. Logsdail SJ, Toone BK. Post-ictal psychoses. British Journal of Psychiatry 1988; 152: 246–252.
12. Hales RH, Yudofsky SC. Textbook of clinical psychiatry. 4th edn. Washington: American Psychiatric Publishing; 2003: 462–463.
13. Boston Collaborative Drug Surveillance Program. Acute adverse reactions to prednisolone in relation to dosage. Clinical Pharmacology Therapy 1972; 13: 694–698.
14. Young BK, Camicioli R, Ganzini L. Neuropsychiatric adverse effects of antiparkinsonian drugs: characteristics, evaluation and treatment. Drugs & Aging 1997; 10: 367–383.
15. Mellor CS. First rank symptoms of schizophrenia. British Journal of Psychiatry 1970; 117: 15–23.
16. Flaum M, Schultz SK. When does amphetamine-induced psychosis become schizophrenia? American Journal of Psychiatry 1996; 153: 812–815.
17. Javitt DC, Zukin SR. Recent advances in the phencyclidine model of schizophrenia. American Journal of Psychiatry 1991; 148: 1301–1308.
18. Abraham HD, Aldridge AM, Gogia P. The psychopharmacology of hallucinogens. Neuropsychopharmocology 1996; 14: 285–298.

19. Hall W. Cannabis and psychosis. Drug Alcohol Review 1998; 17: 433–434.
20. Chopra HD, Beatson JA. Psychotic symptoms in borderline personality disorder. American Journal of Psychiatry 1986; 143: 1605–1607.
21. Butler RW, Mueser KT, Sprock J, et al. Positive symptoms of psychosis in post-traumatic stress disorder. Biological Psychiatry 1996; 39: 839–844.
22. Olshaker JS, Brown B, Jerrard DA, et al. Medical clearance and screening of psychiatric patients in the emergency department. Academic Emergency Medicine 1997; 4: 124–128.
23. Thienhaus OH. Physical evaluation and laboratory tests. In: Hillard JP, ed. Manual of clinical emergency psychiatry. Washington: American Psychiatric Press; 1990.
24. Rock DJ, Wynn Owen P. An investigation of criteria used to indicate cranial CT in males with schizophrenia. Acta Neuropsychiatrica 2003; 15: 284–289.
25. Adams M, Kutcher S, Antonio E, et al. Diagnostic utility of endocrine and neuroimaging screening tests in first-onset adolescent psychosis. Journal of American Academic Child Adolescence Psychiatry 1996; 35: 67–73.

26. Phelan M, Stradius L, Morrison S. Physical health of people with severe mental illness. British Medical Journal 2001; 322: 443–444.
27. Allen MM. Level 1 psychiatric emergency services: the tools of the crisis sector. Psychiatric Clinic of North America 1999; 22: 713–733.
28. Frank R, Fawcett L, Emmerson B. Development of Australia's first psychiatric emergency centre. Australasian Psychiatry 2005; 13: 266–272.
29. Bennett C, Furnall J, Fossey E, et al. Assessing and responding to the needs of people with schizophrenia and related disorders. In: Meadow G, Singh B, eds. Mental health in Australia: collaborative community practice. Melbourne: Oxford University Press; 2001: 283–312.
30. Breslow RE. Structure and function of psychiatric emergency services. In: Allen MH, ed. Emergency psychiatry review of psychiatry. Vol 21. Washington: American Psychiatric Press; 2002: 1–34.

20.6 Pharmacological management of the aroused patient

Mark Monaghan • Simon Byrne

ESSENTIALS

1 Benzodiazepines and atypical antipsychotics are the first-line drugs for sedation of the aroused patient.

2 As much information as possible should be collected before the patient is sedated.

3 The risks involved in giving sedative drugs need to be considered.

4 Dose adjustments are necessary in the older or medically compromised patient.

Introduction

Patients who present to the emergency department (ED) of their own accord with stress-related problems, anxiety, depression and even some patients with psychotic illness can generally be best assisted by verbal reassurance and prompt mental health evaluation. Reducing the waiting time and arriving reasonably quickly at an action plan will in most of these cases provide the best response to the patient's anxiety and agitation. For some acutely distressed patients, high levels of arousal can be relieved with benzodiazepines in conventional doses.

However, it is more difficult to manage patients who have been brought to the hospital reluctantly, by the police, community mental health staff or family. The diagnosis in these patients is usually an acute psychotic episode, a manic episode or a drug-induced psychotic state (often due to amphetamines). In these patients specific differential diagnosis is not the most urgent issue. The immediate need is to gain control of the situation to permit further evaluation, while at the same time ensuring the safety of the patient, the staff and the public.

In these acute emergencies, it is desirable to collect some information about the patient before sedation. The patient should be approached in a calm manner in a safe, observed area of the ED, with security staff in the background if necessary. The patient should be asked about his or her understanding of the problems, and listened to attentively, even if the account is incoherent. This attention will be reassuring to the patient and helps in building rapport. During this process observations can be made about the mental state. Vital signs should be recorded, and if possible a brief physical examination carried out, with particular attention to signs of injury, intoxication or overdose.

In the hostile or frightened uncooperative patient it will often be necessary to proceed to rapid tranquilization. This is a familiar procedure to the emergency physician, and the practice can be enhanced by attention to the basic principles of care, an awareness of the risks and knowledge of the characteristics of the available drugs. The following discussion of these topics is based on experience and a consideration of the published literature.

Pharmacological management should always be tailored to the particular patient. The medically compromised patient will be at greater risk of the complications of sedation. In elderly patients decreased and delayed metabolism and elimination can result in very prolonged therapeutic and adverse effects. Dose adjustments and agents with shorter half-lives and more favourable side effect profiles must be considered for these patients.

General principles of rapid tranquillization

The general principles of care are:

❶ Use sedative benzodiazepines and/or sedative antipsychotics as the first-line agents.

❷ Route of administration depends on the extent to which the patient is cooperative. Should the situation allow, oral dosing is the least distressing approach for patients and staff.

❸ Treating physicians should use agents with which they are familiar. In particular, they should be aware of maximal safe dosing and expected adverse effects.

❹ The endpoint should be a calm cooperative patient. While achieving this endpoint can be difficult and time-consuming, sedation to the point of loss of airway protection is potentially dangerous.

❺ The patient should be nursed in a quiet, calm and gently lit environment if possible.

❻ Sedated patients should be monitored for basic observations, including oximetry, haemodynamics, respiratory rate and blood sugar levels, as clinically indicated.

❼ Supportive care such as hydration, indwelling catheterization, pressure care and deep vein thrombosis prophylaxis are essential for patients requiring ongoing sedation. This is particularly relevant in overcrowded EDs and if patients are detained in the ED for prolonged periods.

❽ Maintenance of patient dignity by using single rooms and limiting visual exposure of the patient to the public is often forgotten but should be a basic standard of care.

Risks of rapid tranquillization

There are inherent risks in attempting to gain control of the aroused patient, including risks of injury to the staff and patient.

If physical restraint is necessary to administer parenteral medication, adequate staff who are trained in restraint procedures should be on hand. Sometimes mechanical (padded strap) restraint may be necessary in the early stages or to limit the dose of medication if the patient is developing toxic effects. Mechanical restraint should not be maintained in the absence of chemical sedation due to the risks of physical injury and rhabdomyolysis, as well as for ethical reasons.

The risks of adverse events from medication administration are well recognized and are summarized in Table 20.6.1.

Over-sedation and resultant respiratory depression and pulmonary aspiration are relatively common and for the most part avoidable with proper care.

Sudden cardiac death, particularly with agents that prolong the QT interval and precipitate torsade des pointes and VT, is a rare but catastrophic complication of rapid tranquilization.[1,2] This risk is heightened in the aroused patient with increased circulating catecholamines and in patients with pre-existing heart disease or conduction disturbance. Antipsychotics combined with other medications that prolong the QT interval pose an increased risk. The agents most associated with risk of sudden death are thioridazine, and clozapine. Droperidol and haloperidol have been associated with QT prolongation and the risk of torsade des pointes. Quetiapine and chlorpromazine are associated with QT prolongation but this is probably less clinically significant than with the above agents. The atypical agent olanzapine appears to be relatively safe from this perspective.

Table 20.6.1 Risks of sedation
Respiratory depression and pulmonary aspiration
Sudden cardiac death
Hypotension
Dystonic reactions
Neurolept malignant syndrome
Anticholinergic effects
Delirium
Lowered seizure threshold
Special problems in the elderly

Hypotension can occur as an idiosyncratic reaction to any sedative, but is especially associated with chlorpromazine (particularly when given intravenously). Dystonic reactions are seen particularly with haloperidol, and much less commonly with atypical agents such as olanzapine. Neurolept malignant syndrome is a risk with any antipsychotic agent, even following a single dose.

Anticholinergic effects such as delirium and urinary retention are risks with all antipsychotics and are generally seen at high doses. Delirium is also caused by high doses of benzodiazepines, particularly diazepam, which accumulates with recurrent dosing. All antipsychotics have the potential to lower the seizure threshold.

Elderly patients are at significantly greater risk of drug accumulation and adverse effects. They are also at far greater risk of delirium, particularly with the combination of possible underlying cognitive impairment and environment change. Age-related reductions in hepatic metabolism and renal function make it reasonable to assume that all agents will have prolonged elimination half-lives in these patients. Even small doses of benzodiazepines can produce significant and prolonged respiratory depression in the elderly. Standard doses of antipsychotics such as haloperidol may result in prolonged extrapyramidal effects that impair mobility for days to weeks post administration.

Specific agents

Benzodiazepines

Midazolam This water-soluble benzodiazepine has major benefits over diazepam in that it produces fewer site reactions and can be given intramuscularly. It has a rapid effect by intramuscular or intravenous injection (2–5 min), with a half-life of 1–3 h. The active metabolite has a similar half-life. The elimination half-life is significantly prolonged in the elderly. The major adverse effect is respiratory depression. It is available in ampoules (5 mg/mL, 15 mg/3 mL, 5 mg/5 mL and 50 mg/10 mL).

Diazepam Can be used orally or intravenously. It is not recommended for intramuscular use due to unpredictable absorption. Diazepam demonstrates biphasic elimination with rapid redistribution of 1–3 h, followed by a prolonged terminal elimination phase of up to 20 h. Hepatic metabolism produces active metabolites and excretion is renal. Elimination is significantly prolonged in the elderly. Major adverse effects are respiratory depression and accumulation causing delirium. It is available in ampoules (10 mg/2 mL), tablets (2 mg and 5 mg) and elixir (10 mg/10 mL).

Clonazepam Can be used by oral, intravenous or intramuscular routes. Clonazepam has a prolonged elimination half-life (20–50 h) with hepatic metabolism and renal excretion. The major adverse effects are excessive sedation and risk of accumulation. It is available in ampoules (1 mg/mL), tabs (0.5 mg and 2 mg) and oral liquid (2.5 mg/mL).

Lorazepam In Australia, lorazepam is only used orally as the parenteral preparation is not available. However, in other countries it is widely used intramuscularly in the sedation of psychotically aroused patients. It is well absorbed orally, with an elimination half-life of 12–15 h. The hepatic metabolites are non-active. The major adverse effect is excessive sedation, but it is less likely to accumulate than diazepam or clonazepam. It is available in tablets (1 mg and 2.5 mg).

Antipsychotics

Haloperidol Can be given by oral, intramuscular or intravenous routes. Peak plasma levels occur 20 min after intramuscular injection and 2–6 h post oral dose. Mean elimination half-life is 20 h, but this includes initial rapid elimination followed by a prolonged elimination over days. Hepatic metabolites are renally excreted. Major adverse effects are extrapyramidal effects that may persist for days (particularly in the elderly), prolongation of QT interval with risk of torsade and neurolept malignant syndrome syndrome. It is available in tablets (0.5 mg, 1.5 mg and 5 mg), liquid (2 mg/mL) and ampoules (5 mg/mL).

Olanzapine Olanzapine is for oral, sublingual (SL) and intramuscular use. It is an atypical antipsychotic that is well absorbed orally with peak plasma levels 2–5 h post oral dose and 30 min post intramuscular injection. It has a half-life of approximately

33 h and is hepatically metabolized to inactive metabolites that are renally and faecally excreted. Major adverse effects include excessive sedation, mild anticholinergic effects and neurolept malignant syndrome (NMS). Extrapyramidal side effects, including dystonias, are rare. Cardiotoxicity is also rare. It is available in tablets (2.5 mg, 5 mg, 7.5 mg and 10 mg), wafers (5 mg and 10 mg) and ampoules (10 mg).

Risperidone Risperidone is for oral and sublingual use. It is an atypical antipsychotic that is well absorbed orally with a peak effect in 1–2 h. It is hepatically metabolized to an active metabolite that is renally excreted. The half-life of the parent compound is 3 h in extensive metabolizers and 17 h in poor metabolizers; the active metabolite' elimination half-life is 24 h. Risperidone's adverse effect profile is benefited by the absence of anticholinergic effects, but includes postural hypotension with initial dosing, extrapyramidal effects and NMS. Extrapyramidal reactions, including dystonias, are less frequent with risperidone than with haloperidol. There has been an increased mortality associated with risperidone and elderly patients on furosemide, so caution should be taken to ensure adequate hydration in these patients. It is available in tablets and sublingual 'quicklets' (0.5 mg, 1 mg, 2 mg, 3 mg and 4 mg) and solution (1 mg/mL).

Chlorpromazine Chlorpromazine is for oral, intramuscular or intravenous use. It has variable and incomplete absorption and a large first-pass metabolism, with peak plasma levels 1–4 h after oral and 30 min after intramuscular administration. Metabolism is hepatic with many metabolites that are renally excreted. Elimination is complicated with early (2–3 h), intermediate (15 h) and late (60 days) elimination phases. Major adverse effects are postural hypotension, strong anticholinergic effects, excessive sedation and the risk of NMS. Extrapyramidal effects are relatively uncommon. It is available in tablets (10 mg, 25 mg and 100 mg), syrup (25 mg/mL) and ampoules (50 mg/2 mL).

Zuclopenthixol acetate ('Acuphase')
This is given intramuscularly. Zuclopenthixol acetate is a medium-acting depot

preparation of a typical thioxanthene antipsychotic. Maximal plasma levels are achieved 24–36 h post intramuscular injection, declining to 30% of maximum levels by day 3. It is hepatically metabolized to inactive metabolites and faecally excreted. Zuclopenthixol acetate should be avoided in neurolept-naïve patients, and those with organic brain disorders, cardiac disease and lowered seizure threshold. This is because any adverse effects, including NMS, will be prolonged because of the slow absorption and elimination.

A rapid tranquillization algorithm
There are a variety of published algorithms for rapid tranquillization.[3–11] The following is a reasonable approach in terms of effectiveness, risk of adverse effects and availability. This algorithm applies to the management of a previously well adult patient. Elderly patients as a general rule should have lower initial doses and smaller daily doses.

First-line treatment
Try to develop rapport with the patient and use oral medication if possible. Oral agents of choice include:

benzodiazepines: diazepam 10 mg, clonazepam 2 mg or lorazepam 2.5 mg (elderly: lorazepam 0.5–1 mg.)

and/or:

antipsychotic: olanzapine 5–10 mg oral/SL (elderly: olanzapine 2.5 mg oral/SL or risperidone 0.25–0.5 mg oral/SL).

Second-line treatment
If oral therapy is not achievable or is not effective, parenteral medications must be given. Agents of choice include:

benzodiazepines: midazolam 2.5–5 mg i.v./i.m. repeated as required to a maximum of around 100 mg (elderly or compromised patients may develop respiratory depression with as little as 1 mg midazolam, so 0.5–1 mg is a safer initial dose, with maximal dose many times lower than 100 mg)

and/or:

antipsychotic: olanzapine 10 mg i.m., which can be repeated up to a maximal daily dose of 30 mg (elderly patients can be given olanzapine in doses of 2.5 mg i.m., but may be better managed with sublingual olanzapine 2.5 mg or sublingual risperidone 0.5 mg).

Third-line treatment

If the maximal doses of the above agents have been reached with the first- or second-line drugs without adequate effect, it is necessary to try other options. Sometimes also the first- or second-line drugs may have to be avoided because of previous adverse effects. The maximum doses described here are based on the likelihood of very limited greater benefit (and the probability of greater adverse effects) of exceeding these doses.

Third-line agents include:

Diazepam 2.5–5 mg i.v., up to a maximum of around 100–150 mg. (risks include accumulation, delirium and respiratory depression; should not be given intramuscularly)

Clonazepam 1–2 mg i.m./i.v., up to a maximum of 8 mg per day. Clonazepam can also be given as an infusion at a rate of 4–6 mg/24 h; the rate of the infusion can be varied according to the arousal level of the patient. (Risks include accumulation, delirium and respiratory depression.)

Haloperidol 2.5–5 mg i.m./i.v., up to a maximum of around 30–50 mg/24 h. (Risks include dystonic reactions, QT prolongation, anticholinergic delirium and NMS.)

Chlorpromazine can also be given as an intravenous infusion, with an initial rate of 6.25–12.5 mg/h to gain initial control and then reduced to a maximum of around 200 mg/24 h. (Risks include anticholinergic effects, hypotension, delirium, accumulation, QT prolongation and NMS.)

Aroused patients with amphetamine intoxication should be managed with benzodiazepines and supportive care, sometimes requiring large doses for initial control. Both intravenous midazolam and oral/intravenous diazepam are reasonable first choices. Severe intoxication with hyperthermia and rigidity requires paralysis and intubation.

In patients who present with paranoid psychosis associated with amphetamine abuse, addition of an antipsychotic such as olanzapine (oral or intramuscular) is appropriate.

Maintenance therapy

Commonly, following initial rapid tranquilization, the patient will remain sedated for several hours. During this time collateral history may be obtained, as well as previous treatment history from hospital records. When the patient awakes, a further psychiatric assessment should be made, especially with a view to deciding whether the patient needs to be admitted to a psychiatric unit.

If the patient does need to remain in hospital, consideration must be given to further appropriate medication. At this stage it may be possible to gain greater rapport with the patient and obtain cooperation with taking oral medication. Sometimes the patient may indicate preferred drugs, which should be offered if clinically appropriate. A general approach is to use benzodiazepines (lorazepam 1 or 2 mg three times a day) or sedative antipsychotics (olanzapine 5 or 10 mg three times a day). It is better to prescribe regular medication (rather than 'as needed') to ensure consistency of dosing. The initial prescription can be made on the basis of the size of the patient and the degree of arousal, and then increased or decreased according to response. The appropriateness of the prescribed medication and the side effects should be reviewed at least daily by the doctor.

If the patient remains uncooperative, intravenous benzodiazepines or intramuscular olanzapine can be used on an as needed basis. If adequate facilities are available for monitoring respiratory function, the use of an infusion of clonazepam or chlorpromazine can help to achieve control. Alternatively, some patients who are likely to remain in the ED for more than 24 h may benefit from a one-off dose of zuclopenthixol acetate. This drug should only be used in patients who have previously been treated with antipsychotics without developing major side effects; the usual dose is 50–100 mg i.m., depending on the size of the patient.

Controversies and future directions

❶ As a result of concerns about QT prolongation and dystonic reactions, some centres actively discourage the use of haloperidol.

❷ The development of more parenteral formulations of atypical antipsychotics will increase the therapeutic options.

❸ Some authorities advocate the use of only benzodiazepines for all aroused patients.

❹ More rapid transfer of patients to psychiatric units reduces the need for prolonged high-dose sedation.

References

1. Abdelmawla N, Mitchell AJ. Sudden cardiac death and antipsychotics. Part 1: Risk factors and mechanisms. Advances in Psychiatric Treatment 2006; 12: 35–44.
2. Abdelmawla N, Mitchell AJ. Sudden cardiac death and antipsychotics. Part 2: Monitoring and prevention. Advances in Psychiatric Treatment 2006; 12: 100–109.
3. McAllister-Williams RH, Ferrier IN. Rapid tranquillisation: time for a reappraisal of options for parenteral therapy. British Journal of Psychiatry 2002; 180: 485–489.
4. MacPherson R, Dix R, Morgan S. A growing evidence base for management guidelines. Advances on Psychiatric Treatment 2005; 11: 404–415.
5. Battaglia J, Moss S, Rush J, et al. Haloperidol, lorazepam or both for psychotic agitation? A multi-centre, double-blind, emergency department study. American Journal of Emergency Medicine 1997; 15: 4335–4340.
6. Atakan Z, Davies T. ABC of mental health: mental health emergencies. British Medical Journal 1997; 314: 1740–1742.
7. Pilowski LS, Ring H, Shine PJ, et al. Rapid tranquillisation: a survey of emergency prescribing in a general psychiatric hospital. British Journal of Psychiatry 1992; 160: 831–835.
8. Alexander J, Tharyan P, Adams C, et al. Rapid tranquillisation of violent or agitated patients in a psychiatric emergency setting: pragmatic randomized trial of intramuscular lorazepam versus haloperidol plus promethazine. British Journal of Psychiatry 2004; 185: 63–69.
9. TREC Collaborative Group. Rapid tranquillisation for agitated patients in emergency psychiatric rooms: a randomized trial of midazolam versus haloperidol plus promethazine. British Medical Journal 2003; 327: 708–713.
10. Currier GW. Atypical antipsychotic medications in the psychiatric emergency service. Journal of Clinical Psychiatry 2000; 61(suppl 14): 21–26.
11. Department of Pharmacy. Clinical management of agitation in the older patient. Fremantle Hospital and Health Service Drug Bulletin 2006; 30: 2.

CHALLENGING SITUATIONS

Edited by **George Jelinek**

21.1 Death and dying

Bryan Walpole

ESSENTIALS

1 Death and dying are an inevitable part of emergency medicine practice.

2 Emergency physicians have a responsibility to initiate grief management.

3 The interview with the family of the recently deceased can be a positive start to successful grieving and recovery.

4 Information about a death should not be given over the telephone.

5 In talking to relatives of the newly deceased, the word 'dead' should be used, as the grieving process can start when there is an acknowledgement of death.

6 Reactions to death include disbelief, numbness, expressive reactions, guilt and displacement activity. There should be no timelines set on recovery.

7 Relatives and their invited friends should be encouraged to view the body.

8 Organ donation services should be offered unless there are clinical contraindications.

9 Caring for the carers is often overlooked.

10 Emergency physicians should regularly self-assess for emotional fatigue.

Introduction

As a truly universal human custom, dying is one of those rare things. We all do it sooner or later, however inexpertly. All societies mark it, some heavily, some lightly. Whole religions have been invented to militate against its all too evident, shocking finality.

It happens more secretly in Western societies than most, but although it happens in every community we do not talk about it as we talk about politics, sex, religion and the economy. Many cultures, not all of them ancient, are on cosier terms with death than us.

Death and dying patients are an inevitable part of emergency medicine practice.

Facing a surviving family, or counselling a dying patient, may for some symbolize failure in the battle against disease. In emergency medicine practice, one does not have the benefit of a long-standing doctor–patient relationship. The support and mutual understanding that are the cornerstones of family practice are missing, and so rapport has to be forged in the heat of the moment. Families need space and time to come to grips with death, but time and space are a precious commodity in the emergency department (ED). Access block and overcrowding should not preclude sensitive, empathetic grief management.

The cold, clean and sterile surroundings of a hospital morgue, or the shambles of a recently deserted resuscitation room, stand in stark contrast to the comfort, soft furnishings and music of the funeral parlour. To follow the heat and adrenaline rush of a difficult resuscitation with the grace and emotional energy required to care for a family, the members of which have now become patients, requires considerable effort. The survivors, however, deserve our care and compassion as much as did the recently deceased.

Similarly, management of the patient brought to the ED in extremis, even when death is anticipated, can be a complex and challenging task, as families, baling

653

out through exhaustion, fear or ignorance, call an ambulance in the few hours prior to death, often in the middle of the night.

Most multicultural societies have no single distinct death ritual, nor a standard way of expressing loss and grief, as in monocultures. This, combined with the fact that most ED deaths are unexpected, places a significant responsibility on emergency physicians to initiate grief management and refer for continuing care.

Quality management of grief states can prevent significant morbidity, as unresolved grief can lead to later problems with physical and mental health.

The death process

Death does not occur at a finite moment. Cardiac death, cerebral death, brainstem death and cellular death form a continuum over minutes or hours. The legal definition of death varies between regions. The diagnosis of brain death can be made accurately and positively by appropriately qualified and experienced people using relatively simple bedside tests.[1] It is imperative, however, that any reversible condition producing depression of the brain must first be excluded. The time of death is the time when brain death is established, not the time when life support is ceased. Persons considered dead may continue to breathe for a considerable length of time, and faint cardiac action that cannot be detected in major vessels, or by auscultation, can continue to provide sufficient oxygen for vital organs to survive for some hours. So it is important that relatives are not informed of death until all breathing and cardiac activity have ceased. A second opinion and cardiac monitor can help verify this.

Illustrative case

A 90-year-old man collapsed in the community and was attended by an emergency physician. Despite 15 min of advanced cardiac life support (including high-dose adrenaline (epinephrine)) the patient remained in persistent asystole, with no respiratory effort. Ambulance staff withdrew, the coroner was notified, but, during family bereavement counselling, the emergency physician noticed the endotracheal tube moving rhythmically against the shroud. Closer inspection revealed good colour, a pulse

and breathing. After 4 days in hospital the patient recovered completely, to live another 2 years and to receive a national award for services to the country. The important principle of waiting 5–10 min before announcing death, and confirming the persistent cessation of vital signs, was not taken into consideration, much to the embarrassment of the doctor concerned.

This period may be used to clean the site, cut off unsightly tubes inside their orifice and tape together or use adhesive on unsightly wounds, prior to family viewing the body. Such activities must be negotiated with forensic services beforehand, so that all requirements of local legislation can be met.

Dying persons

The dying and their families face numerous psychological issues as death draws nigh. Sometimes it can be difficult to counteract the tendency to focus on the physical and tactical needs of care, rather than the emotional, spiritual and cultural dimensions of human experience. A large family may need significant space, which can interfere with the routine work of the ED so a private room should be available. Dying persons can have a deep-seated fear of abandonment, accepting further treatment for the sake of the family or doctor, knowing that it will be of little personal benefit. Open communication and congruent goals for care should be forged early, and links with family doctor, caring specialist teams or hospice care should be established so that everyone feels safe and secure, with the proposed regimen, pending ward admission. Then all can pay special attention to physical comfort, symptom management, privacy and the confidentiality of the patient and family. Extensive references are immediately available on the internet, for staff and family.[2]

Palliative care workers experienced in bereavement care are concerned at the lack of support available particularly after hours in major healthcare institutions, where sudden death, traumatic death and death in unfamiliar and isolated circumstances make more likely the risk of complicated grief for those left behind.

The advent of sophisticated paramedic care has created a new class of patient,

too ill to resuscitate with lethal illness. High (apnoeic) quadriplegia and catastrophic trauma patients can present conscious and in extremis. Early decisions to resuscitate can bring profound distress later and be hard to reverse.

In such cases life-sustaining treatment may legitimately be forgone if it is:

❶ therapeutically futile – open thoracotomy in blunt trauma
❷ overly burdensome to the patient – CPR in the presence of terminal illness
❸ not reasonably available without disproportionate hardship to the patient's carers or others – being transported long distances for marginal treatment
❹ refused by the patient – where an advanced care directive may exist.

In the few minutes after arrival with inadequate information, it is easier to resuscitate first and answer questions afterwards.

Illustrative case

A previously well 84-year-old man was observed by his wife to spontaneously fall, be briefly unconscious and then recover, being very pale with some back pain. Ambulance provided oxygen, fluids and morphine and delivered him to ED grossly hypotensive but talking coherently. From his record, we adduced that he had an inoperable aortic aneurysm. In discussion with him and his family, a morphine and midazolam infusion was started; he died comfortably in ED 3 h later.

Breaking bad news

Most ED deaths are unanticipated, and informing families can be a harrowing experience. If the opportunity presents, it is essential that the family be well briefed during resuscitation and, where practicable, be involved in the process. A member of the family can be invited into the resuscitation room, where the senior emergency physician present should discuss the procedures under way and provide encouragement to touch, speak to and kiss the patient. This is not only reassuring, but the presence of numerous competent staff with an array of sophisticated equipment reassures family members that the healthcare team has not let them down, and this can prevent many doubts and questions later. If the outcome is hopeless this can be discussed with the family members, perhaps asking their permission before abandoning resuscitation. Even if they do not wish to accept such responsibility they will remember these moments for the rest of their lives. Having participated in the resuscitation and in the decision to stop can be helpful, even when the request has been declined.

The interview with the family of the recently deceased can be more difficult than the resuscitation. Handled with sensitivity, however, it can be a positive start to successful grieving and recovery.

Illustrative case

A 5-year-old child was crushed by a falling goalpost during a primary school soccer game. He was brought to hospital with severe (unsurvivable) head injuries and rapidly intubated. His mother arrived shortly afterwards, and despite the gross facial deformation with brain visible, she came to the resuscitation room and had some time with her son before resuscitation was ceased. On the anniversary of his death she came to the ED with flowers and a request to speak to the staff who had been there on the day. She expressed her gratitude for the sensitivity and tact shown in allowing her to be part of his final moments, and stated how much this had supported her, as she knew he had never suffered and that the final words he received prior to death were hers.

The room in which such information is given should be private and comfortable, and contain a telephone. Tea, coffee, iced water and simple food should be readily available. If refreshments arrive soon after the news has been broken, this can help diffuse tension. The offering of food is a time-honoured expression of warmth and comfort, and facilitates communication and the grieving process.

Only in very exceptional cases should any information about death be given over the telephone by hospital staff. Cases abound of misidentification, and of people becoming involved in road trauma while rushing to hospital. A polite request to attend hospital as a relative is ill should bring them in a more orderly, safe fashion. A taxi (paid for on arrival, for indigent persons) should be available.

Illustrative case

A 22-year-old man was killed when bricks being carried in a station wagon crushed his upper torso after a head-on car crash. He was identified from a driver's licence photograph, as his face was grossly distorted. The family was grieving and about to attend the bedside when a brother claimed the deceased must be someone else carrying the licence of his brother, as he had seen his brother in the past hour. It transpired that the deceased was currently suspended for drink-driving and had borrowed a licence.

The emergency physician should greet the family by name, confirm the relationship of each with the patient and shake hands or touch them gently. All parties should be seated, and a helpful way to start is to ask the family members what they know. They may have been present at the scene, where CPR was under way, or have come to hospital independently with no preconceived ideas. Then a short résumé of the resuscitation should be given, such as the following:

'He collapsed at work and his workmates started resuscitation, which was continued in the ambulance. On arrival at hospital he was gravely ill, we were breathing for him, and pumping his heart for almost an hour; however, he has failed to respond to resuscitation. We ceased a short while ago, and I am afraid he is dead'.

or

'She was involved in a car crash on the outskirts of town. She sustained very serious head injuries and on arrival at hospital was completely unresponsive, with severe brain and neck injuries. Shortly after arrival her heart stopped and we were unable to resuscitate her further. She died a few moments ago'.

It is important to use the word 'dead' or 'died'; euphemisms such as 'passed away', 'she's gone' and 'departed this life' are unclear messages that can mislead. The grieving process cannot start until there is acknowledgement of death. A truthful explanation can be comforting.

Reactions

There are a range of responses to the information that a close relative has died. The mode of death can be a guide. Homicide can lead to great distress, along with suicide and unintended injury. Some common reactions are:

- Disbelief: some will immediately deny the event, claiming that it must be somebody else or that they are dreaming. Reinforcement is required.
- Numbness: some sit mute, appearing not to take in the information. They need time to absorb it.
- Expressive: a sudden flood of tears or loud cries (a Latin cultural response) with upsetting or disturbing noises should be allowed to run its course. Such acknowledgement can be a positive response.
- Guilt: particularly with homicide and suicide, such news is often followed by 'if only' or 'why couldn't I have'. Here, gentle repeated reassurance and discussion can be important. These people are at risk of pathological grief reactions and can be helped by seeing the body and talking to it.
- Displacement activity: an immediate call to inform relatives, organize the funeral and discuss family matters is a poor prognostic sign. These people are often seen as mature, rational and born organizers, but they are at serious risk of pathological grief reactions months later. They will need careful follow-up to see that they grieve eventually.

Grief is not like an illness, to be fought and cured as so often is the case in Western medicine. Generalizations can be made about human behavioural tendencies, and time lines can be drawn for predicted recovery, but each person's grieving process is unique.

Some people never get better and nobody survives grief unchanged.

All relatives need time to receive the clear message of death, which they may need to be given again and again. Some need to make meaning of the event, and the clinical art of managing perceptions is paramount.

Viewing the body

Relatives and their invited friends should be encouraged to view the body. By seeing the body, by feeling and touching, the grieving process, separation and rebuilding can start. People should be encouraged to speak to, touch, kiss, stroke, caress, even to argue, negotiate and cajole in private for as long as they wish. Without this time, weeks or months later, delusions can persist that the person might not have died, and conspiracy theories can emerge. The presence of a bereavement or viewing room can make this process much easier as, particularly with children, visiting can go on for several hours. A hospital morgue may be used, some have a purpose-built facility and appropriate staff support. Relatives should be informed of the necessity for police presence if the matter has been referred to the coroner.

Legal issues

By law, in all Australian states a body belongs to the Crown until a death certificate is issued. This is issued by the Registrar General after satisfactory details are supplied by a medical practitioner on the medical certificate as to the reasons for death. This is a legal document and is the source of information for the preparation of national mortality statistics. The quality of these statistics and subsequent public-health interventions depend largely on the ability of doctors to present accurate information.

Euthanasia

Euthanasia (active medical killing of terminally ill patients) is currently illegal in all states of Australia and New Zealand but is under active debate in Western society.[3]

For the proponents of euthanasia, patients are presumed to have endured pain and suffering, which, out of respect for autonomy and compassion, they should be able to relieve by choosing euthanasia.

For opponents of euthanasia this is seen as a potent reason for enhancing access to, and quality of, palliative-hospice care and mental health services. For many, the 'slippery slope', at the end of this is loss of the sanctity of life, a broadening of the criteria for euthanasia, and a gradual change in the values of society and the ethos of medicine frighteningly beckon. The debate highlights the difficulty of clinical decision-making in complex circumstances, which, in themselves, have been neglected in the euthanasia debate with its medical, social, legal and ethical arenas; the law and ethics cannot operate separately from clinical care.

The neutralists emphasize the lack of research into how and where people die and the inadequacies of training programmes for the care of the dying, which lead to calls for euthanasia and draw attention to the complexities and vicissitudes of the communications between patients and doctors.

Finally, clinical educators need to develop programmes that both explore the wider social issues of death and dying and ensure that the circumstances of this inevitable event are compassionate and humane.

Death certificates

Cases where a death must be referred to the coroner are usually detailed on the inside of the death certificate book. Any death suspected to be not entirely from natural causes requires reporting. The coroner's office will assist.

Unless the emergency physician is thoroughly familiar with the patient and the medical history, and saw the patient prior to death, the opinion as to whether a death certificate should be issued should be left to the family practitioner, specialist or hospital unit normally caring for the patient. Where the cause of death is unclear, or no doctor has sufficient information to fill out a death certificate, an autopsy is required. Although this may cause distress to some families (and particular ethnic groups), any bona fide cultural concern can be referred to the coroner, where such matters are usually dealt with sensitively. Under the requirements of the Evidence Act, a body must be under the jurisdiction of the police from as soon as practicable after death until the coroner states that it is no longer required for legal purposes. Thus, any interference with the body is illegal, unless it is with the assent of the police officer in charge. The coroner's office should be notified as soon as practicable after death, so a police officer, if required, can attend.

Organ donation

Although parenchymal organs are generally taken from beating-heart donors, the recently dead can be corneal or occasionally renal donors. Organ donation should be mentioned unless there are clinical contraindications, such as hepatitis B, HIV or malignancy. Relatives can ask later why donation was not suggested, and some really appreciate the opportunity to contribute to the welfare of others. A routine check of the driver's licence or at the donor registry can help clarify the issue. All Australian states have access to professional transplant coordinators to facilitate the process once permission has been obtained.

Bereavement counselling

Most hospitals have qualified practitioners to support the recently bereaved. Referral should be arranged prior to departure if counsellors have not already made contact. Ministers of religion are trained in grief counselling and are usually available after hours. People can feel unprepared to ask for them, and it is not necessary for the deceased to have had any religious affiliation to make use of such counsellors. The family doctor is also a useful resource and should always be informed promptly of the death of a practice patient. Social workers are expert in grief counselling, and many funeral companies now provide counselling services.

Subsequent issues

Permission to leave

Recently bereaved people are sometimes confused, frightened, stunned and at a loss as to what to do next. When forensic issues (identification and statements) and viewing have been completed, they can be given the dead person's possessions and politely given permission to leave the hospital. 'There is nothing more you can do' or 'Can I phone someone or get a taxi to take you home?' may be usefully offered.

Information about contacting a funeral office to arrange for collection of the death certificate and the body, and to discuss burial rites should be in an explanatory leaflet, readily available.

Tranquillizers

Requests for tranquillizers can come from survivors or a third party, who may ask that the bereaved be given sedation. Most experts involved in loss and grief counselling agree that early sedation is contraindicated. It may be part of the management of morbid grief weeks or months later but has no place in early management. Anxiety, sadness and insomnia can be a natural part of early grief.

Follow-up

For most people the normal expectations are that they will live the allotted 3 score years and 10, according to the biblical principle, that parents will predecease their children and that the dying person will be able to deal with any unfinished business and die surrounded by loved ones, as seen on TV, video and film. There is an expectation that death will be natural, peaceful and, for the majority, pain free. In marked contrast to such expectations is the unexpected death of a loved one at an ED, where rape, murder or innocent victims of armed hold-ups, terrorists or love-struck psychopaths are regular realities. The mode of death has major implications for the resolution of grief. Iserson describes four modes of death often referred to as the NASH categories (natural, abuse, suicide and homicide), of which the latter three particularly require careful follow-up for abnormal bereavement reactions. Shame, guilt, morbid hatred, outrage and resignation often follow deaths where there has been violence, violation or other wilful intent. Following receipt of the autopsy report, a follow-up interview can be arranged with the family, when matters surrounding death can be discussed.

Where deaths have been witnessed, post-traumatic stress disorder may occur. This is defined in DSM-III-R as the development of characteristic symptoms following a psychologically distressing event outside the range of usual human experience. Early treatment is controversial and may produce a better outcome, but it is almost always welcome. The concept of trauma debriefing is now well established, not only in the literature but in clinical practice throughout the world. It is a legal requirement in some occupational health and safety legislation. Some organizations offer telephone counselling and meetings.

It is also important to educate significant others in a person's life as to the symptoms of pathological grief, so that appropriate support can be offered.

An ED protocol

Recommended actions for medical and nursing staff in dealing with grieving relatives:

Contacting family
Request family's urgent attendance. Do not inform of death over phone.

Arrival of family
Show to private room with phone. Give prompt update on patient's condition. Offer spiritual or other counsellor.

During resuscitation
Stay with family.
Give regular updates. Allow relatives to be with patient.

After death
Inform family in an unhurried manner. Facilitate grieving. Identify 'at-risk' relatives. Allow deceased to be viewed.

Concluding process
Attend to formalities (e.g. coroner). Give brochure containing useful information and contact numbers. Address final questions.

Follow-up
Contact general practitioner. Send sympathy card.
Make phone call at 1 and 6 weeks, as appropriate. Allow opportunity for interview with treating doctor to address unanswered questions.

Williams et al. have proposed integrating a bereavement management plan to deal sensitively with death in a busy ED.[4] Their evaluation has shown that with educated staff, it is neither overly burdensome, nor confronting, it provides a human side of our role as healers in the face of death.

Professional issues

One of the important aspects of looking after survivors is caring for the carers, who are often overlooked. Those involved in caring for others who have experienced trauma need support and the opportunity to vent thoughts and feelings. Many authorities, including the National Association for Loss and Grief (NALAG), consider it imperative that formal diffusing and debriefing should be provided to any worker involved either at the scene of trauma or with surviving victims, or with family members of victims. The mental health of professionals is an important consideration, and due recognition should be given to this aspect so as to offset possible burnout. ED managers need to give attention to thresholds for adding debriefing to standing orders, as mandated in some hospitals. Junior and rotating staff may be less resistant than professional practitioners of emergency medicine. There is, however, a distinct propensity for those who spend their lives among misery to become cynical and full of black humour. The cultural norms of emergency medicine can become so integrated into personal values that the physician does not even recognize their presence. We should regularly assess our own emotional fatigue, and if there is a significant divergence between our personal values and career activities, we may be motivated to seek support from a trusted source.

Controversies and future directions

❶ The challenge for emergency physicians is to further develop departmental policies and procedures relating to death and dying in the ED, and to ensure that staff are well versed in these procedures. Departments need to work on improving communication with community health practitioners.

❷ There is a growing debate about whether the withholding of information about the death of a loved one over the telephone constitutes medical paternalism and takes away people's autonomy. Currently, however, it is still accepted that such information should be withheld.

❸ Increasingly attention will be paid to ensuring the wellbeing of staff who are constantly exposed to death and dying in the course of their duties.

References

1. Evans DW. Seeking an ethical and legal way of procuring transplantable organs from the dying without further attempts to redefine human death. Philosophy, Ethics, and Humanity in Medicine 2007; 29: 11.
2. www.grieflink.asn.au/links.html (accessed 14/02/08).
3. Vander Weyden MB. Deaths, dying and the euthanasia debate in Australia. Medical Journal of Australia 1997;166: 173.
4. Williams AG, O'Brien DL, Laughton KJ, et al. Medical Journal of Australia 2000; 173: 480–483.

Further reading

Carey G, Sorensen R, eds. The Penguin book of death. Melbourne: Penguin Books, Melbourne University Press; 1997.

Iserson KV. Grave words: notifying survivors about sudden unexpected deaths. Tucson: Galen Press Ltd; 1999.
Plueckhahn VD, Breen KJ, Cordner SM. Law and ethics in medicine for doctors in Victoria. Melbourne: Melbourne University Press; 1994.
Selby H, ed. The aftermath of death. Annandale: Federation Press; 1992.
Tintinalli J, Ruiz E, Krome RL, eds. Emergency medicine: a comprehensive study guide. 4th edn. New York: McGraw-Hill; 1996.

Websites

http://www.findingourway.net/ An American site, extensive links for bereavement information.

http://www.compassionatefriends.org/ An international organisation, offering support for parents that have children die. 'Unconditional love with no timeline'.
http://www.compassionate friendsvictoria.org.au/ The Victorian site for the above. Qld, WA and NSW are linked from the site.
http://www.nalagvic.org.au/ The Victorian site of a national organisation, set up after the Granville train crash. Has a number of good specific links, mostly Australian.
http://www.grief.org.au/ Site for assistance, support, education, claiming to prevent poor outcomes. Partly government funded.

21.2 Sexual assault

Ian Knox • Roslyn Crampton

ESSENTIALS

1 Rape is an assault in which a sexual act is used as a means of humiliating or controlling the victim.

2 The perceived stigma to the victim caused by cultural myths results in under-reporting of this criminal offence.

3 The complex medical, legal and psychological sequelae mandate a team-based approach involving doctors, police and counsellors in a collaborative effort.

4 Management by a sympathetic non-judgemental physician helps the victim to regain control.

5 The medical evaluation is specifically directed at the issues of injury assessment and management, infection risk and emergency contraception.

6 The forensic aspects of the examination require vigilant examination and documentation by the physician to assist in possible legal proceedings.

Introduction

Rape, and all its variations and sub-entities, is an act of violence in which a sexual act is part of the assault. Sexual pleasure, in the way the general community would perceive this pleasure, is not the objective of the rapist. The intention is to subjugate, humiliate or control the victim, and the sexual act is the means by which this is achieved.[1]

The failure to understand this fundamental distinction has allowed a host of misconceptions and myths to arise that not only tend to exonerate the perpetrator but transfer blame to the victim. Over 90% of the victims of adult sexual assault are women and 98% of the offenders are men. Therefore, for the purposes of this review, the victim is referred to as if female and the offender as if male.

Definitions

As the word 'rape' is surrounded by legal and emotional issues, the term 'sexual assault' is preferable. Sexual assault is a physical assault of a sexual nature directed towards another person without their consent. The assault may range from unwanted touching to sexual penetration without consent.

Sexual assault is a crime, with a legal definition, which may vary between states and territories. Each part of this definition has accumulated further legal interpretation and case law. Sexual assault has a number of elements. It is an act of a sexual nature, which is carried out against the will of the victim. The victim does not give consent, is intimidated to consent or is legally incapable of giving consent because of youth or incapacity. It includes attempts to force the victim into sexual activity and also includes rape, attempted rape, aggravated sexual assault (assault with a weapon or infliction of injury), indecent assault (oral or anal intercourse), penetration by objects and forced sexual activity that did not result in penetration. Penetration is not an essential element to sexual assault. Indeed, in many sexual assaults, the assailant is unable to initiate or complete sexual intercourse.[2]

The absence of physical resistance by the victim is not regarded as consent. Consent by intimidation or coercive conduct without physical threat is also a criminal act. Consent requires free agreement and a person may be incapable of consenting because of the influence of drugs or alcohol.

Sexual assault by a carer upon a child is termed sexual abuse. This is sexual activity in which consent is not an issue and involves the child in sexual activity that is either beyond the child's understanding or contrary to accepted community standards. There are legal definitions regarding age, generally in the order of 15–17 years depending on the jurisdiction. Sexual violence involving a disabled person may also be either abuse or assault depending on the nature of the act or the circumstances of the victim.

Epidemiology

In the year 2003, Annual Recorded Crime Statistics[3] indicate 18 237 reports of sexual assault to police in Australia. This represents an increase in reports to police from 12 186 in 1993 and indicates a sexual assault victimization prevalence rate for Australia of 91.7 victims per 100 000 persons. The National Crime and Safety Survey (NCSS) 2002 indicates a prevalence rate for females at 0.4% (33 000 victims) and for males 0.1% (4800 victims).[4]

The reported incidence of sexual assault thus reflects only a fraction of the actual frequency of the crime, although reporting rates are increasing. Victims hesitate to report because of humiliation, fear of retribution, fear they will not be believed, self-blame and lack of understanding of the criminal justice system. Victims are more likely to report sexual assault to police if the perpetrator was a stranger or the victim was physically injured.

Once an incident of sexual assault has been reported to the police, one in four cases result in the perpetrator being charged.[5] The conviction rate is low, with less than 50% of defendants found guilty.[6]

Overwhelmingly, the offender is known to the victim. Recorded Crime Statistics (2002)[3] show that almost three in five female victims of sexual assault report that the offender was known to them. Assaults most commonly occur in the victim or perpetrator's home. The assailant was most likely to be the victim's boyfriend or date (34%), a friend (27%) or a previous partner (21%). The violation of trust that this represents also has a significant effect on the victim. Spousal rape is often more violent and repetitive than other rape and is less commonly reported, in part because of economic dependency.[7] Persons with intellectual disability are at high risk with very few prosecutions. Data collected by survey of 4000 victims of sexual assault in Australia in 2000 revealed one in five victims identified as having a disability.[8]

The victim's response to the assault is also important. NCSS 2002[4] data confirm that four out of five women do not tell police about incidents. Most women look for the support of family, friends, neighbours and workmates. One in five women who suffer a sexual assault does not disclose to anyone, seeks no help and takes no action as a result of the assault.

Rape myths and barriers to care

Any review of the literature on sexual assault will uncover discussions regarding social attitudes and preconceptions, often called rape myths. In general, these myths reflect positions, values or feelings that are not based on fact. Many of the rape myths arise and are perpetuated by socialization processes that specify sex-role behaviours and attitudes towards women. Date rape is thought to be exceedingly under-reported because the victim believes to have contributed to the act because the victim participated in foreplay. Acceptance of these rape myths can convey that victims are responsible for the assault, altering the expectation of jurors, and making it harder to report and recover from sexual assault, reinforcing the victim's guilt and shame. Indeed, the ABS study[5] found that 12.5% of women did not report the assault to the police because of shame and embarrassment.

Emergency physicians and nurses need to be aware of these attitudes that the victim and they themselves may have when approaching the sexual assault victim. A non-judgemental, accepting stance by care providers is essential. The victim will have enough self-doubt without carers adding to that. It is not the health professional's role to make a judgement as to whether the rape occurred; the courts will decide this. False allegations of rape are made, but given the perceived penalties associated with reporting a rape, such a person is likely to be disturbed and in need of help anyway.

Medical care for the victim

The objective for the attending doctor is firstly to provide for the medical needs of the victim and also, if required, to collect forensic evidence to assist in any police investigation. The history taken from the victim must be very specific and questions should be restricted to obtaining information for these purposes only. Questions should not lead into other aspects of the assault which are not relevant to the examining doctor's involvement. It is important not to prolong the examination for the victim. Furthermore, undirected questioning risks bringing inconsistencies into the description of the assault that may hinder subsequent criminal proceedings.

In general terms, there are three matters that need attention when assessing the medical needs of the sexual assault victim. These are the risk of:

❶ physical injury
❷ acquiring an infection
❸ pregnancy.

The literature typically describes about half the victims having some sort of physical injury,[9–13] although less than 5% of victims require admission to hospital for treatment. An analysis of over 1000 cases[14] in the USA revealed that physical examination showed evidence of general body trauma in 64% of victims. Genital trauma was noted in 52%, while 20.4% had no injuries documented. An Australian study confirmed non-genital injuries in 46% of women and genital injury in only 22%.[15] These findings indicate that many sexual assault victims may not have either general or genital trauma on examination, and this absence does not mean that an assault did not occur.

Studies of the genital injuries of victims using colposcopy[16] have revealed that up to 87% of patients have some type of injury. More conventional examination of the premenopausal victim will reveal that only around a third have genital injuries documented, usually cervical erosions, abrasions, bruising and swelling. Generally, such injuries do not require specific treatment with up to one-third being asymptomatic. Nonetheless, they should be assessed and documented. Toluidine blue staining may also increase the detection rate of perineal lacerations in adult victims.[10]

If injuries are photographed, this is best done by a practitioner qualified in forensic photography. The victim may not give an accurate indication of the injuries such may be the emotional impact of the assault. Some victims are unable to recall even if penetration occurred.

Most non-genital injuries are found on the head, neck and face. One-third are on the extremities and 15% on the trunk. Again, the large majority of these injuries require either symptomatic or outpatient care (abrasions, lacerations and minor fractures). Less than 1% are serious enough to warrant admission. Very occasionally, rape may turn into murder. A study from Florida found that one in 1500 sexual assaults resulted in the death of the victim, with asphyxiation being the most common cause of death.[17] While there has been no comparable Australian study, the Australian Institute of Criminology reports that there were 288 homicides committed in Australia in 2003 and a sexual assault was the precipitating factor in 9.[18]

The risk of sexually transmitted diseases following rape is 4–56%, with infection reflecting those organisms that are locally prevalent. One study showed that with baseline testing, 43% of victims had evidence of pre-existing infection.[7] The finding of pre-existing infection is not admissible in court, under Australian law. Baseline screening[19] for the following is worthwhile if follow-up can be arranged:

HIV: HIV antibody
Hepatitis B: hepatitis B surface antigen, HbsAg, core antibody, anti-HBc, and surface antibody, anti-HBs
Syphilis: rapid plasma reagin, RPR, and treponema pallidum haemagglutination assay, TPHA
Chlamydia: PCR endocervical swab, first void urine
Gonorrhoea: endocervical swab, PCR and microscopy culture and sensitivity
Trichomonas: high vaginal swab, microscopy culture and sensitivity.

Poor follow-up rates are the norm and consideration of offering prophylactic antibiotics may be appropriate.

While the risk of acquiring an infection is difficult to define, women generally accept an offer of prophylaxis for infection (Table 21.2), although the effectiveness of

Table 21.2.1   Treatment options for the sexual assault victim
Antibiotic prophylaxis
Ceftriaxone 250mg i.m. plus
Azithromycin 1g po
Antiviral prophylaxis
Protection against hepatitis B or HIV transmission should follow institutional treatment guidelines for occupational exposure to these agents
Emergency contraception
Levonorgestrel 1.5mg as single dose within 72 h with higher protection the earlier the dose

this approach has not yet been fully evaluated. Intramuscular ceftriaxone 250 mg together with 1 g azithromycin orally is the suggested antibiotic regimen for chlamydia and gonorrhoea.[20] Ceftriaxone can be mixed with lignocaine to reduce the pain of the injection.[21]

Given the low prevalence of syphilis in the general community, it may be reasonable not to give benzathine penicillin routinely but to have syphilis serology performed at 3 months, depending on the circumstances and whether follow-up can be assured.

Hepatitis B virus can be transmitted by sexual intercourse[22–24] but the risk of transmission is undefined. By comparison, the risk of infection following a percutaneous needlestick from an HBAg-positive individual to an HBAb-negative recipient is 5–43%.[25] Prophylaxis with hepatitis B vaccine 1 mL IMI is indicated. HBV vaccination and hepatitis B immune globulin (400 IU IMI) should be available where the assailant is either known to be HBV+ve or the woman is considered to be particularly at risk of infection. Hepatitis B vaccination without HBIG is highly effective in preventing HBV infection in sexual contacts of persons who have chronic HBV infection. Persons exposed to an assailant with acute HBV infection additionally require HBIG which prevents 75% of such infections.[26]

It is likely that the victim will be concerned about HIV or will become concerned at a later date. The offer of HIV testing should be made accompanied by the usual full explanation, and written consent needs to be obtained if the test is done. A prospective study from the Royal

London Hospital of 124 victims found one case of HIV seroconversion that could have been a result of a sexual assault.[27] Risk assessment includes the probability that the source is infected, the likelihood of transmission at that exposure, the interval before therapy, the efficacy of the drugs and adherence to therapy. The risk of transmission of HIV following percutaneous needlestick exposure from a known HIV-positive source is considered to be 0.4%. The risk for HIV transmission per episode of receptive penile anal exposure is 0.1–3%. The risk per episode of receptive vaginal exposure is 0.1–0.2%.[28] The risk following exposure to other body fluids is not known but should be lower.

Studies on healthcare workers are not applicable as they have had rapid access to HIV status of the contaminant and access to antiviral agents often within 1–2 hours. Note as many as 35% of healthcare workers do not finish the course due to side effects. However, the circumstances of the victim or the assault may necessitate the consideration of HIV prophylaxis, for example a male rape in a prison setting. Risk is highest for homosexually active men and people from endemic regions such as sub-Saharan Africa.[29] If post-exposure prophylaxis is advisable on the basis of high risk then a starter pack of antiretroviral post-exposure prophylaxis with a three-drug regimen should be started within 72 h,[30] ideally at 1–2 h. Tenofovir 300 mg and emtricitabine 200 mg once daily will be the more appropriate regimen for significant exposures in most cases. These should be dispensed with patient information provided. Urgent follow-up consultation with the local HIV specialist service can be sought.[31] Tetanus prophylaxis must be considered as part of the management of any injuries in the normal way.

The risk of pregnancy following a single unprotected coitus has proven difficult to define. However, a large prospective study from North America rated the risk of pregnancy from rape as 5%.[32]

The progestagen levonorgestrel is used alone for emergency contraception in a dose of 1.5 mg. If this single dose is given within 72 h the proportion of pregnancies prevented was 85% in the WHO multicentre study.[33] The earlier it is given, the more effective it is.

The literature demonstrates that there is poor compliance with follow-up instructions. Arrangements for follow-up testing for pregnancy, sexually transmitted diseases, HIV and hepatitis B vaccination should be supplied as written instructions as victims may subsequently remember little of their interview.

The forensic examination

The forensic examination is carried out at the request of the police for the purpose of obtaining evidence of the rape or assault that could be used in a prosecution. Specific consent should be sought before this examination is undertaken, as therapeutic benefit is not intended. Police services produce kits that give a comprehensive guide to the examinations required for the various aspects of the prosecution. These kits also contain a comprehensive range of swabs, slides and specimen containers for the collection of this evidence. It is important for the examining doctor to be very familiar with the contents of these kits and have an organized approach to collection of all specimens. This familiarization must occur beforehand and should not be left until the time of the examination. Careful documentation of all general and genital injuries is valuable and may be aided by use of a body map. Description of wounds needs to be accurate, comprehensive and use descriptive definitions provided with the police kit to maximize communication across disciplines involved. Grey-Eurom and Seaberg[34] found that evidence of genital and non-genital trauma was significantly associated with successful prosecution.

It is important to recognize that the victim may not be able to make an immediate decision as to whether to proceed to making a formal statement to the police. However, there are time constraints on the collection of forensic evidence. A solution may be to collect the evidence and have the police store it. The victim can then make an unhurried decision over the next few days as to whether the victim wishes to proceed. The forensic examination should also be guided by the history. For example, if anal intercourse has not occurred, there is no point in putting the victim through a rectal examination.

It is always the victim's prerogative as to whether the examination is to occur and whether all parts of the examination are to be performed. The legal concept of 'the chain of evidence' must be followed in the handling of forensic specimens. The chain of evidence does not require a police officer to be present during the examination, but the specimens should be handed to the police after the examination is concluded.

The objectives of the forensic examination are quite specific. They are to collect evidence regarding:

- proof of sexual contact
- consent or the use of force
- the identity of the assailant.

Proof of sexual contact

Proof of sexual contact is established by the detection of spermatozoa or semen either on or within the victim or on the victim's clothes. In general, only 50% of sexual assault cases have seminal evidence recovered, and this rate decreases after 24 h. The likelihood of detecting spermatozoa or semen from the vagina is generally very low by 72 h.[35] However, under some circumstances, spermatozoa may persist for days longer and can be obtained from cervical mucous. The detection of sperm or semen from the rectum or mouth is possible but very dependent on the actions of the victim after the assault. A dry swab and a fresh slide are taken to calculate the number of complete sperm at the time of examination as their concentration may be useful as a guide to the time the assault occurred.

Certain chemicals are detectable in seminal fluid and can be used as proof of sexual contact even when sperm cannot be identified, or after vasectomy. Prostatic acid phosphatase can be detected in significant levels for up to 14 h and sometimes longer in the vagina following sexual intercourse.[36] Acid phosphatase is normally found in vaginal fluid but at levels only 5–10% of seminal fluid. Prostate-specific antigen is a male-specific glycoprotein found in semen and may be detected in the vagina for up to 48 h after intercourse and may be detected when acid phosphatase cannot be found.[37]

It is not necessary to prove sexual contact to prove rape. Legally, penetration is said to have occurred once the tip of the penis has entered the labia majora and ejaculation does not have to occur. A review of 372 female rape victims in Detroit, Tintinalli and Hoelzer found no correlation between the finding of sperm or acid phosphatase activity and the recording of a conviction.[38]

Consent

Evidence of the lack of consent may be found by indications of the use of force. This may be deduced from the state of the victim's clothes or by the presence of injuries. Again, most studies of rape victims record that only about half the victims show any signs of physical injury.

Identification of the assailant

The most accurate laboratory method currently available to identify the assailant is DNA testing.[39,40] The chance of incorrectly identifying an alleged assailant as the source of DNA material is infinitely small, literally one in several trillion. Any sample collected from the victim that contains cellular material from the victim's assailant can be used for DNA testing. This includes spermatozoa, semen if it contains cells, or blood or tissue from under fingernails. DNA evidence left on or in the body of a victim, particularly in moist areas, degrades quickly over 2–10 days. The forensic assessment should thus be made as soon as possible. As DNA degrades quickly if moist, underclothes should be stored in paper not plastic bags.

Stray hair follicles, for example combed from the pubic region of the victim may yield DNA to identify an assailant if the sheath cells are still present. Such hair that also includes the shaft and the follicle can also be used for a direct visual comparison under a microscope with hair from a suspect. As an investigation, however, this has a low return and requires the collection of plucked hair from the head and pubic region of the victim. Plucking the hair from the victim can be done at any time if it becomes important rather than in the aftermath of the assault.

Care must be taken when the victim undresses for the examination. Hair or clothes fibres from the offender or other traces from the crime scene may have adhered to the body or clothes of the victim. The victim should undress standing over a drop sheet, which should then be included in a bag into which her clothes are placed. This becomes part of the physical evidence. The victim should then be able to shower with simple toiletries provided. The victim will need a change of clothes, fresh underwear and loose-fitting comfortable outerwear such as a track suit. Such simple provisions are inexpensive but begin to give the victim the sense of re-establishing control.

Psychological impact of a sexual assault

The predominant psychological reaction of the sexual assault victim is a devastating and profound sense of loss.[41] There are two major causes of this. First, throughout the assault the victim may well be in grave fear for her own survival. It is common knowledge that rapists sometimes murder their victims and the use of actual or threatened violence possibly supported by a weapon is an almost universal feature of rape. Second, the victim suffers a gross invasion of bodily boundaries in a manner that removes her control over that which she holds most personal to her.

As a result, sexual assault survivors are more likely to develop post-traumatic stress disorder than victims of any other crime.[42]

Following a sexual assault, the victim can show a wide range of emotional responses, but these can generally be characterized into one of two broad types: expressed or controlled. In the expressed style, the victim's fear and anxiety may be shown by crying and obvious distress. In the controlled style, the victim will be outwardly calm, even appearing detached or nonchalant. It is important for caregivers to recognize these emotional styles exist and not to make value judgements about victims' credibility on the basis of their emotional presentation.

After this comes a reorganization phase in which the victim attempts to assimilate the event and recover her lifestyle. Continuing counselling can assist the victim during this phase by providing an opportunity for ventilation of feelings, providing reassurance and support of adaptive behaviour and education.

Up to 95% of victims may meet the criteria of post-traumatic stress disorder following the

rape,[43] and as many as 16.5% of victims still show stress-related symptoms 17 years after the attack.[44] Survivors report a variety of emotional changes in the longer term following the assault, including fear, anxiety and depression. Many report sexual dysfunction and disruption of relationships,[41] a finding that has also been noted in male victims.[45] On the other hand, appropriate interventions and support can lead to better outcomes, including changes that could be viewed as positive. One cohort of survivors saw themselves as stronger, more careful, more self-reliant, independent or thoughtful.[46]

Even though emergency physicians play a brief role in the care of the victim, they can also have an important impact on psychological recovery. It has been found that the greater the support the doctor provides to the victim, the better the outcome,[47] and that the victims consider the manner in which the medical examination is performed as more important than other factors such as the gender of the doctor. However, the same study found doctors to be the least supportive in comparison to other health professionals, families, friends and social service agencies.

Sexual assault in special circumstances

Pregnancy

A study from Texas found no difference in the frequency of sexual assault for women who were less than 15 weeks' pregnant.[48] Beyond then, she was less likely to be raped, leading the authors to theorize that being obviously pregnant might be protective against rape or if she was raped, she was less likely to be seriously physically injured. There were no premature deliveries in the 4 weeks following the rape and no adverse fetal effects were detected.

Postmenopausal women

It is one of the myths associated with rape that victims are young and physically attractive or dress or behave in a way which provokes the attacks.[49] The reality is that the victim may be any age, including elderly. This is consistent with the view that rape is an act of subjugation and asserting control rather than of sexual passion. In

terms of physical injury, the injury patterns are similar except that postmenopausal women are significantly more likely to need surgical management and repair of genital injuries than are younger women.[50]

Children

The circumstances regarding children who are the victims of sexual assault differ from those relating to adults. First, the child is likely to have been the victim of chronic abuse rather than an attack by a stranger. Second, almost always the offender will be a man known to the child, often in a position of authority and trust.[51] This introduces the issue of protecting the child from further molestation. The injury pattern is highly variable. Chronic sexual abuse tends to develop as a pattern of behaviour between the victim and the offender beginning with touching and possibly leading to penetrative intercourse. This escalation of activity may evolve over a lengthy period and physical trauma may not be a feature. If the child has been the victim of a stranger assault, the risk of physical injury is greater than for an adult victim.[52] Child sexual assault is ideally managed by a team with specific paediatric expertise.

Men

Male rape outside institutional settings is largely unrecognized and under-reported, but males may comprise up to 10% of rape victims.[53–55] Males may be more likely to suffer significant physical injury during an assault even though their ability to resist may be no different to that of a female victim.[54] Male victims may carry additional burdens of guilt arising from concerns about their sexual orientation, which result from the attack and from the reaction of the police if they report. This concern will be heightened if they find themselves physically sexually stimulated during the assault as can occur with female victims.[46]

In general, the short- and long-term psychological consequences of sexual assault are no different between male and female victims. Apart from the obvious physiological and anatomical differences, there is no difference in the medical consequences of sexual assault for male and female victims.

Drug-facilitated sexual assault

The National Drug Strategy report on Drink Spiking published in 2004[56] revealed between 3000 and 4000 suspected incidents per year in Australia, with approximately one-third involving sexual assault, the most common associated crime. In addition to alcohol, there are three drugs particularly associated with sexual assault: flunitrazepam, γ-hydroxybutyrate and ketamine.

Samples may be evaluated in a therapeutic laboratory, but, if the victim wishes to make a formal complaint, urine and blood samples must be taken under strict collection procedures to ensure the chain of evidence is maintained.

Conclusion

While sexual assault is an act of violence, the consequences for the survivor are primarily emotional and psychological rather than physical. Nonetheless, the emergency physician may well be expected to provide an initial medical assessment and may be asked to assist the police in the collection of forensic evidence. Therefore, this doctor will be amongst the first to attend to the victim in the aftermath of the assault. The doctor must have a clear understanding of the technical aspects of his or her role. It is important for the doctor to have an accepting, non-prejudicial attitude that places the wellbeing of the victim ahead of any other considerations, including apprehension about becoming involved in subsequent legal processes. In this way, survivors may be given the best opportunity to recover from an event that will change their lives.

Controversies and future directions

❶ The continuing challenge for the medical profession and the community is overcoming deeply embedded myths and misconceptions. Some progress has been made and services for most sexual assault victims have improved in the past few years.

❷ Those barriers persist in a number of areas in which the incidence of sexual assault is only starting to become recognized. These areas include institutional and educational settings, including the special problem of sexual assault of the disabled, inmates, military and police recruits in academies, and the general issue of male rape victims.

❸ One of the most challenging areas is the endemic problem of violence, including sexual violence inflicted on indigenous women. Some groups of aboriginal girls and women report that half of them had been the victim of incest or sexual assault.[57]

References

1. Groth AN, Burgess AW, Holmstrom LL. Rape: power, anger and sexuality. American Journal of Psychiatry 1977; 134: 1239–1243.
2. Groth AN, Burgess AW. Sexual dysfunction during rape. New England Journal of Medicine 1977; 297: 764–767.
3. Australian Bureau of Statistics. Recorded Crime Victims, Australia. ABS Catalogue no. 4510.0 Commonwealth of Australia; 2004.
4. Australian Bureau of Statistics. National Crime and Safety Survey. ABS Catalogue no 4509.0 Commonwealth of Australia; 2002.
5. Australian Bureau of Statistics. Sexual assault in Australia: a statistical overview. ABS Catalogue 4523.0 Commonwealth of Australia; 2004.
6. NSW Bureau of Crime Statistics and Research. Crime and Justice Bulletin. No. 92; 2006.
7. Hampton HL. Care of the woman who has been raped. New England Journal of Medicine 1995; 332: 234–237.
8. National Association of Services against Sexual Violence. Report National Data Collection Project. National Association of Services against Sexual Violence, Adelaide; 2000.
9. Rambow B, Adkinson C, Frost TH, et al. Female sexual assault: medical and legal implications. Annals of Emergency Medicine 1992; 21: 727–731.
10. McCauley J, Guzinski G, Welch R, et al. Toluidine blue in the corroboration of rape in the adult victim. American Journal of Emergency Medicine 1987; 5: 105–108.
11. Beebe D. Emergency management of the adult female rape victim. American Family Physician 1991; 43: 2041–2046.
12. Tucker S, Ledray LE, Werner JS. Sexual assault evidence collection. Wisconsin Medical Journal 1990; 89: 407–411.
13. Geist RF. Sexually related trauma. Emergency Medicine Clinics of North America 1988; 6(3): 439–466 .
14. Riggs N, Houry D, Long G, et al. Analysis of 1076 cases of sexual assault. Annals of Emergency Medicine 2000; 35: 358–362.
15. Palmer C. Genital injuries in women reporting sexual assault. Sex Health 2004; 1:55–59.
16. Slaughter L, Brown CR. Colposcopy to establish physical findings in rape victims. American Journal of Obstetrics and Gynecology 1992; 166: 83–86.
17. Deming JE, Mittleman RE, Wetli CV. Forensic science aspects of fatal sexual assaults on women. Journal of Forensic Sciences 1983; 28: 572–576.
18. Australian Institute of Criminology. Homicide in Australia 2003–2004 National Homicide Monitoring Program. Research and Public Policy Series No. 66.
19. Mein J, Palmer C, Shand MC, et al. Management of acute adult sexual assault. Medical Journal Australia 2003; 178(5): 226–230.
20. Workowski KA, Berron SM, STD 2006 Centres for Disease Control and Prevention. Treatment guidelines. Morbidity and Mortality Weekly Report Recommendations and Reports 2006; 55: 1–94.
21. Patel IH, Weinfeld RE, Konikoff J, et al. Pharmacokinetics and tolerance of ceftriaxone in humans after single dose administration in water and lidocaine diluents. Antimicrobial Agents Chemotherapy 1982; 21: 957–962.
22. Szmuness W, Much MI, Prince AM, et al. On the role of sexual behaviour in the spread of hepatitis B infection. Annals of Internal Medicine 1975; 83: 489–495.
23. Schreeder MT, Thompson SE, Hadler SC, et al. Hepatitis B in homosexual men: prevalence of infection and factors related to transmission. Journal of Infectious Diseases 1982; 146: 7–15.
24. Alter MJ, Ahtone J, Weisfuse I, et al. Hepatitis B transmission between heterosexuals. Journal of the American Medical Association 1986; 256: 1307–1310.
25. Gerberding JL, Henderson DK. Management of occupational exposures to blood-borne pathogens: Hepatitis B virus, hepatitis C virus, and human immunodeficiency virus. Clinical Infectious Diseases 1992; 14: 1179–1185.
26. Centre for Disease Control. Post-exposure prophylaxis Hepatitis B. Recommendations and reports. Morbidity and Mortality Weekly Report 1997; 47: 101–104.
27. Estrich S, Forster GE, Robinson A. Sexually transmitted diseases in rape victims. Genitourinary Medicine 1990; 66: 433–438.
28. Centre for Disease Control. Management of possible sexual or injecting drug use or other non occupational exposure to HIV. Morbidity and Mortality Weekly Report 1998; 47: 1–14.
29. National HIV/AIDS Strategy 1999–2000 to 2003–2004 Changes and Challenges. Commonwealth Department of Health and Aging; 2000, pp. 15–17.
30. Winston J, McAllister J, Amin J, et al. The use of triple nucleoside-nucleotide regimen for non occupational HIV PEP. HIV Medicine 2005; 6:191–197.
31. Australian National Council on Aids, Hepatitis C and Related Diseases. ANCAHRD Bulletin No. 28. 2001.
32. Holmes MM, Resnick HS, Kilpatrick DG, et al. Rape-related pregnancy: Estimates and descriptive characteristics from a national sample of women. American Journal of Obstetrics and Gynecology 1996; 175: 320–325.
33. Von Hertzen H, Piaggio G, Pregoudov A, et al. Low dose mifeprostone and two regimes of levonorgestrel for emergency contraception: a WHO multicentre randomised trial. Lancet 2002; 360: 1803–1810.
34. Grey-Eurom K, Seaberg D. The prosecution of sexual assault cases; correlation with forensic evidence. Annals of Emergency Medicine 2002; 39: 39–63.
35. Greydanus DE, Shaw RD, Kennedy EL. Examination of sexually abused adolescents. Seminars in Adolescent Medicine 1987; 3: 59–65.
36. Ricci LR. Prostatic acid phosphatase and sperm in the post-coital vagina. Annals Emergency Medicine 1982; 11: 530–534.
37. Graves HCB, Sensabaugh GF, Blake ET. Post-coital detection of a male-specific semen protein: application to the investigation of rape. New England Journal of Medicine 1985; 312: 338–343.
38. Tintinalli JE, Hoelzer M. Clinical findings and legal resolution in sexual assault. Annals of Emergency Medicine 1985; 14: 447–453.
39. Gill P, Jeffreys AJ, Werrett DJ. Forensic application of DNA fingerprints. Nature 1985; 318: 577–579.
40. Marx JL. DNA fingerprinting takes the witness stand. Science 1988; 240: 1616–1618.
41. Rose DS. Worse than death: Psychodynamics of rape victims and the need for psychotherapy. American Journal of Psychiatry 1986; 143: 817–824.
42. Welch J, Mason F. Rape and sexual assault. British Medical Journal 2007; 334: 1154–1158.
43. Foa EB, Rothbaum BO, Riggs DS, et al. Treatment of post-traumatic stress disorder in rape victims: a comparison between cognitive behavioural procedures and counselling. Journal of Consulting and Clinical Psychology 1991; 59: 715–723.
44. Kilpatrick DG, Saunders BE, Veronen LJ, et al. Criminal victimisation: Lifetime prevalence, reporting to police, and psychological impact. Crime and Delinquency 1987; 33: 479–489.

CHALLENGING SITUATIONS

45. Mezey G, King M. The effects of sexual assault on men: a survey of 22 victims. Psychological Medicine 1989; 19: 205–209.

46. Nadelson CC, Notman M, Zackson H, et al. A follow-up study of rape victims. American Journal of Psychiatry 1982; 139: 1266–1270.

47. Popiel DA, Susskind EC. The impact of the rape: social support as the moderator of stress. American Journal of Community Psychology 1985; 13: 645–676.

48. Satin AJ, Hemsell DL, Stone IC, et al. Sexual assault in pregnancy. Obstetrics and Gynecology 1991; 77: 710–714.

49. Mazelam PM. Stereotypes and perceptions in the victims of rape. Victimology 1980; 5: 121–231.

50. Ramin SM, Satin AJ, Stone IC, et al. Sexual assault in postmenopausal women. Obstetrics and Gynecology 1992; 80: 860–864.

51. Ricci LR. Child sexual abuse: the emergency department response. Annals of Emergency Medicine 1985; 15: 711–716.

52. Cartwright PS, the Sexual Assault Study Group. Factors that correlate with injury sustained by survivors of sexual assault. Obstetrics and Gynecology 1987; 70: 44–46.

53. Kaufman A, DiVasto P, Jackson R, et al. Male rape victims: non-institutionalised assault. American Journal of Psychiatry 1980; 137: 221–223.

54. King MB. Male rape. British Medical Journal 1990; 301: 1345–1346.

55. Lipscomb GH, Muram D, Speck PM, et al. Male victims of sexual assault. Journal of the American Medical Association 1992; 267: 3064–3066.

56. The National Drug Strategy. National Project on Drink Spiking Australian Institute of Criminology; Nov 2004.

57. Atkinson J. Aboriginal and Islander Health Worker 1990; 14: 4–27.

21.3 Domestic violence

Sandra Neate

ESSENTIALS

1 Domestic violence encompasses physical, psychological and sexual violence during childhood, adulthood or both.

2 All forms of domestic violence are inter-related in a complex way. Victims may suffer many forms of violence over their lives.

3 Between 30 and 50% of women and approximately 15% of men experience domestic violence over their lifetime. The incidence is higher in indigenous populations.

4 Domestic violence occurs across all socioeconomic, religious and cultural groups.

5 Predisposing factors for being a perpetrator or victim of violence may begin as early as childhood.

6 Disclosure of violence is uncommon and detection is difficult.

7 Consequences of domestic violence can be physical, psychological, social, economic and forensic. Health outcomes for victims, witnesses of violence and perpetrators are generally poor.

8 Management requires a coordinated approach from health practitioners, social services, the police and the judicial system.

Definition

Domestic violence in its broadest sense includes all types of violence within intimate or family relationships. Domestic violence consists of physical and sexual abuse, threats and intimidation, psychological, emotional and social abuse or financial deprivation and can occur during childhood, adulthood or both. Physical abuse is when physical violence including assault with a weapon is used to control a person. Non-personal physical violence, such as damage to property or brandishing weapons, can be equally intimidating. Sexual violence involves coercing a partner into engaging in sexual activity against his or her will by using intimidation, threats or physical harm.[1] Psychological abuse consists of verbal harassment, ridicule, threats of physical harm and behaviours designed to intimidate, humiliate, control and isolate. Isolation can involve prevention of family contact, attendance at work or contact with medical practitioners. Psychological abuse nearly always precedes physical abuse.[2]

Violence is traditionally assumed to be perpetrated by men against women but may be by women against men or by partners in same-sex relationships. The partnership may be current or past. Other family members related by blood or law may be perpetrators of domestic violence. Indigenous populations often have broader definitions and utilize the term 'family violence.'[3] Domestic violence also includes abuse of the elderly by either spouse or other family member and may involve physical and psychological abuse, neglect and exploitation including financial. Child abuse falls within the spectrum of domestic violence but is often considered a separate issue.

Most studies of domestic violence concentrate on violence between partners in an intimate relationship. In the USA the alternative term of intimate partner violence is frequently used. The common factor in violent intimate relationships is an imbalance of power, with one person exerting coercive control over the other by some means of violence whether physical, psychological or sexual, either actual or threatened. The subjective experience and definition of domestic violence are strongly influenced by cultural beliefs and previous life experiences, and the individual's perceptions of the experience may vary greatly from standard clinical definitions.[4]

Incidence

The prevalence of domestic violence varies according to definition (whether emotional and sexual abuse are included), timing of the abuse (immediate, during adult life or cumulative life time prevalence) and whether the violence is actual or threatened. Prevalence surveys within Australian emergency departments (EDs), where domestic violence was defined as an adult fearing or being the victim of physical violence from a partner, indicate that approximately 30% of women and 15% of men report a lifetime history of domestic violence, with 19–24% of women and 8% of men disclosing a history of domestic violence during adult life.[5–7] US studies report a higher cumulative lifetime prevalence of approximately 50% but include actual and threatened personal and non-personal violence.[8]

The Australian Bureau of Statistics 1996 Women's Safety Survey and 2005 Personal Safety found that 5.8% of women had experienced violence in the preceding 12-month period in 2005 compared with 7.1% in 1996.[9,10] In 2002 in Australia, 408 100 (3% of the population) people were victims of domestic violence, 87% of those were women, 98% of the perpetrators were men, 263 800 children were living with victims of domestic violence and 181 200 had witnessed domestic violence in the 12-month period.[11]

Overall, women have four times the risk of experiencing domestic violence than men and those who have been victims of child abuse have six times the risk of experiencing adult domestic violence. Men and women report similar incidences of approximately 7% of childhood abuse alone.[7] Pregnancy represents a high-risk time for domestic violence. Six per cent of pregnant women are battered during the pregnancy.[12] The incidence of abuse towards women with mental or physical disabilities is between 33 and 83%, depending on the severity of disability and the definition of abuse.[12] In the USA approximately 1 million elderly people per year are physically assaulted, neglected or exploited.[13]

The incidence of violence is generally higher amongst indigenous populations than non-indigenous. A New Zealand general practice survey found 25% of Maori women reported partner violence within the preceding 12 months and 75% reported a lifetime incidence of partner violence.[14] In Australia the rate of family

victimization for indigenous women may be 40 times the rate for non-indigenous women and despite representing just over 2% the total population, indigenous women accounted for 15% of homicide victims in Australia in 2002–2003. Barriers to accurate gathering of data relating to indigenous women are compounded by geographical remoteness and limited resources and indigenous women are often excluded from surveys due to lack of telephones and having no fixed residential address.[15]

Domestic violence rates in women from non-English-speaking backgrounds (NESBs) tend to be lower than those from English-speaking backgrounds for the lifetime incidence of physical, sexual and all forms of violence. NESB women's decreased incidence of reporting violence may be due to perceptions of what constitutes violence and reluctance to report violence due to personal, religious, cultural, informational and language factors.[16]

Overall, approximately 2% of women presenting to EDs have experienced physical violence within the 24 h preceding the presentation.[5,7] The incidence is approximately 10% if psychological abuse is included.[8]

Predictors of domestic violence

Several demographic factors may be associated with an increased risk of being a perpetrator or victim of domestic violence. Characteristics associated with an increased risk of being a male perpetrator of violence are alcohol abuse, drug use, low education standards and unemployment, and being a former rather than current partner. Alcohol abuse is the most identifiable risk factor and has a clear dose–response relationship.[17] One-half of victims report that their male partner was intoxicated at the time of assault. However, the relationship between alcohol and abuse is not necessarily cause and effect. An asymmetric power balance between the perpetrator and victim remains the main determinant of conflict in violent intimate relationships. Within the context of these power-imbalanced relationships the association between alcohol and domestic

violence may be that alcohol abuse makes physical assault more likely.[17]

The greatest risk for being a female victim of domestic violence is having a former partner, with an even higher risk if the woman is living with the former partner. Separated or divorced women are four times more likely to be abused than women who have never married or are married or widowed.[18] Other demographic factors for women do not show statistically significant predictive value for victimization.[17] Male victims of violence in the USA tend to be younger, single and African-American[19] and the perpetrators are more likely to be de facto partners and family members other than spouses.[7] Men who are abused are commonly assaulted by the women whom they abuse.[20]

Despite these trends in demographics, domestic violence occurs across all socio-economic groups, races and religions, and demographic characteristics are not sensitive or predictive indicators of an individual's potential to be a perpetrator or victim of domestic violence.[17,21] Clinical presentations such as injury pattern, specific obstetric and gynaecological symptoms, psychiatric symptoms and substance abuse do not have significant sensitivity or positive predictive value as indicators of domestic violence.[22]

Outcomes

Domestic violence affects the victim's and the family's health in a multitude of physical and psychological ways. Despite the emphasis on physical injury, most presentations to health professionals by domestic violence victims are a complex mix of indirectly related physical and psychological problems and are not trauma related.[8] The perpetrator and particularly the witnesses of violence also experience adverse outcomes.

Physical injury and illness
Physical injuries resulting from domestic violence follow some patterns. Injuries inflicted on females are likely to be contusions, abrasions, lacerations, fractures and dislocations. Women are more likely to be choked, beaten or sexually abused.[7,17] Men have a greater risk of having objects

thrown at them or weapons used against them. Features suggestive of intentional injury are similar to those recognized to suggest non-accidental injury in children and include history inconsistent with the injury, injuries in varying temporal stages, unreasonable delay in presentation and injuries in central rather than peripheral regions of the body. Injuries to defensive areas of the body or to the back, legs, buttocks, back of the head and soles of the feet suggest an attempt at self-protection. Although domestic-violence-related injuries follow certain patterns, injury pattern is of low positive predictive value when attempting to identify domestic violence.[23]

Abuse before, during and after pregnancy represents a threat to mother and fetus. Of women who are victims of physical violence, approximately 40% also experience coercion into non-consensual sex at some stage, highlighting the link between physical and sexual violence. This results in high rates of sexually transmitted disease, unintended and adolescent pregnancy, and elective termination of pregnancy.[24] There is also an established complex link between domestic violence and preterm labour, low-birth-weight babies and postnatal depression.[4,25]

Prevention of access to healthcare by victims of violence, due to the perpetrator's fear of disclosure, is common. A survey of women attending five outpatient hospital-based clinics found that 17% of women who had been abused in the preceding 12 months reported partner interference with accessing healthcare compared with 2% of women who had not been abused. This was found to pose a significant obstacle to healthcare.[26] Prevention of antenatal care is common.

The risks of HIV and being a victim of intimate partner violence are related in a complex manner. Women who reported engaging in sex with an HIV-infected partner or an injecting drug user, having multiple partners in the preceding 12 months and injecting drugs were significantly more likely to have experienced any form of physical or injurious intimate partner violence and any form of sexual intimate partner violence in the preceding 6 months.[27]

Death is the ultimate physical injury. Approximately 25% of US female homicides are domestic-violence related.[28]

One US study examining female homicides over a 5-year period found that 44% of homicide victims had presented to an ED in the 2 years preceding death. Despite 28 injury-related visits and 48 total visits, domestic violence was documented in only two cases and intervention occurred in none.[28]

Psychological impact

Domestic violence is a strong independent risk factor for the development of mental illness. Women experiencing domestic violence have an approximately 11-fold increase of dissociation, 6-fold increase in somatization symptoms, are 5 times as likely to suffer anxiety and 3 times as likely to suffer depression, phobias and drug dependence. Abused women have twice the rates of hazardous alcohol consumption and dependence as non-abused women.[18] A further significant increase in incidence of these psychiatric diagnoses occurs when violence is experienced in both childhood and adulthood.[29] Women experiencing psychological abuse may suffer greater psychological distress and illness than those who experience physical violence. Ridicule and humiliation are particularly responsible for causing low self-esteem in the victim and facilitate the cycle of abuse by contributing to the victim feeling responsible for and deserving of the violence.[2] Seeking treatment for mental health problems can further add to the abused woman's burden, as a psychiatric history may be used against her by the perpetrator in dealings with police or family courts.[20]

Impact on children

The impact on the children living within a household where violence is perpetrated is vast and consists of being the victim of violence, witnessing violence, separations from family members, being placed in foster care, being at risk for future psychiatric illness and drug and alcohol dependence, and becoming a perpetrator of violence themselves. Children who live in violent households are at risk of physical injury. The majority of physical injuries are inadvertent as children are held during the violent episode or as they attempt to intervene to save a parent from harm.[30]

The Australian Bureau of Statistics records that 49–61% of people who had

experienced violence reported that they had children in their care at the time of the violence and 27–36% said that children had witnessed violence.[10] The emotional impact of witnessing family violence is a significant independent factor for lifetime psychiatric diagnoses in women.[29]

Children living in a home where violence is perpetrated against a parent are 15 times more likely to be a victim of abuse or neglect themselves, as domestic violence and child abuse are each predictors of the other.[4] Domestic violence is a risk factor for becoming a perpetrator of homicide in the pre-teenage group.[31] Other flow-on effects include children becoming perpetrators of aggressive behaviour manifest as bullying in childhood.[32]

The outcome of the experience of violence is directly proportional to the duration and frequency of violent episodes. Overall, approximately one-third of the population risk for all psychiatric diagnoses is attributable to domestic violence.[29]

Social

Control by the abuser who fears disclosure by the victim leads to social isolation such as loss of contact with friends and family and prevention from paid employment. Financial dependence on the abuser together with the responsibility of children adds to isolation, loss of choices and difficulties of separation from the abuser. Poverty is prevalent and multifactorial. Separation from or incarceration of the abuser may lead to further loss of income. In the case of the elderly, finances may be improperly used by the legal guardian. For indigenous women or women from NESBs, separation from the perpetrator may require the separation from their community and fragmentation of their identity.[3]

Homelessness may be relative, where there is no sense of safety or security in the home, or absolute where there is need for interim accommodation, emergency shelters or, in extreme cases, families may be living on the streets. Children or elderly people living in violent circumstances may find themselves in foster care or institutionalized by authorities or carers.

Outcomes for male victims of domestic violence differ from outcomes for female victims in several significant ways. Men are more likely to suffer serious physical injury than women. However, male victims express fewer feelings of fear and terror, and less frequently feel trapped and controlled. Men are also generally less constrained by financial dependence. As fear, control, dependence and isolation contribute greatly to the psychological outcomes of domestic violence, women still suffer approximately 95% of the serious physical and psychological consequences of domestic violence.[20]

Economic cost

The costs of domestic violence are vast. Costs include pain, suffering and premature mortality costs, health costs (victim, perpetrator and children), production-related costs (lost productivity), consumption-related costs (property replacement), second-generation costs (childcare and child protection) and administrative (legal and forensic) and transfer costs (income support and lost taxes). The total annual cost of domestic violence in Australia in 2002–2003 was estimated to be AUD $8.1 billion. The lifetime cost per victim was AUD $224 470.[11] International studies estimate costs in the billions of dollars annually.[32]

Barriers to detection and reporting of domestic violence

Detection rates of domestic violence in EDs are low. Only 10% of people presenting with acute domestic-violence-related injuries or issues are directly asked by the attending nurse or physician or volunteer information regarding the violence issue. Documentation of violence in the medical record is rare.[8] After an education programme to promote detection of domestic violence, only 50% of those who reported domestic violence on screening questionnaire had violence documented in the medical record.[33]

Barriers to detection include system and patient factors. System factors include the physical environment such as inadequate privacy and inadequate staffing resulting in time constraints. Further barriers include the health practitioner's lack of time and education, inappropriate attitudes or frustration at the patient's inability to effect

change. Cultural, social and gender issues also contribute. Patient factors include feelings of shame and humiliation, cultural taboos, confidentiality concerns, fear of reprisals from the perpetrator and safety issues, both personal and relating to children.

Rates of reporting of domestic violence to police are low but may be increasing. In Australia 36% of women who experienced physical assault by a male perpetrator reported it to the police in 2005 compared to 19% in 1996, and 19% of women who experienced sexual assault reported it to the police in 2005 compared to 15% in 1996.[9,10] Reluctance to involve the police, children's services and the judicial system may result from fear of removal of children and other legal ramifications.[12]

Indigenous women in Australia report violence rarely. Historical interactions with police such as forcible removal of children and high rates of aboriginal deaths in custody result in indigenous women fearing for the safety of themselves and their families when police or social services are involved.[4] A culture of silence exists in many indigenous communities about these issues. There are barriers in accessibility and cultural appropriateness of legal processes which discourage indigenous women's use of the judicial system.[3]

The elderly may be prevented from reporting by fear of further abuse, neglect or the threat of institutionalization.[4]

Screening

Between 30 and 50% of women presenting to EDs have been the victim of domestic violence in their lifetime, 2–10% within the preceding 24 h. The high prevalence of domestic violence, low positive predictive values of demographic factors and clinical presentations, low detection rates and high incidence of subsequent physical and psychological illness have supported the argument for universal screening. Detection rates without screening are in the order of 0.4%. Opportunistic screening may increase detection rates of domestic violence.[34] Rates of detection rise to approximately 14% with the use of simple direct questioning.[34]

Many methods of screening are described. The use of a single screening question may

be as effective as asking several questions. Screening questions should be simple and direct such as 'Have you been hit, kicked, punched or otherwise hurt by someone in the last year?', 'Do you feel safe at home?' or 'Are you afraid of your partner?'[35,36] Explanation that these questions are routine may improve patient comfort. A computer-based health survey increased screening rates to 99.8%, detection rates to 19%, referral rates to social services to 10% and receiving of services to 4%.[37]

Screening may indicate to the victim that channels of communication are open and that help will be available when he or she is ready to disclose information. It educates victims about violence, its nature and prevalence. Screening may also be important in detection of perpetrators. Approximately 40% of domestic violence perpetrators have sought medical attention in the preceding 6 months with half having attended an ED.[38]

Most women find screening an acceptable practice. Up to two-thirds of medical practitioners and 50% of nurses are not in favour of screening. The most significant potential barriers to screening identified were a lack of education and instruction on how to ask questions about abuse, language barriers between nurses and patients, a personal or family history of abuse and time issues.[39] In the USA the legal implications of mandatory reporting add to reluctance to screen.

Screening may improve detection rates and referral rates to external agencies. However, despite much research into the ideal screening tool and how to implement screening in EDs, currently no evidence exists that screening leads to improved health outcomes for victims.[40,41]

Management

Violence and abuse are criminal matters, but the management of the victim of domestic violence is complex. Common misconceptions include that a woman is best leaving her situation immediately, reporting to police and involving legal services. Simply leaving a violent relationship is no guarantee of safety however. Involvement of police or the judicial system is no guarantee of a positive outcome for the individual. Conversely, leaving and reporting may lead to adverse outcomes such as increased levels of violence. It can be difficult for health practitioners to let go of the need to fix or cure the problem or even know for certain that the problem exists. The goal should not be to persuade the woman to leave the violent relationship. Leaving a violent relationship is a process and not an event, and requires support through all phases. Help may best be offered by expressing concern, listening, providing support and offering a bridge to services.

Understanding

Interviews with survivors of domestic violence have provided a framework for understanding the stages through which a victim must work before being ready to leave a violent relationship.[42] A precontemplative phase, where the victim is not consciously aware of or is in denial about the abuse, occurs first followed by a contemplation phase where the abuse is acknowledged, but the victim is unable to decide to leave. A preparation stage follows where small steps are taken in preparation to leave. This is a period of increased risk of violence and safety is paramount. This may well be the period where the victim faces the greatest obstacles to leaving. The victim may have been isolated from friends and family and may be financially dependent and concerned for her ability to survive and protect her children. The action stage when leaving finally occurs can be prolonged and is typically characterized by relapses with multiple returns to the relationship. After a period of 6 months without return to the relationship the victim is then said to be in a maintenance phase.

Listening and understanding the progress through these phases will assist in assessing readiness for change and guide intervention.[12] The aim is to validate the victim's experience, to emphasize that the victim is not to blame for or deserving of the abuse and to empower the victim and support decision-making, with the emphasis that the victim is in control of her choices. The doctor or nurse is not there to advise the patient what is best.

Referral

There are multiple agencies to assist victims of domestic violence. Community services include hotlines for emergency advice through to counselling services, emergency shelters, police and legal services. Up to 50% of domestic-violence-related ED presentations occur between the hours of 8 pm and 8 am.[31] ED staff should be aware of how to access these community services 24 h a day.

Safety

Immediate action may be required in the form of emergency accommodation. If the victim judges it safe to return home, a safety plan may be organized including readily accessible emergency contact numbers and emergency items such as identification, money, credit cards, legal documents and medication relating to both the woman and her children. Safety is an ongoing issue as a woman in an abusive relationship is at greatest risk of injury as she is leaving the relationship. Seventy per cent of domestic violence murders occur as the woman is leaving or has left the home.[43] Ongoing contact with the perpetrator after separation due to custody arrangements surrounding children makes the risk of abuse a continuing one.

Reporting

Seven states in the USA mandate reporting of injuries resulting from domestic violence. In total, 45 states have laws that require reporting of injuries caused by weapons, major crimes or domestic violence.[44] Reporting of domestic violence is not mandatory in Australasia. Mandatory reporting remains controversial. Arguments in favour of reporting are based on the assumption that reporting will stop the violence. Arguments against reporting are that victims will be deterred from disclosure and that health practitioners will avoid asking about violence due to concerns about their legal responsibility to report even if uncertain.

Documentation

Documentation in the medical record may provide vital legal evidence and should be objective and accurate. Direct quotes should be used rather than paraphrasing, and descriptions of behaviours and appearances rather than interpretation add objectivity. Body maps assist documentation of physical injury. Photographs may be of assistance. When sexual assault is suspected, the involvement of specific sexual-assault-centre staff ensures that legally admissible evidence is obtained.

The perpetrator

Many perpetrators suffer from depression, alcohol and substance dependence, and post-traumatic stress disorder.[38] Some of these conditions may be amenable to treatment. Batterers with antisocial personality disorder are less amenable to treatment. The management of perpetrators of physical and sexual assault still remains largely the domain of the police and criminal justice system.

The management of domestic violence requires a coordinated response from all practitioners and service providers involved from the moment the victim first discloses the violence. This includes the health system, social services and the police and judicial system if the victim chooses to pursue this course of action. At all times, the victim's wishes must be paramount and the service providers should do their utmost to support these wishes.

Conclusion

Domestic violence is a complex issue with risk factors for being a perpetrator or a victim beginning in childhood and continuing through adult life. Factors such as the childhood environment, whether there is violence experienced personally or witnessed, the gaining of self-esteem, education level, drug and alcohol abuse, and mental health and personality issues all impact on an individual's risk of being both a victim or a perpetrator of violence. Domestic violence is extremely common and frequently remains undetected, but interventions aimed at increased detection and referral may not improve outcomes for the individual. ED staff, whilst accepting that identification and referral may not necessarily alter the outcome for the victim, should be aware of the complex nature of the issues surrounding domestic violence and that approximately 2% of the women they see in the ED have experienced domestic violence in the preceding 24 h. Whilst data may not document improved outcomes on a population basis, complacency towards detection should not exist as any one individual may benefit from recognition and support. Expressing concern and willingness to listen, being non-judgemental, supporting and stage-appropriate referral are the mainstays of management.

Controversies and future directions

❶ While there has been considerable research on the ideal screening tool for domestic violence in EDs, there is no evidence that screening leads to improved outcomes for victims of violence. Routine screening for domestic violence in EDs is currently not supported by the literature.

❷ However, improved awareness of the frequent occurrence of domestic violence and education regarding its complex causes and outcomes may aid the practitioner in assisting victims of violence.

❸ Mandatory reporting of violence of all types is controversial. Breach of confidentiality remains a concern.

❹ Encouraging the victim to leave the violent relationship should not be the health practitioner's over-riding concern, although safety is of paramount importance. Support and stage-appropriate referral are the mainstays of management.

References

1. Burke LK, Follingstad DR. Violence in lesbian and gay relationships: theory, prevalence, and correlational factors. Clinical Psychology Review 1999; 19: 487–512.
2. O'Leary KD. Psychological abuse: a variable deserving critical attention in domestic violence. Violence and Victims 1999; 14: 3–23.
3. Calma T. Ending family violence and abuse in Aboriginal and Torres Straight Islander communities. Key issues. An overview by the Aboriginal and Torres Straight Islander Social Justice Commissioner, Canberra; 2006.
4. Astbury J, Atkinson J, Duke JE, et al. The impact of domestic violence on individuals. Medical Journal of Australia 2000; 173: 427–431.
5. Bates L, Redman S, Brown W, et al. Domestic violence experienced by women attending an accident and emergency department. Australian Journal of Public Health 1995; 19: 293–299.
6. de Vries Robbe M, March L, Vinen J, et al. Prevalence of domestic violence among patients attending a hospital emergency department. Australian New Zealand Journal of Public Health 1996; 20: 364–368.
7. Roberts GL, O'Toole BI, Raphael B, et al. Prevalence study of domestic violence victims in an emergency department. Annals of Emergency Medicine 1996; 27: 741–753.
8. Abbott J, Johnson R, Koziol-McLain J, et al. Domestic violence against women. Incidence and prevalence in an emergency department population. Journal of American Medical Association 19995; 273: 1763–1767.
9. Australian Bureau of Statistics. Women's Safety Australia. Canberra; 1996.
10. Australian Bureau of Statistics. Personal Safety Survey; 2005.
11. Access Economics. The Cost of Domestic Violence to the Australian Economy. Canberra Access Economics Pty Ltd; 2004.
12. Kramer A. Domestic violence: how to ask and how to listen. Nursing Clinics of North America 2002; 37: 189–210.
13. Jones J, Dougherty J, Schelbie D, et al. Emergency department protocol for the diagnosis and evaluation of geriatric abuse. Annals of Emergency Medicine 1988; 17: 1006–1015.
14. Koziol-McLain J, Rameka M, Giddings L, et al. Partner violence prevalence among women attending a Maori health provider clinic. Australian New Zealand Journal of Public Health 2007; 31: 12–15.
15. Mouzos J, Segrave M. Homicide in Australia: 2202–2003 National Homicide Monitoring Programme Annual Report. Research and Public Policy Series No. 55. Canberra: Australian Institute of Criminology 2005.
16. Lievore D. Non-reporting and Hidden Recording of Sexual Assault: an International Literature Review. Canberra: Commonwealth Office of the Status of Women; 2003.
17. Kyriacou DN, Anglin D, Taliaferro E, et al. Risk factors for injury to women from domestic violence against women. New England Journal of Medicine 1999; 341: 1892–1898.
18. Roberts GL, Williams GM, Lawrence JM, et al. How does domestic violence affect women's mental health? Women Health 1998; 28: 117–129.
19. Mechem CC, Shofer FS, Reinhard SS, et al. History of domestic violence among male patients presenting to an urban emergency department. Academic Emergency Medicine 1999; 6: 786–791.
20. Frank JB, Rodowski MF. Review of psychological issues in victims of domestic violence seen in emergency settings. Emergency Medicine Clinics of North America 1999; 17: 657–677.
21. Fanslow JL, Norton RN, Robinson EM. One year follow-up of an emergency department protocol for abused women. Australian New Zealand Journal of Public Health 1999; 23: 418–420.
22. Zachary MJ, Mulvihill MN, Burton WB, et al. Domestic abuse in the emergency department: can a risk profile be defined? Academic Emergency Medicine 2001; 8: 796–803.
23. Muelleman RL, Lenaghan PA, Pakieser RA. Battered women: injury locations and types. Annals of Emergency Medicine 1996; 28: 486–492.
24. Campbell JC, Coben JH, McLoughlin E, et al. An evaluation of a system-change training model to improve emergency department response to battered women. Academic Emergency Medicine 2001; 8: 131–138.
25. Gazmararian JA, Petersen R, Spitz AM, et al. Violence and reproductive health: current knowledge and future research directions. Maternity and Child Health Journal 2000; 4: 79–84.
26. McCloskey LA, Williams CM, Lichter E, et al. Abused women disclose partner interference with health care: an unrecognized form of battering. Journal of General Internal Medicine 2007; 22: 1067–1072.
27. El-Bassel N, Gilbert L, Wu E, et al. Intimate partner violence prevalence and HIV risks among women receiving care in emergency departments: implications for IPV and HIV screening. Emergency Medicine Journal 2007; 24: 255–259.
28. Wadman MC, Muelleman RL. Domestic violence homicides: ED use before victimization. American Journal of Emergency Medicine 1999; 17: 689–691.
29. Roberts GL, Lawrence JM, Williams GM, et al. The impact of domestic violence on women's mental health. Australian New Zealand Journal of Public Health 1998; 22: 796–801.
30. Christian CW, Scribano P, Seidl T, et al. Pediatric injury resulting from family violence. Pediatrics 1997; 99: E8.
31. Shumaker DM, Prinz RJ. Children who murder: a review. Clinical Child and Family Psychology Review 2000; 3: 97–115.
32. Laing LBN. Economic costs of domestic violence: Australian Domestic and Family Violence Clearing House. NSW: University of New South Wales, 2002.
33. Roberts GL, Lawrence JM, O'Toole BI, et al. Domestic violence in the Emergency Department: 2. Detection by doctors and nurses. General Hospital Psychiatry 1997; 19: 12–15.
34. Morrison LJ, Allan R, Grunfeld A. Improving the emergency department detection rate of domestic violence using direct questioning. Journal of Emergency Medicine 2000; 19: 117–124.
35. Chescheir N. Violence against women: response from clinicians. Annals of Emergency Medicine 1996; 27: 766–768.
36. Gerard M. Domestic violence. How to screen and intervene. Registered Nurse 2000; 63: 52–56; quiz 58.
37. Trautman DE, McCarthy ML, Miller N, et al. Intimate partner violence and emergency department screening: computerized screening versus usual care. Annals of Emergency Medicine 2007; 49: 526–534.
38. Coben JH, Friedman DI. Health care use by perpetrators of domestic violence. Journal of Emergency Medicine 2002; 22: 313–317.
39. Yonaka L, Yoder MK, Darrow JB, et al. Barriers to screening for domestic violence in the emergency department. Journal of Continuing Education in Nursing 2007; 38: 37–45.
40. Cole TB. Is domestic violence screening helpful? Journal of American Medical Association 2000; 284: 551–553.
41. Ramsay J, Richardson J, Carter YH, et al. Should health professionals screen women for domestic violence? Systematic review. British Medical Journal 2002; 325: 314.
42. Gerbert B, Caspers N, Bronstone A, et al. A qualitative analysis of how physicians with expertise in domestic violence approach the identification of victims. Annals of International Medicine 1999; 131: 578–584.
43. Haywood YC, Haile-Mariam T. Violence against women. Emergency Medical Clinics of North America 1999; 17: 603–615.
44. Houry D, Sachs CJ, Feldhaus KM, et al. Violence-inflicted injuries: reporting laws in the fifty states. Annals of Emergency Medicine 2002; 39: 56–60.

21.4 Alcohol-related illness

Venita Munir • Andrew Dent

ESSENTIALS

1 Acute alcohol intoxication and withdrawal are responsible for many emergency department attendances and carry significant morbidity and mortality.

2 Chronic gastrointestinal and hepatic disease, confusional states, mental illness, central nervous system disease with neuropathy and immunosuppression are common in alcohol-dependent persons, with complications that increase the morbidity and mortality further.

3 Wernicke's encephalopathy is an uncommon but serious illness related to vitamin B1 deficiency. It requires high-dose parenteral thiamine 100 mg i.v. tds.

4 Many serious illnesses mimic alcohol intoxication or are masked by it. Maintain a high index of suspicion in the intoxicated patient with an altered conscious state.

5 Emergency physicians are uniquely placed to screen for high-risk drinking and to offer brief advice or intervention to this group to reduce the burden of recurrent alcohol abuse.

Introduction

Alcohol-related illness is common across the world and has a high prevalence in emergency department (ED) presentations. Alcohol misuse not only places the individual at risk of acute intoxication and injury but also poses significant long-term health issues.

Acute alcohol intoxication causes much morbidity and mortality from all forms of violence from motor vehicle and other accidents, interpersonal to self-harm. Chronic alcohol use contributes to many hospitalizations and deaths due to alcohol-related medical conditions and brain injury, resulting in both physical and psychosocial impairment.

Many acutely intoxicated patients presenting with an altered conscious state have significant comorbidities masked by alcohol, which must be considered on each presentation.

Emergency physicians should not only recognize and treat alcohol-related emergencies, but also intervene in patients at high risk from their alcohol intake who present with other conditions. Early opportunistic screening using recognized alcohol screening tools and standardized brief interventions reduce 'at-risk' drinking and the morbidity and mortality from alcohol-related illness.

Epidemiology

Australia ranks 23rd of 58 countries for alcohol consumption per capita. Australian alcohol consumption per capita is estimated at 9.32 L of pure ethanol per person per annum.[1] At least 44% of Australian drinkers consume more than the National Health and Medical Research Council (NHMRC) recommended levels for preventing chronic harm listed in Table 21.4.1.[2] Alcohol misuse, morbidity and mortality amongst indigenous Australians is appreciably higher than the non-indigenous; certain populations such as in central Northern Territory and north Western Australia experienced double the national alcohol-attributable death rate in 2004.[3] Death rates attributable to alcohol are higher in rural than metropolitan areas. Deaths from acute alcohol-related causes are most common in younger people aged 15–29 years, but chronic alcohol-related deaths mostly occur in those over 45 years.[1]

Alcohol use is implicated in more frequent attendance at EDs[4] with presentations most commonly due to acute intoxication and injuries sustained by violence or motor vehicle trauma. Alcohol consumption is an important reason for repeat ED attendance and is the most common reason for repeat use of an ambulance to attend EDs.[5] In one study, a core group of alcohol-related attendees accounted for 4.3% of ED presentations, but 28% of ambulance transports to ED, 70% of those transports being for episodes of acute intoxication.[5]

Six per cent of young persons attending city hospital EDs are for alcohol-related reasons, with injury significantly more likely among alcohol users than illicit drug users.[6] Amongst young people attending ED, nearly 38% may be drinking harmfully, 18% may have consumed alcohol in the previous 6 h and 15% consider their attendance to be alcohol-related.[7] Up to 45% of injured patients attending ED may have consumed alcohol within the past 24 h, and almost 30% in the last 6 h.[8]

The natural history of alcohol dependence is to remit and relapse, with a relentless progression to early death. Risk factors for alcoholism are a family history of alcohol dependence or total abstention, parental divorce, youngest child, other substance misuse, availability of alcohol and extremes of income.

Pharmacology

Pharmacokinetics

Alcohol is passively absorbed from the entire gastrointestinal tract (GIT), with about 25% from the stomach. Absorption is rapid within 60–120 min of intake and may be slowed by food. Alcohol is distributed throughout body water; females and obese people with lower body water-to-fat ratio reach higher blood alcohol concentrations (BAC) sooner than lean counterparts. Hepatic oxidative metabolism occurs via alcohol dehydrogenase. Alcohol-tolerant people also utilize the hepatic microsomal ethanol oxidizing system, which is upregulated with increasing drinking. First-order elimination kinetics becomes

Table 21.4.1 National Health and Medical Research Council (NHMRC) Australian alcohol guidelines to minimize risks in the longer term and gain any longer-term benefits (2001)[2]

	For risk of harm in the long term:		
	Low risk Standard drinks/day	Risky Standard drinks/day	High risk Standard drinks/day
Males daily	Up to 4	5–6	7 or more
Males weekly	Up to 28	29–42	43 or more
Females daily	Up to 2	3–4	5 or more
Females weekly	Up to 14	15–28	29 or more

National Health and Medical Research Council Australian Alcohol Guidelines: Health Risks and Benefits Endorsed October 2001. Reprinted October 2003.
http://www.nhmrc.gov.au/publications/synopses/_files/ds9.pdf (accessed September 2007)

saturated as the BAC increases, changing to zero-order kinetics and slower sobering at higher BAC.

Pharmacodynamics

Alcohol is thought to act on $GABA_A$ inhibitory neuroreceptors in the brain causing central nervous system (CNS) depression. The characteristic euphoria is thought related to the release of endogenous opioids (endorphins). Rapidly rising BAC causes quicker and more pronounced behavioural changes than the same level achieved over hours. A steady state of absorption to metabolism and excretion can be achieved at about one standard drink per hour. A standard drink is defined as containing 10 g of alcohol. Behavioural intoxication depends on factors such as habituation, food coingestion, body habitus and the concentration of alcohol in the drink.

Measurement of blood alcohol concentration

The blood alcohol concentration may be estimated using a portable breathalyser that estimates BAC after measuring alcohol concentration of alveolar air. This is a useful non-invasive screening tool but relies on a cooperative and awake patient being able to exhale adequately for the reading. There is an approximate difference of 15–20% between breath alcohol readings and serum BAC.[9] Readings are influenced by temperature, hyper- or hypoventilation prior to exhalation, haematocrit level, other substances such as ketones and machine error. Directly measured serum blood alcohol concentration is more reliable. The Australian legal limit for driving is 0.05%, New Zealand's is 0.04%, whilst in the USA and UK it is 0.08%.

Chronic alcohol-related illness

Gastrointestinal

Chronic alcohol use results in disease of the GIT, liver and pancreas. Morbidity most frequently arises from GIT bleeding, liver disease and pancreatopathy.

Gastrointestinal bleeding

The most common causes of alcohol-related GIT haemorrhage are peptic ulcer disease (PUD) and the consequences of portal hypertension such as oesophagogastric varices or subepithelial gastropathy. Mallory–Weiss tears, oesophagitis, and alcoholic gastropathy are less frequent causes of alcohol-related GIT haemorrhage.[10] Heavy alcohol use may be a risk factor for development of PUD, although the exact pathogenesis is poorly understood and the role of alcohol may be additive to the effects of *Helicobacter pylori*, non-steroidal anti-inflammatory drugs (NSAIDs) and tobacco.[11]

Variceal bleeding in portal hypertension results from raised portal blood flow and portal vascular resistance due to hepatic fibrosis.[12] Fifty per cent of cirrhotic patients develop varices, and, once present, variceal bleeding occurs in 10–30% per annum.[13] Variceal bleeding may be catastrophic with a 30% mortality for a first bleed. The 5-year survival was estimated at 26% in one patient series of variceal bleeding, of which 80% were alcohol dependent.[14]

Whilst Mallory–Weiss tears are less common, up to 44% are associated with alcohol use and may have significant morbidity due to blood loss.[15] Alcohol-induced vomiting against a closed glottis can also result in oesophageal rupture (Boerhaave's syndrome).[16]

Management of GIT bleeding Close attention to airway, breathing and circulation is the first priority. Aggressive initial fluid resuscitation is necessary in shock with a crystalloid bolus, progressing to blood transfusion if required. Vitamin K 10 mg i.v. is indicated in patients with known or suspected liver cell failure. Replacement of clotting factors with factor concentrate or fresh frozen plasma and platelets may also be required.

An intravenous proton pump inhibitor such as omeprazole 80 mg stat followed by an infusion at 8 mg/h is often initiated for bleeding from presumed PUD, oesophagitis, gastritis or duodenitis. This decreases hospital length of stay and the need for endoscopic therapy but does not reduce transfusion requirement, rebleeding, the need for surgery or death at 30 days.[17]

Variceal bleeding The acute management of variceal bleeding is best initiated with a bolus of octreotide, a synthetic somatostatin analogue that reduces splanchnic blood flow. Give octreotide 50 µg i.v. stat followed by an infusion of octreotide at 50 µg/h, whilst urgent upper gastrointestinal endoscopy is arranged. Endoscopy is diagnostic for the site of bleeding, as well as being both therapeutic and prognostic. Therapy is usually by banding ligation, sclerotherapy or tissue adhesive. Sclerotherapy with the injection of varices with sclerosant with octreotide is more effective than sclerotherapy alone at controlling bleeding but may not improve longer-term mortality.[18]

Early variceal surgery by oesophageal transection or selective porto-caval shunt or interventional radiology such as transjugular intrahepatic portosystemic shunting (TIPSS) may enhance short- and long-term survival, but both techniques are complicated by the risk of encephalopathy.[19] TIPSS is preferred if liver transplantation is being considered. When the acute episode of variceal bleeding is over, oral propranolol and isosorbide mononitrate are used as maintenance therapy for portal hypertension.

Alcoholic liver disease

Alcoholic liver disease (ALD) comprises a spectrum of disorders from alcoholic fatty liver (steatosis), inflammation (hepatitis) to progressive fibrosis (cirrhosis). These occur from chronic insult to the liver due to oxidative stress, damage from free radicals and the immunogenicity of alcohol metabolites. Many factors are involved in the aetiology of ALD, including chronic viral hepatitis, genetic predisposition, gender, ethnicity, nutrition, obesity, non-alcoholic fatty liver and other liver diseases such as autoimmune.

The duration and amount of alcohol consumed play important roles; drinking at levels above the NHMRC recommendations (Table 21.4.1) is a defined risk for the development of ALD and eventual cirrhosis. Alcohol dependence does not inevitably lead to cirrhosis, as only 10–20% of heavy drinkers progress.[20] Alcoholic fatty liver is a common finding amongst alcohol-dependent patients but is not a frequent cause for presentation to an ED.

Alcoholic hepatitis and cirrhosis

Alcoholic hepatitis may present as acute anorexia, nausea, vomiting, right upper quadrant pain and jaundice. Treatment is supportive and abstinence from alcohol is essential (see Ch. 9.7).

Cirrhosis typically presents late, with subtle malaise, anorexia, weight loss, weakness and fatigue, with a combination of liver cell failure and the development of portal hypertension. Acute decompensation results in symptomatic ascites, jaundice, pruritus, spontaneous bacterial peritonitis (SBP), hepatic encephalopathy, variceal bleeding and coagulopathy.

Ascites Ascites due to hypoalbuminaemia, secondary hyperaldosteronism and portal hypertension is usually recurrent. Sudden exacerbations may be caused by SBP, the development of portal vein thrombosis, a hepatoma or medication non-compliance. Symptoms include abdominal discomfort, girth increase and anorexia. Fever, chills and abdominal pain occur with SBP, or conversely signs of sepsis are minimal but there is sudden worsening of jaundice or encephalopathy.

The long-term treatment of ascites includes sodium restriction and diuretics, especially spironolactone and/or furosemide. Problematic ascites may require fluid restriction, recurrent abdominal paracentesis, and albumin transfusion.[13,21] It is important to exclude SBP by paracentesis and polymorphonuclear (PMN) cell count, with greater than 250 PMN cells/mm^2 being diagnostic. The treatment of SBP includes intravenous broad-spectrum antibiotics such as ceftriaxone 1 g i.v. daily or timentin 3.1 g 6-hourly daily, followed by oral antibiotic prophylaxis with trimethoprim 160 mg and sulphamethoxazole 800 mg tablets once daily.

Coagulopathy and encephalopathy

Coagulopathy results from the failure of hepatic synthesis of coagulation factors, thus administration of vitamin K 10 mg i.v., factor concentrate or fresh-frozen plasma is required in the bleeding cirrhotic patient. Also unrecognized GIT bleeding may precipitate hepatic encephalopathy, with confusion and characteristic asterixis. This potentially reversible decrease in neuropsychiatric function must be distinguished from other causes of an altered conscious level in the cirrhotic patient.

Hepatic encephalopathy is associated with an increased nitrogenous GIT load such as from a gastrointestinal bleed, dehydration, sepsis, certain drugs, hyponatraemia or hypokalaemia, worsening liver function and increasing jaundice. The treatment includes supportive care, GIT cleansing with lactulose (oral and enema) and oral non-absorbable antibiotics such as neomycin to reduce bacterial counts, although their efficacy is unclear.[12,20]

Alcoholic pancreatopathy

Alcoholic pancreatopathy is used to describe a group of pancreatic diseases caused by chronic heavy alcohol intake. It includes acute alcoholic pancreatitis, recurrent abdominal pain or GIT symptoms induced by alcohol, high serum levels of pancreatic enzymes or an abnormal pancreatic ultrasound.[22] Recurrent bouts of acute alcoholic pancreatitis probably precede development of chronic pancreatitis.

Alcohol is the most common aetiology of chronic pancreatitis (70–80%), although as few as 10% heavy drinkers will develop it. Like cirrhosis, its aetiology is multifactorial; other risk factors include tobacco smoking and hyperlipidaemia, which should be addressed if early signs of pancreatopathy are recognized. Acute and chronic alcoholic pancreatitis are managed conservatively, with abstinence from alcohol, intravenous fluids, parenteral analgesia and antibiotics if pancreatic necrosis or an abscess are suspected (see Ch. 7.9).

Chronic pancreatitis Chronic pancreatitis can be debilitating with recurrent cycles of pain and admissions to hospital. Progressive pancreatic calcification, failure of exocrine and endocrine function, and chronic pain can all be mitigated if alcohol is avoided. Recurrent pancreatic insults and chronic pancreatitis increase the risk of pancreatic carcinoma by up to 16 times.[23]

Mental health and mental state issues

Depression and suicidal intent

Alcohol is a recognized risk factor for suicide. Mood expression and self-harm intent are often underestimated in the ED intoxicated patient. A Scandinavian study showed that 62% of 1207 'parasuicides' who presented to an ED involved alcohol use, with even higher rates in young males. Psychiatric referral was less likely if alcohol was involved, yet after 5.6 years 3.3% had completed suicide. This represented a 51-fold increased risk compared to the general population, with the risk of completed suicide being greatest in the first year.[24]

Alcoholic hallucinosis

Alcohol misuse causes psychotic symptoms by several mechanisms, including direct intoxication, alcohol withdrawal, delirium tremens (DTs), Wernicke encephalopathy, Korsakoff psychosis and alcoholic dementia. Alcohol dependence doubles the risk of psychotic symptoms.

Alcoholic hallucinosis is a schizophrenia-like syndrome that differs from the other causes in that it occurs at a younger age, in a setting of clear consciousness and not related to acute withdrawal. There are no associated physical symptoms of autonomic dysfunction as in the DTs and its duration is longer with predominantly auditory hallucinations as opposed to visual.[25] Its chronicity and derogatory auditory hallucinations are similar to schizophrenia, but thought disorder is not a feature.

Alcohol withdrawal states

The alcohol withdrawal syndrome follows prior alcohol dependence. Its clinical importance lies in the potential severity of the symptoms and signs, the need to consider alternative or concomitant pathology, and the likelihood of seizures occurring. The principal symptoms are tremor, agitation, anxiety and autonomic nervous system overactivity with tachycardia, tachypnoea and fever. Sleep disturbance, nausea and vomiting generally begin within 10 h of reduced alcohol intake, with a peak intensity by day 2. The withdrawal syndrome may occur in an individual who usually drinks an 'eye opener' or 'hair of the dog' but is prevented from doing so.

Alcohol withdrawal scales A number of scales measure alcohol withdrawal. One simple one is to rate symptoms as mild (tremulousness), moderate (agitation) and severe (confusion). Most EDs use an alcohol withdrawal scale (AWS) to measure symptoms and predict likelihood of seizure and direct preventative management. The most commonly used AWS is the Clinical Institute Withdrawal Assessment – Alcohol, revised scale (CIWA-R). This scale measures 10 items and was primarily developed for planned detoxification or for use on general medical and psychiatric wards.[26] Surprisingly blood pressure and pulse, although often abnormal, are not included in the scale. A modified version that includes seizures in the AWS is also used.[27] Patients with high scores have an increased risk of seizure if they remain untreated. The higher the score, the greater the relative risk. However, some patients experience complicated withdrawal despite initial low scores.

Benzodiazepine therapy Benzodiazepine (BZD) therapy reduces signs and symptoms of alcohol withdrawal and prevents complications.[28] All BZDs appear to have similar efficacy. Longer-acting agents such

as diazepam used with symptom-triggered dosing (as opposed to regular) decrease the total of drugs given and both shorten and smooth the clinical course. Early treatment is preferred to waiting for advanced withdrawal.

Published data on ideal doses are lacking. High-dose oral diazepam 20 mg 1- to 2-hourly may be needed for symptom control, and up to 160 mg per day may be required to allow for BZD tolerance, which is common in alcohol-dependent patients. Under-dosing for fear of over-sedation is common.

Carbemazepine and other drugs in therapy Carbemazepine is used extensively in Europe and appears as effective as fixed-dose BZDs. β-blockers decrease tremulousness but may worsen delirium and are not anti-convulsant. Clonidine improves symptoms of withdrawal but is not anti-convulsant. Neuroleptics such as haloperidol are sometimes used for behavioural disturbance but lower the seizure threshold. Vigabatrin has shown promise in reducing sedation, BZD use and the total withdrawal treatment time.[29] Large-scale trials using this agent await publication. Ethanol, of course, would 'treat' the symptoms of withdrawal.

Alcohol withdrawal seizures Around 3–5% of those with severe alcohol use disorder experience withdrawal seizures within 48 h of stopping drinking, and 15% will have a seizure in their lifetime. Previous withdrawal seizure is the strongest predictor of recurrent seizure. Most alcohol withdrawal seizures are short lived and self-terminating. Localizing signs or prolonged seizure should prompt a search for alternate pathology. Intravenous BZD such as midazolam 0.1–0.2 mg/kg is given for prolonged seizure. Phenytoin, like alcohol, causes ataxia and drowsiness and is not recommended for alcohol withdrawal seizures.[30]

Delirium tremens DTs is characterized by confusion, altered conscious state and autonomic hyperactivity. The incidence of DTs has been reduced by effective early management of withdrawal, and excluding intercurrent illness. DTs occur in less than one percent during any single withdrawal

episode. The diagnosis is important, as the mortality approaches 15% if untreated. As symptoms usually manifest within 48 h, DTs may be encountered in EDs experiencing access block, or in short-stay observation units.

Risk factors for DTs Five risk factors are associated with the development of the DTs.[31] These include current infection, tachycardia greater than 120 beats/min, signs of alcohol withdrawal accompanied by BAC of more than 0.1%, seizure history and history of delirious episodes. DTs are rare in the absence of these factors. The treatment includes management in an intensive care with regular intravenous BZD such as midazolam 0.1–0.2 mg/kg and a search for underlying conditions such as sepsis.

Wernicke's encephalopathy

The classical features of Wernicke's encephalopathy are ataxia, confusion and ophthalmoplegia, usually lateral rectus palsy. It is caused by thiamine deficiency, but severe deficiency may be present without these signs. In alcohol-dependent persons, oral thiamine absorption is poor. Malabsorption, reduced storage and impaired utilization of thiamine increase the risk of Wernicke's encephalopathy.

Postmortem studies suggest that thiamine deficiency sufficient to cause irreversible brain damage remains undiagnosed antemortem in 80–90% of alcohol-dependent persons. Wernicke's encephalopathy should be considered in all patients in coma, as replacement of depleted brain thiamine is necessary. The mortality approaches 20% if left untreated.

Treatment of Wernicke's encephalopathy High-dose oral thiamine may be ineffective, thus repeated parenteral therapy with thiamine 100 mg i.v. bd or tds is recommended, despite the risk of anaphylaxis.[32] The recommended prophylactic thiamine dosage has been increased to 100 mg parenterally three times daily. Administering glucose acutely further depletes thiamine levels and increases thiamine demand precipitating Wernicke's. Thus, whenever glucose is to be administered to an unconscious patient, give thiamine 100 mg i.v. first.[33]

Other alcohol-related neurological problems

Alcohol is a neurotoxin and chronic heavy use causes CNS damage, peripheral neuropathy, myopathy and movement disorders such as tremor, Parkinsonism, dyskinesias, cerebellar ataxia and asterixis.

Peripheral neuropathy

Peripheral neuropathy is common in alcohol misuse and may have multiple aetiologies. The prevalence amongst chronic drinkers is unclear but is estimated at between 9 and 50%. Other contributing factors are increased age, total lifetime dose of alcohol, nutritional status (malnutrition and thiamine deficiency) and family history of alcohol misuse. Alcoholic peripheral neuropathy is most commonly sensory in the lower limbs.[34]

Alcoholic autonomic neuropathy

Alcoholic autonomic neuropathy is uncommon. It is often asymptomatic or causes erectile dysfunction in males, postural hypotension and/or diarrhoea. It is related to different pathological processes than sensory peripheral neuropathy.[35]

Ataxia

Ataxia is a common presenting symptom and sign and may be due to peripheral neuropathy affecting proprioception, cerebellar degeneration or a combination of both. Cerebellar ataxia is possibly an extension of the insult from thiamine deficiency as in Wernicke's encephalopathy. Whereas in Wernicke's the ataxia may be reversible by thiamine administration, full recovery is rare and permanent damage occurs affecting the superior cerebellar vermis.[36]

Blackouts

Neuronal failure resulting in blackouts and amnesia is a direct toxic result of alcohol on the CNS. This is especially common in binge drinkers. Orthostatic hypotension from autonomic failure is differentiated on the clear relationship to posture.

Respiratory illness in alcohol-dependent persons

Chronic obstructive airways disease

Chronic obstructive airways disease (COAD) is common amongst alcohol-dependent persons, mostly due to the high prevalence of concurrent tobacco smoking (see Ch. 6.5).

Pneumonia

Alcohol dependence increases the risk of community-acquired pneumonia due to immunosuppression, as well as general lifestyle factors such as hygiene and smoking. Typical organisms include *Streptococcus pneumoniae* and *Haemophilus influenzae*. There is also a higher frequency of cavitating disease, empyema and unusual pathogens. Anaerobic and Gram-negative organisms are frequent colonizers of the oropharynx and GIT, and aspiration pneumonia is common.[37] Opportunistic disease such as tuberculosis, *Pneumocystis carinii* pneumonia, now known as *Pneumocystis jiroveci*, and *Legionella* are also more frequent in alcohol-dependent persons.

Metabolic problems with alcohol use

Alcohol use and metabolic acidosis

Alcoholic ketoacidosis There is contention about the existence and frequency of alcoholic ketoacidosis. This refers to high anion gap metabolic acidosis associated with the acute cessation of alcohol on a background of chronic alcohol abuse and relative starvation. Clinical features include nausea, vomiting, abdominal pain, tachycardia, tachypnoea and hypotension, all of which may occur in other alcohol-related emergency presentations.

Chronic alcohol intake can lead to depleted carbohydrate and protein stores in the body due to relative starvation. Reduced hepatic gluconeogenesis from substrates such as lactic acid, glycerol and amino acids can cause hypoglycaemia. In dehydrated states, the combination of hypotension and hypoglycaemia results in reduced insulin production, and raised catecholamines, cortisol, glucagon and growth hormone. These hormones promote utilization of fatty acids for energy, resulting in ketogenesis.

Alcoholic ketoacidosis has been described as 'a common reason for investigation and admission of alcohol dependent patients', although research data appear limited. There may be an increased frequency of sudden death amongst patients who present in this fashion.[38]

Other metabolic acidosis Metabolic acidosis is rare in alcohol intoxication alone. One study of 60 ED patients with BAC greater than 0.1% described seven patients with a raised serum lactate, all of whom had alternative reasons for this such as seizure, hypoxia and sepsis. Only one of these patients had a metabolic acidosis.[39] The treatment of an alcohol-dependent patient with metabolic acidosis is symptomatic with intravenous crystalloid fluid resuscitation and rehydration, thiamine 100 mg i.v., 5% or 10% dextrose for hypoglycaemia, electrolyte replacement (see below) and a search for and treatment of another underlying cause such as sepsis.

Electrolyte disturbance

There are no direct correlations between acute or chronic use of alcohol with specific electrolyte disorders, although certain deficiencies are characteristic such as hypokalaemia, hyponatraemia, hypomagnesaemia and hypocalcaemia. The causes include poor intake, malabsorption, excessive losses from vomiting, diarrhoea and fluid diuresis, reduced renal tubular reabsorption and dilutional changes due to polydipsia.

Electrolyte imbalances result in disturbance of other endocrine systems. Thus hypomagnesaemia suppresses parathyroid hormone release, resulting in hypocalcaemia. Electrolyte disturbances are also related to alcohol-induced illness such as pancreatitis or pneumonia.

Insulin resistance

Acute alcohol ingestion can cause a state of acute insulin resistance. Alcohol-induced post-prandial hyperinsulinaemia occurs without significant decrease in blood glucose levels, consistent with impaired insulin sensitivity. Relative starvation may result in hypoglycaemia and reduced insulin release. Alcohol-induced insulin resistance is important in these patients to recover from hypoglycaemia. Conversely, there is a reduced risk of type II diabetes mellitus in moderate drinkers (18–48 g per day) compared to light or heavy drinkers.[40]

Cardiovascular

Coronary heart disease

There a reduced mortality from coronary heart disease in diabetic moderate drinkers (approximately 28 g per day).[35] However, alcohol use in diabetes increases the risk of retinopathy, peripheral neuropathy and foot ulcers. Coronary protective effects of alcohol are due to influences on increased high-density lipoprotein (HDL) cholesterol, platelet function and fibrinogen.

Hypertension

Acute alcohol intake is a vasodilator, whereas drinking alcohol over the longer term causes systolic hypertension and increased aortic stiffness. An assessment by the World Health Organization Global Burden of Disease 2000 Comparative Risk Analysis attributed 16% of all hypertensive disease to alcohol intake. These findings may be confounded by other lifestyle factors and there are many contrasting effects of alcohol at various intakes, depending on gender and body mass index (BMI). Thus raising HDL cholesterol is cardioprotective, but developing central obesity 'beer gut' is not. Overall any benefits of moderate alcohol consumption on coronary disease are likely to be outweighed by harmful effects.[41]

Cardiac arrhythmias

Heavy alcohol use is associated with an increased risk of sudden cardiac death, most commonly due to ventricular arrhythmias. Atrial arrhythmias including atrial fibrillation occur commonly after heavy binge drinking 'holiday heart' in both acute and chronic drinkers. They are not necessarily associated with cardiomyopathy. The risk of a cardiac arrhythmia is increased by electrolyte abnormalities such as hypokalaemia, hypomagnesaemia and hypocalcaemia, and by the negative inotropic effect of alcohol releasing excess catecholamines.[42]

The treatment of arrhythmias is as recommended by the current Advanced Cardiovascular Life Support guidelines.

Cardiomyopathy

Concentric left ventricular hypertrophy is common in chronic alcohol users. Dilated cardiomyopathy may ensue with progressive dilatation and fibrosis, leading to congestive cardiac failure. This myotoxic process has a worse prognosis than idiopathic dilated cardiomyopathy, particularly if drinking continues. Myocyte function can improve with total abstention.

Aggressive anti-failure therapy should be implemented with dietary measures such as reduced sodium intake, an angiotensin-converting-enzyme inhibitor and other pharmacotherapy, even if total abstention cannot be achieved.[41]

Malignancy

Alcohol has been causally linked to many types of neoplasia, most commonly those of the GIT. Oropharyngeal and other head and neck cancers have a direct link to alcohol. Drinking more than 1.5 bottles of wine daily elevates the risk of oesophageal cancer 100 times. Hepatocellular carcinoma (HCC) is usually preceded by alcoholic cirrhosis in the Western world, although other causes include hepatitis B and C viruses. Progression of cirrhosis to HCC is more rapid if drinking continues. Chronic alcohol consumption is also related to laryngeal, breast, pancreatic and colorectal carcinomas.[43]

Important illnesses to be excluded that mimic alcohol intoxication

It is hard to know when to look for another cause for altered conscious state in the habitual drinker or intoxicated person, as many alternative conditions must be considered that mimic apparent alcohol intoxication (see Table 21.4.2). The mean length of altered conscious state in an ED for intoxication alone has been reported at 3.2 h with a wide standard deviation of 3.6 h, with the likelihood of another pathology being present increasing rapidly after 4 h.[44] Close observation looking for trends in autonomic responses and neurological signs, and detailed examination looking for other pathology are more appropriate than waiting for, or intervening after, a certain period of time.

Metabolic disturbance

There is little evidence that hypoglycaemia occurs with simple alcohol intoxication alone, with one large study of ED patients screened for alcohol use and serum blood glucose finding no linear relation between blood alcohol and glucose levels.[45] The incidence of hypoglycaemia is not increased in alcohol-related ED attendances compared to sober patients. Intravenous glucose administration has not been shown to be useful in changing rates of alcohol elimination or decreasing periods of intoxication.[46] However, it is essential in each patient with an altered mental to measure the blood glucose and treat if it is low. In the intoxicated or alcohol-dependent patient an alternative cause for hypoglycaemia should still be sought.

Hyponatraemia may occur with sepsis and general debility. Diabetic ketoacidosis or hyperglycaemic, hyperosmolar non-ketotic syndrome should also be excluded

Table 21.4.2 Illnesses not to be missed in the presumed intoxicated person	
Metabolic and encephalopathic	Hypoglycaemia Hyperglycaemia Wernicke's (thiamine deficiency) Hyponatraemia Liver failure Renal failure
Head injury	Skull fracture Cerebral contusion Subdural and extradural haematoma
Other intracranial pathology	Infection Cerebrovascular accident Seizure and post-ictal state Space-occupying lesion

Toxicological including
  CNS depressant
  Illicit drugs
 	
  Prescription medications
  Other alcohols
	
	Opioids
	Ecstasy and related drugs, e.g. GHB, ketamine, amphetamines and cocaine
	BZD, anti-depressants and anticonvulsants
	Methanol, ethylene glycol and isopropyl alcohol

Other sepsis	CNS, UTI, pneumonia and aspiration

CNS, central nervous system; GHB, γ-hydroxybutyrate; BZD, benzodiazepine; UTI, urinary tract infection.

(see Ch. 11.2). A homeless alcohol-dependent person may present de novo to an ED with well-established organ failure and encephalopathy, without any prior contact with a primary-care doctor.

Head injury

Head injuries are not only more common in intoxicated and alcohol-dependent persons, they are easily missed due to a presumption that intoxication is the main cause of the altered conscious state. Head injuries may be complicated by coexisting coagulopathy from liver disease, cerebral atrophy and underlying metabolic problems. A computerized tomography (CT) brain scan is essential to rapidly rule out intracranial pathology, particularly cerebral contusion, extradural haematoma, subdural haematoma and base of skull fracture.

Close neurological observation in a monitored resuscitation area is necessary in the intoxicated person with an altered conscious level and a possible head injury. Worsening confusion, deteriorating level of consciousness or focal neurology necessitate an urgent CT brain, which may be challenging in a poorly compliant patient. Intravenous sedation or even endotracheal intubation may be necessary to obtain a CT safely.

Other intracranial pathology

Altered conscious state: differential diagnosis

A patient with any significant intracranial pathology may present with an altered conscious state mimicking alcohol intoxication. The chronic alcohol-dependent patient may present with an unusual cerebral infection such as cryptococcal meningitis, cerebral abscess or herpes encephalitis. Also a cerebrovascular accident either embolic or haemorrhagic is more likely in the habitual drinker, due to comorbid vascular disease and smoking, hypertension and coagulopathy.

An altered conscious state may be due to a seizure from alcohol excess or withdrawal, status epilepticus or a post-ictal state. Cerebral neoplasia, particularly metastases, may present late in this population. Again a CT scan is usually indicated in the alcohol-dependent patient following a seizure,

particularly if there is persisting or deteriorating confusion or focal neurology. A lumbar puncture may be needed to exclude meningitis or a subarachnoid haemorrhage if there is clinical suspicion, even if the CT brain scan was normal.

Other toxicological states in the alcohol-dependent patient

Multiple drug ingestion

Multiple drug ingestion whether prescription or illicit is common in regular drinkers for recreational reasons, due to dependence, to 'come down' from other drug effects, in accidental overdose, or in deliberate self-harm. The most common and important ingested drugs to consider include BZDs, opiates, paracetamol often as over-the-counter analgesics, antidepressants including tricyclics and selective serotonin reuptake inhibitors, Ecstasy and other sympathomimetics such as cocaine, γ-hydroxybutyrate and ketamine.

Other alcohols

Other alcohols such as methanol, ethylene glycol and isopropyl alcohol, although rare, should be considered in the significantly intoxicated, self-harm patient. 'Methylated spirits' bought over the counter in Australia only contains 95% ethanol v/w with no methanol at all, and in New Zealand the methanol content has been reduced to 2% or less, due to deaths attributed to chronic misuse and methanol poisoning there.

Serum drug levels

The only clinically useful serum drug levels are therefore paracetamol, ethanol and perhaps tricylic antidepressants. Other drug levels take hours to days to perform (institution dependent) and thus are not of use at the time. The only safe antidotes to consider are naloxone, thiamine and glucose. Flumazenil is not recommended due to the risk of inducing seizures and then not being able to manage them effectively.

Other sepsis

Sepsis must be considered in any person with an altered conscious state potentially masked by alcohol intoxication and a directed septic work-up carried out.

Treatment of alcohol-related illness

Alcohol intoxication

Intoxication starts with a feeling of well-being and an increasing sense of relaxation, followed by impairment of judgement and incoordination. At BAC of 0.1% dysarthria, ataxia and disinhibition are common. At BAC of 0.2% confusion occurs and new memories are not formed. At BAC of 0.25% cortical depression is seen with the onset of stupor. At BAC of 0.4% most are unconscious and at risk of respiratory depression and death. The mean BAC found in fatal alcohol intoxication is 0.45%.

'Pathological intoxication'

Some people have idiosyncratic responses to alcohol, the so-called 'pathological intoxication', which is more common amongst certain ethnic groups. A clear indicator of alcohol tolerance and neuroadaptation is the recording of high BAC in a person functioning at an otherwise reasonable level, for example the patient capable of normal conversation and gait with a BAC 0.3%. This may follow a continuous prolonged drinking binge.

Treatment of the acutely intoxicated person

The treatment of an acutely intoxicated person is supportive, protecting the at-risk airway and placing in the semi-prone position to reduce the risk of gastric aspiration. Gastric emptying procedures are not recommended under any circumstances.[47] Intravenous fluids in simple alcohol intoxication do not increase the elimination or decrease the BAC.[48] Likewise, i.v. 5% dextrose administration has not been shown to be useful in changing the rates of alcohol elimination or decreasing periods of intoxication.[44]

There remains no antidote to alcohol intoxication. As alcohol affects endogenous opiate GABA receptors, both naloxone and flumazenil have been tried with no effect.[45] Various substances have been tried in animals, but none so far is safe and/or effective.[49] There has been interest in pyridoxine, and more recently its analogue metadoxine in hastening alcohol metabolism and reversing both the biochemical and the clinical symptoms of intoxication, but studies are small.[50]

'Hangover'

It was estimated in Britain in 2003 that £2 billion in lost work value was due to post-alcohol-related headache and malaise 'hangover', which may be a greater economic problem than habitual intoxication. Paradoxically, light or binge drinkers' hangovers cause the most lost work time as the hangover is more common, and the sufferer is more commonly in regular employment than the heavy drinker.

Diagnosis and management

A hangover is distinguished from the alcohol withdrawal syndrome as it follows a defined single episode of intoxication. Symptoms include headache, feeling generally unwell, diarrhoea, anorexia, nausea, tremulousness and fatigue. The presence of two or more of these symptoms following alcohol intake has been used to define a hangover.[51] Acetaldehyde, the dehydrogenated metabolite of alcohol, has been implicated. Alcohol alters cytokine production, and thromboxane B2 is increased, an effect blocked by prostaglandin inhibitors. This may explain why prostaglandin inhibitors such as NSAIDs, including aspirin, may have some limited prophylactic effect on hangover development.

Hangover is not solely dose related. Hangovers are worse with dehydration, no food intake, decreased sleep, increased physical activity while intoxicated and poor general physical condition. Congener by-products of some alcohols including aldehydes, esters, histamine, phenols, tannins, iron, lead and cobalt are found especially in darker liquors, which are associated with an increased severity and incidence of hangover. Clear liquors such as gin, vodka and rum may lead to fewer hangovers. The evidence for hangover treatment and prevention is minimal.[52]

The habitual alcohol-dependent emergency attender

Most EDs particularly in metropolitan areas have a group of recurrent ED attenders who keep presenting with alcohol intoxication and chronic alcohol-related disease. Such people are usually male, aged 30–40 years and often have no fixed place of abode. They usually are well known to neighbouring EDs, community services and police. They tend to attend in cycles, and an absence of attendance may indicate a prison term, a medical illness and/or hospital admission, an attempt at sobriety, use of an adjacent ED or sudden death. Over a year they may accumulate multiple investigations, especially CT scans of the head. This group has an increased mortality over time from assault and other trauma, as well as alcohol-related illness associated with neglect.[53]

The ED as a temporary refuge

The ED provides a temporary refuge in an otherwise chaotic lifestyle, and an opportunity for a health assessment and intervention. It is important to realize that providing care for this group of people is core business for every ED, despite any frustrations felt. Interventions to alter lifestyle and prevent recurrent attendances are successful. ED initiated case management involving community linkages and assistance with accommodation improves health outcomes but may increase ED utilization.[54] Serial inebriate programmes may target this group, often commencing with socialization skills such as personal hygiene and nutrition management.[55] Acceptance to such programmes is often precipitated by the threat of imprisonment. Such programmes have been demonstrated to be cost-effective.

Assessment of alcohol misuse

Alcohol screening tools

Emergency physicians witness daily the effects of lifestyle abuse on ED presentations and thus may find many opportunities to intervene opportunistically to affect the long-term health of the patient, as well as treating the immediate presentation. This is particularly valuable for patients with irregular contact with other medical services, such as the itinerant and the homeless.

Table 21.4.3 CAGE screening questionnaire for alcohol abuse
C = 'Have you ever felt you should **C**ut down on your drinking?'
A = 'Have people **A**nnoyed you by criticizing your drinking?'
G = 'Have you ever felt bad or **G**uilty about your drinking?'
E = 'Have you ever had a drink as an **E**ye-opener first thing in the morning to steady your nerves or help get rid of a hangover?'

'Yes' to two or more indicates probable chronic alcohol abuse or dependence.

Screening for chronic alcohol abuse or dependence

Any screening tool to be of value must have adequate sensitivity and specificity for detecting the illness involved, and there should be an effective, cost-effective intervention available. Many screening tools for chronic alcohol abuse or dependence have been developed for primary care, with the best known being the CAGE questionnaire.[56] This poses four questions on behaviour and a positive answer to two or more indicates probable chronic alcohol abuse (see Table 21.4.3).

Paddington alcohol test

An effective and quick alternative in the time-pressured setting of an ED is the Paddington alcohol test (PAT), which includes 'routine' focused selective screening combined with education, audit and feedback.[57] PAT has reduced screening time to 1 min, simply quantifying the amount of alcohol consumed, how often and whether in the opinion of the patient the reason for ED attendance is due to alcohol.

One study in France that measured γ-glutamyl transferase (GGT) and performed CAGE questionnaire on all patients presenting to an ED with acute alcohol intoxication found 90% were CAGE or GGT positive.[58] This suggests that attendance at an ED with intoxication is itself a marker of a serious drinking problem.

Opportunistic screening and brief intervention

Brief intervention usually consisting of counselling lasting 10–15 min, and a

Table 21.4.4 The top 10 ED presenting conditions associated with alcohol use (see reference[57])	
Falls	Unwell
Collapse	Non-specific gastrointestinal problems
Head injury	Psychiatric-behavioural
Assault	Cardiac
Accident	Repeat attender

To be used with the Paddington alcohol test (PAT).[57] Crawford MJ, Patton R, Touquet R, et al. Screening and referral for brief intervention of alcohol misusing patients in an emergency department: a pragmatic randomised controlled trial. Lancet 2004; 364: 1334–1339.

pamphlet on safe levels of regular alcohol consumption reduce the frequency of dangerous drinking by 30% after ED-initiated PAT screening and trained alcohol health worker follow-up, and recurrent ED attendances by as much as 50%.[57]

Focused PAT screening of high-risk patients (see Table 21.4.4) followed by brief advice and referral for trained alcohol healthworker brief intervention appear the most time- and cost-effective methods of reducing alcohol-related harm and ED attendances.[59] Brief advice consists of informing the patient during the ED 'teachable moment' that they have a drinking problem.[60] This advice increases compliance to attend brief intervention later by 20%. Using PAT to screen all ED attendances as opposed to only those presentations considered at 'high risk' may increase the incidental pick-up of at-risk drinkers but may also decrease the enthusiasm of ED staff to provide screening because of the time required and the many negative screens.[61] Although it has been demonstrated that ED doctors and nurses with empathy and volition can be trained to provide ED-based brief intervention on the spot, the long-term benefit of this type of brief intervention is uncertain.

Pharmacotherapy for alcohol use disorder

Acamprosate

Acamprosate acts on GABA receptors in the CNS to reduce the craving for alcohol after detoxification. It is safe and well tolerated, suitable for use in treatment of alcohol use disorder aimed at maintaining abstinence. The usual dose is 666 mg (two 333 mg tablets) orally three times daily. Mild gastrointestinal side effects may occur, and therapeutic levels take 5–7 days to become established.

Naltrexone

Naltrexone is a partial opioid agonist that is useful in reducing the effects of endogenous opioids. It has had success in opioid addiction treatment, as well as in alcohol use disorder. The usual dose is 50 mg orally daily.

These agents may be used safely in combination, although this has not been shown to have superior effect. Pharmacotherapy produces better results when used in combination with cognitive behavioural therapy and motivational sessions.[62]

Likely developments over the next 5–10 years

- NHMRC Australian alcohol guidelines are currently under review in October 2007. Early recommendations are to reduce the recommended 'safe' intake to two standard drinks per day for *both* males and females, and for zero alcohol consumption in pregnancy.
- ED-initiated screening and intervention for alcohol use disorder are likely to spread to more EDs in the coming years.
- ED-initiated case management of the chronic recurrent alcohol-affected ED attender ('inebriate programmes') is also likely to gain favour.
- Novel pharmacological agents may appear to assist treatment of alcohol intoxication, withdrawal and hangover.

Controversies

❶ The true prevalence and incidence of alcoholic ketoacidosis.

❷ Use of high-dose parenteral thiamine to prevent Wernicke's encephalopathy.

❸ Targeting brief intervention by emergency clinicians for alcohol misuse at high-risk attendances compared to non-selected patients.

References

1. Chikritzhs T, Catalano P, Stockwell TR, et al. Australian Alcohol Indicators, 1990–2001; patterns of alcohol use and related harms for Australian states and territories. Report 2003. Perth: National Drug Research Institute; Fitzroy, Victoria: Western Australia and Turning Point Alcohol and Drug Centre; 2003.
2. National Health and Medical Research Council Australian Alcohol Guidelines. Health Risks and Benefits. Endorsed October 2001. Reprinted October 2003. http://www.nhmrc.gov.au/publications/synopses/_files/ds9.pdf (accessed September 2007).
3. Chikritzhs T, Pascal R, Gray D, et al. Trends in alcohol-attributable deaths among Indigenous Australians, 1998–2004. National Alcohol Indicators, Bulletin 11. Perth: National Drug Research Institute; 2007.
4. Reynaud M, Schwan R, Loiseaux-Meunier MN, et al. Patients admitted to emergency services for drunkenness: moderate alcohol users or harmful drinkers? American Journal of Psychiatry 2001; 158: 96–99.
5. Brokaw J, Olson L, Fullerton L, et al. Repeated ambulance use by patients with acute alcohol intoxication, seizure disorder, and respiratory illness. American Journal of Emergency Medicine 1998; 16: 141–144.
6. Hulse GK, Robertson SI, Tait RJ. Adolescent emergency department presentations with alcohol or other drug-related problems in Perth, Western Australia. Addiction 2001; 96: 1059–1067.
7. Thom B, Herring R, Judd A. Identifying alcohol-related harm in young drinkers: the role of accident and emergency departments. Alcohol 1999; 34: 910–915.
8. Roche AM, Watt K, Mclure R. Injury and alcohol: a hospital emergency department study. Drug Alcohol Review 2001; 20: 155–166.
9. Wikipedia. http://en.wikipedia.org/wiki/Breathalyser (accessed September 2007).
10. Wilcox CM, Alexander LN, Straub RF. A prospective endoscopic evaluation of the causes of upper GI hemorrhage in alcoholics: a focus on alcoholic gastropathy. American Journal of Gastroenterology 1996; 91: 1343–1347.
11. Rosenstock S, Jorgensen T, Bonnevie O. Risk factors for peptic ulcer disease: a population based prospective cohort study comprising 2416 Danish adults. Gut 2003; 52: 186–193.
12. Roberts LR, Kamath PS. Pathophysiology and treatment of variceal hemorrhage. Mayo Clinic Proceeding 1996; 71: 973–983.
13. Heidelbaugh JJ, Bruderly M. Cirrhosis and chronic liver failure: part II. Complications and treatment. American Family Physician 2006; 74: 767–776.
14. Pinto HC, Abrantes A, Esteves AV. Long-term prognosis of patients with cirrhosis of the liver and upper gastrointestinal bleeding. American Journal of Gastroenterology 1989; 84: 1239–1243.
15. Kortas DY, Haas LS, Simpson WG, et al. Mallory–Weiss tear: predisposing factors and predictors of a complicated course. American Journal of Gastroenterology 2001; 96: 2863–2865.
16. Lewis AM, Dharmarajah R. Walked in with Boerhaave's syndrome. Emergency Medicine Journal 2007; 24: e24.
17. Lau JY, Leung WK, Wu JC, et al. Omeprazole before endoscopy in patients with gastrointestinal bleeding. New England Journal of Medicine 2007; 356: 1631–1640.
18. Besson I, Ingrand P, Person B, et al. Sclerotherapy with or without octreotide for acute variceal bleeding. New England Journal of Medicine 1995; 333: 555–560.

19. Orloff MJ, Orloff MS, Orloff SL, et al. Three decades of experience with emergency portacaval shunt for acutely bleeding esophageal varices in 400 unselected patients with cirrhosis of the liver. Journal of American College of Surgery 1995; 180: 257–272.

20. Gramenzi A, Caputo F, Biselli M, et al. Review article: alcoholic liver disease – pathophysiological aspects and risk factors. Aliment Pharmacology and Therapeutics 2006; 24: 1151–1161.

21. Heidelbaugh JJ, Bruderly M. Cirrhosis and chronic liver failure: part I. Diagnosis and evaluation. American Family Physician 2006; 74: 756–762.

22. Sata N, Koizumi M, Nagai H. Alcoholic pancreatopathy: a proposed new diagnostic category representing the preclinical stage of alcoholic pancreatic injury. Journal of Gastroenterology (Tokyo) 2007; 42(suppl 17): 131–134.

23. Mayerle J, Lerch MM. Is it necessary to distinguish between alcoholic and nonalcoholic chronic pancreatitis? Journal of Gastroenterology (Tokyo) 2007; 42(suppl 17): 127–130.

24. Suokas J, Lonnqvist J. Suicide attempts in which alcohol is involved: a special group in general hospital emergency rooms. Acta Psychiatrica Scandinavica 1995; 91: 36–40.

25. Glass IB. Alcoholic hallucinosis: a psychiatric enigma-1. The development of an idea. British Journal of Addiction 1989; 84: 151–164.

26. Sullivan JT, Sykora K, Schneiderman J, et al. Assessment of alcohol withdrawal: the revised clinical institute withdrawal assessment for alcohol scale (CIWA-Ar). British Journal of Addiction 1989; 84: 1353–1357.

27. Williams D, Lewis J, McBride A. A comparison of rating scales for the alcohol withdrawal syndrome. Alcohol and Alcoholism 2001; 36: 104–108.

28. Mayo-Smith MF. Pharmacological management of alcohol withdrawal: a meta-analysis and evidence based guidelines. Journal of the American Medical Association 1997; 278: 144–151.

29. Stuppaeck CH, Deisenhammer EA, Kurz M, et al. The irreversible gamma aminobutyrate inhibitor vigabatrin in the treatment of alcohol withdrawal syndrome. Alcohol and Alcoholism 1996; 31: 109–111.

30. Rathlev NK, D'Onofrio G, Fish SS, et al. The lack of efficacy of phenytoin in the prevention of recurrent alcohol-related seizures. Annals of Emergency Medicine 1994; 23(3): 513–518.

31. Palmstierna T. Model for predicting alcohol withdrawal delirium. Psychiatric Services 2001; 52: 820–823.

32. Thomson AD. Mechanisms of vitamin deficiency in chronic alcohol misusers and the development of the Wernicke-Korsakoff syndrome. Alcohol and Alcoholism 2000; 35(suppl 1): 2–7.

33. Thomson AL, Cook CCH, Touquet R. The Royal College of Physicians report on alcohol: Guidelines for managing Wernicke's encephalopathy in the A and E department. Alcohol and Alcoholism 2002; 37: 513–521.

34. Ammendola A, Tata MR, Aurilio C, et al. Peripheral neuropathy in chronic alcoholism: a retrospective cross-sectional study in 76 subjects. Alcohol and Alcoholism 2001; 36: 271–275.

35. Ravaglia S, Marchioni E, Costa A. Erectile dysfunction as a sentinel symptom of cardiovascular autonomic neuropathy in heavy drinkers. Journal of Peripheral Nervous System 2004; 9: 209–214.

36. Butterworth RF. Pathophysiology of cerebellar dysfunction in the Wernicke–Korsakoff syndrome. Canadian Journal of Neurology Science 1993; 20 (Suppl 3):S123–S126.

37. Moss M, Burnham EL. Alcohol abuse in the critically ill patient. Lancet 2006; 368: 2231–2242.

38. McGuire LC, Cruickshank AM, Munro PT. Alcoholic ketoacidosis. Emergency Medicine Journal 2006; 23: 417–420.

39. MacDonald L, Kruse JA, Levy DB. Lactic acidosis and acute ethanol intoxication. American Journal of Emergency Medicine 1994; 12: 32–35.

40. Zilkens RR, Puddey IB. Alcohol and type 2 diabetes – another paradox? Journal of Cardiovascular Risk 2003; 10: 25–30.

41. Beilin LJ, Puddey IB. Alcohol and hypertension (hypertension highlights). Hypertension 2006; 47: 1035–1038.

42. Spies CD, Sander M, Stangl K, et al. Effects of alcohol on the heart. Current Opinion in Critical Care 2001; 7: 337–343.

43. Poschl G, Seitz HK. Alcohol and cancer. Alcohol and Alcoholism 2004; 39:155–165.

44. Todd K, Berk WA, Welch RD, et al. Prospective analysis of mental status progression in ethanol-intoxicated patients. American Journal of Emergency Medicine 1992; 10: 271–273.

45. Sucov A, Woolard RH. Ethanol-associated hypoglycemia is uncommon. Academic Emergency Medicine 1995; 2: 185–189.

46. Masur J, de Souza ML, Laranjeira RR, et al. Lack of effect of intravenous hypertonic glucose on the intensity of alcohol intoxication induced experimentally and observed in patients of an emergency room. Pharmacology 1983; 26: 54–60.

47. Pollack CV Jr, Jorden RC, Carlton FB, et al. Gastric emptying in the acutely inebriated patient. Journal of Emergency Medicine 1992; 10: 1–5.

48. Li J, Mills T, Erato R. Intravenous saline has no effect on blood ethanol clearance. Journal of Emergency Medicine 1999; 17: 1–5.

49. Saitz R, O'Malley S. Pharmacotherapies for alcohol abuse. Medical Clinics of North America 1997; 81: 881–907.

50. Shpilenya LS, Muzychenko AP, Gasbarrini G. Metadoxine in acute alcohol intoxication: a double-blind, randomized, placebo-controlled study. Alcohol Clinical and Experimental Research 2002; 26: 340–346.

51. Weise JG, Shiplak MG, Browner WS. The hangover. Annals of Internal Medicine 2000; 132: 897–902.

52. Pittler MH, Verster JC, Ernst E. Interventions for preventing or treating alcohol hangover: systematic review of randomised controlled trials. British Medical Journal 2005; 331: 1515–1518.

53. Dent AW, Phillips GA, Chenhall AJ. The heaviest repeat users of an inner city emergency department are not general practice patients. Emergency Medicine (Fremantle) 2003; 15: 322–329.

54. Phillips GA, Brophy DS, Chenhall AJ, et al. The effect of multidisciplinary case management on selected outcomes for frequent attenders at an emergency department. Medical Journal of Australia 2006; 184: 602–606.

55. Greane J. Serial Inebriate programmes: what to do about homeless alcoholics in the emergency department. Annals of Emergency Medicine 2007; 49: 701–793.

56. Nilssen O, Ries RK, Rivara FP. The CAGE questionnaire and the Short Michigan Alcohol Screening Test in trauma patients: comparison of their correlations with biological alcohol markers. Journal of Trauma 1994; 36: 784–788.

57. Crawford MJ, Patton R, Touquet R, et al. Screening and referral for brief intervention of alcohol misusing patients in an emergency department: a pragmatic randomised controlled trial. Lancet 2004; 364: 1334–1339.

58. Reynaud M, Schwan R, Loiseaux-Meunier MN, et al. Patients admitted to emergency services for drunkenness: moderate alcohol users or harmful drinkers? American Journal of Psychiatry 2001; 158: 96–99.

59. Touquet R, Brown A. Alcohol misuse: positive response. Alcohol health work for every acute hospital saves money and reduces repeat attendances. Emergency Medicine Australasia 2006; 18: 103–107.

60. Williams S, Brown A, Patton R, et al. The half-life of the 'teachable moment' for alcohol misusing patients in the emergency department. Drug and Alcohol Dependence 2005; 77: 205–208.

61. Weiland TJ, Dent AW, Phillips GA, et al. Emergency clinician-delivered screening and intervention for high-risk alcohol use: a qualitative analysis. Emergency Medicine Australasia 2008; 20: 121–128.

62. Assanangkornchai S, Srisurapanont M. The treatment of alcohol dependence. Current Opinion in Psychiatry 2007; 20: 222–227.

21.5 The challenging patient

Sandra Neate • Georgina Phillips

ESSENTIALS

1 Many patients characterized as 'challenging' share common characteristics, including complex and chronic medical disease, mental illness, marginalization, poverty, high levels of drug and alcohol use, and lack of social supports, safety and security.

2 An understanding of the issues that contribute to the challenging nature of some patients may assist the practitioner in developing a management approach characterized by sound knowledge, clear and achievable goals and compassion.

3 Management strategies may help to alleviate the dissatisfaction and frustration frequently experienced by the clinician.

4 Allied health and psychiatric services in the emergency department (ED) facilitate multidisciplinary and holistic care for the patient with complex needs.

5 Safety and security for all patients and staff must be assured.

THE HOMELESS PATIENT

ESSENTIALS

1 Multidisciplinary management of the homeless person is required.

2 Discharge planning is difficult and short stay admission is frequently required.

Case 1: A 38-year-old man with MELAS syndrome with a past history of cognitive impairment, refractory epilepsy, psychosis and behavioural disturbance presents with deteriorating behaviour and refusal to eat, drink, take his medications or attend to personal hygiene, with subsequent dehydration, seizures, hallucinations and aggressive behaviour. His elderly parents are no longer able to manage him at home.

Case 2: A 17-year-old male presents locked in the back of a police van with disturbed and aggressive behaviour in the setting of probable drug and alcohol ingestion, with police requesting a psychiatric assessment.

Case 3: A visiting dignitary collapses during a public address and is brought to the ED accompanied by an entourage of assistants, media and public.

Case 4: A prisoner is brought to the department complaining of headache, attempts to escape and is seriously injured by prison officers.

Case 5: A 35-year-old homeless man presents during a long weekend for the third time in 5 days, intoxicated with alcohol and requesting detoxification.

Case 6: A 42-year-old woman presents on a Saturday night with an exacerbation of chronic back pain stating that she is visiting from interstate and has lost her narcotic analgesia, requesting pain relief.

The ED is frequently the easiest or only access to healthcare for patients with multiple and challenging needs. For those impaired due to chronic illness, drugs and alcohol, mental illness or social circumstances, the ED represents a place where services are available 24 h a day or during crisis. The challenges posed by complex patients are compounded by system factors such as after hours' diminution of services, ED overcrowding and access block. Many challenging patients require urgent management for reasons other than medical issues, for example a behaviourally disturbed patient who causes disruption and anxiety within the ED, a VIP who may distract the attention of the staff or someone who poses a security risk. The management of a complex patient in a difficult environment represents a common challenge for the emergency physician. Many doctors find dealing with challenging patients tiring and frustrating and experience feelings of dissatisfaction. Several types of patients are described and discussed, with the aim of understanding the background circumstances that contribute to these presentations and assisting the practitioner to develop an approach to management.

Definition and epidemiology

Definitions of homelessness vary. A homeless person is often considered to be someone living on the streets without shelter. A broader definition includes any person without a conventional home who lacks most of the economic and social supports that a home normally affords. These persons are often cut off from the support of relatives and friends, have few independent resources and often no immediate means and in some cases little prospect of self-support. Homeless people are in danger of falling below the poverty line, at least from time to time.[1] This more inclusive definition accounts for those who are without safety, support and security in their living environment as well as those simply without shelter and includes those who are:

- currently living on the street
- living in crisis or refuge accommodation
- living in temporary arrangements without security of tenure or the legal right to stay (e.g. moving between the residences of friends or relatives, living in squats, caravans or improvised dwellings, or living in boarding houses)
- living in unsafe family circumstances (e.g. families in which child abuse or domestic violence is a threat or has occurred)
- living on very low incomes and facing extraordinary expenses or personal crisis[2]

- living apart from family because of unsuitable accommodation.

Concepts of homelessness vary with culture. People from Aboriginal and Torres Straight Islander cultures may experience homelessness when separated from their spiritual home despite adequate shelter, and conversely may feel a spiritual connection to the land on which they live independent of the presence of shelter. Three broad categories of indigenous homelessness are identified in Australia: those living in public places, those at risk of losing their house and those who are spiritually homeless.[3]

Estimates of prevalence of homelessness are difficult due to variations in definition and methodologies of identification. In the USA approximately 600 000 families and 1.3 million children experience homelessness per year.[4] More than 160 000 Australians experience homelessness each year, one-third of them children, whilst resources allocated in response to homelessness are grossly inadequate. One of every 50 Australian children access homeless services and two in three of them are turned away. One in every 50 women of age 18–19 years experiences homelessness per year, and half of these are unable to access crisis accommodation when needed. Homelessness is more prevalent in women and is closely related to the experience of domestic violence and inequity in general.[5] Other groups are at increased risk of homelessness. The Australian indigenous population comprises 2–3% of the Australian population but accounts for 16% of those accessing homeless services with domestic violence contributing to 40% of homelessness. Ex-prisoners, war veterans (especially in the USA), the mentally and physically ill, youths and people in rural communities experience increased incidence of homelessness.

Clinical features

Homeless patients presenting to the ED exhibit high rates of complex physical and mental illness and substance dependence. Due to poverty and social isolation, access to healthcare is impeded with a subsequent cycle of deterioration in health. Lack of housing stability, social supports and points of reference within the local community lead to a high rate of utilization and

representation to the ED[6] despite the development of outreach programmes or case management strategies.[7] Homeless patients may present to the ED up to 10 times more frequently than the rest of the population.[8]

Representation rates within 28 days of discharge are high and may account for up to 48% of all representation episodes and 23% of all patients who represent to the ED.[8] Certain features such as sociodemographics (age <65 years, receiving government pension), service utilization history (case management and discharge at own risk) and clinical features (primary psychiatric presentation, complex medical history and high numbers of prescribed medications) are highly predictive of representation.[8] Presentations by homeless people are often of low acuity. Triage categories are non-urgent in up to 91% of attendances.[8]

Presentations with infectious diseases (e.g. TB and HIV), penetrating trauma, depression, schizophrenia and ethanol and drug abuse are common.[9] Deliberate self-harm presentations are more frequent and are followed by a higher rate of representation with recurrent self-harm and approximately double the rate of death from successful completion of suicide than in the domiciled population.[10] Homeless patients presenting with deliberate self-harm are more likely to be a recent victim or perpetrator of violence, have a criminal record or a personality disorder, thus highlighting the complex links between these variables.

Management

The management of the homeless patient requires a multidisciplinary approach and an understanding of the social and financial constraints the patient faces. There is no point in prescribing medication that the patient is unable to afford, organizing hospital in the home services when the patient has no home or the services are unwilling to visit the 'home', or suggesting a standard admission to a patient who is unwilling to stay due to drug and alcohol dependence. Allied health services may be able to provide background information or links to established community services, assist with discharge planning or assist with emergency accommodation or other social

services. Discharge planning may be especially difficult and short stay admission for management of simple conditions normally treatable at home or admission to low acuity facilities may assist with improvements in health and other social parameters.[11] A compassionate approach to the homeless patient, where patients were assigned a volunteer who offered food and conversation, was found to significantly decrease rates of representation, dispelling the myth that increasing patient satisfaction encourages homeless patients to reattend.[12]

THE PRISONER

ESSENTIALS

1 The prisoner population is extremely disadvantaged and vulnerable.

2 Prisoners' health needs differ from the general public.

3 Presentations are often injury-related and are generally of high acuity.

4 Security events are uncommon.

Definition and epidemiology

A prisoner is defined as someone who is charged with an offence and remanded in custody or is convicted of a crime, resulting in detention within the prison system. The patient brought to the ED by the police from the community who is under arrest differs somewhat from the patient who is residing in a prison. Both types of patients may pose security issues, but their health needs and demographics may be quite different.

The prisoner poses several challenges when seen in the ED (Table 21.5.1).

The prisoner population is an extraordinarily needy, unhealthy and life-damaged group, and from a health perspective represents a distinct cohort rather than a microcosm of the wider community.[13]

Table 21.5.1 Challenges involving the prisoner in the ED	
Security issues	**Patient care issues**
Perceived threat to safety of staff and other patients	Clinical management of complex illness
Potential for violent incidents	Medical, psychiatric and addiction co-morbidities
Presence of non-hospital security staff	Maintenance of confidentiality
Weapons in the ED	Discharge planning

Demographic points of difference between prisoners and the general population include educational level, employment history, reliance on social welfare, sexual history, nutritional background and marital status. These factors lead to increased rates of prisoner presentation to the ED and contribute to their vulnerability.

The prison population has a high rate of pre-existing mental and physical illness, and issues of dependence and a high rate of hospitalization. Twenty-five per cent of prisoners report having been hospitalized in the preceding year.[13] Prisoners have a high rate of risk-taking behaviours that increase the risk of poor health, such as tattooing and heavy drug, alcohol and tobacco use, and display behaviours with addictive/compulsive orientations and low impulse control. All these factors contribute to the illnesses with which the prisoner may present, the way in which they present, the interactions they have with security, medical and nursing staff, and their approach to the treatments offered.

Prisoners in the ED are in a threatening and embarrassing environment where they can be seen by members of the public to be under guard and restrained. Some prisoners may experience some secondary gain from a visit to the ED; however, most express feelings of distress when removed from their familiar environment. Prisoners are prohibited from having the normal support of friends and family at times of illness. The prison system is overcrowded and prisoners may be kept in many levels of detention right down to sharing a cell in the local police station 'lock up'. Those returning to a cell receive no ongoing observation, medical attention or medication on discharge from the ED.

Clinical features

The mean age of prisoners presenting to the ED is approximately 30 years.[14,15] Presentations are most commonly injury related, with approximately one-third of these self-inflicted injury, one-third accidental and one-third as a result of assault or unclear mechanisms. Seizures are a frequent presenting complaint with diagnoses including alcohol and substance withdrawal, epilepsy and pseudoseizures. Drug withdrawal is implicated in approximately 9% of presentations and 6% of admissions.[14] Prisoners have a high rate of admission to hospital (range 36–49%), which may be due to higher acuity of illness, with approximately 80% of prisoners triaged as category 3 or above, and by the practical and logistical difficulties in managing people in custody. Prisoners have a decreased length of stay in the ED compared with the non-prisoner population.[14]

Whilst most prisoners are cooperative, opportunities do exist for prisoners to attempt escape, as the ED provides an environment that is frequently chaotic and distracting and some circumstances require the removal of restraints. Maintaining a patient's privacy and confidentiality may conflict with security requirements. Episodes of violence are uncommon. The rate of security incidents may be lower than for the non-prisoner population.[14] Perceived threat, and the accompanying stress caused to staff, is something that is yet to be quantified.

The presence of weapons provides the potential for serious injury to the patient if an escape is attempted, or to staff if the patient removes a weapon from security staff. Fatalities have been documented.[14]

Prisoners frequently present after hours, possibly due to unavailability of staff to assess prisoners on-site. In one study, 55% of prisoner attendances occurred after hours.[15] This may compound security issues.

Management

The urgency with which a prisoner is assessed depends on a combination of medical and security issues. Outside of formal triage criteria, the experienced practitioner may elect to prioritize these patients to expedite investigations and decrease length of stay in the ED.

The patient should preferably be assessed by senior staff to enable rapid management decisions to be made. Junior staff should be accompanied by a senior member of staff, particularly if the junior staff member experiences fear or anxiety.

Unless security staff communicate particular security concerns, there should be no enquiry into the reasons for incarceration. However, an enquiry into the length of incarceration may assist assessment as prisoners who have been incarcerated for short periods only may be suffering the effects of substance withdrawal. Drug withdrawal may be the sole reason for presentation or influence the presenting complaint or examination findings and requests for analgesia and other medications.

Confidentiality concerns exist with guards present during assessment. These concerns need to be weighed against security issues. Guidance from security staff as to whether they feel it is safe to leave the cubicle or remove restraints may be helpful. If the clinician feels insecure, security staff should remain within the room. The history obtained in the presence of security guards may be inaccurate. Patients may be fearful of disclosing the mechanism of their injuries due to fears of reprisal or prison guards in attendance overhearing the circumstances of injury.

In many Australian states, psychiatric services are not resourced or mandated to care for prisoners, and mental health acts do not cover those incarcerated under separate forensic laws. This may render the ED care of the mentally unwell prisoner even more difficult, as psychiatric illness may be undiagnosed or undertreated, and access to normal mental health clinicians to aid in assessment and treatment may not be available.

Opportunities for follow-up are difficult. There may be little possibility for observation upon return to the place of detention. Outpatient follow-up is time and resource intensive, and logistically difficult for the prison staff. There is therefore often a need for more extensive investigation whilst in the ED. A low threshold for ruling out potential illnesses and for admission to hospital is generally required.

If the patient is returning to prison, clear written discharge instructions should be formally communicated and discharge medication with dispensing instructions provided. Liaison with the prison nurse or forensic medical officer should establish whether their facilities and staffing can provide the expected management.

THE BEHAVIOURALLY DISTURBED AND VIOLENT PATIENT

ESSENTIALS

1 Complex comorbidities of organic illness, psychosocial issues and substance misuse can manifest as acute behavioural disturbance.

2 Understanding legal and ethical considerations can inform rapid decisions and humane treatment in behavioural emergencies.

3 A safe environment and team approach can maximize containment of disturbed and violent behaviour, whilst respecting the privacy and dignity of patients.

4 A strategic approach to understanding and managing violence in the ED may minimize the harmful effects of violence to staff, patients and carers.

Aetiology and epidemiology

Acute behavioural disturbance has long required urgent medical attention, but it is becoming increasingly common in EDs as psychosocial stressors increase and new substances for potential misuse emerge. Violent and unarmed threats involving patients in the ED have been described with an incidence of between 0.3%[16,17] and 2%.[18] Accurate information on the incidence and subsequent management of acute behavioural disturbance is severely limited by the lack of clarity around what constitutes a behavioural emergency, and significant differences in

treatment response both within and between EDs. Anecdotally, and fuelled by increased media and government scrutiny, the frequency and nature of behavioural disturbance requiring urgent medical care is increasing, as recreational drugs such as 'ice' and the phenomenon of underage alcohol abuse command a high profile in the community. It has also been argued that psychiatric deinstitutionalization and limited community supports have led to an influx of unstable, mentally ill patients to the ED.

Approximately half of the patients presenting with acute behavioural disturbance have an acute flare of a primary mental illness, whilst 40–50% are intoxicated with drugs or alcohol.[16] A smaller number have an organic illness, including dementia, manifesting as a behavioural emergency.[19] A combination of psychiatric illness and substance intoxication commonly occurs. Most patients are male (approximately 65%) and under the age of 40,[16,17] and around 20% are brought to the ED in police custody.[16,20] The majority of unarmed threats occur in the late afternoon, evening and overnight, with a weekly peak on a Saturday.[16] Between 58% and 80% of these require some form of chemical or physical restraint as part of management.[16–18]

Prevention

Whilst there are no validated tools or clinically useful predictive factors for violence and acute behavioural disturbance in the ED, experienced clinicians are able to recognize environmental and individual factors that lead to unstable and dangerous behaviour. Crowded, noisy and brightly lit departments are the antithesis of the calm and stable surrounds that promote controlled behaviour and de-escalate aggression. Fear, confusion and inadequate communication can trigger anger and aggressive behaviour in both patients and carers, whilst long waiting times and negative waiting room environmental factors have been suggested as contributors to violence in the ED.

In order to prevent anger or illness from escalating to a behavioural emergency, recognition of verbal and non-verbal cues is required, as well as an ability to utilize environmental and clinical resources to ensure a calm, controlled situation.

Increasingly, EDs are developing separate rooms or sections that are quiet and private, as sites for the assessment and containment of behavioural disturbance.[21] There is ongoing debate around this and the specialization of EDs as designated 'behavioural centres' in a similar vein to trauma centres.[22] Geographical separation and removal of stimulation may be enough to reverse the trend to increased aggression. Respectful and clear communication with lowered voice tone, eye contact and non-threatening body language may establish a rapport that enhances a therapeutic bond between clinician and patient. Explanation of treatment decisions and the reasons for them may alleviate confusion, whilst bargaining and rewarding compliance can diffuse tension. Allowing a semblance of autonomy and control to the patient, whilst setting clear behavioural limits, is recommended.

A prophylactic 'security response' has been utilized in the ED to contain behaviour when disturbance and aggression have been anticipated. This can be aided by prior police and ambulance notification of the imminent arrival of a patient with a behavioural emergency. A team comprising hospital security service, nursing and medical staff can in itself be a disincentive for increased aggression, when confronting an aroused patient. In the event of violence, the team response carried out in a separate area of the ED can quickly control behaviour safely and thus prevent further episodes or prolongation of aggression.

Clinical features

Whilst the specific clinical features of behavioural emergencies vary according to the aetiology, behavioural disturbance will generally manifest early in the patient's ED presentation, rather than evolve over many hours. The aims of clinical assessment comprise three components: diagnostic, evaluation of risk and assessment of arousal (see Table 21.5.2).

Signs of acute intoxication or withdrawal may follow recognized patterns or drug toxidromes, whilst psychiatric instability may manifest with features of psychosis. Differentiating between organic illness, delirium and substance intoxication, or psychosis

Table 21.5.2 Aims of clinical assessment in acute behavioural assessment	
Diagnosis	What is the aetiology of the behaviour: psychiatric, substance related, organic, personality?
Risk assessment	Can the patient's autonomy be over-ridden?
Arousal assessment	Does the patient require containment?

can be extremely difficult in the initial assessment, and may only be clarified after immediate management and behaviour containment (see Ch. 20.2 Distinguishing medical from psychiatric causes). A breath alcohol can be extremely useful and intravenous puncture sites may suggest substance misuse. In an agitated and aroused patient, the stereotypical act of taking a blood pressure or putting a stethoscope on the chest may be recognized as a familiar and non-threatening action and thus be better tolerated than attempting to get a detailed history or expecting a rational response to verbal requests.

The role of investigations in the behaviourally disturbed patient is controversial. Routine laboratory blood testing is of low yield, and diagnostic evaluation should be directed by history and examination. Urine drug screens have no role in the acute assessment or management. Cognitive abilities should guide the readiness for psychiatric assessment, rather than the suspected presence of drugs or alcohol. A positive breath alcohol should not preclude mental health assessment in the patient who is alert and orientated.[23]

Risk assessments are often made rapidly and intuitively in the highly agitated and aggressive patient. The decision to contain and restrain an aroused patient with extreme behaviour is primarily based around the perceived threat of harm to self or others. If patient competence cannot be assessed, then the assumption of risk of harm and the doctor's duty of care over-ride patient autonomy. Clinical features that are suggestive of high risk include threats or actual self-harm, suicidal behaviour or ideation, threats or actual violence to others, altered conscious state due to

illness, injury or substance intoxication and incompetence. Risk assessments and restraint can only be made within an acute framework (i.e. pertaining to hours rather than weeks or months), as this is the length of time a person can humanely be contained within an ED setting.[24]

Patients with longer-term high-risk behaviours are not suitable for physical or chemical restraint in the ED and may be managed more appropriately in a mental health or forensic setting. Assessment of arousal requires utilization of collaborative and clinical tools, and will inform decisions about urgency and methods of restraint. Information about behaviour immediately prior to ED presentation can be gathered from police and ambulance officers. Physical struggle and violence requiring restraint during transport to the ED is an indication of the need for ongoing restraint. Physical intimidation, threats or acts of violence to self, people or property, attempts to escape, uncontrollable verbal abuse and aggressive acts such as spitting all indicate extreme arousal and the need for immediate containment and restraint. Signs that a patient is increasingly aroused, and that violence may be imminent, include physical agitation and restlessness, pacing, sweating, loss of rational thinking, increased voice tone, swearing or foul language, eye widening and pupil dilation. Early recognition of these prodromal features may prevent the escalation of aggression and ensure the safety of both staff and patient.

Legal and ethical considerations

Sedation and restraint for behaviour containment represent significant deprivations of personal liberty. Australasian law strongly upholds the fundamental principle of individual autonomy, whilst laws pertaining to mental health recognize this with the key concept of 'least restriction' informing all involuntary containment and treatment orders.[25] Emergency physicians must also respect patient autonomy and be mindful of employing the least restrictive practices when making decisions to restrain aroused and aggressive patients.

The ability to detain and treat people without their consent is lawfully recognized in emergency situations, committal under legislation (e.g. mental health acts), suicide prevention, to protect others from harm, self-defence, 'necessity' or 'in best interests' and for incompetent patients.[26] Thus, ED staff are comprehensively protected under the law if they act in good faith and with integrity when managing acute behavioural disturbance. Doctors are also legally required to maintain confidentiality, to take reasonable care, not to take advantage of a patient and to meet professional standards.[27] In highly stressful and potentially dangerous situations involving agitated or violent patients, it is important to be reminded of these duties. Containment and restraint often take place in highly visible sites within the ED, where the patient is exposed to the scrutiny of other staff, patients and visitors, thus undermining personal privacy and confidentiality. Similarly, abusive and aggressive patients may provoke anger and frustration in ED staff, who should be mindful at all times of their legal duties to take care and act professionally.

Competent patients are responsible for their actions and are expected to behave within a reasonable and legal framework. Damage to property and assault to person are crimes which are subject to prosecution if they occur in an ED and towards ED staff. There are occupational health and safety requirements that mandate a safe working environment and can inform structural changes and clinical practices in the management of violence in the ED.

Medical ethics and the law complement each other when recognizing personal autonomy and human rights. A compassionate approach that respects the human dignity of all patients and recognizes the medical duty to provide care is likely to result in both a lawful and an ethical framework for managing patients with behavioural emergencies.

Management

Once the decision to contain and restrain a patient with behavioural disturbance has been made, and preventative, de-escalation measures have been unsuccessful, it is worth determining the desired endpoint of management. Containment methods differ significantly according to the desired outcome, which may range from a calmed, awake patient through to one who is fully tranquillized and shackled. In an ED setting, containing and restraining a patient is not therapeutic and should be viewed as a transient departure from the normal physician–patient collaboration.[28]

Containing a highly aroused and aggressive patient requires a team of trained staff: a minimum of six people comprising hospital security staff and orderlies, with medical and nursing staff to assist with team leadership, documentation, drug administration and subsequent monitoring.[29] Smaller hospitals may need to utilize police in their initial team response, but this is not recommended, given the differing training and aims of hospital- and police-based restraint practices. Police should be involved when a weapon is present, or the violent person is not a patient receiving treatment. The importance of prior planning, regular aggression management training and good communication cannot be overemphasized.

Chemical restraint

The pharmacological management of the acutely aroused patient is discussed in detail elsewhere, but the principles should be emphasized. The least traumatic measures are advocated, depending on the desired endpoint of chemical restraint and the risks to staff and patient in administration.

Oral benzodiazepines are preferred where possible and may allow patients a small sense of control if they are able to choose this option ahead of parenteral sedation. Choice between intramuscular or intravenous administration of sedation depends on perceived risks to staff, ease of obtaining intravenous access, need for blood tests or other intravenous therapy and desired rapidity of sedative effect. Where rapid tranquillization is desired, the intravenous route of administration is required, as the onset of action is within the first 5 min rather than the approximate 15–20 min of intramuscular drugs.[30,31] Commonly used drugs for rapid tranquillization include benzodiazepines (diazepam and midazolam) and neuroleptics (droperidol and haloperidol). Other drugs used for less urgent or longer-term sedation include benzodiazepines administered intramuscular or orally, intramuscular neuroleptics and the newer antipsychotics, including olanzapine.[32] Combinations of these drugs are often used, although the additive sedative effect can result in oversedation. Thus careful monitoring in a high acuity area of the ED is required when chemical restraint is used.

Physical restraint

Physical restraint can initially proceed on the floor and move to a trolley as soon as practical. A five-point hold is recommended, involving securing the head, upper and lower limbs in firm grasps. Personal protective gear of gown, safety goggles and gloves should be worn by all involved, and an oxygen mask or loosely applied towel over the face can be used if the patient is spitting. Whilst it is paramount not to inflict harm on the patient, the safety of staff is also a priority and may justify the use of moderate physical force. Using staff to physically restrain a patient is a temporary measure only and should be followed by more definitive restraint in the form of sedating drugs, physical shackles or both.

Physical restraint with shackles provokes emotional distaste in many clinicians, but it can be used safely and humanely in an ED setting. There have been reported deaths in restrained, agitated patients, described largely in the USA where 'hobble' restraints including prone positioning with hands and feet secured together behind the back are used.[33] Where supine positioning is used, physical shackles have been shown to be safe,[34] although caution should be employed with restraints around the upper chest and neck area. Soft-edged, strong, fabric shackles securing the wrists and ankles of a supine patient to the trolley are recommended. Concomitant chemical sedation is advised with appropriate monitoring. Prolonged shackling is inhumane and carries risks of musculoskeletal injury, respiratory compromise and psychological trauma. Many Australian states have laws that mandate careful and close observation of physically restrained patients, as well as regular review of the need for such ongoing, extreme restraint.

Whilst few EDs have appropriate resources, it may be possible to contain patients with behavioural disturbance in a less restrictive manner by using seclusion rooms. Such areas must be visible to ED staff, be easily accessible to a security response team and have no dangerous furniture or fittings with which patients could potentially harm themselves or others.

Patient perspective

Emergency clinicians rarely consider patient preferences when faced with the need to urgently control aggressive or threatening behaviour, and there is limited evidence to inform this issue. The majority of patients prefer chemical restraint rather than physical for interventions, and seclusion is preferred over physical shackles. Benzodiazepines are the preferred drug for chemical sedation rather than neuroleptics.[35]

Disposition

Behaviourally disturbed patients commonly spend many hours in the ED, both for accurate assessment and for diagnostic purposes. Increasingly, the lack of access to general medical, psychiatric and detoxification inpatient beds means that timely transfer for definitive care is delayed. The result is prolonged, inhumane containment of behaviourally disturbed patients, which is likely to lead to worse therapeutic outcomes. For this reason, ED doctors must be strong advocates on behalf of their patients, as well as maintain vigilant clinical review of physical and mental state, and the need for ongoing restraint. Patients who are transferred to inpatient wards for ongoing care must be alert, have stable vital signs, not require further monitoring and be declared safe for transfer by the most senior available ED clinician. Respiratory depression and death have occurred in patients transferred to psychiatric wards after receiving chemical sedation from the ED (Chief Psychiatrist Victoria, personal communication, 2007); therefore, the time, nature and route of drug administration must be taken into account when considering safety for transfer.

The decision to admit a patient depends on the result of clinical and investigative findings, ongoing mental health and risk assessment and the progress of the patient over time. It is appropriate to keep behaviourally disturbed patients under ED observation for up to 24 h in order to clarify the aetiology of the altered behaviour and determine a safe disposition. Patients with aggression and arousal due to substance intoxication often wake up several hours later with normal behaviour and no recollection of their earlier violent behaviour. This presents a preventative health opportunity to counsel, educate and refer the patient for ongoing drug and alcohol review. Patients should be informed that their substance misuse resulted in dangerous behaviour both for themselves and others, but many will already be socially marginalized and vulnerable as a result of homelessness, substance addiction and psychosocial stressors. A multidisciplinary care-coordination approach optimizes a safe discharge for these patients.

Normal clinical and investigative findings, the absence of substance intoxication and exclusion of acute mental illness mean that the patients do not require further ED care. Such patients may still present a behavioural challenge and, if ongoing risk to self or others exists, then they should be discharged to the care of the police. Collaborative decision-making with mental health clinicians is often required in such situations, as these patients often suffer antisocial or other personality disorders that are difficult to manage in both forensic and health settings. For those discharged to the community, mental health and social work follow-up is recommended.

At all stages in the assessment, containment, restraint and disposition of patients with acute behavioural disturbance, clear documentation is mandatory. The importance of recording management events and the reasons behind containment or discharge decisions protects staff from clinical and legal criticism, as well as aid care in potential future ED presentations.

Violence

The impact of violence is under-recognized in Australasian EDs, although it has been increasingly documented.[36] Whilst aggression and violence most often stem from acutely disturbed patients, violence in the ED can also come from visitors and carers, as well as hospital staff. Internationally recognized as a growing problem, ED violence is also generally poorly documented and under-reported, with limited formal hospital support for those exposed and rare conviction for the perpetrators.[37,38] Whilst conventional definitions of violence centre around the act of intent to cause physical or psychological harm, in an ED setting aggression and violence are commonly a manifestation of underlying illness or substance intoxication. The absence of a malicious intent to cause harm may be a reason why violence has been under-recognized in the hospital environment and has led to an alternative workplace definition: any episode in which staff experience either implicit or explicit challenges to their personal safety, health or sense of wellbeing.[39]

Other reasons for under-reporting of ED violence stem from hospital systems, which act as barriers by burdening staff with excessive and time-consuming paperwork, confusing policies, inadequate confidentiality and lack of peer support.[40] Whilst most episodes of violence in the ED do not result in serious physical injury, staff who experience violence may be traumatized, which can lead to feelings of stress and anger. The cumulative effect of violence may result in clinician 'burnout' and staff attrition.

A strategic approach to managing violence in the ED centres around the key themes of environment and personnel, with a focus on prevention and training. Generally, a comfortable environment with clear visibility that facilitates good communication will have a greater effect on behaviour modification than increasing fortification of waiting rooms, triage and clinical areas in the ED. Violence minimization is assisted by security cameras and televisions at triage so potential aggressors can see that they are being monitored, the visible proximity of security staff, high visibility within the clinical workspace, restricted access areas, minimizing access to potential weapons, widely dispersed and simple-to-use duress alarm devices and security cameras. Weapon searches and metal detectors are rarely used in Australasian EDs, and

the introduction of such measures may compromise the welcoming and therapeutic atmosphere that should characterize an ED. The conflict between the desire to provide care for all people, including those with disturbing and potentially aggressive behaviour, and the need to protect staff and others from potential injury, may result in an environment from which the most vulnerable members of the community are excluded. This contradicts the spirit in which ED clinicians work and promotes inequity within the health system.

Staff training and support is paramount in managing ED violence. Interdisciplinary programmes that involve role-play and real scenario discussions can enhance cooperation between all ED staff, whilst clarifying roles and responsibilities during actual security responses. Peer education sessions can serve to change culture towards a preventative and proactive approach, based on good communication skills and sound knowledge about behavioural emergencies.

In general, ED doctors are required to take a leadership role when managing a violent episode, although collaboration with experienced nursing colleagues improves care. Awareness of personal factors that may impact on the escalation of violence and the subsequent outcomes is therefore essential. Anger, fear and personal insult can lead to interactions with aroused patients that may escalate aggression rather than diffuse tension, and clinicians are advised to remove themselves from situations where their management is compromised by provoked emotions that cannot be controlled. The role of peer support and follow-up in such situations is vital. Similarly, issues of gender, language and culture are often under-recognized as factors influencing the escalation and management of a behavioural emergency. It may be that male staff are more likely to experience higher levels of physical violence than women. Self-awareness and consideration of these issues can optimize management of the violent episode, as well as minimize the potential negative outcomes for staff and others.

The final component of the structured approach to ED violence management is ensuring adequate documentation and follow-up systems which include debriefing and support. Reporting should be incorporated into the standard documentation of any security incident within the ED, rather than the onus of staff who have been victims of violence. As the issue of workplace violence is one of occupational health and safety, follow-up of violent incidents should fall within this framework, thus depersonalizing the impact of aggression and owning violence as an organizational responsibility rather than belonging to the individual.

THE FREQUENT ATTENDER

ESSENTIALS

1 Frequent attenders to the ED have increased morbidity and mortality.

2 Assumptions about inappropriate use of the ED have been shown to be false.

3 Improvements in the psychosocial status of frequent attenders' lives can be made with ED-based multidisciplinary care coordination.

Definition and epidiemiology

Patients who present to hospital EDs more than three times a year can be defined as 'frequent attenders'[41] and represent a particularly vulnerable population.[42,43] Both internationally and within Australasia, the frequent attender population has consistent characteristics that include poverty, homelessness, chronic and complex medical illness, psychiatric illness, and drug and alcohol abuse.[44–46] Frequent attenders also suffer a high mortality, with an increased risk of death from violent causes such as suicide and substance misuse.[47] They are known to use health services in a frequent, chaotic and episodic way,[48] will attend multiple EDs[49] and are difficult to engage in any long-term care.[50] Importantly,

availability and engagement with primary healthcare providers does not alter ED use by frequent attenders.[42,48]

Whilst representing a small number of people, frequent attenders can be responsible for up to 8% or more of annual ED attendances.[51] Demographic details vary according to how the frequent attender population is defined and analysed in the literature, although they are consistently more likely to be male and socially isolated.[7,43] A range of 27–55% have chronic and complex medical illness as the key reason underlying their frequent ED use, whilst the remainder suffer primarily psychiatric, social or drug- and alcohol-related illness.[7,52] Commonly, heavy ED users display a combination of all of these comorbidities. Patterns of attendance generally fall into two categories, with those suffering primarily psychosocial illness or substance abuse sustaining consistently frequent ED use over many years, whilst those with primarily chronic medical illness showing peak ED attendance over 1–2 years.[52] The key pattern over time, however, is the high incidence of death in this population.

Clinical features

There is great variability in the clinical presentation of frequent attenders. Acute exacerbations of underlying chronic medical illness are common, as are traumatic injuries, or injuries and illness sustained through violence or substance misuse, including acute substance intoxication.[53] Infections in the respiratory, gastrointestinal and dermatological systems are frequent. Deterioration in mental state or self-harm and suicide attempts are also common reasons for ED attendance.[51] Compared with the whole population, frequent attenders are represented equivalently across all triage categories but they require longer ED care, including admission to an ED-based observation area. Admissions to inpatient units are fewer in comparison with the general population. Frequent attenders are more likely to discharge themselves from the ED prior to completing their ED care, or self-discharge before assessment after the initial triage process.[51]

There is a pervasive assumption that frequent attenders present to the ED excessively and unnecessarily and are therefore suitable for diversion to general practitioners.[54] Evidence suggests that this belief is false and that the majority of patients presenting frequently for ED care do so appropriately and are unsuitable for diversion to primary-care providers.[51] Patients may be adversely affected if their symptoms are belittled and attendance classified as 'inappropriate'.[55]

Management

Understanding the vulnerability of frequent attenders, and their complex comorbidities, whilst adopting a humane approach are fundamental. Medical care follows standard procedures. Access to past history and information from all healthcare and community services involved in the care of the frequent attender provides an essential context enabling timely, focused and relevant care, without unnecessary duplication of services and investigations. Utilization of ED-based multidisciplinary services for care coordination has been shown to be of benefit when caring for the frequent attender.[7]

Attempts to reduce perceived unnecessary ED attendance have met with varying results. Neither education of patients[56] nor management care plans[57] has reduced the frequency of ED attendance. The most successful international diversion strategies have adopted multidisciplinary approaches, including social worker support.[58,59] ED-based multidisciplinary case management has been shown to increase ED utilization but also to lead to improvement in psychosocial factors such as housing status and engagement with primary- and community-care providers.[7] ED use may need to increase for frequent attenders if psychosocial improvements are desired.

Frequent attenders are a complex, unwell and chaotic population. Diversion away from the ED has no proven patient benefit, therefore it may be that the ED is the best site of care for such vulnerable patients and this can have a role in improving overall wellbeing.

THE PATIENT WITH DRUG-SEEKING BEHAVIOUR

ESSENTIALS

1 Drug addiction can be viewed as a chronic, organic disease.

2 Drug-seeking behaviour is problematic for the patient and the clinician.

3 Physicians managing these patients may experience dissatisfaction, frustration and feelings of manipulation.

Definition and aetiology

Drug abuse is defined as recurrent medication use that occurs outside acceptable standard recommendations and despite adverse consequences. Addiction is defined as a primary, chronic neurobiological disease that develops as a result of genetic, psychosocial and environmental factors and manifests features, including impaired control over use, compulsive use, continuing use despite harmful effects and cravings.[60] In contrast, pseudoaddiction is an often unrecognized iatrogenic syndrome of patient behaviours that occurs when pain is undertreated.[61] Drug-seeking behaviour can be defined as behaviour aimed at obtaining controlled substance prescriptions for reasons of dependence, abuse or illicit use in a manner that is problematic to the prescriber.[62,63] Patients may have a range of underlying disorders such as psychiatric illness, substance misuse, chronic pain and complex medical conditions, which have resulted in drug dependence and institutionalized behaviour on many levels.

The concept of addiction as a disease is useful in modifying the clinician's approach to patients with addiction issues. The illness model has countered the widely held view of addiction as a wilful behaviour with moral implications. Likening addiction to other chronic illnesses such as hypertension and diabetes helps to understand the chronicity of the problem and the vulnerability to relapse. The rehabilitation of patients with substance-abuse problems has, however, been handled largely by non-physicians who work closely with their patients. The ongoing nature of the treatment and the relationship required to effect treatment makes intervention in the ED challenging.

Clinical features

Identification of the patient seeking drugs may be difficult. Features raising suspicion of drug seeking include suspicions of drug seeking previously documented in the medical record, inconsistent history or examination findings, requests for specific narcotic or other drugs of dependence, unwillingness to try simple analgesia, higher than expected analgesia requirements and demanding or aggressive behaviour.[64] Other features that may raise suspicion include complaints of lost or stolen prescriptions or medications, letters from remote medical practices supporting the provision of medications and presentations that are possible to feign such as migraine or ureteric calculus.

Presenting problems of those diagnosed as drug seeking include acute and chronic pain, primary psychiatric disorder or drug and alcohol dependence, or specific request for medication. Patients exhibit a high rate of previous attendances with drug-seeking behaviour and commonly have a past history of mental illness, drug dependence and self-harm.[65]

The possibility of missing organic illness is considerable in patients suspected of drug seeking, as nearly 20% require hospital admission and 17% self-discharge against medical advice. Missed, too, is the opportunity to acknowledge drug dependence and refer appropriately. Of drug-seeking patients seen in the ED, only 11% have a documented discussion around this issue in the medical record, and only 23% are referred to addiction, psychiatric or chronic pain services.[65]

Management

There is considerable individual variation in the management of patients who are drug seeking. Clinicians often find these interactions frustrating and unsatisfying and may feel abused or manipulated. The development of a general approach may assist (Table 21.5.3).

Limit setting requires confidence, experience and familiarity with local laws that limit the prescribing of controlled drugs. A departmental policy regarding the drugs available within the ED available for dispensing after hours and which may be prescribed on an outpatient basis can give guidance. Approaches vary, but a factual and dispassionate explanation about the inability to prescribe controlled substances due to departmental policy or legal requirements may be of assistance.

The physician needs to determine the appropriateness and utility of an open discussion surrounding the perceived problem behaviour. If open discussion is possible, referral for assistance may be more likely to be successful. Opportunities for interdisciplinary discussion of particular patients and an approach to their management with the development of an easily accessible electronically available protocol may assist those in the front line of management.

Table 21.5.3 General approach to the drug-seeking patient
Attempt to develop rapport with the patient
Ensure that new organic pathology does not exist
Determine that genuine pain has been adequately treated
Once the physician has some degree of certainty that problematic drug-seeking behaviour exists, set clear limits regarding medications requested
Consider the possibility of open discussion with the patient regarding the behaviour
Consider referral to appropriate services for ongoing care
Develop management protocols for particular patients if frequent attendance or threatening behaviours develop

THE VERY IMPORTANT PERSON

ESSENTIALS

1 Management of the VIP should be based on the maintenance of standard clinical procedures.

2 Management may be aided by the establishment of a plan resembling a disaster plan aimed at coordination of clinical and administrative issues.

3 Specific issues include security, confidentiality and management of the media.

Definition

A VIP in the ED can be defined as anyone whose presence in the ED may, by virtue of the fame or public position, disrupt normal ED functioning.[66] The care of the VIP unexpectedly arriving in the ED poses challenges of a medical and administrative nature. The attempted assassination of President Reagan and the critical illness of Israel's President Ariel Sharon in 2006 are examples of a person of worldwide repute presenting with a life-threatening illness. However, the patient may also be someone of local fame or importance, such as a prominent staff member. A 'VIP syndrome' has been described where the treating staff become so overwhelmed by the person's presence that they cease to operate in their normal way and the patient's care is compromised.[67] Disaster plans are formulated in hospitals to deal with situations that overwhelm normal ED operations. In a similar manner the formulation of a plan to deal with VIPs, to ensure optimal management of the patient and in the situation where the ED is 'relatively' overwhelmed, may help prevent poor outcomes. Ideally the management of clinical and administrative issues should be individually managed by senior clinical staff.

Management

Medical issues

The most senior clinician should assume control of the clinical issues so that decisions can be made rapidly to ensure optimal management and length of stay. Otherwise, the emphasis in the clinical management of the VIP should be the maintenance of standard clinical procedures. VIPs must be reassured that they will have their medical needs dealt with in the same way as any other patient. Discussions with VIPs regarding their public life or career should be avoided. The clinician should perform a standard clinical evaluation without omitting questioning, examinations or procedures that would normally occur due to other considerations such as embarrassment. Consultation with inpatient specialists should proceed as appropriate and the frequency and timing should reflect standard practice. Deviation from normal procedures, whether in assessment, referral or disposition, invites errors and lack of clarity in management decisions. Healthcare providers function most efficiently when performing their normal roles and nursing staff, junior medical staff and allied health should be involved as appropriate. This was emphasized by the treating physicians involved in the successful resuscitations of Pope John Paul II and President Reagan after assassination attempts.[68,69]

Access to the ED should be restricted after the arrival of the patient. Once information regarding the presence of the VIP circulates, there is a tendency for administrators and clinical heads to attend the ED. Other members of staff and the press may also attempt to enter the ED. Heads of state may be accompanied by their own teams of physicians. The treating clinician should liaise and consult with these physicians when immediate concerns such as resuscitation have been addressed.

EDs are accustomed to managing multiple complex patients at once. However, the presence of a VIP may consume the attention of many staff. The senior medical and nursing clinicians need to ensure that adequate staff are assigned to the management of other patients in the ED and that other patients do not suffer adverse outcomes due to the presence of the VIP.

Different issues arise when treating medical colleagues or their families, other staff members, or friends and relatives who are 'relative' VIPs. Whilst aiming to expedite the management and ensure the comfort of someone who is known to the treating clinician, as with the VIP, the safest pathway for the patients is not to deviate from standard medical care. The clinician may be inclined to take an incomplete history or perform an abbreviated examination, to provide a 'corridor consultation', or to refer to a specialist based on the colleague's own assessment of their symptoms. This risks an incorrect diagnosis and subsequent inappropriate treatment. The chief executive officer of the hospital who attends the ED and requests analgesia for a headache should be triaged and assessed as any other patient. In general, a conservative clinical approach to the VIP is recommended, with a lower than normal threshold for observation or admission.

Administrative issues

The essential administrative issues are security for the VIP and the hospital staff, protection of privacy and confidentiality, containment of the press, timely release of appropriate information, and the administration of a coordinated response to the VIP's needs. If the patient is of national importance, the response may resemble a disaster response and require the appointment of a central coordinator to manage the initial crisis, security control and media liaison.[66] In the case of the protracted illness of Israel's prime minister Ariel Sharon, which involved a 5-month intensive care admission, a forum was formed of all clinicians involved in his care. An intensive care physician was allocated control of the coordination of the medical care and an administrative physician oversaw administrative issues and ensured the ongoing running of routine hospital activities.[70]

Liaison with hospital security is essential with the aim to minimize entry of unnecessary people to the ED and to ensure the safety of the VIP. Assistance from clinical staff may be required to identify those required to enter the ED. Internal security may need to liaise and cooperate with external security teams. The VIP's security team must not impede medical management.

Confidentiality should be respected and consent to release information should be obtained as with any other patient. The VIP should not be discussed within or outside of the hospital and medical records, names on visible computer screens and pathology results should be de-identified and secured. The media's concept of the 'public's right to know' must be balanced with patient confidentiality. Release of information to the media should occur in a graded and accurate manner. Disclosure should occur on two levels: the first is the acknowledgement that the VIP is present and seeking medical attention and the second level involves the graded release of medical information.[66] One senior clinician should be appointed to convey this information. Ideally a centre for the media should be set up on a site remote from the ED.

Whilst the presence of a VIP in the ED may not overwhelm services in the same way as disaster, a similar approach with a pre-formulated plan of management may assist with the management of these rare and unexpected events and assist in attaining positive outcomes for the VIP and all other patients in the ED.

Controversies and future directions

❶ The development of acute behavioural centres similar to trauma centres may assist in streamlining the management of acute behavioural disturbance.

❷ Given the significant deprivations of rights and liberty that are applied when containing those with behavioural disturbance, there is a need to learn more from patients about their experiences.

❸ Management of acute behavioural disturbance is currently not patient focused, but rather centred around the staff and environmental capacities of the ED. A human dignity and rights-based approach would lead to radical differences in ED design and staff practices.

❹ The perception of inappropriate ED use by frequent attenders remains controversial, whilst both healthcare workers and health policy makers continue to assume that frequent attenders can and should be diverted to primary-care providers.

❺ Understanding of drug dependence as a chronic, organic brain disease may reduce stigma and lead to the development of better medical models of treatment that can enhance the behavioural and social therapies currently practised.

References

1. McIntosh G, Phillips J. 'There's No Home-Like Place' – Homelessness in Australia. Canberra: Parliament of Australia; 2000.
2. The Australian Institute of Health and Welfare. Australia's Welfare 1999: Services and Assistance. Canberra: AIHW; 1999.
3. Pinkney S, Ewing S. The Costs and Pathways of Homelessness: Developing Policy – Relevant Economic Analyses for the Australian Homelessness Service System. Melbourne: Institute for Social Research Swinburne University of Technology; 2006: 243.
4. National Alliance to End Homelessness. 2007.
5. Australian Federation of Homelessness Organisations. Homelessness in Australia. Canberra: Parliament of Australia; 2006.
6. Morris DM, Gordon JA. The role of the emergency department in the care of homeless and disadvantaged populations. Emergency Medical Clinics of North America 2006; 24: 839–848.
7. Phillips GA, Brophy DS, Weiland TJ, et al. The effect of multidisciplinary case management on selected outcomes for frequent attenders at an emergency department. Medical Journal of Australia 2006; 184: 602–606.
8. Moore G, Gerdtz M, Manias E, et al. Socio-demographic and clinical characteristics of re-presentation to an Australian inner-city emergency department: implications for service delivery. BMC Public Health 2007; 7: 320.
9. D'Amore J, Hung O, Chiang W, et al. The epidemiology of the homeless population and its impact on an urban emergency department. Academic Emergency Medicine 2001; 8: 1051–1055.
10. Haw C, Hawton K, Casey D. Deliberate self-harm patients of no fixed abode: a study of characteristics and subsequent deaths in patients presenting to a general hospital. Social Psychiatry and Psychiatric Epidemiology 2006; 41: 918–925.
11. Neate S, Dent A. The cottage project: caring for the unwell homeless person. Emergency Medicine Australasia 1999; 11: 78–83.
12. Redelmeier DA, Molin JP, Tibshirani RJ. A randomised trial of compassionate care for the homeless in an emergency department. Lancet 1995; 345: 1131–1134.
13. Department of Justice. Melbourne: Victoria Prisoner Health Study; 2003.
14. Augello M. Patients in custody: why do they present to an emergency department? Australasian College for
Emergency Medicine (Victorian Faculty) Scientific Meeting. Melbourne; 2004.
15. Boyce SH, Stevenson J, Jamieson IS, et al. Impact of a newly opened prison on an accident and emergency department. Emergency Medicine Journal 2003; 20: 48–51.
16. Knott JC, Bennett D, Rawet J, et al. Epidemiology of unarmed threats in the emergency department. Emergency Medicine of Australasia 2005; 17: 351–358.
17. Brookes J, Dunn R. The incidence, severity and nature of violent incidents in the emergency department. Emergency Medicine (Fremantle) 1997; 9: 5–9.
18. Phillips G. Senate 2005 Select Committee on Mental Health (written and oral submissions). Melbourne: Hansard; 2005.
19. Cannon ME, Sprivulis P, McCarthy J. Restraint practices in Australasian emergency departments. Australian New Zealand Journal of Psychiatry 2001; 35: 464–467.
20. Emergency Medicine Research Unit Royal Melbourne Hospital. Mental Health Presentations to the Emergency Department. Melbourne: Department of Human Services, Victorian State Government; 2006.
21. Cowling SA, McKeon MA, Weiland TJ. Managing acute behavioural disturbance in an emergency department using a behavioural assessment room. Australian Health Review 2007; 31: 296–304.
22. Australian Federal Government. Senate Select Committee on Mental Health: recommendations, 2006.
23. Lukens TW, Wolf SJ, Edlow JA, et al. Clinical policy: critical issues in the diagnosis and management of the adult psychiatric patient in the emergency department. Annals of Emergency Medicine 2006; 47: 79–99.
24. Thienhaus OJ, Piasecki M. Of suicide risk. Psychiatric Services 1997; 48: 293–294.
25. Mental Health Act. Victoria; 1986.
26. Wallace M. Health care and the law. 3rd edn. Sydney: Lawbook Company; 2001.
27. Skene L. Law and Medical Practice: Rights, Duties Claims and Defences. 2nd edn. Chatswood; Lexis Nexis Butterworths, 2004.
28. Allen MH. Managing the agitated psychotic patient: a reappraisal of the evidence. Journal of Clinical Psychiatry 2000; 61(suppl 14): 11–20.
29. Brayley J, Lange R, Baggoley C, et al. The violence management team. An approach to aggressive behaviour in a general hospital. Medical Journal of Australia 1994; 161: 254–258.
30. Knott J, Taylor D, Castle D. Randomised clinical trial comparing intravenous midazolam and droperidol for sedation of the acutely agitated patient in the emergency department. Annals of Emergency Medicine 2006; 47: 61–67.
31. Nobay F, Simon BC, Levitt MA, et al. A prospective, double-blind, randomized trial of midazolam versus haloperidol versus lorazepam in the chemical restraint of violent and severely agitated patients. Academic Emergency Medicine 2004; 11: 744–749.
32. Belgamwar RB, Fenton M. Olanzapine IM or velotab for acutely disturbed/agitated people with suspected serious mental illnesses. Cochrane Database Systematic Review 2005; CD003729.
33. Stratton SJ, Rogers C, Brickett K, et al. Factors associated with sudden death of individuals requiring restraint for excited delirium. American Journal of Emergency Medicine 2001; 19: 187–191.
34. Zun LS. A prospective study of the complication rate of use of patient restraint in the emergency department. Journal of Emergency Medicine 2003; 24: 119–124.
35. Sheline Y, Nelson T. Patient choice: deciding between psychotropic medication and physical restraints in an emergency. Bulletin of the American Academy of Psychiatry and the Law 1993; 21: 321–329.
36. Jones J, Lyneham J. Violence: part of the job for Australian nurses? Australian Journal of Advance Nursing 2000; 18: 27–32.
37. Jenkins MG, Rocke LG, McNicholl BP, et al. Violence and verbal abuse against staff in accident and emergency departments: a survey of consultants in the UK and the Republic of Ireland. Journal of Accident and Emergency Medicine 1998; 15: 262–265.
38. Wyatt JP, Watt M. Violence towards junior doctors in accident and emergency departments. Journal of Accident and Emergency Medicine 1995; 12: 40–42.

39. Gerdtz M, Maude P, Santamaria N. Occupational Violence in Nursing: an Analysis of the Phenomenon of Code Grey/Black Events in Four Victorian Hospitals. Published Report. Melbourne: Policy and Strategic Project Division, Victorian Department of Human Services; 2005.

40. Kennedy MP. Violence in emergency departments: under-reported, unconstrained, and unconscionable. Medical Journal of Australia 2005; 183: 362–365.

41. Hunt KA, Weber EJ, Showstack JA, et al. Characteristics of frequent users of emergency departments. Annals of Emergency Medicine 2006; 48: 1–8.

42. Lucas RH, Sanford SM. An analysis of frequent users of emergency care at an urban university hospital. Annals of Emergency Medicine 1998; 32: 563–568.

43. Andren K, Rosenqvist U. Heavy users of an emergency department: psycho-social and medical characteristics, other health care contacts and the effect of a hospital social worker intervention. Social Science Medicine 1985; 21: 761–770.

44. Mandelberg JH, Kuhn RE, Kohn MA. Epidemiologic analysis of an urban, public emergency department's frequent users. Academic Emergency Medicine 2000; 7: 637–646.

45. Helliwell PE, Hider PN, Ardagh MW. Frequent attenders at Christchurch hospital's emergency department. The New Zealand Medical Journal 2001; 114: 160–161.

46. Byrne M, Murphy AW, Plunkett PK, et al. Frequent attenders to an emergency department: a study of primary health care use, medical profile, and psychosocial characteristics. Annals of Emergency Medicine 2003; 41: 309–318.

47. Hansagi H, Allebeck P, Edhag O, et al. Frequency of emergency department attendances as a predictor of mortality: nine-year follow-up of a population-based cohort. Journal of Public Health Medicine 1990; 12: 39–44.

48. Hansagi H, Olsson M, Sjoberg S, et al. Frequent use of the hospital emergency department is indicative of high use of other health care services. Annals of Emergency Medicine 2001; 37: 561–567.

49. Cook LJ, Knight S, Junkins EP Jr, et al. Repeat patients to the emergency department in a statewide database. Academic Emergency Medicine 2004; 11: 256–263.

50. Keene J, Swift L, Bailey S, et al. Shared patients: multiple health and social care contact. Health and Social Care in the Community 2001; 9: 205–214.

51. Dent AW, Phillips GA, Chenhall AJ, et al. The heaviest repeat users of an inner city emergency department are not general practice patients. Emergency Medicine (Fremantle) 2003; 15: 322–329.

52. Kne T, Young R, Spillane L. Frequent ED users: patterns of use over time. American Journal of Emergency Medicine 1998; 16: 648–652.

53. Fuda KK, Immekus R. Frequent users of Massachusetts emergency departments: a statewide analysis. Annals of Emergency Medicine 2006; 48: 9–16.

54. Murphy AW. 'Inappropriate' attenders at accident and emergency departments II: health service responses. Family Practice 1998; 15: 33–37.

55. Olsson M, Hansagi H. Repeated use of the emergency department: qualitative study of the patient's perspective. Emergency Medicine Journal 2001; 18: 430–434.

56. O'shea JS, Collins EW, Pezzullo JC. An attempt to influence health care visits of frequent hospital emergency facility users. Clinical Pediatrics (Philadelphia) 1984; 23: 559–562.

57. Spillane LL, Lumb EW, Cobaugh DJ, et al. Frequent users of the emergency department: can we intervene? Academic Emergency Medicine 1997; 4: 574–580.

58. Okin RL, Boccellari A, Azocar F, et al. The effects of clinical case management on hospital service use among ED frequent users. American Journal of Emergency Medicine 2000; 18: 603–608.

59. Pope D, Fernandes CM, Bouthillette F, et al. Frequent users of the emergency department: a program to improve care and reduce visits. Canadian Medical Association Journal 2000; 162: 1017–1020.

60. Savage SR, Joranson DE, Covington EC, et al. Definitions related to the medical use of opioids: evolution towards universal agreement. Journal of Pain and Symptom Management 2003; 26: 655–667.

61. Weissman DE, Haddox JD. Opioid pseudoaddiction – an iatrogenic syndrome. Pain 1989; 36: 363–366.

62. Boisaubin EV. The assessment and treatment of pain in the emergency room. Clinical Journal of Pain 1989; 5 (suppl 2): S19–S24; discussion S24–S15.

63. Weaver M, Schnoll S. Addiction issues in prescribing opioids in chronic non malignant pain. Journal of Addiction Medicine 2007; 1: 2–10.

64. McNabb C, Foot C, Ting J, et al. Diagnosing drug-seeking behaviour in an adult emergency department. Emergency Medicine of Australasia 2006; 18: 138–142.

65. McNabb C, Foot C, Ting J, et al. Profiling patients suspected of drug seeking in an adult emergency department. Emergency Medicine of Australasia 2006; 18: 131–137.

66. Smith MS, Shesser RF. The emergency care of the VIP patient. New England Journal of Medicine 1998; 319: 1421–1423.

67. Weintraub W. 'The VIP Syndrome': a clinical study in hospital psychiatry. Journal of Nervous and Mental Disorder 1964; 138: 181–193.

68. Breo DL. MDs, hospital ready for Reagan. American Medical News 1981; 24: 1–2, 17.

69. Breo DL. Pope's physicians redeem a request. American Medical News 1981; 24: 1, 7, 14.

70. Weiss YG, Mor-Yosef S, Sprung CL, et al. Caring for a major government official: challenges and lessons learned. Critical Care Medicine 2007; 35: 1769–1772.

22.1 General pain management

Daniel M. Fatovich

ESSENTIALS

1 Acute pain is the most common presenting complaint to an emergency department.

2 Pain is a complex, multidimensional, subjective phenomenon.

3 Patient self-reporting is the most reliable indicator of the presence and intensity of pain.

4 Patients with pain should receive timely, effective and appropriate analgesia, titrated according to response.

5 There is a wide range of pharmacological and non-pharmacological techniques available for the treatment of acute pain. Effective pain relief should always be achievable.

6 Titration of intravenous opioids remains the standard of care for acute severe pain.

Introduction

Pain is defined by the International Association for the Study of Pain as 'An unpleasant sensory and emotional experience associated with actual or potential tissue damage or described in terms of such damage.'[1] Acute pain is defined as 'Pain of recent onset and probable limited duration. It usually has an identifiable temporal and causal relationship to injury or disease.'[2] However, once a patient presents for medical care, severe acute pain has ceased to serve a useful purpose. Whereas in some conditions the nature and progression of the pain may be helpful in making the diagnosis of the underlying pathology, too great a reliance has been placed upon this feature, thereby allowing the patient to suffer needlessly for prolonged periods.[2,3]

When severe pain is inadequately relieved it produces pathophysiological and abnormal psychological reactions that often lead to complications. This is important because acute pain is the most common presenting complaint to an emergency department (ED)[4] and its management forms part of the daily practice of emergency medicine. It should be considered poor patient care not to treat pain while attempting to arrive at a diagnosis. There can be no greater gift to one's neighbour than to practise, teach and discover more effective methods to relieve pain and suffering.[2,3] Unfortunately, the management of acute pain is often not a specific component of medical training.

Physiology

Pain is one of the most complex aspects of an already intricate nervous system.[2] A number of theories have been developed to explain the physiology of pain, but none is proven or complete.

In 1965, the Melzack–Wall 'Gate Control Theory' emphasized mechanisms in the central nervous system that control the perception of a noxious stimulus, and thus integrated afferent, upstream processes with downstream modulation from the brain.[5] However, this theory did not incorporate long-term changes in the central nervous system to the noxious input and to other external factors that impinge upon the individual.[5] Most pain originates when specific nerve endings (nociceptors) are stimulated, producing nerve impulses that are transmitted to the brain. Nociception is the detection of tissue damage by specialized transducers.[5]

It is now recognized that nociceptor function is altered by the 'inflammatory soup' that characterizes a region of tissue injury.[5] The final pain experience is subject to a complex series of facilitatory and inhibitory events that precede pain awareness, such as past experience, anxiety or expectation.[6] There are two types of nociceptors:[7]

❶ Mechanoreceptors, which are present mainly in the skin (also muscle, joints, viscera, meninges) and respond rapidly to pinprick or heat via Aδ, myelinated afferent neurons.

❷ Polymodal, which are widely distributed throughout most tissues and are the nerve endings of unmyelinated C-type afferent neurons. These respond to tissue damage caused by mechanical, thermal or chemical insults, and are responsible for the slow onset, prolonged, poorly localized, aching pain following an injury.

Once transduced into electrical stimuli, conduction of neuronal action potentials is dependent on voltage-gated sodium channels.[2] A number of chemicals are involved in the transmission of pain to the ascending pathways in the spinothalamic tract. These include substance P and calcitonin gene-related peptide, but many others have been identified.[2,8,9] Opioid receptors are present in the dorsal horn, and it is thought that encephalins (endogenous opioid peptides) are neurotransmitters in the inhibitory interneurons.[7]

Phospholipids released from damaged cell membranes trigger a cascade of reactions, culminating in the production of prostaglandins that sensitize nociceptors to other inflammatory mediators, such as histamine, serotonin and bradykinin.[7]

The threshold for the perception of a painful stimulus is similar in everyone, and may be lowered by certain chemicals such as the mediators of inflammation. The discrete cognitive processes and pathways involved in the interpretation of painful stimuli remain a mystery. The cognitive and emotional reactions to a given painful stimulus are variable among individuals, and may be affected by culture, personality, past experiences and underlying emotional state.[2,5,10] In addition, intense and ongoing stimuli further increase the excitability of dorsal horn neurons, leading to central sensitization.[2] With increased excitability of central nociceptive neurons, the threshold for activation is reduced, and pain can occur in response to low intensity, previously non-painful stimuli known as allodynia.[2] Pain is a complex, multidimensional, subjective phenomenon.[10]

Assessment of pain and pain scales

There is no truly objective measurement of pain. Doctors use a variety of methods for determining how much pain a patient feels. These include the nature of the illness or injury, the patient's appearance and behaviour, and physiological concomitants. None of these is reliable.

Pain scales have been developed because there are no accurate physiological or clinical signs to objectively measure pain. Three scales have become popular tools to quantify pain intensity:[11,12] the visual analogue scale (VAS), the numeric rating scale and the verbal rating scale.

Visual analogue scale

The VAS usually consists of a 100-mm line with one end indicating 'no pain' and the other end indicating the 'worst pain imaginable'. The patient simply indicates a point on the line that best indicates the amount of pain experienced. The minimum clinically significant change in patient pain severity measured with a 100-mm visual analogue scale is 13 mm.[13] Studies of pain experience that report less than a 13 mm change in pain severity, although statistically significant, may have no clinical importance.[13]

Numeric rating scale

The patient is asked in the numeric rating scale to choose a number from a range (usually 0–10) that best describes the amount of pain experienced, with zero being 'no pain' and 10 being the 'worst pain imaginable'. This has been used for cardiac ischaemia pain and is also useful in illiterate patients.

Verbal rating scale

The verbal rating scale simply asks a patient to choose a phrase that best describes the pain, usually 'mild', 'moderate' or 'severe'.

The use of pain scales has been restricted predominantly to research, where experimental pain is not associated with the strong emotional component of acute pain. In the clinical setting, anxiety, sleep disruption and illness burden are present.[9] It is difficult to use a unidimensional pain scale to measure a multidimensional process. Using pain intensity alone will often fail to capture the many other qualities of pain and the overall pain experience. The best illustration of this problem is that the same pain stimulus can be applied to two different people with dramatically different pain scores and analgesic requirements.[14] At best the use of pain scales is an indirect reflection of 'real' pain, with patient self-reporting still being the most reliable indicator of the existence and intensity of pain.[15]

Nevertheless, pain scales are simple and easy to use and are now routine in EDs, with some recommending that they should be a standard part of the triage process.[4]

General principles

Patients in pain should receive timely, effective and appropriate analgesia, titrated according to response.[2] Thus, there is essentially no role for the intramuscular route for parenteral analgesia, which simply delays the onset of analgesia. The following points should be stressed:

- The correct analgesic dose is 'enough', that is, whatever amount is needed to achieve appropriate pain relief.
- A patient's analgesic requirements should be reviewed frequently. Do not wait for pain to return to its previous level before re-dosing with analgesia. Larger early doses and more frequent doses of analgesia are associated with lower total doses and shorter duration of analgesic use. Some patients have been misled into believing that pain medicine is dangerous, so it is important to explain the safety and efficacy of this approach.
- EDs should have specific policies relating to pain and analgesia.
- Senior clinicians should lead by example.

Specific agents

Opioids

The term 'opioid' refers to all naturally occurring and synthetic drugs producing morphine-like effects. Morphine is the standard opioid agonist against which others are judged.[16] These drugs are the most powerful agents available in the treatment of acute pain. A number of specific opioid receptors have been identified. They are responsible for a variety of effects, including analgesia, euphoria, respiratory depression and miosis (μ receptor); cough suppression, sedation (κ); dysphoria, hallucinations (σ); nausea and vomiting, and pruritus (δ).[7] Opioids act on injured tissue to reduce inflammation in the dorsal horn to impede transmission of nociception, and supraspinally to activate inhibitory pathways that descend to the spinal segment.[9]

Unfortunately, many doctors use opioids inappropriately and there are particular concerns regarding the risks of respiratory depression and inducing iatrogenic addiction. Less than 1% of patients who receive opioids for pain develop respiratory depression.[17] Tolerance to this side effect develops simultaneously with tolerance to the analgesic effect. If the opioid dose is increased so that at least half the pain is relieved, the chance of respiratory depression is small. Further, naloxone will reverse the effects of opioids. In relation to fears of addiction, large studies have shown that inducing this following opioid analgesia use is exceedingly rare.[18]

From a clinical practice point of view, many patients who require intravenous opioid will also require admission to hospital, as there will be ongoing opioid requirements that can only be administered in hospital. There have been occasions where patients have received opioid analgesia that has relieved their pain, and they have then been discharged without a final diagnosis. This is an unacceptable practice. A patient may present with abdominal pain with vomiting, and, for instance, a provisional diagnosis of gastroenteritis is made. After opioid analgesia is given the patient may feel better and be discharged. A diagnosis such as appendicitis or bowel obstruction has not been excluded.

It is therefore necessary for patients to have an appropriate diagnostic evaluation to confirm a benign cause, and to reassess the patient after the opioid effects have waned. For patients in whom the final diagnosis is certain, such as in anterior shoulder dislocation, discharge is appropriate after a suitable period of observation until the patient is deemed clinically fit for discharge. This is a different scenario from that described previously, as it is a single system problem in which there is no doubt about the diagnosis. In summary, pain that is considered severe enough to warrant intravenous opioid analgesia usually requires a high index of suspicion for significant pathology.

Side effects

All potent opioid analgesics have the potential to depress the level of consciousness, protective reflexes and vital functions. It is mandatory that these are closely monitored during and after administration.[7] Specific side effects include:

- respiratory depression: rare <1%
- nausea and vomiting: nausea occurs in approximately 40% and vomiting in 15%[7]
- hypotension: opioids may provoke histamine release
- constipation
- spasm of the sphincter of Oddi, therefore patients with biliary colic may initially experience more pain. There is no good evidence to suggest that pethidine has any clinically significant advantage at equi-analgesic doses over other opioids for biliary or renal colic[16]
- miosis.

Route of administration

Opioids may be administered by many routes, including oral, subcutaneous, intramuscular, intravenous, epidural, nebulized, intrapleural, intranasal, intra-articular and transdermal. All may have a role in a specific clinical situation.[4] There is a good rationale for the use of the intravenous route in moderate-to-severe pain[4] and titration of intravenous opioids remains the standard of care for acute severe pain.

Morphine The standard intravenous morphine dose is 0.1–0.2 mg/kg or more with a duration of action of 2–3 h. This should be initiated as a loading dose of opioid to provide rapid initial pain relief aiming for an optimal balance between effective pain relief and minimal side effects. This means tailoring the approach to each individual patient. Thus, a young fit healthy man with renal colic may require an initial bolus of 0.1 mg/kg morphine, followed by further increments of 2.5–5 mg. Conversely, a frail elderly patient may only tolerate 1.0–2.5 mg morphine total to begin with. There may also be considerable inter-individual variation in response to analgesia. Procedural pain may require higher-dose opioid analgesia, which has been found to be well-tolerated and safe.[19] Appropriate monitoring and resuscitation

equipment should be available to maximize safety.

Rapid pain relief and titration to effect are obvious advantages. Intramuscular administration results in unreliable and variable absorption, and older routine practices such as prescribing '75 mg pethidine i.m.' are deplorable and take no account of an individual's requirements.[7] Oral opioids tend to be underused in the ED, but are effective for all levels of pain.

Special considerations

Pethidine Pethidine should be used with caution in patients with renal failure, as there is increased risk of central nervous system toxicity due to the toxic metabolite, norpethidine. Norpethidine causes tremor, twitching, agitation and convulsions.[16] Also pethidine is contraindicated in patients receiving monoamine oxidase (MAO) inhibitors, as they interfere with pethidine metabolism, increasing the likelihood of toxicity.[20] Finally, pethidine may trigger the serotonin syndrome if used concomitantly with selective serotonin reuptake inhibitors (SSRIs). Pethidine has approximately one-eighth the potency of morphine and causes the same degree of bronchospasm and increased biliary pressure as morphine.[2] Its use is declining and should continue to be discouraged in favour of other opioids.[2]

Fentanyl Allergic reactions are extremely rare with opioids. Fentanyl does not release histamine, making it ideal for treating patients with reactive airways disease. There are advantages in using fentanyl for brief procedures in the ED because of its short half-life. The intravenous dose of fentanyl is 1–2 µg/kg or more with a duration of action of 30–60 min. High doses of fentanyl may produce muscular rigidity, which may be so severe as to make ventilation difficult, but which responds to naloxone or muscle relaxants. Intranasal fentanyl is an effective analgesic in the ED and in the pre-hospital setting.[2]

Codeine Codeine is the most commonly used oral opioid prodrug. Unfortunately, up to 6–10% of the Caucasian population, 2% of Asians, and 1% of Arabs have poorly functional cytochrome P450 2D6 (CYP2D6), which may render codeine largely ineffective for analgesia in these patients, although some analgesic efficacy may occur via alternate cytochrome P450 pathways.

Prescribed alone in doses as high as 120 mg, codeine has been demonstrated to be no more effective than placebo in both the adult and geriatric populations, while causing increasing gastrointestinal side effects such as nausea, vomiting and constipation with increasing doses.[4] It is frequently given in combination with paracetamol or aspirin.

Tramadol Tramadol is a new opioid, with novel non-opioid properties.[21] Its efficacy lies between codeine and morphine. It has a relative lack of serious side effects such as respiratory depression, and the potential for abuse and psychological dependence is low.[21] Other side effects such as nausea, vomiting, dizziness and somnolence may be troublesome, and there is a risk of seizures.[21,22] Thus, it should be avoided or used with caution in patients who are taking other drugs that reduce the seizure threshold such as tricyclic antidepressants and SSRIs. Also the concomitant administration of tramadol with monoamine oxidase inhibitors, or within 2 weeks of their withdrawal, is contraindicated.[21]

The role of tramadol in emergency medicine is yet to be defined. One review concluded that tramadol does not offer any particular benefits over existing analgesics for the majority of emergency pain relief situations,[22] with oral doses having equivalent analgesic effects in mild-to-moderate severity acute pain compared with currently available analgesics.[22] Intravenous tramadol is less effective than intravenous morphine.[22]

However, tramadol may be useful in certain situations:[22]

- for patients in whom codeine is not effective
- where NSAIDs are contraindicated
- for the treatment of chronic pain.

Non-opioid analgesics

Simple analgesics

Non-steroidal anti-inflammatory drugs

Non-steroidal anti-inflammatory drugs (NSAIDs) are either non-selective cyclo-oxygenase (COX) inhibitors or selective inhibitors of COX-2 (COX-2 inhibitors). NSAIDs are effective analgesic agents for moderate pain, specifically when there is associated inflammation.[4] As with opioids, there are multiple routes of administration available. Unfortunately, their use in acute severe pain is limited by the length of onset time of 20–30 min. There is no clear superiority of one agent over another.

There is up to a 30% incidence of upper gastrointestinal bleeding when NSAIDs are used for over 1–2 weeks. The risk of bleeding in the elderly for short (3–5 days) acute therapy appears to be minimal.[4] NSAID use in pregnancy (especially late) is not recommended. Ibuprofen is considered the NSAID of choice in lactation.

NSAIDs have a spectrum of analgesic, anti-inflammatory and antipyretic effects and are effective analgesics in a variety of pain states.[2] Unfortunately, significant contraindications and adverse effects limit the use of NSAIDs, many of these being regulated by COX-1.[2] NSAIDs are useful analgesic adjuncts and hence NSAIDs are therefore integral components of multimodal analgesia.[2] NSAID side effects are more common with long-term use. The main concerns are renal impairment, interference with platelet function, peptic ulceration and bronchospasm in individuals who have aspirin-exacerbated respiratory disease.[2] In general, the risk and severity of NSAID-associated side effects is increased in elderly people.[2]

Caution is therefore needed in the elderly and in patients with renal disease, hypertension and heart failure, or with asthma. NSAIDs reduce renal cortical blood flow and may induce renal impairment, especially when used in patients already on diuretics. In patients with asthma, 2–20% are aspirin sensitive and there is a 50–100% cross-sensitivity with NSAIDs.

Ketorolac is a parenteral NSAID that is equipotent to opioids, with ketorolac and morphine equivalent in reducing pain. There is a benefit favouring ketorolac in terms of side effects, when ketorolac is titrated intravenously for isolated limb injuries.[23,24] However, the utility of ketorolac in acute pain is limited due to a prolonged onset of action and a significant number of patients (25%) who exhibit little or no response.[25] There is also benefit using ketorolac for acute renal colic.[23,26] A combination of morphine and ketorolac offered pain relief superior to either drug alone and was associated with a decreased requirement for rescue analgesia in patients with renal colic.[27] Rectal NSAIDs are an effective alternative to parenteral NSAIDs in the treatment of renal colic.

Paracetamol

Paracetamol is an effective analgesic for acute pain[2] and has useful antipyretic activity.[28] The addition of an NSAID further improves efficacy.[2] Paracetamol inhibits prostaglandin synthetase in the hypothalamus, prevents release of spinal prostaglandin, and inhibits inducible nitric oxide synthesis in macrophages.[28]

Indications for paracetamol include mild pain, particularly of soft tissue and musculoskeletal origin, mild procedural pain, supplementation of opioids in the management of more severe pain allowing a reduction in opioid dosage, and as an alternative to aspirin.[28] Paracetamol has no gastrointestinal side effects of note and may be prescribed safely in patients with peptic ulcer disease or gastritis.[4] Aspirin has the risk of gastrointestinal side effects, such as ulceration and bleeding. It also has an antiplatelet effect, which lasts for the life of the platelet.

Paracetamol is rapidly absorbed with a peak concentration reached in 30–90 min.[28] The recommended adult dose is 0.5–1 g every 4–6 h to a generally accepted maximum of 4 g per day.[28] Paracetamol has a low adverse event profile and is an excellent analgesic, especially when used in adequate dose. Chronic use of paracetamol alone does not seem to cause analgesic nephropathy.[28] It can be used safely in alcoholics and patients with liver metastases.[28,29]

Combination drugs

Non-opioid agents, e.g. paracetamol, NSAIDs and paracetamol/codeine combinations, are all useful analgesics for mild-to-moderate pain. A systematic review found that paracetamol–codeine combinations in single dose studies produce a slightly increased analgesic effect (5%) compared with paracetamol alone.[30] However, none of the studies reviewed were based in the ED. In multidosage, paracetamol–codeine preparations have significantly increased side effects.[30] However, other reports state that the combination of paracetamol 1000 mg plus codeine 60 mg has a number needed to treat of 2.2.[2] NSAIDs have a higher rate of serious adverse effects.

Other analgesic agents

Nitrous oxide

Nitrous oxide is an inhalational analgesic and sedative which, in a 50% mixture with oxygen (Entonox®), has equivalent potency to 10 mg morphine in an adult.[7] The Entonox® delivery system uses a preferential inhalational demand arrangement for self-administration, which requires an airtight fit between the mask/mouthpiece and face. As the patient holds the mask/mouthpiece their grip will relax if drowsiness occurs, the airtight seal will be lost and the gas flow stops, thereby avoiding overdosage.

This system requires a degree of patient involvement and cooperation, and is useful for patients who have difficult intravenous access or are needle-phobic. Patients who are elderly, young, confused or uncooperative will not find the technique effective. Nitrous oxide increases the volume of a pneumothorax or any other gas-filled cavity, so is contraindicated in patients with pneumothorax or pneumoperitoneum.

Sumatriptan

Sumatriptan is a $5HT_1$ receptor agonist that is effective for the treatment of acute migraine in a high proportion of patients. The dose is 50 mg orally, or 6 mg subcutaneously if the patient is vomiting. Ideally, it should be taken at the onset of headache, but is still effective when the headache is established. In about one-third to one-half of patients the headache returns within 24 h, but is almost always responsive to a second tablet.[31]

Sumatriptan is not an analgesic and should not be used for non-vascular headache, or for migraine aura with early evolving headache, or as a diagnostic test for migraine. Contraindications include pregnancy, ischaemic heart disease or chest pain with previous use, uncontrolled hypertension, ergotamine in the previous 24 h, and current or recent (within 2 weeks) therapy with MAO inhibitors.

Acute migraine headache requires a stepwise approach to the use of pharmacological agents. Moderate-to-severe migraine may warrant the use of specific antimigraine medications such as ergotamine or sumatriptan, unless contraindicated.[2] The combination of aspirin (900 mg) and metoclopramide is as effective as sumatriptan in the treatment of migraine, is better tolerated and also cheaper.[2] Intravenous prochlorperazine is more effective than metoclopramide or rectal prochlorperazine, although is unlicensed for this delivery mode.[2] The use of opioids is not recommended.[2]

Ketamine

Ketamine is an N-methyl-D-aspartate (NMDA) antagonist. It is a unique anaesthetic that induces a state of dissociation between the cortical and limbic systems to produce a state of dissociative anaesthesia, with analgesia, amnesia, mild sedation and immobilization. It does not impair protective airway reflexes, and random or purposeful movements are frequently observed in patients after administration. Side effects include hypersalivation, vomiting, emergence reactions, nightmares, laryngospasm, hypertension, tachycardia and increased intracranial pressure.[32,33]

Unfortunately, there are many potential contraindications to ketamine use including upper or lower respiratory infection, procedures involving the posterior pharynx, cystic fibrosis, age younger than 3 months, head injury, increased intracranial pressure, acute glaucoma or globe penetration, uncontrolled hypertension, congestive cardiac failure, arterial aneurysm, acute intermittent porphyria and thyrotoxicosis.[33] Despite this, ketamine is used increasingly in the EDs as part of procedural sedation (see Ch. 22.3). It is also an effective analgesic especially for opioid resistant pain.

Pain relief in pregnancy

Non-pharmacological treatment options should be considered where possible for pain management in pregnancy, because most drugs cross the placenta.[2] Use of medications for pain in pregnancy should be guided by published recommendations.[2] Paracetamol is regarded as the analgesic of choice.[2] NSAIDs are used with caution in the last trimester of pregnancy and should be avoided after the

32nd week.[2] The use of NSAIDs is associated with increased risk of miscarriage.[2] Overall, the use of opioids to treat pain in pregnancy appears safe.[2]

Non-pharmacological therapies

Although pain perception involves neuro-anatomical processes, the other interrelated component of pain reaction is psychophysiological. The use of non-pharmacological techniques is therefore vitally important. These include empathy, a compassionate approach, a calm manner and reassurance. Immobilization of fractures with splinting is effective, as is the application of ice to a wound. Other techniques, such as hypnosis, transcutaneous nerve stimulation and manipulation have not been widely studied in the ED setting.

Special pain situations and non-analgesic agents

Whilst this chapter has focused on specific analgesic agents, there are many miscellaneous agents that are effective in providing disease-specific analgesia. Examples of these include:

- sumatriptan (see earlier)
- glyceryl trinitrate and beta blockers for acute cardiac ischaemia pain
- redback spider antivenom for latrodectism
- antiviral agents for herpes zoster
- antidepressants or anticonvulsants for neuropathic pain
- oxygen therapy for cluster headache
- calcium gluconate for hydrofluoric acid burns
- hot water (43°C) for venomous marine stings.

In addition, adjuvant therapy with anxiolytics such as midazolam contributes to pain relief. Obtaining a definitive diagnosis allows directed therapy that contributes to pain relief. If specific treatments appear to be ineffective, then the diagnosis should be reconsidered.

Chronic pain

Chronic pain 'commonly persists beyond the time of healing of an injury and frequently there may not be any clearly identifiable cause.[2] Patients with chronic pain attend the ED with exacerbations of their chronic pain. They are often taking multi-modal therapies prescribed by a pain specialist. The main difference between acute and chronic pain is that in chronic pain central sensitization is the main underlying pathophysiology.[34] It is important to avoid a judgemental attitude to these patients as there is a risk of overlooking serious pathology.

Co-analgesics in the setting of chronic pain, especially ketamine, are of particular value in those with poor opioid responsiveness.[2] These patients appear to benefit from several days of a ketamine infusion. Other agents may be useful for neuropathic pain.

The other issue with chronic pain is to be aware of adjuvant therapies for decreasing the likelihood of chronic pain developing. For example, early management of acute zoster infection may reduce the incidence of post-herpetic neuralgia.[2] Aciclovir given within 72 h of onset of the rash accelerates the resolution of pain and reduces the risk of post-herpetic neuralgia.[2] Amitriptyline 25 mg daily in patients over 60 years for 90 days, started at the onset of acute zoster, reduces pain prevalence at 6 months post-zoster infection.[35]

The acute abdomen

Traditionally, it has been held that pain relief masks the clinical signs of pathology in the acute abdomen. However, evidence from randomized controlled trials clearly shows that the early administration of opioids in patients with an acute abdomen does not reduce the detection rate of serious pathology and may facilitate diagnosis. The effect of analgesia on physical signs cannot be used as a diagnostic test.[36–38]

Likely developments over the next 5–10 years

- Further study on the role and utility of various oral analgesics for commonly treated conditions in the ED, including new agents.

- Alternative administration techniques, including needleless systems.
- Better understanding of the pathophysiology of pain.

Controversies

❶ Development of a uniform approach to pain research in order to make meaningful comparisons between studies.

❷ Development of an objective measure of pain.

❸ The effectiveness of codeine combinations in ED patients.

References

1. International Association for the study of pain. Pain terms: a list of definitions and notes on usage. Pain 1979; 6: 249–252.
2. Australian and New Zealand College of Anaesthetists and Faculty of Pain Medicine. Acute pain management: Scientific evidence. 2nd edn. Canberra: Australian Government National Health and Medical Research Council, 2005.
3. Bonica J. Pain management in emergency medicine. Norwalk: Appleton & Lange; 1987.
4. Ducharme J. Emergency pain management: a Canadian Association of Emergency Physicians (CAEP) consensus document. Journal of Emergency Medicine 1994; 12: 855–866.
5. Loeser JD, Melzack R. Pain: an overview. Lancet 1999; 353(9164): 1607–1609.
6. Paris P, Uram M, Ginsburg M. Physiological mechanisms of pain. Norwalk: Appleton & Lange; 1987.
7. Nolan J, Baskett P. Analgesia and anaesthesia. Cambridge: Cambridge University Press; 1997.
8. Besson JM. The neurobiology of pain. Lancet 1999; 353(9164): 1610–1615.
9. Carr DB, Goudas LC. Acute pain. Lancet 1999; 353(9169): 2051–2058.
10. Turk D, Melzack R. The measurement of pain and the assessment of people experiencing pain. New York: Guildford Press; 1992.
11. Ho K, Spence J, Murphy MF. Review of pain-measurement tools. Annals of Emergency Medicine 1996; 27(4): 427–432.
12. Turk DC, Okifuji A. Assessment of patients' reporting of pain: an integrated perspective. Lancet 1999; 353(9166): 1784–1788.
13. Todd KH, Funk KG, Funk JP, et al. Clinical significance of reported changes in pain severity. Annals of Emergency Medicine 1996; 27(4): 485–489.
14. Fatovich D. The validity of pain scales in the emergency setting. Journal of Emergency Medicine 1998; 16: 347.
15. Acute Pain Management Guideline Panel. Acute pain management: operative or medical procedures and trauma: clinical practice guideline. Washington DC, 1992.
16. McQuay H. Opioids in pain management. Lancet 1999; 353(9171): 2229–2232.
17. Miller R. Analgesics. New York: Wiley; 1976.

18. Porter J, Jick H. Addiction rare in patients treated with narcotics. New England Journal of Medicine 1980; 302(2): 123.
19. Barsan WG, Tomassoni AJ, Seger D, et al. Safety assessment of high-dose narcotic analgesia for emergency department procedures. Annals of Emergency Medicine 1993; 22(9): 1444–1449.
20. Meyer D, Halfin V. Toxicity secondary to meperidine in patients on monoamine oxidase inhibitors: a case report and critical review. Journal of Clinical Psychopharmacology 1981; 1(5): 319–321.
21. Bamigade T, Langford R. The clinical use of tramadol hydrochloride. Pain Reviews 1998; 5: 155–182.
22. Close BR. Tramadol: does it have a role in emergency medicine? Emergency Medicine Australasia 2005; 17(1): 73–83.
23. Rainer TH, Jacobs P, Ng YC, et al. Cost effectiveness analysis of intravenous ketorolac and morphine for treating pain after limb injury: double blind randomised controlled trial. British Medical Journal 2000; 321(7271): 1247–1251.
24. Jelinek GA. Ketorolac versus morphine for severe pain. Ketorolac is more effective, cheaper, and has fewer side effects. British Medical Journal 2000; 321(7271): 1236–1237.
25. Catapano MS. The analgesic efficacy of ketorolac for acute pain. Journal of Emergency Medicine 1996; 14(1): 67–75.
26. Holdgate A, Pollock T. Systematic review of the relative efficacy of non-steroidal anti-inflammatory drugs and opioids in the treatment of acute renal colic. British Medical Journal 2004; 328(7453): 1401.
27. Safdar B, Degutis LC, Landry K, et al. Intravenous morphine plus ketorolac is superior to either drug alone for treatment of acute renal colic. Annals of Emergency Medicine 2006; 48(2): 173–181.
28. Therapeutic Guidelines Ltd. Therapeutic Guidelines: Analgesic. North Melbourne: Therapeutic Guidelines Ltd, 2002.
29. Dart RC, Kuffner EK, Rumack BH. Treatment of pain or fever with paracetamol (acetaminophen) in the alcoholic patient: a systematic review. American Journal of Therapeutics 2000; 7(2): 123–134.
30. de Craen AJ, Di Giulio G, Lampe-Schoenmaeckers JE. Analgesic efficacy and safety of paracetamol-codeine combinations versus paracetamol alone: a systematic review. British Medical Journal 1996; 313(7053): 321–325.
31. Goadsby P. Sumatriptan and migraine: breakthrough therapy. Current Therapeutics 1992; 33: 11–18.
32. Terndrup T. Pain control, analgesia and sedation. St Louis: Mosby Year Book; 1992.
33. Green SM, Johnson NE. Ketamine sedation for pediatric procedures: Part 2, Review and implications. Annals of Emergency Medicine 1990; 19(9): 1033–1046.
34. Siddall PJ, Cousins MJ. Persistent pain as a disease entity: implications for clinical management. Anesthesia and Analgesia 2004; 99(2): 510–520.
35. Bowsher D. The effects of pre-emptive treatment of postherpetic neuralgia with amitriptyline: a randomized, double-blind, placebo-controlled trial. Journal of Pain Symptom Management 1997; 13(6): 327–331.
36. Thomas SH, Silen W, Cheema F, et al. Effects of morphine analgesia on diagnostic accuracy in Emergency Department patients with abdominal pain: a prospective, randomized trial. Journal of the American College of Surgeons 2003; 196(1): 18–31.
37. Attard AR, Corlett MJ, Kidner NJ, et al. Safety of early pain relief for acute abdominal pain. British Medical Journal 1992; 305(6853): 554–556.
38. Zoltie N, Cust MP. Analgesia in the acute abdomen. Annals of the Royal College of Surgeons of England 1986; 68(4): 209–210.

22.2 Local anaesthesia

Anthony F.T. Brown • Tor N.O. Ercleve

ESSENTIALS

1 Local anaesthetic nerve blocks should be considered as a supplement to analgesia or as an alternative method of achieving analgesia, particularly where pain is localized.

2 Toxicity may occur with inadvertent rapid intravenous injection, or exceeding the recommended safe maximum dose. Neurological and cardiovascular effects predominate and may be lethal. Resuscitation equipment should always be available when using these agents.

3 Intravenous regional anaesthesia with prilocaine for Bier's block is a simple, safe technique commonly used for reduction of forearm fractures.

Local anaesthesia

Local anaesthetic agents should always be considered for patients presenting to the emergency department (ED) with pain, either to supplement other analgesia or for definitive pain relief. This is particularly appropriate where the pain is quite localized, as in certain fractures and wounds. They may also be used topically mainly in children, and prior to arterial blood gas puncture and insertion of large intravenous cannulae, where contrary to popular perception, they do not increase the likelihood of failing.[1,2]

Pharmacology

Local anaesthetic agents are all weak bases that inactivate intracellular fast sodium channels, temporarily blocking membrane depolarization and preventing nerve impulse transmission. All are vasodilators with the exception of cocaine, hence the use of adrenaline to prolong their duration of activity and to improve safety by delaying absorption and/or by administering lower effective doses.

Amino ester and amino amide local anaesthetics

Local anaesthetic agents containing an ester bond between the intermediate chain and lipophilic aromatic end (amino esters) include cocaine, procaine and amethocaine, are poorly protein bound, and undergo hydrolysis by plasma pseudocholinesterase to para-amino benzoic acid. Amide-type agents containing an amide bond between the intermediate chain and aromatic end (amino amides) include lignocaine, prilocaine and bupivacaine, are highly protein bound, much more stable, and undergo hepatic metabolism.

Local anaesthetics are available in single or multidose vials, with or without dilute adrenaline at 1:200 000 (containing 5 μg adrenaline per millilitre) to prolong the duration of action. Antioxidants such as sodium bisulphite or metabisulphite are added to adrenaline-containing solutions and preservative such as methylparaben to multidose vials, and are implicated in some allergic reactions to the anaesthetics. True allergy to local anaesthetics is extremely rare when verified by progressive challenge testing, and is usually to the amino esters.[3]

The duration of action of local anaesthetics is related to the degree of protein binding, vasoactivity, concentration and possibly pH, although the addition of adrenaline is the most practical way to prolong their effect. Table 22.2.1 gives typical maximum safe doses and duration of action of commonly used agents. Solutions containing adrenaline should not be injected near end arteries, such as in the fingers, toes, nose or penis, even though surprisingly this well-established dogma is not supported by the literature. Normal blood flow is restored to the digit within 60–90 min of inadvertent injection of local anaesthesia with adrenaline (epinephrine) at standard commercial dilutions, without any evidence of harm.[4]

Adverse effects

Systemic toxicity *(Table 22.2.2)*

Systemic toxicity occurs after unrecognized rapid intravenous injection or exceeding the recommended safe maximum dose. Symptoms and signs of toxicity are related to plasma drug levels and progress from circumoral tingling, dizziness, tinnitus and visual disturbance to muscular twitching, confusion, convulsions, coma and apnoea. Cardiovascular effects are also seen with high plasma levels, including bradycardia, hypotension and cardiovascular collapse ultimately with ventricular fibrillation or asystole, which are all exacerbated by associated hypoxia.

Table 22.2.1 Maximum recommended safe dose and duration of action of common local anaesthetics

Drug	Dose (mg/kg)*	Duration (h)
Lignocaine	3	0.5–1
Lignocaine with adrenaline	7	2–5
Bupivacaine	2	2–4
Prilocaine	6	0.5–1.5

*A 1% solution contains 10 mg/mL.

Table 22.2.2 Features of systemic local anaesthetic toxicity (in order of increasing plasma levels)

Circumoral tingling
Dizziness
Tinnitus
Visual disturbance
Muscular twitching
Confusion
Convulsions
Coma
Apnoea
Cardiovascular collapse (highest plasma levels)

The management of systemic toxicity includes immediate cessation of the drug, airway maintenance, supplemental oxygen and incremental doses of an intravenous benzodiazepine such as midazolam 0.05–0.1 mg/kg for seizures. Major reactions may require endotracheal intubation, fluids, vasopressors and inotropic support. As reactions occur immediately or within minutes after local anaesthetic use, medical expertise, resuscitation equipment and monitoring facilities must always be available.

Other reactions (Table 22.2.3)

Other adverse reactions to local anaesthetics involve allergy, including anaphylaxis predominantly to the amino esters (rarely amino amides), catecholamine effects from added adrenaline, vasovagal reactions when the patient is upright, such as during a dental procedure, cytotoxic delayed wound healing, malignant hyperthermia from amino amide use, and methaemoglobinaemia due to prilocaine or benzocaine.

Topical agents

Some agents such as EMLA™ (eutectic mixture of local anaesthetics including 2.5% lignocaine and 2.5% prilocaine) are used topically, particularly to decrease the pain of insertion of cannulae or for lumbar puncture and suprapubic catheter insertion in children. EMLA™ takes up to one hour for maximal effect and paradoxically is a venoconstrictor making vessel puncture harder, thus a superior alternative for cannula insertion is 4% amethocaine (AnGel™), which has a quicker onset and is a vasodilator.[5] Likewise, a mixture of 1:1000 adrenaline,

Table 22.2.3 Adverse reactions to local anaesthetics (other than systemic toxicity)

Allergy
    esters >> amides
    additives such as methylparaben, sodium metabisulphite

Catecholamine effects from added adrenaline
Vasovagal
Delayed wound healing
Malignant hyperthermia
Methaemoglobinaemia – prilocaine, benzocaine

4% lignocaine and 0.5% amethocaine with the acronym ALA (or known as LET in North America standing for lidocaine, epinephrine and tetracaine) may be used inside small wounds instead of, or to reduce the pain of, injecting local anaesthetic prior to closure, again in children or adolescents.

Specific nerve blocks

The following nerve blocks are contraindicated in uncooperative patients, those with local sepsis in the injection zone and in the rare patient with true local anaesthetic allergy. Care must be taken not to exceed the recommended maximum local anaesthetic doses (see Table 22.2.1), and monitoring facilities, resuscitation equipment and medical expertise must be available at all times.

Digital nerve block ('ring block')

Indications

Wound debridement, suturing, drainage of infection, fracture or dislocation reduction around the nail, fingertip and distal finger or toe.

Contraindications

Local sepsis, Raynaud's phenomenon and peripheral vascular disease.

Technique

Use 2% plain lignocaine. Inject 1–1.5 mL using a 25-gauge needle into the palmar aspect of the base of the finger or toe, approaching vertically from the dorsum. Withdraw the needle until subcutaneous and rotate slightly until pointing to the extensor surface of the digit, and inject a further 0.5 mL (Fig. 22.2.1). Perform the same procedure on the other side of the digit. Allow at least 5 min for the block to work.

Complications

Avoid intravascular injection by aspirating prior to injection. Do not use a tourniquet or more than 4 mL total volume, to avoid impairing the circulation due to high local tissue pressures.

Nerve blocks at the wrist

These provide anaesthesia to the hand, particularly for diffuse lesions hard to infiltrate directly such as 'gravel rash', or when the hand is swollen or burned.

Ulnar nerve wrist block (lateral approach)

Indications

Procedures on the medial border of the hand and medial 1.5 digits, or combined with median and radial nerve blocks for hand anaesthesia.

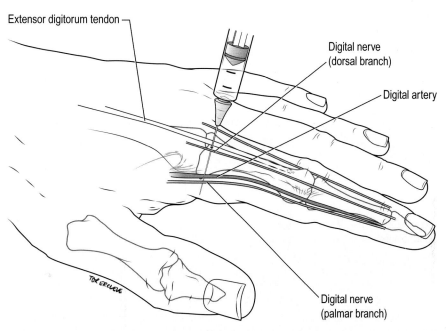

Extensor digitorum tendon

Digital nerve (dorsal branch)

Digital artery

Digital nerve (palmar branch)

Fig. 22.2.1 Digital nerve block.

Contraindications
Local sepsis, neuritis.

Technique
Identify the flexor carpi ulnaris tendon at the proximal palmar crease. Introduce a 25-gauge needle on the ulnar aspect of the tendon, directed horizontally and laterally for 1–1.5 cm under the tendon. Inject 4 mL of 1% lignocaine. Withdraw the needle until subcutaneous then inject 5 mL of 1% lignocaine fanwise to the dorsal midline, to block superficial cutaneous branches (Fig. 22.2.2).

Median nerve wrist block

Indications
Procedures on the lateral border of the hand in the territory supplied by the median nerve, excluding the medial 1.5 digits, or combined with ulnar and radial nerve blocks for hand anaesthesia.

Contraindications
Local sepsis, carpal tunnel syndrome or neuritis.

Technique
Identify the tendons of the flexor carpi radialis and palmaris longus at the proximal wrist crease. Introduce a 25-gauge needle vertically 0.5–1 cm lateral to the palmaris longus (or 0.5 cm medial to the flexor carpi radialis in the 10% of individuals lacking a palmaris longus). Inject 5 mL of 1% lignocaine when the needle gives as it penetrates the flexor retinaculum or paraesthesiae are elicited, at a depth usually of no more than 1 cm to the skin (Fig. 22.2.3). Avoid injecting into the nerve itself, as it may lie more superficial than this.

Radial nerve wrist block

Indications
Procedures on the dorsal radial aspect of the hand, or combined with ulnar and median nerve blocks for hand anaesthesia.

Contraindications
Local sepsis, neuritis.

Technique
Identify the tendon of the extensor carpi radialis, and infiltrate 5–10 mL of 1% lignocaine subcutaneously in a ring around the radial border of the wrist to the area overlying the radial pulse, at the level of the proximal palmar crease (Fig. 22.2.4).

Femoral nerve block

Indications
Analgesia for fractured shaft of femur, especially prior to applying dynamic splintage.

Contraindications
Local sepsis, bleeding tendency.

Technique
Palpate the femoral artery below the midpoint of the inguinal ligament, which extends from the pubic tubercle to the anterior superior iliac spine. Insert a 21-gauge needle 1 cm lateral to this point, perpendicular to the skin. Advance until paraesthesiae are elicited down the leg and withdraw slightly, aspirate to exclude intravascular placement, and inject 10 mL of 0.5% bupivacaine (50 mg). Alternatively, feel for a give as the needle punctures the fascia lata, aspirate, then inject 10 mL of 0.5% bupivacaine fanwise laterally away from the artery (Fig. 22.2.5). Allow up to 15–30 min for onset of maximal anaesthesia.

Complications
Puncture of femoral artery.

Foot blocks at the ankle

Indications
Where local anaesthetic infiltration of the foot is awkward or difficult because of thick sole skin or pain, or when excessive amounts of anaesthetic would otherwise be required.

Contraindications
Local sepsis, peripheral vascular disease.

Technique
Three superficial nerves, the sural, superficial peroneal and saphenous, are blocked by subcutaneous infiltration in a band around 75% of the ankle circumference. Two deeper nerves – the posterior tibial by the posterior tibial artery and the deep peroneal (anterior tibial) nerve by the dorsalis pedis artery – are blocked, usually in combinations with the superficial ones, according to the area of anaesthesia required.

Sural nerve The sural nerve is blocked by injecting 3–5 mL of 1% lignocaine subcutaneously in a band between the Achilles tendon and the lateral malleolus, 1 cm above and posterior to the malleolus

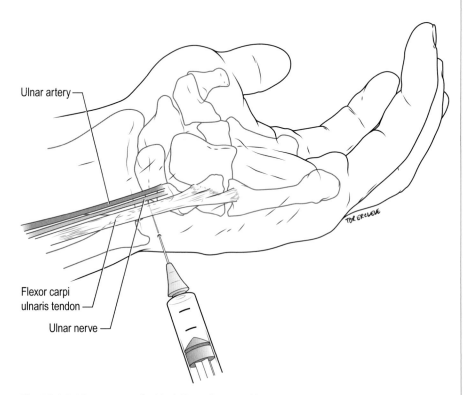

Ulnar artery

Flexor carpi ulnaris tendon

Ulnar nerve

Fig. 22.2.2 Ulnar nerve wrist block (lateral approach).

Posterior tibial nerve The posterior tibial nerve is blocked by infiltrating 3–5 mL of 1% lignocaine immediately lateral to the posterior tibial artery as it passes behind the medial malleolus, at a depth of 0.5–1 cm to the skin (see Fig. 22.2.7). It anaesthetizes the sole of the foot, excluding the posterolateral heel (see sural nerve above), via its medial and lateral plantar branches.

Deep peroneal (anterior tibial) nerve The deep peroneal (anterior tibial) nerve is blocked by infiltrating 1–2 mL of 1% lignocaine just above the base of the medial malleolus, lateral and behind the extensor hallucis longus by the dorsalis pedis pulse at a depth of 0.5 cm (see Fig. 22.2.7). It anaesthetizes the interdigital web between the hallux and second toe.

Complications

Exceeding a total volume of 20 mL of 1% lignocaine local anaesthetic that risks systemic toxicity or poor peripheral perfusion due to raised tissue pressures.

Intravenous regional anaesthesia or Bier's block

Indications

Operative procedures such as debridement, tendon repair and foreign body removal in the forearm and hand. Reduction of fractures and dislocations, typically Colles' fracture of the wrist.

Contraindications

Local anaesthetic sensitivity; peripheral vascular disease, including Raynaud's; sickle cell disease; cellulitis; uncooperative patients, including children; hypertension with systolic blood pressure over 200 mmHg; severe liver disease; and unstable epilepsy.

Technique

Two doctors are required, allowing one to perform the manipulation and the other, with training in the procedure and resuscitation skills, to perform the block. Explain the procedure to the patient and obtain informed consent. Assemble and check all equipment, and apply standard monitoring, including ECG, non-invasive blood pressure and pulse oximetry.

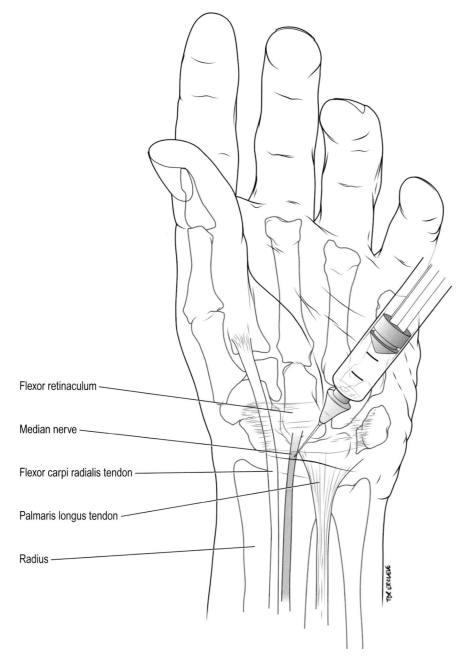

Flexor retinaculum

Median nerve

Flexor carpi radialis tendon

Palmaris longus tendon

Radius

Fig. 22.2.3 Median nerve wrist block.

(Fig. 22.2.6). It anaesthetizes a small strip on the lateral dorsum of the foot at the base of the little toe to the lateral malleolus, and the posterolateral aspect of the ankle and heel.

Superficial peroneal nerves Superficial peroneal nerves are blocked by injecting 4–6 mL of 1% lignocaine subcutaneously in a band between the extensor hallucis longus tendon and the lateral malleolus, on the anterior aspect of the ankle (see Fig. 22.2.6). This block anaesthetizes the dorsum of the foot, save for the lateral aspect (see sural nerve above), and interdigital web between the hallux and second toe (see deep peroneal nerve below).

Saphenous nerve The saphenous nerve is blocked by injecting 3–5 mL of 1% lignocaine subcutaneously above the medial malleolus, laterally until over the tibialis anterior tendon (Fig. 22.2.7). It anaesthetizes the area around the medial malleolus anteriorly and to a lesser degree posteriorly.

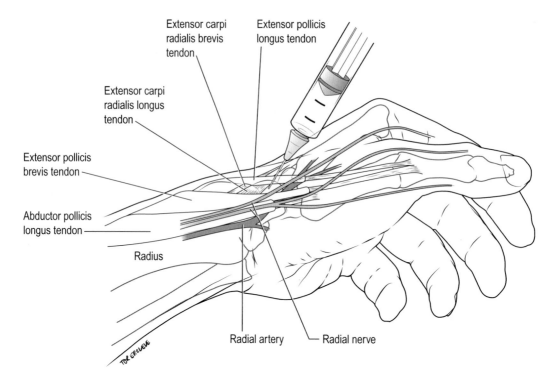

Extensor carpi radialis brevis tendon

Extensor pollicis longus tendon

Extensor carpi radialis longus tendon

Extensor pollicis brevis tendon

Abductor pollicis longus tendon

Radius

Radial artery

Radial nerve

Fig. 22.2.4 Radial nerve wrist block.

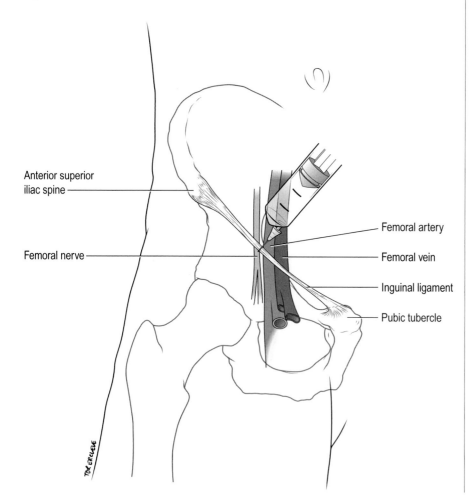

Anterior superior iliac spine

Femoral nerve

Femoral artery

Femoral vein

Inguinal ligament

Pubic tubercle

Fig. 22.2.5 Femoral nerve block.

Use a specifically designed and maintained single 15 cm adult cuff, placed over cottonwool padding to the upper arm.

Double-cuff tourniquets require higher inflation pressures as they are narrower. The upper cuff is inflated first, followed by the lower cuff 15 min later, after injection of the prilocaine, thereby causing less discomfort to the patient. The upper cuff is then released. The use of a double cuff does not always reduce the ischaemia pain, and predisposes to accidental wrong cuff release, so requires additional expertise and understanding.

Insert a small intravenous cannula into the dorsum of the hand of the injured limb and a second cannula in the other hand or wrist as emergency access to the central circulation. Exsanguinate the injured limb by simple elevation and direct brachial artery compression for 2–3 min, carefully supporting the limb at the site of any fracture. An Esmarch bandage may be used instead, in the absence of a painful wrist fracture.

Keep the arm elevated and inflate the cuff to 100 mmHg above systolic blood pressure. The radial artery pulse should now be absent and the veins remain empty. If this is not the case, do not inject

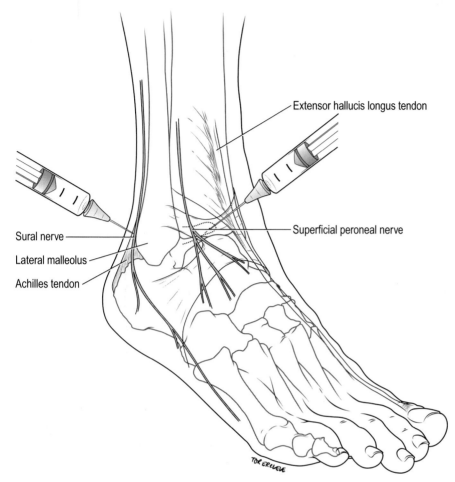

Fig. 22.2.6 Sural and superficial nerve blocks.

Extensor hallucis longus tendon

Superficial peroneal nerve

Sural nerve

Lateral malleolus

Achilles tendon

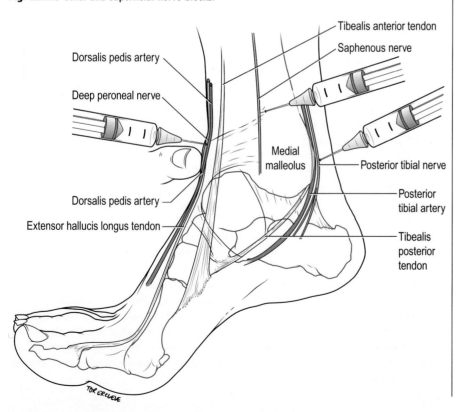

Fig. 22.2.7 Saphenous, posterior tibial and deep peroneal nerve blocks.

Tibealis anterior tendon

Saphenous nerve

Dorsalis pedis artery

Deep peroneal nerve

Medial malleolus

Posterior tibial nerve

Dorsalis pedis artery

Posterior tibial artery

Extensor hallucis longus tendon

Tibealis posterior tendon

anaesthetic but repeat the exsanguination procedure and cuff inflation.

Lower the arm once the radial artery pulse is absent and the veins are empty, and inject 2.5 mg/kg (0.5 mL/kg) of 0.5% prilocaine slowly over 90 sec and record the time.

Continuously monitor the cuff pressure and wait at least 5–10 min to confirm the adequacy of analgesia before removing the cannula on the injured limb. Perform the surgical procedure. Keep the tourniquet inflated for a minimum of 20 min and a maximum of 60 min.

Monitor the patient carefully for any signs of anaesthetic toxicity (see Table 22.2.2) over the next 15 min following cuff release, while organizing discharge from the monitored area.

Complications

No severe cardiac complications, deaths or methaemoglobinaemia have been reported using 0.5% prilocaine at the maximum dose of 2.5 mg/kg (0.5 mL/kg).[6] Discomfort from the cuff is possible, but rarely significant.

Controversies and future directions

❶ There is no evidence that injecting a standard commercial preparation of local anaesthetic with adrenaline (epinephrine) into a digit is harmful (see reference 4).

❷ Necessity for fasting prior to a Bier's block.

References

1. Bates D, Cutting P. Local anaesthetic and arterial puncture. Emergency Medicine Journal 2001; 18: 378.
2. Murphy R, Carley S. Prior injection of local anaesthetic and the pain and success of intravenous cannulation. Emergency Medicine Journal 2000; 17: 406–408.
3. Fisher MM, Bowey CJ. Alleged allergy to local anaesthetics. Anaesthesia and Intensive Care 1997; 25: 611–614.
4. Waterbrook A, Germann C, Southall J. Is epinephrine harmful when used with anesthetics for digital nerve blocks? Annals of Emergency Medicine 2007; 50: 472–475.
5. Boyd R, Jacobs M. EMLA or amethocaine (tetracaine) for topical anaesthesia in children. Emergency Medical Journal 2001; 18: 209–210.
6. Lowen R, Taylor J. Bier's block – the experience of Australian emergency departments. Medical Journal of Australia 1994; 60: 108–111.

22.3 Procedural sedation and analgesia

Anthony Bell • Greg Treston

ESSENTIALS

1 Emergency physicians and nurses should be trained to provide procedural sedation and analgesia in the emergency department.

2 Plan and prepare yourself, and assess the risk–benefit of each individual procedure.

3 Assess the timing and nature of recent oral intake.

4 Determine the safe limit of the targeted depth and duration of sedation.

5 Sedation is a continuum. It is not always possible to predict how an individual will respond or at which point airway reflexes may become jeopardized.

6 Sedative agents should be titrated to clinical endpoints.

7 Embarking on a procedure likely to last more than 20 min under procedural sedation alone is inappropriate.

Introduction and rationale

Procedural sedation and analgesia (PSA) is a core competency for the emergency physician, for the performance of brief, but painful procedures, and has become standard emergency medicine practice. PSA refers to the technique of administering sedatives or dissociative agents, with or without analgesics, to induce a state that allows the patient to tolerate unpleasant or anxiety-provoking procedures, while maintaining cardio-respiratory function.[1,2]

Paediatric patients in particular represent a significant challenge to the emergency physician; children are often frightened when in pain, and their presentation to the hospital disrupts the family's functioning.[3,4] Medical staff underestimate and under-treat pain in children.[5] Procedures may have previously been performed with inadequate sedation or 'oligo-analgesia' for fear of complications, worry about prolonged recovery time or the perception that with the procedure being brief, the child will not remember it.

Painful procedures in the emergency department (ED) are remembered vividly by children, parents and adult patients. Denial of relief from pain that is proportionate to the expressed need for such relief is an unjustified harm and amounts to substandard and unethical medical practice.[6]

Underlying principles

Guidelines

The Australasian College for Emergency Medicine (ACEM),[7] the American College of Emergency Physicians[2] and the Canadian Association of Emergency Physicians[8] have all published on the underlying principles for successful procedural sedation and analgesia within the ED. All guidelines cover pre-sedation preparation and assessment, pre-sedation fasting, physician skills, staffing, equipment and setting, patient monitoring, documentation and post-sedation care.

The ACEM Guidelines require that two medical attendants, one of whom should be a specialist or advanced trainee, be present. Nursing staff are also required and the procedure must be performed in a resuscitation area, as physiological monitoring is mandated during the procedure, extending into the recovery phase.

Although the Australasian guidelines were developed conjointly with the Australian and New Zealand College of Anaesthetists (ANZCA), the Joint Faculty of Intensive Care Medicine and Faculty of Pain Medicine, there is no specific recommendation as to choice of agent, despite the potentially confounding information published by ANZCA relating to the use of intravenous anaesthetic agents.[9]

Depth and duration of sedation

The optimal endpoint of any sedation episode depends on the procedure being performed and the patient's characteristics. Sedation state classification is now well established ranging from minimal sedation (anxiolysis) through moderate sedation (formerly known as conscious sedation), to deep sedation and general anaesthesia. Dissociative sedation is a separate state induced by ketamine.[10] The exact characteristics of respiratory and/or airway reflex depression in relation to the depth of sedation are not well defined.[1]

Titration of drugs and constant verbal and tactile reassessment of the patient reduce the risk of oversedation.[2] Some degree of responsiveness to painful stimuli should indicate preservation of airway reflexes, decreasing the risk of aspiration if vomiting occurs.[11]

Reducing the overall time a patient is sedated reduces the risk of airway compromise or respiratory depression. The duration of sedation is largely determined by the choice and dose of agent used, and the procedure itself as to whether this will be brief such as shoulder dislocation reduction or longer such as a compound scrub, or manipulation of a difficult fracture, with most ED procedures taking less than 20 min.

Indications and patient selection

Patient selection is based on the need for sedation for a brief, painful procedure that will usually facilitate early discharge from the ED. These include but are not limited to fracture and dislocation reduction, incision and drainage of abscesses, and cardioversion.[12] Inherently less painful but anxiety-provoking procedures in children will also be facilitated by the use of dissociative sedation, for example lumbar puncture, suturing, ocular or auditory canal foreign body (FB) removal, or intravenous cannulation under extreme circumstances.[10]

Pre-procedure risk assessment

Age

A young patient's level of anxiety and cooperation will depend upon past medical experiences, anxiety of the parents and the reassurance given by medical staff.[10] Elderly patients, whilst mostly cooperative, may have underlying impairment of cardio-respiratory reserve, and are at greater risk of respiratory depression or hypotension.

ASA classification

The American Society of Anesthesiologists Classification (ASA) system[13] is used to classify the anaesthetic risk of patients (Table 22.3.1). Patients in ASA Class I and ASA Class II are usually preferred as candidates for procedural sedation in the ED. If an ASA Class III patient requires sedation out of necessity, such as emergency cardioversion, this should not be precluded. The management of respiratory depression becomes a more active issue with increasing ASA class in all age groups.[14,15]

Airway assessment

A focused airway assessment with attention to mouth opening, pharyngeal visualization using the Mallampatti score (Fig. 22.3.1), neck movement, thyromental distance and dentition or a known previous troublesome anaesthetic history may signal potential difficulty should active airway intervention be required. An airway assessment checklist predicting difficult endotracheal intubation, should this be needed during or following PSA, is found in Table 22.3.2.

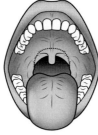
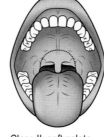

Class I: soft palate, uvula, fauces, pillars visible

No difficulty

Class II: soft palate, uvula, fauces visible

No difficulty

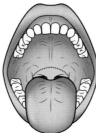
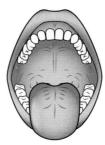

Class III: soft palate, base of uvula visible

Moderate difficulty

Class IV: hard palate only visible

Severe difficulty

Fig. 22.3.1 Mallampatti score, to predict likelihood of difficulty at endotracheal intubation. Perform with the patient sitting.

Table 22.3.2 Airway assessment predictors of a difficult endotracheal intubation	
1	Mallampatti score III & IV
2	Inability to open mouth >4 cm
3	Thyromental distance <6 cm
4	Limitation of neck movement
5	Difficulty in protruding lower jaw
6	History of difficult intubation

Mallampatti score – see Figure 22.3.1.

Past medical history

Some conditions predispose to gastro-oesophageal reflux such as pregnancy or hiatus hernia. Unstable acute medical or neurological conditions, with the exception of a cardiac arrhythmia requiring cardioversion, may carry too high a risk to proceed with PSA. Allergies to any agent in the past preclude use of that agent, as does an egg/soy allergy to the use of propofol in particular.[16]

Table 22.3.1 American Society of Anesthesiologists (ASA) classification	
Class	
1	Healthy patient, no medical problems
2	Mild systemic disease, e.g. hypertension
3	Severe systemic disease, but is not incapacitating
4	Severe systemic disease that is a constant threat to life
5	Moribund expected to live <24 h irrespective of operation

Fasting status

Fasting guidelines

ED patients undergoing urgent PSA are commonly not fasted on presentation or at the time of the procedure. Furthermore, holding a patient in an overcrowded ED to achieve a goal of 6 h of fasting time is impractical if an urgent procedure needs to be performed. Fasting guidelines are consensus, not evidence based.

There are no clinical data to support the consensus view regarding prolonged fasting prior to sedation.[13,17] In fact prolonged pre-procedural fasting has been shown to increase the rate of vomiting when using ketamine.[18,19] The ASA recommends at least 2 h and 6 h from last intake of fluid and food, respectively,[13] despite the lack of evidence regarding these conclusions.

Aspiration risk

The risk of aspiration is low with PSA. Fasting status is just one consideration when individualizing decisions about choice of agent, approach to dosing, desired depth of sedation or even formal referral to the operating theatre.[11,20] PSA does not involve the use of volatile inhalational anaesthetics, which are particularly emetogenic, as occurs during general anaesthesia.[21] In addition ED PSA does not involve pharyngeal manipulation or instrumentation, again a potent stimulus for inducing vomiting.

There is no association between fasting status and adverse events during procedural sedation in the ED for a range of agents including ketamine, midazolam/fentanyl, chloral hydrate, pentobarbital[18,22,23] or nitrous oxide.[16,24] The proportion of unfasted patients in those studies was 53–71%. Recent data looking specifically at patients undergoing PSA with propofol with respect to fasting status showed no difference in adverse events between fasted and unfasted patients.[11] There is only one reported case of aspiration during PSA in the ED literature, which although it probably represents negative reporting bias, is still an extremely low figure.[25]

Post-procedure vomiting

This usually occurs well into the recovery period, when the airway is no longer at risk. Post-procedure vomiting is more common with ketamine or narcotics than it is with propofol or benzodiazepines.[11,26]

Procedural urgency[1]

The endpoint of sedation in the ED should be tailored to the urgency of procedure and availability of appropriate staff.[1,8] Procedures may thus be considered:

- emergency: cardioversion, fractures with neurovascular compromise needing reduction, intractable pain
- urgent: care of dirty wounds or lacerations, dislocation reductions, lumbar puncture (LP), facilitate neuroimaging in trauma
- semi-urgent: foreign body removal, care of clean wounds and lacerations
- elective.

Involvement of parents or carer

Parental cooperation is critical to the success of any procedural intervention in children. ED survey data show the vast majority of parents wish to be present for invasive procedures performed on their child in the ED, with a small drop as the invasiveness of the procedure increases, except for full cardio-pulmonary resuscitation.[27,28]

Despite this, more than one-third of parents were asked to leave the room in one study of children undergoing procedures.[29] This practice of requesting that parents leave the room when their child undergoes a procedure should be abandoned. Parental presence should be welcomed, but ultimately their decision to stay or go should be supported. PSA in children should include ushering the parents to the bedside, not out of the room, with full explanation to both parents and child what is happening and why.[27,30]

Informed consent

Informed consent must be obtained after explanation of the specific risks of both PSA and the procedure itself. In particular, when using ketamine warn parents to expect a staring child with nystagmus, salivation, lacrimation, possible myoclonic jerking and a vomit at the end in 10–15%. This is important to their overall acceptance and experience of their child's procedure. Likewise, the possibility of airway intervention beyond transient support should be raised with propofol, although it is rare.

Documentation

Specific procedural sedation forms or records are recommended. When designed in accordance with current best practice they improve documentation, and may be the focus for educational initiatives and assist in audit, research and quality assurance (QA).[31–33] They can also act as a de facto protocol to ensure safe care during procedural sedation. They increase the chances of compliance with guidelines and ensure essential pre-sedation checks and monitoring are performed. They should include provision for recording adverse events, including vomiting, aspiration or respiratory depression as well as any interventions required.[11]

Choice of agent

The ideal agent for PSA in the ED should have a profile of rapid onset, short duration of action, rapid recovery, minimal side effects and an amnestic effect. The different classes of drugs used alone or in combination in PSA include sedative hypnotics, analgesics, dissociative sedatives, inhalation agents, and antagonists such as flumazenil and naloxone (Table 22.3.3).

Sedative hypnotics

Benzodiazepines

Midazolam Midazolam is one of the most commonly used benzodiazepines with amnestic,[34] anxiolytic and sedative properties. Side effects are dose dependent. Intravenous dosing for PSA ranges from 0.1 mg/kg in younger children to 0.025–0.05 mg/kg in older children and adults. Other routes of administration include intramuscular and intranasal, although the onset of action is slower.[10] Many experienced clinicians have abandoned the use of intranasal midazolam.

Midazolam/opioid combinations were perceived to provide more predictable response and to have a favourable safety profile when compared to propofol, owing to the greater potential with propofol to induce dose-related deep sedation.[35] In fact, there is additive respiratory depression with opiate and midazolam-containing combinations for PSA, with prolonged recovery times when compared to propofol.[36–38]

Diazepam Diazepam is less potent than midazolam, but there is little or no difference in the propensity of the two drugs to produce respiratory depression.[39] Dosing should start at 0.1–0.2 mg/kg with smaller subsequent doses. The antegrade amnestic effect of diazepam is significantly less than that of midazolam.[40,41] Diazepam also causes more pain on injection and a lesser degree of early sedation.[42] The elimination half-lives of benzodiazepines do not necessarily correspond with their sedative pharmacodynamic effects, so there are no clinically important sedative recovery rate differences between midazolam and diazepam.[43,44]

Table 22.3.3	Choice of agent and suggested i.v. drug dosages (adult, 70 kg, normal BMI)		
Drug	*Initial bolus*	*Subsequent titrated i.v. boluses*	*Cumulative maximum dose*
Morphine	2.5 mg	2.5 mg	10–15 mg
Fentanyl	25–50 µg	25 µg	150–200 µg
Midazolam	2 mg	1 mg	10 mg
Diazepam	5 mg	2.5 mg	10 mg
Propofol	40–50 mg	20 mg	150 mg
Ketamine	20–30 mg	10–20 mg	120 mg
Etomidate*	5–7 mg	2 mg	20 mg
'Ketafol'	2–3 mL	1–2 mL	10 mL

These are conservative estimates for a 70 kg adult.
Dose modification is advised where appropriate in the elderly patient (lower doses) and patients with small muscle bulk (lower doses).
'Ketafol' is made with 1 mL of 100 mg/mL ketamine made up to 10 mL with 10 mg/mL propofol in the same syringe giving 10 mg : 9 mg/mL, respectively.
*Etomidate is not available in Australia.
BMI, body mass index.

Short acting agents

Propofol

Propofol is a non-opioid, non-barbiturate sedative hypnotic that acts at gamma amino-butyric acid (GABA) sites within the central nervous system, providing a rapid onset (<1 min) and short duration (5–15 min) of action facilitating rapid recovery times, with an amnestic effect. Propofol is easily titratable and has some antiemetic properties.[17,45] Hypotension is transient when propofol is titrated in euvolaemic patients with normal cardiac function. Propofol has been shown to be safe, when used appropriately, in a wide range of settings including PSA in the ED.[2,46,47]

The optimum dosing regime for propofol in procedural sedation is yet to be defined. Options vary from single bolus,[37,38,48] titration,[15,49–52] bolus and infusion[36,53] or infusion alone.[54–56] Doses recommended include 1 mg/kg initial bolus and 0.5 mg/kg subsequent boluses for PSA in the ED.[38,45,57,58] In children initial doses of 2 mg/kg initial bolus have been used.[59,60] An alternative is to reduce the dose to 0.5–1.0 mg/kg initial bolus followed by 20 mg boluses.[61] Dose reduction is essential in patients over 65 years of age.[53] Higher total mg/kg doses are used in children compared with adults.[61,62]

Sedation times are shorter with propofol and reported respiratory complication rates for propofol are equivalent to midazolam alone,[36] midazolam with or without flumazenil, etomidate,[37] and midazolam plus fentanyl.[38] At excessive doses propofol is associated with greater degrees of oxygen desaturation.[48]

Respiratory depression is seen in up to 50% of ASA Class 1 and Class 2 patients[50,63,64] and 61% in the critically ill (Classes 4 and 5).[14] Apnoea may occur but is transient. It may be seen in up to 22% of patients receiving propofol for PSA.[11,37,57] Transient hypoxia occurs from 6 to 44% of sedation episodes.[14,15,36,37,48–50,52–54,62–64] Supplemental oxygen was not routinely applied during PSA in all studies.[49] The use of propofol becomes increasingly safe as familiarity and experience grow.

Etomidate

Etomidate is a non-barbituate hypnotic currently unavailable in Australia. It is often used for rapid sequence induction (RSI) of endotracheal intubation in the UK and USA, as well as for procedural sedation in the ED. It has a rapid onset <30 s with a duration of action of 5–15 min. The starting dose for PSA is up to 0.1 mg/kg with subsequent boluses of 0.05 mg/kg. It has a similar profile in terms of respiratory depression and duration of sedation to propofol, when compared with midazolam, but is more cardiovascularly stable. Propofol is preferred to etomidate as etomidate has a 20% rate of myoclonus, plus emergence phenomena, higher vomiting rates and a theoretical risk of adrenal suppression.[65–68]

Opiates

The use of opiates before, during and after procedural sedation is common. In addition opiates remain the mainstay of pain control in the ED (see Ch. 22.1). Opiates provide analgesia but have no amnestic or anxiolytic properties.

Fentanyl

Fentanyl is the opiate of choice for ED PSA. It should be titrated up to 2 μg/kg i.v., to avoid respiratory depression from too rapid a push, and should be combined with a pure sedative agent. It may be delivered intranasally. Fentanyl has a rapid onset of action, lack of histamine release, and is cardiovascularly stable when compared to morphine. The duration of action is 30–45 min.

Morphine

Morphine provides a longer duration of analgesia extending to hours, and is useful after a procedure for ongoing analgesia. It may be administered by ambulance officers prior to arrival in hospital. The standard analgesic dose is 0.1 mg/kg i.v.

Ultra short-acting opiates

Newer ultra short-acting opiates such as remifentanil have an increasing role in anaesthesia, and when combined with propofol provide excellent sedation and analgesia with rapid recovery.[69] Experience with this agent in PSA in the ED is limited.

Inhalational agents

Nitrous oxide

Nitrous oxide (N_2O) provides anxiolysis and analgesia. Entonox® is a proprietary mixture of 50% N_2O with 50% O_2 and is widely available in Australia. Entonox® is delivered via a self-administered demand valve mask. It has rapid onset and offset and is safe, but has little or no sedative effect. Entonox® may be useful as an anxiolytic in needle-phobic individuals, particularly children, before definitive intravenous sedation can be provided.

Common side effects include vomiting and dizziness. Airway reflexes are preserved. It is contraindicated in patients with trapped gas disorders such as a pneumothorax.

Dissociative sedative

Ketamine

Ketamine has worldwide use as a dissociative anaesthetic agent, particularly in military situations and third world anaesthesia.[70] Ketamine produces a dose-related 'dissociative anaesthesia' state between deep sedation and general anaesthesia, by dissociating the thalamocortical and limbic systems. It has a rapid on and offset, with preservation of airway reflexes, although it may cause laryngospasm. As it causes an increase in sympathetic tone it is relatively contraindicated in ischaemic heart disease (IHD) and serious head injury, although conversely it finds favour in the hypotense patient.

Ketamine has become a popular drug in the ED given either intravenously or occasionally intramuscularly, particularly in paediatric procedural sedation. It is safe, with preservation of oropharyngeal reflexes and little or no respiratory depression.[6,8,18,71–74] The usual initial intravenous dose is 0.5 mg/kg slowly.

There is some concern with 'emergence delirium'[3,75] also known as 'emergence phenomena'.[72–74,76,77] 'Emergence delirium' has been described as either 'patients are agitated, restless, and combative, and do not seem cognizant of their surroundings. Patients refuse to be comforted, even by their parents',[78] or 'combative, excited, and disoriented behaviour that requires transient physical restraint'.[79] However, 'emergence phenomena' may be something as mild as non-distressing visual hallucinations, or transient diplopia.

Atropine reduces hypersalivation and post-procedure vomiting, used with titrated intravenous ketamine for paediatric procedural sedation in the ED.[80] However, as hypersalivation per se rarely if ever affects the conduct of the procedure, its use is largely unnecessary.

Combinations utilizing ketamine

Midazolam and ketamine

Midazolam (or another benzodiazepine) has traditionally been used in combination with ketamine, in an effort to decrease the incidence of 'emergence delirium', supported by studies reporting lower rates of emergence phenomena/agitation in adults who have received both ketamine and a benzodiazepine, in contrast to ketamine alone. 'Emergence phenomena' are fewer in children anyway than in adults, and the rate of emergence reactions in children is not lowered by adding a benzodiazepine.[81–84]

In addition, recent randomized trials in children show unchanged rates of true emergence delirium with agitation when midazolam is added to ketamine.[85–87] Midazolam use has been associated with higher rates of airway and respiratory compromise during procedural sedation in children.[13] Midazolam as an adjunctive medication with ketamine for PSA does, however, have lower rates of post-procedural emesis.[85,86]

Overall the prophylactic use of adjunctive benzodiazepines with ketamine is not recommended. Furthermore midazolam as a sole sedative agent has been reported to have a rate of emergence agitation of up to 42%.[88–90]

Ketamine and propofol ('Ketafol')

The addition of ketamine to propofol ('Ketafol') has recently been described for procedural analgesia and sedation, and has been used safely in a number of non-ED settings.[91] The combination aims to balance the opposing respiratory and haemodynamic effects of each drug. Additionally, the antiemetic effect of propofol may counteract the vomiting with ketamine, and may minimize the rate of 'emergence', although this is unproven.

In a single ED study the combination was safe and resulted in high staff and patient satisfaction. There are some advantages in the use of ketafol over propofol alone. Modest propofol dose reduction was seen, with a reduced respiratory depression profile. Recovery times remained short, and there were no adverse events that altered patient disposition.[92] As ketamine is analgesic but not dissociative at low doses, targeted depth of sedation is important when using lower doses of propofol.

Prospective trials to compare this combination of ketafol with other agents alone are awaited, and to find the most beneficial ratio of ketamine to propofol balancing synergy with side effect profile.[66] One suggested dilution is to make 1 mL of 100 mg/mL ketamine up to 10 mL with 9 mL of 10 mg/mL propofol in the same syringe, to give a dilution of 10 mg:9 mg/mL respectively.

Preparation and monitoring

Resuscitation area

PSA should always occur in a resuscitation area, with two qualified physician staff; one physician to perform the procedure and one physician to be responsible for the drugs and airway, both assisted by an ED nurse.[7] Supplemental oxygen should be given for the majority of cases of PSA in the ED, with the exception of paediatric PSA with ketamine, when the use of supplemental oxygen by mask is unnecessarily upsetting for the child, prior to commencement of sedation.

Equipment and monitoring

Suction, oxygen, airway adjuncts and resuscitation equipment should be prepared and physiological monitoring applied. Monitoring should include pulse oximetry, non-invasive blood pressure, heart rate, ECG rhythm and respiratory rate. End-tidal carbon dioxide monitoring via nasal prongs is increasingly recommended.[2,11] Intravenous access is mandatory in all cases. See Table 22.3.4 for essential equipment requirements.

Sedation scoring

Monitoring is interactive as verbal and tactile stimulation are used to constantly reassess the depth of sedation. Careful dose titration and subjective evaluation of patient responsiveness throughout the procedure are paramount.[35,46] The Ramsay Sedation Score,[93] or the Motor Component of the Observer's Assessment of Alertness/Sedation Scale (OAA/S)[94] are examples of sedation scores that have been validated for midazolam use. All sedation scoring scales are subject to inter-observer variability and are relatively imprecise, and are not true objective measures of sedation. However, they require little formal training and may be easily incorporated into departmental protocols (Table 22.3.5).

Bispectral EEG analysis

Bispectral EEG analysis (BIS) is not reliably predictive of the conscious state in individual patients.[66] Numerical values (0–100) are assigned to a patient's level of sedation,

Table 22.3.4	Essential equipment requirements for procedural sedation 'SOAPMI'
S	**S**uction equipment (connected and checked) • Wall suction • Yankauer sucker and tubing • Paediatric suction catheters
O	**O**xygen (connected and checked) • Supply • Age appropriate masks including nebuliser attachment • Primed bag-valve-mask
A	**A**irway • Oro- and naso-pharyngeal airways • Laryngoscope and selection of blades (tested) • Appropriate selection of endotracheal tubes • Stylettes and bougies • 'Difficult airway kit' including laryngeal mask airway
P	**P**harmacological agents (accessible but need not be drawn up) • Adrenaline and atropine • Naloxone and flumazenil • Bronchodilators • Drugs for rescue rapid sequence induction endotracheal intubation
M	**M**onitoring equipment • Full non-invasive physiological monitoring • End-tidal CO_2 tubing with transducer (if available)
I	**I**ntravenous access trolley • Selection of cannulae • Crystalloid fluids

Table 22.3.5 Sedation scoring scales

Score	Ramsay sedation scale	Sedation continuum	Score	OAA/S
1	Awake and alert	Minimal	5	Responds readily to name spoken in normal tone
2	Tranquil, purposeful at conversational level	Moderate		
3	Sleepy but purposeful to verbal commands at conversational level		4	Responds only after name called loudly or repeatedly
4	Sleepy and requiring louder voice or tactile stimulus to be purposeful		3	Responds only to mild prodding and shaking
5	Asleep and only purposeful to loud verbal command or harder glabellar tap	Deep	2	Does not respond to mild prodding and shaking
6	Asleep and sluggishly purposeful only to painful stimulus		1	Does not respond to painful stimulus
7	Asleep, reflex response, not purposeful			
8	Unresponsive	Anaesthetised	0	Unresponsive

OAA/S, motor component of the Observer's Assessment of Alertness/Sedation Scale.

but they are a poor measure of analgesia and ineffective when used with ketamine. Correlation with OAA/S[95,96] and Ramsay Sedation Scores[97,98] are poor. Lower BIS scores predict more respiratory depression, but it is unclear whether the use of BIS itself reduces the rate of respiratory depression.[63,64,99]

Capnography

Capnography detects respiratory depression before clinical examination or pulse oximetry.[100–102] Changes in trace character or transient hypercapnia[50,51,103] are the earliest warning signs of hypoventilation or impending upper airway obstruction, of particular importance in children or those with reduced respiratory reserve.[57] Such early detection may avoid further sedation being given, or result in stimulating the patient or repositioning the airway. Only occasionally are airway adjuncts or bag valve mask ventilation required.[11,62] 'Waiting out' respiratory depression for a brief time during propofol sedation in a well pre-oxygenated patient is common.[58]

Post-procedure considerations

Patients should be observed until they have returned to their baseline level of functioning.[2,12,13] The exact time of this will depend on the patient, the drugs administered and the reason for the procedure. One study in children suggested a 30-min rule.[104] There is no need following ketamine use to darken the room or shield a child from the routine background visual and auditory stimuli of a busy ED in an effort to reduce the likelihood of emergence delirium.

Patients receiving propofol do not need prolonged post-procedure monitoring as resedation following propofol use is rare.[61] Once the patient can talk, nursing staff have an endpoint for the cessation of physiological monitoring, knowing that a patient is not likely to develop any adverse events after this point.

This stance is supported by a recent Clinical Practice Advisory statement from the USA.[12] Nursing allocation can be tailored to these less intensive post-procedure monitoring requirements.[105] Written discharge criteria and instructions though do need to be provided (Table 22.3.6).

Likely developments in the next 5–10 years[106]

- Optimal dosing strategies according to procedure type, patient age and depth of sedation required.

Table 22.3.6 Recommended adult discharge criteria and instructions following procedural sedation

1	Patient is alert and oriented, or has returned to pre-procedure state
2	Patient ambulates safely, or has returned to pre-procedure state
3	Patient is comfortable and has discharge analgesia arranged
4	Patient is discharged into care of a responsible adult
5	Driving or the like is banned for a minimum of 8 h
6	Alcohol or other central nervous system depressants are avoided for 12–24 h
7	Patients are warned about the potential for post-procedure pain, unsteadiness or dizziness. Seek medical attention if significant or disabling

- Alternative delivery modalities such as patient-controlled sedation.
- Newer agents or novel combinations that could include alfentanil and remifentanil.
- Increasing use and sophistication of psychological and regional techniques to augment PSA.
- Development of large multicentre trials with standard protocols for adverse event reporting and outcome measures to establish true complication rates.

Controversies

❶ The degree of pre-procedural analgesia impacting upon the amount of sedative required. Inadequate or oligo-analgesia still exists in EDs.[107,108]

❷ Whether lack of recall is a satisfactory justification for patients experiencing pain during a procedure.[106] The place of intraprocedural narcotic analgesia in addition to that given prior remains unclear.

❸ What the overall relationship is between practitioner skill and complications.[109] Implementation of a paediatric procedural sedation credentialling programme results in significant improvement.[110,111]

❹ Optimum definition of procedural sedation success. Should encompass a lack of recall, lack of response to pain, lack of adverse events, lack of interference from the patient during the procedure, and successful completion of the procedure.[106]

❺ Whether the depth or duration of sedation places patients at greater risk for aspiration.

References

1. Green SM, Roback MG, Miner JR, et al. Fasting and emergency department procedural sedation and analgesia: a consensus-based clinical practice advisory. Annals of Emergency Medicine 2007; 49(4): 454–461.

2. Godwin SA, Caro DA, Wolf SJ, et al. Clinical policy: procedural sedation and analgesia in the emergency department. Annals of Emergency Medicine 2005; 45 (2): 177–196.

3. Dean A. Paediatric sedation in Australasian Emergency Departments. Emergency Medicine (Frem) 1998; 10: 324–326.

4. Weisman S, Bernstein B, Schechter N. Consequences of inadequate analgesia during painful procedures in children. Archives of Pediatrics & Adolescent Medicine 1998; 152: 147–149.

5. Wilson J, Pendleton J. Oligoanalgesia in the emergency department. American Journal of Emergency Medicine 1989; 7: 620–623.

6. Walco G, Cassidy R, Schlechter N. Pain, hurt and harm – the ethics of pain control in infants and children. New England Journal of Medicine 1994; 331: 541–544.

7. Statement on clinical principles for procedural sedation. Emergency Medicine 2003; 15(2): 205–206.

8. Innes G, Murphy M, Nijssen-Jordan C, et al. Procedural sedation and analgesia in the emergency department. Canadian Consensus Guidelines. Journal of Emergency Medicine 1999; 17(1): 145–156.

9. Anaesthetists AaNZCo. Guidelines on Conscious Sedation for Diagnostic, Interventional Medical and Surgical Procedures, 2005.

10. Green SM, Krauss B. Procedural sedation and analgesia in children. Lancet 2006; 367: 766–780.

11. Bell A, Treston G, McNabb C, et al. Profiling adverse respiratory events and vomiting when using propofol for emergency department procedural sedation. Emergency Medicine Australasia 2007; 19: 405–410.

12. Miner JR, Burton JH. Clinical practice advisory: emergency department procedural sedation with propofol. Annals of Emergency Medicine 2007; 50(2): 182–187.

13. Practice guidelines for sedation and analgesia by non-anesthesiologists. Anaesthesiology 2002; 96(4): 1004–1017.

14. Miner JR, Martel ML, Meyer M, et al. Procedural sedation of critically ill patients in the emergency department. Academic Emergency Medicine 2005; 12(2): 124–128.

15. Guenther E, Pribble CG, Junkins EP, et al. Propofol sedation by emergency physicians for elective pediatric outpatient procedures. Annals of Emergency Medicine 2003; 42(6): 783–791.

16. Hofer KN, McCarthy MW, Buck ML, et al. Possible anaphylaxis after propofol in a child with food allergy. Annals of Pharmacotherapy 2003; 37(3): 398–401.

17. Bahn EL, Holt KR. Procedural sedation and analgesia: a review and new concepts. Emergency Medicine Clinics of North America 2005; 23(2): 503–517.

18. Treston G. Prolonged pre-procedure fasting time is unnecessary when using titrated intravenous ketamine for paediatric procedural sedation. Emergency Medicine Australasia 2004; 16(2): 145–150.

19. Green SM, Johnson NE. Ketamine sedation for pediatric procedures: Part 2, Review and implications. Annals of Emergency Medicine 1990; 19(9): 1033–1046.

20. Green SM. Fasting is a consideration – not a necessity – for emergency department procedural sedation and analgesia. Annals of Emergency Medicine 2003; 42(5): 647–650.

21. Green SM, Krauss B. Pulmonary aspiration risk during emergency department procedural sedation – an examination of the role of fasting and sedation depth. Academic Emergency Medicine 2002; 9(1): 35–42.

22. Agrawal D, Manzi SF, Gupta R, et al. Preprocedural fasting state and adverse events in children undergoing procedural sedation and analgesia in a pediatric emergency department. Annals of Emergency Medicine 2003; 42(5): 636–646.

23. Roback MG, Bajaj L, Wathen JE, et al. Preprocedural fasting and adverse events in procedural sedation and analgesia in a pediatric emergency department: are they related? Annals of Emergency Medicine 2004; 44(5): 454–459.

24. Babl FE, Puspitadewi A, Barnett P. Preprocedural fasting state and adverse events in children receiving nitrous oxide for procedural sedation and analgesia. Pediatric Emergency Care 2005; 21(11): 736–743.

25. Cheung KW, Watson ML, Field S, et al. Aspiration pneumonitis requiring intubation after procedural sedation and analgesia: a case report. Annals of Emergency Medicine 2007; 49(4): 462–464.

26. Roback MG, Wathen JE, Bajaj L, et al. Adverse events associated with procedural sedation and analgesia in a pediatric emergency department: a comparison of common parenteral drugs. Academic Emergency Medicine 2005; 12(6): 508–513.

27. Isoardi J, Slabbert N, Treston G. Witnessing invasive paediatric procedures, including resuscitation, in the emergency department: a parental perspective. Emergency Medicine Australasia 2005; 217(3): 244–248.

28. Bauchner H, Vinci R, Waring C. Pediatric procedures: do parents want to watch? Pediatrics 1989; 84: 907–909.

29. Bauchner H, Waring C, Vinci R. Parental presence during procedures in an emergency room: results from 50 observations. Pediatrics 1991; 87: 544–548.

30. Ross D, Ross S. Childhood pain: the school-aged child's viewpoint. Pain 1984; 20: 179–191.

31. Nicol MF. A risk management audit: are we complying with the national guidelines for sedation by non-anaesthetists? Journal of Accident and Emergency Medicine 1999; 16(2): 120–122.

32. Law A, Babl F, Priestley D, et al. Pre and post-implementation evaluation of a comprehensive procedural program for children in the emergency department. Journal of Paediatric Child Health (Supplement 8), 2005.

33. Swoboda TK, Munyak J. Use of a sedation-analgesia datasheet in closed shoulder reductions. Journal of Emergency Medicine 2005; 29(2): 129–135.

34. Macken E, Gevers AM, Hendrickx A, et al. Midazolam versus diazepam in lipid emulsion as conscious sedation for colonoscopy with or without reversal of sedation with flumazenil. Gastrointestinal Endoscopy 1998; 47(1): 57–61.

35. Green SM. Propofol for emergency department procedural sedation – not yet ready for prime time. Academic Emergency Medicine 1999; 6(10): 975–978.

36. Havel CJ, Jr., Strait RT, Hennes H. A clinical trial of propofol vs midazolam for procedural sedation in a pediatric emergency department. Academic Emergency Medicine 1999; 6(10): 989–997.

37. Coll-Vinent B, Sala X, Fernandez C, et al. Sedation for cardioversion in the emergency department: analysis of effectiveness in four protocols. Annals of Emergency Medicine 2003; 42(6): 767–772.

38. Taylor D, O'Brien D, Ritchie P. Propofol versus midazolam/fentanyl for reduction of anterior shoulder dislocation. Academic Emergency Medicine 2005; 12: 13–19.

39. Bell GD. Review article: premedication and intravenous sedation for upper gastrointestinal endoscopy. Alimentary Pharmacology and Therapeutics 1990; 4(2): 103–122.

40. Tolia V, Fleming SL, Kauffman RE. Randomized, double-blind trial of midazolam and diazepam for endoscopic sedation in children. Developmental Pharmacology and Therapeutics 1990; 14(3): 141–147.

41. Sanders LD, Davies-Evans J, Rosen M, et al. Comparison of diazepam with midazolam as i.v. sedation for outpatient gastroscopy. British Journal of Anaesthesia 1989; 63(6): 726–731.

42. Wright SW, Chudnofsky CR, Dronen SC, et al. Comparison of midazolam and diazepam for conscious sedation in the emergency department. Annals of Emergency Medicine 1993; 22(2): 201–205.

43. Ariano RE, Kassum DA, Aronson KJ. Comparison of sedative recovery time after midazolam versus diazepam administration. Critical Care Medicine 1994; 22(9): 1492–1496.

44. Mitchell AR, Chalil S, Boodhoo L. Diazepam or midazolam for external DC cardioversion (the DORM Study). Europace 2003; 5(4): 391–395.

45. Symington L, Thakore S. A review of the use of propofol for procedural sedation in the emergency department. Emergency Medicine Journal 2006; 23(2): 89–93.

46. Ducharme J. Propofol in the emergency department: another interpretation of the evidence. Journal of Canadian Association Emergency Physicians 2001; 3: 311–312.

47. Jackson R, Carley S. Towards evidence based emergency medicine: best BETs from the Manchester Royal Infirmary. Use of propofol for sedation in the emergency department. Emergency Medicine Journal 2001; 18(5): 378–379.

48. Godambe SA, Elliot V, Matheny D, et al. Comparison of propofol/fentanyl versus ketamine/midazolam for brief orthopedic procedural sedation in a pediatric emergency department. Pediatrics 2003; 112(1 Pt 1): 116–123.

49. Skokan EG, Pribble C, Bassett KE. Use of propofol sedation in a pediatric emergency department: a prospective study. Clinical Pediatrics (Phila) 2001; 40(12): 663–671.

50. Miner JR, Biros M, Krieg S, et al. Randomized clinical trial of propofol versus methohexital for procedural sedation during fracture and dislocation reduction in the emergency department. Academic Emergency Medicine 2003; 10(9): 931–937.

51. Miner JR, Heegaard W, Plummer D. End-tidal carbon dioxide monitoring during procedural sedation. Academic Emergency Medicine 2002; 9(4): 275–280.

52. Bassett KE, Anderson JL, Pribble CG, et al. Propofol for procedural sedation in children in the emergency department. Annals of Emergency Medicine 2003; 42(6): 773–782.

53. Frazee BW, Park RS, Lowery D. Propofol for deep procedural sedation in the ED. American Journal of Emergency Medicine 2005; 23(2): 190–195.

54. Swanson ER, Seaberg DC, Mathias S. The use of propofol for sedation in the emergency department. Academic Emergency Medicine 1996; 3(3): 234–238.

55. Pershad J, Godambe SA. Propofol for procedural sedation in the pediatric emergency department. Journal of Emergency Medicine 2004; 27(1): 11–14.

56. Frank LR, Strote J, Hauff SR, et al. Propofol by infusion protocol for ED procedural sedation. American Journal of Emergency Medicine 2006; 24(5): 599–602.

57. Green SM, Krauss B. Propofol in emergency medicine: pushing the sedation frontier. Annals of Emergency Medicine 2003; 42(6): 792–797.

58. Krauss B, Green SM. Procedural sedation and analgesia in children 2006; 367(9512): 766–780.

59. Sacchetti A, Cravero J. Sedation in the emergency department. Pediatric Annals 2005; 34(8): 617–622.

60. Barnett P. Propofol for pediatric sedation. Pediatric Emergency Care 2005; 21: 111–114.

61. Bell A, Treston G, Cardwell R, et al. Optimisation of propofol dose shortens procedural sedation time, prevents re-sedation and removes the requirement for post procedure physiologic monitoring. Emergency Medicine Australasia 2007; 19: 411–417.

62. Burton JH, Miner JR, Shipley ER, et al. Propofol for emergency department procedural sedation and analgesia: a tale of three centers. Academic Emergency Medicine 2006; 13(1): 24–30.

63. Miner JR, Biros MH, Heegaard W, et al. Bispectral electroencephalographic analysis of patients undergoing procedural sedation in the emergency department. Academic Emergency Medicine 2003; 10(6): 638–643.

64. Miner JR, Biros MH, Seigel T, et al. The utility of the bispectral index in procedural sedation with propofol in

the emergency department. Academic Emergency Medicine 2005; 12(3): 190–196.

65. Falk J, Zed PJ. Etomidate for procedural sedation in the emergency department. Annals of Pharmacotherapy 2004; 38(7–8): 1272–1277.

66. Green SM. Research advances in procedural sedation and analgesia. Annals of Emergency Medicine 2007; 49(1): 31–36.

67. Van Kuelen S, Burton J. Myoclonus associated with etomidate for ED procedural sedation and analgesia. American Journal of Emergency Medicine 2003; 21: 556–559.

68. Miner JR, Danahy M, Moch A, et al. Randomized clinical trial of etomidate versus propofol for procedural sedation in the emergency department. Annals of Emergency Medicine 2007; 49(1): 15–22.

69. Dunn MJ, Mitchell R, Souza CD, et al. Evaluation of propofol and remifentanil for intravenous sedation for reducing shoulder dislocations in the emergency department. Emergency Medicine Journal 2006; 23(1): 57–58.

70. Guldner GT, Petinaux B, Clemens P, et al. Ketamine for procedural sedation and analgesia by nonanesthesiologists in the field: a review for military health care providers. Military Medicine 2006; 171(6): 484–490.

71. Green SM, Rothrock SG, Lynch EL, et al. Intramuscular ketamine for pediatric sedation in the emergency department: safety profile in 1,022 cases. Annals of Emergency Medicine 1998; 31(6): 688–697.

72. Dachs RJ, Innes GM. Intravenous ketamine sedation of pediatric patients in the emergency department. Annals of Emergency Medicine 1997; 29(1): 146–150.

73. McCarty EC, Mencio GA, Walker LA. Ketamine sedation for the reduction of children's fractures in the emergency department. Journal of Bone and Joint Surgery – American volume 2000; 82-A(7): 912–918.

74. Howes MC. Ketamine for paediatric sedation/analgesia in the emergency department. Emergency Medicine Journal 2004; 21(3): 275–280.

75. Everitt I, Younge P, Barnett P. Paediatric sedation in emergency department: what is our practice? Emergency Medicine (Fremantle) 2002; 14(1): 62–66.

76. Green SM, Kuppermann N, Rothrock SG. Predictors of adverse events with intramuscular ketamine sedation in children. Annals of Emergency Medicine 2000; 35(1): 35–42.

77. Ducharme J. Ketamine: Do what is right for the patient. Emergency Medicine (Freemantle) 2001; 13: 7–8.

78. Wells L, Rasch D. Emergence 'delirium' after sevoflurane anesthesia: a paranoid delusion? Anesthesia & Analgesia 1999; 88: 1308–1310.

79. Uezono S, Goto T, Terui K, et al. Emergence agitation after sevoflurane versus propofol in pediatric patients. Anaesthesia & Analgesia 2000; 91(3): 563–566.

80. Heinz P, Geelhoed GC, Wee C, et al. Is atropine needed with ketamine sedation? A prospective, randomised, double blind study. Emergency Medicine Journal 2006; 23(3): 206–209.

81. Bovill J, Coppel D, Dundee J. Current status of ketamine anaesthesia. Lancet 1971; 297: 1285–1288.

82. Coppel D, Bovill J, Dundee J. The taming of ketamine. Anaesthesia 1973; 28: 293–296.

83. Cartwright P, Pingel S. Midazolam and diazepam in ketamine anaesthesia. Anaesthesia 1984; 39: 439–442.

84. White P, Way W, Trevor A. Ketamine – its pharmacology and therapeutic uses. Anesthesiology 1982; 56: 119–136.

85. Wathen JE, Roback MG, Mackenzie T, et al. Does midazolam alter the clinical effects of intravenous ketamine sedation in children? A double-blind, randomized, controlled, emergency department trial. Annals of Emergency Medicine 2000; 36(6): 579–588.

86. Clinical policy for procedural sedation and analgesia in the emergency department. American College of Emergency Physicians. Annals of Emergency Medicine 1998; 31(5): 663–677.

87. Sherwin TS, Green SM, Khan A, et al. Does adjunctive midazolam reduce recovery agitation after ketamine sedation for pediatric procedures? A randomized, double-blind, placebo-controlled trial. Annals of Emergency Medicine 2000; 35(3): 229–238.

88. Roelofse J, Joubert J, Roelofse G. A double blind randomised comparison of midazolam alone and midazolam combined with ketamine for sedation of pediatric dental patients. Journal of Oral Maxillofacial Surgery 1996; 54: 838–844.

89. Davies FC, Waters M. Oral midazolam for conscious sedation of children during minor procedures. Journal of Accident and Emergency Medicine 1998; 15(4): 244–248.

90. Massanari M, Novitsky J, Reinstein L. Paradoxical reactions in children associated with midazolam use during endoscopy. Clinical Pediatrics 1997; 36: 681–684.

91. Loh G, Dalen D. Low-dose ketamine in addition to propofol for procedural sedation and analgesia in the emergency department. Annals of Pharmacotherapy 2007; 41(3): 485–492.

92. Willman EV, Andolfatto G. A prospective evaluation of 'ketofol' (ketamine/propofol combination) for procedural sedation and analgesia in the emergency department. Annals of Emergency Medicine 2007; 49(1): 23–30.

93. Habibi S, Coursin D. Assessment of sedation, analgesia, and neuromuscular blockade in the perioperative period. International Anesthesiology Clinics 1996; 34: 215–241.

94. Chernik D, Gillings D, Laine H, et al. Validity and reliability of the observer's assessment of alertness/sedation scale: study with intravenous midazolam. Journal of Clinical Psychopharmacology 1990; 10: 244–251.

95. Fatovich DM, Gope M, Paech MJ. A pilot trial of BIS monitoring for procedural sedation in the emergency department. Emergency Medicine Australasia 2004; 16(2): 103–107.

96. Overly FL, Wright RO, Connor FA, et al. Bispectral analysis during pediatric procedural sedation. Pediatric Emergency Care 2005; 21(1): 6–11.

97. Gill M, Green SM, Krauss B. A study of the bispectral index monitor during procedural sedation and analgesia in the emergency department. Annals of Emergency Medicine 2003; 41(2): 234–241.

98. Agrawal D, Feldman HA, Krauss B, et al. Bispectral index monitoring quantifies depth of sedation during emergency department procedural sedation and analgesia in children. Annals of Emergency Medicine 2004; 43(2): 247–255.

99. American Society of Anesthesiologists Task Force on Intraoperative Awareness. Practice Advisory for Intraoperative Awareness and brain function monitoring. Anesthesiology 2006; 104: 847–864.

100. Burton JH, Harrah JD, Germann CA. Does end-tidal carbon dioxide monitoring detect respiratory events prior to current sedation monitoring practices? Academic Emergency Medicine 2006; 13(5): 500–504.

101. Anderson JL, Junkins E, Pribble C, et al. Capnography and depth of sedation during propofol sedation in children. Annals of Emergency Medicine 2007; 49(1): 9–13.

102. Deitch K, Chudnofsky CR, Dominici P. The utility of supplemental oxygen during emergency department procedural sedation and analgesia with midazolam and fentanyl: a randomized, controlled trial. Annals of Emergency Medicine 2007; 49(1): 1–8.

103. McQuillen KK, Steele DW. Capnography during sedation/analgesia in the pediatric emergency department. Pediatric Emergency Care 2000; 16(6): 401–404.

104. Newman DH, Azer MM, Pitetti RD, et al. When is a patient safe for discharge after procedural sedation? The timing of adverse effect events in 1367 pediatric procedural sedations. Annals of Emergency Medicine 2003; 42(5): 627–635.

105. Holger J, Satterlee P, Haugen S. Nursing use between 2 methods of procedural sedation: midazolam versus propofol. American Journal of Emergency Medicine 2005; 23: 248–252.

106. Miner JR, Krauss B. Procedural sedation and analgesia research: state of the art. Academic Emergency Medicine 2007; 14(2): 170–178.

107. MacLean S, Obispo J, Young KD. The gap between pediatric emergency department procedural pain management treatments available and actual practice. Pediatric Emergency Care 2007; 23(2): 87–93.

108. Paris PM, Yealy DM. A procedural sedation and analgesia fasting consensus advisory: one small step for emergency medicine, one giant challenge remaining. Annals of Emergency Medicine 2007; 49(4): 465–467.

109. Cote CJ, Notterman DA, Karl HW, et al. Adverse sedation events in pediatrics: a critical incident analysis of contributing factors. Pediatrics 2000; 105(4 Pt 1): 805–814.

110. Priestley S, Babl FE, Krieser D, et al. Evaluation of the impact of a paediatric procedural sedation credentialing programme on quality of care. Emergency Medicine Australasia 2006; 18(5–6): 498–504.

111. Babl F, Priestley S, Krieser D, et al. Development and implementation of an education and credentialing programme to provide safe paediatric procedural sedation in emergency departments. Emergency Medicine Australasia 2006; 18(5–6): 489–497.

23.1 Emergency department ultrasound

Andrew Haig • Adrian Goudie

ESSENTIALS

1 Ultrasound examination, interpretation and clinical correlation should be available in a timely manner 24 h a day for emergency department patients.

2 Emergency physicians providing emergency ultrasound services should possess appropriate training and hands-on experience to perform and interpret limited bedside ultrasound imaging.

3 Ultrasound imaging by emergency physicians is useful for at least the following clinical indications: traumatic haemoperitoneum, abdominal aortic aneurysm, pericardial fluid, ectopic pregnancy, vascular access, therapeutic diagnostic tests and evaluation of renal and biliary tract disease.

4 Continued research is required in the area of ultrasound imaging and any other known or evolving bedside imaging techniques and modalities.

5 Emergency medicine training programmes should provide instruction and experience in bedside ultrasound imaging for their trainees.

6 The Australasian College for Emergency Medicine supports the use of bedside ultrasound by emergency physicians, as does the American College of Emergency Physicians and the College of Emergency Medicine in the UK.

Background

Clinical ultrasound followed developments in the use of sonar, where the principle that sound waves could be used to locate objects was developed. Initially ultrasound machines were large and cumbersome, but advances in technology have improved image quality while reducing machine size, so that today small machines are able to produce high-quality images. As a result of this improved technology, ultrasound is now available to clinicians and can be performed at the bedside of patients. Although clinician-performed ultrasound has occurred in Europe and Japan for many years, and in the field of obstetrics and gynaecology worldwide, it is a relatively new development in Australasia in emergency departments (EDs).

Clinician-performed ultrasound has a different approach to formal diagnostic ultrasound, such as that performed in radiology departments. Clinician-performed ultrasound is generally limited in scope and targeted to answering a specific question (such as 'Is there an abdominal aortic aneurysm?'), rather than providing a full assessment of an anatomical area. In this regard, it is often viewed more as an extension of the clinical examination than a technique that competes with other imaging techniques (including formal ultrasound).

The Australasian College for Emergency Medicine supports the use of bedside ultrasound by emergency physicians,[1] as does the American College of Emergency Physicians and the College of Emergency Medicine in the UK.[2,3] It is expected that with increasing experience the range of conditions for which ultrasound is used in the ED will increase.

Basic physics of ultrasound

Sound waves are mechanical waves that transmit energy through the vibration of particles. Ultrasound waves are defined as those that are above the usual range of human hearing (20–20 000 Hz). Current diagnostic ultrasound machines are based on the pulse–echo principle, using pulses of sound waves at frequencies of 2–15 MHz that are reflected back. Processing of these reflected echoes creates the ultrasound data and image.[4]

The ultrasound transducer converts electrical impulses into pulses of sound (via the piezo-electrical effect) which are then directed into the body. As the sound wave travels through tissue, it gradually loses energy, termed 'attenuation'. The degree of attenuation differs for different tissues and is also dependent on the frequency of the pulse wave. On reaching a tissue interface, some of the energy is reflected back as an echo, due to the differences in acoustic impedance (gel or other coupling material is used to minimize reflection at the probe/skin surface). This reflected echo then travels back through tissue, undergoing further attenuation, until it reaches the transducer, which converts the energy back to an electrical impulse, which is then amplified and processed. The time taken for the pulse wave to travel to the tissue interface and back is converted into distance using the average speed for sound in tissue. The intensity of the returning wave determines the brightness of the displayed pixel. The returning pulses from the different reflecting surfaces along the path of the ultrasound beam generate a single line of the ultrasound image. The ultrasound beam is steered across the field to generate the multiple lines of information that then form the two-dimensional image (termed 'B mode', for brightness modulation). Alternatively, if the direction of the beam is kept constant and the changing surfaces are mapped over time then an M mode image is generated.

The degree of attenuation is dependent on the frequency of the sound wave, so higher frequency pulses undergo greater attenuation. They also have shorter wavelengths, which improves the resolution of the ultrasound beam (the ability to distinguish two separate objects close together). This leads to one of the most important trade-offs in ultrasound, between resolution and penetration. To obtain high resolution, a high frequency probe can be chosen, but this will be unable to image deep structures.

To form the image, the ultrasound machine makes certain assumptions about the ultrasound beam and sound impulse. Deviations from these behaviours will result in image artefacts, i.e. when the image does not represent the tissue accurately. There are many artefacts, most of which reduce the information available from the image. The most clinically important artefacts, shadowing and enhancement, can also be used diagnostically.

Shadowing occurs when all of the energy of the ultrasound pulse is reflected at a surface (such as air or bone) and there will then be no returning pulses from the tissue distal to the object. This creates a black area on the screen, known as an acoustic shadow. The presence of a shadow behind a brightly reflective surface can thus be used to diagnose a region of calcification, such as a calculus (Fig. 23.1.1). Stones and bones generally give clean shadows, while gas gives 'dirty' or grey shadows due to the superposition of both shadow and reverberation artefact (Fig. 23.1.2).

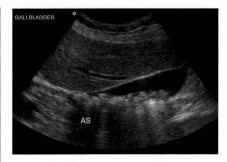

Fig. 23.1.1 Acoustic shadowing from gallstones. AS, acoustic shadow.

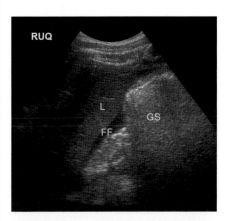

Fig. 23.1.2 Acoustic shadowing from bowel gas in a patient with free fluid. L, liver; FF, free fluid; GS, gas shadow.

Enhancement occurs when an area (such as fluid in a cyst) absorbs less energy than usual. This means that the pulses that have travelled through that area will have more energy, resulting in a bright region behind the image (Fig. 23.1.3). Enhancement is used to confirm the fluid filled nature of lesions.

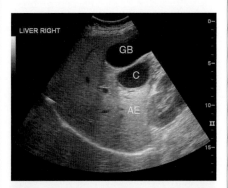

Fig. 23.1.3 Acoustic enhancement from fluid-filled structures. Acoustic enhancement is seen where the ultrasound beam passes through the gallbladder and more prominently where it passes through the gallbladder and pancreatic pseudocyst. GB, gallbladder; C, pancreatic pseudocyst; AE, acoustic enhancement.

Transducers

Different ultrasound transducers are available varying in frequency, the size of the contact area (termed 'footprint') and shape. Transducers may have a small footprint to fit into small areas, such as between ribs, from which the beam spreads in a large arc (e.g. a sector transducer). Alternatively, they may be larger with a flat or slightly curved surface where contact can be maintained, such as a linear probe. Special transducers have been designed for use within body cavities, such as transoesophageal, endovaginal and endo-anal probes. These transducers offer the advantage of reduced distance between the transducer and area of interest, which allows higher frequencies to be used, resulting in improved resolution. Very high frequency transducers have been used for intravascular and superficial ocular scanning.[5,6] The appropriate choice of transducer is important in ensuring the optimal image is obtained.

The scope of emergency department ultrasound

Current indications for emergency ultrasound are given in Table 23.1.1.

Focused assessment by sonography for trauma (FAST)

Descriptions of the use of ultrasound by clinicians to evaluate trauma patients appeared in the European literature in the 1970s.[7] Reports have subsequently appeared from countries around the world[8] and the technique is now well established. With relatively

Table 23.1.1 Current indications for emergency ultrasound
Trauma (haemoperitoneum, haemopericardium, pneumothorax)
Abdominal aortic aneurysm
Early pregnancy complications
Biliary disease
Renal stones and hydronephrosis
Echocardiography in trauma and shock
Proximal deep vein thrombossi exclusion
Procedural
Musculoskeletal

brief training and experience, non-radiologists are able to diagnose haemoperitoneum with a high degree of sensitivity and specificity, although accuracy does improve with experience.[9,10]

Clinical examination in abdominal trauma can be difficult and unreliable.[11] Diagnostic peritoneal lavage (DPL), ultrasound (FAST) and computerized tomography (CT) have been used to further evaluate this group of patients. In most cases, FAST has replaced diagnostic peritoneal lavage as it is non-invasive and does not interfere with subsequent interpretation of CT images. CT scanning is highly accurate for diagnosing both free fluid and solid organ injury, although it is less accurate for hollow viscus and diaphragmatic injury.[11]

Studies of ultrasound scanning in trauma have reported varying sensitivity.[12] Much of this variation is due to differences in the gold standard used for comparison and the definition of 'true positive'. Haematoperitoneum (on further imaging, surgical or post-mortem examination), organ injury and clinical stability have all been used in different studies.[9,12–15] It must be remembered that the primary role of a FAST scan is to detect free fluid in the peritoneal or pericardial spaces, for which it has high sensitivity and specificity.[12,16] Solid organ or retroperitoneal haemorrhage may be detected, but even in expert hands the accuracy is much lower (with as many as two-thirds of injuries being missed).[14,15,17] FAST has been shown to be reliable and useful in both pregnant[18] and paediatric[19] patients.

Technique

FAST scanning evaluates four regions for the presence of free fluid: (1) pericardial, (2) perihepatic, (3) perisplenic and (4) pelvic[8] (Fig 23.1.4). Some authors extend the FAST examination to include examining the pleural spaces postero-laterally for fluid, and anteriorly to exclude pneumothorax.[20] The technique is rapid, generally being completed in under 5 min.[12]

Free fluid appears as an echolucent area (i.e. black) that is generally linear or triangular in shape in the most dependent area of the peritoneal or pericardial space, although blood clots may be seen as echogenic (grey) collections[14] (Figs 23.1.5, 23.1.6, 23.1.7). While fluid is most commonly seen in the perihepatic space, all spaces should be examined before the result can be considered

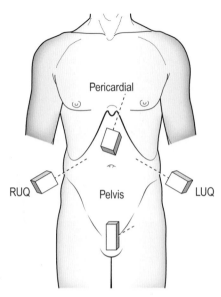

Fig. 23.1.4 Transducer placement for the four views for fast scanning. RUQ, right upper quadrant; LUQ, left upper quadrant.

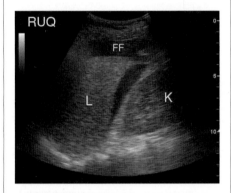

Fig. 23.1.5 Free fluid in the perihepatic view. RUQ, right upper quadrant, L, liver; FF, free fluid; K, kidney.

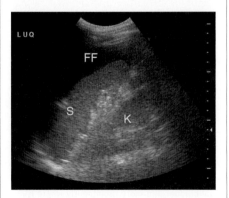

Fig. 23.1.6 Free fluid in the perisplenic view. LUQ, left upper quadrant; S, spleen; FF, free fluid; K, kidney.

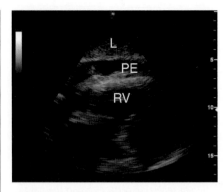

Fig. 23.1.7 Pericardial effusion with clot. L, liver; RV, right ventricle; PE, pericardial effusion with grey blood clots and black (echofree) blood.

negative.[12] Small amounts of fluid (<500 mL) may not be detected.[12]

Limitations and pitfalls[12–14,16]

- User dependent with learning curve.
- Inadequate views occur in up to 10%, especially if the bladder is empty or with subcutaneous emphysema.
- Cannot distinguish between blood and other forms of intra-abdominal or pericardial fluid such as ascites or pericardial effusion.
- Retroperitoneal haemorrhage may be missed.
- Solid organ, hollow viscus or diaphragmatic injuries can occur without free fluid.
- Small amounts of free fluid may not be detected.
- Small amounts of pelvic fluid may be physiological in women.
- Fluid-filled bowel can be misinterpreted as free fluid.
- Pericardial fluid may decompress into the pleural cavity.

Clinical implications and utility[8,12,21–23]

The limitations of ultrasound in excluding all intra-abdominal injuries requiring laparotomy and the increasing use of conservative management of some injuries, even in the setting of intra-abdominal free fluid, have resulted in there being no universally accepted clinical algorithm based on FAST scan results. However, in this regard FAST scanning is no different to any other clinical, laboratory or imaging information about the trauma patient, the results of which

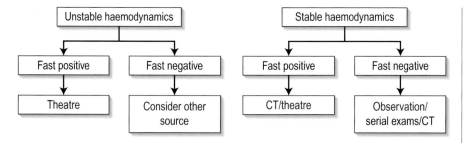

Fig. 23.1.8 Suggested algorithm using FAST results. CT, computerized tomography.

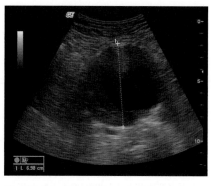

Fig. 23.1.9 Abdominal aortic aneurysm.

are routinely used in combination to determine the management plan. Various algorithms incorporating FAST scanning have been proposed, which generally incorporate haemodynamic stability and FAST scan result, such as in Figure 23.1.8. Some algorithms incorporate a semi-quantitative scoring system to estimate amount of free fluid, with an increased volume of free fluid associated with greater need for therapeutic laparotomy. A positive FAST scan is highly predictive of significant intra-abdominal injury and, based on the clinical condition of the patient, generally indicates the need for CT or surgical exploration. A negative FAST scan, stable haemodynamics and clinical observation have been shown to be highly accurate in excluding significant intra-abdominal injury. Some authors advocate serial FAST examinations in stable patients, suggesting this can reduce the requirement for CT.

In the Australasian setting, FAST is generally accepted as fulfilling a complementary role to CT. Its portability and speed allow it to be used early in the evaluation of trauma patients (e.g. immediately after the primary survey) and this information is then incorporated with other clinical information to risk stratify the trauma patient to help to determine the requirement and timing for either laparotomy or CT. Repeated examinations, particularly if the patient's condition changes, can be valuable. Providing the limitations of the technique are not ignored, it can rapidly provide vital information to assist with patient management.

Abdominal aortic aneurysm

Abdominal aortic aneurysms (AAA), defined as an aortic diameter >3.0 cm, are common, occurring in between 1 and 9% of the population.[24] Clinical assessment of the abdominal aorta is unreliable,[24] and may

be especially difficult in the obese or unstable patient with abdominal pain. Clinical presentation of ruptured abdominal aortic aneurysm can be varied, with only 50% of patients describing the classic presentation of hypotension, back pain and pulsatile mass. Other presentations may include haematuria, abdominal or flank pain, unexplained hypotension, syncope or cardiac failure,[25,26] and AAA should be considered in any of these presentations.

Ultrasound is the primary mode of investigation of the abdominal aorta.[24] Ultrasound performed by emergency clinicians has been shown to be rapid, highly sensitive and highly specific (>95%) in assessing aortic diameter.[27,28] Ultrasound may occasionally detect rupture, but it is not reliable in excluding rupture. In addition to its utility in diagnosing AAA, ED ultrasound is very beneficial in rapidly excluding AAA in the wide variety of presentations listed above.

The risk of rupture of an AAA increases with diameter. Although the risk of rupture if the aneurysm diameter is less than 4 cm is <0.5% per year and 1.5% per year for aneurysms of 4.0–4.9 cm, rupture can still occur.[29,30] Approximately 10% of ruptured aneurysms measure 5 cm or less.[30]

Technique

The aorta should be identified anterior to the vertebral body and to the left of the inferior vena cava (IVC). It should be followed from the epigastric region to its bifurcation, just above the umbilicus, remembering that in elderly patients it may follow an ectactic course rather than following a strictly cranial-caudal course. It must be distinguished from both the superior mesenteric artery (SMA) (which runs anterior to the aorta) and the IVC (ensuring that the venous pulsation of the IVC is not

mistaken for the arterial pulse of the aorta). Measurements should be taken both proximally and distally and, if an aneurysm is present, at the widest point. Measurements from both transverse and longitudinal planes should be taken. Measurements are taken from the outer wall to outer wall, including any mural thrombus (see Fig. 23.1.9). If the renal arteries or SMA origin are identifiable then the relation to the aneurysm should be noted, although in the ED setting this may not be possible. Any periaortic haematoma or peritoneal free fluid should be noted.

Limitations and pitfalls

- Pain or bowel gas may prevent adequate imaging by ultrasound.
- Mistaking the IVC or SMA for the aorta.
- Measuring the lumen without including mural thrombus.
- Attempting to exclude rupture on ultrasound.
- Forgetting that the AAA may be an incidental finding and not the primary cause of the patient's symptoms.

Clinical implications and utility

In the patient with ruptured AAA who is haemodynamically unstable, ED ultrasound allows rapid and accurate diagnosis within the resuscitation area. Rapid diagnosis of these patients is essential to achieve successful treatment. In the stable patient, whose presentation may be atypical, ED ultrasound provides a rapid means of excluding the diagnosis (for example in the elderly patient who presents with 'renal colic'). If an AAA is detected in these patients then further imaging will often be required to determine if the AAA is an incidental finding or the cause of the patient's symptoms. If the

AAA is an incidental finding then formal follow-up should be arranged.

Early pregnancy

Ultrasound is the primary imaging modality for early pregnancy and its complications.[31] In the ED setting, it is most commonly used for the pregnant patient with pain or bleeding. In addition to transabdominal scanning (TAS), transvaginal scanning (TVS) can be performed with patient consent using a specifically designed probe which places the transducer close to the pelvic organs and utilizes higher frequencies to produce images of much higher detail than TAS. It does not require a full bladder and should not be a painful procedure. TAS still has an important role, as it allows a broader field of view that allows better assessment of large amounts of free intraperitoneal fluid and may diagnose other causes of pain. Emergency physician-performed ultrasound for early pregnancy complications has been shown to be safe and reduce the time patients spend in EDs.[32,33]

Technique

TAS is performed initially, preferably when the patient has a full bladder as the pelvic organs will be better visualized. The uterus is identified and examined in both longitudinal and transverse planes (recognizing that the longitudinal axis of the uterus may not necessarily be in a strictly sagittal plane). The endometrial thickness is noted and any fluid collections or gestational sac noted. The adnexa are examined to identify the ovaries and any masses. The pelvis is scanned for free fluid. The upper abdomen can be examined to estimate the volume of free fluid if seen. The kidneys can also be examined to identify any alternate diagnoses.

TVS is performed after the procedure has been explained and consent obtained. A chaperone should be present if the sonographer is male. The patient is asked to empty their bladder and, if possible, the pelvis is elevated slightly off the bed using a foam wedge or similar. The probe is covered with a sterile condom with gel placed inside and outside the condom. The probe is gently inserted into the vagina and advanced. The uterus and adnexa are then examined in both longitudinal and transverse planes as in TAS. After the scan is complete the probe must be cleaned and disinfected.

Limitations and pitfalls

- Confusing a corpus luteum cyst and ectopic pregnancy.
- Misinterpreting a pseudogestational sac for a gestational sac.
- Not considering heterotopic pregnancy in patients receiving fertility treatment.
- Failure to arrange follow-up if an intrauterine pregnancy is not identified, even if an ectopic pregnancy is not seen.
- Failure to recognize an eccentric or low gestational sac could be an interstitial, cervical or scar ectopics.

Clinical implications and utility

The primary aim of ultrasound in evaluating early pregnancy complications in the ED is to locate the gestational sac. Additional information should then be sought for the presence of free fluid, adnexal masses, fetal size and viability. The earliest ultrasound evidence of pregnancy is a small anechoic fluid collection surrounded by an echogenic ring, which can be seen on TVS at approximately 4.5 weeks. A pseudogestational sac (due to fluid within the endometrial cavity), however, can have very similar appearances. Definite signs that the sac is a true gestational sac appear at 5.5 weeks when the yolk sac can be visualized or later when the embryo can be identified.[34] A heartbeat may be visualized from 6.0 to 6.5 weeks onward. TAS will show the same features but 1 to 2 weeks later.

Quantitative human chorionic gonadotrophin (HCG) levels have been used to determine when a gestational sac should be identifiable by ultrasound, termed the 'discriminatory zone'. For TVS, this is usually 1500–2000 IU, and for TAS 4500 IU (varying between institutions and depending on expertise and equipment). Pregnancies that have HCG levels below these levels and are not identified by ultrasound are termed 'pregnancy of unknown location', and most will either fail (miscarry or resolve spontaneously) or progress to normal pregnancy. However, 9–43% will eventually be identified as ectopic pregnancies.[35] As such, they require close follow-up with serial HCG and repeat ultrasound. Ultrasound should still be performed if the HCG is below these levels as it may still show diagnostic findings.[33]

If an intrauterine pregnancy is confirmed, the risk of ectopic pregnancy is very low in spontaneous conceived pregnancies. Heterotopic pregnancy is where both an intrauterine and extrauterine pregnancy coexist, and occurs in up to 1:7000 pregnancies in spontaneous conceived pregnancies,[36] but over 1:100 pregnancies in the setting of fertility treatment.[37] Failure to visualize an intrauterine pregnancy may be due to early dates, failed pregnancy (including miscarriage) or ectopic pregnancy. Other ultrasound findings in ectopic pregnancy include non-specific findings such as pelvic blood and adnexal mass[38] (see Table 23.1.2). Visualization of a gestational sac (with yolk sac or embryo) outside the uterus is diagnostic, but seen only in 8–26% of ectopic pregnancies[31] (see Fig. 23.1.10).

Unusual forms of ectopic pregnancy include interstitial, cervical and scar ectopics. In these cases, a gestational sac may

Table 23.1.2 Ultrasound findings of ectopic pregnancy

Ultrasound finding	Accuracy (%)
Absent IUP	5
Any free fluid (no IUP)	50
Mod-large free fluid (no IUP)	60–85
Adnexal mass (no IUP)	75
Mass + free fluid (no IUP)	97
Ectopic pregnancy seen	100

IUP, intrauterine pregnancy.

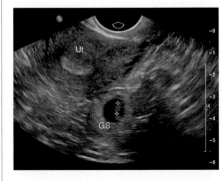

Fig. 23.1.10 Ectopic pregnancy. A gestational sac (GS) containing an embryonic pole is seen outside the uterus (Ut). Image courtesy of Ultrasound Department, King Edward Memorial Hospital, Perth, Australia.

be seen, but not within the uterine cavity. It is recommended that pregnancies that appear low or eccentric should be reviewed by experienced sonographers.

Distinguishing between miscarriage and ectopic pregnancy when no adnexal mass has been identified can be difficult on ultrasound. However, if the clinical symptoms have settled, no free fluid is identified on ultrasound and no adnexal masses have been identified, then it is safe to observe or discharge the patient for formal ultrasound review the following day and subsequent follow-up with repeat ultrasound and quantitative HCG (see Ch. 19.2).

If an intrauterine pregnancy is confirmed, the gestational age can be estimated by measuring the size of the embryo. Most machines will automatically calculate gestational age based on this measurement. Cardiac activity should be identified by TVS once the embryo is approximately 5 mm (9 mm by TAS). Absent cardiac activity when the embryo is above this size suggests fetal demise. Absent yolk sac or embryo on TVS when the gestational sac is 8 or 16 mm (20 and 25 mm, respectively, on TAS) suggests a blighted ovum.[34] Other sonographic signs of poor prognosis for continued pregnancy exist, but they are generally beyond the scope of emergency ultrasound.

RUQ/Gallbladder

Upper abdominal pain due to biliary disease is a common presenting complaint in the ED and includes biliary colic, cholecystitis and ascending cholangitis. Many of the patients suspected of having acute cholecystitis will have alternative diseases, and clinical examination is neither sufficiently sensitive nor specific for these patients.[39] Ultrasound is the primary imaging modality for these patients, where it is used to detect the presence of gallstones (Fig. 23.1.1), other sonographic signs of cholecystitis and bile duct obstruction. It is superior to both scintigraphy and CT for these patients.[40]

Ultrasound has a high sensitivity and specificity for the identification of stones when performed by either radiology or ED staff.[40–42] Some stones may, however, be missed and false positive results also occur.[43] The diagnosis of cholecystitis relies on the associated findings, including sonographic Murphy's sign, gallbladder wall thickening, gallbladder distension and pericholecystic fluid (Fig. 23.1.11). Gallbladder

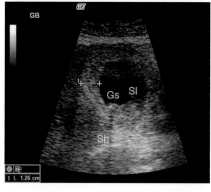

Fig. 23.1.11 Acute cholecystitis. Transverse image of a gallbladder with thickened wall. Within the lumen is a gallstone (Gs), which casts a shadow (Sh), and sludge (Sl), which does not.

wall thickening and pericholecystic fluid are both non-specific findings and may be seen in other hepatic or generalized diseases as well as in acalculous cholecystitis. Fasting can cause gallbladder distension. The common bile duct, if visualized, should be measured and examined for stones, although this is technically more difficult and may be beyond the scope of a focused gallbladder examination.

Technique

The gallbladder is usually identified by scanning under the costal margin in a longitudinal plane. Positioning the patient in the left lateral decubitus position and/or deep inspiration may assist. The gallbladder should be scanned throughout its length in both longitudinal and transverse planes. The sonographic Murphy's sign is assessed by pressing with the ultrasound probe over the gallbladder. Wall thickness should be measured in the transverse plane. Gallstones will appear as brightly echogenic masses with an acoustic shadow that are mobile (unless impacted in the neck or cystic duct). Care should be taken to examine the neck of the gallbladder and cystic duct carefully as stones may be missed in this location. Sludge and polyps will also appear echogenic but will not shadow. If seen, the common bile duct diameter should be measured.

Limitations and pitfalls

- Misinterpreting an incidental finding of gallstones as the cause of the patient's symptoms.
- Misinterpreting gas in the duodenum as gallstones in the gallbladder.

- A gallbladder that is contracted or full of stones can appear as an echogenic mass without any lumen, similar to duodenal gas.
- Stones in the neck or cystic duct may be missed.
- Small stones (<3 mm) may not cast shadows.
- Misinterpreting sludge or polyps as stones.
- Misinterpreting other causes of gallbladder wall thickening as cholecystitis.

Clinical implications and utility

In a patient with abdominal pain, the finding of gallstones with a positive sonographic Murphy's sign is strongly predictive of cholecystitis. The more sonographic signs of cholecystitis that are seen, the more likely the diagnosis. However, asymptomatic gallstones are common and may therefore represent an incidental finding, especially if the sonographic Murphy's sign is absent. In elderly, diabetic or critically ill patients, 5–10% of cholecystitis can be acalculous.[40] In those patients thought to have biliary colic or cholecystitis, a negative ultrasound should prompt a search for alternative diagnoses or consideration of further imaging, either formal ultrasound or, if an alternate diagnosis is believed likely, CT.

Renal ultrasound

The primary focus of renal ultrasound in the emergency setting is the detection of hydronephrosis in the presence of acute renal failure or renal colic.[44] In this context it is rapidly available to confirm or exclude the presence of obstruction.

Technique

The kidneys are paired retroperitoneal organs lying on either side of the spine between T12 and L4. They have a convex lateral border and a concave medial border and hilum. The normal adult kidney is 9–12 cm in length, 2.5–4 cm thick and 4–6 cm wide. The kidney itself is composed of two distinct areas, the renal parenchyma and the renal sinus.

The adult kidney is scanned using a curvilinear 3.5–5 MHz transducer and a renal pre-set that provides the best contrast resolution and grey map for imaging the kidneys. The patient may be supine, although the kidneys are usually best seen with the patient in a lateral decubitus position. A combination of subcostal and intercostal approaches is often necessary to fully evaluate the kidneys. The kidneys should be imaged in at least two planes, including the sagittal or coronal plane, and the transverse plane (Figs 23.1.12, 23.1.13 and 23.1.14). On ultrasound the kidney can be identified by its elliptical shape

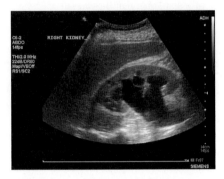

Fig. 23.1.12 Sagittal image of right kidney demonstrating moderate hydronephrosis.

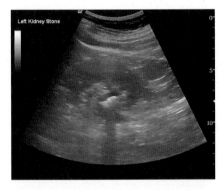

Fig. 23.1.13 Coronal image of left kidney demonstrating a calculus in the renal pelvis with acoustic shadowing.

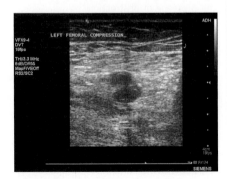

Fig. 23.1.14 Transverse image of the left femoral vein and artery with incomplete collapse of the femoral vein with compression indicating intraluminal thrombus.

with a thin brightly echogenic capsule. Normal renal parenchyma is slightly decreased or equal in echogenicity relative to the hepatic or splenic parenchyma, although this is age dependent, with it being comparatively hyperechoic in the elderly. The central renal sinus is echodense due to the fat and fibrous tissue content. The renal pelvis and infundibulum are usually collapsed and not seen except in the setting of hydronephrosis, when they become filled with urine, appearing anechoic. The bladder should be full and examined in both the sagittal and transverse planes to complete the study. It should be noted that an excessively full bladder may cause mild dilatation of the pelvicalyceal system, but this will return to normal following micturition.

Hydronephrosis is the dilatation of the renal pelvis and calyces and may be secondary to an anatomical obstruction or may be functional in nature (such as with ureteric reflux). Obstructive hydronephrosis may be intrinsic or extrinsic. Depending on the level of obstruction it may be unilateral or bilateral with or without associated hydroureter. When hydronephrosis is identified, the cause for the obstruction should be sought. Common intrinsic obstructive causes seen in the ED include obstructive or partially obstructive renal or ureteric calculi, and bladder outlet obstruction due to prostatic hypertrophy. Extrinsic masses in the pelvis should also be considered.

Hydronephrosis may be described as mild, moderate or severe depending on the extent of dilatation of the renal collecting system:

Mild: dilatation limited to the renal pelvis

Moderate: dilatation extending into the pelvicalyceal system with splitting and distension of the calyces

Severe: marked pelvicalyceal dilatation with clubbed calyces and associated cortical thinning.

Limitations and pitfalls

- Assuming hydronephrosis and obstruction are synonymous.
- Evaluation before hydronephrosis has had time to develop, particularly in the dehydrated patient.
- Not recognizing that hydronephrosis can persist after obstruction is relieved.
- Mistaking an extra-renal pelvis for hydronephrosis.
- Mistaking parapelvic renal cysts for hydronephrosis.

Clinical implications and utility

Whilst ultrasound is less sensitive than plain films and CT in detecting renal calculi as small stones may often be obscured by the echogenic renal sinus and be hard to detect if they have a weak posterior acoustic shadow, stones in the kidney that are greater than 5 mm in size have been shown to be detected with 100% sensitivity sonographically.[45] Renal stones appear as bright echogenic foci with sharp distal acoustic shadowing. Ureteric calculi are far more difficult to visualize due to the retroperitoneal position of the ureters being obscured by overlying bowel. A normal-appearing kidney and the failure to visualize a calculus therefore does not exclude a ureteric calculus that is non-obstructing or where hydronephrosis has not yet developed.

Deep vein thrombosis

The primary focus of ED ultrasound in the assessment of deep vein thrombosis (DVT) is in the diagnosis or exclusion of a proximal lower limb DVT.

The clinical assessment of DVT is unreliable and inaccurate.[46,47] Positive findings on sonographic examination of only 11% have been reported for patients referred for suspected acute DVT on the basis of clinical features.[48]

Technique

Ultrasound is the imaging modality of choice for assessing for DVT. The technique relies primarily on grey-scale imaging with intermittent venous compression, with the main diagnostic criteria used to exclude a DVT being complete collapse of the vein with apposition of the anterior and posterior walls of the vessel.

A broadband linear array transducer with a centre frequency of about 5 MHz is used to examine the femoral, popliteal and calf veins. In larger patients the curved linear array transducer with a centre frequency of 3.5 MHz (as used for abdominal studies) may be substituted. The curved linear array transducer is also used to examine the iliac veins. The machine should be configured to use the lower limb venous pre-set and the use of harmonic imaging may improve the contrast resolution between the vessel and surrounding tissue. Transducer compression of the interrogated vessel should be in the transverse imaging plane. Starting at the level of the groin, with the patient in a supine position, the common femoral vein is identified lying medial to the common femoral artery and the vein is compressed to demonstrate patency extending distally in a stepwise fashion and the vein compressed every 2–3 cm. The popliteal vein is best examined with the patient in a lateral or prone position with the knee slightly flexed. Colour and spectral Doppler may be used to supplement the findings from intermittent compression. Emergency physicians who had undergone standardized training to identify clots in the femoral or popliteal veins have shown an accuracy comparable to formal vascular studies.[49]

Limitations and pitfalls
- Mistaking the saphenous vein for the superficial femoral vein.
- Not recognizing that the superficial femoral vein is a deep vein.
- Sensitivity of ultrasound for calf DVT detection is much lower than proximal DVT.
- Not recognizing a duplicated popliteal vein with one patent and one thrombosed.
- Misdiagnosing a chronic clot for a fresh clot.

Clinical implications and utility
The accuracy of compression ultrasonography is highest in symptomatic patients, with studies comparing venography with compression ultrasound demonstrating an average sensitivity of 95% and specificity of 98%.[50] For proximal lower limb DVT this technique has demonstrated sensitivity of up to 100%.[51] The use of colour and spectral Doppler to assess for vessel filling defects and flow patterns has not been shown to significantly increase the sensitivity for proximal DVT detection in the lower limb.[51–54] It has also been suggested that an abbreviated technique, using only two compression points (the saphenofemoral junction and the lower popliteal vein), has adequate sensitivity, provided repeat examination is performed in 5–7 days.[53,55,56] The accuracy of ultrasound in detecting isolated calf DVT, especially when applied to bedside emergency ultrasound, is low, with success rates as low as 40% reported.[57]

Thus, the aim of focused ED ultrasound in the assessment of DVT is generally to confirm or exclude the presence of a clot in the proximal deep veins of the lower limb. A negative compression ultrasound study of the proximal lower limb significantly reduces the likelihood of DVT and discharge from the ED without anticoagulation with outpatient follow-up for a definitive study can be considered.[50,58–60]

Emergency echocardiography

Focused use of echocardiography in the ED represents one of the most valuable uses of ultrasound in emergency medicine. Applications include its use in cardiac arrest, undifferentiated hypotension, suspected pericardial effusion and tamponade, chest pain, pulmonary embolus and ultrasound guided procedures. The use of cardiac ultrasound in emergency medicine is likely to increase significantly as more emergency physicians learn the technique and look to apply it increasingly in the clinical environment.

Echocardiography provides direct structural and functional information on cardiac structures only inferred by clinical examination, which has been shown to have limited accuracy, and with greater sensitivity and specificity than indirect tests such as electrocardiogram (ECG) and chest radiograph.[61–63]

Technique
Modern general ultrasound machines can provide good quality transthoracic echocardiography capability. A broadband phased array transducer with a centre frequency of 3.5 MHz and a small footprint to improve access between the ribs should be used. Standard echocardiographic windows and views are described. These include the parasternal long- and short-axis views obtained at the left sternal edge in the second to fourth rib spaces, the apical four-, five-, three- and two-chamber views that are obtained at the cardiac apex, and the subcostal views obtained from a sub-xiphoid position. The standard examination involves a two-dimensional assessment of cardiac structure and function using B mode supplemented by the use of colour and spectral Doppler to assess valvular function and measure transvalvular pressure gradients using the windows described above.

Emergency physicians have been shown to be accurate in assessing left ventricular function in the hypotensive patient.[64]

Limitations and pitfalls
- Good views may not be obtainable in a supine patient, especially if ventilated.
- Confusing pleural and pericardial effusions.
- Cannot exclude pulmonary embolism (PE).
- Difficult to distinguish acute pulmonary hypertension from PE and chronic pulmonary hypertension.

Clinical indications and utility
In cardiac arrest the aim of echocardiography is to assess left ventricular activity. In the setting of cardiac arrest, cardiac standstill on initial presenting echocardiographic assessment has important prognostic implications, irrespective of presenting electrical rhythm. Blaivas et al. demonstrated that no patients out of 136 presenting with cardiac standstill on initial echocardiographic assessment survived to leave the ED irrespective of presenting rhythm, findings supported by Salen et al. in a study of 102 patients presenting in cardiac arrest.[65,66]

Echocardiography is very useful in determining the cause of undifferentiated hypotension and shock. The primary aim of focused emergency echocardiography in this setting is to assess left ventricular systolic function and differentiate between a primary cardiac and a non-cardiac aetiology. In shock due to hypovolaemia, echocardiography demonstrates a small left ventricular end-systolic volume with hyperdynamic left ventricular motion. Conversely, if the cause of the shock is primarily cardiac, then echocardiography may demonstrate a dilated left ventricle and/or atrium with hypokinesis, akinesis or dyskinesis of the left ventricle wall or wall segments.

A pericardial effusion is seen as an anechoic collection of fluid between the visceral and parietal pericardium (Fig. 23.1.15), although an inflammatory pericardial effusion or haemopericardium may exhibit internal echoes. In differentiating between a pericardial effusion and a pleural effusion, a pericardial effusion tapers towards the descending aorta and may extend a short distance between the aorta and left atrium,

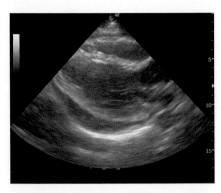

Fig. 23.1.15 Parasternal long-axis view of the heart demonstrating a moderately sized pericardial effusion.

whereas a pleural effusion will accumulate and extend behind the descending aorta. When a pericardial effusion is identified, its location and size should be documented and any evidence of tamponade looked for. The size of an effusion can be described as small, moderate or large. A small effusion is equal to 1 cm in thickness and may be localized. A moderately sized effusion is between 1 and 2 cm and is generally circumferential unless loculated. A large effusion is described as being >2 cm. In a group of 515 patients at high risk for pericardial effusions (103 of whom had pericardial effusions) emergency physicians were able to detect an effusion with an overall sensitivity of 96%, specificity of 98% and accuracy of 97%.[67]

The risk of tamponade is more a function of the rate of accumulation than total volume. The echocardiographic diagnosis of tamponade is more difficult and controversial. The most frequently used echocardiographic finding to support a diagnosis of tamponade is collapse of the right heart chambers during mid-to-late diastole and specifically right ventricular diastolic collapse. This can be difficult to appreciate and may be more easily appreciated using M-mode through the right ventricular free wall and timing the collapse with the ECG. However, pericardial tamponade remains a clinical diagnosis, and in a patient with a known pericardial effusion the focus of emergency echocardiography in this setting remains the identification of the pericardial effusion that can then be interpreted in the clinical context.

In the patient with chest pain due to acute coronary syndrome echocardiography is more sensitive than ECG for acute cardiac ischaemia. Focal wall motion abnormalities occur within a couple of minutes of the onset of ischaemia. When two-dimensional echocardiography is performed on patients with possible ischaemic chest pain and no focal wall motion abnormality is detected, myocardial infarction or ischaemia is very unlikely. However, the detection of focal wall motion abnormalities requires high levels of training and experience, and is likely to remain outside of the practice of emergency medicine physicians.

Transthoracic echocardiography lacks sensitivity for diagnosing PE. Echocardiography missed 16 out of 39 patients presenting to an ED with PE diagnosed by other modalities in a prospective observational study.[68] However, there are echocardiographic features associated with PE that when identified and put into clinical context can be highly suggestive or diagnostic. These include right ventricular dysfunction or dilatation, paradoxical septal motion, acute tricuspid regurgitation and the presence of a clot in the right heart. Whilst echocardiography may be a poor tool for diagnosing PE it may be useful in assessing right ventricle (RV) function caused by PE and may have a role in risk stratifying patients and influencing the decision to use thrombolytic therapy. RV dysfunction is associated with a significantly higher mortality,[69] and thrombolysis may be considered in this setting, although the specific criteria for the use of thrombolytic therapy to treat PE remain controversial.

Ultrasound guided vascular access

Traditionally, central venous access has been secured using the landmark technique, where surface anatomical features are used to predict the location of the internal jugular, subclavian and femoral veins. However, access using this technique has been associated with a 20% failure rate and a 10% complication rate, including inadvertent arterial puncture, excessive bleeding, vessel laceration, pneumothorax and haemothorax.[70,71] Improved success rates and decreased complication rates have been described using ultrasound-guided central venous access, including reduction in needle puncture time, increased overall success, reduction in carotid puncture, reduction in pneumothorax and a reduction in catheter related infection.[72,73] National guidelines from the UK[74] and the USA[75] support the use of ultrasound guidance for central venous catheter placement.

Ultrasound guidance can also be useful in aiding peripheral vascular access. The basilic and cephalic veins are frequently not visible but are readily cannulated using ultrasound guidance. Basilic vein cannulation has been shown to be very successful in the ED setting in patients in whom other peripheral access was difficult.[76]

Technique

A medium to high frequency broad bandwidth linear array transducer with a centre frequency of 7.5–10 MHz is used with a sterile cover. The pre-set that best visualizes the needle should be chosen for the machine, usually breast or musculoskeletal. Patient preparation is as per the landmark technique. Two techniques have been described. The static technique is used to locate the vessel, its location, dimensions and depth below the skin. The vessel is then centred on the screen and the skin marked at the centre of the transducer that corresponds to the vessel's subcutaneous position. This mark is then used for the puncture site without ultrasound visualization of the needle as it enters the vessel. The dynamic technique uses real-time ultrasound guidance visualizing the needle tip as it enters the vessel. Higher success rates have been demonstrated with the dynamic technique than with the static technique.[77]

Both transverse and longitudinal transducer orientation relative to the vessel have been described. The transverse orientation is an easier footprint to obtain and provides information related to adjacent structures, but the needle tip is less clearly seen. The longitudinal orientation is a more difficult footprint to obtain but provides information related to vessel orientation and slope and provides visualization of the needle tip as it enters the vessel.

Ultrasound-guided central vascular access should become an expected standard of care and should be included as part of the training curriculum for emergency medicine.

Miscellaneous applications

Scrotal ultrasound

Patients may present to the ED with scrotal or testicular pain, a scrotal mass or following scrotal trauma. Acute scrotal pain in the absence of trauma may be due to testicular torsion or epididymo-orchitis. Scrotal swelling may be due to hydronephrosis, hernia or testicular mass. Scrotal trauma may be associated with testicular rupture and associated testicular ischaemia. Ultrasound is the imaging modality of choice for assessing for testicular pathology and injury. The scrotum is examined using a high resolution linear array transducer with the patient in a supine position with the scrotum supported by a towel between the patient's legs. In testicular torsion the testis rotates on its axis, leading to twisting of the spermatic cord with compromise of both venous drainage and arterial supply. To diagnose torsion it is important to demonstrate normal flow within the normal testis and absent flow in the affected side.[78] However, it should be noted that flow may be very difficult to identify in normal paediatric testes and with intermittent torsion–detorsion blood flow may appear normal or even increased in the affected testis.

Epididymo-orchitis is the most common cause of scrotal pain in postpubertal men. Sonographically the epididymis is characteristically thickened with increased blood flow demonstrated with colour Doppler in the epididymis or testis or both. A reactive hydrocele is common.

Appendicitis

Misdiagnosis of appendicitis on clinical assessment is associated with a negative appendectomy rate of 15%, with rates as high as 40–50% reported in some series.[79] Delays in intervention can result in appendiceal perforation with associated increased morbidity and mortality.[80] The aim in assessing a patient with clinically suspected appendicitis is to adequately identify the appendix to confirm or refute the diagnosis, identify complications such as perforation or to identify other causes of the patient's presentation. The appendix is identified as a blind-ending, tubular aperistaltic structure arising from the postero-medial caecum 1–2 cm distal to the ileo-caecal junction. The patient should be examined in a supine position using a high-frequency linear array transducer to optimize image resolution. The normal appendix is compressible with a wall thickness equal to or less than 3 mm.[81] Increased wall thickness

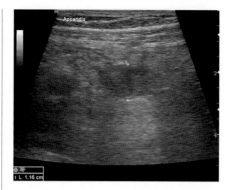

Fig. 23.1.16 Acute appendicitis. Transverse view across the appendix demonstrating wall thickening and loss of definition of the layers of the appendiceal wall.

to greater than 6 mm with loss of compressibility (Fig 23.1.16), loss of definition of the mucosa, submucosa and muscularis propria, and the visualization of an appendicolith support a diagnosis of appendicitis. Additionally the detection of peri-appendiceal inflammatory changes in the presence of an abnormal appendix increases the likelihood of appendicitis.[82] Failure to identify the appendix is common and does not exclude appendicitis.

Musculoskeletal applications

There are numerous musculoskeletal applications for diagnostic ultrasound in emergency medicine. These include foreign body identification, evaluation of suspected tendon tears (Fig. 23.1.17), muscle tears and haematomas, joint effusions (Fig. 23.1.18) and fractures. Most musculoskeletal imaging is done using a broadband, high resolution, linear array transducer with centre frequency of about 10 MHz.

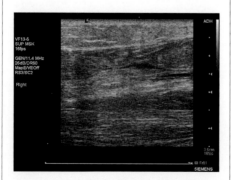

Fig. 23.1.17 Longitudinal view of the tendo-Achilles showing full thickness tear at the level of the musculotendinous junction.

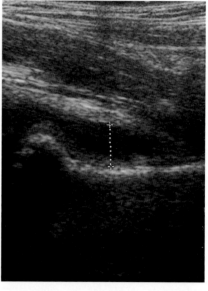

Fig. 23.1.18 Longitudinal view of right hip demonstrating joint effusion.

Ultrasound-guided procedures

Ultrasound is a useful modality for identifying fluid collections and guiding diagnostic or therapeutic aspiration, including thoracocentesis, paracentesis and arthrocentesis.

Training and credentialing

In Australasia both the Australasian College for Emergency Medicine (ACEM) and the Australasian Society for Ultrasound in Medicine (ASUM) make recommendations and provide credentialling pathways in emergency ultrasound. ASUM provides the nationally recognized qualifications: the Diploma in Diagnostic Ultrasound (DDU) and the Certificate in Clinician-Performed Ultrasound (CCPU).

In 1999, ACEM proposed a policy supporting the use of ultrasound by emergency physicians for at least the detection of traumatic haemoperitoneum, abdominal aortic aneurysm, pericardial fluid, ectopic pregnancy, and renal and biliary disease.[1] The subsequently published policy document supported a credentialling process for training in FAST and AAA studies, and included recommendations on training requirements. These requirements mandated a minimum of 25 FAST examinations with at least five positive scans for intraperitoneal, pleural or pericardial fluid, and 15 AAA examinations of which five should demonstrate an aneurysm for credentialling purposes. All of these training examinations should be confirmed by another study or direct supervision of a suitably qualified physician or sonographer.[83] The requirements also include attendance at an ultrasound workshop that covers the basic information for an emergency physician to perform and interpret FAST and AAA studies. Guidelines for the minimum criteria for ultrasound workshops were published by ACEM in 2000.[84] These policies were reviewed in 2006 and are current at the time of publication.

The ASUM is the recognized national training, qualifying and credentialling body in medical ultrasound. ASUM offers two qualifications to medical practitioners performing ultrasound: the CCPU and the DDU. Both of these qualifications are endorsed by ACEM for the purposes of training and credentialling in emergency ultrasound and describe a scope of practice that extends beyond that described by the college. Further details can be obtained from the ASUM website.[85,86]

In 2005 the Royal College of Radiologists in the UK, in consultation with the clinical colleges, published a document entitled *Ultrasound Training Recommendations for Medical & Surgical Specialties*.[87] This document defines three levels of competency, with suggested training and practice requirements for each level and has been endorsed by the College of Emergency Medicine (UK).

The 2001 American College of Emergency Physicians (ACEP) policy statement *Emergency Ultrasound Guidelines* reviewed the previous criteria for achievement of competency to perform focused clinical ultrasound. These recommendations included a 16-hour introductory course and a minimum of 25 ultrasound examinations for each defined primary modality.

Although the minimum training requirements for emergency physicians to become proficient in focused emergency ultrasound remain unclear, the recommendations from ACEP, ACEM, ASUM (for the CCPU) and the training recommendations of the Royal College of Radiologists (UK) for clinical ultrasound are similar, providing some international consensus.

The increasing technological sophistication, portability and affordability of ultrasound machines has led to an increasing demand for ultrasound as a diagnostic tool to be devolved to the clinician managing the patient. This is no more so than in emergency medicine, where ultrasound has the potential of establishing a broad range of applications and indications that extend beyond FAST and AAA detection, as described by the training curricula and guidelines above. The challenge now lies in developing adequate training and supervision networks to allow these skills to be learnt and maintained.

Controversies and future directions

❶ The scope of practice of emergency ultrasound is likely to expand out of the resuscitation room to integrated diagnostic algorithms to aid risk stratification and disposition decisions in broader and more clinically stable patient populations. The major rate-limiting step is likely to be initial access and supervision of training.

❷ Paradoxically, skill maintenance in the so-called advanced applications of emergency ultrasound may be easier to achieve given that the majority of emergency physicians have far greater exposure to these patient groups than those with suspected haemoperitoneum in the setting of trauma or ruptured AAA.

❸ The amount of training required by clinicians to achieve competency and to maintain the sensitivity and specificity of an ultrasound study remains to be determined.

References

1. ACEM. Policy on the use of bedside ultrasound by Emergency Physicians: Australasian College for Emergency Medicine; 2006.
2. ACEP. ACEP Policy Statement – Emergency Ultrasound Guidelines: American College of Emergency Physicians; 2001.
3. UK C. College of Emergency Medicine – Specialised skills training. 2006 [cited 27 July 2007]; Available: http://www.emergencymed.org.uk/CEM/Training/Specialised%20Skills%20Training.asp.
4. Hangiandreou NJ. AAPM/RSNA physics tutorial for residents. Topics in US: B-mode US: basic concepts and new technology. Radiographics 2003; 23(4): 1019–1033.
5. Coleman DJ, Silverman RH, Daly SM, et al. Advances in ophthalmic ultrasound. Radiologic Clinics of North America 1998; 36(6): 1073–1082, x.
6. Kopchok GE, Donayre CE, White RA. Principles and devices. Seminars in Vascular Surgery 2006; 19(3): 128–131.
7. McGahan JP, Wang L, Richards JR. From the RSNA refresher courses: focused abdominal US for trauma. Radiographics 2001; 21 Spec No: S191–S199.
8. Scalea TM, Rodriguez A, Chiu WC, et al. Focused assessment with sonography for trauma (FAST): results from an international consensus conference. Journal of Trauma 1999; 46(3): 466–472.
9. Hsu JM, Joseph AP, Tarlinton LJ, et al. The accuracy of focused assessment with sonography in trauma (FAST) in blunt trauma patients: experience of an Australian major trauma service. Injury 2007; 38(1): 71–75.
10. Jang T, Sineff S, Naunheim R. Residents should not independently perform focused abdominal sonography for trauma after 10 training examinations. Journal of Ultrasound Medicine 2004; 23(6): 793–797.
11. Marx JA, Isenhour J. Abdominal trauma. In: Marx JA, ed. Rosen's emergency medicine: concepts and clinical practice. Elsevier: Philadelphia; 2006.
12. Rose JS. Ultrasound in abdominal trauma. Emergency Medicine Clinics of North America 2004; 22(3): 581–599, vii.
13. Brooks A, Davies B, Smethhurst M, et al. Prospective evaluation of non-radiologist performed emergency abdominal ultrasound for haemoperitoneum. Emergency Medicine Journal 2004; 21(5): e5.
14. McGahan JP, Richards J, Fogata ML. Emergency ultrasound in trauma patients. Radiologic Clinics of North America 2004; 42(2): 417–425.
15. Shanmuganathan K, Mirvis SE, Sherbourne CD, et al. Hemoperitoneum as the sole indicator of abdominal visceral injuries: a potential limitation of screening abdominal US for trauma. Radiology 1999; 212(2): 423–430.
16. Rozycki GS, Feliciano DV, Ochsner MG, et al. The role of ultrasound in patients with possible penetrating cardiac wounds: a prospective multicenter study. Journal of Trauma 1999; 46(4): 543–551, discussion 51–2.
17. Rozycki GS, Knudson MM, Shackford SR, et al. Surgeon-performed bedside organ assessment with sonography after trauma (BOAST): a pilot study from the WTA Multicenter Group. Journal of Trauma 2005; 59(6):1356–1364.
18. Ormsby EL, Geng J, McGahan JP, et al. Pelvic free fluid: clinical importance for reproductive age women with blunt abdominal trauma. Ultrasound Obstetrics and Gynecology 2005; 26(3): 271–278.
19. Soudack M, Epelman M, Maor R, et al. Experience with focused abdominal sonography for trauma (FAST) in 313 pediatric patients. Journal of Clinical Ultrasound 2004; 32(2): 53–61.
20. Kirkpatrick AW, Sirois M, Laupland KB, et al. Hand-held thoracic sonography for detecting post-traumatic pneumothoraces: the extended focused assessment with sonography for trauma (EFAST). Journal of Trauma 2004; 57(2): 288–295.
21. Rose JS, Richards JR, Battistella F, et al. The fast is positive, now what? Derivation of a clinical decision rule to determine the need for therapeutic laparotomy in adults with blunt torso trauma and a positive trauma ultrasound. Journal of Emergency Medicine 2005; 29(1): 15–21.
22. Sirlin CB, Brown MA, Andrade-Barreto OA, et al. Blunt abdominal trauma: clinical value of negative screening US scans. Radiology 2004; 230(3): 661–668.
23. Lee BC, Ormsby EL, McGahan JP. The utility of sonography for the triage of blunt abdominal trauma patients to exploratory laparotomy. Ajr 2007; 188(2): 415–421.
24. Sakalihasan N, Limet R, Defawe OD. Abdominal aortic aneurysm. Lancet 2005; 365(9470): 1577–1589.
25. Lederle FA, Simel DL. The rational clinical examination. Does this patient have abdominal aortic aneurysm? Journal of the American Medical Association 1999; 281(1): 77–82.
26. Barkin AZ, Rosen CL. Ultrasound detection of abdominal aortic aneurysm. Emergency Medicine Clinics of North America 2004; 22(3): 675–682.
27. Tayal VS, Graf CD, Gibbs MA. Prospective study of accuracy and outcome of emergency ultrasound for abdominal aortic aneurysm over two years. Academic Emergency Medicine 2003; 10(8): 867–871.
28. Kuhn M, Bonnin RL, Davey MJ, et al. Emergency department ultrasound scanning for abdominal aortic

aneurysm: accessible, accurate, and advantageous. Annals of Emergency Medicine 2000; 36(3): 219–223.

29. Brown LC, Powell JT. Risk factors for aneurysm rupture in patients kept under ultrasound surveillance. UK Small Aneurysm Trial Participants. Annals of Surgery 1999; 230(3): 289–396, discussion 96–97.

30. Nicholls SC, Gardner JB, Meissner MH, et al. Rupture in small abdominal aortic aneurysms. Journal of Vascular Surgery 1998; 28(5): 884–888.

31. Eyvazzadeh AD, Levine D. Imaging of pelvic pain in the first trimester of pregnancy. Radiologic Clinics of North America 2006; 44(6): 863–877.

32. Shih CH. Effect of emergency physician-performed pelvic sonography on length of stay in the emergency department. Annals of Emergency Medicine 1997; 29(3): 348–351, discussion 52.

33. Adhikari S, Blaivas M, Lyon M. Diagnosis and management of ectopic pregnancy using bedside transvaginal ultrasonography in the ED: a 2-year experience. American Journal of Emergency Medicine 2007; 25(6): 591–596.

34. Morin L, Van den Hof MC. SOGC clinical practice guidelines. Ultrasound evaluation of first trimester pregnancy complications. Number 161. International Journal of Gynaecology and Obstetrics 2006; 93(1): 77–81.

35. Condous G, Okaro E, Bourne T. Pregnancies of unknown location: diagnostic dilemmas and management. Current Opinion in Obstetrics & Gynecology 2005; 17(6): 568–573.

36. Barrenetxea G, Barinaga-Rementeria L, Lopez de Larruzea A, et al. Heterotopic pregnancy: two cases and a comparative review. Fertility and Sterility 2007; 87(2): 417, e9–15.

37. Johnson N, McComb P, Gudex G, et al. Heterotopic pregnancy complicating in vitro fertilization. Australian & New Zealand Journal of Obstetrics & Gynaecology 1998; 38(2): 151–155.

38. Brown DL, Doubilet PMS. Transvaginal sonography for diagnosing ectopic pregnancy: positivity criteria and performance characteristics. Journal of Ultrasound Medicine 1994; 13(4): 259–266.

39. Trowbridge RL, Rutkowski NK, Shojania KG. Does this patient have acute cholecystitis? Journal of the American Medical Association 2003; 289(1): 80–86.

40. Hanbidge AE, Buckler PM, O'Malley ME, et al. From the RSNA refresher courses: imaging evaluation for acute pain in the right upper quadrant. Radiographics 2004; 24(4): 1117–1135.

41. Rosen CL, Brown DF, Chang Y, et al. Ultrasonography by emergency physicians in patients with suspected cholecystitis. American Journal of Emergency Medicine 2001; 19(1): 32–36.

42. Kendall JL, Shimp RJ. Performance and interpretation of focused right upper quadrant ultrasound by emergency physicians. Journal of Emergency Medicine 2001; 21(1): 7–13.

43. Rubens DJ. Hepatobiliary imaging and its pitfalls. Radiologic Clinics of North America 2004; 42(2): 257–278.

44. Noble VE, Brown DF. Renal ultrasound. Emergency Medicine Clinics of North America 2004; 22(3): 641–659.

45. Middleton WD, Dodds WJ, Lawson TL, et al. Renal calculi: sensitivity for detection with US. Radiology 1988; 167(1): 239–244.

46. Cranley JJ, Canos AJ, Sull WJ. The diagnosis of deep venous thrombosis. Fallibility of Clinical Symptoms and Signs. Archives of Surgery 1976; 111(1): 34–36.

47. Barnes RW, Wu KK, Hoak JC. Fallibility of the clinical diagnosis of venous thrombosis. Journal of the American Medical Association 1975; 234(6): 605–607.

48. Lewis BD. The peripheral veins. In: Rumack CM, R WS, Charboneau W, Johnson J, eds. Diagnostic ultrasound. 3rd edn. St Louis, MO: Elsevier Mosby; 2004.

49. Blaivas M, Lambert MJ, Harwood RA, et al. Lower-extremity Doppler for deep venous thrombosis – can

emergency physicians be accurate and fast? Academic Emergency Medicine 2000; 7(2): 120–126.

50. Cronan JJ. Venous thromboembolic disease: the role of US. Radiology 1993; 186(3): 619–630.

51. Lensing AW, Doris CI, McGrath FP, et al. A comparison of compression ultrasound with color Doppler ultrasound for the diagnosis of symptomless postoperative deep vein thrombosis. Archives of Internal Medicine 1997; 157(7): 765–768.

52. Trottier SJ, Todi S, Veremakis C. Validation of an inexpensive B-mode ultrasound device for detection of deep vein thrombosis. Chest 1996; 110(6): 1547–1550.

53. Poppiti R, Papanicolaou G, Perese S, et al. Limited B-mode venous imaging versus complete color-flow duplex venous scanning for detection of proximal deep venous thrombosis. Journal of Vascular Surgery 1995; 22(5): 553–557.

54. Birdwell BG, Raskob GE, Whitsett TL, et al. The clinical validity of normal compression ultrasonography in outpatients suspected of having deep venous thrombosis. Annals of Internal Medicine 1998; 128(1): 1–7.

55. Heijboer H, Buller HR, Lensing AW, et al. A comparison of real-time compression ultrasonography with impedance plethysmography for the diagnosis of deep-vein thrombosis in symptomatic outpatients. New England Journal of Medicine 1993; 329(19): 1365–1369.

56. Cogo A, Lensing AW, Koopman MM, et al. Compression ultrasonography for diagnostic management of patients with clinically suspected deep vein thrombosis: prospective cohort study. British Medical Journal (Clinical research edition) 1998; 316(7124): 17–20.

57. Eskandari MK, Sugimoto H, Richardson T, et al. Is color-flow duplex a good diagnostic test for detection of isolated calf vein thrombosis in high-risk patients? Angiology 2000; 51(9): 705–710.

58. Frazee BW, Snoey ER, Levitt A. Emergency department compression ultrasound to diagnose proximal deep vein thrombosis. Journal of Emergency Medicine 2001; 20(2): 107–112.

59. Jang T, Docherty M, Aubin C, et al. Resident-performed compression ultrasonography for the detection of proximal deep vein thrombosis: fast and accurate. Academic Emergency Medicine 2004; 11(3): 319–322.

60. Cronan JJ. Controversies in venous ultrasound. Seminars in Ultrasound, CT, and MR 1997; 18(1): 33–38.

61. Mangione S, Nieman LZ. Cardiac auscultatory skills of internal medicine and family practice trainees. A comparison of diagnostic proficiency. Journal of the American Medical Association 1997; 278(9): 717–722.

62. Kontos MC, Arrowood JA, Paulsen WH, et al. Early echocardiography can predict cardiac events in emergency department patients with chest pain. Annals of Emergency Medicine 1998; 31(5): 550–557.

63. Thomas JT, Kelly RF, Thomas SJ, et al. Utility of history, physical examination, electrocardiogram, and chest radiograph for differentiating normal from decreased systolic function in patients with heart failure. American Journal of Medicine 2002; 112(6): 437–445.

64. Moore CL, Rose GA, Tayal VS, et al. Determination of left ventricular function by emergency physician echocardiography of hypotensive patients. Academic Emergency Medicine 2002; 9(3): 186–193.

65. Blaivas M, Fox JC. Outcome in cardiac arrest patients found to have cardiac standstill on the bedside emergency department echocardiogram. Academic Emergency Medicine 2001; 8(6): 616–621.

66. Salen P, O'Connor R, Sierzenski P, et al. Can cardiac sonography and capnography be used independently and in combination to predict resuscitation outcomes? Academic Emergency Medicine 2001; 8(6): 610–615.

67. Mandavia DP, Hoffner RJ, Mahaney K, et al. Bedside echocardiography by emergency physicians. Annals of Emergency Medicine 2001; 38(4): 377–382.

68. Jackson RE, Rudoni RR, Hauser AM, et al. Prospective evaluation of two-dimensional transthoracic

echocardiography in emergency department patients with suspected pulmonary embolism. Academic Emergency Medicine 2000; 7(9): 994–998.

69. Ribeiro A, Lindmarker P, Juhlin-Dannfelt A, et al. Echocardiography Doppler in pulmonary embolism: right ventricular dysfunction as a predictor of mortality rate. American Heart Journal 1997; 134(3): 479–487.

70. Sznajder JI, Zveibil FR, Bitterman H, et al. Central vein catheterization. Failure and complication rates by three percutaneous approaches. Archives of Internal Medicine 1986; 146(2): 259–261.

71. Mansfield PF, Hohn DC, Fornage BD, et al. Complications and failures of subclavian-vein catheterization. New England Journal of Medicine 1994; 331(26): 1735–1738.

72. Hudson PA, Rose JS. Real-time ultrasound guided internal jugular vein catheterization in the emergency department. American Journal of Emergency Medicine 1997; 15(1): 79–82.

73. Karakitsos D, Labropoulos N, De Groot E, et al. Real-time ultrasound-guided catheterisation of the internal jugular vein: a prospective comparison with the landmark technique in critical care patients. Critical Care 2006; 10(6): R162.

74. NICE. NICE technology appraisal guidance No 49: guidance on the use of ultrasound locating devices for placing central venous catheters. London: National Institute for Clinical Excellence; 2002.

75. Rothschild JM. Ultrasound guidance of central vein catheterization. In: Shojania KG, Duncan BW, McDonald KM, et al, eds. Making health care safer: A critical analysis of patient safety practices. Evidence report/technology assessment no 43. Rockville, MD: Agency for Healthcare Research and Quality; 2001.

76. Keyes LE, Frazee BW, Snoey ER, et al. Ultrasound-guided brachial and basilic vein cannulation in emergency department patients with difficult intravenous access. Annals of Emergency Medicine 1999; 34(6): 711–714.

77. Nadig C, Leidig M, Schmiedeke T, et al. The use of ultrasound for the placement of dialysis catheters. Nephrology, Dialysis, Transplantation 1998; 13(4): 978–981.

78. Howlett DC, Marchbank ND, Sallomi DF. Pictorial review. Ultrasound of the testis. Clinical Radiology 2000; 55(8): 595–601.

79. Flum DR, Morris A, Koepsell T. Has misdiagnosis of appendicitis decreased over time? A population-based analysis. Journal of the American Medical Association 2001; 10: 286(14): 1748–1753.

80. Wilson EB. Surgical evaluation of appendicitis in the new era of radiographic imaging. Seminars in Ultrasound, CT, and MR 2003; 24(2): 65–68.

81. Simonovsky V. Normal appendix: is there any significant difference in the maximal mural thickness at US between pediatric and adult populations? Radiology 2002; 224(2): 333–337.

82. Vignault F, Filiatrault D, Brandt ML, et al. Acute appendicitis in children: evaluation with US. Radiology 1990; 176(2): 501–504.

83. ACEM. Policy on credentialling for ED Ultrasonography: Trauma examination and suspected AAA. Melbourne: Australasian College for Emergency Medicine; 2006.

84. ACEM. Guidelines on minimum criteria for ultrasound workshop. Melbourne: Australasian College for Emergency Medicine; 2006.

85. ASUM. Diploma of diagnostic ultrasound handbook. Sydney: Australasian Society for Ultrasound in Medicine; 2007.

86. ASUM. Certificate in Clinician-Performed Ultrasound for Point of Care Limited Ultrasound Examination; 2007 [cited 7 August 2007]. Available: http://www.asum.com.au/open/home.htm

87. RCR. Ultrasound Training Recommendations for Medical and Surgical Specialties. London: Royal College of Radiologists; 2005.

24.1 Research methodology

David McD Taylor

ESSENTIALS

1 Research projects should be designed and undertaken in a structured, predetermined fashion.

2 During the study design phase, assistance from a statistician is highly recommended.

3 The study protocol should be written well in advance of data collection and adhered to throughout the project.

4 Most research mistakes relate to inadequate sample size calculations and selection bias in subject recruitment.

5 Ethical issues related to research are becoming more important, especially since the introduction of new privacy legislation. Ethics committee authorization should be sought prior to study commencement.

Introduction

The basic strategy of clinical research is to compare groups of people. These might be different groups or the same group pre- and post-intervention. The methods used are mainly non-experimental, that is observational. They are based on what we can observe and compare in groups of people within populations. By comparing the characteristics (such as behaviours and exposures) and the health experiences of these groups of people, it is possible to identify associations that might be responsible for the cause of a disease.

Initiating the research project

The research question

The research question forms the basis of every research study and is the reason that it is undertaken. It is the scientific, clinical, practical or hypothetical question that, when answered, will allow the researcher to apply newly found knowledge for some useful purpose. The researcher should always aim to undertake studies that will impact upon clinical practice.

The research question may be generated from many sources, including questions raised by clinical observations, the published medical literature, scientific conferences, seminars and discussions, or the effectiveness of currently used or new treatment.

For example:

• Is drug A better than drug B?

The study hypothesis

A hypothesis is a bold statement of what we think the answer to the research question is. Essentially, it is our best guess of what the underlying reality is. As such, it has a pivotal role in any study. The purpose of a research study is to weigh the evidence for and against the study hypothesis. Accordingly, the hypothesis is directly related to the research question.

For example:

- directional hypothesis: drug A is *better* than drug B
- null hypothesis: drug A is *as good as* drug B.

In expressing a hypothesis, the researcher needs to be very specific about who or what is to be observed and under what conditions. A failure to define clearly the study groups and the study endpoints often leads to sloppy research.

The study aims

The aims of a study are a description of what the researcher hopes to do in order to weigh up the evidence regarding the study hypothesis.

For example:

- We aim to determine which is the better drug, drug A or drug B.

Just as the research question begs the hypothesis, the hypothesis begs the study aims. The examples above demonstrate clearly the natural progression from research question through to the study aims. This is a simple, yet important, process and time spent defining these components will greatly assist in clarifying the study's objectives. These concepts are discussed more fully elsewhere.[1,2]

Assembling the research team

All but the smallest of research projects are undertaken as collaborative efforts with the co-investigators each contributing in their area of expertise. Co-investigators should meet the criteria for co-authorship of the publication reporting the study's findings.[3]

Usually, the person who has developed and wishes to answer the research question takes the role of principal investigator (team leader) for the project. Among the first tasks is to assemble the research team. Ideally, the principal investigator determines the areas of expertise required for successful completion of the project (e.g. biostatistics) and invites appropriately skilled personnel to join the team.[1] It is advisable to keep the numbers within the team to a minimum. In most cases, three or four people are adequate to provide a range of expertise without the team becoming cumbersome. It is recommended that nursing staff be invited to join the team, if this is appropriate. This may foster research interest among these staff, improve departmental morale and may greatly assist data collection and patient enrolment.

All co-investigators are expected to contribute time and effort to the project, although the extent of this contribution will vary. The temptation to include very senior staff or department heads simply to bolster the profile of the project should be avoided if possible. It is recommended that personality and track record for 'pulling one's weight' be considered when assembling the team. There is little more frustrating than having poor contributors impede the progress of a study. Assigning specific responsibilities, in writing, to each member of the team is a useful tactic in preventing this potential problem. However, care should be taken to ensure that the timelines for assignment completion are reasonable.

The importance of good communication within the research team cannot be overemphasized. This is usually the responsibility of the principal investigator and may involve regular meetings or reports. At the risk of flooding each co-investigator with excessive or trivial communications (e.g. e-mail), selected important communications should be forwarded as they appear, for instance notification of ethics committee approval and updates on enrolment.

Development of the study protocol

The protocol is the blue print or recipe of a research study. It is a document drawn up prior to commencement of data collection that is a complete description of study to be undertaken.[4] Every member of the study team should be in possession of an up-to-date copy. Furthermore, an outside researcher should be able to pick up the protocol and successfully undertake the study without additional instruction.

Purpose of the study protocol

Research protocols are required:

- for the ethics committee application
- for applications for research funding
- to facilitate the smooth and efficient running of the study through the provision of well-researched and documented information
- for the basis of the Introduction and Methods sections of the final research report.

Protocol structure

The protocol should be structured largely in the style of a journal article's Introduction and Methods sections.[4] Hence, the general structure is as follows:

Introduction

- Background, including a brief summary of the literature
- Research question
- Hypothesis
- Aims
- Need for the proposed research, that is the purpose of the study.

Methods

- Study design – a simple description of the design of the proposed study, e.g. randomized clinical trial, cohort study, cross-sectional survey
- Study setting and period – a description of where and when the study will take place
- Study subjects – inclusion and exclusion criteria and a description of how participants are to be recruited
- Procedures and interventions – the nature of any interventions to be used, including information on safety, necessary precautions and rationale for the choice of dose(s)
- Study endpoints (outcome variables) – variables that are impacted upon by the factors under investigation e.g. those that are affected by a study intervention
- Data-collection instruments, e.g. questionnaires, proformas, equipment
- Data-collection procedures – including quality-control procedures to ensure integrity of data

- Data management – including a description of how data will be handled, how privacy concerns will be addressed and how storage and back-up of data will be undertaken
- Bias and confounding control – sources of bias and variability, and measures to be taken to address them
- Ethical issues – subject confidentiality, safety, security and access to data
- Statistical analysis

    (a) sample size: a description of calculations used to determine sample size and assumptions included in this process should be included. This should include calculations, where appropriate, to ensure that it is clear that the study can recruit a sufficient number of patients to achieve a significant result

    (b) data analysis: this should include a description of the primary variables to be analysed, a specification of any a priori subgroup analyses and the statistical methods to be used. Few researchers are adequately trained in research statistical methods to undertake their own data analysis. It is highly recommended that a statistician be consulted during protocol development and data analysis.

This general plan should be followed in the preparation of any study protocol. However, the final protocol will vary from study to study.

Study design

Study design, in its broadest sense, is the method used to obtain data to prove or disprove the study hypothesis. Many factors influence the decision to use a particular study design and each design has important advantages and disadvantages. For a more extensive discussion on study design the reader is referred elsewhere.[1,5]

Observational studies

In general, research studies examine the relationship between an exposure or risk factor (e.g. smoking, obesity, vaccination) and an outcome of interest (e.g. lung cancer, cardiac disease, protection from infection).

In observational (non-experimental) studies, the principal challenge is to find a naturally occurring experiment, i.e. a comparison of two or more populations that enables the investigator to address a hypothesis about the outcome of interest.

Cross-sectional studies

Cross-sectional studies examine the present association between two variables. For example, within a population you could take a single random sample of all persons, measure some variable of interest (e.g. lung function) and then correlate that characteristic with the presence or absence of lung cancer. Data are often collected in surveys and the information on exposure and outcome of interest is collected from each subject at one point in time. The main outcome measure obtained from a cross-sectional study is prevalence.

Ecological studies

Ecological studies relate the rate of an outcome of interest to an average level of exposure that is presumed to apply to all persons in the population or group under investigation. So, for example, we could determine the association between the average amount smoked per capita in different countries and the incidence of lung cancer in each country.

Cohort studies

In a cohort study, a group of individuals, in whom the personal exposures to a risk factor have been documented, are followed over time. The rate of disease that subsequently occurs is examined in relation to the individuals' exposure levels. For example, within a population you could take a sample (cohort) of healthy individuals, document their personal past and ongoing smoking history, and relate that to the subsequent occurrence of lung cancer in that same sample. Although not as powerful a study design as clinical trials (see below), cohort studies are able to provide valuable data relating to the causation of disease.

Case-control studies

Case-control studies involve a comparison between a representative sample of people with an outcome of interest (cases) and another sample of people without the

outcome (controls). If an antecedent feature (exposure) is found to be more common in the cases than the controls, this suggests an association between that exposure and the development of the outcome. The frequencies of past exposures to risk factors of interest are compared in each group. Case-control studies provide only medium level evidence of an association between exposure and outcome of interest.

Case reports and case series

This study design is often employed in emergency medicine research. The clinical details (history, management, outcome) of interesting or similar patients are described. This study design provides weak evidence for an association between exposure and outcome of interest and is best employed for hypothesis generation. For example, a series of patients who all developed skin necrosis after being bitten by a certain spider would reasonably lead to the hypothesis that the venom of the spider of interest contained a particular tissue necrosis factor. However, this hypothesis would need to be proven by the isolation of the factor and experimental demonstration of its effects.

Data for case reports/series are often extracted from medical record reviews or existing databases. This is one reason for the weakness of this study design insofar as the data were most likely collected for purposes other than the research study. Accordingly, such data are often of low quality and may suffer from inaccuracies, incompleteness and measurement bias.

Experimental studies

In an experimental study, the researcher is more than a mere observer, and actively manipulates the exposure of study subjects to an exposure of interest (risk) and measures the effects (outcomes) of this manipulation.

The preferred form of experimental study is currently the randomized, controlled trial, in which the intervention is randomly assigned at the level of the individual study subject. Although this is the most scientifically rigorous design, other study designs must often be used for a number of reasons including:

- the state of knowledge about a disease process
- real-world opportunities

- logistics and costs
- ethical considerations.

For ethical reasons, we cannot easily use experimental studies to study factors that are thought to increase the risk of disease in humans. For example, you could not do a study where you ask half of the group to smoke for 10 years and half of the group to remain non-smokers.

Types of clinical trials

- Parallel group trials – these are the most common type of clinical trial and involve two or more groups of patients treated separately, but concurrently.
- Two-period crossover trial – patients are treated for two periods using a different treatment in each period. Patients are randomly allocated to the two possible orders of treatment so that half the patients receive the treatments in the sequence AB and the other half in the sequence BA.
- Other types – factorial trials, N-of-one trials and sequential trials– are used much less frequently.

Key features of clinical trials

Randomization Randomization is a process by which patients are allocated to one of two or more study groups, purely by chance. The overwhelming advantage of randomization is that it prevents any manipulation by the investigators or treating doctors in the creation of the treatment groups. This prevents a situation whereby a doctor can, for example, allocate the sicker (or not so sick) patients to a new treatment. Randomization also has the benefit of producing study groups comparable to one another with respect to known, as well as unknown, risk factors and guarantees that statistical tests will have valid significance levels. The most convenient methods of randomizing patients are random number tables in statistical textbooks or computerized random-number-generating programs.

A fundamental aspect of randomization is that it must only take place after the commitment to participate has been made (enrolment has taken place). Another important principle is that randomized patients are irrevocably committed to follow-up and must not be excluded from, or lost to, follow-up, regardless of their subsequent compliance or progress ('intention to treat analysis').

Blinding Blinding is the most effective method of minimizing systematic error (bias) in clinical trials. In single-blinded studies, patients participating in the trial are unaware which treatment they are receiving but the investigators do know. In double-blind studies, neither the subjects nor the investigators know which patient is receiving which treatment. This type of study is usually only feasible with drug studies where it is possible to provide identically appearing medication. This is often achieved using the double dummy approach in which patients receive two medications, one active and the other placebo. The alternative treatment involves a swap-over of the active and placebo medications. Even in apparently blinded studies, there may be various indicators that allow the patient or investigator to determine which treatment they are receiving. In this circumstance, additional methods of bias control may be needed.

Concepts of methodology

Validity and repeatability of the study methods

It is essential that the study uses valid and repeatable methods, that is measurements that measure what they purport to measure. Ideally, the validity of each of the measurements used in any study should be tested, during the design stage of the study, against another method of measuring the same thing that is known to be valid.

Two types of validity are described:

- Internal validity means that, within the confines of the study, the results appear to be accurate, the methods and analysis used bear scrutiny, and the interpretation of the investigators appears supported.
- External validity is the extent to which the results of a study can be generalized to other samples or situations.

Again, for all types of study, it is important that repeatable methods are used, for example measurements that are closely similar when repeated under the same circumstances. Thus, if someone is asked the same question twice about a characteristic that has not changed in the meantime (such as their height), it would be said to be repeatable if they always (or almost always) answered in the same way. Repeatability of the question should be tested during the design phase, though it is also useful to monitor it during the main study. A good example would be a haemoglobinometer that consistently measured the haemoglobin level 2 g/dL too low. Although the haemoglobin measurements would be repeatable, they would be wrong (invalid).

Response rate

Non-response is a problem for many types of observational study. Almost invariably, people who participate in a study (responders) have different characteristics from those who do not (non-responders). This can introduce substantial selection bias into the prevalence estimates of a cross-sectional study. In order to minimize this bias, as large a sample as possible is required. To this end, investigators undertaking cross-sectional surveys aim for at least 70% of invited participants to actually respond. Unfortunately, a target response rate of 70% is often not met and low response rates are likely to impact significantly upon bias and validity of the study.

Study variables

A variable is a property or parameter that may vary from patient to patient. The framework for the study hypothesis is the independent variable. This variable is often the factor that is thought to affect the measurable endpoints, or dependent variables, in the study. For example, cigarette smoking causes lung cancer. In this example, cigarette smoking is the independent variable and lung cancer is the dependent variable, as its incidence and nature depends upon cigarette smoking.

Study endpoints

Study endpoints are variables that are impacted upon by the factors under investigation. It is the extent to which the endpoints are affected, as measured statistically, that will allow us to accept or reject the hypothesis. For example, a researcher wishes to examine the effects of a new anti-hypertensive drug. It is known that this drug has minor side effects of impotence and nightmares. A study of this new drug would have a primary endpoint of blood pressure drop and secondary endpoints of the incidence of the known side effects.

A good hypothesis predicts what we would find if we were to measure certain endpoints. The testing of the hypothesis involves seeing whether or not the endpoint measurements confirm these predictions. Accordingly, the careful selection of appropriate endpoints is of vital importance, as is the accurate measurements of those endpoints.

Essentially, all forms of investigation involve counting or measuring to quantify the study endpoints. In doing so, there is always the opportunity for error, either in the measurement itself or in the observer who makes the measurement. Such errors (measurement bias) can invalidate the study findings and render the conclusions worthless.

Sampling study subjects

There are several important principles in sampling study subjects:

- The sample must be representative of the study population. If the study population comprises all people living in a certain area, the study sample should include a representative sample of all members of the population. Certain groups are frequently left out (for instance the homeless, squatters, people in institutions or people with no telephone). Such groups must be thought of in advance, and steps taken to ensure their inclusion. Otherwise, selection bias may be introduced.
- The sample must be derived from the population randomly. The way in which the sample is drawn from the study population is critical to how well the sample represents that population. This determines how 'generalizable' the results will be. Although there are many alternative ways to maximize sample representativeness, as a general rule, a random sample is preferred. A random sample is one in which each member of the population has an equal likelihood or probability of being selected.

- Loss to follow-up. The researcher must avoid loss of members from the sample once it has been taken, for two reasons. First, loss of subjects will effectively decrease the study sample size and may impact adversely on the power of the study to generate statistically significant results. Second, if subjects lost to follow-up differ in important ways from subjects who remain in the study, then the study results may be affected by selection bias.

Sampling frame

This is a list of all members (for instance persons, households, businesses) of the target population that can be used as a basis for selecting a sample. For example, a sampling frame might be the electoral roll, the membership list of a club, or a register of schools. It is important to ensure that the sampling frame is complete, that all known deficiencies are identified and that flaws have been considered (omissions, duplications, incorrect entries).

Sampling methodology

Probability sampling

When every member of the population has some known probability of inclusion in the sample, we have probability sampling. There are several varieties:

Simple random sampling: in this type of sampling, every element has an equal chance of being selected and every possible sample has an equal chance of being selected. This technique is simple and easy to apply when small numbers are involved, but requires a complete list of members of the target population and it is very cumbersome to use with large populations.

Systematic sampling: this employs a fixed interval to select members from a sampling frame. For example, every twentieth member can be chosen from the sampling frame. It is often used as an alternative to simple random sampling as it is easier to apply and less likely to make mistakes. Furthermore, the cost is less, its process can be easily checked and it can increase the accuracy and decrease the standard errors of the estimate.

Stratified sampling

A stratified sample is obtained by separating population elements into non-overlapping groups (strata) and by selecting a single random (or systematic) sample from each stratum. This may be done to:

- gain precision – this is possible by dividing a heterogeneous population into strata in such a way that each stratum is internally homogeneous
- accommodate administrative convenience – field work is organized by strata, which usually results in cost savings
- obtain separate estimates for each stratum
- accommodate different sampling plans in different strata, e.g. over-sampling.

However, the strata should be designed so that they collectively include all members of the target population, each member must appear in only one stratum and the definitions or boundaries of the strata should be precise and unambiguous.

Non-probability sampling

Convenience sampling is an example of non-probability sampling. This technique is used when patients are sampled during periods convenient for the investigators. For example, patients presenting to an emergency department after midnight are much less likely to be sampled if research staff are not present. This technique is less preferred than probability sampling, as there is less confidence that a non-probability sample will be representative of the population of interest or can be generalized to it. However, it does have its uses, such as in in-depth interviews for groups difficult to find, and for pilot studies.

Data-collection instruments

Surveys

Surveys are one of the most commonly used means of obtaining research data. While seemingly simple in concept, the execution of a well-designed, questionnaire-based survey can be difficult.

Designing a survey

From a practical point of view, the following points are suggested:

Before a survey

- Define the research question(s) to be answered.
- Determine the sampling strategy.
- Design, test and revise the questionnaire (validation).
- Train the data collectors.
- Determine the technique for cross-validation.
- Define the methods of data analysis.

During the survey

- Verify and cross-validate the questionnaire.
- Check timetables and budget.

After the survey

- Cross-check all the data again.
- Perform the main data analysis.
- Perform any other exploratory data analysis.
- Write the report.

If possible, incorporate commonly asked questions into your questionnaire. One good source of such questions is standard surveys (such as Australian Bureau of Statistics). There are many other sources of pre-validated questions (for instance measures on quality of life, functional ability and disease-specific symptoms). The scientific literature, accessible through MEDLINE and other databases is a good start. This is particularly important if you want to compare the sample with other surveys or, in general, if you want to be able to compare the sample's responses to previously completed work.

Also, previously used questionnaires for similar topics are very helpful and often can be used directly. The advantage to doing this is that these questionnaires' reliability and validity are established.

The wording of a question can affect its interpretation. Attitude questions with slightly different wordings can elicit differing responses, so several questions on the same topic may be helpful to be certain that the 'true attitude' of the respondent is obtained. This technique can enhance internal validity and consistency.

Pre-testing of a questionnaire is most important. Consider the following points:

- Assess face validity of all questions.
- Is the wording clear?
- Do different people have similar interpretations of questions?

- Do closed questions have appropriate possible answers?
- Does the questionnaire give a positive impression?
- Is there any bias in the questions?

It is always worth checking with your colleagues to determine whether the questionnaire will answer the study question. Also, test the questionnaire on a cross-section of potential respondents of differing reading levels and background. There can be a few surprises, and several revisions may be required before the final questionnaire is determined.

Data-collection proformas

These documents are generally used to record individual case data that are later transferred to electronic databases. These data may be obtained from the patient directly (e.g. vital sign measurements) or extracted from the medical records or similar source.

While simple in concept, careful design of a data-collection proforma should be undertaken. First, a list of the data required should be drafted and translated into data fields on the proforma. These fields should be clearly laid out and well separated. Prior to data collection, the proforma should be trialled on a small selection of subjects. In such an exercise, it is commonly found that the data fields are not adequate for the collection of the required data. Hence, revision of the proforma is often required.

Consideration should be given to the ease of data entry and extraction from the proforma. Data entry should progress logically from the top to the bottom of the document without interruption. This is particularly important for data extraction from medical records. Data extracted from the front of the record should be entered at the top of the proforma and so on. Consideration should also be given to later translation of the data to an electronic database. This should follow the same principles as described above. If possible, design a proforma that will allow data to be scanned directly into an electronic database.

Bias and confounding

Study design errors

In any study design, errors may occur. This is particularly so for observational studies. When interpreting findings from an observational study, it is essential to consider how much of the association between the exposure (risk factor) and the outcome may have resulted from errors in the design, conduct or analysis of the study.[5] The following questions should be addressed when considering the association between an exposure and outcome:

- Could the observed association be due to bias (systematic errors) in the way subjects were selected for the study or in the way information was obtained from them?
- Can the result be explained by confounding factors?
- Could the result be due to chance?

Systematic error (bias)

Bias in the way a study is designed or carried out can result in an incorrect conclusion about the relationship between an exposure (risk factor) and an outcome (such as a disease) of interest.[5] Small degrees of systematic error may result in high degrees of inaccuracy. It is important to note that systematic error is not a function of sample size. Many types of bias can be identified:

- Selection bias occurs when there is a difference between the people selected for a study (study sample) and those who are not, for instance employed versus unemployed. Only proportional representation of all groups can, in a way, indicate the absence of selection bias.
- Non-response bias is a function of two components: the non-response rate and the extent to which non-respondents systematically differ from respondents. We may need to ask why the question was not answered. Is it not clear? Is it too personal? Is there a negative interaction with the interviewer? Is the subject afraid of answering 'yes'? Non-response bias may be a type of selection bias.
- Measurement bias may result from faulty methods to measure study endpoints. These may include poorly calibrated machines or stretched measuring tapes, for example. Strictly speaking, the following examples of bias are all types of measurement bias.
- Prevarication bias relates to subjects purposely giving incorrect answers and may result from threatening or insensitive questions.
- Interviewer bias results from the incorrect interpretations by the interviewer of the

responses made by the interviewee. This is often an unconscious process, but may result if the interviewer expects, or would like, certain responses.

- Interpretation bias may result from questions that are not clear enough or that the subject does not understand. Some subjects may 'interpret' the question differently from others; for instance, does 'teeth' include 'dentures'?
- Recall bias may result when asking about events that happened a long time ago. For example, 'Were you ever vaccinated against tetanus?' Every effort to avoid historical questions should be made.

Confounding

This is not the same as bias. A confounding factor can be described as one that is associated with the exposure under study and independently affects the risk of developing the outcome.[5] Thus, it may offer an alternative explanation for an association that is found and, as such, must be taken into account when collecting and analysing the study results.

Confounding may be a very important problem in all study designs. Confounding factors themselves affect the risk of disease and if they are unequally distributed between the groups of people being compared, a wrong conclusion about an association between a risk factor and a disease may be made. A lot of the effort put into designing non-experimental studies is in addressing potential bias and confounding. For example, in an often-cited case-control study on the relationship between coffee drinking and pancreatic cancer, the association between exposure and disease was found to be confounded by smoking. Smoking is a risk factor for pancreatic cancer; it is also known that coffee drinkers are more likely to smoke than non-coffee drinkers. These two points create a situation in which the proportion of smokers will be higher in those who drink coffee than in those who do not. The uneven distribution of smokers then creates the impression that coffee drinking is associated with an increased rate of pancreatic cancer when it is smoking (related to those who drink coffee and to pancreatic cancer) that underlies the apparent association.

Common confounders

Common confounders that need to be considered in almost every study include age, gender, ethnicity and socioeconomic status. Age is associated with increased rates of many diseases. If the age distribution in the exposure groups differs (such as where the exposed group is older than the non-exposed group) then the exposed group will appear to be at increased risk for the disease. However, this relationship would be confounded by age. Age would be the factor that underlies the apparent, observed, association between the exposure and disease. Although age is a common confounder, it is the biological and perhaps social changes that occur with age that may be the true causes that increase the rate of disease.

There are several ways to control for the effect of confounding. To control for confounding during the design of the study, there are several possible alternatives:

- Randomization – random assignment into treatment groups, the cornerstone of a randomized, controlled trial, randomly distributes potential confounding factors between the control and intervention groups.
- Restriction – restricting the participants to one level of a potentially confounding variable is another method used in the design of a study to control for confounding, for instance only enrolling patients aged 60 years or more.
- Matching – matching subjects on potential confounding variables ensures that these variables are evenly distributed between cases and controls, especially in case-control studies.

In the analysis phase of a study, one can use:

- Stratification – during the analysis phase of a study, the effect of potential confounders can be assessed within separate strata of the confounding variable.
- Statistical modelling – regression models offer the benefit of controlling for multiple confounders simultaneously.

Principles of clinical research statistics

Sample size

The sample must be sufficiently large to give adequate precision in the prevalence estimates obtained by the study for the purposes required. On the other hand, any increase in the sample size increases the study's cost, so an excessive sample size, though a much rarer event, should also be avoided.

The most common mistake made by inexperienced researchers is to under-estimate the sample sizes required for their study. As a result, the sample sizes used may be too small and not representative of the population that the sample is meant to represent. This usually leads to outcome measures that have very wide 95% confidence intervals and, hence, statistically significant differences between study groups may not be found.

To ensure that a study has adequate sample sizes to show statistically significant differences, if they are there, sample sizes should be calculated prior to the study commencement. In reality, sample size is often determined by logistic and financial considerations, that is to say a trade-off between sample size and costs.

Study power

The power of a study is the chance of correctly identifying, as statistically significant, an effect that truly exists. If we increase the sample size, we increase the power. As a general rule, the closer the power of a study is to 1.0, the better. This means that the type II error will be small and there will be only a small chance of not finding a statistical difference when there really is one. Usually, a power of 0.8 or more is sufficient.

Statistical versus clinical significance

To determine statistical significance, we can obtain a P value, relative risk or some other statistical parameter that is indicative of a difference between study groups. However, a statistical difference (e.g. $P < 0.05$) between groups may be found if the study is highly powered (many subjects), even though the absolute difference between the groups is very small and not a clinically significant or meaningful difference.

This difference is important for two reasons. First, it forms the basis of sample size calculations. These calculations include consideration of what is thought to be a clinically significant difference between study groups. The resulting sample sizes adequately power the study to demonstrate a statistically and clinically significant difference between the study groups, if one exists. Second, when reviewing a research report, the absolute differences between the study groups should be compared. Whether or not these differences are statistically significant is of little importance if the difference is not clinically relevant. For example, a study might find an absolute difference in blood pressure between two groups of 3 mmHg. This difference may be statistically significant, but too small to be clinically relevant.

Databases and principles of data management

The fundamental objective of any research project is to collect information (data) to analyse statistically and, eventually, produce a result or report. Data can come in many forms (laboratory results, personal details) and is the raw material from which information is generated. Therefore, how data are managed is an essential part of any research project.[4]

Defining data to be collected

Many a study has foundered because the wrong data were collected or important data were not collected. Generally, data fall into the following groups with examples:

- Identification data: personal information needed to link to the appropriate patient.
- Research data: provides the information that is analysed to answer the study question, i.e. endpoints.
- Administrative data: initials of the data collector, the study centre if multi-centred trial.

Collect only the research data that are essential to answer the study aims. It is important to avoid collecting data that will not be of use. This is time-consuming, expensive and may detract from the quality of the remaining data. However, there will usually be a minimum of data that must be collected. If these data are not collected, then the remaining data may not be analysed adequately. This relates particularly to data on confounding factors.

Database design

A database is a specific collection of data that is organized in a structured fashion. In other words, database software provides us with a way of organizing the data we collect from a research project in a systematic way.

Good database design will:

- reduce repetitiveness, for instance entering in an address or age for a patient many times
- include validation
- have data in a convenient form for analysis
- be pilot tested.

Data entry

This refers to the entry of data into the electronic database, e.g. Access®, Excel®. Even if the study design and the data collection have been well done, the final data set may contain inaccurate data if the data-entry process is inadequate. This relates particularly to manually entered data where mistakes are bound to happen.

Data entry can be achieved in many ways:

- Manual data entry – this may be single entry undertaken by one person. Alternatively, double entry involves two independent people entering the same data. Any differences between the two are reconciled. This is a form of double-checking but is clearly more time-consuming and, therefore, expensive.
- Direct data entry – this can be achieved by having database forms (proformas) on a computer screen. Direct entry of data via an Internet web page is one form of direct data entry. Alternatively, scannable forms can be fed into a scanner, avoiding the need for manual transcription.

Data validation

Effectively, this is a quality assurance process that confirms the accuracy of the data during its various phases of the study. Data validation can be done in the following ways:

- Visual review: matching data on questionnaires with medical records (source data)

- Value range checks: cholesterol levels should be >0 and <20 mmol/L (i.e. do the numbers in the database make sense?)
- Field type checks: text should not be entered into numerical field
- Logical checks (if, then): if classed as a non-smoker, then cigarettes per day should be zero.

Research ethics

Participation in a clinical trial involves a sacrifice, by the participant, of some of the privileges of normal medical care for the benefit of other individuals with the same illness. The privileges forgone might include:

- the right to have treatment decided entirely on the basis of the treating doctor's judgement rather than by random allocation
- the right to have concomitant therapy according to requirements, rather than be standardized for all trial participants.

Participation also requires the discomfort and inconvenience associated with additional investigations and the potential incursion on privacy. Without the willingness of some individuals to make the sacrifices associated with participation in clinical trials, progress in clinical medicine would be greatly impaired. Most individuals who now expect to receive safe and effective medical care are benefiting by the sacrifices previously made by other individuals.

Some have argued in contrast, that enrolment into clinical trials ensures the absolute best care currently available, with greater involvement and scrutiny by attending healthcare teams.

If one accepts that clinical trials are morally appropriate, then the ethical challenge is to ensure a proper balance between the degree of individual sacrifice and the extent of the community benefit. However, it is a widely accepted community standard that no individual should be asked to undergo any significant degree of risk regardless of the community benefit involved, that is the balance of risks and benefits must be firmly biased towards an individual participant. According to the Physician's Oath of the World Medical Association 'concern for the interests of the subject must always prevail over the interests of science and society'.

Because of the trade-offs required and because of the spectrum of views about the degree of personal sacrifice that might be justified by a given community benefit, it is accepted that all clinical trials should be reviewed by an ethics committee that should have as a minimum:

- sufficient technical expertise to quantify the risks and benefits involved
- adequate community representation so that any decisions are in keeping with community standards.

Scientific value

It is unethical to request individuals to undergo the risks, inconvenience and expense of a study that is unlikely to provide a scientifically worthwhile answer. It is also unethical to request sacrifices from volunteers that are out of keeping with the value of the research being undertaken. In keeping with this principle, studies that suffer from substantial design errors or are susceptible to serious bias in event recording or measurement should not be approved until these deficiencies are remedied.

It is unethical to allow scientifically invalid studies to proceed. Sample-size calculations should be scrutinized because of the ethical undesirability of including too few subjects to provide an answer or many more than is needed to provide a convincing answer. Another safeguard to ensure that the research will be valuable is that the investigator should be qualified, experienced and competent, with a good knowledge of the area of study, and have adequate resources to ensure its completion.

Benefits forgone

It is unethical to require any patient to forgo proven effective treatment during the course of a trial. It follows that clinical trials should only be undertaken when each of the treatments being compared is equally likely to have the more favourable outcome.

Very commonly, however, there is an expectation that one or other treatment is the more beneficial before a trial is commenced. This may be based on results of uncontrolled studies or even on biochemical or physiological expectations. The large number of times such expectations have been proven wrong can still provide strong justification for a trial.

If such an expectation of benefits is held strongly by an individual, it is probably not ethical for that individual to participate in a study. Furthermore, it is the responsibility of an ethics committee to assess the strength of the presumptive evidence facing one or other treatment, and consider whether any substantial imbalance in likely outcome exists. This must be considered in relation to the importance of the question being addressed.

Informed consent

Participants in clinical trials have a fundamental right to be fully informed about the nature of a clinical trial and to be free to choose whether or not to take part. Ethical principles also dictate that prospective participants be:

- told they are taking place in a clinical trial and have an unambiguous right to decline to participate or to withdraw at any time
- provided with a full explanation about the discomforts and inconvenience associated with the study, and a description of all risks that may reasonably be considered likely to influence the decision whether or not to participate.[4]

It is usual practice to provide prospective participants with a Plain Language Statement that provides a simple, easy to understand account of the purposes, risks and benefits associated with participation in the study. Ethics committees are required to review these statements and confirm that they provide a reasonable account.

In practice the procedures involved in obtaining informed consent are often problematic. Considering the dependence of sick patients on the health system, their anxiety

and their desire to cooperate with their physicians, it is doubtful whether informed consent is ever freely given. When ethics committees identify situations where this scenario is likely to be a particular problem, the involvement of an independent uninvolved person to explain the study may be useful.

Controversies and future directions

❶ The issue of consent of patients requiring resuscitation raises serious ethical issues. In this circumstance, the patient is clearly unable to give consent and some argue that this automatically precludes their enrolment. Others disagree and note that such a position would terminate much research in this difficult area.

❷ In response to perceived difficulties in the passage of research through the ethical approval process, ethics committee streamlining is occurring in some jurisdictions and standardization of application forms has begun at state level.

❸ Substantial clinical research requires skilled personnel, time, funding and a supportive infrastructure. Emergency medicine in Australasia has established a respected clinical practice. However, among its present challenges is the establishment of a culture of research with the resources to support and promote it.

References

1. Taylor DMcD. Practical issues in the design and execution of an emergency medicine research study. Emergency Medicine 1999; 11: 167–174.
2. Hall GM, ed. How to write a paper. 2nd edn. London: British Medical Journal Publishing; 1999.
3. Uniform requirements for manuscripts submitted to biomedical journals. Available: http://www.jama.ama-assn.org/info/auinst_req.html (accessed March 2002).
4. Good Research Practice Committee, eds. A guide to good research practice. Melbourne: Department of Epidemiology and Preventive Medicine, Monash University, 2001.
5. Jekel JF, Katz DL, Elmore JG, eds. Epidemiology, biostatistics, and preventive medicine. 2nd edn. Philadelphia: WB Saunders; 2001.

24.2 Writing for publication

Anne-Maree Kelly

ESSENTIALS

1 Check and follow the journal's suggested format and length. Pay particular attention to format of abstract, text and references.

2 Make sure that the objectives, methods, results and conclusions are logically consistent.

3 Be clear and concise.

Introduction

Sharing of knowledge and experience through publication is an important way of improving clinical practice. Communication may be by way of an original research publication, brief report, case report or letter to the editor. Each of these has different requirements in terms of content, format and length, and these requirements may vary between journals. It is useful to choose the intended journal for publication early on. While impact factor may be a consideration in this choice, most authors are more concerned with publishing in a journal that has the appropriate target audience for the subject matter of the paper. It is important to check the *Instructions for Authors* for the chosen journal to ensure that your submission matches that journal's requirements. Failure to do so reduces the chances of acceptance considerably.

Although journals may have differences in format and style, all prefer clear and concise communications. In particular, it is important for the material to be arranged logically so that clear relationships can be seen between the objective of the study or communication, the evidence and any conclusions drawn.

Manuscript preparation

Original research manuscripts

Original research manuscripts are usually divided into five sections: Abstract, Introduction (or Background), Methods, Results and Discussion. In addition, some journals prefer a separate concise Conclusion, although many prefer this as the last paragraph of the Discussion. A few journals have additional section headings such as Theoretical Concept and Limitations, although this is uncommon. It is very important to check the journal's preferred format for each section and ensure the manuscript complies. Most manuscripts also require a key word list of up to five words or phrases to assist with indexing.

Abstract

This is a summary of the paper, usually under the headings 'Objectives', 'Methods', 'Results' and 'Conclusions'. The usual word limit is 250 words. It is wise not to exceed this word count, not only to comply with the journal's requirements, but also because indexing services such as PubMed truncate abstracts at 250 words and information may be lost to readers who search electronically. There is considerable variation between journals about how the abstract section is set out. Some prefer a single paragraph without sub-headings but many of the major journals are moving to structured abstracts requiring particular sub-headings usually detailed under *Instructions for Authors*.

With the easy availability of electronic searching, the abstract is the most commonly accessed part of a manuscript so must contain all the key data. In particular, the specific aims, methods, outcomes of interest, main results (with numbers) and conclusions should be clear enough to be understood without the support of the text. It is important that no data or conclusions appear in the abstract that have not been presented in the main body of the paper.

Introduction

Shorter introductions are often more effective. The aim is to convince the reader why the area of study is important, what this study adds to the body of knowledge and the specific aims of the study. A lengthy review of the literature should be avoided unless it is imperative to put the study in context. A concise review of the literature is more appropriately reported in the Discussion. The last paragraph should explicitly state the aims of the study.

Methods

The Methods sections should address a number of headings. Some journals like this done explicitly, while others are happy for it to be rolled into logical paragraphs.

- *Study design:* What type of study is it?
- *Setting:* Where was it conducted? What are the special features of this setting?
- *Selection of patients:* What are the inclusion and exclusion criteria? How were patients identified? Was anything extra done to ensure that no patients were missed?
- *Data collected:* This should describe all the data collected.
- *Outcomes measures:* What was the primary outcome of interest? Were there secondary outcomes sought?
- *Sample size:* How was the number of subjects chosen? A power calculation is often helpful to justify the numbers.
- *Data analysis:* What types of analyses were used? This refers to the types of tests used rather than the name of a software program.
- *Ethics approval:* There should be a statement saying that the study was approved and by whom or whether it was deemed a quality activity.

Results

It is important for the results to be presented logically and for the relationships with the objectives and methods to be obvious.

A useful structure is to start by describing the study population. This should include how it was derived (a summary figure such as a Consolidated Standards of Reporting Trials (CONSORT) diagram may be very effective for this) and its features such as gender, age, and so on.

This should be followed by descriptions of the results with respect to stated outcomes of interest: primary outcome first then secondary outcomes. These should align with the stated objectives. Any subgroup or other analysis should follow this. All results should give the appropriate statistics with confidence intervals (if appropriate) and the type of test used. A significant proportion of journals are moving away from P values as a way of expressing statistical significance, instead preferring effect size with confidence intervals (or similar). It is important to avoid any comments on what the results might mean or why they might have occurred. Interpretation of the results belongs in the Discussion section.

Tables and figures can be very effective ways of communicating results. They should not repeat what can be described adequately in the text. All tables and figures should be self-explanatory, with clear descriptive headings. Tables should be constructed so that the main comparisons of interest are horizontal and left-to-right, with number of subjects clearly shown for each column. Graphs or figures should be used to convey patterns and details that cannot be succinctly conveyed in tables or text. Figures that show the distribution of data (scatterplots, box plots, etc.) are more effective than those simply summarizing data (bar graphs, pie charts, etc.). Axes must be clearly labelled. Tables and figures should be kept to the minimum number needed to convey the information, and should be numbered in the convention of the journal.

Discussion

A well-constructed discussion adds significantly to the impact of a paper, but keeping it concise and to the point can be challenging. This structure may assist.

- Summarize the principal findings.
- Comment on how it compares with other research. Where does it agree? Disagree?
- Taken together with the other available evidence, comment on possible explanations and implications, avoiding the temptation to over-state the significance of the findings.
- Discuss any other results that are worthy of comment.
- Describe any unanswered questions or directions for future research.
- Describe the limitations of the study. This is important as it is an opportunity to acknowledge limitations and give rationale for some of these. A good limitations section adds to the quality of the paper rather than detracting from it.
- State a summary or conclusion. This should be a few sentences only and should not overstate the findings. Some journals prefer this as a separate heading.

All statements throughout the Introduction, Methods and Discussion that make an assertion or refer to other evidence or methods must be referenced. Ensure that referencing is in the journal's preferred style. Selective referencing should be avoided, that is choosing references that agree with the study findings, or worse, citing mostly the authors' own work. Journal referees are likely to be aware of the breadth of references around the subject.

In general, as long as the key elements are included, shorter is better than longer in manuscripts. If in doubt, shorten the Introduction and Discussion rather than Methods or Results. Stephen Lock, former Editor of the British Medical Journal states: 'A good paper has a definite structure, makes its point, and then shuts up'.

An alternative to the full original research manuscript is the short report. This form has a word limit of 1000–1500 words and usually has some minor formatting differences. It is, however, indexed the same as a full original research manuscript and for many studies is a good format.

Case reports

Fewer journals are accepting case reports. Those accepted for publication tend to have an exceptional element or important clinical message, either in terms of an unusual diagnosis, an innovative use of tests or treatments or an unusual adverse event. It is not enough for a case to simply be 'interesting'.

The usual structure for a case report is an abstract of about 100–150 words summarizing the case and the clinical messages, the case report itself and a discussion. The case should be described in sufficient detail for the reader to be confident of the evidence. This usually requires two or three paragraphs of moderate length. The Discussion is the key element of a case report. It usually includes a review of the literature and uses the case to draw out important clinical messages. It needs to be logical in idea development and well referenced.

Letter to the editor

These are short communications, usually 500–600 words in length. Most often they comment on a recently published paper in the journal concerned, but they may also be used to report a case or case series or an observation. For most journals they are an important method of 'secondary' peer review, where the general medical community has a chance to comment on a paper that may have only been assessed by two or three experts in the field to date.

Manuscript submission

More and more journals are moving to online submission of manuscripts. This is good for authors as it significantly reduces turn-around time, but can take a bit of getting used to. The sites vary in the way they want material entered, so it is important to check this.

A manuscript must only be under consideration by one journal at a time. Authors will be required to attest to this and to the fact that appropriate ethics approvals were obtained. Authors will also be required to provide a statement of any conflicts of interest.

The cover letter

Whether manuscripts are submitted electronically or in hard copy, a cover letter is usually required. This is often quite short and includes a request for consideration for publication in the journal concerned, a statement that the paper has not been published and is not under consideration by another journal, a statement regarding ethics approvals and a note of the presence or absence of author conflicts of interest.

The cover letter is also an opportunity to alert the editor to other issues that may be important. For example, if the manuscript overlaps with previously published work or another manuscript such that there might be a possibility of redundant publication, it allows the editors to assess any overlap for themselves. Alternatively, it also provides the opportunity to identify potential reviewers that the authors believe should be avoided, usually because of actual or perceived conflicts of interest.

Feedback from journals

It is quite rare for manuscripts to be accepted 'as is'. Usually, some revision is required and in some cases manuscripts are rejected. Neither of these necessarily implies that the study or material is without worth. It may simply be that the editors consider the journal not appropriate for the subject matter of the paper. Seriously consider the comments given, which are often detailed, and decide whether the issues

can be addressed. If so, it is important to undertake a revision and re-submit expeditiously. After all the effort of undertaking the research and preparing the paper, it is a waste to miss the opportunity to publish the findings, and indeed, is probably unethical if the study involved consenting human subjects. If the journal requested revision and the concerns can be addressed, re-submit to that journal, otherwise submit to another journal after notifying the initial journal that the paper will not be re-submitted to them.

Post acceptance issues

There are usually several actions required post-acceptance. These include completion of assignment of copyright forms and checking the proofs of the paper. The publisher will usually manage these processes.

Scientific misconduct

There are a few important principles regarding standards of scientific conduct that must be respected when submitting material for publication. They cover issues including plagiarism, ethical approvals of research, data veracity and handling, disclosure of conflicts of interest and redundant publication. Details can be found in the material cited in the further reading section. If in doubt, particularly regarding potential conflicts of interest or redundant publication, this should be notified to or discussed with the editor of the journal.

Further reading

1. Committee of Publication Ethics. Guidelines on Good Publication Practice. Available: http://www.publicationethics.org.uk/guidelines. (accessed July 2007).

24.3 Principles of medical education

Andrew Dent • Debbie Paltridge

ESSENTIALS

1 The emergency department (ED) provides a rich learning environment despite the constraints of service provision and time pressure.

2 Applying adult learning principles, acknowledging prior learning experiences, the need for self-evaluation, the preference for problem-based and experiential learning, and the desire for feedback assist the effectiveness of the ED teacher.

3 Setting clear learning objectives at the beginning and summarizing the learning experience at its conclusion enhances any form of teaching.

4 A learner-centred approach allows the learner to determine learning objectives, actively engage in learning opportunities and participate in evaluation.

5 Characteristics of a 'good' ED teacher include providing a role model, tailoring teaching to the learner and situation, involving the learner in problem-solving, actively seeking opportunities to teach and giving timely feedback.

Introduction

George Bernard Shaw famously quipped, 'He who can, does. He who cannot, teaches'. However, the emergency physician can rarely teach without doing. The tradition

for doctors to teach their colleagues and students goes back to the Hippocratic Oath, where the duties of a doctor to students are outlined: '... to teach them this art, if they want to learn it, without fee or indenture'.[1]

Emergency physicians have been taking an increasing role in teaching and education, in part because of the need for all doctors to learn and refresh emergency skills, but also because emergency physicians are usually full time and hospital-based and have access to students, patients and teaching resources. In addition, they have a unique opportunity of seeing students progress in their chosen specialty and may have multiple inputs vertically over several years in a younger doctor's career. This can be very satisfying and also very motivating.

The emergency environment is one of constant new learning experiences while at the same time being the location for patient care and critical decision-making. Barriers to teaching in hospitals in general, but applicable to emergency departments (ED), have been summarized by Lake in her 'Teaching on the Run' series as lack of time, lack of knowledge, lack of training in teaching, criticism of teaching when given, and lack of rewards, either materially or by recognition.[1]

In addition, teaching in the pressure cooker environment of an ED gives further layers of difficulty, both logistically and ethically. Challenges include:

- shifts, requiring teaching at all hours of the day and night
- junior medical staff from a variety of specialties and backgrounds with varying needs
- numbers of junior medical staff and rostering effecting continuity for teacher and learner
- huge variation in workloads from shift to shift
- administration pressures to reduce waiting times
- physical restraints in many ED environments caused by overcrowding.[2]

The ED is a teaching environment, not only for physicians at various levels, but also for nurses, allied health workers, paramedics and others. A significant component of ED teaching is procedural. It is suggested that most patients believe they should be informed if it is the first time a doctor is performing a procedure on them, but less than half of patients feel comfortable about themselves being the first patient ever for suturing (49%), intubation (29%) or lumbar puncture (15%) for a resident.[3] For non-procedural medicine the evidence is that most patients enjoy being part of the teaching process, in outpatient and ambulatory settings at least, and that no extra negative effects on patients occur from teaching.[4,5]

An added component of complexity in teaching in the ED is the potential for slowing patient processing by having to stop and supervise a junior. It is often so much quicker just to do it yourself. Supervising a lumbar puncture, for example, may take both the teacher and the taught away from seeing new patients for half an hour. However, as far as it has been researched, teaching in academic EDs does not appear to slow down patient care but in fact improves quality of care.[6] Doctors who are seen by their juniors as good teachers are just as likely to see as many patients per shift as those who are not.[7]

ED crowding can be seen to have positive and negative effects on emergency teaching. On the one hand, if crowding is due to patients staying for longer periods of time, it may provide increased patient contact and teaching opportunities over that time. On the other, the emergency doctors may have less time for teaching if the crowding is due to increased throughput and production pressure is high.[8]

All emergency physicians are teachers at some stage in their career at various levels, and, as in Hippocrates' time, are mostly unpaid for it. Although most doctors become teachers, the majority of prevocational doctors in Australia have had no exposure to learning how to teach.[9] Here we present the principles of teaching and learning to assist emergency physicians, whether they are involved with medical students, residents, registrars or other health professionals.

Adult learning principles

Contemporary medical education needs to be couched in terms of contemporary education theory. Adult learning principles should underpin educational practice from the bedside, through the clinical skills laboratory to the seminar room. In addition, these principles are relevant to the education of the undergraduate, prevocational (first 2 years' postgraduate), and vocational registrar years, as well as the continuing professional development of the mature medical practitioner.

Malcolm Knowles first introduced the notion of andragogy or adult learning in the early 1970s.[10] He described five assumptions regarding how adults learn:

❶ As people mature they move from being dependent to being self-directing. This transition allows them to determine their own learning needs.
❷ Adults bring a wide range of experiences accumulated over their lifetime to the learning situation. These experiences provide both a context and a resource for new learning.
❸ Adults' readiness to learn (or motivation) is linked to the applicability of the learning to their current life/employment.
❹ Adults are more problem-centred, that is they want learning relating to a problem they may encounter in everyday life.
❺ Adults are motivated to learn by internal factors such as desire to succeed, personal goals, etc. as compared to external factors such as rewards.

Knowles and other authors have since developed principles of adult learning that can be used to guide education activities:[11-15]

- An effective educational climate is one that allows learners to feel safe. They should be encouraged to express themselves without fear of judgement.
- Establishment of learning needs requires learner participation so that their intrinsic motivation to learn is engaged. The process of developing learning needs helps to assist learners' self-reflection and establish relevancy for them.
- Once a need has been identified learners should be involved in determining specific learning objectives for the educational intervention.
- Designing the educational intervention should be collaborative, ensuring communication between the learner and teacher/facilitator. This will ensure that the methodology chosen will be relevant to the learner's needs.
- Learners should be encouraged to identify appropriate resources to assist their achievement of learning objectives. This will ensure that activities are learner-centred and self-directed as required by adult learners.
- Facilitators should assist learners to implement their learning plans so that objectives are achieved.
- Learners should be involved in evaluating their learning.

However, these principles of adult learning are irrelevant to the emergency physician educator unless they are actively applied to the education of their postgraduate charges. The question remains of how these principles are put into practice. Table 24.3.1 outlines some examples of how these principles may be incorporated into education within the ED.

Learner-centred education

Many traditional medical education experiences are teacher-centred. The teacher is the expert and determines what, how, when and where much is learnt. The teacher is the active participant and the learner is the passive recipient.[16] However, a more effective approach to education is the learner-centred approach. Learner-centred

Table 24.3.1 Application of Adult Learning Principles and Assumptions in the ED environment

Adult Learners	Application to ED teaching
Have prior learning and experience	Even the most junior doctors (e.g. interns) bring experiences with them to the ED. They may have specific experience relevant to the condition that they are treating (e.g. they saw similar patients in their undergraduate course) or it may be life experience (e.g. they had relatives with that experience). Open questioning techniques (requiring a more detailed answer from the learner as opposed to a closed question requiring a yes/no answer) can be used to promote reflection on past experiences and practices. A case study with short answer questions to facilitate this reflection could be used in a small group tutorial situation. Small group discussions can also provide opportunities for learners to draw on their own experiences and to learn from each other as well as the facilitator.
Are self directed learners	At the commencement of a rotation in the ED, junior staff should be asked as part of their orientation, what it is they specifically want to get out of this rotation. This allows the identification of personal learning goals. This is relevant to new senior staff as well. Orientation is also very important for establishing expectations of both learner and facilitator, and ground rules for how education will be carried out within the ED rotation. Learners should also be offered a choice of learning activities. This will allow learners to choose activities which will address their individual learning objectives and which will address their specific learning requirements and styles. For example, one intern may want to watch a lumbar puncture before performing one under supervision, another may want to practise a lumbar puncture on a manikin first before performing one.
Learn most effectively when they perceive a need for learning	The ED educator needs to help learners recognise the relevance of a learning experience. This will significantly impact on their motivation to learn. Sharing of experiences eg a case example from real life, can help to establish relevancy for a learner. Additional methods may include; documentation of ED presentations, participation in unit audit meetings or presentations of cases
Prefer problem-centred approaches	ED presentations require sophisticated problem-solving techniques. The undifferentiated patient is the norm. Modelling of clinical reasoning from experienced practitioners can assist the novice to understand problem-solving approaches. Evidence suggests that the experienced practitioner does this subconsciously, however verbalisation is necessary to promote collaborative problem-solving by the less experienced. Unit case-based discussions also encourage shared problem solving.
Practice self evaluation	Adults require an opportunity for "reflection-on-action"[1] or self-evaluation. Self-evaluation opportunities can be incorporated formally by: • Use of case studies in a tutorial setting • End of shift review of cases • Trolley-side reflection opportunities using open questions
Require feedback	Opportunities for feedback on performance should be incorporated into the ED term both formally (as part of a requirement of training eg mid and end of term feedback) and informally from supervisors or peers. Written and verbal feedback can be used.
Value experiential ("hands on") learning opportunities	There are numerous opportunities for hands on experience within the ED. Educators need to involve learners in case based discussions and problem solving activities. However, procedural skills may need to be practised away from patients until competence is determined. Then practice under supervision will be appropriate.

1. Schön, D. (1983) The Reflective Practitioner. How professionals think in action, London: Temple Smith.

medical staff require an orientation for a number of practical workplace reasons, such as awareness of policies and procedures, occupational health and safety, rostering, pay, etc. However, this is an important opportunity from an educational perspective. The orientation can allow exploration of the junior doctor's learning goals and objectives, past experiences, confidence with procedural tasks and expectations of their ED rotation. The orientation allows the educational supervisor the opportunity to establish ground rules in terms of educational interactions, when feedback will be given and how education with patients will occur. The ED supervisor can acknowledge barriers to learning which are more specific to the ED environment and discuss how these will be overcome.

• Ask the resident to select a patient to present rather than dictating which patient or topic will be discussed.

• Ask residents about past experiences to assist in determining their confidence in managing certain conditions independently. Obviously, supervision will be required until this is determined first hand, but demonstrating insertion of an intravenous cannula (i.v.) to an intern who has previously inserted numerous i.vs may not be the most appropriate and you will not know unless you ask!

• Present junior medical staff with suggested topics for in-service education and ask them to prioritize.

• Ask junior medical staff to present a case to their peers. Let them determine the format they want to use and resources they require.

Junior medical staff are not a homogeneous group. They differ in how they learn, what they need to learn, and why they want to learn. By involving learners in the planning, implementation and evaluation of their learning experiences, both relevance and motivation to learn will be facilitated.

education refers to educational events that place the learner in the pivotal position, responsible for determining learning objectives, actively engaging in learning opportunities and participating in evaluation.[17] This is more in line with adult learning principles.

So how does the ED physician become a learner-centred educationalist? The following suggestions are provided to assist:

• Orientation – to the unit, to the department, to the rotation. Junior

What makes a good ED teacher?

The challenges facing the emergency physician educator, including environmental, patient characteristics, administrative and

ACADEMIC EMERGENCY MEDICINE

production imperatives and resource availability, cannot be overstated. However, despite this, there is a consistent commitment to education by emergency physicians. What then makes a good ED teacher? Bandiera and colleagues used a qualitative research design to investigate experienced ED teachers and establish the behaviours that made them good teachers.[2]

Twelve strategies were identified:

❶ Tailor teaching to the learner – taking time to get to know the learner was seen to increase the efficacy of the teaching and learning interaction.

❷ Optimize the teacher–learner interaction – this refers to making the teaching more directed and efficient by listening to the learner and using what you know about them.

❸ Tailor teaching to the situation – this relies on being adaptable to the situation and changing strategies accordingly, for example by adjusting teaching amounts, types and timing to the time of day, workload and case mix.

❹ Actively involve the learner – involve the junior doctor in problem-solving, give them responsibility and some autonomy.

❺ Actively seek opportunities to teach – sometimes it is necessary to seek out learners. The junior doctor may be busy with an administrative task when an interesting teaching case arrives. The teacher needs to recognize the potential for learning and bring this to the junior doctor's attention.

❻ Agree on expectations – this can be done at the orientation, when learning objectives and ground rules for interactions are established.

❼ Demonstrate a good teacher attitude – this is about being an approachable supervisor/teacher.

❽ Make additional teaching resources – this may involve collecting sample cardiographs, X-rays or blood gases for a resource file. It may be writing up some interesting case-generated problems for future review or development of evidence-based clinical guidelines.

❾ Use teaching methods beyond patient care. With the advent of interest in clinical skills training and simulation there are opportunities to take the teaching away from the bedside on occasion. Use of standardized patients and role-plays may also be appropriate.

❿ Be a role model. This is about demonstrating and practising the principles that you are trying to teach.

⓫ Provide and encourage feedback – adult learners require feedback for motivation and for learning.

⓬ Improve the environment – the competing demands within an ED environment make this difficult, but the effective teacher identifies ways in which to enhance the learning environment, for example by creating space and time in a crowded ED.

These findings are supported further in the literature with what learners want. Additional suggestions include:

• using teachable moments well
• taking the time to teach
• challenging the learner
• treating the junior doctor as a colleague.[18]

The factors reported by ED teachers and ED learners reflect what is required according to adult learning theory and reinforce the applicability within the ED environment.

Types of teaching in the ED

There are a number of teaching and learning strategies available for use within the ED environment. These can include spot electronic searches on active clinical problems, formal quarantined tutorials, case discussions, demonstrations of procedures or techniques, audit meetings, self-directed learning opportunities such as reading medical literature, online learning programmes, and so on. This section deals with three strategies: 'trolley-side' teaching, teaching procedural skills which most ED physicians are familiar with and perform regularly, and simulation, which is developing an emergent role within teaching and learning in the ED.

'Trolley-side' teaching

Interactions with patients at the bedside are a crucial component for learning in medicine, the traditional apprenticeship model relying on this methodology. Bedside teaching can provide an opportunity for the experienced clinician to explain clinical reasoning and role model appropriate communication, including listening, patient questioning and respect, supervising the more junior clinicians as they practise these skills, assessing the junior clinicians' interaction with the patient and providing feedback to them.[19] However, with the numerous environmental constraints within the ED there is a need to look at bedside teaching and determine how best to conduct this activity. In addition, the care of the patient remains paramount and ensuring that this is maintained and that the junior doctor–patient relationship is not undermined is an additional challenge.

The benefits of orientation have previously been mentioned in terms of adult learning principles and learner-centred instruction. However, they are crucial to establishing the expectations from both the learner and the teacher's perspectives in regards to bedside teaching. Establishing up front how bedside teaching will be conducted, while remaining patient-centred, will enable the learner's needs to be met. Briefing the patients beforehand and getting them involved in the teaching process enhances patient comfort and participation and may provide enjoyment. Expectations of patient-based teaching may include:

❶ Number of bedside teaching opportunities per shift. The supervisor may want to ensure one bedside teaching interaction per shift, identified by either the supervisor or the learner. Alternatively, the supervisor may prefer to be less prescriptive and more opportunistic, identifying bedside opportunities as they arrive, accepting that some shifts may have none and others numerous.

❷ Type of bedside teaching. This involves discussing the types of teaching and learning the supervisor is prepared to undertake, for example a procedural skill or history taking or interaction with relatives.

❸ What will happen by the trolley-side? It is important to discuss what will and won't happen by the trolley-side. For example, the history and physical examination will be done at the bedside, but discussion of clinical reasoning may occur away from the patient. This is important to consider, especially if the junior doctor is to have an ongoing professional relationship with the patient. Feedback as to the resident's performance should also be conducted away from the patient. The supervisor should establish whether or not the resident will be asked questions at the bedside so that this is understood prior to the interaction at the bedside.

❹ Outline specific teaching approaches. There are a number of models of bedside teaching that can be used. Lake and Ryan[20] describe the use of set, dialogue and closure. This technique involves an introduction, outlining the objectives of the session (set), a discussion in which questioning techniques are used to elicit information from the learner and to discuss reasoning/rationales (dialogue), and a summation in which the main learning points are discussed and further learning required (closure). An alternative to this is the SNAPPS model described by Wolpaw et al.,[21] in which the learner:

- Summarizes the case history and their findings
- Narrows the differential diagnosis usually to two or three possibilities
- Analyses the different diagnoses by comparing and contrasting them
- Probes the supervisor/teacher for opinions or any information on which they require clarification
- Plans the patient's management
- Selects an issue for self-directed learning later on.

This model was piloted and tested within the outpatient setting. However, it has relevance and application for a number of clinical settings. It would require the experienced clinician to explain and possibly model the process in the first instance.

Procedural skill teaching

Management of patients in the ED often involves the practitioner performing procedural skills. Some of these are to assist in formulating diagnoses in the undifferentiated patient, for example performance of bedside ultrasound, others are for treatment of patient conditions, for example application of a plaster to a fracture. Ideally, in this day and age, procedural skills should be practised in a clinical skills setting prior to implementation on a 'real' patient.[22] However, observation by a junior doctor of an experienced clinician performing a task is also valuable and can sometimes be overlooked in the busy ED department. Sometimes it is done before you realize you could have shown a junior doctor.

The educational theories relevant to teaching clinical skills are drawn from psychomotor theories. There are seven basic principles of the psychomotor domain,[23] including:

❶ conceptualization – where the learner needs to understand the background knowledge element of the skill, that is the cognitive components – this involves a knowledge of why the skill should be done, when to do it, precautions and contraindications, etc.
❷ visualization – where the learner needs to see the skill demonstrated to get a clear picture of what the skill looks like
❸ verbalization – where the learner needs to hear the steps of the skill verbalized
❹ practice – where the learner gets the chance to practise the skill
❺ correction and reinforcement – where feedback is given to reinforce performance
❻ skill mastery – where the learner can perform the skill independently in the learning environment
❼ skill autonomy – where the learner can perform the skill independently in a variety of real life situations.

Similarly, Gagne[24] describes three phases in instructional design relevant to teaching a technical skill, including a cognitive phase where the learner is developing cues from the facilitator, an associative phase where the learner is integrating the component parts and an autonomous phase where the skill has become automatic for the learner.

The issue of the relationship of the learner to the experienced clinician is further investigated within the cognitive apprenticeship model.[25,26] The emphasis in this model is on the requirement that the thinking of the expert be made visible and brought to the surface for the learner. Underpinning this model is the ability of the teacher to assess/recognize the level of the learner.

Another debate in the literature is around the issue of whole skill training versus part skill training. Evidence would suggest that the part skill training method be used for the more complex skills while whole skill training be used for the relatively straightforward skills. This requires the facilitator to analyse the skills to be taught and determine the level of complexity of that specific skill. Additionally, what is the whole skill? It can be argued that procedural skills do not occur in isolation. Rather, communication skills are required along with the technical expertise, and should be taught together rather than in isolation to reflect the requirement in reality.[27,28]

So what do these theories mean for the ED physician wanting to assist a learner in developing a procedural skill? The important requirements are:

- Background knowledge is required – why, what, how.
- Demonstration by, or observation of an experienced clinician is an important component of learning a psychomotor skill.
- Verbalization of steps – this requires breaking the skill down into steps.
- Feedback on performance by the expert.
- Opportunities for repeated practice under supervision, to allow for feedback and self-reflection.
- Teaching the skill in context not in isolation.

A dedicated skills area within the ED is most beneficial, as this can be used in quarantined or quieter times for supervised or independent practice (once the learner is deemed relatively competent in the skill, to avoid practising incorrect technique). Highlighting the need for practice and observation for all the experienced clinicians assists in identifying these opportunities for the learner within the ED environment.

Simulation

Simulation is an emergent teaching methodology within the ED environment. In its broadest sense it refers to any situation in which the real situation is emulated. It may involve actors playing the role of patients, who are often described as standardized patients, or manikins with computer-generated physiological responses.[29,30]

The underpinning educational theory behind simulation comes from a number of theories, including adult learning. However, experiential learning theory is probably of most relevance. Experiential learning theory as espoused by Kolb[31] describes experiential learning activities as opportunities for learners to acquire and apply knowledge, skills and attitudes in an immediate and relevant setting. A four-point continuous learning cycle is described:

❶ concrete experience
❷ observation and reflection
❸ forming abstract concepts
❹ testing in new situations.

Simulation in healthcare education is clearly an example of experiential learning. It provides the learners with a relevant and realistic patient problem to manage. Following this experience, the learners are able to observe their performance and reflect, whilst exploring with a facilitator hypotheses and new concepts. They can then test this experience by repeat simulations.

There are a number of ways in which ED physicians can incorporate simulation opportunities into their teaching in ED. It may be that paper-based simulations are used to explore clinical reasoning. This involves developing case scenarios and structured questions. Role-playing, using peers or expert clinicians, can be used to practise difficult communication skills such as breaking bad news. Simple part-task trainers can be incorporated into a more complex scenario involving the practice of the skill whilst interacting with a patient. Kneebone and colleagues[28] describe integrating a urinary catheter manikin with an actor to ensure that the technical and communication skills are taught concurrently.

Where higher level manikins are available, whole patient scenarios can be conducted. Teams of junior medical staff can practise rarer critical situations and explore not only technical skills but non-technical skills such as teamwork. Use of audio-visual aids to capture performance is important for providing feedback after such activities. It also allows an opportunity for reflection and peer feedback.

Not all EDs have the luxury of the highly technical simulation 'gadgetry', but this should not put them off using simulation as a teaching methodology. Determining the content areas appropriate for using simulation and how this fits into the overall curriculum will be important to ensure that resources are used rationally.[32]

Feedback to learners

Feedback is a crucial requirement for learning, and the importance of positive feedback for learning has been established.[33] Feedback should provide the learner with information that offers 'insight into what he or she did as well as the consequences of his or her actions'.[34] It should allow the learner to know what went well and what could be improved or changed next time. Feedback is part of the formative assessment process that occurs throughout the learning period, rather than as a summative assessment that is to determine a grade or make a final judgment.

Effective feedback has a number of characteristics.[35,36] It should be given in a suitable environment to allow privacy and maintain confidentiality for the learner. There should be adequate time to allow the learner and the facilitator to explore the observed behaviour or skill. There should be clear goals established at the beginning of the learning so that feedback can be related to these goals. The feedback should come from direct observation of the learner's performance where possible.

Providing learners with feedback is a specific skill in itself and requires practise to develop. A model to assist the emergency physician to give feedback is suggested from Pendleton's[37] work as:

- Ask the learner how he or she felt.
- Ask the learner what went well and why.
- As the facilitator/teacher to say what went well and why.
- Ask the learner what could have been done better and why.
- Ask the facilitator/teacher to say what could have been done better and why.
- Ask the facilitator/teacher to summarize the strengths and up to three things to concentrate on.

Feedback, when delivered effectively, is a strong motivator to the adult learner and encourages ongoing performance review and reflection by the learner.

Conclusion

Juggling the demands of a being a busy emergency physician requires balancing clinical, administrative and teaching duties.

Time is often limited and yet the rewards of being involved in teaching are obvious. Apart from personal satisfaction gained from interacting with junior colleagues, the ability to keep up to date and the opportunity to reflect on one's own performance are enhanced. Reviewing performance as a teacher and practising education techniques to improve the effectiveness of the facilitation motivate the teacher to continue to teach and improve the satisfaction from teaching. Structuring learning experiences, considering learner needs and providing effective feedback are essential for learners in the ED environment.

Likely developments over the next 5–10 years

- Increasing numbers of medical students and junior medical staff seeking learning in the ED may lead to the need for specific emergency physician educators to orientate and supervise them in the ED.
- Expansion of scenario-based simulation and skills centres may lead to more opportunities for ED team-based interdisciplinary education.
- Increasing patient participation in decision making will necessitate more detailed consent when procedures are performed by the inexperienced.

Controversies

❶ Teaching procedural skills should no longer be 'see one, do one, teach one' on surprised patients, although some find it difficult to break out of this mould.

❷ Communication skills should be practised during a procedure, with a building of skills involving conceptualization of the skill, visualization, verbalization, practice, correction and reinforcement, with eventual skill mastery and skill autonomy.

❸ Should patients be informed of the level of experience of those providing care or performing a procedure?

References

1. Lake FR. Teaching on the run tips: doctors as teachers. Medical Journal of Australia 2004; 180(8):415–416.
2. Bandiera G, Lee S, Tiberius R. Creating effective learning in today's emergency departments: how accomplished teachers get it done. Annals of Emergency Medicine 2005; 45:253–261.
3. Santen S, Hemphill R, McDonald F, et al. Patients' willingness to allow residents to learn to practice medical procedures. Academic Medicine 2004; 79:144–147.
4. Simons R, Imboden E, Mattel J. Patient attitudes toward medical student participation in a general internal medicine clinic. Journal of General Internal Medicine 1995; 10(5):251–254.
5. Simon S, Peters A, Christiansen C. Effect of medical student teaching on patient satisfaction in a managed care setting. Journal of General Internal Medicine 2000; 15(7):457–461.
6. Berger TJ, Ander DS, Terrell ML, et al. The impact of the demand for clinical productivity on student teaching in academic emergency departments. Academic Emergency Medicine 2004; 11: 1364–1367.
7. Denninghoff KR, Moye PK. Teaching students during an emergency walk-in clinic rotation does not delay care. Academic Medicine 1998; 73:1311.
8. Atzema C, Bandiera G, Schull MJ. Emergency department crowding: the effect on resident education. Annals of Emergency Medicine 2005; 45:276–281.
9. Dent AW, Crotty B, Cuddihy H, et al. Learning opportunities for Australian prevocational hospital doctors: exposure, perceived quality and desired methods of learning. Medical Journal of Australia 2006; 184:436–440.
10. Knowles M. The adult learner: a neglected species. Houston: Gulf Publishing; 1973.
11. Cantillon P, Hutchinson L, Wood D. ABC of learning and teaching in medicine. London: British Medical Journal Publishing; 2003.

12. Knowles M. The modern practice of adult education: from pedagogy to andragogy. 2nd edn. New York: Cambridge Books; 1980.
13. Kaufman D, Mann K. Teaching and learning in medical education: How theory can inform practice. Edinburgh: Association for the Study of Medical Education; 2007.
14. Peyton J. Teaching and learning in medical practice. Great Britain: Manticore Europe; 1998.
15. Brookfield S. Understanding and facilitating adult learning. Buckingham: Open University Press; 1986.
16. Gunderman R, Williamson K, Frank M, et al. Learner-centered education. Radiology 2003; 227:15–17.
17. Weimer M. Learner centred teaching. New York: Jossey-Bass; 2002.
18. Thurger L, Bandiera G, Lee S. What do emergency medicine learners want from their teachers? A multicentre focus group analysis. Academic Emergency Medicine 2005; 12:856–861.
19. Celenza A, Rogers I. Qualitative evaluation of a formal bedside clinical teaching programme in an emergency department. Emergency Medicine Journal 2007; 23:769–773.
20. Lake F, Ryan G. Teaching on the run tips 4: Teaching with patients. Medical Journal of Australia 2004; 181:158–159.
21. Wolpaw T, Wolpaw D, Papp K. SNAPPS: a learner centred model for outpatient education. Academic Medicine 2003; 78:893–898.
22. De Young S. Teaching psychomotor skills. In: Teaching strategies for nurse educators. United Kingdom: Prentice Hall Health; 2003:201–215.
23. George J, Doto F. A simple five-step method for teaching clinical skills. Family Medicine 2001; 33:577–578.
24. Gagne R. The conditions of learning. 4th edn. New York: Holt, Rinehart & Winston; 1985.
25. Collins A, Brown J, Newman S. Cognitive apprenticeship: teaching the crafts of reading, writing and mathematics. In: Resnick L, ed. Learning and instruction: essays in honor of Robert Glaser. New Jersey: Lawrence Erlbaum; 1989: 453–494.

26. Woolley N, Jarvis Y. Situated cognition and cognitive apprenticeship: a model for teaching and learning clinical skills in a technologically rich and authentic learning environment. Nurse Education Today 2007; 27:73–79.
27. Kneebone R, Kidd J, Nestel D, et al. An innovative model for teaching and learning clinical procedures. Medical Education 2002; 36:628–634.
28. Kneebone R, Nestel D, Yadollahi F, et al. Assessing procedural skills in context: exploring the feasibility of an integrated procedural performance instrument (IPPI). Medical Education 2006; 40:1105–1114.
29. Ker J, Bradley P. Simulation in medical education. Edinburgh: Association for the Study of Medical Education; 2007.
30. Good M. Patient simulation for training basic and advanced clinical skills. Medical Education 2003; 37 (suppl):14–21.
31. Kolb D. Experiential learning. Englewood Cliffs. NJ: Prentice Hall; 1984.
32. Binstadt E, Walls R, White B, et al. A comprehensive medical simulation education curriculum for emergency residents. Annals of Emergency Medicine 2007; 49:495–504.
33. Kilminster S, Jolly B, van der Vleuten C. A framework for effective training for supervisors. Medical Teacher 2002; 24:385–389.
34. Ende J. Feedback in clinical medical education. American Medical Association 1983; 250:777–781.
35. Schwenk T, Whitman N. The physician as teacher. Baltimore: Williams & Wilkins; 1987.
36. Vickery A, Lake F. Teaching on the run tips 10: Giving feedback. Medical Journal of Australia 2005; 183: 267–268.
37. Pendleton D, Schofield T, Tate P, et al. The consultation: an approach to teaching and learning. Oxford: Oxford University Press; 1984.

24.4 Undergraduate teaching in emergency medicine

Geoffrey Couser

ESSENTIALS

1 Medical student teaching should be considered core business of an emergency department.

2 The specialty of emergency medicine has a unique body of knowledge that can contribute much to an undergraduate curriculum.

3 To be effective, emergency physician educators need to adopt a strategic and comprehensive approach to curriculum development, delivery and assessment.

4 It is essential that goals and objectives of student education in emergency medicine be clearly defined so that a consistent and integrated curriculum is delivered.

5 The specialty will play an increasingly important role in medical student education in the next 10 years as numbers of students rapidly increase and models of healthcare continue to change.

Introduction

Emergency medicine now plays a central role in medical curricula in undergraduate and postgraduate medical schools in Australia and New Zealand. This is not unexpected, as the principles and practice of the specialty have much in common with contemporary medical education: it is problem-focused, interdisciplinary, and integrates many aspects of community-based and hospital-based clinical practice. Clinical practice easily integrates and builds upon the basic medical sciences traditionally taught early in the medical course. Much growth in academic emergency medicine has occurred in the last 10 years, with the establishment of academic departments and dedicated university positions. However, the majority of medical student teaching is performed by emergency physicians in clinical practice in public, and an increasing number of private, emergency departments (EDs). This chapter will address the issues surrounding medical student teaching at the departmental and the broader faculty level.

Overview of undergraduate medical education in Australia

It is important for emergency physicians interested in teaching medical students to be aware of recent trends and developments in medical education in Australasia. The last 15 years have seen the establishment of graduate schools of medicine and a massive reform of the traditional undergraduate curricula. The CanMEDS 2000 Project and the World Health Organization, among others, have listed the key outcomes expected of a doctor.[1] These outcomes have been adopted by many schools worldwide as a basis for reform and reorganization, and are listed in Table 24.4.1. In more detail, the Australian Medical Council has listed 40 attributes of medical graduates to guide faculties with curriculum design and subsequent accreditation.[2] Many schools have organized their curricula into themes, or domains, so that these outcomes can be vertically integrated, tracked and assessed throughout the course. Some schools have adopted problem-based learning as a tool to achieve these educational outcomes, with others using case-based and outcomes-based learning to place content in a clinical context.

These changes have not been without controversy, with some critics concerned that this has been at the expense of basic science teaching and the teaching of sound clinical

practice.[3] Curriculum reform has occurred in parallel with significant changes in the health system, with a growth in information technology, changing patient expectations and a massive increase in medical knowledge. Models of healthcare delivery are changing, with increased pressures on public hospitals such as access block, declining numbers of inpatient beds and the increasing complexity of medical conditions. The shift to the home and community management of many conditions has altered the patient mix available for student teaching. University salaries have not kept pace with the growth in public and private medical salaries, which has contributed to a decline in numbers of academic faculty and core medical school functions shifting to specialists within the public hospital system. Despite this, there has been an increasing number of medical students and medical schools, with over 3000 graduates per year predicted to require intern posts by the middle of the next decade.[4] It is in this changing environment that emergency medicine has established itself as a key part of any modern medical curriculum. With a growing number of medical students, emergency physicians and patients, the specialty is poised to play an even greater role in the training of future doctors. Both the need and the opportunity exist for such expansion.

The importance of medical student teaching

This is an important point to consider, as many feel that the provision of clinical care is the core business of an ED and hence may not be willing to allocate resources for teaching students. Similarly, university medical schools may not be aware of the growth of emergency medicine as a specialty and hence may not be aware of what it can offer students. However, once established, a strong academic presence can contribute to departmental morale and performance. Table 24.4.2 lists the benefits of emergency medicine teaching to students, EDs and medical schools. These points may be used to argue for an increased presence and accompanying resources within a curriculum.[5] Resources and a formal place in the curriculum often come only after years of hard work in establishing the bona fides of emergency medicine. This may require much time and effort from a dedicated individual.

Table 24.4.1 Essential roles and key competencies of specialist physicians – The CanMEDS criteria[1]
Medical expert
Communicator
Collaborator
Manager
Health advocate
Scholar
Professional

Table 24.4.2 Benefits of medical student teaching in emergency departments
Benefits to students
• Usually an enjoyable term with unparalleled pathology and clinical experience
• Integrates theoretical knowledge with the workplace
• Learns acute care resuscitation skills
• The opportunity to see patients before anyone else in the system
• Emergency medicine is the embodiment of an equitable and accessible healthcare system
Benefits to the emergency department and hospital
• Students gain a positive view of the specialty and this may influence subsequent career choice
• May improve subsequent intern performance
• Improves the overall professionalism and reputation of the department
• Teaching is a core business of a hospital and should be embraced
• May assist with recruitment and retention of staff with an interest in teaching
• Students can assist with procedures and may improve patient flow in some circumstances
Benefits to the medical school
• Allows access to a large number of patients with a broad range of clinical conditions otherwise not available for teaching
• Allows access to a large pool of medical and nursing staff otherwise not available for teaching
• Emergency medicine can teach knowledge and skills not readily taught by other disciplines, such as resuscitation, health systems and time management

Curriculum development

Medical student teaching in EDs has, until recent years, been largely a passive and opportunistic affair. Inpatient units would send groups of hapless students 'down to "cas"' to see if there was 'anything interesting going on'. As such, exposure to emergency medicine was ad hoc, unstructured and highly selective, in that clinical exposure was based around what the students themselves thought was interesting and useful. With the growth of the specialty in recent years departments have been able to take a more active role in education, control student entry to the department, ensure appropriate orientation and attempt to take advantage of the rich and broad clinical experience on offer. As faculties have become aware of the learning opportunities on offer in EDs, as well as the teaching abilities of staff, emergency physicians have been able to negotiate a greater role in university affairs and integrate emergency medicine into the broader undergraduate curriculum.

Table 24.4.3 Minimum requirements for developing student placements in emergency departments

- Nominate one person to be the term coordinator and liaison with the university
- Understand the rules and regulations which govern student placements in your hospital and at the affiliated university
- Develop a clear orientation package for students and make it clear that students will not be allowed into the department until they have received orientation
- Develop a clear curriculum statement providing a broad overview of goals and objectives for the term (see Table 24.4.4)
- Define specific learning objectives for students, e.g. 'At the end of this placement you will be able to describe the assessment of the patient presenting with chest pain'
- Consider how students will be assessed and clearly describe this prior to the commencement of the term
- Consider who will supervise the students – for this reason it is essential to engage with all levels of staff within the department and to provide them with support, training and guidance

With this comes a responsibility for emergency physicians to understand the function of universities, and the requirements which come with running an academic term. Table 24.4.3 provides suggestions for developing a university teaching presence.

It is essential that once a department has decided that medical student teaching should be a part of its function then a curriculum needs to be considered. Both the Australasian College for Emergency Medicine and the American College of Emergency Physicians have produced documents with varying degrees of detail concerning this,[6,7] and a growing number of papers are being published providing guidance to curriculum developers.[8–10] Most core curriculum statements contain elements which reflect the clinical practice of emergency medicine, and an example of such a list is provided in Table 24.4.4. This provides a framework around which specific topics can then be taught. The teaching programme will need to be modified and adapted accordingly depending upon the expertise of and time available to specialists within the department.

An often overlooked but essential component to consider is that of the 'hidden curriculum'. This is less well understood, but relates to what students learn by being exposed to the practice of medicine. It can cover aspects such as professionalism, ethics and physician behaviour. As the vanguard of a fair and equitable health system, emergency medicine can teach important attitudes to the next generation of doctors.

Table 24.4.4 Suggested core curriculum topics in emergency medicine

| Assessment and management of the undifferentiated patient |
| Key practical skills: basic life support skills and basic procedural skills |
| Recognition and management of the seriously ill and injured patient |
| The assessment and management of common clinical problems in emergency medicine |
| Assessment and management of the unwell child |
| Acute pain management |
| Assessment and management of the poisoned patient |
| Toxinology |
| Health systems management |
| Critical thinking and clinical decision making |
| Safety and quality in healthcare: medical error and handover |
| Professional issues: teamwork, communication, time management |

Different ways to teach emergency medicine

Once teaching content is decided upon, then it is worth spending time considering which format is the best way to deliver the material. Until recently, undergraduate emergency medicine has largely been taught in the workplace and no other teaching options have existed. However, with the growth of the specialty and the increased need for teachers, the specialty has been able to attract resources and play a greater role in all years of the medical course in some universities. Therefore, depending upon available time and resources, different formats of teaching should be considered for different situations. For example, resuscitation skills may be best taught using simulation and practice, once basic concepts have been covered by lectures or online modules.

In all formats, teachers should consider the basic principles of adult learning and teach accordingly. When delivering material, teachers should remember that adults learn best when the topic is meaningful, linked to experience and pitched at the correct level, and the students are motivated, have clear goals, are actively involved, receive regular feedback and have time for reflection.[11] Utilizing

a range of methods means that material can be delivered in a meaningful way and optimal learning conditions can be achieved. It is essential that the physician taking responsibility for undergraduate teaching within a department takes a leadership role and provides ongoing training and support for both junior and senior colleagues in effective teaching methods.

Whichever teaching method is chosen, evaluation of the process by the participants is an essential part of the quality improvement cycle. This may be in the form of a brief questionnaire or standardized form, such as a part of a student evaluation of teaching and learning (SETL) programme. Evaluation helps ensure teaching is meeting students' learning needs, identifies areas where teaching can be improved, and provides feedback and encouragement for teachers.[12] Documenting evaluations can form part of a teaching portfolio, which can be used in academic job applications as tangible evidence of a clinician's commitment to and proficiency in teaching. Importantly, from a student's perspective, being asked to evaluate a teaching session and then seeing the comments acted upon provides a strong sense that their participation is valued and as a result may improve the learning process overall.

Some basic pedagogical theory should be considered when choosing and applying methods of teaching: many educators refer to Miller's triangle of clinical competence[13] and the concept of a spiral curriculum[14] when designing curricula. Figure 24.4.1 is a schematic representation of how emergency medicine as a subject could ideally progress through a 5-year course utilizing these theories of curriculum design. Most departments will only be in a position to offer clinical exposure in the final years of the course, but much progress has been made across the region in penetrating all years. The following delivery methods could be used in this framework to deliver a comprehensive and effective emergency medicine curriculum.

Lecture based

Lectures can be delivered at any stage of the medical course, but to maximize their effectiveness they need to be developed in an integrated fashion and linked to other components of the course. Emergency medicine can be used effectively as a vehicle to illustrate

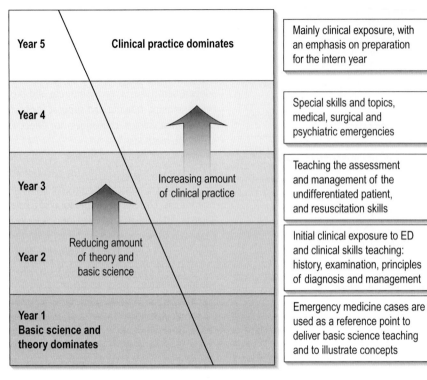

Fig. 24.4.1 A suggested overview of the progression of emergency medicine in an integrated 5-year curriculum.

basic science concepts to junior medical students.[15] Case-based learning is a popular method to use in this setting, as learning objectives and concepts can be illustrated in a 'real-world' setting. For example, rather than delivering a lecture on ischaemic heart disease, an emergency medicine lecture would be entitled 'I've got pain in my chest' and the lecturer would engage with students to create a genuine feel for this common emergency presentation. The content would need to be modified depending upon the seniority of students, for example junior medical students would use the case as a reference point to illustrate anatomy and physiology, whilst more senior students may use the same scenario to learn about clinical decision making and evidence-based medicine.

Lectures need not be didactic and overloaded with content – they can be an efficient means of transmitting information to large groups. In general, lectures should add value. There is little point simply repeating content from a text, as students can gather information themselves in their own time. In this sense, prospective lecturers should remind themselves of the qualities of an effective educator: expertise in the subject area, enthusiasm for the topic and the task, and capacity to engage the learners.[16] By utilizing these qualities, educators can turn a lecture into a valuable learning experience.

Tutorials and small-group learning

Tutorials are small group sessions, with opportunities for interaction and reflection. This model of teaching is well-suited to emergency medicine, as individual cases and experiences can be presented and discussed in a comfortable environment. The learners can lead the discussion and take the topics into new and previously unconsidered areas. Nevertheless, providing a structure to the tutorial will help ensure that the time is spent wisely and learning opportunities are maximized. These are usually easily implemented in a department, as they can be integrated with other departmental activities and can run independently of any broader curriculum. This is often the only way that the specialty can deliver its core curriculum in a school without a formal emergency medicine presence.

Web-based

This is growing in popularity as schools rely more on information technology to deliver content, but few emergency physicians have had the time or the access to moderate and upload content and hence maximize the opportunities this mode of teaching can present. At a basic level, bulletin boards, web logs (blogs) and email are useful ways to maintain regular communication with students and to distribute journal articles and policies, and orientation manuals can be posted online.[17]

However, with faster internet conditions and a new generation of students increasingly familiar with technology, new opportunities are appearing: virtual worlds and the operation of a 'Second Life' ED (http://secondlife.com) may become useful tools for education.

Work-based

This is the original method of medical student education: at the bedside of the patient. Medicine has been taught this way for thousands of years, and reinforces the point that medical students are essentially apprentices in a trade. Emergency medicine excels in this area because of the broad range of experiences on offer in a department. Challenges exist, as not all students will be exposed to the same conditions during a rotation. Achieving a uniform experience for students is difficult,[18] and so workbooks have been developed to guide students through their rotation, alerting them to the broad range of undifferentiated conditions which regularly present. Utilizing junior staff can be helpful in the education of medical students: pairing a student with a resident or registrar allows the students to see how a doctor works, and it involves junior doctors in teaching at an early stage of their careers. It helps with rostering, in that students can be allocated to medical staff with a pre-existing timetable. Medical schools offer clinical academic titles to doctors involved in teaching, and all staff should be encouraged to apply for such titles.

Teaching by the bedside is an important activity and opportunities abound for clinical teaching. Clinicians being aware of a broader curriculum can be of assistance, as it can be difficult to think on the spot when confronted with a 'teachable moment.' Some guidelines exist to maximize the value of bedside teaching and the well-developed principles of 'set, dialogue and closure'[19] are explained and listed with an example in Table 24.4.5.

Table 24.4.5	Planning a teaching episode	
Concept	Components	Example in practice
Set	Roles – trainers, learners, patients Objectives – what are they going to learn? Linkages – to other learning events Environment – seating, lighting, distractions	Gather the students in a quieter part of the department where distractions will be minimal, and make it clear what the session is about: 'I'd like to talk about ways we assess headaches in the emergency department'
Dialogue	Questions – use often Understanding Eyes – two-way contact Stimulation – make it interesting Timing – finish on time	Check what the students know about the topic, and ask an open question to start, e.g. 'What are the worrying signs of a headache?' Encourage discussion, use first names in the discussion
Closure	Review – ask for questions, check understanding Eyes – contact with learner Summary Termination	Summarize the discussion, check that the students have understood it, terminate with a comment (e.g. 'Thunderclap headaches are a feature of subarachnoid haemorrhage, and later we'll talk about the role of a lumbar puncture')

You have just assessed a young male with a severe headache. You realize that this is an ideal teaching opportunity for the medical students present.

Simulation

Simulation is a growing field which has been embraced by emergency physicians and the Australasian College for Emergency Medicine. A large knowledge base has been developed, and as such it will not be discussed at length here. However, the main barrier to utilizing simulation for undergraduate teaching is cost and the available time of emergency physicians. Fortunately, universities are starting to recognize the value of this method of teaching and opportunities are being created.

Clinical skills teaching

Emergency medicine has long had a reputation amongst students for 'being the place where you get to do useful things'. Whilst proponents of the specialty in universities are keen to promote the other features of emergency medicine in an educational setting, this statement is still undoubtedly true. Many skills can be taught in the ED or a skills laboratory, and emergency physicians are ideally placed to teach them. Whether it is junior medical students examining patients for the first time or learning practical skills such as venesection and suturing, emergency physicians have a lot to offer in this regard. Like most teaching, there are useful techniques that can be employed to improve learning.[20]

Assessment principles

Assessment should be considered as a tool which drives learning, and should be developed in parallel with the curriculum rather than considered at the end. It is essential that the appropriate form of assessment be matched to the subject matter. Assessment tools selected should be valid, reliable and practical, and have an appropriate impact on student learning.[21] For instance, when assessing competency in advanced cardiac life support, it would be more valid to use a practical-based assessment process such as an observed objective structured clinical examination (OSCE) rather than a written examination. Figure 24.4.2 provides a graphical representation of matching assessment processes to skills and knowledge. A large number of assessment methods exist and educators should possess at least a basic

understanding of their use and application. It is essential to understand that all universities have rules which govern the assessment of students, and failure to strictly adhere to these rules exposes a department to academic appeals and complaints of unfairness and bias.

Likely developments over the next 5–10 years

Emergency medicine will continue to play a significant role in medical student education and is poised to make greater contributions in coming years. This will occur both by design and necessity: as described, the increase in student numbers is coinciding with the growth and maturation of the specialty in Australia and New Zealand. Emergency medicine will continue to expand throughout medical curricula rather than being the practice-based pre-intern term it currently occupies in the latter years of most medical courses. A recent shift in focus in the tertiary sector towards teaching ability rather than purely a research output will create opportunities for emergency medicine to gain a stronger foothold in universities. Teaching programmes will expand to deliver material, not just unique to emergency medicine, but the specialty will be opportunistic and be called upon to teach where significant gaps exist at an undergraduate level. In many universities there is no academic presence in surgical subspecialties such as ear, nose and throat, ophthalmology, and orthopaedics. It will be left to emergency physicians to teach students the basics of these specialties, just as we currently manage many common acute conditions in these areas without specialist input.

It is now time for the specialty to move beyond just the provision of training in acute medicine as envisaged by the landmark Macy

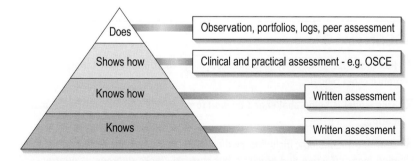

Fig. 24.4.2 The learning assessment pyramid.[21] OSCE, objective structured clinical examination.

report in 1994.[22] The specialty will develop its own body of knowledge and curriculum in important but under-represented areas of medical education such as clinical decision-making, medical error and health systems design and management. Emergency physicians need to take a leading role in the development and delivery of curricula in these areas. There is much to suggest that the increased sub-specialization of medicine has led to fragmentation of the health system, with the subsequent inability of society to achieve coherent and sustainable outcomes in health policy. Emergency medicine as a specialty has the opportunity to take a leading role in training doctors and other health professionals capable of understanding the key challenges facing the health system in the 21st century.

Controversies

❶ There is much debate about the effectiveness of current methods of medical student training, but emergency medicine as an academic specialty is adaptable and capable of working within any number of curricular styles.

❷ EDs will struggle to handle increased numbers of students without additional dedicated support from universities and may need to consider withholding access until appropriate sustainable resources can be provided.

❸ Emergency physicians still have much to do in creating a coordinated undergraduate curriculum that is vertically integrated with prevocational and specialist training in the specialty.

❹ It is inevitable that more academic departments of emergency medicine will be created but first the specialty must clearly define its core curriculum and its role in the health education system

❺ Changes in the health workforce with a re-definition of the role of the doctor and an evolution of the other health professions will necessitate that the specialty apply its knowledge base to broader health science training, including that of evolving positions such as physician assistants.

References

1. The Royal College of Physicians and Surgeons of Canada. Can MEDS 2000 Project skills for the new millennium: Report of the societal needs working group. Ontario: 1996.
2. Australian Medical Council. Goals and objectives of basic medical education. http://www.amc.org.au/GoalsBasicMed.asp (accessed 13 August 2007).
3. Van der Weyden M. Medical education and hard science. Medical Journal Association 2003; 180(12): 601.
4. Crotty B, Brown T. An urgent challenge: new training opportunities for junior medical officers. Medical Journal Association 2007; 186(7): S25–S27.
5. Russi CS, Hamilton GC. A case for emergency medicine in the undergraduate medical school curriculum. Academic Emergency Medicine 2005; 12(10): 994–998.
6. Australasian College for Emergency Medicine. Policy on the emergency medicine component of the undergraduate medical curriculum. http://www.acem.org.au (accessed 13 August 2007).
7. ACEP Academic Affairs Committee. Guidelines for Undergraduate education in emergency medicine. http://www.acep.org/webportal/PracticeResources/issues/acad/prepemundergradguideeduc.htm (accessed 9 August 2007).
8. Task Force on National Fourth Year Medical Student Emergency Medicine Curriculum Guide. Report of the Task Force on National Fourth Year Medical Student Emergency Medicine Curriculum Guide. Annals of Emergency Medicine 2006; 47: E1–E7.
9. Pacella CB. Advanced opportunities for student education in emergency medicine. Academic Emergency Medicine 2004; 11(10): 9–12.
10. Coates WC, Gendy MS, Gill AM. Emergency medicine subinternship: Can we provide a standard clinical experience? Academic Emergency Medicine 2003; 10: 1138–1141.
11. Lake F, Ryan G. Teaching on the run tips 2: educational guides for teaching in a clinical setting. Medical Journal Association 2004; 180(10): 527–528.
12. Morrison J. ABC of learning and teaching in medicine: evaluation. British Medical Journal 2003; 326: 385–387.
13. Miller GE. The assessment of clinical skills/competence/performance. Academic Medical Journal 1990; 65: 563–567.
14. Harden RM, Stamper N. What is a spiral curriculum? Medical Teacher 1999; 21: 141–143.
15. Walls J, Couser GA, Gennat H, et al. Clinical cases in emergency medicine: a physiological approach. Sydney: McGraw-Hill; 2006.
16. Arnold R. The theory and principles of psychodynamic pedagogy. Forum of Education 1994; 49(2).
17. McKimm J, Jollie C, Cantillon P. ABC of learning and teaching: web based learning. British Medical Journal 2003; 326: 870–873.
18. Coates WC, Gendy MS, Gill AM. Emergency medicine subinternship: can we provide a standard clinical experience? Academic Emergency Medicine 2003; 10: 1138–1141.
19. Lake F, Ryan G. Teaching on the run tips 3: planning a teaching episode. Medical Journal Association 2004; 180(12): 643–644.
20. Lake F, Hamdorf J. Teaching on the run tips 5: Teaching a skill. Medical Journal Association 2004; 181(6): 327–328.
21. Shumway JM, Harden RM AMEE Guide No. 25: The assessment of learning outcomes for the competent and reflective physician. Medical Teacher 2003; (25)6: 569–584.
22. Josiah Macy Jr Foundation. The role of emergency medicine in the future of American medical care. Annals of Emergency Medicine 1995; 25: 230–233.

24.5 Postgraduate emergency medicine teaching and simulation

Victoria Brazil

ESSENTIALS

1 Postgraduate emergency medicine teaching traditionally has followed an apprenticeship model.

2 This model is being challenged by workforce trends and innovations in medical education.

3 Learning technology, including medical simulation, has the potential to make training more effective and efficient, but currently lacks rigorous evaluation.

Introduction

Emergency departments (EDs) provide many learning opportunities for postgraduate doctors. The varied clinical case mix, procedural nature of practice and flexibility of work attract doctors to vocational training. Postgraduate emergency medicine teaching has traditionally followed an apprenticeship model, with the underlying assumption that patient care experience and opportunistic bedside teaching from clinical experts provided the knowledge, skills and attitudes requisite for emergency medicine practice. This model is currently being challenged by contemporary workforce issues, changed service provision models, improved technology and advances in medical education.

Current training pathways in postgraduate emergency medicine

In those countries where emergency medicine has been recognized as a specialty, with a model and scope of practice, formalization of postgraduate training has followed. In Australasia, Canada, South Africa and the UK, specialist colleges have been responsible for accreditation and standards for emergency medicine training.[1-3] The American Board of Emergency Medicine (ABEM)[4] in the USA fulfils a similar role. In other jurisdictions, tertiary institutions (Malaysia) or professional societies (many European countries) provide the educational framework for vocational training.

These formal training programmes provide a structured educational experience for vocational trainees. The length of training varies from 3 to 7 years, generally uses graduated patient care responsibility as the primary learning experience, and requires a range of rotations through emergency medicine and other clinical experience such as anaesthesia, intensive care, psychiatry and paediatrics.[5] Most programmes involve both in-training assessment and formal examinations during the period of training. Many programmes also require logbooks or portfolios of clinical experience.

The regulatory frameworks continue to evolve. The UK has recently reconfigured postgraduate training in the 'Modernising Medical Careers' initiative,[6,7] resulting in the NHS taking on roles previously held by specialist colleges. In Australia there are calls for shorter 'non-specialist' training programmes for career emergency doctors, particularly to address rural and regional workforce challenges.[8] In developing countries, there is variable progress toward formal postgraduate training.

The inconsistency in programme requirements, together with traditional protectionist policies in some countries, has meant that there exists minimal mutual recognition of emergency medicine qualifications internationally.

Challenges for contemporary emergency medicine education

There are growing pressures on postgraduate medical education in emergency medicine (Table 24.5.1). The impact of these trends can be observed in emergency medicine curricula, teaching and learning processes, learning technology, assessment and accreditation, and faculty development.

Curricular trends

There has been a global trend in postgraduate medical education toward 'outcomes based' curricular models. This has resulted in a shift from curricula defining a knowledge base to be acquired, to 'outcome' concepts of roles and competencies for specialist physicians.

The CanMEDS model, developed in Canada and adopted by the Australasian College for Emergency Medicine (ACEM), requires training be oriented toward preparing emergency physicians (and other specialist trainees) for

---

Table 24.5.1 Pressures leading to change in delivery of postgraduate education in emergency medicine

- An international medical workforce shortage,[9] increasing pressure to produce qualified practitioners in a shorter time, and with a more 'work ready' focus
- Changing workforce roles, with challenges to traditional emergency physician scope of practice from nurse practitioners, physician assistants and other extended role practitioners
- Increased service provision expectations of clinicians, as a result of rising healthcare costs throughout the developed world, decreasing the time available for teaching and learning in the clinical arena
- The patient safety agenda and societal expectations mean that 'learning by doing' and practising skills on patients is less acceptable
- The expectations of GenerationY, in which trainees expect flexibility in training delivery and a practice model that provides work–life balance
- Learners' changing expectations of teaching processes, as a result of exposure to innovations in undergraduate medical education

---

their roles as medical expert, communicator, collaborator, manager, health advocate, scholar and professional.[10]

The Accreditation Council for Graduate Medical Education (ACGME) in the USA defines six core competencies required of specialist trainees: medical knowledge, patient care, practice-based learning and improvement, interpersonal and communication skills, professionalism, and systems-based practice. These general competencies have been translated into specific emergency medicine curricular objectives.[11]

Integral to this curricular trend has been increased recognition of communication and professional domains of practice. Concepts of teamwork, leadership, patient safety, quality improvement, and communication with patients and peers have been specified in recent curricula.[12] New domains of learning, such as medical informatics and evidence based medicine, have become explicit curricular content.

Innovation in teaching and learning

Bedside teaching, or 'teaching on the floor', remains the foundation of most ED trainees' educational experience. It provides the opportunity to reflect upon clinical and professional aspects of emergency medicine practice in an integrated manner. It should be facilitated by a graduated increase in patient care responsibility throughout the training programme. However, the quality of this experience is dependent on the availability and skill of clinical supervisors, and on time constraints in busy EDs. In this environment, clinical teaching can remain 'education by random opportunity', and learners may not be exposed to rare but important conditions or procedures.

Didactic elements of specialist training vary in format but most programmes or institutions provide a structured element of training that consists of trainee- and supervisor-delivered presentations, procedural skill sessions, journal clubs and lectures by visitors or outside specialists. Following the trend towards competency-based curricular models, there is a general trend toward these teaching activities becoming more standardized and structured.

Reflective practice is an important learning skill for postgraduate trainees. Clinical audit[13] and portfolios[14] can facilitate this, and most training programmes also encourage participation in critical incident review, trauma review meetings and morbidity and mortality rounds.

Recent innovations in training incorporate interprofessional and team-based learning, following recognition of the team approach required for effective clinical practice. This includes multidisciplinary formal educational sessions and team-based simulation experiences.[15] Such activities are focused on communication and professional domains of competence, and provide trainees with a broader perspective on systems-based practice in emergency medicine.

Learning technology

Technology provides many potential applications for teaching and learning in emergency medicine, but frequently is adopted without critical review of educational value.

Content-based technological adjuncts such as textbooks on CD ROMs have made published references more available and more easily updated. Electronic formats also allow replication of high quality images and videos. These adjuncts do not fundamentally change the way trainees learn.

Web-based content for emergency medicine has exploded over recent years. A Google search for 'emergency medicine' reveals more than 64 million web pages. As a result, the emergency medicine trainee requires effective information retrieval and quality analysis skills. Recent literature suggests that public access search engines such as Google Scholar have now replaced traditional Medline database searches as the preferred method of information retrieval by trainees.[16]

Procedural skill training has been enhanced by the use of manikins, part trainers, and virtual reality systems,[17] reducing the use of animal labs and cadavers. There is evidence that this approach is more effective than traditional procedural skills training on patients.[18] Video-based instruction of procedures allows demonstration of procedural performance under ideal conditions, with rehearsed teaching scripts. Many of these are now available on personal digital assistants for 'just-in-time learning' for trainees. More comprehensive e-learning packages for procedural skills training use a problem-based approach, informed by known complications and high risk situations, and often complemented by hands-on sessions.[19]

Clinical decision support software provides educational opportunities in conjunction with solutions to clinical problems. Many of these programmes have extensive resource materials embedded that can be utilized in clinical practice or for primarily educational purposes.

The internet has also provided opportunities for the formation of virtual learning communities in emergency medicine. Informal discussion boards and weblogs foster collaborative networking and debate. Formal training activities can also be conducted via asynchronous learning networks,[20] and specialized software platforms can enhance interactivity and promote user-generated content for more active e-learning experiences.[21]

Videoconferencing and tele-education have sought to answer the challenges of distance in emergency medicine education.[22] This technology has been successfully employed in the continuing medical education (CME) arena,[23] but improvements in technology and bandwidth potentially provide greater access to interactive educational activities at all levels of emergency medicine training. It may help to relieve the teaching workload in smaller or more remote EDs.

Simulation-based learning for emergency medicine

Medical simulation encompasses any kind of simulated patient interaction, manikin or virtual-reality-based procedural skill performance, or simulated complex emergency medicine scenario. It involves technology as simple as standardized human patients with a role play script, and as complex as high fidelity simulators designed to provide realistic tactile, auditory and visual stimuli. The varied dimensions of simulation and its wide application to professional practice offer potential solutions to many healthcare educational challenges.[24]

The critical issue for simulation-based learning is an understanding of the educational objectives. These may range from knowledge acquisition, procedural skill proficiency, applied physiology and pharmacology, to complex teamwork skills and behaviours inherent in crisis resource management. The educational objective should then determine the nature of the equipment used, scenario design, the level of fidelity required, and the approach to debriefing.

Simulators, equipment and fidelity

Manikin technology continues to improve. The most technologically complex full body simulators currently cost more than $A400 000. They operate via detailed physiological modelling software, and can manifest pulses, breathing, blinking and vocalization, together with an ability to alter lung mechanics and compliance, and cardiovascular parameters. Less complex simulators can manifest many of these same features without the strict adherence to physiological modelling, but with the benefit of lower cost and increased portability.

Manufacturers have classified manikins as high or low fidelity based on their technological complexity. However, the fidelity of the simulation experience as perceived by the learner is far more complex. The authenticity of the scenario presented, including clinical, professional and communication challenges, the realism of the team composition and the physical environment all appear to be more important to both the learners' perception of fidelity and the learning outcomes achieved.[25,26]

Combining simple 'part trainers' with standardized patients has been successfully used to integrate a procedural skill with communication performance, for instance an actor wearing a synthetic skin pad with a laceration and responding to a junior doctor suturing the wound.

Teamwork and communication skills training using medical simulation

Crisis resource management (CRM) training in emergency medicine using human patient simulation[27] draws on parallels between acute patient care and the aviation and military industries, where it has been recognized that human factors are crucial to team performance.

A typical scenario might involve a team of medical and nursing participants managing a man with chest pain, who is accompanied by his wife in the ED, and who then develops a life-threatening arrhythmia. Participants need to identify and manage clinical issues, while engaging in the communication, teamwork and leadership activities inherent in real clinical practice. The scenario is then followed by video-assisted, expert debrief to reflect upon individual and team performance. This experiential learning approach enables cross-domain training in which cognitive, procedural and affective domains of practice are authentically integrated. The interprofessional nature of the learning experience provides a unique opportunity for increased understanding of the role of other healthcare disciplines.

Educational benefits

Simulation enables 'efficient' learning through standardized exposure to clinical challenges which may be infrequent in clinical practice. It allows practice and failure in a safe environment, without risk to patients.

Advanced manikin and audiovisual technology, together with logistic expertise, mean that these learning experiences can be provided in the practitioner's own ED. The use of the authentic work environment allows very high levels of fidelity to be achieved, as the team uses its own equipment and clinical processes. The other key advantage of this approach is that the usual work team can engage in learning together, without the cost and logistical barriers of travelling to a synthetic environment. Provision of the simulation-based experience and group debriefing via videoconferencing and remote control of equipment is at the boundary of present technological capacity.

In addition to their role in learning, human patient simulators can be used for competency assessment, which is made reliable by standardized challenges. However, it is important that assessment activities are clearly distinguished from those whose objective is learning, as key differences in simulation performance are observed.

This reproducibility also provides opportunities to study the effect of fatigue or expertise level on emergency physician or trainee performance, and for testing new medical equipment or clinical systems.

Limitations

There are limitations to simulation-based training. There are significant costs in equipment and trained personnel to run programs. Critical care situations, especially cardiac and airway emergencies, can be simulated with a high degree of fidelity, but many other emergency medicine clinical challenges are not suitable. Negative training is a recognized risk. Allowing the participants to not wear gloves or lead aprons, or simulating overly positive clinical responses to medical interventions, can allow poor behaviour patterns to develop, or train learners to have unrealistic expectations in the real clinical environment.

Training for providers

Educators using simulation-based modalities require proficiency in technological issues, experiential learning principles and small group process. Training for providers of simulation-based emergency medicine education is varied. Short courses exist at many simulation centres, and most providers run their own 'in-house' quality assurance process to ensure a standardized approach to scenario design, delivery and group debriefing. However, there is a lack of agreed standards in this area.

Evidence for simulation-based learning

Evidence for clinical practice improvement is currently lacking, despite intuitive appeal.[28] There are methodological challenges in the reliable measurement of teamwork and communication performance, and attribution issues involved in any demonstration of patient outcome improvement. Professional associations in the field are working towards international consensus on learning objectives, methodology and evaluation.

Assessment and performance appraisal

Trainee assessment formats in formal postgraduate emergency medicine training programmes are diverse. These formats have usually been determined by national training and accreditation bodies (see Chapter 27.5). There is considerable variation in the domains of performance formally assessed, the definition of 'professional competence' required and in the standardization of assessment processes undertaken.

In-training assessment by clinical supervisors is a core element in most programmes, but this may be provided by one designated supervisor of training or many clinical supervisors in a group-based assessment. Literature suggests that in-training assessment is a valid tool (i.e. measures the right thing),[29] but the potentially subjective nature of supervisor assessments continues to raise questions as to reliability.

Most programmes also have formal examination components, generally developed and administered externally by the national training body. A variety of formats exist, including multiple-choice questions, written tests, structured interviews and clinical examination vivas.

Workplace-based assessment is becoming more prevalent, with use of tools such as clinical simulations, portfolios, standardized patients and multisource '360 degree feedback' assessment that involves assessment by patients, peers, nursing staff and others.[30] Patient care quality outcomes have been suggested as an assessment tool.[31] These formats encourage the trend toward specific assessment of communication and professional competence, which mirror the shift in curricular content.

Faculty development in emergency medicine

Many emergency physicians are enthusiastic clinical teachers. However, there is now recognition that these clinician educators require specific preparation for their teaching role. Specific training for educators in emergency medicine is variable, including Masters level courses, short workshops,[32] and institution-based group professional development activities. These courses typically cover topics such as curriculum development, teaching and learning processes, and assessment and feedback skills.

Programmes are more formally developed in the USA, where a number of teaching fellowships exist in emergency medicine and the Society for Academic Emergency Medicine (SAEM) has published a *Faculty Development Handbook*.[33] These initiatives have been reinforced by the emergence of 'clinician educator tracks' in academic institutions to provide an academic career structure for clinical teachers.

Non-vocational teaching in emergency medicine

Pre-vocational education

In Australasia, the UK and other countries where prevocational doctors exist, the emergency medicine term has been recognized for learning acute care skills, management of the undifferentiated patient, and professional skills such as teamwork and communication. These competencies and domains of learning have been formalized recently in consensus statements such as the Australian Junior Doctor Curriculum Framework.[34]

Continuing medical education

There is a societal expectation in developed countries that physicians maintain their skills and competence to manage patients in their speciality. This concept has led to certification processes that require participation in learning activities after specialist qualification has been achieved. The extent and complexity of these systems vary, but mostly require periodic assimilation of a portfolio of attendance at conferences and workshops, together with demonstration of participation in teaching, quality assurance activities, research or other special interests. Some jurisdictions require update examinations.

The provision of CME is a significantly more deregulated market than vocational training. Government health departments, hospitals, private companies and tertiary institutions are all active in providing CME activities.

The effectiveness of current CME offerings, as measured by changes in physician behaviour, appears lacking,[35] raising questions about the design and educational value of many of these courses. However, it is recognized that many CME activities also provide a political and social function.

Controversies and future directions

❶ Workforce issues will create pressure to shorten and standardize vocational training, including that in emergency medicine, around the world. The Australian and UK governments in particular have been proactive in reviewing postgraduate training models to address workforce challenges. This may result in a significantly more deregulated training environment in which tertiary institutions and private providers play a greater role.

❷ Adoption of advances in educational methodology should continue to make teaching and learning processes more efficient, effective and outcome orientated. However, this process depends upon financial support, models for which vary between countries.

❸ Societal expectations will likely require increased transparency and reliability in assessment methods.

❹ Technology and web-based modalities have an enormous potential to facilitate collaboration, distance learning, and to compensate for the inefficiencies inherent in clinical exposure, but require critical analysis of educational benefit.

References

1. Steiner IP. Emergency medicine practice and training in Canada. Canadian Medical Association Journal 2003; 168(12): 1549–1550.
2. Australasian College for Emergency Medicine. Online. http://www.acem.org.au (accessed 5 August 2007).
3. College of Emergency Medicine South Africa (CMSA). Online. http://www.collegemedsa.ac.za/view_college.asp?Type=Link and CollegeID=5 5 (accessed August 2007).
4. American Board of Emergency Medicine. Online. http://www.abem.org/public/ (accessed 5 August 2007).
5. Taylor DM, Jelinek GA. A comparison of Australasian and United States emergency medicine training programs. Academic Emergency Medicine 1999; 6(4): 324–330.
6. How is medical training changing? Modernising medical careers. Online. Available: http://www.mmc.nhs.uk/download/What%20is%20changing%20at%20MMC.pdf (accessed 9 August 2007).
7. McGowan A. Modernising medical careers: educational implications for the emergency department. Emergency Medicine Journal 2006; 23(8): 644–646.
8. Arvier PT, Walker JH, McDonagh T. Training emergency medicine doctors for rural and regional Australia: can we learn from other countries? Rural & Remote Health 2007; 7(2): 705.
9. Brooks P, Lapsley H, Butt D. Medical workforce issues in Australia: 'Tomorrow's doctors – too few, too far'. Medical Journal of Australia 2003; 179: 206–208.
10. Frank JR, ed. The CanMEDS 2005 physican competency framework. Better standards. Better physicians. Better care. Ottawa: The Royal College of Physicians and Surgeons of Canada. Online. Available: http://rcpsc.medical.org/canmeds/CanMEDS2005/index.php (accessed 6 August 2007).
11. Chapman DM, Hayden S, Sanders AB, et al. Integrating the Accreditation Council for Graduate Medical Education core competencies into the model of the clinical practice of emergency medicine. Annals of Emergency Medicine 2004; 43(6): 756–769.
12. Leonard M, Graham S, Bonacum D. The human factor: the critical importance of effective teamwork and communication in providing safe care. Quality and Safety in Health Care 2004; 13: 85–90.
13. Brazil V. Audit as a learning tool in postgraduate emergency medicine training. Emergency Medicine Australasia. 2004; 16(4): 348–352.
14. Cook RJ, Pedley DK, Thakore S. A structured competency based training programme for junior trainees in emergency medicine: the 'Dundee model'. Emergency Medicine Journal 2006; 23(1): 18–22.
15. Shapiro MJ, Morey JC, Small SD. Simulation based teamwork training for emergency department staff: does it improve clinical team performance when added to an existing didactic teamwork curriculum? Quality Safety Health Care 2004; 3: 417–421.
16. Giustini D. How Google is changing medicine. British Medical Journal 2005; 331: 1487–1488.
17. Vozenilek J, Huff JS, Reznek M, et al. See one, do one, teach one: advanced technology in medical education. Academic Emergency Medicine 2004; 11(11): 1149–1154.
18. Seymour NE, Gallagher AG, Roman SA, et al. Virtual reality training improves operating room performance: results of a randomized, double-blinded study. Annals of Surgery 2002; 236(4): 458–464.
19. Med-e-serv. Insertion of chest tubes and management of chest drains in adults. Online. Available: http://learning.medeserv.com.au/products/MES2020/MES2020_brochure.cfm (accessed 14 August 2007).
20. Ashton A, Bhati R. The use of an asynchronous learning network for senior house officers in emergency medicine. Emergency Medicine Journal 2007; 24(6): 427–428.
21. Moodle. Online. Available: http://moodle.org/ (accessed August 16 2007).
22. Sweetman G, Brazil V. Education links between the Australian rural and tertiary emergency departments: Videoconference can support a virtual learning community. Emergency Medicine Australasia 2007; 19(2): 176–177.
23. Allen M, Sargeant J, Mann K, et al. Videoconferencing for practice-based small group continuing medical education: feasibility, acceptability, effectiveness, and cost. Journal of Continuing Education in the Health Professions 2003; 23: 38–47.
24. Gaba D. The future vision of simulation in health care. Quality and Safe Health Care 2004; 13: 2–10.
25. Rehmann A, Mitman R, Reynolds M. A handbook of flight simulation fidelity requirements for human factors research. Technical Report No. DOT/FAA/CT-TN95/46 Wright Patterson Air Force Base, Ohio: Crew Systems Ergonomics Information Analysis Centre; 1995.
26. Beaubien JM, Baker DP. The use of simulation for training teamwork skills in healthcare: how low can you go? Quality Safe Health Care 2004; 13: 51–56.
27. Reznek M, Smith-Coggins R, Howard S, et al. emergency medicine crisis resource management (EMCRM): pilot study of a simulation-based crisis management course for emergency medicine. Academic Emergency Medicine 2003; 10: 386–389.
28. Issenberg SB, McGaghie WC, Petrusa E, et al. Features and uses of high-fidelity medical simualtions that lead to effective learning: a BEME systematic review. Medical Teacher 2005; 27(1): 10–28.
29. Epstein R. Assessment in medical education. New England Journal of Medicine 2007; 356: 387–396.
30. Rodgers KG, Manifold C. 360-degree feedback: possibilities for assessment of the ACGME core competencies for emergency medicine residents. Academic Emergency Medicine 2002; 9: 1300–1304.
31. Swing SR, Schneider S, Bizovi K, et al. Using patient care quality measures to assess educational outcomes. Academic Emergency Medicine 2007; 14(5): 463–473.
32. Sherbino J, Frank J, Lee C, et al. Evaluating "ED STAT!": a novel and effective faculty development program to improve emergency department teaching. Academic Emergency Medicine 2006; 13: 1062–1069.
33. Faculty Development Handbook, Society for Academic Emergency Medicine. Online. Available: www.saem.org (accessed 20 August 2007).
34. Graham IS, Gleason AJ, Keogh GW, et al. Australian curriculum framework for junior doctors. Medical Journal of Australia 2007; 186(7): S14–S19.
35. Davis D, Thomson M, O'Brien K, et al. Do conferences, workshops, rounds, and other traditional continuing education activities change physician behavior or health care outcomes? Journal of the American Medical Association 1999; 282: 867–874.

EMERGENCY MEDICINE AND THE LAW

Edited by **George Jelinek**

25.1 Mental health and the law: the Australasian and UK perspectives

Georgina Phillips • Suzanne Mason • Simon Baston

ESSENTIALS

1 The emergency department is frequently the point of access to the mental health system.

2 Emergency physicians need to be able to distinguish between patients with physical and those with psychiatric illness.

3 Patients should only be committed involuntarily to an approved hospital if they have a mental illness requiring immediate treatment for their own health or safety or the protection of others, and if adequate treatment cannot be obtained in a less restrictive manner.

4 Emergency physicians need to have a sound working knowledge of mental health legislation as it relates to their practice and to the jurisdiction in which they work.

Introduction

The ED is frequently the interface between the community and the mental health system. In recent years changes in health policy have resulted in 'mainstreaming' of mental health services, so that stand-alone psychiatric services are less common and services are more likely to be provided in a general hospital setting. Linked to this has been a move away from managing long-term psychiatric patients in institutional settings, so that many of these former patients are now living in the community with or without support from mental health services.

Traditionally, by virtue of their accessibility, EDs have been a point of access to mental health services for persons with acute psychiatric illness, whether this be self or family referral or by referral from ambulance, police or outside medical practitioners. An important function of an ED is to differentiate between those who require psychiatric care for a psychiatric illness, and those who present with a psychiatric manifestation of a physical illness and who require medical care. Admission of a patient with a psychiatric manifestation of a physical illness to a psychiatric unit may result in further harm to or death of the patient.

In the UK and Australasia, doctors in general are empowered by legislation to detain a mentally ill person who is in need of treatment. Mental illness, particularly its manifestation as self-harm, is a common ED presentation (in the UK, making up around 1–2% of new patient attendances, and up to 5% of attendances in Australasia), and emergency physicians require not only the clinical skills to distinguish between those who require psychiatric or medical intervention, but also a sound working knowledge of the mental health legislation and services relevant to the state where they practise. This ensures that patients with psychiatric illness are managed in the most appropriate way, with optimal utilization of mental health resources and with the best interests and rights of the patient and the community taken into consideration.

Whilst there are variations in mental health legislation between the UK, Australia and New Zealand, all legislation recognizes fundamental common principles that respect individual autonomy and employ least restrictive management practices. The World Health Organisation (WHO) advises 10 basic principles of mental healthcare law, including enshrining geographical, cultural and economic equity of access to mental health care, acceptable standards of clinical assessment, facilitating self-determination, minimizing restrictive treatment and enshrining regular and impartial decision-making and review of care.[1] These themes are all present in Australasian and UK law, and awareness of such principles aids the clinician in delivering humane and ethical treatment for mentally unwell patients who seek emergency care.

Variations in practice

Mental health legislation in England and Wales

The National Service Framework for Mental Health

The National Service Framework for Mental Health produced by the Department of Health in the UK (1999) is aimed at improving quality and addresses the mental health needs of working age adults up to 65 years. It states as one of its standards that:

'Any individual with a common mental health problem should be able to make contact round the clock with the local services necessary to meet their needs and receive adequate care.'

Although EDs do not provide the ideal environment for a mental health assessment, they are likely to continue to provide an entry point for people with mental health problems. Easy access to the ED can lead to individuals with acute mental health problems seeking help directly, making up to perhaps 5% of ED attenders.

Two pieces of legislation cover the care and treatment of patients with disorders of the brain or mind. The Mental Health Act (1983) deals with compulsory assessment and treatment of people with mental illnesses, while the Mental Capacity Act (2005) deals with people who are unable to make decisions about their medical treatment for themselves for various reasons.

Mental Health Act

Definition of mentally ill or mental illness According to the 1983 Mental Health Act, mental illness is undefined. However, in practice it includes conditions such as schizophrenia, bipolar disorder, depression, psychosis and organic brain syndromes. Mental impairment is defined as 'a state of arrested or incomplete development of mind which includes significant impairment of intelligence and social functioning and is associated with abnormally aggressive or seriously irresponsible conduct on the part of the person concerned'. A psychopathic disorder is defined as 'a persistent disorder or disability of mind which results in abnormally aggressive or seriously irresponsible conduct on the part of the person concerned'. The Act does not cover promiscuity or other immoral conduct, or sexual deviancy, which in the past could result in incarceration in psychiatric hospitals or dependence on drugs or alcohol.

Detention of patients with mental illness The Mental Health Act 1983 provides legislation with regard to the management of patients with a mental illness unwilling to be admitted or detained in hospital voluntarily, where this would be in the best interests of the health and safety of patients and others. For the purposes of the Act, patients in the ED are not considered inpatients until they are admitted to a ward. In order for legislation to be imposed it is necessary for two conditions to be satisfied: the patient must be suffering from a mental illness and emergency hospital admission is required because the patient is considered to be a danger to themselves or others.

Detention under the Mental Health Act does not permit treatment for psychiatric or physical illness. Treatment can be given under common law where the patient is considered to pose a serious threat to themselves or others. Otherwise all treatment must be with the patient's consent.

Section 2 of the Mental Health Act facilitates compulsory admission to hospital for assessment and treatment for up to 28 days. The application is usually made by an approved social worker or the patient's nearest relative and requires two medical recommendations, usually from the patient's general practitioner and the duty senior psychiatrist (who is approved under Section 12 of the Mental Health Act). In the ED, the responsibility for coordinating the procedure often lies with the emergency physician.

Section 3 of the Mental Health Act covers compulsory admission for treatment. Once again, recommendations must be made by two doctors, one of whom is usually the general practitioner and the other a psychiatrist approved under Section 12 of the Act. The application is usually made by an approved social worker or the patient's nearest relative. Detention is for up to 6 months but can be renewed.

Section 4 of the Mental Health Act covers emergency admission for assessment and attempts to avoid delay in emergency situations when obtaining a second recommendation could be dangerous. It requires the recommendation of only one doctor, who may be any registered medical practitioner who must have seen the patient within the previous 24 h. The order lasts for 72 h. Application can be made by the patient's nearest relative or an approved social worker. In practice, the application of Section 4 of the Mental Health Act rarely happens. Usually Section 2 or 3 is the preferred option.

Section 5 (2) – doctors holding power and Section 5 (4) – nurses holding power of the Act allow the detention of patients who are already admitted to hospital until a more formal Mental Health Act assessment can take place. Unfortunately, presence in the ED is not considered to constitute admission to hospital, and this section is, therefore, not applicable to the ED.

A new draft Mental Health Bill published in 2002 was opposed by professional and patient groups alike. It aimed to introduce a new legal framework for the compulsory treatment of people with mental disorders in hospitals and the community. The new procedure involved a single pathway in three stages: a preliminary examination, a period of formal assessment lasting up to 28 days and treatment under a Mental Health Act order. In order for the compulsory process to be used, four conditions needed to be satisfied: the patient must have a mental disorder, the disorder must warrant medical treatment, treatment must be necessary for the health and safety of the patient or others, and an appropriate treatment for the disorder must be available. The draft Bill made provision for treatment without consent as it is justified under the European Convention on Human Rights Article 8 (2) in the interests of public safety or to protect health or moral standards.

The resulting debate saw much of the draft Bill being scrapped in favour of amendments being made to the existing Mental Health Act. This included the creation of community treatment orders and a broader definition of mental disorder.

Police powers

Section 136 of the Act authorizes the police to remove patients who are believed to be mentally disordered and causing a public disturbance to a place of safety. The place of safety referred to in the Act is defined in Section 135 as 'residential accommodation provided by a local authority under Part III of the National Assistance Act 1948, or under Paragraph 2, Schedule 8 of the National Health Service Act 1977, a hospital as defined by this Act, a police station, a mental nursing home or residential home for mentally disordered persons or any other suitable place, the occupier of which is willing temporarily to receive the patient'. In practice, the police often transport these patients to local EDs. The patient must be assessed by an approved social worker and a registered doctor. The order lasts for 72 h.

Section 135 allows the police to enter premises to remove a patient believed to be suffering from a mental disorder to a place of safety for up to 72 h. The patient is then assessed as above.

Mental Capacity Act

The Mental Capacity Act relates to decision-making, for those whose mental capacity is in doubt, on any issue from what to wear to the more difficult issues of medical treatment, personal finance and housing.

Lack of capacity can occur in two distinct ways. Firstly, that capacity is never achieved – for example someone with a severe learning difficulty. Secondly, capacity can be lost either as a result of long-term conditions such as dementia or for a short period because of a temporary factor such as intoxication, shock, pain or emotional distress.

It is also important that decision-making is task specific. An individual may be able to make decisions about simple matters such as what to eat or wear but may be unable to make more complex decisions, for example about medical care.

Assessment of capacity   To have capacity about a decision the patient should be able to comply with the following four steps:

- Understand the information relevant to the decision.
- Retain the information for the period of decision-making.
- Use or weigh that information as part of the process of making a decision.
- Communicate their decisions.

Every effort needs to be made to enable people to make their own decisions.

The Act points out that people should be allowed to make 'eccentric' or 'unwise' decisions, as it is their ability to decide that is the issue not the decision itself.

Advance directives   The Act makes provision for advance directives to be made at a time when the patient has capacity. These directives need to make specific reference to the medical treatments involved and include the statement 'even if life is at risk'. The validity of any advance decision needs to be clearly documented.

Advocates   Although family and friends have no legal powers (unless specified in advance) to make decisions for the incapacitated patient, the Act recognizes their role in acting as an advocate. An independent mental capacity advocate is available to represent those with no close family or friends.

Emergency treatment   Treatment can be given to patients who lack capacity but several factors need to be considered:

- Any action must be in the best interest of the patient.

- Anything done must be the least restrictive of the patient's rights and freedoms.
- Where time can be afforded every effort should be made to enable the patient to make his or her own decision.
- Treatment should not be delayed while attempts are made to establish the validity of any advance decision.
- Medical staff have a duty of care to the incapacitated patient.

Use of sedation or physical restraint   This is covered in detail elsewhere (Chapters 20.6 and 21.5). From the perspective of the mental health legislation, there are occasions where physical or pharmacological restraint is needed. Sedation or restraint must be the minimum that is necessary to prevent the patient from self-harming or harming others. Generally, a patient committed involuntarily is subject to treatment necessary for their care and control, and this may reasonably include the administration of sedative or antipsychotic medication as emergency treatment. Transporting these patients to a mental health service should be done by suitably trained medical or ambulance staff, and not delegated to police officers or other persons acting alone.

Mental health legislation in Australasia

In Australia mental health legislation is a state jurisdiction, and among the various states and territories there is considerable variation in the scope of mental health acts, and between definitions and applications of the various sections. Since the National Mental Health Strategy in 1992, there has been an effort in Australia to adopt a consistent approach between jurisdictions, with an emphasis on ensuring legislated review mechanisms and a broad spectrum of treatment modalities.[2] Nevertheless, key differences apply between mental health acts and therefore specific issues should be referred to the Act relevant to the emergency physician's practice location.

The Australian and New Zealand mental health acts referred to in this chapter are the following:

ACT – Mental Health (Treatment and Care) Act 1994 and amendments 2007
New South Wales – Mental Health Act 1990 and amendments (to be repealed by the commencement of the Mental Health Act 2007)
New Zealand – Mental Health (Compulsory Assessment and Treatment) Act 1992 and the 1999 Amendment
Northern Territory – Mental Health and Related Services Act 1998 and amendments 2005
Queensland – Mental Health Act 2000
South Australia – Mental Health Act 1993 and amendments
Tasmania – Mental Health Act 1996
Victoria – Mental Health Act 1986 and incorporating amendments as at 1 July 2007
Western Australia – Mental Health Act 1996.

Sections of the various mental health acts relevant to emergency medicine include those dealing with:

- the definition of mentally ill
- indigenous and cultural acknowledgment
- the effects of drugs or alcohol
- criteria for detention and admission as an involuntary patient
- involuntary admission
- persons unable to recommend a patient for involuntary admission
- physical restraint and sedation
- emergency treatment
- powers of police
- prisoners with mental illness
- amendment of documents
- offences in relation to documents
- information and patient transfer between jurisdictions
- deaths.

Definition of mentally ill or mental illness

For the purposes of their respective mental health acts, New Zealand and all the Australian states and territories define mental illness or disorder as follows.

Australian Capital Territory

The Australian Capital Territory (ACT) Act defines a psychiatric illness as a condition that seriously impairs (either temporarily or permanently) the mental functioning of a person and is characterized by the presence in the person of any of the following symptoms: delusions, hallucinations, serious disorder of thought form, a severe disturbance of mood or sustained or repeated irrational behaviour indicating the presence of these symptoms.

The ACT Mental Health Act also defines 'mental dysfunction' as a 'disturbance or defect, to a substantially disabling degree, of perceptual interpretation, comprehension, reasoning, learning, judgement, memory, motivation or emotion'.

New South Wales

The New South Wales Act defines mental illness in the same way as the ACT, but in addition distinguishes between a mentally ill person and a mentally disordered person.

A person is mentally ill if suffering from mental illness and, owing to that illness, requires care, treatment or control in order to protect the patient or others from serious physical harm. A person is also considered to be mentally ill if suffering from a mental illness that is characterized by a severe disturbance of mood or sustained or repeated irrational behaviour and requires care, treatment or control to protect the person from serious financial harm or damage to the person's reputation. There is also an acknowledgement of chronicity and the effects of likely deterioration, which should be taken into account when determining whether a person has mental illness.

A person (whether or not the person is suffering from mental illness) is mentally disordered if the person's behaviour for the time being is so irrational as to justify conclusion on reasonable grounds that temporary care, treatment or control of the person is necessary for the person's own protection from serious physical harm, or for the protection of others from serious physical harm.

New Zealand

In New Zealand, the Mental Health Act defines a mentally disordered person as possessing an abnormal state of mind, whether continuous or intermittent, characterized by delusions or by disorders of mood, perception, volition or cognition to such a degree that it poses a danger to the health or safety of the person or others, or seriously diminishes the capacity of the person to take care of themselves.

Northern Territory

In the Northern Territory, mental illness means a condition that seriously impairs, either temporarily or permanently, the mental functioning of a person in one or more of the areas of thought, mood, volition, perception, orientation or memory and is characterized by the presence of at least one of the following symptoms: delusions, hallucinations, serious disorders of the stream of thought, serious disorders of thought form or serious disturbances of mood. A mental illness is also characterized by sustained or repeated irrational behaviour that may be taken to indicate the presence of at least one of the symptoms mentioned above. The Northern Territory Act goes further, to specify that the determination of mental illness is only to be made in accordance with internationally accepted clinical standards and makes special mention of the World Health Association and both UK and American mental disorder classification guidelines.

Similar to the New South Wales Act, there is a provision in the Northern Territory for those who are 'mentally disturbed', which means behaviour of a person that is so irrational as to justify the person being temporarily detained under the Act.

Queensland

The Queensland Act defines mental illness in a similar way to Victoria, in that it is a condition characterized by a clinically significant disturbance of thought, mood, perception or memory, in accordance with internationally acceptable standards.

South Australia

In the South Australian Act mental illness means any illness or disorder of the mind.

Tasmania

A mental illness is a mental condition resulting in serious distortion of perception or thought, or serious impairment or disturbance of the capacity for rational thought. Also included in the Tasmanian definition is a serious disorder of mood, or involuntary behaviour or serious impairment of the capacity to control behaviour.

Victoria
A person is mentally ill if they have a mental illness, being a medical condition characterized by a significant disturbance of thought, mood, perception or memory.

Western Australia
Persons have a mental illness if they suffer from a disturbance of thought, mood, volition, perception, orientation or memory that impairs judgement or behaviour to a significant extent.

Indigenous and cultural acknowledgement
Cultural differences in the understanding and experiences of mental illness can impact greatly on the ability to provide adequate care. Whilst there are some cursory references to acknowledging special cultural and linguistic needs when interpreting the various mental health acts, only the Northern Territory in Australia and the New Zealand Mental Health Acts make specific mention of indigenous people, who are known to be a particularly vulnerable group.[3]

The Northern Territory Act states that there are fundamental principles to be taken into account when caring for Aborigines and Torres Strait Islanders. Treatment and care needs to be appropriate to the cultural beliefs and practices of the person, their family and community, and involuntary treatment for an Aborigine is to be provided in collaboration with an Aboriginal health worker.

New Zealand stipulates that powers are to be exercised in relation to the Mental Health Act with proper respect for cultural identity and personal beliefs, and with proper recognition of the importance and significance to the persons of their ties with family, whanau, hapu, iwi and family group. Interpreters are to be provided if the first or preferred language is not English, with special mention of Maori and New Zealand Sign Language.

Safeguards against prejudice
New Zealand and all Australian states, except South Australia, include a number of criteria that, alone, cannot be used to determine that a person has a mental illness and requires involuntary admission. These generally include the expression of or refusal to express particular religious, political and philosophical beliefs; cultural or racial origin; sexual promiscuity or preference; intellectual disability; drug or alcohol taking; economic or social status; immoral or indecent conduct; illegal conduct; and antisocial behaviour. The Northern Territory and Queensland also include past treatment for mental illness and past involuntary admission under these criteria.

Effects of drugs or alcohol
In most Australian states and New Zealand the taking of drugs or alcohol cannot, of itself, be taken as an indication of mental illness. However, the mental health acts of New South Wales and Victoria specify that this does not prevent the serious temporary or permanent physiological, biochemical or psychological effects of alcohol or drug taking from being regarded as an indication that a person is mentally ill. The Queensland Act acknowledges that a person may have a mental illness caused by taking drugs or alcohol.

The remaining states do not specifically exclude the temporary or permanent effects of drugs or alcohol but use definitions of mental or psychiatric illness that are broad enough to cover this. Generally, when a person is so mentally and behaviourally disordered as a result of drug or alcohol use that adequate assessment is impossible and risk of harm to self or others is high, then detaining them for the purposes of assessment and treatment is possible under all Australian and New Zealand mental health acts.

Criteria for admission and detention as an involuntary patient
All states require that an involuntary patient has a mental illness that requires urgent treatment while detained in an inpatient setting for the health (mental or physical) and safety of that patient or for the protection of others. Victoria, Western Australia, Queensland, the Northern Territory and the ACT also require that the patient has refused or is unable to consent to voluntary admission. It is also emphasized that appropriate treatment must be available and cannot be given in a less restrictive setting.

Both New South Wales and Western Australia include the protection of the patient from self-inflicted harm to the patient's reputation, relationships or finances as grounds for involuntary admission.

In New Zealand the doctor must have reasonable grounds for believing that the person may be mentally disordered and that it is desirable, in the interests of the person, or of any other person or of the public, that assessment, examination and treatment of the person are conducted as a matter of urgency.

Involuntary admission
The process of involuntary admission varies quite markedly across the states. It is variously known as recommendation, certification or committal. All jurisdictions require doctors to examine patients and carefully document on prescribed forms the date and time of examination as well as the particular reasons why the doctor believes that the person has a mental illness that requires involuntary treatment. In addition, patients or their advocates are to be informed of the decisions made about them and their rights under the law at all stages of the involuntary admission process.

Act
In the ACT a medical or police officer is able to apprehend a mentally ill person who requires involuntary admission and is able to use reasonable force and enter premises in order to do so. The officer is required, as soon as possible, to provide a written statement to the person in charge of the mental health facility giving patient details and the reasons for taking the action.

A doctor employed by the mental health facility must examine the patient within 4h of arrival and may authorize detention for up to 3 days. The doctor must inform the Community Advocate and Mental Health Tribunal of the patient's admission within 12h, and the patient must receive a physical and psychiatric examination within 24h of detention.

New South Wales
The Mental Health Act in New South Wales allows for a patient requiring involuntary admission to be detained in hospital on the certificate of a doctor who has personally examined the patient immediately or shortly before completing the certificate.

For a mentally ill patient the certificate is valid for 5 days from the time of writing, whereas for a mentally disordered patient the certificate is valid for 1 day. Mentally disordered patients cannot be detained on the grounds of being mentally disordered on more than three occasions in any 1 month.

Part of the certificate, if completed, directs the police to apprehend and bring the patient to hospital and also enables them to enter premises without a warrant.

An involuntary patient must be examined by the 'medical superintendent' as soon as practicable, but within 12 h of admission. The patient cannot be detained unless further certified mentally ill or disordered. This doctor cannot be the same doctor who requested admission or certified the patient. After their own examination, the 'medical superintendent' must arrange for a second examination as soon as practicable, this time by a psychiatrist. If neither doctor thinks that the person is mentally ill or disordered, then the person must be released from the hospital.

A patient who has been certified as mentally disordered, but not subsequently found to be mentally ill, cannot be detained for more than 3 days and must be examined by the 'medical superintendent' at least once every 24 h and discharged if no longer mentally ill or disordered, or if appropriate and less restrictive care is available.

New Zealand

In New Zealand, a person aged 18 years or over may request an assessment by the area mental health service if it has seen the person within the last 3 days and believes the person to be suffering from a mental disorder. The request may be accompanied by a certificate from a doctor who has examined the 'proposed patient' within the preceding 3 days and who believes that the person requires compulsory assessment and treatment. The medical certificate must state the reasons for the opinion and that the patient is not a relative. The area mental health service must then arrange an assessment examination by a psychiatrist or other suitable person forthwith. If the assessing doctor considers that the patient requires compulsory treatment, the patient may be detained in the 'first period' for up to 5 days. Subsequent assessment may result in detention for a 'second period' of up to 14 more days, after which a 'compulsory treatment order' must be issued by a family court judge.

Northern Territory

Any person with a genuine interest in or concern for the welfare of another person may request an assessment by any medical practitioner to determine if that person is in need of treatment under the Northern Territory Mental Health Act. The assessment must then occur as soon as practicable, and a subsequent recommendation for psychiatric examination made if the doctor believes that the person fulfils the criteria for involuntary admission on the grounds of mental illness or mental disturbance. The person may then be detained by police, ambulance officers or the doctor making the recommendation and taken to an approved treatment facility, where the person may be held for up to 12 h. The Northern Territory Act acknowledges that delays in this process are likely and enshrines a process to account for this, including the use of interactive video conferencing. A psychiatrist must examine and assess the recommended person at the approved treatment facility and must either admit as an involuntary patient or release the patient if the criteria for involuntary admission are not fulfilled.

A patient admitted on the grounds of mental illness may be detained for 24 h or 7 days if the recommending doctor was also a psychiatrist. Patients admitted on the grounds of mental disturbance may be detained for 72 h or have that extended by 7 days if two examining psychiatrists believe that the person still requires involuntary treatment and cannot or will not consent. Frequent psychiatric reassessment of detained and admitted patients is required to either extend admission or release patients who do not fulfil involuntary criteria.

Queensland

In Queensland the recommendation for involuntary assessment of a patient must be made by a doctor who has personally examined the patient within the preceding 3 days and is valid for 7 days from the time the recommendation was made. The recommendation needs to be accompanied by an 'application' for assessment made by a person over the age of 18 years who has seen the patient within 3 days. The person making the application cannot be the doctor making the recommendation or be a relative or employee of the doctor. The

recommendation enables the health practitioner, ambulance officer or police, if necessary, to take the patient to a mental health service or public hospital for assessment. Once there, or if the recommendation was made at a hospital, the assessment period lasts for no longer than 24 h.

The patient must be assessed by a psychiatrist (who cannot be the recommending doctor) as soon as practicable, and if the treatment criteria apply, will have the involuntary status upheld through an involuntary treatment order. The assessment period can be extended up to 72 h by the psychiatrist after regular review.

South Australia

In South Australia, a doctor who considers that a patient requires involuntary admission is required to fill in the appropriate order for admission and detention in an approved treatment centre. This is valid for 3 days, unless revoked, and requires that the person is examined by a psychiatrist as soon as practicable but within 24 h. The psychiatrist may revoke the order or may order further detention of up to 21 days.

The South Australian Mental Health Act enables police to enter premises, apprehend and convey a mentally ill person to a medical practitioner for examination. It also enables ambulance officers to convey, using reasonable force if necessary, a mentally ill person to a place for assessment or care.

Tasmania

In Tasmania, an application for involuntary admission of a person may be made by close relative or guardians, or an 'authorized officer'. A medical practitioner must then assess the person and, if satisfied that the criteria are met, make an order for admission and detention as an involuntary patient in an approved hospital. This initial order is valid for 72 h and gives authority for the patient to be taken to the hospital and detained, whereupon a psychiatric assessment must be carried out within 24 h and the initial order confirmed or discharged. A further order for the continuing detention of a person as an involuntary patient can be made if the appropriate criteria are met and after two doctors (at least one a psychiatrist and neither having written the initial order) have examined the patient. A continuing care order can be valid for up to 6 months.

Victoria

A person may be admitted to and detained in an approved mental health service once the 'request' and the 'recommendation' have been completed. The request can be completed by any person over 18 years of age, including relatives of the patient, but cannot be completed by the recommending doctor. The recommendation is valid for 3 days after completion, and the recommending doctor must have personally examined or observed the patient.

The request and recommendation are sufficient authority for the medical practitioner, police officer or ambulance officer to take the person to a mental health service or to enter premises without a warrant and to use reasonable force or restraint in order to take the person to a mental health service. Prescribed medical practitioners (psychiatrists, forensic physicians, doctors employed by a mental health service, the head of an ED of a general hospital or the regular treating doctor in a remote area) are also enabled to use sedation or restraint to enable a person to be taken safely to a mental health service.

Once admitted, the patient must be seen by a medical practitioner employed by the mental health service as soon as possible, but must be seen by a registered psychiatrist within 24 h of admission. The admitting doctor must make an involuntary treatment order, which allows for the detention of the patient until psychiatrist review and the urgent administration of medication if needed. The psychiatrist can then either authorize further detention, a community treatment order, or discharge the patient.

Western Australia

In Western Australia a patient who requires involuntary admission is referred, in writing, for examination by a psychiatrist in an authorized hospital (all public and certain private hospitals). The referring doctor must have personally examined the patient within the previous 48 h. If no suitable alternatives are available and the condition of the patient requires their involvement, the referring doctor may direct police to apprehend the patient, by writing a 'transport order'. This enables police to apprehend, enter premises, and search the patient or premises. The transport order lapses 72 h after it was made, or at the end of the seventh day after the initial referral was made.

The referral for assessment is valid for 7 days; however, the patient must be examined by a psychiatrist within 24 h of admission and cannot be detained further if not examined. The patient can be detained for further assessment for up to 72 h after initial admission on the order of the psychiatrist, after which time the patient is formally admitted as an involuntary patient, discharged on a community treatment order or released.

Persons unable to recommend a patient for involuntary admission

New Zealand and most states, except for the ACT, specify that certain relationships prevent a doctor from requesting or recommending a patient for involuntary admission.

The recommending doctor cannot be a relative (by blood or marriage) or guardian of the patient, and, in addition, in the Northern Territory, Queensland, Tasmania and Western Australia, the doctor cannot be a business partner or assistant of the patient. In Queensland and Tasmania, the recommending doctor cannot be in receipt of payments for the maintenance of the patient.

In New South Wales, the doctor must declare, on the schedule, any direct or indirect pecuniary interest, or those of their relatives, partners or assistants, in an 'authorized hospital'. In Tasmania, the doctor cannot be on the staff of a private hospital to which the patient will be admitted, and, in Western Australia, the doctor cannot hold a licence from or have a family or financial relationship with the licence holder of a private hospital in which the patient will be treated, nor can the doctor be a board member of a public hospital treating the patient.

Use of sedation or physical restraint

From time to time a patient may need to be sedated or even restrained. The various mental health acts vary considerably in dealing with this issue, and accepted clinical practice has evolved differently in each jurisdiction and does not necessarily reflect subtleties within the legislation.

Generally, patients committed involuntarily are subject to treatment necessary for their care and control, and this may reasonably include the administration of sedative or antipsychotic medication as emergency treatment. In general, sedation or restraint must be the minimum that is necessary to prevent the patient from self-harming or harming others, and careful documentation of the reasons for restraint and the types of restraint is required.

Patients who are physically or pharmacologically restrained must be closely supervised and not left alone or in the care of persons not trained or equipped to deal with the potential complications of these procedures. Transporting these patients to a mental health service should be done by suitably trained medical or ambulance staff and not delegated to police officers or other persons acting alone.

The ACT specifies that sedation may be used to prevent harm, whereas Western Australia specifies that sedation can be used for emergency treatment without consent, and that the details must be recorded in a report to the Mental Health Review Board. Queensland allows a doctor to administer medication for recommended patients without consent to ensure safety during transport to a health facility.

Victoria specifically permits the administration of sedative medication by a 'prescribed medical practitioner' to allow for the safe transport of a patient to a mental health service. There is a schedule to complete if this is undertaken.

The legislation is more specific with regard to the use of physical restraint or seclusion. In the ACT this can be done to prevent an immediate and substantial risk of harm to the patient or others, or to keep the patient in custody.

Queensland requires that restraint used for the protection of the patient or others can only be done on an 'order' but is permissible for the purposes of treatment if it is clinically appropriate. Tasmania permits its use, on the approval of the responsible medical officer, for the medical treatment or protection of the patient, other persons or property. Victoria permits the restraint of involuntary patients for the purposes of medical treatment and the prevention of injury or persistent property destruction. Victoria also allows the use of restraint by ambulance officers, police or doctors in order to safely transport the patient to a mental health service, but this must be documented in the recommendation schedule.

Both the Northern Territory and Western Australia permit the use of restraint for the purposes of medical treatment and for the protection of the patient, other persons or property. In Western Australia this authorization must be in writing and must be notified to the senior psychiatrist as soon as possible, whilst in the Northern Territory, it must be approved by a psychiatrist or the senior nurse on duty in the case of an emergency.

The New Zealand Mental Health Act makes minimal specific reference to restraint or sedation but enables any urgent treatment to protect the patient or others and allows hospitals and police to take all reasonable steps to detain patients for assessment and treatment. Authority is given to administer sedative drugs if necessary, but the Act mandates a record of this for the area mental health service.

Emergency treatment and surgery

On occasions, involuntary patients may require emergency medical or surgical treatment. New Zealand and most states, except for Queensland and Tasmania, make provision for this in their legislation, in that patients can undergo emergency treatment without consent, but usually only with the approval of the relevant mental health authorities or treating psychiatrist. In New Zealand, treatment that is immediately necessary to save life, prevent serious damage to health or prevent injury to the person or others can be undertaken without consent.

Victoria has the most specific reference to this treatment by making special allowance for a patient requiring treatment that is life sustaining or preventing serious physical deterioration to be admitted as an involuntary patient to a general hospital or ED for the purposes of receiving treatment. The patient is deemed to be on leave from the mental health service, and all the other provisions of the Act apply.

Apprehension of absent involuntary patients

Involuntary patients who escape from custody or who fail to return from 'leave' are considered in most state mental health acts to be 'absent without leave' (AWOL) or

'unlawfully at large', although the ACT Act makes no reference to this. In the remaining states and the Northern Territory, authorized persons, including staff of the mental health service and police, have the same powers of entry and apprehension as for other persons to whom a recommendation or certificate relates. In Tasmania these powers exist for 28 days from the time of going AWOL, whereas in Victoria they apply for 12 months, after which time the patient is automatically discharged unless the chief psychiatrist considers it appropriate for the patient to remain, theoretically at least, in custody. Queensland, New South Wales, the Northern Territory, South Australia and Western Australia do not specify a time limit for the return of AWOL patients.

In New Zealand any compulsory patient who becomes AWOL may be 'retaken' by any person and taken to any hospital within 3 months of becoming absent. If not returned after 3 months the patient is deemed to be released from compulsory status.

Powers of the police

The police in all states and New Zealand have powers in relation to mentally ill persons who may or may not have been assessed by a doctor. For someone who is not already an involuntary patient and who is reasonably believed to be mentally ill, a risk to self or others and requiring care, police are able to enter premises and apprehend, without a warrant, and to use reasonable force if necessary, in order to remove the person to a 'place of safety'. Generally, this means taking the person to a medical practitioner or a mental health service for examination without undue delay.

South Australia and Queensland specifically include ambulance officers within this legislation and acknowledge that they often work together with police to detain and transport people for mental health assessment. In Tasmania, people may only be held in protective custody for the purposes of medical assessment for no longer than 4 h and then released if no involuntary admission order has been made.

Some states (ACT, New South Wales and Victoria) make special mention of a threatened or actual suicide attempt as justification for police apprehension and transfer to a health facility. New South Wales

allows police discretion, after a person who appears mentally disordered has committed an offence (including attempted murder), to determine whether it is beneficial to their welfare to be detained under the mental health act rather than under other criminal law. The Victorian Act, in contrast, acknowledges that police do not need clinical judgement about mental illness but may exercise their powers based on their own perception of a person's appearance and behaviour that may be suggestive of mental illness.

In New Zealand, detention by police is limited to 6 h, by which time a medical examination should have taken place. Ideally, police should not enter premises without a warrant, if it is reasonably practicable to obtain one.

The same powers apply to involuntary patients who abscond or are absent without leave, although some states have specific schedules or orders to complete for this to be done. In general, once police become aware of the patient they are obliged to make attempts to find and return them to what can be viewed as lawful custody.

Prisoners with mental illness

Mental illness amongst people in prison is extremely prevalent, either as a cause or as a result of incarceration. New Zealand and most Australian states and territories include provisions for prisoners with mental illness within their mental health legislation. Whilst the health care of prisoners is generally managed within regional forensic systems, EDs in rural and less-well-resourced areas can become a site of care for prisoners with acute psychiatric illness.

The New Zealand Act states that prisoners with mental illness who require acute care can be transferred to a general hospital for involuntary psychiatric treatment, if the prison is unable to provide that care. Australian Acts in New South Wales, the Northern Territory and Victoria all include similar specific provisions for mentally ill prisoners to be able to access involuntary care in public hospitals if needed. The Victorian Act is most detailed in this matter, although in practice rarely relies on public hospitals due to the development of a stand alone forensic psychiatric hospital. Both Queensland and Western Australia enshrine the same principle of allowing prisoners access to general psychiatric treatment, although their legislation is less specific, whilst the Tasmanian, South Australian and ACT Acts do not mention prisoners at all. In all jurisdictions, there is significant overlap with other laws such as Crimes and Prisons Acts, which also mention health needs of prisoners.

Amendment of documents

New South Wales, Tasmania, Victoria, the Northern Territory and Western Australia specify that the amendment or correction of documents in relation to the admission of an involuntary patient is permissible, without the patient being discharged or returned to the recommending doctor or their status being changed. Western Australia does not specify a time limit for this to be done, but in Tasmania it must be done within 14 days, in Victoria and the Northern Territory within 21 days and in New South Wales within 28 days. The documents must be amended by the person who signed the original and not compromise the sufficiency of the grounds on which the involuntary order was made. The New Zealand Act makes no reference to the amendment of documents.

Offences in relation to certificates

Most states and New Zealand specify in their respective mental health acts that it is an offence to wilfully make a false or misleading statement in regard to the certification of an involuntary patient.

Some states (New South Wales, South Australia, the Northern Territory and Victoria), except in certain circumstances, also regard failure to personally examine or observe the patient as an offence.

Protection from suit or liability

New Zealand and all Australian states specify in their mental health acts that legal proceedings cannot be brought against doctors acting in good faith and with reasonable care within the provisions of the Mental Health Act relevant to their practice.

Information and patient transfer between jurisdictions

All Australian states and territories except for South Australia include special provisions for the apprehension, treatment and transfer of mentally ill patients from other jurisdictions. State governments can enter into agreements to recognize warrants or orders made under 'corresponding law' in other states or territories, as long as appropriate conditions are met within their own law. Thus, a patient under an involuntary detention or community treatment order in another state can be apprehended and treated under the corresponding law in a different jurisdiction. Authority is given to police and doctors to detain such patients, and information to facilitate assessment and treatment can be shared between states.

Deaths

Involuntary patients should be considered to be held in lawful custody, whether in an ED, as an inpatient in a general hospital or psychiatric hospital or as an AWOL. As such, the death of such a patient must be referred for a coroner's investigation.

Controversies and future directions

United Kingdom

❶ The provision of mental health services to EDs varies widely across the UK. Responsiveness of services remains an issue of contention, particularly in light of national 4 h targets for treatment in EDs. Representatives of the various Royal Colleges are currently writing a national strategy, which aims to set standards for what they describe as 'emergency psychiatry'.

❷ In the UK the most commonly used places of safety for individuals deemed to be a danger to themselves or the public are EDs, police stations and psychiatric units. Concern exists about the suitability of EDs for acting as places of safety. The Royal College of Psychiatrists jointly with the British Association for Emergency Medicine stated in 1996 that EDs were inappropriately staffed and equipped to supervise such individuals. However, the National Service Framework on Mental Health states that hospitals should be used in preference to police stations. To date, there has been no national consensus on the future use of the ED as a place of safety. Currently, individual departments are entering into local policy agreements with other agencies on their use.

❸ As the specialty of emergency medicine expands, health professionals such as emergency nurse practitioners and paramedics are increasingly making clinical decisions about patients. This presents a challenge to the specialty in ensuring that all are appropriately trained and informed of the law relating to patients with mental health problems. It is vital that training and education continues to be central to delivering an appropriate service in often difficult circumstances.

❹ In 2004, the National Institute for Health and Clinical Excellence (NICE) published a guideline on the treatment and prevention of self-harm focusing on care in the ED. It stressed the importance of staff attitudes towards these patients. Patients who have self-harmed reported frequently being treated not only with a lack of respect, as 'time wasters', but at times receiving punitive treatment at the hands of ED staff.

Australasia

❶ Greater uniformity between the mental health legislation of Australian states and territories is desirable from both a patient's and a healthcare provider's perspective. Whilst there has been some move towards commonality with recognition of 'corresponding laws', great disparity still exists in some areas between jurisdictions. These differences could be overcome without compromising the fundamental principles of mental health legislation in the Australasian region.

❷ More legal recognition of cultural and language difference is required as Australia and New Zealand become home to increasingly diverse populations. In particular, refugees and people from areas exposed to warfare and torture have specific mental health needs that should be accounted for within progressive legislation. Better acknowledgement of indigenous mental health issues is also an area requiring legislative improvement.

❸ Police are given great powers within Australasian laws to apprehend and detain mentally unwell people, yet lack a sophisticated knowledge of mental illness. Greater education and collaborative work between police and healthcare providers, especially those working in EDs, should lead to more humane and patient-focused provision of care.

❹ The use of physical restraints as a means of detaining mentally unwell people varies greatly in EDs throughout the region. Whilst many jurisdictions allow for physical restraints, the interpretation and practice of the law in various regions show remarkable disparity. From a human rights perspective, there needs to be some uniformity in the approach to physical restraint. This would incorporate flexibility and reflective practice and give primacy to 'least restrictive' principles.

References

1. World Health Organisation. Mental Health Care Law: Ten Basic Principles. World Health Organisation, Division of Mental Health and Prevention of Substance Abuse, Geneva; 1996.
2. Forrester K, Griffiths D. Essentials of law for health professionals. 2nd edn. Sydney: Elsevier, 2005.
3. Australian Human Rights and Equal Opportunity Commission. Human Rights and Mental Illness. Report of the national inquiry into the human rights of people with mental illness. Canberra: Australian Government Publishing Service; 1993.

Further reading

Mental Capacity Act (2005). http://www.opsi.gov.uk/acts/acts2005/20050009.html.
Jones R. Mental Health Act manual. 8th edn. London: Sweet and Maxwell; 2002.
Jones R. Mental Capacity Act manual. 2nd edn. London: Sweet and Maxwell; 2007.
Wallace M. Health care and the law. 2nd edn. Sydney: The Law Book Company Ltd; 1995.
WHO. Resource Book on Mental Health, Human Rights and Legislation. Geneva: World Health Organisation; 2005.

25.2 The coroner: the Australasian and UK perspectives

Simon Young • Helen L. Parker

AUSTRALASIA

ESSENTIALS

1 The function of the coroner is to investigate and report on a person's death. Where possible, the coroner must determine the identity of the deceased, the circumstances surrounding the death, the medical cause of death and the identity of any person who contributed to that death. The coroner may also comment on matters of public health and safety.

2 Each jurisdiction has a number of defined circumstances in which a death must be reported to the coroner. Commonly these are when the death appears to have been caused by violent, unnatural or accidental means or has occurred in suspicious circumstances or when the cause is unknown.

3 Preparation for a coronial investigation starts as soon as someone dies in reportable circumstances. The body, medical notes and details of all investigations and procedures may be required by the coroner. Accurate and complete medical notes are an essential part of this process.

4 A coronial inquest is a public inquiry into a death to which a medical practitioner may be subpoenaed. The doctor may be required to give evidence of fact regarding what happened or expert opinion.

5 The findings of a coronial inquest in which the performance of an emergency physician or department has been examined should be carefully scrutinized. They may contain important statements regarding the practice of the emergency physician, the functioning of the emergency department and the emergency medical system as a whole.

6 Coronial findings may be used constructively to effect positive change within a department, institution or system.

Introduction

The function of the coroner is to investigate and report the circumstances surrounding a person's death. A coronial inquest is a public inquiry into one or more deaths conducted by a coroner within a court of law. Legislation in each Australian state and territory defines the powers of this office and the obligations of medical practitioners and the public towards it. The process effectively puts details concerning a death on the public record and is being increasingly used to provide information and recommendations for future injury prevention.

As many people die each year either in an ED or having attended an ED during their last illness, it is almost inevitable that emergency physicians will become involved in the coronial process at some stage during their career. Such involvement may be brief, such as the discharge of a legal obligation by reporting a death, or may extend further to providing statements to the coroner regarding deaths of which they have some direct knowledge. Later, the coroner may require them to appear at an inquest to give evidence regarding the facts of the case, and possibly their opinion. Occasionally, the coroner requires a suitably experienced emergency physician to provide an expert opinion regarding aspects of a patient's emergency care.

Although the inquisitorial nature of the coronial process is sometimes threatening to medical practitioners, their involvement is a valuable community service. In addition, they may obtain important information regarding aspects of a patient's clinical diagnoses and emergency care.

Legislation

The office of the coroner, and its functions, procedures and powers, is created by state and territory legislation. The legislation also creates obligations on medical practitioners to notify the coroner of reportable deaths, and to cooperate with the coroner by providing certain information in the course of an inquiry. The normal constraints of obtaining consent for the provision of clinical information to a third party do not apply in these circumstances.

The coroner is vested with wide-ranging powers to assist in obtaining information. In practice, the police are most commonly used to conduct the investigation. Under the various Coroners Acts they have the power to enter and inspect buildings or places, take possession of and copy documents or other articles, take statements and require people to appear in court. The coroner has control of a body whose death has been reported and may direct that an autopsy be performed.

As each Australian state and territory legislation is different, emergency physicians must be familiar with the details in their particular jurisdiction. The current legislation in each state and territory is the following:

Australian Capital Territory – Coroners Act 1997
New South Wales – Coroners Act 1980
New Zealand – Coroners Act 1988
Northern Territory – Coroners Act 1993
Queensland – Coroners Act 1958–1977
South Australia – Coroners Act 1975
Tasmania – Coroners Act 1995
Western Australia – Coroners Act 1996
Victoria – Coroners Act 1985.

Reportable deaths

Most deaths that occur in the community are not reported to a coroner and, consequently, are not investigated. The coroner has no power to initiate an investigation unless a death is reported. If a medical practitioner is able to issue a medical certificate of the cause of death, the Registrars-General of that state or territory may issue a death certificate and the body of the deceased may be lawfully disposed of without coronial involvement.

In general, to issue a certificate of the cause of death, a doctor must have attended the deceased during the last illness, and the death must not be encompassed by that jurisdiction's definition of a reportable death. It is essential that every medical practitioner has a precise knowledge of what constitutes a reportable death within the jurisdiction.

It is uncommon for a doctor who is working in an ED to have had prior contact with a patient during the last illness. Therefore, even if sure of the reason why the patient died, the doctor is often unable to complete a medical certificate of the cause of death. It is quite permissible, and even desirable, under these circumstances, to contact the patient's treating doctor to inquire as to whether that doctor is able to complete the certificate. This process reduces the number of deaths that must be reported and assists families who may be distressed about coronial involvement.

All Australian Coroners Acts contain a definition of the deaths that must be reported. Although the precise terminology varies, there are many similarities between them. In general, each Act has provisions for inquiring into deaths that are of unknown cause or that appear to have been caused by violent, unnatural or accidental means. Many Acts also refer to deaths that occur in suspicious circumstances, and some specifically mention killing, drowning, dependence on non-therapeutic drugs and deaths occurring while under anaesthesia. The Tasmanian Act goes further, to specify deaths that occur under sedation.

As an example, the Victorian Coroners Act 1985 defines a reportable death as one (1) where the body is in Victoria; (2) that occurred in Victoria; (3) the cause of which occurred in Victoria; (4) of a person who ordinarily resided in Victoria at the time of death; (5) that appears to have been unexpected, unnatural or violent, or to have resulted, directly or indirectly, from accident or injury; (6) that occurs during an anaesthetic; (7) that occurs as a result of an anaesthetic and is not due to natural causes; (8) that occurs in prescribed circumstances; (9) of a person who immediately before death was a person held in care; (10) of a person whose identity is unknown; (11) that occurs in Victoria where a notice under Section 19(1)(b) of the Registration of Births Deaths and Marriages Act 1959 has not been signed; or (12) that occurs at a place outside Victoria where the cause of death is not certified by a person who, under the law in force in that place, is authorized to certify that death.

Despite the seemingly straightforward definitions given in the various Acts, there are many instances where it may not be clear whether a death is reportable or not. Emergency physicians are often faced with situations where there is a paucity of information regarding the circumstances of an event, and where the cause of death may be difficult to deduce. Correlation between the clinical diagnoses recorded on death certificates and subsequent autopsies has been consistently shown to be poor. What exactly constitutes unexpected, unnatural or unknown is open to debate and may require some judgement. In all cases the coroner expects the doctor to act with common sense and integrity. If at all in doubt it is wise to discuss the circumstances with the coroner or assistant, and to seek advice. This conversation and the advice given must be recorded in the medical notes.

The process of reporting a death is generally a matter of speaking to the coroner's assistants (often referred to as coroner's clerks), who will record pertinent details and, if necessary, investigate. The report should be made as soon as practicable after the death. A medical practitioner who does not report a reportable death is liable to a penalty.

Even though coroners' offices and the police work closely together, reporting a death to the coroner is not necessarily equivalent to reporting an event to the police. If it is possible that a person has died or been seriously injured in suspicious circumstances, then it is prudent to ensure that the police are also notified.

A coronial investigation

After a death has been reported, the coroner or designated assistant may initiate an investigation. This is most commonly conducted by the police assisting the coroner, with an autopsy conducted by a forensic pathologist.

The body, once certified dead, becomes part of that investigation and should be left as far as possible in the condition at death. If the body is to be viewed by relatives immediately it is often necessary to make it presentable. This must be done carefully, so as to not remove or change anything that

may be of importance to the coroner. If a resuscitation was attempted all cannulae, endotracheal tubes and catheters should be left in situ. All clothing and objects that were on (or in) the deceased should be collected, bagged and labelled. All medical and nursing notes, radiographs, electrocardiographs and blood tests should accompany the body if it is to be transported to a place as directed by the coroner.

Medical notes taken during or soon after the activity of a busy resuscitation are often incomplete. It is not easy to accurately recall procedures, times and events when the main task is to prevent someone from dying. Similarly, after death there are many urgent tasks, such as talking to relatives, notifying treating or referring doctors, and debriefing staff. It is essential, however, that the documentation is completed as accurately and thoroughly as possible. The notes must contain a date and time and clearly specify the identity of the author. If points are recalled after completing the notes, these may be added at the end of the previous notes, again with a time and a date added. Do not under any circumstances change or add to the body of the previous notes.

In addition to completing the medical notes, a medical practitioner may be requested to provide a statement to the coroner regarding the doctor's involvement with the deceased and an opinion on certain matters. Such a statement should be carefully prepared from the original notes and written in a structured fashion, using non-medical terminology where possible. The statement often gives the opportunity for the medical practitioner to give further information to the coroner regarding medical qualifications and experience, the position fulfilled in the department at the time of the death, and a more detailed interpretation of the events. If a statement is requested from junior ED staff, it is strongly advisable for these to be read by someone both clinically and medicolegally experienced.

Providing honest, accurate and expeditious information to relatives when a death occurs assists in preventing misunderstandings and serious issues arising in the course

of a coronial investigation. Relatives vary enormously in the quantity and depth of medical information they request or can assimilate after an unexpected death. It is wise not only to talk to the relatives present at the death but also to offer to meet later with selected family members. Clarification with the family of what actually occurred, what diagnoses were entertained and what investigations and procedures were performed is not only good medical practice but can allay concerns regarding management.

If a significant diagnosis was missed or inappropriate or an inadequate treatment given, or a serious complication of an investigation or procedure occurred, assistance and advice from the hospital insurers and medical defence organizations should be sought before talking to the family. However difficult it may be, it is far better that the family is aware of any adverse occurrences before the inquest than for them to harbour suspicions or to get a feeling something is being covered up. The coroner is far more likely to be sympathetic to a genuine mistake or omission when it has been discussed with the family and the hospital has taken steps to prevent a recurrence.

Expert opinion

Having gathered all the available information regarding a death the coroner may decide that expert opinion is necessary on one or more points. Commonly, this involves the standard of care afforded to the deceased. It may, however, also include issues such as the seniority of doctors involved, the use of appropriate investigations, the interpretation of investigations and the occurrence of complications of a procedure. The coroner relies heavily on such opinions for the findings, and the selection of an appropriate expert is essential.

The person selected by the coroner to give this opinion should possess postgraduate specialist medical qualifications and be broadly experienced in the relevant medical specialty. For events occurring in the ED, a senior emergency physician with over

5 years of experience is usually most appropriate. The specialist medical colleges may be requested to nominate such a person.

The emergency physician requested to give expert opinion must have access to be able to review all of the available relevant information. Such persons must also consider themselves adequately qualified and experienced to provide an opinion and to answer any specific questions the coroner may have requested to be addressed. The doctor must have the time and ability to provide a comprehensive statement and to appear as a witness at the inquest if requested and to act impartially. The doctor should decline involvement if an interest in the outcome of the case could be implied.

A coronial inquest

A coronial inquest is a public inquiry into one or more deaths. Deaths may be grouped together if they occurred in the same instance, or in apparently similar circumstances. The purpose of the inquest is to put findings on the public record. These may include the identity of the deceased, the circumstances surrounding the death, the medical cause of death, and the identity of any person who contributed to the death. The coroner may also make comments and recommendations concerning matters of health and safety. In some jurisdictions these are termed 'riders'. In addition, as His Honour B. R. Thorley pointed out, the inquest serves to:

... include the satisfaction of legitimate concerns of relatives, the concern of the public in the proper administration of institutions and matters of public and private interest ...

The inquest does not serve to commit people for trial or to provide information for a subsequent criminal investigation.

With broad terms of reference, and the ability to admit testimony that may not be allowed in criminal courts, inquests interest many people, not only those who may have been directly involved. They are often highly publicized media events and may provoke political comment, especially where government bodies are involved. A medical practitioner served a subpoena to attend should prepare carefully, both individually and in conjunction with the hospital.

Preparation for an inquest begins at the time of the death. Complete and accurate medical notes, together with a carefully considered statement, provide a solid foundation for giving evidence and handling any subsequent issues. Statements containing complex medical terminology, ambiguities or omissions only serve to create confusion. Discuss the case with colleagues who are not directly involved, the hospital medical administration and a medical defence organization. Legal advice and representation are essential to any doctor appearing in an inquest, even though the case may appear straightforward. It is wise for any areas of damaging evidence or potential conflict to be identified and managed accordingly.

Appearing at an inquest can be a stressful event, especially if on a review of the circumstances a doctor's actions or judgement may be called into question. Professional peer support, as well as legal advice, should be offered to all medical staff. Simple actions, such as a briefing on court procedures and some advice on how to deal with cross-examination, can be of immense value.

A coroner's court is conducted with a mix of 'inquisitorial' and 'adversarial' legal styles. It is inquisitorial in that the coroner may take part in direct proceedings and can question witnesses and appoint court advisers. It is adversarial in that parties with a legitimate interest can be represented in proceedings and can challenge and test witnesses' evidence, especially where it differs from what they would like presented. The 'rules of evidence' are more relaxed in the coroner's court than in a criminal court. Hearsay evidence – that is, evidence of what someone else said to a witness – is generally admissible. Despite these differences, it is important to remember that it is no less a court than a criminal court and demands the same degree of respect and professional conduct one would accord to the latter.

Coronial findings

At the conclusion of an inquest the coroner makes a number of findings directed at satisfying the aims of that inquest. These findings are made public and are often of interest to those who are directly involved, as well as to a wider audience.

The findings of an inquest in which the conduct of a particular emergency physician, ED or hospital have been scrutinized will be of particular interest. Although it is always pleasing to have either positive or a lack of negative comment delivered in the finding, criticism of some aspect of the conduct of an individual, department, hospital or the medical system in general is not uncommon. Unfortunately, it is often this criticism that attracts the most public attention and, somewhat unfairly, the public perception of our acute healthcare system is shaped by the media's attention to coronial findings.

In the recent past, coroners have commented on inadequate training, experience and supervision of junior doctors, inadequate systems of organization within departments and poor communication between doctors and family members.

Although adverse or critical findings have no legal weight or penalties attached to them, they are in many respects a considered community response to a situation in which the wider population has a vested interest. Used constructively, they can be extremely useful in convincing hospital management that a problem exists and beginning a process for effecting positive change within a department or institution.

UK

ESSENTIALS

1 The coroner, or procurator fiscal in Scotland, is responsible for the investigation of circumstances surrounding death in particular situations.

2 Emergency physicians should be familiar with the types of death which require referral to the coroner/procurator fiscal. These include deaths due to any trauma, poisoning or other unnatural causes, deaths related to medical procedures and deaths whose cause is unknown. Deaths that occur whilst detained under the Mental Health Act or in custody of police should also be reported. Several other specific circumstances exist, and, in doubtful cases, discussion with the district coroner's office should occur.

3 The body remains under the control of the coroner once death has been reported. Medical devices should be left in situ and the body should receive minimal handling, particularly in suspicious or violent deaths, in order to preserve forensic trace evidence.

4 Concise documentation of the clinical circumstances surrounding the death may direct the pathologist towards a detailed examination of the relevant organ or system and acts as a solid basis for the emergency physician for the preparation of a subsequent statement and examination at an inquest.

5 Emergency physicians should seek assistance from senior colleagues and legal advice when asked to prepare a statement for the coroner or attend an inquest.

Table 25.2.1 Reasons for an inquest (according to the Broderick Committee)

- To determine the medical cause of death
- To allay rumours or suspicion
- To draw attention to the existence of circumstances which, if unremedied, might lead to further deaths
- To advance medical knowledge
- To preserve the legal interests of the deceased person's family, heirs or other interested parties[2]

Introduction

The investigation into circumstances surrounding deaths is an important part of civilized society. Accurate recording of cause of death serves many purposes including accurate disease surveillance, the detection of secret homicide and the detection of potentially avoidable factors that have contributed to a death. Various death investigation systems exist around the world. The UK uses the coronial system, Scotland the procurator fiscal. By virtue of the patient population encountered by emergency physicians, and the types of deaths that are subject to investigation, emergency physicians may expect to find themselves in contact with either the coroner or the procurator fiscal system during their working lives, thus necessitating an understanding of the workings of these systems.

History of the coroner

The history of the coroner's office is an interesting reflection of events that shaped our civilization and is in constant evolution. The Shipman Inquiry is the most recent event that will shape the coroner's role. The office of the coroner was established in 1194 and its primary function then was that of protection of the crown's pecuniary interests in criminal proceedings. The coroner was involved when a death was sudden or unexpected or a body was found in the open; however, aside from the duty to ensure the arrest of anyone involved in homicide, the coroner held a significant role in the collection of the deceased's chattels and collection of various fines.[1]

Introduction of the Births and Deaths Registration Act in 1836, mandated registration of all deaths before burial could legally occur. This may have arisen out of concern regarding the accurate statistical information concerning deaths, but also concern about hidden homicide. Another Act introduced the same year enabled coroners to order a medical practitioner to attend an inquest and perform an autopsy in equivocal cases. The Coroners Act of 1887 saw a shift of emphasis from protection of financial interests to the emphasis that remains today – the medical cause of death and its surrounding circumstances with eventual community benefit in mind.

The Broderick committee was appointed in 1965 to review death certification in response to adverse publicity about inquests and pressures to improve death certification. Their report published in 1971 contained 114 recommendations, many of which were enacted. Table 25.2.1 lists the reasons the Broderick Committee considered the purpose of an inquest.[2]

The current Coroners Act (1988) states that a coroner shall hold an inquest into a death when there is '... reasonable cause to suspect that the deceased has died a violent or unnatural death, has died a sudden death of which the cause is unknown, or has died in prison or in a such place or circumstances as to require an inquest under any Act.'[3]

Structure of the coroner system in the UK

Coroners are independent judicial officers who mostly have a legal background (some also have a medical background) and must possess at least 5 years of postqualification experience. They are responsible only to the Crown, this being an important safeguard for society; however, their administration is largely the responsibility of the Home Office. They must work within the laws and regulations that apply to them: The Coroners Act 1988, Coroners Rules 1984 and the Model Coroners Charter. There are approximately 148 coroner's districts throughout England

and Wales, and each district has a coroner and a deputy and possibly several assistant deputy coroners. Coroners are assisted in their duties by coroner's officers, who are frequently police officers or ex-police officers, whose work is dedicated solely to coronial matters. This follows long-established practice and has probably arisen because of the significant proportion of cases in which police are the notifying agent. The nature of a coronial investigation also frequently requires a person to possess knowledge about legal matters and skill in information gathering. From a practical viewpoint, the coroner's assistants may be responsible for performing such duties as attending the scene of a death, arranging transport of the body to the mortuary, notification of the next of kin and obtaining statements from relevant parties. Clearly, variation in the structure of the service between regions is inevitable and reflects the size, composition and workload within the district.[4]

Overview of the coronial process

Upon notification of a death, the coroner makes initial inquiries and may direct a pathologist to perform a postmortem. Sometimes it becomes clear at this early point that the death is a natural one and does not fall within the Coroners Act, thus no inquest is required and a death certificate is issued. In other circumstances, further investigations occur and relevant information is gathered. If the coroner is subsequently satisfied that the death is natural, again no inquest is required. In other cases, or in certain prescribed circumstances, an inquest is held. At the conclusion of an inquest, a finding or verdict is delivered. This verdict must not be framed in a way that implies civil or criminal liability.

Reportable deaths

There is no statutory obligation in the UK for a doctor or any member of the public to report certain deaths to the coroner. However, an ethical responsibility exists and it is recognized practice to do so in particular circumstances. A 1996 letter from the Deputy Chief Medical Statistician to all doctors outlined these circumstances (Table 25.2.2).[5]

Each booklet of medical death certificates also contains a reminder of the deaths that a coroner needs to consider. The list is not exhaustive. Other circumstances include where the deceased was

Table 25.2.2 Circumstances in which a death should be reported to the coroner
• The cause of death is unknown
• The deceased was not seen by the certifying doctor either after death or within the 14 days before the death
• The death was violent or unnatural or suspicious
• The death may be due to an accident (whenever it occurred)
• The death may be due to self-neglect or neglect by others
• The death may be due to an industrial disease or related to the deceased's employment
• The death may be due to an abortion
• The death occurred during an operation or before recovery of the effects of an anaesthetic
• The death may be a suicide
• The death occurred during or shortly after detention in police or prison custody

detained under the Mental Health Act, the death may be related to a medical procedure or treatment, or there is an allegation of medical mismanagement.

Scotland

In Scotland, the role of death investigation is undertaken by the procurator fiscal's office, which is also responsible for the investigation and prosecution of crime. The spectrum of deaths investigated is essentially the same as in England and Wales; however, more specific guidelines regarding deaths possibly related to medical mismanagement are provided (Table 25.2.3).

Table 25.2.3 Specific guidelines regarding deaths related to medical management in Scotland
• Deaths that occur unexpectedly having regard to the clinical condition of the deceased prior to receiving medical care
• Deaths that are clinically unexplained
• Deaths seemingly attributable to a therapeutic or diagnostic hazard
• Deaths that are apparently associated with lack of medical care
• Deaths that occur during the actual administration of general or local anaesthetic

How to report a death

Having determined that a death is reportable, the emergency physician should contact the district coroner's office and notify the details of the deceased. Where doubt exists about the necessity or, otherwise, to report a death, a doctor should contact that office to discuss the matter further. This may avoid undue distress to relatives should the death be subsequently referred by the registrar of births and deaths. The discussion and subsequent decision should be recorded in the patient's clinical notes. A death certificate should not be written.

Handling the body

There appear to be no official guidelines in place regarding handling of the body once death has been reported to the coroner; however, this aspect may be an important component of the subsequent investigation. Any therapeutic and monitoring devices such as endotracheal tubes, intercostal catheters and intravascular catheters should be left in situ, as determination of their correct placement or otherwise may be relevant to the death investigation. In a similar line, it may be important to isolate any equipment (e.g. intravenous infusion pump devices) suspected of being faulty and contributing to the death. In circumstances of suspicious, or violent deaths in particular, the body should be not be handled unnecessarily, nor should the body be washed. Important trace evidence that may be crucial for subsequent criminal proceedings could conceivably be lost. For example, in deaths involving firearms, it may be useful for a forensic scientist to swab the deceased's hands for gunshot residue to help confirm or refute the notion of a self-inflicted injury.

Clothing removed from the deceased during resuscitation efforts should be set aside and preferably placed into individual paper bags. Any remaining clothing on the deceased should be left in situ.[6] Blood taken during resuscitation attempts, regardless of whether it was processed or not, should not be discarded, but kept refrigerated and its existence indicated to the coroner. The examination of antemortem blood samples can provide valuable information, particularly with respect to electrolyte and glucose concentrations, drug concentrations and in deaths possibly attributable to anaphylaxis, tryptase assay.[7]

Documentation

The clinical record of the deceased will usually accompany the body to the mortuary and is frequently perused by the pathologist. Clinical information is crucial in consideration of the cause of death and may help direct the pathologist towards an appropriately detailed examination of the relevant system or organ. The guidelines for appropriate documentation in reportable cases are really the same that apply in medical record-keeping in general. They should be made contemporaneously, or as close to as is possible in a resuscitation environment. Each entry should be dated and the time recorded. They must be legible, objective and the sources of information identified. Any errors made should be crossed out, dated and signed. Likewise, if information comes to hand or is recalled at a later date, that entry should be dated and timed. Never add an entry or alter notes without identifying that it is, indeed, so. Finally, the author's name and designation should be clear, and all entries signed.

Information for families

The next-of-kin of the deceased must be informed that the death has been reported to the coroner and the requirement or reasons for doing so. It is important to inform them that police may be involved in the investigation of the death on behalf of the coroner, but that this does not imply a criminal wrongdoing. An information leaflet explaining the coroner's work and rights of the next-of-kin is available from the Home Office[8] and should be available in every ED to pass on to bereaved families. Another useful publication written for bereaved families provides information regarding postmortems and is available from the Royal College of Pathologists.[9]

Postmortems

The coroner may decide upon the initial report of a death that a postmortem is necessary in order to determine the cause of death or resolve an issue relevant to a coronial inquiry. In the year 2000, postmortem examinations were conducted in 62% of cases reported to the coroner, continuing a steady downward trend in the proportion of postmortems conducted out of reported cases.[10] Having decided upon the necessity for a postmortem, the coroner directs a pathologist to conduct a postmortem. The Coroners Act states that, in fact, the coroner may 'direct any legally qualified medical practitioner' to conduct the postmortem; however, the Coroners Rules 1984 direct that they should be performed 'whenever practicable by a pathologist with suitable qualifications and experience', and, in practice, most are conducted by Home Office accredited forensic pathologists. Clearly, if the standard of medical care provided by the hospital in which the death occurred is in question, it is inappropriate for a pathologist employed by that hospital to conduct the postmortem.

Consent from relatives to conduct the postmortem is not required in coroner's cases. In the event that relatives object to the postmortem examination, the coroner may delay it to allow them time to obtain legal advice. However, if the death does fall within the coroner's jurisdiction, and is deemed to be necessary, their objection would be over-ridden. Relatives may request a second postmortem; however, this seldom occurs in practice.

The coroner must, in theory, notify certain persons, including the usual medical attendant of the deceased or the hospital in which the death occurred, of the time and date of the postmortem (Rule 7, The Coroners Rules 1984). In practice, this tends to occur when a desire to be represented at the examination has been expressed to the coroner, and in that instance a nominated, medically qualified representative (not a doctor whose practice may be in question) may be present to observe the postmortem.

The issue of tissue retention at autopsy has received recent worldwide attention. Rule 9 of the Coroners Rules 1984 is quite broad, allowing the pathologist to retain 'material which in his opinion bears upon the cause of death, for such a period as the Coroner sees fit'. Guidelines issued by The Royal College of Pathologists[11] recommend that, in coroner's cases, clear protocols between the coroner and the pathologist should exist, and retention of tissues outside of the above-mentioned context should occur with the agreement of both the relatives of the deceased and the coroner.

Preparing a statement for the coroner

The coroner may request a statement from a doctor involved in the care of the deceased and, while there is no obligation to comply with this request, it is generally in the doctor's interest to do so. The coroner, otherwise, has no option but to compel the doctor to attend court and answer questions. A statement, therefore, that has been carefully prepared with due thought to any issues identified may, indeed, avert the need for an inquest or at least will act as a solid base upon which the examination in court will occur. It is important that the doctor writing the statement understands the circumstances of the death; thus, access to the postmortem report is often vital and is allowable under Rule 57 of the Coroners Rules. It is generally advisable, except perhaps in circumstances where it is clear that simple, factual background information only is required, to seek legal advice early when requested to provide a statement or attend an inquest.

The statement should be typewritten and contain the author's qualifications, work experience and current employment post. The sources from which the report is prepared (e.g. clinical notes and pathology reports) should be acknowledged, and it should be set out in a logical manner in chronological order. Technical terms should be qualified with an explanation readily understood by a lay person. It is advisable to have a senior colleague review the statement before submission to the legal representative for final review. The final statement should be dated and signed, and a copy kept for future reference.

Inquest

An inquest is a public hearing at which the identity of the deceased and how, when and where the deceased came by his/her death are to be determined. In the year 2000, only 12% of reported deaths proceeded to inquest, the remainder being examined 'in chambers'. Inquests (or fatal accident inquiries in Scotland) are mandatory in certain prescribed circumstances, including deaths in prison or police custody, and deaths resulting from workplace incidents. In certain circumstances, inquests are held with a jury that is responsible for the final verdict.

The inquest is inquisitorial in nature, where the truth surrounding the circumstances of the death is sought, rather than adversarial, where two or more parties have a particular claim to prove. As with the preparation of a statement for the coroner, it is wise for a medical witness to seek legal advice and possibly representation prior to attendance at an inquest. The legal arena in which they are held is unfamiliar territory to most doctors and they frequently attract intense media scrutiny; thus, involvement in an inquest may be a daunting and stressful experience requiring support from colleagues and friends.

Controversies and future directions

❶ The current coronial system in the UK is under fundamental review.

References

1. Knapman P, Powers M. The law and practice on coroners. Chichester: Barry Rose; 1985.
2. Cordner S, Loff B. 800 years of coroners: have they a future? Lancet 1994; 344: 799–801.
3. Coroners Act 1988 (c.13). www.hmso.gov.uk.
4. Tarling R. Coroner Service Survey: A Research and Statistics Directorate Report. London: Home Office; 1998.
5. Dorries C. Coroner's courts – a guide to law and practice. Chichester: Wiley; 1999.
6. Dimond B. Death in accident and emergency. Accident and Emergency Nursing 1995; 3: 38–41.
7. Burton J, Rutty G. The hospital autopsy. 2nd edn. London: Arnold; 2001.
8. Home Office. When sudden death occurs – coroners and inquests. London: Home Office; 2002.
9. The Royal College of Pathologists. Examination of the body after death – information about post-mortem examination for relatives. London: The Royal College of Pathologists; 2000. www.rcpath.org.
10. Allen R. Deaths reported to coroners England and Wales 2000. London: Home Office Research Development and Statistics Directorate; 2000.
11. The Royal College of Pathologists. Guidelines for the retention of tissues and organs at post-mortem examination. London: The Royal College of Pathologists; 2000. www.rcpath.org.

25.3 Consent and competence – the Australasian and UK perspectives

Edward Brentnall • Helen L. Parker

ESSENTIALS

1 Patient consent is essential for medical treatment.

2 Consent may be implied, verbal or written.

3 Consent must be informed, specific and freely given, and must cover that which is actually done.

4 The patient must be competent to give the consent or to refuse.

5 In the emergency department it is often necessary to give treatment without waiting for consent, for instance when the patient is unconscious.

Consent

All medical treatment is based on law and ethical principles. The four basic ethical principles in medicine are often quoted as follows:

- Beneficence: the duty to do the best for the patient.
- Autonomy: the right of individuals to make decisions on their own behalf.
- Non-maleficence: the duty to do no harm to the patient.

- Justice: the fair distribution of resources, incorporating the notion of responsibility to the wider community.

There is therefore a requirement that patients consent to treatment, provided they are competent to do so. In situations where an intervention is proposed, agreement of the patient should therefore be sought. The term 'informed decision-making' is preferred by some to 'informed consent' as it reflects consideration of patient autonomy.[1] It is also important to consider consent as a two-way process, with an exchange of knowledge between a patient and a doctor.[2] The concepts of competence, provision of adequate information and the voluntariness with which consent is given are crucial in the consideration of obtaining valid consent or seeking an informed decision. Technically, treatment without consent may be considered an assault. This makes it extremely important that consent is obtained before treatment starts.

The patient has the right to self-determination. Consent lies at the heart of the medical contract between the doctor and the patient. Medical investigation and treatment are essentially voluntary acts, which the patient consents to the doctor performing. Great attention has been placed on the issue of consent since the *Rogers v Whittaker* case (High Court of Australia 1992) in which consent given by the patient was held to be invalid. The issue revolved around whether or not disclosure by the surgeon was sufficiently detailed to allow the consent to be informed.

Consent may be given in several ways: implied, verbal or written.

If the patient voluntarily presents to the emergency department then some degree of consent is implied. If a doctor says 'put your arm out straight because I need to take some blood for a test' then this may be taken as *implied consent*. However, this would not cover the insertion of an intercostal catheter, for instance, a much more invasive procedure. Such a procedure would usually need some explanation in order that the patient understood what was to be done before the consent was given. This would be *verbal consent*.

Written consent is often sought before more serious or prolonged procedures, such as surgery under anaesthesia. Written consent is not more valid than verbal, just easier to prove. However, it must be given after full explanation of what is to be done, the expected results, risks and the consequences if it is *not* done. In some ways, written consent is the most difficult to establish. It is impossible to cover every outcome. The difficulties lie with being specific and with the patient being informed. For simpler procedures, it may be better to have implied or verbal consent, rather than written consent.

Consent must be informed, specific and freely given and must cover that which is actually done. Informed consent (or decision-making) requires that clear, accurate and relevant information must be given to the patient. Legal judgements have defined the importance of considering what may be 'material' or 'significant' to that particular individual when disclosing information. Essentially, the patient should be provided with information regarding (1) treatment options, (2) the foreseeable consequences and side effects of any proposed treatment or intervention, and (3) the consequences of not proceeding with the advised treatment. This information should be conveyed in unambiguous terms and in a manner that is likely to be understood by the patient. Language and other communication needs must be met, and there must be an opportunity for the patient to ask questions and to reflect on the information given. The information should be given by the doctor responsible for providing the intervention or a delegate who is suitably qualified and has sufficient knowledge of the proposed intervention.

It is appropriate for a doctor to give advice as to the best clinical options and for the reasons for this professional opinion. Such an opinion is frequently expected and desired by patients and cannot be considered as coercive unless the information has been presented in a manipulative fashion in order to elicit a particular choice.

Competence

The patient must be competent to give the consent or to refuse.

For consent to be valid it must be given by a person who has the capacity to make that decision. The assessment of the competence, or capacity of adults to make decisions on their own behalf, is a functional one that requires more than cognitive testing with a tool such as the mini-mental status examination, although this should be performed and documented as part of the assessment process. Assessment of competence should be sought and conducted by the doctor proposing the treatment or investigation. The essential elements required to demonstrate competence are:

- the ability to maintain and communicate a choice
- the ability to understand the relevant information
- an ability to appreciate the situation and its consequences
- the ability to manipulate the information in a rational fashion.[3]

Questions that may be of assistance in assessing competence are listed in Tables 25.3.1 and 25.3.2. Third parties, such as relatives, are unable to legally provide consent, although it is frequently assumed that they are. However, it is a long-established practice and frequently a useful exercise to involve relatives in the process of determining what the patient would have wanted in a particular circumstance. They may also provide valuable information during the process of competence assessment regarding a person's set of values and beliefs, and usual behaviour, particularly if the patient appears to have elected a path at odds with a previously expressed wish or one that might appear imprudent or irrational. A list of people considered to have parental responsibility is provided in Table 25.3.3.

Table 25.3.1 Questions for determining competence
Comprehension
Ask patient to recall and paraphrase information related to proposed treatment, including risks and benefits of treatment, alternative treatment and consequences of no treatment at all. Retest later to check for stability
Belief
Tell me what you really believe is wrong with your health now
Do you believe that you need some kind of treatment?
What is the treatment likely to do for you?
Why do you think it will have that effect?
What do you believe will happen if you are not treated?
Why do you think the doctor has recommended this treatment for you?
Weighing
Tell me how you reached the decision to accept (reject) treatment
What things were important to you in reaching the decision?
How do you balance those things?
Choice
Have you decided whether to go along with your doctor's suggestion for treatment?
Can you tell me what your treatment decision is?

Table 25.3.2 Simplified questions for assessing competence
What is your present physical condition?
What is the treatment being recommended for you?
What do you and the doctor think might happen to you if you decide to accept the treatment?
What do you and your doctor think might happen if you decide not to accept the recommended treatment?
What are the alternatives available (including no treatment) and what are the possible consequences of accepting each?

Patients may make an advance statement or living will detailing their wishes for medical treatment should they become incapacitated at a later date. This may take the form of a written document or

Table 25.3.3 People considered to have parental responsibility
The child's parents if married to each other at the time of conception or birth
The child's mother, but not the father, if they were not so married, unless the father has acquired parental responsibility via a court order or a parental responsibility agreement or the couple subsequently marry
The child's legally appointed guardian
A person in whose favour the court has made a residence order concerning the child
A local authority designated in a care order in respect of the child
A local authority or other authorized person who holds an emergency protection order in respect of the child

witnessed oral statement. It is legally binding provided the patient is an adult and was competent at the time made and the statement clearly applies to the current circumstances.[4] If doubt exists about its validity, a court ruling should be sought.

Patients who might not be able to consent

Children and adolescents

The legal age of consent in Australasia has changed in the last quarter of a century from 21 to 18 years and in some circumstances to 16 years or less. This has occurred against a background of differing ages at which persons may vote, buy tobacco or alcohol, drive cars or engage in sexual activity.

The most important factor to be considered by the emergency physician is the competence of the patient to understand what is wrong and what the treatment entails. This has more to do with intellectual and emotional maturity than chronological age. It would be reasonable for a 14-year-old girl to consent to appendicectomy, but quite unreasonable to expect the same person to understand the consequences of a hysterectomy.

In a genuine emergency the care of the patient is the most important factor and the absence of a parent or guardian is not a bar to an emergency procedure. Should treatment of a minor be required and valid consent not obtainable, the emergency physician must document the steps taken

to obtain consent and the reason why the treatment must be carried out. If at all possible the opinion of a second doctor should also be attached, provided that the second doctor approximates the first in seniority. Many hospitals require that in such circumstances the director of clinical services or delegate give 'approval'. This is simply a means of ensuring that the hospital is aware of the situation and accepts responsibility.

A special situation occurs for children whose parents hold religious beliefs that proscribe blood transfusion or the administration of blood products. This creates a situation where the child is incompetent and the parents do not consent. There is now almost standard legislation that allows the attending doctors to certify that blood transfusion is required to sustain life, and to then administer the treatment in the face of active opposition from the parents. The relevant legislation protects the doctor who acts out of a duty of care to the patient.

Intellectually impaired

For consent to be valid, the patient must be able to understand the nature of the condition, the options available and the treatment being recommended. In addition there must be an understanding of the material risks and the possible outcome of any potential treatments. The mildly disabled may be able to satisfy these criteria, but the more severely disabled will not be in a position to give valid consent. In the latter situation the guardian or Guardianship Board would have to be involved in all but the most urgent cases.

In every state and territory of Australia there is legislation that covers the protection and administration of incompetent patients. All of these bodies are available to give timely help and, if necessary, hold a formal hearing. Whenever possible, this avenue of assistance should be used. The boards have the authority to conduct hearings, receive evidence and make decisions on behalf of incompetent persons. These decisions have the authority of law and provide protection for the patient and the doctor. Emergency physicians should ensure that they are aware of how to contact their local Board, both in and out of working hours.

Mentally ill

A diagnosis of mental illness does not automatically preclude a patient from giving consent. The attending doctor must decide on the competence of the patient to consent. The attending psychiatrist may be in a position to assist. If the patient is not competent then the relevant mental health legislation must be considered. In an emergency where life or quality of life is seriously threatened and time is of the essence, the facts should be recorded and treatment commenced. A sound knowledge of the mental health and guardianship legislation relevant to the region is essential.

Patient disabled by drugs or alcohol

When a patient is temporarily disabled by drugs or alcohol the situation is less clear. In some Australian states persons who have committed serious assault may escape conviction because the law considers them incapable of forming the intention to commit the act. Legal and medical opinions do not always agree, especially in respect of 'capacity' and blood alcohol readings. The absolute legal position is unclear as to whether an intoxicated person can give consent, but there is no doubt that any doctor who acts in the best interest of the patient will always be on solid ground in the event of an action (see Box 25.3.1).

Restraint may be justified in order to prevent patients taking their own discharge when that might have adverse medical results. There are no simple rules, but it is worth considering whether it is better to be sued for assault and wrongful imprisonment or to be sued for the damage that followed to the patient who was allowed to leave. It may be possible to ask the Guardianship Board for help, but there will be occasions in which immediate decisions must be taken, and the best rule is to do whatever will be the best for the patient in the longer term. Again, documentation at the time, and the signatures of witnesses, will help if the court is involved.

The emergency patient

There has been little written about the patient who requires emergency care but is temporarily incapable of providing consent. The overriding principle, however, is one of

BOX. 25.3.1 Practical advice for difficult issues related to consent and competence

A useful and practical take on this subject from an emergency physician's point of view is encapsulated by the four Ds: *the dumb dedicated documenting doctor*.

If one is faced with a difficult decision in the emergency department, it is usually at a time when there is no easily obtainable advice. The medical director is away, the hospital lawyer is not around at 2.00 am, and the problem must be solved now. The practical choice is between only two options. Do I let the patients discharge themselves (for example), or do I restrain them and treat them without their consent?

If one does the latter, the patient may sue for wrongful imprisonment, assault etc. If, however, he discharges himself against advice (possibly because he is drunk) and sustains harm, he will then inevitably sue for breach of duty of care, and claim damages. Then suppose the doctor faces court. Which charge can be defended most easily? If the doctor restrained the patient, the (four Ds) doctor can speak to the court, saying in effect: 'Your Honour, I don't understand all the legal niceties. I am not a lawyer. But all I did was for the patient's welfare and health, and I wrote it all down, at the time.' What can the physician say if the physician allows the patient to self-discharge?

The more one thinks about it, the less likely it is that the doctor will be convicted in the former circumstance. Even if the doctor was to lose the case, the damages would be tiny compared with the damages for suffering and so on in the other case. Sensible restraint to allow duty of care to be satisfied undoubtedly provides a more satisfactory outcome for all concerned, with little chance of litigation.

Table 25.3.4 Factors to be considered when acting in the patient's best interests without consent

The patient's own wishes and values (where these can be ascertained) including any advance statement
Clinical judgement about the effectiveness of the proposed treatment, particularly in relation to other options
Where there is more than one option, which option is least restrictive of the patient's future choices
The likelihood and extent of any degree of improvement in the patient's condition if treatment is provided
The views of the parents if the patient is a child
The views of people close to the patient, especially close relatives, partners, carers or proxy decision-makers about what the patient is likely to see as beneficial
Any knowledge of the patient's religious, cultural and other non-medical views that might have an impact upon the patient's wishes

the 'duty of care' owed by the doctor to the patient. This duty is to provide appropriate care at a standard commensurate with the skill and experience of the doctor. There is also an obligation to explain to the patient what has been done as early as is reasonable in the recovery phase.

The emergency physician must know the five essentials of consent and the differences between implied, verbal and written consent. A sound knowledge of mental health and guardianship legislation is required. It is of the greatest importance that there is adequate and contemporaneous documentation of decisions. The doctors' primary responsibility to their patients is their duty of care. If it is clear that the doctors were acting in the best interests of their patient, it is highly unlikely that they will be successfully sued.

Unique considerations for the emergency department

Emergency physicians work in an environment where multiple simultaneous demands are placed upon them. Particularly with respect to critically ill and injured patients, detailed information regarding their presentation, past history and usual level of functioning is often lacking, incomplete and may, in fact, be wrong. A physician may suspect that a patient might be impaired but have little time to make a detailed assessment before a treatment decision is required. Similarly, the information available to the physician at a point in time might suggest that a particular diagnosis and a course of action are warranted, and this might change markedly upon receipt of further information.

In short, the emergency physician must frequently make complex decisions at short notice with little background information. In situations where decisions have been made on behalf a patient who is felt to be incompetent, it is important to document carefully the information available to the physician, and the possible diagnoses and their sequelae entertained at that time, and the reasons for the course taken. It is good practice also to seek the assistance and advice of a colleague where the competence of a patient is in doubt and significant interventions are deemed necessary. Factors to be considered when acting in the patient's best interests without consent are listed in Table 25.3.4.

Controversies and future directions

❶ English medical law is likely to be influenced in the future by the recent introduction of the Human Rights Act 1998, with courts having to take into consideration case law of the European Court of Human Rights.

❷ Case law on the issue of what is considered appropriate information to give to patients regarding treatment options is evolving.

❸ One philosopher proposed that patients in emergency departments already have their freedom of choice restricted because they have not chosen their site of treatment, and treatment choices are restricted to institutional policies.

References

1. Skene L, Nisselle P. High Court warns of the 'retrospectoscope' in informed consent cases: Rosenberg v. Percival. Medicine Today 2001; October: 79–82.
2. Alderson P, Goodey C. Theories of consent. British Medical Journal 1998; 317: 1313–1315.
3. Miller S, Marin D. Assessing capacity. Emergency Medicine Clinics of North America 2000; 18: 233–242.
4. British Medical Association. Consent Tool Kit Card 9 Advance Statements.

Further reading

Annas GJ, Densberger JE. Competence to refuse medical treatment: autonomy vs. paternalism. Toledo Law Review 1984; 15: 561–592.

Appelbaum P, Grisso T. Assessing patients' capacities to consent to treatment. New England Journal of Medicine 1988; 319: 1635–1658.

Biegler P, Stewart C. Assessing competence to refuse medical treatment. Medical Journal of Australia 2001; 174: 522–525.

Breen K, Plueckhahn V, Cordner S. et al. Ethics Law and Medical Practice. Allen and Unwin, St Leonard's British

Medical Association Consent Tool Kit Card 5 Assessment of Competence; 1997.

British Medical Association. Assessment of Mental Capacity. BMA and the Law Society. Chapter 10. On www.bma.org.uk (1995).

General Medical Council. 0–18 Years: . The General Medical Council; London, Sept 2007.

Medical Practitioners Board of Victoria. Medico-Legal Guidelines. Medical Practitioners Board of Victoria; Melbourne, March 2006.

Moskop J. Informed consent in the emergency department. Emergency Medicine Clinics of North America 1999; 17: 327–339.

Oats L. The courts' role in decisions about medical treatment. British Medical Journal 2000; 321: 1282–1284.

Pownall M. Doctors should obtain informed consent for intimate body searches. British Medical Journal 1999; 318: 1310A.

Savulescu J, Kerridge I. Competence and consent. Medical Journal of Australia 2001; 175: 313–315.

World Medical Association Declaration on the Rights of the Patient. www.net/e/policy/17-h e.html. Accessed Sept. 2008.

World Medical Association International Code of Medical Ethics. www.wma.net/e/policy/17-a e.html. Accessed Sept. 2008.

25.4 Privacy and confidentiality

Allen Yuen

ESSENTIALS

1 Privacy and confidentiality issues can be related to the physical environment in which care is given or to the personal health information involved in the patient's care.

2 Breaching confidentiality of personal health information now breaks Australian federal and state legislation introduced in 1988 (public sector) and 2001 (private health providers).[1–3] The relevant New Zealand legislation was introduced in 1994, and revised in 2005.[4]

Introduction

An individual's right to privacy and confidentiality has gained increasing recognition over the past decade. In an emergency setting, where patients are more vulnerable because of illness or injury, staff are often provided with confidential family and legal information, which would otherwise not be divulged, trusting that this will only be used to assist in the care of the patient.

Physical privacy

Emergency departments (EDs) are necessarily designed in an open plan to increase efficiency, observation and communication, but these requirements do intrude on privacy, particularly if cubicles are separated by curtains rather than solid walls. Consultations may be overheard during history taking, and when discussing patients with other medical staff or specialists, either directly or by telephone.

Patient privacy incidents occur frequently in an ED, risk factors being length of stay and absence of a walled cubicle. Patients who have their conversations overheard are more likely to withhold information and less likely to have their expectations of privacy met.[5] Privacy and confidentiality are challenged by physical design, crowding, visitors, film crews, communication and other factors.[6]

Prior permission should be obtained from the patient to allow students, nurses, other medical officers to be present during history taking, examination and procedures. This applies both in public and private hospitals. Some aspects of privacy in healthcare in the

ED relate to confidentiality while being assessed (being overheard, being seen, being exposed and being embarrassed), which relate to ED design, staff awareness, sensitivity and care. ED staff may be unaware how their routine behaviour may infringe on patient privacy.[7]

Staff bays are now often enclosed by glass screens to prevent others from hearing details on a patient's history or to prevent patients from becoming unnecessarily alarmed by discussion of serious differential diagnoses, which may need to be excluded. Inappropriate or unprofessional comments by staff may also be heard.[8]

When the patient is an adolescent, privacy needs may exclude communication with a parent. An understanding of the relevant informed consent law relating to minors is required.[9] The federal Privacy Act does not specify an age at which a child is considered of sufficient maturity to make his or her own privacy decisions. Doctors need to address each case individually, having regard to the child's maturity, degree of autonomy, understanding of the circumstances and the sensitivity of the information being sought.[3]

It is only within the last 5 years that the almost universal 'whiteboard' has virtually disappeared. This was a popular and useful management tool in EDs, displaying the patients' names, working diagnoses, locations and management plans. They were easily visible to anyone who came into the department. To preserve privacy and confidentiality, it was inevitable that they were withdrawn despite strong opposition from ED staff, claiming that this would lead to disruptions in patient care, coordination and flow. These problems did occur during the change-over period, but staff adapted well, and the advent of patient-tracking computer systems means that each monitor now provides more clinical information than the whiteboard ever did.

Well-known people (VIPs, politicians, media personalities and sports stars) need even more privacy than others, since they may be accompanied by support staff and, perhaps, a bevy of reporters who may be difficult to control, armed with video cameras and portable recorders. They cannot be restricted until the patient is actually inside the hospital building, after which security is in charge. Even when outside the building, most will accept advice to remain in a provided access zone where they may use their cameras or microphones without intruding on the privacy of other patients or their subject of interest. Hospital staff involved in the care of such patients may also wish to have their own privacy protected. Most hospitals now have media relations officers to take on the role of providing regular updated bulletins.

Healthcare providers

There is also the important matter of privacy for health providers. Whether full names should be displayed on identity badges is debatable. Details of contact numbers and home addresses of consultants, medical staff and nurses must be kept confidential, as there are cases of disgruntled or psychotic patients harassing and stalking clinical staff. Even if the request for contact details is innocent, it is an invasion of a healthcare worker's privacy for that information to be released without consent.

Mandatory reporting

Mandatory reporting overrides privacy laws where they are for the purpose of protection of the health of individuals or communities. Examples are:

- notification of communicable infectious diseases[10]

- child abuse
- elder abuse
- domestic violence.

This becomes more difficult when there is merely a suspicion, but doctors are protected if they report on this basis only. The laws vary between jurisdictions.

Police

Assistance must be given to the police when a criminal offence has been committed. In such cases, patient name, date of birth, address, nature of incident, description of injuries and conscious state may be released. An opinion of causation must not be stated.

If an injured patient is suspected of being a crime victim or perpetrator and may be a danger to that patient's or another's life, it is the doctor's civic duty to inform police of the circumstances.[11]

If a police enquiry is made by telephone, record the name, station, contact number and request and advise that the information will be obtained and provided. The given contact number must be checked to ensure if it is genuine before providing information, heeding the principles of confidentiality.

With police statements, the doctor should state credentials and experience before giving details of alleged history and physical findings. It is important to be objective, and to avoid venturing opinions outside a doctor's area of expertise. It is preferable for all police statements to be written by the ED director, so that a confidential record is kept of all statements issued.

Assistance is also given to help police identify missing or deceased persons.

Blood samples may need to be collected by law for drug or alcohol screening for patients involved in motor vehicle accidents. These are provided to police for testing.

Forensic issues

All deaths from unknown, unexpected, unnatural, accidental, violent or suspicious causes must be reported to the state coroner. This also includes cases of unknown identity, during or after surgery, in custody, a ward of the state, requested by next of kin or where unable to issue a death certificate.

Patient health information

Privacy of patients' health information refers to:

- their medical and social conditions
- their medical record
- any images (still, video or diagnostic imaging)
- results of investigations
- their treatments
- their treating doctors
- specialist and medicolegal reports.

Legislation

Confidentiality of health information has been the focus of legislation over recent years.

The Privacy Act 1988[1] applied only to the Australian Commonwealth public sector, but steps were taken early on to introduce it to the private sector, resulting in the Privacy Amendment (Private Sector) Act 2000 becoming law to cover the private (and public) health sector in December 2001.[2]

In New Zealand, the Privacy Act was enacted in 1993 and was used to develop the Health Network Code of Practice and Health Information Privacy Code 1994, which was further modified by the Health Information Standards Organisation in 2005.[5]

National privacy principles

The Privacy Act offers privacy protection to patients, while balancing this with the need for health service providers to share information, where necessary, for the provision of quality healthcare. The National Privacy Principles (NPPs) applicable to hospitals are summarized in Table 25.4.1.

NPP1

Patients or their relatives should be informed of the main consequences, if all relevant information is not provided. Information is collected primarily from the patient, but where collected from other sources, such as specialist or imaging reports, the patient should be told this. In an emergency, one may obtain from or provide information to another health organization or health practitioner without patient consent.

When collecting demographic data, this is best done by providing a patient with

Table 25.4.1	National Privacy Principles (applicable to hospitals)
NPP1	Collection Only collect information necessary to deliver the health service Obtain consent (this may not be possible with some emergency department patients, in which case, consent is implied)
NPP2	Use and disclosure Explain how the information will be used To whom the information may be disclosed, e.g. other treating clinicians and health carers, pathology, radiology and pharmacy By law, to courts, when subpoenaed
NPP3	Data quality Set standards to keep information accurate, complete and up to date
NPP4	Data security Protect and secure from loss, misuse and unauthorized access
NPP5	Openness Explain how health information is handled
NPP6	Access and correction Gives patients right of access to their own records and the right to correct it
NPP7	Identifiers Hospital must have its own identifier such as a Unit Record number, and must not use Commonwealth identifiers such as Medicare or Veteran Affairs numbers
NPP8	Anonymity Where lawful or practicable, patients must have the option of using health services without identifying themselves
NPP9	Transborder data flows Obligations regarding transfer of health information to another country
NPP10	Sensitive information Health information is sensitive information and must not be collected or disclosed without the patient's consent, except when required by law or under certain specified limited circumstances, such as serious or imminent threat to life or health, medical defence, for research relevant to public health or safety (preferably de-identified) Includes racial or ethnic origin, religious beliefs, sexual preferences or criminal record

documents to complete, rather than asking patients at an open desk in a waiting room. Triage should be performed in a private area. Taking of family histories can be done without their consent, as this helps in diagnosis, and is part of good clinical practice.

NPP2

The 'primary purpose' is to use the information for the patient's healthcare. The primary purpose must be aligned with the patient's expectations. A 'secondary purpose' may be to use it for research, for which specific consent must be obtained. When information is provided to a third party, that should be recorded in the unit record. It is standard practice to send a discharge summary to a patient's usual general practitioner (GP), unless the patient has requested otherwise.

NPP3

In EDs, it is sometimes difficult to obtain an accurate history, due to the patients' anxiety about their presenting symptoms. More accurate information may become available after

they have had a chance to collect their thoughts, or to affirm areas of their history with family or other witnesses. It is useful to recheck details that may not fit a working diagnosis.

Medication histories are often also inaccurate, since the patient may not be responsible for self-administration or may obtain tablets from a prepackaged dispensing system. Computerized GP letters often have all medications ever prescribed for that patient by the GP practice, and to be accurate, every medication should be checked with the patient or carer to ensure their currency.

NPP4

Patient records must not be left within reach of, or viewed by, others.

Any documents, notes on scrap paper or labels containing identifiable patient details must be disposed of securely, e.g. shredded, and not left in general waste paper bins.

Patient details on a computer screen should not be visible to other patients or visitors. Screen savers are useful if the screen is unattended. Computerized patient

data must only be accessible to authorized personnel by password-protected access.[10]

NPP6

Patients do have a right to access opinion as well as factual material, including a specialist's report, whether or not the report states that it is not to be shown to the patient without the patient's consent.[3] Patients are not obliged to give their reason for requesting access. Patients do not have immediate right to investigation results. The doctor ordering the tests must be given the opportunity to assess and discuss the results; otherwise there is the risk of misinterpretation.

NPP8

In some settings such as counselling in HIV/AIDS or sexual health, there are instances where anonymity is requested and granted. In the case of public or private hospital EDs, for providing a safe health service, and for billing and rebate purposes, doctors are required to record the identity of the patient.[3]

NPP9

Hospitals may transfer health information to countries where similar privacy laws exist. Consent needs to be obtained from the patient when in doubt, or when sending to countries where no such protection exists.

NPP10

The original 10th NPP was titled 'Sensitive Information'. In some revisions of this principle, it has been split into NPP10 'Limits on Use of Personal Information' and NPP11 'Limits on Disclosure of Personal Information'. The Federal Privacy Act 1988 has recently been amended to permit disclosure of genetic information to an *at-risk* relative when there is a serious (although not necessarily imminent) threat to the person's life, health or safety. It applies only to doctors and other health professionals in the private sector and does not cover those in state public hospitals or Commonwealth government agencies.[12,13] Why this is so needs further consideration.

New Zealand

New Zealand implemented its Privacy Act in 1993, with 12 principles that are similar to the Australian NPPs.[4] The Privacy Act has 12 information privacy principles:

Principles 1–4 govern the collection of personal information. This includes the reasons why personal information may be collected, where it may be collected from, and how it is collected.

Principle 5 governs the way personal information is stored. It is designed to protect personal information from unauthorized use or disclosure.

Principle 6 gives individuals the right to access information about themselves.

Principle 7 gives individuals the right to correct information about themselves.

Principles 8–11 place restrictions on how people and organizations can use or disclose personal information. These include ensuring information is accurate and up to date and that it is not improperly disclosed.

Principle 12 governs how 'unique identifiers' (such as IRD numbers, bank client numbers, driver's licence and passport numbers) can be used.

In 2005, the Ministry of Health released the Health Information Strategy for New Zealand,[4] with an emphasis on security of electronic data, and maintenance of trust in, and integrity of, communication. They developed a Privacy, Authentication and Security (PAS) guide, which brought all the existing relevant documents together.[14]

Implementation

Most hospitals now provide brochures to patients on arrival, outlining these privacy issues. These are important whether the hospital is public or private.[15,16] ED staff must be aware that some patients will require more detailed explanation before they are prepared to reveal all relevant information, and a sensitive approach is needed. Complaints about alleged breaches of privacy may be made and, if necessary, may be referred to the state health ombudsman or the state or federal privacy commissioner.

Communications

In this electronic era, sending information by facsimile, e-mail or telephone messaging can breach security, and ED staff need to take great care to ensure that there is a responsible person receiving the data, or that with telephone messages, only the caller's contact details are left. Health details should only be discussed directly with the patient, or parent in the case of a minor.

Medicolegal reports

Medical reports can only be provided to lawyers, after written consent is obtained from the patient. Such reports are the intellectual property of the doctor writing the report. While a patient has a right to view them, there is no right for a copy to be supplied, unless an appropriate fee for preparation of the report is paid.

Where a lawyer requests copies of medical records, rather than a report, the doctor must check the records to ensure that information collected is not sensitive information and does not contain information about others. Payment may be requested for the costs of reviewing and photocopying.

Research and quality assurance

Patients must be asked for consent before participating in research or quality assurance studies and must be de-identified in any reports. They must be fully informed of the reasons for, and the possible side effects of, the study.

Complaints and non-compliance

Doctors are advised to obtain their own independent legal advice and notify their medical indemnity/insurance company, if they are investigated by the privacy commissioner as the result of a complaint that privacy may have been breached. Monetary fines or imprisonment may result from non-compliance.[17]

Retrospectivity

In general, the principles apply to information collected on or after 21 December 2001 in Australia but may apply before then, if referred to, used or disclosed later. If compliance poses an unreasonable administrative burden or expense, then a summary is an option. This refers to NPP 5, 6, 7 and 9.[3] There is no obligation by a doctor to provide access to information which is not in use collected prior to 21 December 2001.

State, territory and New Zealand privacy laws

The 10 NPPs apply throughout Australia. While these are generally accepted, some states have rewritten them. The differences are not significant in content.

New South Wales has 15 health privacy principles, which came into effect on 1 September 2004. They are a more detailed expansion of the NPPs.[18] In Victoria, the Health Records Act 2001 came into operation on 1 July 2002, and this becomes the relevant date for 'old' versus 'new' information.[19] In Queensland, there is no separate privacy law. Queensland Health requires compliance with the 10 NPPs.[20] In Western Australia, there is currently no legislative privacy regimen, but an Information Privacy Bill was introduced in March 2007.[14] South Australia has a Code of Fair Information Practice based on the NPPs.[21] Tasmania has superseded its previous privacy principles with the Personal Information and Protection Act 2004.[22] The Northern Territory has a Health Information Privacy website issued in March 2002.[23] The Australian Capital Territory uses a slightly amended version of the Federal Privacy Act, which is administered by the Federal Privacy Commissioner on behalf of the ACT government.[24]

New Zealand implemented its Privacy Act in 1993, with 12 principles that are similar to the Australian NPPs.[4] In 2005, the Ministry of Health released the Health Information Strategy for New Zealand,[4] with an emphasis on security of electronic data, and maintenance of trust in, and integrity of, communication. They developed a PAS guide, which brought all the existing relevant documents together.[25]

Controversies

❶ Release of information on adolescents to parents.

❷ Protection of staff privacy – should full names be displayed on identity badges?

❸ The extent to which information may be provided to the police or other authorities.

❹ Whether reporting of elder and domestic abuse should be mandatory in all regions.

❺ Whether the security on current computer systems is sufficient to protect personal health information.

References

1. Office of the Federal Privacy Commissioner. National Privacy Principles. The Privacy Act 1988. http://www.privacy.gov.au.
2. Office of the Federal Privacy Commissioner. Guidelines on Privacy in the Private Health Sector. 9 Nov 2001. http://www.privacy.gov.au/publications/hg_01.html (Accessed Sept. 2008.)
3. Phelps K, Mudge T. Privacy resource handbook. Canberra: Australian Medical Association; 2002.
4. Health Information Standards Organisation. Health Information Strategy for New Zealand; 2005. www.moh.govt.nz.
5. Karro J, Dent AW, Farish S. Patient perceptions of privacy infringements in an emergency department. Emergency Medicine of Australasia 2005; 17: 117–123.
6. Geiderman JM, Moskop JC, Derse AR. Privacy and confidentiality in emergency medicine: obligations and challenges. Emergency Medical Clinics of North America 2006; 24: 633–656.
7. Knopp RK, Satterlee PA. Confidentiality in the ED. Emergency Medical Clinics of North America 1999; 17: 385–396.
8. Olsen JC, Sabin BR. ED patient perceptions of privacy and confidentiality. Journal of Emergency Medicine 2003; 25: 329–333.
9. Baren JM. Ethical dilemmas in the care of minors in the ED. Emergency Clinics of North America 2006; 24: 619–631.
10. Privacy Legislation and Notifiable Infectious Diseases. Melbourne: Department of Human Services; June 2002. http://www.dhs.vic.gov.au/phd/.
11. Frampton A. Some legal and ethical issues surrounding breaking patient confidentiality. Emergency Medicine Journal 2005; 22: 84–86.
12. Otlowski MFA. Disclosure of genetic information to at-risk relatives. Medical Journal of Australia 2007; 187: 398–399.
13. Skene L. Patient's rights or family responsibilities? Two approaches to genetic testing. Medical Law Review 1998; 6: 1–41.
14. Information Privacy Bill March 2007. Western Australia Legislative Assembly.
15. Treatment of Patient Information at Epworth Hospital: 2001.
16. Know your rights and responsibilities: Private patients hospital charter. Commonwealth of Australia 2006.
17. Privacy an ongoing concern. Pamela Burton, Legal Counsel, Federal AMA, Australian Medicine 18 Mar 2001.
18. Health Records and Information Privacy Act 2002. Office of the New South Wales Privacy Commissioner.
19. Information to Private Health Service Providers. Health Services Commissioner, Victoria; April 2004. http://www.health.vic.gov.au/hsc/.
20. Queensland Government Information Standard (IS42A). Queensland Department of Health; Sep 2001.
21. Code of Fair Information Practice. South Australian Department of Health. http://www.publications.health.sa.gov.au/ainfo/1/
22. Personal Information and Protection Act 2004. Tasmanian Ombudsman. http://www.thelaw.tas.gov.au.
23. Northern Territory Government. Health Information Privacy website:http://www.nt.gov.au/health/org-supp/legal/privacy/health.
24. Health Records (Privacy and Access) Act 1997. Australian Capital Territory.
25. The Privacy, Authentication and Security Guide. Ministry of Health; New Zealand 2005.

26 EMERGENCY MEDICAL SYSTEMS

Edited by **George Jelinek**

26.1 Pre-hospital emergency medicine

Stephen Bernard

ESSENTIALS

1 Ambulance dispatch is increasingly becoming computerized and this allows for medical determination of response speed and skill set, as well as telephone instructions for cardiopulmonary resuscitation and first aid.

2 Ambulance care of the critically ill or injured patient is similar to initial evaluation by the emergency physician, with emphasis on basic life-support measures.

3 The role of advanced life-support measures such as endotracheal intubation and intravenous fluid therapy in severe trauma and cardiac arrest is uncertain.

4 Patients with chest pain and suspected ST-segment elevation myocardial ischaemia should be triaged to a centre with facilities for interventional cardiology.

5 Ambulance officers have effective treatments for medical emergencies, including respiratory distress, seizures, hypoglycaemia and anaphylaxis.

Introduction

Ambulance services have the primary role of providing rapid stretcher transport of patients to an emergency department (ED). Increasingly, ambulance officers are trained to administer emergency medical care prior to hospital arrival in a wide range of life-threatening illnesses with the expectation that earlier and/or more advanced treatment will improve outcomes.

Dispatch

Many countries now have a single telephone number for immediate access to the ambulance service in cases of emergency, such as 911 in North America, 999 in the UK and 000 in Australasia. However, the accurate dispatch of the correct ambulance skill set in the optimal time frame is complex. It is inappropriate to dispatch all ambulances on a 'code 1' (lights and sirens) response, since this entails some level of risk to the ambulance officers and other road users. On the other hand, it may be difficult to accurately identify life-threatening illnesses or injuries using information gained from telephone communication alone, especially from bystanders. Also, it is inappropriate to dispatch ambulance officers with advanced life-support training to routine cases where these skills are not required.

In order to have consistent, accurate dispatch of the appropriate skill set in the optimal time frame, many ambulance services are now using computer-aided dispatch programs. These computer programs have structured questions for use by call-takers with some limited medical training. Pivotal to accurate dispatch is identification of the chief complaint, followed by subsequent structured questions to determine the severity of the illness. The answers to these questions allow the computerized system to recommend the optimal skill set and speed of response. This computer algorithm is medically determined according to local protocols and practices and provides consistency of dispatch.

Most ambulance services generally have at least four dispatch codes. A code 1 (or local equivalent terminology) is used for conditions that are considered immediately life-threatening. For these, emergency warning devices (lights and sirens) are routinely used. The possibility of life-saving therapy arriving as soon as possible is judged as outweighing the potential hazard of a rapid response. In a code 2 (or equivalent) response, the condition is regarded as being urgent and emergency warning devices are used only when traffic is heavy. In a code 3 response, an attendance by ambulance within an hour is deemed medically appropriate. Finally, non-emergency or 'booked' calls are transports arranged at a designated time negotiated by the caller and the ambulance service.

Despite continuous developments in computer algorithms, accurate telephone identification of life-threatening conditions may be difficult. For example, identification of patients who are deceased (beyond resuscitation),[1] in cardiac arrest[2] or suffering acute coronary syndrome[3] has been shown to lack the very high sensitivity and specificity that might be expected.

The dispatch centre also has a role for telephone instructions on bystander cardio-pulmonary resuscitation[4] and first aid.

Clinical skills

Ambulance service protocols vary considerably around the world. Since there are few randomized controlled trials to provide high-quality evidence-based guidance for pre-hospital care, there is still much controversy and considerable variation in the ambulance skill set in different ambulance services worldwide.

Many ambulance services provide a number of levels of skill set, dispatching ambulance officers trained in basic life support (including defibrillation) to non-emergency or urgent cases and more highly trained ambulance officers (designated as advanced life-support paramedics or intensive-care paramedics) to patients with an immediately life-threatening condition for which advanced life-support skills may be

appropriate. In addition, ambulance services may correspond with other emergency services (such as fire fighters) to provide rapid-response defibrillation.

The rationale for common pre-hospital interventions is outlined in the following sections.

Trauma care

Pre-hospital trauma care may be considered as either basic trauma life support (clearing of the airway, administration of supplemental oxygen, control of external haemorrhage, spinal immobilization, splinting of fractures and the administration of inhaled analgesics) or advanced life support including intubation of the trachea, intravenous (i.v.) cannulation and fluid therapy, and the administration of i.v. analgesia.

Basic trauma life support

On arrival at the scene of the patient with suspected major trauma, ambulance officers are trained to perform an initial 'DR-ABCDE' evaluation, which is similar to the approach that has been developed for physicians, namely consideration of dangers, response, airway, breathing, circulation, disability and exposure. Of particular importance in the pre-hospital trauma setting are dangers to ambulance officers from passing traffic, electrical wires and fire from spillage of fuel.

The initial assessment of the airway and breathing includes the application of cervical immobilization in patients who have a mechanism of injury that suggests a risk of spinal column instability. Although decision instruments have been developed to identify patients in the ED who require radiographic imaging,[5] the accuracy of these guidelines in the pre-hospital setting is uncertain. On the other hand, spinal immobilization of many patients with minimal risk of spinal cord injury is uncomfortable, mandates transport and possibly leads to unnecessary radiographic studies.[6] Therefore, ambulance officers are generally instructed to immobilize the neck in all cases of suspected spinal-column injury based largely on mechanism of injury.

Accurate triage of major trauma patients is an important component of trauma care in cities with designated major trauma

centres. Triage tools based on vital signs, injuries and modifying factors such as age, comorbidities and mechanism of injury are used.[7] Paramedic judgement may also have a role, although some injuries such as occult intra-abdominal injuries are difficult to detect on clinical grounds.[8]

Advanced trauma life support

Advanced trauma life support (ATLS) by ambulance paramedics, particularly intubation of the trachea and i.v. cannulation for fluid therapy, is controversial. Although these interventions are routinely used after hospital admission, studies to date indicate that the provision of ATLS provided by paramedics does not improve outcomes.[9,10] On the other hand, few studies conducted to date have been sufficiently rigorous to allow definitive conclusions, and many were conducted in cities with predominantly penetrating trauma rather than blunt trauma. Many ambulance services therefore continue to authorize advanced airway management and i.v. fluid resuscitation in selected trauma patients.

Intubation

Following severe head injury, many unconscious patients have decreased oxygenation and ventilation during pre-hospital care, and this secondary brain injury is associated with worse neurological outcome.[11] In addition, a depressed gag or cough reflex may lead to aspiration of vomit and this may cause a severe pneumonitis, which may be fatal or result in a prolonged stay in an intensive-care unit. To prevent these complications of severe head injury, endotracheal intubation may be performed. This facilitates control of oxygen and carbon dioxide, provides airway protection and is recommended for patients with Glasgow Coma Score <9 following severe head injury.[12] However, most patients with severe head injury maintain a gag or cough reflex, and successful intubation requires the use of drugs to facilitate laryngoscopy and placement of the endotracheal tube.

The usual approach involves rapid sequence intubation (RSI), which is the administration of both a sedative drug and a rapidly acting muscle relaxant such as suxamethonium. It is unclear from the literature as to whether RSI should be performed pre-hospital by ambulance paramedics or be performed in an ED by appropriately trained physicians.

There is some evidence that pre-hospital intubation in head injury is beneficial.[13,14] In a study of 671 patients with severe head injury, intubation in the field using RSI was associated with a decrease in mortality rate from 56% to 36%.[13] In another study of 799 patients with severe head injury, patients intubated using RSI in the field were compared with those not intubated.[14] When adjusted for confounding variables, the RSI patients were more likely to survive (odds ratio, 0.63; 95% confidence interval, 0.41–0.97; $P = 0.04$) and have a good outcome (odds ratio, 1.7; 95% confidence interval, 1.2–2.6; $P = 0.006$) than those in the no-RSI group.

However, two studies have suggested that pre-hospital intubation may be associated with worse outcome in head trauma patients.[15,16] In a review of registry data of patients admitted to an urban trauma centre with severe head injury, patients were stratified by pre-hospital methods of airway management (not intubated, intubated or unsuccessful intubation).[15] This study showed that patients requiring pre-hospital intubation or in whom intubation was attempted had an increased mortality (81% and 77%, respectively) when compared with non-intubated patients (43%).

In a second study, RSI was introduced as a protocol for adult patients with severe head injury in San Diego, USA, and the effect on outcome was assessed compared with historical controls.[16] Each study patient was hand-matched to three non-intubated historical controls from a trauma registry using the following parameters: age, sex, mechanism of injury, trauma centre and AIS score for each body system. The study enrolled 209 trial patients who were hand-matched to 627 controls. Both groups were similar with regard to all matching parameters, admission vital signs, frequency of specific head injury diagnoses and incidence of invasive procedures. Mortality was significantly increased in the RSI cohort versus controls for all patients (33.0% versus 24.2%, $P < 0.05$).

Given the limited evidence of benefit and potential for harm with intubation in head injury, it has been proposed that intubation not be introduced into paramedic practice until prospective randomized, controlled trials have been conducted.[17]

Intravenous fluid

Intravenous fluid resuscitation has been shown to worsen outcome in patients with penetrating trauma and hypotension.[18] However, this finding has recently been questioned.[19] In any case, most major trauma in Australasia and Europe is blunt rather than penetrating and few patients require urgent surgical control of haemorrhage. The issue of pre-hospital i.v. fluid for the treatment of hypotension therefore remains the subject of debate.

Supporters of pre-hospital i.v. fluid therapy suggest that this treatment is intuitively beneficial and that any delay of this therapy increases the adverse effects of prolonged hypotension, which may result in end-organ ischaemia, leading to multiorgan system failure and increased morbidity and mortality. In particular, hypotension after severe head injury is associated with an adverse outcome and should be promptly treated.[20]

Opponents of pre-hospital i.v. fluid therapy suggest that this therapy prior to surgical control in patients with uncontrolled bleeding increases blood loss due to increased blood pressure, dilution coagulopathy and hypothermia from large volumes of unwarmed fluid. Any additional blood loss would increase transfusion requirements and could be associated with increased morbidity and mortality. Also, ambulance paramedic training and skills maintenance in pre-hospital fluid therapy is costly and may not be justified without some evidence of patient benefit.

There is no evidence from clinical trials for benefit of the administration of i.v. fluid to bleeding patients in the pre-hospital setting. Studies to date suggest that pre-hospital i.v. fluid does not improve outcomes.[8,9] Nevertheless, if i.v. fluid is given to patients with hypotension and severe head injury, crystalloid rather than colloid should be given.[21]

Analgesia

The administration of effective analgesia in the pre-hospital setting for traumatic pain remains a difficult issue for ambulance services. Many ambulance officers are not trained to administer i.v. therapy, and treatment options are, therefore, limited to inhaled therapy.

Inhaled analgesic treatments include methoxyflurane and oxygen/nitrous oxide. However, while the former is reasonably effective,[22] there are concerns with the administration of these in enclosed spaces such as ambulances because of the perceived risk of repeated exposures of these analgesics to the ambulance officers.

Alternatively, the training of ambulance officers in the insertion of an i.v. cannula and administration of small increments of i.v. morphine is increasingly regarded as a feasible alternative to inhalation analgesia. Alternative routes of narcotic administration such as intranasal administration are the subject of current studies. For example, the use of intranasal fentanyl has been shown to be equivalent to i.v. morphine.[23]

Cardiac care

Cardiac arrest

In 1967, external defibrillation was introduced into pre-hospital care and this led to the development of mobile coronary care units in many countries for the delivery of advanced cardiac care for the patient with suspected myocardial ischaemia. This approach was subsequently extended to rapid response for defibrillation of patients in cardiac arrest. Protocols for the management of pre-hospital cardiac arrest are based on the concept of the 'chain of survival', which includes an immediate call to the ambulance service, the initiation of bystander CPR, early defibrillation and advanced cardiac life support (intubation and drug therapy).

The patient in cardiac arrest represents the most time-critical patient attended by ambulance services. For the patient with ventricular fibrillation, each minute increase from time of collapse to defibrillation is associated with an increase in mortality of approximately 10%. However, most ambulance services have urban response times that average 8–9 min. Since there may be 2 min between collapse and dispatch, and 1 min between arrival at the scene to delivery of the first defibrillation, total time from collapse to defibrillation would usually be approximately 12 min, therefore current survival rates for witnessed cardiac arrest due to defibrillation in urban areas are low[24] and there are even fewer survivors in rural areas.[25]

The most effective strategy to improve outcomes would be to decrease ambulance response times. However, this would require very significant increases in ambulance resources and would be an expensive strategy in terms of cost per life saved. Alternatively, response times to cardiac arrest patients may be reduced with the use of co-response by first responders equipped with defibrillators. Such first responder programmes have been introduced in Melbourne, Australia,[26] and Ontario, Canada,[27] with promising results.

The role of advanced life support (intubation and i.v. drug therapy) during cardiac arrest remains controversial. When these skills were introduced into Ontario, Canada, there was an increase in the numbers of patients with return of spontaneous circulation (10.9% versus 14.6%, $P < 0.001$) but the rate of survival to hospital discharge did not significantly increase (5.0% versus 5.1%, $P = 0.83$).[28]

Acute coronary syndromes

Most ambulance services have protocols for the management of the patient with chest pain where the cause is suspected as an acute coronary syndrome. These protocols usually include supplemental oxygen, administration of sublingual trinitrates and aspirin, followed by rapid transfer to an ED for definitive diagnosis and management. In addition, pain relief using i.v. morphine may be given by advanced life-support paramedics. Whilst these interventions may decrease symptoms, more recent strategies to improve outcomes involve triage of patients with ST-segment elevation myocardial ischaemia (using 12-lead electrocardiography) by paramedics to centres for interventional cardiology.[29]

Cardiac arrhythmias

Some patients with an acute coronary syndrome develop a cardiac arrhythmia during ambulance care. Pulseless ventricular tachycardia is treated with immediate defibrillation, and amiodarone is recommended for ventricular tachycardia where a pulse is palpable.[30] However, the pre-hospital drug treatment of supraventricular tachycardia is more controversial. Whilst the use of verapamil or adenosine appears to be equivalent in efficacy,[31] many ambulance services require the patient to be transported for 12-lead electrocardiography and management of the tachyarrhythmia in an ED.

Pulmonary oedema

During myocardial ischaemia, the patient may develop pulmonary oedema and in these patients the use of oxygen and glyceryl trinitrates is regarded as useful.[32] Despite common use in the ED, pre-hospital continuous positive airways pressure for acute pulmonary oedema has not been widely adopted, since the equipment is expensive, oxygen consumption is high and there is no proven benefit with pre-hospital administration of continuous positive airways pressure at this time.

Other medical emergencies

Hypoglycaemia

The patient with hypoglycaemia due to relative excess of exogenous injected insulin will suffer neurological injury unless the blood glucose level is promptly corrected. Treatment involves orally or intravenously administered dextrose. For ambulance officers who are not trained to insert i.v. cannulae, or where i.v. access is not possible, the administration of intramuscular glucagon is also effective, although this is associated with an increase in the time to full consciousness.[33]

Narcotic overdose

Patients who inject narcotic drugs may suffer coma and respiratory depression which is readily reversed by naloxone. However, the administration of i.v. naloxone by paramedics is somewhat problematic, since i.v. access may be difficult and the half-life of i.v. naloxone (approximately 20 min) may be shorter than the injected narcotic. If the patient awakens and leaves medical care, there may also be a recurrence of sedation. Many ambulance services therefore administer naloxone via the intramuscular or subcutaneous route. Whilst the absorption via this route may be slower, overall the time to return of normal respirations is equivalent. To avoid the use of needles, naloxone may also be administered via the intranasal route and this has an equivalent onset time to intramuscular naloxone.[34]

Anaphylaxis

Many patients with known severe anaphylaxis are prescribed adrenaline (epinephrine) by their physician for self-administration. The use of intramuscular adrenaline (epinephrine) by ambulance officers is a safe and effective pre-hospital therapy.[35]

Seizures

Out-of-hospital status epilepticus is also regarded as a time critical medical emergency. The first-line treatment of status epilepticus is usually a benzodiazepine. There are supportive data on the use of intramuscular midazolam, which may have an initial success rate of 80%.[36] Intravenous benzodiazepines may given if seizures persist.

Controversies and future directions

❶ Computer-aided dispatch algorithms require further improvement to increase the sensitivity and specificity for the detection of life-threatening emergencies.

❷ Advanced life support, including intubation and i.v. fluid therapy, by ambulance paramedics for the severe trauma and cardiac arrest patient is unproven and expensive. Randomized controlled trials are required to justify these interventions.

❸ Patients with chest pain and ST-segment elevation myocardial ischaemia should be identified with 12-lead electrocardiography and triaged to a centre with facilities for interventional cardiology.

References

1. Harvey L, Woollard M. Outcome of patients identified as dead (beyond resuscitation) at the point of the emergency call. Emergency Medicine Journal 2004; 21: 367–369.
2. Flynn J, Archer F, Morgans A. Sensitivity and specificity of the medical priority dispatch system in detecting cardiac arrest emergency calls in Melbourne. Prehospital and Disaster Medicine 2006; 21: 72–76.
3. Deakin CD, Sherwood DM, Smith A, et al. Does telephone triage of emergency (999) calls using Advanced Medical Priority Dispatch (AMPDS) with Department of Health (DH) call prioritisation effectively identify patients with an acute coronary syndrome? An audit of 42,657 emergency calls to Hampshire Ambulance Service NHS Trust. Emergency Medicine Journal 2006; 23: 232–235.
4. Vaillancourt C, Verma A, Trickett J, et al. Evaluating the effectiveness of dispatch-assisted cardiopulmonary resuscitation instructions. Academic Emergency Medicine 2007; 14: 877–883.
5. Hoffman JR, Mower WR, Wolfson AB, et al. Validity of a set of clinical criteria to rule out injury to the cervical spine in patients with blunt trauma. National Emergency X-Radiography Utilization study (NEXUS) Group. New England Journal of Medicine 2000; 343: 94–99.
6. Armstrong BP, Simpson HK, Crouch R, et al. Prehospital clearance of the cervical spine: does it need to be a pain in the neck? Emergency Medicine Journal 2007; 24: 501–503.
7. Markovchick VJ, Moore EE. Optimal trauma outcome: trauma system design and the trauma team. Emergency Medicine Clinics of North America 2007; 25: 643–654.

8. Mulholland SA, Gabbe BJ, Cameron P. Victorian State Trauma Outcomes Registry and Monitoring Group (VSTORM). Is paramedic judgement useful in prehospital trauma triage? Injury 2005; 36: 1298–1305.
9. Isenberg DL, Bissell R. Does advanced life support provide benefits to patients? A literature review. Prehospital Disaster Medicine 2005; 20: 265–270.
10. Liberman M, Mulder D, Lavoie A. Multicenter Canadian study of prehospital trauma care. Annals of Surgery 2003; 237: 153–160.
11. Chi JH, Knudson MM, Vassar MJ, et al. Prehospital hypoxia affects outcome in patients with traumatic brain injury: a prospective multicenter study. Journal of Trauma 2006; 61:1134–1141.
12. www.braintrauma.org/prehospital (accessed January 2008).
13. Winchell RJ, Hoyt DB. Endotracheal intubation in the field improves survival in patients with severe head injury. Archives of Surgery 1997; 132: 592–597.
14. Bulger EM, Copass MK, Sabath DR. The use of neuromuscular blocking agents to facilitate prehospital intubation does not impair outcome after traumatic brain injury. Journal of Trauma 2005; 58: 718–723.
15. Murray JA, Demetriades D, Berne TV, et al. Prehospital intubation in patients with severe head injury. Journal of Trauma 2000; 49: 1065–1070.
16. Davis DP, Hoyt DB, Ochs M, et al. The effect of paramedic rapid sequence intubation on outcome in patients with severe traumatic brain injury. Journal of Trauma 2003; 54: 444–453.
17. Bernard SA. Paramedic intubation of patients with severe head injury: a review of current Australian practice and recommendations for change. Emergency Medicine of Australasia 2006; 18: 221–228.
18. Bickell W, Pepe P, Mattox K, et al. Immediate versus delayed fluid resuscitation for hypotensive patients with penetrating torso injuries. New England Journal of Medicine 1994; 331: 1105–1108.
19. Yaghoubian A, Lewis RJ, Putnam B. Reanalysis of prehospital intravenous fluid administration in patients with penetrating truncal injury and field hypotension. American Surgicals 2007; 73: 1027–1030.
20. Chesnut RM, Marshall LF, Klauber MR, et al. The role of secondary brain injury in determining outcome from severe head injury. Journal of Trauma 1993; 34: 216–222.
21. SAFE Study Investigators. Saline or albumin for fluid resuscitation in patients with traumatic brain injury. New England Journal of Medicine 2007; 357: 874–884.
22. Buntine P, Thom O, Babl F, et al. Prehospital analgesia in adults using inhaled methoxyflurane. Emergency Medicine Australasia 2007; 19: 509–514.
23. Rickard C, O'Meara P, McGrail M, et al. A randomized controlled trial of intranasal fentanyl vs intravenous morphine for analgesia in the prehospital setting. American Journal of Emergency Medicine 2007; 25: 911–917.
24. Fridman M, Barnes V, Whyman A, et al. A model of survival following pre-hospital cardiac arrest based on the Victorian Ambulance Cardiac Arrest Register. Resuscitation 2007; 75: 311–322.
25. Jennings PA, Cameron P, Walker T, et al. Out-of-hospital cardiac arrest in Victoria: rural and urban outcomes. Medical Journal of Australia 2006; 185: 135–139.
26. Smith KL, McNeill JJ, The Emergency Medical Response Steering Committee. Cardiac arrests treated by ambulance paramedics and fire fighters. Medical Journal of Australia 2002; 177: 305–309.
27. Stiells IG, Wells GA, Field BJ, et al. Improved out-of-hospital cardiac arrest survival through the inexpensive optimization of an existing defibrillation program. Journal of American Medical Association 1999; 281: 1175–1181.
28. Stiell IG, Wells GA, Field B, et al. Advanced cardiac life support in out-of-hospital cardiac arrest. New England Journal of Medicine 2004; 351: 647–656.
29. Le May MR, Davies RF, Dionne R, et al. Comparison of early mortality of paramedic-diagnosed ST-segment elevation myocardial infarction with immediate transport to a designated primary percutaneous coronary intervention center to that of similar patients transported to the nearest hospital. American Journal of Cardiology 2006; 98: 1329–1333.
30. Morley PT, Walker T. Australian Resuscitation Council. Australian Resuscitation Council: adult advanced life support (ALS) guidelines 2006. Critical Care and Resuscitation 2006; 8: 129–131.
31. Madsen CD, Pointer JE, Lynch TG. A comparison of adenosine and verapamil for the treatment of supraventricular tachycardia in the prehospital setting. Annals of Emergency Medicine 1995; 25: 649–655.
32. Stiell IG, Spaite DW, Field B, et al. Advanced life support for out-of-hospital respiratory distress. New England Journal of Medicine 2007; 356: 2156–2164.
33. Howell MA, Guly HR. A comparison of glucagon and glucose in prehospital hypoglycaemia. Journal of Accident Emergency Medicine 1997; 14: 30–32.
34. Kelly AM, Kerr D, Dietze P, et al. Randomised trial of intranasal versus intramuscular naloxone in prehospital treatment for suspected opioid overdose. Medical Journal of Australia 2005; 182: 24–27.
35. Kane KE, Cone DC. Anaphylaxis in the prehospital setting. Journal of Emergency Medicine 2004; 27: 371–377.
36. Vilke GM, Sharieff GQ, Marino A. Midazolam for the treatment of out-of-hospital pediatric seizures. Prehospital Emergency Care 2002; 6: 215–217.

26.2 Retrieval

Garry J. Wilkes

ESSENTIALS

1 Retrieval medicine involves the transport of specialized medical personnel and equipment to remote areas to stabilize and transport critically ill or injured patients to more central hospitals.

2 Retrieval supplements are in cooperation with the pre-hospital ambulance service.

3 Transfers and time in transit are times of greatest risk to patients.

4 Retrieval systems aim more to minimize transit times and numbers of transfers than to simply reduce overall time from incident to arrival at a tertiary centre, therefore exposing patients to the least possible risk.

5 The decision on the mode of transport can only be made by staff familiar with the various modalities available and the local conditions.

6 All procedures necessary or likely to be in transit should be performed prior to departure, all lines firmly secured and redundant vascular access available in the event of an emergency.

7 Early consultation with the retrieval team and discussion between the sending and receiving doctors facilitates the transfer process and identifies preparation and treatment that can be completed before the arrival of the retrieval team.

8 Aerial transport is associated with specific problems and is potentially hazardous. The safety of the crew is of primary importance. The final decision as to whether or not a flight is safe will always rest with the pilot.

Introduction

Retrieval medicine is a term used to describe the branch of emergency medicine involved with the retrieval and transport of patients from remote locations to primary hospital treatment sites. Retrieval is the process whereby medical teams are transported from central hospitals to peripheral areas with the intention of treating, stabilizing and transporting patients back to these centres. The most common form is a secondary retrieval where the patient is transferred from one healthcare facility to another. A primary retrieval is where the patient is retrieved direct from the scene or incident. However, the clinical distinction between primary and secondary retrieval becomes less clear in smaller healthcare settings where staff are unfamiliar with management of critically ill or injured patients.

Retrieval is more than simply retrieving patients. The process more importantly encompasses the transportation of personnel and expertise from a tertiary centre to a peripheral location. It would not be cost-effective to place specialists from every field in every rural location even if the workforce was available. In addition, the volume of suitable work in each location would be insufficient to adequately maintain specialist skills. Transporting specialist services to the rural patient when needed is more economical than supplying each rural area with a fixed, dedicated specialist service and allows these specialists to maintain skills. The general concepts of a retrieval service also include provision of rural areas with an information and advice network that can be accessed at any time, a bed-finding facility at receiving institutions and activation of the retrieval team when required. The rural practitioner therefore has the capacity to gain expert advice or the means for transporting patients when necessary from a single phone call. The alternative of the remote practitioner having to make multiple phone calls to find a bed as well as simultaneously managing the patient is not an accepted standard of care. This provision of an information and support network is more essential than the transport itself. The term 'retrieval' unfortunately focuses upon the transport itself, distracting from the other vital system components.

Principles of transport

Speed of transport is not the prime consideration in retrieval medicine. The overriding principle is to provide the best possible care whilst exposing the patient to the least possible risk. The times of greatest risk are during transit and transfer. Every transfer is an opportunity for line disconnection, interference with monitoring equipment, injury to patients and staff and loss of information if escorts are changed. Difficulties associated with transit are discussed below. Reducing the number of transfers and spending as little time as possible in transit minimize the time the patient is exposed to the greatest risk.

Another principle of retrieval is that the level of medical care should be maintained or increased at each stage of transfer from the peripheral to central institution. This principle has been adopted in the recommendations of the specialties involved in critical care transport in Australasia.[1] In general the retrieval team can provide a level of care above that available at the referring hospital whereas a team sent from the peripheral hospital will be unable to provide the same level of care in transit as in their own hospital. Utilizing peripheral location staff as transport escorts may also significantly affect the level of care available at that location. For smaller locations this effect may be critical.

Organization structure and staffing

Physicians involved in retrieval medicine are typically from the critical care specialties of emergency medicine, intensive care and anaesthesia. Specific training in the retrieval environment is essential for familiarization of the different equipment and vastly different environments of noisy, moving vehicles, limited patient access, altitude and prolonged periods without on-site assistance.

Retrieval systems vary greatly in organizational structure. Some are run out of single departments. Others are hospital-based units and others again are external non-government and/or charitable organizations employing clinicians directly. Each system has advantages and disadvantages, with the selected model strongly influenced by workforce supply and funding structures.

Modes of transport

The mechanism by which the medical team is transported varies with individual circumstances. Road transport is the most readily available and requires the least resources. Transport by helicopter is more expensive and takes time to activate but enables greater distances to be covered in a shorter time period. If helicopters can land at each location there is no need for secondary ambulance transfers. Fixed-wing aircraft share similar drawbacks, can cover even greater distances but require special landing strips and the need for secondary transfers to and from airstrips. Loading and unloading patients in appropriately configured aircraft is almost identical to land ambulance transfers. Issues specific to altitude will be addressed later.

When road transport can be achieved in less than 1–2 h this is normally the cost-effective choice. Transport by air has the disadvantages of increased cost and problems associated with altitude. The greatest benefit of aerial transport is in reducing the time spent in transit and therefore minimizing the time at greatest risk. Figure 26.2.1 shows the time differences between road and

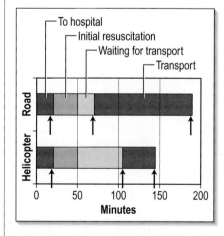

Fig. 26.2.1 Comparison of road and helicopter transport times. Times of high risk are shown as red (in transit) and arrows (transfers). Although helicopter transport does not significantly reduce overall time, it significantly reduces the high-risk time in transit without increasing the number of transfers.

helicopter transport. Overall time from incident to arrival at a central hospital may not be significantly reduced by use of a helicopter if road transport is immediately available. The time spent in transit, however, and therefore the time the patient is exposed to maximum risk is significantly reduced. The time taken for the retrieval team to reach a patient is also minimized by use of helicopter transport where road distances are prolonged. The choice between helicopter and fixed wing is a balance between avoiding secondary transfers with helicopters and more rapid flight with fixed wings. Beyond helicopter flight times of 1 h (~250 km), fixed wing becomes increasingly preferable. Helicopter use beyond 400 km is unusual. The transport distance, terrain covered and the specific condition of the patient all influence the decision on the mode of transportation. It is inappropriate to transport some patients by air whilst others require pressurization to ground level in order to be transported safely. The final decision will rest with the retrieval team familiar with the options available. The team should be contacted early in order to arrange the most appropriate transport as quickly as possible.

Preparation for transport

It is very difficult to perform even simple tasks in a moving vehicle. Planes and helicopters are particularly noisy, with unexpected movements and light fluctuations. Listening to heart sounds, respiratory sounds or even taking a pulse may be impossible. Despite this there are several examples in the literature of the successful performance of intubation, i.v. cannulation and other procedures in aircraft.[2,3] Although this is reassuring, it should be considered a failure of pre-flight preparation to be put in the position where such a procedure becomes necessary in transit. If a procedure is considered to be likely or possibly needed before arrival at the destination, serious consideration should be given to performing that procedure prior to departure. It is essential to have lines secured, redundant lines operational in case of emergencies and contingency plans prepared for common and potentially serious complications. In practice this means checking that each vascular access is patent, operational and sufficiently secured to withstand sudden turbulence. Some lines may require suturing to achieve this. It is prudent to have at least one i.v. line that is patent but not in use in order to provide access in an unexpected emergency. Wherever practicable, a single port at a secure site can be used for several infusions, thus freeing up other ports.

Conscious patients should be asked how they feel about aerial transport as early as possible. Urinary catheters may be needed for long flights if patients are unable to void before or likely to need to do so in flight. Antiemetics should be administered early and anxious patients may require sedation. Unconscious patients require gastric and urinary catheterization and confirmation of position, and the patency and security of endotracheal tubes and other invasive devices must be checked before departure. Medical gases are dry, and heat–moisture exchangers or other forms of humidification for ventilated patients are essential to reduce tube occlusion from dried secretions.

Restless, anxious or combative patients are a danger to themselves and everyone else in the confines of an ambulance or aircraft. Sedation should be liberally used. It may even be necessary to intubate some patients for safety reasons prior to departure. Careful discussion with conscious patients prior to departure will usually reveal anxieties related to air transport. Reassurance and pharmacotherapy are more effective the earlier they are given.

Patient comfort in transport is important. The type of mattress used should be considered well in advance. The most comfortable and practical solutions are beanbag-filled vacuum mattresses. Multiple commercial brands are available, all sharing the same design characteristics. The mattresses are insufflated with air and the patient is allowed to settle in comfortably. Air is then evacuated by wall suction or with a hand pump whilst the mattress is moulded to the patient. Moulding to the head and neck and around splinted limbs is possible. Most mattresses are covered in waterproof material, have handles for ease of transfer and are radiolucent. Plain radiography and computerized tomography (CT) scanning can be performed without the need to transfer the patient. The stiffness of the evacuated mattress and the carry handles may make transfer for procedures such as CT scanning easier than with conventional methods. Some emergency departments use these vacuum mattresses routinely in major resuscitation bays.

A final check with the patient and relatives is wise prior to departure. Contact details for and of significant others as well as informed estimations of arrival times help to reduce communication difficulties. Time should be set aside for answering any questions prior to departure. Written information detailing where the patient is to be taken, the names of the transporting crew and phone numbers for further information relieves much anxiety on the part of relatives and friends.

Common problems in transit

Estimating transport time is difficult. Assumptions by non-transport personnel are generally half to one-third of actual times. Considerable time is required for familiarization with the patient and in transferring from one transport modality to the next. Hasty transfers without adequate familiarization increase complications. Oxygen supplies are crucial in longer transports. The amount needed should be calculated to last for at least twice and preferably triple the estimated journey time. If a minimum supply only is taken, any complication or delay may prove fatal. It is also wise to have several cylinders and a spare regulator as a safeguard in the event of equipment failure.

Monitoring and equipment used in transport should be in accordance with recommended standards. Detailed guidelines are available.[1] Most patients require continuous ECG, pulse oximetry and blood pressure monitoring as a minimum. Equipment must be selected carefully. Display screens must be visible in daylight and battery life must be appropriate for duration of transport with a large capacity for additional work. It should always be assumed that the next task will occur immediately without the opportunity to recharge batteries. Consideration should be given to the placement of invasive lines for potentially unstable patients. Use of arterial lines significantly reduces battery requirements for non-invasive blood pressure monitoring. Equipment alarms must be clearly visible as auditory alarms are difficult or impossible to hear in moving vehicles, especially helicopters.

Infusions may be delivered by pumps or syringe drivers. Infusion pumps are more accurate and are essential for critical infusions such as inotropes. However, they are relatively heavy and require specific tubing. Syringe drivers are lighter and require no specialized tubing. However, they are less accurate, must be shielded from sunlight to prevent rubber plungers drying and seizing when exposed and therefore should only be used for less critical infusions.

Loading and unloading are critical times. The combination of patient, stretcher and equipment can be very heavy. Injuries to patients and personnel may occur unless extreme care is taken. Equipment and lines can be damaged or dislodged. The concentration required easily distracts attention from the patient, monitor alarms may not be heard and critical incidents can occur most easily at these times. For all these reasons transfers are considered the most at-risk time for the patient. Reducing the number of transfers is a priority in care.

Defibrillation in moving vehicles creates some special problems. Movement artefact may make it impossible to synchronize for cardioversion or may make rhythm interpretation difficult. Positioning and operating a standard defibrillator can be almost impossible in a moving vehicle. Patients should be assessed prior to departure for likelihood of the need for defibrillation in-flight and this possibility discussed with the pilot. High-risk patients, such as those with acute myocardial infarction or those with known arrhythmias, can be prepared before the journey. All contact with metal should be avoided by wrapping the patient in blankets and sheets, with special attention paid to stretcher edges. Self-adherent defibrillation pads should be applied to the thorax prior to transport. This improves signal quality as well as providing good insulation. A major problem is with residual current leakage. If DC shock is indicated in-flight the pilot must be consulted prior to any attempt. Current leakage and microshocks have the potential to damage and disable electronic equipment. The pilot may elect to allow the DC shock, to turn off electronic equipment first or not permit the procedure. The final decision in these circumstances is a balance between the treatment of the patient and the safety of the aircraft and crew. Only the pilot can make this decision. A pre-informed pilot may be able to avoid situations where defibrillation would be denied.

Special problems associated with travelling at altitude

All transport is associated with motion sickness. Staff tend to become accustomed whilst first-time travellers (including patients) are most affected. Antiemetics should be discussed and administered early whenever possible. Another related condition reducing performance of medical attendants is the sopite syndrome. This condition is characterized by yawning, drowsiness, disinclination for either physical or mental work and lack of participation in group activities.[4] It is not directly related to the degree of turbulence, is not responsive to anti-motion-sickness medications and, unlike motion sickness, there appears to be little adaptation with time. As many as two-thirds of air attendants are affected to some degree, making this condition an important cause of reduced performance during transport.[5]

Travelling at altitude exposes patients and crew to reduced atmospheric pressure. The two most important consequences of this are hypoxia and expansion of gases. Most fixed-wing aircraft can pressurize the interior of the craft to sea level or above, making these complications avoidable. Medical helicopters do not have the option of pressurization but may elect to fly at low altitudes. Pressurization to sea level causes excessive fuel demand and additional stress on the aircraft. As a compromise, most commercial and medical aircraft will pressurize to an equivalent altitude of 5000–7000 ft whilst travelling at 30 000–40 000 ft. At this cabin altitude ambient PO_2 is reduced to 60 mmHg and trapped gases expand by one-third of their volume. Breathing cabin air produces an $Sa–O_2$ of 90% under these conditions. For healthy individuals this poses no problem. For unwell or oxygen-dependent patients, however, being on the shoulder of the $Hb–O_2$ dissociation curve can be dangerous with only small decreases in PO_2 from this point inducing large falls in $Sa–O_2$. Supplemental O_2 or increased pressurization may be required.

Expansion of trapped gas can produce disastrous consequences. All pneumothoraces, no matter how small, require venting prior to elevation to altitude. Heimlick valves are preferable to underwater seal drains during transport as underwater seal apparatus is disturbed by movement and is at greater risk of damage and breakage. Air trapped in small bowel (for instance in ileus) can produce considerable discomfort. Gas at either end of the gastrointestinal tract can vent spontaneously. Middle ear gas can be particularly painful on ascent and descent. Patients should be taught equalization techniques such as the Valsalva, Frenzel or Toynbee manoeuvres. The Valsalva manoeuvre reduces cardiac venous return and may be associated with syncope. The most effective technique is the Frenzel manoeuvre, which is carried out with the mouth, nostrils and epiglottis closed. Air in the nasopharynx is then compressed by the action of the muscles of the mouth and tongue. This technique not only generates higher nasopharyngeal pressures than the Valsalva manoeuvre, it opens the eustachian tubes at lower pressures. The easiest taught technique is the Toynbee manoeuvre, which raises pharyngeal pressure by swallowing with the mouth closed and nostrils occluded. In babies and young children, the angle of entry of the eustachian tubes into the nasopharynx is less acute and hence ear problems in flight are less common. Older children and some adults are unable to learn the various techniques.[6] Nasal decongestants prior to departure or sweets to suck on during descent may be of benefit. If a patient is unable to clear the ears, pain increases until the tympanic membrane ruptures with sudden relief of discomfort.

Expansion of gases has consequences for medical equipment. Air in an endotracheal tube cuff expands, increasing cuff pressure on ascent. Although modern high-volume, low-pressure cuffs minimize this effect, the increased pressure may cause tracheal damage if left unchecked for long periods. On descent the volume falls, making tube displacement more likely and increasing the likelihood of leakage around the cuff. Loss of ventilatory volumes and aspiration may result. The cuff pressure should be monitored on ascent and descent and adjusted as necessary. An alternative practice is to fill the cuff with sterile fluid such as normal saline. This makes it impossible to monitor the pressure in the cuff and is not necessary if the air-filled cuff is monitored appropriately.

Ascent to altitude may cause or increase the symptoms of decompression illness. The use of portable hyperbaric chambers or pressurization to sea level may be required. In aircraft where pressurization is not possible the lowest safe altitude is the next best alternative. These requirements must be discussed with the pilot as soon as they are known and certainly well prior to departure.

Decisions on flight safety

At times a choice must be made whether or not it is safe to fly. The decision is based on meteorological conditions and other circumstances. The final decision must always rest with the pilot. Crew safety is under the direction of the pilot whose decision is absolute. No patient is worth more than the crew.

Future directions

Medical equipment is becoming more complex as well as smaller and lighter. Sophisticated ventilators, multilumen infusion devices and complicated equipment such as intra-aortic balloon pumps can already be transported in surface and aerial craft. Non-invasive pressure-monitoring equipment has been developed, enabling beat-to-beat measurement of arterial and other pressures and real-time cardiac output monitoring. This evolution of equipment will continue, making it possible to transport increasingly complex cases with greater safety and less need for invasive interventions.

The capacity for interactive communication with remote areas is increasing at an accelerated rate. Multimedia communications allow teleconferencing, data transmission of electrocardiograms, and radiological images and video viewing of patients with increasing clarity. Pilot systems have already been developed whereby surgeons can perform operations with the aid of video cameras and remote control devices without the need to leave the central institutions. The further development of this technology will greatly reduce the need to transfer patients and allow comprehensive management in rural locations.

Controversies

❶ The appropriateness of helicopter transport for trauma patients in a metropolitan area has been questioned. Trauma is unlike other major illnesses in being more dependent on time to definitive treatment than level of care in transport. Helicopter transport in an urban system may improve survival for major trauma (injury severity score >15) but has no proven benefit for head-injured patients.[7] Further study is underway.

❷ The nature of medical staff for retrieval systems differs widely and is a source of debate. Various mixes of nurses, paramedics and doctors have been described with equally successful outcomes. It appears more important to have dedicated and appropriately trained staff than to focus on the professional group from which they arise.

References

1. Joint Faculty of Intensive Care Medicine and Australasian and New Zealand College of Anaesthetist and Australasian College for Emergency Medicine. Minimum Standards for the Transport of Critically Ill Patients. http://acem.org.au/media/policies_and_guidelines/min_standard_crit_ill.pdf (updated February 2003; accessed August 2007).
2. Boyle MF, Hatton D, Sheets C. Surgical cricothyrotomy performed by air ambulance flight nurses: a 5-year experience [see comments]. Journal of Emergency Medicine 1993; 11(1): 41–45.
3. Harrison T, Thomas SH, Wedel SK. In-flight oral endotracheal intubation. American Journal of Emergency Medicine 1997; 15(6): 558–561.
4. Graybiel A, Knepton J. Sopite syndrome: a sometimes sole manifestation of motion sickness. Aviation, Space Environmental Medicine 1976; 47(8): 873–882.
5. Wright MS, Bose CL, Stiles AD. The incidence and effects of motion sickness among medical attendants during transport. Journal of Emergency Medicine 1995; 13(1): 15–20.
6. Harding MH, Mills FJ. Aviation Medicine. 2nd edn. British Medical Association, London; 1988.
7. Nicholl JP, Brazier JE, Snooks HA. Effects of London helicopter emergency medical service on survival after trauma [see comments]. British Medical Journal 1995; 311(6999): 217–222.

26.3 Medical issues in disasters

Richard J. Brennan • David A. Bradt • Jonathan Abrahams

ESSENTIALS

1 The incidence of both natural and technological disasters has increased significantly over the past three decades.

2 Effective disaster planning requires knowledge of a community's major hazards, vulnerabilities, capabilities, disaster history, and disaster-associated patterns of morbidity and mortality.

3 An all-hazards environment, including natural hazards, technological hazards, communicable disease and acts of terrorism, must be considered in updated disaster plans.

4 While emergency medical care is the main focus of emergency physicians, public health interventions become high priorities following disasters that disrupt environmental health infrastructure (e.g. water supply and sewerage), disasters that result in significant population displacement and disasters that involve the unintentional or deliberate release of chemical, biological or radiological agents.

5 Emergency physicians and other health professionals have a vital role across the spectrum of disaster management arrangements including preparedness, prevention, mitigation, response and recovery operations.

6 Emergency physicians are most likely to respond to disasters associated with multiple casualties. Effective management of mass casualty incidents requires knowledge of the regional disaster plan, scene assessment issues, site management, communications, casualty flow plans, field triage and the clinical management of unique clinical entities, including crush injury and blast injury.

Introduction

Disaster preparedness and response involve a complex, multidisciplinary process of which emergency medicine comprises one component. Government agencies, fire fighters, law enforcement, ambulance services, civil defence, the Red Cross and other aid organizations may all have a role to play. The health and medical management of disasters can also cut across professional disciplines and require contributions from emergency medicine, public health, primary care, surgery, anaesthetics and intensive care.

From the health perspective, different types of disasters are frequently associated with well-described patterns of morbidity and mortality. The clinical and public health needs of an affected community will, therefore, also vary according to the type and extent of disaster. Emergency physicians should understand the health and medical consequences of the various types of disasters in order to determine their own roles in preparedness and response. In practice, emergency physicians will be most actively involved in the response to an acute-onset disaster that involves multiple casualties, such as a transportation incident. Several other types of disasters, including floods and cyclones, are generally associated with few, if any, casualties. The health and medical needs in these settings usually involve augmenting public health and primary-care services.

The aims of this chapter are to familiarize emergency physicians with disaster epidemiology and disaster management arrangements, and to provide an overview of the medical response to a disaster involving multiple casualties. While the chapter focuses on health and medical issues, it should be remembered that the effects of disasters are often widespread and long term. Disasters cause significant social, economic and environmental losses that can have a devastating effect on the general wellbeing of the affected community.

Definitions and classification

There is no internationally accepted definition of disaster or disaster classification. There are, however, increasingly consistent uses of terms among stakeholder organizations. Common to most definitions is the concept that following a disaster the capacity of the impacted community to respond is exceeded and there is, therefore, a need for external assistance. The World Health Organization characterizes a disaster as a phenomenon that produces large-scale disruption of the normal healthcare system, presents an immediate threat to public health and requires external assistance for response. The Australian Emergency Manual defines disaster as an event that overwhelms normal community and organizational arrangements and requires extraordinary responses to be instituted. The Center for Research on the Epidemiology of Disasters (CRED), which compiles the data behind the annual World Disasters Report of the International Federation of Red Cross and Red Crescent Societies, stipulates a quantitative surveillance definition involving one of the following: 10 or more people killed, 100 or more people affected, declaration of state of emergency or an appeal for international assistance.[1]

Disaster management is the range of activities designed to establish and maintain control over disaster and emergency situations, and to provide a framework for helping at-risk populations avoid or recover from the impact of a disaster. It addresses a much broader array of issues than health alone, including hazard identification, vulnerability analysis and risk assessment. Disaster medicine can be defined as the study and application of clinical care, public health, mental health and disaster management to the prevention, preparedness, response and recovery from the health problems arising from disasters.[2] This must be achieved in cooperation with other agencies and disciplines involved in comprehensive disaster management. In practice, emergency medicine and public health are the two specialties most intimately involved in disaster medicine.

A mass casualty incident is an event causing illness or injury in multiple patients simultaneously through a similar mechanism, such as a major vehicular crash, structural collapse, explosion or exposure to a hazardous material.

Disasters are commonly classified as natural versus technological/human-generated (Box 26.3.1).[1] Disasters may also be classified according to other characteristics, including acute versus gradual onset, short versus long duration, unifocal versus multifocal distribution, common versus rare and primary versus secondary. Classifications of disaster magnitude exist for selected natural hazards, such as earthquakes and hurricanes/cyclones; however, there is currently no standard classification of severity of disaster impact.

Epidemiology

Globally, the types of disasters associated with the greatest numbers of deaths are complex emergencies (CEs). These are crises characterized by political instability, armed conflict, large population displacements, food shortages and collapse of public health infrastructure. Because of insecurity and poor access to the affected population, aggregate epidemiological data for CEs are somewhat limited. However, between 1998 and 2004 in the eastern region of the Democratic Republic of Congo, 3.9 million people lost their lives due to the consequences of the major humanitarian crisis afflicting that country.[3] Incredibly, this was more than three times the total number of deaths globally due to natural and technological disasters during the decade of the 1990s. Based on United Nations definitions, there were 27 ongoing CEs in 2007, involving over 30 countries and impacting on the lives of hundreds of millions of people.[4] Thirteen (44%) of these crises were ongoing in Africa, with 10 (37%) occurring in Asia.

According to information compiled by the International Federation of the Red Cross, there has been a significant increase in the total number of natural and technological disasters worldwide during the past 30 years. From 1996 to 2005, an average of approximately 641 such disasters was documented annually, peaking at 801 in 2000. While the total number of people killed by natural and technological disasters is approximately 93 000 per year, there is a wide annual range (21 888 in 2000 to 251 768 in 2004 due to the Indian Ocean tsunami). Moreover, the total number affected has almost trebled over the past three decades. It is estimated that approximately 250 million people are directly affected on an annual basis. Selected data are presented in Figures 26.3.1 and 26.3.2.

The commonest types of disasters across the globe are transportation incidents, floods, windstorms, industrial incidents, building collapses, droughts/famines and earthquakes/tsunamis (see Fig. 26.3.1). Asia is the region of the world most prone to natural and technological disasters, recording 41% of such incidents between 1996 and 2005. It is followed by Africa (22%), the Americas (20%), Europe (14%) and Oceania (3%). Compared with other regions of the world, Australasia and Oceania clearly have a relatively low incidence of disasters. Over the past 10 years the commonest causes of natural disasters in Australia have been floods, severe storms and cyclones. Nationally, an average of 33 lives are lost per year due to disasters in Australia. In addition, over 68 000 people are affected annually, through injury, displacement, financial loss, damage or loss of homes and businesses. Historically, the leading causes of death from natural disasters have been heatwaves, followed by cyclones, floods and bushfires. Human-generated disasters resulting in multiple casualties have occurred more frequently in Australia in recent years. The

BOX 26.3.1 Classification of disasters

Natural	Human-generated
Acute onset	Technological
Hydrometeorological	*Industrial accidents*
Avalanches, landslides	Explosions
Bush fires, forest fires	Fires
Extreme temperatures	Hazardous material
Floods	releases
Windstorms	Structural collapses
	Transportation crashes
Geophysical	Air
Earthquakes	Rail
Tsunamis	Road
Volcanic eruptions	Water
Other	Terrorism
Epidemics	
Gradual/chronic onset	War/Complex emergencies
Desertification	
Droughts/famines	
Insect/pest infestations (e.g. locusts)	

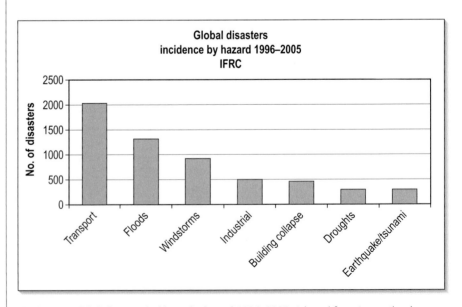

Fig. 26.3.1 Global disasters incidence by hazard 1996–2005. Adapted from: International Federation of the Red Cross. World Disasters Report 2006: Focus on neglected crises. IFRC, Geneva; 2006.

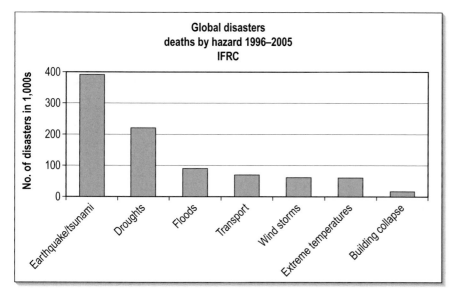

Fig. 26.3.2 Global disasters deaths by hazard 1996–2005. Adapted from: International Federation of the Red Cross. World Disasters Report 2006: Focus on neglected crises. IFRC, Geneva; 2006.

commonest causes of mass casualty incidents have been bus crashes, structural fires, mining incidents, aviation incidents and train crashes.

The impact of disasters has been less in New Zealand, where only 28 lives were lost among 9040 persons affected over the last decade. The pattern of natural disasters also differs, with the commonest major events being floods, earthquakes and landslides. The North Island of New Zealand has six active volcanoes, with the last attributed loss of life occurring in 1953.

Data reporting on the incidence of terrorism has recently been complicated by changing definitions and political motivations of the reporting agencies. In spite of the controversies and complexities surrounding the reporting, the number of international terrorist attacks has increased significantly since 2000, following a steady decline during the latter half of the 1990s.[5] There were on average 229 international terrorist attacks between 1997 and 2006, with a peak of 395 in 2004. Over that period, an average of 694 persons per year were killed, with a peak of 3184 in 2001 (including 2982 deaths due to the September 11 attacks by Al Qaeda in the USA). This is just a very small fraction of the total number deaths attributed to natural and technological disasters and CEs. The regions documenting the highest number of international terrorist attacks over that period have been the Middle East (51%), Western

Europe (13%), South Asia (11%), Africa (6%), and Southeast Asia and Oceania (4%).

Disaster epidemiology globally, including the Australasian region, is being impacted by climate change. Global warming has already been associated with an increase in the frequency and unpredictability of weather-related disasters, such as heatwaves, floods and droughts. There is also evidence of increased intensity of tropical cyclones,[6] as has been reflected by recent experience with hurricane Katrina (2005) and cyclone Larry (2006). Rising temperatures have already been implicated in the spread of infectious disease vectors, including malaria-carrying mosquitoes. Other important diseases are also sensitive to changing temperatures and rainfall, including dengue, malnutrition and diarrhoea. The health-related and other impacts of climate change will not be evenly distributed. Disasters associated with global warming are particularly likely to threaten the lives and livelihoods of coastal communities, those living in low-lying islands (e.g. due to rising sea levels), and in arid and high mountain zones.

Socioeconomic impact

Disasters have the potential for major socioeconomic impact, costing the international community billions of dollars annually. In

developing countries, years of development work and investment can be devastated by a single disaster. During the 10 years to 2005, disasters caused a global average of approximately US$73.4 billion damage per year. Windstorms were the costliest disaster over the decade, accounting for 43% of disaster-associated costs, led by hurricane Katrina at US$125 billion, which caused 40% of all windstorm damage. Terrorist attacks on major financial centres, such as the World Trade Center in New York have demonstrated the potential for tens of billions of direct economic impact, enormous social consequences and political repercussions for mismanaged disaster response. These figures may be overshadowed by pandemic disease, such as from avian influenza, for which economic cost estimates range to upwards of US$1 trillion.[7]

In Australia, disasters have cost an average of A$ 1.14 billion annually. Over the past 30 years, floods, storms, then cyclones have caused the greatest disaster-related economic losses in Australia. The most economically costly disasters were cyclone Tracy (1974), the Newcastle earthquake (1989) and the Sydney hailstorm (1999).

Economic estimates, of course, are unable to reflect the true scale of human suffering associated with disasters. While we can often document the mortality, morbidity and financial losses associated with disasters, it is impossible to quantify the associated personal, psychological, social, cultural and political losses.

Disaster management/emergency management

As emergency physicians play a vital role in the medical aspects of disaster management, they should be familiar with the four underlying concepts on which these arrangements are based.

All agencies (integrated) approach

The basis for the Australian system for managing disasters is a partnership between the Commonwealth, state/territory and local governments, and the community. Under legislation, state and territory governments have the primary responsibility for coordinating disaster-management activities. The major role of the Australian Federal Government is to assist state and territory governments in developing their capacity to deal with disasters, for example by providing training courses and developing manuals of best practice. The Commonwealth also provides physical assistance to a state or territory in the event that a disaster exceeds that state or territory's response capability. Federal assistance in the area of health would most likely be medical resources provided by the Australian Defence Force (ADF). The ADF also has special expertise in the management of incidents involving chemical and biological agents.

Comprehensive approach

The comprehensive approach to disaster management encompasses prevention, preparedness, response and recovery. Health and medical professionals contribute most significantly to disaster preparedness and response. Prevention activities include regulatory and physical measures that prevent or mitigate the effects of disasters. Preparedness involves arrangements to ensure that resources and services which may be needed can be rapidly mobilized and deployed. Response activities are those actions taken during and immediately after impact to ensure that the disaster's effects are minimized. Recovery involves strategies and services that support affected communities in reconstructing their physical infrastructure and restoration of their social, economic, physical and emotional wellbeing.

All hazards approach

Different types of disasters can cause similar problems, therefore disaster management plans are based on a core set of arrangements and measures that can be applied to all hazards. Many risks, however, including acts of terrorism, will also require specific prevention, preparedness, response and recovery measures.

The prepared community

The prepared community is the focus of Australia's disaster management arrangements. Local governments, voluntary organizations and individuals all play a critical role in this area. Experience has demonstrated that individual and community self-help can often provide the most immediate, decisive and effective relief following a disaster, as it cannot be assumed that assistance from external sources will always arrive promptly, particularly in remote area communities.

Disaster planning

Disaster planning is the process by which a community develops a comprehensive strategy to effectively manage and respond to disasters. It is a collaborative effort that requires cooperation between government agencies, community services and private organizations. The ultimate goals of the planning process include clarification of the capabilities, roles and responsibilities of responding agencies, and the strengthening of emergency networks. Other operational issues, such as emergency communications and public warning systems, will also be addressed.

A critical concept in disaster planning is the graduated response. The initial response to an event begins at the local level. More resources can subsequently be requested from regional, state or national levels, as required, to supplement those of the local providers. Compatibility between plans at the different levels is therefore necessary. A hierarchy of disaster management plans exists in which plans at lower levels dovetail with those of the next highest level. Command and control arrangements, as well as the roles and responsibilities described in a particular plan, must be compatible with the other plans to which it relates. Emergency physicians must be aware of these requirements if they are to constructively contribute to the development of state, regional and hospital disaster plans.

Several high-profile terrorist events (e.g. World Trade Center attack in New York) and important gatherings (e.g. APEC Leaders Meeting in Sydney) have highlighted the need for specific planning for terrorist events. Such planning will frequently involve collaboration with relevant military, security and intelligence agencies, and a consideration of the tactics used by terrorists. Over the past decade 73% of international terrorist attacks have used conventional weapons, including explosives and small arms. Other terrorist tactics include assassinations, hijacking and kidnapping. Unconventional attacks, including those that using jet airliners as weapons of mass destruction, or chemical, biological and radiological weapons have constituted only 0.5% of international terrorist attacks. Nonetheless, prudent planning for these types of incidents is also required, observing the all-hazards approach.

Disaster exercises must be conducted regularly to test the response and recovery aspects of the plan. Exercises range from desktop simulations to realistic scenarios with moulaged patients in the field. If conducted appropriately, they should effectively test whether the objectives of the plan have been met and provide the opportunity for disaster response training. Disaster planning is a continuous process, and plans need to be regularly reviewed and updated. Disaster exercises may provide insights into areas in which the plan needs to be improved.

Planning and responding for international disasters have become more relevant for Australasian health professionals in light of the recent terrorist attacks in Bali (2002 and 2005), the Indian Ocean tsunami (2004) and the earthquake in Pakistan and India (2005). Such planning and response can be advised by the internationally recognized Sphere Minimum Standards in Disaster Response[8] and in collaboration with important international agencies, such as the United Nation's Office for Coordination of Humanitarian Affairs. Sphere specifies standards in six sectors of disaster response: water and sanitation, food security, food aid, nutrition, shelter and health services. These standards are relevant for all disasters and represent an extremely useful reference to guide planning and response for domestic incidents as well.

Disaster response activities

Incident management

Scene assessment and stabilization
The initial scene assessment will be conducted by first responders, such as police or ambulance personnel. It is important for the first medical responder, generally an ambulance officer, to rapidly report findings to the Ambulance Communications Centre. An accurate, timely assessment is critical to initiating an appropriate and effective response. Key information that should be related from the scene includes the nature and magnitude of the disaster, the presence of ongoing

hazards, the estimated number of deaths and injuries, the need for further assistance, and the most appropriate routes of access to the scene. In large-scale disasters that affect entire populations, such as cyclones or earthquakes, a rapid health assessment followed by broader epidemiological assessments will be required, including an evaluation of the impact on the health infrastructure, public utilities and shelter.

Site security and safety procedures must be observed to ensure that rescuers and bystanders do not become victims. This is particularly relevant when a terrorist incident is suspected because of the threats posed by a secondary attack on responders or the potential use of weapons of mass destruction. The police should establish a perimeter around the scene of a multiple casualty incident and allow access only to authorized personnel. If a hazardous material is involved, rescuers may be required to wear specialized personal protective equipment to protect their airways, eyes and skin. Electrical hazards, fires, explosions, leaking gases and unstable structures may all pose significant threats to rescue personnel. These hazards must be eliminated or controlled prior to initiating rescue operations.

Hazard-specific issues

While the all-hazards approach remains fundamental to disaster management, a unifying approach for undifferentiated hazards has been developed for the management of incidents involving chemical, biological or radiological agents. Basic principles of awareness include recognition of potential terrorist events, avoidance of the affected area, isolation of the affected area and notification of proper authorities. Basic principles for first responders include the four do nots: do not become a victim, do not rush in, do not TEST (taste, eat, smell and touch) anything and do not assume anything. Only properly trained and equipped hazardous material personnel should be in contaminated areas.

Site arrangements

Regardless of the nature of the incident, a forward command post should be set up at or near the disaster site at the beginning of the emergency operation. The command post will have representatives from the major responding services and report back to the regional or state emergency operations centre. The function of the command post is to coordinate the activities of the various services during the rescue operations. It also provides a central point for the submission of requests for assistance by each of the responding services. Medical and ambulance commanders will be located at the command post to direct and coordinate medical care to victims at the scene, patient transportation, hospital communications, provision of medical supplies and medical air operations.

Communications

Good communications are vital to ensure appropriate command, control and coordination during a disaster. Communication problems are often cited as a major cause of suboptimal disaster response. There are many factors that may contribute to poor communications at the scene. Damaged equipment and overloaded telephone systems indicate the need for back-up systems, including cellular phones. The use of different radio frequencies by different agencies may lead to poor coordination and an inability to communicate vital information. Compatible frequencies need to be identified and utilized. Megaphones may be required to overcome noise at the scene due to heavy extrication equipment, helicopters and general rescue activities. Information overload may also hamper the rescue effort. Radio and telephone reports should be kept brief, relevant and succinct. Professional jargon is frequently misunderstood or misinterpreted by other agencies and is best avoided.

Hospitals must also have reliable communications systems. Designated phone lines, cellular phones and back-up radio networks may augment the existing system during a disaster. It is essential for hospitals to remain in regular contact with the incident medical director, to provide information regarding medical capabilities, bed capacity and bed availability.

Medical management

Personnel

Provider roles in disasters continue to evolve. Dedicated disaster medical response teams have been extensively studied.[9] These teams form an integral part of national response plans in many developed countries notwithstanding lack of data attesting to any reduction in disaster-associated mortality associated with their deployments.[10] Considerations of such teams for Australia are presently under discussion at Commonwealth level.

Emergency responders generally respond best when their disaster roles are similar to their daily professional practice. Medical and nursing personnel are best suited to staffing emergency rooms and hospitals, where they have the advantage of working in a familiar, more stable environment. Ambulance personnel have more experience in pre-hospital settings and are usually responsible for conducting the initial medical assessment and triage. In situations where there are multiple casualties, it may be appropriate to send a hospital team to the scene of a disaster, where their main functions will be to perform primary and secondary triage and to provide medical care at the patient treatment post. The science and practice of disaster medicine have progressed significantly over the past decade. Therefore, only doctors and nurses specifically trained to work in the field environment and familiar with the relevant best practices and standards should be deployed to the disaster scene, as inexperienced personnel may well hinder the medical response.

Casualty-flow plan

Disaster epidemiology has refined the expectations of casualty flow plans. Current epidemiological evidence indicates that 50–80% of people acutely injured in a mass casualty disaster will arrive at the closest medical facilities generally within 90 min after the event.[11] Moreover, the vast majority of disaster-affected patients will self-evacuate without benefit of prehospital triage, transport or decontamination. A casualty-flow plan remains crucial to optimize patient care and transportation of those remaining at the scene. A casualty collection area should be established at a site that is close enough to the disaster scene to allow easy access, but far enough away to ensure protection from potential hazards. Patients are assembled and triaged here prior to transfer to a nearby patient treatment post, where they are once again triaged, and basic medical care provided. An ambulance loading point and ambulance holding point also need to be clearly marked so that patient transportation is conducted efficiently, and to ensure that scene convergence and congestion is minimized. Landing zones for helicopters are established away from the incident site for safety reasons, to limit noise and to reduce downwash from rotor blades. A temporary morgue may need to be established in a nearby area when many fatalities have occurred.

Triage

The aim of triage is to allocate medical resources, including personnel, supplies and facilities, in a manner that provides the greatest good to the greatest number of patients. The emphasis is not on providing optimal care to each individual patient, but rather on directing limited medical resources to those who are most likely to benefit. Triage is the single most important medical activity at the disaster site. It is a dynamic, ongoing process that occurs at every stage of patient management, from the disaster site to the casualty collection area, patient treatment post and again at the hospital. Patients are rapidly assessed and categorized according to priority of treatment and transport. The condition of patients frequently changes, and repeated examinations are required so that patients may be moved up or down in the order of priority. Triage is a learned skill and should be conducted by the most experienced medical or ambulance officer at the scene.

Different triage systems have emerged in different parts of the world. In British and Australasian health systems, 'sieve and sort' triage processes have become the preferred approach through major incident medical management and support (MIMMS) training courses.[12] In North America, 'start and save' triage processes have become incorporated into the national disaster medical system.[13] More recently, a national disaster life support consortium in the USA has promulgated a triage approach based on 'move, assess, sort and send'.[14] These different systems rely on different assessment approaches with different vital sign thresholds to assign triage priority.

In general, most systems recognize that there are categories of patients who require immediate care, delayed care and minimal care, and those who are expectant or unsalvageable. Patients requiring immediate care are individuals who are in critical condition, but to whom simple life-saving procedures may be successfully applied,

such as the manual clearing of the airway. Patients classified as requiring delayed care may have significant injuries but are likely to survive if treatment is postponed for several hours. Minimal care patients are generally ambulatory and their treatment may be delayed until other patients have been appropriately treated. Expectant or unsalvageable patients are those who have acutely life-threatening injuries requiring advanced resuscitation, or those who have non-survivable injuries, such as massive head trauma. Advanced life-support measures, such as cardiopulmonary resuscitation, are rarely indicated at a scene with multiple casualties. Instead, these patients generally receive palliative care, but only after patients in the immediate category have received appropriate treatment.

Stabilization

Following triage of the affected patients, rapid stabilization of airway, breathing and circulation is provided to those with the greatest potential for survival. Definitive care is not generally provided at the scene. On-scene medical care concentrates on securing the airway, administration of oxygen, external pressure to control haemorrhage and insertion of intravenous catheters for volume expansion prior to hospital transportation. Medical care should generally be provided at the patient treatment post, but during prolonged rescues resuscitative procedures may be required prior to extrication. Appropriate use of analgesia, including parenteral narcotics and regional nerve blocks, may assist with the extrication of trapped individuals. Special on-scene procedures are sometimes required for those with crush injury, blast injury, burns or hypothermia. Amputation of a mangled limb, although rarely indicated, may be a life-saving procedure for an entrapped patient.

Decontamination

Chemical, biological, radiological and nuclear (CBRN) agents have the potential to contaminate individuals, property and the general environment. In practice, industrial accidents represent by far the most common cause of exposure to hazardous materials that may require decontamination. A small number of high-profile chemical-biological terrorist incidents over the past 15 years have also prompted medical as well as lay attention to

this potential threat. Regardless of the cause, the principles guiding the process of decontamination remain consistent. Decontamination is the process of removing or neutralizing a hazard from the victim or environment. Detailed management protocols exist for these hazards.[15–17] Fundamental principles involve:

❶ staff and site preparation with establishment of hot/warm/cold zones
❷ casualty, staff and crowd protection
❸ decontamination procedures
❹ clinical treatment of contaminated patients and transport to definitive care
❺ recovery of environment.

Removal of contaminated clothes should be conducted as a matter of urgency. Rapid decontamination of the skin is especially necessary following exposure to the liquid or aerosolized form of an agent. It is most useful when conducted within 1 min of exposure, but in practice this is rarely possible. When indicated, decontamination should be conducted close to the scene (i.e. in the 'warm zone') and, ideally, prior to transportation. Commonly used agents for decontamination include soap and water, and hypochlorite (household bleach) in concentrations of 0.5–2.0%. Steps must be taken to ensure that emergency responders, health personnel and other patients are not at risk of secondary exposure to the chemical agent. Decontamination after exposure to a biological agent is less important, as most biological agents are not dermally active. However, decontamination may be an effective way to limit the spread of the agent from potential secondary aerosolization.

Transportation

Efficient and rational transportation of patients to appropriate health facilities is dependent on good communications between hospitals and the incident transport officer. Capabilities of the affected community's hospitals should be identified and documented in the regional disaster plan. Hospitals will be required to regularly update the incident commander and transport officer of their bed availability status. The closest hospitals are often flooded by 'walking wounded' who have made their own way from the scene, and by victims transported by well-meaning civilians. This has the potential of overwhelming local emergency departments, and the transport officer must take this into consideration when determining the appropriate distribution of patients. It is essential that the disaster not be relocated to the nearest hospitals.

A number of factors need to be considered when determining the most appropriate hospital for a particular patient, including the patient's triage category, the hospital's capabilities (e.g. trauma, burns), transportation times, distance from the scene and the available transportation modalities. Medical helicopters may be able to transport patients to more distant hospitals to relieve pressure on nearby facilities.

Hospitals

Generic hospital plans for disaster management have become widely available from the World Health Organization[18] as well as domestic stakeholders.[19] Emergency physicians are expected to be familiar with their own hospital disaster plan and have contributed significantly to its development. The plan should address both internal and external disasters.

It is the responsibility of hospital administration to establish a control centre with adequate communication resources. The emergency department needs to be cleared of non-critical patients, and steps taken to expedite appropriate discharge of stable ward patients, so that bed capacity may be optimized. The emergency department should be well stocked with supplies. A recall system for additional medical and nursing staff mobilized in a disaster needs to be incorporated into the plan. Extra security staff should be on standby to assist with the control of patients, families, friends, onlookers and the media.

Patients require re-triage by a senior medical officer as they arrive at the emergency department. Those with acutely life-threatening injuries are immediately resuscitated. Less severely injured patients need to be regularly reviewed while awaiting definitive care, to monitor for a potential deterioration in their condition. Expectant, unsalvageable patients are provided appropriate palliative care, and their condition clearly explained to their families. Documentation is kept succinct and should generally be limited to the essential points about each patient's condition and treatment.

Urban search and rescue

Urban search and rescue (USAR) is the science of locating, reaching, treating and safely extricating survivors who remain trapped following a structural collapse. Search and rescue response capabilities have increased significantly in recent years, due to advances in rescue technology and in emergency services.

In the period immediately following a structural collapse, many survivors are rescued by uninjured bystanders. Those who remain trapped generally require the assistance of specially trained and equipped units from fire, ambulance or police services in order to be safely extricated. Medical members of search and rescue teams are tasked to provide medical care to the victims and medical support to the rescuers. They are not involved in the actual extrication process. Potential hazards to victims and rescuers are numerous, and scene safety is of critical importance. The identification and extrication of victims following a major structural collapse is one of the most physically and emotionally challenging tasks of any rescue operation. The shock of dealing with scenes of carnage and mutilation may render some rescue personnel ineffective. These teams must therefore be trained and prepared to deal with the emotional strains of working in such a demanding environment.

Mental health

It is easy to overlook the mental health needs of affected individuals during the emergency response, when rescue and life-saving interventions receive top priority. Emergency physicians should be aware of the significant psychological impact of disasters on victims, families and rescue personnel. Psychological support is recommended as first-level assistance to disaster-affected communities and personnel.[20] Mental health consequences, such as depression, anxiety states and post-traumatic stress syndrome, are well described following disasters and need to be considered when developing the disaster plan. Crisis counselling may play an important role in the overall medical care provided to patients following a disaster. In addition, rescue personnel may well suffer psychological consequences from their own involvement in the disaster response and

should therefore be provided with access to appropriate services, including critical incident debriefing.

Mass gatherings

Social and cultural events can result in the gathering of many people in one place at a particular time, sometimes over several days. Common examples include rock concerts, sporting events, fairs and parades. The organization of medical services for mass gatherings is generally designed to address minor medical needs but must also take into consideration medical emergencies, such as cardiac arrests and disaster planning, for incidents such as fire, structural collapse or terrorism. Medical services developed for the mass gathering must be linked to local emergency medical systems. Public health and occupational health regulations, including food safety and environmental health measures, must be observed.

Public health issues in disasters

Public health professionals are involved in all phases of the disaster cycle, and it is important for emergency physicians to understand the role of public health in disaster medicine and disaster management. Epidemiological studies that have identified risk factors for illness and injury following disasters have contributed greatly to disaster planning, mitigation, response and recovery. These investigations have been central to the development of the science of disaster medicine. They have led to key strategies that have been effective in reducing disaster-related morbidity and mortality.

Public health interventions become high priorities following disasters that disrupt the social infrastructure (for instance cyclone, flooding and earthquake), and disasters that result in significant population displacement (such as CEs). Priorities for the affected population include the provision of adequate water quantity and quality, sanitation, food, shelter, infectious disease control and disease surveillance. The role of public health following a mass casualty incident includes injury control, occupational health and safety measures for responders, and injury surveillance.

The interface between emergency medicine and public health becomes increasingly important following technological disasters or terrorist events involving biological, chemical or nuclear agents. The terrorist attacks with anthrax in the USA during 2001 and their aftermath demonstrated the vital importance of key public health tools such as disease surveillance and outbreak investigation and control. Following incidents with chemical or radiological agents, public health officials may be required to provide guidance on issues such as evacuation of the public, mass decontamination and the mass distribution of iodine. Emergency physicians should become more familiar with the skills, roles and responsibilities of their public health colleagues, especially as they relate to disaster management and infectious disease control.

Conclusion

Emergency physicians contribute most significantly to the preparedness and response aspects of disaster management. Emergency physicians should plan and build capacities for disasters based on an assessment of the major risks which their communities face and those which are most likely to result in multiple casualties. These include natural disasters and technological hazards. The increased risks posed by climate change and terrorists require the continuing review and revision of disaster risk-assessment processes and disaster planning. Disasters associated with multiple casualties provide unique challenges to the health and medical communities. Curative medical skills and public health principles are both critical to the comprehensive management of a community affected by a disaster.

Controversies and future directions

❶ Over the past decade the field of disaster response has professionalized dramatically. There are now clearly established standards and best practices for most aspects of disaster response. Impressive advances have been made in the areas of rapid assessment, data collection and analysis, triage, mass casualty care, control of communicable diseases and other public health interventions. Emergency physicians should familiarize themselves with these developments so that they are better able to respond to both small- and large-scale disasters.

❷ Acts of terrorism, including those due to chemical and biological agents, have contributed to a major increase in interest in disaster preparedness and response. Some experts and authorities have emphasized chemical and biological incidents to a level that has been out of proportion to their demonstrated level of threat. Disaster planning and preparedness must address the most common hazards and vulnerabilities within a community, while still including a prudent approach to low-probability, high-consequence events. The all-hazards approach provides appropriate guiding principles for such planning. The threat of pandemic influenza and other potential epidemics must now also be considered in disaster planning and preparedness. Emergency physicians should increase their familiarity with important concepts such as infectious disease surveillance, case detection, and outbreak investigation and response. They should also become more familiar with the skills, roles and responsibilities of their public health colleagues, especially as they relate to disaster management and infectious disease control.

References

1. International Federation of Red Cross and Red Crescent Societies. World Disasters Report. International Federation of Red Cross and Red Crescent Societies, Geneva; 2006: 197.
2. Murray V, Clifford J, Seynaeve G, et al. Disaster health education and training: a pilot questionnaire to understand current status. Prehospital and Disaster Medicine 2006; 21(3): 156–167.
3. Coghlan B, Brennan RJ, Ngoy P, et al. Mortality in the Democratic Republic of Congo: a nationwide survey. Lancet 2006; 367: 44–51.
4. United Nations Office for the Coordination of Humanitarian Affairs. http://www.reliefweb.int (accessed 8 October 2007).
5. Memorial Institute for the Prevention of Terrorism. http://www.tkb.org/chwiz1.jsp (accessed 13 September 2007).
6. Intergovernmental Panel on Climate Change. Climate Change 2007: The Physical Science Basis. Contribution of Working Group I to the Fourth Assessment Report of the Intergovernmental Panel on Climate Change, 5 February 2007. Available at: http://www.ipcc.ch/SPM2feb07.pdf (accessed 8 October 2007).
7. Brahmbhatt M. Economic Impacts of Avian Influenza Propagation. Available from URL: http://web.worldbank.org/WBSITE/EXTERNAL/NEWS/0,contentMDK:20978927~menuPK: 34472~pagePK:34370~piPK:34424~theSitePK:4607,00.html (accessed August 2006).
8. Sphere Project. Humanitarian Charter and Minimum Standards in Disaster Response., Oxford: Sphere Project; 2004.
9. Anton Breil Centre for Public Health and Tropical Medicine, James Cook University. Disaster Medical Assistance Teams: a literature review. Available from the Health Protection Group, Department of Health, Western Australia, Australia; 2006.
10. Bradt DA. Site management of health issues in the 2001 World Trade Center disaster. Academic Emergency Medicine 2003; 10: 650–660.
11. US Centers for Disease Control and Prevention. Mass trauma casualty predictor. http://www.cdc.gov/masstrauma/preparedness/predictor.htm (accessed January 2007).
12. Advanced Life Support Group. Major incident medical management and support – the practical approach. London: BMJ Publishing,1998.
13. Benson M, Koenig KL, Schultz CH. Disaster Triage: START, then SAVE – a new method of dynamic triage for victims of a catastrophic earthquake. Prehospital Disaster Medicine 1996; 11: 117–124.
14. National Disaster Life Support Education Consortium. Basic Disaster Life Support Provider Manual. Available from the NDLSEC, Chicago: American Medical Association, 2003.
15. Agency for Toxic Substances and Disease Registry. Hospital emergency departments: a planning guide for the management of contaminated patients. In: Managing Hazardous Materials Incidents. Vol. 2 revised. September 2001. CD-ROM available from ATSDR, Atlanta, GA, http://www.atsdr.cdc.gov.
16. US Army Medical Research Institute of Infectious Diseases. Medical Management of Biological Casualties Handbook. 6th edn. April 2005. Available from http://www.usamriid.army.mil/education/bluebookpdf/USAMRIID%20BlueBook%206th%20Edition%20-%20Sep%202006.pdf (accessed August 2007).
17. US Army Medical Research Institute of Chemical Defense. Medical Management of Chemical Casualties Handbook. 3rd edn. July 2000. Available from www.gmha.org/bioterrorism/usamricd/Yellow_Book_2000.pdf (accessed August 2007).
18. World Health Organization Western Pacific Region. Field manual for capacity assessment of health facilities in responding to emergencies. Available from the WHO Western Pacific Regional Publications Office, WHO Regional Office for the Western Pacific; 2006.
19. Qureshi K, Gebbie KM, Gebbie EN. Public Health Incident Command System: A Guide for the Management of Emergencies or Other Unusual Incidents within Public Health Agencies. Vol. 1 & 2. 1st edn. October 2005. Available from http://www.ualbanycphp.org/pinata/phics/guide/default.cfm
20. Interagency Standing Committee. IASC Guidelines on Mental Health and Psychosocial Support in Emergency Settings. Geneva: IASC; 2007.

26.4 Triage

Drew Richardson

ESSENTIALS

1 Triage is the ongoing process of sorting patients on the basis of the urgency of their need for medical care.

2 Urgency is distinct from both severity and complexity.

3 Triage categorization has been found to strongly relate to both resource use and patient outcome.

4 The five-level Australasian Triage Scale (ATS) forms the basis of emergency department triage in Australasia.

5 The ATS is also used in casemix funding models and important performance measures.

6 Similar triage scales have been developed and adopted in other jurisdictions.

Introduction

Provision of high-availability quality medical care is expensive and has been traditionally limited to the very wealthy or to situations of great demand, such as the military in battle. Even today, well-organized emergency medical systems are concentrated in societies sufficiently affluent to spend 5% or more of gross domestic product on health. Some form of rationing is required whenever an expensive resource is coupled with fluctuating demand. Price, queuing and denial are all used in different areas of medicine. Simple application of any of these methods in emergency medicine would not be efficient or equitable, so the majority of emergency medical systems use a triage process to sort patients into a number of queues.

Triage, the sorting of patients on the basis of urgency, is an ongoing process that nevertheless requires formal structures at different points within the continuum of care. In the emergency department (ED) setting, there is considerable evidence that urgency can be assigned reliably and distinctly on a five-level scale and that this categorization is applicable and useful beyond the concept of 'urgency' into other aspects of hospital care.

Origins of triage

The word 'triage', arising from the French *trier* meaning 'to sort' has its origins in Latin. It has entered English at least three times: from the 18th century wood industry, the 19th century coffee industry and 20th century emergency medicine. The process understood today as triage was first described by Baron Dominique Jean-Larrey (1766–1842),[1] the surgeon to Napoleon, who also developed the ambulance volante, the first field ambulance. This delivered large numbers of injured but salvageable cases to medical units, mandating a more efficient system than treatment in order of military rank. Jean-Larrey's 'order of dressing and arrangement' by urgency was also in keeping with the egalitarian spirit of the French revolution, although there is no evidence that he actually used the word triage. His concept was embraced and refined by military surgeons over the next 150 years, usually with the primary intent of returning soldiers to battle in the most efficient manner.

Civilian triage developments

There was certainly some sorting of patients from the moment 'casual wards' opened in 19th century hospitals, but the first systematic description in civilian medicine was by E. Richard Weinerman in Baltimore in 1966.[2] Since that time, there has been a huge growth in emergency medicine as a specialty and a number of workers have undertaken formal investigation of triage, particularly in Australasia. The Australasian experience formed the basis of ED triage development in Canada and the UK, whilst some other jurisdictions have developed systems independently.

Process of triage

The underlying principles of triage are those of equity (or justice) and efficiency. EDs experience potentially overwhelming demand from patients with an enormous range of conditions. Equity demands that the distribution of resources for treatment is fair in the broadest sense. The concept of urgency is well understood by the population who generally accept that it is fair to treat those in the greatest need ahead of those who arrived before them. Efficiency demands that best use is made of available resources. In the setting of ED, cost and resource pressures prevent all demand being satisfied simultaneously. The overall philosophy of 'doing the greatest good for the greatest number' requires resource allocation on the basis of need, which in turn requires a process to identify and prioritize the needs of the presenting population.

In the ED, urgency is distinct from severity, prognosis, complexity and casemix, although a correlation exists. Some urgent problems (for example upper airway obstruction) have a poor outcome without rapid intervention but are not severe in the sense of requiring long-term care, other severe problems (for example life-threatening malignancy) may not require any treatment in the ED time frame. Complexity is reflected in the number of interventions such as investigations or consultations required, whereas casemix is an indication of the resources required to provide care.

Triage is an ongoing process that may change in response to alterations in patient status and resource availability, but it is efficient to undertake a formal process once, early in the patient's encounter, and then review only as necessary. ED triage is normally undertaken by trained nursing staff at the time of arrival, and the assigned urgency is then used to guide treatment order. The overall efficiency and effectiveness of such a system depends not only on the allocated priority but also on the treatment strategy, that is, the way in which the next patient is chosen from the different queues. A more urgent case should wait less time than a less urgent case, but when resources become available to treat the next patient, choice may still be required between a new arrival and a slightly less urgent patient who has already been waiting for some time.

Australasian triage development

The first Australasian description was of the Box Hill Triage Scale by Pink and Brentnall in 1977.[3] They used verbal descriptions without time consideration and classified patients into five categories: immediate, urgent, prompt, non-urgent and routine. Fitzgerald modified this scale in 1989,[4] to produce the Ipswich Triage Scale. This used five colours to categorize patients according to the question: 'This patient should under optimal circumstances be seen within....' The five categories were seconds, minutes, an hour, hours and days. Fitzgerald found his triage scale to have good interobserver reliability on formal testing and to be a practical predictor of ED outcome and length of intensive care stay, but a relatively poor predictor of outcome at hospital discharge.

Jelinek[5] investigated the relationship between the Ipswich Triage Scale and resource use in a stratified sample of 2900 presentations. He observed a strong correlation between triage categorization and overall use of resources in the ED and validated possible funding models. He proposed two possible casemix classifications: urgency and disposition groups (UDGs – 12 groups), and urgency-related groups (URGs – 73 groups) based on urgency, disposition and diagnosis. After trimming for outliers, these were found to account for 47% and 58% of the cost variance in large hospitals.

In 1994, the Australasian College for Emergency Medicine formalized the National Triage Scale (NTS),[6] derived from

the Ipswich Triage Scale. This used colours, names or numerical categories to represent five groups, based on the answer to the question: 'This patient should wait for medical care no longer than....' The categories were immediate, 10 min, 30 min, 1 h and 2 h. The definition document also proposed Jelinek's concept[5] of performance indicators based on the proportion of patients whose care fell within the desired time threshold, and audit by means of admission rates and sentinel diagnoses. It influenced treatment strategies by indicating the need to achieve performance indicators in a high proportion of patients in every category (higher in the more urgent) and it clearly established the need for EDs to employ systematic, accountable and audited triage processes.

Over the next few years the NTS was widely accepted and recognized by all Australian State Governments as an appropriate measure of access to emergency care. It was also adopted in the performance indicators promulgated by the Australian Council on Healthcare Standards.[7] Research repeated the findings of Fitzgerald and Jelinek with reference to the new five-point scale and investigated many more of the subtleties of triage scale use.

The Australasian triage scale

The ATS[8] is the current refinement of the NTS. It has been jointly developed by the Australasian College for Emergency Medicine, emergency nursing organizations and other interested parties. For practical purposes the scale concept itself is unchanged, but the ATS uses numeric classification only, better defines waiting time and includes associated implementation guidelines and educational material, partly derived from work on the NTS in areas such as mental health triage.[9]

The ATS categorizes patients presenting to EDs in response to the question: 'This patient should wait for medical assessment and treatment no longer than...' (Table 26.4.1).

Other triage scales

The concept of desirable waiting time must include some subjective component but has nevertheless been found to be reliable and

Table 26.4.1 ATS categorization of patients presenting to EDs	
ATS category	Treatment acuity (maximum waiting time)
ATS 1	Immediate
ATS 2	10 min
ATS 3	30 min
ATS 4	60 min
ATS 5	120 min

reproducible. Achievement of ATS waiting times has proven to be a useful performance indicator but remains a measure of process rather than ED outcome. Concerns have been expressed in some jurisdictions about the medicolegal implications of a time-based threshold which will not always be met, and other systems have taken different approaches in development of their own ED triage systems. Nevertheless, most have developed five-level triage systems along the Australasian model. Major validated triage scales include the following:

- the Canadian Emergency Department Triage and Acuity Scale (CTAS):[10] derived from the ATS but using a 15 min threshold in Category 2
- the Manchester Triage Scale:[11] uses an algorithmic approach to the UK Triage Scale, similar to the ATS but with longer thresholds in the lower acuity categories
- the ESI Triage algorithm:[12] developed in the USA without any time thresholds, but using a simple approach to classifying urgency.

Use beyond waiting time

Triage is based on a brief assessment, and an individual triage categorization can reflect only the probability of certain outcomes. Large populations of triaged patients, however, exhibit predictable patterns. There is a very strong, almost linear relationship between triage category and total rate of admission, transfer, or death, ranging from 80–100% in ATS 1 to 0–20% in ATS 5. This pattern is repeated across hospitals of different size and different patient mix.[13] Admission rates by triage category follow the pattern of overall admission rates in relation to age, giving a flattened U-shaped distribution. The inter-rater reliability studies performed using the Ipswich Triage Scale have been repeated using the NTS/ATS, which has been found to be slightly better.[14] Further, admission rates by triage category have been shown to be constant over time in individual institutions.[15]

The NTS/ATS has been extensively studied as a casemix tool. ED outcome (admission/transfer/death versus discharge) accounts for the largest variance in cost, but triage categorization comes a close second, with age third. The mean cost of care for a Category 1 patient is approximately 10 times that of a Category 5 patient. UDGs, described by Jelinek using the Ipswich Triage Scale, have been validated using the NTS by Erwich on 17 819 attendances.[16,17] Age has been included to derive urgency, disposition, and age groups (UDAGs – 32 groups), which account for 51% of the cost variance and are not susceptible to different diagnostic approaches.[14] These studies may not be valid in the era of overcrowding and access block, because staff costs for admitted patients reflect length of time in the ED, which may now be driven by outside factors. Furthermore, the costs for discharged patients are skewed by increased pressure to keep complex patients out of hospital.

Triage categorization is a very strong predictor of ED outcome and a good predictor of utilization of critical care resources. However, it is a relatively poor predictor of outcome at hospital discharge.[18,19] Many patients with chronic or subacute conditions that frequently cause death are triaged to less urgent categories because there is no benefit from earlier treatment within the time scales available in the ED.

Attainment of performance indicators for patients seen within triage thresholds has been shown to be a measure of resource allocation within the ED. A longitudinal comparative study has demonstrated a significant improvement with an increase in ED staff and funding.[20]

Triage categorization alone is insufficient to direct patients to fast-track services designed for low-complexity patients, but triage staff are appropriate and are able to assess complexity.[21]

Structure and function of a triage system

The exact requirements for triage vary with the role, location and size of the hospital, but effective systems share a number of important features, mostly derived from experience:

- A single point in the ED near the entrance where triage is undertaken so that all patients will be exposed to the nurse undertaking triage.
- Appropriate facilities for undertaking brief assessment and limited treatment (first aid) including relevant equipment and washing facilities for staff and patients.
- A balance between competing concerns of accessibility, confidentiality and security.
- A means of recording assessment and triage categorization that will 'follow' the patient through their time in the ED and be available for review afterwards. In most large departments this is now a computerized information system.
- Contemporary data on the state of the ED and the expected patients, such as the information system and ambulance and police radio systems.

Pre-hospital triage

The principle of making best use of available resources to maximize patient outcome remains the basis of triage in any setting. Relatively less therapeutic options are available to pre-hospital providers and patient disposition is generally limited to transport and sometimes choice of hospitals. The initial pre-hospital phase, the travel to the patient, must be undertaken on the basis of minimal information. Allocation of resources through a structured triage system remains important, but data may not be sufficient for a five-level scale, although this is currently being studied in Western Australia. Most pre-hospital systems are strongly protocol-driven and tend towards three- or four-level assessment: rapid response (lights and sirens), immediate response, routine response or no transport.

Military and disaster triage

In situations of overwhelming imbalance between resources and demand, triage remains critical in ensuring that available resources are used to achieve the greatest good. The principles of rapid assessment, documentation and multiple queues for care remain the same, but competing demands on resources may mean triaging cases to receive minimal or no care, or treating first those who can return to work or duty. The need for both human and physical resources for more important tasks may profoundly limit individual patient care.

Military and disaster triage require seniority and experience (which by definition is rarely available), the ability to make and defend rapid decisions and a successful liaison with other players outside the medical or nursing hierarchy. Senior personnel with significant experience and preferably with additional training should be chosen for this role if possible. Formal triage and documentation must be brief and will use different scales from those appropriate in the ED.

Controversies and future directions

The research base undertaken on the NTS showed it to be relatively reliable and reproducible but identified some areas for improvement. The Australasian Triage Scale and its associated guidelines and educational materials were designed to address some of the recognized problems with the NTS, but revision and improvement of the scale will continue. Further study is required to assess the impact of the ATS on issues including:

❶ variation in implementation between sites, particularly hospitals of different role delineation[13]

❷ variation associated with activity or overcrowding – there is evidence of consistency in some hospitals,[15] but changes in others[22]

❸ variation in approach to paediatric triage, especially between mixed and paediatric EDs[23]

❹ marked differences in education practice for triage nurses.[24]

The role of the ATS is still under assessment in pre-hospital and disaster triage, and the process of triage in EDs continues to evolve. The importance of triage as a management tool and the demand for greater reliability and consistency will continue to increase in line with the pressure of ED workload.

References

1. Larrey DJ. In: Mercer JC, transl. Surgical memoirs of the campaigns in Russia, Germany, and France. Carey and Lea, Philadelphia; 1832. Cited in Winslow G. Triage and Justice. University of California Press; 1982.
2. Weinerman ER, Ratner RS, Robbins A. Yale studies in ambulatory care V. Determinants of use of hospital emergency services. American Journal of Public Health Nations Health 1966; 56(7): 1037–1056.
3. Pink N. Triage in the accident and emergency department. Australian Nurses Journal 1977; 6(9): 35–36.
4. Fitzgerald GJ. Emergency department triage. Doctor of Medicine Thesis, University of Queensland; 1989.
5. Jelinek GA. Casemix classification of patients attending hospital emergency departments in Perth, Western Australia. Doctor of Medicine Thesis, University of Western Australia; 1995.
6. Australasian College for Emergency Medicine. National Triage Scale. Emergency Medicine (Australia) 1994; 6(2): 145–146.
7. Australian Council on Healthcare Standards. Clinical indicators – a user's manual. Zetland, NSW: ACHS; 1996.
8. Australasian College for Emergency Medicine. Australasian Triage Scale. Emergency Medicine (Australia) 2002; 14: 335–336.
9. Smart D, Pollard C, Walpole B. Mental health triage in emergency medicine. Australian and New Zealand Journal of Psychiatry 1999; 33: 57–66.
10. Beveridge R, Ducharme J, James L, et al. Beaulieu S, Walter S. Reliability of the Canadian Emergency Department Triage and Acuity Scale: interrater agreement. Annals of Emergency Medicine 1999; 34(2): 155–159.
11. Manchester Triage Group. London: Emergency triage. Publishing Group; 1997.
12. Wuerz RC, Milne LW, Eitel DR. Reliability and validity of a new five-level triage instrument. Academic Emergency Medicine 2000; 3: 236–242.
13. Whitby S, Ieraci S, Johnson D, et al. Analysis of the process of triage: the use and outcome of the National Triage Scale. Liverpool, NSW: Liverpool Health Service; 1997.
14. Jelinek GA, Little M. Inter-rater reliability of the National Triage Scale over 11 500 simulated occasions of triage. Emergency Medicine (Australia) 1996; 8: 226–230.
15. Richardson DB. No relationship between emergency department activity and triage categorization. Academic Emergency Medicine 1998; 5: 141–145.
16. Erwich MA, Bond MJ, Phillips DG. The identification of costs associated with emergency department attendances. Emergency Medicine (Australia) 1997; 9: 181–187.
17. Erwich MA, Bond MJ, Baggoley CJ. Costings in the emergency department. Report to the Commonwealth Department of Health and Human Services (Australia); 1996.
18. Dent A, Rofe G, Sansom G. Which triage category patients die in hospital after being admitted through emergency departments? A study in one teaching hospital. Emergency Medicine (Australia) 1999; 11: 68–71.
19. Doherty SR, Hore CT, Curran SW. Inpatient mortality as related to triage category in three New South Wales regional base hospitals. Emergency Medicine (Australia) 2003; 15(4): 334–340.
20. Rogers IR, Evans L, Jelinek GA. Using clinical indicators in emergency medicine: documenting performance improvements to justify increased resource allocation. Journal of Accident and Emergency Medicine 1999; 16: 319–321.
21. Vance J, Sprivulis P. Triage nurses validly and reliably estimate emergency department patient complexity. Emergency Medicine Australasia 2005; 17(4): 382–386.
22. Richardson DB, Kelly AM, Baggoley CJ, et al. Variation in triage categorisation: does daily activity make a difference? [abstract]. Academic Emergency Medicine 1999; 6: 397–398.
23. Durojaive L, O'Meara M. A study of triage in paediatric patients in Australia. Emergency Medicine (Australia) 2002; 14: 67–76.
24. Kelly AM, Richardson D. Training for the role of triage in Australasia. Emergency Medicine (Australia) 2001; 13: 230–232.

26.5 Refugee health

Aled Williams • Mark Little

ESSENTIALS

1 The worldwide refugee problem is massive and likely to increase.

2 Overall responsibility for refugees lies with the United Nations High Commission for Refugees (UNHCR) although numerous other organizations also assist.

3 The most familiar scenario is the movements of large populations across a border into a 'refugee camp'.

4 The response to a refugee crisis consists of an emergency phase where acute needs are met and a post-emergency phase when mortality levels in the camp approach those of the local area.

5 The basics of nutrition, shelter, clean water and sanitation are always the most important.

6 There are well-documented standards in all areas of refugee care.

7 For individual refugees the outcomes are resettlement in their country of origin, integration into the new host country or resettlement into a third country.

8 Ultimately, solutions to refugee movements are political.

Introduction

Increasingly over the past few years Australian health professionals, including emergency medicine staff, have responded to refugee crises due to conflict or natural disasters in our region.

Caring for refugees is not a new problem. Since World War II up to 100 000 000 civilians have been forced to flee their homes due to unrest. The major factors that cause people to flee their country, conflict, political repression and persecution, are as old as humanity. In 1573, the term 'refugee' was first used for Calvinists fleeing political repression in the Spanish-controlled Netherlands. Refugee numbers are now higher than ever and seem to be relentlessly increasing. The United Nations High Commission for Refugees (UNHCR) is currently responsible for the welfare of some 33 million refugees and other persons of concern

(January 2007 figures). These consist mostly of internally displaced persons (refugees inside their country of origin), asylum seekers and recently returned refugees. This equates to about 1:200 persons on the planet. The problem is massive.

The solution to any refugee problem is, ultimately, political and non-medical. Even in the acute phases of refugee movement the most important things are simple, such as food, shelter and clean water. Physicians, however, can play a considerable role, especially if they are adaptable and able to use simple cheap and effective solutions to problems.

This chapter provides an understanding of the issues and possible solutions to the refugee health problem, a bibliography for further reading, an outline of the essential attributes of refugee doctors and links to appropriate organizations for the interested reader.

Responsibility for refugee care

Until the end of the World War I, the response to refugees was from philanthropic sections of the community. The formation of the League of Nations began the process of the international community assuming responsibility for refugees. In 1921 a High Commission for Refugees was established with a mandate to look after refugees fleeing the Russian and Armenian wars. Its first Commissioner was Fridtjof Nansen, who established a special identity document, the 'Nansen Passport', as refugees frequently had no means of identification.

In the wake of World War II, the United Nations (UN) established the International Refugee Organization to assist the millions of displaced persons in Europe. Between 1947 and 1951 it helped 1.6 million people, mainly Germans and Austrians.

The modern response to refugees started in 1951 with the establishment of the UNHCR and the Convention Relating to the Status of Refugees, which has the force of law and has been ratified by 120 countries. With some fine-tuning over the years this remains the cornerstone of International Refugee Law. It defines a refugee as:

> ... any person who, owing to a well founded fear of being persecuted for reasons of race, religion, nationality, member of a particular social group or political opinion, is outside the country of his nationality and is unable or, owing to such a fear, unwilling to avail himself of the protection of that country.

The UNHCR also encourages countries to receive refugees and to provide them with assistance and protection. One of the major points of the Convention is the principle of 'non-refoulement', which means that refugees cannot be forcibly returned to their countries of origin.

Refugee camps

Persons fleeing war or persecution escape in many different ways and may live in host countries in several different arrangements, for instance integration with local community or staying with relatives. The typical image of refugees is of mass movements of populations across borders into temporary accommodations or 'refugee camps'. It is under these circumstances that refugees are most at risk. Importantly, the populations in refugee camps do not exist in isolation. There are always interactions with the local population, and these may not always be beneficial. Also important are political and ethnic factors within the refugee population. These can lead to tensions or even violence in the camps, as was demonstrated tragically in the post-Rwandan holocaust camps in 1994. Camps themselves can even sustain conflict in some areas, for instance in the West Bank or in the camps on the Thai–Cambodian border, which were used by the Khmer Rouge as refuges from which to carry on a war.

Emergency phase

As a result of a crisis, due to either war or acts of nature, large populations can be displaced from their normal environment. This often results in large numbers of people, with minimal or none of the basic life needs, descending on a region. Where the people congregate is usually where refugee camps evolve. Most population movements into refugee camps occur in third-world countries, which have limited resources to deal with them. Preplanning by aid agencies and governments is, therefore, essential so that humanitarian responses can be quick and coordinated. Considerable expertise in responding to refugee emergencies has been gained and the main priorities are now well recognized. These are outlined below, as per Médecins Sans Frontières (MSF) guidelines.

Initial assessment

A rapid assessment of the population structure, their medical and other needs is essential in the very early stages to enable planning and appropriate delivery of resources.

Measles immunization

Conditions in refugee camps can facilitate large-scale measles epidemics, which in an at-risk population can have devastating consequences. In a 5-month period, in 1992 in the Tuareg refugee camp, Mauritania, 40% of the paediatric deaths were due to measles. Mass vaccination of all children from 6 months to 15 years is essential and is usually combined with administration of vitamin A, which reduces the under 5 years mortality rate and the measles case fatality rate.

Water and sanitation

Poor water supply and sanitation play a major role in the spread of diarrhoeal diseases. Well-defined standards that can be checked with simple kits now exist for acceptable water quality. Standards for quantity are 5 L/person/day initially rising to 15 L/person/day when possible. Similarly set standards apply to the location, type and number of latrines and washing facilities.

Food and nutrition

Malnutrition is common in refugee populations, especially in the at-risk young and elderly groups. The initial food ration recommended is 2100 kcal/person/day. It is also important to undertake surveys for specific nutritional deficiencies such as scurvy or pellagra and treat accordingly.

Assessment of nutrition in the population is an ongoing process and special feeding programmes may need to be set up for at-risk groups. Generally, there are specific agencies such as the UN World Food Program, which specialize in this area.

Shelter and site planning

Proper shelter and adequate clothing are essential early priorities. Overcrowding can lead to or worsen disease outbreaks as well as affecting the mental health of refugees. Protection from the elements is also essential for wellbeing, especially in extreme climates. Again well-defined standards for living space and shelter construction exist. Planning the location of the camp is also essential. A good site needs to be large enough and secure and have adequate infrastructure like good road or air access. It should also have access to water supply and be relatively protected from the elements.

General healthcare

Organizing a system to deal with common infections and diseases is essential. There may be numerous organizations involved in the refugee camp and so there is a need for coordination. Medical needs of the population are rapidly assessed and locally occurring diseases taken into account. Experience has led to the creation of medical kits intended to cover the needs of 1000 refugees for a 3-month period. There are also manuals and guidelines available.

Control of infectious disease

The four most frequent infectious diseases in the emergency phase are diarrhoea, malaria, respiratory infections and measles. Providing good basic living conditions will help ward off these and other illnesses, but once an outbreak has occurred there is potential for high mortality rates so aggressive treatment and decisive public health measures are essential. As diarrhoea is a major cause of death, early establishment of oral rehydration centres is essential.

Public health surveillance

Collecting epidemiological data on a daily basis provides essential information to those in charge of a camp so that interventions can be planned and disease outbreaks rapidly recognized. The most useful health indicator is the daily crude mortality rate (CMR), which is normally expressed as deaths/10 000 population/day. A CMR of over 1 is an indicator of an emergency situation. Disease-specific mortality rates may also be useful.

Human resources and training

Administering a refugee camp is very complex and requires a variety of skilled personnel including doctors, water/sanitation experts, nutritionist, logisticians and others. First, the need for different types of personnel needs to be assessed and then their activities need to be coordinated and managed. Local staff and some of the refugees need to be trained to help in essential tasks.

Coordination

Any refugee action may have a large number of agencies assisting. There may be UN agencies, military forces, international non-government organizations (NGOs), such as MSF, Oxfam and local agencies like the national Red Cross societies. The host country's government and local authority also have an important role to play. Coordinating many diverse agencies, some of whom have conflicting agendas, is a huge challenge and means that one agency needs to take on a leadership role, good communication needs to be established early and overall goals must be established.

Post-emergency phase

This phase begins when the basic needs of the population are met (food, shelter, water and so on) and the CMR is less than 1 per day, which is roughly similar to that of the local population. The situation in the post-emergency phase is complex and fluid. Some of the refugees may become quite settled and start to work locally or farm some land. The health and nutritional status of refugees may even surpass those of local population because of large amounts of overseas aid. This may lead to resentment. Complex political issues may arise. Descent back into the emergency phase may occur with an epidemic outbreak or fresh influx of refugees.

In general, however, the post-emergency phase is concerned with consolidation of what has been achieved, preparation for possible new emergencies and sustainability.

There needs to be continuing monitoring of water quality, public health and nutritional status. Healthcare issues in the post-emergency phase are complex. Some of the issues that may need to be addressed include:

- standardization of training, supervision and delivery of health services
- curative healthcare services
- reproductive healthcare, including antenatal and delivery, postnatal family planning, sexually transmitted diseases (STDs) and HIV/AIDS
- child health activities such as expanded programmes of immunization (EPIs)
- specific HIV/AIDS/STD programmes
- tuberculosis programmes
- psychosocial and mental health.

Permanent solutions

There are three possible solutions to any refugee situation: repatriation, integration or resettlement in another country.

Repatriation is the preferred option but is often quite complex. First, there needs to be a solution to the problem that caused the refugees to leave initially. This may take years. Persons returning need a lot of extra support in order to rebuild their lives. Some refugees remain in the host countries and integrate into local communities. This was commonplace in African nations but is increasingly difficult, especially when African governments look at the reluctance of affluent Western countries to accept refugees.

The minority of refugees who cannot return are resettled in third (mostly Western) countries. Many countries have quotas and will only admit once a person is assessed by the UNHCR as having a valid claim. In 2001 the number resettled was 100 000. Of these, the USA took 68 500, Canada took 12 200 and Australia received 6500.

Past problems

In the past there have been important problems with the response to a refugee crisis. Often these have their root in poor coordination between the agencies that respond to a particular crisis, which may lead to inappropriate interventions and even frank competition. Often in a dramatic disaster such as an earthquake, which has considerable media coverage, there is a frenzy of intervention as agencies attempt to get their image across to international viewers to assist in fundraising. In the 2001 earthquake in Gujarat province, India, it was estimated that there were as many as 200 different government and non-government agencies in the field. There is no doubt that this has resulted in unnecessary death, most notably in the great lakes region of Africa following the Rwandan genocide.

Innovations in refugee care

Overcoming the problems of lack of planning and coordination has been the major thrust of more recent developments. Importantly, in 1997 it was decided to establish a set of minimum standards and rights to which refugees were entitled. The collaborative project called Sphere involved numerous organizations involved in humanitarian care including Red Cross, MSF and Oxfam. It produced a manual that is available at no cost from the website www.sphere.org. Individual organizations, such as MSF, have several excellent manuals describing in detail the approach to humanitarian emergencies.

The UN in conjunction with other agencies has been refining its disaster response capabilities. Through the Office for the Coordination of Humanitarian Affairs (OCHA) there is now a system of stockpiling supplies, cash reserves and ability for rapid assessment and deployment. The UN works in partnership with several NGOs and the Federation of Red Cross and Red Crescent Societies who have also been developing rapid response field assessment and coordination teams (FACTs). There is now a system of coordination through the Field Coordination Support Section (FCSS) of OCHA and the ability to appoint 'lead agency' status to a particular organization.

The Internet and electronic media are also being increasingly used in innovative ways by humanitarian agencies. It is now possible to follow evolving disasters on several websites (e.g. UN affiliated sites, Red Cross sites and MSF sites) and explore what that particular organization is doing. OCHA is also exploring the use of a Virtual Operations Coordination Center, which is an online resource that can be accessed by registered users from various agencies to coordinate their approach to a particular disaster.

Attributes of a refugee doctor

Working under the special conditions imposed by a refugee camp demands special qualities. It is certainly not a glamorous job and often much of what has been learned from training and practice in the West either is not relevant or needs much modification to suit local conditions and resources. In general the main requirements are:

- flexibility, versatility and ability to improvise
- ability to work independently
- ability to work under extreme circumstances
- cultural sensitivity
- getting on with all types of people
- ability to follow leadership and direction
- acceptance of security and health risks
- a family willing to accept risks.

Controversies and future directions

❶ There is often a lack of coordination between agencies involved in refugee care, leading to adverse outcomes. The challenge is to coordinate the response and maximize efficiencies and outcomes.

❷ There is often a reluctance by Western countries to accept refugees from the developing world.

❸ Improving standards and training in refugee care is a high priority.

❹ Arguably, the response would be considerably improved with the formation of rapid assessment and deployment teams.

❺ There is a need for better coordination between the UN and other agencies.

❻ Much could be gained from increased preparedness of the international community in holding cash reserves and humanitarian stockpiles.

Further reading

Emergency Relief Items. Vol. 1 & 2. United Nations Development Program; 2000.
Hospitals for War Wounded 1998 International Committee of the Red Cross. Available: www.refiefweb.int. This is the entry point into the UN agencies such as OCHA and its various branches. Also publishes situation reports of evolving disasters.
www.unhcr.org. Refugee facts, figures and histories.
Humanitarian Charter and Minimum Standards in Disaster Response. Available free on website www.sphereproject.org; 2004.
www.ifrc.org. International Federation of Red Cross and Red Crescent societies.
www.icrc.org. International Committee of the Red Cross site. This is more concerned with war zones.
www.msf.org. The MSF website, which is a very useful resource with several free publications on refugee healthcare.
www.oxfam.org.
www.sphere.org, from which you can download the sphere manual.
www.redcross.org.au. The Australian Red Cross site for information on where Australians are currently posted overseas. www.msf.org.au has similar data for MSF.
Médecins Sans Frontières. Refugee health, an approach to emergency situations. McMillan Education Ltd.; 1997. This and many other invaluable MSF texts on treatment protocols, basic kits are all available free on the MSF website: www.msf.org.

26.6 Emergency department observation wards

Aled Williams

ESSENTIALS

1 Observation wards (OWs) are an integral part of modern emergency departments (EDs).

2 They are run by ED staff according to strict policies and protocols.

3 The spectrum of conditions considered suitable for OW care is increasing.

4 Intensive treatment, frequent reassessment and rapid turnover lead to great efficiency in patient care.

5 Overall effects are to reduce admission length of stay for conditions suitable for OW treatment.

6 Inappropriate discharges from the ED are reduced.

7 The overall standing of the ED is enhanced.

Introduction

An observation ward (OW) is an essential part of a modern emergency department (ED). OWs are a valuable tool in the safe and efficient management of patients and are rapidly being embraced by EDs worldwide. In a 1989 survey it was found that of 44 EDs in major Australian hospitals 50% had beds designated as an OW. A further 25% expressed an intention to establish one.[1] Although there is much local variability, OWs are defined by the following general characteristics:

- They are run and staffed by ED personnel.
- They are separate from main patient assessment and treatment areas but remain either attached or in close proximity to the main body of the ED.
- Specific policies exist as to the type of patients who can and cannot be admitted.
- Admitting rights lie with ED staff only.
- Admissions are time limited, after which patients are either discharged or transferred to the care of another specialist team.

- Frequent ward rounds by senior medical staff are conducted.
- OW patients have preferential access to acute diagnostic, referral and paramedical services.

The primary role of OWs is to provide rapid turnover intensive observation and treatment to patients with suitable medical conditions. This increases efficiency of both the EDs and the hospital overall. OWs have additional benefits, which may include improving patient flow through a busy ED by providing a temporary 'holding area' for admissions, temporary accommodation for patients for whom discharge at an antisocial hour would be inappropriate (such as the elderly) or acute situational crises at antisocial hours. They may also function as a 'safety net' for patients seen at night by junior medical staff who are uncertain of the diagnosis for review by senior staff in the morning, thus possibly reducing inappropriate discharges.

OW policies and protocols

OWs function well under the umbrella of firm policies and protocols. These of course vary according to the institution, the number of beds in the OW, medical and nursing staff levels and the main perceived functions of the OW in a particular ED. In general, however, the following issues need to be addressed.

Admission process

To avoid confusion, requests for admission to the OW should go through a specific doctor nominated on each shift to have overall responsibility for OW patients. All patients need to have a clear treatment plan with defined objectives for the admission. Any treatment to be given during the admission such as intravenous fluids or medications needs to be clearly documented. If the patient is admitted for observation then what is required should also be clearly documented as well as action to be taken if there is any deterioration.

Admission criteria

Only some types of patients are suitable for OW management. The list below is not comprehensive and varies from institution to institution. The general principle is that the admitting doctor expects that the patient will be admitted for a definite and limited time (usually 24 h).

Time-limited intensive treatment:

- analgesia for renal colic
- mild-to-moderate asthma
- rehydration after gastroenteritis
- migraine headache
- some cases of envenoming, e.g. red back spider, brown snake envenoming with coagulopathy only
- analgesia and mobilization after soft-tissue injuries
- commencement of therapies that are to be continued out of hospital by either the patient's GP or home care nurses (e.g. intravenous antibiotics for cellulitis or fractionated heparin for deep vein thrombosis).

Patients requiring a period of observation before a decision about final disposition is made:

- post minor head injury with Glasgow Coma Scoe (GCS) of 14–15
- possible snakebite victims with no evidence of envenoming who are awaiting repeated blood tests
- post procedure, e.g. lumbar puncture or Bier's block
- many toxicology patients if ventilation or specific intensive care procedures are not required
- alcohol intoxication
- abdominal pain without specific signs in otherwise well patients.

Patients for whom discharge is inappropriate for social or other reasons:

- elderly isolated or vulnerable patients at antisocial hours
- acute situational crises out of hours that could benefit from social work or psychiatric input in the morning.

'Safety net' for junior staff working out of hours:

- There are some patients in whom junior staff may be unclear as to a diagnosis, but there is no definite indication to admit, inpatient teams refuse admission or the junior doctor 'is just not sure'. Such patients can be admitted and observed overnight for review by senior staff in the morning. As well as being a useful teaching exercise, the potential for 'missing' a diagnosis is reduced, but a clear management plan needs to be in place and the patient regularly reviewed so that deterioration is not missed.

'Bed management' issues:

- 'Holding bay' for patients admitted to other wards where there is a delay in availability of the bed. This can ease congestion in the ED.
- Patients awaiting an investigation, e.g. CT or ultrasound where there is an expected delay.

Special 'institution-specific' cases:

- Some institutions may develop more complex uses for OWs in order to capitalize on their efficiencies. Some examples are:

- chest pain assessment units
- toxicology units for treatment of more complex overdoses, e.g. paracetamol toxicity requiring NAC, prolonged anticholinergic delirium, etc.

Exclusion criteria

In order for the OW to work efficiently it is also necessary to have exclusion criteria for some types of patient. Again these vary from institution to institution but in general terms should include the following.

Patients who will clearly need >24 h admission:

- patients who should be admitted to inpatient wards, e.g. those with complex medical problems
- greater than one problem, especially in the elderly
- patients who cannot be given a clear treatment plan.

Patients who require intensive nursing care:

- Because of the nature of OWs nursing time is at a premium. Patients who are a heavy nursing load are therefore not suitable. For similar reasons, as well as safety issues, OWs are generally not suitable for psychotic, violent or disruptive patients.

Admission means that proper assessments are not done:

- 'Can't you just put them in the OBS ward and I'll see them in the morning' is a frequently heard plea from tired inpatient registrars. Although, at times, some flexibility is needed, this practice can be dangerous if appropriate intervention is delayed. The decision to admit to the OW should always lie with ED staff only.

Efficiency of patient care

Efficiency is essential if an OW is to maintain rapid patient turnover and treat patients within defined time criteria. This is achieved by a combination of factors:

- Frequent reassessments are complemented by regular ward rounds with senior staff such as experienced registrars or consultants. This results in

rapid decision-making and referral if necessary. Frequency and seniority of ward rounds are not affected by weekends or public holidays as is often the case in other inpatient wards. Typically ward rounds are conducted at shift change times when the responsibility for the patients in the ward is passed from one senior doctor to another (e.g. at commencement of morning, afternoon and night shifts).
- There is preferential access to diagnostic services such as radiology to expedite diagnosis and treatment.
- Typically, a large number of OW patients require the services of a social worker, alcohol and drug counsellor or other paramedical service. Streamlining the referral process to these services greatly increases the efficiency of the OW. Ideally, this is done by their attendance on morning ward rounds.
- Depending on criteria for admission and discharge about 10–20% of patients admitted to the OW need to be referred to another specialist team for admission and others may need a specialist opinion before discharge. Again preferential access is important to ensure smooth and efficient patient flow. Because in general a large proportion of OW patients require psychiatric input (e.g. post minor overdose and situational crisis), it is especially important to have an arrangement with the psychiatry department.

Staffing

OWs are staffed by ED personnel. As mentioned, a senior doctor is nominated to have responsibility for the ward during each shift. It is preferable to allocate nursing staff from each shift to the OW from the general ED pool of nurses rather than employ nurses only for the OW. This leads to increased flexibility with staffing and demonstrates that the OW is an integral part of the ED. The nursing establishment of an ED needs to take into account commitment to the OW and will need to be increased when it is initially set up. Some units, however, find that a stable, OW-experienced nursing workforce responsible for the ward facilitates greater efficiency. This is a matter for individual units.

Audit and feedback

As with any other medical activity auditing admissions to the OW and monitoring adverse events is important. Results can then be fed back through ED doctors as a quality improvement exercise. Firm key performance indicators for OWs have not been established yet but data worth collecting and analysing might include numbers of OW admissions subsequently admitted under an inpatient team (internationally 10–20% is considered acceptable[2]), patients discharged who re-present within 48 h, and adverse events and outcomes.

Overall impact of observation wards

OWs are generally well accepted by ED staff who easily see the benefits to efficient functioning of the department. The improved efficiency, however, goes beyond the ED and can affect the hospital as a whole. In a recent study performed in a major Australian ED[3] it was found that the introduction of an OW had significant effects on the hospital as a whole. Using diagnostic related grouping (DRG) codes for the most frequently admitted OW patient types a comparison on numbers admitted to OW and inpatient wards was done. Total inpatient days for these groups were also analysed. It was found that the introduction of an OW resulted in a decrease of these patients admitted to the inpatient wards associated with an increase in admissions to the OW. Overall the total numbers of patients increased, but, despite this increase, the total number of bed days decreased. Effectively, more patients were treated using fewer days in hospital, a clear indication of increased efficiency throughout the hospital.

The safety net function in reducing inappropriate discharges and picking up missed diagnoses has an effect on patient well-being as well as potentially reducing litigation and adverse publicity against the hospital. Less tangible results are an increase in staff satisfaction, an increase in patient satisfaction because of fewer days in hospital and an improvement in the public image of the ED within the hospital.

Short-stay medicine

Much of the difference between emergency physicians and their colleagues lies in their approach to a patient or a problem. To some extent, emergency medicine is a method of practice rather than a set of skills and clinical knowledge. A similar comparison can be drawn between standard inpatient wards and an OW. The main difference is in the high-efficiency, rapid turnover, problem-based approach. The 'technique' of observation medicine can be applied to situations other than EDs. The examples of chest pain assessment units and toxicology units as an extension of OWs have already been mentioned.

In the increasing drive for efficiency and cost-effectiveness it is likely that more variations on the technique of 'OW' medicine will appear. Medical acute assessment units and short-stay wards have already made an appearance in some Australasian hospitals and it is likely that their numbers will increase. What role there will be for emergency physicians in this treatment model remains to be seem, but there is a large potential for at least some expansion of emergency medicine beyond its traditional boundaries with positive effects on both job satisfaction and professional longevity.

Controversies and future directions

❶ There is potential for expansion of the OW concept to increase hospital efficiency, and many hospitals now have short-stay medical wards (acute assessment units and emergency medicine units) modelled on these wards.

❷ This provides new roles for emergency physicians in chest-pain units, toxicology units and other short-stay areas.

❸ There is a gradual blurring of the boundaries between the ED and inpatient units as a result.

References

1. Brillman J, Mathers-Dunbar L, Graff L, et al. Management of observation units. American College of Emergency Physicians. Annals of Emergency Medicine 1995; 25: 823–830.
2. Jelinek GA, Galvin GM. Observation wards in Australian hospitals. Medical Journal of Australia 1989; 151: 509–511.
3. Williams A, Jelinek GA, Rogers IR. The effect of establishment of an observation ward on hospital admission profiles. Medical Journal of Australia 2000; 173: 411–414.

26.7 Emergency department overcrowding and access block

Drew Richardson

ESSENTIALS

1 Overcrowding is the situation where emergency department (ED) function is impeded primarily by the excessive number of patients needing or receiving care.

2 Access block is excessive delay in accessing appropriate inpatient beds and in Australasia is defined as the proportion of patients with longer than 8 h total ED time.

3 Access block is the principal cause of overcrowding.

4 Although multiple different definitions have been used in studying overcrowding and access block, there is clear evidence that both are associated with diminished quality of care and worse patient outcomes.

5 Changes to ED structure and function including senior staffing, increased size, fast-track observation units and multidisciplinary discharge procedures can to some extent improve the function of the ED in the face of overcrowding, but do not address the underlying causes, and are easily overwhelmed by increasing access block.

6 The causes of overcrowding and hence the solutions lie largely outside the ED, especially in managing hospital bedstock in such a way that inpatient beds remain available.

Introduction

Wherever human beings gather there are fluctuations in number, and, without outside control, numbers occasionally exceed the efficient maximum for a given purpose. Emergency departments (EDs) are designed largely for ongoing flow of patients rather than gathering, but even in systems designed purely for flow (such as roads) there are peaks and troughs of activity, and occupancy sometimes exceeds the number able to move safely and smoothly.

Overcrowding to the point of dysfunction has gradually become the norm in Australasian EDs since the mid-1990s. The greatest contributing factor has been access block, the inability of patients requiring inpatient admission to access appropriate beds in a timely fashion, a phenomenon which is generally called 'boarding' in North America. There has additionally been some increase in demand on EDs in both number and complexity of patients resulting from

the enlarging, aging population and the growth in diagnostic and therapeutic choices. This has not been matched by growth in other services, especially outside working hours, increasing the burden on EDs.

Theoretical basis of overcrowding

Queuing theory indicates that the length of a queue and hence the waiting time to treatment is determined by the arrival rate, the treatment rate and the baulk rate (did not wait to be seen rate, which is usually dependent on the length of the queue). An individual patient's access to emergency care is dependent firstly on the urgency (assuming the patient is triaged to the correct queue), secondly on the number of similar patients already waiting ahead and thirdly on the rate and strategy of treatment. Treatment rate is dependent on

staffing and on the number of patients already being treated (occupancy), which determines physical availability of resources and the competing demands on staff. On a daily basis, patient flow is significantly dependent on occupancy because even a small decrease in treatment rate has a cumulative effect: it further increases the number waiting ahead of each new arrival.

EDs can be considered as overcrowded when treatment is dysfunctional, that is the treatment rate is reduced or the treatment quality suffers. This has been termed the 'cardiac analogy' model,[1] where ED function is regarded as a starling curve, which increases to a peak but then starts to decrease with overwhelming workload. Some authorities consider that an ED can be purely overcrowded with patients waiting to be seen whilst the treatment function remains optimal, others regard this situation as a 'surge' – a subset of disaster medicine, rather than an overcrowding problem.

Definition of overcrowding

The Australasian College for Emergency Medicine (ACEM) defines ED overcrowding[2] as the situation where ED function is impeded primarily because the number of patients waiting to be seen, undergoing assessment and treatment, or waiting for departure exceeds either the physical or the staffing capacity of the ED. Access block is quantified as the proportion of admissions to hospital, transfers to other hospitals, and deaths that have a total ED time of greater than 8 h.[2]

The American College of Emergency Physicians defines crowding[3] as occurring when the identified need for emergency services exceeds available resources for patient care in the ED, hospital, or both, a definition deliberately closer in spirit to that of disaster medicine. Most research on the subject, however, is concerned with the balance between daily fluctuations and ED occupancy, rather than the response to mass-casualty surges.

'Crowding' might be the more descriptive term, but 'overcrowding' is in common use, and researchers have used multiple definitions in attempts to quantify the phenomenon. All major recognized definitions incorporate occupancy with patients under treatment, but many also include subjective factors and outcomes such as ambulance bypass, which are not applicable to all EDs.

Retrospectively identified episodes of overcrowding tend to be reliable for research but are of only strategic significance in ED management. Real-time assessments may be correlated with patient service (number of patients waiting correlates well with waiting time for new arrivals) but are only useful if there is a managerial commitment to intervening. Predictive algorithms based on the number being treated suffer from false positives and again are only justified if interventions exist to prevent deterioration in flow.

There are multiple scales proposed and used to define overcrowding:[4,5] EDWIN,[6] NEDOCS,[7] READI[8] and Work score.[9] Validation studies are difficult and many rely on ambulance diversion as an outcome measure, which is only suitable for multi-ED urban centres. The few Australasian studies have not shown them to be clinically useful in real time.[10]

Causes of overcrowding

The single most important factor affecting ED overcrowding is the availability of inpatient beds.[11,12] ED overcrowding is best seen as a marker of whole-of-hospital dysfunction which requires a whole-of-hospital response.[13,14] Bed availability depends not only on the number of physical beds but also on the way the bedstock is managed.

Hospitals providing a local service in areas of significant demographic change, such as a large aging cohort or rapid growth, may experience ED overcrowding simply through the pressure of presenting numbers exceeding appropriate ED changes.

Development of new diagnostic approaches and therapies has contributed to increases in total ED time in some groups. Chest pain 'rule-out' protocols using delayed marker measurements and increasing use of computerized tomography (CT) scans for conditions such as abdominal pain are two examples. These are partly mitigated by shorter, protocol-driven care of other conditions, for example routine CT for minor head injury with immediate discharge after a normal result rather than observation.

Results of overcrowding

Adverse effects of hospital overcrowding have been described since the birth of modern medicine,[15] and ED overcrowding had been seen as undesirable since before the recognition of emergency medicine as a specialty.[16] In Australasia, access block was recognized as a quality issue from 1998,[17] first shown to be associated with decreased ED function in 2000[18] and defined by the ACEM from 2002.[2] Worldwide, properly conducted research started in 2001 and since that time multiple studies in different centres have found an association between overcrowding and reduced access to care, decreased quality measures and lesser outcomes.

Associations between overcrowding and outcomes demonstrated in peer-reviewed studies are shown in the Table 26.7.1. Whilst there is probably some publication bias, there remain no published studies equating overcrowding with improvements in care. The association between overcrowding and poor outcomes is accepted to be causative by most medical authorities.[11,12]

Strategies to deal with overcrowding

EDs have an obligation to reduce overcrowding and to mitigate its effects. As noted, any reduction in overcrowding will be largely achieved through whole-of-hospital changes. Long time-series suggest that, in the absence of hospital-wide changes, access block tends to continue to increase even after mitigation efforts within the ED.[39,40]

Increases in the number and seniority of ED staff are associated with improvements in process measures[41,42] and are a widely used initial response to overcrowding. Physical rebuilding is used to increase patient care spaces but changes in flow dynamics are highly dependent on the rest of the hospital.[43] Analysis of flow and system redesign can allow better use of existing resources.[44] Deployment of senior medical staff to assist early in the patient's journey through ED (at triage) reduces total ED time.[45] None of these responses can be used indefinitely if access block keeps increasing.

Discretionary, low-complexity presentations by patients who might reasonably be managed elsewhere, often incorrectly called 'GP-type' patients, constitute a significant number but an insignificant workload in most EDs.[46,47] Such presentations have a short assessment and treatment time and do not need fixed capacity spaces such as resuscitation rooms, so their contribution to occupancy with patients under treatment is low. However, being of lower triage urgency their contribution to the number waiting at any given time is relatively high.

Telephone advice services have not been shown to reduce ED workload in Australasia[48,49] but are highly regarded by the public. Dedicated ED fast-track areas[50] address the management of low-complexity patients in an efficient manner and thus tend to improve overall waiting time performance and staff and patient satisfaction. Their contribution to reducing occupancy with patients under treatment, and hence improving ambulance offload, is low.

EDs also have a small but significant role in reducing hospital occupancy. Observation medicine within the ED is a useful adjunct or alternative to formal inpatient admission.[51] Multidisciplinary assessment and discharge is effective at reducing representation at least in the elderly.[52]

Conclusions

Overcrowding has changed the nature of emergency medicine practice. Access block represents a useful simple description of overcrowding because the fundamental issue is the availability of inpatient beds. There is sufficient evidence to convince most authorities that the relationship between overcrowding and worse patient outcomes is causal. Emergency physicians have a role to play in maintaining patient care function in the face of overcrowding, but most of the solutions lie outside the ED.

Table 26.7.1 Adverse outcomes associated with overcrowding

Type	Outcome	Overcrowding definition	Reference
Process measures	Increased ambulance bypass	Access block	19
	Ambulance delay in chest pain	Divert status (time series)	20
	Increased left without being seen rate	NEDOCS	21
		Staff subjective	22
	Worse waiting time performance	ED access block	23
Quality measures	Decreased patient satisfaction	Staff subjective	22
	Missed myocardial infarction	ED volume	24
	Delay to reperfusion	Network diversion	25
	Reduced adherence to myocardial protocols	Simultaneous trauma cases	26
		Patient ED LOS	27
	Delay to antibiotics in pneumonia	Administrative cycle time and performance data	28
		ED volume and number needing admission	29
		Multiple measures at triage	30
	Inadequate analgesia (#NOF)	ED census >120%	31
	Lower quality pain management	Multiple measures at triage	32
Outcome measures	Increased reinfarction rate	Patient ED LOS	27
	Increased incidence of pneumonia in ventilated patients	Patient ED LOS	33
	Increased admission length of stay	Patient access block	34,35
		≥6 h in ED (ICU survivors)	36
	Increased short term mortality	≥6 h in ED (ICU patients)	36
		ED occupancy	37
		ED and hospital occupancy	38

NEDOCS, National Emergency Department Overcrowding Scale; LOS, length of stay; #NOF, fractured neck of femur; ICU, intensive care unit.

Controversies/future directions

❶ Political dimension: ED overcrowding is the product of hospital overcrowding, that is lack of available inpatient beds. Hospital overcrowding is likely to continue whilst hospital funding schemes favour electives over emergencies and utilization over efficiency.

❷ Financial dimension: Demand for healthcare is effectively unlimited, but demand for current levels of care will grow as the cohort of 'baby boomers' age, meaning significant rationing is inevitable if health spending remains contained. Although EDs have a role to play in reducing admissions, the major change needs to be in increasing early discharges, as the inpatient bed-day is the largest driver of acute hospital costs.

❸ Ethical dimension: Emergency physicians are comfortable with rationing on the basis of need – it is the foundation of the triage system. However, rationing by queuing becomes fundamentally inefficient once the time in the queue starts to approach the time course of the disease. The current institutional culture of the majority of hospital units

does not accept rationing of care to ward inpatients even when other patients with clearly greater medical needs are waiting for immediate access. These differences partly reflect ethical conflict between the principles of justice for all patients and beneficence for individual patients.

References

1. Richardson SK, Ardagh M, Gee P. Emergency department overcrowding: the Emergency Department Cardiac Analogy Model (EDCAM). Accident and Emergency Nursing 2005; 13: 18–23.
2. Australasian College for Emergency Medicine. Policy document – standard terminology. Emergency Medicine (Australia) 2002; 14: 337–340.
3. American College of Emergency Physicians. Crowding. Annals of Emergency Medicine 2006; 47(6): 585.
4. Hwang U, Concato J. Care in the Emergency Department: How crowded is overcrowded? Academic Emergency Medicine 2004; 11(10): 1097–1101.
5. Jones SS, Allen TL, Flottemesch TJ, et al. An independent evaluation of four quantitative emergency department crowding scales. Academic Emergency Medicine 2006; 13(11): 1204–1211.
6. Bernstein SL, Verghese V, Leung W, et al. Development and validation of a new index to measure emergency department crowding. Academic Emergency Medicine 2003; 10(9): 938–942.
7. Weiss SJ, Derlet R, Arndahl J, et al. Estimating the degree of emergency department overcrowding in academic medical centers: results of the National ED Overcrowding Study (NEDOCS). Academic Emergency Medicine 2004; 11(1): 38–50.
8. Reeder TJ, Burleson DL, Garrison HG. The overcrowded emergency department: a comparison of staff perceptions. Academic Emergency Medicine 2003; 10: 1059–1064.
9. Epstein SK, Tian L. Development of an emergency department work score to predict ambulance diversion. Academic Emergency Medicine 2006; 13(4): 421–426.

10. Raj K, Baker K, Brierley S, et al. National Emergency Department Overcrowding Study tool is not useful in an Australian emergency department. Emergency Medicine Australasia 2006; 18(3): 282–288.
11. Hostetler MA, Mace S, Brown K, et al. Subcommittee on Emergency Department Overcrowding and Children, Section of Pediatric Emergency Medicine, American College of Emergency Physicians. Emergency department overcrowding and children. Pediatric Emergency Care 2007; 23(7): 507–515.
12. Trzeciak S, Rivers EP. Emergency department overcrowding in the United States: an emerging threat to patient safety and public health. Emergency Medical Journal 2003; 20(5): 402–405.
13. Cameron PA. Hospital overcrowding: a threat to patient safety? Managing access block involves reducing hospital demand and optimising bed capacity. Medical Journal of Australia 2006; 184(5): 203–204.
14. Richardson DB. Reducing patient time in the Emergency Department. Medical Journal of Australia 2003; 179(10): 516–517.
15. Nightingale F. Notes on Hospitals. 3rd edn. Longman, Green, Longman, Roberts and Green, London; 1863.
16. Shah CP, Carr LM. Triage: a working solution to over crowding in the emergency department. Canadian Medical Association Journal 1974; 110: 1039–1043.
17. Baggoley C. President's message. Emergency Medicine (Australia) 1998; 10: 169–271.
18. Richardson DB. Quantifying the effects of access block [abstract]. Emergency Medicine (Australia) 2001; 13: A10.
19. Fatovich DM, Nagree Y, Sprivulis P. Access block causes emergency department overcrowding and ambulance diversion in Perth, Western Australia. Emergency Medicine Journal 2005; 22(5): 351–354.
20. Schull MJ, Morrison LJ, Vermeulen M, et al. Emergency department overcrowding and ambulance transport delays for patients with chest pain. Canadian Medical Association Journal 2003; 168: 277–283.
21. Weiss SJ, Ernst AA, Derlet R, et al. Relationship between the National ED Overcrowding Scale and the number of patients who leave without being seen in an academic ED. American Journal of Emergency Medicine 2005; 23(3): 288–294.
22. Vieth TL, Rhodes KV. The effect of crowding on access and quality in an academic ED. American Journal of Emergency Medicine 2006; 24(7): 787–794.
23. Dunn R. Reduced access block causes shorter emergency department waiting times: an historical control observational study. Emergency Medicine (Australia) 2003; 15(3): 232–238.

24. Schull MJ, Vermeulen MJ, Stukel TA. The risk of missed diagnosis of acute myocardial infarction associated with emergency department volume. Annals of Emergency Medicine 2006; 48: 647–655.

25. Schull MJ, Vermeulen MJ, Slaughter G, et al. Emergency department crowding and thrombolysis delays in acute myocardial infarction. Annals of Emergency Medicine 2004; 44(6): 577–585. Erratum in Annals of Emergency Medicine 2005; 45(1): 84.

26. Fishman PE, Shofer FS, Robey JL, et al. The impact of trauma activations on the care of emergency department patients with potential acute coronary syndromes. Annals of Emergency Medicine 2006; 48(4): 347–353.

27. Diercks DB, Roe MT, Chen AY, et al. Prolonged emergency department stays of non-ST-segment-elevation myocardial infarction patients are associated with worse adherence to the American College of Cardiology/American Heart Association guidelines for management and increased adverse events. Annals of Emergency Medicine 2007; 50(5): 489–496.

28. Pines JM, Hollander JE, Localio AR, et al. The association between emergency department crowding and hospital performance on antibiotic timing for pneumonia and percutaneous intervention for myocardial infarction. Academic Emergency Medicine 2006; 13(8): 873–878.

29. Fee C, Weber EJ, Maak CA, et al. Effect of emergency department crowding on time to antibiotics in patients admitted with community-acquired pneumonia. Annals of Emergency Medicine 2007; 50(5): 501–509, 509.e1.

30. Pines JM, Localio AR, Hollander JE, et al. The impact of emergency department crowding measures on time to antibiotics for patients with community-acquired pneumonia. Annals of Emergency Medicine 2007; 50: 510–516.

31. Hwang U, Richardson LD, Sonuyi TO, et al. The effect of emergency department crowding on the management of pain in older adults with hip fracture. Journal of the American Geriatrics Society 2006; 54: 270–275.

32. Pines JM, Hollander JE. Emergency department crowding is associated with poor care for patients with severe pain. Annals of Emergency Medicine 2008; 51(1): 1–5; discussion 6–7. Epub 2007 Oct 25.

33. Carr BG, Kaye AJ, Wiebe DJ, et al. Emergency department length of stay: a major risk factor for pneumonia in intubated blunt trauma patients. Journal of Trauma 2007; 63(1): 9–12.

34. Richardson DB. The access block effect: relationship between delay to reaching an inpatient bed and inpatient length of stay. Medical Journal of Australia 2002; 177: 492–495.

35. Liew D, Liew D, Kennedy MP. Emergency department length of stay independently predicts excess inpatient length of stay. Medical Journal Australia 2003; 179: 524–526.

36. Chalfin DB, Trzeciak S, Likourezos A, et al. DELAY-ED study group. Impact of delayed transfer of critically ill patients from the emergency department to the intensive care unit. Critical Care Medicine 2007; 35(6): 1477–1483.

37. Richardson DB. Increase in patient mortality at 10 days associated with emergency department overcrowding. Medical Journal of Australia 2006; 184: 213–216.

38. Sprivulis PC, Da Silva JA, Jacobs IG, et al. The association between hospital overcrowding and mortality among patients admitted via Western Australian emergency departments. Medical Journal of Australia 2006; 184(5): 208–212.

39. Richardson DB. Responses to access block in Australia: Australian Capital Territory. Medical Journal of Australia 2003; 178(3): 103–104.

40. Fatovich DM. Responses to access block in Australia: Royal Perth Hospital. Medical Journal of Australia 2003; 178(3): 108–109.

41. Rogers IR, Evans L, Jelinek GA, et al. Using Clinical indicators in emergency medicine: documenting performance improvements to justify increased resource allocation. Journal of Accidents and Emergency Medicine 1999; 16: 319–321.

42. Cardin S, Afilalo M, Lang E, et al. Intervention to decrease emergency department crowding: does it have an effect on return visits and hospital readmissions? Annals of Emergency Medicine 2003; 41: 173–185.

43. Han JH, Zhou C, France DJ, et al. The effect of emergency department expansion on emergency department overcrowding. Academic Emergency Medicine 2007; 14: 338–343.

44. King DL, Ben-Tovim DI, Bassham J. Redesigning emergency department patient flows: application of Lean Thinking to health care. Emergency Medicine Australasia 2006; 18: 391–397.

45. Holroyd BR, Bullard MJ, Latoszek K, et al. Impact of a triage liaison physician on emergency department overcrowding and throughput: a randomized controlled trial. Academic Emergency Medicine 2007; 14: 702–708.

46. Schull MJ, Kiss A, Szalai JP. The effect of low-complexity patients on emergency department waiting times. Annals of Emergency Medicine 2007; 49: 257–264.

47. Sprivulis P, Grainger S, Nagree Y. Ambulance diversion is not associated with low acuity patients attending Perth metropolitan emergency departments. Emergency Medicine Australasia 2005; 17(1): 11–15.

48. Graber DJ, Ardagh MW, O'Donovan P, et al. A telephone advice line does not decrease the number of presentations to Christchurch Emergency Department, but does decrease the number of phone callers seeking advice. New Zealand Medical Journal 2003; 116(1177): U495.

49. Sprivulis P, Carey M, Rouse I. Compliance with advice and appropriateness of emergency presentation following contact with the HealthDirect telephone triage service. Emergency Medicine Australasia 2004; 16(1): 35–40.

50. O'Brien D, Williams A, Blondell K, Jelinek GA. Impact of streaming 'fast track' emergency department patients. Australian Health Review 2006; 30(4): 525–532.

51. Williams AG, Jelinek GA, Rogers IR, et al. The effect on hospital admission profiles of establishing an emergency department observation ward. Medical Journal of Australia 2000; 173(8): 411–414.

52. Caplan GA, Williams AJ, Daly B. A randomized, controlled trial of comprehensive geriatric assessment and multidisciplinary intervention after discharge of elderly from the emergency department-the DEED II study. Journal of American Geriatrics Society 2004; 52(9):1417–1423.

26.8 Patient safety

Peter Sprivulis

ESSENTIALS

1 Approximately 1 in 10 hospital patients experiences an adverse event, of which half may be attributed to clinical error and a third result in significant harm or death.

2 Emergency medicine faces particular challenges to safe patient care, due to the undifferentiated and potentially unstable patient casemix, high staff turnover, staff inexperience and fatigue, and distractions, noise and overcrowding in the clinical care environment.

3 Clinical errors in emergency medicine may include errors of patient identification, hospital-acquired infections due to poor procedure asepsis and patient isolation procedures, medication errors, misdiagnosis and failure of follow-up of investigation and imaging abnormalities, communication errors, physical care errors and mis-triage.

4 Improving patient safety in emergency departments (EDs) requires an understanding of the ED environment and a methodical stepwise approach to improving safety based upon

    a. fostering reporting of clinical incidents, including 'near misses'

    b. evaluating reported incidents using accepted methodologies such as root cause analysis

c. treating the risk; this is rarely achieved by exhorting staff to 'try harder' or removing the offending individual. Rather, risk reduction usually requires process redesign to make the 'right' thing easier to do and an error less likely.

5 Patient safety should be monitored proactively in order to ascertain risks and assist assessment and refinement of interventions to improve patient safety.

6 An open, communicative, culture that promotes reporting and minimizes blame supports patient safety improvement.

Introduction

Patient safety, or the freedom from accidental injury due to medical care or from medical error, is increasingly being recognized as a critical consideration in the delivery of acute and emergency healthcare.[1] Several OECD countries have examined the proportion of acute care admissions during which an adverse event (an unexpected medical problem that happens during treatment with a drug or other therapy) is identifiable using a standard medical chart review. They typically report that 1 in 10 admitted patients experiences an adverse event, of which half are considered preventable with the current state of medical knowledge (i.e. are due to medical error).[1] Typically, a third of adverse events lead to moderate, or greater, disability or death.[1] An important consideration for the emergency care of admitted patients is that the day of greatest risk of an adverse event is usually the first day of admission to hospital. This is when knowledge of the patient's clinical condition is often incomplete, the clinical condition is least stable and when most patients experience the greatest number of procedures and interventions.[2]

Specific emergency department factors that may compromise patient safety

Safe patient care is challenged by several specific emergency department (ED) factors that include:

- *Staff factors*: ED staffing profiles, particularly in public EDs, typically include a high proportion of junior medical and nursing staff who are still in training. Safety improves with experience. In addition, there is usually a scheduled high turnover of staff, as staff are rotated between alternate training positions. These high levels of rotation can corrode 'memory' of safe and desirable processes and systems of care. ED staff are usually rostered to work shifts spanning 24 h a day. Poorly designed rosters may contribute to fatigue.[3,4]
- *Clinical factors*: ED patients have an inherently high severity of illness, placing them at greater risk of serious adverse sequelae if a medical error occurs. In addition, the undifferentiated nature of illness and injuries cared for, often coupled with the incomplete clinical information, creates clinical uncertainty, increasing risk.[4,5]
- *Physical environment*: EDs are noisy, busy work spaces, with frequent intrusions from alarms, pages, telephone calls and personal consultations, all of which create distractions, increasing the risk of error.[6]
- *Linkages to other care systems*: Emergency care is reliant upon a complex set of relationships between the ED, referring practitioners, pre-hospital carers, other hospital services and other services responsible for aftercare or following up after discharge from the ED. Poor linkages or communication between the ED and any of these other services can result in errors or omissions in information transfer that compromise patient safety.[7]
- *Overcrowding*: EDs have little control over patient attendance and increasingly suffer overcrowding as a consequence of poor access to beds downstream of the ED for admitted patients. This is associated with overcrowding and increased mortality, most likely due to a combination of resource effects (incorrect or insufficient resources or attempting procedures or monitoring in inappropriate locations) and delays in time to critical care.[4,8]

Common safety problems encountered in emergency departments

The factors described above interact to create a wide range of risks to patients needing emergency care.[4] Some of the errors observed in the emergency setting include:

- *Patient identification errors*: Errors in patient identification, incorrect labelling of laboratory requests and mislabelled samples may result in delays, misdiagnosis and incorrect treatment such as transfusion errors.
- *Hospital-acquired infection*: The conduct of simple procedures, such as peripheral intravenous line insertion, by inexperienced staff using suboptimal asepsis techniques in inappropriate or crowded locations, increases the risk of hospital acquired infection. Poor screening or compromise of isolation procedures due to overcrowding can pose genuine life threats to other patients.
- *Incorrect interpretation or failure to follow up pending imaging or laboratory investigations*: Incorrect interpretation of radiographs or failure to check for a pending laboratory result can result in incorrect or delayed diagnosis.
- *Medication errors*: Illegible, incomplete and verbal drug prescriptions, dosing errors (particularly in *children*) and compromise of medication administration procedures increase the risk of adverse drug events.
- *Communication errors*: Omissions in the handover of care between clinicians within the ED at the change of shift, upon transfer to inpatient teams or upon

discharge/transfer may cause serious delays in both diagnosis and the follow-up of urgently needed investigations or treatment.

- *Physical care errors*: The care of elderly patients for extended periods in a bright, noisy environment, in the era of access block, increases the risk of confusion and falls.
- *Triage errors*: Triage is known to be an imperfect art; however, in the era of overcrowding, which may result in significant delays in care for low-priority patients, a triage error may result in significant delays in diagnosis or initiation of treatment.

Improving safety in the emergency department

Specific actions to improve patient safety should be undertaken in the context of a comprehensive organizational framework for clinical governance and quality improvement.[1] The development of a programme of safety improvement for an ED should be undertaken methodically, in accordance with existing Australasian and international standards that usually encompass the following process elements:

- *Understand the environment*: Initially, it is essential that the specific environment of emergency care, including the characteristics of EDs and emergency patients that impair safety and the types of errors encountered in emergency care, are fully understood.
- *Identify specific risks*: Risk identification is usually undertaken with the aid of clinical incident reporting systems that encourage the structured reporting of clinical incidents that resulted, or could have resulted, in unexpected harm to the patient (e.g. the Australian Incident Monitoring System). These reports are usually collated both at the ED level and also at the hospital or organization level and even at the jurisdictional or national level.
- For every thousand prevented or no-harm incidents there may be a hundred of the same type that cause minor to moderate

harm, ten that cause severe harm and one that causes death. Therefore it is important to learn from the prevented or no harm incidents to reduce the chance of the single death incident happening. Often, employees are more willing to report near misses. The importance of including near misses in the incident reporting systems cannot be overemphasized.[1]

- *Analyse and evaluate the risks*: Risk analysis should be undertaken using an accepted methodology with the support of staff trained in its use. Two common forms of analysis are root cause analysis and failure modes and effects analysis. Root cause analysis is conducted 'after the event' and aims to identify what happened, why and what can be done to prevent it in the future by attempting to identify systems problems that contributed to the clinical event. Failure modes and effects analysis can be conducted in the absence of specific clinical events. It uses a proactive and systematic approach to evaluate common clinical processes in order to identify where and how they might fail and to assess the relative impact of different failures in order to identify the parts of the process that are most in need of change. This approach is particularly useful in evaluating a new process prior to implementation and in assessing the impact of a proposed change to an existing process.
- *Treat the risks*: Two common preconceptions that can stand in the way of an effective remedy include the 'perfection myth' – if we try hard enough we will not make any errors – and the 'punishment myth' – if we punish people when they make errors they will make fewer of them. In reality, at least 80% of errors may be attributed to poorly designed care systems and processes that fail to account for human fallibility. Unfortunately, the mere publication of a new clinical guideline rarely results in a sustained change in practice. For these reasons, the preferred approach to reducing risk is to use the principles of reliability engineering and process redesign that substitute clumsy,

unreliable and dangerous processes or systems with standardized and sustainable processes that make errors more difficult to perform, make the 'right' thing to do the easiest thing to do and aid the detection and correction of errors if they do occur (e.g. replacement of vials of similar appearing drugs with well-labelled, prefilled syringes on a resuscitation trolley).[1]

At all times:

- *Monitor and review*: The improvement of patient safety is a continuous process and information concerning safety should be collated systematically and routinely and evaluated at scheduled intervals in order to detect changes in patient safety trends as early as possible. Additionally, the impact of any changes to processes to improve patient safety should be monitored and evaluated in order to determine the effectiveness of the changes in reducing errors and to identify any unintended consequences that necessitate further refinement.
- *Communicate and consult*: Patient safety is a team activity that requires communication of the approach to improving safety and its high priority to all members of an ED's staff. An open and fair culture, rather than a blame culture, must be promoted in order to yield the benefits of reporting systems. Participation in wider hospital and regional or national reporting systems offers the opportunity to learn from the mistakes of others. Expert help should be sought in attempting to evaluate patient risks or design interventions to improve safety. In the event of an adverse event, being open and honest with patients and with other staff improves the prospect of learning and the prevention of further errors.

Conclusion

Patients seeking emergency care are at significant risk of harm, in part due to their clinical situation and in part due to the challenges of delivery of emergency care itself. Improving patient safety in the ED

requires a systematic approach to risk identification, risk analysis and evaluation and
the implementation of safer processes of
care. Monitoring is an essential component
of patient safety improvement. An open,
communicative culture that promotes
reporting and minimizes blame supports
patient safety improvement.

References

1. Botwinick L, Bisognano M, Haraden C. Leadership Guide to Patient Safety. Cambridge, MA: Institute for Healthcare Improvement; 2006.
2. Weissman J, Rothschild J, Bendavid E, et al. Hospital workload and adverse events. Medical Care 2007; 45: 448–455.
3. Feddock CA, Hoellein AR, Wilson JF, et al. Do pressure and fatigue influence resident job performance? Medical Teacher 2007; 29(5): 495–497.
4. Croskerry P, Sinclair D. Emergency medicine: a practice prone to error? Canadian Journal of Emergency Medicine 2001; 3(4): 271–276.
5. Brown AF. Do we realize when we do not know? Recognizing uncertainty in clinical medicine. Emergency Medicine of Australasia 2005; 17(5–6): 413–415.
6. Brixey JJ, Tang Z, Robinson DJ, et al. Interruptions in a level one trauma center: a case study. International Journal of Medical Informatics 2007; 77:235–241.
7. Bomba DT, Prakash R. A description of handover processes in an Australian public hospital. Australia Health Review 2005; 29(1): 68–79.
8. Sprivulis PC, Da Silva JA, Jacobs IG, et al. The association between hospital overcrowding and mortality among patients admitted via Western Australian emergency departments. Medical Journal of Australia 2006; 184(5): 208–212.

26.9 The medical emergency team

Daryl Andrew Jones

ESSENTIALS

1 Up to 17% of hospitalized ward patients suffer serious adverse events (SAEs), including cardiac arrest.

2 These events are often preceded by signs of physiological derangement for up to 24 h prior to the event.

3 Medical emergency teams (METs) are designed to review ward patients in the early phases of this deterioration.

4 Single-centre studies have demonstrated a reduction in cardiac arrests and unplanned admissions to the intensive care unit.

5 A multicentre study of METs in Australia did not confirm these benefits.

6 Future research needs to focus on patient related and hospital system related factors that lead to MET calls and strategies to improve their outcome.

Introduction and definitions

Medical emergency teams (METs) are composed of doctors and nurses that review
acutely unwell hospital ward patients in an
attempt to reduce cardiac arrests and other
serious adverse events (SAEs). The team
should have a number of competencies,
including abilities in the following areas:[1]

❶ prescription of therapies
❷ advanced airway management skills
❸ insertion of invasive vascular lines
❹ commencement of intensive care level
of care at the bedside.

The term 'rapid response system' (RRS)
has been proposed to represent an entire
system that provides both an 'afferent' component to identify patient deterioration and
an 'efferent' component to assess and treat
the patient. The most common efferent
component is the MET. Other types of review
team include the rapid response team (RRT)
and critical care outreach team (CCO), which
differ in their staff composition, skill set and
mechanism of activation.[1] The remainder of
this chapter will focus on the MET, which is
the predominant team used in hospitals in
Australia and New Zealand.

Additional components of the RRS include
quality improvement and clinical governance
arms, which permit audit and evaluation of
SAEs and implementation of hospital-wide
strategies to prevent their recurrence.[1]

Epidemiology and principles underlying the MET

Several principles underpin the MET and
RRS. In summary, SAEs are common in hospitalized patients and these are often preceded by a period of instability of up to
24 h. The MET is summoned to review
patients in the early phases of deterioration in an attempt to prevent further deterioration, morbidity and mortality.

SAEs are common in hospitalized patients

Studies in Australia,[2] New Zealand,[3,4] England,[5] and Canada[6] have assessed the incidence of SAEs in hospitalized patients.
These studies defined an SAE as 'unintended
injury or complication resulting from medical
management rather than the underlying disease process'. They reported an incidence of
SAEs ranging between 7.5% and 16.6%
and suggested that 36.9–51% were
preventable.

A recent single-centre study in an Australian hospital[7] found that 16.9% of
1125 patients undergoing major surgery
suffered at least one of 11 predefined SAEs
(which included myocardial infarction,
stroke, arrest and respiratory failure).

SAEs are preceded by signs of clinical instability

At least four studies[8–11] have demonstrated
that patients suffering SAEs develop new

complaints, deterioration of commonly measured vital signs or derangement in laboratory investigations in up to 84% of cases prior to the event. It is for this reason that common triggers for MET activation are based on derangements in vital signs. More importantly, three studies[12-14] have confirmed that patients who develop vital signs that satisfy MET criteria are at increased risk of death.

Deterioration of the MET patient is typically gradual

Unexpected out-of-hospital cardiac arrest is usually sudden and due to cardiac arrhythmias, pulmonary embolism or major vascular catastrophe. In contrast, progression to in-hospital cardiac arrests and other SAEs is typically gradual.[8] This allows sufficient time for intervention and, potentially, prevention of the event.

Early intervention improves outcome

One of the tenets underlying the MET principle is that early intervention in the course of critical illness is associated with improved outcome. This observation has been made in patients suffering trauma,[15,16] myocardial infarction[17] and in resuscitation of patients presenting to the emergency department (ED) with sepsis.[18]

Skilled staff already exist in the hospital

METs are usually composed of critical care staff with skills in advanced airway management, insertion of invasive vascular lines, and with knowledge of therapies commonly used in acute care medicine (Table 26.9.1). Staff need to be available 24 h per day, 7 days a week to manage acutely unwell patients anywhere in the hospital.[19]

How MET services and RRS work

Different roles of the MET

The MET was originally described in 1995 when Lee and coworkers reported the introduction of a MET service into Liverpool Hospital in Sydney, Australia.[19] The MET superseded the existing cardiac arrest team

Table 26.9.1 MET staff members and their roles	
Staff member	**Roles**
Intensive care registrar	• Knowledge of acute care medicine and physiological basis of acute deterioration • Skill in advanced resuscitation and insertion of invasive vascular lines • Skill in airway management and advanced cardiac life support
Intensive care nurse	• Knowledge of delivering advanced resuscitation • Provision of ongoing information and advice to ward nurses for patients remaining on the ward following MET call • Liaising with intensive care unit regarding potential for patient admission
Medical registrar	• Skill in diagnosis and management of underlying aetiology of medical condition • Follow-up and ongoing management of patients remaining on ward following MET call
Ward nurses and doctors	• Knowledge of patients' nursing issues since admissions and leading up to MET call

and was modelled on rapid detection and correction of abnormal vital signs indicative of trauma teams. In this model, the MET is merely an expansion of the existing cardiac arrest team and reviews all medical emergencies including arrests.

In other hospitals[20,21] two separate RRTs operate: a cardiac arrest team to review patients who have suffered cardiorespiratory arrest and a MET that reviews all medical emergencies other than cardiac arrest.

Activation of the MET – the afferent ARM

The MET service is activated when one or more predefined criteria are reached. Typical criteria involve derangement of commonly measured vital signs (Table 26.9.2). Other criteria include conditions such as uncontrolled seizures or chest pain. Finally, some hospital MET criteria contain a 'staff member worried' criterion

Table 26.9.2 Commonly used MET calling criteria	
System	**Criteria**
Airway	Stridor Threatened airway
Breathing	Acute change in RR <8 or >30 bpm Acute change in saturation <90% despite oxygen Difficulty breathing Noisy breathing
Circulation	Acute change in heart rate <40 or >130 bpm Acute change in systolic BP <90 mmHg Uncontrolled chest pain
Neurology	Acute change in conscious state Agitation or delirium
Other	Staff member is worried about the patient Acute change in UO to <50 mL in 4 h

RR, respiratory rate; BP, blood pressure; UO, urine output.

to permit activation of the MET service for any possible medical emergency.

Composition of the MET – the effector ARM

The precise composition of each MET varies between hospitals. Each member will have a predefined role (Table 26.9.1), and simulation or mock sessions may be held as part of their training.[22] The teams typically bring their own equipment to the MET call, either on a trolley or in a carry bag, which includes equipment needed for endotracheal intubation, invasive vascular access and medicines and fluids used in advanced resuscitation.

Clinical features of MET patients

Characteristics of triggers leading to MET activation

A number of studies[13,21,23] have reported the relative frequency of MET call criteria leading to MET calls (Table 26.9.3). Variations between hospitals are likely to represent differences in the limits of the criteria as well as differences in local case mix. Hypoxaemia, hypotension and altered

Table 26.9.3   Relative frequency (%) of MET triggers leading to MET calls

Criteria	Bellomo et al (2003) (n = 99)	Buist et al (2004) (n = 564)	Jones et al (2006) (n = 400)
Hypoxia	37	51	41
Respiratory rate	19	≅7	14
Hypotension	35	17.3	28
Tachycardia	20	≅7	19
Altered conscious state	28	≅7	23
Oliguria	2	Not assessed	8
Worried	46	Not assessed	Not assessed

conscious state were the commonest causes of MET calls in these studies.

Medical conditions leading to MET calls

The clinical cause of MET calls has also been assessed in a number of studies, and the concept of 'MET syndromes' (e.g. the 'hypoxic MET syndrome') has recently been raised.[23,24] Again, variations in case mix and MET calling criteria are likely to account for these differences. In the original description of the MET, Lee and coworkers reported that acute respiratory failure, status epilepticus, coma and pulmonary oedema were the most common causes of MET calls.[19] In a district general hospital, Daly and coworkers reported that chest pain, respiratory distress, seizures and cardiopulmonary arrest caused most MET calls.[25] Finally, a study of 400 MET calls at the Austin hospital[23] revealed that infections, pulmonary oedema and arrhythmias caused 53% of all MET calls.

Management of MET call patients

One of the most underinvestigated aspects of the MET system is the details of the management undertaken by the staff during a MET call. De Vita and coworkers have recently reported that use of a detailed curriculum and a computerized human patient simulator resulted in increased task completion rate and improved survival of the simulated patient.[22]

An analysis of the MET syndromes associated with 400 MET calls and an approach to their management has been reported.[23]

The 'A to G' approach described can be used to manage any possible medical emergency and can be used in the management of specific MET syndromes (Table 26.9.4).

Other issues – the MET and the ED

MET services involving the ED

In the original description of the MET system, the ED was one of the hospital areas serviced by the MET.[19] This approach involves review of ED patients by intensive care unit (ICU) staff and is most appropriate during periods when there are limited senior emergency medical staff, particularly out of hours. In contrast, Daly and coworkers described a MET model for a district general hospital in which staff from the ED formed the core of the MET and reviewed patients in the general wards when the MET service was activated.[25]

The MET philosophy in the ED

The MET involves a coordinated multidisciplinary approach to the management of acute deterioration of hospital ward patients.[1] As outline above (Table 26.9.1), each member has a designated role which is coordinated by the team leader. This is similar to the team-based approach to trauma management seen in most EDs and trauma centres (Table 26.9.5).

The MET system principle is equally applicable in the ED as it is on the hospital ward. For example, a multidisciplinary programme was shown to reduce the hospital mortality rate of patients presenting to a community hospital with non-traumatic shock.[26]

Table 26.9.4   A to G approach to management of a hypoxic MET call

Step of A to G approach	Approach for hypoxic MET call
Ask	How can I help Why was the MET called
Assess for aetiology	Pulmonary oedema, atelectasis, pneumonia, asthma, sepsis and pulmonary embolism
Begin Basic investigations Basic resuscitation	Chest X-ray, sepsis screen, ECG and cardiac enzymes and arterial blood gas; consider V/Q scan Apply oxygen and monitor arterial saturation CCF – loop diuretic, morphine, nitrates, oxygen and upright posture COAD – bronchodilators, hydrocortisone and non-invasive ventilation Atelectasis – chest physiotherapy and humidified oxygen Pulmonary embolism – anticoagulation or thrombolysis
Call for help (if needed)	SaO_2 <90% despite 10 L inspired oxygen Respiratory rate >40, elevated $PaCO_2$, altered conscious state
Discuss Decide Document	With parent unit, patient and next of kin, intensive care consultant Where the patient is most appropriately managed If limitations of therapy should be instituted The cause, management and follow-up of the call
Explain	To the patient, nursing and junior medical staff The cause, management and follow-up of the call
Follow-up	Clearly indicate who will follow up the patient and when this will occur
Graciously thank the staff	

MET, medical emergency team; ECG, electrocardiogram; CCF, congestive cardiac failure; COAD, chronic obstructive airways disease.

Table 26.9.5 Similarities and differences between MET services and trauma teams

Variable	Trauma team	MET service
Location of patient	Emergency department or trauma centre	Hospital ward
Team leader	Typically emergency department doctor	Typically intensive care unit registrar
Patient profile	Young with few comorbidities	Elderly with multiple comorbidities
Presenting problem	Trauma	Hypoxia, hypotension and tachycardia
Need for early intervention	Concept of 'golden hour'	Shown for sepsis and myocardial ischemia

Controversies

The MET service and deskilling of ward staff

The increasing use of MET services to manage acutely unwell hospital ward patients has the potential to deskill ward nursing and medical staff.[27] However, in a survey conducted at a hospital with a well-established MET service, most of the nurses questioned stated that the MET actually taught them how to better manage sick ward patients.[28]

Improved outcome is demonstrated only in single-centre studies

Reduction in cardiac arrests, unplanned ICU admission and other SAEs following introduction of MET services and RRSs has been shown in a number of single-centre studies.[20,21,29–31] A cluster randomized trial of 23 Australian hospitals was recently reported in which 12 hospitals introduced a MET system and 11 continued with usual care.[32] The study did not demonstrate that introduction of a MET service reduced the incidence of cardiac arrests, unplanned ICU admissions or unexpected deaths. While this finding may suggest that MET services do not improve the outcome of acutely unwell ward patients, the negative result is at least in part due to other factors. First, the education period preceding introduction of the MET was brief (4 months), and the subsequent call rate was only 8.3 calls/1000 admissions.[32] At the Austin hospital, a 1-year education period resulted in a progressive increase in the use of the MET to a call rate of >40 calls/1000 admissions.[33]

Most importantly, only 30% of the patients admitted to the ICU who had MET criteria actually received a MET call.[32] Combined, these findings suggest that the negative result of the MERIT study is at least in part due to a failure of MET use as opposed to a failure of the process of MET review.

Other controversies

A number of other problems of the MET service have been proposed[27,34] including inappropriate patient management because the MET is unfamiliar with the patient, diversion of attention away from adequate ward staffing and development of other strategies that might benefit acutely ill ward patients, diversion of critical care staff from their usual duties and conflict between MET staff and the ward staff caring for the patient.

Likely future developments

Despite the absence of level I evidence of the effectiveness of MET services, RRSs have been introduced into thousands of hospitals worldwide. RRSs are a key component of the Institute of Health Improvement's 100k campaign, which aims to save 100 000 lives across American hospitals.[35] For theses reasons, it is unlikely that further randomized trails will be conducted to assess the effectiveness of METs in improving the outcome of acutely unwell hospitalized patients.

The most important questions that need addressing regarding rapid responses systems and MET services in the near future include:

❶ Why do patients need MET calls? – clinical, disease state and system factors.

❷ What is the outcome of MET calls?

❸ What are barriers to MET activation?

❹ How can MET be most effectively used to review patients that are most likely to benefit from MET service intervention?

References

1. Devita MA, Bellomo R, Hillman K, et al. Findings of the first consensus conference on medical emergency teams. Critical Care Medicine 2006; 34(9): 2463–2478.
2. Wilson RM, Runciman WB, Gibberd RW, et al. The quality in Australian health care study. Medical Journal of Australia 1995; 163(9): 458–471.
3. Davis P, Lay-Yee R, Briant R, et al. Adverse events in New Zealand public hospitals I: occurrence and impact. New Zealand Medical Journal 2002; 115(1167): U271.
4. Davis P, Lay-Yee R, Briant R, et al. Adverse events in New Zealand public hospitals II: preventability and clinical context. New Zealand Medical Journal 2003; 116(1183): U624.
5. Vincent C, Neale G, Woloshynowych M. Adverse events in British hospitals: preliminary retrospective record review. British Medical Journal 2001; 322(7285): 517–519.
6. Baker GR, Norton PG, Flintoft V, et al. The Canadian Adverse Events Study: the incidence of adverse events among hospital patients in Canada. Canadian Medical Association Journal 2004; 170(11): 1678–1686.
7. Bellomo R, Goldsmith D, Russell S, et al. Postoperative serious adverse events in a teaching hospital: a prospective study. Medical Journal of Australia 2002; 176(5): 216–218.
8. Buist MD, Jarmolowski E, Burton PR, et al. Recognising clinical instability in hospital patients before cardiac arrest or unplanned admission to intensive care. A pilot study in a tertiary-care hospital. Medical Journal of Australia 1999; 171(1): 22–25.
9. Hodgetts TJ, Kenward G, Vlackonikolis I, et al. Incidence, location and reasons for avoidable in-hospital cardiac arrest in a district general hospital. Resuscitation 2002; 54(2): 115–123.
10. Nurmi J, Harjola VP, Nolan J, et al. Observations and warning signs prior to cardiac arrest. Should a medical emergency team intervene earlier? Acta Anaesthesiologica Scandinavica 2005; 49(5): 702–706.
11. Schein RM, Hazday N, Pena M, et al. Clinical antecedents to in-hospital cardiopulmonary arrest. Chest 1990; 98(6): 1388–1392.
12. Bell MB, Konrad D, Granath F, et al. Prevalence and sensitivity of MET-criteria in a Scandinavian University Hospital. Resuscitation 2006; 70(1): 66–73.
13. Buist M, Bernard S, Nguyen TV. Association between clinically abnormal observations and subsequent in-hospital mortality: a prospective study. Resuscitation 2004; 62(2): 137–141.
14. Goldhill DR, White SA, Sumner A. Physiological values and procedures in the 24 h before ICU admission from the ward. Anaesthesia 1999; 54(6): 529–534.
15. Hedges J, Adams A, Gunnels M. ATLS practices and survival at rural level trauma hospitals, 1995–1999. Prehospital Emergency Care 2002; 6: 299–305.
16. Nardi G, Riccioni L, Cerchiari E, et al. Impact of an integrated treatment approach to the severely injured patients (ISS > 16) on hospital mortality and quality of care. Minerva Anesthesiology 2002; 68: 25–35.
17. Fresco C, Carinci F, Maggioni AP, et al. Very early assessment of risk for in-hospital death among 11,483 patients with acute myocardial infarction. GISSI investigators. American Heart Journal 1999; 138(6 Pt 1): 1058–1064.
18. Rivers E, Nguyen B, Havstad S, et al. Early goal-directed therapy in the treatment of severe sepsis and septic shock. New England Journal Medicine 2001; 345(19): 1368–1377.
19. Lee A, Bishop G, Hillman KM. The medical emergency team. Anaesthesia and Intensive Care 1995; 23(2): 183–186.
20. Bellomo R, Goldsmith D, Uchino S, et al. Prospective controlled trial of effect of medical emergency team on postoperative morbidity and mortality rates. Critical Care Medicine 2004; 32(4): 916–921.
21. Bellomo R, Goldsmith D, Uchino S, et al. A prospective before-and-after trial of a medical emergency team. Medical Journal of Australia 2003; 179(6): 283–287.
22. De Vita M, Schaefer J, Lutz J, et al. Improving medical emergency team (MET) performance using a novel curriculum and a computerized human simulator. Quality and Safe Health Care 2005; 14: 326–331.

23. Jones D, Duke G, Green J, et al. Medical emergency team syndromes and an approach to their management. Critical Care 2006; 10(1): R30.
24. DeVita M. Medical emergency teams: deciphering clues to crises in hospitals. Critical Care 2005; 9(4): 325–326.
25. Daly FF, Sidney KL, Fatovich DM. The medical emergency team (MET): a model for the district general hospital. Australian New Zealand Journal of Medicine 1998; 28(6): 795–798.
26. Sebat F, Johnson D, Musthafa A, et al. A multidisciplinary community hospital program for early and rapid resuscitation of shock in non-trauma patients. Chest 2005; 127: 1729–1743.
27. Brown D, Bellomo R. Are medical emergency teams worth the cost? In: DeVita MA, Hillman K, Bellomo R, eds. Medical emergency teams: a guide to implementation and outcome measurement. New York: Springer; 2006.
28. Jones D, Baldwin I, McIntryre T, et al. Nurses' attitudes to a medical emergency team service in a teaching hospital. Quality & Safety in Health Care 2006; 15: 427–432.
29. Bristow PJ, Hillman KM, Chey T, et al. Rates of in-hospital arrests, deaths and intensive care admissions: the effect of a medical emergency team. Medical Journal of Australia 2000; 173(5): 236–240.
30. Buist MD, Moore GE, Bernard SA, et al. Effects of a medical emergency team on reduction of incidence of and mortality from unexpected cardiac arrests in hospital: preliminary study. British Medical Journal 2002; 324(7334): 387–390.
31. DeVita MA, Braithwaite RS, Mahidhara R, et al. Use of medical emergency team responses to reduce hospital cardiopulmonary arrests. Quality and Safe Health Care 2004; 13(4): 251–254.
32. Hillman K, Chen J, Cretikos M, et al. Introduction of the medical emergency team (MET) system: a cluster-randomised controlled trial. Lancet 2005; 365(9477): 2091–2097.
33. Jones D, Bates S, Warrillow S, et al. Effect of an education programme on the utilization of a medical emergency team in a teaching hospital. Internal Medicine Journal 2006; 36(4): 231–236.
34. Joyce C, McArthur C. Rapid response systems: have we MET the need? Critical Care Resuscitation 2007; 9: 127–128.
35. Overview of the 100,000 Lives Campaign [cited 2007 16th January]. Available from: http://www.ihi.org/IHI/Programs/Campaign/100kCampaignOverviewArchive.htm (cited 16 January 2007).

EMERGENCY MEDICAL SYSTEMS

27.1 Emergency department staffing

Sue Ieraci

ESSENTIALS

1 An appropriate emergency department staff mix is required to provide both high-quality and timely clinical care while maintaining sustainable working conditions for staff.

2 Clinical work for senior medical staff includes not only direct patient care, but also supervision and teaching of junior staff, coordination of patient flow and liaison with other clinicians.

3 Senior medical staff profile should provide protected time for administrative, educational and research roles.

4 In calculating staff numbers required, it is essential to consider not only the hours of extent of senior cover required, but also the volume of the clinical and non-clinical workload.

5 Precise numbers and types of staff required depend on individual and institutional work practices, and hospital roles.

General principles

Patients requiring emergency care have the right to timely care by skilled staff. The aim of staffing an emergency department (ED) is ultimately to provide care in an acceptable time according to the patient's clinical urgency (triage category). Staff working in the department also have the right to safe and manageable working conditions and reasonable job satisfaction.

As the activity of an ED fluctuates in both volume and acuity, a threshold level of staffing and resources is required in order to be prepared for likely influxes of patients. In addition, the staffing number and mix needs to take account of the important teaching role of EDs.

The precise number and designation of medical and other staff employed will be determined by the local work practices (what tasks are carried out and by whom). This chapter discusses staffing requirements under the current Australasian model of ED work practices. This includes a major supervisory and teaching role for consultants, and a significant proportion of specialist trainees and junior medical staff in the medical workforce, with a range of tasks, including venepuncture, test requisitioning and written documentation. In addition, roles are expanding into wider realms such as toxicology and observation medicine.

In the UK, there is a move away from the traditional model of staffing based on enthusiastic and committed, but relatively inexperienced, senior house officers, towards more care being delivered by senior medical staff: consultants, registrars, staff grades and associate specialists. There is significant expansion under way in the numbers of registrar training posts and consultants in EDs.

This expansion will ensure that more care is delivered by experienced medical staff in conjunction with nursing colleagues, particularly in the enhanced nurse practitioner role. The concept is of an experienced team of clinicians delivering care.

Calculating clinical workload

ED case-mix and costing studies have sought to measure the medical time commitment for various clinical conditions. Table 27.1.1 describes the approximate average medical time commitment for each of the Australasian Triage Scale categories:[1]

- The direct clinical workload can be calculated from census data (number of presentations by the triage category).
- Additional staffing will need to be added to cover the requirements of short stay units or other services.
- The workforce should be resourced and organized so that patients are treated within the benchmark times for their clinical acuity (triage category). The Australasian College for Emergency Medicine (ACEM) has defined benchmarks for waiting time by triage category (see Table 27.1.2).[2]
- Staffing should be adequate to achieve benchmark clinical performance, as well as providing for the various clinical and non-clinical medical roles that supplement direct patient care.

Medical staff

The medical workforce of Australasian EDs currently includes the following categories:

- consultants (specialist emergency physicians), including a medical director
- registrars (specialist trainees)
- senior non-specialist staff: experienced hospital medical officers
- junior medical staff: interns and resident medical officers who have not yet started specialty training.

Table 27.1.1 Australasian Triage Scale Categories

NTS category	Medical time (min)
Category 1	160
Category 2	80
Category 3	60
Category 4	40
Category 5	20

Table 27.1.2 Benchmarks for waiting time by triage category

	Category 1	Category 2	Category 3	Category 4	Category 5
Treatment acuity	Immediate	Within 10 min	Within 30 min	Within 60 min	Within 120 min
Benchmark performance	98%	95%	90%	90%	85%

The specialist practice of emergency medicine includes non-clinical roles (including departmental management and administration, planning, education, research and medico-political activities) as well as clinical roles. The non-clinical workload of an individual department varies with its size and role, the structure of its staffing and the other management systems within the institution. For senior staff, clinical work generally includes coordination of patient flow, bed management and supervision, and bedside teaching of junior staff, in addition to direct patient care. Some emergency physicians may have other particular roles, such as retrieval and hyperbaric medicine or toxicology services. The increasing number of academic staff may have major research and teaching commitments.

To cover these roles, the ACEM recommends a minimum of 30% non-clinical time for consultants (more for directors of departments) and 15% non-clinical time for registrars.

In 2003, the Australian Medical Workforce Advisory Committee (AMWAC) revised its initial recommendations for the emergency medicine specialist workforce (AMWAC Report 2002–2012, September 2003). The review recognized that greater numbers than previously recommended will be required to provide a 24-h, 7-day consultant cover for major referral hospitals, and a 16-h, 7-day consultant cover for urban district and major rural/regional centres. Throughout Australasia, EDs are experiencing increasing levels of activity. The calculation of medical staff numbers required for a particular department must include not only the extent of consultant cover required, but also the clinical workload and performance, local work practices, and the nature of clinical and non-clinical roles. Because of variations in roles and work practices between sites, it is not possible to devise a staffing profile that is

universally appropriate. Other recent changes in staffing patterns include employment across a network, increasing part-time work and sessional contract arrangements. Many emergency physicians are diversifying their practice profile to achieve a balanced and sustainable career, combining salaried and contract work, different types of hospitals and part-time work with a range of other interests.

Ancillary staff

Clerical, paramedical and other ancillary staff are essential to the efficient provision of emergency medical services. They should be specifically trained and experienced for ED work. Clerical staff have a crucial role, encompassing reception, registration, data entry and communications within and outside the department, as well as maintenance of medical records. Dedicated paramedical staff, including therapists and social workers, are important in providing thorough assessment and management of patients, including participating in disposition decisions and discharge support. Other staff, such as porters and ward assistants, play an important role in releasing clinical staff from non-clinical roles.

Optimizing work practices

Traditional hospital work practices involve systems and tasks that are inefficient for the smooth running of modern, busy EDs. In a work environment with a rapid patient throughput and large numbers of staff, efficient work practices are crucial in optimizing clinical performance as well as job satisfaction. A review of staff numbers and seniority cannot provide maximum benefit without consideration of the way the work is done, what tasks are done and by whom.

A review of ED work practices can encompass the following principles:

- re-allocation or deletion of inefficient tasks
- optimal use of ancillary and technical staff
- an extended clinical nursing role
- use of communication technology and data systems.

As the ED workforce develops greater seniority and specialization, and the demands of patient care increase, it is no longer possible to justify outdated work practices. Local research has shown that it is possible to improve clinical service provision by reorganizing roles and tasks in a sustainable way.[3] The opportunity exists to create a work environment that both delivers good clinical service and is rewarding and satisfying for staff.

Controversies and future directions

❶ The role of junior medical staff in Australasian EDs continues to evolve in the effort to balance clinical care and service provision with teaching and training. The ratio of senior to junior staff is crucial in maintaining safety and performance.

❷ Many urban and rural EDs rely on experienced doctors who have not completed specialist training in emergency medicine. As trained specialists begin to be employed in these EDs, hospitals should also aim to retain the expertise of other senior doctors.

❸ The role and cost-effectiveness of the nurse practitioner in urban EDs is a source of controversy. While there is ample scope for extended nursing practice, which is largely treatment-focused, the role of independent nursing practice within an ED staffed with senior doctors is still being evaluated.

References

1. Bond MJ, Erwich-Nijout MA, Phillips D, et al. Urgency, disposition and age groups: a case-mix model for emergency medicine. Emergency Medicine 1998; 10: 103–110.
2. Australasian College for Emergency Medicine Policy. P06, March 2006.
3. Morris J, Ieraci S, Bauman A, et al. Emergency department work practice review project: introduction of work practice model and development of clinical documentation system specifications. In: Emergency Department Work Practice Review Project, 2001.

27.2 Emergency department layout

Matthew W. G. Chu • Robert Dunn

ESSENTIALS

1 The layout of the emergency department should maximize access to every space with the minimum of cross-traffic.

2 The triage location should enable staff to directly observe and gain access to both the ambulance entry and the patient waiting areas.

3 The acute treatment area should be open, with all spaces directly observable from the staff station.

4 Supporting areas, such as the clean and dirty utilities, the medication room and equipment stores, should be centrally located.

5 Areas often poorly planned include office, clinical spaces and tutorial rooms. The number of data and telephone entry points and the amount of storage space required are often underestimated.

6 Planning should consider the implications on night staffing when minimal staff are on duty.

7 The security of staff and patients is paramount in planning an emergency department.

undifferentiated conditions which may be critical to semi-urgent in nature. The ED may contribute between 15 and 75% of the hospital's total number of admissions. It plays an important role in the hospital's response to trauma, and in the reception and management of disaster victims. To optimize its core function, the department should be purpose-built, providing a safe environment for both patients and staff. The physical environment includes an effective communication system, appropriate signposting, adequate ambulance access and clear observation of relevant areas from the triage area. There should be easy access to the resuscitation area, and quiet and private areas should cater to patients and relatives. Adequate staff facilities and tutorial areas should be available. Clean and dirty utilities and storage areas are also required.

Introduction

The emergency department (ED) is a core clinical unit within a hospital. The experience and satisfaction of patients attending the ED are significant contributors to the public image of the hospital. Its primary function is to receive, triage, stabilize and provide emergency care to patients who present with a wide range of

Design considerations

The design of the department should promote rapid access to every area with the minimum of cross-traffic. There must be proximity between the resuscitation and

Table 27.2.1 Configurations for clinical areas

	Resuscitation	Acute treatment	Specialty plaster/ procedure	Consultation room
Oxygen outlets	3	2	2	1
Medical air outlets	2	1	1	-
Suction outlets	3	2	1	1
Nitrous oxide	1	1	1	-
Scavenging unit	1	1	1	-
Power outlets	16	8	8	4

the acute treatment areas for non-ambulant patients. Supporting areas, such as clean and dirty utilities, the pharmacy room and equipment stores, should be centrally located to prevent staff traversing long distances. The main aggregation of clinical staff will be at the staff station in the acute treatment area. This is the focus around which the other clinical areas should be grouped.

Lighting should conform to national standards and clinical care areas should have exposure to daylight whenever possible to minimize patient disorientation. Climate control is essential for the comfort of both patients and staff. Each clinical area needs to be serviced with medical gases, suction, scavenging units and power outlets. The minimum suggested configuration for each type of clinical area is outlined in Table 27.2.1.

Medical gases should be internally piped to all patient care areas, and adequate cabling should ensure the availability of power outlets to all clinical and non-clinical areas. Although patient and emergency call facilities are often considered, there is often inadequate provision for telephone and information technology ports. Emergency power must be available to all lights and power outlets in the resuscitation and acute treatment areas. All computer terminals in the department should have access to emergency power, and emergency lighting should be available in all other areas. The electricity supply should be surge protected to protect electronic and computer equipment, physiological monitoring areas should be cardiac protected, and other patient care areas should be body protected.

Approximately 35–45% of the total area of the department is circulation space. An example of this would be the provision of corridors wide enough to allow the easy passage

of two hospital beds with attached intravenous fluids. Although circulation space should be kept to a minimum, functionality, fire safety, and occupational health and safety requirements also need to be considered. The floor covering in all patient care areas should be durable and non slip, easy to clean, impermeable to water and body fluids, and with properties that reduce sound transmission and absorb shocks. Areas accommodating the administrative functions, interviewing and distressed relatives should be carpeted.

Size and composition of the emergency department

The appropriate size of the ED depends on a number of factors: the census, patient mix and acuity, the admission rate, the desired performance level manifested in waiting times, the length of stay of patients in the ED and the role delineation of the department. Departments of inadequate size are uncomfortable for patients, often function inefficiently, and may significantly impair patient care. Overcrowding of patients increases the risk of infectious disease transmission and increases harmful cognitive stimulation for patients with mental disturbance. For the average Australasian ED with an admission rate of approximately 25–35%, its total internal area (excluding departmental radiology facilities and observation/holding ward) should be approximately 50 m^2/1000 yearly attendances. The total number of patient treatment areas (excluding interview, plaster and procedure rooms) should be at least 1/1100 yearly attendances, and the number of resuscitation areas should be at least one for every 15 000 yearly attendances. It is recommended

that, for departments with average patient acuity, at least half the total number of treatment areas should have physiological monitoring available.

Clinical areas

Individual treatment areas

The design of individual treatment areas should be determined by their specific functions. Adequate space should be allowed around the bed for patient transfer, assessment, performance of procedures and storage of commonly used items. The use of modular storage bins or other materials employing a similar design concept should be considered.

To prevent transmission of confidential information, each area should be separated by solid partitions that extend from floor to ceiling. The entrance to each area should be able to be closed by a movable partition or curtain.

Each acute treatment bed should have access to a physiological monitor. Central monitoring is recommended and monitors should ideally be of the modular type, with print and monitoring modules. The minimum monitored physiological parameters should include SpO$_2$, NIBP (non-invasive blood pressure), electrocardiogram (ECG), and temperature. Monitors may be mounted adjacent to the bed on an appropriate pivoting bracket, or be movable.

All patient care areas, including toilets and bathrooms, require individual patient call facilities and emergency call facilities, so urgent assistance can be summoned when required. In addition, an examination light, a sphygmomanometer, ophthalmoscope and otoscope, waste disposal and footstool should all be immediately available. Basins for hand washing should be readily available.

Resuscitation area

This area is used for the resuscitation and treatment of critically ill or injured patients. It must be large enough to fit a standard resuscitation bed, allow access to all parts of the patient and allow movement of staff and equipment around the work area. As space must also be provided for equipment, monitors, storage, wash-up and disposal facilities, the minimum suitable size for such a room is usually 35 m^2 (including storage area), or 25 m^2 (excluding storage area) for each bed space in a multi-bedded room. The area should also have visual and auditory privacy for both the occupants of the room and other patients and their relatives. The resuscitation area should be easily accessible from the ambulance entrance and the staff station, and be separate from patient circulation areas. In addition to standard physiological monitoring, invasive pressure and capnography monitoring should be available. Other desirable features include a ceiling-mounted operating theatre light, a radiolucent resuscitation trolley with cassette trays, overhead X-ray and lead lining of walls and partitions between beds.

Acute treatment area

This area is used for the assessment, treatment and observation of patients with acute medical or surgical illnesses. Each bed space must be large enough to fit a standard mobile bed, with adequate storage and circulation space. The recommended minimum space between beds is 2.4 m and each treatment area should be at least 12 m^2. All of these beds should be positioned to enable direct observation from the staff station and easy access to the clean and dirty utility rooms, procedure room, pharmacy room and patient shower and toilet.

Single rooms

These rooms should be used for the management of patients who require isolation, privacy, or who are a source of visual, olfactory or auditory distress to others. Deceased patients may also be placed there for the convenience of grieving relatives. These rooms must be completely enclosed by floor-to-ceiling partitions but allow controlled visual access and have a solid door. Each department should have at least two such rooms. The isolation room is used to treat potentially infectious patients. The isolation room should be located in an area which does not allow cross infection to other patients in the emergency department. Each isolation room should have negative-pressure ventilation, an ante room with change and scrub facilities and be self-contained with en-suite facilities. A decontamination area should be available for patients contaminated with toxic substances. In addition to the design requirements of an isolation room, this room must have a floor drain and contaminated water trap. The decontamination area should be directly accessible from the ambulance bay and be located in an area

which will prevent the ED from being contaminated in the event of a chemical or biological incident. Single rooms should otherwise have the same requirements as acute treatment area bed spaces.

Acute mental health area

This is a specialty area designed specifically for the assessment, protection and containment of patients with actual or potential behavioural disturbances. Ideally, each unit comprises two separate but adjacent rooms allowing for interview and examination/treatment functions. Each room should have two doors large enough to allow a patient to be carried through, and must be lockable only from the outside. One of the doors may be of the 'barn door' type, enabling the lower section to be closed while the upper section remains open. This allows direct observation of and communication with the patient without requiring staff to enter the room. Each room should be squarely configured and be at least 16 m^2 in size to enable a restraint team of five members to contain a patient without the potential of injury to a staff member. The examination/treatment room will facilitate physical examination or chemical restraint when indicated. The unit should be shielded from external noise, located as far away as possible from external sources of stimulation (e.g. noise, traffic) and must be designed in such a way that direct observation of the patient by staff outside the room is possible at all times. Services such as electricity, medical gases and air vents or hanging points should not be accessible to the patient. It is preferable that furniture be made of foam rubber and no materials be accessible that could be used as weapons or for inflicting self-harm. A smoke detector should be fitted, and closed-circuit television may be used in addition to direct visual monitoring.

Consultation area

Consultation rooms are provided for the examination and treatment of ambulant patients who are not suffering a major or serious illness. These rooms have similar space requirements to acute treatment area bed spaces. In addition, they are equipped with office furniture, radiological viewing panel and a basin for hand washing. Consultation rooms may be adapted and equipped to serve specific functions, such as ENT or ophthalmology treatment, or as part of a

fast track area to treat patients with non-complex single system diseases.

Plaster room

The plaster room allows for the application of splints, plaster of Paris and for the closed reduction of displaced fractures or dislocations, and should be at least 20 m^2 in size. Physiological equipment to monitor the patient during procedures involving regional anaesthesia or sedation is required. Specific features of such a room include a storage area for plaster, splints and bandages; X-ray viewing panels; provision of oxygen and suction; a nitrous oxide delivery system; plaster trolley with plaster instruments; and a sink and drainer with a plaster trap. Ideally, a splint and crutch store should be directly accessible in the plaster room.

Procedure room

A procedure room(s) may be required to undertake procedures such as lumbar puncture, tube thoracostomy, thoracocentesis, diagnostic peritoneal lavage, bladder catheterization or suturing. It requires noise insulation and should be at least 20 m^2 in size.

Staff station

A single central staff area is recommended for staff servicing the different treatment areas, as this enables better communication between, and coordination of, staff members. The staff station in the acute treatment area should be the major staff area within the department. The staff area should be of an 'arena' or 'semi-arena' design, whereby the main areas of clinical activity are directly observable. The station may be raised in order to give uninterrupted vision of patients, and should be centrally located. It should be constructed to ensure that confidential information can be conveyed without breach of privacy. Sliding windows and adjustable blinds may be used to modulate external stimuli, and a separate write-up area may be considered. Sufficient space should be available to house an adequate number of telephones, computer terminals, printers and data outlets, and X-ray viewing panels/digital imaging systems; dangerous drug/medication cupboards; emergency and patient call displays; under-desk duress alarm; valuables storage area; police blood alcohol sample safe; photocopier and stationery store;

and write-up areas and workbenches. Direct telephone lines, bypassing the hospital switchboard, should be available to allow staff to receive admitting requests from outside medical practitioners or to participate in internal or external emergencies when the need arises. A dedicated line to the ambulance and police service is essential, as is the provision of a facsimile line. A pneumatic tube system for transporting specimens to pathology and transferring medical records and imaging requests may also be located in this area.

Short-stay unit

Many EDs operate short-stay units that support the function of the department. The purpose of these units is to manage patients who would benefit from extended treatment and observation but have an expected length of stay of less than 24 h. It is considered that the minimum functional unit size is eight beds. It is configured along similar lines to a hospital ward with its own staff station. The capacity is calculated to be 1 bed per 4000 attendances per year and its size will be influenced by its function and case mix. As short stay units are usually high volume users of mental health, social work, physiotherapy, drug and alcohol and community support services, appropriate space should be allocated to allow these services to operate.

Medical assessment and planning unit

A medical assessment and planning unit is an inpatient hospital unit which may either be co-located or built near an ED. It is managed by inpatient medical teams. The purpose is to facilitate the assessment and treatment of patients who require coordinated multidisciplinary team interventions minimizing length of stay and optimizing health outcomes. Its configuration and function is determined by case mix and local operational policies. It is usually configured up to 30 beds along similar lines to a hospital ward.

Clinical support areas

The clean utility area requires sufficient space for the storage of clean and sterile supplies and procedural equipment, and bench tops to prepare procedure trays. The dirty utility should have sufficient space to house a

stainless steel bench top with sink and drainer, pan and bottle rack, bowl and basin rack, utensil washer, pan/bowl washer/sanitizer, and slop hopper and storage space for testing equipment (such as for urinalysis). A separate store room may be used for the storage of equipment and disposable medical supplies. A common design fault is to underestimate the amount of storage space required for a modern department. A pharmacy/medication room may be used for the storage of medications used by the department, and should be accessible to all clinical areas. Entry should be secure with a self-closing door, and the area should have sufficient space to house a refrigerator for the storage of heat-sensitive drugs. Other design features should include spaces for a linen trolley, mobile radiology equipment, patient trolleys and wheelchairs. Beverage-making facilities for patients and relatives, a blanket-warming cupboard, disaster equipment store, a cleaners' room and shower and toilet facilities also need to be accommodated. An interview room may be designated for the interviewing or counselling of relatives in private. It should be acoustically treated and removed from the main clinical area of the department. A distressed relatives' room should be provided for the relatives of seriously ill or deceased patients. Consideration for two such rooms should be given in larger departments to allow the separation of relatives of patients who have been protagonists in violent incidents or clashes. They should be acoustically insulated and have access to beverage-making facilities, a toilet and telephones. A single-room treatment area should be in close proximity to these rooms to enable relatives to be with dying patients, and should be of a size appropriate to local cultural practices.

Non-clinical areas

Waiting area

The waiting area should provide sufficient space for waiting patients as well as relatives or escorts, and should be open and easily observed from the triage and reception areas. Seating should be comfortable and adequate space should be allowed for wheelchairs, prams, walking aids and patients being assisted. There should be an area where children may play, and support facilities such as television should be available. Easy access

from the waiting room to the triage and reception area, toilets and baby change rooms, and light refreshment should be possible. Public telephones should be accessible and dedicated telephones with direct lines to taxi firms should be encouraged. The area should be monitored to safeguard security and patient well-being, and it is desirable to have a separate waiting area for children. The waiting area should be at least 5 m²/1000 yearly attendances, and should contain at least one seat per 1000 yearly attendances.

Reception/triage area

The department should be accessed by two separate entrances: one for ambulance patients and the other for ambulant patients. It is recommended that each contain a separate foyer that can be sealed by the remote activation of security doors. Access to treatment areas should also be restricted by the use of security doors. Both entrances should direct the patient flow towards the reception/triage area, which should have clear vision to the waiting room and the ambulance entrance. The triage area should have access to a pulse oximeter, a computer terminal, a hand basin, examination light, telephones, chairs and desk, and patient weighing scales, and should have adequate storage space for bandages, medical equipment and stationery.

Reception/clerical office

Staff at the reception counter receive patients arriving for treatment and direct them to the triage area. After assessment there, patients or relatives will generally be directed back to the reception/clerical area, where clerical staff will conduct registration interviews, collate the medical record and print identification labels. When a decision to admit has been made, clerks also interview patients or relatives at the bedside or at the reception counter to finalize admission details. The counter should provide seating and be partitioned for privacy at the interview. There should be direct communication with the reception/triage area, the staff station in the acute treatment area, and the design should take due consideration of the safety of staff. This area should have access to an adequate number of telephones, computer terminals, printers, facsimile machines and photocopier. It should also have sufficient storage space for stationery and medical records.

Tutorial room

This room provides facilities for formal undergraduate and postgraduate education and meetings. It should be in a quiet, non-clinical area near the staff room and offices. Provision should be made for a DVD/VCR, television, projectors and screen, whiteboard, power outlets, tube X-ray viewer or picture archiving communication system, telephone and examination couch.

Telemedicine area

Departments using telemedicine facilities should have a dedicated, fully enclosed room with appropriate power and communications cabling. This room should be of suitable size to allow simultaneous viewing by members of multiple service teams, and should, ideally, be close to the staff station.

Offices

Offices provide space for the administrative, managerial, quality assurance, teaching and research roles of the ED. The number of offices required will be determined by the number and type of staff. In a large department, offices may be needed for the director, deputy director, nurse manager, academic staff, staff specialists, registrars, nurse consultants/practitioners, nurse educator, secretary, social worker/mental health crisis worker, information support officer, research and projects officers and clerical supervisor. Larger departments may consider the incorporation of a meeting room into the office area.

Staff facilities

A room should be provided within the department to enable staff to relax during rest periods. Food and drink should be able to be prepared and appropriate table and seating arrangements should be provided. It should be located away from patient care areas and have access to natural lighting and appropriate floor and wall coverings. A staff changing area with lockers, toilets and shower facilities should also be provided.

Likely developments over the next 5–10 years

Over the last 20 years EDs have been providing care of an ever-increasing complexity. Changes in technology have enabled the management of greater numbers of patients in the community who would previously have required hospitalization. As financial pressures on hospitals have also increased, the importance of the ED has grown considerably, and modern departments have significantly expanded facilities. Future design considerations are likely to centre on advances in the areas of information technology, telecommunications and new non-invasive diagnostic modalities. In addition to these technologically driven changes, it is likely that a greater emphasis will be placed on developing ED design configurations that maximize efficient work practices. Computerized patient tracking systems using electronic tags and built-in sensors will provide additional information that may further improve operational efficiency. The electronic medical record will make detailed medical information immediately available and will greatly facilitate quality improvement and research activities. Digital radiography, personal communication devices, voice recognition systems and expanded telemedicine facilities will make the ED of the future as reliant on electricity and cabling as it is on oxygen and suction.

The increasing age of the population needs also to be considered when designing an ED. Older patients are more likely to have poor mobility, vision and balance as well as being at increased risk of delirium due to underlying disease or hospitalization. They are likely to require greater space for the use of mobility aids and require greater shielding from sources of cognitive overstimulation than other patients. Standard hospital trolleys may pose a falls risk and contribute to the development of pressure areas so consideration should be given to the use of more comfortable 'reclining lounge chair' style seating or hospital beds for this group of patients. Adequate lighting and the maintenance of a normal diurnal 'night-day' light pattern should be considered for elderly patients who spend prolonged periods of time in the emergency department.

Controversies

❶ Expert opinion significantly differs in the design of security features. Some experts argue that the use of physical barriers to isolate potentially violent people may cause further aggravation to those people, and this may have the paradoxical effect of increasing the incidence of violence. Others argue that protective physical features are of significant benefit, as staff feel less vulnerable to physical attack and are, therefore, better able to diffuse potentially violent situations.

❷ Another area of debate relates to how patient privacy can be protected while still maintaining the ability to closely monitor patients within the department. Advocates of the direct observation of all patients believe that the resultant loss of privacy is a small price to pay to prevent the deterioration of a small number of patients with unrecognized severe illness. Opponents of this view believe that a significant number of patients in emergency departments do not require constant observation, and that 'open-plan' departments inhibit good communication and create a noisy and distressing environment. A satisfactory solution that meets the requirements of each group can be obtained by the use of solid partitions between treatment areas while leaving the entrance to each area open. Ceiling baffles installed in the staff station significantly reduces noise transmission. If the treatment areas are also arranged in such a way that they surround the staff base, direct observation of each area is still possible.

Further reading

A look at our new emergency department series, Journal of Emergency Nursing, 1992–6.

American Institute of Architects/Facilities Guidelines Institute. Guidelines for Design and Construction of Health Care Facilities; 2006.

Christie C. Waiting for Health – Strategies and Evidence for Emergency Waiting Areas, Inform ED Program; 2005.

Emergency Unit Design Guidelines. Health Department of Western Australia Facilities Unit; 1995.

Guidelines on Emergency Department Design. Australasian College for Emergency Medicine; 2007.

Huddy J. Emergency Department Design – A Practical Guide to Planning for the Future, American College of Emergency Physicians; 2002.

Huddy J, McKay JI. The Top 25 problems to avoid when planning your new emergency department, Journal of Emergency Nursing 1996; 22(4): 296–301.

McKay JI. Building the Emergency Department of the Future: Philosophical, operational and physical dimensions, Nursing Clinics of North America 2002; 37(1): 111–22, vii.

http://www.akhdem.co.nz/newed.htm (accessed 5 Oct 2008). Pictorial tour of major ED.

http://www.qehae.dircon.co.uk/gallery/tour.htm (accessed 5 Oct 2008).

www.healthcaredesignmagazine.com (accessed 5 Oct 2008 but no longer accessible).

27.3 Quality assurance/quality improvement

Diane King

ESSENTIALS

1 Quality management plays a pivotal role in the running of an emergency department and in patient safety.

2 All staff must be engaged in the process of quality improvement.

3 Data and performance measures are an integral part of the quality cycle.

Introduction

A primary role of the emergency department (ED) is to deliver the best possible care to presenting patients. In order to deliver optimal care, a system of quality management must be part of the culture for all staff and must be applied to all functions of the department. Quality management requires effective leadership, organizational vision, strategic development, commitment to improving processes and systems, accountability, communication, support for staff development and commitment to analysis, change and review. Quality management is a continuous cycle, with measurement and monitoring required to establish that change is required, planning and implementation of the change and re-evaluation and monitoring to ensure the change has the desired effect. Consumer involvement is a fundamental part of quality management. In the emergency setting, consumers include patients, staff and the other clinical and hospital staff who interface with the ED.

History

The traditional approach of quality assurance involves a number of retrospective attempts to police various activities of the ED. The types of tools used in this approach are pathology result checking, missed fractures, medical record reviews, death audits and patient complaints. Although these checks are essential, it must be recognized that the traditional quality-assurance (QA) philosophy involves crisis management and implies 'fault', and the apportioning of blame. The trend currently involves movement from the QA model to the philosophy of total quality improvement and total quality management (TQM).[1] This management system has been adopted from industrial models, and applied to hospitals.[2] Much of the change has been triggered by the climate of accountability and clinical governance.

Definitions

- Quality – 'doing those things necessary to meet the needs and reasonable expectations of those we service, and doing those things right every time.'[2]
- Quality assurance (QA) – 'a system used to establish standards for patient care, to monitor how well standards of care are met, and to correct unwarranted deviations from the standards.'[3]
This implies intervention to correct deficiencies, and is often externally driven.
- Quality improvement (QI) – raising quality performance to ever increasing levels.
- Continuous quality improvement (CQI) – a management approach that focuses on providing a service that meets the 'customers' needs in such a fashion that the process itself leads to continuous improvement. This uses data collection, statistical tools and team dynamics to develop quality processes.
- Total quality management (TQM) – uses the management approach of continuous quality improvement, and implies the commitment of the whole organization to the implementation of a quality plan. This involves the crossing of boundaries, and traditional spheres of activity.
- Clinical indicators – measures of the clinical outcomes of care. They are population-based screens that help point to potential problems. They also allow comparative data to be collected nationally and benchmarking to occur.
- Clinical guidelines – are reference tools that help guide clinical practice. They provide a focus for standardization and a reference point for peer review.
- Benchmarking – comparing performance with others, and the use of the best practices in a field to act as a marker and goal for improvement.[4]
- Credentialling – a formal process to recognize and verify an individual's qualifications to enable a view of their capacity to perform safely in relation to a particular field or task

Continuous quality improvement

The Deming cycle (described by WE Deming) is a fundamental tool for the approach to quality in any system. The PDCA (plan, do, check, act) cycle should incorporate the important sequential steps of planning, staff engagement, implementation, measurement, re-measurement and re-evaluation, followed by an improved plan and so on.

A QI system covers a number of dimensions. These are:

- access, e.g. waiting times and access to inpatient beds
- safety, e.g. body fluid exposures, work-related injury, stress
- acceptability, e.g. complaint rates, staff and patient satisfaction surveys
- effectiveness, e.g. time to thrombolysis, unplanned representations, appropriate antibiotic prescribing

- continuity, e.g. discharge letters to GPs, wound, plaster and head-injury advice.

There are a number of vital characteristics of a CQI programme that are necessary for its successful operation.[1] A CQI programme:

- requires leadership (management) commitment and strategic planning
- is 'customer' focused. Customers include patients primarily, but also relatives, staff, other departments within the hospital, students, ambulance personnel, and anyone who is involved with the functioning of the ED
- is performance-based. This requires accurate and relevant performance measures, monitoring and benchmarking
- focuses around clear governance structures and accountability
- has effective communication and change management
- focuses on systems first, and individuals second. This acknowledges the fact that a perfect world does not exist, but that quality can always be improved within a system (improving the norm), and takes the emphasis away from apportioning blame
- incorporates a risk management framework, with risk analysis and monitoring, risk mitigation and where possible risk avoidance
- includes sound credentialling processes.

A more detailed outline of TQM is beyond the scope of this book; however, the recent literature abounds with discussion on the various tools used, pitfalls in introduction, and so on.[5-14]

National bodies

The push to TQM has been facilitated by various bodies, including The Australian Council on Healthcare Standards (ACHS), that in 1997 introduced its Evaluation and Quality Improvement Program (EQuIP) as a framework for hospitals to establish quality processes.[15] This is a requirement for accreditation with the ACHS. In 2006, the Australian Commission for Safety and Quality of Health Care was established to oversee improvements in the Australian context (previously the Australian Council

for Safety and Quality). In the USA, the Joint Commission on Accreditation of Healthcare Organizations (JCAHO) and the Institute for Healthcare Improvement have led the way in the move from QA to QI.[16-17]

The Australasian College for Emergency Medicine, the American College of Emergency Physicians and the British Association for Accident and Emergency Medicine are facilitating the process of QI by their training role, introduction of clinical indicators, policy development and standards for EDs.[18-19] In Australasia, the introduction of the Australasian Triage Scale, which has been widely adopted in EDs, has been used in the process of benchmarking, and the development of standards.[20]

Quality in the ED

The ED is a complex environment, which involves close interaction with the rest of the hospital and the community. The inputs are uncontrollable and unregulated, and the 'customers' are under a high level of stress because of the nature of their problems, the unfamiliarity of the environment and the lack of control they perceive at a time when they are feeling personally vulnerable.

The ED is dealing simultaneously with life-threatening illness and minor complaints. It is an area under a high level of scrutiny from all quarters, the patients, the families and friends, the other departments in the hospital, and the wider community – both medical and non-medical. This in itself is stressful, and is compounded by the fact that many of the staff working in the ED are rotating through the department for relatively short periods of time, are often relatively junior and are undergoing training themselves. This training role is of critical importance in most EDs, and must not be forgotten in any process dealing with quality issues. All these aspects of an ED make the maintenance of quality difficult and all the more imperative. In order to establish a system where quality care can be delivered with any degree of reliability, it is important that all staff are committed to the process, and that management provide appropriate leadership and resources. The delivery of quality involves a continuing

process of data collection (performance measures), analysis, feedback and introduction of strategies to improve the system, followed by re-analysis of the performance measures (the quality cycle).

Common measures of clinical performance or outcome

The following are commonly used measures:

- time to thrombolysis or percutaneous coronary intervention (PCI)
- waiting time by triage category
- death audits – and morbidity or adverse event reviews
- admission rates by triage category
- access block measures
- chart audits for specific complaints
- total ED treatment time
- time to analgesia, or time to antibiotic for sentinel diagnoses such as febrile neutropenia
- trauma audits – missed cervical fractures, delay in craniotomy
- patient satisfaction surveys
- staff satisfaction surveys
- X-ray and pathology report follow-up
- patient complaints audits
- equipment functioning and supply
- safety of the working environment including for example, electrical safety or violent incidents
- staff retention or sick leave.

The first three of these are the current ACHS/ACEM Clinical Indicators for Emergency Medicine.[17]

It is clear from the list that the measures are potentially innumerable, that local factors must dictate those areas of special interest and that this will vary from hospital to hospital. In deciding which areas should be measured it is important to focus on areas that have been targeted as requiring improvement.

It is also evident that all EDs have common areas where there is high potential for problems to develop, and that these areas should be routinely monitored. The mechanism for doing this will vary from institution to institution.

Another aspect of the measuring of performance is that the process is one in evolution.

Not only should the quality of the service improve as the measures are improved and re-assessed, but the areas for attention can change and develop with the whole system. Peeling off layers as problems are addressed, exposes new things to improve. Again, this process must be internally driven to be effective. There is little point in collecting an enormous amount of data, unless the process is useful to the improved functioning of the whole system. Those best able to make those improvements should be an integral part of the system.

Likely developments over the next 5–10 years

- There will be more of a focus on credentialling for practice
- Practice is likely to be increasingly standardized. Standardization is the platform from which quality care is delivered.
- Patient safety will be a growing priority.

- There will be increasing professional accountability and public access to performance measure and benchmarks.
- Information technology will be used to support quality and safety.

References

1. O'Leary DS, O'Leary MR. From quality assurance to quality improvement. The Joint Commission on Accreditation of Healthcare Organizations and Emergency Care. Emergency Medicine Clinics of North America 1992; 10(3): 447–491.
2. Mayer TA. Industrial models of continuous quality improvement. Implications for emergency medicine. Emergency Medicine Clinics of North America 1992; 10 (3): 523–447.
3. American College of Emergency Physicians. Quality assurance manual for emergency medicine. Dallas: American College of Emergency Physicians; 1986.
4. American College of Emergency Physicians. Benchmarking in emergency medicine: an information paper. Dallas: American College of Emergency Physicians; 1997.
5. Juran JM. The quality trilogy: a universal approach to managing for quality. Quality Progress. 1986 August; 19: 19–24.
6. Allison EJ. Continuous quality improvement in emergency medicine. Dallas: American College of Emergency Physicians News; 1992: pp. 4–5.
7. Carlin E, Carlson R, Nordin J. Using continuous quality improvement tools to improve pediatric immunization rates. Journal on Quality Improvement 1996; 22: 277–287.
8. Fernades C, Christenson J. Use of CQI to facilitate patient flow throughout the triage and fast-track areas

of an ED. Journal of Emergency Medicine. 1995; 13(6): 847–855.
9. Howland R, Decker M. Continuous quality improvement and hospital epidemiology: common themes. Quality Management in Health Care 1992; 1: 9–12.
10. Kaissier JP. The quality of care and the quality of measuring it. New England Journal of Medicine 1993; 329: 1263–1264.
11. Brown MG, Hitchcock DE, Willard ML. Why TQM Fails. Toronto: Irwin Publishing; 1994.
12. Berwick DM. Quality comes home. Annals of Internal Medicine 1996; 125: 839–843.
13. Berwick DM. Continuous improvement as an ideal in health care. New England Journal of Medicine 1989; 320: 53–56.
14. Kennedy MP, Cleaton PGA, Harrington AP, et al. Quality assurance to continuous quality improvement: development of an emergency department system. Emergency Medicine 1997; 9: 247–253.
15. Australian Council on Healthcare Standards. The Australian Council on Healthcare Standards EQuIP Standards. 4th edn. Melbourne: Australian Council on Healthcare Standards; May 2006.
16. Joint Commission on Accreditation of Health Care Organizations. Accreditation manual for hospitals. Joint Commission on Accreditation for Health Care Organizations; 1991.
17. Institute for Healthcare Improvement. http://www.ihi.org.
18. The Australian Council on Healthcare Standards Clinical indicators, a users' manual. Emergency medicine indicators, version 3. The Australian Council on Healthcare Standards, Melbourne.
19. Australasian College for Emergency Medicine Policy Document. Quality Management in Emergency Medicine. P28 July 2002.
20. Standards Committee Australasian College for Emergency Medicine. National Triage Scale. Emergency Medicine 1994; 6: 145–146.

27.4 Business planning

Richard H. Ashby

ESSENTIALS

1 The business plan is an important multipurpose document developed annually by the emergency department (ED) management group, to inform the organization about the agreed performance dimensions of expenditure, activity, efficiency and quality of services proposed for the next financial year.

2 The basic content of the business plan should include a projection and analysis of the current year's performance, together with proposed budget, activity, efficiency and quality targets and indicators for the next financial year. Additional issues which may require inclusion are capital expenditure, information and communication technology and special projects.

3 Once approved by the hospital executive, the ED management group should regularly monitor actual outcomes against the targets and take remedial action where necessary.

Introduction

Emergency departments (EDs) in public sector health services in Australasia are typically mid-sized clinical units within the organizational structures of hospitals. Staff numbers may range from 20 to over 200 and expenditure budgets from $1m to over $20m per annum. ED efficiency directly affects the global efficiency of the healthcare process in the hospital, and purchasers are therefore increasingly interested in the value and performance of emergency medicine services. ED managers are being required to report on the dimensions of cost, output, quality and efficiency through a business planning process and other reporting mechanisms in order to justify their level of resourcing.

Types of plans

ED plans are relatively low in the hierarchy of planning instruments that begin with national and state health policy, health departments' strategic and corporate plans, regional and hospital strategic and business plans and, finally, the business and project plans of individual clinical units and departments. Strategic plans describe how organizations propose to respond to changing technology, altered demographics, shifting paradigms of care and industrial and regulatory reform, as well as issues associated with the cost, quality and accessibility of health care. These plans typically look 5–10 years into the future, and the ED should reasonably expect to have input at a variety of levels into the strategic planning process.

Project plans, on the other hand, are highly focused on a particular objective outcome to be achieved within a given timeframe, and with a specified level of resources. Project plans may need to be created by an ED for the implementation of a new and significant piece of technology, major refurbishment or redevelopment, or some types of work practice reform. However, the most important planning instrument for an ED is its annual business plan.

The business plan

The business plan is an important multipurpose document that needs to be developed by the ED management group, in consultation with hospital management, on an annual basis. At one level, the business plan represents a management contract between the executive of the hospital and the ED. At another level, the business plan provides information to the staff of the department about the agreed targets for expenditure, activity, efficiency and quality of services to be provided in the next financial year.

Planning process

The plan should be developed by the medical director, business manager and nurse manager of the ED. It is often useful to include a representative from the hospital's financial services department early in the process, so that there is a clear understanding of the financial framework for the plan. It is vitally important that the process be informed with as much useful data as possible, including accurate and up-to-date financial and activity statistics, and quality and efficiency indicators. The premises, or context, of the business plan need to be established. Unless there are specific reasons for change, it can usually be assumed that hospital managers will require that the business plan be based on management of the same level of activity at a similar quality to the previous year. Other assumptions, relating to estimated wages growth, non-labour cost escalations, leave requirements and so on, should be stated.

The timing of business plan development depends on the government budget cycle for public sector EDs and the timing of the financial year for private sector EDs. In most jurisdictions this process needs to commence in early January, with the draft business plan available for the hospital executive by the end of February. The process may need to begin much earlier if significant additional or special funding is being sought. Such requests are best handled as separate submissions, which will then need to pass through the various evaluation and approval steps to be finally included in the government's forward estimates and budget. It is uncommon for special projects requiring substantial funds to be approved and funded within one budget cycle.

A typical business planning cycle is illustrated in Figure 27.4.1.

Business plan content

The ED business plan must address, as a minimum, each of the dimensions of performance, that is, expenditure, activity, quality and efficiency. A typical index is illustrated in Table 27.4.1. Some hospitals may require that their own format be used.

The introduction to the business plan should be brief. It is often useful to re-state the role and objectives of the ED, and of any of its subunits. The executive summary should present an overview of the business plan, including a general perspective on the integrity of the budget and activity targets for the current year, and outlining any premises used in the creation of the current plan. Special issues may be highlighted.

Budget

The projected financial outcomes for the current financial year should have been

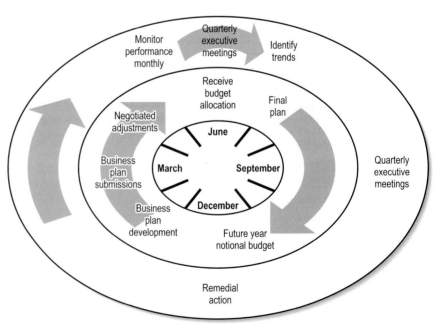

Fig. 27.4.1 Business plan cycle.

carefully estimated. This projected end-of-year position should be shown in a tabular format against the agreed targets from the previous year's business plan, as well as the actual outcomes of the previous year. In government organizations, adherence to budget is the highest priority and, therefore, the budget details should be presented first. The management group should have a detailed understanding of every variance from the budget that has occurred in the current year, and a note of explanation of variance on every line item should be provided. Because the high fixed costs associated with operating an ED are related to the labour intensity of the service, it is useful to include a section tracking paid full-time equivalent staff, by month, for the current year compared to the previous financial year. This is especially important if there has been an overrun in the labour budget, as the hospital executive will wish to be reassured that this is not due to the employment of excess staff.

Activity

The activity of the ED may be shown as total attendances and attendances by category of the Australasian Triage Scale. The admission rate by triage category should also be shown, and all values should be tabulated against the previous year's activity levels. Where an ED operates a short-stay ward or observation unit, the top 20 diagnosis-related groups by volume should be shown, together with the number of total separations, weighted separations and the case-mix index. This information should be available from the financial services department. Again, the data should be benchmarked to the previous year. Additional relevant activity data, such as inter-hospital transfers, retrievals and so on, should be included.

Quality

Waiting time by triage category is the key quality and efficiency indicator for an ED. The average waiting time per patient in each triage category should be shown, together with the percentage of patients in each triage category who are seen within the timeframe specified by the Australasian Triage Scale. These data should be benchmarked against the previous year's performance and, ideally, also against benchmarking data from similar hospitals elsewhere. Performance against clinical indicators recommended by the Australian Council on Healthcare Standards should also be reported. Additional access indicators include the frequency and duration of ambulance bypass (occasions per month), and admission access block (percentage of total admitted patients spending longer than 8 h in the ED) should be provided. Some units use additional quality indicators, such as the percentage of correct diagnoses made on admitted patients by the ED, and the mortality rate of sentinel diagnoses (for instance poisoning and overdose, major trauma), among others.

The written complaint rate (per 10 000 attendances) about ED services should be known and reported.

It is appropriate in the section on 'quality' that research and educational achievements should be succinctly reported, together with any innovative projects.

Projections

Having summarized the current year's performance, the remainder of the business plan should be used to present the ED's projections and estimates for the next financial year. Again, the projected budget should be presented first. This is best done in a tabular format and compared to the previous year's budget and projected actual expenditure. Any premises, assumptions or caveats related to the projected budget should be included as footnotes to the table. The most common premise relates to the volume and quality of services to be provided, and the usual approach is iso-volume/iso-quality; this should not be varied in the business plan unless previously agreed by the hospital executive. Periodically, circumstances will dictate that a hospital vary the desired quality of services, perhaps as part of a strategic initiative to develop the ED, or the volume of services in response to changing demographic projections. Apart from anticipated wages growth, it is important for the management group to make reasonable enquiries about predictable leave (such as sabbaticals or long-service leave), and these should be appropriately costed. In the non-labour budget, possible variations in the cost of overseas-sourced clinical supplies or pharmaceuticals due to revaluation of the currency should be considered, although in some jurisdictions non-labour increments are specified, for budget purposes, across the whole of government.

Realistically, most hospital executives will reject a budget proposal that exceeds the previous year's expenditure, escalated by projected wages growth, unless there are special mitigating factors, or a source of funds for the predicted additional expenditure has been identified. For this reason, it is often useful to have three additional sections in the business plan addressing equipment needs, facility maintenance needs, and a projects summary.

Equipment

The ED management group should canvass widely among the staff about perceived equipment needs. It is important that the totality of clinical and non-clinical equipment needs is understood and equitably prioritized in order to optimize the efficiency of the whole department. Most hospitals require that equipment requests be stratified according to cost, with items less than $5000 typically being met from a global allocation to the department. Apart from tabulating the need for this lower-priced equipment, a few lines of narrative about each item often assists the executive in ensuring the reasonableness of the request. The table should indicate whether the equipment is new or replacement. High-cost equipment (e.g. ultrasound machines, computerized tomography scanners or arterial blood gas machines) will almost always require the presentation of a full business case and economic analysis in line with all government procurement instructions.

Facility maintenance

All but the newest departments will require some expenditure on maintenance each year. Again, it is useful for the ED management group to undertake a focused tour of all areas of the department to establish an inventory of maintenance needs. Reasonably accurate costings can be obtained from hospital engineering services or external contractors.

Projects

This final section can be used to describe and cost small or large projects to enhance the ED facilities, infrastructure or services. For example, there may be a proposal to establish a 10-bed short-stay unit adjacent to the ED, involving facility redevelopment, the acquisition of clinical and non-clinical equipment (including information systems), staff resourcing and business process reform. This is best presented in a project format, including a clear description of the business need (supported by all available, relevant data), a business case outlining all the costs and benefits and, if possible, additional material such as architects' sketches and a project implementation plan, including a project timetable.

Private EDS

The overview of business planning presented above is equally relevant to EDs in private hospitals. However, private EDs also need to develop a revenue budget and marketing plan appropriate to their circumstances. The marketing plan will usually be a part of the hospital's overall arrangements, but the ED should be in a position to report on any changes in referral pattern or on any opportunities to expand the business.

Business plan implementation and monitoring

Soon after the hospital receives its global budget and activity targets from government, a short process of negotiation between the hospital executive and the ED management group should take place. This will fine-tune the business plan and, ultimately, permit authorization of the plan and the appropriate delegation for its implementation.

The ED management group should meet at least monthly to review actual performance against the outcomes predicted by the plan. Any variance from the budget in particular should be studied and understood. Remedial action should be taken wherever possible to maintain budget integrity. In many places, the ED management group would meet with the hospital executive at least quarterly to review department performance and to deal with any variation that may have occurred.

27.5 Accreditation, specialist training and recognition in Australasia

Wayne Hazell • Allen Yuen • Andrew Singer

ESSENTIALS

1 Specialist training in emergency medicine (EM) in Australia and New Zealand is the responsibility of the Australasian College for Emergency Medicine (ACEM).

2 International medical graduates with specialist qualifications or overseas-trained specialists (OTS) also require recognition from either the Australian Medical Council or the Medical Council of New Zealand.

3 OTS must undergo an assessment by ACEM in order to be recognized as specialist emergency physicians in either country.

4 Specialist training in EM under ACEM occurs in three phases: basic, provisional and advanced training. Provisional trainees must complete the ACEM Primary Examination and advanced trainees, the Fellowship Examination. Advanced trainees must complete a minimum paediatric requirement, as well as a research component.

5 ACEM training accreditation is awarded to hospitals if they satisfy minimum threshold criteria and the majority of the criteria that are set for the minimum level of accreditation.

6 There are three levels of accreditation which pertain to the maximum amount of advanced training that a trainee can complete in these departments: 6 months, 12 months and 24 months.

7 Accreditation criteria are set by the ACEM and transparent comprehensive guidelines were introduced in 2006 with a 1-year transition period designed to give accredited departments time to meet new minimum threshold criteria.

8 Hospitals are inspected at regular 5-year intervals to determine whether standards are being maintained to allow continuation of accreditation. This is supplemented by an annual accreditation survey. Progress is being made towards mandatory on-line trainee feedback about each training rotation.

9 Following an accreditation inspection, recommendations are made and fed back to the hospital and emergency department. The accreditation process is an important component in improving ACEM training performance.

Specialist recognition and registration

Specialist recognition in New Zealand and Australia is handled by the respective medical councils in each country – the Medical Council of New Zealand (MCNZ) and the Australian Medical Council (AMC). In New Zealand, MCNZ handles both specialist recognition (termed vocational registration) and general medical registration. In Australia, the AMC has responsibility for specialist recognition of overseas-trained specialists (OTS) and the accreditation of specialist medical colleges. Medical registration (both general and specialist where applicable) is the responsibility of the eight state and territory medical boards. All International Medical Graduates (IMG) must be both recognized by the AMC and registered with the medical board of the state or territory in which they are practising.

Medical registration is also required for specialist training. State and territory medical boards have provision for temporary registration for training purposes under an occupational training visa, which allows up to 4 years of training in Australia. These require sponsorship by an Australian employing hospital, as well as the ACEM.

Specialist training in emergency medicine

Specialist medical training is the responsibility of the various specialist medical colleges. Most of these organizations cover both Australia and New Zealand. They are accredited by the AMC. Specialist training in emergency medicine (EM) is covered by the ACEM which was accredited by the AMC in 2007.

The college provides the framework, standards and supervision for specialist training in EM, and successful trainees are granted Fellowship of the ACEM (FACEM).

Training occurs in hospitals and rotations accredited by ACEM for training. Each accredited emergency department (ED) appoints a Director of Emergency Medicine Training (DEMT). This is the college Fellow with the responsibility of running the training programme in that department and hospital. The description below of the training programme reflects the situation in July 2007. The training programme undergoes regular review and revision.

Specialist training in EM is divided into three phases:

- basic training
- provisional training
- advanced training.

Basic training

This usually consists of the pre-registration year of practice (internship in Australia or post graduate year 1 (PGY 1) in New Zealand) and the second year of practice following a doctor's primary medical degree. It must occur in a variety of clinical rotations, and be signed off by the administration of the employing institution.

Provisional training

This usually occurs in the third postgraduate year or beyond. There are three requirements of provisional training:

- Completion of 12 months of training in approved rotations. At least 6 months of this must be in EM. Each rotation is assessed and signed off at its completion by the DEMT or local supervisor for non-ED rotations.

- Successful completion of the ACEM primary examination. The ACEM primary examination is a basic science examination covering four subjects: anatomy, pathology, physiology and pharmacology. Each subject consists of a 90-minute multiple-choice examination and a 10-minute viva-voce examination. The examination is conducted twice a year in a number of locations across Australia and New Zealand. Each subject may be attempted multiple times, but each subject must be passed to successfully complete the examination.

- Provision of three structured references and completion of the trainee selection process. Each trainee must obtain three structured references (as supplied by the ACEM). These assess the trainee's potential for a career in EM and are reviewed by the Trainee Selection Committee.

Advanced training

Advanced training occurs once the trainee has completed all the requirements of provisional training. ACEM has a detailed curriculum outlining the knowledge and skills required by the completion of advanced training. The main elements are ED training, non-ED advanced training, the minimum paediatric requirement, a research component and completion of the fellowship examination.

ED training

Trainees must complete 30 months of training in accredited EDs. Each accredited ED is allowed to provide training for an individual trainee up to a specified maximum amount of time (6, 12 or 24 months).

Training must be in a minimum of 3-month rotations. Each rotation is assessed and signed-off at its completion by the DEMT.

Hospitals are also assigned a role delineation (major referral, urban district, rural/regional) when they are inspected for training accreditation. Trainees must complete at least 6 months in a major referral hospital and either an urban district or rural/regional hospital. There is some political pressure to have trainees rotated to rural regional areas but at present there are limited numbers of these departments that meet current accreditation standards.

Non-ED training

Trainees must complete 18 months of training in approved non-ED rotations. These are usually in hospitals accredited for training by the respective college for that specialty. It is required that at least 6 months be spent in critical-care rotations (anaesthesia and intensive care). Experience can be gained in designated special skills rotations, such as retrieval, toxicology, rural critical care, research, academic EM and general practice.

Minimum paediatric requirement

This is gained concurrently during ED and non-ED advanced training. Trainees must log at least 400 substantive encounters with paediatric (aged 15 years and under) patients, as well as complete a number of procedures on paediatric patients under supervision. EDs are given specific accreditation for this minimum paediatric requirement.

Research component

Each trainee must publish or present research to the satisfaction of ACEM. A review of this regulation has begun and it may be in the future that trainees can meet the learning objectives of this research requirement in a number of ways.

Fellowship examination

Trainees may attempt the fellowship examination when they are within 1 year of completion of their training. The examination consists of three written sections (multiple choice, short-answer questions and visual aid questions) and three clinical sections (long case, short cases and structured clinical examination). It is run twice a year in various locations across Australia and New Zealand.

Variations to training

Recognition of prior learning can be applied for in line with regulations and upon registration. Up to 2 years of advanced training (up to 1 year of which can be in EM) can be gained overseas, with the prior approval of the ACEM.

Training can also be completed on a part-time basis (at least 20 h per week), and can be suspended for up to 2 years.

Dual training

Dual training programmes in paediatric EM (in conjunction with the Royal Australasian College of Physicians) and intensive care medicine (in conjunction with the Joint Faculty of Intensive Care Medicine) are now operational.

Recognition of specialist training obtained outside of the ACEM

This can essentially be divided into two groups: (i) training in EM and (ii) training obtained outside of EM.

OTSs in EM must apply for specialist recognition from either AMC or MCNZ. In both cases, once the documentation and English language status have been confirmed, the OTS is referred to the ACEM for assessment. The ACEM reviews the applicant's training, qualifications and experience on paper. If these appear potentially substantially comparable, the ACEM conducts a structured interview for further clarification. The three senior FACEMs on the interview panel review the applicant's qualifications and experience, and determine their level of confidence in the following areas: undergraduate training, basic training, advanced training, postgraduate experience, research and publication profile, education and training experience and administration. Additionally, three topical issues are discussed.

The ACEM then makes a recommendation to the AMC or MCNZ for either specialist recognition, or further supervision or further training.

Those applicants with training within Australia or New Zealand but outside of the ACEM must apply to the ACEM for recognition. The ACEM reviews the applicant's training qualifications and experience and may conduct an interview. The college then makes a ruling on the required further training and assessment, if any.

The ACEM has a comprehensive website (http://www.acem.org.au) that provides up-to-date information on all aspects of training and other college matters. The AMC (http://www.amc.org.au) and MCNZ (http://www.mcnz.org.nz) also have websites with useful information for overseas-trained doctors wishing to work in either country.

Accreditation

Hospitals seeking accreditation for defined purposes such as service provision or training must comply with set standards determined by external institutions which oversee the criteria applicable to such hospitals.

In the case of hospitals overall, the Australian Council on Healthcare Standards (ACHS) determines the service standards of patient care provided by a hospital and its individual departments.[1,2] The process focuses on improving performance, continuum of care, leadership and management, human resource management, information management, safe practice and environment, utilizing audits and key performance indicators.

The learned colleges, including the ACEM, separately accredit hospitals for their ability to provide postgraduate training, taking the above criteria into account, but placing greater emphasis on the quality of experience, education and supervision for trainees. The items that the ACEM considers and takes into account in any accreditation decision are outlined in the following list from the ACEM guidelines:[3]

- The level and numbers of emergency physicians and senior staff capable of providing adequate and appropriate supervision for trainees of all levels of experience and at all times.
- An appropriate number and case-mix of emergency patients to provide adequate clinical experience and with trainees having an adequate and appropriate level of involvement at an assessment, procedural and management level.
- There will be an adequate specialist workforce. In considering the adequacy of the specialist workforce, regard will be given to the appropriateness of rosters, safe hours,

access to leave, overall department performance and benchmarks.
- Appropriate levels of staffing with respect to medical, nursing, secretarial and other personnel.
- Design and equipment of the department appropriate to the provision of emergency care and training.
- An appropriate range and level of support services.
- An appropriate education programme, including lectures, case presentations, mortality and morbidity review, discussions, audit and review. There should be a strong emphasis on activities that encourage adult learning, reflection, self-evaluation, discussion and collaborative learning. There should be emphasis placed on interactive teaching. There should be appropriate provisions in the education programme to meet the needs of trainees sitting the primary or fellowship examination.
- The opportunity for trainee research and the infrastructure supporting this.
- Accreditation of an appropriate range of specialties within the hospital by their respective colleges and the opportunity for rotations which will provide relevant clinical experience for EM.
- Evaluation of ED function and level of access block so as to determine how this may impact on training and registrar wellbeing.

The accreditation process plays an important role in the identification of problems and guiding subsequent corrective actions.[2]

Accreditation guidelines

Transparent comprehensive ACEM guidelines for mixed and adult EDs seeking training accreditation were introduced in 2006 with a 1-year transition period designed to give accredited departments time to meet new minimum threshold criteria. These guidelines can be viewed on the ACEM website.[3]

The rationale for the minimum threshold relates to the minimum number of specialists required to provide a combination of leadership; mentorship; off-floor training, feedback and assessment and on-floor clinical supervision and feedback.

The minimum threshold criteria that must be met before an ED can be considered for

ACEM training accreditation are: 1 full-time equivalent (FTE) FACEM as Director of Emergency Medicine; 0.5 FTE FACEM as DEMT and 2.5 FTE total FACEMs inclusive of the Director and DEMT.[4] In addition to this minimum threshold, departments must meet mandatory criteria as outlined below before any level of accreditation can be considered:[3]

- Appropriate and acceptable standards of patient care.
- Documented management, admission, discharge and referral policies.
- A functional electronic patient information management system.
- A formal system of quality management. Trainees are expected to participate in these activities.
- A formal orientation programme for new staff.
- Educational programmes for all grades of medical and nursing staff.
- Adequate EM textbooks, journals, management guidelines and protocols available on site. There should also be access to electronic sources of medical information.
- Access to advice or information which facilitates trainees seeking mentorship if they wish to do so.

College procedure

The ACEM conducts regular (at least 5-yearly) inspections of ACEM training-accredited EDs, to ensure that standards are maintained and that the various criteria for accreditation are met.[5,6]

The completed hospital information questionnaire, minimum criteria checklist and any accompanying documents supplied to the inspection team before the inspection are carefully studied. Interviews with administration, department heads, specialists, trainees, nurse managers and educators contribute significantly to the decisions made.

The minimum criteria checklist is a checklist against the minimum threshold, mandatory criteria, and a number of specific criteria per level of accreditation currently held or desired in the future. An example of these specific criteria for a 24-month department is illustrated below:[3]

- There should be at least 30 000 presentations per year to the ED, which are primarily attended to by ED staff.

- The ED should have a comprehensive case-mix, which may include major trauma, critically ill patients, a broad range of complex patients and acute cardiology. It is important to ensure that with increasing experience trainees are able to provide immediate care and assume increased responsibility for these patients, while at the same time receiving appropriate levels of supervision.
- The ED should have an admission rate of >25%.
- The ED should have one FTE Nurse Unit Manager, or equivalent, who is supernumerary to the clinical staffing needs of the department.
- The ED should have at least one FTE Nurse Educator.
- The ED should display a willingness and capacity to host or co-host the fellowship clinical examinations and to contribute invigilators for the primary and fellowship examinations.

With respect to the level of supervision of trainees, the ED requires:

- One FTE FACEM as Director of Emergency Medicine who should ideally be supernumerary to the clinical staffing needs of the department. If this is not possible, the Director of Emergency Medicine should be provided with at least 50% non-clinical time.
- One FTE FACEM as Director of Emergency Medicine Training. The Director of Emergency Medicine Training should ideally be provided with at least 50% non-clinical time. It is recommended that this one FTE, including 0.5 FTE of non-clinical time, be satisfied by the appointment of a single FACEM. However, two part-time FACEMs could combine to wholly satisfy this one FTE which must include 0.5 FTE of non-clinical time.
- A minimum of a further six FTE FACEMs. Each FACEM should ideally be provided 25% non-clinical time for approved teaching, research or administrative activities.
- The presence of a FACEM exclusively rostered to clinical duties for at least 98 h every week.

- A minimum of 60% of trainee time to be under the direct clinical supervision of a FACEM.

With respect to the structure of the training programme, the ED requires:

- An educational programme, which includes access to teaching for both the primary and fellowship examination. For EDs seeking a continuation of accreditation, there should be demonstrated proven performance in a) assisting trainees to pass both the primary and fellowship examination and b) the development of highly regarded emergency physicians who practise good clinical care.
- There must be protected teaching time for trainees of 4 h per week. Additional non-clinical time should be provided to allow trainees to complete other non-clinical duties specified by the department.
- Formal arrangements for the rotation of trainees to other specialty areas. Adult-only departments should be able to demonstrate that they can offer assistance to trainees wishing to access appropriate paediatric terms, either emergency- or ward-based.
- There should be at least one FACEM formally responsible for the provision of advice, supervision and support of trainee's planning, executing, presenting or publishing the research component of their training. They should also be responsible for providing critical review of the trainee's final manuscript to ensure it is suitable for submission for presentation or publication.

These specific criteria are repeated for 6- and 12-month accreditation but the numbers or threshold for each criterion are devised such as to be appropriate to these lower levels of accreditation.[3]

Prior to the inspection, the department does a self-assessment on the minimum criteria checklist and indicates which criteria it meets or does not meet. Uncertainty about meeting or not meeting a criterion can be indicated. At the end of an inspection, the inspection team revisits the checklist and performs its own criteria assessment. Any variance between

the department's assessment and the inspectors' assessment can then be discussed to clarify items of confusion, error or misunderstanding.

Levels of accreditation

There are three levels of accreditation awarded: 6 months, 12 months or 2 years. These periods refer to the amount of accredited time recognized as a part of a trainee's advanced EM training in that particular ED. The trainee may spend more time in the department, but the extra time will not count towards training requirements. The trainee may spend more time within the same hospital accruing non-ED time in accredited rotations in other specialties relevant to EM.

Since the period of advanced training is 4 years after success in the primary examination, the above periods of accreditation ensure that trainees rotate through at least two hospitals, benefiting from the particular strengths of each.

Rationale for the accreditation criteria

The Board of Censors and Council have discretion on how the criteria are applied. This is for a number of reasons. Firstly, the criteria are not comprehensive and factors not listed in the criteria may weigh positively or negatively on the outcome. Not all criteria necessarily need to be met as great strengths in some criteria may outweigh concerns of not meeting another. Any criteria that are clearly not met are at least fed back as a concern.

The criteria were themselves developed by a panel of experts, who were essentially FACEMs from the Board of Censors and Council. Each individual criterion was debated and it is certainly possible that opinions may vary about each criterion within the fellowship at large.

The rationales for the mandatory criteria are fairly self-explanatory. Standards required for acceptable patient care and wellbeing of staff are paramount. ACEM would not wish to put a trainee at risk in an environment where this was jeopardized.

A functional electronic patient information management system has posed a challenge as some departments do not have this. Systems such as these are important

for training as trainees are able to instantaneously have an overview of what is happening in a department at any one time. This is extremely important if they have supervisory duties. These systems aid education in a number of ways. Instantaneous vision with regard to other interesting or informative cases in the department at any one time, access to laboratory results, past health event information, electrocardiograph storage, radiographic image storage and the ability to generate reports for audit and research are highly beneficial for trainees.

Access to a mentoring system is also mandatory and is an AMC requirement of colleges. The ACEM has sent out an information package to all DEMTs, and addresses this issue in a DEMT course. Trainees need to have the opportunity to seek a mentor although it is not an obligation of the department to have a mentor for each trainee. Some departments run a supervisor system to aid the DEMT but, as supervisors participate in assessment; these are different from mentor systems.

With regard to specific criteria per level of accreditation, adequate senior staffing with emergency physicians is essential. Trainees must be well-supervised, particularly after-hours and during busy evening and weekend periods. As the level of accreditation increases FACEM minimum numbers and the overlap of FACEMs working directly on the floor with trainees increases also. The number of FACEM FTE required increases from 2.5 to 5 to 8, the hours of the week 'FACEM to trainee overlap' increases from 50 h to 80 h to 98 h, and the minimum percentage of trainee time under the direct supervision of a FACEM increases from 30% to 40% to 60%; respectively per 6-, 12- and 24-month level of accreditation criteria.

At the same time, trainees need to be given increasing levels of responsibility, including administrative, as they advance in their training, as some may be appointed to director positions at smaller hospitals, soon after attaining their specialist qualification.[6,7]

Excellent leadership is a requirement for a well functioning department and training environment, hence the FACEM Director requirement and, as clinical leadership in the ED goes hand in hand with nursing leadership, the nurse unit manager requirement.

One FTE of both medical and nursing leadership is required for all levels of accreditation.

Educators are of course an absolute requirement and medical and nursing education should be closely linked. Nurses can be a great source of trainee education and trainees can gain experience by participating in nurse education. Inspectors take note of the interaction between medical and nursing staff education and it becomes easily apparent whether these are well integrated or separate entities. The DEMT and nurse educator requirements are less with lower levels of accreditation as such departments are likely to have a lower number of trainees.

Education programmes, particularly for 24-month accredited departments, must show the full spectrum of education. These should include on-floor clinical teaching; fellowship exam-specific programmes; primary exam-specific programmes and departmental general education sessions. These programmes may be shared between a network of hospitals and trainees must be rostered dedicated teaching time to allow them to attend education sessions. The culture for education and training can also be demonstrated by the quality and standard of resident and undergraduate education programmes, as well as FACEM university academic appointments. It is expected that the registrars, as advanced trainees, will be involved in student and resident teaching. Access to simulation training is becoming more widespread and available. FACEM commitment to assisting in college exam processes is a requirement for higher levels of accreditation and again is a marker of enthusiasm and educational culture.

The ability of a hospital to provide rotations for EM trainees to training positions at registrar level in such terms as medicine, surgery, cardiology, anaesthesia, intensive care, paediatrics, retrieval medicine, psychiatry and toxicology enhances a hospital's chances of attaining full accreditation.

Research and quality assurance projects provide a framework for improving performance, and the College examines the department's commitment to research.[8] Smaller 6-month departments may not have great research infrastructure but 24-month accredited departments must have at least an individual or a few individuals to assist trainees in their research component.

Case-mix and attendance can, of course, ultimately limit or maximize a training experience and this also varies in stipulation per level of accreditation. As many departments now are trying to limit admissions and providing hospital-in-the-home services, required admission rates are perhaps lower than they would have been 10 years ago.

Recommendations

Following an accreditation inspection, a detailed report is forwarded to the College's Board of Censors and Council for discussion.

Recommendations are then made regarding level of accreditation, suitability for paediatric training, accreditable rotations, and the number of trainee positions the particular ED can sustain.

Identified concerns are listed, and it is expected the hospital will address these. Interestingly over 90% of the recommendations made by ACHS surveyors prior to 1990 were implemented.[2]

If standards for the level of existing accreditation are not met departments receive 12–months' notice that the accreditation status may be reduced to a lower level. A further inspection in 12 months' time is conducted to determine the outcome. If any hospital at inspection fails to meet the minimum threshold criteria accreditation is immediately lost without any notice period.

Implications

The accreditation process is comprehensive, fair and important but it can also be intimidating.[9] Hospitals will retain their accreditation as long as they maintain the desired standards. Inspections by either the ACHS or college can highlight a department's or hospital's shortcomings to administrators, so that attention can be paid to correcting the deficiencies.[2,4]

While there has been criticism that a single visit may not be sufficient, there has been, in fact, little disagreement with the recommendations made. Where there has been dispute, changes have been implemented within the hospital or department to allow early re-inspection to determine whether the desired accreditation level can be restored.

Loss of accreditation can occur at any time if departments fall below the minimum threshold. Losing accreditation can have adverse long-term consequences in terms of loss of reputation and lack of good applicants for positions in these departments.

In order to protect the trainees at an institution that loses accreditation, or has a reduction in accreditation status, trainees are allowed to continue having training accredited up to the end point of the current employment contract or change in training year.

Success with accreditation ensures a continuation or upgrading of an ED's reputation and makes that hospital more attractive for prospective trainees and staff specialists. Hospitals therefore have strong incentives to maintain high standards in their EDs.

Accreditation of paediatric-only departments

In 2007, accreditation guidelines for paediatric-only departments were jointly finalized by ACEM and the RACP (Royal Australian College of Physicians) through the Joint Training Committee in Paediatric EM. These guidelines reflect ACEM training requirements and also reflect the accreditation criteria for joint training. They follow a very similar format and structure to the adult and mixed guidelines but have a paediatric-specific theme. The first accreditation inspection using these guidelines was considered at the July 2007 Board of Censors and Council meetings after an inspection team from both ACEM and the RACP provided a recommendation.

Accreditation of overseas rotations

ACEM regulations are relatively flexible and trainees are encouraged to work in a variety of hospitals, both in Australia and New Zealand as well as overseas. Overseas terms are preferably in centres with respective college specialist training accreditation and prior approval needs to be sought from ACEM. So far most of these overseas accredited terms have been in the UK and USA.[10,11]

Accreditation in the future

Work is currently being done by the Australian Health Workforce Secretariat, in consultation with the learned colleges and jurisdictions, with regard to generic accreditation guidelines across all colleges and disciplines. At this stage, eight generic standards have been proposed with the concept of colleges developing their own particular criteria under each standard. To date the proposed standards are as follows:

❶ education and training programme
❷ clinical experience
❸ clinical and infrastructure support
❹ resources to support education and training
❺ supervision
❻ organization support
❼ institutional responsibilities
❽ quality and safety.

It may be in the future that colleges have to construct and/or map their guidelines to each of these standards. ACEM should not have any difficulty achieving this.

One of the most important areas of the accreditation process is the interview with trainees and their feedback. Unfortunately at present, annual feedback from trainees via survey achieves poor response rates. From 2008, it is hoped to have mandatory web-based trainee feedback linked to web-based submission of in-training assessment. The concept is that a trainee does not have assessment and feedback unless feedback is simultaneously provided to the college about a rotation. This will of course achieve 100% feedback. This opens the possibility to automatically generated reports fed back to the Board of Censors and the departments themselves. Rankings or percentiles via overall feedback and individual domains would be possible, allowing some degree of norm referencing and corrective action to take place.

A combination of 5-yearly routine inspections; more frequent inspections if required; department self-assessment in the form of an annual DEMT survey; and 100% feedback from trainees should provide a very robust system.

Jurisdictional and trainee representation on accreditation inspections and processes may be a requirement in the future.

As more data are collected by the new hospital information questionnaire and annual DEMT survey, as more inspections are done using the new guidelines and perhaps as generic guidelines become a requirement, there will likely be some adjustment or review of the guidelines in the future.

Controversies

❶ There is some political pressure to have trainees rotated to rural regional areas but at present there are limited numbers of these departments meeting accreditation standards.

❷ The research component of training has always been controversial within the college. A research component is likely to always be present but in the future, a plurality of ways of meeting this requirement may be possible. A major review has now commenced.

❸ There is considerable debate over whether a fair accreditation assessment can be made on the basis of a single inspection. Many argue that a single snapshot of an ED in time cannot adequately represent the complex pattern of functions and activities going on within that department and that a longer inspection over a period of time may be necessary. This has to be balanced against the drain on college resources this would entail. The annual DEMT survey and trainee feedback initiatives are a possible compromise.

❹ Generic accreditation processes and criteria may occur across colleges in the future.

❺ Jurisdictional and trainee representation on accreditation inspections and processes may be a requirement in the future.

References

1. Australian Council on Healthcare Standards. The EquIP Guide 1998 Standards and guidelines for the ACHS evaluation and quality improvement program.
2. Holt PE, Darby DN. ACHS surveyor recommendations: recent trends in the accident and emergency service. Australian Clinical Reviews 1992; 12(1): 29–30.
3. Australasian College for Emergency Medicine. G01 Guidelines for Adult and Mixed EDs Seeking Training Accreditation, http://www.acem.org.au, 2007. (Accessed Sept. 2008).
4. Australasian College for Emergency Medicine. Training and Examination Handbook Melbourne, ACEM ; The College; 2007.
5. Yuen A. A review of Australasian College for Emergency Medicine accreditation: 1986–1995. Emergency Medicine 1996; 8(3): 152–162.
6. Gaudry PL. Did you pass accreditation? Emergency Medicine 1992; 4(1): 29.
7. Baggoley C. Emergency medicine. Where to from here? The College. Emergency Medicine 1999; 11: 234–237.
8. O'Leary DS, O'Leary MR. From quality assurance to quality improvement. The Joint Commission on Accreditation of Healthcare Organizations and Emergency Care. Emergency Medicine Clinics of North America 1992; 10(3): 477–492.
9. Taylor DMcD, Jelinek GA. A comparison of Australasian and United Sates emergency medicine training programmes. Emergency Medicine 1999; 11(1): 49–56.
10. Hamilton G. Emergency medicine: Where to from here? Overseas viewpoint. Emergency Medicine 1999; 11: 229–233.
11. Vinen J. Accreditation - was it worth it? Emergency Medicine 1992; 4(1): 30.

27.6 Specialist training and recognition in emergency medicine in the United Kingdom

Alastair McGowan

ESSENTIALS

1 Postgraduate medical training in the UK has been in a state of flux.

2 Changes to immigration rules are also occurring in response to insufficient training opportunities for UK and European graduates, although it should still be relatively easy for graduates from Australia, New Zealand, Hong Kong, Singapore, South Africa and the West Indies to undertake postgraduate training in the UK.

3 The Postgraduate Medical Education and Training Board (PMETB), established in 2003, sets standards for the curricula and training programmes of the royal colleges and faculties.

4 The route to specialist recognition in the UK is by completing a full PMETB-approved programme of training, or for relevant College and PMETB approval of training, qualifications and experience gained elsewhere.

5 The PMETB will be assimilated into the General Medical Council by 2010.

6 The Modernizing Medical Careers (MMC) Programme began in 2003 with the aim of improving postgraduate training in the UK. The system is, however, at present in a state of flux, and emergency medicine (EM) in England, Wales and Northern Ireland, but not in Scotland, has uncoupled and re-introduced a competitive appointment process, re-instating the concept of basic and higher training, now known as core and specialist.

7 EM training lasts for 6 years comprising a 3 year core training programme, successful completion of which results in Membership of the College of Emergency Medicine (CEM) at examination, followed by a 3-year specialist training programme leading to Fellowship of the CEM by exit examination.

Introduction

Postgraduate medical training in all specialties in the UK has been in a state of flux in recent years. Changes to the structure of training and recruitment thereto have proved problematic. Many changes have been introduced very quickly and not always with reference to each other.

An understanding of UK training in emergency medicine (EM) cannot be

gained without some knowledge of the new regulatory bodies and systems that have been put in place since 2003, relating to the regulation of training, the shape of training and the content of training.

Regulation of training

General Medical Council (GMC)

Anyone who wishes to practise medicine in the UK must be registered with the General Medical Council (GMC). The GMC introduced a new registration framework in Oct 2007. This framework simplifies registration to either 'full' or 'provisional'. Provisional registration allows newly qualified doctors to

undertake general clinical training in the UK as a Foundation Year 1 doctor (see below) in posts specifically approved for this purpose. Full registration allows doctors to undertake unsupervised medical practice.

Those new to full registration or those who have been away from UK practice for 5 years or more, must work for 1 year in an 'approved practice setting'. A list of these placements can be found on the GMC website. They meet defined standards for training, support and management of doctors.

For either provisional or full registration, non-European Economic Area (EAA) applicants will need to demonstrate to the GMC that they:

- hold an acceptable primary medical qualification
- have the requisite knowledge and skills for registration
- have no impairment to their fitness to practise
- have the necessary knowledge of English.

This can be done by:

- a pass in the PLAB test (Professional and Linguistic Assessments Board)*
- sponsorship by a medical Royal College (or other sponsoring body)
- an acceptable postgraduate qualification
- eligibility for entry to the specialist or GP register.

Doctors applying for full registration must also supply evidence that they have had a period of postgraduate experience equivalent to the general clinical training of the Foundation Year 1.

New immigration rules

New immigration rules have been introduced that will restrict access to UK postgraduate medical education (PGME) for international medical graduates (IMG). This was driven by the concern that there may

---

*Graduates from Australia, New Zealand, Hong Kong, Singapore, South Africa, West Indies (and Malaya before 31/12/89) and who hold or have held provisional registration since before 19/10/07 do not need to take PLAB.

be insufficient training opportunities for UK and EEA graduates.

The Department of Health's (DoH's) preferred option is that IMGs be considered for training posts only if there are no suitable UK or EEA applicants. This stance has been challenged in the Court of Appeal and found to be unlawful. The DoH's appeal against this decision is currently being heard in the House of Lords. It is likely that a points system will be developed that will stratify entitlement to apply for training posts.

Postgraduate Medical Education and Training Board (PMETB)

The PMETB was established in 2003 as an independent regulatory body for PGME. It has significant statutory powers which it uses to:

- set and secure standards for PGME
- certify doctors for specialist and GP registers
- develop and promote PGME.

It sets standards for the curricula devised by the royal colleges and their faculties and has approved 57 of these so far. It also sets standards for and approves the assessment processes and programmes of training used by royal colleges, and defines equivalence routes to registration as a specialist or GP.

Specialist registration

Doctors who are fully registered with the GMC and who wish to practise as a substantive consultant or GP in the NHS must be on the specialist or GP register. The usual route for registration is to complete a full PMETB approved programme of training. Such doctors may then apply via their royal college for a Certificate of Completion of Training (CCT).

A second route ('Article 14' of the standing order which brought PMETB into existence) is available to doctors who have not completed a full PMETB approved training programme but who wish their training, qualifications and experience, wherever gained, to be considered for eligibility to be entered on to the specialist or GP register. Application forms, portfolios and other documentary evidence of what the doctor has achieved are sent by PMETB to the relevant college for consideration and for a recommendation to be made with regard to registration. It is important to note that PMETB is not bound by that recommendation.

If successful, such doctors are issued with a Certificate of Eligibility for Specialist Registration (CESR) which entitles them to apply for inclusion on the UK register but does not confer EEA registration privileges. The process tends to be slow and an application currently costs £1250.

As a consequence of the review of Modernizing Medical Careers (see below) PMETB is to be assimilated into the GMC to form a single regulatory body by 2010.

Modernizing medical careers

This is the name given to a national programme of reform of PGME instigated by the four UK health departments in 2003. Its aim has been to review and adapt the processes of PGME in the UK to supply doctors better equipped to meet the future needs of the NHS. It proposed that:

- more medical care should be provided by fully trained doctors than by trainees
- national standards for training be established (see PMETB above)
- competency-based curricula be devised and trainee acquisition of those competencies be regularly assessed
- trainers and supervisors be better trained and resourced for their roles.

As a consequence of MMC, the shape of PGME in the UK has been substantially altered. Foundation programmes of 2 years' duration have been introduced; they are designed to allow general clinical training, a broader experience and the acquisition and verification of generic competencies. Thereafter, those who have successfully completed such programmes and those doctors from other countries who can provide evidence of equivalent experience and competence (and who satisfy immigration rules) can apply for specialist training programmes. These programmes vary in their duration and pattern according to the specialty but lead to the award of a CCT.

Those doctors who do not obtain a place on such a programme can apply for Fixed Term Specialty Training Appointments (FTSTAs) which are PMETB approved and count towards training for either 2 or 3 years depending on the specialty. If after this period such doctors still have not obtained a place on a specialist training programme, it is expected that they will take up a service post and, if

they wish, continue to progress towards specialist registration by the CESR route.

In 2007, all specialist training programmes were 'run through' so that those appointed would progress through training without further competition for employment until the point where a CCT could be issued, provided satisfactory progress against the curriculum was being made.

Concerns about the lack of flexibility of such arrangements, lack of confidence within the profession of the selection tools being used and major systematic failures of the supporting recruitment infrastructure led to an independent inquiry into the MMC programme. This inquiry, led by Sir John Tooke, made 47 recommendations, the vast majority of which attracted the support of the profession as a whole. Forty-two of these recommendations (including the assimilation of PMETB into the GMC) were accepted by the government. Five are still under consideration.

The fallout from MMC and the inquiry into it is ongoing. MMC still exists and is seeking to re-establish its reputation and re-emphasize its very laudable aims.

Some specialties, such as psychiatry, obstetrics and gynaecology and paediatrics, have elected to continue with run through training.

Others, including EM in England, Wales and Northern Ireland but not in Scotland, have decided to 'uncouple' and re-introduce a competitive appointment process after year 2 or 3 of the programme thus re-instating the concept of basic and higher training – now known as core and specialist.

Training in EM in the UK

EM in the UK took advantage of the opportunities offered by MMC and PMETB to re-write the curriculum, re-design assessment processes and re-structure training programmes. EM training in the UK now lasts for 6 years after Foundation and broadly comprises a 3-year core training programme, successful completion of which is marked by gaining membership of the College of Emergency Medicine (CEM) at examination, followed by a 3-year specialist training programme leading to fellowship of the CEM to those successful in the exit examination. Transition from core to specialist training is by competition (other than in Scotland where it is still 'run through').

The first 2 years of Core Training (CT) are a 'common stem', with trainees from intensive care medicine, anaesthesia and acute medicine (AM). Each will spend 1 year doing EM and AM and another year doing anaesthesia and ICM. For those wishing to pursue a career in EM, CT year 3 comprises 6 months of trauma and orthopaedics (either in an orthopaedic department or in an ED where the educational emphasis is on trauma) and 6 months of paediatric EM.

Specialty training (ST) years 4–6 will be spent in a series of EDs. Year to year progression is dependent on satisfactory assessment and appraisals, mostly conducted in the workplace. In the final year of training, candidates who are supported by their local programme are eligible to sit for the FCEM examination, successful completion of which is necessary for eligibility for a CCT.

Sub-specialty training

Paediatric EM is a recognized CCT subspecialty of both EM and of paediatrics. EM trainees who hold a CCT may undertake additional training in the care of children. The format and content of this training has been agreed upon by CEM and the Royal College of Paediatrics and Child Health (RCPCH) and will last for at least one year. There are currently 18 departments accredited for such training in the UK with about 40 training slots available each year. Pathways for dual accreditation in acute medicine and intensive care medicine have also been agreed with other relevant authorities.

Conclusion

Recent years have been difficult for all involved in PGME in the UK. Well-intentioned changes have had unintended consequences. Much work remains to be done before a stable pattern of postgraduate training, which enjoys the confidence of all involved, is re-established across the whole gamut of medicine in the UK.

Despite the problems that became apparent as the national picture unfolded, the pattern of EM training which emerged, attracted positive comment and has proven popular with trainees. Both EM and its new college have survived these tribulations better than most. Anyone interested in EM training in the UK is advised to make frequent visits to the websites of CEM, PMETB and MMC. The report of the inquiry into MMC by Sir John Tooke is a forensic analysis of the work of committees and government bodies and is a rich rewarding experience for anyone who reads it.

Controversies and future directions

❶ A generation of young doctors has felt itself under-valued by the system and let down by its seniors, following the introduction of dramatic and rapidly changing structures for postgraduate training in the UK. The future shape of postgraduate medical training in the UK is by no means clear.

❷ While laudable, the Modernizing Medical Careers Programme has been something of a disaster with many colleges, including EM, in all parts of the UK except Scotland, withdrawing from their recommended programmes and re-introducing their own competitive programmes. The lack of stability engendered by these changes is proving enormously disruptive to young doctors in the UK.

27.7 Complaints

Allen Yuen

ESSENTIALS

1 Complaints occur in every emergency department.

2 They indicate dissatisfaction with some aspect of a patient's attendance.

3 The majority of complaints are, at least partly, justified.

4 They warrant acceptance, apology and investigation.

5 A timely report of findings and recommendations must follow.

6 The complaint should be resolved satisfactorily.

7 Lessons learnt should be audited and used in quality improvement.

Introduction

Complaints are inevitable in the setting of busy emergency departments (EDs) and high patient expectations. Senior ED staff are well aware of what constitutes optimal care. However, EDs are areas where there is little control over the cases which present and the timing and volume of new arrivals, where unexpected scenarios can develop at any time, where caseload and case-mix are completely unpredictable, and where there is a mixture of staff with different levels of experience. For these reasons and others (Table 27.7.1), complaints are common. Improvements in clinical care resulting from advances in emergency medicine (EM) and nursing have set new standards, with which the public has become familiar through the media.

Patients and their relatives have much higher expectations of EDs than previously. They are better informed, and more litigious, encouraged by legal firms advertising to patients that they have a right to complain and to take legal advice if they have any cause for dissatisfaction.

Table 27.7.1 Contributing factors and reasons for complaints
Unpredictability of case-mix and caseload
Variation in attendance rates
Long waiting times
Insufficient staffing for unexpected peaks
Junior staff with variable experience and supervision
Deficiencies in treatment (real or perceived)
Inadequate assessment and missed diagnosis (real or perceived)
Poor attitudes, lack of professionalism
Poor communication, lack of information or consent
Interruptions, multiple concurrent tasks
Delays in investigations, consultations
Access block to inpatient beds
No appropriate follow-up
Inappropriate or premature discharge
Unmet expectations
Invasion of privacy
Fees in private hospital EDs
Litigation for compensation

Nevertheless, many patients, who may have legitimate cause for complaint, do not. The frequency of complaints is not an accurate gauge of patient satisfaction.

Patients have a right to complain if they feel dissatisfied about any aspect of their attendance, and it is appropriate to acknowledge this, note the complaint, apologize for the disappointment and take any corrective measure that will help at the time. If there is no immediate remedial action available, then the complainant should be given an undertaking that the problem will be investigated with those involved, and any appropriate actions taken. Once it is decided what measures are needed, the complainant is contacted to resolve the matter satisfactorily. If this cannot be achieved for whatever reason, wider consultation may be required, and this will often involve the hospital's legal advisers and the doctor's medical defence organization.

Incidence
Complaint rates vary from 0.26 to 3.8 complaints/1000 patients.[1,2] Some hospitals only record written complaints, while others also include verbal complaints in their data. Often the complaints refer to more than one issue. More complaints relate to paediatric patients, and more may be made by the literate.

In a recent Victorian study of 2419 ED-related complaints from 36 hospitals over 5 years, 37% were made by the patient while 48% were from relatives. Friends accounted for 3%, and the rest included GPs, specialists, government representatives and lawyers. ED complaints were 14.3% of the total 16 901 hospital complaints.[1]

It is likely that all reports of rate of complaints are underestimates.

Reasons

There were four main reasons for complaint: problems relating to care, inadequate treatment, diagnosis or follow-up (33.5%), poor communication skills, rudeness and discourtesy (31.5%), delays (26%), and administrative deficiencies such as incorrect documentation, inability to obtain previous records, lack of privacy or confidentiality and loss of property (7%).[1] In private hospitals, fees are an increasing source of complaint.

Complaints may be classified into two main groups. The first involves problems in clinical care, including alleged medical negligence, in which compensation may be sought and litigation threatened. Second are those in which the patient or relative has a grievance for a variety of reasons, for which they seek assurance that corrective measures will be made to ensure that no-one else has a similarly unpleasant experience.[3]

Problems in clinical care
About 50% of complaints claiming inadequate medical assessment and treatment are substantiated.[2] Inadequate physical examination followed by a missed diagnosis found on a later visit may be a source of complaint and can only be refuted if relevant positives and negatives, found at the initial visit, are documented accurately.

Medicine is not an exact science, and the early clinical features may be atypical or overlap with other causes which seem unlikely at initial presentation. To try to explain this to an anxious patient who simply wants a quick diagnosis and symptom relief can pose difficulties to a busy doctor. Still, efforts need to be made to help the patient to understand.

'Missed' fractures are the most frequent (some cannot even be picked by experts on initial imaging), but some 'misdiagnoses' as perceived by patients may result from poor communication, with lack of explanation by the treating doctor of possible causes, and what to do if there is no improvement, such as to attend their local doctor or to have an outpatient appointment arranged.[2]

Lack of treatment includes insufficient or no analgesia, lack of X-rays, blood tests, urine culture or antibiotics (where an initial presentation, particularly in a child, may have suggested a viral illness with eventual progression to a bacterial infection), and lack of a splint for a 'soft tissue injury', which is subsequently diagnosed as a fracture.

Rough, unskilled or incompetent treatment still occurs despite advances in training of both doctors and nurses. A heavy workload is not an acceptable excuse for this. With the reduction in allowable weekly labour hours for hospital-employed doctors, EDs rely to some extent on junior staff and locums, under variable levels of senior supervision on some rosters.

Unprofessional conduct and refusal to refer to a specialist or to a previous treating doctor are unacceptable causes of complaint. Cases of sexual misconduct are very rare in EDs, and would be referred to a medical board.

Communication problems
Failures of communication feature prominently in most complaints.[4] Failure of doctors to introduce themselves and to explain the reasons for examination, investigations, treatment, admission or discharge, referrals or delays are all easily avoidable causes of complaints.[2]

Abruptness, rudeness, discourtesy, insensitivity, absence of caring and other aspects of poor attitude used to be the main reason for complaints, but no longer, perhaps because the public is now more accustomed to this, as standards in general society have changed. However, in EDs, when people are rightfully anxious about their medical condition, such attitudes should not be tolerated.

Failure to obtain consent in the case of minors, to gain informed consent for procedures and to warn about risks, occurs commonly in EDs, where it is assumed that their attendance gives implied consent, but this can be challenged if the patient is brought to hospital by ambulance or other means.

Incorrect documentation is a significant cause for complaint, particularly when it results in the wrong treatment. Doctors may miss significant clues, if they ignore aspects of a patient's history which do not fit in with a presumed working diagnosis. This may also occur if the history is rushed and overly brief.

Reliance on referring letters or ambulance sheets, without checking with the patient, often results in transcribing incorrect past history, medication charts and allergies. It cannot be assumed that referral details or old case histories are correct.

Conflicting, wrong and misleading information may be related to differences in the information supplied by various sources, but is more reason for being meticulous in ensuring their accuracy. Sometimes this is impossible to do, because reliable sources cannot be contacted. At times, it is due to 'doctor-shopping', a trend which sees patients attend the most convenient bulk-billing family medicine clinic, where their past history is unknown, hoping for a quick cure for acute problems, while reserving attendances at their usual general practitioner for their more complicated ongoing illnesses.

Clinical staff in EDs are commonly faced with excessive communication loads. The combination of interruptions and multiple concurrent tasks resulted in 36 communication events an hour in one study, and this may produce clinical errors by disrupting memory processes.[5]

Problems with delays

Difficulty with access to healthcare is a worldwide problem, even in first world countries, where economic rationalism and changing government policies have resulted in closure of hospital beds, mental health institutions and community resources. Life style and industrial issues have decreased the numbers of medical and nursing staff in hospitals, particularly after hours.

Diminished outpatient services mean that patients need to be referred to private consultants' rooms where appointments may not be readily available. Fewer general practices open in the evenings or weekends. Some patients want a one-stop service for their medical consultation, their laboratory tests and their radiology. These social reasons make unnecessary use of scarce resources, despite strategies such as telephone triage services and hospital-run after hours GP clinics. All the above have contributed to increased ED attendances.

Delays in triage, time seen by doctor, treatment, investigations, consultations, admission or discharge therefore occur. Measures to decrease these are only partially successful, because there is generally no excess of staff or resources to call upon when there are unexpected peaks in workload. Steps to improve waiting times, increase throughput of short-stay patients, and decrease misdiagnosis of fractures have resulted in fewer complaints.[8]

Particularly in the case of children, long delays cannot be easily tolerated, and a significant number 'walk out' without being seen. The majority of these do not generate a complaint, but some lead on to increased morbidity.[9] The elderly are less likely to complain, but suffer in silence, such that any pain they have may be unrecognized and untreated until late in the management.[10]

Administrative problems

Incorrect documentation by clerical, nursing or medical staff, lack of privacy or confidentiality, loss of valuables, poor cleaning or other environmental issues and queries regarding billing in private hospitals comprise the majority of administrative complaints.[1,2]

Errors are made by doctors in giving advice regarding a patient's right to claim compensation, since the full circumstances cannot easily be ascertained at the time of consultation. Doctors should not advise patients regarding entitlements to worker's or traffic accident compensation, but should complete the necessary documentation objectively. Care should be taken with accuracy in completing medical certificates. Poor department design, lack of an accessible staff room or little adherence to departmental policy may cause complaints about staff socializing, eating or drinking.

Their laughter is seen by some patients as inappropriate, but by others as a sign of good staff morale.

Lack of formality, addressing older patients by their given name and casual dress standards without identification have become the accepted norm in many Australasian hospitals, but still upset some of our senior citizens and immigrants. The Federal Privacy Act 1988 was recently amended, and became effective in December 2001.[6,7] It has resulted in removal of prominent whiteboards detailing patient information in view of other patients and visitors. Computers are now used in most departments, but even these may be visible to passersby.

The Federal Privacy Act gives patients a general right of access to information held about them (see Chapter 25.4 Privacy and Confidentiality). However, the doctor still has ownership of his clinical notes and specialists have legal rights over their reports. While patients have right of access, they must obtain consent from the doctors for further reproduction of the material. Ethics are involved, in that relevant material must be made available to another doctor. Refusal of access must be based on reasonable grounds, such as that access would pose a serious threat to the life or health of any person.[7] In contrast, information on a patient must not be divulged to third parties without patient consent, unless compelled by law, such as with mandatory reporting of child abuse. Disputes may need to be settled in court.

Unmet expectations

Patient satisfaction surveys have ranked waiting times, symptom relief, a caring and concerned attitude and correct diagnosis as their priorities when attending an ED. However, there is a mismatch when compared with staff, who agree with the same priorities, but rank waiting time fourth.[11]

Patients expect ED doctors to identify serious or dangerous conditions and to treat these appropriately. Explanation and reassurance is needed. They expect investigations and admission as indicated.[3]

Pressure for litigation and compensation

Legal firms now advertise in the lay press that patients dissatisfied with any aspect of their healthcare should seek legal advice as they may be entitled to compensation, and some recent large awards may encourage more patients to take this course. While progression to litigation is relatively rare, this has resulted in increasing rates of medical indemnity insurance and has contributed to the practice of 'defensive medicine'.[4]

Responding to complaints

All verbal complaints need to be responded to (Table 27.7.2) immediately by the person to whom the complaint is made, and subsequently by a senior person, the department director, nurse unit manager, or, in the case of financial disputes, the business manager. An appropriate immediate response is preferable, as this helps to defuse any anger. The complainant should be interviewed in a private office or cubicle away from distractions. The ability to respond satisfactorily to formal complaints is a necessary part of emergency medical practice.[12]

The basis of the patient's grievance must be fully understood, and addressed. It may be that one has to deal with a patient's misperception of what has happened. Empathy is more likely to lead to a successful outcome than an aggressive denial.[13] How to do this without further alienating the patient will require good rapport and skill.

Table 27.7.2 Suggested procedure for response to complaints
Accept the complaint
Apologize for the complainant's dissatisfaction
Defuse any anger
Record the details
Undertake to investigate
Arrange follow-up
Investigate
Discuss with staff
Inform administration
Consider legal implications
Follow-up with complainant
Resolve complaint
Lessons to be learnt

Understanding and patience is required in handling complaints. Verbal complaints must be listened to attentively, and a record made of the complainant's name and contact details, the nature of the complaint, the patient's name and other relevant information. If the complainant is abusive, there is no point in reacting likewise, as this will only escalate the hostility. State that you would like to help, but can only do so if you are permitted to record the details, without undue pressure.

For written complaints, a written acknowledgement of the complaint together with an apology for their dissatisfaction should be sent within 3 days with an undertaking to have the matter investigated and measures taken to address the problem.

Some experienced directors thank patients for their complaints, on the basis that these provide an opportunity for improving the service. An initial apology that they have been dissatisfied acknowledges the complaint; it does not admit error. Nor does it admit that the complaint is correct; it recognizes that the complainant is aggrieved, and that the complaint will be investigated and appropriate action taken to address the grievance.

If the complaint is of an obviously serious nature, such as a fatal outcome, an apology, such as 'I'm terribly sorry that you have lost your wife/father', does not admit liability, but empathizes with the relative and allows you to undertake to investigate the circumstances, and then to discuss the matter further after obtaining additional information, so as to be able to help in understanding the cause of death or in establishing if management was appropriate. Respect the grief and the need to know as much as possible about the circumstances. It may be that the grief reaction includes a need to blame. Counselling support may be offered (pastoral care, social work, stress psychologists etc).[11] Arrangements for a follow-up appointment, telephone call or letter should be made.

If there is a ready explanation, then this can be given, and may often be sufficient. Complaints about waiting times may be easily dealt with in most instances by a courteous explanation of the triage process, the current caseload, the priorities within the department, the staffing, cubicle and bed availability and reassurance that they will be seen as soon as possible. If they are not satisfied, then alternatives such as attending another ED or medical centre can be offered.

Complaints relating to 'misdiagnosis', may be due rather to natural progression of a disease, such as with meningococcal septicaemia, which may present in its early stages as a non-specific viral-like illness, only to deteriorate rapidly and sometimes fatally over the next few hours, or subarachnoid haemorrhage which does not always present with classical sudden onset of headache with neck stiffness and photophobia, or even more frequently, pulmonary embolism which can be present without the usual classical features. The patients themselves, previously relatively young and healthy, tend to deny their symptomatology, and may not give a full history, making it extremely difficult for the doctor to make an accurate diagnosis.

Failure to spot a borderline fracture or pneumonia on a film may not be classed as negligent, but failure to follow up on a positive radiological report most certainly is.[13]

While some complaints may appear trivial, the underlying reasons for the complaints must be investigated, and causes identified, so that corrective measures can be taken to prevent recurrences. Patients must feel that their complaints are taken seriously, and appropriate action taken. Making flimsy excuses without looking properly into the matter will not help. The responses must not be seen as arrogant, defensive or dismissive; any of these could merely exacerbate the problem. The concept of establishing an adult–adult relationship with the complainant is a good basis for continuing useful discussion.

If a complaint has medicolegal implications, then the medical director, chief executive or hospital legal liaison officer need to be informed and the matter discussed with a view to appropriate responses.

If the complaint has come indirectly from the Health Complaints Commissioner (or its equivalent), a legal firm, a parliamentarian or the medical board, these usually go to the medical director or the chief executive, seeking information for their client, so that they can decide whether the matter could be resolved by mediation or conciliation, rather than proceeding to litigation.[4]

Any doctor involved should decide whether their medical defence/indemnity insurance organization needs to be informed, and where doubt exists, they should.

Check with the involved staff, record notes and charts. Establish facts regarding assessment, treatment and follow-up. If it is established that there is justification for the complaint, then involved staff may need debriefing and counselling.[14] This is often overlooked, and doctors and nurses have left clinical medicine or nursing following a complaint, even though they may not have been directly responsible for the outcome.

When the complaint is a result of human error, the doctor or nurse must accept that no-one can function at optimal capacity at all times in such an unpredictable area as an ED, nor can they be responsible for unexpected changes or serious deterioration in a patient's illness. There are many mitigating circumstances in patient care that can affect outcome, such as distractions, simultaneous care of patients, other priorities, inability to contact the patient's usual doctor to obtain important information, etc.

Once the facts have been established and a report formulated, contact the complainant for further discussion. This must be a factual interview with a frank discussion of the situation, and the actions which are recommended.

Resolution

In the Victorian study, about 75% of complaints were resolved,[1] usually by explanation or apology. As a result, changes in procedure or policy occurred (2%). Remedial action took place in 5% of cases. Only a small percentage (less than 1%) proceeded to the courts. Compensation was rare (0.2%). The complaint was not upheld, was unsubstantiated, was frivolous or vexatious or lapsed in up to 15% of cases. In 1% there was not enough detail to investigate. Fees were refunded, waived or reduced in less than 1% of cases, but this could well rise with changes in societal expectations. The majority of complainants who go to State Health Complaints Commissioners are not seeking revenge or compensation. Most of their cases are resolved

by enquiry, assessment and investigation of the complaint, and then conciliation with the affected parties.[4]

Prevention

A well-equipped ED which has adequate numbers of senior staff supervising junior staff with strict lines of responsibility will have fewer adverse events and complaints.

Verbal and printed explanations of triage, department assessment procedure and investigation turn-around times must be provided to patients, particularly when waiting times are excessive. Children and psychiatric patients are the ones who tolerate long waits least well, and need to be seen earlier. If the situation changes, triage staff should give updated waiting times to patients who have still not been seen.[2] If the doctor makes a point of describing, to the patient, the findings during the examination, and records this in the notes, this overcomes complaints that certain areas were not examined. Patients may be unaware of, or not remember, which areas have been examined. Patient notes should be contemporaneous, but if additions or alterations are appropriate in order to clarify a matter, they may be added and dated as such. Guidelines and protocols of recommended management should be available in all EDs to ensure maintenance of standards.[13]

When an adverse event occurs, medical defence organizations now advise that staff should disclose it fully, apologize early and sincerely, with a statement of genuine and empathic regret and acknowledgement of the patient or relative's distress,[15] and then discuss the circumstances with them giving an undertaking to take corrective measures. They should not be seen as avoiding the patient, otherwise anger and suspicion will arise.[4] An apology is much more likely to defuse rather than inflame the situation. Early crisis counseling and psychological support may be offered to patient, relatives and affected staff.[12]

Staff should be encouraged to report any incident or adverse outcome which might generate a complaint, so that the appropriate manager can investigate with staff, prepare a report and convey lessons to be learnt to prevent a recurrence. If the expected complaint then eventuates, a

ready response may well reassure the complainant that this hospital takes its work seriously, and may find the actions already taken as adequate to address the issues.

Addressing senior citizens by their prefixed surname may avert complaints of lack of respect or over-familiarity. These patients and many of those from overseas still prefer doctors to wear white coats, but changing attitudes to professional attire allows neatness and an identification badge to suffice.[14]

Better communication by either or both medical and nursing staff of reasons for delays, examination, investigations, treatment, consultations, admission or discharge, referrals and choice of specialist will prevent a large proportion of the complaints relating to actual patient care.

Good documentation may provide the only means to resolve a dispute, as stressed patients are not good listeners, the use of medical jargon tends to confuse patients and the drama and trauma of the emergency can distort perceptions of what actually occurred.[4] Systems must be in place to check and take appropriate action on abnormal pathology and imaging results, which often return after the treating doctor has finished a rostered shift. Misdiagnoses need to be audited and used as educational tools. Care with department design is a necessity, so that the waiting and resuscitation areas are visible, patient privacy is maintained, temperature is comfortable, rest rooms are accessible and staff have tea and tutorial rooms adjacent to the main clinical area (See Chapter 27.2).

The lessons to be learnt after investigation of a complaint should be discussed with all those concerned, and then presented to all staff to reinforce the issues and solutions. In doing so, anonymity of patient and staff involved should be preserved. Specific training on how to relate to patients in the pressures of the ED environment should be incorporated into orientation and graduate programmes for both doctors and nurses.[1]

An understanding of patient expectations assists in the prevention of complaints.[17] Complaints are opportunities for learning, as few lessons are better learnt than those which threaten one's self-esteem. Debriefing and counselling should be offered to affected staff. Objective and supportive feedback will facilitate improved staff performance.[2]

All complaints should be audited, and the results summarized for presentation at a department meeting for discussion. These would form part of a quality improvement programme.

Controversies

❶ There is still controversy about whether an apology should be made, particularly amongst lawyers and hospital administrators. However, the evidence strongly suggests that apology, without admission of liability, actually reduces the risk of litigation, and more often results in patient satisfaction.[18]

❷ The question of how to approach an abusive complainant is difficult. Self-protection and empathy are important aspects of a successful negotiation.

References

1. Taylor DMcD, Wolfe R, Cameron PA. Complaints from emergency department patients largely result from treatment and communication problems. Emergency Medicine 2002; 14: 43–49.
2. Brookes J. Complaints. In: Dunn R, ed. The emergency medicine manual. 2nd edn. Adelaide: Venom Publishing 2000: 27–29.
3. Bartley B, Cameron PA. QUEST: Questionnaire relating to patients' understanding and expectations of their symptoms and treatment. Emergency Medicine 2000; 12: 123–127.
4. Wilson B. Using complaints constructively. Australasian Journal of Emergency Care 1998; 5(4): 269.
5. Coiera A, Jayasuriya R, Hardy J, et al. Communication loads on clinical staff in the emergency department. Medical Journal of Australasia 2002; 176: 415–418.
6. Burton P. Privacy an ongoing concern. Australasia Medicine 2002; 10.
7. Federal Privacy Commissioner. Guidelines on privacy in the private health sector. 8 November 2001.
8. Jelinek GA, Mountain D, O'Brien D, et al. Re-engineering an Australian emergency department. Journal of Quality Clinic Practices. 1999; 19(3): 133–138.
9. Hanson R, Clifton-Smith B, Fasher B, et al. Patient dissatisfaction in a paediatric accident and emergency department. Journal of Quality Clinic Practices 14: 137–143.
10. Nerney M, Chin M, Lei Jin, et al. Factors associated with older patients' satisfaction with care in an inner-city emergency department. Annals of Emergency Medicine 2001;38: 140–145.
11. Holden D, Smart D. Adding value to the patient experience in emergency medicine: What features of the emergency department visit are most important to patients? Emergency Medicine 1999; 11(1): 3–8.
12. Doig G. Responding to formal complaints about the emergency department. Emergency Medicine Australasia 2004; 16(4): 353–360.
13. Bryce G. Complaints – How to deal with them. Journal of Accident and Emergency Medicine 1998; 14: 63–64.
14. Valent P. Treating helper stresses and illnesses. In: Valent P, (ed.) Trauma and fulfillment therapy. Brunner/Mazel; 1998: 153–156.
15. Nisselle P. Crisis management: honest and open disclosure. Australian Medicine 2002; April 1: 9.
16. Hertzberg S. Attitudes to dress standards of medical officers (Abstract). Emergency Medicine 2000; March 12: A10.
17. Stuart PJ, Parker S, Rogers M. A qualitative study of consumer expectations for the emergency department. Emergency Medicine 2003; 15 (4):369–375.
18. Schwartz LR, Overton DT. The management of patient complaints and dissatisfaction. Emergency Medical Clinics of North America 1992; 10: 557–572.

27.8 Clinical risk management in the emergency department

John Vinen

ESSENTIALS

1 Awareness by all emergency department (ED) staff of the concept of patient safety and factors affecting the delivery of safe care is an essential component of the ED's clinical risk management (CRM) strategy.

2 The delivery of safe and effective patient care is reliant on a culture of safety within the ED.

3 To be effective and not intrusive, CRM strategies must be incorporated into every aspect of ED operations.

4 The use of common definitions and data sets is essential, if factors compromising patient safety in the ED are to be understood and preventative strategies introduced.

5 To monitor, analyse incidents and introduce preventative strategies occurring in the ED, a thorough understanding of the process of patient care in the ED is essential.

6 Quality indicators facilitate the monitoring of patient safety in the ED and assist in the establishment of benchmarks.

7 A range of factors, particularly overcrowding due to access block, has been shown to increase adverse events; poorly managed handover rounds have also been identified as contributing to error rates.

Introduction

The emergency department (ED) environment is complex, time-pressured and dynamic. The random presentation of a broad spectrum of undifferentiated conditions of varying acuity, from trivial to immediately life-threatening is unique to the practice of emergency medicine (EM). Nowhere else in medical practice are staff required to make (often critical) decisions with high levels of uncertainty, minimal information and significant time pressure. Attending to multiple patients simultaneously in a noisy ever-changing environment with constant interruptions and the frequent need to interrupt what one is doing in order to attend to a new arrival or the sudden deterioration of an existing patient leads to the creation of an environment of error.

The ED is a recognized high-risk environment 'perfectly designed' for errors to occur.[1,2] Clinical risk management (CRM) of necessity needs to be part of the day-to-day activities within the ED. CRM needs to be incorporated into all aspects of the delivery of emergency care if it is to be effective and not intrusive. CRM is a comprehensive yet focused strategy aimed at the three components of the delivery of care in the ED; the system, the process and the individual. CRM is aimed at ensuring the delivery of safe error-free patient care.[3]

To be effective, CRM also requires a culture of safety rather than a culture of blame. CRM encompasses the entire 'episode of care' involving all phases of emergency care (Fig.27.8.1).[2]

The extent of the problem

In order to understand both the need and the focus of a CRM programme, it is necessary to understand the extent and nature of problems related to patient safety in the ED. In the USA, medical error in the ED compromises an estimated 21.9% of medical liability based on location of the incident. Failure to diagnose myocardial infarction is the fifth most costly, based on average cost with the majority of cases involving serious injury or death. Risk increases after-hours, with the majority of cases involving patients discharged from the ED, of whom 50% fulfilled the criteria for admission.[4–7]

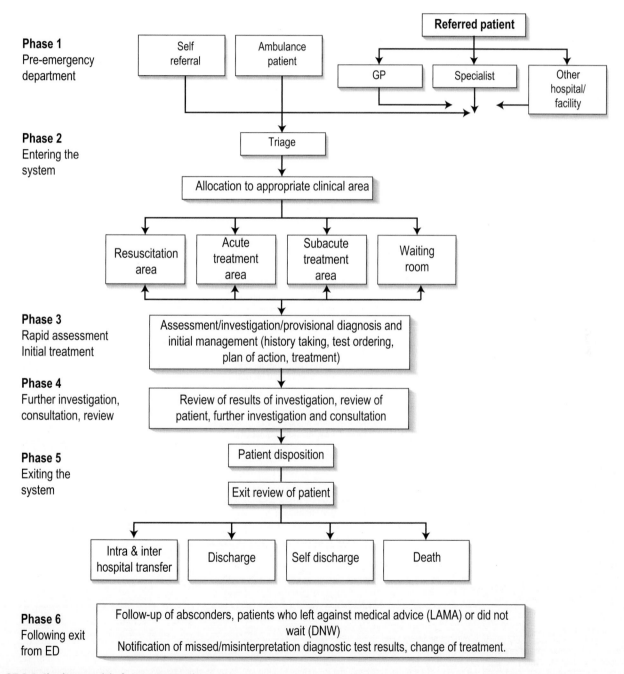

Phase 1
Pre-emergency department

Self referral

Ambulance patient

Referred patient

GP

Specialist

Other hospital/ facility

Phase 2
Entering the system

Triage

Allocation to appropriate clinical area

Resuscitation area

Acute treatment area

Subacute treatment area

Waiting room

Phase 3
Rapid assessment
Initial treatment

Assessment/investigation/provisional diagnosis and initial management (history taking, test ordering, plan of action, treatment)

Phase 4
Further investigation, consultation, review

Review of results of investigation, review of patient, further investigation and consultation

Phase 5
Exiting the system

Patient disposition

Exit review of patient

Intra & inter hospital transfer

Discharge

Self discharge

Death

Phase 6
Following exit from ED

Follow-up of absconders, patients who left against medical advice (LAMA) or did not wait (DNW)
Notification of missed/misinterpretation diagnostic test results, change of treatment.

Fig. 27.8.1 Six-phase model of emergency patient care.

Studies utilizing differing methodologies (retrospective criteria-based chart review, study of closed claims, longitudinal surveys and prospective anonymous privileged incident reporting) identified that the majority of incidents occurring in the ED are preventable with a high risk of an adverse outcome (AO) and with a significant chance of legal action being taken.[1,8–13] The Critical Incident Monitoring Study (CIMS) study in Australia found that the majority of incidents involved junior inexperienced staff, when the ED was busy, after-hours when senior experienced staff were not available to supervise.[5]

Recognition of problem areas in the ED from the literature facilitates the recognition and implementation of corrective strategies (Table 27.8.1).

CIMS evaluated data from six Australian EDs, and found that 78% of reported incidents were due to 'systems' factors, ranging from 54% for medication errors to 96.2% for 'failure to admit'. Nearly all (96.6%) of the incidents in the CIMS study were considered to be preventable. The Quality in Australian Health Care Study (QAHS) found that 70% of adverse events were due to systems factors and demonstrated high preventability, with preventability higher than average for family practice, internal medicine, and EM.

CIMS determined that four system factors are associated with the incidents: junior or very junior medical and nursing staff, on night duty or on duty on the weekend with no senior cover (i.e. staff with wider clinical

Table 27.8.1 Examples of incidents/errors

Problem	Corrective strategy
Phase 1:	Pre-Emergency Department
• Failure to accept/transfer care	Direct line to ED Admitting Officer (Duty Consultant) and pre-determined transfer agreement
• Delayed transfer/acceptance	
• Incorrect medical advice	
– EMS	
– other hospitals/facilities	
– family practitioners	
– phone advice to patient/relatives	
• Incidents involving external medical teams	
– Medical emergency on campus (e.g. cardiac arrest team)	
– Mass Casualty Incident [Disaster] teams	
Phase 2:	**Entering the System**
• Failure to triage	Backup staff for busy periods
• Delayed triage	Experienced trained triage nurse at all times
• Incorrect triage [under triage]	
• Incorrect allocation to Clinical Area	
• Vital signs not done	
Phase 3:	**Rapid Assessment / Initial Treatment**
• Delayed assessment	Trauma Team/activation criteria
• Failure to adequately manage airway	Priority assessment process for patients presenting with chest pain/ACS
• Inadequate fluid administration	
Phase 4:	**Further Investigation, Consultation and Review**
• Failure to order required investigation	Senior experienced staff on duty
• Failure to consult	Senior experienced staff on duty
• Delayed consultation	Senior experienced staff on duty
Phase 5:	**Exiting the System**
• Failure to admit / inappropriate discharge	EGAIRT Nurse
• No discharge instructions	Appointment made prior to discharge
• Failure to refer	followed by reminder contact
Phase 6:	**Following exit from the ED**
• Failure to follow-up	Patient contact ASAP after leaving
– LAMA	
– DNW	
• Failure to ensure follow-up	Patient contact ASAP after leaving
– Timely	Recalled for treatment
– At all	
• Failure to notify missed abnormality	
– X-ray	Patient contacted to arrange change in therapy
– Pathology	
– ECG	
• Failure to contact re:	
– Change of treatment - resistant organisms	
– Delayed return of abnormal result	

All phases
• Medication error
• Incorrect/failure to accurately interpret diagnostic test/X-ray
• Failure to act on abnormal result
• Inadequate documentation
In order to improve patient safety and the quality of care it is first essential to understand the issues by studying the problems utilizing standard definitions and a defined minimum data set followed by analysis of the findings looking at causation with the aim of introducing corrective strategies.

experience on whom they could call) and a busier than usual ED and where there was a comparative shortage of senior and experienced ED staff.[5]

Incidents, errors, adverse events and adverse outcomes

In order to ensure consistency and to allow for accurate data collection, analysis and interpretation, standard definitions and data sets must be used (Table 27.8.2).

To identify, monitor and correct problem areas it is essential that all EDs incorporate into their CRM programme an incident reporting and analysis process. An incident reporting system is essential because:

- it draws attention to the problems that are occurring
- data are essential for an effective CRM system

Table 27.8.2 Standard definitions and data sets
Definitions
Incidents: ... are 'any unintended event which is inconsistent with routine hospital practice or of the quality of patient care which has had or could have had a demonstrable adverse outcome for a patient. Incidents may or may not result in an adverse event.'[2]
Adverse Event: ... is 'where an incident has resulted in a demonstrable impact on the quality of patient care. An adverse event in turn may or may not result in an adverse outcome.'[2]
Adverse Outcome: ... is 'where an incident has occurred and resulted in an undesirable event (adverse event) leading to harm to the patient.'[2]
Medical Errors: ... are 'failure of a planned action to be completed as intended (error of execution) or use of a wrong plan to achieve an aim (error of planning)'.[14] It may be a simple mistake or due to lack of expertise, negligence or other cause.
Malpractice/Negligence: 'Negligence' is the failure to use reasonable care under the circumstances as determined by the courts. It is doing, or not doing, something that a reasonably prudent doctor would do (or not do) under the same circumstances. It is a deviation, or departure, from accepted practice. 'Malpractice' is professional negligence, with medical malpractice the negligence of a doctor.[15] The term 'medical negligence' or 'malpractice' should not be used to describe an incident, adverse event, or adverse outcome unless judgement on a particular case has been handed down.

- it highlights to staff that patient safety is important, that it is a focus of the department and that action is being taken to address the problems.[2,5]

Cause and effect

It needs to be clearly understood that rarely is there only one cause of an incident. Most of the incidents have multiple causes, the majority of which involve system failures (Fig. 27.8.2).

The vast majority of incidents do not result in actual harm, (adverse event (AE) or adverse outcome (AO)). Because of the potential for an AE or AO from each and every incident no incident can be considered to be trivial (Fig. 27.8.3).

Incidents are indicators of a failure in patient safety and should be treated as such. Incidents are also frequent, and most go unnoticed or are accepted as part of doing business in the ED. Unless documented and analysed, problem areas cannot be readily identified. Trends are important.

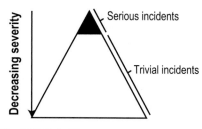

Fig. 27.8.3 Incidents.

Practical application of CRM strategies

CRM strategies can be practically applied based on the system, process, and individual, and the phase of care (Fig. 27.8.1). System strategies for applying CRM are detailed in Table 27.8.3. Process strategies are listed in Table 27.8.4. Individual strategies are noted in Table 27.8.5. Strategies for applying CRM based on phase of care can be found in Table 27.8.6.

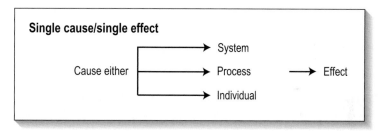

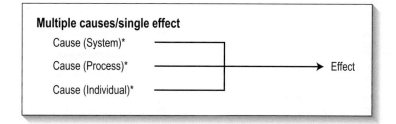

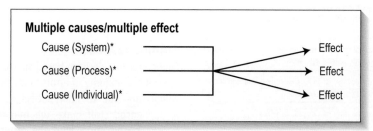

* Any combination possible

Fig. 27.8.2 Cause and effect of incidents.

Table 27.8.3   System strategies

- Adequate resourcing
- Adequate facilities
- Equipment – checklist/maintenance and replacement programme
- Staffing (numbers and seniority)
  - extended hours cover by consultants
- Reference databases/decision support systems
  - protocols/guidelines/algorithms
- Communication process/system
  - communication clerk
- Effective and efficient patient processing system
- Environmental
  - temperature, light and noise
- Emergency Department Information System (EDIS)
  - system
  - alerting
  - overview of department activity
  - patient tracking
  - fully interfaced IT system [PMI, pathology, radiology, pharmacy, etc]
- Support systems (diagnostic radiology, pathology, supplies department, bed management, etc.)
  - need to be responsive/responsible with agreed performance criteria
- Crisis response process
  - access block, major incidents/disasters
- Standardization
  - equipment, processes
- Teamwork
  - shift times/formal handover/transfer of care
- Essential power supply
- Needleless system/sharps disposal system

Table 27.8.4   Process strategies

- Direct line to ED Admitting Officer (AO), cordless phone
- 'Patient expects' database (patients referred/transferred to the ED)
- Triage process:
  - Utilization of the Australasian Triage Scale (ATS)[16]
  - Backup for busy periods
  - Allocation to appropriate clinical area
- Patient senior staff review process
- Structured handover process for each and every patient
- Pre-exit review of all patients
  - the 'EGAIRT' (Reverse Triage) Nurse (Table 27.7.8)
- Senior staff real time review of ECGs, X-rays, abnormal pathology results
- Timely review of post discharge and transfer radiology/pathology results
- Timely review of DNWs, LAMAs
- Proforma
  - assessment/admission, ODs, chest pain, traumas.

Table 27.8.5   Individual strategies

- Recruitment/selection/appointment
- Orientation
- Credentialling and accreditation
- Training – 'error training' – increased awareness of problems/high risk conditions/situations, recurrent incidents and corrective strategies ('share the lesson').
- Supervision
- CME/MOPS
- Performance appraisal

Staffing issues

Emergency is a decision-based specialty; as a result the majority of errors made by individuals are due to poor decision-making. Inexperienced staff make the majority of decision-based errors with the result that one of the most effective ways of reducing errors in the ED is to ensure junior staff

are adequately supervised with each and every patient reviewed by a medical officer of at least advanced trainee level.

Training programmes need to incorporate the process of critical thinking and clinical decision making.

Role of the 'reverse triage' nurse

An important part of the CRM process is the role of the 'EGAIRT' or reverse triage nurse (Table 27.8.7). This pre-exit review ensures all patients leave the ED with minimal potential for adverse events and outcomes.

CRM and major incidents/disaster response

In order for the ED to respond to major incidents, (internal and external) a number of requirements need to be met (Table 27.8.8).

Clinical guidelines/reference databases

The use of assessment and management charts utilizing clinical guidelines has been demonstrated to improve clinical decision-making and documentation.

On-line reference databases (with a down-time manual backup system) facilitate clinical decision-making and drug administration. The availability of comprehensive up-to-date information on the range of conditions presenting to the ED is now a reality. Not only should this information and the technology to support it be available, staff should be required to use it (e.g. MIMS on-line, New South Wales DOH Clinical Information Access Program (CIAP) website,[17] etc.).

High-risk issues

High risk can be applied to reasons for presentation/diagnoses, situations and personal factors (human factors). High risk patients include the very young, the elderly, immunosuppressed patients, those intoxicated with alcohol and/or drugs, people from non-English speaking backgrounds, patients with psychiatric conditions and those on anticoagulants. Specific complaints or diagnoses associated with high risk include chest pain, headache and fever in children.

High risk situations include new staff unfamiliar with the environment, high

Table 27.8.6 Phase of care strategies

Phase 1
- Referral/transfer agreements
- Medical advice policies and protocol
- Medical emergency team(s):
  – policies and protocols
  – training

Phase 2
- 24/7 trained triage nurse available
- Back up triage staff for busy periods
- Link triage category with clinical area role
- Measurement and documentation of vital signs
- Availability of medical records
- Immediate availability of MRN/labels

Phase 3
- Immediate bed availability for all triage category 1 & 2 patients
- Triage category 1/trauma/cardiac arrest team

Phase 4
- Timely senior staff review of all patients post-assessment by junior staff
- Regular review of status of all patients in the ED by senior staff on duty

Phase 5
- Pre-exit review all patients by senior (EGAIRT) nurse and MO
- Appropriate referral of discharged patients
- Written discharge instructions, all discharged patients

Phase 6
- Timely review of all discharged patients – radiology, ECG and pathology results
- Review of LAMAs, and DNWs

All Phases
- Documentation
- Incident/error reports
- Complaints
- Documentation of interpretation of ECG/X-ray findings
- Date and signing each and every diagnostic report form indicating that it has been reviewed in a timely manner

QA/Audit/CRM review

In order to ensure that all aspects of ED operations are monitored as part of a comprehensive CRM programme, a range of structured activities is essential.

The activities that are required to be monitored on a continuous basis range from overall ED efficiency in managing patients to ensuring individual patients receive the care that they require. The focus of these strategies is patients' safety and the delivery of timely appropriate care.[19,20]

Indicators/benchmarks

The utilization of performance and quality indicators (QIs) to monitor performance and measure quality allows for benchmarking and the identification of problem areas and trends.

All indicators are inter-related as a result of the complexity of care in the ED with a number of indicators functioning as both performance indicators (PIs) and quality indicators (QIs) (Table 27.7.9).

Indicators and audit

A number of the data elements utilized in studying incidents, AEs, error and ED per-

Table 27.8.7 Role of the 'EGAIRT' (reverse triage) nurse

E	ducation of patient
G	uarantee that treatment is complete
A	dmission not indicated
I	nformation (documentation) complete
R	eview (follow-up) arranged
T	ransport arranged

Table 27.8.8 Essentials for CRM in Mass Casualty Incidents

- Entire ED on essential power supply/backup via generator
- Key support services (pathology, diagnostic imaging, operating theatres, lift (at least one), etc. also need to be on essential power supply service
- Bottled oxygen cylinders to be available for supply failure
- Back-up suction equipment essential
- Non-PABX communication system
- Back-up manual patient registration and tracking system

Table 27.8.9 Performance and quality indicators

Performance indicators
- Triage waiting times
- Treatment time
- Access block (a hospital bed management PI)

Quality indicators
- Time to 1st ECG for patient with chest pain
- Measurement and documentation of vital signs
- Pregnancy test for female patient of child-bearing age with abdominal pain
- Time to thrombolysis or angioplasty/stenting for patients with AMI
- Weight (in Kg) measured for all children

Failure to:
- Investigate
- Interpret X-rays correctly
- Act on abnormal results

Delay in:
- Administering
  – thrombolysis
  – antibiotics for
    - meningitis
    - sepsis
    - compound fractures

workload situations, ED overcrowding and frequent interruptions. Human factors include inexperience, fatigue, stress and shiftwork.

Risk factors are additive, with error rates increasing significantly for each additional risk factor.

Facilities

The ED should be purpose-designed and built, large enough to meet peak period demand and comply with the Australasian College for Emergency Medicine Emergency Department Design Guidelines.[18] Environmental and other services need to comply with Australian Standards. A communication system separate from the PABX should also be available. Security and Occupational Health and Safety Standards (OHSS) requirements should be in place.

formance/operations can be used as quality indicators.[21]

QIs are a subset of safety indicators, and measure and monitor the quality of care in the ED. QIs must meet the requirement of an indicator, reflect the environment, be directly relevant to clinical practice and reflect the quality of care in the ED no matter what the circumstances (resource constraint, overcrowding, etc.).

QIs assist in improving quality through a number of mechanisms (Table 27.8.10). Few QIs are pure. All ED QIs are impacted by external (to the ED) factors.

Some QIs can be considered to be relatively pure (Table 27.8.11).

There is also an overlap of many indicators. Triage waiting times are both PIs and QIs. When used as PIs, triage waiting times measure the system's ability to attend to the medical assessment of new arrivals based on the urgency for medical care (based on the ATS). When used as QIs triage waiting times measure the quality of care of a range of medical conditions where there is good evidence that outcome (morbidity and mortality) is directly influenced by time to medical treatment (Table 27.8.12).

QIs can be categorized in several ways. They can be indicators of system, process or individual aspects of care (Table 27.8.13), indicators of phase of care (Table 27.8.14), or indicators of the problem (disease specific) (Table 27.8.15). Because of the complexity of the ED, studying QIs by phase of care allows for identification of causal factors in a manageable way.

Access block is a hospital PI and not an ED PI, but has a very significant impact on ED PIs and QIs.

ED overcrowding due to access block has been demonstrated to increase AEs.[23,24] Problems associated with poor handover of patients have been recognized as a significant risk factor for AEs.[25,26]

The audit process, whilst time-consuming is an essential component of the ED's CRM program. Some of the important operations that need to be audited function as QIs (Table 27.8.16).

Table 27.8.10 Mechanisms by which QIs improve quality

- Providing a better understanding of the process of care
- Increasing understanding of the variation that exists in a process and measuring the variation
- Monitoring a process over time
- Providing a common reference point and allowing comparisons/benchmarking
- Allowing the documentation and analysis of failures in the quality of care and facilitating the development of preventative strategies aimed at reducing the frequency of quality of care failure
- Seeing the effect of change in a process
- Establishing a more accurate basis for further research

Table 27.8.11 Pure ED QIs

Arrival time to:
- Medical assessment/resuscitation for triage category 1
- Initial ECG in chest pain/suspected AMI
- Administration of aspirin and thrombolysis/angioplasty for AMI
- Administration of antibiotics in:
  - suspected bacterial meningitis
  - compound fractures[20]
- Defibrillation for VF
- Ventilation for respiratory arrest
- Airway management for GCS = 8

Table 27.8.12 Triage waiting times QIs

- Time to thrombolysis/angiogram for AMI
- Time to intervention for compromised airway
- Time to DC shock for VF

Table 27.8.13 System, process and individual aspects of care indicators

System
- Triage waiting times
- Senior staff review of all patients

Process
- Triage process/accuracy
- Patient tracking during treatment
- Measurement of vital signs

Individual
- Errors
- Failure to consult
- Failure to refer
- Failure to admit

Table 27.8.14 Phase of care indicators

Phase 1
- Failure to accept urgent transfer
- Delayed transfer
- Failure to give treatment advice (administer penicillin for suspected meningitis)
- Increased transport time/patient taken to inappropriate facility because ED on bypass status

Phase 2
- Failure to triage
- Delayed triage
- Incorrect triage (under-triage)
- Incorrect allocation of treatment area

Phase 3
- Delayed assessment/treatment
  - excessive waiting time
- Failure to protect/establish airway
- Inadequate resuscitation fluids

Phase 4
- Required investigation not done
- Failure to consult
- Incorrect diagnosis
- Missed diagnosis
- Missed injuries

Phase 5
- Failure to admit
- LAMA
- DNW

Phase 6
- Death after discharge
- Recalls
- No or delayed follow-up
- Failure to refer
- Inappropriate escort during transfer
- Incorrect mode of transport during transfer
- Failure to notify re missed abnormality
- Failure to contact re required change of treatment

All Phases
- Died in the ED
- Misinterpretation or failure to act on abnormal diagnostic investigation findings
- Incident reports
- Medication errors
- Failure to document
- Complications of procedures

Table 27.8.15 Problem (disease specific) indicators

Problem/Disease Specific
- Failure to use spirometric based management of acute asthma
- Pre-eclampsia – failure to:
  - Measure BP
  - Examine for oedema
  - Examine for proteinuria
- Time to thrombolysis/angioplasty
- Time to antibiotic administration
  - Meningitis
  - Compound fractures
- Pregnancy test
  - Females with abdominal pain

Table 27.8.16	Potential targets for audit

- Accuracy of triage category allocation
- Accuracy of allocation to clinical areas
- Chart audits:
  - adequacy of documentation
  - documentation of:
    - vital signs
    - weight in Kg (children)
- Review of results of diagnostic investigations
- Representations within 7 days
- LAMAs
- DNWs
- Deaths (DIED)
- Recalls for:
  - treatment
  - admission

Future directions

❶ It is likely that greater awareness and understanding of the extent of the problem and what preventative strategies are required will develop over the next decade.

❷ There is also likely to be greatly improved ED staffing with a focus on senior staffing, aiming at 24/7 cover.

❸ There needs to be increased awareness of taking human factors into consideration in relation to rostering practices in particular.

❹ The use of decision support tools is likely to become widespread.

❺ Universal implementation of an integrated hospital-wide IT system ('paperless system') is likely in the near future.

❻ Improved training with a focus on critical thinking and use of simulators will have an impact on error rates.

Controversies

❶ Causation of error in the ED is well-understood, with local preventative strategies widely implemented with some success, but little has been done system-wide for a number of reasons, including resistance to change, bureaucratic inertia, lack of political will and inadequate funding.

❷ Access block leading to serious ED overcrowding continues to grow as a major problem and contributes to sometimes serious adverse events.

❸ There is still not a consensus on patient safety terminology. The commonly used term 'error' is judgemental and a process of attribution based on outcome. Its use compromises staff commitment to incident reporting activities.

❹ Hindsight bias remains a problem even with those that are supposedly well informed.

❺ It remains to be proved whether incident reporting and the implementation of many CRM strategies actually reduce the frequency of incidents and increase patient safety.

❻ It is increasingly clear that lessons learned from other high risk industries can be used to improve the safety of patient care.

❼ Research into patient safety in the ED is in its infancy. What is required is a concerted effort to study the relationship between the unique environment in the ED and factors compromising patient safety.

References

1. Brennan TA, Leape LL, Laird NM, et al. Incidence of adverse events and negligence in hospitalized patients: results of the Harvard Medical Practice Study I. New England Journal of Medicine 1991: 324: 370–376.
2. Vinen JD. Incident monitoring in emergency departments: an Australian model. Applied and Environmental Microbiology. 2000; 7: 1290–1297.
3. Australasian College for Emergency Medicine Policy on Quality 2002 Improvement in Emergency Medicine www.acem.org.au/open/documents/quality.pdf
4. Annual Report to Policy Holders: Physicians and Surgeons 1991. St Paul: MN St Paul Fire and Marine Insurance Company.
5. Vinen JD, Gaudry PL, Ashby R. Critical incident monitoring study in emergency medicine (CIMS) interim report. Sydney: Australasian College for Emergency Medicine and Commonwealth Department of Human Services and Health;1994.
6. Rusnak RA, Stair TO, Hansen K. Litigation against the emergency physician: common features in cases of missed myocardial infarction. Annals of Emergency Medicine 1989; 1029–1034.
7. Trautlein JJ, Lambert RL, Miller J. Malpractice in the emergency department – review of 200 cases. Annals of Emergency Medicine 1984; 13: 709–711.
8. Leape LL, Breanan, TA, Laird NM, et al. The nature of adverse events in hospitalized patients: results of the Harvard Medical Practice Study II. New England Journal of Medicine 1991; 324: 377–384.
9. Thomas EJ, Studdert DM, Burstin HR, et al. Incidence and types of adverse events and negligent care in Utah and Colorado in 1992-2000. Medicine Care 1992–2000; 38: 261–271.
10. California Medical Association Medical Feasibility Study. In: Mills DH, Boxden JS, Rubsamen, PS (eds). San Francisco: Sutter; 1977.
11. Wilson R McL, Runciman WB, Gibberd RW, et al. The quality in Australian Health Care Study. Medical Journal of Australia 1995; 163: 458–471.
12. Thomas EJ, Studdert DM, Runciman WB, et al. A comparison of iatrogenic injury studies in Australia and the USA, I: context, methods, case-mix, population, patients and hospital characteristics. International Journal of Quality Health Care. 2000; 12: 371–378.
13. Runciman WB, Webb RK, Helps SC, et al. A comparison of iatrogenic injury studies in Australia and the USA II. Reviewer behaviour and quality of care. International Journal of Quality Health Care 2000; 12: 379–378.
14. Kohn LT, Corrigan JM, Donaldson MS, eds. To err is human: building a safer health system. Institute of Medicine Report. Washington, DC : National Academy Press; 1999.
15. Mackauf SH. Neurologic malpractice. Neurological Clinics 1999; 17: 345–353.
16. Australasian College for Emergency Medicine National Triage Scale. Emergency Medicine 1994; 6: 145–146.
17. www.ciap.health.nsw.gov.au/index.html
18. www.acem.org.au/open/documents/ed-design_htm
19. Hendrie J, Sammartino L, Silvapulle MJ, et al. Experience in adverse events detection in an emergency department: Nature of events. *** 2007; 19: 9–15.
20. Hendrie J, Sammartino L, Silvapulle MJ, et al. Experience in adverse events detection in an emergency department: Incidence and outcome of events. 2007; 19: 16–24.
21. Vinen JD. Time to initiation of thrombolysis after myocardial infarction: quality indicators. Emergency Medicine 2002; 32: 125–126.
22. McCaskill ME, Little DG. Time to definitive management of open fractures of long bones. Emergency Medicine 1993; 5: 272–275.
23. Pines JM, Hollander JE. The impact of emergency department crowding on cardiac outcomes in ED patients with potential acute coronary syndromes. Annals of Emergency Medicine 2007; 50: S3.
24. Sprivulis PC, Da Silva JA, Jacobs IG, et al. The association between hospital overcrowding and mortality among patients admitted via Western Australian emergency departments. Medical Journal of Australia 2006; 184: 208–212.
25. Ye K, Taylor D McD, Knott JC, et al. Handover in the emergency department: Deficiencies and adverse effects. Emergency Medicine 2007; 19: 433–441.
26. Perry S. Transitions in care: studying safety in emergency department signovers. National Patients Safety Foundation 2004; 7: 1–3.

28.1 Heat-related illness

Ian Rogers • Aled Williams

ESSENTIALS

1 Heat exhaustion and exercise-associated collapse are largely manifestations of intravascular volume depletion and usually respond simply to rest and oral fluids.

2 Heatstroke is a true medical emergency, where rapid cooling using tepid spraying, fanning and ice packs is essential to minimize morbidity and mortality.

3 Iced water immersion may cool patients more rapidly but is not always practical in an emergency department setting.

4 Patients with drug-related hyperthermia die from the complications of the high temperature, not from direct drug toxicity. Early and aggressive treatment of hyperthermia before complications occur is vital.

Introduction

Heat-related disorders have a broad range of potential aetiologies and manifestations. In some the primary disorder is a failure of thermal homoeostasis, whereas in others the hyperthermia is secondary to other processes. The major heat-related illnesses to consider are heat exhaustion and exercise-associated collapse (EAC), heatstroke, neuroleptic malignant syndrome, serotonin toxicity and malignant hyperthermia. Although of different aetiologies they share much common ground, particularly with regard to complications and treatment.

Epidemiology and pathophysiology

Heat exhaustion and EAC are the most common heat-related illnesses presenting to emergency departments (EDs). Heat exhaustion occurs where substantial losses of fluid and electrolytes as sweat are inadequately replaced, and is most commonly observed in athletes and manual workers. The primary pathophysiological mechanisms are dehydration and intravascular volume depletion, but may include electrolyte loss and exercise-induced respiratory alkalosis. EAC manifests at the end of a race when muscle pump

enhanced venous return ceases and cardiac output drops. This leads to collapse, often with a brief loss of consciousness.

The other, more serious, heat-related disorders are all associated with hyperthermia, which if not treated promptly results in similar pathophysiology at a cellular and organ system level. A core body temperature greater than 41°C results in progressive denaturing of a number of vital cellular proteins, failure of vital energy-producing processes and loss of cell membrane function. At a cellular level the exact mechanisms leading to loss of cell membrane function and cell death in heat illness remain uncertain. At an organ system level these changes may manifest as rhabdomyolysis, acute pulmonary oedema, disseminated intravascular coagulation, cardiovascular dysfunction, electrolyte disturbance, renal failure, liver failure and permanent neurological damage.[1] Any or all of these complications must be expected in severe heat illness.

Heatstroke shares some aetiological similarities with heat exhaustion but the hallmark of heatstroke is failure of the hypothalamic thermostat, leading to hyperthermia and the associated additional pathophysiological features described above. Clinically, heatstroke can be divided into 'exertional heatstroke' due to exercise in a thermally stressful environment, and 'classic heatstroke', which occurs in patients with impaired

Table 28.1.1 Heatstroke risk factors

Behavioural
Army recruits
Athletes
Exertion
Inappropriate clothing
  Elderly
Inappropriate exposure
  Babies left in cars
Manual workers
Pilgrims

Drugs
Anticholinergics
Diuretics
Phenothiazines
Salicylates
Stimulants/hallucinogens

Illness
Delirium tremens
Dystonias
Infections
Seizures

Table 28.1.2 Drugs causing severe serotonin toxicity

Antidepressants
Buspirone
Lithium
Monoamine oxidase inhibitors (MAOIs)
Selective serotonin reuptake inhibitors (SSRIs)
Selective serotonin and noradrenaline reuptake inhibitors (SSNRIs)
Trazodone
Tricyclics

Analgesics
Fentanyl
Pethidine
Tramadol

Antiparkinsonian agents
L-Dopa
Bromocriptine

OTC preparations
Dextromethorphan

Recreational drugs
Amphetamines
Methylenedioxymethamphetamine (MDMA, 'Ecstasy')

Table 28.1.3 Risk factors for neuroleptic malignant syndrome

Patient factors
Agitation
Dehydration
Male sex (male:female = 2:1)
Organic brain disease

Drug dosing factors
Depot neuroleptics
High initial neuroleptic dose
High-potency neuroleptic (e.g. haloperidol)
Rapid dosage increase

NB: Duration of drug exposure and toxic overdose are not related to risk of developing NMS.

thermostatic mechanisms. Common risk factors for heatstroke are listed in Table 28.1.1.

Certain drugs produce hyperthermia by mechanisms in addition to interference with thermostatic function. In severe serotonin toxicity and neuroleptic malignant syndrome, increased motor activity and central resetting of the hypothalamic thermostat combine to produce hyperthermia. In the case of serotonin toxicity these effects are a consequence of a relative excess of central nervous system serotonin, whereas in neuroleptic malignant syndrome dopamine depletion or dopamine receptor blockade is responsible.

The elevation of central nervous system serotonin in serotonin toxicity is usually associated with combinations of serotoninergically active drugs, taken either therapeutically or in overdose. The incidence of serotonin toxicity when such combinations are taken is not known, but is low, and there is much individual variation in susceptibility.[2] The syndrome is rarely precipitated by a single serotoninergic agent. Drugs associated with the serotonin syndrome are listed in Table 28.1.2. The most commonly implicated combinations are MAOI with SSRI, MAOI with tricyclics, and MAOI with pethidine.

Neuroleptic malignant syndrome (NMS) is a rare idiosyncratic reaction to neuroleptic agents with an incidence of between 0.02% and 3.0%, depending on the diagnostic criteria used. It occurs in response to a single agent, usually at therapeutic dosage.

In individuals, the occurrence may be dose-related. Certain at-risk groups have been identified and are listed in Table 28.1.3.

Malignant hyperthermia is a genetically inherited disorder in which triggering agents cause a release of sarcoplasmic Ca^{2+} stores. The resulting elevation of myoplasmic Ca^{2+} stimulates many intercellular processes, including glycolysis, muscle contraction and an uncoupling of oxidative phosphorylation. This leads to hyperthermia that, in contrast to neuroleptic malignant and serotonin syndromes, is purely peripheral in origin.

Prevention

Prevention of exertional heatstroke should focus on the education of at-risk groups.

Dehydration limits the body's cooling ability, so the value of maintaining adequate but not excessive fluid intake during extreme exertion should be stressed. As high ambient temperatures and high humidity predispose to exertional heatstroke, exertion in these environments should be limited.

Clinical features

Heat exhaustion and exercise-associated collapse

The clinical presentation of heat exhaustion will be familiar to all emergency practitioners as it mirrors that of dehydration from any other cause. Patients complain of headache, nausea, vomiting, malaise and dizziness. There may be a history of collapse, and there is likely to be a tachycardia and (orthostatic) hypotension. The orthostatic hypotension may manifest at the end of physical exertion (such as running) by collapse with brief loss of consciousness that is typical of EAC. In these syndromes, and in distinction to heatstroke, the core temperature will be less than 40°C and neurological function will rapidly return to normal once the patient is lying down.

Heatstroke

The classic clinical features of heatstroke are neurological dysfunction, core temperature above 41°C and hot, dry skin. However, relying on this classic triad to make the diagnosis will result in a number of cases being missed. Loss of consciousness is a constant feature of heatstroke,[1] but by the time of ED presentation conscious state may be improving, although some neurological abnormality will persist. Temperature readings may be misleadingly low, due either to effective pre-hospital care or to measurements at inappropriate sites, such as the oral cavity or axilla. Profuse sweating is a common feature.[1] Other clinical features may include tachycardia, hyperventilation, seizures, vomiting and hypotension.

Serotonin toxicity

Serotonin syndrome is characterized by CNS, autonomic and motor dysfunction (Table 28.1.4). It develops after a latent period, which is normally a few hours but may be as long as several days.[4] The spectrum of illness produced is broad.

Table 28.1.4 Features of the serotonin toxicity
Central nervous system
Agitation
Anxiety
Confusion
Decreased level of consciousness
Seizures
Motor
Clonus
Hyperreflexia
Hypertonia
Incoordination
Myoclonus
Tremor
Autonomic
Diaphoresis
Diarrhoea
Hypertension
Hyperthermia
Tachycardia

Most patients are only mildly affected and may escape clinical detection. Only the most serious develop hyperthermia severe enough to produce the complications of rhabdomyolysis, disseminated intravascular coagulation and renal failure. Most cases will resolve within 24–48 h once the precipitating agents are withdrawn. Even in severe cases, the underlying biochemical abnormality rapidly improves. The morbidity and mortality in these cases is caused by the complications that develop while the syndrome is active.

Neuroleptic malignant syndrome

This syndrome manifests in patients who have recently been started on neuroleptic treatment, or in whom the dose of a neuroleptic agent has been increased. It has also been reported in patients in whom a dopaminergic agent has been rapidly withdrawn (e.g. in parkinsonism). There is a latent period of several days. Characteristically, there are four classic signs: fever, rigidity, altered mental state and autonomic instability. In practice, it may be difficult to distinguish clinically from serotonin toxicity unless a good drug history is obtained. As in serotonin toxicity, the spectrum of severity may be very broad, with only the more severe cases developing hyperthermia and its complications.[5]

Malignant hyperthermia

This occurs when a triggering agent is given to a susceptible individual, usually in the context of an anaesthetic. Triggering agents identified include inhalational anaesthetic agents such as halothane, isoflurane and enflurane, as well as succinylcholine and ketamine. The first signs are failure to achieve muscle relaxation following succinylcholine, tachyponea and tachycardia. If not recognized and treated, acidosis, rhabdomyolysis and hyperthermia will ensue. In some cases signs and symptoms may be delayed, or even reappear after apparently successful treatment, so that malignant hyperthermia may even present as a postoperative fever. Untreated, the mortality is as high as 70%, but this can be reduced tenfold by appropriate management.

Clinical investigation

Diagnosis of the hyperthermic disorders is based on the history, clinical picture and exclusion of alternative diagnoses. Investigations are thus directed towards excluding other possible causes of temperature elevation (e.g. infection, metabolic disorders) and evaluation of the specific complications of hyperthermia.

Patients with a presumed clinical diagnosis of heat exhaustion or EAC should still have serum electrolytes and creatine kinase measured, together with a dipstick urinalysis. Measurement of serum electrolytes will detect dilutional hyponatraemia and other electrolyte disorders. In heat exhaustion there should be no myoglobin in the urine and, at most, only minor elevation of serum muscle enzymes.

All other heat disorders warrant a far more extensive laboratory and radiological workup, as multiorgan system dysfunction is the rule.[6] Tests should include an ECG (electrocardiograph), serum electrolytes, arterial blood gases, disseminated intravascular coagulation (DIC) screen, liver function tests, muscle enzyme assays, renal function and urinalysis, serum glucose and a chest X-ray.

Treatment

Heat exhaustion and exercise-associated collapse

Heat exhaustion and EAC respond rapidly to rest and fluids. Oral fluids such as commercial glucose/electrolyte solutions are ideal if they can be tolerated. Intravenous normal saline will provide more rapid recovery in severe cases but is rarely required. Heat exhaustion is a diagnosis of exclusion: should any doubt exist the patient should be treated as for heatstroke.

Heatstroke

This is a true medical emergency. Early recognition and aggressive therapy in the field and in hospital can prevent substantial morbidity and mortality. The key management is aggressive cooling. Cooling rates of at least 0.1°C/min should be achievable. Several cooling methods have been proposed, including evaporative cooling, iced water immersion, ice slush, cool water immersion, iced peritoneal lavage and pharmacological methods.[7] A combination of methods is most widely used in EDs. All of the patient's clothing should be removed and the patient sprayed with a fine mist of tepid water while gentle fanning is commenced (a ceiling fan is ideal). At the same time, areas with vascular beds close to the surface (neck, axillae and groins) should be packed with ice bags. This technique facilitates patient access and monitoring when compared to methods such as ice-bath immersion even though an iced bath may offer more rapid cooling.

In hospital, shivering, seizures and muscle activity may need to be controlled with pharmacological agents such as chlorpromazine, benzodiazepines and paralyzing agents. Aspirin and paracetamol are ineffective and should be avoided. Intravenous fluids need to be used cautiously and may need titrating to central venous or pulmonary capillary wedge pressures. High-flow oxygen should be routine and ventilatory support may be required. Urine flow needs to be maintained with initial volume loading, and later with mannitol or furosemide, to prevent secondary renal injury, especially from rhabdomyolysis. Electrolyte, acid–base and clotting disturbances should be closely monitored and treated by standard measures.

Serotonin toxicity

Treatment of the drug-related hyperthermia involves both specific pharmacological therapy and full supportive and cooling measures, as described above. The objective is to recognize and treat before serious complications occur. In mild cases of the serotonin syndrome, benzodiazepines may be all that is required while awaiting spontaneous resolution. In severe cases, neuromuscular paralysis should be considered early, especially in cases of altered mental state. Specific antiserotoninergic drugs that can be used include chlorpromazine (12.5–50 mg i.m./i.v.),[8,9] and cyproheptadine (4 mg orally 4-hourly, max. 20 mg in 24 h).[2]

Neuroleptic malignant syndrome

Again early recognition and full supportive care, combined with specific therapy, is the mainstay of treatment. Dopamine agonists such as bromocriptine may reduce the duration of the syndrome that, in contrast to serotonin syndrome, takes several days to resolve spontaneously. It can be administered orally or by nasogastric tube at an initial dose of 2.5–10 mg tds.[3]

Malignant hyperthermia

Dantrolene is the specific agent used in the treatment of malignant hyperthermia and should be given in addition to full supportive care and discontinuing the triggering agents. The dose is 1–2 mg/kg i.v. initially, repeated up to a maximum of 10 mg/kg/24 h if needed. It acts by inhibiting release of Ca^{2+} from the sarcoplasmic reticulum.

Prognosis and disposition

In heatstroke both the maximum core temperature and the duration of temperature elevation are predictors of outcome.

Prolonged coma and oliguric renal failure are poor prognostic signs.[1] Mortality is still of the order of 10%, but most survivors will not suffer long-term sequelae.[1] Any patient with suspected heatstroke should routinely be referred to the intensive care unit for ongoing care. Most cases of heat exhaustion and EAC will be suitable for short-stay ED treatment.

Prognosis in the drug-related group of hyperthermia is dependent largely on the degree to which the complications have progressed before definitive and aggressive treatment is begun. Again, early referral to intensive care is indicated. Even with appropriate treatment, mortality for malignant hyperthermia approaches 7%. After recovery, the patient's medication regimen will need to be reassessed, although in the case of neuroleptic malignant syndrome it may be possible to slowly reintroduce a neuroleptic agent at a lower dose. With malignant hyperthermia future anaesthesia will need to be modified to avoid precipitating agents. In addition, family members should be tested for susceptibility.

Controversies

❶ Although debate is likely to continue about the most effective cooling therapy in heatstroke, this is largely of academic interest as all methods seem to achieve the desired outcome of rapid temperature drop. Of more interest will be research that focuses on the cellular mechanisms of the damage seen with hyperthermia. Such research may lead to the development of pharmacological agents that can prevent or treat heatstroke and other heat-related illnesses.

❷ There are still no prospective trials comparing the various antiserotoninergic drugs available for the treatment of serotonin toxicity.

References

1. Shapiro Y, Seidman DS. Field and clinical observations of exertional heat stroke patients. Medicine and Science in Sports and Exercise 1990; 22: 6–14.
2. Isbister GK, Buckley NA, Whyte IM. Serotonin toxicity: a practical approach to diagnosis and treatment. Medical Journal of Australia 2007; 187: 361–365.
3. Heimann-Patterson TD. Neuroleptic malignant syndrome and malignant hyperthermia. Medical Clinics of North America 1993; 77: 477–492.
4. Sternbach H. The serotonin syndrome. American Journal of Psychiatry 1991; 148: 705–713.
5. Bristow MF, Kohen D. How malignant is the neuroleptic malignant syndrome? British Medical Journal 1993; 307: 1223–1224.
6. Dematte JE, O'Mara K, Buescher J, et al. Near fatal heat stroke during the 1995 heat wave in Chicago. Annals of Internal Medicine 1998; 130: 173–181.
7. Smith JE. Cooling methods used in the treatment of exertional heat illness. British Journal of Sports Medicine 2005; 39: 503–507.
8. Gillman P. Successful treatment of serotonin syndrome with chlorpromazine. Medical Journal of Australia 1996; 165: 345.
9. Chan BSH, Graudins A, Whyte IM, et al. Serotonin syndrome resulting from drug interactions. Medical Journal of Australia 1998; 169: 523–525.

ENVIRONMENTAL

28.2 Hypothermia

Ian Rogers

ESSENTIALS

1 Hypothermia is categorized into mild (32–35°C), moderate (29–32°C) and severe (<29°C) on the basis of a rectal core temperature reading.

2 Moderate-to-severe hypothermia produces progressive delirium and coma, hypotension, bradycardia and failure of thermogenesis.

3 The electrocardiograph will often show slow atrial fibrillation and an extra positive deflection in the QRS (the J or Osborn wave) in leads II and V_3–V_6 with worsening hypothermia.

4 Endotracheal intubation is safe in hypothermia. Ventilation and acid–base status should be manipulated to maintain uncorrected blood gases within the normal range.

5 Endogenous rewarming should form part of all rewarming protocols. In most cases of moderate-to-severe hypothermia rewarming can be achieved with forced-air rewarming blankets without the need to resort to more aggressive techniques.

6 In the arrested hypothermic patient rewarming should be with cardiopulmonary bypass or warm left pleural lavage.

Introduction

Hypothermia is defined as a core temperature of less than 35°C. This can be measured at a number of sites (including oesophageal, right heart, tympanic and bladder). Rectal remains the routine in most emergency departments (EDs), despite concerns at how rapidly it equilibrates to and reflects true core temperature. Conventionally, hypothermia is divided into three groups: mild (32–35°C), moderate (29–32°C) and severe (<29°C) on the basis of measured core temperature. In a field setting, where core temperature measurements may not be possible, moderate and severe are often grouped together as they typically share the clinical features of absence of shivering and altered mental state. These categorization systems can be used both out of and in hospital as a guide to selecting rewarming therapies and prognosis. Mild hypothermia is considered the stage where thermogenesis is still possible; moderate is characterized by a progressive failure of thermogenesis; and severe by adoption of the temperature of the surrounding environment (poikilothermia) and an increasing risk of malignant cardiac arrhythmia. Nevertheless, there are substantial differences between individuals in their response to hypothermia.

Epidemiology and pathophysiology

Hypothermia may occur in any setting or season.[1] True environmental hypothermia occurring in a healthy patient in an adverse physical environment is less common in clinical practice than that secondary to an underlying disorder. Common precipitants include injury, systemic illness, drug overdose and immersion, and are outlined in more detail in Table 28.2.1. The elderly are at greater risk of hypothermia because of reduced metabolic heat production and impaired responses to a cold environment.[2] Alcohol is a common aetiological factor and probably acts by a number of mechanisms, including cutaneous vasodilatation, altered behavioural responses, impaired shivering and hypothalamic dysfunction. Hypothermia in the ED setting is often associated with underlying infection.[3]

Clinical features

Despite substantial individual variations it is still possible to describe the typical patient in each category of hypothermia. The clinical manifestations of hypothermia also depend on the underlying aetiology and any associated features. To guide management in a field setting, where rectal temperature measurements are impractical or dangerous, moderate and severe hypothermia are often grouped together.[4]

Mild hypothermia manifests clinically as shivering, apathy, ataxia, dysarthria and tachycardia. Moderate hypothermia is typically marked by a loss of shivering, altered mental state, muscular rigidity, bradycardia and hypotension. In severe hypothermia signs of life may become almost undetectable, with coma,

Table 28.2.1	Hypothermia aetiologies
Environmental	Cold, wet, windy ambient conditions Cold water immersion Exhaustion
Trauma	Multitrauma (entrapment, resuscitation, head injury) Minor trauma and immobility (e.g. #NOF, #NOH) Major burns
Drugs	Ethanol Sedatives (e.g. benzodiazepines) in overdose Phenothiazines (impaired shivering)
Neurological	CVA Paraplegia Parkinson's disease
Endocrine	Hypoglycaemia Hypothyroidism Hypoadrenalism
Systemic illness	Sepsis Malnutrition

fixed and dilated pupils, areflexia and profound bradycardia and hypotension. The typical cardiac rhythm of severe hypothermia is slow atrial fibrillation. This may degenerate spontaneously, or with rough handling, into ventricular fibrillation or asystole.

Many complications may also manifest as part of a hypothermia presentation, although at times it may be difficult to separate cause from effect. These include cardiac arrhythmias, thromboembolism, rhabdomyolysis, renal failure, disseminated intravascular coagulation and pancreatitis.

Clinical investigation

Mild hypothermia with shivering and without apparent underlying illness needs no investigation in the ED.

Moderate or severe hypothermia mandates a comprehensive work-up to seek common precipitants and complications that may not be clinically apparent.

Biochemical and haematological abnormalities are frequently associated with hypothermia,[1] although there is no consistent pattern. Blood tests that are indicated include sodium, potassium, glucose, renal function, calcium, phosphate, magnesium, amylase, creatine kinase, ethanol, full blood count, clotting profile and arterial blood gases. Blood gas results should be accepted at face value, rather than adjusting for the patient's temperature.[5]

Impaired ciliary function, stasis of respiratory secretions or aspiration may be expected in moderate-to-severe hypothermia, so chest radiography should be routine. Other radiology may be indicated if a trauma-related aetiology is suspected.

A 12-lead electrocardiograph (ECG) and continuous ECG monitoring should be routine in moderate-to-severe hypothermia. The typical appearance is slow atrial fibrillation, with J or Osborn waves most prominent in leads II and V_3–V_6 (Fig. 28.2.1). The J wave is the extra positive deflection after the normal S wave, and is more obvious and more commonly seen with increasing severity of hypothermia.

Treatment

General

The general and supportive management of hypothermia victims largely follows that of other critically ill patients. However, some syndrome-specific issues demand careful attention.

Muscle glycogen is the substrate preferentially used by the body to generate heat by shivering. All hypothermics, therefore, need glucose. In mild cases this can be given orally as sweetened drinks or easily palatable food. With more severe hypothermia gastric stasis and ileus are common, and glucose should be given intravenously: 5% dextrose can be

infused at 200 mL/h. Additional volume resuscitation with normal saline or colloid should be gentle, bearing in mind the contracted intravascular space in severe hypothermia, and that hypotension that would be classified as severe at a core temperature of 37°C is a normal physiological state at 27°C. All intravenous fluids should be warmed to minimize ongoing cooling. Current opinion is that endotracheal intubation by a skilled operator is safe in severe hypothermia. Intubation is indicated as in any other clinical condition to provide airway protection or to assist in ventilation.

Ventilatory support and, where necessary, manipulation of acid–base status, should be titrated to maintain uncorrected blood gas pH and PCO_2 within the normal range.

The slow atrial fibrillation so common in more severe hypothermia is a benign rhythm and requires no chemical or electrical correction. It will revert spontaneously with rewarming. Pulseless ventricular tachycardia and ventricular fibrillation should largely be managed along conventional lines. However, if initial DC shocks are unsuccessful, then others are unlikely to be so until the patient is warmer. Repeat countershocks are generally reapplied with every 1°C increase in core temperature.

Magnesium may be the antiarrhythmic drug of choice in hypothermia.

The pharmacokinetics and dynamics of most drugs are substantially altered at low

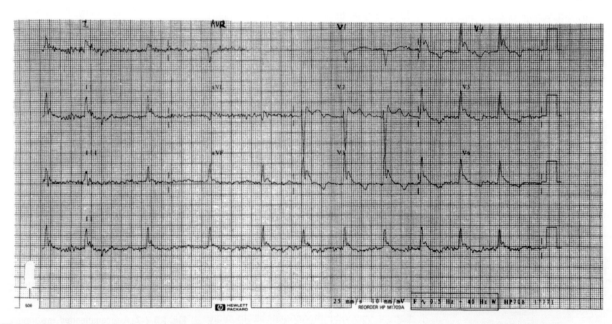

Fig. 28.2.1 ECG in hypothermia: slow atrial fibrillation and J waves in leads II, V_3–V_6 in a patient with a core temperature of 23.9°C.

body core temperatures. Indeed, for many of the common drugs used in an ED they are unknown. Insulin is known to be inactive at <30°C. Hyperglycaemia, due in part to loss of insulin activity, is common in hypothermia, but should probably be managed expectantly until sufficient rewarming has occurred to ensure full endogenous insulin activity.

Rewarming therapies

Rewarming therapies in hypothermia have generated substantial debate. Unfortunately, there are only limited clinical trials on which to base recommendations. Although more invasive and rapid techniques are advocated for more severe hypothermia, there is little evidence to support this advice. The traditional concern of afterdrop (a paradoxical initial drop in core temperature with rewarming) is probably of little or no relevance in a clinical setting.[6]

Rewarming therapies are broadly divided into three groups: endogenous rewarming, which allows the body to rewarm by its own endogenous heat production; external exogenous rewarming, which supplies heat to the outside of the body; and core exogenous rewarming, which applies the heat centrally. The classification of the common rewarming therapies is outlined in Table 28.2.2.

Endogenous rewarming is a mandatory component of any ED rewarming protocol. It consists of drying the patient, covering them with blankets, placing them in a warm and wind-free environment, and warming any intravenous or oral fluids that are administered. Endogenous rewarming alone can be expected to rewarm at a rate of about 0.75°C/h. For most patients above 32°C (the level at which shivering

thermogenesis is typically preserved), endogenous rewarming is the only therapy required. The exception is the exhausted patient in whom shivering has ceased at a core temperature higher than expected. Although more sophisticated techniques, such as bath immersion, will more rapidly rewarm a mildly hypothermic patient, there is no evidence that an increased rewarming rate improves prognosis in this group.

In moderate hypothermia, endogenous heat production is likely to progressively fail and more aggressive exogenous rewarming therapies are indicated. Hot-bath immersion has the theoretical disadvantage of causing peripheral vasodilatation, with shunting of cool blood to the core and convective heat loss. This might be expected to increase core afterdrop and produce circulatory collapse. In fact, rewarming rates of at least 2.5°C/h with minimal afterdrop have been achieved using baths at 43°C.[7] Nevertheless, substantial practical difficulties are obvious with monitoring a more seriously ill patient immersed in a bath. This method of rewarming can only be recommended for otherwise healthy patients who are expected to make a rapid recovery from accidental environmental hypothermia (e.g. immersion in very cold water).

The two therapies that have been best studied and are widely used in moderate hypothermia are forced-air rewarming and warm humidified inhalation.[8] Forced-air rewarming is achieved by covering the patient with a blanket filled with air at 43°C. These devices direct a continuous current of air over the patient's skin through a series of slits in the patient surface of the blanket. This method produces minimal, if any, afterdrop, is apparently without complication and, combined with warm humidified inhalation, should produce rewarming at about 2.5°C/h. The value of warm humidified inhalation is probably by preventing ongoing respiratory heat loss. Given its widespread availability and lack of complications, it seems reasonable to combine it with forced-air rewarming in moderate hypothermia.[9] Body-to-body contact and chemical heat packs are often recommended as field treatments for all degrees of hypothermia. In mild hypothermia it seems that the benefit of any heat they deliver is negated by an inhibition of shivering thermogenesis. In more severe cases, where shivering is absent, it

may be that even the small amount of exogenous heat they deliver is beneficial, but this remains unproven.

In severe hypothermia more aggressive exogenous rewarming therapies may be indicated in order to rapidly achieve core temperature above 30°C, the threshold below which malignant cardiac arrhythmias may occur spontaneously. When available, full cardiopulmonary bypass achieves rewarming rates of about 7.5°C/h without core afterdrop. Pleural lavage using large volumes of fluid warmed to 40–45°C through an intercostal catheter may be nearly as effective. Both techniques are clearly invasive and carry associated risks. These risks are certainly acceptable in a hypothermic arrest, but in the non-arrested patient a slower rate of rewarming using forced-air and warm humidified inhalation may be more appropriate.

A suggested rewarming algorithm based on the evidence available to date is reproduced in Fig. 28.2.2.

Prognosis and disposition

Attempts at developing a valid outcome prediction model for hypothermia are likely to be frustrated by its multifactorial aetiology. Recovery with appropriate treatment is likely from accidental environmental hypothermia when there is no associated trauma. To date, the coldest patient to

Table 28.2.2 Rewarming therapy classification	
Endogenous rewarming	Warm, dry, wind-free environment Warmed intravenous fluids
External exogenous rewarming	Hot bath immersion Forced-air blankets Heat packs Body-to-body contact
Core exogenous rewarming	Warmed, humidified inhalation Body cavity lavage -peritoneal -pleural Extracorporeal

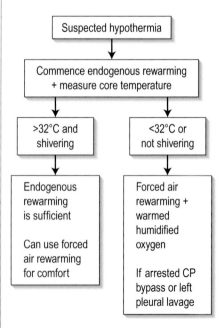

Fig. 28.2.2 A recommended rewarming algorithm in hypothermia.

survive accidental hypothermia neurologically intact had an initial measured temperature of 13.7°C.[10] Although increasing severity of hypothermia does worsen prognosis, the major determinant of outcome is the precipitating illness or injury. Reported mortality rates vary from 0 to 85%.

Mild hypothermics without associated illness or injury can be safely managed at home in the care of a responsible adult. Moderate hypothermia may be treatable in a short-stay observation ward, but often requires a longer inpatient stay to manage underlying illness or injury. Severe hypothermics are at risk of multiorgan system complications and should be considered for admission to an intensive care unit.

Controversies

❶ Many questions remain unanswered in hypothermia, the major one being which rewarming therapy to use. This will only be answered when the focus moves to randomized clinical trials measuring clinically relevant outcomes, such as morbidity and mortality, rather than surrogate markers such as rewarming rate and core afterdrop.

❷ Future research may confirm a role for induced mild hypothermia for more conditions other than that already shown post cardiac arrest.[11–13]

References

1. Danzl DF, Pozos RS, Auerbach PS, et al. Multicentre hypothermia survey. Annals of Emergency Medicine 1987; 16: 1042–1055.
2. Weinberg AD. Hypothermia. Annals of Emergency Medicine 1993; 22: 370–377.
3. Delaney KA, Vasallo SU, Larkin GL, Goldfrank LR. Rewarming rates in urban patients with hypothermia: prediction of underlying infection. Academic Emergency Medicine 2006; 13: 913–921.
4. Forgey WM (ed.). Wilderness Medical Society Practice Guidelines for Wilderness Emergency Care. 5th edn. Guilford: Globe Pequot; 2006.
5. Danzl DF. Accidental hypothermia. In: Marx JA, et al., eds. Rosen's emergency medicine: concepts and clinical practice. 6th edn. Philadelphia; Mosby; 2005.
6. Rogers IR. Which rewarming therapy in hypothermia? A review of the randomised trials. Emergency Medicine Australasia 1997; 9: 213–220.
7. Hoskin RW, Melinshyn MG, Romet TT, Goode RC. Bath rewarming from immersion hypothermia. Journal of Applied Physiology 1986; 61: 1518–1522.
8. Steele MT, Nelson MJ, Sessler DI, et al. Forced air speeds rewarming in accidental hypothermia. Annals of Emergency Medicine 1996; 27: 479–484.
9. Giesbrecht GG. Emergency treatment of hypothermia. Emergency Medicine Australasia 2001; 13: 9–16.
10. Gilbert M, Busund R, Skogseth A, et al. Resuscitation from accidental hypothermia of 13°C with circulatory arrest. Lancet 2000; 355: 375–376.
11. Alzaga AG, Cerdan M, Varon J. Therapeutic hypothermia. Resuscitation 2006; 70: 369–380.
12. Bernard SA, Gray TW, Buist M, et al. Treatment of comatose survivors of out-of-hospital cardiac arrest with induced hypothermia. New England Journal of Medicine 2002; 346: 557–563.
13. The Hypothermia after Cardiac Arrest Study Group. Mild therapeutic hypothermia to improve neurologic outcome after cardiac arrest. New England Journal of Medicine 2002; 346: 549–555.

ENVIRONMENTAL

28.3 Dysbarism

David R. Smart

Introduction

This chapter focuses on medical problems that develop secondary to breathing gases at higher than normal atmospheric pressure (dysbarism). This usually occurs in the context of scuba (self-contained underwater breathing apparatus) diving, a popular recreational activity in Australasia. Diving is generally very safe, and serious decompression incidents occur approximately 1: 10 000 dives. However, because of a high participation rate, between 300 and 400 cases of decompression illness are treated in Australia each year.[1] It is estimated that 10 times that number of divers experience less serious health problems after diving. Emergency physicians are often the first medical staff to assess the diver after a diving accident and it is essential they understanding the risks and potential injuries.

Diving physics and physiology

An understanding of pressure and some gas laws is essential to understand the pathophysiology of diving injuries. Absolute pressure at sea level is 1 atmosphere (ATA). Multiple units are used to measure pressure (Table 28.3.1). For every 10 m a diver descends in sea-water, the pressure increases by 1 ATA. This pressure change impacts on gas spaces within the body according to Boyle's Law.

Boyle's Law states that at a constant temperature the volume of a gas varies inversely to the pressure acting on it:

$$PV = k$$

where P = pressure, V = volume and k = constant.

The proportionate change in volume is greatest near the surface (Table 28.3.2).

Dalton's law states that the total pressure (P_t) exerted by a mixture of gases is equal to the sum of the pressures of the constituent gases (P_x, P_y, P_z):

$$P_t = P_x + P_y + P_z$$

Therefore, as divers breathe air at increasing atmospheric pressure, the partial pressures of nitrogen and oxygen increase:

Surface = 1 ATA
= 0.8 ATA N_2 + 0.2 ATA O_2

10 m = 2 ATA
= 1.6 ATA N_2 + 0.4 ATA O_2

40 m = 5 ATA
= 4.0 ATA N_2 + 1.0 ATA O_2

A diver breathing air at 40 m is inhaling a gas with a partial pressure of oxygen equivalent to breathing 100% oxygen at the surface. At partial pressures above 3 ATA, the PN_2 affects coordination and judgement ('nitrogen narcosis'). Oxygen

Table 28.3.1 Atmospheric pressure at sea level in various units
1 Atmosphere absolute (ATA)
101.3 kPa (SI units)
1.013 Bar
10 m of sea water (MSW)
760 mm of mercury (mmHg)
14.7 pounds per square inch (PSI)

Table 28.3.2 Depth vs pressure and gas volume (Boyle's law)

Depth (m)	Absolute pressure (ATA)	Gas volume (%)
0	1	100
10	2	50
20	3	33
30	4	25
40	5	20

may also become toxic at partial pressures greater than 1 ATA. Recreational scuba diving generally has a limit of 40 m because of these effects.

Henry's law states that at a constant temperature the amount of a gas that will dissolve in a liquid is proportional to the partial pressure of the gas in contact with the liquid:

$$Q = kP_{gas}$$

where Q = volume of gas dissolved in a liquid, k = constant and P_{gas} = partial pressure of the gas.

Henry's law is relevant in diving illness in that it is the basis of decompression illness (DCI). As the ambient pressure increases, the diver is exposed to increasing partial pressures of nitrogen, which dissolves in bodily fluids. The amount of nitrogen absorbed depends on both the depth (which determines the partial pressure of nitrogen) and the duration of the dive. Tissues also take up nitrogen at different rates depending on their blood supply and permeability. Eventually, the tissues become saturated with nitrogen and no further absorption occurs. As the diver ascends and ambient pressure decreases, the partial pressure of nitrogen in some tissues will exceed ambient pressure, resulting in tissue supersaturation. If the diver ascends slowly enough, nitrogen diffuses out of the tissues and is transported, safely dissolved in the blood, to the lungs for elimination. This is known as 'off-gassing'.

If the diver ascends too rapidly, sufficient nitrogen bubbles will form in their body to cause decompression illness. Oxygen does not cause problems because it is rapidly metabolized by the tissues.

Barotrauma

Barotrauma occurs when changes in ambient pressure lead to expansion or contraction of gas within enclosed body cavities. The change in gas volume distorts or tears adjacent tissue. Injury by this mechanism may occur to the middle ear, inner ear, sinuses, lungs, eyes and, rarely, the gut. Different injury patterns occur in breath-hold divers (snorkellers) compared to those breathing compressed air. Both breath-hold and scuba divers may experience injury of the middle and inner ear, sinuses and eyes if they do not equalize pressures in the gas spaces as they descend. Breath-hold divers are unlikely to injure their lungs as their lung volumes reduce as they descend and return to their original volume as they ascend to the surface by the increasing ambient pressure.

Middle-ear barotrauma

Pathophysiology

Middle-ear barotrauma (MEBT), the most common medical disorder of diving,[2] usually occurs during descent. Increased ambient pressure results in a reduction of middle-ear volume. If equalization of the volume via the eustachian tube is inadequate, a series of pathological changes results. The tympanic membrane (TM) is deformed inwards, causing inflammation and haemorrhage. Middle-ear mucosal oedema is followed by vascular engorgement, effusion, haemorrhage and rarely, TM rupture.

Clinical features

Symptoms of middle-ear barotraumas include ear pain, tinnitus and conductive hearing loss. Mild vertigo may also be experienced. More severe vertigo and pain occur if water passes through a perforated TM. Severe vertigo and significant sensorineural hearing loss should alert the emergency physician to possible inner-ear barotrauma (IEBT) (see below). MEBT severity is graded by visual inspection of the TM (see Table 28.3.3). An audiogram is useful to document any hearing loss.

Table 28.3.3 Grading of severity of middle-ear barotrauma

Grade 0	Symptoms without signs
Grade 1	Injection of TM along handle of malleus
Grade 2	Slight haemorrhage within the TM
Grade 3	Gross haemorrhage within the TM
Grade 4	Free blood in middle ear
Grade 5	Perforation of TM

TM, tympanic membrane

Treatment

Treatment of MEBT consists of analgesia, decongestants, and ear, nose and throat (ENT) referral if there is TM perforation, or suspected IEBT. Antibiotics are indicated for TM rupture because of potential contamination with water. The patient should not dive again until symptoms and signs have resolved, any TM perforation has healed, and the eustachian tube is patent.

Inner-ear barotrauma

Pathophysiology

Sudden pressure changes between the middle and inner ears can cause rupture of the round or oval windows, or a tear of Reissner's membrane. This usually occurs during rapid descent without equalizing or forceful Valsalva manoeuvres.

Clinical features

Symptoms include sudden onset of tinnitus, vertigo, nausea and vomiting, vestibular symptoms and profound hearing loss, which may not be apparent until the diver has left the water.[3] Onset of symptoms after the dive while performing an activity that increases intracranial pressure (e.g. heavy lifting) suggests IEBT. Coexistent middle-ear barotrauma is absent in about one-third of cases.[3]

The main differential diagnosis is DCI involving the inner ear or vestibular apparatus. Inner-ear DCI usually occurs on deep dives using helium and oxygen mixtures (heliox), and is typically accompanied by other symptoms or signs of DCI. Frequently it is difficult to distinguish between IEBT and vestibular DCI. Isolated inner-ear DCI has been reported in sports divers breathing air.[4,5]

Treatment

Treatment of IEBT consists of avoidance of activities that increase intracranial pressure and urgent (same day) ENT referral for more detailed assessment and audiometry. Surgical repair may be undertaken when vertiginous symptoms are severe. Vomiting should be treated with anti-emetics, and the diver kept supine with their head on a pillow. If DCI is excluded, then a 45° semi recumbent position is preferred. If DCI cannot be excluded, the diver should have a trial of recompression. In one series, exposure to pressure did not worsen the diver's condition.[2] The benefit of steroids in IEBT has not been confirmed.

It was thought that further diving was contraindicated after IEBT, but recent case data suggests that diving might be possible following full recovery of hearing.[6]

External ear barotrauma

Ear-canal barotrauma is very rare and only occurs if there is a complete obstruction of the canal (usually by wax or ear plugs), creating a non-communicating gas cavity between the obstruction and the TM. Treatment is symptomatic. ENT specialist referral may be necessary if the TM cannot be visualized.

Sinus barotrauma

Pathophysiology

Mucosal swelling and haemorrhage occur if the communication of the sinuses with the nasopharynx is blocked, and equalization of sinus pressure is not possible during descent. The frontal sinuses are most commonly involved.

Clinical features

Sinus pain usually develops during descent. Maxillary sinus involvement can refer pain to the upper teeth or cheek. There may be resolution of the pain at depth, due to mucosal oedema and blood filling the volume deficit left by gas compression. Pain and epistaxis may occur as the diver ascends. The pain usually persists after diving. Tenderness will be noted over the affected sinus. In doubtful cases, a sinus CT (computerized tomography) scan will assist the diagnosis.

Treatment

Treatment includes analgesia, decongestants and recommendations to avoid diving until asymptomatic. Antibiotics may be required if secondary infection occurs.

Mask squeeze

If divers fail to exhale air into their masks on descent, the reduced volume inside the mask can cause pain, petechiae and conjunctival haemorrhage. In assessing these divers it is important to confirm that they have normal visual acuity. Treatment is with analgesia alone.

Gastrointestinal barotrauma

Expansion of gas within the gastrointestinal tract on ascent can occasionally cause colicky abdominal pain. Rupture of the stomach is rare but has occurred where panic or equipment failure has led to air swallowing and rapid ascent.[7] Presentation is with abdominal pain and distension. Shoulder pain may be due to diaphragmatic irritation or coexisting DCI.[8] Sub-diaphragmatic free air may be visible on an erect chest X-ray. The differential diagnosis includes pulmonary barotrauma, because air can enter the peritoneum via the mediastinum and oesophageal or aortic openings in the diaphragm.[7] The diagnosis is confirmed with endoscopy, and surgical repair is necessary.

Dental barotrauma

Severe tooth pain may occur with descent or ascent if air is trapped under a decaying tooth or recent filling. Percussion of the involved tooth is painful. Treatment is with analgesia and dental repair.

Pulmonary barotrauma

Pathophysiology

Breathing compressed air at depth, the diver's lungs contain greater amounts of gas than they would on the surface. Divers are trained to breathe continuously during ascent or to exhale continuously if they have lost their air supply. Pulmonary barotrauma results when a diver ascends without exhaling adequately and the expanding gas in the lungs exceeds the lung's elasticity, tearing alveoli. This occurs most commonly when a diver runs out of air, panics and ascends too rapidly.[9] The change in pressure over 1 m near the surface is sufficient to cause lung barotrauma. It has been reported in student divers training in swimming pools[10] and in helicopter escape training.[11] It can also occur with a normal ascent if there is a localized area of lung that does not empty properly, as is possible in people with asthma, reduced pulmonary compliance or air trapping.[12]

The resultant clinical syndromes depend on the sites at which the air escapes, and include pneumomediastinum, pneumothorax, and arterial gas embolism (AGE).

Clinical features

Onset of symptoms is usually rapid. If pneumomediastinum or pneumothorax is detected after diving it is essential to look for features consistent with associated gas embolism. These include impairment or loss of consciousness, cognition impairment including loss of memory, or neurological abnormalities. Sometimes the abnormalities are subtle, and tests of cognition and memory should be performed in addition to a detailed history and thorough examination.

Treatment

If AGE is suspected, then urgent recompression treatment is required. Management of AGE is discussed under the heading of decompression illness. Lung barotrauma is regarded as the cause of AGE; however, in early studies, only about 5% of divers with AGE had radiographic evidence of a pneumothorax on plain chest X-ray.[12,13] Subtle signs of extra-alveolar air suggesting pulmonary barotrauma are present in nearly half with more sophisticated imaging such as CT.[14–16]

The reverse also applies. If divers present with a pneumomediastinum or pneumothorax, then they may have up to 50% chance of AGE.[14] The signs of AGE in these circumstances may be subtle with only a brief period of loss of memory or dizziness.

Pneumomediastinum and subcutaneous emphysema can usually be managed conservatively. If symptoms are severe, 100% oxygen can accelerate resolution of the trapped gas. If recompression is required for coexistent AGE, then the pneumomediastinum does not require any specific additional management unless a pneumothorax is present.

Isolated pneumothorax resulting from pulmonary barotrauma is very uncommon. Pneumothorax from pulmonary barotrauma should be managed in the same way as non-diving-related causes, and recompression is not necessary. If recompression is required for coexisting AGE, a chest tube with a Heimlich valve should be placed before commencing treatment, because the size of any remaining pneumothorax will increase markedly on depressurization.

Once the acute management of pneumomediastinum and pneumothorax has occurred, the divers should be referred to a diving medical specialist for long-term follow up, because the conditions will impact upon their future diving fitness.

Decompression illness

Classification and criteria for diagnosis

Diving accidents involving bubbles are traditionally divided into *decompression sickness* (DCI; due to nitrogen bubbles coming out of tissue) and *arterial gas embolism* (AGE; due to pulmonary barotrauma releasing air into the circulation). DCS is then classified as type I or II. Type I DCS involves the joints or skin only; type II involves all other pain, neurological injury, vestibular and pulmonary symptoms.

In the 1990s the term 'decompression illness' (DCI) was proposed to include both DCS and AGE, for the following reasons:[2,17]

- It can be difficult to distinguish clinically between cerebral arterial gas embolism (CAGE) and neurological DCS.
- AGE can be caused by arterialization of venous bubbles released from tissues.
- Pre-hospital and emergency management prior to recompression is identical.
- The division of DCS into type I and type II is inadequate for research purposes, and divers classified as type I have been found to have subtle sub-clinical neurological manifestations.
- Symptomatic classification is adequate to guide management.

The current classification system describes DCI in terms of four components:

❶ Onset (acute/chronic)
❷ Evolution of symptoms (spontaneously resolving/static/progressive/relapsing)
❸ Body system affected (musculoskeletal/cutaneous/lymphatic/neurological/vestibular/cardiorespiratory)
❹ Presence/absence of barotrauma.

For example, a diver may be classified as having acute progressive neurological DCI with no evidence of barotrauma. The new classification has been generally adopted in Australia and New Zealand, but not in North America. DCI is a satisfactory term from a management perspective, but from a scientific perspective it does not describe differing aetiologies and pathophysiology.

Pathophysiology

DCI occurs if excessive nitrogen comes out of solution to form bubbles which gain access to the venous and lymphatic systems or if bubbles form within tissues themselves. The formation of bubbles requires tissues to be supersaturated with nitrogen and for ascent to be excessively rapid. As bubbles form in tissues they distort tissue architecture, which results in impaired function, pain and inflammation and is probably responsible for most musculoskeletal symptoms.

Many bubbles entering the venous system do not cause symptoms. In fact, using ultrasonic detection methods, intravascular micro-bubbles are detected after approximately 60% of routine dives. It appears that these bubbles are safely filtered by the lung and diffuse into the alveoli.

Bubbles entering the arterial system are more likely to cause serious problems. This can occur under several circumstances. Large volumes of bubbles may overwhelm the pulmonary filter and arterialize. Bubbles may also bypass the lungs via a right-to-left shunt. Up to one-third of the population may have a patent foramen ovale.[18] Under normal circumstances, the valve over the foramen is kept closed by the pressure difference between the left and right atria. However, during diving the pressure differential may reverse during a Valsalva manoeuvre or with acute increases in right-sided pressures associated with a large pulmonary gas load.

Alternatively gas can enter the circulation following pulmonary barotrauma. Air entering the pulmonary arterial system is carried to the pulmonary capillaries, where it is trapped and reabsorbed by the alveoli. Air entering the pulmonary venous system, however, will pass through the heart and result in AGE.

Gas bubbles entering the circulation (either from tissues or barotrauma) cause both mechanical and biochemical abnormalities. Trapping in the pulmonary circulation may result in elevation of right heart and pulmonary pressures, leading to increased venous pressures, reduced cardiac output and impairment of tissue microcirculation. Arterial bubbles can cause end-organ ischaemia, although most pass through the capillaries and into the venous system. Most of the deleterious effects are a consequence of secondary inflammation of the vascular endothelium.

Bubble-endothelial interaction activates complement, kinin and coagulation systems, and precipitates leukocyte adherence. This results in increased vascular permeability, interstitial oedema and microvascular sludging.[2,19] The end result is ischaemia and haemoconcentration. Increased vascular permeability of the cerebral circulation will produce cerebral oedema. Vasospasm and reduced flow occurs approximately 1–2 h after bubbles have passed through the arterial tree. This explains the commonly observed clinical course of a diver with a cerebral AGE experiencing an initial deterioration (bubble emboli), followed by spontaneous improvement (bubbles pass through the cerebral capillaries) and then a subsequent secondary deterioration. Animal studies have demonstrated that bubbles travel against arterial flow because of their buoyancy, and lodge in the highest point of the body.

Prevention

A number of dive tables and computer algorithms have been developed in an attempt to avoid nitrogen supersaturation of tissues and improve diver safety. Limits are placed on depth, time and ascent rates to allow safe decompression after diving. However, as with all mathematical models which attempt to predict biological behaviour, the dive tables are far from perfect. One series has shown that 39% of DCI cases were within the limits of the table they were using, and 24% within the limits of the conservative Canadian Defence and Civil Institute of Environmental Medicine (DCIEM) tables.[20] Historically, it was assumed that DCI could not occur after dives shallower than 10 m but it is now known that this can occur particularly if there has been more than one dive per day, or multiple ascents.[21] The occurrence of DCI is a probabilistic event where risk increases with increasing depth, time, numbers of dives, numbers of ascents and rates of ascent.[22]

Flying after diving can precipitate DCI. Even if there are no bubbles at the end of the dive, excess nitrogen remains in the tissues and is slowly off-gassed. Further reduction in ambient pressure at altitude can cause bubbles, or enlarge pre-existing asymptomatic ones. Current guidelines advise against flying for 12 h after a single short no-decompression dive, and 24 h following multiple or decompression dives.[23]

Clinical features

Onset of any symptoms during or in the hours after diving should be regarded as DCI until proven otherwise. Failure to recognize and treat milder cases can lead to permanent morbidity because the disease can progress as the bubble load increases with time. Early onset of symptoms or signs (up to 1 h), especially those that are neurological in nature, indicates a serious decompression emergency, and recompression is a time-critical treatment. Milder syndromes of decompression illness may develop up to 24 h after a dive, or even later if there is a precipitant such as heavy exercise or ascent to altitude (e.g. flying).[24]

In general, pulmonary barotrauma that results in AGE has a dramatic clinical presentation, and the onset of major neurological symptoms and signs occurs within seconds to minutes after the dive. DCI caused by intravascular bubbles from barotrauma can be rapidly fatal and has a mortality of 5% in sport divers who reach a recompression chamber alive.[9] In Australia, it is the second most common cause of diving-related death, after drowning.[2] The brain is the organ most commonly affected, probably because of the vertical positioning of the diver on ascent. Cerebral gas emboli can cause sudden loss of consciousness, convulsions, visual disturbances, deafness, cranial nerve palsies, memory disturbance and asymmetric multiplegias. Hemiplegia is much less common than asymmetric multiplegias.[9] Symptoms almost always begin within 10 min of surfacing. Sudden loss of consciousness on surfacing should be assumed to be due to cerebral gas emboli. Spontaneous improvement may occur with first aid measures, but relapse is common.

Coronary arterial emboli rarely may present as acute myocardial infarction or arrhythmia. Abdominal organs and skin may also be embolized. Elevation of serum creatine kinase (predominantly from skeletal muscle), serum transaminase and lactate dehydrogenase levels in divers with AGE suggests that emboli are distributed more extensively than previously recognized.[25,26] Peak CK may be a marker of the degree and severity of AGE.[25,26]

Onset of DCI due to gas bubbles coming out of solution can be equally as dramatic (especially after rapid ascents from deep dives), but frequently evolves over hours post dive. DCI caused by bubbles released from tissues usually causes symptoms within 1 h of completing a dive, and 90% of cases have symptoms within 6 h.[2,24] Common symptoms include profound fatigue, myalgia, periarticular pain and headache. Shoulders and elbows are the joints most commonly involved. The pain is usually a dull ache, which may initially be intermittent and migrate from joint to joint, but later becomes constant. Movement aggravates the pain, but local pressure with an inflated sphygmomanometer cuff may improve it. Paraesthesia and numbness may accompany the pain suggesting concomitant neurological disease.

Neurological DCI may present as personality change, headache, memory loss, visual defects, convulsions, confusion and altered level of consciousness. A flat affect may be the only symptom. The vestibular system can also be involved, with dizziness, vertigo, vomiting, nystagmus and ataxia.

Spinal-cord involvement occurs in up to 60% of cases of neurological DCI.[24] The exact cause of spinal DCI is still debated. It may be a result of venous infarction of the cord due to obstruction of the epidural vertebral venous plexus.[19] Other explanations include ischaemia and inflammation from bubble emboli or the formation of local bubbles within the spinal cord (autochthonous bubbles). Symptoms include back pain, paraesthesia and paraplegia, with bowel and bladder involvement. It is potentially disastrous to misdiagnose back pain coming on a few minutes after a dive as musculoskeletal pain and not consider spinal cord DCI.

If the bubble load overwhelms the pulmonary filter a diver can present with a syndrome known as 'the chokes'. The symptoms of this syndrome include dyspnoea, pleuritic substernal chest pain, cough, pink frothy sputum, cyanosis and haemoptysis. It is usually self-limiting but indicates the diver has sustained a large intravascular gas load, so a careful inquiry about other symptoms of DCI is mandatory. Diving related pulmonary oedema and salt-water aspiration syndrome are the major differential diagnoses.

A variety of rashes may be caused by cutaneous bubbles; however, these syndromes affect less than 10% of divers. The most common presentations are pruritis with no rash, a scarlatinaform rash with pruritis, and cutis marmorata. Cutis marmorata begins as a spreading erythema but subsequently develops a marbled appearance of pale areas surrounded by cyanotic mottling.

Assessment of the injured diver

The injured diver requires simultaneous assessment and treatment. One hundred per cent oxygen treatment should be continued during the assessment. If the history suggests AGE, the patient should not be moved from the horizontal position to avoid re-embolization. If symptoms are progressing rapidly, the examination should be brief but thorough so as to ensure rapid access to recompression. In serious cases, some of the historical information may be obtained once the diver is receiving treatment in the recompression chamber.

The diagnosis of DCI is made on history and examination. A full dive history must be obtained, in addition to the medical history. Important details include the number of dives over recent days, depth, bottom time (the time from beginning descent to beginning direct ascent), performance of any decompression or safety stops, dive complications such as rapid ascents, surface interval between dives and the time interval between completing the dive and onset of symptoms. Previous dive experience, equipment used and gases breathed should also be recorded. A history of using surface supply equipment (the 'Hookah' apparatus) should alert the examining physician to the possibility of carbon monoxide poisoning and carboxyhaemoglobin measurement is required. Cold water, hard exercise during the dive, increasing age, multiple ascents and repetitive dives are predisposing factors in the development of DCI. Any exposure to altitude (>300 m) or heavy exercise post dive should be recorded.

A thorough examination, particularly of the neurological system, to detect subtle abnormalities is required. It is also helpful to perform basic tests of cognitive function such as the mini-mental state examination. For milder static DCI syndromes with delayed presentation, the sharpened Romberg test provides useful information.[27] It is performed by asking the patient to stand heel-to-toe with open palms on opposite shoulders. The patient is stable. They are then asked to close their eyes and timed until they lose balance or achieve 60 s. A score of less than 60 s is suggestive of DCI in an injured diver. This test should not be performed if the history was suggestive of AGE, or if there are neurological symptoms or signs.

Clinical investigation

Recompression should only be delayed for investigations if they will directly alter management.

A full blood count and electrolytes are useful in that intravascular fluid depletion is common in severe DCI and the degree of haemoconcentration may correlate with eventual neurological outcome.[28] Serum CK and LFTs may be indicators of gas embolism, however these do not influence clinical management.[25] The blood glucose level should be checked in divers with impaired consciousness. A chest X-ray is indicated if pulmonary barotrauma is suspected, because a pneumothorax requires treatment before recompression. A dilemma occurs if the diver has a neurological presentation, because they should not be moved from the horizontal position until they are recompressed. If CAGE is suspected and CT is available, a supine CT scan of the thorax is preferable to a chest X-ray to diagnose pneumothorax or pneumomediastinum. Magnetic resonance imaging has no role in the acute investigation of DCI.

Treatment

First aid

One hundred per cent oxygen provides the maximum gradient for diffusion of nitrogen out of the bubbles. It should be administered in the pre-hospital setting and continue until and during recompression. Failure to improve on oxygen does not rule out DCI. Conversely, complete improvement on oxygen does not obviate the need for recompression. The diver should be supine or in the left lateral position if unable to protect their airway. Traditionally, the Trendelenburg position was advocated to reduce bubble embolization to the brain,

but is now thought to increase the risk of cerebral oedema and should only be used if required to maintain blood pressure.[29] The diver should be prevented from sitting or standing up, to avoid bubbles redistributing from the left ventricle to the brain. Initial resuscitation is along standard basic and advanced life support protocols. If intubation is required, the endotracheal tube cuff should be filled with saline prior to recompression to avoid a change in volume and a tube leak as ambient pressure increases.

Intravenous isotonic crystalloids should be commenced and titrated to response. Glucose-containing fluids are to be avoided because they may exacerbate CNS injury. Divers who present after several days with mild symptoms may be adequately managed with oral fluids. A urinary catheter should be inserted for spinal cord DCI with bladder involvement. Hypothermia should be corrected.

Retrieval

Long-distance retrieval can either be by air transport pressurized to 1 ATA or by portable recompression chambers. There is little debate that the longer the delay in recompression of severe DCI, the worse the outcome. However, Australian experience suggests that the number of cases where a portable chamber would have made a difference is so small that their use is unwarranted, largely because of the time required to prepare and transport portable chambers.[30,31] Commercial aircraft are pressurized to 0.74 ATA (2440 m) and not appropriate to retrieve DCI patients, unless arrangements can be made to fly lower and pressurize to sea level. Road retrieval is not suitable over great distances, or where an altitude of 300 m will be exceeded. Consultation with a hyperbaric physician should occur if retrieval is difficult.

Recompression

Recompression in a hyperbaric chamber is indicated even if the diver becomes asymptomatic with first aid, because otherwise many will relapse. The relapse may be more severe than the original presentation, due to the pathophysiological changes already initiated by bubbles in the microvasculature and tissues, or redistribution of bubbles. Response to recompression is

determined by time to recompression and the initial severity of injury. Recompression should always occur as soon as possible. It is particularly urgent for severe cases where treatment commenced later than 4 h after injury is associated with a poor response. Mild cases often respond despite longer delays to recompression.[32]

Two types of hyperbaric chamber are available to administer recompression treatment:

- *Multiplace* chambers can accommodate more than one person, including a clinician attendant, and are compressed on air while the patient breathes 100% oxygen via a head hood, demand regulator or endotracheal tube. Air breaks to lessen the risks of oxygen toxicity are provided by removing the head hood in a multiplace chamber. Full monitoring and mechanical ventilation are possible. All hyperbaric facilities in Australasia use multiplace chambers.
- *Monoplace* chambers accommodate one patient only and are usually compressed with 100% oxygen. These are more frequently used to treat non-diving medical illness; however, in other countries they may be used for definitive treatment of divers.

Hyperbaric oxygen has the following beneficial effects:

- Reduction in bubble size in accordance with Boyle's law. Increased pressure also increases the partial pressure of nitrogen within the bubble. There is no nitrogen outside the bubble because of the 100% oxygen. This markedly increases the outward diffusion gradient for nitrogen. This relieves the obstruction caused by intravascular bubbles and the tissue distortion of extravascular bubbles.
- Reduction of endothelial inflammation caused by the bubbles.[33]
- Relief of ischaemia and hypoxia.

There are no published randomized trials comparing recompression protocols, and hence no international agreement on how to manage DCI. The general consensus is that initial treatments should begin with a standard 18 m (2.8 ATA) table breathing 100% oxygen. Recent studies have suggested a benefit from initially recompressing deeper, however this procedure is not universally accepted and subject to considerable debate.[34]

The identical Royal Navy 62 (RN62) and US Navy 6 have become the standard of care for initial treatment of diving accidents in Australia and New Zealand. These are 18 m tables, lasting 4.75 h to 7.25 h (see Figure 28.3.1). Recompression is followed by gradual decompression. A response to treatment is usually evident by the second air break. If there is a partial response then there is the option of extending the table at 18 m. If there is minimal or no response and there is no doubt about the diagnosis, then it is reasonable to proceed to a deeper table (most units use the Comex 30 table). Because of the risks of oxygen toxicity at greater than 18 m, a combination of helium and oxygen (heliox) is used. Anecdotal evidence suggests that this technique is particularly effective for severe spinal cord DCI.[35,36] In-water recompression is dangerous and difficult and should only be considered if retrieval is impossible. Hypothermia and oxygen toxicity pose serious risks during treatment and supervision by an experienced hyperbaric physician is essential.

Adverse effects of hyperbaric oxygen

Adverse effects of hyperbaric oxygen are uncommon.[1] Even in non-divers, significant middle-ear barotrauma interrupting treatment occurs in 1/170 treatments. Claustrophobia is even rarer at 1/910 treatments.

The most serious adverse effect is oxygen toxicity, and the attendant must continually watch for signs of its development. Toxicity is due to the formation of oxygen free radicals, which overwhelm the body's antioxidants. It can affect the brain and the lung.

Cerebral oxygen toxicity can occur with brief exposures to 2 ATA oxygen, and pulmonary toxicity may occur with prolonged exposure to 0.5 ATA or higher. The most common presentation of cerebral oxygen toxicity is muscle twitching, particularly of the lips and face. Other possible symptoms include apprehension, vertigo, visual disturbance, nausea, confusion and dizziness. If the oxygen is removed at this stage, progression to generalized convulsions may be avoided. Convulsions can, however, occur without premonitory symptoms. Treatment is as for any generalized convulsion, although removal of the oxygen will almost always stop it. Decompression should not be attempted during the convulsion as this may cause pulmonary barotrauma. Oxygen can be safely reinstituted 15 min after all symptoms have resolved. Predisposing factors to cerebral oxygen toxicity include fever, steroids, a past history of epilepsy, and carbon monoxide poisoning. Incidence is directly proportional to time of exposure and inspired oxygen partial pressure. The incidence of convulsions in divers treated at 2.8 ATA on the RN62 is less than 1%.

Pulmonary oxygen toxicity manifests initially as an asymptomatic reduction in vital capacity, followed by cough and retrosternal pain. The symptoms usually abate when treatment is completed. Up to 10% reduction in vital capacity has been measured during extended treatments, which reverses within 24 h of completing treatment.[2]

Adjuvant therapies for DCI

Recent research in the use of lignocaine infusions in patients undergoing open-heart surgery has demonstrated a significant benefit for the lignocaine group in terms of the incidence of post-operative neuropsychiatric abnormalities.[38] The mechanism of injury in open-heart surgery is likely to be gas emboli and therefore provides a useful model for divers with AGE. There is now sufficient evidence to recommend a 48-h lignocaine infusion at standard anti-arrhythmic doses to divers with unequivocal CAGE. A recent randomized clinical trial demonstrated a reduction in symptoms after treatment for decompression illness if tenoxicam was administered to divers in the recovery phase. There was a reduction in total recompression requirements.[39]

Prognosis after treatment

Relapses may occur after initial recompression, and all neurological cases should be observed in hospital to allow immediate recompression if deterioration occurs. Further daily recompression is carried out until the patient stops improving or becomes asymptomatic, and then one additional treatment is performed. Follow-up treatments are usually at 18 m, using either the RN61 table (18 m for 45 min, ascent to 9 m over 30 min, 9 m for 30 min then ascent over 30 min) or the 18:60:30 table (18 m for 60 min then ascent over 30 min).

Residual symptoms occur in up to 30% of cases[20,37] and are more likely where recompression is delayed. Delays to treatment are not unusual with a mean time to recompression of 68 h in one series.[20] It is not known whether there is a delay interval after which recompression is ineffective, and therefore any diver with unexplained symptoms after diving should be referred to a diving medicine specialist. Many divers with DCI still respond to treatment even when delayed for 7–10 days.

Flying after treatment and return to diving

Recommendations for flying and diving after treatment for DCI vary greatly and are not

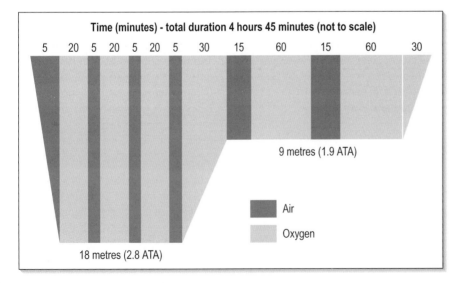

Fig. 28.3.1 US Navy Treatment Table 6.

evidence based. Flying should be avoided for at least 1 week after treatment to avoid relapse. It is reasonable to permit resumption of diving after 4 weeks if there are no residual symptoms or signs. Because of the risk of recurrence, further diving is contraindicated if the DCI is thought to be due to pulmonary barotrauma, or where there are residual neurological signs or symptoms.

Other issues

Vertigo and headache in divers

These two symptom complexes are challenging to assess and diagnose. There are several possible causes of vertigo in divers. Vertigo developing while the diver is underwater is extremely dangerous: it can induce panic and lead to a rapid ascent. It can disorientate the diver so that they do not know which way the surface is, and is often associated with vomiting.

The most common cause, alternobaric vertigo, begins just as divers commence their ascent, and is caused by a unilateral pressure difference between the middle and inner ears. It usually lasts only a few minutes. Middle-ear barotrauma can also cause mild vertigo. Other causes include inner-ear DCI, inner-ear barotrauma and TM rupture. Any persistent vertiginous symptoms may indicate a more serious cause such as neurological decompression illness or inner-ear barotrauma. Headache occurring during or after diving has a number of possible diving related causes such as sinus and mask squeeze, carbon dioxide accumulation, carbon monoxide toxicity, decompression illness, patent foramen ovale, ill-fitting wetsuits, and marine envenomation. It is recommended that for all divers presenting with vertigo or headache, there is early consultation with a diving medicine specialist.

Oxygen toxicity

Cerebral oxygen toxicity in the diver underwater causes the same problems as in the hyperbaric chamber. Divers are more likely to develop toxicity underwater than in the chamber because immersion, exercise and carbon-dioxide retention increase the risk. The use of oxygen-enriched gases such as nitrox increases the risk of cerebral oxygen toxicity. Enriched-air divers should ensure they stay below an oxygen partial pressure of 1.4 ATA.

Nitrogen narcosis

Described by Jacques Cousteau as 'rapture of the deep', nitrogen narcosis is due to the anaesthetic effect of nitrogen dissolved in lipid membranes. Symptoms are similar to those of alcohol intoxication. Some divers experience it at 30 m and almost all by 50. Loss of consciousness occurs at 90 m. This condition will not present to the emergency department because it is immediately reversible on ascent. However, it may result in other diving accidents, such as rapid ascent or near-drowning. Those planning to dive deeper than 50 m should use an alternative to air, such as heliox.

Gas contamination

Contaminants may be in the air before compression, added during compression, or already in the tanks. Common contaminants include carbon dioxide, carbon monoxide and oil. Increasing partial pressures of the contaminant gases at depth may result in toxicity. Contamination is rare but must always be included in the differential diagnosis of injured divers, particularly those presenting with headache, shortness of breath or loss of consciousness at depth.

Diving-related pulmonary oedema

Pulmonary oedema in the diver may be caused by DCI, near-drowning or immersion itself. Pre-existing cardiovascular disease, increasing age (>40), hypertension and beta blockade appear to be risk factors for immersion-induced pulmonary oedema. Symptoms often begin while the diver is still at depth, distinguishing it from DCI. There may also be episodes occurring when immersed but not diving (e.g. swimming). Treatment is supportive and recompression is not required provided DCI can be excluded. However, if detected, the occurrence of pulmonary oedema as a result of diving has long-term ramifications for future diving fitness.[40]

Controversies

❶ *What position is best for managing the injured diver?* There are no controlled trials assessing the best position to manage an injured diver. The current recommendation is to maintain a supine position for all suspected or confirmed neurological presentations, based on expert opinion and known pathophysiology.

❷ *Should intravenous or oral fluids be administered?* Based on expert consensus, and known pathophysiology, the injured diver is usually dehydrated. Fluid management is regarded as an important adjunct to recompression. In an acute diving accident <12 h, where consciousness or airway reflexes are impaired, or where there is nausea and vomiting, i.v. salt based crystalloids should be administered, due to the need for 100% oxygen and the possible risk of oxygen toxicity during the initial treatment phase at 2.8 ATA. In the less acute presentation of static DCI, oral fluids may be acceptable, although there are some risks if an oxygen toxicity seizure occurs during treatment at 2.8 ATA.

❸ *Should we compress divers deeper than 2.8 ATA during treatment?* This is very controversial, with recent reports of deep tables being used successfully in Hawaii. To date, there are no completed randomized controlled trials comparing outcomes of different treatment pressures.

Important phone numbers

24-h services offering advice on management, retrieval and location of the nearest hyperbaric facility:

Australia
Divers Alert Network 1800 088 200
+61 8 8212 9242 (outside Australia)

New Zealand
DES 0800 4337 111

USA
Diving Accident Network (DAN) (919) 6848111

UK
Aberdeen Royal Infirmary 01224 681818
Diving Diseases Centre, Plymouth 01752 261910
Institute of Naval Medicine 02392 768026

References

1. Hyperbaric Technicians and Nurses Association and Australian and New Zealand Hyperbaric Medicine Group. Papers and Proceedings from the Tenth Annual Scientific Meeting of the Hyperbaric Technicians and Nurses Association and the Australian and New Zealand Hyperbaric Medicine Group 2002, Christchurch, New Zealand.

2. Edmonds C, Lowry C, Pennefather J, et al. Diving and subaquatic medicine. 4th edn. London: Arnold Publishers;2002.

3. Edmonds C. Inner ear barotrauma: a retrospective clinical series of 50 cases. South Pacific Underwater Medicine Society Journal 2004; 34(1): 11–14.

4. Shupak A, Doweck I, Greenberg E, et al. Diving related inner ear injuries. Laryngoscope 1991; 101: 173–179.

5. Wong R, Walker M. Diagnostic dilemmas in inner ear decompression sickness. South Pacific Underwater Medicine Society Journal 2004; 34(1): 5–10.

6. Roydhouse N. Round window membrane rupture in scuba divers. South Pacific underwater Medicine Society Journal 1997; 27(3): 148–151.

7. Molenat FA, Boussuges AH. Rupture of the stomach complicating diving accidents. Undersea and Hyperbaric Medicine 1995; 22(1): 87–94.

8. Schriger DL, Rosenberg G, Wilder RJ. Shoulder pain and pneumoperitoneum following a diving accident. Annals of Emergency Medicine 1987; 16: 1281–1284.

9. Kizer KW. Dysbaric cerebral air embolism in Hawaii. Annals of Emergency Medicine 1987; 16: 535–541.

10. Weiss LD, Van Meter KW. Cerebral air embolism in asthmatic scuba divers in a swimming pool. Chest 1995; 107: 1653–1654.

11. Benton PJ, Woodfine JD, Westwood PR. Arterial gas embolism following a 1 metre ascent during helicopter escape training: a case report. Aviation Space and Environmental Medicine 1996; 67(1): 63–64.

12. Williamson J. Arterial gas embolism from pulmonary barotrauma: what happens in the lung? South Pacific Under Water Medicine Society Journal 1988; 18(3): 90–92.

13. Gorman D. 1984 Arterial gas embolism as a consequence of pulmonary barotrauma. South Pacific Under Water Medicine Society Journal 1984; 14(3): 8–16.

14. Tetzlaff K, Beuter B, Leplow B, et al. Risk factors for pulmonary barotrauma in divers. Chest 1997; 112(3): 654–659.

15. Leitch D, Green R. Pulmonary barotrauma in divers and the treatment of cerebral arterial gas embolism. Aviation Space and Environmental Medicine 1986; 57: 931–938.

16. Harker CP, Neuman TS, Olson K, et al. The roentographic findings associated with air embolism in sport scuba divers. Journal of Emergency Medicine 1993; 1(4): 443–449.

17. Francis TJR, Mitchell SJ. Manifestations of decompression disorders. In: Brubakk AO, Neuman TS, eds. Bennett and Elliott's physiology and medicine of diving. 5th edn. London: Harcourt Publishers; 2003: 578–599.

18. Hagen PT, Scholz DG, Edwards WD. Incidence and size of patent foramen ovale in the first ten decades of life: an autopsy study of 965 normal hearts. Mayo Clinic Proceedings 1984; 59: 17–20.

19. Hallenbeck JM, Bove AA, Elliot DH. Mechanisms underlying spinal cord damage in decompression sickness. Neurology 1975; 25: 308–316.

20. Gardner M, Forbes C, Mitchell S. One hundred divers with DCI treated in New Zealand during 1995. South Pacific Under Water Medicine Society Journal 1996; 26(4): 222–226.

21. Goble SJ. 1997 Is DCS possible if diving shallower than 10 metres? Proceedings 5th Annual Scientific Meeting Hyperbaric Technicians and Nurses Association and the Australian and New Zealand Hyperbaric Medicine Group, Sydney.

22. Survanshi SS, Parker EC, Thalmann ED, et al. Statistically based decompression tables XII. (Volume 1) Repetitive decompression tables for air and constant 0.7 ATA PO2 in N2 using a probabilistic model. Technical report of the naval medical research institute, Bethesda, MD: Network of Minority Research I; 1997: 97–136.

23. Standards Australia. Occupational Diving Operations. Part 1. Standard operational practice AS/NZS 2299.1; 2007.

24. Divers Alert Network. Report on diving accidents and facilities. Durham, NC; 2006.

25. Smith RM, Neuman TS. 1994 Elevation of serum creatine kinase in divers with arterial gas embolism. New England Journal of Medicine 1994; 330(1): 9–24.

26. Smith RM, Neuman TS. Abnormal serum biochemistries in association with arterial gas embolism. Journal of Emergency Medicine 1997; 15(3): 285–289.

27. Fitzgerald B. A review of the sharpened Romberg test in diving medicine. South Pacific Under Water Medicine Society Journal 1996; 26(3): 142–146.

28. Smith RM, Van Hosen KB, Neuman TS. Arterial gas embolism and haemoconcentration. Journal of Emergency Medicine 1994; 2(2): 1147–1153.

29. Moon RE, Sheffield PJ. Guidelines for treatment of decompression illness. Aviation Space and Environmental Medicine 1997; 8: 234–243.

30. Butler C. Hyperbaric retrievals in Townsville: is a portable chamber useful? South Pacific Under Water Medicine Society Journal 1996; 26(2): 66–70.

31. Oxer HF. Is transport of diving casualties under pressure worth it? Proceedings IX International Congress on Hyperbaric Medicine: Sydney. Flagstaff: Best Publishing; 1987: pp. 137–138

32. Ball R. Effect of severity, time to recompression with oxygen and retreatment on outcome in 49 cases of spinal cord decompression. Undersea and Hyperbaric Medicine 1993; 20(2):133–145.

33. Zamboni WA, Roth AC, Russell RC, et al. The effect of hyperbaric oxygen on the microcirculation of ischaemic skeletal muscle. Undersea Biomedical Research 1990; 17(Supplement): 26.

34. Smerz RW, Overlock RK, Nakayama H. Hawaiian deep treatments: efficacy and outcomes 1983–2003. Undersea and Hyperbaric Medicine 2005; 32(5): 363–373.

35. Kol S, Adir Y, Gordon CR, Melamed Y. Oxy-helium treatment of severe spinal decompression sickness after air diving. Undersea and Hyperbaric Medicine 1993; 20(2): 47–54.

36. Douglas JDM, Robinson C. Heliox treatment for spinal decompression sickness following air dives. Undersea Biomedical Research 1988; 15(4): 315–319.

37. Gorman DF, Pearce A, Webb RK. Dysbaric illness treated at the Royal Adelaide Hospital 1987: a factorial analysis. South Pacific Under Water Medicine Society Journal 1988; 18: 95–101.

38. Mitchell SJ, Pellett O, Gorman DF. Cerebral protection by lidocaine during cardiac operations. Annals of Thoracic Surgery 1999; 67: 1117–1124.

39. Bennett M, Mitchell S, Dominquez A. Adjunctive treatment of decompression illness with a non-steroidal antiiflammatory drug (tenoxicam) reduces recompression requirement. Undersea and Hyperbaric Medicine 2003; 30(3): 195–205.

40. Hampson, NB, Dunford, RG. Pulmonary edema of scuba divers. Undersea and Hyperbaric Medicine 1997; 24: 29–33.

28.4 Radiation incidents

Paul D. Mark

ESSENTIALS

1 Radiation accidents are rare but require well-planned protocols for successful management. The principal challenge will be managing anxious patients who are potentially contaminated with radioactive particulate material.

2 Effective triage is based on early clinical symptoms and lymphocyte counts.

3 The management of life-threatening illness or injury always takes precedence over the radiation aspects of the patient's condition.

4 The principles of contamination control are little different from those dealing with patients contaminated with chemical or biological material

5 Contamination with radioactive material should be distinguished from exposure to ionizing radiation. Except in nuclear detonations or reactor accidents it is very uncommon for both to occur in the same victim.

6 Removing the patient's clothing and washing exposed skin and hair can reduce the level of external contamination by up to 90%.

7 The risks to hospital personnel are minimal provided appropriate precautions are taken.

8 The presence of a qualified radiation physicist with appropriate radiation monitoring equipment is invaluable when dealing with (potentially) contaminated patients.

9 Following whole-body irradiation, survival is likely only from the haemopoietic and milder gastrointestinal syndromes.

10 Blocking and chelating agents can successfully reduce the incorporation of radioactive substances into body tissues if they are given early.

11 The advent of bone marrow transplant can increase the survival rates of more severely affected patients but resources around the nation are limited.

Introduction

Historically, radiation incidents have been the result of accidental exposures. In August 1945, the first atomic fission bombs were detonated above the Japanese cities of Hiroshima and Nagasaki with devastating effects. A further 120 fatalities from radiation accidents were documented worldwide from 1946 to 2000.[1] The most serious incident occurred in 1986 at Chernobyl in the former Soviet Union when a nuclear reactor unit exploded, dispersing radioactive material over a wide area. One hundred and thirty six people developed acute radiation syndrome, of which 28 died.

A dramatic increase in thyroid cancers was observed amongst those who were either very young or in utero.[1] Most other accidents have involved small numbers of people and many have occurred as a result of deliberate bypassing of safety procedures.[2]

Much of our knowledge of the long-term effects of ionizing radiation comes from the study of people who survived the Chernobyl and Japanese incidents.

In Australia, the Australian Radiation Incidence Registry records all accidents where exposures occur that are not 'within the limits known to be normal for the particular source of radiation and for the particular use being made of it'. Very few accidents are recorded in which individuals received exposure or contamination significant enough to cause health concerns.[3] Strict licensing and control systems, coupled with improving technology and training, have helped to minimize the number of Australian radiation incidents.

The advent of terrorism might increase the risk of multiple casualty incidents particularly from the use of radiation dispersal devices. Significant acute irradiation from such a device is unlikely but victims may present with a variety of clinical syndromes, and their management requires a multidisciplinary approach and close liaison between clinical staff and health physicists.[4]

Decontamination is essential for all patients to avoid the delayed effects of continuing low dose radiation.

Radiation sources and incidents

Worldwide, the most common radiation sources are:

- X-ray equipment: used for medical diagnosis and treatment, industrial and commercial inspections, quality control techniques, irradiations and research.
- Accelerators: used for medical treatments, industrial irradiation, the production of radioisotopes and research.
- Radioactive materials: used for medical diagnosis and treatment, industrial radiography, quality control and tracing techniques, soil density and moisture tests, and research. Radioactive material may be unsealed or contained within sealed containers.
- Nuclear processing and reactor plants: used for processing uranium and plutonium for fuel purposes and nuclear weapons, power production and research.

With X-ray equipment and accelerators the victim may be exposed to radiation but this does not make the tissues radioactive. These patients pose no threat to others, including medical attendants.

Unsealed radioactive material has the potential to cause radioactive contamination. This may be external on clothing or skin, or internal following inhalation, ingestion or absorption through body orifices, mucous membranes and wounds. Following internal contamination radioactive material may become incorporated into the patient's tissues.

Other than for accidents involving nuclear processing and reactor plants, accidents usually lead to either exposure or contamination. Contaminated patients rarely suffer significant radiation exposure, and exposed patients are seldom contaminated.[3]

There are no nuclear reactors in Australia except for the occasional visiting nuclear powered warship. These vessels are closely monitored whilst in Australian ports. In the unlikely event of a reactor accident, there would be a risk of direct radiation exposure for several kilometres especially at right angles to the vessel. A plume of steam containing radioactive material, especially iodine, could spread downwind for many kilometres contaminating the air, pastures and crops.

Terrorism

The most likely means for terrorist organizations to deploy radiation is a radiation dispersal device (RDD) or 'dirty bomb'. These weapons use conventional explosives such as trinitrotoluene, ammonium nitrate or other explosive material to spread radioactive substances. A variety of substances could be used including americium, caesium, cobalt, iodine, phosphorous, plutonium, strontium, tritium and uranium. Only some of these are available in Australia.

RDDs are sometimes called 'weapons of mass disruption' because of the fear they engender in the population, multiple casualties, contamination of widespread areas and the economic cost.[5] Immediate injuries are generally the result of blast or thermal effects. Few contain sufficient material to cause acute radiation injury. Only those trapped near the site of detonation run this risk. However, radioactive material will be spread over a large area and many people might be exposed to the risks of low dose radiation. Hospital staff treating the victims of RDD explosions are at negligible risk provided they wear appropriate protective equipment. Unlike surface burst nuclear weapons, RDDs do not cause fallout downwind of the detonation. Radioactive material without the explosive component could potentially be hidden in a crowded space such as a theatre where it could cause occult irradiation.

Measuring radioactivity

Radioactivity of an isotope is expressed as the average number of atoms that disintegrate per second. The Becquerel (Bq) is the SI unit for one nuclear disintegration per second. The activity of a given mass of a radioactive substance with a short half-life will decrease with time.

Ionization in air can be measured by portable dosimeters to give an estimate of the levels of radioactivity at the site of an incident. This is used to calculate the exposure level of a patient with acute radiation illness. The units used are Roentgens. Dosimeters are also used in hospitals to measure the level of radiation to which staff members have been exposed or to monitor patients during decontamination.

The absorbed dose of radiation is the amount of ionization energy deposited in matter by ionizing radiation. One Gray (Gy) is equivalent to one joule per kilogram. The effect of a given dose of radiation depends on the type of radiation emitted and the tissue type irradiated.

Type of radiation emitted

Different types of ionizing radiation transfer energy to tissue at different rates. The Sievert (Sv) is the international unit of effective radiation dose and is obtained by multiplying the absorbed dose measured in Gray (Gy) by a quality factor to reflect the different effects of each radiation type and their potential biological damage. For beta and gamma radiation 1 Sv = 1 Gy. Alpha and neutron radiation deposit more energy in tissue so the quality factor is higher.

Alpha particles, composed of two protons and two neutrons, do not penetrate the dermis but may cause local damage if ingested, inhaled or absorbed through open wounds. Beta radiation, consisting of electron-like particles, travels about a metre through the air and is stopped by clothing. It often causes radiation injury to exposed skin. Gamma particles have no mass and are similar to X-rays, penetrating the body freely and causing the acute radiation syndrome if the trunk is involved. Neutrons are produced only during nuclear detonations and whilst they can technically make an irradiated victim emit radiation this is not clinically significant.[6]

The average natural background radiation is 2 mSV per annum in Australia. The Australian National Occupational Health and Safety Commission's standard for a worker is a maximum effective dose of 50 mSv in any year (or 20 mSv per year averaged over 5 years).

Pathophysiology

Radiation damages tissue both directly and indirectly by the production of free radicals from water molecules. Direct damage to cell membranes may cause changes in permeability and the release of lysosomes. Germinal, haemopoietic and gastrointestinal epithelial cells are relatively radiosensitive. The cells of bone, liver, kidney, cartilage, muscle and nerve tissue are relatively radioresistant. The delayed effects of radiation depend on whether the dose is lethal or sublethal to the tissue involved.

Lethal (deterministic) injuries are threshold dependent. Cells are killed when they receive a radiation dose, which varies with different tissues. Clinical expression occurs when the amount of cell killing cannot be compensated for by proliferation of viable cells. The acute and chronic radiation syndromes are deterministic. The earliest delayed effect of acute radiation injury, cataract formation at about 10 months, is an example of this type of injury.

For sublethal (stochastic) injuries there is no threshold level of radiation and the consequence is based on statistical probability. Sublethal injury to chromosomes is the most important effect of ionizing radiation. Double-strand breaks are not easily reparable, especially if the damage occurs simultaneously to both strands. This results in broken chromosomes with no template for repair. The exposed ends of chromosome fragments may join up at random, resulting in morphological chromosomal abnormalities. Sublethal damage to chromosomes is implicated in the development of tumours. Children are more prone to radiation-induced carcinogenesis. Although the incidence of malignancy in adults is increased by radiation exposure, the age at which malignancies are clinically expressed does not change. The estimated increase in lifetime risk of fatal cancer is 0.008% per milligray of gamma radiation exposure.[7] Therefore, an individual who is exposed to 100 milligrays (twice the acceptable Australian occupational annual exposure) has a 0.8% increase in the lifetime risk of fatal cancer.

Radiation exposure to the gonads may produce temporary or permanent infertility in men depending on the dose. With temporary infertility there is preservation of the secondary sexual characteristics. In the female, however, all ova are present at birth and larger radiation doses are required to produce sterility. Radiation-induced infertility in females is associated with premature menopause. Unlike animals, in humans gonadal exposure to radiation does not affect future generations.[8]

The fetus may receive less radiation than the mother when exposed to external radiation. However, when internal contamination occurs it is possible for the fetus to receive a higher dose as material excreted in the urine collects in the maternal bladder. Exposures during organogenesis (weeks 3 to 7) may cause malformations. Exposure during weeks 8 to 25 causes decreasing IQ with increasing dose. There is a small increased risk of childhood cancers and possibly leukaemia.

Chronic radiation exposure

Chronic radiation exposure was first described in Russia following the exposure of workers in the plutonium enrichment programme to excessive doses of radiation over a period of time. Persons at risk have been exposed to radiation well above occupational health and safety standards for at least three years and have received a dose of 1 Gy or more to the bone marrow. Symptoms include sleep and appetite disturbance, easy fatiguability, impaired concentration and memory, vertigo, ataxia, paraesthesia, bone pain and hot flushes. Clinical findings include localized bone and muscle tenderness, tremor, hyperreflexia and underdeveloped secondary sexual characteristics. Investigations may reveal

pancytopenia and bone dysplasia. Following cessation of exposure symptoms may slowly resolve.

Acute radiation exposure

Radiation exposure accidents usually involve penetrating radiation such as high-energy X-rays or gamma rays. The effects are primarily due to the loss of cells in the body. Acute exposure is more dangerous than chronic, as it does not allow time for cell replacement or tissue recovery. Clinically, radiation exposure may produce a generalized acute radiation syndrome or a localized irradiation injury.

The Acute Radiation Syndrome

The Acute Radiation Syndrome refers to the effects of radiation on one or more body systems. The haemopoietic tissue alone is affected at doses of 1 to 4 Gy and produces pancytopenia with its consequent risks of infection, bleeding and anaemia.[9] Above 6 Gy, gastrointestinal effects are also manifest and the prognosis is poorer. The neurovascular syndrome occurs with doses above 20 Gy and is manifest by leaky capillaries, hypotension and a progressive decline in mental function with eventual death in weeks to months. The symptoms depend on the part of the body irradiated, the dose, and the time over which it is delivered.

Clinical features

The course of the illness can be divided into four phases. The higher the dose, the shorter the duration of each phase and the more severe the symptoms:

- the prodromal phase, which generally lasts up to 48 h
- a latent period, lasting hours to weeks
- the manifest illness period
- death or recovery; the latter may take up to 10 weeks.

The prodromal symptoms are due to the effects of radiation on cell membranes and the release of vasoactive amines. The symptoms are non-specific, with anorexia, nausea, vomiting, weakness, fever, conjunctivitis, erythema and hyperaesthesia. The time to emesis, presence of diarrhoea and duration of symptoms are markers of the

severity of the exposure.[10] Vomiting, however, may be psychogenic.

The phase of manifest illness corresponds to the loss of cells.[11] The haemopoietic syndrome occurs alone with whole-body radiation doses of between 1 and 4 Gy. It is due to loss of stem cells in the bone marrow. At these doses, some stem cells survive and recovery is therefore possible. The latent period lasts from 2 to 20 days and is followed by a rapid fall in the number of white blood cells and platelets. Recovery commences about 30 days after exposure, regardless of the exact dose.

The gastrointestinal syndrome predominates with radiation doses greater than 6 Gy. The prodromal symptoms are more severe. Early bloody diarrhoea suggests death within 2 weeks. The gastrointestinal symptoms recur during the manifest illness phase and can be very severe leading to dehydration and electrolyte imbalance. This syndrome is due to the loss of stem cells in the intestinal mucosal crypts. It is superimposed upon the haemopoietic syndrome with both occurring after a short latent period of under a week.

The neurovascular syndrome occurs with doses of greater than 20 Gy and is characterized by leakage of fluid into tissues and hypotension. The latent period is just a few days. Leakage into the brain causes neurological symptoms. These effects are superimposed on those due to gastrointestinal and haemopoietic damage. At very high doses, greater than 30 Gy there is incapacitation usually within the first few minutes and certainly within 40 min. The effects are largely due to disruption of cell membranes and electrochemical inactivation of neurons. Death can be anticipated within hours.

Whole body irradiation also produces visible changes in the skin. Hair epilation occurs at 3 Gy, erythema at 6 Gy, dry desquamation at 10 Gy and wet desquamation at 20 Gy. The erythema may come and go and occurs earlier with higher doses but rarely within 24 h.

Patients presenting after definite or presumed exposure to ionizing radiation can be triaged based on symptoms and lymphocyte counts. Less than 10% of people vomit if the radiation dose is less than 1 Gy, whereas most vomit if the dose is more than 2 Gy. Onset of emesis in less than

4 h suggests a dose of at least 2 Gy. For exposures of less than 6 Gy, emesis will usually cease within 24 h without treatment.

Treatment

The threshold for admission on initial presentation will depend on the number of casualties but in general patients who do not vomit within 6 h can be managed as outpatients.

Supportive treatment includes maintenance of fluid and electrolyte balance, nutritional supplementation, antiemetics and antidiarrhoeals. Control of infection commences in the prodromal phase, with identification and aggressive treatment of any potential infection, so that the patient is in optimal condition to survive a period of manifest haemopoietic depression. To reduce the infection risk, patients may be kept home during the latent period and admitted to hospital when neutropenia develops. Hospital management involves strict isolation and lamina airflow units. The prophylactic administration of antibacterial, antiviral, antifungal and antihelminthic therapy is reserved for the most severely neutropenic. Non-absorbable agents are commonly used to sterilize the gastrointestinal tract. Anaerobic agents should be included if there is gut injury.[12]

Management of neutropenia follows the principles established in the management of bone marrow suppression secondary to chemotherapeutic agents. Fever is investigated and managed with empirical therapy in the first instance. If as many as 10% of the stem cells remain intact, the blood cells will repopulate. Therapeutic modalities include platelet transfusion and colony stimulating factors which must be commenced early. The role of stem cell transplantation is evolving. Early oral feeding is encouraged to maintain the immunological and physiological integrity of the gut.

Clinical investigation

Acute radiation exposure is confirmed by laboratory investigation.[13] A lymphocyte count of 1000/mm^3 at 24 h suggests a dose of at least 2 Gy and the eventual development of the haemopoietic syndrome. A count of 500/mm^3 suggests a radiation dose of 6 Gy and the subsequent development of both the gastrointestinal and haemopoietic syndromes. If lymphocytes

disappear within 6 h the dose is likely to be fatal.[14]

Lymphocyte counts every 6–12 h for 48 h are useful for admitted patients to further refine the likely dose and clinical course.[15]

- No symptoms and lymphocytes >1500/mm^3 after 48 h – unlikely to require clinical support but should be observed periodically.
- Nausea, vomiting, erythema and lymphocytes between 800 and 1500/mm^3 at 48 h – probable serious injury, which will require clinical support.
- Pronounced nausea, vomiting, diarrhoea, erythema and lymphocytes between 100 and 800/mm^3 at 48 h – probable life-threatening injury, which will require maximal clinical support.
- Early vomiting and bloody diarrhoea, erythema and lymphocytes <100/mm^3 at 48 h – lethal injury.

The lymphocyte count may be less useful if there is significant concomitant trauma or at low levels of exposure.

Cytogenetic studies using blood collected at 48 h in a lithium heparin tube examine the number and structure of chromosomes. Radiation dose is reflected in the number of excess acentric and dicentric forms.[16] T lymphocytes are relatively long-lived and reliable dose estimates can be made up to 5 weeks after collection of the sample. Few laboratories can perform this test, which takes 48 h to give an initial result but many weeks for a full analysis. A newer method involves electron spin resonance of tooth enamel, and can detect very low doses (0.1 Gy).[17]

Prognosis

The LD$_{50/60}$ is the dose at which half the victims succumb within 60 days. Without treatment, the LD$_{50/60}$ is 3.5 Gy. With supportive care, antibiotics and colony stimulating factors the LD$_{50/60}$ is almost doubled up to around 7 Gy. Bone marrow transplantation may be used in patients exposed to 8–10 Gy.

Survival from the cardiovascular and neurovascular syndromes does not occur.

Combined injuries

Combined injury occurs when there is additional trauma, either physical or thermal, in addition to the radiation injury. The effects

of the radiation exposure may become apparent earlier and may be more severe when other injuries are present. Healing of tissues including callus formation at fracture sites will be delayed even with subclinical radiation doses. Radiation exposure increases the probability of mortality when combined with other injuries or pre-existing conditions that result in immunosuppression, blood loss and danger of infectious complications. All administered blood products should be irradiated to remove the T-cell population and minimize graft-versus-host reactions. Platelets should be transfused if the platelet count falls below 20×10^9/L and, if surgery is anticipated, it should be maintained higher than 75×10^9/L. Emergency surgery including the excision of dead tissue and the closure of wounds should be completed within 48 h while some white blood cells remain. For thermal burns, early excision of potentially septic tissue and skin grafting are indicated. Wound closure is an important means of reducing vulnerability to infection. Non-urgent surgery should wait until any bone marrow suppression resolves.

Early reintroduction of enteral nutrition is important to maintain gastric acidity and prevent infectious organisms spreading from the gut to the respiratory system. Medication should be prescribed to reduce the risk of stress ulceration. Radiation pneumonitis may develop some time following the exposure and be confused with ARDS.

Local irradiation injuries

The majority of local irradiation injuries occur when operators of X-ray diffraction units inadvertently place their fingers or hands in the direct X-ray beam. Other accidents have occurred when radioactive sources, often from industrial radiography equipment, are detached and then picked up and placed in the pockets of workers. There have been mis-administrations of radiation to patients undergoing radiotherapy. The higher the dose, the greater the severity and the earlier the onset of the local injury. The smaller the area irradiated, the higher the dose required to produce a particular change.

Clinical features

Symptoms may include tenderness, itching, tingling, and a changed sensitivity to heat and cold. Skin changes include epilation, erythema, dry desquamation, wet desquamation, blisters and radionecrotic lesions. If the area irradiated includes the epigastrium, nausea and vomiting may also occur. The degree of radiosensitivity of the skin depends on the thickness of the epidermis. The most sensitive areas are those that are also moist and subject to friction, such as the axillae, groins and skin folds. The least sensitive areas are the nape of the neck, scalp, palms and soles.

Erythema may not appear for some days. If it occurs within 48 h the lesion will probably progress to ulceration. If irradiated skin appears normal at 72 h, the lesion is likely to be less severe but may still ulcerate in 1 or 2 weeks. Erythema may be delayed for up to 30 days. Pain is minimal unless ulceration occurs or the dose is extreme. Late effects include progressive tissue atrophy, fibrosis and chronic radiodermatitis with tissue breakdown. There may be stiffness and tenderness and decreased sensitivity to temperature change.

Treatment

Mild injuries may be simply observed. An effort should be made to protect the area from additional trauma. For more severe injuries, particularly with pain, local debridement and skin grafting may be necessary but should be delayed until the full extent of the lesion is known.[18] Amputation is reserved for gangrene. Skin grafts are indicated for areas of exposed cartilage or bone, or for severe scarring. Topical antibiotics are often prescribed in an attempt to reduce infection. Hyperbaric oxygen therapy may be useful.[19] In the long term, the irradiated area must be watched for the possible development of neoplastic change.

Occult radiation exposure

Occult exposure to radiation without an explosion might result in unsuspecting patients presenting with delayed symptoms. It should be in the differential diagnosis of the following especially if associated with a 2- to 3-week prior history of nausea and vomiting.

- Unexplained bone marrow suppression (neutropenia, lymphopenia and thrombocytopenia).

- Immunological dysfunction with secondary infections.
- An unexplained tendency to bleeding.
- Acute onset of alopecia.
- Thermal burn like skin changes or desquamation with no history of thermal injury.

Contamination with radioactive material

The care of individuals who are contaminated with radioactive material requires similar preparation and precautions as for those contaminated with hazardous chemicals. Radioactive contamination has the advantage that it can be readily detected by instruments when on the skin. With the exception of Chernobyl, survivors of radiation accidents have not been sufficiently contaminated so as to pose a threat to emergency or hospital personnel using appropriate precautions and procedures.[11]

Prevention

All staff using shielded or unshielded radiation sources in their daily work must be thoroughly trained in their safe use. Facilities using unshielded radioactive material must have procedures in place to deal with spillage and other accidents, and all workers must be adequately trained in emergency procedures.

Preparedness

Emergency equipment must include appropriate monitors for detecting ionizing radiation or contamination, facilities for decontaminating victims, and plastic bags for biological and other samples. Appropriate blocking or chelating agents should be stocked at the facility.[20] Emergency planning must include early warning of the receiving hospital so that adequate preparations can be made prior to the arrival of patients.

Scene management

For incidents involving small numbers of patients, members of the rescue team should put on the protective clothing normally used by personnel working with radioactive material at that site. This includes gloves, facemask and cap. Gowns may be covered with large plastic aprons

to make them waterproof. Additional measures, such as taping plastic bags over shoes, may be used if the normal protective clothing is judged inadequate. The implementation of life-saving procedures may make it necessary to forgo some of this protection. Contamination of the rescuer will be low and decontamination can be carried out later.

Serious illness or injury is not due to radiation per se, and should be treated on its own merits. Unless the patient's condition is serious, external decontamination begins at the scene so as to minimize internal contamination and incorporation of the radionuclide into the body tissues, and to reduce the risk of contaminating other persons and the hospital environment. As much as 80% of contaminating material may be on the clothing.[21] Accordingly, the victim's outer clothing should be removed at the earliest practicable stage. If monitoring is not available, it should be assumed that all outer clothing is contaminated. Clothing is cut from head to toe and down the sleeves, folded back over itself as it is cut, and then rolled up. The person removing the contaminated clothing must wear protective clothing and limit contact with the outside of the victim's clothing. The victim is then wrapped in plain sheets and transferred to hospital.[22] If small contamination spots on the skin cannot be easily removed at the scene, they should be dressed and the victim transported to hospital.

At larger incidents, it may also be necessary to establish a controlled area, the periphery of which is located just beyond the region where contamination is detected above background levels. Rescue team members should wear the maximum level of personal protective equipment available. This should be removed at the perimeter of this area prior to both patient and rescuers leaving. Monitoring of all personnel leaving the area should be undertaken if facilities are available.[23]

Portable vacuum units with high efficiency particulate air filters have reportedly been used to facilitate rapid decontamination outdoors.

Emergency department

The elements of planning for the management of radiation accident patients are similar to those for other types of emergencies, namely prevention, preparedness, response and recovery.

Facilities using unsealed radioactive sources should be identified in advance. These include nuclear medicine departments, scientific laboratories and nuclear facilities. An emergency department (ED) response plan should be developed and emergency response team membership designated. Equipment for monitoring, decontamination and contamination control should be in place. Regular practice is essential.[24]

A decontamination area must be designated and be itself capable of adequate decontamination. Ambulant patients and lower acuity stretcher bound patients should be decontaminated outside the ED. Waste water may be legally discharged into normal draining systems if it does not exceed specified limits. In the clinical setting of a few patients, this is unlikely. Incidents involving contaminated or possibly contaminated patients rapidly deplete a receiving hospital's emergency response. If multiple patients with possible contamination are being managed, the hospital may need to defer where possible the arrival of other patients.

Hospital protocols should include plans for dealing with relatives, the press and the public. The timely release of appropriate information is important. Persons issuing this information should be well versed in radiation medicine, as the avoidance of questions and confusion in answers may generate public uncertainty and panic. Security personnel will be required to restrict the entry of unauthorized persons to the treatment area.

Decontamination process

Life-saving procedures resulting from trauma or burns should take priority over consideration of the radiation aspects of the patient's condition, even if preparations to minimize the spread of contamination have not been completed. A radiation physicist with appropriate monitoring equipment should be present in the ED. However, if patients arrive before monitoring is available, treatment of severe injury should proceed immediately and subsequent decisions regarding decontamination should be based on the patient's likely exposure.

In the ideal situation, all patients should be monitored at triage and, if found to be contaminated, those without severe injury should be showered and re-monitored prior to admission to the ED. This is especially so if whole-body contamination has occurred, for example from a gaseous plume from a reactor accident.[3] Washing starts with the hair and works downwards. Wounds should be covered with a waterproof dressing before showering to avoid washing contaminated water into them.

Because some patients with severe injury will require immediate admission to the ED, adequate preparations are necessary.[25] The floor of the entry and some treatment cubicles should be covered with plastic and any non-essential items removed. Access to this controlled area must be strictly supervised and there should preferably be a buffer zone. Disposable fluid-repellent gowns are ideal but surgical gowns covered by plastic aprons are satisfactory. Lead aprons as used in X-ray departments are not satisfactory; these prevent exposure but not contamination and are heavy and hot to wear. Plastic bags are taped over the shoes and the cuffs of overalls should be taped and secured to the outsides of overshoes. Facemasks are required to protect against airborne contamination but they do not protect the face from being touched by contaminated hands. N95 masks may be superior to standard surgical masks.[26] Trauma masks with clear plastic visors are the best option. Two pairs of gloves should be worn. The inner ones should be surgical gloves taped to the sleeves. The outer gloves are not taped down and should be changed frequently. Hair cover is desirable. Rubbish bins lined with garbage bags serve as waste receptacles and should be emptied promptly to minimize the amount of radiation in the department.

Once the patient is in the controlled area, all clothing should be removed and other medical conditions assessed and treated. Blocking agents can be administered if they have not already been given. All mucosal surfaces should be swabbed to aid in the assessment of likely internal contamination. These include nostrils and ears, the mouth and rectum. The swabs should be placed in sealed labelled plastic bags and sent for radiation assessment and identification of the chemicals involved. Blood samples should be drawn for a baseline complete blood count, differential and absolute lymphocyte counts, and later cytogenic analysis. A serum amylase is also useful as the parotid is very sensitive to radiation.

External decontamination utilizes the principles of barrier nursing and contamination control. Staff should stand back from the patient except when actually examining them or performing procedures. Radiation exposure is inversely proportional to the distance from the source squared. Hospital personnel should be rotated during the decontamination procedure to minimize the perceived risk to any one individual. Pregnant staff should not be involved. Each staff member should shower following completion of their turn in decontamination.

The priority areas for external decontamination are wounds and orifices, as it is through these that the risk of subsequent internal contamination is greatest. Other priority areas include the hands, face and head, as early contamination removal reduces spread. Decontamination of intact skin is the last priority.

Following removal of clothing, decontamination starts at the periphery of a contaminated area and works inwards. The skin is washed initially with warm water and mild soap. If this is ineffective, progressively stronger detergents can be used. If the skin becomes damaged or red and sore, cleansing should be discontinued. Wounds are decontaminated in the same manner as when removing dirt or bacteria. Deeper wounds should be opened up and thoroughly irrigated. Burnt areas also should be carefully irrigated. Metal fragments should be removed with forceps. Deep debridement and excision of a wound is rarely necessary in extreme cases where highly toxic material is embedded in the tissues. The mouth is decontaminated by gentle irrigation and frequent rinsing with 30% hydrogen peroxide solution. Brushing of the teeth with toothpaste is helpful, as toothpaste contains chelating agents. External ear canals should be irrigated, and nasal douches can be effective. The eyes are rinsed by directing a stream of water or saline from the inner canthus to the outer canthus, so that material is not forced into the lacrimal duct. Hair should be shampooed several times with the head deflected backwards over a basin to keep water from the eyes and ears. A hair dryer is used to dry the hair. Clipping of hair may occasionally be necessary.

Decontamination efforts should continue until the radiation level is at background levels or there is minimal reduction with further washing.

If contamination is only discovered after patients are admitted to an ED, the entire area through which they have passed should be taped off, surveyed with the help of a radiation physicist and, if necessary, decontaminated. Staff should put on protective clothing and remove nearby patients so as to create a spacious treatment area. Following a radiation incident, all equipment, instruments and work areas used in treating contaminated patients must be thoroughly cleaned.

Monitoring decontamination

Radiation physicists should check the background level of radiation in the ED from time to time so that they have a baseline from which to assess each patient's exposure. Scanning should occur slowly to avoid missing radiation. Headphones should be used or the sound turned off to avoid alarming patients.

Internal contamination

Internal contamination causes no acute clinical effects and it is usually not feasible to confirm its presence before commencing treatment directed at the reduction of absorption, prevention of incorporation into tissues and promotion of elimination. Significant internal contamination has traditionally occurred through wounds or body orifices in small-scale accidents. It could readily occur on a wider scale following the explosion of an RDD, a reactor accident or a nuclear detonation. Absorption would be by inhalation of contaminated air and / or ingestion of foodstuffs contaminated by fallout. Radionuclides, which have short effective half-lives such as technetium used in nuclear medicine ($t_{1/2} = 5$ h) pose no danger. For isotopes with effective half-lives measured in days, the decision to treat will depend on the likely intake especially via the lungs, whether the drug is concentrated in tissue such as iodine in the thyroid or uranium or americium in bone, whether the emission is high energy as with cobalt and whether the chemical itself is toxic. The effective half-life combines radioactive and chemical properties and describes the rate of elimination without decontamination. For maximal effectiveness, internal decontamination should commence within 24 to 48 h of pulmonary exposure.

Table 28.4.1 describes the radioisotopes most likely to be available in Australia, their common uses, emissions, toxicity, effective half-life and treatment.

To assist in the determination of the extent of internal contamination a 24-h urine sample should be collected. If gastrointestinal contamination is suspected a 24-h stool sample should also be collected.

Selection of the appropriate technique or drug depends on knowledge of the radionuclide involved and its physical form.[27] For example, uranium is found in order of increasing radioactivity in depleted uranium used in artillery shells, natural uranium, fuel rods and weapons grade enriched uranium. The first two are not significant radiation hazards but the latter two can emit significant levels of gamma radiation if sufficient quantity is present.

Uptake by the various organs can be reduced by the use of blocking agents, dilution techniques or chelating agents. Administration of stable iodine in the form of potassium iodate or potassium iodide tablets will reduce uptake by the thyroid gland by up to 90% if given less than 2 h after intake, and by about 50% if in less than 3 h. Chelating agents and mobilizing agents may be useful for up to 2 weeks. Mobilizing agents, such as antithyroid drugs, increase the natural rate of turnover of a biological molecule and thereby increase excretion. Gastrointestinal decontamination is unusual but an enema might be used to empty the bowel. In the absence of external contamination this would be

| Table 28.4.1 Isotopes likely to cause internal contamination in Australia ||||||||
Element	Emissions	Primary toxicity	Effective $t_{1/2}$[a]	Common use	Detection[b]	Absorption	Treatment
Americium[241]	Alpha Gamma	Marrow suppression	Years	Smoke detector	Yes	Lung, skin	DTPA or EDTA i.v.
Caesium[137]	Beta Gamma	Whole body irradiation	70 days	Medical radiology	Yes	Lung. GI tract, wounds	Prussian blue orally
Cobalt[60]	Gamma Beta	Whole body irradiation	10 days	Medical radiology Commercial food irradiation	Yes	Lung	Penicillamine orally
Iodine[131]	Beta Some gamma	Thyroid	8 days	Nuclear medicine therapy	Yes	Lung	Iodine orally[c]
Tritium[3]	Beta	No significant hazard	12 days	Signs	No	Lung[d]	Increase fluids
Uranium[235/238]	Alpha	Kidney	Can be permanent in bone	Fuel rods for reactors[e]	Yes	Lung	NaHCO$_3$ Tubular diuretics

[a]Effective half-life combines radioactive and chemical properties and describes rates of elimination without decontamination.
[b]Detection by standard radiation detection equipment.
[c]Iodine dose in adults 130 mg daily.
[d]Tritium is not a significant radiation hazard except perhaps in closed spaces.
[e]Natural and depleted uranium are not serious irradiation threats.
GI, gastrointestinal.

the only circumstance in which internal contamination posed any risk to hospital staff.

References

1. Gusev I, Guskova A, Mettler F. Medical management of radiation accidents. Boca Raton, FL: CRC Press; 2001.
2. Cardis E. Epidemiology of accidental radiation exposures. Environmental Health Perspectives 1996; 104(3)supplement: 643–649.
3. Swindon T. Manual on the medical management of individuals involved in radiation accidents. Australian Radiation Laboratory; 1991.
4. Ricks RC. Guidance for Radiation Accident Management. Radiation Emergency Assistance Centre/Training Site (REAC/TS) Oak Ridge Institute for Science and Education; 2002.
5. Levi M, Kelly H. Weapons of mass disruption. Scientific American 2002; 287(5): 77–81.
6. Reeves G. Radiation Injuries. Critical Care Clinics 1999; 15(2): 457–473.
7. Beir V. National Research Council. Health effects of exposure to low levels of ionizing radiation. Washington, DC: National Academy Press; 1990: p 6.
8. Rytoman T. Ten years after Chernobyl. Annals of Medicine 1996; 28(2): 83–87.
9. Directorate of Military Medical Operations. Emergency Radiation Medicine Response Pocket Guide. Armed Forces Radiation Research Institute. Bethesda, MD. www.afrri.usuhs.mil (accessed 1 October 2007).
10. Berger M, Christensen D, Lowry P, et al. Medical management of radiation injuries: current approaches. Occupational Medicine 2006; 56(3): 162–172.
11. Mettler FD. Emergency management of radiation accidents. Journal of the American College of Emergency Physicians 1978; 7: 302.
12. Waselenko J, MacVittie T, Blakely W, et al. Medical management of the acute radiation syndrome: recommendations of the Strategic National Stockpile Radiation Working Group. Annals of Internal Medicine 2004; 140: 1037–1051.
13. Swindon T. The management of individuals involved in radiation accidents. Emergency Medicine 1991; 3(3) suppl: 131–135.
14. Goans RE, Holloway EC, Berger ME, Ricks RD. Early dose assessment following severe radiation accidents. Health Physics 1997; 72(4): 513–518.
15. Anno GH, Baum SJ, Withers HR, et al. Symptomatology of acute radiation effects in humans after exposure to doses of 0.5-30 Gray. Health Physics 1989; 56: 821–838.
16. Salassidis K, Schmid E, Peter RU, et al. Dicentric and translocation analysis for retrospective dose estimation in humans exposed to ionizing radiation during the Chernobyl nuclear power plant accident. Mutation Research 1994; 311(1): 39–48.
17. Baranov AE, Guskova AK, Nadejini NM, Nugis Yyu. Chernobyl experience: biological markers of exposure to ionizing radiation. Stem Cells 1995; 13(1)suppl: 69–77.
18. Oliveira AR, Brandao-Mello CE, Valverde NJ. Localized lesions induced by 137 Cs during the Goiania accident. Health Physics 1991; 60: 25-29.
19. Berger ME, Hurtado R, Dunlap J, et al. Accidental radiation injury to the hand: anatomical and physiological considerations. Health Physics 1997; 72(3): 343–348.
20. Lincoln TA. Importance of initial management of persons internally contaminated with radionuclides. Journal of the American Industrial Hygiene Association 1976; 37: 16–21.
21. Hugner KF, Fry SA, eds. The Medical Basis for Radiation Accident Preparedness. New York: Elsevier; 1980.
22. Ricks RC. Transport of irradiated or radioactively contaminated patients to the hospital. Bulletin of the New York Academy of Medicine 1983; 59: 1108–1118.
23. Hubner KF. Symposium on the health aspects of nuclear power plant incidents. Decontamination procedures and risks to health care personnel. Bulletin of the New York Academy of Medicine 1983; 59: 1119–1128.
24. Fong F, Schrader DC. Radiation disasters and emergency department preparedness. Emergency Medicine Clinics of North America 1996; 14(2): 349–370.
25. Leonard RB, Ricks RD. Emergency department radiation accident protocol. Annals of Emergency Medicine 1980; 9: 462–470.
26. Sansom G. Emergency department personal protective equipment requirements following out-of-hospital chemical, biological or radiological events in Australasia. Emergency Medicine Australasia 2007; 19: 86–95.
27. Zarzycki W, Zonenberg A, Telejko B, et al. Iodide prophylaxis in the aftermath of the Chernobyl accident in the area of Senjy in north-eastern Poland. Hormone and Metabolic Research 1994; 26(6): 293–296.

Further reading

Armed Forces Radiobiology Research Institute. Medical management of radiological casualties. Bethesda, MD: 2003. http://www.afrri.usuhs.mil.
Daly F, Inglis T, Robertson A. Protocols for the hospital management of chemical, biological and radiological external incidents. Perth: Western Australian Department of Health; 2005.
NCRP and Disaster Mortuary Operational Response team guidelines. www.dmort.org.
Radiation Emergency Action Centre / Training Site. www.orau.gov/reacts.
US Centre for Disease Control and Prevention. www.bt.cdc.gov/radiation.

28.5 Drowning

David Mountain

ESSENTIALS

1 The incidence of drowning requiring medical assessment is estimated to be 2 to 20 times greater than fatal drowning.

2 The highest rates of drowning occur in children from 1 to 4 years of age and young adult males. Alcohol or intoxicants are associated with many adult deaths.

3 10 to 20% of drownings have minimal aspiration with asphyxia probably due to laryngospasm, shunting and mucus plug formation. Experimental differences between fresh and salt water drowning have been demonstrated but are unimportant for management.

4 Hypothermia following warm-water ($>10°C$) drowning carries a poor prognosis. Hypothermia following cold-water ($<10°C$) drowning may be associated with intact neurological outcome after prolonged resuscitation.

5 Initiation of good-quality CPR within 10 min of witnessed drowning or any attempts at breathing before hospital arrival are associated with good outcomes. Initial management on the side for airway drainage is recommended in the spontaneously breathing but lung drainage procedures and the Heimlich manoeuvre are no longer recommended.

6 Positive end-expiratory pressure/continuous positive airway pressure are useful therapies in hospital. Newer therapies, such as artificial surfactant and inhaled nitric oxide, have so far shown equivocal results. Extracorporeal membrane oxygenation is used in some centres.

Introduction

Australia, the driest inhabited continent, has the one of the highest reported incidences of drowning in the developed world.[1] It is a major cause of death in those under 30 years of age.[1,2] Good outcome is mainly determined by pre-hospital factors, but an accurate history, a well-run resuscitation and informed judgement on prognosis will optimize outcome and aid management of the patient and their family.

In many groups/regions, preventative and educative measures have reduced fatality rates in the last 20 years.[3,4] Emergency physicians should be strong advocates of these initiatives.

Epidemiology

Overall, there is a marked preponderance of male over female deaths from drowning, and in adults, the ratio has been reported as high as 9:1.[5,6] This ratio seems to have declined in recent years with fewer male deaths and drownings being reported.[4] Groups with high rates of drowning include: infants (particularly males), young adult males (15–30 years), epileptics, overseas visitors and the mentally retarded. In young adult males, bravado, inexperience and alcohol lead to many deaths. Alcohol is found in 14–50% of adult drownings and the majority of male adult drownings are related to recreational activities in some series.[5–8] In the elderly, underlying medical illnesses and suicide attempts are common. Most of these factors (except age) are associated with worse outcomes. Cold water is associated with worse outcomes overall although some younger patients may survive prolonged immersions.

The ratio of initially survived to fatal drowning is not accurately known because of differences in nomenclature, definitions and the inability to collect all attendances related to drowning, but is estimated at between 2 and 20:1.[7] In a well-conducted study from the Netherlands, the ratio of patients admitted to the intensive care unit (ICU) following drowning compared to those who died before admission was 2:1.[5]

Prevention

Prevention of drowning is a major area for ongoing research and it is important that emergency physicians act as advocates for preventative strategies of proven benefit.

Patrolled beaches and early CPR are associated with better outcome.[9,10] Important public educational initiatives include beach safety, CPR training, protective fencing, raising public awareness of the dangers of mixing alcohol and water activities and wearing of life vests and safety equipment.[6] Enforcement of alcohol laws on the water and safety regulations pertaining to providers of water activities are also important.

Definitions and terminology

Much confusion has been caused in research and management by imprecise definitions of drowning. Phrases commonly used have been near-drowning, dry, wet, active, passive or silent, late or secondary drowning, immersion, submersion, suffocation and asphyxia. Modell historically gave succinct definitions with drowning defined as death due to suffocation (asphyxia) after submersion in a liquid medium.[11] It was further divided into 'dry' or 'wet', depending on the presence or absence of aspirated fluid in the lungs. Near-drowning was defined as survival of any length after suffocation (asphyxia) due to submersion in a liquid medium.

In 2002 ILCOR (International Liaison Committee on Resuscitation) provided updated and internationally agreed Utstein style nomenclature for drowning.[12] The system simplifies the definition of drowning to '...a process resulting in primary respiratory impairment from submersion/immersion in a liquid medium.' Implicit in this definition is that a liquid/air interface is present at the entrance of the victim's airway, preventing the victim from breathing air.

The distinction between 'near-drowning' and 'drowning' is now redundant as they are both regarded as drowning events, irrespective of the outcome. Similarly, there is no longer any distinction between 'wet' and 'dry' drownings; all drowning is wet by definition and almost all have some degree of aspiration. Descriptions of 'active' and 'passive' or 'silent' drowning (determined by bystander descriptions of activity in the water) have been replaced by 'witnessed' and 'unwitnessed' drowning which are defined according to whether or not entry to water was observed. The term 'secondary drowning' has been used to describe both associated problems causing drowning (e.g. intoxication, injury, illness, etc.) or death after a drowning event due to secondary problems (e.g. lung problems, hypoxic encephalopathy, etc.). This description is inherently confusing and it is preferable to specifically describe associated precipitating factors and sequelae. Immersion describes any situation when the airway is below a fluid/air interface whilst submersion implies the whole body is covered in water.

Pathophysiology

The sequential pathophysiology of drowning is well described:[7,9,13]

- Initial submersion or immersion leads to voluntary apnoea except where drowning is due to initial loss of consciousness such as occurs in patients with genetic predisposition to prolonged QT syndrome or other catastrophic illness.[14] Unless submersion is voluntary, most adult victims panic and struggle. This is associated with increases in blood pressure and pulse rate. Slowing of the pulse secondary to the primitive dive reflex or cold-induced reflex bradyarrhythmias, particularly seen in children and accentuated by alcohol in adults, may be observed.[13,15]

- After an interval that depends on pre-submersion oxygenation, intoxication, injury or illness, fitness levels and the degree of panic and struggle, the synergistic effects of hypercapnia and hypoxia lead to an involuntary breath. This is known as the 'breaking point'. During this stage, large quantities of water are often swallowed. If an individual hyperventilates before diving, plasma CO_2 concentrations may remain so low that unconsciousness from hypoxia occurs before the breaking point is reached.

- The initial inhalation of fluid leads to a sudden increase in airway pressure, bronchoconstriction, pulmonary hypertension and shunting. In 10–20% of cases laryngospasm reduces further aspiration, and a plug of mucus and foam forms (previously known as 'dry drowning').
- Secondary apnoea occurs and is closely followed by loss of consciousness. Vomiting of swallowed fluid is common and frequently results in pulmonary aspiration.
- Involuntary gasping respirations lead to flooding of the lungs and alveolar injury, surfactant loss, increased ventilation/perfusion (V/Q) mismatch and hypoxia.
- Hypoxia leads to marked bradycardia, hypotension and irreversible brain injury within 3–10 min (except occasionally in rapid hypothermia in very cold water), and culminates in cardiopulmonary arrest.

In patients who drown, the average amount of fluid retrieved from the lungs is from 3 to 4 mL/kg, or less than 10% of total lung volume. However, the effect on the lungs is dramatic. Experimentally, fresh water and sea-water cause lung injury by different mechanisms. Fresh water denatures surfactant and damages the alveolar cells. Sea-water tends to draw in fluid, wash out surfactant and lead to foam formation. The aspiration of vomitus and chemicals in the water further complicates the clinical picture. Soap and chlorine in water do not appear to affect outcome. Clinically, the type of fluid inhaled rarely makes a difference, unless grossly polluted. Electrolyte disturbances are normally minimal and transient except in prolonged arrests, owing to the small volumes aspirated (more than 20 mL/kg are required for major disturbances).[9,13]

Clinical features and organ-specific effects

Lungs

The major features are intense bronchospasm and laryngospasm, pulmonary hypertension and marked V/Q mismatch with physiological shunt. Even in patients without respiratory embarrassment after near drowning, shunts of up to 70% may

occur and take up to 1 week to resolve. In the alveoli, there is surfactant loss, formation of protein-rich exudate and injury to alveolar cells, often exacerbated by pneumonitis from gastric aspiration and secondary infection.[13,16,17] These changes result in a marked reduction in pulmonary compliance and hypoxia.

Brain

The major effects on the brain are secondary to hypoxia and are the major cause of death in drownings. Cerebral oedema, convulsions and persistent vegetative states are all observed. The possibility of trauma or an underlying medical complaint should always be considered in the differential diagnosis of an altered mental state especially in unwitnessed events, the intoxicated and the elderly.

Cardiovascular

Most drowning patients are haemodynamically stable after resuscitation. Hypothermic patients may develop any arrhythmia and should be gently handled and aggressively rewarmed (see Ch. 28.2). In older patients underlying ischaemic heart disease should be considered. Congenital long QT syndrome may be associated with arrhythmia in some cold water immersions.[10,14,16]

Haematological

Haemolysis occurs occasionally in freshwater drownings.[7]

Renal

Acute tubular necrosis or tubular injury from hypoxia may occur. Electrolyte disturbances are rarely significant.[3,16]

Gastrointestinal

Vomiting is frequently observed (up to 80% in some series).[18,19] It is secondary to ingestion of large volumes of water and may be associated with aspiration. Diarrhoea is less frequent except with grossly polluted water.

Orthopaedic

Cervical spine injury should always be considered and excluded in drownings related to diving injuries. Coexistent trauma may complicate recreational drowning particularly if alcohol related.[6,17]

Treatment

Pre-hospital

Hypoxia to the brain is the major cause of mortality and morbidity in drownings. Rapid institution of effective pre-hospital care (particularly supplemented breathing/oxygenation) and emergency service activation are the most important factors in determining good outcome following near-drowning.[10,18–20] All patients seen alive within 1 h of removal from cold water (<5–10°C) should be transported for definitive care.[17,19,21] The level of pre-hospital care required varies with the clinical severity of the case, which may range from asymptomatic to cardiopulmonary arrest. Initial assessment of the airway, breathing and circulation may be done with the patient on their side to assist in draining fluid from the airway followed by institution of cardiopulmonary resuscitation if respirations or pulse are absent.[19] There is little role for in-water resuscitation except when performed by expert retrievers using snorkel equipment and who can get to shore easily.[17–19] Lung drainage procedures (e.g. abdominal compressions) and the Heimlich manoeuvre are dangerous because they increase the risk of aspiration. The Heimlich manoeuvre is only indicated for removal of a foreign body.[7,17–19] Victims often vomit upon resumption of spontaneous respiration, and obtunded, spontaneously breathing patients should be transported on their side to minimize the risk of aspiration.[18,19] Wet clothing should be removed and the patient wrapped to minimize further heat loss. If associated trauma is possible, the cervical spine should be immobilized.[17–19] All symptomatic patients should be given supplemental high-flow oxygen. Early access to emergency medical systems is essential to minimize time to definitive care.[18,19,22,23] A person with knowledge of the patient or witness to the drowning should be encouraged to go directly to the hospital or travel in the ambulance.[3,10]

Emergency department

History

Important factors in the history include duration of submersion (or time since last seen), time to institution of CPR, first spontaneous breath and return of spontaneous cardiac output. A collateral history regarding previous health problems (including psychiatric issues),

Initial resuscitation

Initial assessment and resuscitation, continuing the priorities established in the pre-hospital setting, is directed towards the assessment and maintenance of airway, breathing and circulation. Monitoring should include cardiac rhythm, blood pressure, pulse oximetry and core temperature (urinary or rectal probes are fine).

Airway management may simply involve clearing and positioning the airway and the provision of supplemental oxygen via a non-rebreathing mask. Endotracheal intubation is indicated if respiration is ineffective or the patient is comatose. Patients who cannot maintain a P_aO_2 greater than 90 mmHg on a non-rebreathing mask should be considered for intubation, although continuous positive airway pressure (CPAP) ventilation is an alternative in the cooperative patient. Patients with bronchospasm should be treated with nebulized β agonists. In the unconscious patient a nasogastric tube should be placed early after intubation to minimize the risk of pulmonary aspiration.[3,10] All intubated patients require positive end-expiratory pressure (PEEP) and end-tidal CO_2 monitoring.

Cardiac complications should be managed according to standard treatment regimens except in patients with core temperatures less than 33°C. These hypothermic patients must be handled gently and administration of anti-arrhythmic drugs avoided if possible until rewarming has taken place. All rhythms without output require CPR.[10,18,19] In general, asystole following drowning has the same dire prognosis as from other causes. Hypotension is managed with inotropes and fluids, together with invasive monitoring if required.[3,16] This is particularly important in patients with pulmonary oedema.[3,22]

The management of hypothermia is described elsewhere in this book. Where cervical spine injury is a possibility (especially following diving and water sports accidents), cervical spine immobilization should be maintained until the injury can be excluded radiologically.

Ongoing management

Patients who require intubation for near-drowning, especially if pulmonary changes are present on chest X-ray, should be given PEEP. Commence with low pressures (5–7.5 cmH$_2$O) and then increase until adequate oxygenation is achieved or hypotension or high airway pressures prevent further increases. Pressure-controlled ventilation may be added. These modalities improve outcome for near-drowning patients with secondary lung injury. Ventilatory weaning should begin as soon as possible in order to minimize the risk of barotrauma.[3,10,16] Maintenance of normothermia, normoglycaemia, normovolaemia, normocarbia, seizure control and avoidance of hypoxia and hypotension are important in optimizing cerebral outcome. Dehydration and prolonged hyperventilation are dangerous.

Experimental therapies

A number of other therapeutic modalities have been trialled in an effort to improve the outcome of lung and brain injuries caused by near-drowning. These include the following.

- Induced hypothermia. Popularized by Conn, this therapy offers the theoretical advantage of cerebral protection but is no longer recommended.[3,16] However, recent trials of hypothermia in cardiac arrest have renewed interest in this area but there are no specific data for drowning patients as they were excluded from these studies.[18]
- Pharmacological cerebral protection. Barbiturate infusions, steroids and chlorpromazine have all been trialled. None have been shown to be of benefit and all may have deleterious effects.[10,16,18]
- Intracranial pressure monitoring. Its use is controversial and lacking in outcome data, and depends on which ICU cares for the patient.[3,10,16]
- Prophylactic antibiotics. These are of no value except following drowning in polluted water. In such cases, a second-generation cephalosporin is recommended. Drownings in hot spas and tubs may require anti-pseudomonal cover.[7,16]
- Hyperbaric oxygen therapy and nitric oxide therapy are of unproven benefit.
- Exogenous surfactant therapy. No proven benefit and recent animal research has suggested that it may increase lung injury.
- Extracorporeal oxygenation. Has been used successfully in some centres for severe lung injury particularly in hypothermic children.[7,18,22]

Clinical investigation

Ordering of investigations in the emergency department is guided by the clinical status of the patient, in particular, mental status. Using the Modell/Conn classification of mental status (Table 28.5.1),[24,25] patients in group A only require a chest X-ray and oximetry. Patients in group B also require a full blood count, electrolytes and creatinine, blood sugar, arterial blood gases and an ECG. If they do not improve rapidly after arrival and supplemental oxygen they should be investigated and managed like group C patients. Patients in group C should also have liver function tests, creatine kinase and troponin at 6 h, coagulation profile, alcohol level, consideration for a drug screen, urine dipstick and microscopy, along with a computerized tomography (CT) scan of the head if coma persists. Cervical spine X-rays and other trauma films are indicated if trauma is suspected.

Table 28.5.1 Modell/Conn classification of mental status following drowning

Grade	Description of mental status	Equivalent GCS	Expected likelihood of good outcome (neurologically intact) (%)
A	Awake/alert	14–15	100
B	Blunted	8–13	100
C	Comatose	6–7	>90
C1	Decerebrate	5	>90
C2	Decorticate	4	>90
C3/4	Flaccid coma or arrest	3	<20

Prognosis

Mortality rates of 15–30% and persistent severe neurological deficit rates of up to 25% are reported in series of patients admitted to hospital following drowning events. Potential prognostic features in drowning have been extensively evaluated in an effort to reduce the number of neuro-vegetative survivors, avoid prolonged CPR, and provide relatives and medical personnel with early accurate prognostic information.

The most useful predictors relate to the initial resuscitation (field predictors). Factors associated with good outcome include witnessed drowning and time to retrieval of less than 5 min, good-quality CPR provided within 10 min, first spontaneous breath within 30 min of retrieval from the water, and return of spontaneous circulation before arrival at hospital.[10] The last two are associated with very good neurological outcome, provided secondary lung injury does not supervene. Pre-hospital factors associated with poor outcome include male sex, unwitnessed or prolonged submersion, asystole, fresh water, cold water submersion and prolonged resuscitation before arrival at hospital.[3,7,10] However, absolute field predictors of poor outcome have not been identified and all patients who arrive in the emergency department following drowning deserve assessment for full resuscitation efforts.[18,19]

Emergency department prognostic factors have also been identified, but again no combination of factors reliably predicts all patients who will do badly. Emergency department prognostic factors associated with good outcome are pupillary response on arrival, perfusing cardiac rhythm on arrival,[20] or any motor response to pain on arrival.[22,23] Asystole is predictive of very poor outcome and except in paediatric/young adults cold water drowning should lead to early cessation of CPR in the emergency department.[3,5,11] Hypothermia has been described as a favourable prognostic indicator but is debatable. Although this may be true following near drowning of children in cold water, hypothermia is generally a marker of prolonged submersion and, as such, is associated with a poor prognosis in near drowning in warm water and in adults.[5,26]

In-hospital factors associated with poor outcome include Glasgow Coma Score less than 5 on transfer to intensive care (less than 20% intact survival), fixed dilated pupils at 6 h, and any abnormality on CT scan in the first 36 h. However, a normal CT scan is of no prognostic value.

Disposition

All drowning victims should be carefully observed for a minimum of 6 h.[7,10] Monitoring during that time should include pulse oximetry. Any patient with an abnormal chest X-ray or respiratory examination or significant hypoxaemia after 6 h should be admitted. Those requiring intubation, with a history of cardio-respiratory arrest, persistently altered mental status or significant hypoxaemia should be admitted to intensive care. Truly asymptomatic patients may be discharged home after 6 h of observation, but should be instructed to return to hospital if they develop respiratory symptoms.[3,10]

Controversies

❶ The development of accurate prognostic indicators that decrease the burden of patients surviving in persistent vegetative states is very important. Most authorities agree that all but the obviously dead should be aggressively resuscitated. However, of those patients admitted to ICU, up to 15% survive in a persistent vegetative state.[22]

❷ The role of new treatment modalities for secondary lung injury, including nitrous oxide, artificial surfactant and extracorporeal oxygenation, individually or sequentially, is yet to be defined.

References

1. Peden M, McGee K, Sharma G. The injury chart book: a graphical overview of the global burden of injuries. Geneva: World Health Organization [E1]; 2002.
2. Pearn J, Nixon J, Wilkey I. Freshwater drowning and near-drowning accidents involving children: a five year total population study. Medical Journal of Australia 1976; 2: 942–946.
3. Pearn J. The management of near drowning. British Medical Journal 1985; 291: 1447–1452.
4. Report of the New South Wales Chief Health Officer 2006: Injury and poisoning; Drowning deaths and hospitalizations. http://www.health.nsw.gov.au/public-health/chorep/inj/inj_drowndthhos.htm (accessed September 2007).
5. Bierens JJLM, van der Velde EA, van Berkel M, et al. Submersion cases in the Netherlands. Annals of Emergency Medicine 1989; 18(4): 366–373.
6. Plueckhahn VD. Alcohol and accidental drowning. A 25 year study. Medical Journal of Australia 1984; 141: 22–25.
7. Braun R. Near drowning. Emergency Medicine Clinics of North America 1997; 15(2): 461–464.
8. Driscoll TR, Harrison JA, Steenkamp M. Review of the role of alcohol in drowning associated with recreational aquatic activity. Injury Prevention 2004; 10: 107–113.
9. Martin TG. Near drowning and cold water immersion. Annals of Emergency Medicine 1984; 13: 263–273.
10. Olshaker JS. Near drowning. Emergency Medicine Clinics of North America 1992; 10(2): 339–350.
11. Modell JH. Drown versus near-drown: a discussion of definitions. Critical Care Medicine 1981; 9(4): 351–352.
12. Idris, AH, Berg, RA, Bierens, JJ, et al. Recommended guidelines for uniform reporting of data from drowning. Circulation 2003; 108: 2565–2574.
13. Pearn J. Pathophysiology of drowning. Medical Journal of Australia 1985; 142: 586–588.
14. Ackerman MJ, Tester DJ, Porter CJ. Swimming, a gene-specific arrhythmogenic trigger for inherited long QT syndrome. Mayo Clinical Proceedings 1999; 74(11): 1088–1094.
15. Gooden BA. Why some people do not drown. Hypothermia versus the diving response. Medical Journal of Australia 1992; 157: 629–632.
16. Oh TE. Near-drowning. Intensive care manual, 4th edn. Oxford: Butterworth-Heinemann; 1997: 617–621.
17. Ornato JP. The resuscitation of near-drowning victims. Journal of the American Medical Association 1986; 256(1): 75–77.
18. American Heart Association Guidelines for Cardiopulmonary Resuscitation and Emergency Cardiovascular Care Part 10.3: Drowning. Circulation. 2005; 112: IV-133, IV-135.
19. Australian Resuscitation Council, Guideline 8.7 resuscitation of the drowning victim. http://www.resus.org.au/public/guidelines/section_8/resuscitation_of_drowning_victim.htm (accessed September 2007).
20. Quan L, Kinder D. Paediatric submersions: Prehospital Predictors of Outcome. Pediatrics 1992; 90(6): 909–913.
21. Wyatt JP, Tomlinson GS, Busuttil A. Resuscitation of drowning victims in south-east Scotland. Resuscitation 1999; 41(2): 101–104.
22. Maguire JE. Advances in cardiac life support: sorting the science from the dogma. Emergency Medicine 1997; 9(4 Supplement): 1–21.
23. Quan L. Drowning issues in resuscitation. Annals of Emergency Medicine 1993; 22(2): 366–399.
24. Conn AW, Montes JE, Barker GA, et al. Cerebral salvage in near-drowning following neurological classification by triage. Canadian Anaesthetic Society Journal 1980; 27(3): 211–221.
25. Modell JH, Graves SA, Kuck EJ. Near-drowning: correlation of level of consciousness and survival. Canadian Anaesthetic Society Journal 1980; 27(3): 211–215.
26. Kemp AM. Outcome in children who nearly drown: a British Isles study. British Medical Journal 1991; 302: 931–933.

28.6 Electric shock and lightning injury

Daniel Fatovich

ESSENTIALS

1 Death from electric shock is due to ventricular fibrillation, the lethal arrhythmia occurring at the time of the exposure. Routine admission for ECG monitoring is unnecessary.

2 Most deaths are caused by low-voltage (<1000 V) exposures.

3 The amount of current passing through the body is determined mainly by tissue resistance, which is dramatically reduced by moisture.

4 Electrical injury resembles a crush injury more than a burn. The tissue damage below skin level is invariably more severe than the cutaneous wound would suggest.

5 There is a diversity of clinical manifestations seen with electrical injury.

6 Lightning injury is different from high-voltage electrical injury and has a unique range of clinical features. The management is predominantly expectant.

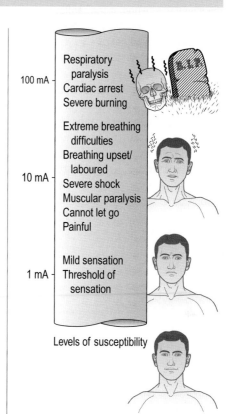

100 mA	Respiratory paralysis, Cardiac arrest, Severe burning
10 mA	Extreme breathing difficulties, Breathing upset/laboured, Severe shock, Muscular paralysis, Cannot let go, Painful
1 mA	Mild sensation, Threshold of sensation

Levels of susceptibility

Fig. 28.6.1 The levels of electric shock and their effects.

ELECTRIC SHOCK

Introduction and epidemiology

Electricity is an integral part of our everyday world and electric shock is common. Patients may present to the emergency department (ED) with resulting injuries that range from trivial to fatal (termed electrocution). Although permanent disability can occur, it is reassuring to note that if the initial exposure is survived, subsequent death is unlikely. For each death caused by electricity there are two serious injuries and 36 reported electric shocks.[1]

There are approximately 20–30 electrical fatalities each year in Australia. Victims are predominantly male and relatively young. Death is just as likely to occur at home as in the workplace, most often in summer. Electricians and linesmen are most at risk. The ratio of low-to-high-voltage deaths ranges from 3:1 to 7:1. The presence of water is associated with fatality.[1,2] Electrical burns represent 3–5% of admissions to burns units.[3]

Physics of electricity and pathophysiology of electrical Injury

Electrical current passing through the body can cause damage in two ways:

❶ thermal injury
❷ physiological change.[4]

The threshold for perception of an electrical current is 1 mA, which results in a tingling sensation. Current greater than 10 mA can induce muscular tetany and prevent the patient letting go of the current source. Above about 50 mA, extreme breathing difficulty and pain are experienced. The threshold for ventricular fibrillation is 100 mA (Fig. 28.6.1).[5,6] The maximum 'safe' current tolerable for 1 s is 50 mA.[5]

Ohm's law is fundamental to the understanding of the physics of electricity. This states that:

The amount of current passing through the body is directly proportional to voltage and inversely proportional to resistance (current (amperes) = voltage (volts)/resistance (ohms)].[4]

Factors that determine the effects of an electrical current passing through the body are:

- type of current
- voltage
- tissue resistance
- current path
- contact duration.

Type of current

The vast majority of serious electrical injuries result from alternating current (AC), which is approximately three times as dangerous as direct current (DC).[5] Alternating current can produce tetanic contraction of muscle such that the victim may not be able to let go of the current source. This is not a feature of direct current shock.[4]

Human muscular tissue is sensitive to frequencies between 40 and 150 Hz. As the frequency increases beyond 150 Hz, the response decreases and the current is less dangerous. In Australia, a frequency of 50 Hz is used for household current because this is optimal for the transmission and use of electricity, and also has advantages in terms of generation.[1] As such, household current lies directly within the dangerous frequency range. It also spans the vulnerable period of the cardiac electrical potential, and is thus capable of causing ventricular fibrillation.

Voltage

Voltage is the electromotive force in the system. In general terms, the greater the voltage the more extensive the injury, but it must be remembered that the amount of current passing through the body will also be determined by resistance (Ohm's law). High voltage is defined as greater than 1000 V. Household voltage in Australia is 240 V. Voltages less than 50 V (50 Hz) have not been proved hazardous.[5] Survival has been reported following shocks of greater than 50 000 V.[4]

Resistance

Different tissues provide differing resistances to the passage of electrical current. Bone has the highest resistance, followed by, in decreasing order, fat, tendon, skin, muscle, blood vessels and nerves. Importantly, however, skin resistance varies greatly according to moisture, cleanliness, thickness and vascularity.[4] Moist skin may have a resistance of 1000 Ω and dry, thick, calloused skin a resistance of 100 000 Ω. By Ohm's law, dry skin resistance to a contact with a 240 V potential results in a current of about 2.4 mA, which is just above the threshold for perception. However, the resistance of wet or sweat-soaked skin drops to 1000 Ω, increasing the current flow to 240 mA, which is easily enough to induce ventricular fibrillation. Not surprisingly, moisture has been identified as a key factor in over half of electrocutions.[1]

Current path

Prediction of injuries from a knowledge of the current path is unreliable. Mortalities of 60% for hand-to-hand (transthoracic) and 20% for head-to-foot passage of current are quoted,[4] but have not been verified. When current passes hand-to-hand (or hand-to-foot), only about 5% of the total current passes through the heart.[7] If current passes leg-to-leg, no current traverses the heart.[7]

Contact duration

The longer the duration of contact, the greater the potential for injury. Fortunately, most contacts are brief and frequently result in the victim being thrown back from the current source. This may result in a secondary injury, especially if the victim falls from a height.

Unfortunately, exposures to more than 10 mA of alternating current can induce sweating. Moisture decreases skin resistance and increases current flow, thereby reducing the ability to release the current source. This can progress to a fatal exposure.[5]

Prevention

All members of the community must be encouraged to treat electricity with respect and to practice electrical safety. Licensed electrical contractors should be used to carry out any electrical repairs or installations. Water and electricity should never be mixed.[20]

Residual current devices are useful in providing an additional level of personal protection from electric shock. These devices continuously compare current flow in both active and neutral conductors of an electrical circuit. If current flow becomes sufficiently unbalanced, then some of the current in the active conductor is not returned through the neutral conductor, and leaks to earth. These devices operate within 10–50 ms and disconnect the electricity supply when they sense harmful leakage, typically 30 mA.[5]

Clinical features

Electrical injury resembles a crush injury more than a burn. Invariably, the damage below skin level is more severe than the cutaneous wound suggests. The current passing through low-resistance structures produces massive necrosis of muscles, vessels, nerves and subcutaneous tissues.[4]

The clinical manifestations differ from thermal burns in the following ways:

- There are direct effects on the heart and nervous system.
- Electrical injury classically involves deep structures.

- The small entry and exit wounds do not accurately indicate the extent or depth of tissue damage.
- A diversity of clinical manifestations is seen with electrical injury.

Burns

As electricity traverses the skin, energy is converted to heat. The smaller the area of contact, the greater the current density, heat production, and the consequent skin and adjacent tissue destruction.

Electrothermal burns are best characterized by arc burns, which result from the external passage of current from the contact point to the ground. These may be associated with extensive damage to skin and underlying tissue. Secondary flame burns may occur when the current arc ignites clothing or nearby combustibles.[4]

Electrical burns may range from first degree to third degree. The typical appearance is of a central depressed charred black area surrounded by oedema and erythema. Single or multiple exit wounds may be present.

Cardiac

Ventricular fibrillation is the usual cause of immediate death from electric shock, and occurs at the time of the shock.[1] Delayed arrhythmia resulting in death is exceptionally rare.[8] Sinus tachycardia is common, and non-specific ST- and T-wave changes may be observed. Atrial fibrillation occurs infrequently and usually resolves spontaneously. Acute myocardial infarction following electric shock has been reported.[9]

Nervous system

Both acute and delayed neurological sequelae have been described following electric shock. Acute complications include respiratory arrest, seizures, altered mental state, amnesia, coma, expressive dysphasia and motor deficits.[4] Reported delayed complications include spinal cord injury (myelopathy) with local amyotrophy and long tract signs, and reflex sympathetic dystrophy.[4]

Peripheral nerve injury is usually associated with significant soft-tissue injury. It has also been reported in the absence of soft-tissue injury, and such cases appear to have a good prognosis.[10]

Renal

Acute renal failure may occur secondary to myoglobinuria. Electric shock results in disruption of muscle cells with the release of myoglobin and creatine phosphokinase, similar to a crush injury. Transient oliguria, albuminuria, haemoglobinuria and renal casts are common, and there have been reports of high-output renal failure.[4,11]

Vascular

Large and small vessel arterial and venous thrombosis is responsible for the tissue damage in electrical injury. Vascular complications have included immediate and delayed major vessel haemorrhage, arterial thrombosis and deep vein thrombosis.[4,11,12]

Musculoskeletal

Tetanic muscle contractures can result in compression fractures of vertebral bodies, fractures of long bones and dislocations of joints. Injuries may also result from a secondary fall, rather than from the electric shock.[4,11]

Other

Numerous complications involving other systems, including the eye (especially cataracts) have been reported following electric shock.[4,11]

Electric shock in pregnancy

Reports of electric shock in pregnancy are rare and the true incidence is unknown. A high mortality has been reported in the literature.[13] However, this may represent publication bias and a prospective cohort study concluded that in most cases, accidental electric shocks during pregnancy do not pose a major fetal risk.[14]

If there was an immediate problem, the mother may notice a sudden cessation of fetal movements. However, there is no preventative action possible in the ED. Other reported fetal complications of electric shock include intrauterine growth retardation, oligohydramnios and abortion.[13]

Fortunately, therapeutic electric shocks such as DC cardioversion and electroconvulsive therapy are known to be safe in pregnancy. The critical factor is current path: accidental electric shocks include the uterus, whereas therapeutic shocks do not.[15–17]

Treatment

Pre-hospital

Everyone should be aware of the pre-hospital management of electric shock.[4] Most importantly, the rescuer should avoid becoming a further victim. The victim can be separated from the electrical source by using rubber, a wooden handle, a mat or any other non-conductive substance or, if possible, by turning off the electricity supply. Cardiopulmonary resuscitation (CPR) should begin immediately, if indicated, and help summoned. Ventricular fibrillation is the most common lethal arrhythmia after electric shock, and early defibrillation provides the greatest chance for survival.[1]

Emergency department

The majority of patients who present to the ED after electric shock are relatively well. Following appropriate assessment to exclude primary or secondary injury, an ECG should be performed. Cardiac monitoring is not indicated if the patient is asymptomatic and has a normal ECG.[6,18] Most patients are able to be reassured and discharged directly from the ED. Measurement of creatine phosphokinase levels is not required. It should be remembered that exposure to an electric shock is a very unpleasant experience and this should be acknowledged. Tetanus status should be checked.

Many patients have a degree of muscle pain following electric shock owing to the tetanic nature of alternating current. Simple analgesia is appropriate. Any secondary injury, such as fractures or loss of consciousness, should be treated as dictated by the injury.

If an arrhythmia is present it will usually resolve spontaneously and not require specific treatment. Delayed lethal arrhythmias have not been reported in patients without initial arrhythmias.[8]

Severe electrical injury with extensive soft-tissue damage should be managed as a crush injury. This is more likely following high-voltage exposure, which results in a large exudation and sequestration of fluids in the damaged area. Emergency management includes adequate volume replacement, and treatment of acidosis and myoglobinuria.[4,11]

Emergency physicians should be aware of the low potential for fetal harm following electric shock in pregnancy. Publication bias suggests that apparently minor exposures can have profound effects.[13] It would be prudent to adopt a conservative approach of performing a fetal heart doppler assessment with obstetric follow-up including ultrasound.[18,19]

Prognosis

The prognosis for the majority of patients surviving the initial shock is excellent. Those with significant soft-tissue injury or secondary injury may be left with long-term deficits.

Disposition

The majority of patients presenting to the ED following an electric shock will be suitable for discharge home following assessment and reassurance as detailed above. Those suffering muscle pain secondary to tetanic contractions should be given simple analgesia and instructed to follow-up with their general practitioner.

Patients with cardiac arrhythmias require admission for observation until the arrhythmia resolves. Those with evidence of neuropathy should be referred to a neurologist, as nerve conduction studies may be required.[10]

Severe electrical injuries with extensive soft-tissue damage require admission to hospital, and sometimes to an intensive care unit. All patients with electrical burns should be reviewed by a burns specialist, and referral to a specialist burns unit may be indicated. Minor burns may be suitable for elective review.

Secondary injuries such as loss of consciousness or fractures should be admitted or referred on their merits.

The Taser

The Taser is a development of the stun gun. It is used by the police service to fill the operational gap between the baton and the gun for controlling potentially dangerous and violent suspects. 'Tasered' victims are occasionally brought to the ED for assessment.[21]

The device is a battery operated unit resembling a hand gun that fires two barbed electrodes on 7 m long copper wires at 60 m/s.[21] The barbs attach to the subject's skin or clothing and deliver up to 50 000 V of electricity in rapid pulses over 5 s. The current can cross up to 5 cm of clothing.[21]

Electricity delivered by a taser is neither pure AC nor pure DC, and is probably akin to rapid-fire low-amplitude DC shocks.[21] The output is believed to stay near the surface of the body in the skin and muscles and does not penetrate into the internal organs.[22] There is no evidence to date that this form of electrical delivery interfered with cardiac or neurological function in the 30 000 volunteers or in the reported operational uses.[21]

One author concluded that the pre-existing injuries and toxic conditions leading to the patient being tasered are the most important problems requiring medical treatment after taser use. It seems that the device is essentially safe on healthy people.[21] Suggestions for management of these patients attending EDs are:[21]

- Most healthy subjects may be safely discharged after barb removal and routine history and examination.
- Important points in the history include known cardiac disease including implanted pacemaker or defibrillator, pregnancy, drug or alcohol intoxication, bizarre behaviour at the time of arrest, other psychiatric disturbance, or coincidental medical problems.
- Look closely for direct injury from the barbs or indirect injury from falls.
- An ECG is appropriate in the assessment of those with chest pain, palpitations, or cardiac history.
- Most patients will complain of muscle aches and anxiety.
- There are likely to be small puncture wounds and minor burns at the barb sites. On occasion, medical intervention will be required if the barbs are not easily removed, if the barb tip breaks off in the skin, or if the barbs have

struck vulnerable areas (e.g. mouth, eyes, neck, and groin).

It is clear that, properly used as a method of restraining violent people, tasers are less likely than guns to cause injury and death of the target (and of the police officer).[22] They are also generally more effective than other methods of restraint. The deaths that have followed taser use have occurred in people who were out of control and who had taken potentially fatal drugs. It is likely that the deaths would have occurred whether or not the taser was used.[22]

LIGHTNING INJURY

Introduction and epidemiology

There are two or three deaths each year in Australia from lightning. For each death, there are five injuries. These events are always prominent and emergency physicians should be familiar with the pathophysiology. In addition, about 60 people each year report injuries caused by lightning surges while using the telephone during thunderstorms.[23,24]

Many myths surround lightning injury;[25] they include:

- Lightning strike is invariably fatal. In fact, the mortality is 30%. In addition, the probability of long-term impairment after recovery is low.
- A victim of lightning is charged and dangerous to touch. This false notion has led to the withholding of CPR, with fatal results.
- Lightning should be treated in the same way as high-voltage electrical injury. This is incorrect.[25]

Physics

Lightning occurs most commonly during thunderstorms. Particles moving up and down in a thunderstorm create static electricity, with a large negative charge building up at the bottom of clouds. Electrical discharge (lightning) occurs as a result of the great charge difference between the negatively charged thundercloud underside and the positively charged ground.[4] The duration of the lightning stroke is between 1 and 100 ms.

Lightning strike is very different from high-voltage electric shock (Table 28.6.1)[25] and produces different clinical effects, requiring a different management approach.

An interesting phenomenon called 'flashover' seems to save many victims from death by lightning. Current passes around and over, but not through the body. The victim's clothing and shoes may be blasted apart. Only cutaneous flame-type burns result.[4]

Clinical features

Immediate

- Cardiac arrest. This takes the form of asystole, as opposed to the ventricular fibrillation of high-voltage electrical injury.[25] The heart is thought to undergo massive depolarization. Although primary lightning-induced arrest may revert quickly, it can be followed by secondary hypoxic arrest.
- Chest pain and muscle aches.
- Neurological deficits. A person struck by lightning may be rendered unconscious. On first regaining consciousness, they may be mute and unable to move. This is transient and usually resolves within minutes, but may take up to 24 h.
- Contusions from shock waves.
- Tympanic membrane rupture.

Table 28.6.1 Lightning versus high-voltage injury		
Factor	Lightning	High voltage
Time of exposure	Brief instantaneous	Prolonged tetanic
Energy level	100 million V 200 000 A	Usually much lower
Type of current	Direct	Alternating
Shock wave	Yes	No
Flashover	Yes	No

(Adapted from: Cooper MA 1983 Lightning injuries. In: Auerbach P, et al (eds) Management of wilderness and environmental emergencies. New York: Macmillan; 500–21)

Delayed

- Keraunoparalysis.[25] Lightning-induced limb paralysis is extremely common. Flaccidity and complete loss of sensation of the affected limb are observed. Peripheral pulses are generally impalpable and the affected limb takes on a mottled, pale, blue appearance. The mechanism is unclear, but may be lightning-induced vasospasm. The condition is self-limiting and resolves within 1–6 h.
- 'Feathery' cutaneous burns (Lichtenberg flowers). These burns, pathognomonic of lightning injury, may appear immediately but more often become visible a few hours after injury. Burns may be severe but heal remarkably easily.
- Cataracts. Occur more commonly than following electrical injuries.
- Myoglobinuria and haemoglobinuria are rare.

Other

- Sensorineural deafness
- Vestibular dysfunction
- Retinal detachment
- Optic nerve damage.

Reports of lightning strike in pregnancy reveal a high rate of fetal death in utero, despite maternal survival.[13]

Treatment

Pre-hospital

The important principle is that those who appear dead should be resuscitated first. Immediate institution of basic cardiopulmonary resuscitation in the field for those in asystole prevents secondary hypoxic cardiac arrest during the interval until cardiac function resumes spontaneously. Fixed dilated pupils should not be taken as an indicator of death after lightning strike.

Emergency department

Most lightning strikes are unwitnessed, and diagnosis may be difficult in the unconscious or confused patient. The diagnosis should be considered where such patients were found outdoors in stormy weather. The presence of multiple victims, exploded clothing, linear or punctuate burns, keraunic markings or tympanic membrane rupture all add weight to the diagnosis. The differential diagnosis includes cerebrovascular event, seizure disorder, spinal cord injury, closed-head injury, Stokes–Adams attack, myocardial infarction and toxin effects.[25]

Standard trauma resuscitation measures should be adopted. Examination of the ears for tympanic rupture and eyes for lens/corneal defects, retinal detachment and optic nerve injury is especially important. If the conscious state deteriorates after arrival, cranial computerized tomography scan is indicated. Examination of the cardiovascular system should include an ECG.

Burns are rarely more than superficial and are managed expectantly using standard treatments. Tetanus prophylaxis should be arranged.[25]

Treatment of lightning-induced limb paralysis is expectant. If it does not resolve within a few hours, other causes should be considered.[25] Fasciotomy is unnecessary.

Standard therapy for ocular complications such as retinal detachment or cataracts is indicated. Baseline visual acuity should be documented for future reference.

Prognosis and disposition

For survivors of the initial strike the prognosis is excellent, unless significant secondary trauma has occurred. Admission for observation is indicated for those with abnormal mental status or ECG, or with significant burns or traumatic complications. The burns usually heal well and grafting is rarely required.[25] For those with ocular complications, long-term ophthalmic follow-up is necessary.[25]

Controversies

❶ Timing and extent of development of tissue necrosis associated with electrical injury.

References

1. Fatovich DM. Electrocution in Western Australia, 1976–1990. Medical Journal of Australia 1992; 157 (11–12): 762–764.
2. Fatovich D. Electrocution in Western Australia, 1991 to 2004. Journal of Occupational Health and Safety in Australia, New Zealand 2006; 22: 19–20.
3. Walpole BG. Electric shock. Australian Family Physician 1989; 18(10): 1252–1256.
4. Kobernick M. Electrical injuries: pathophysiology and emergency management. Annals of Emergency Medicine 1982; 11(11): 633–638.
5. Standards Association of Australia (SEM 36–91). Residual Current Devices. North Sydney, 1991.
6. Fatovich DM, Lee KY. Household electric shocks: who should be monitored? Medical Journal of Australia 1991; 155(5): 301–303.
7. Bruner JMR, Leonard PF. Electricity, safety and the patient. Chicago: Yearbook Medical Publishers; 1989.
8. Fatovich D. Delayed lethal arrhythmia after an electrical injury. Emergency Medicine Journal 2007; 24(10): 743.
9. Kinney TJ. Myocardial infarction following electrical injury. Annals of Emergency Medicine 1982; 11(11): 622–625.
10. Fatovich D. Neuropathy from household electric shock. Emergency Medicine 1992; 4: 63–65.
11. Dixon GF. The evaluation and management of electrical injuries. Critical Care Medicine 1983; 11(5): 384–387.
12. D'Attellis N, Luong V, Grinda JM. A shocking injury. Lancet 2004; 363(9427): 2136.
13. Fatovich DM Electric shock in pregnancy. Journal of Emergency Medicine 1993; 11(2): 175–177.
14. Einarson A, Bailey B, Inocencion G, et al. Accidental electric shock in pregnancy: a prospective cohort study. American Journal of Obstetrics and Gynecology 1997; 176(3): 678–681.
15. Abrams R. Electroconvulsive therapy. Oxford: Oxford University Press; 1988.
16. Finlay AY, Edmunds VDC. Cardioversion in pregnancy. British Journal of Clinical Practice 1979; 33(3): 88–94.
17. Schroeder JS, Harrison DC. Repeated cardioversion during pregnancy. Treatment of refractory paroxysmal atrial tachycardia during 3 successive pregnancies. American Journal of Cardiology 1971; 27(4): 445–446.
18. Fish RM. Electric injury, part III: cardiac monitoring indications, the pregnant patient, and lightning. Journal of Emergency Medicine 2000; 18(2): 181–187.
19. Jaffe R, Fejgin M. 1997 Accidental electric shock in pregnancy: a prospective cohort study. American Journal of Obstetrics and Gynecology 1997; 177(4): 983–984.
20. Fatovich D. Household electric shocks. Medical Journal of Australia 1991; 155: 852–853.
21. Bleetman A, Steyn R, Lee C. Introduction of the Taser into British policing. Implications for UK emergency departments: an overview of electronic weaponry. Emergency Medicine Journal 2004; 21(2): 136–140.
22. Fish RM, Geddes LA. Effects of stun guns and tasers. Lancet 2001; 358(9283): 687–688.
23. Andrews CJ. Telephone-related lightning injury. Medical Journal of Australia 1992; 157(11-12): 823–826.
24. Andrews CJ, Darveniza M. Telephone-mediated lightning injury: an Australian survey. Journal of Trauma 1989; 29(5): 665–671.
25. Andrews CJ, Darveniza M, Mackerras D. Lightning Injury – a review of clinical aspects, pathophysiology and treatment. Advances in Trauma 1989; 4: 241–288.

28.7 Anaphylaxis

Anthony F. T. Brown

ESSENTIALS

1 Anaphylaxis describes both IgE, immune-mediated reactions and non-allergic, non-immunologically triggered events. Comorbidities such as asthma or infection, exercise, alcohol or stress and concurrent medications such as β blockers, angiotensin converting enzyme inhibitors and aspirin increase the risk ('summation anaphylaxis').

2 Parenteral penicillin, hymenopteran stings and foods are the most common causes of IgE, immune-mediated fatalities. Radiocontrast media, aspirin and other non-steroidal anti-inflammatory drugs are the most common causes of non-allergic fatalities.

3 Deaths occur by hypoxia from upper airway asphyxia or severe bronchospasm, or by profound shock from vasodilatation and extravascular fluid shift.

4 Oxygen, adrenaline (epinephrine) and fluids are first-line treatment.

5 The role of H_1 and H_2 antihistamines, steroids, glucagon and salbutamol is unclear. They should only be considered once cardiovascular stability has been achieved with first-line agents.

6 Discharge may follow a period of observation from 4 to 6 h after full recovery. A clear discharge plan, and referral to an allergist for all significant, recurrent, unavoidable or unknown stimulus reactions are essential. Patient education is important to successful, long-term care.

Introduction

Anaphylaxis represents the most catastrophic of the immediate-type generalized hypersensitivity reactions and remains the quintessential medical emergency. It usually occurs unheralded in otherwise healthy people following exposure to a trigger. It presents as a dynamic continuum from mild to severe, gradual in onset to fulminant, and may involve multiple organ systems or cause isolated shock or wheeze. Prompt clinical recognition and treatment with oxygen, adrenaline and fluids to restore cardiorespiratory stability is essential to ensuring a favourable outcome. Careful discharge planning, including allergy referral where appropriate, protects against further attacks of anaphylaxis.

Definition

The term 'anaphylaxis' was introduced by Richet and Portier in 1902, literally meaning *against protection*. It is currently used to describe the rapid, generalized and often unheralded immunologically mediated events that follow exposure to certain foreign substances in previously sensitized persons, known as antigen-induced, or immune-mediated, allergic anaphylaxis.

An identical clinical syndrome known as non-allergic anaphylaxis follows non-immunological mechanisms, with the release of identical inflammatory mediators. Non-allergic anaphylaxis may occur on first exposure to an agent, and does not require a period of sensitization. The term 'non-allergic anaphylaxis' is preferred to the older one of an 'anaphylactoid reaction'.[1] This chapter will use the clinical term 'anaphylaxis' to describe *both* of these syndromes, despite their important aetiological differences.

Surprisingly, there is still no international agreement on the classification, diagnosis or severity grading of anaphylaxis.[2] Following international meetings convened in the USA in 2004 and 2005, the National Institute of Allergy and Infectious Disease (NIAID) and the Food Allergy and Anaphylaxis Network (FAAN) recommended the brief, broad definition: 'Anaphylaxis is a serious allergic reaction that is rapid in onset and may cause death'. The full definition suggested was considerably longer but more complete, aiming to capture over 95% of clinical cases within three diagnostic criteria (see Table 28.7.1).[3] Criterion 1 was to identify at least 80% of anaphylaxis cases, even if the allergic status of the patient and potential cause of the

---

Table 28.7.1 Definition of anaphylaxis: clinical criteria for diagnosis

Anaphylaxis is highly likely when any *one* of the following three criteria are fulfilled:

1. Acute onset of an illness (minutes to several hours) with involvement of the skin, mucosal tissue, or both (e.g. generalized hives, pruritus or flushing, swollen lips-tongue-uvula).
and at least one of the following:
   - Respiratory compromise (e.g. dyspnoea, wheeze–bronchospasm, stridor, reduced PEF, hypoxaemia)
   - Reduced BP or associated symptoms of end-organ dysfunction (e.g. hypotonia (collapse), syncope, incontinence)

2. Two or more of the following that occur rapidly after exposure to a *likely allergen for that patient* (minutes to several hours):
   - Involvement of the skin-mucosal tissue (e.g. generalized hives, itch–flush, swollen lips-tongue-uvula)
   - Respiratory compromise (e.g., dyspnoea, wheeze-bronchospasm, stridor, reduced PEF, hypoxaemia)
   - Reduced BP or associated symptoms (e.g. hypotonia (collapse), syncope, incontinence)
   - Persistent gastrointestinal symptoms (e.g. crampy abdominal pain, vomiting)

3. Reduced BP after exposure to *known allergen for that patient* (minutes to several hours):
   - Infants and children: low systolic BP (age-specific) or greater than 30% decrease in systolic BP*
   - Adults: systolic BP of less than 90 mmHg or greater than 30% decrease from that person's baseline

PEF, peak expiratory flow; BP, blood pressure.
*Low systolic blood pressure for children is defined as less than 70 mmHg from 1 month to 1 year; less than (70 mmHg + [2 × age]) from 1 to 10 years; and less than 90 mmHg from 11 to 17 years.
Reproduced with permission from Journal of Allergy and Clinical Immunology.[3]

Table 28.7.2   A severity grading system for generalized hypersensitivity reactions

Grade	Defined by
1: Mild[a] (skin and subcutaneous tissues only)	Generalized erythema, urticaria, periorbital oedema, or angio-oedema
2: Moderate[b] (features suggesting respiratory, cardiovascular, or gastrointestinal involvement)	Dyspnoea, stridor, wheeze, nausea, vomiting, dizziness (presyncope), diaphoresis, chest or throat tightness, or abdominal pain
3: Severe[b] (hypoxia, hypotension, or neurological compromise)	Cyanosis or $SpO_2 \leq 92\%$ at any stage, hypotension (SBP <90 mmHg in adults), confusion, collapse, LOC, or incontinence

SBP, systolic blood pressure; LOC, loss of consciousness; SpO_2, oxygen saturation on pulse oximetry.
[a]Mild reactions can be further sub-classified into those with and those without angio-oedema.
[b]Only Grades 2 and 3 constitute true anaphylaxis.
Reproduced with permission from Journal of Allergy and Clinical Immunology.[5]

reaction may be unknown, as the majority of anaphylactic reactions include skin symptoms. Criterion 2 was to identify anaphylaxis in the absence of cutaneous features such as in children with food allergy, or insect sting allergy, but requires a known allergic history and possible exposure. Gastrointestinal symptoms are included. Criterion 3 was to capture the rare patient with an acute hypotensive episode after exposure to a known allergen.[3] This inclusive definition for anaphylaxis should be used by researchers unless and until refined by future prospective data.[4]

Severity grading

No validated grading system exists that prospectively links the clinical features of anaphylaxis with severity, urgency, treatment or outcome. One system based on retrospective multivariate analysis of over 1000 clinically diagnosed generalized hypersensitivity reactions defined three grades (see Table 28.7.2).[5] Generalized allergic reactions confined to the skin and subcutaneous tissues were considered as mild grade, but the moderate and severe grades with multisystem involvement that correlated with the need for adrenaline represented true anaphylaxis according to the NIAID/FAAN criteria. Again this grading system should be used as a starting point by researchers for descriptive purposes, until prospective data in the future refine the criteria.

Aetiology

Important clinical categories of anaphylaxis include anaphylaxis related to medications, biologics and vaccines, as well as to insect stings, food, anaesthesia, latex exposure,

exercise and idiopathic anaphylaxis (see Table 28.7.3).[6]

Drug-induced anaphylaxis

Penicillin is the most common cause of drug-induced anaphylaxis. Around 1:500 patient courses have an apparent allergic reaction, mostly urticaria alone.[7] True allergic cross-reactivity to cephalosporins occurs in under 4%, and is largely with the first-generation cephalosporins.

Aspirin and non-steroidal anti-inflammatory drugs (NSAIDs) are the next most common cause of drug-induced anaphylaxis. Reactions appear to be medication-specific, as there is no clinical cross-reactivity with structurally unrelated NSAIDs.

Valid tests for IgE-mediated reactions are unavailable for most drugs or biologics, with the exception of the penicillins.

Insect sting anaphylaxis

Reactions to stings from bees, wasps and ants of the order *Hymenoptera* are second only to drug-induced anaphylaxis and occur in up to 3% of the population. Non-anaphylactic toxic, large local or late serum sickness-like reactions also occur following a sting.

Food-induced anaphylaxis

This is most common in the young, particularly following peanuts, tree nuts such as walnuts and pecans, shellfish, fin fish, milk and egg ingestion. Cross-reactivity with other foods is unpredictable, or reactions may occur to additives such as carmine, metabisulphite and tartrazine. Mislabelling and contamination during manufacturing or at home cause inadvertent exposure, and associated factors such as exercise after food must be recognized (see later).

Although fatalities are rare and usually associated with pre-existing asthma, biphasic reactions are seen, as with all the other causes, when symptoms subside then recur several hours later. Patient and carer education is paramount, with schools in particular prepared to respond with auto-injector

Table 28.7.3   Causes of anaphylaxis

IgE-dependent mechanisms
   Drugs, chemicals and biologic agents:
      penicillins, cephalosporins, sulphonamides, muscle relaxants, vaccines, insulin, thiamine, protamine, gamma globulin, antivenoms, formaldehyde, ethylene oxide, chlorhexidine, semen
   Foods:
      peanuts, tree nuts, shellfish, fin fish, milk, egg, fruits, vegetables, flour
   Hymenopteran sting venom, insect saliva, other venoms:
      bees, wasps, ants, hornets, ticks, triatomid bugs, snakes, scorpions, jellyfish
   Latex
   Environmental:
      pollen, horse dander, hydatid cyst rupture

Non-IgE-dependent mechanisms
   Physical factors:
      exercise, cold, heat
   Medications and biologic agents:
      opiates, aspirin and NSAID, ACEI, vancomycin, radiocontrast media, N-acetylcysteine, fluorescein
   Food additives:
      metabisulphite, tartrazine,

Idiopathic

NSAID, non-steroidal, anti-inflammatory drugs; ACEI, angiotensin converting enzyme inhibitors
Note:
Cross-reactivity occurs, and both IgE-dependent and non-IgE-dependent reactions may happen with the same agent.
Several mechanisms may coexist such as exercise-induced following food.
Non-IgE-dependent mechanisms include complement activation, kinin production or potentiation, and direct mediator release.
ACEI use is an important cause of unexplained angio-oedema, occurring in up to 1:200 patients on these drugs, and may develop at any interval after starting (most commonly early on).

adrenaline (epinephrine) in an emergency, such as the EpiPen™ or EpiPen Jr™.

Anaesthesia-related anaphylaxis

Neuromuscular blocking drugs, latex, antibiotics and induction agents cause most cases, but opioids, colloids, blood products, radiocontrast dye, isosulphan or methylene blue, methylmethacrylate, chlorhexidine and protamine may be responsible for 'perioperative anaphylaxis'. The incidence ranges from 1:3500 to 1:20 000 anaesthetics, with up to 4% of reactions fatal.[8]

General anaesthesia reactions are due to muscle relaxants in 60% of cases, with suxamethonium in the highest-risk group. Reactions to suxamethonium and other relaxants can occur in the absence of prior use suggesting cross-reactivity, and rendering large-scale pre-operative testing unfeasible.

Latex-induced anaphylaxis

Healthcare workers, children with spina bifida and genitourinary abnormalities, and occupational exposure are the highest-risk groups for latex allergy. Reactions may follow direct contact, parenteral contamination or aerosol transmission.

Patients at known risk need treatment in a latex-free environment with glass syringes and non-latex containing gloves, stethoscope, breathing-system, blood pressure cuff, intravenous tubing and administration ports. Every emergency department (ED) should have the capacity to support an unexpected case of latex allergy, perhaps by sharing with the anaesthesia department access to a 'latex allergy resuscitation cart' containing relevant non-latex equipment.

Exercise-induced anaphylaxis

Anaphylaxis occurs with a variety of physical activities, although up to 50% of exercise-induced reactions occur following the ingestion of a food, or with prior aspirin or NSAID use. Mast cell degranulation appears to be triggered by cross-linking of allergen-specific IgE combined with neuropeptide release by adjacent nerve endings.

The severity of symptoms is generally influenced by the amount of food ingested, the vigour of the exercise and the lapse of time between the two, with more severe reactions occurring with exercise soon after food ingestion. Prophylactic medication is not effective, unlike prophylactic salbutamol or sodium cromoglycate to prevent exercise-induced asthma.

Idiopathic anaphylaxis

This is defined as anaphylaxis in which no discernible causative allergen or inciting physical factor can be identified. The diagnosis is by exclusion, with the majority of cases seen in adults, but it does occur in children.

Summation anaphylaxis

Comorbidities and concurrent medications increase the risk of anaphylaxis, giving rise to the concept of 'summation anaphylaxis'.[9] These include asthma, intercurrent infection, psychological stress, exercise, alcohol and drugs such as β-adrenergic blockers, angiotensin converting enzyme inhibitors (ACEIs), NSAIDs, and to a lesser extent angiotensin II receptor blockers (ARBs) and α-adrenergic blockers. Summation anaphylaxis may explain the unpredictable response of some individuals to recurrent antigen exposure.

Epidemiology

The true incidence of anaphylaxis is unknown. Data are unreliable with the lack of a standard definition, and are mostly derived from retrospective case collections from sources as diverse as the ED, perioperatively or the allergist-immunologist's office. Under-reporting is common as the diagnosis may have been missed, or when there is spontaneous recovery, pre-hospital treatment or a fatality. However, despite this, all anaphylaxis data from Western countries show that the incidence is increasing.[10]

Emergency department anaphylaxis

ED anaphylaxis presentations in adults have an annual incidence from 1:439 to 1:1100 ED cases, representing up to one adult presentation per 3400 population per year.[11] The annual incidence of paediatric anaphylaxis is around 1:1000 ED presentations, although generalized allergic reactions in children (that is, without multisystem involvement) are nearly ten times more common than this.[12]

The causative agent is suspected in 75% of ED anaphylaxis cases, recognized from a previous reaction or by close temporal association with symptom onset. The most frequent causes in adults are drug-related and hymenopteran stings, whereas in children food-induced or drug-related predominate. Respiratory features appear more common in paediatric anaphylaxis, and cardiovascular features in adults.[12]

Fatal anaphylaxis

Deaths follow hypoxia from upper airway swelling with asphyxia, bronchospasm and mucus plugging, and from shock related to vasodilatation, extravascular fluid shift and direct myocardial depression. Tachycardia is usual in shock, but bradycardia related to a neurocardiogenic, vagally-mediated mechanism (Bezold–Jarisch reflex) has occasionally been observed. This may respond to atropine if adrenaline fails (see under Management, second-line agents).

Fatalities are rare at less than one per million population per year. When they do happen, fatal reactions are rapid with a median time to cardiorespiratory arrest of just 5 min if iatrogenic, 15 min for venom and 30 min following foods. Adrenaline is given in only 14% cases prior to arrest, and not at all in 38% of fatalities.[13] In a recent review of fatal food-induced anaphylaxis in the UK, 43 of 48 cases had associated asthma usually with suboptimal daily inhaled steroid use, and over half had only ever had mild previous food reactions. This suggested that the severity of subsequent reactions cannot be predicted from the reaction history, and that sound professional advice was often inadequate or absent.[14]

Pathophysiology

Triggering events

Most cases of immune-mediated, allergic anaphylaxis are IgE- or occasionally IgG$_4$-mediated. Reaginic antibodies are released into the circulation by plasma cells derived from B lymphocytes, under the influence of helper T cells following previous exposure to an antigen (quite why this happens is unknown). These antibodies then bind to glycoprotein receptors on bloodborne basophils or tissue mast cells, sensitizing them. A huge variety of substances induce IgE antibody formation, ranging from drugs, chemicals and biologic agents, foods, hymenopteran sting venom, insect saliva and other venoms, to latex and environmental allergens (see Table 28.7.3).

Non-IgE-dependent, non-allergic anaphylactic reactions are caused by mediator release triggered independently of reaginic antibodies, leading to complement activation, the direct pharmacological release of mediators, or coagulation/fibrinolysis system activation. Physical factors, medications, biologic agents and food additives may trigger these non-IgE reactions (see Table 28.7.3).

Cellular events

Mast cells and basophils release inflammatory mediators following the binding of multivalent allergen cross-linking the surface, high-affinity IgE Fc receptors (FcεRI), or from cell membrane perturbation. This coupled with the mobilization of Ca^{2+} in the endoplasmic reticulum leads to release of pre-formed granule-associated mediators by exocytosis, or to the de novo synthesis of lipid mediators based on arachidonic acid metabolism, and the activation of genes for various cytokines and chemokines.[15]

Mast cell and basophil inflammatory mediators

The preformed mediators include histamine, proteases such as tryptase, chymase and carboxypeptidase A, and proteoglycans such as heparin and chondroitin sulphate E. Newly synthesized lipid mediators include prostaglandin D_2 and thromboxane A_2 via the cyclo-oxygenase pathway, and the leukotrienes LTC_4, LTD_4 and LTE_4 via the lipoxygenase pathway. The cytokines released include TNF-α, various interleukins such as IL-3, IL-4, IL-5, IL-6, IL-8, IL-13 and IL-16 and GM-CSF. Finally, chemokines include platelet activating factor, neutrophil chemotactic factor and eosinophil chemotactic factor, plus macrophage inflammatory protein Iα.[16]

At the cellular level mediator release is modulated by the steady-state resting intracellular cyclic AMP (cAMP) levels. Substances that elevate cAMP, such as adrenaline, inhibit mediator release, partly explaining its essential role in treatment. Also, from knowledge of the complex array of mediators involved it is self-evident why antihistamines cannot form the first line of therapy.

Mediator pharmacology

Mediators act to induce vasodilatation, increase capillary permeability and glandular secretion, cause smooth muscle spasm particularly bronchoconstriction and to attract new cells such as eosinophils, leukocytes and platelets. Positive feedback mechanisms amplify and perpetuate reactions recruiting further effector cells to release increasing amounts of mediators in a 'mast cell–leukocyte cytokine cascade' effect.[17] Conversely, other anaphylactic reactions self-limit, with spontaneous recovery related to endogenous compensatory mechanisms including increased adrenaline and angiotensin II secretion.[18]

Clinical features

Anaphylaxis is characteristically a disease of fit patients, and is rarely seen or described in critically ill or shocked patients, other than asthmatics. The speed of onset relates to the mechanism of exposure, and the severity of the reaction. Parenteral antigen exposure may cause life-threatening anaphylaxis within minutes, whereas symptoms can be delayed for some hours following oral or topical exposure.

Cutaneous and generalized allergic reactions

A premonitory aura, tingling or warm sensation, anxiety and feeling of impending doom precede generalized erythema, urticaria with pruritus, and angio-oedema of the neck, face, lips and tongue. Rhinorrhoea, conjunctival injection and tearing are seen.

Eighty to ninety-five per cent of patients with anaphylaxis have cutaneous features, which assist the prompt, early diagnosis.[11,12] However, alerting cutaneous features may be absent because of pre-hospital treatment or their spontaneous resolution, be subtle clinically and missed, or the onset of other life-threatening systemic complications such as laryngeal oedema or shock may precede them.

Systemic reactions

The hallmark of anaphylaxis is the precipitate onset of multisystem involvement with respiratory, cardiovascular, gastrointestinal and or neurological system dysfunction (see Table 28.7.4).

Table 28.7.4 Clinical features of anaphylaxis

Cutaneous
- Tingling or warmth, erythema (flushing), urticaria, pruritus (itch), angio-oedema
- Rhinorrhoea, conjunctival injection, lacrimation

Respiratory
- Throat tightness, cough, dyspnoea, hoarseness, stridor, aphonia
- Tachypnoea, wheeze, $SpO_2 \leq 92\%$,[a] cyanosis[a]

Cardiovascular and neurological
- Tachycardia (rarely bradycardia), hypotension,[a] arrhythmias, cardiac arrest[a]
- Light-headedness, sweating, incontinence,[a] syncope,[a] confusion,[a] coma[a]

Gastrointestinal
- Odynophagia (difficult or painful swallowing), abdominal cramps, nausea, vomiting, diarrhoea

Non-specific
- Premonitory aura, anxiety, feeling of impending doom
- Pelvic cramps

SpO_2, oxygen saturation on pulse oximetry.
[a]Indicative of a severe reaction. (See Table 28.7.2 for grading system).

Respiratory manifestations

Throat tightness and cough precede mild to critical respiratory distress due to oropharyngeal or laryngeal oedema with dyspnoea, hoarseness, stridor even aphonia; or related to bronchospasm with tachypnoea and wheeze. Hypoxia with an oxygen saturation less than 92% on pulse oximetry and central cyanosis indicate severe anaphylaxis and the need for immediate treatment (see severity grading Table 28.7.2).

Cardiovascular and neurological manifestations

Light-headedness, sweating, incontinence, syncope or coma may precede or accompany cardiovascular collapse with tachycardia, hypotension and cardiac arrhythmias again heralding severe anaphylaxis. These arrhythmias may appear seemingly benign supraventricular rhythms, particularly in children, but can progress to an impalpable pulse requiring external cardiac massage (see severity grading Table 28.7.2).

Gastrointestinal manifestations

Difficult or painful swallowing, nausea, vomiting, diarrhoea and abdominal cramps may be associated with a severe reaction, but are usually overshadowed by more immediately life-threatening features.

Differential diagnosis

The protean manifestations of anaphylaxis have a potentially vast differential diagnosis, although the rapidity of onset, accompanying cutaneous features, and the relationship to a likely or known potential trigger suggest the true diagnosis in most cases. The following differential diagnoses should be considered.

Wheeze and difficulty breathing

Bronchial asthma, cardiogenic pulmonary oedema, foreign body inhalation, irritant chemical exposure and tension pneumothorax are distinguished by the history, comorbidity and associated presenting features.

Light-headedness and syncope

An anxiety or vasovagal reaction should be considered where there is a history of exaggerated fear of an impending reaction; or in the context of a painful procedure such as an injection or local anaesthetic infiltration with collapse. Bradycardia, sweating and pallor without urticaria, erythema or itch, associated with a brief prodrome and rapid response to the recumbent position favour a vasovagal reaction over anaphylactic shock.

Other forms of shock

Other types of distributive shock such as septicaemia, spinal denervation, epidural or spinal block, hypovolaemic shock from haemorrhage or fluid loss, cardiogenic shock from primary myocardial dysfunction and obstructive shock from cardiac tamponade or tension pneumothorax should all be apparent from the history and examination. Cutaneous and respiratory features other than tachypnoea are absent in these non-anaphylactic causes of shock.

Facial swelling or angio-oedema

Bacterial or viral infections usually have fever and or pain, and traumatic or anticoagulant-related bleeding causes recognizable bruising. Angio-oedema in the absence of urticaria can be caused by actual or functional C_1 esterase inhibitor deficiency. This may be hereditary autosomal dominant, with a positive family history, an absence of pruritus, prominent abdominal symptoms and a history of recurrent attacks related to minor stress.

Alternatively, C_1 esterase inhibitor deficiency may be acquired in lymphoproliferative and some connective tissue disorders. A rapid, inexpensive screening test for serum C4 should be performed, and if low, be followed by the more specific C1 esterase inhibitor assay to confirm the diagnosis. Management is with C1 esterase inhibitor concentrate in a serious attack, or with fresh frozen plasma in its absence.

Flushing

Scombroid poisoning following spoiled-fish ingestion, carcinoid syndrome, alcohol and systemic mastocytosis all produce flushing, and require a careful history and investigation to differentiate.

Clinical investigation

The diagnosis of anaphylaxis is clinical. No immediate laboratory or radiological test confirms the process, and must never delay immediate management. The measurement of electrolytes and renal function, blood glucose, chest X-ray and an ECG are indicated if there is a slow response to treatment, or when there is doubt about the diagnosis.

Disease progress may be monitored by pulse oximetry, haematocrit level which may rise with fluid extravasation, and arterial blood gases to look for a respiratory or metabolic acidosis.

Laboratory testing

Mast cell tryptase

Despite initial promise, a serum mast cell tryptase taken from 1 to 6 h after a suspected episode cannot be solely relied upon to diagnose anaphylaxis, as it is not elevated consistently, particularly following food allergy. Conversely a mast cell tryptase assay may be elevated postmortem in non-anaphylactic deaths. However, measuring serial levels, or specific allelic subtypes such as mature β tryptase may improve the value of this test.[6,19]

Histamine

Histamine levels are impractical to measure as they are unstable and evanescent, only remaining elevated for 30 to 60 min maximum.

Treatment

Stop immediately any potential causative agent such as an intravenous drug or infusion. Manage the patient in a monitored resuscitation area, including at least a pulse oximeter, non-invasive blood pressure device and ECG tracing.

Obtain a brief history of possible allergen exposure and perform a rapid assessment of the extent and severity of the reaction. Look particularly for signs of upper airway swelling, bronchospasm or circulatory shock.

The primary objective is to achieve stabilization of cardiorespiratory status by administration of oxygen, adrenaline (epinephrine) and fluids to the supine patient. Antihistamines and steroids play no role until after this has been achieved, and even then their value is debatable (see Table 28.7.5).[3,6]

Oxygen and airway patency

Give oxygen by face mask to all patients, aiming for an oxygen saturation above 92%. Place the patient supine, preferably with the legs elevated to optimize venous return. Elevate the head and torso if respiratory distress is prominent or worsened. Prepare for active airway intervention including opening the difficult airway kit, if there are signs of impending airway obstruction or rapidly progressive respiratory failure.

Table 28.7.5 Treatment of anaphylaxis

Initial Treatment
- Stop delivery of any potential causative agent
- Call for senior help
- Give adrenaline (epinephrine) 0.01 mg/kg i.m. into upper lateral thigh, to maximum 0.5 mg, e.g. 0.3–0.5 mL of 1:1000 adrenaline (epinephrine) i.m.
  - may be repeated every 5–15 min
  - or use patient's EpiPen™ if readily available – may be given through clothing
- Lay supine (or elevate legs) for shock
- Give high-flow oxygen
- Insert large-bore i.v. cannula (14-g or 16-g) and give crystalloid fluid bolus of 10–20 mL/kg

Deteriorating rapidly or failure to respond
- Start 1:100 000 adrenaline (epinephrine) infusion with 1 mL (1 mg) of 1:1000 adrenaline in 100 mL normal saline at 60–120 mL/h (10–20 µg/min) titrated to response:
  - *must* be on ECG monitor
  - give faster in cardiopulmonary collapse/ arrest
- Consider assisted ventilation and endotracheal intubation by a skilled emergency doctor (may be technically challenging)

Cyanosis and exhaustion indicate imminent respiratory arrest. Never give sedative or muscle relaxant drugs unless well trained in the management of the difficult airway, as endotracheal intubation and mechanical ventilation may be extremely challenging. Perform a surgical airway via the cricothyroid membrane as a last resort, before hypoxic cardiac arrest occurs.

Adrenaline (epinephrine)

Adrenaline is the drug of choice for acute anaphylaxis, whether allergic IgE-mediated or non-allergic. Give adrenaline in all but the most trivial cases and certainly if there is progressive airway swelling, bronchospasm or hypotension. It has α-, β_1- and β_2-adrenergic effects to counteract the profound vasodilatation, mucosal oedema and bronchospasm. Equally important is that adrenaline triggers a rise in intracellular cyclic AMP inhibiting further mast cell and basophil mediator release.

Adrenaline (epinephrine) dose

The dose of adrenaline is 0.01 mg/kg up to a maximum of 0.5 mg intramuscularly, repeated every 5–15 min as necessary. Give this as 0.01 mL/kg of 1:1000 aqueous adrenaline, or 0.3–0.5 mL (0.3–0.5 mg) into the upper outer thigh. The adrenaline may be injected through clothing in an emergency, including when self-administered pre-hospital using an EpiPen™.

Adrenaline (epinephrine) route

Intramuscular adrenaline is recommended when anaphylaxis is treated early, progressing slowly, venous access is difficult or delayed, or in the unmonitored patient. The intramuscular route is superior to subcutaneous, and the vastus lateralis muscle in the thigh is preferred to the deltoid muscle in the arm.

Intravenous adrenaline is only necessary if there is rapidly progressive vascular collapse with shock, imminent airway obstruction or critical bronchospasm. The patient must have ECG monitoring and an experienced emergency physician in charge. Administer the intravenous adrenaline slowly with extreme care, suitably diluted, and titrated to response to avoid potentially lethal complications such as cardiac arrhythmias, myocardial ischaemia and cerebrovascular accident.[13,20,21]

Adrenaline (epinephrine) infusion

Although 1:10 000 adrenaline containing 100 µg/mL is readily available, for instance as the Min-I-Jet™ preparation, it is impossible to give slowly enough at 10 µg/min, in the small initial quantities of 0.75–1.5 µg/kg (ie. 50–100 µg) necessary.

Therefore, make up an infusion of adrenaline by putting 1 mg in 100 mL normal saline (that is 1:100 000 adrenaline with 10 µg/mL) and start at 60–120 mL/h via an infusion device, to deliver 10–20 µg/min and titrate to response. Be prepared to continue the infusion for anything up to 60 min after resolution of all the symptoms and signs of anaphylaxis, then wean over the next 30 min and stop, watching closely for any recurrence.[22] Patients with persistent symptoms (protracted anaphylaxis) require a maintenance infusion of 5–10 µg/min and admission to a monitored intensive care area.

Adrenaline (epinephrine) nebuliser

Give patients nebulized adrenaline 5 mg, as 5 mL of undiluted 1:1000 adrenaline particularly for upper airway oedema and bronchospasm, whilst parenteral adrenaline is being prepared as above.

Fluid replacement

Insert a large-bore intravenous cannula as soon as possible in patients showing signs of shock. Administer an initial fluid bolus of 10–20 mL/kg normal saline, up to 50 mL/kg total to counter the massive intravascular fluid shifts and peripheral vasodilatation that occurs in minutes with anaphylactic shock. There are no outcome data favouring colloids over crystalloids.

Second-line agents

Once oxygen, adrenaline and fluids have been given to optimize the cardiorespiratory status and tissue oxygenation, the following drugs may be administered in a support role.

H_1- and H_2- antihistamines

Reserve antihistamines for the symptomatic relief of skin symptoms such as urticaria, mild angio-oedema and pruritus. They must never be relied upon as sole therapy in significant anaphylaxis. Side effects of sedation, confusion and vasodilatation with the H_1-antihistamines can be troublesome, particularly when given parenterally.

The combination of an H_2-antihistamine with an H_1-antihistamine is better at attenuating the cutaneous manifestations of a generalized allergic reaction than an H_1-antagonist given alone. Choose a non-sedating H_1-antihistamine such as loratadine 10 mg daily, especially on discharge, if the patient wishes to continue working, or driving a vehicle (see Discharge oral medication).

Corticosteroids

As with the antihistamines, there are no placebo-controlled trials to confirm the effectiveness of steroids in significant anaphylaxis, despite their many theoretical benefits on mediator release and tissue responsiveness. Most clinicians give prednisone 1 mg/kg up to 50 mg orally or hydrocortisone 1.5–3 mg/kg i.v. particularly in patients with airway involvement and bronchospasm, based purely on their important role in asthma. Side effects including sodium and potassium ion flux changes and anaphylaxis itself are more likely with the intravenous route for steroid delivery.

It is also possible that steroids prevent a biphasic reaction with recrudescence of symptoms following recovery, but again supporting data are unconvincing (see Disposition). Steroids are, however, essential in the management of recurrent idiopathic anaphylaxis.

Glucagon, atropine and salbutamol

Patients taking β blockers have more severe and/or treatment-refractory anaphylaxis. Give glucagon from 1–5 mg intravenously, followed by an infusion at 5–15 µg/min titrated to response, if adrenaline has been ineffective. Glucagon raises cyclic AMP by a non-adrenergic mechanism, but may cause nausea and vomiting.

As mentioned earlier, some patients with anaphylactic shock develop a bradycardia resistant to adrenaline, possibly mediated by a neurocardiogenic vagal reflex. Atropine 0.6 mg intravenously up to 0.02 mg/kg has been successful in this situation.[20]

Finally, give nebulised salbutamol in addition to adrenaline for resistant bronchospasm, which has the advantage of familiarity.

Other vasopressors

Vasopressors such as noradrenaline, metaraminol, phenylephrine and vasopressin have anecdotally treated hypotension resistant to initial adrenaline and fluid therapy.

Pretreatment

There is no convincing justification for pretreatment, in particular the practice of routine prophylactic corticosteroids and/or antihistamines to reduce the risk of serious iodinated contrast media reactions during radiological procedures is neither reliable, nor supported by the literature, and should be abandoned.[23]

Disposition

Patients with systemic anaphylactic reactions, including all those who receive adrenaline, should be kept under observation for at least 4 to 6 h after apparent full recovery. Keep patients with reactive airways disease a little longer, because most deaths from anaphylaxis occur in this group.[4] Observation is safely performed in the ED if a suitable holding area exists, and ECG monitoring is not necessary.[11,12]

Most anaphylactic reactions are uniphasic and respond rapidly and completely to treatment. Some patients develop protracted reactions with an incomplete response to adrenaline, or deteriorate on attempted adrenaline weaning. Keep these patients with unstable vital signs monitored and admit to an intensive care area.

Biphasic anaphylaxis

Relapse after an apparent complete resolution of all initial symptoms and signs, known as biphasic anaphylaxis, is reported in 1–5% of cases. It is unknown if more severe presenting features, delayed or inadequate doses of adrenaline, or the non-use of steroids predispose to, or predict the biphasic response.[24]

Discharge policy

Discharge the patient following observation and consider the need for take-home medication, self-injectable adrenaline, and allergist-immunologist referral.

Discharge oral medication

There are no data to support the common practice of prescribing a two- or three-day discharge supply of combined H_1- and H_2-antihistamines plus oral steroids to prevent early relapse. However, consider loratadine 10 mg once daily, ranitidine 150 mg 12-hourly and prednisolone 50 mg once daily

in adults with predominant cutaneous features following a generalized allergic reaction, or bronchospasm.

Self-injectable adrenaline (epinephrine)

The quandary of who to prescribe self-injected adrenaline to and what to write in an anaphylaxis action plan is well described.[25] Attitudes vary as to whether the emergency physician or general practitioner should initiate EpiPen™ use, rather than waiting for specialist allergist–immunologist review and formulation of an individualized anaphylaxis action plan. As a guide, consider self-injectable adrenaline for the patient with anaphylaxis after known allergen exposure outside of a medical setting, patients with food allergy particularly to nuts or peanuts, and for those in whom the reaction was severe and or the cause unknown.

The EpiPen™ with 0.3 mg (300 μg) of adrenaline, and the EpiPen Jr™ containing 0.15 mg (150μ μg) are approved for self-administered intramuscular use. They are now available on the Pharmaceutical Benefits Scheme (PBS) Schedule as an initial supply on an Authority script for a patient who: 'has been discharged from hospital or an emergency department after treatment with adrenaline for acute allergic reaction with anaphylaxis' or as a continuing supply for patients who have previously been issued with an Authority prescription.[26]

If an EpiPen™ is dispensed in the ED, it is essential to explain and demonstrate exactly how to use the device, and to educate both the patient and another caregiver, particularly with children. Teach the patient and carer to recognize the symptoms and signs of anaphylaxis, and encourage the actual use of the device particularly if distant from a healthcare facility. Tell recipients self-injectable adrenaline has a relatively short shelf-life of around one year, and how to look after it.[27]

Allergist-immunologist referral

Disappointingly few patients who suffer an episode of anaphylaxis are referred from the ED for specialist allergist–immunologist follow-up. Refer anyone prescribed a self-injectable adrenaline (epinephrine) device, patients following a wasp or bee sting suitable for immunotherapy, suspected food-, drug-induced or exercise-induced anaphylaxis, and patients

with severe reactions without an obvious trigger.[28]

Give the patient a letter detailing the nature and circumstances of the anaphylactic reaction, the treatment given, and the suspected causative agent(s). Ask the patient to also write a brief diary of the events in the 6 to 12 h preceding the reaction, particularly when the cause is unclear. Ask them to include all foods ingested, drugs taken including non-proprietary, cosmetics used and activities performed outside as well as indoors. Later recall of events at specialist allergist–immunologist review will be flawed unless documented contemporaneously.

Drug and allergen avoidance

Patients at risk of recurrent anaphylaxis with hypertension or ischaemic heart disease should ideally be taken off β blockers, and care taken not to substitute an ACE inhibitor. Discuss this with the patient's other specialists to be certain the overall risk-benefit favours medication change.

Advise patients to reduce allergen exposure risk by destroying nearby wasp nests and removing allergenic foods in the house, plus to avoid insect sting with appropriate clothing, and certain foods by checking the manufacturer's label.

IgE skin testing, in vitro testing and challenge testing

Skin or blood tests for specific IgE antibodies should only be done by those trained in their performance and interpretation. Skin prick testing is the more sensitive and when possible, standardized extracts should be used with correct technique. In addition, an experienced physician such as a specialist allergist–immunologist should supervise as occasional severe reactions occur.[10] They are not appropriately performed by an emergency physician.

In vitro testing for allergen-specific IgE is less sensitive, and depends on clinical correlation and the availability of specific assays. Over 500 different allergens are available for testing with the ImmunoCAP™ system (Phadia AB, Uppsala, Sweden), or clinicians may use a radio-allergosorbent (RAST) technique.

Finally, challenge testing may help diagnose non-allergic anaphylaxis. False positive and false negative reactions do occur but are much less likely than with skin prick or in vitro testing, but again experienced specialist allergist–immunologist supervision is essential.[18]

Controversies

❶ The exact mechanisms which underly IgE antibody formation in response to such a myriad of different substances, and why this happens in one individual but not another.

❷ There remains no single internationally agreed definition or grading system for anaphylaxis.

❸ The symptoms or signs which most reliably predict the risk of severe anaphylaxis.

❹ The utility of laboratory testing in confirming and quantifying the severity of an anaphylactic reaction.

❺ Most effective drug doses in acute treatment.

❻ Predictors of biphasic reactions.

❼ The utility of discharge medications.

References

1. Johansson SGO, Bieber T, Dahl R, et al. Revised nomenclature for allergy for global use: Report of the Nomenclature Review Committee of the World Allergy Organization, October 2003. Journal of Allergy and Clinical Immunology 2004; 113: 832–836.
2. Galli SJ. Pathogenesis and management of anaphylaxis: Current status and future challenges. Journal of Allergy and Clinical Immunology 2005; 115: 571–574.
3. Sampson HA, Munoz-Furlong A, Campbell RL, et al, Second symposium on the definition and management of anaphylaxis: Summary report – Second National Institute of Allergy and Infectious Disease/Food Allergy and Anaphylaxis Network symposium. Journal of Allergy and Clinical Immunology 2006; 117: 391–397.
4. Sampson HA, Munoz-Furlong A, Bock SA, et al. Symposium on the definition and management of anaphylaxis: Summary report. Journal of Allergy and Clinical Immunology 2005; 115: 584–591.
5. Brown SGA. Clinical features and severity grading of anaphylaxis. Journal of Allergy and Clinical Immunology 2004; 114: 371–376.
6. Lieberman P, Kemp SF, Oppenheimer J, et al. The diagnosis and management of anaphylaxis: An updated practice parameter. Journal of Allergy and Clinical Immunology 2005; 115: S483–S523.
7. Sicherer SH, Leung DYM. Advances in allergic skin disease, anaphylaxis, and hypersensitivity reactions to food, drugs, and insects. Journal of Allergy and Clinical Immunology 2005; 116: 153–163.
8. Axon AD, Hunter JM. Anaphylaxis and anaesthesia - all clear now? British Journal of Anaesthesia 2004; 93: 501–504.
9. Ring J, Darsow U. Idiopathic anaphylaxis. Current Allergy Asthma Reports 2002; 2: 40–45.
10. Douglass JA, O'Hehir RE. Diagnosis, treatment and prevention of allergic disease: The basics. Medical Journal of Australia 2006; 185: 228–233.
11. Brown AFT, McKinnon D, Chu K. Emergency department anaphylaxis: A review of 142 patients in a single year. Journal of Allergy and Clinical Immunology 2001; 108: 861–866.
12. Braganza SC, Acworth JP, McKinnon DRL, et al. Paediatric emergency department anaphylaxis: Different patterns from adults. Archives of Disease in Childhood 2006; 91: 159–163.
13. Pumphrey RSH. Lessons for management of anaphylaxis from a study of fatal reactions. Clinical and Experimental Allergy 2000; 30: 1144–1150.
14. Pumphrey RSH, Gowland MH. Further fatal allergic reactions to food in the United Kingdom, 1999-2006. Journal of Allergy and Clinical Immunology 2007; 119:1018–1019.
15. Chang TW, Shiung Y-Y. Anti-IgE as a mast cell-stabilizing therapeutic agent. Journal of Allergy and Clinical Immunology 2006; 117:1203–1212.
16. Prussin C, Metcalfe DD. IgE, mast cells, basophils, and eosinophils. Journal of Allergy and Clinical Immunology 2006; 117: S450–S456.
17. Brown SGA, Mullins RJ, Gold MS. Anaphylaxis: Diagnosis and management. Medical Journal of Australia 2006; 185: 283–289.
18. Simons FER. Anaphylaxis, killer allergy: Long-term management in the community. Journal of Allergy and Clinical Immunology 2006; 117: 367–377.
19. Caughey GH. Tryptase genetics and anaphylaxis. Journal of Allergy and Clinical Immunology 2006; 117:1411–1414.
20. Brown SGA, Blackman KE, Stenlake V, et al. Insect sting anaphylaxis: Prospective evaluation and treatment with intravenous adrenaline and volume resuscitation. Emergency Medicine Journal 2004; 21: 149–154.
21. Brown AFT. Anaphylaxis gets the adrenaline going. Emergency Medicine Journal 2004; 21:128–129.
22. Brown SGA. Anaphylaxis: Clinical concepts and research priorities. Emergency Medicine Australasia 2006; 18: 155–169.
23. Tramèr MR, von Elm E, Loubeyre P, et al. Pharmacological prevention of serious anaphylactic reactions due to iodinated contrast media: Systematic review. British Medical Journal 2006; 333: 675–678.
24. Lieberman P. Biphasic anaphylactic reactions. Ann Allergy, Asthma Immunology 2005; 95: 217–226.
25. Sicherer SH, Simons FER. Quandaries in prescribing an emergency action plan and self-injectable epinephrine for first-aid management of anaphylaxis in the community. Journal of Allergy and Clinical Immunology 2005; 115: 575–583.
26. Australian Government – Department of Health and Ageing. Information in the PBS Schedule about Epipen™. http://www.pbs.gov.au/html/healthpro/product/restrictions?code=8697 (accessed September 2007).
27. Australasian Society of Clinical Immunology and Allergy. Anaphylaxis. ASCIA Education Resources. Information for Health Professionals. http://www.allergy.org.au/aer/infobulletins/hp_anaphylaxis.htm (accessed September 2007).
28. Leung D, Schatz M. Consultation and referral guidelines citing the evidence: How the allergist-immunologist can help. Journal of Allergy and Clinical Immunology 2006; 117: S495–S523.

28.8 Altitude illness

Ian Rogers • Debra O'Brien

ESSENTIALS

1 The high-altitude syndromes – acute mountain sickness (AMS), high-altitude cerebral oedema (HACE) and high-altitude pulmonary oedema – are all clinical diagnoses, where management may need to be undertaken without access to diagnostic testing.

2 AMS and HACE represent stages along a continuum owing to cerebral vasodilatation and cerebral oedema.

3 Early recognition and descent are the keys to successful management.

4 Pharmacological agents are available to assist in the prevention and management of altitude syndromes, but are generally considered to be second line to physical therapy.

5 Prevention is best achieved by controlled ascent, with adequate time for acclimatization.

6 Low-dose acetazolamide provides effective prophylaxis against AMS.

Introduction

Altitude illness comprises a number of syndromes that can occur on exposure to the hypobaric hypoxic environment of high altitude. At any altitude, the partial pressure of inspired oxygen (P_iO_2) is equal to 0.21 times the barometric pressure minus water vapour pressure of 47 mmHg. At an altitude of 5500 m, barometric pressure is halved. On the summit of Mount Everest (8850 m), the P_iO_2 is only 43 mmHg, and a typical climber without oxygen can be expected to have a PaO_2 of <30 mmHg and a $PaCO_2$ of about 7.5 mmHg.[1] In addition to the hypoxic stress of altitude, a subject may also be exposed to cold, low humidity, fatigue, poor diet and increased ultraviolet radiation. For the emergency physician, the unique feature of altitude illness is that it requires recognition and treatment in the field, frequently without access to sophisticated diagnostic and imaging techniques, and often without access to rapid evacuation.

Epidemiology and pathophysiology

The human body has the capacity to acclimatize to hypoxic environments. This is principally achieved by increasing ventilation (the hypoxic ventilatory response effected by the carotid body), increasing numbers of red blood cells (via stimulation of erythropoietin), increasing the diffusing capacity of the lungs (resulting from increased lung volume and pulmonary capillary blood volume), increasing vascularity of the tissues, and increasing the tissues' ability to use oxygen (possibly owing to increased numbers of mitochondria and oxidative enzyme systems).

In some individuals, exposure to low PO_2 initiates a sequence of pathophysiological changes, which result in oedema formation in the brain and lungs. The altitude illness syndromes, acute mountain sickness (AMS), high-altitude cerebral oedema (HACE) and high-altitude pulmonary oedema (HAPE), are the result of this oedema formation. The exact mechanism of these pathophysiological changes is still debated but vasodilatation is a key part.

In the brain, the development of oedema causes intracranial pressure (ICP) to rise.

Initially, this is partially compensated for by displacement of cerebrospinal fluid (CSF) into the spinal space, and adjustment of the balance between production and absorption of CSF. However, once these compensatory mechanisms are overwhelmed, ICP can rise beyond the cerebral perfusion pressure. Without intervention, cerebral blood flow ceases and the patient dies.

In the lung, non-cardiogenic pulmonary oedema develops. A significant rise in pulmonary artery pressure appears to be a crucial pathophysiological factor.[2] Recent work suggests that impaired sodium driven clearance of alveolar fluid may contribute to HAPE.[3] Patients with a history of HAPE have an exaggerated pressor response to hypoxia, with increased secretion of noradrenaline (norepinephrine), adrenaline (epinephrine), renin, angiotensin, aldosterone and atrial natriuretic peptide. It has been postulated that uneven pulmonary vasoconstriction increases the filtration pressure in non-vasoconstricted lung areas, worsening the interstitial and alveolar oedema.

The tendency to develop altitude illness is idiosyncratic. The major predisposing factors are the rate of ascent and the altitude reached. It is not related to physical fitness or gender. Individuals vary in their ability to compensate for changes in ICP, and in their pressor responses to hypoxia. This may explain the reproducibility of AMS, HACE and HAPE in susceptible individuals, and why some, and not others, develop symptoms at the same altitude. The risk is higher in those who have an impaired ventilatory response to hypoxia in normobaric conditions, and with dehydration, vigorous exercise and the use of depressant drugs.

Prevention

The best form of prevention is gradual ascent to allow sufficient time for acclimatization. Although individuals vary in how quickly they acclimatize, a sensible recommendation is sleeping no more than 500 m higher than the previous day once above 2500 m. Keeping warm, avoiding alcohol, keeping well hydrated and eating a high-carbohydrate diet to improve the respiratory quotient, will all decrease the incidence of altitude illness. Modest exercise on acclimatization days should be encouraged.

Acclimatization is not always practical or possible, and so pharmacological agents may be required to enhance the physiological process. Acetazolamide reduces the incidence and severity of AMS/HACE when used prophylactically in subjects experiencing rapid ascent.[9] Doses recommended have decreased as a result of ongoing research.[10] Chemoprophylaxis can be achieved with 125 mg bd, starting on the day of ascent and continued for 2 days after reaching high altitude. Dexamethasone 4 mg qid may be equally effective, and may be more so when a rapid onset is required, such as in unacclimatized personnel involved in high-altitude rescue missions. Nifedipine 20 mg slow-release tds may provide protection against HAPE in susceptible individuals, but the wisdom of re-exposing patients to such an environment is questionable. Although gingko biloba has now been shown to be ineffective for AMS prophylaxis,[11,12] other research suggests a role for sumatriptan.[13] Current research focuses on the value of salmeterol[3] and dexamethasone and phosphodiesterase-5 inhibitors such as tadalafil[14] in prevention of HAPE.

Clinical features

AMS is common, occurring in about 30% of subjects exposed to moderate altitude (3500 m). HACE and HAPE are much less common, but a study in pilgrims at 4300 m reported AMS in 68%, HACE in 31% and HAPE in 5% of subjects.[4] The diagnosis is usually made on clinical assessment and setting.

Acute mountain sickness

AMS is primarily a neurological syndrome, associated with some degree of respiratory compromise. The onset is usually 6–24 h after arrival at high altitude. The majority of patients present in the early stages when the symptoms are like those of a hangover, and include headache, nausea, anorexia, weakness and lassitude. In the early stage of AMS, there are no abnormalities on physical examination, and the oxygen saturation, if measured, should be no lower than that expected for a given altitude. Mild AMS is usually benign and self-limiting.

If the illness progresses, the more severe form of AMS is characterized by dyspnoea at rest, nausea and vomiting, altered mental state, headache and ataxia. Ataxia is the most useful sign of progression to serious illness. Retinal haemorrhages and venous dilatation may be seen on fundoscopy. Left untreated, severe AMS may progress to life-threatening HACE or HAPE.

AMS can be scored using the Lake Louise AMS score.[5] This consists of five symptom groups: headache, gastrointestinal distress, fatigue or weakness, dizziness or light headedness, and difficulty sleeping. Each symptom is scored on a scale from 0 (not present) to 3 (severe or incapacitating) and the totals of the five symptom groups are summed. A total score of 3 or more is considered diagnostic of AMS.

High-altitude cerebral oedema

HACE is the progression of neurological signs and symptoms in the setting of AMS. There is a progressive decline in mental status and truncal ataxia is a prominent physical finding. Focal neurological signs, such as third and sixth cranial nerve palsies, may develop as a result of raised intracranial pressure. Unrecognized and untreated, there may be rapid progression to coma and death due to raised intracranial pressure.

High-altitude pulmonary oedema

HAPE occurs in susceptible individuals who may have no underlying pulmonary or cardiac disease. It most commonly manifests on the second night at high altitude. In the early stages, the oedema is interstitial, and the patient may only have a dry cough and decreased exercise tolerance. Few abnormalities will be seen on examination at this stage. As more fluid accumulates, the patient develops tachycardia, increasing dyspnoea, marked weakness, cough productive of frothy sputum, and cyanosis. Pulse oximetry, if available, confirms profound hypoxia. A chest X-ray will demonstrate widespread interstitial and alveolar infiltrates. It may occur in conjunction with AMS/HACE, or as an isolated clinical syndrome.

Treatment

Early recognition is an essential component of the management of all acute altitude

Table 28.8.1 Key treatments in severe altitude syndromes

HACE/Severe AMS	HAPE
Descent	Descent
Oxygen	Oxygen
Hyperbaric therapy (e.g. Gamow bag)	Hyperbaric therapy (e.g. Gamow bag)
Dexamethasone 8 mg stat then 6-hourly	Nifedipine 10–20 mg 6-hourly

HACE, high-altitude cerebral oedema; AMS, acute mountain sickness; HAPE, high-altitude pulmonary oedema.

syndromes. Developing symptoms in a party member may have substantial impact on route planning choices, particularly whether to halt ascent or descend. The goal is to stop the pathophysiological process (Table 28.8.1).

Acute mountain sickness and high-altitude cerebral oedema

A patient presenting with symptoms of mild AMS should be advised to halt ascent to allow time for acclimatization. They should rest, as physical exertion aggravates symptoms, and take simple analgesics and antiemetics if desired. It is important that the patient be closely observed for progression of symptoms.

With moderate symptoms the management is the same as for mild AMS, with the addition of oxygen 2–4 L/min and, possibly, pharmacological agents. Acetazolamide, a carbonic anhydrase inhibitor, aids the normal process of ventilatory acclimatization by reducing the renal reabsorption of bicarbonate, resulting in metabolic acidosis and compensatory hyperventilation. It relieves symptoms, improves arterial oxygenation, and prevents further impairment of pulmonary gas exchange.[6] It also helps to maintain cerebral blood flow despite hypocapnia, and opposes the fluid retention of AMS. The recommended treatment dose is 125–250 mg orally bd. Acetazolamide is a sulpha drug and contraindicated in those with allergy. Dexamethasone may also be used as it improves oxygen saturation and provides symptomatic relief.[7] This benefit may be derived from reduced capillary permeability and ICP. It does not aid in acclimatization. It may be given as an alternative, or in addition to acetazolamide.

The dose recommended is 8 mg orally initially, followed by 4 mg every 6 h.

If a patient shows signs of severe AMS progressing to HACE, then rapid and controlled descent is the highest priority. Oxygen 2–4 L/min should be administered. Additional therapy may be required if the illness is severe, the patient's condition must be improved to allow descent, or where immediate descent is not possible. Additional therapeutic options include dexamethasone 8 mg orally, i.m. or i.v., and hyperbaric therapy using a portable fabric hyperbaric chamber (e.g. Gamow bag). This device simulates descent and provides short-term relief for 1–3 h. Long-term benefits have yet to be established.[8] The bags are expensive and need to be pumped continuously, but have the advantage of using air rather than oxygen. Acetazolamide does not have a role in the setting of severe AMS and HACE.

High-altitude pulmonary oedema

Rapid and controlled descent, with oxygen, is the mainstay of management in a patient suffering from HAPE. In a large proportion of cases this is sufficient. Oxygen flow should be titrated to maintain adequate oxygen saturation. Continuous positive airway pressure may be required. The patient should be rested and kept warm, as cold may further increase pulmonary hypertension through sympathetic stimulation.

Nifedipine should be considered as adjunctive therapy when oxygen is not available and descent is not possible. A calcium channel blocker, it lowers the raised pulmonary artery pressure that characterizes HAPE and results in clinical improvement, better oxygenation and progressive clearing of alveolar oedema on chest X-ray. The recommended dosage is 10–20 mg orally 6-hourly.

Controversies

❶ The effectiveness of acetazolamide and dexamethasone in AMS prophylaxis is now generally well accepted. Which agent is more effective and in which circumstances they should be used is less clear. The side effects of acetazolamide at recommended doses can mimic AMS and, conversely, the euphoriant effects of dexamethasone can interfere with a subject's ability to accurately report symptoms. Dexamethasone and acetazolamide appear to differ in their effectiveness when trialled in field conditions compared to simulated conditions in hypobaric chambers. The dose of each drug used is not the same across trials. The rate of ascent appears to influence the effectiveness of pharmacological prophylaxis. The current recommendation is that dexamethasone be used when individuals are required to ascend immediately and unexpectedly (e.g. for mountain rescues) and that acetazolamide be used when prophylaxis can be commenced greater than 24 h prior to the ascent.

❷ Further research is required to clarify the role of new preventive strategies for both AMS and HAPE.

References

1. Windsor JS, Rodway GW. Research at the extremes: Lessons from the 1981 American Medical Research Expedition to Mt Everest. Wilderness Environmental Medicine 2007; 18: 54–56.
2. Bartsch P. High altitude pulmonary edema. Respiration 1997; 64: 435–443.
3. Sartori C, Allemann Y, Duplain H, et al. Salmeterol for the prevention of high altitude pulmonary edema. New England Journal of Medicine 2002; 346: 1631–1636.
4. Basnyat B, Subedi D, Sleggs J, et al. Disorientated and ataxic pilgrims: an epidemiological study of acute mountain sickness and high altitude cerebral edema at a sacred lake at 4300 m in the Nepal Himalayas. Wilderness Environmental Medicine 2000; 11: 89–93.
5. Roach RC, Bartsch P, Hackett PH, Oelz O. (Lake Louise AMS Scoring Consensus Committee). The Lake Louise acute mountain sickness scoring system. In: Sutton JR, Houston CS, Coates G, eds. Hypoxia and molecular medicine. Burlington, VT: Queen City Printers; 1993: 272–274.
6. Grissom CK, Roach RC, Sarnquist FH, et al. Acetazolamide in the treatment of acute mountain sickness: clinical efficacy and effect on gas exchange. Annals of Internal Medicine 1992; 116: 461–465.
7. Ferrazzini G, Maggiorini M, Kriemler S, et al. Successful treatment of acute mountain sickness with dexamethasone. British Medical Journal 1997; 294: 1380–1382.
8. Bartsch P. Treatment of high altitude diseases without drugs. International Journal of Sports Medicine 1992; 13: S71–S74.
9. Hackett PH, Rennie D. The incidence, importance, and prophylaxis of acute mountain sickness. Lancet 1976; 2: 1149–1155.
10. Basnyat B, Gerstsch JH, Holck PS, et al. Acetazolamide 125 mg BD is not significantly different from 375 mg BD in the prevention of acute mountain sickness: the prophylactic acetazolamide dosage comparison for efficacy (PACE) trial. High Altitude Medicine & Biology 2006; 7: 17–27.
11. Gertsch JH, Basnyat B, Johnson EW, et al. Randomized, double blind, placebo controlled comparison of gingko bilboa and acetazolamide for prevention of acute mountain sickness among Himalayan trekkers: the prevention of high altitude illness trial (PHAIT). British Medical Journal 2004; 328: 797–801.
12. Chow T, Browne V, Heilson HL, et al. Gingko bilboa and acetazolamide prophylaxis for acute mountain sickness: a randomized, placebo-controlled trial. Archives of Internal Medicine 2005; 165: 296–301.
13. Jafarian S, Gorouhi F, Salimi S, et al. Sumatriptan for prevention of acute mountain sickness: Randomised clinical trial. Annals of Neurolology 2007; 62: 273–277.
14. Maggiorini M, Brunner-La Rocca HP, Peth S, et al. Both taldalafil and dexamethasone may reduce the incidence of high-altitude pulmonary edema: a randomized trial. Annals of Internal Medicine 2006; 145: 497–506.

TOXICOLOGY

Edited by **Lindsay Murray**

29.1 Approach to the poisoned patient

Lindsay Murray

ESSENTIALS

1 Self-poisoning is a manifestation of an underlying psychiatric, drug and alcohol or social disorder.

2 A wide range of clinical manifestations of toxicity may be observed following drug overdose.

3 An accurate risk assessment predicts the likely clinical course and informs planning for subsequent investigation, management and disposition.

4 The mainstay of management is timely institution of an appropriate level of supportive care.

5 The role of gastrointestinal decontamination is controversial. Except in select cases, it is unlikely that these procedures have a significant impact on clinical outcome when performed more than 1 h following ingestion.

6 Specific antidotes and techniques of enhanced elimination are rarely indicated, but their timely use may be life saving in specific instances.

Introduction

Drug overdose in adults usually occurs in the context of self-poisoning, which may be either recreational or an act of deliberate self-harm.

Deliberate self-poisoning is one of the commonest reasons for general hospital admission in the UK[1] and accounts for 1–5% of all public hospital admissions in Australia.[2,3] The bulk of the medical management of cases presenting to hospital is carried out in the emergency department (ED), and the emergency physician is expected to be expert in the field. Although the management must vary considerably according to the nature and severity of the poisoning, some general principles apply.

Above all, it must be remembered that the acute overdose presentation is only a discrete time-limited event in the course of the underlying condition, which is usually psychiatric or social in origin.

Pathophysiology and clinical features

The effects of ingestion of pharmaceuticals or illicit drugs range from the non-toxic to the life-threatening and may involve any system. Poisoning is a dynamic presentation and the patient may present at varying points in the time course of the poisoning. Consequently, rapid clinical deterioration or improvement may be observed after the initial presentation and assessment.

Acute morbidity and mortality from poisoning is usually a consequence of the cardiovascular, respiratory or central nervous system (CNS) complications of the poisoning. Less commonly, hepatic, renal or metabolic effects are potentially life-threatening.

The most frequent life-threatening respiratory complication of poisoning is ventilatory failure, which is usually a consequence of CNS depression. Less commonly, it is secondary to ventilatory muscle paralysis. The frequency and depth of respirations are reduced. Respiratory failure may also be caused by direct pulmonary toxicity, or complications such as pulmonary aspiration or non-cardiogenic pulmonary oedema (Table 29.1.1).

Cardiovascular manifestations of poisoning include tachycardia, bradycardia, hypertension, hypotension, conduction defects and arrhythmias (Table 29.1.2). Bradycardia is relatively rarely observed and is associated with a number of potentially life-threatening ingestions. Tachycardia is commonly observed and is usually benign. It may be due to intrinsic sympathomimetic or anticholinergic effects of a drug, or a reflex response to hypotension or hypoxia. Hypotension is also commonly observed and may be due to a number of different causes (Table 29.1.2). Hypertension is unusual. Severe hypertension is usually associated with illicit drug use and is important because it may produce complications such as intracerebral haemorrhage.

CNS manifestations of poisoning include decreased level of consciousness, agitation or delirium, seizures and disordered temperature regulation. A decreased level of consciousness is a common presentation of poisoning and is associated with many drugs,

some of which are listed in Table 29.1.1. Although usually a direct drug effect, CNS depression is occasionally secondary to hypoglycaemia, hypoxia or hypotension. Common causes of agitation or delirium following overdose are listed in Table 29.1.3. Toxic seizures are potentially life-threatening, and important causes are listed in Table 29.1.4.

Hypothermia is usually a complication of environmental exposure secondary to a decreased level of consciousness or altered behaviour. Hyperthermia is a direct toxic effect and causes are listed in Table 29.1.5. Severe hyperthermia is rapidly lethal if not corrected.

Metabolic and other manifestations of poisoning include hyper- and hypoglycaemia, hyper- and hyponatraemia, acidosis and alkalosis and hepatic failure.

Acute poisoning is distinguished from many other forms of acute illness in that, given appropriate supportive care over a relatively short period, a full recovery can usually be expected. A small number of potentially fatal poisonings may demonstrate progressive toxicity despite full supportive care. These are the so-called cellular toxins, and include colchicine, iron, salicylate, cyanide, paracetamol, theophylline and digoxin. In some of these cases early aggressive gastrointestinal decontamination, timely administration of antidotes

or the institution of techniques of enhanced elimination may be life saving.

Mortality or morbidity may also result from specific complications of a poisoning. These include trauma, pulmonary aspiration, adult respiratory distress syndrome, rhabdomyolysis, renal failure and hypoxic encephalopathy. These complications usually occur prior to arrival in the ED.

Pulmonary aspiration frequently complicates a period of decreased level of

---

Table 29.1.1 Toxic causes of respiratory failure

Central nervous system depression
Alcohols
Anticonvulsants
Antidepressants
Antihistamines
Barbiturates
Baclofen
Clonidine
Opioids
Phenothiazines
Sedative-hypnotics

Weakness of ventilatory muscles
Botulism
Carbamate pesticides
Muscle relaxants
Organophosphorus pesticides and warfare agents
Snakebite
Strychnine

Pulmonary
ARDS
Cardiogenic pulmonary oedema
Non-cardiogenic pulmonary oedema
Pulmonary aspiration and pneumonitis
  • Activated charcoal
  • Gastric contents
  • Hydrocarbons
Paraquat

Table 29.1.2 Cardiovascular effects of poisoning

Tachycardia
Anticholinergics
  • Antihistamines
  • Benztropine
  • Phenothiazines
  • Tricyclic antidepressants
Reflex response to hypotension
Sympathomimetics
  • Amphetamines
  • Caffeine
  • Cocaine
  • Theophylline

Bradycardia (includes AV block)
β-Blockers
Calcium channel blockers
Clonidine
Digoxin

Hypotension
Fluid loss/third spacing
Myocardial depressants
  • β-Blockers
  • Calcium channel blockers
Peripheral vasodilators

Hypertension
Anticholinergics
Sympathomimetics
  • Amphetamines
  • Cocaine
  • MAO inhibitors

Rhythm/ECG abnormalities
QRS prolongation (fast sodium channel blockade)
  • Class 1a and 1c antiarrhythmics
  • Thioridazine
  • Tricyclic antidepressants
  • Propranolol
QT prolongation/torsades de pointes
  • Amisulpride
  • Chloroquine
  • Citalopram
  • Quinine
  • Thioridazine
  • Tricyclic antidepressants
Ventricular tachycardia/fibrillation
  • Amphetamines
  • Chloral hydrate
  • Cocaine
  • Digoxin
  • Theophylline
  • Tricyclic antidepressants

Ischaemia/infarction
Cocaine
Complication of hypoxia or hypotension

Table 29.1.3 Toxic causes of agitation or delirium

Alcohol

Anticholinergic syndrome

Antidepressants
- Bupropion
- Venlafaxine

Atypical antipsychotic agents
- Olanzapine

Benzodiazepines and other sedative-hypnotics

Cannabis

Hallucinogenic agents

Serotonin syndrome

Sympathomimetic syndrome
- Amphetamines
- Cocaine

Theophylline

Withdrawal syndromes

Table 29.1.4 Toxic causes of seizures

Amphetamines

Bupropion

Carbamazepine

Chloroquine

Cocaine

Isoniazid

Mefanamic acid

Theophylline

Tramadol

Tricyclic antidepressants

Venlafaxine

Table 29.1.5 Toxic causes of hyperthermia

Amphetamines

Anticholinergics

Cocaine

MAO inhibitors

Salicylates

Serotonin syndrome

consciousness or a seizure. It is a leading cause of in-hospital morbidity and mortality following overdose. This complication is characterized by rapid onset of dyspnoea, cough, fever, wheeze and cyanosis.

Rhabdomyolysis occurs as a direct toxic effect (rare) or secondary to excessive muscular hyperactivity, seizures, hyperthermia or prolonged coma with direct muscle compression. The urine is dark and acute renal failure can develop secondary to tubular deposition of myoglobin.

Assessment

Risk assessment

A risk assessment should be made as soon as possible in the management of the poisoned patient. Only resuscitation is a greater priority (see Table 29.1.6). Risk assessment is a distinct quantitative cognitive step through which the clinician attempts to predict the likely clinical course and potential complications for the individual patient at that particular presentation.[4] An accurate risk assessment allows informed decision-making in regard to all subsequent management steps including duration and intensity of supportive care and monitoring, screening and specialized testing, decontamination, enhanced elimination, antidotes and disposition. Factors that are taken into account when formulating this risk assessment include: the agent(s), the dose, the time since ingestion, the clinical features present and patient factors (Table 29.1.6). Specialized

Table 29.1.6 Risk assessment-based approach to poisoning

Resuscitation
- Airway
- Breathing
- Circulation
- Control seizures
- Correct hypoglycaemia
- Correct hyperthermia
- Consider resuscitation antidotes

Risk assessment
- Agent
- Dose
- Time since ingestion
- Clinical features and course
- Patient factors

Supportive care and monitoring

Investigations
- Screening: 12-lead ECG, paracetamol
- Specific

Decontamination

Enhanced elimination

Antidotes

Disposition

Reproduced from Toxicology Handbook. Murray L, Daly F, Little M, Cadogan M. Elsevier, Sydney 2007.

testing may refine risk assessment. Access to specialized poisons information in the form of a poisons information centre or in-house databases is often necessary to formulate an accurate risk assessment.

History

Every effort should be made to obtain information as to the type and dose of drug ingested, the time of ingestion and the progression of symptoms since ingestion. History provided by the patient, if they are awake, is usually reliable and should not be dismissed.

Physical examination

The focused physical examination of the poisoned patient aims to:

- identify any immediate threats to life and the need for intervention
- establish a baseline clinical status
- corroborate the history
- identify intoxication syndromes
- identify possible alternative diagnoses
- identify any complications of the poisoning.

The initial physical examination of the overdose patient in many ways parallels the primary survey of the trauma patient. The airway, breathing and circulation are assessed and stabilized as necessary. The level of consciousness should be assessed, the presence of seizure activity noted and the blood glucose and temperature measured.

A more complete examination is carried out when the patient is stable. This should include a full neurological examination, including assessment of the level of consciousness and mental status, pupil size, muscle tone and movements and the presence or absence of focal neurological signs. Poisoning normally causes global CNS depression, and focal signs suggest an alternative diagnosis or a CNS complication such as cerebral haemorrhage.

Other features that should be specifically sought are any evidence of associated trauma, the state of hydration, the condition of the skin, in particular the presence of pressure areas, the presence or absence of bowel sounds and the condition of the urine.

Several toxic autonomic syndromes, or 'toxidromes', have been described in relation to poisoning. The principal ones are listed in Table 29.1.7. Identification of these syndromes may narrow the differential diagnosis in cases of unknown poisoning.[5]

Table 29.1.7 Toxic autonomic syndromes or 'toxidromes'

Toxidrome	Features	Common causes
Anticholinergic	Agitated delirium Tachycardia Hyperthermia Dilated pupils Dry flushed skin Urinary retention Ileus	Antihistamines Benztropine Carbamazepine Phenothiazines Plant poisonings Tricyclic antidepressants
Mixed cholinergic	Brady- or tachycardia Hypo- or hypertension Miosis or mydriasis Sweating Increased bronchial secretion Gastrointestinal hyperactivity Muscle weakness Fasciculations	Organophosphates Carbamates
Mixed α- and β-adrenergic	Hypertension Tachycardia Mydriasis Agitation	Amphetamines Cocaine
β-Adrenergic	Hypotension Tachycardia Hypokalaemia Hyperglycaemia	Caffeine Salbutamol Theophylline
Serotonin	Altered mental status Autonomic dysfunction Fever Hypertension Sweating Tachycardia Motor dysfunction Hyperreflexia Hypertonia (esp. lower limbs) Myoclonus	Amphetamines Antihistamines Monoamine oxidase inhibitors NSSRIs SSRIs Tricyclic antidepressants (Usually combined overdose)

NSSRI, non-selective serotonin re-uptake inhibitor; SSRI, selective serotonin re-uptake inhibitor.

Table 29.1.8 Supportive care measures for the poisoned patient

Airway	Endotracheal intubation
Breathing	Supplemental oxygen Ventilation
Circulation	Intravenous fluids Inotropes Antihypertensives Antiarrhythmics Defibrillation/cardioversion Cardiac pacing Cardiopulmonary bypass
Metabolic	Hypertonic dextrose Hypertonic saline Insulin/dextrose Calcium salts Sodium bicarbonate
Agitation/ delirium	Benzodiazepines Butyrophenones
Seizures	Benzodiazepines Barbiturates
Body temperature	External rewarming External cooling
Impaired renal function	Rehydration Haemodialysis

Poisons information

Information on the clinical course and toxic doses of specific pharmaceutical and non-pharmaceutical poisons is available on a 24 h basis throughout Australia by telephoning 131126. The poison information centres are staffed by pharmacists and are also able to refer cases to clinical toxicologists for consultation.

Treatment

The management of poisoning should be approached in a systematic way. Following initial resuscitation, further treatment is informed by the risk assessment (Table 29.1.6).

Resuscitation, supportive care and monitoring

Supportive care is the key element in the management of poisoning. The vast majority of poisonings result in temporary dysfunction of one or more of the body systems. If appropriate support of the system in question is instituted in a timely fashion and continued until the toxic substance is metabolized or excreted, a good outcome can be anticipated. In severe poisonings supportive care may be very aggressive, and possible interventions are listed in Table 29.1.8.

The specific supportive management of a number of manifestations or complications of poisoning warrants further mention insofar as it may differ from the standard management of such conditions with other aetiologies.

Cardiopulmonary arrest from poisoning should be aggressively resuscitated. Direct current cardioversion is rarely successful in terminating toxic arrhythmias and should not take precedence over establishing adequate ventilation and oxygenation, cardiac compressions, correction of acidosis or hypovolaemia and the administration of specific antidotes. Resuscitative efforts should be continued beyond the usual timeframe. In cardiac arrest due to drugs with direct cardiac toxicity, the use of cardiopulmonary bypass or extracorporeal membrane oxygenation (ECMO) until the drug is metabolized may be life-saving.

In general, intravenous benzodiazepines are the drugs of choice for control of toxic seizures. Large doses may be required. Hypoxia and hypoglycaemia must be corrected if they are contributory factors. Patients with toxic seizures do not generally need long-term anticonvulsant therapy. Isoniazid-induced seizures are not controlled without administration of an adequate dose of the specific antidote, pyridoxine.

The management of pulmonary aspiration is essentially supportive, with supplemental oxygenation and intubation and mechanical ventilation if necessary. Neither prophylactic antibiotics nor corticosteroids have been shown to be helpful in the management of this condition, which is essentially a chemical pneumonitis.

Toxic hypertension rarely requires specific therapy. Most cases are mild and simple observation is sufficient. Agitation or delirium is a feature of many intoxications associated with hypertension, and adequate sedation with benzodiazepines usually lowers the blood pressure. Severe toxic hypertension is most likely in toxicity from cocaine or amphetamine-type drugs, and treatment may be indicated to avoid complications such as cardiac failure or intracerebral haemorrhage. The drug of choice in this situation is sodium nitroprusside by intravenous infusion. The extremely short duration of action of this vasodilator allows accurate control of hypertension during the toxic phase, and avoids the development of hypotension once toxicity begins to wear off.

Management of rhabdomyolysis consists of treatment of the causative factors, fluid resuscitation and careful monitoring of fluids and electrolytes. The role of mannitol and urinary alkalinization in reducing the risk of renal failure is not clear. Established acute renal failure requires haemodialysis, often for up to 6 weeks.

Decontamination

The aim of decontamination of the gastro-intestinal tract is to bind or remove ingested material before it is absorbed into the circulation and able to exert its toxic effects. This is a very attractive concept and has long been considered one of the fundamental interventions in management of the overdose patient.

However, gastrointestinal decontamination should not be regarded as a routine procedure in the management of the patient presenting to the ED following an overdose. The decision to perform gastrointestinal decontamination and the choice of method should be based on an assessment of the likely benefit, the likely risk and the resources required. Gastrointestinal decontamination should only be considered where there is likely to be a significant amount of a significantly toxic material remaining in the gut. It is never indicated when the risk assessment predicts a benign course. Efforts at decontamination technique should never take precedence over the institution of appropriate supportive care.

Three basic approaches to gastrointestinal decontamination are available: gastric emptying, administration of an adsorbent and catharsis.

Gastric emptying can be attempted by the administration of an emetic, most commonly syrup of ipecac, or by gastric lavage. In volunteer studies both of these techniques removed highly variable amounts of marker substances from the stomach even if performed immediately after ingestion, and the effect diminished rapidly with time to the point of being negligible after one hour.[6,7] Clinical outcome trials have failed to demonstrate improved outcome as a result of routine gastric emptying in

Table 29.1.9	Materials that do not bind well to activated charcoal

Alcohols
- Ethanol
- Ethylene glycol
- Isopropanol
- Methanol

Corrosives
- Acids
- Alkalis

Hydrocarbons

Metals and their salts
- Iron
- Lead
- Lithium
- Potassium

addition to administration of activated charcoal, except, perhaps, in patients presenting unconscious within 1 h of ingestion.[8–10]

The principal adsorbent available to clinicians is activated charcoal (AC), which effectively binds most pharmaceuticals and chemicals, and is currently the decontamination method of choice for most poisonings. Materials that do not bind well to charcoal are listed in Table 29.1.9.

Charcoal is 'activated' by treatment in acid and steam at high temperature. This process removes impurities and greatly increases the surface area available for binding. Activated charcoal is packaged as a 50 g dose premixed with water or sorbitol, which is likely to be sufficient for the majority of ingestions. Adult patients are usually able to drink AC slurry from a cup. If the level of consciousness is too impaired to allow this, they should be intubated first. Administration of AC is absolutely contraindicated unless the patient has an intact or protected airway.

Volunteer studies demonstrate that the effect of AC diminishes rapidly with time and that the greatest benefit occurs if it is administered within 1 h. There is as yet no evidence that AC improves clinical outcome.[11]

There is no evidence to suggest that the addition of a cathartic such as sorbitol to AC improves clinical outcome.[12,13]

Apart from rarely employed endoscopic and surgical techniques, whole-bowel irrigation (WBI) is the most aggressive form of gastrointestinal decontamination. Polyethylene glycol solution (Golytely™) is administered via a nasogastric tube at a rate of 2 L/h until a clear rectal effluent is produced. This usually takes about 6 h and requires one-to-one nursing. In volunteer studies, this technique reduced the absorption of slow-release pharmaceuticals and so may be of benefit in life-threatening overdoses of these agents.[13,14] Again, clinical benefit has not yet been conclusively demonstrated.[15] The use of WBI has also been reported in the management of potentially toxic ingestions of iron, lead and packets of illicit drugs. Whole-bowel irrigation is contraindicated if there is evidence of ileus or bowel obstruction, and in patients who have an unprotected airway or haemodynamic compromise.[16]

Enhanced elimination

A number of techniques are available to enhance the elimination of toxins from the body. Their use is rarely indicated, as only a very few drugs capable of causing severe poisoning have pharmacokinetic parameters that render them amenable to these techniques (Table 29.1.10).

Repeat-dose AC (25–50 g every 3–4 h) may enhance drug elimination by interrupting the enterohepatic circulation or by 'gastrointestinal dialysis'. Gastrointestinal dialysis is the movement of a toxin across the gastrointestinal wall from the circulation into the gut down a concentration gradient that is maintained by charcoal binding. For this technique to be effective, a drug must undergo considerable enterohepatic circulation or, in the case of 'gastrointestinal dialysis', have a small volume of distribution, small molecular weight, low protein binding, slow

Table 29.1.10	Techniques of enhanced elimination
Technique	**Suitable toxin**
Repeat-dose activated charcoal	Carbamazepine Dapsone Phenobarbitone Phenytoin Salicylate Theophylline
Urinary alkalinization	Phenobarbitone Salicylate
Haemodialysis	Ethylene glycol Lithium Methanol Salicylate Theophylline
Haemoperfusion	Theophylline

endogenous elimination and bind to charcoal.[16,17] The advantages of this technique are that it is non-invasive and simple to carry out.

Alkalinization of the urine enhances urinary excretion of drugs that are filtered at the glomerulus and are unable to be reabsorbed across the tubular epithelium when in an ionized form at alkaline pH. For elimination to be effectively enhanced by this method, the drug must be predominantly eliminated by the kidneys in the unchanged form, have a low pKa, be distributed mainly to the extracellular fluid compartment and be minimally protein bound.[18]

Haemodialysis (HD) and haemoperfusion (HP) are both very invasive techniques and for that reason are reserved for potentially life-threatening intoxications. Only a small number of drugs that have small volumes of distribution, slow endogenous clearance rates, small molecular weights (HD) and bind to charcoal (HP) will have their rates of elimination significantly enhanced by these procedures.

Antidotes

Very few drugs have effective antidotes. Occasionally, however, timely use of an antidote may be life saving or substantially reduce morbidity, time in hospital or resource requirements. Antidotes that may be indicated in the ED setting are listed in Table 29.1.11. However, it must be remembered that antidotes are also drugs, and are frequently associated with adverse effects of their own. An antidote should only be used where a specific indication exists, and then only at the correct dose, by the correct route, and with appropriate monitoring. Because many antidotes are so infrequently used, obtaining sufficient supplies when the need arises can be difficult. Every ED must review its stocking of antidotes and have a plan for obtaining further supplies should the need arise.

Differential diagnosis

It is essential to exclude important non-toxic diagnoses in the patient presenting with coma or altered mental status presumed to be due to drug overdose. These diagnoses include head injury, intracerebral haemorrhage or infarction, CNS infection, hyponatraemia, hypoglycaemia, hypo- or hyperthermia, postictal states and psychiatric disorders.

Table 29.1.11	Useful emergency antidotes
Poisoning	**Antidote**
Atropine	Physostigmine
Benzodiazepines	Flumazenil
Cyanide	Dicobalt edetate, hydroxocobalamin
Digoxin	Digoxin-specific Fab fragments
Insulin	Dextrose
Iron	Desferoxamine
Isoniazid	Pyridoxine
Methaemoglobinaemia	Methylene blue
Methanol and ethylene glycol	Ethanol, fomepizole
Organophosphates and carbamates	Atropine, oximes
Opioids	Naloxone
Paracetamol	N-acetyl cysteine
Sulphonylureas	Dextrose, octreotide
Tricyclic antidepressants	Sodium bicarbonate
Warfarin, brodifacoum	Vitamin K

Clinical investigation

Investigations should only be performed if they are likely to affect the management of the patient. They are employed as either screening tests or for specific purposes.

In poisoning, screening tests aim to identify occult toxic ingestions for which early specific treatment might improve outcome. The recommended screening tests for acute poisoning are the 12-lead ECG and the serum paracetamol level. The ECG is used to exclude conduction defects, which may predict potentially life-threatening cardiotoxicity. The serum paracetamol is useful to ensure that paracetamol poisoning is diagnosed within the time available for effective antidotal treatment.

Other specific investigations may be indicated to exclude important differential diagnoses, confirm a specific poisoning for which significant complications might be anticipated, assess the severity of intoxication, assess response to treatment or assess the need for a specific antidote or enhanced elimination technique.

The patient with only minor manifestations of poisoning may require no other blood tests apart from a screening paracetamol level. Pregnancy should be excluded in women of childbearing age by serum or urine β-HCG if necessary. More seriously ill patients may require electrolyte, renal and liver function tests and a full blood count, creatine kinase and arterial blood gases. Urinalysis reveals myoglobinuria in significant rhabdomyolysis.

Routine qualitative drug screening of urine or blood in the overdose patient is rarely useful in planning management.

Measurement of serum drug concentrations is only useful if this provides important diagnostic or prognostic information, or assists in planning management. Some drug levels that may be useful are listed in Table 29.1.12. For most cases, drug overdose management is guided by clinical findings and not by drug levels. Some drugs commonly taken in overdose for which serum concentrations are of no value in planning management are listed in Table 29.1.13.

Radiology has a limited role in the management of overdose. A chest X-ray is indicated in any patient with a significantly decreased level of consciousness, seizures or hypoxia. It may show evidence of pulmonary aspiration. A computerized tomography scan of the head may be indicated to exclude other intracranial pathology in the patient with an altered mental status. The abdominal X-ray is useful in evaluating overdose of radio-opaque metals including iron, lithium, potassium, lead and arsenic.

Table 29.1.12 Drug levels that may be helpful in the management of selected cases of overdose
Carbamazepine
Digoxin
Dilantin
Lithium
Iron
Paracetamol
Phenobarbitone
Salicylate
Theophylline
Valproate

Table 29.1.13 Drug levels that are not helpful in the management of overdose

CNS drugs	Cardiovascular drugs
Antidepressants	ACE inhibitors
Benzodiazepines	Beta-blockers
Benztropine	Calcium channel blockers
Cocaine	Clonidine
Newer antipsychotics	
Opiates	
Phenothiazines	

Disposition

Both the medical and the psychiatric disposition of the overdose patient must be considered. A good risk assessment is essential to determining timely and safe disposition.

The majority of overdose patients who remain stable at 4–6 h after the ingestion do not need further close monitoring and may be admitted to a non-monitored bed until manifestations of toxicity completely resolve. An emergency observation ward is ideal for this purpose.

Any patient who develops clinical manifestations of intoxication severe enough to require the institution of specific supportive care measures requires admission to an intensive care environment. A few patients will require admission for prolonged monitoring based on the history of the ingestion. For example, anyone with a history of ingestion of colchicine, organophosphates, slow-release theophylline or slow-release calcium channel blockers requires admission because of the possibility of delayed onset of severe toxicity.

Psychiatric evaluation of deliberate self-poisoning cases is indicated as soon as the patient's medical condition permits. All such patients must be continuously supervised until the psychiatric evaluation has taken place.

Controversies

❶ The role of, choice of method, and indications for gastric decontamination remain controversial. These procedures are no longer regarded as routine, but there are likely to be subgroups of overdose patients who may derive clinical benefit from gastrointestinal decontamination. These groups have not yet been precisely identified.

❷ The clinical and economic utility of establishing specialized toxicology treatment centres.[19,20]

References

1. Hawton K, Fagg J. Trends in deliberate self-poisoning and self-injury in Oxford. British Medical Journal 1992; 304: 1409–1411.
2. McGrath J. A survey of deliberate self-poisoning. Medical Journal of Australia 1989; 150: 317–322.
3. Pond SM. Prescription for poisoning. Medical Journal of Australia 1995; 162: 174–175.
4. Murray L, Daly F, Little M, Cadogan M, eds. Toxicology handbook. Sydney: Elsevier; 2007.
5. Kulig K. Initial management of ingestion of toxic substances. New England Journal of Medicine 1992; 326: 1677.
6. Krenzelok EP, McGuigan M, Lheureux P. Position statement: ipecac syrup. American Academy of Clinical Toxicology; European Association of Poisons Centres and Clinical Toxicologists. Journal of Toxicology – Clinical Toxicology 1997; 35(7): 699–709.
7. Vale JA. Position statement: gastric lavage. American Academy of Clinical Toxicology; European Association of Poisons Centres and Clinical Toxicologists. Journal of Toxicology – Clinical Toxicology 1997; 35(7): 711–719.
8. Kulig K, Bar-Or D, Kantrill SV, et al. Management of acutely poisoned patients without gastric emptying. Annals of Emergency Medicine 1990; 14: 562–567.
9. Merigian KS, Woodard M, Hedges JR, et al. Prospective evaluation of gastric emptying in the self-poisoned patient. American Journal of Emergency Medicine 1990; 8: 479–483
10. Pond SM, Lewis-Driver DJ, Williams G, et al. Gastric emptying in acute overdose: a prospective randomised controlled trial. Medical Journal of Australia 1995; 163: 345–349.
11. Chyka PA, Seger D. Position statement: single-dose activated charcoal. American Academy of Clinical Toxicology; European Association of Poisons Centres and Clinical Toxicologists. Journal of Toxicology – Clinical Toxicology 1997; 35(7):721–741.
12. Barceloux D, McGuigan M, Hartigan-Go K. Position statement: cathartics. American Academy of Clinical Toxicology; European Association of Poisons Centres and Clinical Toxicologists. Journal of Toxicology – Clinical Toxicology 1997; 35(7): 743–752.
13. Kirshenbaum LA, Mathew SC, Sitar DS, et al. Whole-bowel irrigation versus activated charcoal in sorbitol for the ingestion of modified-release pharmaceuticals. Clinical Pharmacology Therapy 1989; 46: 264–271.
14. Smith SW, Ling LJ, Halstenson CE. Whole-bowel irrigation as a treatment for acute lithium overdose. Annals of Emergency Medicine 1991; 20: 536–539.
15. Tenenbein M. Position statement: whole bowel irrigation. American Academy of Clinical Toxicology; European Association of Poisons Centres and Clinical Toxicologists. Journal of Toxicology – Clinical Toxicology 1997; 35(7): 753–756.
16. Pond SM. Role of repeated oral doses of activated charcoal in clinical toxicology. Medical Toxicology 1986; 1: 3–11.
17. Chyka PA. Multiple-dose activated charcoal and enhancement of systemic drug clearance: summary of studies in animals and human volunteers. Clinical Toxicology 1995; 33: 399–405.
18. Winchester JF. Active methods for detoxification. In: Haddad LM, Shannon MW, Winchester JF, eds. Clinical management of poisoning and drug overdose. 3rd edn. Philadelphia: WB Saunders; 1998.
19. Whyte IM, Dawson AH, Buckley NA, et al. A model for the management of self-poisoning. Medical Journal of Australia 1997; 167: 142–146.
20. Lee V, Kerr JF, Braitberg G, et al. Impact of a toxicology service on a metropolitan teaching hospital. Emergency Medicine 2001; 13: 37–42.

29.2 Cardiovascular drugs

Betty Chan • Lindsay Murray

ESSENTIALS

1 Many cardiovascular medications, including the calcium channel blockers, the β-blockers and digoxin, are associated with potentially life-threatening toxicity.

2 The key to the management of calcium channel blocker and β-blocker toxicity rests with aggressive supportive care of the circulation including early use of hyperinsulinaemia euglycaemia therapy.

3 The onset of toxicity following overdose with slow-release formulations of calcium channel blockers may be delayed.

4 Early aggressive decontamination with whole-bowel irrigation is important in the management of slow-release calcium channel blocker overdose.

5 Early identification of patients presenting with potentially severe digoxin toxicity and appropriate use of the specific Fab fragment antibody is life saving.

6 The management of clonidine poisoning is largely supportive.

CALCIUM CHANNEL BLOCKERS AND β-BLOCKERS

Introduction

The calcium channel blockers (CCBs) and β-blockers are widely prescribed in the community. In overdose, they present with similar clinical pictures of potentially life-threatening impairment of cardiac function. The management of both types of overdose is similar and they are discussed together.

Pharmacokinetics

Standard CCB preparations are rapidly absorbed from the gastrointestinal tract, with onset of action occurring within 30 min.[1] Pharmacokinetic parameters are shown in Table 29.2.1. Verapamil and diltiazem undergo significant first-pass hepatic clearance. Verapamil is metabolized to norverapamil, which possesses 15–20% of verapamil's pharmacological activity and is renally excreted. Diltiazem is metabolized to deacetyldiltiazem, which has half the potency of the parent compound and undergoes biliary excretion. The elimination half-lives of all

CCBs may be prolonged following massive overdose. Amlodipine has a longer plasma half-life (30–50 h) than other CCBs.

Importantly, slow-release preparations of both verapamil and diltiazem are widely prescribed and are associated with much longer times to peak plasma concentration and clinical effect.

Absorption of β-blockers is rapid, with peak clinical effects occurring within 1–4 h. Pharmacokinetic parameters of the principal β-blockers are detailed in Table 29.2.2. Agents with high lipid solubility, such as propranolol, penetrate the blood–brain barrier better than the water-soluble agents, and hence cause greater central nervous system (CNS) toxicity.

Pathophysiology

CCBs antagonize the entry of extracellular calcium into cardiac and smooth muscle, but not skeletal muscle. Upon entry into cells, calcium participates in mechanical, electrical and biochemical reactions. It is involved in excitation–contraction of cardiac and smooth muscles, as well as phase 0 depolarization in the sinus and atrioventricular

Table 29.2.1 Pharmacological profiles of the calcium channel blockers			
Class	*Phenylalkylamines*	*Benzothiazepines*	*Dihydropyridines*
Prototype	Verapamil	Diltiazem	Nifedipine
Hours to peak plasma concentration (NR/SR)	1.5/5–7	2.3/5–11	0.5/5
Half-life (h)	3–7/10–12	3–5/6–7	2–5/5–7
Half-life in massive overdose (h)	10–12	8–9	7–8
Absorption (%)	>90	>90	>90
Vd (L/kg)	4	5	1.2
Protein binding (%)	90	80–90	90
Predominant excretion route	(1) Hepatic (2) Renal	Hepatic	Renal
Active metabolite	Yes (20%)	Yes (25–50%)	No
Heart rate (%)	−10	−15	+10
Systemic vascular resistance (%)	−10	−10	−20
AV node conduction velocity (%)	−20	−25	+10

NR, normal release; SR, slow release.
(Adapted from: Kerns W II, Kline J, Ford MD β-blocker and calcium channel blocker toxicity. Emergency Medicine Clinics of North America 1994; 12:365–389.)

Table 29.2.2 Pharmacological profiles of the β-blockers

Agent	β_1 selective	Membrane stabilization	Absorption (%)	Protein binding (%)	Volume of distribution (L/kg)	Elimination/ half-life (h)	Lipophilic
Atenolol	Yes	No	50	<5	0.6–1.1	Renal/6–9	Weak
Carvedilol	No	Yes	25	98	2	Hepatic/6	Weak
Esmolol	Yes	No	NA	55	3.4	Blood esterase 9 min	Weak
Labetalol	No	No	90	50	5.1–9.4	Hepatic/3–4	Weak
Metoprolol	Yes	No	90	12	5.6	Hepatic/3–4	Moderate
Oxyprenolol	No	Yes	90	80	1.2	Hepatic/2–3	Moderate
Pindolol	No	Yes	90	57	1.2–2	Renal/3–4	Moderate
Propranolol	No	Yes	90	93	3.4–6	Hepatic/3–4	High
Sotalol	No	No	70	0	0.23–0.7	Renal/9–10	Weak
Timolol	No	No	90	10	1.3–3.6	Renal/4–5	Weak

(Adapted from: Kerns W II, Kline J, Ford MD β-blocker and calcium channel blocker toxicity. Emergency Medicine Clinics of North America 1994; 12:365–389.)

(AV) nodes by calcium influx through channels.[2] CCBs affect myocardial contractility and slow conduction through the sinus and AV nodes. Contraction of smooth muscle is mediated by calcium influx, which is inhibited by CCBs. This results in vasodilatation and secondary reflex tachycardia from an increase in sympathetic activity.

The different classes of CCB have somewhat different pharmacological and toxic effects, as a consequence of their different binding characteristics to the dihydropyridine (DHP) receptors. Verapamil, a phenylalkylamine, produces more profound cardiac conduction defects and equal reductions in systemic vascular resistance when compared with other CCBs on a mg/kg basis.[1] Verapamil is more likely to produce symptomatic decreases in blood pressure, heart rate and cardiac output than diltiazem, a benzothiazepine. The DHPs, which include amlodipine, felodipine, lercanidipine and nifedipine preferentially bind to vascular smooth muscle and predominantly decrease systemic and coronary vascular resistance. With the exception of felodipine, they also produce a reflex tachycardia by the unloading of baroreceptors.

β-blockers prevent the binding of catecholamines to β receptors (β_1, β_2). β_1 receptors are located in the myocardium, kidney and eye, and β_2 receptors in adipose tissue, pancreas, liver and both smooth and skeletal muscle. β_1 stimulation produces increased chronotropy and inotropy in the heart, increased renin secretion in the kidney and increased aqueous humor production. β_2 stimulation relaxes smooth muscle in the blood vessels, bronchial tree, intestinal tract and uterus.

Blockade of β receptors results in increased intracellular cAMP concentrations, with a resultant blunting of the metabolic, chronotropic and inotropic effects of catecholamines. Some β-blockers, especially propranolol, may also impede sodium entry via myocardial fast inward sodium channels, thus slowing phase 0 of the action potential. This results in a prolonged QRS duration on the electrocardiogram and produces cardiotoxicity in overdose more like that of the tricyclic antidepressants.

The different β-blockers have slightly differing pharmacological properties, including selectivity for β adrenoreceptors, intrinsic sympathomimetic activity and membrane-stabilizing activity. The relative affinity for β adrenoreceptors may influence expression of toxicity. Atenolol, esmolol and metoprolol are β_1-selective agents, and therapeutic use of these drugs is less likely to produce the peripheral vasoconstriction, bronchospasm and disturbances in glucose homoeostasis that result from β_2 inhibition. However, pharmacological specificity decreases with increasing dose.[3] Several β-blockers have partial agonist activity such that, although they block the β receptor to catecholamines, they also weakly stimulate the receptor. This partial agonist activity may have a protective effect in overdose.

Clinical features

Calcium channel blockers

The severity of toxicity is determined by a number of factors, including the amount and characteristics of the drug ingested, the underlying health of the patient, co-ingestants and delay until treatment. The majority of serious cases result from the ingestion of verapamil or diltiazem, the most toxic of the CCBs. Elderly patients and those with congestive cardiac failure are more prone to develop CCB poisoning. The principal clinical features are shown in Table 29.2.3. Ingestion of toxic amounts of standard preparations typically

Table 29.2.3 Clinical features of CCB overdose

Central nervous system
- Lethargy, slurred speech, confusion, coma
- Respiratory arrest
- Coma

Gastrointestinal
- Nausea, vomiting

Cardiovascular
- Hypotension
- Bradycardia and other arrhythmias
- Sinus bradycardia
- Accelerated AV nodal rhythm
- 2° AV block
- 3° AV block with AV nodal or ventricular escape rhythm
- Sinus arrest with AV nodal escape rhythm
- Asystole

Metabolic
- Hyperglycaemia
- Lactic acidosis

produces symptoms within 2 h, although maximal toxicity may not occur for up to 6–8 h. The slow-release preparations can produce significant toxicity, with onset of symptoms more than 6 h post ingestion. The major threats to life are myocardial depression and hypotension. Nifedipine produces tachycardia with normal blood pressure during the first 30 min, followed later by hypotension and bradycardia in large ingestions (>10 mg/kg). With verapamil and diltiazem poisoning, nausea, vomiting, hyperglycaemia and metabolic acidosis can develop. All CCBs can cause symptoms of cerebral hypoperfusion, such as syncope, lethargy, lightheadedness, dizziness, altered mental status, seizures and coma.

β-blockers

In one large series of patients with β-blocker overdose, 30–40% of patients remained asymptomatic and only 20% developed severe toxicity.[4] Toxicity is more likely to develop after ingestion of propranolol, in patients with pre-existing cardiac disease or where there is co-ingestion of other drugs with effects on the cardiovascular system, especially CCBs and cyclic antidepressants.[4,5] If β-blocker toxicity is to develop, it is usually observed within 6 h of ingestion.[5,6]

Sinus node suppression and conduction abnormalities and decreased contractility are typical. First-degree AV block, AV dissociation, right bundle branch block and intraventricular conduction delay have been reported.

Propranol overdose is characterized by cardiotoxicity including prolongation of the QRS interval and ventricular arrhythmias that more closely resemble tricyclic antidepressant overdose; a consequence of the sodium channel blocking effects.

Sotalol has both β-blocker activity and class III antiarrhythmic properties. Class III drugs lengthen the duration of the QT interval owing to prolongation of the action potential in His-Purkinje tissue. Therefore, ventricular arrhythmias are more common with sotalol.

Hypotension occurs as a result of negative inotropic effect. In addition, CNS effects, such as depressed conscious level and seizures, can occur, especially with the more lipid-soluble and membrane-depressant agents such as propranolol. Hypoglycaemia is reported following atenolol overdose.

Clinical investigation

The ECG is essential in evaluating and monitoring toxic conduction defects. Serum drug levels are unhelpful in management. Patients with severe toxicity require monitoring of serum electrolytes and glucose. Serum calcium must be closely monitored if calcium salts are administered therapeutically.

Treatment

The primary aim in both β-blocker and CCB toxicity is to restore perfusion to vital organs by increasing cardiac output, and the methods used are similar.

Supportive management may include airway and ventilatory support, intravenous fluid administration, transcutaneous or transvenous pacing and administration of inotropes. Severe cases may require placement of a Swan–Ganz catheter and invasive blood pressure monitoring.

Oral-activated charcoal should be administered as soon as practicable to all patients presenting within 2–4 h of ingestion, and to all those presenting after ingestion of slow-release preparations. More aggressive decontamination, with whole-bowel irrigation, is indicated following overdose with slow-release CCBs.[7]

A number of drugs play a role in the management of significant CCB or β-blocker poisoning, although none is a completely effective antidote. Suggested doses are shown in Table 29.2.4.

Calcium, an inotropic agent, is the initial drug of choice for CCB toxicity. Administration must be closely monitored, with ionized calcium measured 30 min after commencing the infusion, and then second-hourly.[8] Catecholamines are useful in attempting to restore adequate tissue perfusion.

Glucagon, a polypeptide hormone of pancreatic origin, enhances myocardial performance by increasing intracellular cAMP concentrations. This increase in cAMP triggers the release of cAMP-dependent protein kinase, which activates the calcium channels, causing an increase in heart rate and myocardial contractility. It works independently from that of the β-adrenoreceptor stimulation of the heart. Use of glucagon is supported only by case reports and some animal studies. There are no clinical trials supporting its efficacy in either calcium channel or beta-blocker poisoning and its role in management of these poisoning is questioned.[9] It is frequently difficult to source adequate stocks of glucagon for use as an inotropic agent.

Hyperinsulinaemic euglycaemia therapy (HIET) is increasingly advocated as therapy for hypotension unresponsive to fluids, calcium salts and inotropes. This therapy is supported by animal work[10,11] and promising initial human case reports[12] but again clinical trials are lacking. Insulin administration switches cardiac cell metabolism from fatty acids to carbohydrates. It restores calcium fluxes and improves myocardial contractility. The recommended initial dose of actrapid is 1 U/kg i.v. followed by an infusion of 0.5–1 U/kg/h. This should be accompanied by an initial bolus dose of 50 mL 50% dextrose followed by an infusion to maintain euglycaemia.[13]

Table 29.2.4 Useful drugs in the management of CCB and β-blocker toxicity		
	CCBs	**β-Blockers**
Calcium	0.5–1 g (5–10 mLs) calcium chloride or 1–2 g (10–20 mLs) calcium gluconate i.v. over 5–10 minutes. Repeat every 10–15 minutes as required. Further administration guided by serum calcium concentrations.	
Catecholamines	Adrenaline (epinephrine) infusion started at 1 µg/kg/min and titrate to maintain organ perfusion.	Isoprenaline or adrenaline (epinephrine) infusion titrated to maintain organ perfusion.
Glucagon	A bolus dose of 5–10 mg followed by an infusion of 1–5 mg/h.	A bolus dose of 5–10 mg followed by an infusion of 1–5 mg/h.
Hyperinsulinaemia euglycaemia	Actrapid 1 U/kg i.v. bolus followed by 0.5–1 U/kg/hr infusion. Give with 50% dextrose 50 mL followed by infusion to maintain euglycaemia.	Actrapid 1 U/kg i.v. bolus followed by 0.5–1 U/kg/hr infusion. Give with 50% dextrose 50 mL followed by infusion to maintain euglycaemia.

Severe propranolol toxicity is usually due to sodium channel blockade and treatment as for tricyclic antidepressant poisoning, including intubation, ventilation and sodium bicarbonate, is appropriate.

There are no clinically effective methods of enhancing the elimination of CCBs or β-blockers.

Disposition

Following overdose of β-blockers or standard CCBs, patients should be observed in a monitored environment for at least 6 h. Overdoses of slow-release CCBs require monitoring for at least 16 h from the time of ingestion. All symptomatic patients should be admitted to a monitored environment until toxicity resolves.

DIGOXIN

Introduction

Both chronic and acute digoxin toxicity are potentially life-threatening presentations to the emergency department (ED). Early recognition and administration of the specific Fab fragment antidote, if indicated, usually results in a good outcome.

Pharmacokinetics

Digoxin is moderately well absorbed following oral administration, with a bioavailability in the range of 50–80%. The initial volume of distribution is relatively small, but it is then slowly redistributed, predominantly to skeletal muscle, to give a relatively large volume of distribution of approximately 8 L/kg. Digoxin is excreted predominantly unchanged by the kidney, with an elimination half-life of about 36 h.

Pathophysiology

At a subcellular level digoxin inhibits the function of Na-K ATPase, which leads to intracellular depletion of potassium and accumulation of sodium and calcium ions. Alteration of ionic fluxes affects cell membrane conduction. At toxic concentrations of digoxin, the effects on the cardiac conducting system produce decreased conduction velocity throughout the system, increased refractoriness at the AV node and enhanced automaticity of the Purkinje fibres. Vagal tone is also enhanced. In acute digoxin poisoning the sudden loss of Na-K ATPase function produces hyperkalaemia.

Clinical features

Two distinct clinical presentations of digoxin toxicity are observed: acute and chronic. Both are characterized by cardiac arrhythmias, and virtually all types of arrhythmia have been reported in the context of digoxin toxicity.[14]

Acute digoxin overdose in adults is usually intentional. The therapeutic margin for digoxin is relatively narrow, and any ingestion with suicidal intent is regarded as potentially life-threatening.

The non-cardiac manifestations of toxicity are nausea and vomiting and hypokalaemia. Nausea and vomiting occur early and may be the presenting complaint. The most common cardiac manifestations are sinus bradycardia, sinoatrial node arrest and first-, second- or third-degree heart block. Ventricular tachycardia and fibrillation may occur. In significant acute overdose progressive worsening of the conduction disturbance over a period of hours is usually observed.

Chronic digoxin toxicity may be precipitated by therapeutic errors, intercurrent illnesses that decrease renal elimination of digoxin or by drug interactions. Common drug interactions include those with quinidine, CCBs, amiodarone and indometacin. The patient is commonly elderly. Reduced muscle mass and reduced renal function in the elderly mean that both the volume of distribution and rate of elimination of digoxin may be substantially reduced.

Nausea and vomiting are also common manifestations of chronic digoxin toxicity and are frequent presenting symptoms. Neurological manifestations are characteristic of chronic toxicity and include visual disturbances, weakness and fatigue. The most common cardiovascular manifestations of chronic digoxin toxicity are arrhythmias, and these may be sinus bradycardia, atrial fibrillation with slowed ventricular response or a junctional escape rhythm, atrial tachycardia with block and ventricular tachycardia and fibrillation.

Death from digoxin toxicity results from pump failure, severe cardiac conduction impairment or ventricular arrhythmia.

Clinical investigation

The most important investigations are the ECG, serum electrolytes and creatinine and serum digoxin concentration.

The ECG is invaluable in documenting the type and severity of any cardiac conduction defect. Serial ECGs may demonstrate worsening of the cardiac conduction defects as toxicity progresses.

In acute poisoning the serum potassium rises as Na-K ATPase function is progressively impaired. Hyperkalaemia denotes significant acute digoxin toxicity. Prior to the availability of a specific antidote for digoxin poisoning, a serum potassium concentration >5.5 mEq/L was associated with a high probability of lethal outcome.[16] Hyperkalaemia is not usually observed in chronic digoxin toxicity. In fact, these patients are frequently hypokalaemic and hypomagnesaemic secondary to chronic diuretic use. Both these electrolyte disorders are important as they exacerbate digoxin toxicity.

Serum digoxin concentrations are extremely useful in assessing and confirming toxicity, but must be carefully interpreted in the context of the clinical presentation. They do not accurately correlate with clinical toxicity. Therapeutic concentrations are usually quoted as 0.6–2.3 nmol/L (0.5–1.8 μg/L). Significant chronic toxicity may be associated with relatively minor elevations of the serum digoxin concentration. This is particularly the case in the presence of pre-existing cardiac disease, hypokalaemia or hypomagnesaemia. Following acute overdose the serum digoxin concentration is relatively high compared to tissue concentrations, until distribution is completed by 6–12 h post ingestion. However, early concentrations greater than 15 nmol/L indicate serious poisoning.

Treatment

The best outcome is associated with early recognition of digoxin toxicity.

For chronic toxicity with minimal symptoms, management may involve no more than observation, cessation of digoxin administration, correction of hypokalaemia and hypomagnesaemia and appropriate management of any factors that contributed to the development of toxicity. However, presence of any cardiovascular system effects, particularly in elderly patients, is an indication for the administration of Fab fragments of digoxin-specific antibodies. The potential lethality of chronic digoxin poisoning is often underestimated with the result that digoxin antibody fragments are inappropriately withheld.[16] From a purely economic view, the reduction in length of stay as a result of treatment with digoxin-specific antibodies outweighs the expense of the therapy.[17]

Following acute overdose the patient should be initially managed in a monitored area with full resuscitative equipment available. Immediate attention to the airway, breathing and circulation may be required. Intravenous access should be established and blood sent for urgent electrolytes and serum digoxin concentration. Although digoxin is well bound by charcoal, administration is usually difficult because of repetitive vomiting, and attempts should not detract from other interventions.

The specific antidote to digoxin poisoning is Fab fragments of digoxin-specific antibodies, which should be administered as soon as possible in any potentially life-threatening digoxin intoxication. Commonly accepted indications for the administration of Fab fragments are listed in Table 29.2.5.

Fab fragments of digoxin-specific antibodies

These are derived from IgG antidigoxin antibodies produced in sheep. Removal of the Fc fragments of the antibodies greatly reduces the potential for hypersensitivity reactions and contributes to the remarkable

safety profile of the product. Intravenously administered Fab fragments bind digoxin in the intravascular space on a mole-for-mole basis. As binding continues, digoxin moves down a concentration gradient from the tissue compartments to the intravascular compartment. Bound digoxin is inactive. A clinical response is usually observed within 20–30 min of administration. The Fab–digoxin complexes are excreted in the urine.

The extraordinary clinical efficacy of digoxin-specific fragments has been well documented in a multi-centre study.[17] The same study also demonstrated the safety of the product, with the only adverse reactions reported being hypokalaemia (4% incidence) and worsening of congestive cardiac failure (3%).

The correct dose of Fab fragments may be calculated on the basis that 40 mg (one vial) will bind 0.6 mg of digoxin. If the dose ingested is unknown and/or a steady-state serum digoxin concentration is not available, dosing of Fab fragments must be empiric. Following acute overdose a reasonable approach to empiric dosing is to give five vials initially and then repeat until a clinical response is observed. Smaller doses (two vials) are usually sufficient to reverse the effects of chronic toxicity.

It is important that ED staff are aware of the amount and location of supplies of Fab fragments within their own institution, and know the most rapid way to acquire further stocks should the need arise.

Serum digoxin concentrations will be extremely high following the administration of Fab fragments because most assays measure both bound and unbound digoxin.

Disposition

Patients with mild, chronic digoxin toxicity (gastrointestinal symptoms only) may be discharged after cessation of digoxin therapy provided there are no significant electrolyte disturbances, renal failure or other precipitating medical conditions. Following administration of Fab fragments, cases of chronic toxicity with conduction defects usually require medical admission for observation and treatment of intercurrent illness.

Acute overdoses require close observation for at least 12 h. Those that develop

toxicity require admission and an appropriate level of monitoring. Following successful administration of digoxin-specific Fab fragments, patients must be carefully monitored for hypokalaemia and worsening of any underlying medical conditions for which digoxin may have been prescribed therapeutically. All intentional ingestions require psychiatric evaluation prior to medical discharge.

CLONIDINE

Introduction

Clonidine, an imidazoline derivative, is a central alpha$_2$ adrenergic agonist. It was first developed in the 1960s as a nasal decongestant. It is currently used for the management of hypertension, attention deficit hyperactivity disorder (ADHD) as well as withdrawal symptoms from drug and alcohol addiction, tobacco withdrawal and Tourette's syndrome. Clonidine toxicity often mimics that of opioids.

Pharmacokinetics

Clonidine is well absorbed with a bioavailability of almost 100%. The peak concentration in plasma and effect is observed within 1–3 h. The elimination half-life is 6–24 h with a mean half-life of 12 h. Half of the administered dose is excreted unchanged by the kidney.[19]

Pathophysiology

Clonidine activates central α_2 receptors. This results in a reduction in CNS sympathetic outflow at the vasomotor centre in the medulla oblongata. Clonidine is thought to reduce blood pressure through a reduction in cardiac output as well as its weak peripheral alpha adrenergic antagonist properties. Clonidine also stimulates parasympathetic outflow and this may contribute to the slowing of heart rate as a consequence of increased vagal tone. Paradoxically, clonidine overdose can result in an initial hypertension from its partial α_1 adrenergic agonist effect. It is suggested

---

Table 29.2.5 Indications for administration of Fab fragments of digoxin-specific antibodies following acute overdose

Hyperkalaemia ($K > 5.0$ mmol/L) associated with digoxin toxicity
History of ingestion of more than 10 mg of digoxin
Haemodynamically unstable cardiac arrhythmia
Cardiac arrest from digoxin toxicity
Serum digoxin concentration greater than 15 nmol/L

that clonidine's inhibition of sympathetic outflow is mediated through endogenous opiate release.

Clinical features

Clonidine can cause transient hypertension from initial vasoconstriction with parenteral administration followed by hypotension. In addition to bradycardia and conduction defects, it can cause a central chlorpromazine-like effect with sedation. Other CNS symptoms include coma, seizure, miosis, reduced respiration and hypothermia.[20] The median onset of symptoms following clonidine ingestion is 30 min and patients are usually symptomatic on arrival at the ED.[20] Symptoms usually resolve by 24 h.[21]

Investigations

The ECG is essential in evaluating and monitoring for bradycardia and conduction defects.

Treatment

The management of clonidine poisoning is primarily supportive. Hypotension usually responds to intravenous fluids. Atropine has been shown to abolish bradycardia in some case reports. Occasionally inotropes may be required to maintain haemodynamic stability. Hypertension is usually short-lived and rarely requires treatment. Patients are usually symptomatic on arrival and the benefits of administering activated charcoal are unlikely to outweigh the risk of aspiration.

Disposition

Patients should be observed in hospital until they are asymptomatic and bradycardia has resolved. They do not require ongoing cardiac monitoring for a stable sinus bradycardia.

Controversies

❶ The advantages of glucagon over other inotropic agents in the management of CCB and beta-blocker overdose are questionable. It is now rarely used as a first-line agent.

❷ The indications for initiation of hyperinsulinaemia euglycaemia therapy in CCB and beta-blocker overdose are not well defined. This therapy is being advocated as first-line therapy for toxic hypotension.

❸ There are reports of the successful use of cardiopulmonary bypass to maintain an adequate cardiac output until such time as hepatic metabolism of the drug occurs following severe β-blocker overdose.[22] Techniques such as this and extracorporeal membrane oxygenation may play a role in the management of otherwise fatal cases of cardiovascular collapse.

❹ As experience with the use of digoxin-specific fragments increases, the threshold for administration has lowered. In the past, concerns about the safety and expense of treatment have limited their use. The cost of the fragments should be weighed against the costs of additional in-hospital care that may be incurred if they are withheld.

❺ A clinical response to naloxone may occur in up to 31% of cases of clonidine toxicity[20] but the clinical value of this intervention is doubtful.

References

1. Robertson RM, Robertson D. Drugs used for the treatment of myocardial ischaemia. In: Gilman AG, Hardman JG, Limbird LE, et al., eds. Goodman and Gilman's: The pharmacological basis of therapeutics, 9th edn. New York: Pergamon Press; 1996: p. 770.
2. Antman EM, Stone PH, Muller JE, et al. Calcium channel blocking agents in the treatment of cardiovascular diseases: Part E Basic and clinical
3. Lewis RV, McDevitt DG. Adverse reactions and interactions with beta-adrenoreceptor blocking drugs. Medical Toxicology 1986; 1: 343–361.
4. Taboulet P, Cariou A, Berdeaux A, et al. Pathophysiology and management of self-poisoning with beta-blockers. Journal of Toxicology and Clinical Toxicology 1993; 31: 531–551.
5. Reith DM, Dawson AH, Epid D, et al. Relative toxicity of beta blockers in overdose. Journal of Toxicology and Clinical Toxicology 1996; 34: 273–278.
6. Love J, Howell JM, Litovitz TL, et al. Acute beta blocker overdose: factors associated with the development of cardiovascular morbidity. Journal of Toxicology and Clinical Toxicology 2000; 38: 275–281.
7. Buckley N, Dawson AH, Howarth D, et al. Slow release verapamil poisoning. Use of polyethylene glycol whole bowel lavage and high dose calcium. Medical Journal of Australia 1993; 158: 202.
8. Pertoldi F, D'Orlando L, Mercante WP. Electromechanical dissociation 48 hours after atenolol overdose: usefulness of calcium chloride. Annals of Emergency Medicine 1998; 31: 777–781.
9. Bailey B. Glucagon in beta-blocker and calcium channel blocker overdoses: a systematic review. Journal of Toxicology Clinical Toxicology 2003; 41: 595–602.
10. Kline JA, Leonova E, Raymond RM. Beneficial myocardial metabolic effects of insulin during verapamil toxicity in the anesthetized canine. Critical Care Medicine 1995; 23: 1251–1263.
11. Holger JS, Engerbretsen KM, Fritzlar SJ, et al. Insulin versus vasopressin and epinephrine to treat b-blocker toxicity. Clinical Toxicology 2007; 45: 396–401.
12. Yuan I, Kerns WP, Tomaszewski CA, et al. Insulin glucose as adjunctive therapy for severe calcium channel antagonist poisoning. Journal of Toxicology Clinical Toxicology 1999; 37: 463–474.
13. Megarbane B, Karyo S, Baud FJ. The role of insulin and glucose (hyperinsulinaemia/euglycaemia) therapy in acute calcium and beta-blocker poisoning. Toxicology Reviews 2004; 23(4): 214–222.
14. Moorman JR, Pritchett ELC. The arrhythmias of digitalis intoxication. Archives of Internal Medicine 1985; 145: 1289–1292.
15. Bismuth C, Gaultier M, Conso F, et al. Hyperkalemia in acute digitalis poisoning: prognostic significance and therapeutic implications. Clinical Toxicology 1973; 6: 153–162.
16. Marik PE, Fromm L. A case series of hospitalised patients with elevated digoxin levels. American Journal of Medicine 1998; 105(2): 110–115.
17. DiDomenico RJ, Walton SM, Sanoski CA, et al. Analysis of the use of digoxin immune Fab for the treatment of non-life-threatening digoxin toxicity. Journal of Cardiovascular Pharmacology & Therapeutics 2000; 5(2): 77–85.
18. Antman EM, Wenger FL, Butler VP, et al. Treatment of 150 cases of life threatening digitalis intoxication with digoxin specific Fab antibody fragments: final report of multicenter study. Circulation 1990; 81: 1744–1752.
19. Seger D. Clonidine Toxicity Revisited. Clinical Toxicology 2002; 40(2): 145–155.
20. Nichols MH, King WD, James LP. Clonidine poisoning in Jefferson County, Alabama. Annals of Emergency Medicine 1997; 29: 511–517.
21. Erickson SJ, Duncan A. Clonidine poisoning – an emerging problem: Epidemiology, clinical features, management and preventative strategies. Journal of Paediatrics and Child Health 1998; 34(3): 280–282.
22. McVey FK, Corke CF. Extracorporeal circulation in the management of massive propranolol overdose. Anaesthesia 1991; 46: 744–746.

electrophysiological effects. Annals of Internal Medicine 1980; 93: 875–885.

29.3 Central nervous system drugs

George Braitberg • Fergus Kerr

ESSENTIALS

1 Benzodiazepines have a wide safety margin, and death from isolated overdoses is very rare. The treatment is supportive.

2 Certain non-benzodiazepine sedatives and hypnotics exhibit toxicity profiles quite different from those of the benzodiazepines.

3 The antipsychotics, at therapeutic doses, are associated with numerous adverse effects, including extrapyramidal movement, neuroleptic malignant syndrome, seizures, hypotension, agranulocytosis and priapism. They are generally associated with low lethality in overdose. Management is supportive.

4 The newer atypical antipsychotics have an improved adverse effect profile and are relatively benign in overdose although central nervous system (CNS) depression may be significant enough to require intubation.

5 Overdose of extended-release bupropion is associated with dose-related delayed onset of seizures.

6 Tricyclic antidepressant (TCA) overdose produces severe CNS and cardiovascular toxicity and remains a major cause of morbidity and death.

7 The specific treatment of TCA cardiotoxicity is sodium bicarbonate.

8 The selective serotonin reuptake inhibitors are associated with the serotonin syndrome, both following overdose and as an interaction with other serotonergic drugs.

9 The anticonvulsants, carbamazepine and sodium valproate, have specific toxicity and are potentially life-threatening in overdose.

Introduction

Pharmaceuticals used to treat CNS and psychiatric conditions are frequently taken in overdose. The manifestations of toxicity include systems other than the CNS. This chapter discusses those agents from this group most frequently taken in overdose including the sedative-hypnotics, antipsychotics, antidepressants and anticonvulsants.

BENZODIAZEPINES

Pharmacology

Benzodiazepines possess a shared structure comprising a benzene ring fused to a diazepine ring. The pharmacologically significant benzodiazepines also demonstrate a 5-aryl substituent.

Most benzodiazepines are highly lipid soluble and rapidly absorbed following oral administration. The more water-soluble agents, such as temazepam and oxazepam, are more slowly absorbed. Following ingestion, peak plasma concentrations are reached within 90 min for midazolam and diazepam, compared to 120–180 min for temazepam and oxazepam. Following intramuscular injection absorption of benzodiazepines is often erratic, except for lorazepam and midazolam.

Plasma protein binding is variable. Diazepam has the highest (99%) and alprazolam the lowest (70%) plasma protein binding. The unbound fraction is able to cross the blood–brain barrier and interact with specific receptors in the CNS. Benzodiazepines are widely distributed to the body tissues, with volumes of distribution ranging from 0.3 to 5.5 L/kg.

The duration of action for benzodiazepines depends on a number of factors, including the rate of redistribution from the CNS compartment to the body tissues, the metabolism and excretion of the drug and the sensitivity of the benzodiazepine receptor to its agonist. Drugs that are lipophobic tend to have a shorter measured plasma half-life but a longer duration of action. This reflects slower redistribution from the CNS compartment. Lipophilic drugs rapidly redistribute to body fat and muscle and, therefore, have a rapid onset but relatively short duration of CNS effect together with relatively longer plasma half-lives. Repeated dosing eventually saturates peripheral body stores and this 'stored' drug may then leach out resulting in prolonged pharmacological activity.

The metabolism of most benzodiazepines includes both phase I oxidative and phase II conjugative processes, with phase I producing pharmacologically active metabolites. The major metabolite of diazepam is desmethyldiazepam, which is pharmacologically active and has a longer half-life than its parent compound. Lorazepam, temazepam and oxazepam only undergo phase II metabolism.

Gamma-aminobutyric acid (GABA) is an inhibitory neurotransmitter found predominantly in the basal ganglia, the hippocampus, hypothalamus, cerebellum and the dorsal horn of the spinal cord.[1] GABA interacts with two receptors, GABA-A and GABA-B, resulting in the influx of chloride through a ligand-gated ion channel. The former receptor is the predominant site of benzodiazepine action. By binding to the GABA-A receptor complex at a specific site, benzodiazepines enhance the binding of GABA at GABA-A, which in turn opens more chloride channels, and hence produces their sedative, hypnotic, anxiolytic and anticonvulsant effects. GABA-B is mainly involved in feedback mechanisms and the control of muscle tone. GABA receptor subunits have been identified, and the sensitivity and specificity of individual benzodiazepines is determined by their interaction with these subunits. Tolerance develops to most of the effects of benzodiazepines, and may be associated with downregulation of GABA receptors.

Clinical features

Adverse effects

The various benzodiazepines share a common adverse effect profile. These effects vary in severity between individuals and tend to be more pronounced in the elderly. Common adverse effects include drowsiness, motor incoordination, amnesia, headache, nausea, vomiting and blurred vision. Long-acting agents such as diazepam may produce more residual lethargy and drowsiness. Conversely, rebound insomnia is associated with short-acting benzodiazepines such as temazepam. More unusual side effects include the unmasking of disinhibited and sometimes violent behaviour. Long-term use of benzodiazepines may also be associated with irreversible deficits in cognition. Parenteral administration of benzodiazepines has been associated with life-threatening reactions, including respiratory arrest, cardiac arrest and hypotension. This usually occurs following too-rapid parenteral administration of an excessive dose. It may also be partly related to the propylene glycol diluent found in these preparations.

Overdose

Death as a result of pure benzodiazepine overdose is very uncommon.[2] When death is reported, it is usually in the setting of a mixed overdose including other CNS depressants such as alcohol, antidepressants, phenothiazines and narcotics. The most common manifestation of overdose is drowsiness, which may progress to stupor depending on patient characteristics, co-ingestants and dose. Coma is uncommon. Other features characteristic of benzodiazepine overdose are respiratory depression, hypothermia and hypotension, though these are not usually life-threatening.[3] The duration of effect varies from 6 to 36 h, depending on the drug.

Respiratory insufficiency in the setting of benzodiazepine overdose may be due to an increase in upper airway resistance and work of breathing rather than central apnoea.[4]

The duration of benzodiazepine effect varies between 6 and 36 h depending on the agents(s) involved. The effects on the CNS are exacerbated if there is co-ingestion of other CNS depressants such as alcohol, antidepressants, phenothiazines or narcotics. A fatal outcome is more likely in this setting. Acute alcohol ingestion tends to delay benzodiazepine metabolism whereas chronic alcohol ingestion induces metabolic pathways and may increase clearance rates of these drugs.[5]

Treatment

The management of benzodiazepine overdose is supportive, with careful attention to the patient's airway, ventilation and circulatory status. Patients should be assessed for the presence of co-ingestants, including paracetamol, alcohol and antidepressants. Those who are able to walk safely and who have normal vital signs can be medically cleared at 4–6 h post ingestion, providing there are no complicating factors such as aspiration. Hypotension, if present, is usually mild and responds to intravenous fluid replacement.

The role of flumazenil, a specific benzodiazepine receptor antagonist, in the management of overdose is limited. Recovery from benzodiazepine overdose is usually uncomplicated with simple supportive care and the use of flumazenil may precipitate acute withdrawal syndrome in benzodiazepine-dependent patients and seizures in those with co-ingestants which lower the seizure threshold.[6] Flumazenil does have a role as a diagnostic agent to confirm benzodiazepine overdose, in the reversal of postoperative benzodiazepine-induced sedation and those patients with a pure benzodiazepine overdose, who would otherwise require intubation.

Clinical investigation

Specific quantitative laboratory assays for individual benzodiazepines are available in some large centres, but they offer no clinical utility and should not be routinely performed. Clinical effects correlate very poorly with blood levels. Qualitative urine screens are readily available but are subject to a relatively high false negative rate. They do offer some assistance in the setting of an unknown overdose or an unconscious patient.

Pharmacology

Sedative and hypnotic effects are thought to be regulated through the GABA receptor complex, particularly GABA-A receptors. Agonist action at the GABA-A receptor results in longer and/or more frequent opening of the ligand-gated chloride ion channels. The subsequent influx of chloride hyperpolarizes the neuron suppressing electrical excitability.

Barbiturates

Like benzodiazepines, barbiturates exert their action at the GABA-A receptor complex. However, barbiturates increase the length of time the chloride channel remains open, rather than increasing the frequency of opening. The CNS-depressant effect of barbiturates is stronger than that of the benzodiazepines. In combination these two types of drug have a synergistic effect.

Preparations of barbiturates are usually alkaline salts, which in turn dictates that the primary site of absorption is the small intestine. The more lipid-soluble barbiturates are taken up into the CNS more rapidly and produce a more rapid effect. Plasma protein binding varies from a high 80% for thiopentone to only 50% for phenobarbitone. The volume of distribution ranges from 0.6 to 2.6 L/kg, depending on the agent. Elimination half-lives vary considerably, from only 6 h for thiopentone to up to 100 h for phenobarbitone.

Chloral hydrate

The sedative effects of chloral hydrate are thought to be mediated through GABA-A receptors. Chloral hydrate is rapidly absorbed from the gastrointestinal tract and widely distributed throughout the body. A pro-drug, it is metabolized almost entirely by alcohol dehydrogenase in the liver and red blood cells, with a half-life of only 4 min. Its active metabolite, trichloroethanol, begins to have a therapeutic effect within 30 min of dosing with the parent drug. Trichloroethanol is metabolized to an inactive compound via alcohol dehydrogenase and aldehyde dehydrogenase, with a half-life of approximately 8 h.

Zopiclone

Zopiclone also acts on the GABA-A receptor complex, but at a separate site to that of the benzodiazepines and barbiturates. Furthermore, unlike the benzodiazepines where the binding to GABA-A receptors is modulated by the presence of GABA itself, the binding of zopiclone is not. It is also suggested that zopiclone binds to the same receptor site as benzodiazepines, but the resulting conformational change is different.

Zopiclone is rapidly absorbed, with peak plasma concentrations occurring at about one hour post ingestion. Its volume of distribution is approximately 1.5 L/kg, with a plasma protein binding of only 45%. Only 5% of an ingested dose is excreted unchanged by the kidneys, with most of the drug undergoing hepatic metabolism. The plasma elimination half-life varies between 4 and 7 h.

Zolpidem

This drug is structurally unrelated to the other sedative-hypnotics, belonging to the imidazopyridine group. It selectively binds to the ω-1 receptor subtype of the GABA-A receptor complex in contrast to the benzodiazepines which bind all 3 ω subtypes. The modulation of the chloride anion channel at this receptor allows preservation of deep sleep. Zolpidem's effects are reversed by flumazenil. The elimination half-life of zolpidem is approximately 2.5 h, with pharmacological effect lasting up to 6 h. The volume of distribution is 0.5 L/kg, smaller in the elderly. The main cytochrome P450 enzyme involved in the hepatic biotransformation of zolpidem is CYP3A4. Its metabolites are pharmacologically inactive and are eliminated in the urine and faeces.

Clinical features

Barbiturates

Typical effects of barbiturate overdose include a depressed conscious state of varying degrees, including profound coma. Respiratory depression, hypotension, hypothermia and miosis are also observed. Cutaneous bullous lesions may be evident.

Chloral hydrate

As well as CNS and respiratory depression, overdose with chloral hydrate may produce severe gastrointestinal irritation, with haematemesis, gastric ulceration and oesophageal stricture formation. More importantly, chloral hydrate overdose characteristically produces cardiac rhythm disturbances, including simple ventricular ectopics, ventricular tachycardia, torsades de pointes and ventricular fibrillation. Fatalities continue to be reported.[7]

Zopiclone

Overdose with zopiclone produces CNS depression and potentially respiratory depression. First-degree heart block[8] and fatalities are reported.[9,10]

Zolpidem

As with the other sedative-hypnotics, the primary clinical effects observed following zolpidem overdose are CNS and respiratory depression. Pure ingestions of <400 mg in adults tend to produce sedation and amnesia only.[11] Fatalities have been ascribed to zolpidem overdose on the basis of postmortem toxicological analyses.[12]

Treatment

As with the benzodiazepines, the most important aspect of management for patients presenting following an overdose of the other sedative-hypnotic drugs is good supportive care. Careful attention must be paid to maintaining an adequate airway, ventilation and blood pressure. Hypotension usually responds to intravenous fluid administration, but may require administration of inotropes. Activated charcoal can be considered if patients present within 1–2 h of ingestion. Specific medications may be of use with certain types of overdose. Flumazenil has been shown to reverse the effect of zopiclone, and its use in pure zopiclone overdoses with respiratory depression that might otherwise require intubation should be considered.[13–15] In the setting of chloral hydrate overdose, ventricular arrhythmias may be resistant to usual therapies but will often respond to the use of β-blockers, such as intravenous propranolol.[16,17] Hypoxia and electrolyte disturbances should also be corrected.

Techniques to enhance elimination, such as haemodialysis and haemoperfusion, have been used in the past to manage barbiturate and chloral hydrate overdose. However, with more effective intensive care such techniques are rarely indicated. Urinary alkalinization and repeat-dose activated charcoal enhance the elimination of phenobarbitone and may be useful in management of significant overdose of this drug.

ANTIPSYCHOTIC DRUGS

Pharmacology

This large group of drugs can be classified as typical or atypical (Table 29.3.1), according to structure (Table 29.3.2) or according to neuroreceptor-binding affinity. The latter may offer the most reliable prediction of the risk of toxicity.[18]

Atypical drugs are defined as such on clinical and pharmacological grounds. Clinically, they produce fewer extrapyramidal side effects and tardive dyskinesias. For this reasons the newer atypical antipsychotic agents have largely replaced the traditional agents as first-line treatment of schizophrenia. Pharmacologically, they may be regarded as atypical for a variety of reasons including low D_2-dopamine receptor potency, low D_2-receptor occupancy in the mesolimbic and nigrostriatal areas and high affinities for M_1-muscarinic, D_1- and D_4-dopamine and 5-HT1A- and 5-HT2A-serotonin receptors.[19] This produces three broad functional groups of atypical antipsychotics: the D_2-, D_3-receptor antagonists such as amisulpiride, the D_2, α_1, 5-HT2A-receptor antagonists such as risperidone, and the broad-spectrum multiple receptor

Table 29.3.1 Typical and atypical antipsychotic drugs

Typical	Atypical
Chlorpromazine	Mesoridazine
Fluphenazine	Thioridazine
Perphenazine	Clozapine
Prochlorperazine	Olanzapine
Trifluoperazine	Risperidone
Haloperidol	Remoxipride
Thiothixene	Loxapine
Molindone	Quetiapine

Table 29.3.2 Structural classification of the antipsychotics

Structural class	Generic name
Phenothiazines	
Aliphatic	Chlorpromazine Triflupromazine Promethazine
Piperazine	Fluphenazine Perphenazine Prochlorperazine Trifluoperazine
Piperidine	Mesoridazine Thioridazine
Butyrophenone	Haloperidol
Thioxanthene	Droperidol Chlorprothixene Thiothixene
Dihydroindolone	Molindone
Dibenzoxazepine	Loxapine Clozapine Olanzapine
Diphenylbutylpiperidine	Pimozide
Benzisoxazole	Risperidone
Benzamides	Sulpiride Remoxipride

antagonists such as clozapine, quetiapine and olanzapine.[19]

The therapeutic and predominant toxic effects of these drugs are related to their blockade of the D_2-subtype dopamine receptors. These are located throughout the brain in the basal ganglia, hypothalamus, pituitary, medulla and the mesocortical and mesolimbic pathways. The antipsychotic effect of a drug is mediated by its blockade of D_2 receptors in the mesocortical and mesolimbic pathways. The development of extrapyramidal effects is closely related to a drug's affinity with D_2 receptors in the basal ganglia. D_2-receptor blockade in the pituitary can cause elevated prolactin levels, with resulting galactorrhoea and gynaecomastia. Blockade of D_2 receptors in the hypothalamus affects body temperature regulation: hypothermia or hyperthermia may result. The strong antiemetic effect of some antipsychotic agents is regulated through D_2-receptor blockade in the medulla.

The blockade of other neuroreceptors and the relative ratio to D_2-receptor blockade predicts the likelihood of adverse effects at therapeutic dosing and in overdose. Blockade of α_1-adrenergic receptors results in postural hypotension of varying

degrees, depending on binding affinity. Significant α_2-receptor blockade occurs with clozapine but the clinical importance of this is not clear. H_1-histamine receptor blockade correlates with sedation and, to a lesser extent, hypotension. Sedation, along with delirium, hallucinations, mydriasis, flushing, dry skin, urinary retention and ileus, is seen with M_1-acetylcholine receptor blockade. Agents that possess a relatively higher anticholinergic activity compared to dopaminergic activity have a lower risk for inducing extrapyramidal side effects. Examples include chlorpromazine, thioridazine, clozapine and olanzapine. The reverse is also true: those drugs with a higher dopaminergic effect in relation to their anticholinergic activity have a higher risk of inducing extrapyramidal side effects, e.g. fluphenazine, prochlorperazine and haloperidol. Serotonin antagonism may be an important mechanism in the antipsychotic action and responsible for the low incidence of extrapyramidal side effects seen with the newer atypical antipsychotics such as clozapine and olanzapine. These drugs, which tend to have a high 5-HT2A antagonism in relation to D_2 antagonism, can be given in smaller doses to produce the same therapeutic effect.

Phenothiazine antipsychotics also have a quinidine-like effect and can produce a variety of ECG changes, both at therapeutic doses and in overdose. Thioridazine and mesoridazine are considered to be the most cardioactive, and also possess calcium channel blocking ability, which may contribute to the cardiotoxicity observed in overdose of these agents.

Generally, the pharmacokinetics of this heterogeneous group of drugs are similar. They are rapidly and well absorbed after oral administration. Peak plasma concentrations occur between 1 and 6 h following oral administration and from 30 to 60 min following intramuscular administration. Those agents that possess a considerable anticholinergic effect may show delayed absorption after ingestion. Most antipsychotics exhibit a relatively high plasma protein binding of between 75% and 99%, are widely distributed to the tissues and have high volumes of distribution, ranging from 10 to 40 L/kg. Clozapine and risperidone are exceptions with smaller volumes of distribution (2 and 1 L/kg respectively). Only about 1% of an ingested dose is

excreted unchanged in the urine, with the majority of drugs undergoing extensive hepatic metabolism, some with significant enterohepatic circulation.

Clinical features

Adverse effects

Adverse effects following therapeutic dosing may be idiosyncratic or dose-related, and may occur after initiation of the medication in question or late into a course of treatment.

Extrapyramidal movement disorders

Up to 90% of patients receiving antipsychotic medication will experience some extrapyramidal side effects, and these often result in the cessation of treatment.[20] Of the four recognized extrapyramidal syndromes, acute dystonia, parkinsonism and akathisia are reversible and tend to occur early in a course of treatment. Tardive dyskinesia is irreversible but occurs after months to years of treatment. Clozapine, olanzapine and quetiapine are not associated with extrapyramidal syndromes.[19]

The pathophysiology of acute dystonic reactions is not fully understood, but involves disruption of the dopaminergic-cholinergic-GABA balance in the basal ganglia. Reactions are idiosyncratic and equally frequent following a single therapeutic ingestion or an overdose. Risk factors for developing an acute dystonic reaction following antipsychotic medication are the use of antipsychotic drugs with a high D_2-dopaminergic, low M_1-muscarinic and low 5-HT2A-serotonergic receptor binding affinity; young and male patients; the use of depot preparations and the recent use of alcohol.[21,22] Reactions may present in varied forms and may be spasmodic or sustained, but are always involuntary. The muscles of the face, trunk and neck are commonly involved, but other sites may also be affected. About half of all cases occur within 48 h of dosing.[20] The overall incidence of acute dystonic reactions varies considerably: rates of 3.5% have been reported for chlorpromazine, and 16% for haloperidol.[21]

Akathisia is dose-related, can occur at any age, and tends to appear some days after beginning treatment. It is thought to be due to D_2-dopaminergic blockade in the mesocortical pathways.[23] Drug-induced parkinsonism is more common in the elderly and tends to be seen with high-potency agents that block the postsynaptic D_2-dopaminergic receptors in the nigrostriatal area. Tardive dyskinesia appears after months or years of antipsychotic treatment. It is seen with all antipsychotics except clozapine, and has a prevalence of between 27% and 35% in patients on long-term therapy.[24] It is thought to be the result of an increased number and sensitivity of dopaminergic receptors in the nigrostriatal area of the brain, a response to long-term blockade.

Seizures

Antipsychotic drugs lower the seizure threshold.[25] They also produce EEG changes that vary depending on the agent.[26] Organic brain disease, epilepsy, drug-associated seizures and polypharmacy are risk factors for the development of seizures. They are more likely with chlorpromazine, clozapine and loxapine.

Cardiovascular

Postural hypotension and ECG changes can occur with therapeutic dosing of antipsychotics. Postural hypotension is multifactorial, with α_1-adrenergic blockade, central vasomotor reflex depression and direct myocardial depression all playing a part. ECG changes can be diverse, with QRS and QT prolongation, a right axis shift, ST segment depression and T-wave inversion/flattening. QT prolongation is less evident with the newer atypical antipsychotics.[27] Torsades des pointes is reported following high therapeutic dosing with haloperidol, thioridazine and mesoridazine.

Neuroleptic malignant syndrome

This idiosyncratic adverse reaction to antipsychotic medication therapy is rare. It occurs early in the treatment course or after changes in dose. Neuroleptic malignant syndrome (NMS) has been reported with all typical antipsychotics but is particularly associated with higher potency drugs such as haloperidol and fluphenazine. In the atypical group, NMS has been reported with clozapine, olanzapine and risperidone.[28–30] Pooled data studies suggest the incidence is somewhere between 0.07% and 0.2%, although some have described incidences of up to 12.2%.

Typically, patients are male (male : female ratio 2 : 1), with symptoms developing over 1–3 days. Risk factors associated with the development of NMS include the use of high-potency agents and depot preparations, organic brain disease, past history of NMS, dehydration and interactions with other drugs such as lithium and anticholinergics.[31] The characteristic clinical features are a temperature $\geq 38°C$, muscle rigidity, altered consciousness and autonomic dysfunction. Other features that may be seen are an elevated creatine kinase, leukocytosis, elevated hepatic transaminases, renal failure and metabolic acidosis. There is no specific test to confirm or exclude the diagnosis, which is reliant upon clinical and historical data. Alternative diagnoses must be excluded, especially infection (including meningitis and encephalitis). Other differential diagnoses include heat stroke, thyrotoxicosis, intracranial haemorrhage, phaeochromocytoma, tetanus, serotonin syndrome, drug overdose (MAOI, sympathomimetics and lithium), substance/alcohol withdrawal and malignant hyperthermia. The mortality rate has been reduced from 30% to 5–11% mainly as a result of improved intensive supportive care.[32] Death is usually secondary to respiratory or cardiovascular failure; however, renal failure secondary to myoglobinuria, arrhythmias, pulmonary embolism and disseminated intravascular coagulation are also reported.

Other

Clozapine is associated with idiosyncratic agranulocytosis. The incidence is between 0.6% and 2.0% and usually occurs within the first 18 weeks of therapy. The mortality rate of clozapine-induced agranulocytosis, once established, is up to 85%.[18] Other phenothiazines have also been associated with agranulocytosis, but with a much lower incidence.

Other unusual adverse effects seen with some phenothiazines include priapism, dermatitis, photosensitivity and cholestatic jaundice.

Overdose

Most patients with serious poisoning display manifestations of cardiovascular and/or CNS toxicity. Isolated antipsychotic overdose is rarely fatal. Peak toxicity is usually seen from 2 to 6 h following ingestion but may be delayed especially after thioridazine overdose.[33] Delayed onset of life-threatening cardiotoxicity is also reported following amisulpride overdose.[34] CNS effects vary greatly, depending on individual susceptibility, dose ingested and the presence of co-ingestants. Lethargy is common to most patients, with effects potentially progressing to confusion, ataxia, coma and seizures. Ingestion of more than 300 mg of olanzapine or 3 g of quetiapine is likely to cause CNS depression significant enough to require intubation. Seizures are more often seen following overdose with loxapine or clozapine, and are usually generalized.[35] Paradoxically, agitation may also be observed, especially in the setting of mixed overdose, and following overdose with clozapine, olanzapine or thioridazine.

Life-threatening cardiotoxicity is unusual, except in the setting of piperidine phenothiazine overdoses, e.g. thioridazine, which is associated with QRS widening, QT prolongation, ventricular tachycardia and torsade des pointes.[36,37] Torsades des pointes is also reported in large haloperidol overdoses, either following deliberate self-poisoning or in the setting of excessive intravenous therapy in critically ill patients.[38] More common cardiovascular effects are hypotension (initially postural) and tachycardia. Uncommon effects are hypertension and bradycardia. ECG abnormalities are not unusual in significant overdoses and can range from simple ventricular ectopics to conduction abnormalities, QRS widening, ventricular tachycardia and torsades des pointes. QT prolongation has been reported in the setting of thioridazine overdose and more recently quetiapine and amisulpride ingestions.[34,39–41] The prolonged corrected QT observed in a number of reported quetiapine overdoses may be the result of the underlying sinus tachycardia observed, rather than an indicator of significant cardiotoxicity.[39,40] Amisulpride overdose can result in severe cardiotoxicity, characterized by intraventricular conduction abnormalities, QT prolongation and torsades des pointes.[34]

Temperature abnormalities may also occur, and commonly manifest as mild hypothermia. Hyperthermia may be seen in the setting of a high environmental temperature and seizures. Following ingestions of aliphatic and piperidine phenothiazines, clozapine and olanzapine, significant anticholinergic toxicity may occur.

The diagnosis of antipsychotic drug overdose is based on a history of ingestion and the presence of symptoms and signs in keeping with the expected findings, as outlined above. Qualitative serum and urine drug screening can be used to detect the presence of many of the antipsychotic drugs, but a high false–negative rate makes these screens notoriously unreliable. Quantitative levels may also be performed, but the results do not correlate with clinical findings and do affect management. The differential diagnosis of antipsychotic drug overdose includes meningitis and other CNS infections, stroke and head injury, as well as other drug toxicities, including tricyclic antidepressants, sedatives, alcohols, anticholinergic drugs and anticonvulsants. Many other agents have also been reported as causing acute dystonic reactions, including tricyclic antidepressants, antihistamines and anticonvulsants.

Treatment

The management of antipsychotic drug overdose is essentially supportive. Patients should undergo an initial resuscitation period with a careful airway assessment and, if necessary, endotracheal intubation. Ventilation should be supported with supplemental oxygen and mechanical ventilation if indicated. Hypotension should be treated with Trendelenburg positioning, intravenous fluids and, if resistant, inotropic agents, preferably with some α-agonist properties. All patients should be placed on a cardiac monitor, have a 12-lead ECG recorded and an intravenous cannula inserted, with blood being drawn for full blood examination, electrolytes, creatine kinase and renal function. If paracetamol overdose is suspected appropriate levels should be measured.

Administration of activated charcoal should be considered unless there has been considerable delay in presentation. Multidose charcoal has not been shown to be of benefit in antipsychotic drug overdose. The use of extracorporeal blood purification techniques to enhance drug elimination is not effective, owing to the large volume of distribution and high tissue-protein binding of these drugs.

Seizures should be treated with benzodiazepines such as diazepam or clonazepam as the first-line agents. For resistant seizure activity phenobarbitone may be needed.

Cardiac arrhythmias should be treated according to advanced cardiac life support protocols. However, type IA antiarrhythmics should be avoided in the setting of QRS widening or conduction abnormalities, as they may exacerbate the toxicity. Serum alkalinization, to a pH of 7.45–7.55, should be performed in the presence of significant QRS widening or life-threatening arrhythmias. Intravenous magnesium and chemical or electrical overdrive pacing may be required to control torsades des pointes.

Acute dystonia

Acute dystonia is generally reversed by the use of an intravenous or intramuscular anticholinergic agent such as benztropine (1–2 mg i.v. or i.m.) or diphenhydramine (1 mg/kg i.v. or i.m.). Symptoms and signs usually resolve within 10–15 min. Repeated doses may be required for resistant cases. Following acute resolution of symptoms in the emergency department (ED) the patient should be discharged on oral medication for 2–3 days.

Neuroleptic malignant syndrome

NMS is a diagnosis of exclusion, with a CT brain scan, lumbar puncture and routine blood analyses essential to exclude other pathology, especially CNS infection. Empiric antibiotics are often necessary until a clearer picture can been gleaned and culture results have returned. Aggressive supportive care is life-saving. Neuroleptic agents and other drugs, which may be contributing to the condition, should of course be ceased.

BUPROPION

Pharmacology

In Australia, bupropion is supplied in a slow-release preparation and is approved only for use in smoking cessation. In other countries it has been marketed for many years as an atypical antidepressant with a relatively safe cardiovascular profile.

Bupropion is a monocyclic antidepressant with structural similarities to amphetamine and diethylpropion. It is a selective inhibitor of the reuptake of catecholamines with minimal effect on the reuptake of serotonin. It also possesses mild anticholinergic activity.[42] Bupropion is metabolized to hydroxy-bupropion, with plasma protein binding of 84% and 77%, respectively. The elimination half-life of bupropion is between 13 and 20 h, while that of hydroxy-bupropion is approximately 20 h. Bupropion is widely distributed with an apparent volume of distribution of approximately 2000 L.[43]

Clinical features

Adverse effects

The adverse effects of bupropion are relatively mild compared to other antidepressants. Mild hypertension has been noted, but has usually occurred in the already hypertensive.[44] Postural hypotension has also been observed in sporadic patients.[45] QRS or QT prolongation is not seen with bupropion at therapeutic doses.[46] Neurological side effects occur more commonly with headache, insomnia, agitation and seizures being reported.[47,48] Minor gastrointestinal irritation and priapism are also reported.

Overdose

The most significant clinical feature of overdose of the sustained release product is seizures and, importantly, the onset of the first seizure is commonly delayed until 6 to 8 h following ingestion. In a series of 59 overdoses, 19 of which involved sustained-release bupropion alone, the clinical effects noted were sinus tachycardia (83%), hypertension (56%) and seizures (37%). Seizures were dose-dependent, occurring in 30% of patients ingesting <4.5 g, in 50% of those ingesting 4.5–9 g and in 100% of cases involving >9 g (n = 2).[49]

Cardiotoxicity is rarely reported following overdose but may occur following massive ingestion (>9 g).[50,51] It is suggested that QTc prolongation (>440 ms) observed following bupropion overdose is an overcorrection of the QTc due to the tachycardia, rather than a change indicative of cardiotoxicity.[52]

Fatalities are reported following bupropion overdose. In one case a 26-year-old male who ingested 23 g of bupropion became hypoxic following recurrent seizure activity and died despite resuscitation after a cardiac arrest.[54]

Treatment

The management of bupropion overdose is essentially supportive. Patients should be managed in an area equipped for cardiore-spiratory monitoring and resuscitation. Close observation for at least 12 h and until the patient is asymptomatic is essential. Staff should be prepared to recognize and treat seizures. Intravenous benzodiazepines are the agent of choice. Prophylactic administration of titrated intravenous benzodiazepines to patients with agitation or tachycardia may be useful.

Administration of activated charcoal is likely to be useful in the patient who presents within two hours but the decision to decontaminate by this method must take into account the risk of subsequent seizures and aspiration of charcoal. Whole-bowel irrigation whilst offering theoretical benefits entails similar risks.

TRICYCLIC ANTIDEPRESSANTS

Tricyclic antidepressants (TCAs) have long been the leading cause of death from prescription drug overdose. However, they are increasingly being replaced in clinical practice by newer agents, which appear to be significantly safer in overdose. The TCAs currently available in Australia are listed in Table 29.3.3. Reported mortality rates for intentional TCA overdose range from 2% to 5%.[54] The vast majority of successful TCA suicides do not reach hospital but die at home.[55] The ingestion of 10 mg/kg or more of a TCA is potentially fatal, though there are differences in toxicity within the group. In Australia, doxepin is associated with the greatest lethality.[56]

Table 29.3.3 Tricyclic antidepressants available in Australia
Amitriptyline
Clomipramine
Dothiepin
Doxepin
Imipramine
Nortriptyline
Trimipramine

Pharmacology

TCAs have a distinct chemical structure, comprised of three aromatic rings. TCAs are non-selective agents that exhibit a large number of pharmacological effects. The therapeutic effect is most likely due to the inhibition of amine reuptake in the CNS, particularly serotonin and dopamine.[57] This effect is not responsible for the toxicity of TCA overdose, but forms the basis of the role of TCAs in the development of serotonin syndrome.[58]

The major features of TCA overdose are related to the following pharmacological actions:

- anticholinergic effects
- antihistaminic effects
- anti-α-adrenergic effects
- anti-GABAminergic effects
- sodium channel-blocking effects
- potassium channel-blocking effects.

TCAs bind to inactivated sodium channels, producing a rate-dependent inhibition of fast sodium channel function. This is thought to be the principal mechanism of TCA-induced cardiotoxicity. Inhibition of sodium entry slows phase 0 depolarization in His-Purkinje and myocardial tissue, and this is reflected in widening of the QRS complex on the 12-lead ECG. This disturbed depolarization, if severe, can lead to cardiac rhythm disturbances and impaired myocardial contractility. TCAs also slow repolarization and phase 4 repolarization, and this is reflected in prolongation of the QT interval on the 12-lead ECG. Peripheral α-adrenergic blockade results in vasodilatation and contributes to the hypotension observed in TCA overdose.

Clinical features

The clinical features of TCA overdose include anticholinergic, cardiovascular and CNS effects. The type and severity of clinical manifestations are dose-related (Table 29.3.4) Onset is usually rapid and, following large ingestions, rapid deterioration in clinical status within 1–2 h is characteristic.

The clinical features of central and peripheral anticholinergic toxicity are described elsewhere in this book. Anticholinergic delirium is most commonly observed following a modest TCA overdose or early in the course

Table 29.3.4 Tricyclic antidepressants: dose-related risk assessment	
Dose	Effect
<5 mg/kg	Minimal symptoms
5–10 mg/kg	Drowsiness and mild anticholinergic effects Major toxicity not expected
>10 mg/kg	Potential for all major effects to occur within 2–4 h of ingestion
>30 mg/kg	Severe toxicity with pH-dependent cardiotoxicity and coma expected to last >24 h

Adapted from Toxicology Handbook. Murray L, Daly F, Little M, Cadogan M (eds), Sydney: Elsevier; 2007.

of more significant ingestions. Large overdoses usually lead to coma, which obscures any evidence of anticholinergic delirium. Seizures are characteristic of TCA overdose and usually occur early in the clinical course. Overall the rate is quoted to be 3–4%.[59] Myoclonic jerking is also associated with TCA overdose.

Sinus tachycardia is commonly observed following TCA overdose and is usually due to the anticholinergic effects of the TCA, rather than sodium channel blockade. More serious cardiac arrhythmias can develop as a consequence of the effects on the fast sodium channels and cardiac depolarization and conduction. These include supraventricular tachycardia (with or without aberrancy), ventricular tachycardia, torsades des pointes (augmented by potassium channel blocking effects) and ventricular fibrillation. Junctional or idioventricular rhythms, second- or third-degree heart block or asystole can also occur.[60] Hypotension is commonly observed and is due to both peripheral vasodilatation and impaired myocardial contractility.

Clinical investigation

Serum TCA concentrations correlate poorly with the clinical severity of TCA intoxication. The single most important investigation in assessing the patient following a TCA overdose is the 12-lead ECG. The degree of prolongation of the QRS interval is predictive of the risk of both ventricular arrhythmias and seizures.[61] The positive and negative predictive values of ECG changes in TCA poisoning in one study were 66% and 100%, respectively.[62] A QRS duration of >120 ms in the setting of a TCA overdose indicates cardiotoxicity. A terminal R wave >3 mm in lead aVR may be a more useful predictor of seizures or arrhythmias than QRS duration.[63] A patient may exhibit significant CNS toxicity despite a normal ECG.

Treatment

The management of TCA poisoning is largely supportive. In particular, it involves maintenance of the airway, ventilation and blood pressure and control of ventricular arrhythmias and seizures.

The potential for rapid deterioration in clinical status must be appreciated and patients with a history of recent TCA overdose should be managed in a closely monitored environment. Intravenous access should be established, supplemental oxygen administered and cardiac monitoring commenced on arrival. There should be a relatively low threshold for performing endotracheal intubation in the patient with deteriorating mental status because hypoxia and acidosis exacerbate cardiotoxicity. Patients with a decreased level of consciousness or anticholinergic symptoms should undergo urinary catheterization.

Oral activated charcoal should be administered to all patients with significant ingestions after the airway is secured (if necessary). All the TCAs have very large volumes of distribution, and so techniques of enhancing elimination are not helpful.

Hypotension should initially be managed with i.v. fluids. If blood pressure fails to respond to infusions of crystalloid or colloid, then sodium bicarbonate should be tried even in the presence of a normal QRS. If there is still no response inotropes should be started. The ideal inotrope is one that will overcome α-adrenergic blockade and have little stimulatory effect on β receptors. For these reasons, noradrenaline (norepinephrine) is usually regarded as the inotrope of choice. Dopamine is best avoided as it stimulates β receptors (and may lead to a paradoxical decrease in blood pressure) and, as an indirectly acting sympathomimetic, it will become ineffective when neuronal stores of noradrenaline (norepinephrine) are depleted in the presence of a potent reuptake pump inhibitor such as TCAs.[64]

Seizures, delirium and hyperthermia should be controlled using standard techniques.

Flumazenil should be avoided in the setting of a TCA overdose because its action may precipitate refractory seizures and increase morbidity and mortality.[65]

Sodium bicarbonate

Sodium bicarbonate is regarded as a specific antidote in the management of TCA poisoning. It offers a hypertonic source of sodium, which competitively overcomes sodium channel blockade. It appears that the pH alteration also contributes to improved sodium channel function.[66,67] However, manipulation of pH by hyperventilation is not reliably effective in reducing QRS duration.

Sodium bicarbonate is absolutely indicated in the presence of cardiac arrhythmia and may be indicated as a prophylactic measure in the presence if significant widening of the QRS. Bolus doses of 2 mmol/kg should be repeated until cardiovascular stability is achieved. This can be followed by an infusion of 20–100 mmol/h (while maintaining PCO_2 below 40 mmHg with appropriate ventilation settings). Care must be taken to monitor sodium level and arterial blood gases. If arrhythmias persist despite adequate bicarbonate therapy, standard advanced cardiac life support (ACLS) management should be instituted.

Disposition

Patients with a history of TCA ingestion and who have received oral-activated charcoal but show no signs of toxicity after 6 h of observation are safe for medical discharge and ready for psychiatric evaluation.[68] Those with significant cardiovascular or CNS toxicity should be admitted to an intensive care environment. Those with mild CNS manifestations only should be observed in hospital until these resolve.

SELECTIVE SEROTONIN REUPTAKE INHIBITORS (AND ATYPICAL ANTIDEPRESSANTS)

The selective serotonin reuptake inhibitors (SSRIs) have now replaced the TCAs as the first-line drug therapy for depression, bringing with them the advantages of fewer

Table 29.3.5 Seletive serotonin reuptake inhibitors and atypical antidepressants available in Australia

Selective serotonin reuptake inhibition
  Fluoxetine
  Fluvoxamine
  Paroxetine
  Sertraline

Serotonin, noradrenaline (norepinephrine) and dopamine reuptake inhibition
  Citalopram
  Escitalopram
  Venlafaxine

Serotonin reuptake inhibition with α₂-adrenergic antagonism
  Mirtazipine

adverse effects and relative safety in overdose. These drugs are also used in the treatment of obsessive-compulsive disorder, panic disorders and eating disorders including bulimia nervosa. Currently available SSRIs together with the atypical antidepressants that modulate serotonin neurotransmission are listed in Table 29.3.5.

Pharmacology

SSRIs raise synaptic concentrations of serotonin by inhibiting serotonin uptake into presynaptic neurons. In addition, serotonin release from neurons, like other biogenic amines, is subject to autoregulation by presynaptic serotonin receptors that mediate negative feedback. SSRIs desensitize presynaptic serotonin autoreceptors, resulting in increased serotonin release. The rise in synaptic serotonin concentration and resultant stimulation of serotonin receptors (at least 14 different receptors discovered to date) is thought to explain SSRIs' antidepressant activity.[69]

The atypical antidepressants have other effects apart from those on serotonin neurotransmission and these are listed in Table 29.3.5. The SSRIs and atypical antidepressants are generally rapidly and well absorbed after oral administration. Importantly, an extended release formulation of venlafaxine is widely prescribed. These drugs display diverse elimination patterns and have numerous active metabolites, which results in an extended therapeutic effect but also prolongs the time during which drug interactions and adverse effects can occur.

Clinical features

Adverse effects

The most common adverse effects attributed to the SSRIs are gastrointestinal symptoms, sexual dysfunction, headache, insomnia, jitteriness, dizziness and fatigue.[70] Inappropriate antidiuretic hormone secretion is also reported, particularly in the elderly.[71] The adverse effect most likely to result in presentation to the ED is the development of serotonin syndrome (see below) as a result of an interaction between two drugs that enhance serotonergic activity or where there has been an insufficient 'wash-out' period between ceasing one such drug and commencing another.

Overdose

Overdose of the SSRIs and atypical antidepressant generally follows a relatively benign course with the vast majority of patients remaining asymptomatic or experiencing minor self-limiting symptoms only. Venlafaxine with its significant noradrenaline reuptake inhibitor properties is an exception. It is associated with seizures and, in large doses (>4.5 g), cardiotoxicity. Citalopram is associated with QT prolongation although this is rarely of clinical significance.[73,74] For most SSRIs the major concerns are the adverse interactions and serotonin syndrome.

Serotonin syndrome

Previously known as serotonin behavioural syndrome, this was first described in the late 1960s and early 1970s when rats, after being given a combination of a non-selective monoamine oxidase inhibitor and L-tryptophan, developed resting tremor, rigidity and abnormal limb, tail and head movements. Subsequent experiments showed that any drug capable of increasing synaptic levels of serotonin could induce a similar syndrome in larger animals. Human reports of recognized serotonin syndrome first appeared in the literature in the early 1980s.[75,76]

Clinically relevant drugs that can increase synaptic serotonin levels and have been implicated in the development of serotonin syndrome are listed in Table 29.3.6. The mechanisms by which these agents increase synaptic serotonin levels in the cortex, lower brain stem and spinal cord regions are variable and described elsewhere. The postsynaptic receptor subtype 5-HT$_{1A}$ appears to be mainly responsible.[69]

Table 29.3.6 Serotonergically active drugs by mechanism

Increased serotonin production
  Tryptophan

Increased release of stored serotonin
  Amphetamines (including, 'ecstasy')
  Bromocriptine
  Cocaine
  L-dopa

Impaired reuptake of serotonin into presynaptic nerve
  Dextromethorphan
  Mirtazipine
  Nefazadone
  Pethidine

Serotonin reuptake inhibition
  Citalopram
  Fluoxetine
  Fluvoxamine
  Paroxetine
  Sertraline
  Tricyclic antidepressants
  Venlafaxine

Inhibition of serotonin metabolism
  Monoamine oxidase (MAO) inhibitors
    Moclobemide
    Non-selective MAO inhibitors
      Phenelzine
      Tranylcypromine

Enhanced post-synaptic serotonin receptor stimulation
  Lithium
  Lysergic acid diethylamide (LSD)

Symptoms usually begin shortly after the commencement of a serotoninergic drug, or the administration of two different classes of drugs that increase serotonin levels synergistically, for example lithium and fluoxetine. In addition, potential drug interaction may arise when the appropriate 'change-over' period between drugs is not observed.[77] A severe form of the syndrome may develop some hours following overdose with an SSRI or, more commonly, following overdose with multiple serotonergically active drugs.[78–80]

The diagnosis of serotonin syndrome is clinical and based upon the presence of the triad of alteration in behaviour-cognitive ability, autonomic function and neuromuscular activity. A grading system has been proposed.[81] In its most benign form the patient experiences anxiety and apprehension, but altered sensorium with confusion occurs in 50% of reported cases.[69] Seizures may occur.[79] Abnormal neuromuscular activity, caused by increased brainstem and spinal-cord serotonin levels, manifests as increased rigidity (more in the lower than the upper limbs), hyperreflexia, involuntary jerks and resting extremity tremor. Hyperthermia,

secondary to increased muscle activity is a common feature and may lead to confusion with NMS. Diaphoresis, diarrhoea and rigors are common. Cardiovascular instability may occur. Although most patients recover, fatalities are reported.[79,80] There is no correlation with drug levels, and serotonin syndrome remains a clinical diagnosis.[69] The differential diagnosis includes NMS, acute dystonia, hyperadrenergic states (e.g. cocaine toxicity), anticholinergic syndrome and malignant hyperthermia. Decision algorithms have been developed to help the clinician distinguish serotonin syndrome from other conditions.[82]

Treatment

The management of most SSRI and atypical antidepressant overdose is supportive. This usually consists of simple observation, particularly for clinical evidence of serotonin syndrome. Venlafaxine overdose may require more aggressive intervention to ensure control of seizures and cardiotoxicity. Overdose of extended-release preparations of venlafaxine mandates observation for at least 12 h and until symptom-free.

Management of the serotonin syndrome is directed towards withdrawal of the causative agent and the administration of benzodiazepines to decrease muscular rigidity. Benzodiazepines have been reported to nonspecifically inhibit serotonin neurotransmission. If hyperthermia is severe more aggressive treatment may be warranted, including neuromuscular paralysis. Seizures should be treated with benzodiazepines or barbiturates.

Non-specific 5-HT$_1$ and 5-HT$_2$ antagonists such as propranolol, cyproheptadine, chlorpromazine and olanzapine have been tried.[83–85] There are no controlled trials using these agents, but anecdotally cyproheptadine appears to be effective without the adverse effects of the other drugs.[58] A dose of 4–8 mg 8-hourly is recommended.

ANTICONVULSANTS

Anticonvulsants are frequently taken in deliberate self-poisoning. Toxicity resulting in ED attendance also results as a consequence of therapeutic administration. The benzodiazepines and phenobarbitone are discussed earlier in this chapter. This section discusses the traditional anticonvulsants, carbamazepine, phenytoin and sodium valproate – all of which have important toxic syndromes, and the newer anticonvulsants.

Carbamazepine

Pharmacology

Carbamazepine is a carbamylated derivative of iminostilbene. It is structurally related to the TCAs but does not share the same cardio-toxicity profile. An extended-release preparation is widely prescribed.

Absorption from the gastrointestinal tract is slow and erratic because of the insoluble lipophillic nature of the drug. Peak concentrations usually occur at 4 to 8 h but can be greatly delayed after over-dose, particularly of the extended-release preparation. The volume of distribution is from 0.8 to 2.0 L/kg. Metabolism occurs in the liver with an active primary metabolite. The drug or metabolites may undergo enterohepatic circulation. Elimination half-life is normally 18–55 h but may be longer following large overdoses.

Therapeutic carbamazepine concentrations are frequently quoted as 4–12 µg/mL (17–51 µmol/L) and are achieved after an oral loading dose of 18 mg/kg. Thus overdoses of greater than this amount may produce toxicity and ingestions of more than 100 mg/kg are likely to be associated with severe toxicity.

Clinical features

Onset of clinical features of carbamazepine toxicity may be delayed many hours following overdose due to delayed absorption.[86,87] The clinical features are predominantly neurological and include CNS depression which may progress to coma, drowsiness, ataxia, nystagmus and dystonia. Paradoxical seizures are also reported in severe poisoning.[88,89] Carbamazepine toxicity may also manifest as the anticholinergic syndrome, although the delirium may be masked by coma as the intoxication progresses.

Minor ECG changes may be observed in severe carbamazepine poisoning but significant cardiovascular effects are rare.[90]

Treatment

Management of carbamazepine toxicity is primarily supportive and in severe cases involving coma this will include intubation and ventilation. The potential for delayed absorption and deterioration must be considered when determining the period of observation and monitoring following carbamazepine overdose. Serial carbamazepine levels are very useful in determining that absorption is complete and that clinical deterioration will not take place. Carbamazepine levels are also useful in confirming the diagnosis of carbamazepine poisoning. Any elevation above the therapeutic range is significant and levels about 40 mg/L are usually associated with coma. Naturally, a low level early after presentation does not exclude carbamazepine overdose.

Administration of activated charcoal is indicated even after delayed presentation and repeat dose charcoal should be considered as it may enhance elimination of carbamazepine and shorten the duration of toxicity and medical care. Patients who present after carbamazepine overdose should be observed for at least 8 h and have declining carbamazepine levels documented. They may then be medically cleared if asymptomatic. Patients with clinical evidence of poisoning require admission for further observation or supportive care as dictated by the clinical manifestations of poisoning.

Phenytoin

Pharmacology

Phenytoin, also known as diphenylhydantoin, is relatively slowly absorbed from the small intestine with peak levels occurring at about 8 h after a single therapeutic dose but much later following overdose. The volume of distribution is from 0.4 to 0.6 L/kg and the drug is highly bound to plasma proteins. Metabolism occurs in the liver to form inactive metabolites and this metabolism is saturated at relatively low serum concentrations with the result that elimination half-lives are extremely variable.

Clinical presentation

Chronic toxicity

With a relatively low therapeutic index and multiple drug interactions phenytoin toxicity occurs relatively frequently with therapeutic dosing. This is most likely to occur after injudicious dose adjustment.[91,92] These patients usually present with neurological disturbance characterized by ataxia, dysarthria and nystagmus.

Overdose

Similar neurological disturbances are observed following acute overdose, although following large overdoses, a more severe neurological disturbance and even progressive CNS depression may develop. Paradoxical seizures may also occur.[93]

Oral phenytoin overdose is not associated with cardiovascular effects of clinical significance. Cardiotoxicity in the form of hypotension, dysrhythmias and death is only reported followed over-rapid administration or excessive doses of intravenous phenytoin.[94] This cardiotoxicity is thought to be due to the propylene glycol diluent rather than the phenytoin per se.

Treatment

Management of chronic phenytoin toxicity consists of simply withdrawing the drug and maintaining the patient in a safe environment until toxicity resolves.

The management of phenytoin overdose is principally supportive. A single dose of activated charcoal should be administered in the patient who presents early. Cardiac monitoring is not required where phenytoin is the only agent ingested. Serial phenytoin levels may be useful to confirm the diagnosis and guide therapy. Therapeutic levels are 40–80 µmol/L (10–20 mg/L). Progressive toxicity albeit with much individual variation is seen as levels extending above that range (Table 29.3.7).

Valproic acid

Pharmacology

Valproic acid is a simple monocarboxylic acid, chemically unrelated to any other class of antiepileptic drug. Its mechanism

Table 29.3.7 Correlation between serum phenytoin concentration and clinical features	
Phenytoin concentration (µmol/L)	Clinical features
80–120	Horizontal nystagmus
120–160	Vertical nystagmus, ataxia, dysarthria
>160	CNS depression, coma, seizures

of action is thought to involve but not be limited to a decrease in breakdown of GABA-A and increased conversion of GABA from glutamate.[95]

Oral absorption of valproic acid is rapid with peak levels usually occurring within 4 h but this may be delayed following overdose.[96] The volume of distribution is very small at 0.13–0.23 L/kg and there is extensive plasma protein binding which may be saturated in overdose. The drug undergoes extensive hepatic metabolism and has active metabolites. The elimination half-life of 7–15 h may be prolonged in overdose.[97]

Clinical presentation

The clinical course following valproate overdose is dose-dependent. Ingestions of less than 200 mg/kg are usually asymptomatic or result in minor drowsiness only.[98] For ingestions >200 mg/kg, coma may develop and, for ingestions >400 mg/kg, there is a risk of prolonged profound coma and metabolic disorders including hyperammonaemia, hypernatraemia, hypocalcaemia and bone-marrow depression.[99] Death from cerebral oedema is reported.

Treatment

Management is primarily supportive. Minor ingestions can usually be simply observed until drowsiness resolves. Ingestions of more than 200 mg/kg should be decontaminated with oral-activated charcoal if they present early and then observed closely for CNS depression. This should occur within 4 h. It is useful to monitor serum levels until falling. Peak levels >500 mg/L (3500 μmol/L) are usually associated with coma. Patients who develop coma will require intubation and intensive care management with careful attention to monitoring electrolytes, renal function, blood counts and haemodynamics. The coma may persist days after valproate levels fall and in this instance, CT scanning of the head is indicated to look for cerebral oedema.

Haemodialysis greatly enhances elimination of valproate and should be considered whenever life-threatening systemic toxicity is anticipated. Although precise indications for haemodialysis remain controversial, reasonable guidelines are an ingestion of >1000 mg/kg with a serum level >7000 μmol/L (1000 mg/L) or a serum level of >10 400 μmol/L (1500 mg/L) at any time.

L-carnitine

L-carnitine is an amino acid carrier molecule used to transport long-chain fatty acids across to mitochondria. It is synthetized chiefly in liver and kidney. It is available in oral and intravenous forms and appears to have an acceptable safety profile.[100] It is postulated that L-carnitine could provide benefit in patients with concomitant hyperammonemia encephalopathy and/or hepatotoxicity as there is some evidence that it reduces ammonia concentrations in acute valproate overdose.[101,102] While L-carnitine has been used in a number of case reports definitive evidence of efficacy is lacking.

Newer antiepileptic drugs

A number of new antiepileptic drugs with differing pharmacokinetic properties and mechanisms of action have been introduced into clinical practice over the last decade. These include oxcarbazepine, gabapentin, felbamate, vigabatrin, topiramate and tiagabine. The toxicity profiles of these drugs in overdose are not yet well established. Gabapentin, felbamate and lamotrigine are reported to cause only minor CNS effects in overdose.[99–103] Vigabatrin overdose has resulted in severe agitation.[104]

Controversies

❶ The role of flumazenil, a specific benzodiazepine receptor antagonist, remains controversial.

❷ The use of specific agents, such as bromocriptine and dantrolene in the treatment of neuroleptic malignant syndrome is controversial. Given the rarity of NMS, prospective controlled trials have not been, and are unlikely to be, conducted.

❸ The indications (if any) for the administration of sodium bicarbonate therapy as prophylaxis against TCA-induced cardiac arrhythmias remain controversial.

❹ Physostigmine, an acetylcholinesterase inhibitor that crosses the blood–brain barrier, can dramatically reverse the anticholinergic effects of TCA overdose. However, its use in this setting is usually regarded as contraindicated because of an association with significant adverse effects, including seizures, bradycardia, and even asystole.

❺ Fab fragments have been produced and used experimentally to treat TCA toxicity in animals but are not yet commercially available.

❻ The role of cyproheptadine and other serotonin antagonists in the management of serotonin syndrome is yet to be clearly defined.

❼ Haemodialysis enhances the elimination of valproate but indications for its implementation are not yet well defined.

❽ L-carnitine has been proposed as an antidote to valproate poisoning but again clinical value has not been established.

❾ Toxicity profiles for the newer anticonvulsants are yet to be established.

References

1. Goodchild CS. GABA receptors and benzodiazepines. British Journal of Anaesthesia 1993; 71: 127–133.
2. Greenblatt DJ, Allen MD, Noel BJ, et al. Acute overdosage with benzodiazepine derivatives. Clinical Pharmacology and Therapy 1977; 21: 497–514.
3. Busto U, Kaplan HL, Sellers EM. Benzodiazepine-associated emergencies in Toronto. American Journal of Psychiatry 1980; 137: 224–227.
4. Gueye PN, Lofaso F, Borron SW, et al. Mechanism of respiratory insufficiency in pure or mixed drug-induced coma involving benzodiazepines. Clinical Toxicology 2002; 40: 35–47.
5. Tanaka E. Toxicological interactions between alcohol and benzodiazepines. Clinical Toxicology 2002; 40: 69–75.
6. Haverkos GP, DiSalvo RP, Imhoff TE. Fatal seizures after flumazenil administration in a patient with mixed overdose. Annals of Pharmacotherapy 1994; 28:1347–1349.
7. Gaulier JM, Merle G, Lacassie E, et al. Fatal intoxications with chloral hydrate. Journal of Forensic Sciences 2001; 46: 1507–1509.
8. Regouby Y, Delomez G, Tisserant A. First-degree heart block caused by voluntary zopiclone poisoning. Therapie 1990; 45: 162.
9. Bramness JG, Arnestad M, Karinen R, et al. Fatal overdose of zopiclone in an elderly woman with bronchogenic coma. Journal of Forensic Sciences 2001; 46: 1247–1249.
10. Boniface PF, Russel SG. Two cases of fatal zopiclone overdose. Journal of Analytical Toxicology 1996; 20: 131–133.
11. Meram D, Descotes J. Acute poisoning with zolpidem. Revue Medicine Interne 1989; 10: 466.

12. Gock SB, Wong SHY, Nuwayhid N, et al. Acute zolpidem overdose – report of two cases. Journal of Analytical Toxicology 1999; 23: 559–562.

13. Ahmad Z, Herepath M, Ebden P. Diagnostic utility of flumazenil in coma with suspected poisoning. British Medical Journal 1991; 302: 292.

14. Lheureux P, Debailleul G, De Witte O, et al. Zolpidem intoxication mimicking narcotic overdoses: response to flumazenil. Human and Experimental Toxicology 1990; 9: 105–107.

15. Lheureux P. Continuous flumazenil for zolpidem toxicity – commentary. Clinical Toxicology 1998; 36: 745–746.

16. Graham SR, Day RO, Lee R, et al. Overdose with chloral hydrate: a pharmacological and therapeutic review. Medical Journal of Australia 1988; 149: 686–688.

17. Zahedi A, Grant MH, Wong DT. Successful treatment of chloral hydrate cardiac toxicity with propranolol. American Journal of Emergency Medicine 1999; 17: 490–491.

18. Black JL, Richelson E, Richardson JW. Antipsychotic agents: a clinical update. Mayo Clinic Proceedings 1985; 60: 777.

19. Burns MJ. The pharmacology and toxicology of atypical antipsychotic agents. Clinical Toxicology 2001; 39: 1–14.

20. Casey DE, Keepers GA. Neuroleptic side effects: acute extrapyramidal syndromes and tardive dyskinesia. In: Casey DE, Christensen AV, eds. Psychopharmacology: current trends. Springer-Verlag; 1988: 74–83.

21. Rupniak NJ, Jenner P, Marsden CD. Acute dystonia induced by neuroleptic drugs. Psychopharmacology 1986; 88: 403.

22. Swett C. Drug induced dystonia. American Journal of Psychiatry 1975; 132: 532.

23. Marsden CD, Jenner P. The pathophysiology of extrapyramidal side effects of neuroleptic drugs. Psychological Medicine 1980; 10: 55.

24. Yassa R, Ananth J, Cordozo S, et al. Tardive dyskinesia in an outpatient population: prevalence and predisposing factors. Canadian Journal of Psychiatry 1983; 28: 391.

25. Marks RC, Luchins DJ. Antipsychotic medications and seizures. Psychiatric Medicine 1991; 9: 37.

26. Logothetis J. Spontaneous epileptic seizures and electroencephalographic changes in the course of phenothiazine therapy. Neurology 1967; 17: 869.

27. Reilly JG, Ayis SA, Ferrier IN, et al. QTc-interval abnormalities and psychotropic drug therapy in psychiatric patients. Lancet 2000; 355: 1048–1052.

28. Kariagianis JL, Phillips LC, Hogan KP, et al. Clozapine-associated neuroleptic malignant syndrome: two new cases and a review of the literature. Annals of Pharmacotherapy 1999; 3(5):623–630.

29. Levin GM, Lazowick AL, Powell HS. Neuroleptic malignant syndrome with risperidone. Journal of Clinical Psychopharmacology 1996; 16: 192–193.

30. Burkhard PR, Vingerhoets FLG. Olanzapine-induced neuroleptic malignant syndrome (letter). Archives of General Psychiatry 1999; 56:101–102.

31. Nierenberg D, Disch M, Manheimer E, et al. Facilitating prompt diagnosis and treatment of the neuroleptic malignant syndrome. Clinical Pharmacology and Therapy 1991; 50: 580.

32. Shalev A, Hermesh H, Munitz H. Mortality from neuroleptic malignant syndrome. Journal of Clinical Psychiatry 1989; 50: 18.

33. Blaye IL, Donatini B, Hall M, et al. Acute overdosage with thioridazine: a review of the available clinical exposure. Veterinary and Human Toxicology 1993; 35:147–150.

34. Isbister GK, Murray L, John S, et al. Amisulpride deliberate self-poisoning causing severe cardiac toxicity including QT prolongation and torsades de pointes. Medical Journal of Australia 2006; 184: 354–356.

35. Haag S, Spigset O, Edwardsson H, et al. Prolonged sedation and slowly decreasing clozapine serum concentrations after an overdose. Journal of Clinical Psychopharmacology 1999; 19: 282–284.

36. Buckley NA, Whyte IM, Dawson AH. Cardiotoxicity is more common in thioridazine overdose than with other neuroleptics. Clinical Toxicology 1995; 33: 199–204.

37. Schmidt W, Lang K. Life-threatening dysrhythmias in severe thioridazine poisoning treated with physostigmine and transient atrial pacing. Critical Care Medicine 1997; 25: 1925–1930.

38. Sharma ND, Roman HS, Padhi D, et al. Torsades de pointes associated with intravenous haloperidol in critically ill patients. American Journal of Cardiology 1998; 81: 238–240.

39. Ward DI. Two cases of amisulpride overdose: A cause for prolonged QT syndrome. Emergency Medical Association 2005; 17: 274–276.

40. Balit CR, Isbister GK, Hackett PL, et al. Quetiapine Poisoning: A Case Series. Annals of Emergency Medicine 2003; 42:751–758.

41. Hunfeld NGM, Westerman EM, Boswijk DJ, et al. Quetiapine in overdosage. a clinical and pharmacokinetic analysis of 14 cases. Therapeutic Drug Monitoring 2006; 28: 185–189.

42. Bryant SG, Guernsey BG, Ingrim NB. Review of bupropion. Clinical Pharmacology 1983; 2: 525–537.

43. Lai AA, Schroeder DH. Clinical pharmacokinetics of bupropion: a review. Journal of Clinical Psychiatry 1983; 44: 82–84.

44. Roose SP, Dalack GW, Glassman AH, et al. Cardiovascular effects of bupropion in depressed patients with heart disease. American Journal of Psychiatry 1991; 148: 512–516.

45. Szuba MP, Leuchter AF. Falling backward in two elderly patients taking bupropion. Journal of Clinical Psychiatry 1992; 53: 157–159.

46. Wenger TL, Stern WC. The cardiovascular profile of bupropion. Journal of Clinical Psychiatry 1983; 44: 176–182.

47. Settle EC, Stahl SM, Batey SR, et al. Safety profile of sustained-release bupropion in depression: results of three clinical trials. Clinical Therapeutics 1999; 21: 454–463.

48. Davidson J. Seizures and bupropion: a review. Journal of Clinical Psychiatry 1989; 50: 256–261.

49. Balit CR, Lynch CN, Isbister GK. Bupropion poisoning: a case series. Medical Journal of Australia 2003; 178: 61–63.

50. Druteika D, Zed PJ. Cardiotoxicity following bupropion overdose. Annals of Pharmacotherapy 2002; 36: 1791–1795.

51. Biswas AK, Zabrocki LA, Mayes KL, et al. Cardiotoxicity associated with intentional ziprasidone and bupropion overdose. Journal of Toxicology, Clinical Toxicology 2003; 41: 101–104.

52. Isbister GK, Balit CR. Bupropion overdose: QTc prolongation and its clinical significance. Annals of Pharmacotherapy 2003; 37: 999–1002.

53. Harris C, Gualtieri J, Stark G. Fatal bupropion overdose. Clinical Toxicology 1997; 35: 321–324.

54. Mills KC. Tricyclic antidepressants. In: Tintinalli JE, Ruiz E, Krome RL, eds. Emergency medicine: a comprehensive study guide. 4th edn. Ohio: McGraw Hill. 1996: 740.

55. Buckley NA, Dawson AH, Whyte IM, et al. Six years of self-poisoning in Newcastle: 1987–1992. Medical Journal of Australia 1995; 162: 190–193.

56. Buckley NA, Dawson AH, Whyte IM, et al. Greater toxicity of dothiepin in overdose than of other tricyclic antidepressants. Lancet 1994; 343: 159–162.

57. Curry SC. Neurotransmitter principles. In: Goldfrank LR, Weissman RS, Flomenbaum NE, Howard MA, Lewin NA, Hoffman RS, eds. Goldfrank's toxicologic emergencies. 5th edn. Norwalk, Connecticut: Appleton and Lange; 1994: pp. 231–257.

58. Chan BC, Graudins A, Whyte IA, et al. Serotonin syndrome resulting from drug interactions. Medical Journal of Australia 1998; 169: 523–525.

59. Wedin GP, Odra GM, Klein-Schwartz W, et al. Relative toxicity of cyclic antidepressants. Annals of Emergency Medicine 1986; 15: 797.

60. Dzuikas LJ, Vohra J. Tricyclic antidepressant poisoning. Medical Journal of Australia 1991; 154: 344–350.

61. Boehnert MT, Lovejoy FH. Value of the QRS duration versus the serum drug level in predicting seizures and ventricular arrhythmias after an acute overdose of tricyclic antidepressants. New England Journal of Medicine 1985; 313: 474–479.

62. Niemann JT, Benson HA, Rothstein RJ, et al. Electrocardiographic criteria for tricyclic antidepressant cardiotoxicity. American Journal of Cardiology 1986; 57: 1154–1159.

63. Liebelt EL, Francis PD, Woolf AD. ECG lead aVR versus QRS interval in predicting seizures and arrhythmias in acute tricyclic antidepressant toxicity. Annals of Emergency Medicine 1995; 26: 195–201.

64. Buchamn AL, Dauer J, Giederan J. The use of vasoactive agents in the treatment of antidepressant overdose. Journal of Clinical Psychopharmacology 1990; 10: 409–413.

65. Spivey WH. Flumazenil and seizures: Analysis of 33 cases. Clinical Therapy 1992 14(2): 292–305.

66. Nattel S, Mittleman M. Treatment of ventricular tachyarrhythmias from amitriptyline toxicity in dogs. Journal of Pharmacology and Experimental Therapy 1984; 1231: 430–435.

67. Nattel S, Keable H, Sasyniuk BI. Experimental amytriptyline intoxication: electrophysiologic manifestations and management. Journal of Cardiovascular Pharmacology 1984; 6: 83–89.

68. Callaham M, Kassel D. Epidemiology of fatal tricyclic antidepressant ingestion: implications for management. Annals of Emergency Medicine 1985; 14: 1–9.

69. Mills K. Serotonin toxicity: a comprehensive review for emergency medicine. Topics in Emergency Medicine 1993; 15: 54–73.

70. Woodrum ST, Brown CS. Management of SSRI-induced sexual dysfunction. Annals of Pharmacotherapy 1998; 32: 1209–1215.

71. Kirchner V, Silver LE, Kelly CA. Selective serotonin reuptake inhibitors and hyponatremia: review and proposed mechanisms in the elderly. Journal of Psychopharmacology 1998; 12: 396–400.

72. Whyte IM, Dawson AH, Buckley NA. Relative toxicity of venlafaxine and selective serotonin reuptake inhibitors in overdose compared to tricyclic antidepressants. Quarterly Journal of Medicine 2003; 96: 369–374.

73. Isbister GK, Bowe SJ, Dawson A, et al. Relative toxicity of selective serotonin re-uptake inhibitors (SSRIs) in overdose. Clinical Toxicology 2004; 42: 277–285.

74. Isbister GK Fridberg LE, Duffull SB. Application of pharmacokinetic-pharmacodynamic modelling in the management of QT abnormalities after citalopram overdose. Intensive Care Medicine 2006; 32: 1060–1065.

75. Insel TR, Roy BF, Cohen RM, et al. Possible development of the serotonin syndrome in man. American Journal of Psychiatry 1982; 139: 954–955.

76. Sternbach H. The serotonin syndrome. American Journal of Psychiatry 1991; 148: 705–714.

77. DeVane DL. Pharmacokinetics of the selective serotonin reuptake inhibitors. Journal of Clinical Psychiatry 1992; 53(Supplement):13–19.

78. Kaminski CA, Robbins MS, Weibley RE. Sertraline intoxication in a child. Annals of Emergency Medicine 1994; 23: 1371–1374.

79. Kline SS, Mauro LS, Scala-Barnett DM, et al. Serotonin syndrome versus neuroleptic malignant syndrome as a cause of death. Clinical Pharmacology 1989; 8: 510–514.

80. Power BM, Pinder M, Hackett LP, et al. Fatal serotonin syndrome following a combined overdose of moclobemide, clomipramine and fluoxetine. Anaesthetics and Intensive Care 1995; 23: 499–502.

81. Dunkley EJ, Isister GK, Sibbritt D, et al. The Hunter Serotonin Toxicity Criteria: simple and accurate diagnostic decision rules for serotonin toxicity. Quarterly Journal of Medicine 2003; 96: 635–642.

82. Boyer EW, Shannon M. The serotonin syndrome. New England Journal of Medicine 2005; 352: 1112–1120.

83. Graudins A, Aaron CK. Delayed peak serum valproic acid in massive divalproex overdose – treatment with charcoal hemoperfusion. Journal of Toxicology, Clinical Toxicology 1996; 34: 335–341.

84. Guze BH, Baxter LR. The serotonin syndrome: case responsive to propranolol (letter). Journal of Clinical Psychopharmacology 1986; 6: 119–120.

85. Geer SC, Baldessarini RJ. Motor effects of serotonin in the central nervous system. Life Sciences 1980; 27: 1435–1451.

86. Sandyk R.. L dopa induced 'serotonin syndrome' in a parkinsonian patient on bromocriptine (letter). Journal of Clinical Psychopharmacology 1980; 6: 194–195.

87. Sullivan JB, Rumack BH, Peterson RG. Acute carbamazepine toxicity resulting from overdose. Neurology 1981; 31: 621–624.

88. Sethna M, Solomon G, Cedarbaum J, et al. Successful treatment of massive carbamazepine overdose. Epilepsia 1989; 30: 71–73.

89. Hojer J, Malmlund HO, Berg A. Clinical features in 28 consecutive cases of laboratory confirmed massive poisoning with carbamazepine alone. Clinical Toxicology 1993; 3: 449–458.

90. Tibballs J. Acute toxic reaction to carbamazepine: clinical effects and serum concentrations. Journal of Pediatrics 1992; 121: 295–299.

91. Apfelbaum JD, Caravati EM, Kerns WP, et al. Cardiovascular effects of carbamazepine toxicity. Annals of Emergency Medicine 1995; 25: 631–635.

92. Morgan F. Fortnightly review: drug treatment of epilepsy. British Medical Journal 1999; 318: 106–109.

93. Maloteaux EG. Pharmacological management of epilepsy. Mechanism of action, pharmacokinetic drug interactions, and new drug discovery possibilities. International Journal of Clinical Pharmacology and Therapeutics 1988; 36: 181–184.

94. Peruca E, Gram L, Avanzi G, Dulac O. Antiepileptic drugs as a cause of worsening seizures. Epilepsia 1998; 39: 5–17.

95. Russell MA, Bousvaros G. Fatal results from diphenylhydantoin administered intravenously. Journal of the American Medical Association 1968; 20: 2118–2119.

96 Curry SC, Mills KC, Graeme KA. Neurotransmitters In: Goldfrank LR, ed. Goldfranks toxicologic emergencies. 7th edn. New York: McGraw-Hill. 2002: pp. 133–165.

97. Brubacher JR, Dahghani P, McKnight D. Delayed toxicity following ingestion of enteric-coated divalproex sodium (Epival). Journal of Emergency Medicine 1999; 17: 463–467.

98. Garnier R, Boudignat O, Fournier PE. Valproate poisoning. Lancet 1982; 2: 97.

99. Anderson GO, Ritland S. Life-threatening intoxication with sodium valproate. Clinical Toxicology 1995; 33: 279–284.

100. LoVecchio F, Shriki J, Samaddar R. L-carnitine was safely administered in the setting of valproate toxicity. Am J Emerg Med 2005; 23(3): 321–322.

101. Yehya N, Saldarini CT, Koski ME, et al. Valproate-induced hyperammonemic encephalopathy. [Case Reports. Letter] Journal of the American Academy of Child & Adolescent Psychiatry. 2004; 43(8): 926–927.

102. Perez A, McKay CA. Role of carnitine in valproic acid toxicity. Journal of Toxicology Clinical Toxicology 2003: 1901–2100.

103. Nagel TR, Schunk JE. Felbamate overdose: a case report and discussion of a new antiepileptic drug. Pediatric Emergency Care 1995; 11: 369–371.

104. O'Donnel J, Bateman ND. Lamotrigine overdose in an adult. Clinical Toxicology 2000; 38: 659–660.

29.4 Lithium

Mark Monaghan • Lindsay Murray

ESSENTIALS

1 Chronic lithium toxicity is associated with significant morbidity and mortality especially where diagnosis and treatment are delayed. Acute lithium overdose, unless massive, has a more benign course.

2 Chronic lithium poisoning presents with neurological dysfunction. Acute lithium overdose presents with gastrointestinal dysfunction.

3 Consider the diagnosis of lithium intoxication and check a serum lithium concentration in any patient on lithium therapy who presents unwell.

4 Chronic lithium intoxication usually develops because of impaired lithium excretion. The underlying factors must be identified and corrected.

5 Serum lithium levels correlate with central nervous system (CNS) levels and clinical severity in chronic but not acute intoxication.

6 Haemodialysis effectively enhances lithium elimination but is rarely required in patients with normal renal function. This intervention is more likely to be necessary in chronic intoxication than acute overdose.

Introduction

Lithium, the metal with the lowest molecular weight, is usually dispensed as the carbonate salt. It is widely used in the therapy of bipolar disorder and a number of other conditions. Both immediate-release and sustained-release preparations are available. This drug has a relatively narrow therapeutic index and chronic intoxication develops relatively frequently. Acute overdose is less common.

Pharmacokinetics

Standard lithium preparations are rapidly and completely absorbed after oral administration with peak serum levels occurring at 2–4 h. Absorption and time to peak level is delayed after administration of sustained-release preparations and following overdose. Once absorbed, lithium is slowly redistributed from the intravascular space to the total body water. Lithium is not metabolized and its elimination is almost exclusively renal.

Lithium is freely filtered at the glomerulus but, under normal circumstances, approximately 80% of filtered ions are reabsorbed in the proximal tubule and only 20% are excreted in the urine. Under these circumstances, renal clearance of lithium is approximately 10–40 mL/min and its elimination half-life is 20–24 h. The renal elimination of lithium is greatly affected by sodium and water balance and by the presence of drugs that affect renal tubular reabsorption of sodium. In the early stages following acute overdose, renal elimination is much greater because lithium is relatively concentrated in the intravascular compartment and available for filtration at the glomerulus.

Clinical features

Chronic lithium toxicity

Chronic lithium toxicity may develop in association with prolonged excessive dosing or, more commonly, as a result of impaired lithium excretion due to intercurrent illness or a drug interaction. Lithium excretion is impaired in renal failure and congestive cardiac failure because of reduced filtration at the glomerulus and also in water or sodium depletion states because of increased reabsorption of sodium (and lithium) in the proximal tubule. A number of drugs including nonsteroidal anti-inflammatory drugs (NSAIDs), selective serotonin reuptake inhibitors (SSRIs), angiotesin converting enzyme (ACE) inhibitors, thiazide diuretics and topiramate may also impair lithium excretion.

The clinical features of chronic lithium toxicity are almost exclusively neurological and the following severity grading system is widely used:[1]

- Grade I (mild): nausea, vomiting, tremor, hyperreflexia, agitation, muscle weakness, ataxia
- Grade II (serious): stupor, rigidity, hypotonia, hypotension
- Grade III (life threatening): coma, seizures, myoclonia, cardiovascular collapse.

The differential diagnosis for this presentation is broad and includes non-convulsive status epilepticus, serotonin and neuroleptic malignant syndromes, electrolyte abnormalities and CNS pathologies such as sepsis.

Lithium toxicity is generally not associated with significant cardiovascular effects although delayed onset of conduction disturbances is reported.[2] Minor benign ECG changes are more commonly observed.[3]

Chronic lithium therapy is also associated with nephrogenic diabetes insipidus and hypothyroidism, which may complicate the clinical presentation of toxicity.

Acute lithium overdose

Patients who take a significant overdose of lithium carbonate as with any other metal salt, develop rapid onset of gastrointestinal toxicity characterized by nausea, vomiting, abdominal pain and diarrhoea. This gastrointestinal disturbance can be very severe and may result in significant fluid and electrolyte losses. It is usually observed where more than 25 g are ingested but can occur following smaller doses. Gastrointestinal upset is not a prominent feature of chronic lithium toxicity.

Acute lithium overdose is much less likely to result in significant neurotoxicity than is chronic lithium toxicity.[4] Neurotoxicity could theoretically slowly develop following acute overdose if renal clearance were sufficiently impaired so as to allow redistribution of sufficient lithium from the intravascular compartment to tissue compartments before it could be excreted. This situation may develop if there is pre-existing renal failure or if inadequate fluid resuscitation leads to dehydration, sodium depletion or renal impairment as a consequence of the fluid losses from gastrointestinal toxicity.

Clinical investigation

Essential laboratory investigations in the assessment of lithium toxicity are serum electrolytes, renal function and serum lithium concentration. Serial serum lithium concentrations are often required. Other investigations are performed as indicated to evaluate and manage intercurrent disease processes and to exclude important differential diagnoses.

Therapeutic serum lithium concentrations are generally quoted as 0.6–1.2 mEq/L, although clinical evidence of lithium toxicity can be observed at concentrations within this range, particularly in the elderly.[5] More commonly in cases of chronic intoxication, mild toxicity is observed at lithium concentrations of 1.5–2.5 mEq/L, severe toxicity at concentrations of 2.5 to 3.5 mEq/L, and life-threatening toxicity at concentrations >3.5 mEq/L. Following acute overdose, serum lithium concentrations do not correlate with clinical severity as they do not reflect CNS concentrations; however, when performed serially, they are useful in guiding management. Peak serum lithium concentrations >4.0 mEq/L are frequently observed following acute overdose in patients who do not go on to develop neurotoxicity.

Treatment

Chronic lithium toxicity

The diagnosis of lithium toxicity should be considered in any individual on lithium therapy who presents to the emergency department unwell, in particular with evidence of neurological dysfunction. The diagnosis should be confirmed or excluded by ordering a serum lithium concentration as part of the initial work-up. A precipitating illness that has resulted in impaired lithium excretion will usually be present and require assessment and treatment on its own merits.

Appropriate supportive care measures should be instituted on arrival. Once the diagnosis of chronic lithium toxicity is confirmed, further care is oriented towards management of the precipitating medical condition and enhancing lithium excretion by optimizing renal function and correcting any water or sodium deficits with intravenous normal saline. Therapy with lithium

carbonate and any drugs contributing to lithium toxicity should be immediately discontinued.[6]

Enhanced elimination of lithium by haemodialysis may be attempted in severe or worsening chronic lithium neurotoxicity. The aim of this intervention is to minimize the duration of neurological dysfunction and avoid permanent neurological sequelae. Lithium has physicochemical and pharmacokinetic properties that render it very suitable for enhancing elimination by haemodialysis: low molecular weight, high water solubility, small volume of distribution, no plasma protein binding and an endogenous renal clearance rate much lower than that achieved by haemodialysis.[7] There is, however, no evidence that haemodialysis improves clinical outcome or survival rates.

The indications for haemodialysis are difficult to define. It should be considered in any patient with an elevated serum lithium concentration and severe or life-threatening neurotoxicity. It may be considered in the patient with less severe toxicity in whom adequate renal function and a falling lithium concentration are unable to be established with initial fluid resuscitation. Once instituted haemodialysis should be continued until the serum lithium is <1 mEq/L. Some rebound in serum lithium may be noted after intermittent haemodialysis is discontinued, which may be avoided if continuous arterio-venous (AV) or veno-venous (VV) haemodiafiltration is sustained for >16 h.[8,9] The decision to dialyse can usually be made some 8–12 h after admission.[7]

Acute lithium overdose

In contrast to chronic toxicity, the vast majority of acute poisonings can be managed solely with good supportive care. Intravenous access should be established and infusion of normal saline commenced during the initial assessment. Administration should be sufficient to correct any sodium or water deficits arising as a result of the toxic gastroenteritis and to ensure a good urine output. Excessive administration of normal saline or attempts at forced diuresis do not further enhance lithium excretion.[10] A serum lithium concentration, renal function and electrolytes should be performed as part of the initial assessment and repeated as necessary to guide further management. In particular, the serum lithium should be followed until falling and <2 mEq/L.

Activated charcoal does not bind lithium well and need not be administered unless there has been a significant co-ingestion. Sodium polystyrene sulfonate has been proposed as an effective alternative absorbent but is not widely used and repeated administration can cause hypokalaemia.[11] On the basis of a single volunteer study, whole-bowel irrigation has been recommended for overdose of extended-release preparations[12] but the gastrointestinal upset renders this intervention technically difficult in patients with large ingestions.

Haemodialysis is rarely indicated following acute overdose in the patient with normal renal function who receives good supportive care. It may be necessary in the presence of renal failure or in the patient who goes on to develop neurotoxicity in the presence of a slowly falling serum lithium concentration.

Disposition and prognosis

Patients with chronic lithium intoxication require admission for management of their fluid and electrolyte status, monitoring of renal function and serum lithium concentration and management of intercurrent illnesses. Ideally, admission should be to an institution with a capacity to perform haemodialysis where toxicity is moderate or severe. Following haemodialysis, neurological recovery may be delayed well beyond the removal of lithium and permanent neurological deficits are reported.[13,14]

Acute lithium overdose usually has an excellent outcome with good supportive care and may be admitted to a non-monitored setting for intravenous fluids and monitoring of fluid and electrolytes and lithium concentrations. The asymptomatic patient with normal renal function and lithium level falling to below 2 mEq/L is fit for medical discharge. This usually occurs within 24 h. Psychiatric evaluation is mandatory and may take place whilst waiting for lithium levels to fall.

Controversies

❶ The indications for and preferred method of gastrointestinal decontamination following acute lithium overdose remain undefined.

❷ Precise criteria for haemodialysis in chronic lithium intoxication remain undefined.

❸ Continuous arterio- or venovenous haemofiltration have been proposed as alternatives to haemodialyis for enhancement of lithium elimination. Although lower clearances are achieved with these methods, they are often easier to institute and may minimize rapid transcellular fluid and electrolyte shifts.[11] At the moment they can only be recommended where haemodialysis is not available.

References

1. Hansen HE, Amdisen A. Lithium intoxication. Quarterly Journal of Medicine 1978; 47: 123–144.
2. Waring WS. Delayed cardiotoxicity in chronic lithium poisoning: discrepancy between serum lithium concentrations and clinical status. Basic and Clinical Pharmacology and Toxicology 2007; 100(5): 353–355.
3. Tilkian AG, Schroeder JS, Kao JJ. Cardiovascular effects of lithium in man: a review of the literature. American Journal of Medicine 1976; 61: 665–667.
4. Oakley PW, Whyte IM, Carter GL. Lithium toxicity: an iatrogenic problem in susceptible individuals. Australian & New Zealand Journal of Psychiatry 2001; 35: 833–840.
5. Strayhorn JM, Nash JL. Severe neurotoxicity despite 'therapeutic' serum lithium levels. Diseases of the Nervous System 1977; 38: 107–111.
6. Eyer F, Pfab R, Felgenhauer N, et al. Lithium poisoning: pharmacokinetics and clearance during different therapeutic measures. Journal of Clinical Psychopharmacology 2006; 26(3): 325–330.
7. Jaeger A, Saunder P, Kopferschmidt J, et al. When should dialysis be performed in lithium poisoning? A kinetic study in 14 cases of lithium poisoning. Clinical Toxicology 1993; 31(3): 429–447.
8. LeBlanc M, Raymond M, Bonnardeau A, et al. Lithium poisoning treated by high-performance continuous arteriovenous and venovenous hemodiafiltration. American Journal of Kidney Disease 1996; 27: 365–372.
9. Waring WS. Management of lithium toxicity. Toxicology Reviews 2006; 25(4): 221–230.
10. Amidsen A. Clinical features and management of lithium poisoning. Medical and Toxicological Adverse Drug Experiences 1988; 3: 18–32.
11. Roberge RJ, Martin TG, Schneider S. Use of sodium polystyrene sulfonate in a lithium overdose. Annals of Emergency Medicine 1993; 22: 1911–1915.
12. Smith S, Ling L Halstenson C. Whole-bowel irrigation as a treatment for acute lithium overdose. Annals of Emergency Medicine 1991; 20: 536–539.
13. Verdoux H, Bougeois M. A case of lithium neurotoxicity with irreversible cerebellar syndrome. Journal of Nervous and Mental Disorders 1990; 178: 761.
14. Shou M. Long lasting neurological sequelae after lithium intoxication. Acta Psychiatrica Scandinavica 1984; 70: 594.

29.5 Antihistamine and anticholinergic poisoning

Andis Graudins • Naren Gunja

ESSENTIALS

1 Anticholinergic toxicity is a relatively common and often unrecognized toxicological problem in the emergency department.

2 H_1-receptor antagonists are readily accessible and a common cause of anticholinergic poisoning.

3 Significant central nervous system and cardiovascular toxicity may infrequently complicate large ingestions of first-generation H_1-receptor antagonists.

4 H_2-receptor antagonist overdose rarely produces any significant clinical effects.

Introduction

Anticholinergic toxicity is a common side effect of many pharmaceutical agents, natural remedies and plants, both in therapeutic dosing and in overdose (see Table 29.5.1). Symptoms and signs may range from mild manifestations of the syndrome (e.g. dry mouth and blurred vision) to severe anticholinergic delirium with agitation, hallucinations and aggressive behaviour.

The antihistamine agents are a diverse group of drugs that can be broadly classified, based upon receptor specificity, into H_1- and H_2-receptor antagonists. The H_1-receptor antagonists are widely used in the treatment of allergic conditions and nasal congestion, as over-the-counter sleep aids and as antiemetics. This group can be further divided into the 'first-generation' agents, which tend to be more lipophilic

Table 29.5.1 Anticholinergic agents
Pharmaceuticals
Anticholinergic agents
Atropine
Benzhexol
Benztropine
Scopolamine
Antipsychotic agents
Clozapine
Olanzapine
Phenothiazines
Quetiapine
Risperidone
Cyclic antidepressants
Amitriptyline
Chlormipramine
Dothiepin
Doxepin
Imipramine
Nortriptyline
First-generation H_1-receptor blockers
Cetirizine
Chlorpheniramine
Cyproheptadine
Dexchlorpheniramine
Diphenhydramine
Diphenylpyraline
Doxylamine
Pheniramine
Promethazine
Others
Amantadine
Carbamazepine
Botanicals
Datura *spp.*
Jimson weed or thorn apple
Angel's trumpet
Atropa belladona – deadly nightshade

and are more sedating, and the 'second-generation' or non-sedating agents. The H_2-receptor antagonists are primarily used in the treatment of peptic ulcer disease and gastro-oesophageal reflux, but are also used in conjunction with H_1 antagonists in the treatment of severe allergic reactions.

Antihistamine agents are relatively easy to obtain and frequently used in overdose for attempted suicide and abused recreationally for their sedating and anticholinergic effects. The incidence of antihistamine poisoning and abuse in Australia is not well characterized. Other prescription drugs may also result in anticholinergic toxicity both in therapeutic dosing and in overdose. These may also be intentionally abused for their anticholinergic effects.[1-4] Chinese and traditional herbal medicines may result in anticholinergic toxicity either directly from the herbal agent ingested or as a result of contamination with anticholinergic agents such as atropine or scopolamine.[5-7] The intentional abuse of botanicals (e.g. *Datura* spp.) may also present with anticholinergic toxicity.[8-10] In view of the easy availability of many of these pharmaceutical and herbal agents, the emergency physician should include a detailed drug history in the evaluation of any patient presenting with evidence of mental status change and anticholinergic symptoms and signs. In particular, polypharmacy and drug interactions between multiple agents with the potential for anticholinergic effects should be included in the differential diagnosis of elderly patients presenting with mental status changes.

Pharmacodynamics and pharmacokinetics

The H_1-antagonists are a diverse group of agents that reversibly block the action of histamine at H_1 receptors. High lipid solubility results in central nervous system (CNS) penetration and sedation. The first generation agents also block muscarinic, α-adrenergic and serotonergic receptors. Local anaesthetic effects due to sodium channel blockade may mimic the antiarrhythmic properties of class 1A antiarrhythmic agents.[11] Diphenhydramine, dimenhydrinate and cyproheptadine, in particular, may prolong the cardiac muscle cell action potential duration by this mechanism.[12,13]

The second generation H_1-antagonists (fexofenadine, loratadine) have much less CNS penetration and are more histamine receptor specific with little or no effect at other receptor subtypes.[11]

All the H_1-antagonists are well absorbed orally with peak serum concentrations occurring within 2 to 4 h. Absorption may be delayed in overdose due to anticholinergic effects seen with the first-generation agents. Bioavailability is limited by significant first-pass metabolism. Some agents may be converted to active metabolites (e.g. hydroxyzine). Volume of distribution and protein binding are generally high. Elimination half-lives for the first generation agents are between 2 and 6 h.[11] The second generation agents generally have longer half-lives (e.g. loratadine 8.3 h).[11]

The H_2-antagonist agents are generally well tolerated with few side effects with therapeutic dosing. Cimetidine inhibits hepatic microsomal enzyme metabolism and reduces the metabolism of drugs eliminated by this pathway. This may result in increased serum concentrations and clinical effects of co-ingested medications.

All drugs with anticholinergic side effects have the potential to slow gastric emptying and produce gastrointestinal ileus when taken in overdose. As a result, absorption of these agents may be slowed and result in the potential for prolonged toxicity.

Clinical features

The anticholinergic toxidrome is usually manifest by a combination of peripheral and central muscarinic, cholinergic receptor blockade. Peripheral effects may include sinus tachycardia, cutaneous vasodilatation and flushing, low-grade temperature, warm dry skin with an absence of axillary sweat, dry mucous membranes, gastrointestinal ileus and urinary retention. CNS effects include mydriasis with blurred vision due to the inhibition of visual accommodation, delirium, confusion, visual hallucinations, incoherent speech, agitation, combativeness, aggression and coma.[14] Patients presenting with anticholinergic syndrome will often have an impaired perception of their environment. This may result in behaviour that could injure the patient. Anticholinergic symptoms and signs may be prominent with ingestion of first-generation antihistamines.[15–17] Even therapeutic doses of some of the H_1-antagonist agents may be sufficient to produce an anticholinergic delirium in susceptible individuals (especially the elderly and children). Topical use of these agents, particularly on broken skin surfaces, may also result in anticholinergic delirium.[18,19]

In patients who present to hospital several hours following poisoning with an anticholinergic agent, the peripheral features of the toxidrome may be absent.[20–22] This may also occur in elderly people with mild-to-moderate anticholinergic delirium resulting from the side effects of therapeutic drug administration.[22]

Other manifestations of H_1-antagonist toxicity may include CNS and cardiovascular effects, and rhabdomyolysis. Overdose of first-generation agents commonly produces drowsiness, sedation, confusion, agitation and ataxia. Large ingestions may result in coma.[23,24] Seizures may also occur. Pheniramine, a commonly abused antihistamine in Australia, appears to be more proconvulsant than other agents following overdose, with a reported incidence of seizures of 30%.[17] Seizures have been reported with other first-generation H_1-antagonists, such as diphenhydramine, in doses as small as 150 mg in children.[23,25] Fatal doses of diphenhydramine in adults range from 20 to 40 mg/ kg.[26] Doxylamine poisoning may result in non-traumatic rhabdomyolysis.[27,28] Hypotension, due to α-receptor blockade, can occur following large ingestions of first-generation agents. Conduction defects are infrequent following poisoning with first-generation H_1-antagonists. Diphenhydramine and dimenhydrinate poisoning can result in QRS-interval prolongation, broad-complex tachycardia and ventricular arrhythmias similar to that seen in cyclic antidepressant poisoning.[12,13] This effect has not been reported with other first-generation H_1-antagonists.

Overdose with H_2-antagonists, such as cimetidine, usually results in little or no evidence of toxicity. Doses of up to 15 g have failed to produce clinical toxicity.[29]

Clinical investigation

A 12-lead electrocardiograph should be performed to check for the presence of sinus tachycardia, QRS and QT-interval duration. Bedside blood glucose testing is indicated in all patients with altered mental status. Blood for serum electrolytes and paracetamol level should be collected. In patients with mental status changes not easily explained by drug intoxication, other organic causes for cognitive impairment should be ruled out. Serum antihistamine levels are not readily available and do not influence patient management. Standard 'drugs-of-abuse' urine screens do not detect antihistamines or most other agents with anticholinergic toxicity.

Treatment

The mainstay of therapy for poisoning with anticholinergic agents is supportive care in a safe environment. Comatose or hypoventilating patients should have appropriate airway intervention and ventilatory support. Hypotension should be treated initially with intravenous crystalloid boluses. Hypotension refractory to fluids may necessitate the use of pressor agents such as noradrenaline. Agitation and seizures can be controlled using parenteral benzodiazepines in the first instance. Barbiturates (thiopentone, phenobarbitone) may be considered in refractory cases.

Gastrointestinal decontamination, if indicated, should be performed with a single-dose of oral activated charcoal. The benefit of activated charcoal in patients presenting with minimal or no signs of toxicity more than 2 h following ingestion is doubtful. Methods of enhancing elimination of antihistamines are ineffective because of their large volumes of distribution and high protein binding.

The reversible acetylcholinesterase inhibitor physostigmine has been used in the management and diagnosis of anticholinergic agitation and delirium.[30–32] Physostigmine rapidly reverses the effects of anticholinergic delirium and may prevent the need for escalating doses of benzodiazepines to control agitation. Physostigmine may decrease the need for other interventions such as cerebral computerized tomography scanning and lumbar puncture in patients with suspected anticholinergic delirium.[31]

When using physostigmine, an initial test dose 0.5 mg i.v. is followed by 1.0–2.0 mg over the following 3–5 min in an adult. A partial response may necessitate further 0.5–1.0 mg boluses. Clinical effects may last from 30 to 120 min. Caution should be exercised in using physostigmine in patients with suspected acute cyclic antidepressant poisoning or ECG evidence of cardiac conduction delay because of the risk of precipitating cardiac asystole.[33,34]

Broad-complex tachycardia resulting from severe poisoning with diphenhydramine or dimenhydrinate should be treated with serum alkalinization with intravenous sodium bicarbonate boluses (0.5–1.0 mmol/kg) as for severe cyclic antidepressant poisoning.[12,13] Symptomatic bradycardia and high degree atrioventricular block should be initially treated with atropine. Unresponsive cases may need cardiac pacing or inotropic support. Class-1a, -1c or -3 anti-arrhythmic agents should be avoided in cases of antihistamine-induced arrhythmias.

Disposition

Patients who present with minimal or no signs of toxicity require 4–6 h of observation and monitoring. They may be medically cleared if, at the end of this period, they are alert and awake with a normal ECG. Patients with persistent mental status changes require further observation but, if the ECG is normal, do not require further cardiac monitoring. The duration of anticholinergic delirium may be from 12 h to several days depending on the agent and dose ingested. Severe toxicity, if it is to develop, will be evident within 2–3 h of ingestion. Those patients with poisoning complicated by coma, seizures or CVS toxicity require admission and observation in an intensive-care or high-dependency setting.

All patients with intentional ingestions or suspicion of self-harm require psychiatric assessment prior to discharge.

Controversies

❶ The precise indications/ contraindications for use of the anticholinesterase inhibitor, physostigmine, are yet to be clearly delineated in the management of anticholinergic delirium.

References

1. Acri AA, Henretig FM. Effects of risperidone in overdose. American Journal of Emergency Medicine 1998; 16: 498–501.
2. Fisher RS, Cysyk B. A fatal overdose of carbamazepine: case report and review of literature. Journal of Toxicology – Clinical Toxicology 1988; 26: 477–486.
3. Graudins A, Peden G, Dowsett RP. Massive overdose with controlled-release carbamazepine resulting in delayed peak serum concentrations and life-threatening toxicity. Emergency Medicine (Fremantle) 2002; 14: 89–94.
4. Yang CC, Deng JF. Anticholinergic syndrome with severe rhabdomyolysis – an unusual feature of amantadine toxicity. Intensive Care Medicine 1997; 23: 355–356.
5. Chan TY. Anticholinergic poisoning due to Chinese herbal medicines. Veterinary & Human Toxicology 1995; 37: 156–157.
6. Chan JC, Chan TY, Chan KL, et al. Anticholinergic poisoning from Chinese herbal medicines. Australian & New Zealand Journal of Medicine 1994; 24: 317–318.
7. Chan TY, Tang CH, Critchley JA. Poisoning due to an over-the-counter hypnotic, Sleep-Qik (hyoscine, cyproheptadine, valerian). Postgraduate Medical Journal 1995; 71: 227–228.
8. Finlay P. Anticholinergic poisoning due to Datura candida. Tropical Doctor 1998; 28: 183–184.
9. Hanna JP, Schmidley JW, Braselton WE. Datura delirium. Clinical Neuropharmacology 1992; 15: 109–113.
10. Mahler DA. Anticholinergic poisoning from Jimson weed. Journal of the American College of Emergency Physicians 1976; 5: 440–442.
11. Rimmer SJ, Church MK. The pharmacology and mechanism of action of histamine H1 antagonists. Clinical and Experimental Allergy 1990; 20: 3.

12. Clark RF, Vance MV. Massive diphenhydramine poisoning resulting in a wide-complex tachycardia: successful treatment with sodium bicarbonate. Annals of Emergency Medicine 1992; 21: 318–321.
13. Farrell M, Heinrichs M, Tilelli JA. Response of life threatening dimenhydrinate intoxication to sodium bicarbonate administration. Journal of Toxicology – Clinical Toxicology 1991; 29: 527–535.
14. Feldman MD. The syndrome of anticholinergic intoxication. American Family Physician 1986; 34: 113–116.
15. Jones IH, Stevenson J, Jordan A, et al. Pheniramine as an hallucinogen. Medical Journal of Australia 1973; 1: 382–386.
16. Jones J, Dougherty J, Cannon L. Diphenhydramine-induced toxic psychosis. American Journal of Emergency Medicine 1986; 4: 369–371.
17. Buckley NA, Whyte IM, Dawson AH, et al. Pheniramine- a much abused drug. Medical Journal of Australia 1994; 160: 188–192.
18. Schipior PG. An unusual case of antihistamine intoxication. Journal of Pediatrics 1967; 71: 589–591.
19. Reilly JF, Jr., Weisse ME. Topically induced diphenhydramine toxicity. Journal of Emergency Medicine 1990; 8: 59–61.
20. Ruprecht J, Dworacek B. Central anticholinergic syndrome in anesthetic practice. Acta Anaesthesiologica Belgica 1976; 27: 45–60.
21. Koppel C, Hopfe T, Menzel J. Central anticholinergic syndrome after ofloxacin overdose and therapeutic doses of diphenhydramine and chlormezanone. Journal of Toxicology – Clinical Toxicology 1990; 28: 249–253.
22. Feinberg M. The problems of anticholinergic adverse effects in older patients. Drugs Aging 1993; 3: 335–348.

23. Koppel C, Ibe K, Tenczer J. Clinical symptomatology of diphenhydramine overdose: an evaluation of 136 cases in 1982 to 1985. Journal of Toxicology – Clinical Toxicology 1987; 25: 53–70.
24. Koppel C, Tenczer J, Ibe K. Poisoning with over-the-counter doxylamine preparations: an evaluation of 109 cases. Human Toxicology 1987; 6: 355–359.
26. Krenzelok EP, Anderson GM, Mirick M. Massive diphenhydramine overdose resulting in death. Annals of Emergency Medicine 1982; 11: 212–213.
27. Mendoza FS, Atiba JO, Krensky AM, et al. Rhabdomyolysis complicating doxylamine overdose. Clinical Paediatrics 1987; 26: 595–597.
28. Frankel D, Dolgin J, Murray BM. Non-traumatic rhabdomyolysis complicating antihistamine overdosage. Clinical Toxicology 1990; 27: 493.
29. Krenzelok EP, Litovitz T, Lippold KP, et al. Cimetidine toxicity: an assessment of 881 cases. Annals of Emergency Medicine 1987; 16: 1217–1221.
30. Beaver KM, Gavin TJ. Treatment of acute anticholinergic poisoning with physostigmine. American Journal of Emergency Medicine 1998; 16: 505–507
31. Burns MJ, Linden CH, Graudins A, et al. A comparison of physostigmine and benzodiazepines for the treatment of anticholinergic poisoning. Annals of Emergency Medicine 2000; 35: 374–381.
32. Mendelson G. Pheniramine aminosalicylate overdosage. Reversal of delirium and choreiform movements with tacrine treatment. Archives of Neurology 1977; 34: 313.
33. Pentel P, Peterson CD. Asystole complicating physostigmine treatment of tricyclic antidepressant overdose. Annals of Emergency Medicine 1980; 9: 588–590.
34. Suchard JR. Assessing physostigmine's contraindication in cyclic antidepressant ingestions. Journal of Emergency Medicine 2003; 25: 185–191.

29.6 Paracetamol

Andis Graudins

ESSENTIALS

1 Paracetamol poisoning is one of the most common toxicological presentations to Australasian emergency departments.

2 The decision to treat patients with antidotal therapy following acute single ingestions should be made using the paracetamol treatment nomogram.

3 N-acetylcysteine (N-ac) is an effective and safe antidote for paracetamol poisoning.

4 The efficacy of antidotal treatment decreases with time. Patients presenting more than 8 h post-ingestion should have N-ac commenced whilst waiting for the return of serum paracetamol concentrations and liver function tests.

5 The paracetamol treatment nomogram cannot be used to assess the risk of hepatotoxicity following repeated supra-therapeutic ingestions.

6 Paracetamol overdose should be excluded in all patients with deliberate self-poisoning and anyone with evidence of unexplained hepatic impairment on liver function studies.

7 Sustained-release formulations of paracetamol are available in Australia and should be considered when taking the drug history.

Introduction

Paracetamol is the most widely used over-the-counter analgesic and antipyretic medication in Australia. As a result, poisoning with paracetamol is common in Australia, as well as other western countries. Paracetamol exposure is the most common reason for calls to the New South Wales Poisons Information Centre.[1] In the USA, over 100 000 potential paracetamol poisonings are reported annually to the American Association of Poison Control Centres.[2] In the UK paracetamol poisoning accounts for up to 43% of poisoning exposures presenting to emergency departments.[3]

Pharmacokinetics and pathophysiology

Paracetamol (N-acetyl para-aminophenol, acetaminophen) is rapidly absorbed from the GI tract in therapeutic doses with peak plasma concentrations occurring within 30–60 min with tablet formulations and less than 30 min with liquid preparations.[4] Bioavailability increases with size of the dose, ranging from 68% following 500 mg to 90% following 1–2 g orally.[5] Time to peak plasma concentration may be delayed in the presence of co-ingestants which delay gastric emptying such as dextro-propoxyphene, antihistamines and anticholinergic agents.[5–7] The volume of distribution for paracetamol is approximately 1 L/kg, with protein binding of less than 50%. Metabolism occurs primarily in the liver with small amounts also metabolized in the kidneys. Metabolites are renally excreted with less than 4% excreted unchanged in the urine.[8] Elimination half-life is approximately 1.5–2.5 h following therapeutic dosing.[8] Paracetamol is metabolized by three mechanisms. With therapeutic dosing, approximately 60% is conjugated to glucuronide metabolites and 35% to sulphate metabolites.[5,8] Less than 5% of paracetamol is metabolized by microsomal enzymes. CYP2E1 is the major isoenzyme but CYP2A and CYP1A2 are also significant. Microsomal metabolism produces a reactive intermediary metabolite, N-acetyl-para-benzoquinoneimine (NAPQI). This is rapidly conjugated with glutathione to produce non-toxic mercapturic acid and cysteine metabolites that are renally excreted.[8] Elimination half-life is the same for adults, children and elderly patients but may be slightly elevated in neonates.[9]

A sustained-release formulation of paracetamol (Panadol Extend™) was introduced in Australia for the management of arthritis pain in 2002. This formulation contains 665 mg of paracetamol in a bilayer tablet with one-third being immediate-release and two-thirds sustained-release. It has been designed to release paracetamol slowly and maintain a therapeutic drug level for up to 8 h.[10] Human volunteer data in simulated overdose suggests a delay to, and reduction in, peak paracetamol concentration.[11] Comparison with immediate-release paracetamol at similar doses showed reduction in peak paracetamol concentration and area under the curve by more than 50% and delay to peak paracetamol concentration from 1 to 3 h.[11] To date, clinical overdose with Panadol Extend™ has not been reported in the medical literature. Unpublished pharmacokinetic data following deliberate self-poisoning with this formulation suggests that clinical overdose follows a similar pharmacokinetic profile to that seen in the volunteer study and that there may be a dose-dependent delay in peak levels.

In overdose, glucuronidation and sulphation pathways are rapidly saturated, resulting in increased metabolism of paracetamol by the microsomal enzyme pathway. When glutathione stores are depleted by more than 70%, NAPQI begins to accumulate in the liver. NAPQI binds to hepatocytes producing cell death and a predominantly centrilobular hepatic necrosis.[12]

Microsomal metabolism of paracetamol may be enhanced by barbiturates, carbamazepine, oral contraceptives, chronic alcohol ingestion or starvation.[13] Inhibition of microsomal metabolism may occur in the presence of acute alcohol ingestion and with the administration of 4-methylpyrazole. Therapeutic doses of cimetidine do not decrease excretion of mercapturate metabolites of paracetamol following therapeutic doses in humans.[14] There are no human studies to support the use of cimetidine in prevention of hepatotoxicity following paracetamol poisoning.

An isolated small rise in INR has been observed in patients with paracetamol poisoning in the absence of hepatic impairment. Mild elevations in INR and reduced levels of functional factor VII occurred in 66% of patients with an extrapolated 4-hour paracetamol concentration greater or equal to 1000 μmol/L (150 mg/L).[15] This effect appears to be related to inhibition of vitamin K dependent activation of coagulation factors.[15]

Clinical features

The clinical features of early paracetamol poisoning are non-specific and do not permit diagnosis on clinical grounds. Classically, untreated poisoning progresses through four stages of toxicity.[12] Stage 1 lasts about 24 h and is a subclinical period where the patient may exhibit only mild nausea, vomiting and malaise. During this period paracetamol is being metabolized, glutathione stores are being depleted and hepatotoxicity is in its early stages. In severe poisoning, mild elevations of hepatic aminotranferases may be apparent as early as 16 h post-ingestion.[16] In stage 2, nausea and vomiting resolve. Patients may develop right upper quadrant pain and hepatic tenderness 24–48 h post-ingestion. Liver function begins to deteriorate, with increasing aminotransferases, bilirubin and prothrombin time. Stage 3 is essentially a continuum of the above between 72 and 96 h post-ingestion. Hepatic function deteriorates and chemical hepatitis, jaundice and encephalopathy may develop. Peak aminotransferases are seen around 72 h post-ingestion.[16] Stage 4 is either the stage of resolution and fall in aminotransferase concentrations or, less commonly, the development of fulminant hepatic failure. Renal failure may also develop as a consequence of paracetamol toxicity. This may either be the result of direct hepatoxicity due to renal microsomal enzymatic metabolism of paracetamol to NAPQI or as a consequence of liver failure induced hepatorenal syndrome.[17]

Other manifestations of acute paracetamol poisoning may include coma and myocardial damage. Coma results from massive ingestion of paracetamol and is independent of any hepatic impairment. Serum paracetamol concentrations greater than 10 000 μmol/L (1000 mg/L) may present with coma.[18] Similarly, massive overdose may result in cardiac changes such as ST–T wave changes, bundle-branch block and sinus bradycardia.[19]

In general, most patients recover from paracetamol toxicity. The overall untreated mortality is less than 1% and that of untreated patients with hepatotoxicity around 3.5%.[19]

There are a number of 'over-the-counter' cough and cold preparations containing paracetamol in combination with other agents. These include sympathomimetics such as pseudoephedrine, antihistamines such as diphenhydramine, or cough suppressants such as dextromethorphan. Patients may present with symptoms and signs of an acute toxidrome from one or more of these agents. Compound analgesics may also be ingested. These may result in the development of salicylate and/or opioid toxicity. Ingestion of large amounts paracetamol/dextro-propoxyphene-containing analgesics may also result in propoxyphene-induced cardiotoxicity.

Assessment of risk of hepatotoxicity

The risk of hepatotoxicity following acute ingestion of paracetamol is dose-dependent. In healthy adults, hepatotoxicity may result from ingestion of more than 200 mg/kg or 10 g, whichever is the least.[20] In children less than 6 years old, ingestion of more than 200 mg/kg may result in toxic serum concentrations.[21] The threshold for toxicity may be less in patients with underlying hepatic impairment (e.g. chronic alcoholic liver disease, chronic active hepatitis), severe malnutrition or in the presence of microsomal enzyme inducing agents.[13,22–24]

The Rumack–Matthews nomogram shows a clear relationship between the serum paracetamol concentration and the potential for subsequent hepatotoxicity.[12] The nomogram begins at 4 h post-ingestion to allow for absorption and distribution of paracetamol. Serum concentrations taken less than 4 h post-ingestion may be unreliable in predicting the potential for hepatotoxicity. The risk of hepatotoxicity from untreated acute paracetamol ingestion can be estimated from this nomogram. Patients with a serum concentration falling above a line from 1300 μmol/L (200 mg/L) at 4 h post-ingestion to 170 μmol/L (25 mg/L) at 16 h post-ingestion (the 'probable toxicity' line) will have a 60% chance of developing hepatotoxicity (AST > 1000 IU/L) if left untreated.[25] This risk increases to 87% in untreated patients with paracetamol concentrations above 2000 μmol/L (300 mg/L) 4 h post-ingestion.[25] A third 'possible hepatotoxicity', 1000 μmol/L (150 mg/L) at 4 h post-ingestion to 125

μmol/L (16 mg/L) at 16 h post-ingestion was introduced to allow for errors in calculation of the time of ingestion. The efficacy and safety of dosing N-ac according to this 1000 μmol/L at 4 h nomogram line has been demonstrated in the U.S. in over 11 000 patients, where no patients treated with N-ac within 15 h of ingestion died.[26] In contrast, use of the higher line (1300 μmol/L at 4 h) has been demonstrated to be safe in smaller patient cohorts,[25] but there are reports of untreated patients with concentrations below this line that died from acute hepatic failure.[27]

With the recognition that there are numerous 'at risk' groups that may have a lower threshold for hepatotoxicity it has previously been recommended that the treatment line be dropped by 50% of the 'probable toxicity line'. It must be noted that lowering of the treatment threshold was purely empiric in these cases and there have been no studies to confirm this approach.

Australasian Poisons Information Centres have adopted a single-nomogram line approach to the management of paracetamol poisoning.[28] This aims to reconcile the problems associated with risk stratifying patients and misinterpreting previous guidelines using two lines on the nomogram by using a single nomogram line to simplify decision-making. The new nomogram (Fig. 29.6.1) lowers the previous Australasian nomogram line by 25% (thus it starts at 1000 μmol/L (150 mg/L at 4 h) and parallels the treatment approach practised in North America. This

provides an additional margin of safety for patients that may possess risk factors, provides a small margin of error for estimation of time of ingestion and obviates the need for potentially confusing additional lines.[28] It is also the treatment threshold with the largest volume of clinical data supporting its safety.[26]

Repeated supratherapeutic dosing with paracetamol may be associated with a risk of hepatotoxicity, particularly in those with the hepatic risk factors. Liver failure has been reported in retrospective case series with chronic use of as little as 4 g a day in patients with underlying acute illnesses with associated decreased oral intake. However, prospective evaluation of the risk of liver failure with therapeutic doses of paracetamol in chronic alcoholics does not provide any indication that there is an increased susceptibility to liver failure in this subset of patients.[29] It is important to note that the Rumack–Matthew's nomogram is not useful in the assessment of hepatotoxic risk in these patients. In alcoholic patients, raised hepatic aminotransferases into the thousands are suggestive of a toxin-induced hepatitis as seen with paracetamol. Both alcoholic hepatitis and viral hepatitis rarely produce aminotransferase that rises above 1000 IU/L.[22]

Antidotal therapy with N-acetylcysteine

N-acetylcysteine (N-ac) has been shown to be effective at preventing the development

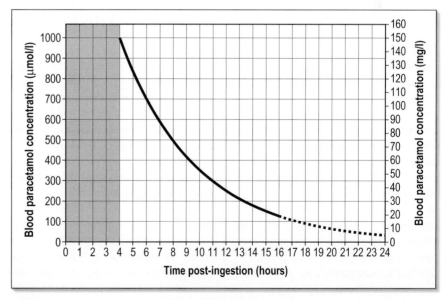

Figure 29.6.1 Paracetamol treatment nomogram. For use in the risk assessment of acute paracetamol ingestion at a single point in time.[26,28]

of hepatotoxicity following paracetamol poisoning.[25,26,30,31] N-acetylcysteine is metabolized to cysteine in the liver. It is a precursor to glutathione, necessary for the inactivation of the toxic metabolite NAPQI. Additionally, N-ac may be used as a substrate for hepatic sulphation, thus reducing the amount of paracetamol being shunted to the microsomal pathway of metabolism. In Australia, N-ac is usually administered according to the 20-hour intravenous protocol described by Prescott (150 mg/kg over 15 min, 50 mg/kg over 4 h, 100 mg/kg over 16 h).[25] There is no need to empirically commence N-ac therapy in patients presenting within 8 h of ingestion. The incidence of hepatotoxicity following institution of therapy within 8 h of ingestion is very low (1–6%) and independent of the route of dosing (i.v. versus oral) or length of N-ac protocol.[25,26,30,31] The incidence of hepatotoxicity increases to 40% if N-ac is delayed from 10 to 16 h following ingestion and may be as high as 87% if delayed from 16 to 24 h in patients treated with the 20 h intravenous protocol.[25] However, N-ac probably limits the degree of hepatic damage even in late presenting patients.

Adverse reactions to intravenous N-ac are limited to anaphylactoid, allergic type phenomena such as urticaria, bronchospasm and hypotension usually occurring during or soon after the administration of the intravenous loading dose.[31,32] Reactions have also been reported following administration of oral N-ac. These are not IgE-mediated but anaphylactoid histamine release reactions, dose-dependent in nature and usually responding to slowing or cessation of the infusion for a short period. Occasionally, administration of antihistamines and adrenaline may be necessary. The incidence of anaphylactoid reactions may be as high as 20%.[31,33,34] A prospective study varying the rate of infusion of the N-ac loading dose did not find any significant difference in the incidence of anaphylactoid reactions when comparing the standard 15 min loading-dose rate to a 1 h loading-dose rate.[34] The occurrence of previous reactions to N-ac does not preclude its use in the event of subsequent presentations for paracetamol poisoning. Life-threatening reactions are rare but have uncommonly been reported in patients with pre-existing asthma.

Treatment

Management of paracetamol poisoning is tailored according to the specific clinical scenario.

Acute overdose presenting within 8 h of ingestion

GI decontamination with activated charcoal (AC) should be performed in the cooperative patient presenting within 1–2 h of ingestion. Early administration of AC may prevent the development of a toxic 4-h paracetamol concentration and the need for subsequent antidotal therapy.[35] Administration of AC more than 2 h post-ingestion is unlikely to affect serum paracetamol concentrations.[36] Antidotal therapy with N-ac is commenced if the serum paracetamol concentration falls above the nomogram toxicity line. Patients treated within 8 h of ingestion do not require blood tests at the end of their 20-h N-ac infusion if they are clinically well.

Pregnant patients are treated in a similar fashion to other patients. Paracetamol crosses the placenta and in overdose may result in an increased risk of spontaneous abortion.[37] Cord blood samples taken from newborns of mothers being treated with N-ac for paracetamol poisoning have shown that therapeutic serum N-ac concentrations are found in the fetal circulation.[38]

Acute overdose presenting 8–24 h post-ingestion

In view of the increased incidence of hepatotoxicity with delayed antidote administration, these patients should have N-ac therapy commenced on presentation. Blood should be taken for serum paracetamol concentration and liver function tests (LFTs). Antidotal treatment may be ceased if the paracetamol level is non-toxic and liver function is normal. Otherwise, a full 20-h course of N-ac is administered.

Acute overdose presenting more than 24 h post-ingestion

Patients presenting more than 24 h following paracetamol ingestion may still benefit from antidotal therapy with N-ac. Therapy should be commenced if the patient has a detectable serum paracetamol level, evidence of aminotransferase elevation suggesting paracetamol hepatic injury or clinical evidence of paracetamol hepatotoxicity

(nausea, vomiting, right upper quadrant pain). Patients may benefit from prolonged duration of N-ac therapy if serum aminotransferases and/or prothrombin time continue to rise after 24 h of therapy.[26,31,39,40] NAC should be continued at a rate of 100 mg/kg/12 h until prothrombin time and liver function begins to normalize or the patient requires liver transplantation.[40]

Acute overdose with unknown time of ingestion

The time of ingestion of a single overdose of paracetamol may be unknown, especially in patients with altered mental status from co-ingestants or other causes. N-acetylcysteine should be commenced empirically in these patients to avoid delayed therapy. Serum paracetamol, LFTs and prothrombin time should be collected. In view of the inherent safety of N-ac as an antidote, the most practical approach to management in this setting is to empirically treat patients with unknown ingestion times with the standard 20-h N-ac protocol. A more accurate history of overdose may be elicited when the patient is awake. Treatment may be ceased based on accurate history or if aminotransferase enzymes and INR are normal at the end of 20 h of N-ac therapy.

The staggered acute overdose

In patients presenting with a history of more than one paracetamol overdose over several hours, a worse case scenario can be adopted. An assumption is made that the whole dose of paracetamol has been ingested as a single dose at the earliest possible time. The serum paracetamol concentration is plotted on the nomogram based on this time point. Treatment is initiated if it is above the nomogram line.

Repeated supra-therapeutic ingestion

Current consensus guidelines suggest that in adults and children over 6 years of age with normal liver function, the risk of hepatic injury is increased if more than 200 mg/kg or 10 grams (whichever is the least) are ingested over 24 h, or more than 150 mg/kg or 6 g are ingested per 24 h for the preceding 48 h, or, in patients with underlying liver impairment, more than 100 mg/kg or 4 g a day is ingested per 24 h.[20,28] (See Table 29.6.1.) In these groups, a biochemical

Table 29.6.1 Paracetamol dosing associated with hepatic injury in adults and children over 6 years of age	
Acute single ingestion	>200 mg/kg or 10 g (whichever is lower) over a period of <8 h
Repeated supra-therapeutic ingestion (RSI)	>200 mg/kg or 10 g (whichever is lower) over a single 24-h period
	>150 mg/kg or 6 g (whichever is lower) per 24-h period for the preceding 48 h
	>100 mg/kg or 4 g/day (whichever is less) in patients with pre-disposing risk factors (see text)

Adapted from Dart RC et al, 2006.[21]

risk assessment should be made. If serum paracetamol is less than 70 μmol/L and serum aminotransferases are less than 50 IU/L no treatment is required. If either assay is elevated N-ac should be commenced. LFTs can be reassessed in 12 h time. If they are not rising and the patient is well, N-ac therapy may be ceased. Otherwise the full 20-h course should be administered or continued further until aminotransferases begin to fall.[41] Static aminotransferases suggest an alternative cause for hepatic pathology. The reason for analgesic overuse should also be sought and patients counselled regarding their analgesic strategies for their condition.

Paracetamol-induced hepatic failure

The development of hepatic failure is uncommon following paracetamol poisoning. The risk is greater in late presenting patients. Patients with evidence of developing fulminant hepatic failure following paracetamol poisoning will exhibit clinical signs of encephalopathy and liver failure. Poorer prognosis is associated with a number of biochemical abnormalities including INR more than 2 at 24 h or more than 3 at 48 h, INR increasing between day 3 and 4, serum creatinine greater than 200 mmol/L, pH < 7.3 sdespite fluid resuscitation, or high serum lactate.[42–44]

Prolonged NAC therapy may be of benefit in these patients along with supportive care in a specialized liver unit. A lower mortality may be seen in patients with hepatic failure treated with NAC. Early consultation with a liver transplantation unit should be sought.[40]

Sustained-release paracetamol ingestion

Minimal data exist in overdose with the Australian sustained-release formulation of paracetamol (Panadol Extend™). Human volunteer data in simulated overdose suggests that this product will produce delayed peak paracetamol concentrations.[11] This may translate to delayed peak levels and delayed crossing of the nomogram line in clinical overdose. N-ac should be commenced if the ingested dose is greater than 200 mg/kg or 10 g (whichever is the least). Serum paracetamol concentration should be estimated for 4 or more hours post-ingestion and a second level taken 4 h after the first. If both levels fall below the nomogram line treatment may be discontinued, otherwise N-ac should be administered in the full dose.[28] Large ingestions (>30 g) of this formulation have the potential to produce prolonged paracetamol absorption. Serial paracetamol estimations may be useful in this setting to ascertain when the concentration is falling to an insignificant level. The administration of AC more than 2 h post-ingestion may be of benefit in view of the sustained-release nature of this product.

Controversies

❶ The optimal nomogram treatment line for different patient groups. Most recommendations are conservative.

❷ The clinical significance of suggested 'risk factors' for hepatotoxicity. Most of the suggested factors are theoretical and have never been validated. Current treatment guidelines should be able to be applied without taking these factors into account.

References

1. Kirby J. 2006 Annual Report of the New South Wales Poison Information Centre. Sydney: The New Children's Hospital; 2007.
2. Watson WA, Litovitz TL, Rodgers GC, et al. 2004 Annual Report of the American Association of Poison Control Centers Toxic Exposure Surveillance System. American Journal of Emergency Medicine 2005; 23(5): 589–666.
3. Thomas SH, Horner JE, Chew K, et al. Paracetamol poisoning in the north east of England: presentation, early management and outcome. Human and Experimental Toxicology 1997; 16(9): 495–500.
4. Rawlins MD, Henderson DB, Hijab AR. Pharmacokinetics of paracetamol (acetaminophen) after intravenous and oral administration. European Journal of Clinical Pharmacology 1977; 11(4): 283–286.
5. Forrest JA, Clements JA, Prescott LF. Clinical pharmacokinetics of paracetamol. Clinical Pharmacokinetics 1982; 7(2): 93–107.
6. Bizovi KE, Aks SE, Paloucek F, et al. Late increase in acetaminophen concentration after overdose of tylenol extended relief. Annals of Emergency Medicine 1996; 28(5): 549–551.
7. Tighe TV, Walter FG. Delayed toxic acetaminophen level after initial four hour nontoxic level. Journal of Toxicology – Clinical Toxicology 1994; 32(4): 431–434.
8. Prescott LF. Kinetics and metabolism of paracetamol and phenacetin. British Journal of Clinical Pharmacology 1980; 10(2): 291S–298S.
9. Peterson RG, Rumack BH. Pharmacokinetics of acetaminophen in children. Pediatrics 1978; 62: 877–879.
10. GlaxoSmithKline. Panadol Extend Product Information; 2002.
11. Tan C, Graudins A. Comparative pharmacokinetics of Panadol Extend and immediate-release paracetamol in a simulated overdose model. Emergency Medicine of Australasia 2006; 18(4): 398–403.
12. Rumack BH, Matthew H. Acetaminophen poisoning and toxicity. Pediatrics 1975; 55(6): 871–876.
13. Whitcomb DC, Block GD. Association of acetaminophen hepatotoxicity with fasting and ethanol use. Journal of American Medical Association 1994; 272(23): 1845–1850.
14. Burkhart KK, Janco N, Kulig KW, Rumack BH. Cimetidine as adjunctive treatment for acetaminophen overdose. Human and Experimental Toxicology 1995; 14(3): 299–304.
15. Whyte IM, Buckley NA, Reith DM, et al. Acetaminophen causes an increased International Normalized Ratio by reducing functional factor VII. Therapy in Drug Monitoring 2000; 22(6): 742–748.
16. Singer AJ, Carracio TR, Mofenson HC. The temporal profile of increased transaminase levels in patients with acetaminophen-induced liver dysfunction. Annals of Emergency Medicine 1995; 26(1): 49–53.
17. Eguia L, Materson BJ. Acetaminophen-related acute renal failure without fulminant liver failure. Pharmacotherapy 1997; 17(2): 363–370.
18. Flanagan RJ, Mant TG. Coma and metabolic acidosis early in severe acute paracetamol poisoning. Human Toxicology 1986; 5(3): 179–182.
19. Hamlyn AN, Douglas AP, James O. The spectrum of paracetamol (acetaminophen) overdose: clinical and epidemiological studies. Postgraduate Medical Journal 1978; 54(632): 400–404.
20. Dart RC, Erdman AR, Olson KR, et al. Acetaminophen poisoning: an evidence-based consensus guideline for out-of-hospital management. Clinical Toxicology 2006; 44(1): 1–18.
21. Mohler CR, Nordt SP, Williams SR, et al. Prospective evaluation of mild to moderate pediatric acetaminophen exposures. Annals of Emergency Medicine 2000; 35(3): 239–244.
22. Kumar S, Rex DK. Failure of physicians to recognize acetaminophen hepatotoxicity in chronic alcoholics. Archives of Internal Medicine 1991; 151(6): 1189–1191.
23. Lauterburg BH, Velez ME. Glutathione deficiency in alcoholics: risk factor for paracetamol hepatotoxicity. Gut 1988; 29(9): 1153–1157.
24. Bentur Y, Tannenbaum S, Yaffe Y, Halpert M. The role of calcium gluconate in the treatment of hydrofluoric acid eye burn. Annals of Emergency Medicine 1993; 22(9): 1488–1490.
25. Prescott LF, Illingworth RN, Critchley JA, et al. Intravenous N-acetylcysteine: the treatment of choice for paracetamol poisoning. British Medical Journal 1979; 2(6198): 1097–1100.
26. Smilkstein MJ, Knapp GL, Kulig KW, Rumack BH. Efficacy of oral N-acetylcysteine in the treatment of acetaminophen overdose. Analysis of the national multicenter study (1976 to 1985) [see comments]. New England Journal of Medicine 1988; 319(24): 1557–1562.

27. Bridger S, Henderson K, Glucksman E, et al. Deaths from low dose paracetamol poisoning. British Medical Journal 1998; 316: 1724–1725.

28. Daly FFS, Fountain J, Graudins A, et al. Consensus Statement: New Guidelines for the Management of Paracetamol (Acetaminophen) Poisoning in Australia and New Zealand – Explanation and Elaboration. Medical Journal of Australia; 2008; 188(1): 296–301.

29. Palmer RB, Bogdan GM, Dart RC. Alcohol–acetaminophen syndrome: Maxim or myth? (abstract). Journal of Toxicology – Clinical Toxicology 2002; 40(5): 649–650.

30. Rumack BH, Peterson RC, Koch GG, Amara IA. Acetaminophen overdose. 662 cases with evaluation of oral acetylcysteine treatment. Archives of Internal Medicine 1981; 141(3 Spec No): 380–385.

31. Smilkstein MJ, Bronstein AC, Linden C, et al. Acetaminophen overdose: a 48-hour intravenous N-acetylcysteine treatment protocol. Annals of Emergency Medicine 1991; 20(10): 1058–1063.

32. Prescott LF, Donovan JW, Jarvie DR, Proudfoot AT. The disposition and kinetics of intravenous N-acetylcysteine in patients with paracetamol overdosage. European Journal of Clinical Pharmacology 1989; 37(5): 501–506.

33. Brotodihardjo AE, Batey RG, Farrell GC, Byth K. Hepatotoxicity from paracetamol self-poisoning in western Sydney: a continuing challenge. Medical Journal of Australia 1992; 157(6): 382–385.

34. Kerr F, Dawson AH, Whyte IM, et al. The Australasian clinical toxicology investigators collaboration randomized trial of different loading infusion rates of N-acetylcysteine. Annals of Emergency Medicine 2005; 45(4): 402–408.

35. Buckley NA, Whyte IM, O'Connell DL, Dawson AH. Activated charcoal reduces the need for N-acetylcysteine treatment after acetaminophen (paracetamol) overdose. Journal of Toxicology – Clinical Toxicology 1999; 37(6): 753–757.

36. Yeates PJ, Thomas SH. Effectiveness of delayed activated charcoal administration in simulated paracetamol (acetaminophen) overdose. British Journal of Clinical Pharmacology 2000; 49(1): 11–14.

37. Riggs BS, Bronstein AC, Kulig K, et al. Acute acetaminophen overdose during pregnancy. Obstetric Gynecology 1989; 74(2): 247–253.

38. Horowitz RS, Dart RC, Jarvie DR, et al. Placental transfer of N-acetylcysteine following human maternal acetaminophen toxicity. Journal of Toxicology – Clinical Toxicology 1997; 35(5): 447–451.

39. Harrison PM, Keays R, Bray GP, et al. Improved outcome of paracetamol-induced fulminant hepatic failure by late administration of acetylcysteine. Lancet 1990; 335(8705): 1572–1573.

40. Keays R, Harrison PM, Wendon JA, et al. Intravenous acetylcysteine in paracetamol induced fulminant hepatic failure: a prospective controlled trial. British Medical Journal. 1991; 303(6809): 1026–1029.

41. Murray L, Daly FFS, Little M, Cadogan M. Paracetamol: repeated supratherapeutic ingestion. In: Murray L, Daly FFS, Little M, Cadogan M, eds. Toxicology handbook. Sydney: Churchill Livingstone – Elsevier; 2007: 267–269.

42. Bernal W, Donaldson N, Wyncoll D, Wendon J. Blood lactate as an early predictor of outcome in paracetamol-induced acute liver failure: a cohort study. Lancet 2002; 359: 558–563.

43. Bernal W, Wendon J. Acute liver failure; clinical features and management. European Journal of Gastroenterology and Hepatology 1999; 11: 977–984.

44. Bernal W, Wendon J. More on serum phosphate and prognosis of acute liver failure. Hepatology 2003; 38: 533–534.

29.7 Salicylate

Andis Graudins • Digby Green

ESSENTIALS

1 Salicylate pharmacokinetics are complex and alter markedly following overdose.

2 Therapeutic serum salicylate concentrations range from 1.1 to 2.2 mmol/L (15 to 30 mg/dL).

3 Treatment and disposition decisions cannot be made on the basis of a single serum salicylate concentration.

4 The Done nomogram is unreliable and should not be used in the management of salicylate poisoning.

5 Urinary alkalinization is an effective method for enhancing elimination of salicylate. Haemodialysis is rarely indicated.

6 Chronic salicylate poisoning is an insidious condition, mostly seen in the elderly, manifested by an unexplained metabolic acidosis that may be incorrectly attributed to another medical condition.

Introduction

Salicylate poisoning is currently rather an infrequent presentation to Australian emergency departments. In 2006, less than 0.3% of calls to the New South Wales Poison Information Centre related to salicylate exposure.[1] This change largely reflects the change to paracetamol as the over-the-counter analgesic of choice. However, salicylates remain widely available as pharmaceutical preparations and as over-the-counter herbal products, cough and cold remedies, ointments and topical rubefacients. The emergency physician must be able to recognize and manage significant salicylate poisoning, particularly in the very young or elderly patient because of its significant morbidity and mortality.

Pharmacology and pathophysiology

Aspirin (acetylsalicylic acid, ASA) is rapidly absorbed from the gastrointestinal (GI) tract, predominantly the upper small intestine,[2] and then undergoes rapid hydrolysis to form salicylic acid.[3] Peak serum salicylate levels usually occur within 2 h of therapeutic dosing but may be delayed for up to 6 h following administration of enteric-coated formulations.[2] Following overdose, absorption may be erratic and delayed. This may be partly accounted for by pylorospasm and pharmacobezoar formation. Overdose with sustained-release or enteric-coated preparations may result in peak serum levels being delayed for up to 24 h.[4]

Following therapeutic doses, salicylate is highly protein bound (85–90%) with a very small apparent volume of distribution (0.1–0.2 L/kg). Salicylic acid has a pKa of 3.0 and exists predominantly in the unionized form at a pH of 7.4. Following overdose, plasma protein binding is saturated and free salicylate concentrations rise. As pH falls, a greater proportion of salicylate exists in the unionized form, and movement into the extravascular compartments, including the central nervous system (CNS), is enhanced with resulting increases in the volume of distribution and tissue toxicity.[5]

Salicylic acid is metabolized in the liver and kidney to form salicyluric acid, glycine, glucuronic, acyl and salicyl phenolic conjugates. These conjugates are excreted renally along with small amounts of free salicylate. The elimination half-life following therapeutic dosing is around 4 h. Salicylate metabolism is saturated when plasma salicylate concentrations rise above therapeutic levels and the kinetics change from first-order to zero-order. As a consequence, elimination half-life increases dramatically.

Urinary excretion of unchanged salicylate is minimal when the urine pH is in the acidic range. As urine pH increases, a greater proportion of filtered salicylate is in an ionized state and is unavailable for reabsorption in the proximal convoluted tubule. An increase in urine pH from 5.0 to 8.0 results in an up to 1000-fold increase in ionized salicylate excretion. [2]

At therapeutic doses, salicylate acts as an analgesic, antipyretic, anti-platelet and anti-inflammatory agent primarily by way of its inhibitory effects on prostaglandin synthesis mediated by irreversible inhibition of cyclo-oxygenase enzymes one and two (COX-1 and COX-2). In overdose, the major toxic effects are on the CNS, acid–base balance, cellular metabolism, coagulation, lungs and the GI tract.

CNS effects include an initial direct stimulation of the medullary respiratory centre producing an increase in rate and depth of respiration and a corresponding primary respiratory alkalosis, tinnitus, deafness and confusion. In severe poisoning, where systemic acidaemia enhances cerebral penetration of unionized salicylate, coma, convulsions and cerebral oedema occur.[6]

Metabolic effects include direct uncoupling of oxidative phosphorylation and inhibition of Krebs cycle enzymes leading to systemic acidaemia, hyperglycaemia, hyperthermia, derangement of carbohydrate, amino acid and lipid metabolism.[2,7] Increased oxygen consumption and carbon dioxide production are also apparent. Dehydration results from increased insensible respiratory and cutaneous fluid losses, as well as from nausea and vomiting due to GI irritation. Inhibition of platelet aggregation as well as vitamin-K-sensitive clotting factor function may produce a mild coagulopathy. Haemorrhage rarely occurs in humans or animals following severe salicylate poisoning.[8] Salicylate-induced non-cardiogenic pulmonary oedema is also reported in association with severe poisoning.[9]

Clinical features

The degree of clinical toxicity following acute ingestion of salicylate is dose-related and may be predicted from the reported dose ingested. The most useful features in assessing the patient are the clinical signs and symptoms, the acid–base status and serum salicylate concentrations.

Acute ingestion of less than 150 mg/kg of salicylate is unlikely to produce significant toxicity. Ingestion of 150–300 mg/kg produces mild-to-moderate symptoms and signs including hyperpnoea, tinnitus, nausea and vomiting. Ingestion of greater than 300 mg/kg is associated with severe toxicity including marked dehydration, hyperpyrexia, agitation, confusion and mental status depression, which may progress to coma, seizures and respiratory depression. Ingestion of greater than 500 mg/kg may be fatal.[7] Cerebral and pulmonary oedema have been reported in association with severe acute poisoning but are more common with chronic salicylate intoxication.

The diagnosis of chronic salicylate poisoning, most common in the elderly, is often missed. Recurrent dosing with aspirin, usually in the context of a viral illness or chronic pain condition, results in accumulation of plasma salicylate and prolongation of the elimination half-life. Patients may present with non-specific symptoms or signs suggesting inflammatory or infective aetiology, such as confusion, delirium, fever, dehydration or hyperglycaemia. The history of excessive salicylate ingestion may not be elicited and the clinical findings erroneously attributed to other conditions such as septicaemia, cardiogenic pulmonary oedema, cerebrovascular accidents or diabetic ketoacidosis. The presence of an unexplained metabolic acidosis may be the vital clue leading to the diagnosis.[10] Delay in the diagnosis of chronic salicylate poisoning is associated with an increased morbidity and mortality.[11,12]

Clinical investigation

Salicylate intoxication should be suspected in any patient with clinical signs suggestive of poisoning, an unexplained respiratory alkalaemia or metabolic acidosis.[13] Patients in whom the diagnosis is suspected should have blood drawn for serum electrolytes, urea, creatinine, blood glucose, prothrombin time, paracetamol and salicylate concentration. An arterial or venous blood gas is necessary to assess acid–base status and urine pH should be checked.

A qualitative screening test is available to assess the presence of salicylate in the urine. Addition of Trinder's reagent (ferric nitrate 0.1 molar, hydrochloric acid 0.1 molar and mercuric chloride) in equal volumes with urine results in a deep purple discolouration of the urine in the presence of even trace quantities of salicylate. A negative test rapidly excludes the presence of salicylate in the urine in patients with unexplained metabolic acidosis. As the test is qualitative, the colour change is the same regardless of the amount of aspirin in the urine. A positive test indicates the need for a serum salicylate estimation.[14]

Patients with mild or early poisoning may present with a pure respiratory alkalosis due to respiratory centre stimulation and hypokalaemia. Urine pH may initially be alkaline as a response to hyperventilation. Adult patients with moderate-to-severe poisoning may present with a mixed acid–base disturbance of respiratory alkalosis and metabolic acidosis. Urine pH is commonly acidic in this setting due to increased excretion of hydrogen ions. A metabolic acidosis with normal or falling serum pH signifies development of potentially severe salicylate poisoning. Co-ingestion of sedatives may depress respiratory drive leading to loss of respiratory compensation for the metabolic acidosis and an earlier deterioration in acid–base status.

The Done nomogram was developed in 1960 in an attempt to relate peak serum salicylate concentration to clinical severity of salicylate poisoning.[15] This nomogram cannot be used to reliably make a risk assessment for salicylate toxicity.[8] Combined use of serial clinical observation, blood–gas estimations and serial salicylate measurements to monitor for ongoing absorption of aspirin, will give the best indication of the degree of toxicity and response to treatment.[15]

Treatment

Patients presenting following salicylate ingestion should have intravenous access established, blood drawn for serum salicylate levels, electrolytes and blood sugar level. In moderate-to-severe poisoning these should be repeated every 2 to 3 h in view of the potential erratic salicylate absorption. Intravenous rehydration is often necessary in view of the increased insensible fluid losses due to hyperventilation and pyrexia, and vomiting from GI irritation. Strict attention to fluid balance should be observed particularly in the very young, elderly or those with cardiac disease. Occasionally, central venous and arterial pressure monitoring may be necessary as well as urinary catheterization and hourly urine measures.

Gastrointestinal decontamination with oral-activated charcoal should be performed on presentation. It should not be withheld even when patients present several hours following ingestion in view of the potential for delayed aspirin absorption. Whole-bowel irrigation with polyethylene glycol-electrolyte solution may be considered in patients with ingestion of sustained-release formulations of aspirin. Repeat doses of activated charcoal may be of benefit where there is evidence of ongoing absorption of salicylate on serial serum levels. Multiple-dose activated charcoal does not enhance salicylate elimination but may inhibit ongoing GI absorption from pharmacobezoars or aspirin concretions.[16,17]

Pulmonary oedema should be treated with continuous positive pressure ventilation by mask or endotracheal intubation.[6,18,19] Ensure that acidaemia is not exacerbated by institution of controlled ventilation. Salicylate poisoning normally results in high minute volumes and respiratory alkalosis. Neuromuscular paralysis and controlled ventilation may reduce minute volume and worsen acidosis resulting in clinical deterioration. Seizures should be treated with parenteral benzodiazepines and/or barbiturates.

Urinary salicylate excretion can be enhanced by urinary alkalinization which may reduce salicylate elimination half-life from 20 to 5 h. The aim of urinary alkalinization is to increase urine pH above 7.5 to enhance the trapping of ionized salicylate in the urine. Indications include the presence of symptoms, acid–base abnormalities or serum salicylate levels greater than 2.2 mmol/L (30 mg/dL). In patients with clinical symptoms and signs of salicylate toxicity, urinary alkalinization can be commenced whilst awaiting the results of drug assays and electrolyte concentrations. Urinary alkalinization is accomplished by initially giving a bolus of intravenous sodium bicarbonate (0.5 to 1.0 mmol/kg) followed by an infusion of 100–150 mmol of sodium bicarbonate in 1 L of 5% dextrose solution at a rate of 100–250 mL/h adjusted to urine pH. Urine output should be maintained between 1 and 2 mL/kg/h. Serum potassium should be maintained within normal limits by the addition of supplemental potassium to the bicarbonate infusion (30 mmol per bag). In the presence of systemic hypokalaemia, the potassium ions are retained in the renal tubules in preference to hydrogen. This makes it extremely difficult to achieve urinary alkalinization. Serial serum electrolytes, salicylate concentrations and urinary pH should be measured every 2–4 h. The endpoint for therapy is a serum salicylate concentration within the therapeutic range (1.1–2.2 mmol/L or 15–30 mg/dL), resolution of clinical signs of toxicity and normalization of acid–base status.

Extracorporeal removal of salicylate is infrequently required and the accepted clinical indications are listed in Table 29.7.1. Intermittent high-flow haemodialysis (HD) is the preferred option as it can rapidly normalize acid–base, fluid balance and electrolyte abnormalities as well as remove salicylate from the blood.[20]

Severe cases of salicylate intoxication may require endotracheal intubation and ventilation as a direct result of toxicity or co-ingestants. In such circumstances, urinary alkalinization, followed by haemodialysis is essential to prevent a worsening metabolic acidosis as ventilatory manipulation is often insufficient to maintain alkalosis.

Table 29.7.1 Indications for haemodialysis in salicylate poisoning

Metabolic acidosis refractory to optimal supportive care and urinary alkalinization
Evidence of end-organ injury (i.e. seizures, rhabdomyolysis, pulmonary oedema)
Renal failure and fluid overload
Serum aspirin concentration >6.0 mmol/L or 100 mg/dL in acute poisoning
Serum aspirin concentration >4.0 mmol/L or 60 mg/dL in chronic poisoning

Note: In elderly patients, with chronic salicylate toxicity, the suggested serum threshold for haemodialysis is lower at 2.2–4.4 mmol/L (30–60 mg/dL).

Disposition

In view of the potential for delayed and erratic salicylate absorption, patients require serial salicylate concentrations and observation for a minimum of 12 h. Salicylate estimations earlier than 6 h post-ingestion do not usually reflect peak serum concentrations.

Patients without clinical evidence of salicylate toxicity may be medically cleared in the presence of normal arterial blood gas and two falling serum salicylate levels in the therapeutic range (1.1–2.2 mmol/L; 15–30 mg/dL) 3–4 h apart. Patients with evidence of acid–base abnormalities, end-organ dysfunction or requiring urinary alkalinization should be admitted to a high dependency or intensive care unit. Transfer to a tertiary referral centre with facilities for haemodialysis should be considered if criteria for severe toxicity are present.

Controversies

❶ The threshold for initiating urinary alkalinization is not well defined. Many clinicians now prefer to alkalinize any symptomatic patient with a view to minimizing the duration of medical admission.

❷ Although there is minimal case-controlled evidence supporting the use of continuous arterio-venous or veno-venous HD in severe salicylate poisoning, newer high-flow continuous veno-venous haemodialysis units may be able to remove larger amounts of salicylate and provide an alternative to intermittent high-flow dialysis in selected cases.

References

1. Kirby J. 2006 Annual Report of the New South Wales Poison Information Centre. The Children's Hospital at Westmead, Westmead, NSW; 2007.
2. Notarianni L. A reassessment of the treatment of salicylate poisoning. Drug Safety 1992; 7: 292–303.
3. Kershaw RA, Mays DC, Bienchine JR. Disposition of aspirin and its metabolites in the semen of man. Journal of Clinical Pharmacology 1987; 27: 304–309.
4. Wortzman DJ, Grunfeld A. Delayed absorption following enteric-coated aspirin overdose. Annals of Emergency Medicine 1987; 16: 434–436.
5. Hill JB. Salicylate intoxication. New England Journal of Medicine 1973; 288: 1110–1113.
6. Thisted B, Krantz T, Strom J, et al. Acute salicylate self-poisoning in 177 consecutive patients treated in ICU.

Acta Anaesthesiologica Scandinavica 1987; 31: 312–316.

7. Temple AR. Acute and chronic effects of aspirin toxicity and their treatment. Archives of Internal Medicine 1981; 141: 364–369.

8. Yip L, Dart RC, Gabow PA. Concepts and controversies in salicylate toxicity. Emergency Medicine Clinics of North America 1994; 12: 351–364.

9. Heffner JE, Sahn SA. Salicylate-induced pulmonary edema. Clinical features and prognosis. Annals of Internal Medicine 1981; 95: 405–409.

10. Chalasani N, Roman J, Jurado RL. Systemic inflammatory response syndrome caused by chronic salicylate intoxication. Southern Medical Journal 1996; 89: 479–482.

11. Anderson RJ, Potts DE, Gabow PA, et al. Unrecognized adult salicylate intoxication. Annals of Internal Medicine 1976; 85: 745–748.

12. Gabow PA, Anderson RJ, Potts DE, et al. Acid-base disturbances in the salicylate-intoxicated adult. Archives of Internal Medicine 1978; 138: 1481–1484.

13. Chan TYK, Chan AYW, Ho CS. The clinical value of screening for salicylates in acute poisoning. Veterinary and Human Toxicology 1995; 37: 37–38.

14. Asselin WM, Caughlin JD. A rapid and simple color test for detection of salicylate in whole hemolyzed blood. Journal of Analytical Toxicology 1990; 14: 254–255.

15. Dugandzic RM, Tierney MG, Dickinson GE, et al. Evaluation of the validity of the Done nomogram in the management of acute salicylate intoxication. Annals of Emergency Medicine 1989; 18: 1186–1190.

16. Johnson D, Eppler J, Giesbrecht E, et al. Effect of multiple-dose activated charcoal on the clearance of high-dose intravenous aspirin in a porcine model. Annals of Emergency Medicine 1995; 26: 569–574.

17. Mayer AL, Sitar DS, Tenenbein M. Multiple-dose charcoal and whole-bowel irrigation do not increase clearance of absorbed salicylate. Archives of Internal Medicine 1992;152: 393–396.

18. Cohen DL, Post J, Ferroggiaro AA, et al. Chronic salicylism resulting in noncardiogenic pulmonary edema requiring hemodialysis. American Journal of Kidney Diseases 2000; 36: E20.

19. Woolley RJ. Salicylate-induced pulmonary edema: a complication of chronic aspirin therapy. Journal of the American Board of Family Practice 1993; 6: 399–401.

20. Jacobsen D, Wiik-Larsen E, Bredesen JE. Haemodialysis or haemoperfusion in severe salicylate poisoning? Human Toxicology 1998; 7(2): 161–163.

29.8 Antidiabetic drugs

Jason Armstrong

ESSENTIALS

1 Deliberate self-poisoning with insulin or sulphonylureas may lead to life-threatening hypoglycaemia requiring prolonged observation and treatment over several days.

2 Octreotide blocks endogenous insulin secretion and is indicated in the management of symptomatic sulphonylurea toxicity.

3 Central venous access is usually required following deliberate insulin overdose to facilitate treatment with concentrated glucose solutions.

4 Metformin is associated with life-threatening lactic acidosis. It does not cause significant hypoglycaemia in overdose.

Introduction

Diabetes mellitus (DM) is a chronic metabolic condition caused by an absolute (type I) or relative (type II) lack of insulin. In Australia, over one million people have diabetes and 100 000 people are diagnosed every year with the condition. Aboriginal and Maori populations in Australasia have some of the highest rates of type II diabetes in the world.[1] For these reasons, antidiabetic medications are readily available and frequently taken in overdose by both diabetic and non-diabetic individuals.

The three major groups of antidiabetic medications are insulin, sulphonylureas and biguanides, all of which have been used for over 50 years. Toxicity can result from intentional overdose, but also from decreased clearance of the medication at therapeutic dosing, due to underlying hepatic or renal disease.

A number of newer agents have been developed recently, including thiazolidinediones, alpha-glucosidase inhibitors, glinides and dipeptidyl peptidase-IV (DPP-IV) inhibitors.[2] Overdose with these medications is less likely to cause significant clinical effects.

Insulin

Pharmacology and pathophysiology

Insulin is synthesized by the pancreatic β islet cells as a pro-hormone packaged inside secretory vesicles. It is secreted primarily in response to elevated serum glucose levels and becomes metabolically active when pro-insulin is cleaved by serum proteases to form insulin and C-peptide. Exogenous insulin, administered therapeutically in the management of type I and II DM, does not contain C-peptide.

Insulin is eliminated by hepatic metabolism (60%) and renal clearance (40%). A number of preparations are available and these have varying durations of action. However, following overdose the usual pharmacokinetic properties of insulin may be altered because the injected dose forms a subcutaneous or intramuscular depot. Slow and erratic release of insulin from the depot can result in a markedly extended duration of action (up to several days) even with short-acting preparations.[3,4]

Insulin promotes the intracellular movement of glucose, potassium, magnesium and phosphate, as well as decreasing ketone production from the breakdown of fatty acids. It inhibits the breakdown of fat and protein to release glucose (gluconeogenesis), and stimulates the synthesis of glycogen, protein and triglycerides.

In overdose, the principal effect of clinical significance is that of hypoglycaemia, which may be prolonged and profound following self-administration of large doses subcutaneously or intramuscularly.[4,5] Hypoglycaemia tends to be more profound and prolonged in non-diabetic patients.[5] Insulin toxicity also causes electrolyte abnormalities, the most important of which is hypokalaemia, secondary to intracellular shift of potassium. Hypophosphataemia and hypomagnesaemia are also reported.[6]

Clinical features

The clinical features of insulin toxicity are the neuropsychiatric and autonomic manifestations of hypoglycaemia. Autonomic symptoms and signs include diaphoresis, tremor, nausea, palpitations and tachycardia; neuropsychiatric features are confusion, agitation, seizures, coma and focal neurological deficits. These manifestations are usually evident within hours of self-administration of an insulin overdose and the patient frequently presents in coma. The suspicion of deliberate overdose is entertained when recurrent profound hypoglycaemia occurs following an initial response to dextrose administration. If the history of deliberate overdose is known at the time of presentation, then profound prolonged hypoglycaemia should be anticipated.

Prolonged severe hypoglycaemia can cause permanent neurological sequelae or death.

Clinical investigation

Serial measurement of blood glucose concentrations, usually at the bedside, allows titration of dextrose administration. Serial measurements of electrolytes are necessary to monitor hypokalaemia and potassium replacement. Serum magnesium and phosphate levels may also be affected.

If surreptitious or malicious administration is suspected, assays of insulin and C-peptide levels can be useful to provide objective evidence of the presence of exogenous insulin, as endogenous insulin levels should always be suppressed in the presence of hypoglycaemia unless an insulinoma is present.

Treatment

Management of insulin overdose is essentially supportive and involves administration of sufficient concentrated dextrose solution so as to maintain euglycaemia until all the insulin is absorbed from the depot site and its hypoglycaemic action terminated. After initial correction of hypoglycaemia with 50% dextrose, a 10% dextrose infusion should be commenced at 100 mL/h and blood sugar levels followed closely. Further boluses of dextrose and titration of the infusion rate are implemented as necessary. Very large dose of dextrose may be required, sometimes over days.[3–5]

Frequently it is necessary to administer a 50% dextrose infusion to maintain euglycaemia and this requires placement of a central venous line because concentrated dextrose solutions are irritating to veins.

Hypokalaemia due to intracellular shifts should be anticipated, and supplemental K^+ administered (e.g. 20–40 mmol/h i.v. in adults), guided by serial monitoring. Hyponatraemia and volume overload are other complications of hypertonic dextrose therapy.

Disposition

Patients who report an overdose of insulin should be admitted and observed with bedside blood glucose assays for at least 8 h after self-administration. They are medically fit for discharge if they remain asymptomatic and euglycaemic at this stage. Those who develop hypoglycaemia requiring dextrose therapy should be admitted to a high-dependency or intensive unit for ongoing dextrose infusion, potassium supplementation and close monitoring of blood sugar and electrolytes.

The duration of therapy required is variable. Dextrose therapy may be withdrawn by halving the rate of infusion every 2–4 h once hyperglycaemia develops, guided by regular bedside assessments of serum glucose. This minimizes the risk of precipitous hypoglycaemia. It may be particularly difficult to wean dextrose infusions in non-diabetic patients, as the large load of infused dextrose tends to stimulate endogenous insulin secretion after the effects of the initial overdose have worn off. In these cases a slower weaning regimen may be required to prevent hypoglycaemia. It is sensible to avoid withdrawing dextrose infusions overnight when clinical features of hypoglycaemia are less easily recognized.

Patients are medically fit for discharge if they remain asymptomatic and euglycaemic 6 h after dextrose therapy is ceased. All intentional overdoses require psychiatric assessment once their medical condition has stabilized.

Sulphonylureas

Pharmacology and pathophysiology

Sulphonylureas are the most commonly prescribed oral hypoglycaemics in Australasia.

Currently available agents include glibenclamide, gliclazide, glimepiride and glipizide. These agents bind to and block outgoing K^+ channels on the pancreatic β cells leading to depolarization of the cell membrane, which opens voltage-gated Ca^{2+} channels and causes insulin release secondary to Ca^{2+} influx.[7] The result is a hyperinsulinaemic state. Although in therapeutic dose the duration of action is usually from 12 to 24 h, this can be prolonged following overdose. They all undergo hepatic metabolism and have a combination of active and inactive metabolites, which are excreted renally. An exaggerated therapeutic effect can therefore occur when these agents accumulate in patients with coexistent hepatic or renal disease.

Clinical features

Sulphonylurea-induced hypoglycaemia may occur as a complication of therapy, inadvertent administration to a non-diabetic patient or as a consequence of deliberate self-poisoning. The hypoglycaemia after intentional ingestion is likely to be particularly profound and prolonged.

Treatment

Hypoglycaemia should be corrected immediately once identified with bedside blood glucose testing, or suspected on clinical grounds. An initial bolus of 50 mL 50% dextrose followed by an infusion of 10% dextrose at 100 mL is appropriate for hypoglycaemia secondary to deliberate self-poisoning with sulphonylureas. However, hypoglycaemia is frequently refractory to dextrose supplementation in this setting and early use of octreotide is then indicated to maintain euglycaemia (see below).

Activated charcoal can be administered to patients who present within a few hours of intentional ingestion of sulphonylureas but does not take precedence over resuscitation and correction of hypoglycaemia.

Elderly patients with sulphonylurea-induced hypoglycaemia often have intercurrent medical illnesses that require treatment. Euglycaemia may be relatively easy to maintain with intravenous or oral dextrose supplementation.

Octreotide

Octreotide is a synthetic octapeptide analogue of the naturally occurring foregut hormone somatostatin. It suppresses insulin release from pancreatic β cells by binding to Ca^{2+} channels on the cell membrane, inhibiting Ca^{2+} influx and subsequent insulin release.[8]

Octreotide is indicated as antidotal therapy in patients with hypoglycaemia secondary to sulphonylurea overdose. Early administration of octreotide may greatly reduce or abolish the dextrose requirement, obviate the need for central access and greatly facilitate subsequent management and disposition.[8–12] Therapy can be initiated with an initial bolus of 50 μg i.v. followed by an infusion of 25 μg/h. An alternative dosing regimen is 100 μg by intramuscular or subcutaneous injection every 6 h. Once initiated, octreotide therapy should be continued for at least 24 h before withdrawal is attempted. Octreotide is well tolerated, with nausea and vomiting only occasionally reported.[9]

For the treatment of therapeutic accumulation, a single dose of octreotide 25–50 μg subcutaneously may be adequate to prevent recurrent hypoglycaemia.[13]

Disposition

Patients with a history of sulphonylurea overdose should be admitted and observed with bedside blood glucose assays for at least 8 h after ingestion, or up to 12 h if a slow-release preparation. They are medically fit for discharge if they remain asymptomatic and euglycaemic at this stage.

Patients who require treatment for hypoglycaemia need admission, usually for several days. Discharge can occur once they are tolerating a normal diet, and their blood glucose level remains normal 6 h after cessation of glucose and/or octreotide therapy.

Patients who develop hypoglycaemia on therapeutic doses of sulphonylureas should be admitted for at least 24 h to monitor serum glucose and to review their medication regimen.

Metformin

Pharmacology and pathophysiology

Metformin is the only biguanide currently available in Australasia. It is rapidly absorbed from the gastrointestinal (GI) tract, minimally metabolized and is excreted almost entirely by the kidneys. The major antidiabetic effect is to inhibit gluconeogenesis, as well as to increase tissue sensitivity to insulin, thereby improving HbA_1C control. It does not cause hypoglycaemia at therapeutic doses and even following massive overdose; clinically significant hypoglycaemia is rarely observed. Metformin is however associated with life-threatening lactic acidosis because it is thought to interfere with intracellular oxidative pathways leading to increased anaerobic metabolism. Lactic acidosis occurs during therapeutic dosing when impaired renal function leads to drug accumulation. It is also reported after massive overdose. The threshold for this effect is not well characterized but is probably over 10 g.[14] The risk of toxicity from an acute ingestion will be exacerbated by other agents that cause hypotension or decreased renal perfusion.

Clinical features

The majority of metformin overdoses are associated with only minor or no symptoms. In particular, hypoglycaemia is not a feature of the presentation. Where the clinical progress is complicated by lactic acidosis, an insidious onset of non-specific symptoms such as nausea, malaise and lethargy may be observed. As lactate levels rise, the patient's condition will deteriorate with progressive tachypnoea, cardiovascular instability and altered mental state.[16–18]

Patients who develop lactic acidosis whilst on therapeutic metformin may present very unwell.

Lactic acidosis is associated with a mortality as high as 50% if it is not recognized and treated effectively.[8,19]

Clinical investigation

Urgent electrolytes, renal function and lactate levels are indicated in any patient on metformin therapy who presents unwell or in any patient who becomes symptomatic whilst being observed following deliberate self-poisoning with metformin.

Treatment

Most cases of metformin overdose can be managed supportively. Maintenance of euvolaemia is imperative, and i.v. crystalloid should be given to ensure effective renal clearance. If lactate levels are elevated, serial estimations of pH and lactate must be performed until they return to the normal range. If lactate rises above 10 mmol/L, or worsening acidosis, renal dysfunction and clinical deterioration occur, immediate treatment with lactate-free haemodialysis is indicated.[15–17] This not only corrects the acid–base disturbance, but also rapidly removes metformin from the circulation. Either intermittent or continuous dialysis techniques can be used, as long as flow rates are adequate to ensure effective clearance.[20]

Temporary improvement in acidosis can be achieved by infusion of $NaHCO_3$ whilst organizing dialysis but this does not address ongoing metformin toxicity, and progressive deterioration is likely without definitive therapy.

Disposition

Patients can be discharged following metformin overdose if they remain clinically well with normal haemodynamic parameters. Those who develop lactic acidosis require intensive care admission and consideration for haemodialysis. All patients on therapeutic metformin who develop lactic acidosis require admission for careful clinical and biochemical monitoring and consideration for haemodialysis.

Other agents

Thiazolidinediones (Rosiglitazone) are used in type II DM. They improve insulin sensitivity in skeletal muscle and adipose tissue via the receptor peroxisome proliferator-activated receptor gamma (PPAR-γ), and also inhibit hepatic gluconeogenesis. They improve insulin resistance and thereby act to decrease circulating insulin levels. They do not stimulate insulin secretion, and are not associated with hypoglycaemia. A recent meta-analysis has suggested an increased risk of cardiac mortality in patients treated with these agents – further prospective studies are underway to clarify this concern.[21]

Alpha-glucosidase inhibitors (Acarbose) are oligosaccharide agents that inhibit the activity of enzymes in the GI endoluminal brush border. Their action decreases the breakdown of complex sugars to monosaccharides, thereby decreasing the postprandial rise in blood glucose levels. They are not absorbed to any significant degree and do not cause hypoglycaemia or other systemic effects in overdose.

Glinides (Repaglinide) are not commonly available in Australasia, but are prescribed more frequently in other countries. Their mode of action is to stimulate insulin secretion from the pancreas, but via a different part of the membrane receptor than sulphonylurea agents.[22] There are limited data available on overdose presentations, but there is potential for hypoglycaemia requiring therapy with i.v. dextrose. Because of the short half-life of glinides in comparison to sulphonylureas, prolonged toxicity is unlikely to result.

Controversies

❶ Glucagon is sometimes given pre-hospital for symptomatic hypoglycaemia. It can raise serum glucose due to enhanced breakdown of hepatic glycogen stores, but this effect is short-lived and unreliable. It does not have a role in the management of deliberate self-poisoning with insulin or sulphonylureas.

❷ Surgical excision of insulin depot stores has been attempted but is not indicated as medical management is effective in dealing with all clinical manifestations of insulin overdose.

❸ The optimal dose and route of administration of octreotide in sulphonylurea overdose is not well-defined. Recommendations are empiric. Greater doses than those quoted above might be necessary following massive overdose of sulphonylureas in non-diabetic patients.

❹ The role of insulin assays in determining ongoing requirement for octreotide therapy in sulphonylurea toxicity needs to be explored. Currently, insulin levels are not routinely monitored in this setting.

References

1. AusDiab Report. International Diabetes Institute, Melbourne. http://www.diabetes.com.au (accessed 4 February 2008).
2. Nathan DM. Finding new treatments for diabetes – how many, how fast… how good?. New England Journal of Medicine 2007; 356: 437–439.
3. Arem R, Zoghbi W. Insulin overdose in eight patients: insulin pharmacokinetics and review of the literature. Medicine Baltimore 1985; 64: 323–332.
4. Samuels MH, Eckel RH. Massive insulin overdose: detailed studies of free insulin levels and glucose requirements. Clinical Toxicology 1989; 27: 157–168.
5. Haskell RJ, Stapczynski JS. Duration of hypoglycaemia and need for intravenous glucose following intentional overdoses of insulin. Annals of Emergency Medicine 1984; 13: 505–511.
6. Matsumura M, Nakashima A, Tofuku Y. Electrolyte disorders following massive insulin overdose in a patient with type 2 diabetes. Internal Medicine 2000; 39: 55–57.
7. Bosse GM. Antidiabetic and hypoglycaemic agents. In: Goldfrank LR, Flomenbaum NE, Lewin NA, et al., eds. Goldfrank's toxicological emergencies. 7th edn,. New York: McGraw Hill; 2002. pp593–605.
8. McLaughlin SA, Crandall CS, McKinney PE. Octreotide: an antidote for sulphonylurea induced hypoglycaemia. Annals of Emergency Medicine 2000; 36: 133–138.
9. Krentz AJ, Boyle PJ, Justice KM, et al. Successful treatment of severe refractory sulphonylurea-induced hypoglycaemia with octreotide. Diabetes Care 1993; 76: 752–756.
10. Boyle PJ, Justice K, Krentz AJ, et al. Octreotide reverses hyperinsulinaemia and prevents hypoglycaemia induced by sulfonylurea overdoses. Journal of Clinical Endocrinology and Metabolism 1993; 76: 752–756.
11. Hung O, Eng J, Ho J, et al. Octreotide as an antidote for refractory sulfonylurea hypoglycemia. Journal of Toxicology – Clinical Toxicology 1997; 25: 540–541.
12. Graudins A, Linden CH, Ferm RO. Diagnosis and treatment of sulfonylurea induced hyperinsulinemic hypoglycemia. American Journal of Emergency Medicine 1997; 15: 95–96.
13. Braatvedt GD. Octreotide for the treatment of sulphonylurea induced hypoglycaemia in type 2 diabetes. New Zealand Medical Journal 1997; 110: 189–190.
14. Barr ELM, Magliano DJ, Zimmett PZ, et al. Metformin. In: Murray L, Daly F, Little M, Cadogan M, eds. Toxicology handbook. Sydney: Churchill Livingstone; 2007 pp235–237.
15. Gjedde S, Christiansen A, Pedersen SB, et al. Survival following a metformin overdose of 63 g: a case report. Pharmacology & Toxicology 2003; 93: 98–99.
16. Teale KFH, Devine A, Stewart H, et al. The management of metformin overdose. Anaesthesia 1998; 53: 691–701.
17. Harvey B, Hickman C, Hinson G, et al. Severe lactic acidosis complicating metformin overdose successfully treated with high-volume venovenous hemofiltration and aggressive alkalinization. Critical Care Medicine 2005; 6: 598–601.
18. Heaney D Majid A, Junor B. Bicarbonate haemodialyis as a treatment of metformin overdose. Nephrology Dialysis Transplantation 1997; 12: 1046–1047.
19. Bailey CJ, Turner RC. Metformin. New England Journal of Medicine 1996; 334: 574–579.
20. Barrueto F, Meggs W, Barchman M. Clearance of metformin by hemofiltration in overdose. Clinical Toxicology 2002; 40: 177–180.
21. Home PD, Pocock SJ, Beck-Nielsen H, et al. Rosiglitazone evaluated for cardiovascular outcomes –an interim report. New England Journal of Medicine 2007; 357(28): 1–11.
22. Frandsen KB, Tambascia MA. Repaglinide and prandial glucose regulation: the rational approach to therapy in type 2 diabetes? Arquivos Brasileiros de Endocrinologia & Metabologia 1999; 43(5): 325–335.

29.9 Colchicine

Lindsay Murray

ESSENTIALS

1 All deliberate self-poisonings with colchicine should be regarded as potentially life-threatening.

2 May present asymptomatic or with gastrointestinal symptoms only.

3 Consider the diagnosis in patients presenting with gastrointestinal symptoms followed by development of multiorgan failure.

4 The key points in management are early recognition of the potential severity of this intoxication, early gastrointestinal decontamination and aggressive supportive care.

Introduction

Colchicine is an alkaloid extracted from the plant *Colchicum autumnale*. It has traditionally been widely used in the treatment of acute gout but has also been prescribed for conditions, including familial Mediterranean fever, scleroderma, primary biliary cirrhosis and recurrent pericarditis.

Colchicine poisoning is relatively rare, most commonly occurring in the context of deliberate self-poisoning or therapeutic overdose. Severe toxicity from therapeutic administration of oral colchicine is unusual, but can occur in the elderly or patients with renal or hepatic disease. In this situation the appearance of gastrointestinal symptoms usually acts as a safety mechanism, and results in discontinuation of the drug before the appearance of more severe symptoms. Poisoning is also reported from ingestion of *Colchicum autumnale* itself.[1]

It is important for the emergency physician to be familiar with the recognition and management of colchicine poisoning because it is associated with high mortality, and the potential seriousness of the intoxication is often underestimated at initial presentation.

Pharmacokinetics

Colchicine is rapidly absorbed following oral administration, with peak levels occurring from 0.5 to 2 h post ingestion.[2] Absorption is not significantly delayed following overdose.[3] Bioavailability following oral administration ranges from 25 to 40% because of extensive first-pass hepatic metabolism.[4,5] Following absorption, colchicine rapidly distributes from plasma to tissues, where it binds with high affinity to intracellular binding sites. The distribution half-life is from 45 to 90 min and the apparent volume of distribution is 21 L/kg in patients with toxicity.[3] Terminal elimination half-lives in toxic patients range from 10.6 to 31.7 h, elimination being via renal excretion, hepatic metabolism via CYP3a4 and enterohepatic circulation.[6]

Pathophysiology

Colchicine binds to tubulin and prevents its polymerization to form microtubules.[7] Microtubules are not only essential components of the cell cytoskeleton during mitosis, but are also integral to other cellular processes such as endocytosis, exocytosis, phagocytosis, cell motility and protein assembly in the Golgi apparatus. In toxic doses, colchicine causes mitosis to arrest in metaphase with serious consequences for the rapidly dividing cells of the gut mucosa and bone marrow. As colchicine-induced microtubular disruption continues it affects cell shape, intracellular transport and the secretion of hormones, enzymes

and neurotransmitters, resulting in toxicity to virtually every cell in the body.[8]

Clinical features

Severe colchicine poisoning presents as a relatively distinct clinical syndrome characterized by early onset of gastrointestinal symptoms followed by delayed onset of multiorgan toxicity and a high incidence of mortality.

In the largest reported series of colchicine poisoning (69 cases), ingestions estimated at <0.5 mg/kg were associated with gastrointestinal symptoms and coagulation disturbances only, and a mortality of 0%. Ingestions of 0.5–0.8 mg/kg were associated with bone-marrow aplasia and a mortality of 10%, and ingestions >0.8 mg/kg with cardiovascular collapse and 100% mortality at 72 h.[9] However, a number of fatalities have been reported following ingestions of doses <0.5 mg/kg,[10–13] therefore any overdose of colchicine should be regarded as potentially serious.

It is convenient to divide the clinical course of colchicine toxicity into three sequential (and usually overlapping) stages (Table 29.9.1). Less severe cases may not progress beyond the first stage. The most severe cases die during the second stage.

Following a significant acute oral overdose the patient may remain asymptomatic for between 2 and 24 h. The toxic patient then develops severe nausea, vomiting, diarrhoea and abdominal pain. This symptomatology corresponds to gastrointestinal mucosal damage and impairment of secretion of normal mucosal enzymes.[14] During this stage, fluid losses from vomiting and diarrhoea may be significant enough to result in hypovolaemic shock.

Multisystem organ failure is characteristic of the second stage, with onset from 24 to 72 h following ingestion. Respiratory, neurological, renal, haematological and cardiovascular involvement is typical. Acute adult respiratory distress syndrome may be a consequence of hypovolaemic shock or sepsis, or occur as a result of direct damage to the pulmonary vasculature.[15] Bone marrow suppression is heralded by lymphopenia, followed by granulocytopenia, reticulocytopenia and thrombocytopenia, reaching a nadir at 4–8 days following ingestion.

Sepsis may complicate this stage of toxicity.[9] Disseminated intravascular coagulopathy was noted to be a frequent complication in one large series of patients with colchicine toxicity.[9] Fever occurs commonly, and may be a direct drug effect or a sign of complicating infection.[16] Shock, frequently observed during this phase, is cardiogenic and/or hypovolaemic in origin, and is strongly associated with death.[13,17] Cardiac rhythm disturbances, including sinus bradycardia and sinus arrest,[18] complete atrioventricular block[14] and sudden cardiac arrest[8] have been reported. Renal failure in acute colchicine toxicity is multifactorial and related to

Table 29.9.1 Clinical stages of significant colchicine toxicity	
Stage 1: Gastrointestinal phase Time of onset: 2–24 h post-ingestion	Nausea, vomiting, diarrhoea, abdominal pain Intravascular volume depletion Peripheral leukocytosis
Stage 2: Multiorgan failure phase Time of onset: 24–72 h post-ingestion	Adult respiratory distress syndrome Bone marrow suppression Cardiac arrhythmias, failure, arrest Consumptive coagulopathy Fever Hypomagnesaemia Hyponatraemia Hypocalcaemia Hypophosphataemia Ileus Metabolic acidosis Mental status changes Neuromuscular abnormalities Oliguric renal failure Secondary sepsis Seizures
Stage 3: Recovery phase Time of onset: 6–8 days post-ingestion	Resolution of organ system derangements Rebound leukocytosis Alopecia

prolonged hypotension, hypoxia, sepsis and rhabdomyolysis.[8] Metabolic derangements described include metabolic acidosis, hyperglycaemia, hypokalaemia, hypocalcaemia, hypophosphataemia and hypomagnesaemia.[19] Neurological disturbances include delirium, coma, seizures, transverse myelitis and ascending paralysis.[8,20] Death is common during this period and usually occurs as a result of profound cardiogenic shock, sudden cardiac arrest or sepsis. Cardiac arrest has been observed as early as 36 h following acute colchicine ingestion.[18]

In those who survive stage two, a rebound leukocytosis occurs at 7 or more days after initial symptoms and corresponds to the recovery of bone-marrow function. Alopecia commonly occurs at about this time. Complete recovery is the rule in patients surviving stage two.

Myopathies and neuropathies have been observed as a reversible toxic reaction to long-term colchicine therapy.[21]

Differential diagnosis

The diagnosis of colchicine poisoning is usually evident when the history and clinical features are taken into account. Difficulties and delayed diagnosis occur when the history of colchicine ingestion is not obtained. Colchicine poisoning should be considered whenever progressive multiple organ dysfunction, especially with bone marrow depression, develops following predominantly gastrointestinal symptoms.[22,23]

Clinical investigation

Given the potential for severe multisystem organ failure as described above, extensive baseline laboratory studies should be performed upon presentation. These include electrolytes, full blood count, coagulation profile, renal function tests, liver function tests, electrocardiography and chest radiography. These studies need to be repeated during a hospital admission at intervals dictated by the patient's clinical course. Although colchicine concentrations in biological fluids can be measured, they are not readily available and not useful in the management of colchicine poisoning.

Treatment

The key points in the management of acute colchicine toxicity are early recognition of the potential severity of this intoxication, early gastrointestinal decontamination and aggressive supportive care.

Decontamination of the gut by the administration of oral-activated charcoal is the management priority for the patient presenting in the first (asymptomatic) stage of colchicine intoxication; prevention of absorption of even small amounts may favourably affect the severity of the intoxication and the ultimate outcome. In patients who present later (during the second stage) resuscitative efforts take precedence over gastrointestinal decontamination.

Careful monitoring of vital signs and cardiac rhythm should be instituted upon arrival. An i.v. cannula should be placed and i.v. fluid therapy commenced in any symptomatic patient. In those patients who present with substantial delay, immediate resuscitative measures may be required. Baseline laboratory studies as outlined above should be performed.

All patients with colchicine overdose require admission to hospital for a minimum of 24 h observation. Careful monitoring, not only of vital signs and cardiac rhythm but also of fluid and electrolyte status and blood cell counts, is mandatory. Further supportive therapy is dictated by clinical status, and may include intravenous crystalloid rehydration, plasma expansion, inotropes, artificial ventilation, correction of electrolyte and acid–base disturbances, correction of coagulation disorders and antibiotic treatment of infectious complications.

Because of colchicine's large volume of distribution and high affinity to intracellular binding sites, attempts to enhance elimination by repeat-dose activated charcoal, haemodialysis or haemoperfusion are unlikely to be effective.

Disposition

All patients in whom colchicine toxicity is diagnosed or even suspected require admission. The asymptomatic patient should be observed for a minimum of 24 h. If no symptoms of intoxication (diarrhoea, vomiting or abdominal pain) are evident at the end of

that period, colchicine toxicity may be confidently excluded and the patient discharged. The symptomatic patient should be admitted to an intensive care unit for careful monitoring and supportive care as outlined above.

Prognosis

As noted above, a relatively high mortality is associated with colchicine overdose. Prognosis is to a large extent determined by the dose ingested. Early resuscitation and provision of excellent supportive care improve prognosis. Patients who present late, in whom the diagnosis is delayed or where the potential seriousness of the presentation is underestimated initially do worse. In patients who survive stage two a complete recovery can be anticipated. The alopecia observed during the recovery phase is not permanent, with hair growth commencing after the first month.

Controversies

❶ The bone-marrow suppression associated with colchicine toxicity has been reported to respond to the administration of granulocyte colony-stimulating factor.[24–27] However, it is unclear whether these reports represent a true therapeutic response or the natural course of recovery.

❷ Colchicine-specific Fab fragments have been produced in goats immunized with a conjugate of colchicine and serum albumin, and effectively reverse colchicine toxicity in mice.[28] When administered to a patient with severe colchicine toxicity, rapid improvement in haemodynamic parameters and ultimate survival were observed.[29] Unfortunately, colchicine-specific Fab fragments are not yet commercially available.

References

1. Brvar M, Ploj T Kozel G, et al. Case report: fatal poisoning with colchicum autumnale. Critical Care 2004; 8(1): R56–59.
2. Wallace SL, Ertel NH. Plasma levels of colchicine after administration of a single dose. Metabolism 1973; 22: 749–753.
3. Rochdi M, Sabouraud A, Baud FJ, et al. Toxicokinetics of colchicine in humans: analysis of tissue, plasma and

urine data in ten cases. Human Experimental Toxicology 1992; 11: 510–516.

4. Hunter AL, Klaassen CD. Biliary excretion of colchicine. Journal of Pharmacology and Experimental Therapy 1974; 192: 605–607.

5. Thomas G, Girre C, Scherrmann JM, et al. Zero-order absorption and linear disposition of oral colchicine in healthy volunteers. European Journal of Clinical Pharmacology 1989; 37: 79–84.

6. Ferron GM, Rochdi M, Jusko WJ, et al. Oral absorption characteristics and pharmacokinetics of colchicine in healthy volunteers after single and multiple doses. Journal of Clinical Pharmacology 1996; 36: 874–883.

7. Borizy GG, Taylor EW. The mechanism of action of colchicine: binding of colchicine-H^3 to cellular protein. Journal of Cell Biology 1967; 34: 525–533.

8. Stapczynski JS, Rothstein RJ, Gaye WA, et al. Colchicine overdose: report of two cases and a review of the literature. Annals of Emergency Medicine 1981; 10: 364–369.

9. Bismuth C, Gautier M, Conso F. Aplasie médullaire après intoxication aiguë á la colchicine. Nouvelle Presse Medicale 1977; 6: 1625–1629.

10. MacLeod JG, Phillips L. Hypersensitivity to colchicine. Annals of Rheumatological Diseases 1947; 6: 224–229.

11. Harris R, Gillet M. Colchicine poisoning – overview and new directions. Emergency Medicine 1998; 10: 161–167.

12. Van Heyningen C, Watson ID. Troponin for prediction of cardiovascular collapse in acute colchicine

overdose. Emergency Medicine Journal 2005; 22: 599–600.

13. Mullins ME, Carrico EA, Horowitz BZ. Fatal cardiovascular collapse following acute colchicine ingestion. Journal of Toxicology – Clinical Toxicology 2000; 38: 51–54.

14. Stemmermann GN, Hayashi T. Colchicine intoxication. A reappraisal of its pathology based on a study of three fatal cases. Human Pathology 197; 12: 321–332.

15. Heaney D, Derghazarian CB, Pineo GF, et al. Massive colchicine overdose: report on the toxicity. American Journal of Medical Science 1976; 271: 233–238.

16. Baldwin LR, Talber TL, Sampler R. Accidental overdose of insufflated colchicine. Drug Safety 1990; 5: 305–312.

17. Sauder P, Kopferschmitt J, Jaeger A, et al. Haemodynamic studies in eight cases of acute colchicine poisoning. Human Toxicology 1983; 2: 169–179.

18. Stahl N, Weinberger A, Benjamin D, et al. Fatal colchicine poisoning in a boy with familial Mediterranean fever. American Journal of Medical Science 1976; 278: 77–81.

19. Putterman C, Ben-Cherit E, Caraco Y, Levy M. Colchicine intoxication: clinical pharmacology, risk factors, features and management. Seminars in Arthritis and Rheumatism 1991; 3: 143–155.

20. Naidus R, Rodvien R, Nielke C. Colchicine toxicity. A multisystem disease. Archives of Internal Medicine 1977; 137: 394–396.

21. Kuncl RW, Duncan G, Watson D, et al. Colchicine myopathy and neuropathy. New England Journal of Medicine 1987; 316: 1562–1568.

22. Blackham RE, Little M, Baker S, et al. Unsuspected colchicine overdose in a female patient presenting as an acute abdomen. Anaesthesia and Intensive Care 2007; 35(3): 437–439.

23. Miller MA, Hung YM, Haller C, et al. Colchicine-related death presenting as an unknown case of multiple organ failure. Journal of Emergency Medicine 2005; 28(4): 445–448.

24. Katz R, Chuang LC, Sutton JD. Use of granulocyte colony-stimulating factor in the treatment of pancytopenia secondary to colchicine overdose. Annals of Pharmacotherapy 1992; 26: 1087–1088.

25. Folpini A, Furfori P. Colchicine toxicity – clinical features and treatment. Massive overdose case report. Clinical Toxicology 1995; 33: 71–77.

26. Harris R, Marx G, Gillett M, Kark A. Colchicine-induced bone marrow suppression: treatment with granulocyte colony-stimulating factor. Journal of Emergency Medicine 2000; 18: 435–440.

27. Yoon KH. Colchicine induced toxicity and pancytopenia at usual doses and treatment with granulocyte colony-stimulating factor. Journal of Rheumatology 2001; 28: 1199–1200.

28. Sabouraud A, Urtizberea M, Grandgeorge M, et al. Dose-dependent reversal of acute murine colchicine poisoning by goat colchicine-specific Fab fragments. Toxicology 1991; 68: 121–132.

29. Baud FJ, Sabouraud A, Vicaut E, et al. Brief report: treatment of severe colchicine overdose with colchicine-specific Fab fragments. New England Journal of Medicine 1995; 332: 642–645.

29.10 Theophylline

Lindsay Murray

ESSENTIALS

1 Theophylline toxicity is associated with life-threatening seizures and cardiac arrhythmias.

2 Serum theophylline levels are useful in assessing and managing acute theophylline toxicity.

3 Onset of maximal toxicity may be significantly delayed following overdose of sustained-release preparations.

4 Techniques of enhancing drug elimination play an important role in the management of severe theophylline toxicity.

5 Early identification of high-risk patients allows the institution of enhanced elimination techniques before life-threatening complications develop.

Introduction

Theophylline, a methylxanthine derivative related to caffeine, has long been used in the treatment of asthma and chronic airflow limitation. Although the use of the drug has declined in recent times, both acute and chronic theophylline toxicity continue to result in potentially life-threatening presentations to the emergency department (ED).

Therapeutic blood concentrations of theophylline are generally regarded as being between 55 and 110 µmol/L (10 and 20 mg/L). A single ingestion of more than 10 mg/kg of theophylline by an adult is capable of producing a blood concentration above this range.

Pharmacokinetics

Theophylline is well absorbed orally, with a bioavailability of almost 100%. The rate of absorption depends on the pharmaceutical formulation. The most commonly prescribed preparations are sustained-release, and following overdose of these preparations peak absorption may be delayed up to 15 h.

Once absorbed, theophylline is rapidly distributed with a relatively small volume of distribution (0.3–0.7 L/kg). Theophylline is metabolized via the cytochrome P450 system to produce active and inactive metabolites. Only about 10% of absorbed theophylline is excreted unchanged in the urine. The rate of metabolism is extremely variable and decreases with time. Theophylline metabolism exhibits saturable (Michaelis–Menten) kinetics. At higher doses of theophylline, relatively small increments in dose are associated with disproportionate increases in serum concentration.[1] In cases of severe intoxication, endogenous elimination of theophylline is very slow.

Pathophysiology

The precise mechanisms of toxicity of theophylline are unknown. Proposed mechanisms include inhibition of phosphodiesterase leading to elevated concentrations of intracellular cAMP, augmented plasma catecholamine activity, competitive antagonism of adenosine and changes in intracellular calcium transport.[2]

Clinical features

Two different clinical syndromes of theophylline poisoning are recognized: acute and chronic. Both are potentially life-threatening, although the chronic form is associated with a greater incidence of morbidity and mortality.[3]

Chronic intoxication is the most common clinical presentation and occurs when excessive doses of theophylline are administered repeatedly, or where intercurrent illness or drug interaction interferes with hepatic metabolism. Theophylline has a notoriously narrow therapeutic index, and up to 15% of patients with a serum theophylline concentration in the therapeutic range have clinical manifestations of toxicity. Acute intoxication is usually the result of deliberate overdose with suicidal intent, but is occasionally observed following inadvertent iatrogenic overdose.

The clinical manifestations of theophylline intoxication are numerous and principally affect the gastrointestinal, cardiovascular, central nervous, musculoskeletal and metabolic systems.

The gastrointestinal tract is particularly sensitive to theophylline toxicity, the most prominent symptom being vomiting. This is usually severe and frequently refractory to treatment with antiemetics.

Sinus tachycardia is an almost universal manifestation of theophylline toxicity. However, severe intoxication is also associated with more unstable rhythms, including supraventricular tachycardia, atrial fibrillation, atrial flutter, multifocal atrial tachycardia and ventricular tachycardia.[4] Refractory hypotension may occur in severe toxicity as a result of β_2-mediated peripheral vasodilation.

Central nervous system manifestations most commonly consist of anxiety and insomnia. With more severe intoxication, tachypnoea from respiratory centre stimulation and seizures occur. Seizures can develop suddenly, may be repetitive, are difficult to treat and are associated with poor outcome.

Metabolic complications of theophylline poisoning include hypokalaemia, hypophosphataemia, hypomagnesaemia, hyperglycaemia and metabolic acidosis.[5] Hypokalaemia is frequent following acute overdose, occurs early and is a consequence of intracellular shift of potassium secondary to catecholamine excess.[6,7] Musculoskeletal manifestations include muscle aches, increased muscle tone and myoclonus.

Chronic intoxication usually occurs in elderly patients and is associated with vomiting and tachycardia. The metabolic abnormalities are less frequently observed. Seizures and cardiac arrhythmias occur more frequently and at much lower serum theophylline concentrations than in acute intoxication.[8,9]

Following acute overdose, especially where sustained-release preparations are involved, the clinical manifestations of severe toxicity may be delayed up to 12 h. These patients usually present with severe vomiting before the onset of more severe toxicity, including seizures and arrhythmias.

Clinical investigation

The diagnosis of theophylline toxicity is suspected on history and clinical presentation, and confirmed by documentation of a significant serum theophylline concentration. The serum theophylline concentration is also invaluable in the assessment of severity and ongoing management of theophylline poisoning. Although theophylline is readily measured, it is not detected on routine drug screens.

Patients with acute theophylline overdose generally exhibit signs of minor toxicity at serum concentrations from 110 to 220 μmol/L (20–40 mg/L), moderate toxicity with concentrations from 220 to 440 μmol/L (40–80 mg/L) and severe toxicity with concentrations greater than 440 μmol/L (80 mg/L). Serum theophylline concentrations of greater than 550 μmol/L (100 mg/L) are frequently fatal.[10] After an acute overdose serum theophylline should be measured every 3 h or so until a falling concentration is documented.

In chronic theophylline poisoning, serious toxicity is observed at lower serum concentrations and the measured concentration is not predictive of the severity of poisoning.[11] Seizures, arrhythmias and fatalities can occur at concentrations as low as 220–330 μmol/L (20–30 mg/L).[12] In these patients the best predictor of poor outcome is age over 60 years.[13]

Other useful laboratory studies include electrolytes and creatinine, glucose, liver function tests (LFTs) and electrocardiogram (ECG).

Treatment

The initial management of theophylline poisoning follows the principles of general supportive care. Specific attention may need to be directed towards control of the airway, hypotension, tachyarrhythmias and seizures.

Hypotension usually responds to intravenous fluid administration. A noradrenaline (norepinephrine) infusion may be necessary in resistant cases. Supraventricular arrhythmias can be treated with a β-blocker such as propranolol or esmolol intravenously,[14] but this may induce bronchospasm in susceptible individuals. Seizures must be treated aggressively with high-dose benzodiazepines. If this fails, phenobarbitone and even general anaesthesia may be required. Phenytoin is ineffective and contraindicated. Metabolic disturbances do not generally require specific therapy. Severe hypokalaemia should be corrected with potassium supplementation.

Following acute overdose, oral-activated charcoal should be administered, even if presentation is delayed. Antiemetics are usually required for successful administration.

The pharmacokinetic properties of theophylline, especially the small volume of distribution, lend themselves to methods of enhanced elimination. Theophylline is relatively efficiently removed by haemodialysis, charcoal haemoperfusion and administration of repeat-dose activated charcoal.[15]

Theophylline clearance rates of 100 mL/min have been reported with multiple-dose activated charcoal.[15] Again, aggressive antiemetic therapy may be necessary if this non-invasive method of enhancing drug elimination is to be effective. Administration of a selective serotonin antagonist such as ondansetron has proved particularly effective in this setting.[16,17]

Both charcoal haemoperfusion and haemodialysis greatly increase the elimination of theophylline and are highly effective in achieving a good clinical outcome.[3,18] Such invasive methods are only indicated in potentially life-threatening theophylline toxicity. Commonly accepted indications include acute intoxication, where the serum theophylline is greater than 550 µmol/L; chronic intoxication, where it is greater than 220–330 µmol/L or in any patient with intractable hypotension, ventricular ectopy or resistant seizures.[8,10] Ideally, patients at greatest risk of developing arrhythmias or seizures should be identified early and haemodialysis or haemoperfusion instituted before these complications develop. Continuous venovenous haemofiltration has been successfully used as an alternative to standard intermittent haemodialysis in the treatment of severe theophylline poisoning with a reduction in the elimination half-life to 5.87 h reported.[19]

Disposition

All patients with symptomatic theophylline toxicity require admission to hospital. Patients with acute overdose of sustained-release preparations should be admitted for monitoring and serial serum theophylline concentrations. Patients with moderate-to-severe theophylline toxicity require admission to a monitored bed.

Controversies

❶ Although charcoal haemoperfusion has been recommended as the most effective way to enhance theophylline elimination, it has not yet been shown to be associated with any additional improvement in clinical outcome compared to haemodialysis.

❷ Continuous renal replacement therapies offer a number of advantages over standard intermittent dialysis as a method of enhancing theophylline elimination. They are easily set up and run in most intensive care units and can be run 24 h a day. However, clearance rates are slower and these techniques are not currently recommended except where standard dialysis is not available or unfeasible because of haemodynamic instability.

❸ Based on sound pharmacodynamic principles, adenosine infusion has been proposed as an antidote to theophylline toxicity. There are as yet no data to support the use of this therapy.[20]

References

1. Weinberger M, Ginchansky E. Dose-dependent kinetics of theophylline disposition in asthmatic children. Journal of Pediatrics 1977; 91: 820.
2. Haddad L, Shannon MW, Winchester JF, eds. Clinical management of poisoning and drug overdose. 3rd edn. Philadelphia: WB Saunders; 1998.
3. Shannon MW. Comparative efficacy of hemodialysis and hemoperfusion in severe theophylline intoxication. Academic Emergency Medicine 1997; 4: 674–678.
4. Bender PR, Brent J, Kulig K. Cardiac arrhythmias during theophylline toxicity. Chest 1991; 100: 884–886.
5. Hall KW, Dobson KE, Dalton JG, et al. Metabolic abnormalities associated with intentional theophylline overdose. Annals of Internal Medicine 1984; 101: 457–462.
6. Amitai Y, Lovejoy FH. Hypokalaemia in acute theophylline poisoning. American Journal of Emergency Medicine 1988; 6: 214–218.
7. Shannon M, Lovejoy FH. Hypokalemia after theophylline intoxication. The effects of acute vs chronic poisoning. Archives of Internal Medicine 1989; 149: 2725–2729.
8. Olson KR, Benowitz NL, Woo OF, Pond SM. Theophylline overdose: acute single ingestion versus chronic repeated overmedication. American Journal of Emergency Medicine 1984; 3: 386–394.
9. Shannon M. Life-threatening events after theophylline overdose: a 10-year prospective analysis. Archives of Internal Medicine 1999; 159: 989–994.
10. Sessler C. Theophylline toxicity: clinical features of 116 consecutive cases. American Journal of Medicine 1990; 88: 567–576.
11. Shannon M, Lovejoy F. Effect of acute versus chronic intoxication on clinical features of theophylline poisoning in children. Journal of Pediatrics 1992; 121: 125.
12. Bahls F, Ma KK, Bird TD. Theophylline-associated seizures with 'therapeutic' or low toxic serum concentrations: risk factors for serious outcome in adults. Neurology 1991; 41: 1309.
13. Shannon M. Predictors of major toxicity after theophylline overdose. Annals of Internal Medicine 1993; 119: 1161–1167.
14. Seneff M, Scott J, Friedman B, Smith M. Acute theophylline toxicity and the use of esmolol to reverse cardiovascular instability. Annals of Emergency Medicine 1990; 19: 671–673.
15. Kulig KW, Bar-Or D, Rumack BH. Intravenous theophylline poisoning and multiple-dose charcoal in an animal model. Annals of Emergency Medicine 1987; 16: 842.
16. Brown S, Prentice D. Ondansetron in the treatment of theophylline overdose. Medical Journal of Australia 1992; 156: 512.
17. Sage TA, Jones WN, Clark RF. Ondansetron in the treatment of intractable nausea associated with theophylline toxicity. Annals of Pharmacotherapy 1993; 27: 584–585.
18. Heath A, Knudsen K. Role of extracorporeal drug removal in acute theophylline poisoning – a review. Medical Toxicology 1987; 2: 294.
19. Henderson JH, McKenzie CA, Hilton PJ, Leach RM. Continuous venovenous haemofiltration for the treatment of theophylline toxicity. Thorax 2001; 56: 242–243.
20. Blery JC, Kauflin MJ, Mauro VF. Adenosine in acute theophylline intoxication. Annals of Pharmacotherapy 1995; 29: 1285–1287.

29.11 Iron

Zeff Koutsogiannis

ESSENTIALS

1 Acute iron poisoning is a potentially life-threatening condition.

2 The risk of severe toxicity is determined by the dose of elemental iron ingested not the weight of the iron salt.

3 Iron poisoning has both local (gastrointestinal) and systemic effects.

4 Early effective gastrointestinal decontamination, usually with whole-bowel irrigation, is important in the management of high-risk cases.

5 Chelation therapy with intravenous desferrioxamine is the definitive treatment for severe poisoning.

6 Generally, most patients recover, although presence of shock or coma indicates a poor prognosis.

7 Long-term sequelae are gastrointestinal scarring and obstruction.

Introduction

Although the majority of exposures to iron occur in small children, significant iron ingestions also occur in adults as a result of deliberate self-poisoning. It is one of the most commonly ingested agents in self-poisoning during pregnancy as a result of its ready availability to obstetric patients.[1] Iron supplements are often considered by patients and parents to be innocuous dietary supplements, leading to careless storage and handling, and delays in seeking medical care following ingestions.

Pathophysiology

Iron is an essential element in red blood cell production, haemoglobin and myoglobin oxygenation, cytochrome function and many enzyme cofactor catalytic activities.[2,3] Under normal circumstances, absorption of iron from the gastrointestinal (GI) tract is finely regulated according to the requirements of the body. After absorption across the GI mucosa in the ferrous form (Fe^{2+}), iron is oxidized to the ferric state (Fe^{3+}) and then stored bound to ferritin or transported across the cell membrane into the blood, where it binds to transferrin.[2] Iron is extracted from transferrin in the bone marrow and used for haemoglobin synthesis. It is also removed from transferrin by the reticuloendothelial system and hepatocytes and stored as haemosiderin and ferritin.[4] Total iron binding capacity (TIBC) is a measurement of the total amount of iron that transferrin can bind and normally exceeds serum iron by two- to threefold.[3] Ferritin is a large storage protein that reversibly binds to iron. When an iron deficit exists, iron is transported from ferritin and the GI tract to the liver, spleen and bone marrow where it is incorporated into appropriate molecules.[5] If the body's iron requirements have been met, iron remains stored in the intestinal cell rather than bound to transferrin. Eventually, the intestinal cell dies and sloughs off into the lumen for elimination.[3] This is the main mechanism limiting excessive iron absorption and the mechanism by which the body regulates iron balance.[5]

Iron rarely exists as an unbound or 'free' element.[5] It is free iron that is toxic to cellular processes. Iron toxicity manifests as both local (GI) and systemic effects.

Local effects

Iron preparations, like other metal salts, have a direct corrosive effect on the GI mucosa. In overdose this can lead to irritation, ulceration, bleeding, ischaemia, infarction and perforation.[6] Associated profound fluid losses can result in hypotension, shock and lactate formation leading to metabolic acidosis. The long-term sequelae of this corrosive action include GI scarring and obstruction.[6,7] As the mucosal surface is disrupted iron is absorbed, passively down concentration gradients.[3,7] When the transferrin binding capacity is exhausted, free iron becomes available.

Systemic effects

Free iron is an intracellular toxin and localizes in the mitochondria, which in turn catalyses free radical formation, disrupts oxidative phosphorylation and lipid peroxidation.[8] The resultant mitochondrial dysfunction and destruction lead to cell death and can occur in any organ. Other systemic findings of iron poisoning include cardiovascular collapse, anion-gap metabolic acidosis, coagulopathy and encephalopathy.[3,8] The cardiovascular collapse has been attributed to decreased intravascular volume from GI haemorrhage, third space losses from increased capillary membrane permeability and iron-induced venodilation.[7] Metabolic acidosis persisting after correction of hypovolaemia and hypoperfusion is probably a result of mitochondrial toxicity.[8] Coagulopathy developing early in iron poisoning results from inhibition of serum proteases while in the later stages it is due to hepatic dysfunction.[9]

Toxic dose

In general, the risk of developing iron toxicity can be predicted from the dose of elemental iron ingested per kilogram body weight (Table 29.11.1).[8,10] It essential to calculate the dose of elemental iron rather than dose of iron salt.

Prevention

Iron poisoning is a major cause of unintentional poisoning death in young children. In a pre-intervention–post-intervention study there was a decrease in the incidence of non-intentional ingestion by young children and decrease mortality following the introduction of unit-dose packaging.[11] This, together with

Table 29.11.1 Risk assessment based on dose of elemental iron ingested

Risk assessment	Dose ingested (mg/kg)
Asymptomatic	<20
Local (GI) symptoms only	20–60
Risk of systemic iron poisoning	60–120
Potentially lethal	>120

education may further decrease the incidence of toxicity and late presentations.

Clinical features

The clinical course of iron poisoning is traditionally described as comprising five stages.[7,12,13] Not all patients will experience all stages; they can die at any stage; can present at any stage and the time frames for each stage are imprecise and may overlap.

A more practical approach is to consider iron poisoning as comprising two clinical stages with a pathophysiological basis: GI toxicity and systemic toxicity.

Stage 1 (0–6 h)

This stage is dominated by symptoms and signs of GI injury particularly vomiting, but also abdominal pain, diarrhoea and GI bleeding. In severe cases, hypovolaemic shock secondary to GI losses can develop.[8] The failure to develop any GI symptoms within 6 h of ingestion effectively excludes significant iron poisoning.[3,14,15]

Stage 2 (2–24 h)

Also known as the 'latent' or 'quiescent' phase, this stage represents the period between resolution of GI symptoms and appearance of overt systemic toxicity. It is not always seen and, indeed, may represent a failure to recognize development of toxicity rather than a true quiescent phase. Most patients will recover and not progress to Stage 3. Those with significant poisoning remain clinically ill with subtle signs and progress to Stage 3.

Stage 3 (6–48 h)

This is the stage of systemic toxicity characterized by shock and multiorgan system failure. By definition, it represents severe toxicity. The shock is multifactorial arising from hypovolaemia, vasodilation and poor cardiac output. There is evidence of poor peripheral perfusion, worsening acidosis and acute renal failure. A coagulopathy may develop and lead to recurrent GI bleeding. Central nervous system effects include lethargy, coma and convulsions.

Stage 4 (2–5 days)

This is the hepatic phase of iron toxicity and is relatively uncommon.[2] It is characterized by acute hepatic failure with jaundice, hepatic coma, hypoglycaemia, coagulopathy and elevated transaminase and ammonia levels. It has a high mortality.[16]

Stage 5 (2–6 weeks)

This stage is relatively rare and represents the delayed sequelae from the corrosive effects of iron resulting in GI scarring. This results in gastric outlet and small bowel obstructions.

Clinical investigation

Acute iron poisoning is a clinical diagnosis and all symptomatic patients require treatment regardless of the iron level or results of other tests. However serum iron levels, abdominal X-rays and other tests do play a role in determining management.

Serum iron concentration

Normal serum iron concentrations are between 10 and 30 µmol/L. Peak iron levels usually occur between 2 and 6 h after overdose, although they may sometimes be delayed.[3,17] Frequent levels may need to be taken to determine the true peak. Nevertheless, iron levels have been used to determine toxicity and direct management.[7] A serum iron concentration greater than 90 µmol/L at 4–6 h after an overdose is associated with a greater risk of subsequently developing systemic iron toxicity. However, it is intracellular and not serum iron that is responsible for systemic toxicity and thus during Stages 2 or 3, the iron level may be decreasing or even normal while the patient deteriorates. In the presence of desferrioxamine, the serum iron level is artificially lowered.

The TIBC is falsely elevated in the presence of high iron concentrations or desferrioxamine and is no longer regarded as useful in the assessment of iron poisoning.[18]

Plain abdominal X-rays

Most iron preparations are radio-opaque and an early abdominal X-ray is useful in confirming ingestion of iron, and in subsequently guiding gastric decontamination and the risk of continued iron absorption. A negative X-ray does not exclude iron ingestion as the tablets may have disintegrated or not be radio-opaque.

Other laboratory tests

Although leukocytosis and hyperglycaemia are frequently observed in iron poisoning they are not useful in terms of diagnosis or management.[15] The presence of an anion gap metabolic acidosis is a useful marker of systemic iron poisoning. Other tests that are useful in managing patients with established iron poisoning include serum electrolytes, renal function, liver function, arterial blood gases, cross match and clotting profile.

Treatment

The approach to management of a patient presenting following an iron overdose is determined by the initial assessment of the risk of iron poisoning. This risk assessment is based on the dose ingested and the presence or absence of GI and/or systemic features of iron poisoning. For most patients, a period of observation and good supportive care, often including intravenous fluids will be sufficient. In those patients at risk of systemic poisoning or who present with established iron poisoning, aggressive decontamination measures and chelation therapy may be necessary to achieve a good outcome. The aim is to prevent the development of systemic toxicity in those patients at risk.

Observation and supportive care

All patients demonstrating signs and symptoms consistent with clinical toxicity of Stages 1, 2 or 3 warrant further treatment. Enthusiastic fluid replacement with isotonic fluid is essential. An initial bolus of 20 mL/kg should be given, followed by boluses as needed to replace fluid losses and maintain urine output. Patients with established iron poisoning may require more advanced supportive care including inotropic support, blood transfusions, correction of coagulopathy with fresh frozen plasma and correction of acidosis.

Gastrointestinal decontamination

Iron is not well adsorbed to activated charcoal. Other modalities designed to reduce iron absorption from the GI tract including oral bicarbonate, phosphate, magnesium hydroxide, oral calcium disodium EDTA and sodium polystyrene sulphonate are equally ineffective.[19–22] Thus, alternative methods of GI decontamination must be considered in patients who present following ingestion of more than 60 mg/kg of elemental iron, especially where unabsorbed iron is evident on abdominal X-ray.

Inducing emesis with syrup of ipecac is not recommended because it may mask the symptoms produced by iron and can lead to an underestimation of the severity of the toxicity.[10] Gastric lavage may be a useful option if performed early but is often technically difficult in that the tablets tend to clump together, form pharmacobezoars and attach to the gastric mucosa.[2] Endoscopy has been used to remove large iron loads but this is also technically difficult.[8] Surgical removal is reported.[23,24]

Whole-bowel irrigation (WBI) is widely advocated as the GI decontamination method of choice in the setting of iron poisoning, although there are no controlled trials.[25] It should be initiated in any patient who has ingested more than 60 mg/kg of elemental iron and still has iron present in the GI tract on X-ray. The procedure is continued until there is a clear rectal effluent and no visible iron on X-ray. As iron has a direct corrosive effect on the GI mucosa, caution is therefore advised with the use of WBI in late presenters who may have sustained mucosal damage.

Chelation therapy

Desferrioxamine is the parenteral chelating agent of choice for iron poisoning. It binds Fe^{3+} to form ferrioxamine which is water soluble, red-to-orange in colour and renally excreted.[3] Desferrioxamine binds free iron and iron in transit between transferrin and ferritin thus effecting a redistribution of iron from tissue sites back into plasma. It does not chelate iron bound to transferrin, haemoglobin, myoglobin or cytochrome enzymes.[3]

Chelation therapy is indicated in any patient with established systemic iron toxicity or at risk of developing such toxicity. Clinical features and laboratory results may be useful in identifying these patients. The presence of GI bleeding, coma, shock or metabolic acidosis are indications for immediate desferrioxamine therapy irrespective of iron levels. Serum iron levels greater than 90 µmol/L are generally regarded as being predictive of subsequent systemic toxicity and an indication to commence chelation therapy.

Ferrioxamine's red-to-orange colour is responsible for the classically described *vin rose* urine in patients given desferrioxamine but this colour change is an insensitive marker of the presence of free iron and the desferrioxamine intramuscular challenge test is no longer used.[26]

Desferrioxamine is given as a continuous intravenous infusion starting slowly and aiming for a rate of 15 mg/kg/h.[7,10] Administration rate may be limited by hypotension, the principal adverse effect. Intramuscular administration is not recommended as it is painful, requires multiple injections, has erratic absorption and higher side effect profile.[10] The precise endpoints for chelation therapy are unclear but therapy can be safely discontinued once the serum iron level is normal or low, the patient clinically well, the anion gap resolved and there is no further urine colour change.[3,27] Except under exceptional circumstances, desferrioxamine should not be continued for longer than 24 h because of the risk of pulmonary toxicity and ARDS.[28]

The approach to iron poisoning is not altered in the pregnant patient. Symptomatic iron overdose in pregnancy is associated with preterm labour, spontaneous abortion and maternal death.[1] Desferrioxamine does not cause perinatal complications or fetal toxicity and is potentially life saving.[29] It is therefore indicated in iron intoxication in pregnancy with clinical evidence of moderate to severe toxicity. The dose is based on the pre-pregnancy weight of the patient.

Disposition

Patients who have ingested less than 60 mg/kg of elemental iron and remain asymptomatic at 6 h may be medically discharged. Those with GI symptoms or requiring WBI because of large ingestion require admission for supportive care and ongoing observation and monitoring. Those with systemic toxicity and/or requiring chelation therapy require intensive care admission. All patients where deliberate self-poisoning is suspected require psychosocial assessment.

Prognosis

Most patients with iron overdose remain asymptomatic or develop minor GI toxicity only and do well with supportive care. Those with large ingestions should have an excellent outcome if recognized early, and appropriate and timely decontamination and/or chelation therapy is instituted. Patients presenting late with established severe systemic toxicity have a poorer prognosis.[2] Gastrointestinal stricture formation is a potential long-term sequela.

Controversies

❶ Continuous arterio-venous haemofiltration may be useful to remove iron in the presence of acute renal failure.[30]

❷ N-Acetylcysteine may protect against iron-induced hepatotoxicity.[31]

❸ New oral chelating agents, such as deferiprone (effective in patients with chronic iron overload states such as thalassaemia)[32] and the hexadentate phenolic aminocarboxylate iron chelator sodium N,N'-bis(2-hydroxybenzyl) ethylenediamine-N,N'-diacetic acid (HBED) ligand[33] have been shown to improve survival and enhance iron excretion in animal studies, but no human data are as yet available.[33,34]

❹ Modifications of desferrioxamine, such as conjugation with dextran or hydroxyethyl starch, have shown the potential for enhanced efficacy and improved patient tolerability.[35] Additional research must be conducted to determine the role of these agents.

References

1. Tran T, Wax JR, Philput C, et al. Intentional iron overdose in pregnancy-management and outcome. Journal of Emergency Medicine 2000; 18(2): 225–228.
2. Gruber J. Acute iron and lead poisoning. In: Rosen P, Barkin R, eds. Emergency medicine. St Louis: Mosby; 1998: 1367–1378.
3. Mills KC, Curry SC. Acute iron poisoning. Emergency Medical Clinics of North America 1994; 12(2): 397–413.
4. Henretig FM, Temple AR. Acute iron poisoning in children. Emergency Medical Clinics of North America 1984; 2(1): 121.
5. Finch CA, Huebers H. Perspectives in iron metabolism. New England Journal of Medicine 1982; 306: 1520.
6. Tenenbein M, Littman C, Stimpson RE, et al. Gastrointestinal pathology in adult iron overdose. Journal of Toxicology – Clinical Toxicology 1990; 28: 311–320.
7. Banner W, Tong TG. Iron poisoning. Pediatrics Clinics of North America 1986; 33: 393–409.
8. Rella JG, Nelson LS. Iron. In: Tintinalli, et al. eds. Emergency medicine. New York: McGraw Hill; 1997: 1159–1162.
9. Tenenbein M, Israels SJ. Early coagulopathy in severe iron poisoning. Journal of Pediatrics 1988; 113: 695.
10. Curry SC. Iron. In: Reisdorff EJ, et al. eds. Paediatric emergency medicine, Philadelphia: WB Saunders; 1993: 673–679.
11. Tenenbein M. Unit-dose packaging of iron supplements and reduction of iron poisoning in young children. Archives of Pediatric and Adolescent Medicine 2005; 159(6): 557–560.
12. Jacobs J, Greene H. Acute iron intoxication. New England Journal of Medicine 1965; 273: 1124–1127.
13. Schauben JL, Augenstein WL, Cox J, et al. Iron poisoning: Report of 3 cases and review of therapeutic intervention. Journal of Emergency Medicine 1990; 8: 309–319.
14. Chyka PA, Butler AY. Assessment of acute iron poisoning by laboratory and clinical observations. American Journal of Emergency Medicine 1993; 11: 99.
15. Palatnick W, Tenenbein M. Leukocytosis, hyperglycaemia, vomiting, and positive X-rays are not indicators of severity of iron poisoning. American Journal of Emergency Medicine 1996; 14: 454–455.
16. Tenenbein M. Hepatotoxicity in acute iron poisoning. Journal of Toxicology – Clinical Toxicology 2001; 39(7): 721–726.
17. Ling LJ, Hornfeldt CS. Absorption of iron after experimental overdose of chewable vitamins. American Journal of Emergency Medicine 1991; 9: 4–26.
18. Siff JE, Meldon SW. Usefulness of the total iron binding capacity in the evaluation and treatment of acute iron overdose. Annals of Emergency Medicine 1999; 34(1): 567–568.
19. Czajka PA, Konrad JD, Duffy JP. Iron poisoning: An in vitro comparison of bicarbonate and phosphate lavage solutions. Journal of Pediatrics 1981; 98: 491–494.
20. Dean BS, Krenzelok EP. In vivo effectiveness of oral complexation agents in the management of iron poisoning. Clinical Toxicology 1987; 25: 221–230.
21. Matteucci MJ, Habibe M, Robson K, et al. Effect of oral calcium disodium EDTA on iron absorption in a human model of iron overdose. Clinical Toxicology 2006; 44(1): 39–43.
22. Shepherd G, Klein-Schwartz W, Burstein AH. Efficacy of the cation exchange resin, sodium polystyrene sulfonate, to decrease iron absorption. Clinical Toxicology 2000; 38(4): 389–394.
23. Foxford R, Goldfrank L. Gastrotomy: a surgical approach to iron overdose. Annals of Emergency Medicine 1985; 14: 1223–1226.
24. Peterson CD, Fifeld GS. Emergency gastrotomy for acute iron poisoning. Annals of Emergency Medicine 1980; 9: 262–264.
25. Tenenbein M. Position statement: whole bowel irrigation. American Academy of Clinical Toxicology; European Association of Poisons Centres and Clinical Toxicologists. Journal of Toxicology – Clinical Toxicology 1993; 35(7): 753–762.
26. Yatscoff RW, Wayne EA, Tenenbein M, et al. An objective criterion for the cessation of deferoxamine therapy in the acutely iron poisoned patient. Journal of Toxicology – Clinical Toxicology 1991; 29: 1–10.
27. Howland MA. Risks of parenteral deferoxamine for acute iron poisoning. Journal of Toxicology – Clinical Toxicology 1996; 35(5): 491–497.
28. Tenenbein M, Kowalski S, Stenko A, et al. Pulmonary toxic effects of continuous administration in acute iron poisoning. Lancet 1992; 34: 485–489.
29. Tran T, Wax JR, Steinfeld, et al. Acute intentional overdose in pregnancy. Obstetrics and Gynecology 1998; 92: 678–680.
30. Banner W, Vernon DD, Ward R, et al. Continuous arterio-venous haemofiltration in experimental iron intoxication. Veterinary and Human Toxicology 1988; 30: 755.
31. Sumanth R, Hayashi, PH. Acute liver failure due to iron overdose in an adult. Southern Medical Journal 2005; 98(2): 241–244.
32. Diav-Citrin O, Koren G. Oral iron chelation with deferiprone. Pediatric Clinics of North America 1997; 44 (1): 236–247.
33. Bergeron R, Wiegand J, Brittenham G. HBED ligand: preclinical studies of a potential alternative to deferoxamine for treatment of chronic iron overload and acute iron poisoning. Blood 2002; 99: 3019–3026.
34. Berkovitch M, Livne A, Lushkov G, et al. The efficacy of oral deferiprone in acute iron poisoning. American Journal of Emergency Medicine 2000; 18(1): 36–40.
35. Dragsten PR, Hallway PE, Hanson GJ, et al. First human studies with a high-molecular-weight iron chelator. Journal of Laboratory and Clinical Medicine 2000; 135: 57–65.

29.12 Drugs of abuse

Frank Daly

ESSENTIALS

1 The diagnosis of intoxication by drugs of abuse is clinical.

2 Good supportive care ensures optimal outcome for the majority of cases.

3 Intoxication with amphetamine-related agents is common. Hyperthermia, decreased level of consciousness, headache, focal neurological signs or chest pain indicate severe intoxication or life-threatening complications and warrant aggressive management and investigation.

4 Benzodiazepines are important in the management of the central nervous and cardiovascular manifestations of sympathomimetic intoxication.

5 Predisposing factors for heroin overdose include co-ingestion of other central nervous system (CNS) depressant drugs, poor tolerance, high street purity and reluctance to seek medical care.

6 Naloxone, a short-acting opioid antagonist, is a useful adjunct in the management of airway and ventilation in opioid overdose.

7 Gamma hydroxybutyrate is a sedative-hypnotic drug of abuse causing CNS depression. Management is supportive.

8 Presentation to the emergency department following overdose with an illicit drug provides an important opportunity for intervention. Education to avoid future overdoses and referral to agencies specializing in drug detoxification and rehabilitation is appropriate.

OPIOIDS

Introduction and epidemiology

Opioids are derivatives of the opium poppy, *Papaver somniferum*, which contains approximately 20 alkaloids, including morphine, codeine and thebaine.[1]

Recent data suggest that 38% of Australians aged over 14 have used illicit drugs during their lifetime, with 1.4% using heroin.[2] In the period 1998–2004 the proportion of the Australian population over the age of 14 years reporting heroin use in the previous 12 months declined from 0.8% to 0.2%. Deaths from accidental opioid overdose in Australia peaked in 1998 at 102 deaths per million persons, and declined to 31 deaths per million in 2004.[2] Forensic data indicate that 77% of opioid-related deaths in Western Australia are due to heroin (diacetylmorphine).[3]

Overseas longitudinal studies suggest that illicit drug abuse in teenagers is associated with mortality rates of 10–20 times that of their peers,[4] while heroin users have an annual mortality rate between 1% and 3%, 6–20 times that of their peers.[5] The predominant cause of this excess mortality is overdose, rather than trauma, infectious disease or suicide.[4,5]

Factors that contribute to non-fatal and fatal opioid overdose include the co-ingestion of other central nervous system (CNS) depressant drugs,[5–7] poor tolerance,[6] high street purity[8] and reluctance to seek medical care.[5]

Heroin overdose is a common occurrence among Australian heroin users, with 68% experiencing overdose and 86% witnessing an overdose in one study.[6] Overdose occurred in experienced addicts who used multiple drugs. Sixty per cent reported using alcohol or benzodiazepines at the time of their last overdose. In a study of heroin-related deaths in New South Wales, two or more drug classes were detected in 71% of subjects.[7]

Pharmacology and pathophysiology

Most opioids are well absorbed across mucous membranes and from subcutaneous and intramuscular sites. Opioids absorbed from the gastrointestinal (GI) tract are subject to extensive first-pass metabolism. They are converted to polar metabolites and excreted in the urine. Tissue hydrolysis (diacetylmorphine/heroin to morphine) also occurs in addition to glucuronidation (morphine), demethylation (a minor pathway) and oxidative metabolism in the liver. Active metabolites (e.g. morphine-6-glucuronide) may accumulate in renal failure. The demethylated metabolite of pethidine may accumulate and cause seizures.[1]

Opioids produce their effects by binding to specific receptors found in the brain and spinal cord, and are classified as agonists, partial agonists or antagonists. The receptors are classified as μ (mu), δ (delta) and κ (kappa). The principal effects of opioids on the CNS, such as analgesia, euphoria, sedation and respiratory depression, are due to their action on μ receptors. All opioids cause miosis, to which tolerance does not develop. Other CNS effects include cough suppression, nausea and vomiting. Opioids also cause constipation, increased gastric tone, contraction of biliary smooth muscle and prolongation of labour.[1]

Clinical features

Patients may present to the emergency department (ED) with acute opioid intoxication, symptoms of opioid withdrawal or with complications of illicit opioid use. Illicit opioid abusers may use the parenteral, inhalational, oral or rectal routes. Venepuncture ('track') marks are not always evident.

The clinical signs of pure opioid intoxication are related to their well-known effects on the CNS. With increasing dose euphoria, miosis, sedation, coma, respiratory depression and apnoea occur. Death is due to respiratory depression.

The signs of opioid intoxication are altered by co-ingested drugs, trauma or medical complications. Alcohol, benzodiazepines, amphetamines and hallucinogenic agents may cloud the clinical picture. The purity of heroin may vary from less than 20 to greater than 50%, and the drug is 'cut' with a variety of adulterant agents,[5] which may have their own clinical effects.

Hypoxia, hypercarbia and acidaemia may lead to tachycardia, hypertension and variable pupillary responses. Finally, bradycardia, hypotension and cardiac arrest occur as terminal events.

The pharmacokinetics of each opioid agent effect the clinical presentation and thus management. Morphine and heroin (diacetylmorphine) taken parenterally reach peak clinical effect within minutes, and have a relatively short half-life of 3 h. In contrast, methadone and slow-release morphine preparations taken orally have slow and erratic absorption, reach peak plasma concentrations after several hours and have long durations of effect. The duration of clinical CNS depression also depends on co-ingested drugs.

Diagnosis

The diagnosis of opioid intoxication is clinical, based on history and examination. A Glasgow Coma Scale less than 12 associated with respirations of 12 breaths/min or less, miotic pupils or circumstantial evidence of drug use had a sensitivity of 92% and specificity of 76% for diagnosing opioid overdose in one cohort of patients.[9]

A thorough physical examination is usually adequate to exclude complications such as aspiration, non-cardiogenic pulmonary oedema and compartment syndrome.

Investigations are directed at excluding alternative diagnoses and complications as clinically indicated.

The differential diagnosis is that of any patient with an altered level of consciousness, and includes toxicological and metabolic causes, sepsis, neurotrauma, stroke and post-ictal state. The presence of fever without localizing symptoms and signs should raise the suspicion of bacteraemia secondary to parenteral drug abuse.

Complications

The complications of opioid abuse are classified into three main groups: those due to direct opioid effect, those secondary to the general intoxicated state and those due to poor injection technique. The prevalence of complications in patients who present to EDs with non-fatal opioid intoxication is not known, but recent Australian research suggests it is underestimated.[10] A high index of suspicion is required.

Loss of airway protective reflexes may lead to aspiration pneumonitis or pneumonia. Respiratory depression may lead to hypoxic encephalopathy.

Dependent areas may suffer peripheral neuropathy, compartment syndrome or rhabdomyolysis, which in turn may combine with hypovolaemia and hypoxia to produce renal failure and hyperkalaemia. Hypothermia or hyperthermia may occur depending on prevailing environmental conditions. Trauma must be considered in all intoxicated patients.

Heroin-induced non-cardiogenic pulmonary oedema is an infrequent complication of heroin overdose. It is usually recognized in the context of resuscitation from severe respiratory depression or apnoea, when hypoxia, high levels of catecholamines and other metabolic derangements are present. Symptoms are present within four hours of presentation and only a minority require mechanical ventilation.[11]

Complications of poor injection technique include cellulitis, thrombophlebitis, inadvertent intra-arterial injection and possible embolization, mycotic aneurysm, staphylococcal pneumonia, endocarditis, anaerobic clostridial infection and viral infections such as hepatitis B, C and HIV.

Treatment

Initial care is directed at assessing and managing the immediate threats to airway, breathing and circulation in a conventional manner. All patients should receive oxygen and have a bedside blood glucose estimation. Patients with an altered level of consciousness should be closely monitored in a resuscitation area, positioned to minimize the probability of aspiration, and moved frequently to prevent dependent injuries.

Physical examination and investigations are directed toward exclusion of complications and alternative diagnoses, as detailed above. Intravenous access plus laboratory and radiological investigation are reserved for those in whom they are clinically indicated.

Naloxone is a short-acting opioid antagonist useful in the management of opioid intoxication. It has a role as an adjunct to the support of airway and ventilation. It may be given via the intravenous, intramuscular, subcutaneous or endotracheal routes. Naloxone is safe and rarely associated with serious complications. There are case reports of cardiac arrest following the administration of naloxone to deeply comatose patients.[12] However, such reports probably represent the complications of hypoxia rather than the naloxone itself.

Bolus therapy (e.g. 0.4–2.0 mg intravenously or intramuscularly in an adult; 0.01 mg/kg in a neonate or child) quickly reverses the respiratory depression of opioid intoxication, but may be complicated by rapid wakening, agitation and, rarely, an acute withdrawal state.

An alternative approach to bolus therapy is the use of small intravenous doses (e.g. 0.1 mg) titrated to achieve airway control and adequate ventilation while avoiding abrupt emergence and behavioural difficulties. Intravenous doses of naloxone are usually effective within a few minutes. Note that the serum half-life of naloxone (approximately 1 h) is less than that of most opioids, therefore patients must be carefully monitored for resedation.[13]

Naloxone infusions may be useful in carefully selected patients who are intoxicated by long-acting opioids, to prevent airway compromise or intubation. The rate of infusion must be carefully titrated to maintain clinical effect. Naloxone infusions must not generate a false sense of security in those monitoring the patient: absorption and elimination of opioids may be unpredictable, and undulating levels of CNS depression may occur despite continuous naloxone infusion. All patients must be closely observed.

Disposition

The duration of observation in the ED and the need for admission depends on the opioid involved, route of administration, the influence of coingested drugs and the presence of comorbidity or complications. Accidental or deliberate self-poisoning with long-acting opioids will generally require observation for a minimum of 12 h and discharge should not occur at night. Following overdose with short-acting agents, patients can be safely discharged when they are ambulant and competent. Following naloxone, patients may be considered for discharge after one hour if they are ambulant, alert, have normal vital signs and normal oxygen saturation.[14]

Heroin overdose is a life-threatening event and indicates ongoing hazard. Australian data suggest that the 18-month mortality following presentation to an ED with non-fatal opioid overdose may be as high as 20% for recidivist patients.[15] Presentation to an ED provides an opportunity for preventative intervention. Patients should be counselled regarding strategies to avoid future overdose, including minimizing coingestion of other CNS depressants, not using heroin alone, awareness of tolerance levels, and early activation of emergency medical services. In addition, the patient can be referred to agencies specializing in drug detoxification and rehabilitation.

Opioid withdrawal syndrome

The development of physiological dependence with repeated doses of opioid agonists leads to an abstinence or withdrawal syndrome when opioids are ceased. The symptoms represent the reverse of the central and peripheral effects of opioid administration, and may include anxiety, insomnia, apprehension, hyperventilation, mydriasis, nausea, vomiting, diarrhoea and abdominal pain. Opioid withdrawal is not associated with delirium, seizures or high fever unless there is concomitant pathology, such as alcohol/benzodiazepine withdrawal or sepsis. The onset of symptoms depends on the half-life of the opioid used. Symptoms usually occur 12 h after the last dose of morphine or heroin, reach a peak at approximately 2 days and abate after approximately 5 days. Withdrawal from methadone may take several weeks. Psychological craving for opioids may persist for months.

Unlike the benzodiazepine and alcohol withdrawal syndromes, seizures do not occur and the prognosis is good, even without medical intervention. Patients in opioid withdrawal may present to EDs seeking symptomatic relief. A multifaceted approach should include an attempt to exclude concomitant pathology, treatment of dehydration, palliation of symptoms and referral to agencies specializing in withdrawal services.

The short-term use of small doses of benzodiazepine may alleviate anxiety and hyperventilation. Clonidine, an α_2-receptor adrenergic agonist, has been used to decrease symptoms of autonomic dysfunction.[16] An initial dose of 1–2 μg/kg, 2–3 times per day, can be increased depending on tolerance of side effects, such as dry mouth and orthostatic hypotension.

Methadone is a long-acting opioid used in the management of withdrawal and maintenance therapy. Methadone maintenance programmes decrease long-term mortality rates by 25%.[17] Patients in such programmes are less likely to die of heroin overdose or suicide, but methadone maintenance does not seem to have a measurable effect on the risk of death from non-heroin overdose, violence, trauma or natural causes. Buprenorphine is a partial opioid agonist also used in opioid replacement regimens. The doses of methadone or buprenorphine are tapered over many weeks.

Naltrexone is a long-acting opioid antagonist. Rapid detoxification programmes using combinations of naltrexone, buprenorphine and clonidine have been successful in selected patients.[18] Ultra-rapid opioid detoxification programmes precipitate rapid opioid withdrawal, frequently under general anaesthetic. This technique remains controversial.

COCAINE

Introduction and epidemiology

Coca leaves have been chewed by the natives of the South American Andes for approximately 1200 years, and were first exported to Europe in 1580. The local anaesthetic properties of cocaine were recognized in the second half of the 19th century. Cocaine has been used as a local anaesthetic with vasoconstrictive properties for over a century.

In Australia the prevalence of cocaine abuse is low, with 4.7% of the population aged over 14 reporting cocaine use in their lifetime, and 1% reporting use in the last 12 months.[2]

Pharmacology and pathophysiology

Cocaine hydrochloride, or benzoylmethylecgonine hydrochloride, is a fine white powder prepared from the leaves of the *Erythroxylon coca* plant. This form of cocaine is not heat stable and cannot be smoked. 'Freebase' cocaine is an alkaloid that melts at 98°C and can be smoked. It is prepared by mixing cocaine hydrochloride, water and baking soda. The precipitate is separated by a filter or by dissolution in ether or ethanol. If the solvent is allowed to evaporate pure cocaine crystals remain, known as 'rock' cocaine or 'crack' because of the sound they make when they are heated.[19]

Cocaine reaches the cerebral circulation 6–8 s after smoking, 16–20 s after intravenous injection and 3–5 min after nasal insufflation.[19] Gastrointestinal peak absorption may be delayed for up to 90 min.[20]

Cocaine is an ester-type local anaesthetic and is hydrolyzed by plasma and liver cholinesterases to produce an active metabolite, ecgonine methyl ester.[20] 5–10% of cocaine is excreted in the urine unchanged.[20] The half-life of cocaine in the blood is 60–90 min.[19] In animal models cocaine is metabolized in the presence of ethanol to ethylecgonine. This is a myocardial depressant more potent than the sum of the depressant effects of cocaine and ethanol alone.[21]

The pathophysiology of cocaine is complex and incompletely understood. It is a CNS stimulant acting via enhanced release of noradrenalin, plus blockade of noradrenalin, dopamine and serotonin reuptake. Cocaine is also a local anaesthetic that blocks fast sodium channels.

With increasing doses, euphoria is followed by dysphoria, agitation, seizures and coma. Considerable tachyphylaxis may occur. Cocaine stimulates the medullary vasomotor centre resulting in hypertension and tachycardia. Small doses may produce transient bradycardia (rarely clinically significant) owing to a vagotonic effect on the cardiovascular system.[20] At high levels the medullary centres may be depressed, leading to respiratory depression. In severe toxicity hypotension may occur and is probably due to a direct toxic effect on the myocardium mediated by sodium channel blockade.

Peripherally, cocaine inhibits the reuptake of adrenalin and noradrenalin, while at the same time stimulating the presynaptic release of noradrenalin. This leads to a sympathomimetic response mediated through both α- and β-adrenoreceptors, leading to tachycardia, diaphoresis, vasoconstriction and hypertension.

A model to explain the clinical effects of cocaine toxicity and provide a rationale for management has been proposed.[20] CNS stimulation leads to seizures, hyperthermia and increased sympathetic drive. This sympathetic drive is augmented by the peripheral synaptic effects of cocaine, and produces many of the cardiovascular manifestations of cocaine toxicity. The exaggerated peripheral sympathetic response in turn also has a positive feedback effect on the brain, increasing the likelihood of hyperthermia and seizures.

Increased psychomotor activity, vasoconstriction and direct hypothalamic toxicity, possibly mediated by dopamine receptors, contribute to hyperpyrexia.[22]

Cocaine-induced myocardial ischaemia and infarction may occur. The pathophysiology is complex, but it appears that cocaine increases myocardial oxygen demand while decreasing myocardial oxygen supply. Contributing factors include immediate or delayed coronary artery vasospasm, increased platelet aggregation, accelerated atherosclerosis and dilated cardiomyopathy.[20]

Wide complex tachyarrhythmias, including ventricular tachycardia and fibrillation, are observed with cocaine toxicity. There are reports of prolongation of QRS and QT intervals, plus terminal right axis deviation (large R wave in aVR), implicating sodium channel blockade in addition to the sympathomimetic, ischaemic and cardiomyopathic factors mentioned above.[20,23] Transient arrhythmias may account for the syncope noted by some patients not attributable to seizures.

Clinical features

The predominant symptoms are those of CNS excitation and peripheral sympathomimetic response. The wide variety of manifestations and complications may include palpitations, agitation, altered mental state, chest pain, syncope, seizures, dyspnoea, abdominal pain, transient focal neurological signs, urticaria, intracranial haemorrhage and cardiac arrest.[24]

The spectrum of neurological changes may include euphoria, apprehension, agitation, altered mental state, seizures and coma. Tachypnoea, mydriasis, tremor, diaphoresis and hyperpyrexia may also be seen. Cardiovascular manifestations may include tachycardia, hypertension, any supraventricular or ventricular tachydysrrhythmia, syncope and chest pain. Rhabdomyolysis complicated by renal failure and hyperkalaemia is reported.[20,25]

Chest pain may be due to musculoskeletal, pulmonary or cardiovascular causes. A retrospective study of patients intoxicated with cocaine presenting with chest pain consistent with ischaemia found that 6% suffered acute myocardial infarction.[26]

Aortic dissection associated with cocaine use is reported.[27]

Smoking cocaine may lead to a number of respiratory complications, including thermal airway injury, pneumothorax and pneumomediastinum, non-cardiac pulmonary oedema, interstitial pneumonitis and bronchiolitis obliterans.[19]

Several CNS complications have been attributed to cocaine, in addition to the phenomena described above. Cerebral infarction, transient ischaemic attacks, subarachnoid haemorrhage, cerebral vasculitis and migraine-like headache are described.[20] Contributing pathophysiological mechanisms include hypertension, vasoconstriction, vasculitis, increased coagulability, altered cerebrovascular autoregulation and embolization of particulate matter. Mesenteric vasoconstriction and vasculitis may lead to bowel ischaemia and infarction.[20]

Diagnosis

The diagnosis of cocaine intoxication is clinical, based on history or clinical suspicion, the presence of sympathomimetic symptoms and signs, and the exclusion of other life-threatening conditions. The differential diagnosis includes other sympathomimetic agents such as amphetamines or hallucinogenic agents, anticholinergic delirium, serotonin syndrome, monoamine oxidase inhibitors, theophylline, alcohol and benzodiazepine withdrawal, sepsis, hypoglycaemia, thyrotoxicosis and phaeochromocytoma.

Rapid qualitative urine screening tests are commercially available to identify the presence of drugs of abuse. They should be interpreted with caution, as metabolites may be present for several days and not be relevant to the patient's presentation. Most commercially available urine qualitative tests detect metabolites of cocaine. The tests rarely alter management in emergencies, and may give false negative results in cases where the cocaine was taken only a short time before the test is performed.

Physical examination and investigations should be directed at excluding complications and alternative diagnoses, as detailed above. Laboratory and radiological investigations should be reserved for those patients in whom they are clinically indicated. All patients with altered vital signs should have ECG monitoring in the ED, and all patients should have at least one 12-lead ECG.

Treatment

Initial care is directed towards the assessment and management of immediate threats to airway, breathing and circulation, in a conventional manner. All patients should receive oxygen and have a bedside blood glucose estimation. Patients with an altered level of consciousness should be closely monitored in a resuscitation area.

A direct relationship between the neuropsychiatric and cardiovascular complications of cocaine toxicity has been proposed.[20] Patients exhibiting CNS agitation or sympathomimetic cardiovascular effects should receive an intravenous benzodiazepine titrated to achieve sedation. This will control most manifestations of cocaine toxicity in the majority of patients. Seizures should be managed in the standard manner. Benzodiazepines are considered as first-line therapy, followed by barbiturates, general anaesthesia and paralysis if required.

Atrial tachycardia and hypertension usually also respond to sedation with benzodiazepines. If titrated benzodiazepine sedation fails to adequately control blood pressure, vasodilators such as intravenous nitrates, nitroprusside or phentolamine have been recommended. Atrial tachyarrhythmias are usually benign and rarely require specific treatment other than benzodiazepine sedation. The use of β-adrenergic receptor blockers in cocaine intoxication is controversial and not recommended. There are no experimental data to show improved mortality in animal models with their use. In addition, there is the potential to produce 'unopposed' α-adrenergic receptor effects, leading to paradoxical hypertension.

Ventricular arrhythmias should be treated according to advanced cardiac life support guidelines. Those occurring within minutes of cocaine use are presumed to be secondary to excess catecholamines, direct cocaine-mediated myocardial sodium channel blockade and myocardial ischaemia. The use of lignocaine in this setting is controversial. In addition to defibrillation or cardioversion, immediate intravenous bolus bicarbonate (1–2 mEq/kg) and benzodiazepine sedation are used in this setting. Ventricular arrhythmias occurring after the acute phase are presumed to be secondary to myocardial ischaemia and should therefore be treated in a standard manner.[20]

If myocardial ischaemia or infarction is suspected, investigation should be as for ischaemic chest pain of non-toxicological aetiology. Benzodiazepine sedation, nitrates and verapamil are recommended to decrease heart rate, reduce hypertension and reduce cocaine-induced coronary vasoconstriction,[28] but β-adrenergic blocking agents should be avoided as they increase coronary vasospasm.[29] Primary angioplasty is considered the treatment of choice for cocaine-induced acute myocardial infarction.[28] Thrombolytic therapy may be considered if angioplasty is not available, maximal medical management has failed and there is no evidence of intracranial haemorrhage.[28] In patients with non-diagnostic electrocardiograms short-term admission may be required to exclude myocardial infarction.

Hyperthermia is an important contributing factor to morbidity and mortality following cocaine intoxication.[22] A core temperature should be measured in all patients and core temperature monitoring is recommended if the temperature is elevated. Mild-to-moderate hyperthermia (<39°C) often responds to benzodiazepine sedation and fluid resuscitation. If this is unsuccessful, then cooling by convection, ice packs and intubation and paralysis are indicated. Further study is required to delineate the role of dopamine receptor antagonists in the management of hyperthermia. There is no evidence that dantrolene has a role in the management of hyperthermia associated with psychostimulants.[22]

Disposition

The duration of observation in the ED and the need for admission depend on the severity of toxicity, the influence of co-ingested drugs and the presence of comorbidity or complications. Patients with mild intoxication (without severe hyperthermia or ischaemic chest pain) may be observed in the ED and discharged when the patient is asymptomatic with normal vital signs and mental status.

Presentation to an ED provides an opportunity for preventative intervention. Patients should be counselled and offered strategies to avoid future toxicity or overdose. Alternatively, the patient may be referred to agencies specializing in drug detoxification and rehabilitation.

AMPHETAMINE AND RELATED 'DESIGNER DRUGS'

Introduction and epidemiology

Amphetamine refers to β-phenylisopropylamine, but the term 'amphetamines' refers to a broad group of related derivatives characterized clinically by CNS stimulatory and peripheral sympathomimetic responses. Amphetamine was first synthesized in 1887, and marketed as a nasal decongestant in 1932.[30] The potential for abuse was recognized as people became dependent on the euphoric and stimulant effects of these drugs.

The use of amphetamine as a drug of abuse has been prevalent since its introduction. Amphetamine, amphetamine derivatives and fentanyl derivatives (together often called the 'designer drugs'), plus the hallucinogenic drugs, have become increasingly popular in the recent past. The 2004 National Drug Strategy Household Survey reported that 9% of Australians over 14 reported using amphetamine–methamphetamine in their lifetime, and 3% in the previous 12 months. 3,4-methylenedioxymethamphetamine (MDMA; ecstasy) use was also common, with 8% of people over age 14 reporting use in their lifetime and 3% reporting use in the previous 12 months.[2] The use of amphetamines–methamphetamine and MDMA appears to have remained stable in recent years.

The piperazine-based psychoactive compounds have similar clinical effects to the amphetamines. They are popular in New Zealand where 1-benzylpiperazine (BZP) and trifluoromethylphenylpiperazine (TFMPP) are sold as herbal party pills.

Pharmacology and pathophysiology

Amphetamine is structurally related to ephedrine and resembles the catecholamines, but is effective when given orally.[30] The amphetamine group are characterized by substitutions on the basic structure of amphetamine, and include methamphetamine ('ice', 'speed'), 3,4-methylenedioxy-methamphetamine (MDMA, 'Ecstasy', 'Adam' or 'E'), 3,4-methylenedioxyethamphetamine (MDEA, 'Eve'), and 3,4-methylenedioxyamphetamine (MDA, 'love drug') and para-methoxyamphetamine (PMA).[31]

Amphetamines may be ingested, smoked, insufflated or injected parenterally. All are absorbed from the GI system, with peak serum levels within 3 h. They are weak bases, 20% bound to plasma proteins and tend to have large volumes of distribution. Half-lives vary from 8 to 30 h, with hepatic transformation being the major route of elimination. However, up to 30% of amphetamine and methamphetamine may be eliminated in the urine.[31]

Amphetamines enhance the release of catecholamines and block their subsequent reuptake. This causes increased stimulation of central and peripheral adrenergic receptors, leading to CNS excitation and a sympathomimetic syndrome. Higher doses also lead to central serotonin release. Increased dopaminergic action in the mesolimbic system leads to automatic behaviours, altered perception and psychosis. Movement disorders such as choreoathetosis are reported.[32]

Different substitutions on the basic amphetamine structure (the amphetamine derivatives) alter the relative hallucinogenic, behavioural and cardiovascular effects of the drugs at low doses. At high doses, the toxic effects of the group are more uniform and can be discussed as a single entity.

Considerable tolerance may develop, so that patients take increasing doses to achieve euphoria and a stimulant effect. An acute organic psychosis, similar to paranoid schizophrenia, may develop during and after these binges.[31]

Severe hyponatraemia associated with cerebral oedema is reported following MDMA use.[33,34] Mechanisms contributing to hyponatraemia include psychogenic polydipsia[34] and inappropriate secretion of antidiuretic hormone.[34,35]

Animal models of MDMA abuse demonstrate destruction of serotonergic and dopaminergic neurons.[36] This has also been reported in humans and raises the concern of permanent neurological damage associated with chronic MDMA use, which in turn carries enormous public health implications.[37]

Clinical features

In an Australian study, patients with amphetamine-related problems represented 1.2% of all presentations to an urban ED. The patients had high acuity: 67% had triage scores 1–3, 20% presented with an agitated delirium, 12% had acute psychosis and 4% presented with seizures. The admission rate was 40%, and 37% required psychiatric evaluation.[38] Patients presenting to a New Zealand ED following piperazine abuse had anxiety, vomiting, headache, confusion and collapse. Seizures occurred in 18% of presentations.[39]

The clinical signs, symptoms and complications of amphetamine intoxication are similar to those of cocaine. However, amphetamine effects may last up to 24 h. In addition, the spectrum of signs and symptoms is influenced by co-ingested agents such as opioids, alcohol, benzodiazepines or cannabis.

The predominant symptoms are those of CNS excitation and peripheral sympathomimetic response. Following euphoria, apprehension, agitation, altered mental state, seizures and coma may ensue. Tachypnoea, mydriasis, tremor, diaphoresis and hyperpyrexia may also be seen. After acute intoxication, with or without delirium, amphetamine-induced psychosis may occur[40] with frightening visual and tactile hallucinations, severe agitation and paranoia. MDMA-induced hyponatraemia may present with decreased level of consciousness and seizures.

Death is secondary to hyperpyrexia, seizures, arrhythmia or intracerebral haemorrhage.[30] Myocardial infarction,[41] aortic dissection,[42] rhabdomyolysis, acidosis, acute cardiomyopathy,[43] shock, renal failure[22] and coagulopathy[30] are documented.

Parenteral amphetamine abuse may be complicated by cellulitis, thrombophlebitis, inadvertent intra-arterial injection and possible subsequent embolization, mycotic aneurysm, staphylococcal pneumonia, endocarditis, anaerobic clostridial infection and viral infections such as hepatitis B, C and HIV. In addition, chronic abuse of amphetamines may be complicated by a necrotizing vasculitis that leads to a characteristic beading of small and medium arteries on angiography. The vasculitis may involve multiple organ systems and lead to renal failure, myocardial ischaemia and cerebrovascular disease.[31]

Amphetamine dependence and withdrawal is recognized. Withdrawal is characterized by numerous neurasthenic symptoms, including somnolence and intense cravings for amphetamines.[31,44]

Diagnosis

The diagnosis of amphetamine intoxication is clinical, based on history or clinical suspicion, the presence of sympathomimetic symptoms and signs, and the exclusion of other life-threatening conditions. In overdose it may be impossible to distinguish the exact amphetamine derivative involved, but this is unlikely to be clinically significant. Intoxication by an amphetamine derivative may not be discernible clinically from cocaine, except for the increased propensity for psychotic features and the longer duration of action. The differential diagnosis includes cocaine intoxication, anticholinergic delirium, serotonin syndrome, monoamine oxidase inhibitors, theophylline, alcohol and benzodiazepine withdrawal, sepsis, hypoglycaemia, thyrotoxicosis and phaeochromocytoma.

Physical examination and investigations should be directed at excluding complications and alternative diagnoses, as detailed above. Laboratory and radiological investigations should be reserved for those in whom they are clinically indicated.

Treatment

Initial attention must be directed at assessing and managing immediate threats to airway, breathing and circulation in a conventional manner. All patients should receive oxygen and have a bedside blood glucose estimation. Close monitoring of the patient in a quiet area away from excessive stimulation may be advantageous.

Patients exhibiting psychomotor acceleration or psychosis should be managed with an intravenous benzodiazepine titrated to achieve adequate sedation.

As with cocaine, hyperthermia, seizures and fluid resuscitation should be managed aggressively. The organ-specific effects of amphetamines are similar to those of cocaine, and management should follow that detailed above. Following resolution of the acute intoxication phase, patients with persistent psychotic features may respond to an antipsychotic agent such as olanzapine.[44,45]

Disposition

The duration of observation in the ED and the need for admission will depend on the severity of intoxication, the influence of co-ingested drugs and the presence of comorbidity or complications. Patients with mild intoxication (e.g. without severe hyperthermia or ischaemic chest pain) may be observed in the ED and discharged when vital signs and mental status have returned to normal. The longer half-lives of the amphetamines may dictate inpatient care if symptoms or abnormal vital signs do not resolve within a few hours.

Presentation to an ED provides an opportunity for preventative intervention. Patients should be counselled and offered strategies to avoid future toxicity or overdose. Alternatively, the patient may be referred to agencies specializing in drug detoxification and rehabilitation.

GAMMA-HYDROXYBUTYRATE

Introduction and epidemiology

Gamma-hydroxybutyrate (GHB) (4-hydroxybutanoate; sodium oxybate) is a sedative-hypnotic agent causing significant CNS depression. It has significant psychotropic effects and is associated with addiction and significant withdrawal. GHB was originally developed as a short-acting anaesthetic agent in the 1960s, but lost favour due to poor analgesic properties and a propensity to cause seizure-like activity at the onset of coma.[46] GHB has also been used as a treatment for opioid withdrawal,[47] alcohol dependence and narcolepsy.[48,49]

GHB and its congeners gamma-butyrolactone (GBL) and 1,4-butanediol, have become popular recreational drugs advocated for body building, euphoria, sleep enhancement and sexual stimulant. Street names for GHB include 'grievous bodily harm', 'fantasy', 'scoop', 'liquid X', 'liquid E' and 'somatomax'.[50] Although forensic data are scarce, GHB has also been implicated as a 'date rape' agent.[51] Recreational use of GHB in Australia appears to be uncommon. The 2004 National Drug Strategy Household Survey reported that 0.5% of Australians over 14 reported using GHB in their lifetime, and 0.1% reported use in the previous 12 months.[2] However, small reports of epidemics of GHB use and anecdotal reports of ED presentations suggest that its use in Australia may be increasing.[52]

Pharmacology and pathophysiology

GHB is a short-chain fatty acid that occurs naturally in the brain and possibly acts as a neurotransmitter. It is one of the breakdown products of gamma-aminobutyric acid (GABA), the primary inhibitory neurotransmitter in the CNS. The mechanism by which GHB causes its effects are unclear, but it may be a combination of intrinsic effects via specific GHB receptors and effects mediated through GABA-B receptors.[51] GHB also has dopaminergic activity, increases acetylcholine and serotonin levels, and may interact with endogenous opioids.[51]

GHB is usually ingested as a liquid and is rapidly absorbed by the GI tract; peak plasma levels occur within 15–45 min. It is rapidly metabolized to succinate, which then enters the Krebs cycle. The average half-life is usually 20–50 min.[51]

Clinical features

Most patients present to the ED following acute GHB intoxication. The major clinical signs of GHB intoxication are related to its effects on the CNS. With increasing dose there is euphoria, then agitation followed rapidly by sedation and coma. Co-ingestion of ethanol or other illicit drugs is common.[46,53] Respiratory depression and apnoea may occur following GHB ingestion, but this is usually reported in the context of multiple co-ingestants (e.g. alcohol or ketamine). Profound coma may occur but the patient may resist instrumentation of the airway or rouse when stimulated, only to relapse again when the stimulus is removed. The duration of CNS depression is usually short. Most patients recover abruptly within 1–2 h.

Agitation, myoclonus and generalized seizures are reported, although generalized seizures have not been seen during electroencephalographic (EEG) monitoring of human volunteers given sedative doses of GHB.[47] In animal studies, GHB causes an abnormal EEG pattern similar to that seen in absence seizures, and GHB has been used as a tool for the study of the neurophysiological mechanisms of this disorder.[54] It is possible that the seizures noted in some patients represent the clonic movements commonly seen with GHB intoxication, or they may be generalized seizures due to hypoxia or a co-ingested agent.[51,55]

Severe degrees of CNS depression may be associated with mild bradycardia and/or hypotension. There does not appear to be any consistent pattern of ECG changes seen with GHB intoxication.[51] GHB intoxication may be associated with vomiting in up to 40% of cases.[51]

Diagnosis

The diagnosis of GHB intoxication is clinical. Abrupt resolution of coma within 1–2 h of presentation is characteristic of GHB intoxication. However, other agents are frequently co-ingested (ethanol, amphetamines, cannabis, opiates, ketamine) and may cloud the clinical picture. A thorough physical examination is usually adequate to exclude complications such as pulmonary aspiration. Investigations are directed at excluding alternative diagnoses and complications as clinically indicated. The differential diagnosis is that of any patient with an altered level of consciousness, and includes toxicological and metabolic causes, sepsis, neurotrauma, stroke and post-ictal state.

Treatment

Initial care is directed at assessing and managing the immediate threats to airway, breathing and circulation in a conventional manner. All patients should receive oxygen and have a bedside blood glucose estimation. Patients with an altered level of consciousness should be closely monitored in a resuscitation area, positioned to minimize the probability of aspiration and moved frequently to prevent dependent injuries. Physical examination and investigations are directed toward exclusion of complications and alternative diagnoses, as detailed above. Intravenous access plus laboratory and radiological investigation should be reserved for those in whom they are clinically indicated. Persistent CNS depression beyond 6 h should prompt a search for alternative causes.

Activated charcoal is not routinely indicated as GHB is rapidly absorbed, associated with rapid onset of coma, has a short clinical effect and good prognosis with thorough supportive care.

There is no specific antidote for GHB. Naloxone does not appear to reverse the CNS depression or respiratory depression associated with GHB intoxication.[51] Physostigmine has been advocated in the management of GHB intoxication,[56] but is not indicated as it may be accompanied by unwanted side effects. Moreover, GHB has a short clinical effect and has good prognosis with thorough supportive care, thus the routine use of physostigmine is not recommended.[51,57,58]

Disposition

The duration of observation in the ED or the need for admission will depend on the need for intubation, coingested agents or the presence of complications. Most patients recover within a few hours and may be safely discharged from the ED when they are ambulant and competent.[51]

Although patients may be medically fit for early discharge, presentation to an ED also provides an opportunity for preventative intervention. Patients should be counselled regarding strategies to avoid future overdose. In addition, the patient may be referred to agencies specializing in drug detoxification and rehabilitation.

'BODY-PACKERS' AND 'BODY STUFFERS'

Body-packers and body-stuffers are people who conceal illicit drugs within body cavities. Patients may ingest many times the lethal dose of an illicit drug, conceal the nature of their problem and appear completely asymptomatic at presentation. In addition, there is a paucity of data regarding the efficacy of various imaging, decontamination and treatment modalities.

A body-packer attempts to conceal a large quantity of an illicit drug inside a body cavity, usually the GI tract, in an attempt to smuggle it across an international border. The drugs are usually carefully packaged in plastic, latex, condoms or balloons, and often layered with wax. By the time these patients reach the ED almost all of the packets will have entered the small or large intestine, making decontamination problematic. The vagina and rectum are less popular sites to conceal packets as they are more likely to be discovered on physical examination.

A body-stuffer hurriedly ingests smaller quantities of illicit drugs just before apprehension by the authorities in order to avoid conviction. The package is likely to be poorly constructed and is more likely to leak. Time from ingestion to hospital arrival is usually short and the drug may still be within the stomach at the time of presentation. The vagina and rectum are alternative sites for drug concealment in the body-stuffer.

In view of the potential sudden lethality of both these practices, regardless of presenting symptoms or signs, all patients should receive a high triage priority and be managed in a resuscitation setting. They should receive supplemental oxygen and intravenous access.

Police may bring the patient to the ED and request physical examination and/or investigation. When a history is taken in the presence of police many patients deny the practice and resist treatment. The emergency physician should remember the potential threat to the patient's life, and his or her primary duty of care to the patient.

Whenever possible a detailed history should be obtained, noting the exact type and amount of drug ingested, the method of packaging, symptoms of drug intoxication and any factors that may increase the likelihood of bowel obstruction or ileus. A thorough physical examination should include careful speculum examination of the vagina, digital examination of the rectum and a search for any signs of drug intoxication.

Heroin, cocaine, amphetamine, methamphetamine, MDMA and cannabis are all reported in body-packers and -stuffers. Up to 1 kg of drug may be packaged in a body-packer in 50–150 packages.

Cooperative patients should immediately receive activated charcoal to adsorb intraluminal drug.[59]

Abdominal radiographs of body-stuffers are unlikely to show packages clearly,[60] and a negative abdominal radiograph does not exclude the diagnosis. Fortunately, most patients remain asymptomatic or exhibit only mild symptoms, although deaths are reported.[61] Qualitative urine drug screens do not change management and are not routinely indicated. Following a dose of activated charcoal, asymptomatic body-stuffers should be observed in the ED or emergency observation unit for a minimum of 8 h. Those who

remain asymptomatic at the end of the observation period may be discharged. If a patient becomes symptomatic they should be treated as outlined above for the individual substance.

Imaging of the potential body-packer is controversial. Abdominal radiographs are positive in a higher percentage of body-packers, where multiple package–air interfaces may be seen. The sensitivity and specificity of plain abdominal films in large series is reported to be 85–90%.[62] Importantly, plain radiographs do not exclude the diagnosis, so oral contrast and abdominal computerized tomography (CT) scanning has been recommended, although sensitivity is not 100%.[33] Given the need to confidently exclude the diagnosis of body-packing and the imperfect sensitivity of these modalities it has been suggested two imaging modalities (e.g. plain abdominal radiograph plus abdominal CT scanning) be used to exclude the diagnosis.[30]

Gastrointestinal decontamination of suspected body-packers is also controversial. Whole bowel irrigation with polyethylene glycol has been recommended. However, recent experience suggests that asymptomatic patients may be managed conservatively, with close observation, laxatives and light diet until all packets are retrieved. In such circumstances the rates of late-onset drug intoxication, bowel obstruction, laparotomy or death are less than 5%.[61]

All body-packer patients, even the asymptomatic, should remain in an environment where they can be closely monitored, either in the ED, observation unit or intensive care unit, until there is satisfactory evidence that all packages have been retrieved. Staff should be aware of potential signs of intoxication and be available 24 h a day to intervene if required. Asymptomatic patients may ambulate.

Evidence of drug intoxication, either at presentation or during decontamination, represents a medical emergency, and requires aggressive management. Initial care must be directed at assessing and managing immediate threats to airway, breathing, circulation and the control of seizures in a standard manner. If a cocaine body-packer exhibits toxicity, immediate surgical exploration to remove all packages has been advocated.[60,62] A similar approach is also indicated if amphetamines

are involved. Such interventions may also be indicated if there is evidence of bowel or gastric outflow obstruction, concretion formation, ileus or bowel perforation.[62] Surgical management is probably not necessary in the heroin body-packer manifesting signs of opioid intoxication, as adequate resuscitation, supportive care and antidote therapy should ensure a favourable outcome.

Patients are observed until all packages have been accounted for and there have been three normal package-free stools. Repeat radiology is performed to confirm no further packages.

Controversies

❶ Optimal sedation regimes for cocaine and amphetamine-intoxicated patients.

❷ Role and optimal method of gastrointestinal decontamination in body-packers.

❸ Optimal imaging modality for evaluation of known or suspected body-packer.

References

1. Katzung BG. Basic and clinical pharmacology. 7th edn. Sydney: Prentice Hall; 1998.
2. Australian Institute of Health and Welfare. Statistics on drug use in Australia 2006. Drug Statistics Series No. 18. Cat. no. PHE 80. Canberra: AIHW; 2007.
3. Swensen G. Mortality caused by opioids Western Australia 1996. Task Force on Drug Abuse, Statistical Bulletin No 2; 1996.
4. Oyefeso A, Ghodse H, Clancy C, et al. Drug abuse-related mortality: a study of teenage addicts over a 20-year period. Social Psychiatry and Psychiatric Epidemiology 1999; 34(8): 437–441.
5. Darke S, Zador D. Fatal heroin 'overdose': a review. Addiction 1996; 91(12): 1765–1772.
6. Darke S, Ross J, Hall W. Overdose among heroin users in Sydney, Australia: I. Prevalence and correlates of non-fatal overdose. Addiction 1996; 91(3): 405–411.
7. Zador D, Sunjic S, Darke S. Heroin-related deaths in New South Wales, 1992: toxicological findings and circumstances. Medical Journal of Australia 1996; 164: 204–207.
8. Darke S, Ross J, Hall W. Overdose among heroin users in Sydney, Australia: II. Responses to overdose. Addiction 1996; 91(3): 413–417.
9. Hoffman JR, Schriger DL, Luo JS. The empiric use of naloxone in patients with altered mental status: a reappraisal. Annals of Emergency Medicine 1991; 20: 246–252.
10. Warner-Smith M, Darke S, Day C. Morbidity associated with non-fatal heroin overdose. Addiction 2002; 97(8): 927–928.
11. Sporer KA, Dorn E. Heroin-related noncardiac pulmonary edema: a case series. Chest 2001; 120(5): 1628–1632.
12. Osterwalder JJ. Naloxone for intoxications with intravenous heroin and heroin mixtures – harmless or

hazardous? A prospective clinical study. Clinical Toxicology 1996; 34(4): 409–416.

13. Watson WA, Steele MT, Muelleman RL, Rush MD. Opioid toxicity recurrence after an initial response to naloxone. Journal of Toxicology – Clinical Toxicology 1998; 36(1–2): 11–17.

14. Christenson J, Etherington J, Grafstein E, et al. Early discharge of patients with presumed opioid overdose: development of a clinical prediction rule. Academic Emergency Medicine 2000; 7(10): 1110–1118.

15. Morgan D, Daly FFS, Fatovich DM, et al. Eighteen-month mortality in a cohort of patients presenting to an emergency department with non-fatal opioid overdose (abstract). Emergency Medicine 2002; 14(1): A23.

16. Kosten TR, O'Connor PG. Management of drug and alcohol withdrawal. New England Journal of Medicine 2003; 348: 1786–1795.

17. Caplehorn JRM, Dalton MSYN, Haldar F, et al. Methadone maintenance and addicts risk of fatal heroin overdose. Substance Abuse and Misuse 1996; 31(2): 177–196.

18. O'Connor PG, Carroll KM, Shi JM, et al. Three methods of opioid detoxification in a primary care setting: a randomized trial. Annals of Internal Medicine 1997; 127: 526–530.

19. Haim DY, Lippmann ML, Goldberg SK, Walkenstein MD. The pulmonary complications of crack cocaine, a comprehensive review. Chest 1995; 107(1): 233–240.

20. Goldfrank LR, Hoffman RS. The cardiovascular effects of cocaine. Annals of Emergency Medicine 1991; 20(2): 165–175.

21. Henning RJ, Wilson LD, Glauser JM. Cocaine plus ethanol is more cardiotoxic than cocaine or ethanol alone. Critical Care Medicine 1994; 2(12): 1896–1906.

22. Callaway CW, Clark RF. Hyperthermia in psychostimulant overdose. Annals of Emergency Medicine 1994; 24(1): 68–76.

23. Kerns W, Garvey L, Owens J. Cocaine-induced wide complex dysrhythmia. Journal of Emergency Medicine 1997; 15(3): 321–329.

24. Derlet RW, Albertson TE. Emergency department presentation of cocaine intoxication. Annals of Emergency Medicine 1989; 18(2): 182–186.

25. Skluth HA, Clark JE, Ehringer GL. Rhabdomyolysis associated with cocaine intoxication. Drug Intelligence and Clinical Pharmacy 1988; 22: 778–780.

26. Zimmerman JL, Dellinger RP, Majid PA. Cocaine associated chest pain. Annals of Emergency Medicine 1991; 20(6): 611–615.

27. Perron AD, Gibbs M. Thoracic aortic dissection secondary to crack cocaine ingestion. American Journal of Emergency Medicine 1997; 15: 507–509.

28. Lange RA, Hillis LD. Medical progress: cardiovascular complications of cocaine use. New England Journal of Medicine 2001; 345(5): 351–358.

29. Lange RA, Cigarroa RG, Flores ED, et al. Potentiation of cocaine-induced coronary vasoconstriction by beta-adrenergic blockade. Annals of Internal Medicine 1990; 112: 897–903.

30. Goldfrank LR, Flomenbaum NE, Lewin NA, et al., eds. Goldfrank's toxicologic emergencies. 7th edn. New York: McGraw-Hill; 2002.

31. Morgan JP. Amphetamine and metamphetamine during the 1990s. Paediatric Review 1992; 13(9): 330–333.

32. Downes MA, Whyte IM. Amphetamine-induced movement disorder. Emergency Medicine Australasia 2005; 17: 277–280.

33. Maxwell DL, Polkey MI, Henry JA. Hyponatraemia and catatonic stupor after taking 'ecstasy'. British Medical Journal 1993; 307(6916): 1399.

34. Sue YM, Lee, YL, Huang, JJ. Acute hyponatremia, seizure and rhabdomyolysis after ecstacy use. Journal of Toxicology – Clinical Toxicology 2002; 40(7): 931–932.

35. Henry JA, Fallon JK, Kicman AT, et al. Low-dose MDMA ('ecstasy') induces vasopressin secretion. Lancet 1998; 351(9118): 1784.

36. Ricuarte G, Yuan J Hatzidimitriou G, et al. Severe dopaminergic neurotoxicity in primates after a common recreational dose regimen of MDMA ('ecstasy'). Science 2002; 297: 2260–2263.

37. McCann UD, Szabo Z, Scheffel U, et al. Positron emission tomographic evidence of toxic effect of MDMA ('Ecstasy') on brain serotonin neurons in human beings. Lancet 1998; 352(9138): 1433–1437.

38. Gray SD, Fatovich DM, McCoubrie DL, Daly FF. Amphetamine-related presentations to an inner-city tertiary emergency department: a prospective evaluation. Medical Journal of Australia 2007; 186: 336–339.

39. Gee P, Richardson S, Woltersdorf W, Moore G. Toxic effects of BZP-based herbal party pills in humans: a prospective study in Christchurch, New Zealand. New Zealand Medical Journal 2005; 118(1227): U1784.

40. Murray JB. Psychophysiological aspects of amphetamine-methamphetamine abuse. Journal of Psychology 1998; 132(2): 227–237.

41. Waksman J, Taylor RN Jr, Bodor GS, et al. Acute myocardial infarction associated with amphetamine use. Mayo Clinic Proceedings 2001; 76(3): 323–326.

42. Dihmis WC, Ridley P, Dhasmana JP, Wisheart JD. Acute dissection of the aorta with amphetamine misuse. British Medical Journal 1997; 314(7095): 1665.

43. O'Connor AD, Rusyniak DE, Bruno A. Cerebrovascular and cardiovascular complications of alcohol and sympathomimetic drug abuse. Medical Clinics of North America 2005; 89: 1343–1358.

44. Landabaso MA, Iraurgi I, Jimenez-Lerma JM, et al. Ecstasy-induced psychotic disorder: six-month follow-up study. European Addiction Research 2002; 8(3): 133–140.

45. Clinical guidelines: management of acute amphetamine related problems. Western Australia Department. http://www.dao.health.wa.gov.au (accessed 10 December 2007).

46. Miró, Nogué S, Espinosa G, et al. Trends in illicit drug emergencies: the emerging role of gamma-hydroxybutyrate. Journal of Toxicology – Clinical Toxicology 2002; 40(2): 129–135.

47. Gallimberti L, Schifano F, Forza G, et al. Clinical efficacy of gamma-hydroxybutyric acid in treatment of opiate withdrawal. European Archives of Psychiatry and Clinical Neuroscience 1994; 244(3): 113–114.

48. Li J, Stokes SA, Woeckener A. A tale of novel intoxication: seven cases of g-hydroxybutyric acid overdose. Annals of Emergency Medicine 1998; 31(6): 723–728.

49. Anonymous. A randomized, double blind, placebo-controlled multicenter trial comparing the effects of three doses of orally administered sodium oxybate with placebo for the treatment of narcolepsy. Sleep 2002; 25(1): 42–49.

50. Chin RL, Sporer KA, Cullison B, et al. Clinical course of g-hydroxybutyrate overdose. Annals of Emergency Medicine 1998; 31(6): 716–722.

51. Mason PE, Kerns WP. Gamma-hydroxybutyrate (GHB) intoxication. Academic Emergency Medicine 2002; 9(7): 730–739.

52. Harrayway T, Stephenson L. Gamma hydroxybutyrate intoxication: The Gold Coast experience. Emergency Medicine 1999; 11: 45–48.

53. Kim SY, Anderson IB, Dyer JE, et al. High-risk behaviours and hospitalizations among gamma hydroxybutyrate (GHB) users. American Journal of Drug and Alcohol Abuse 2007; 33(3): 429–438.

54. Snead OC. Gamma-Hydroxybutyrate model of generalized absence seizures: further characterization and comparison with other absence models. Epilepsia 1988; 29(4): 361–368.

55. Daly FFS. Gamma hydroxybutyrate (letter). Emergency Medicine 1999; 11(4): 300.

56. Caldicott DG, Kuhn M. Gamma-hydroxybutyrate overdose and physostigmine: teaching new tricks to an old drug? Annals of Emergency Medicine 2001; 37: 99–102.

57. Traub SJ, Nelson LS, Hoffman RS. Physostigmine as a treatment for gamma-hydroxybutyrate toxicity: a review. Journal of Toxicology – Clinical Toxicology 2002; 40(6): 781–787.

58. Zvosec DL, Smith SW, Litonjua R, Westfal REJ. Physostigmine for gamma-hydroxybutyrate coma: inefficacy, adverse events, and review. Clinical Toxicology 2007; 45(3): 261–265.

59. Tomaszewski C, McKinney P, Phillips S, et al. Prevention of toxicity from oral cocaine by activated charcoal in mice. Annals of Emergency Medicine 1993; 22(12): 1804–1806.

60. Hoffman RS, Smilkstein MJ, Goldfrank LR. Whole bowel irrigation and the cocaine body-packer: a new approach to a common problem. American Journal of Emergency Medicine 1990; 8(6): 523–527.

61. June R, Aks SE, Keys N, Wahl M. Medical outcome of cocaine bodystuffers. Journal of Emergency Medicine 2000; 18(2): 221–224.

62. Traub SJ, Hoffman RS, Nelson LS. Body packing – the internal concealment of drugs. New England Journal of Medicine 2003; 349: 2519–2526.

29.13 Methaemoglobinaemia

Robert Edwards

ESSENTIALS

1 Consider the diagnosis of methaemoglobinaemia in patients with cyanosis unresponsive to oxygen.

2 Multiple presentations can occur following incidents involving contamination of food or water. Early clinical recognition allows institution of treatment and prevention of further cases.

3 Pulse oximetry is misleading in methaemoglobinaemia. Readings do not usually fall below 85%.

4 Administer methylene blue to symptomatic patients with elevated methaemoglobin levels and to unstable patients with a history of exposure to an agent known to cause methaemoglobinaemia.

5 Methylene blue can cause haemolysis and methaemoglobinaemia if given to patients who do not have methaemoglobinaemia or who are G6PD deficient, or if more than 5 mg/kg is used.

6 Failure to respond to methylene blue may result from too small or too large a dose, congenital enzyme or haemoglobin defects or an incorrect diagnosis.

Introduction

Although it is an uncommon presentation, the emergency physician must be able to diagnose methaemoglobinaemia because it is potentially fatal and can be readily treated with the antidote, methylene blue.

Aetiology and pathophysiology

Under normal conditions, methaemoglobin is continuously produced from haemoglobin by the oxidation of the iron molecule from the ferrous (Fe^{2+}) to the ferric (Fe^{3+}) state. In the normal physiological state, less than 1% of haemoglobin is methaemoglobin because it is continuously being reduced, predominantly by the enzyme NADH methaemoglobin reductase (see Fig. 29.13.1).

Excessive methaemoglobinaemia causes tissue hypoxia because methaemoglobin is incapable of carrying oxygen[1] and causes a shift of the oxygen haemoglobin dissociation curve to the left.[2]

Methaemoglobinaemia may be acquired or congenital. Congenital methaemoglobinaemia is due either to a deficiency of the enzyme NADH methaemoglobin reductase (a rare autosomal recessive condition) or the haemoglobinopathy, haemoglobin M (Milwaukee). The latter is transmitted with an autosomal inheritance. Homozygotes usually do not survive and heterozygotes live with a methaemoglobin level of around 15–30%.[3,4]

Acquired methaemoglobinaemia in adults arises as a consequence of accidental or intentional exposure to a therapeutic drug or other oxidizing agent. Oxidants that commonly result in excessive methaemoglobin production are listed in Table 29.13.1.

Nitrates, nitrites and local anaesthetics are the culprits most commonly reported in the medical literature. Recreational use of amyl, butyl or isobutyl nitrite can cause severe methaemoglobinaemia.[1,5] Transdermal absorption of industrial nitrate solutions, ingestion of food and water contaminated with nitrates and the intravenous use or inhalation of nitrates may all cause methaemoglobinaemia.[6] Sodium nitrite is commonly used commercially as a food preservative, colouring agent or corrosion inhibitor.

Therapeutic use of glyceryl trinitrate (GTN) has been reported to increase methaemoglobin levels up to 38% but it is more likely to cause severe hypotension before methaemoglobinaemia develops. Prolonged use of high doses of GTN ($>10\,\mu g/kg/min$) and the presence of renal or hepatic dysfunction make this complication more likely.[7]

Local anaesthetics, prilocaine and benzocaine in particular, can cause methaemoglobinaemia even when applied topically and administered in standard doses.[8,9] Risk factors for the development of methaemoglobinaemia from topically applied local anaesthetics include excessive dosing, a break in the mucosal barrier and a partial deficiency of the enzyme NADH methaemoglobin reductase.[9]

Dapsone therapy can cause both haemolytic anaemia and methaemoglobinaemia.

Aniline (aminobenzene) and its major metabolite, phenylhydroxylamine, are potent methaemoglobin forming agents, even after transdermal exposure.[10] Aniline and related compounds such as nitrobenzene are used widely in industry, especially the chemical and rubber industries.

Clinical features

The symptoms and signs of methaemoglobinaemia are attributable to the effects of cellular hypoxia on the CNS and the heart. At levels between 25% and 40%, headache, weakness, anxiety, lethargy, syncope, tachycardia and dyspnoea are observed. Further elevations are associated

$$NADH + Methaemoglobin \longrightarrow NAD^+ + Haemoglobin$$

NADH methaemoglobin reductase

Fig. 29.13.1 Major pathway for reduction of methaemoglobin under physiological conditions.

Table 29.13.1 Agents causing acquired methaemoglobinaemia[1]

Nitrites
- Amyl nitrite
- Isobutyl nitrite

Nitrates
- Glyceryl trinitrate
- Nitrate food preservatives
- Silver nitrate burns treatments
- Sodium nitrate
- Water contaminated with nitrates

Local anaesthetics (including topical)
- Benzocaine
- Lidocaine
- Prilocaine

Aniline dyes and related compounds
- Aniline
- Nitroethane
- Toluidine

Antimicrobial agents
- Dapsone
- Quinones (chloroquine, primaquine)
- Sulphonamides

Others
- Cetrimide
- Chlorates
- Combustion products
- Copper sulphates
- Methylene blue
- Naphthalene

with decreasing level of consciousness (45–55%) leading to coma, seizures, arrhythmias and cardiac conduction disturbances (55–70%). Levels above 70% are associated with mortality but deaths can occur at lower levels.[11,12]

With accidental exposures (either ingestion or cutaneous), multiple presentations of either family members of co-workers can be encountered after common exposure to the offending agent. It is not unusual in these circumstances for the relationship between the toxic substance and the presentations to be unclear initially.

The hallmark of methaemoglobinaemia is a deep cyanosis that is unresponsive to oxygen therapy. The cyanosis may be so deep that it is more brown than blue and has been termed chocolate cyanosis.[5] A useful diagnostic clue is the classic chocolate brown appearance of the patient's blood. This may be observed at methaemoglobin levels as low as 15–20% and is best appreciated by placing a drop of blood on filter paper and comparing to a normal sample.

Clinical investigation

The diagnosis of methaemoglobinaemia is confirmed by spectrophotometric measurement of methaemoglobin. The result is expressed as a percentage of the total haemoglobin level. Analysis of the sample should be performed as soon as possible because methaemoglobin levels fall with time.[13] The indications for spectrophotometry are:

- cyanosis unresponsive to oxygen
- tachypnoea or other features of hypoxia and history of exposure to methaemoglobin-inducing agents
- normal or raised PaO_2 and low SaO_2 on pulse oximetry
- chocolate brown appearance of arterial blood.

Arterial blood gas analysis often demonstrates a metabolic acidosis with a normal oxygen tension. Other important investigations include a chest X-ray to exclude pulmonary pathology that might contribute to hypoxia and an ECG to assess cardiac rhythm and look for evidence of myocardial ischaemia or infarction. A full blood count to check haemoglobin and electrolytes, urea, creatinine and liver function tests should also be performed.

Pulse oximetry

Methaemoglobin interferes with the accuracy of pulse oximetry. With increasing levels of methaemoglobin, pulse oximetry readings approach 85% (at around 30% methaemoglobin) and remain in the mid-eighties range.[8,13] Methaemoglobin has a maximal light absorption at a wavelength similar to that of oxyhaemoglobin (660 nm) and is therefore not differentiated from oxyhaemoglobin.[14]

A newer generation of pulse co-oximeters which measure more than the standard two wavelengths of light, can distinguish not only methaemoglobin but also carboxyhaemoglobin and, if available, can confirm the diagnosis of methaemoglobin by direct transcutaneous measurement.[15]

Treatment

Initial management includes assessment of the airway, breathing and circulation and institution of appropriate measures of care. Administration of oxygen therapy is often not associated with any clinical benefit but the presence of cyanosis not responsive to oxygen is a diagnostic clue.

Decontamination of the GI tract or skin may be indicated.

Methylene blue (tetramethylthionine) is a specific antidote for methaemoglobinaemia. Whilst under normal conditions, 95% of methaemoglobin is reduced by the NADH methaemoglobin reductase system, a greater proportion is reduced by a second enzyme system, NADPH methaemoglobin reductase when methylene blue is present acting as a cofactor to methaemoglobin reductase.

NADPH is produced by the Embden–Myerhoff pathway and requires adequate G6PD activity. Thus, in states of G6PD deficiency, methylene blue may not be as effective.

Methylene blue is indicated for symptomatic patients with an elevated methaemoglobin level. Patients who are blue but asymptomatic do not require methylene blue. Symptoms can normally be expected in patients with levels greater than 15%, less if the patient is anaemic.

The dose of methylene blue is 1–2 mg/kg intravenously over 5 min. Unstable patients with cyanosis unresponsive to high flow oxygen and a history of oxidant exposure or 'chocolate brown' blood should be given methylene blue even if the methaemoglobin level is not available. A reduction in the methaemoglobin level and accompanying clinical improvement usually occur over 30–60 min. A further dose of 1 mg/kg can be given after 1 h if the methaemoglobin level remains elevated. Factors that may result in failure to respond are listed in Table 29.13.2.

The side effects of methylene blue include dyspnoea, a feeling of pressure on the chest, restlessness, apprehension, tremor, nausea and vomiting.[16] Paradoxically, methaemoglobin itself can oxidize haemoglobin to methaemoglobin if given in high doses (>5–7 mg/kg).[17] Adverse effects are minimized if the correct dose is used.[18] Methylene blue occasionally causes persistent blue discolouration of the patient or haemolytic anaemia.[19] G6PD-deficient patients should not be given methylene blue as it may precipitate massive haemolysis.

Table 29.13.2 Reasons for failure of methaemoglobinaemia to respond to methylene blue
Excessive oxidant
• Ongoing exposure
• Inadequate decontamination
Insufficient methylene blue
• Inadequate dose
Excessive methylene blue
• Excessive methylene blue acts as an oxidant in high doses (>7 mg/kg)
Methylene blue ineffective
• G6PD deficiency
• NADPH metHb reductase deficiency
• Haemoglobin M
Incorrect diagnosis
• Sulphaemoglobinaemia
• Carbon monoxide poisoning
• Cyanosis unresponsive to oxygen: cardiac shunt

Exchange transfusion is indicated for patients with G6PD deficiency or where there is failure to respond to methylene blue.[6,10,13,20,21]

Continuous infusion of methylene blue has been used to treat prolonged methaemoglobinaemia formation associated with dapsone.[20]

Controversies

❶ Hyperbaric oxygen treatment has been recommended as an alternative to methylene blue. The partial pressure of oxygen can be increased to such a degree so as to ensure adequate oxygen transport in the absence of functioning haemoglobin.

❷ Adjuvant treatment with ascorbic acid (vitamin C) has been recommended. It has a direct effect in reducing methaemoglobin, but this effect is too slow for it to be used as a primary treatment. The dose is 0.5–1.0 g 6-hourly, either orally or intravenously.[2]

References

1. Edwards RJ, Ujma J. Extreme methaemoglobinaemia secondary to recreational use of amyl nitrite. Journal of Accident and Emergency Medicine 1995; 12: 134–137.
2. Curry S. Methemoglobinemia. Annals of Emergency Medicine 1982; 11: 214–221.
3. Stucke AG, Riess ML, Connolly LA. Hemoglobin M (Milwaukee) affects arterial oxygen saturation and makes pulse oximetry unreliable. Anesthesiology 2006; 104: 887–888.
4. Babbit CJ, Garret JS. Diarrhea and methemoglobinemia in an infant. Pediatric Emergency Care 2000; 16: 416–417.
5. Forsythe RJ, Moulden A. Methaemoglobinaemia after ingestion of amyl nitrite. Archives of Disease in Children 1991; 66: 152.
6. Harris JC, Rumack BH, Peterson BG, McGuire BM. Methemoglobinemia resulting from absorption of nitrates. Journal of American Medical Association 1979; 242: 2869–2870.
7. Bojar RM, Rastegar H, Payne DP, et al. Methemoglobinemia from intravenous nitroglycerin. A word of caution. Annals of Thoracic Surgery 1987; 43: 332–334.
8. Anderson ST, Hadjucek J, Barker SJ. Benzocaine induced methemoglobinemia. Anaesthesia and Analgesia 1988; 67: 1096–1098.
9. Dineen SF, Mohr DN, Fairbanks VF. Methemoglobinemia from topically applied anaesthetic spray. Mayo Clinical Proceedings 1994; 69: 886–889.
10. Mier RJ. Treatment of aniline poisoning with exchange transfusion. Clinical Toxicology 1988; 26: 357–364.
11. Gowans WJ. Fatal methemoglobinemia in a dental nurse. A case of sodium nitrite poisoning. British Journal of General Practice 1990; 40: 470–471.
12. Shesser R, Dixon D, Allen Y, et al. Fatal methemoglobinemia from butyl nitrite ingestion. Annals of Internal Medicine 1980; 92: 131–132.
13. Shimelman MA, Soler JM, Muller HA. Methemoglobinemia: Nitrobenzene. Journal of American College of Emergency Physicians 1978; 7: 406–408.
14. Reider HU, Frei FJ, Zbinden AM, Thomson DA. Pulse oximetry in methaemoglobinaemia. Failure to detect low oxygen saturation. Anaesthesia 1989; 44: 326–327.
15. Barker SJ, Curry J, Redford D, Morgan S. Measurement of carboxyhemoglobin and methemoglobin by pulse oximetry. A human volunteer study. Anesthesiology 2006; 105: 892–897.
16. Rosen PL, Johnson C, McGehee WG. Failure of methylene blue in toxic methaemoglobinaemia. Association with glucose-6-phosphate dehydrogenase deficiency. Annals of Internal Medicine 1971; 75: 83–86.
17. Bodansky O. Methaemoglobinaemia and methaemoglobin producing compounds. Pharmacological Review 1951; 3: 144–196.
18. Harvey JW, Keith AS. Studies of efficacy of methylene blue therapy in aniline induced methaemoglobinaemia. British Journal of Haematology 1983; 54: 29–41.
19. Goluboff N, Wheaton R. Methylene blue induced cyanosis and acute haemolytic anaemia complicating treatment of methaemoglobinaemia. Journal of Paediatrics 1961; 58: 86–90.
20. Berlin G, Brod AB, Hilden JO, et al. Acute dapsone intoxication: a case treated with continuous infusion of methylene blue, forced diuresis and plasma exchange. Clinical Toxicology 1984; 22: 537–548.
21. Kellet PB, Copeland CS. Methemoglobinemia associated with benzocaine containing lubricant. Anesthesiology 1983; 59: 463–464.

29.14 Cyanide

George Braitberg

ESSENTIALS

1 Cyanide is a metabolic poison associated with a high mortality.

2 Cyanide toxicity is characterized by rapid onset of central nervous, respiratory and cardiovascular effects and by metabolic acidosis.

3 Cyanide exposure correlates well with serum lactate levels.

4 Prompt administration of antidotes may be life-saving; a number of alternative agents are available.

5 Cyanide poisoning from smoke inhalation is often overlooked and treatment is complicated by the potential coexistence of carboxy and methaemoglobinaemia.

Introduction and epidemiology

Cyanide is used in a variety of commercial processes including metal extraction and recovery, metal hardening and in the production of agricultural and horticultural pest control compounds. Exposure can also occur to hydrogen cyanide (HCN) gas, produced when inorganic cyanide comes in contact with mineral acids as in electroplating, or accidentally when cyanide solutions are poured into acid waste containers. Cyanide off-gassing in house fires is well documented with significant blood levels being reported in 59% of smoke inhalation victims.[1]

Death from cyanide poisoning is one of the most rapid and dramatic seen in medicine, and antidotal therapy must be given early to alter outcome. A dose of 200 mg of ingested cyanide, or 3 min exposure to HCN gas, is potentially lethal.[2]

Fortunately, serious acute cyanide poisoning is rare. Of 2 424 180 human poison exposures reported to the American Association of Poison Control Centers during 2005, only 214 involved cyanide poisoning. Of the 118 cases in which clinical outcome is known, only six were reported to develop major symptoms, and only six patients died.[3] However, the incidence of cyanide poisoning may be significantly underestimated. Blood cyanide concentrations greater than 40 µmol/L were found in 74% of victims found dead at the scenes of fires.[1]

Toxicokinetics and pathophysiology

The uptake of cyanide into cells is rapid and follows a first-order kinetic simple diffusion process. The half-life of cyanide is from 2 to 3 h.

While the precise in vivo action of cyanide is yet to be determined, it is thought that its major effect is due to binding with the ferric ion (Fe^{3+}) of cytochrome oxidase, the last cytochrome in the respiratory chain. This results in inhibition of oxidative phosphorylation, leading to a net accumulation of hydrogen ions, a change in the NAD:NADH ratio and greatly increased lactic acid production. Other enzymatic processes, involving antioxidant enzymes, catalase, superoxide dismutase and glutathione, may contribute to toxicity.[4] Cyanide is also a potent stimulator of neurotransmitter release, in both the central and the peripheral nervous systems.[5]

Humans detoxify cyanide by transferring sulphane sulphur, R–Sx–SH, to cyanide to form thiocyanate (SCN). The availability of R–Sx–SH is the rate-limiting step. This reaction is thought to be catalyzed by the liver enzyme rhodanese. However, other enzymes, such as β-mercaptopyruvate sulphur

transferase, may be important. Other routes of biotransformation include oxidative detoxification.[4]

Clinical features

Cyanide toxicity is characterized by effects on the central nervous system (CNS), respiratory and cardiovascular systems, and by metabolic acidosis.[2]

CNS manifestations, in order of increasing severity of cyanide exposure, are headache, anxiety, disorientation, lethargy, seizures, respiratory depression, CNS depression and cerebral death. An initial tachypnoea gives way to respiratory depression as CNS depression develops.

Cardiovascular manifestations include hypertension followed by hypotension, tachycardia followed by bradycardia, arrhythmias, atrioventricular block and cardiovascular collapse. The classic finding of bright red skin and blood is not observed if significant myocardial, respiratory or CNS depression has already occurred; in these situations the patient may appear cyanotic. Other cardiovascular parameters of interest include decreased systemic vascular resistance, increased cardiac output and decreased arterio-venous oxygen gradient.

Clinical investigation

Arterial blood gas analysis and serum lactate measurements reveal metabolic acidosis with a raised lactate. Concentration decay curves suggest that serum lactate concentration is closely related to blood cyanide concentration. In smoke-inhalation victims without severe burns, plasma lactate concentrations above 10 mmol/L correlate with blood cyanide concentrations above 40 µmol/L, with a sensitivity of 87%, a specificity of 94% and a positive predictive value of 95%.[6]

Cyanide is concentrated ten-fold by erythrocytes and whole-blood cyanide concentrations are used as the benchmark when comparing levels. A level of 40 µmol/L is considered toxic, and a level of 100 µmol/L potentially lethal. Symptomatic intoxication starts at levels of about 20 µmol/L.[7]

Treatment

Attention to airway, breathing, circulation and other resuscitative measures must be instituted immediately.

In the case of cyanide poisoning from smoke inhalation or self-poisoning with clinical signs and associated lactic acidosis and where cyanide poisoning is suspected to be the cause of coma or cardiovascular instability, antidote administration is indicated. A number of antidotes are available (see discussion below) but the regime below is recommended if available:

- 5–15 g of hydroxocobalamin i.v. over 30 min (but may be given as i.v. push if needed). Repeat if needed.
- plus
- sodium thiosulphate 12.5 g i.v. (50 mL of a 25% solution at 2.5–5.0 mL/min).

Cyanide antidotes

Dicobalt edetate (Kelocyanor®)

This inorganic cobalt salt was introduced as a cyanide antidote in the late 1950s. It complexes with cyanide to form cobalt cyanide, thus removing cyanide from the circulation and reducing toxicity. However, unless cyanide is forced into the extracellular fluid, tissue levels are minimally affected.

Adverse effects are considerable and may be life-threatening.[7] Severe hypotension, cardiac arrhythmias, convulsions and gross oedema are reported.[8] These effects are exacerbated when drug is administered to an individual who is not cyanide poisoned. In life-threatening situations where cyanide poisoning is suspected the antidote is a must. The treating physician therefore faces a significant dilemma when presented with a critically ill patient in whom the history of exposure is unclear. A semiquantitative bedside test for cyanide in blood is available and may be helpful in determining the need for antidotal therapy when time permits.[9] The recommended initial dose of dicobalt edetate is 300 mg i.v.. Further doses may be required. Therapeutic endpoints are improvement in conscious state, haemodynamic stability and improvement in metabolic acidosis.

Hydroxocobalamin

Hydroxocobalamin (vitamin B_{12A}) is the cyanide antidote most widely used in Europe. It complexes with cyanide, on a mole-for-mole ratio, to form cyanocobalamin. Antidotal doses of hydroxocobalamin are approximately 5000 times the physiological dose.

Hydroxocobalamin and cyanocobalamin are excreted by the kidney. The half-life of hydroxocobalamin in cyanide-exposed patients is 26.2 h.[10] As the half-life of cyanide in smoke inhalation victims is calculated to be between 1.2 and 3.0 h, it is suggested that hydroxocobalamin can be satisfactorily used as single-dose therapy. The amount of cyanocobalamin formed after a dose of 5 g hydroxocobalamin correlates linearly until a blood cyanide level of 40 µmol/L is reached. At higher blood cyanide concentrations there is little further rise in plasma cyanocobalamin, and it is suggested that the rate-limiting step in the formation of cyanocobalamin is the availability of antidote, not the absence of cyanide ions.[11]

Extensive research has demonstrated the safety of this drug.[12] In healthy adult smokers, 5 g of i.v. hydroxocobalamin is associated with a transient reddish discolouration of the skin, mucous membranes and urine, and a mean elevation in systolic blood pressure of 13.6%, with a concomitant 16.3% decrease in heart rate. No other clinical adverse effects are noted.[13] Allergic reactions are rare.[14] There is substantial experimental evidence to support the efficacy of hydroxocobalamin at lower levels of toxicity.[10,12] Hydroxocobalamin has been shown to be safe and efficacious in mild-to-moderate cyanide poisonings with levels up to 150 µmol/L and has been given successfully to patients with severe cyanide toxicity.[15] In cases of ingestion of cyanide with suicidal intent (where blood cyanide levels may be >150 µmol/L or plasma lactate concentrations >20 mmol/L), the usual dose of 5–10 g may be insufficient.

There are no data comparing the efficacy of hydroxocobalamin with dicobalt edetate so it is not possible to make any definitive conclusion about which antidote is best. However, in the emergency situation hydroxocobalamin appears to offer a greater margin of safety.

Limited volunteer studies suggest a synergistic effect of hydroxocobalamin and thiosulphate. Thiosulphate used on its own is limited by a slow onset of action and thus cannot be used alone as a first-line antidote. Case reports document successful outcomes in patients with extremely high levels of cyanide (494 µmol/L) with combination therapy.[15]

Hydroxocobalamin has been recommended as the treatment of choice for mass casualty chemical disasters where cyanide poisoning is suspected.[16]

Eli lilly cyanide kit

Administration of sodium nitrite followed by sodium thiosulphate is a long-accepted antidote for cyanide poisoning. The current Eli Lilly Cyanide kit was devised in 1970 and contains:

- amyl nitrite perles
- sodium nitrite 10 mL (30 mg/mL)
- sodium thiosulphate 50 mL (250 mg/mL).

The kit is based upon the premise that humans can tolerate up to 30% methaemoglobinaemia.[17,18] Conversion of haemoglobin to methaemoglobin promotes the movement of cyanide out of the cytochrome system; 4 mg/kg of sodium nitrite takes 30 min to achieve 7–10.5% methaemoglobin.[15] The formation of sodium thiocyanate allows for the reformation of Hb^{2+}, restoring the oxygen-carrying capacity of haemoglobin. Cellular respiration can continue as normal with cyanide removed from the respiratory chain. The observation that dramatic improvements in symptoms have occurred well before methaemoglobin levels have peaked has led many authors to suggest different mechanisms of action, such as vasodilatation and extracellular redistribution of cyanide.[7,14] In smoke inhalation victims with suspected combined carbon monoxide and cyanide poisoning, the availability of an antidote that will not exacerbate any oxygen carriage or delivery problem, or cause toxicity by its own action, is highly desirable. The combination of 10% methaemoglobin with carboxyhaemoglobin has synergistic detrimental effects on the oxyhaemoglobin dissociation curve.

Controversies

❶ The choice of antidote in cyanide poisoning is extremely controversial and different agents are favoured in different parts of the world. The current recommended treatment in Australia is dicobalt edetate, Kelocyanor®. However, European data suggest that hydroxocobalamin is a far superior and safer antidote.

❷ Hyperbaric oxygen (HBO) has been proposed as a therapeutical modality in cyanide poisoning but remains controversial with conflicting animal data. In most published human reports HBO is offered after a combination of modalities, and it is not possible to determine the treatment effect specific to each.[19]

References

1. Baud FJ, Barriot P, Toffis V, et al. Elevated blood cyanide levels in victims of smoke inhalation. New England Journal of Medicine 1991; 325: 1761–1766.
2. Gonzales J, Sabatini S. Cyanide poisoning: pathophysiology and current approaches to therapy. International Journal of Artificial Organs 1989; 12(6): 347–355.
3. Lai MW, Klein-Schwartz, Rodgers, GC, et al. Annual report of the American Association of Poison control Centers' National Poisoning and Exposure Database. Clinical Toxicology 2006; 44: 803–932.
4. Curry SC. Hydrogen cyanide and inorganic salts. In: Sullivan JB, Krieger GR, eds. Hazardous materials toxicology. Clinical principles of environmental health. Philadelphia Williams and Wilkins; 1992: 698–670.
5. Isom GE, Borowitz JL. Modification of cyanide toxicodynamics mechanistic based antidote development. Toxicology Letters 1995; 82/83: 795–799.
6. Baud FJ, Borron SW, Bavoux E, et al. Relationship between plasma lactate and blood cyanide concentrations in acute poisoning. British Medical Journal 1996; 312: 26–27.
7. Marrs TC. Antidotal treatment of acute cyanide poisoning. Advances in drug reaction. Acute Poisoning Review 1988; 4: 179–206.
8. Dodds C, McKnight C. Cyanide toxicity after immersion and the hazards of dicobalt edetate. British Medical Journal 1985; 291: 785–786.
9. Fligner CL, Luthi R, Linkaityle-Weiss F, et al. Paper strip screening method for detection of cyanide in blood using the CYANOTESTMO test paper. American Journal of Forensic Medical Pathology 1992; 13(1): 81–84.
10. Houeto P, Borron SW, Sandauk P, et al. Pharmacokinetics of hydroxocobalamin in smoke inhalation victims. Clinical Toxicology 1996; 34(4): 397–404.
11. Houeto P, Hoffman JR, Imbert M, et al. Relation of blood cyanide to plasma cyanocobalamin concentration after a fixed dose of hydroxocobalamin in cyanide poisoning. Lancet 1995; 346: 605–608.
12. Riou B, Baud FJ, Borron SW, et al. *In vitro* demonstration of the antidotal efficacy of hydroxocobalamin in cyanide

poisoning. Journal of Neurosurgical Anaesthetics 1990; 2(4): 296–304.

13. Forsyth JC, Mueller PD, Becker CE, et al. Hydroxocobalamin as a cyanide antidote: safety, efficacy and pharamacokinetics in heavily smoking normal volunteers. Journal of Toxicology and Clinical Toxicology 1993; 31: 277–294.

14. Borron SW, Baud FJ. Acute cyanide poisoning: clinical spectrum, diagnosis and treatment. Arhiv za Higijenu Rada i Toksikologiju (Zagreb) 1996; 47: 307–322.

15. Tassan H, Joyon D, Richard T, et al. Potassium cyanide poisoning treated with hydroxocobalamin. Annales Françaises d'Anesthésie et Réanimation 1990; 4: 383–385.

16. Sauer SW, Keim ME. Hydroxocobalamin: improved public health readiness for cyanide disasters. Annals of Emergency Medicine 2001; 37: 635–641.

17. Kirk MA, Gerace R, Kulig KW. Cyanide and methaemoglobin kinetics in smoke inhalation victims treated with the cyanide antidote kit.

Annals of Emergency Medicine 1993; 22: 1413–1418.

18. Kiese M, Weger N. Formation of ferrihaemoglobin with aminophenols in the human for the treatment of cyanide poisoning. European Journal of Pharmacology 1969; 7: 97–105.

19. Hart GB, Strauss MB, Lennon PA, et al. Treatment of smoke inhalation by hyperbaric oxygen. Journal of Emergency Medicine 1985; 3: 111.

29.15 Corrosive ingestion

Robert Dowsett

ESSENTIALS

1 Symptomatic patients may have burns to the airway or supraglottic tissues.

2 Decontamination has limited utility; care should be taken not to make patients vomit, and no attempt should be made to neutralize corrosives.

3 Serious injuries to the oesophagus or stomach may occur in the absence of visible burns to the lips, mouth or throat.

4 Admit all symptomatic patients.

5 Upper gastrointestinal endoscopy is the best guide to prognosis and management.

6 The major acute complications are perforation and necrosis, which may involve other intra-abdominal organs.

7 The major long-term complication is oesophageal stricture.

Introduction

Corrosives cause injury by an acid–base reaction with tissues. Strong solutions, capable of causing significant injury, are those with a pH of less than 2 or greater than 12 (Table 29.15.1). The pH of a solution is dependent on the concentration and dissociation constant (pK_a) of the chemical. Strong acids have a $pK_a \leq 0$ and strong alkalis have a $pK_a \geq 14$ (Table 29.15.2). The extent of injury also depends on the volume ingested, contact time and viscosity.

Domestic hypochlorite bleaches and ammonia products are the commonest substances ingested, but severe injury generally does not occur unless large amounts are swallowed.[1] Death results mainly from the ingestion of drain or toilet cleaners. Powdered automatic dishwasher detergents are also capable of causing severe injuries.[2,3]

Pathophysiology

Acid–base reactions cause injury by disrupting organic macromolecules. Heat generation may cause thermal burns. Highly exothermic reactions occur between strong acids and bases, or between light metallic compounds and water. Chemical reactions may also result in the production of other compounds that can cause additional injury to the gastrointestinal (GI) tract and lungs (Table 29.15.3).

Alkalis cause 'liquefactive' necrosis, a process that involves saponification of fats, dissolution of proteins and emulsification of lipid membranes. Disruption of cellular membranes enhances penetration of alkali through the tissues.

Acids cause 'coagulative' necrosis, a process that involves denaturation of protein. The denatured protein forms a hard eschar that may limit further penetration of the acid.

In both settings, tissue injury progresses rapidly and can continue for several hours following ingestion. Granulation tissue develops after 3–4 days, but collagen deposition may not begin until the second week, making the healing tissue extremely fragile during this period. Complete repair of the epithelium may take weeks. From the third week newly deposited collagen begins to contract and may produce strictures of the oesophagus, stomach and affected bowel.

Hydrocarbon compounds can produce injury by dissolving lipids and coagulating proteins. Other chemicals can injure tissues by redox reactions and alkylation.

Following corrosive ingestion tissue inflammation, necrosis and infection can result in hypovolaemia, acidosis and organ failure.

Table 29.15.1 Approximate pH of some common solutions

Solution	pH
Battery acid (1% solution)	1.4
Domestic toilet cleaner (1%)	2.0
Bleach (1% solution)	9.5–10.2
Automatic dishwasher detergents	10.4–13
Laundry detergents	11.6–12.6
Domestic ammonium cleaners	11.9–12.4
Drain cleaner (containing NaOH, KOH)	13.3–14

Table 29.15.3 Chemical reactions resulting in the production of further toxic chemicals

Chemical	Plus	Produces
Chlorine	Water	Hydrochloric acid Hypochlorous acid Oxygen radicals Heat
Ammonia	Water	Ammonium hydroxide Heat
Nitrogen dioxide	Water	Nitric acid Nitrous acid
Ammonia	Hypochlorite	Chloramine gas (NH_2Cl and $NHCl_2$)
Hypochlorite	Acid	Chlorine gas Hydrogen Sulphide
Sulphur compounds (e.g. plaster casts)	Acid	Sulphur oxide

Table 29.15.2 pKa of some common corrosives

Chemical	pKa	Highly corrosive?
Hydrochloric acid	−3	Yes
Bromic acid	<1	Yes
Nitric acid	<1	Yes
Sulphuric acid	1.9	
Arsenic acid	2.3	
Nitrous acid	3.3	
Hydrofluoric acid	3.4	
Ammonia	9.3	
Ammonium hydroxide	9.3	
Magnesium hydroxide	10	
Zinc hydroxide	11	
Calcium hydroxide	11.6	
Lithium hydroxide	>14	Yes
Potassium hydroxide	>14	Yes
Sodium hydroxide	>14	Yes
Calcium oxide	>14	Yes
Sodium carbonate	>14	Yes
Potassium carbonate	>14	Yes
Sodium hypochlorite	>14	Yes

Narrowings in the GI tract are most at risk from corrosive ingestion: the cricopharyngeal area, the diaphragmatic oesophagus, antrum and pylorus.[4] Up to 80% of patients have injuries at multiple sites.[5] Alkalis are more likely to produce oesophageal injury than are acids, which typically injure the stomach.[4,6–11] Solid corrosives are more likely to affect the mouth, pharynx and upper oesophagus, and to cause deeper burns.

The main acute complications of corrosive ingestion are haemorrhage, perforation and fistula formation. These result from severe burns causing full-thickness necrosis.

Full-thickness necrosis of the stomach may be associated with injury to the transverse colon, pancreas, spleen, small bowel, liver and kidneys. Perforation of the upper anterior oesophagus may lead to the formation of a tracheoesophageal fistula. Formation of a tracheoesophago-aortic fistula is a rapidly lethal complication.

Clinical features

Symptoms and signs associated with significant alkali ingestion include mouth and throat pain, drooling, pain on swallowing, vomiting, abdominal pain and haematemesis.[7] If the larynx is involved, local oedema may produce respiratory distress, stridor and a hoarse voice.[9,12,13]

Extensive tissue injury may be associated with fever, tachycardia, hypotension and tachypnoea.

Inspection of the oropharynx may reveal areas of mucosal burn. The absence of visible burns to the lips, mouth or throat does not imply an absence of significant burns to the oesophagus.[3,5,7,9–11,14–17]

Symptoms and signs associated with the life-threatening complications of oesophageal perforation and mediastinitis include chest pain, dyspnoea, fever, subcutaneous emphysema of the chest or neck and a pleural rub. Perforation of the abdominal oesophagus or stomach is associated with the clinical features of chemical peritonitis, including abdominal pain, fever and ileus.[5,6,10,18] Septic shock, multiorgan failure and death may develop rapidly if perforation is not recognized.

The systemic effects of large acid ingestion include hypotension, metabolic acidosis, haemolysis, haemoglobinuria, nephrotoxicity, pulmonary oedema and hypotension. Features of systemic toxicity can result from the ingestion of arsenic, cyanide and other heavy metal salts, fluoride, ammonia, hydrazine, hydrochloric acid, nitrates, sulphuric acid and phosphoric acid. Ingestion of ammonia can cause coma, hypotension, acidosis, pulmonary oedema, liver dysfunction and coagulopathy.[19] Systemic effects of phenol and related compounds include haemolysis and renal failure.[20]

Long-term complications

The major late complication of corrosive ingestion is the development of an oesophageal stricture. All patients with full-thickness necrosis of the oesophageal wall develop strictures, as do 70% of those with deep ulceration.[5,10] Symptoms of oesophageal narrowing (principally dysphagia) may develop within 2 weeks; 80% occur within the first 2 months. Early onset of symptoms is associated with a more rapidly progressive and severe obstruction. Strictures do not develop in areas of superficial mucosal ulceration.[6,11,18,21-25] Strictures can also affect the mouth, pharynx and stomach. Only 40% of gastric outlet strictures become symptomatic.[5,10,11] A very late complication of alkali ingestion is the development of oesophageal carcinoma, reported to develop 22–81 years after exposure.[26]

Clinical investigation

Initial investigations in symptomatic patients should include an ECG, arterial blood gas, blood count, type and cross-match, coagulation profile, serum electrolytes, blood glucose and liver and renal function.

Chest and upright abdominal X-rays should be assessed for evidence of mediastinal widening, pleural effusions, pneumomediastinum, pneumothorax and subphrenic gas.

All patients who are symptomatic or have visible oropharyngeal burns should undergo upper GI endoscopy within 24 hours. Endoscopy should also be considered in any patient who has intentionally ingested a strong acid or alkali. Endoscopy is the only way to fully assess the extent of injury to the GI tract, and the findings are the best guide to prognosis and subsequent management. The entire upper GI tract may be safely examined with a small-diameter flexible endoscope, provided it is not retroflexed or forced through areas of narrowing.[4,5,27] It is not necessary to terminate the examination at the first circumferential or full-thickness lesion. The cricopharynx should be assessed initially to identify any laryngeal burns. If laryngeal oedema or ulceration is encountered, endotracheal intubation may be necessary before continuing with endoscopy.

Oesophageal burns can be graded according to the depth of ulceration and the presence of necrosis, as determined at endoscopy (Table 29.15.4). Some parallel grading systems are used for thermal skin burns; others differentiate several levels of ulceration and necrosis. Injuries can be divided into three main groups:

- Mucosal inflammation or superficial ulceration only. These injuries will heal completely and are not at risk of stricture formation.
- Areas of deep ulceration or discrete areas of necrosis or circumferential ulceration of any depth. Stricture formation may occur.
- Deep circumferential burns or extensive areas of necrosis. These patients are at high risk of perforation and stricture formation.

Contrast oesophagography with a water-soluble contrast agent is useful for the detection of perforation, but is less sensitive than endoscopy in evaluating ulceration.[28]

Treatment

Patients should initially be assessed for the presence of any symptomatic airway burns or respiratory distress. The need for urgent intubation should be considered in any patient with stridor or hypoxia.

Efforts at decontamination must not induce vomiting, as this may exacerbate the oesophageal injury. The mouth should be rinsed thoroughly with water. Dilution of an ingested solid chemical by drinking 250 mL of water or milk is recommended. The value of administering oral fluids following ingestion of a liquid corrosive is controversial.[8,29] Patients should otherwise be given nothing by mouth. Neutralization, aspiration and administration of activated charcoal are all contraindicated.

Patients with persistent symptoms should be admitted for observation and undergo endoscopy 12–24 h later. Further management is dictated by the findings at endoscopy.

Patients with endoscopic evidence of superficial injury can be managed on a general medical ward with supportive care only. Complete healing can be expected. Patients with deep discrete ulceration, circumferential ulceration or isolated areas of necrosis should be admitted to high-dependency or the intensive care unit and kept nil by mouth. Intravenous fluid replacement, accurate fluid and electrolyte balance and symptom control are the mainstays of therapy. These patients may require prolonged i.v. access, and parenteral feeding and central venous access should be considered.

If perforation or penetration is suspected clinically or documented by endoscopy or contrast radiography, urgent laparotomy with or without thoracotomy must be considered. Early excision of areas with extensive full-thickness necrosis has been proposed, but this needs to be weighed against mortality rates of 40–50% for patients undergoing such emergency surgery.

Prophylactic broad-spectrum antibiotics are only indicated where there is evidence of GI tract perforation.

Strictures are dilated by endoscopy 3–4 weeks after ingestion. Reconstructive surgery may be required if the oesophageal lumen becomes completely obstructed, or if perforation occurs.

Disposition

Asymptomatic patients can be discharged after observation. They should be instructed to return if they develop pain, respiratory

Table 29.15.4	Classification of gastrointestinal corrosive burns	
Grade I Mucosal inflammation	**First-degree** Mucosal inflammation, oedema or superficial sloughing
Grade IIA Haemorrhages, erosions and superficial ulceration	**Second-degree** Damage extends to all layers of, but not through, the oesophagus
Grade IIB Isolated discrete or circumferential superficial ulceration	
Grade IIIA Small scattered areas of necrosis	**Third-degree** Ulceration through to perioesophageal tissues
Grade IIIB Extensive necrosis involving the whole oesophagus	

symptoms or difficulty swallowing. Symptomatic patients should be admitted for endoscopy with subsequent disposition dependent on the findings, as detailed above.

Controversies

❶ The use of corticosteroids to prevent oesophageal strictures following corrosive ingestion is controversial. Clinical trials show contradictory results.[22,23,30,31] Steroids do not decrease stricture formation following extensive or deep ulceration or necrosis, and may increase the risk of perforation.

References

1. Litovitz TL, Klein-Schwartz W, White S, et al. 2000 annual report of the American Association of Poison Control Centers Toxic Exposure Surveillance System. American Journal of Emergency Medicine 2001; 19: 337–395.

2. Clausen JO, Nielsen TL, Fogh A. Admission to Danish hospitals after suspected ingestion of corrosives. A nationwide survey (1984–1988) comprising children aged 0–14 years. Danish Medical Bulletin 1994; 41: 234–237.

3. Kynaston JA, Patrick MK, Shepherd RW, et al. The hazards of automatic-dishwasher detergent. Medical Journal of Australia 1989; 151: 5–7.

4. Sugawa C, Lucas CE. Caustic injury of the upper gastrointestinal tract in adults: a clinical and endoscopic study. Surgery 1989; 106: 802–806.

5. Zargar SA, Kochhar R, Mehta S, et al. The role of fiberoptic endoscopy in the management of corrosive ingestion and modified endoscopic classification of burns. Gastrointestinal Endoscopy 1991; 37: 165–169.

6. Estrera A, Taylor W, Mills LJ. Corrosive burns of the esophagus and stomach: a recommendation for an aggressive surgical approach. Annals of Thoracic Surgery 1986; 41: 276–283.

7. Gorman RL, Khin-Maung-Gyi MT, Klein-Schwartz W, et al. Initial symptoms as predictors of esophageal injury in alkaline corrosive ingestions. American Journal of Emergency Medicine 1992; 10: 189–194.

8. Penner GE. Acid ingestion: toxicology and treatment. Annals of Emergency Medicine 1980; 9: 374–379.

9. Vergauwen P, Moulin D, Buts JP, et al. Caustic burns of the upper digestive and respiratory tracts. European Journal of Pediatrics 1991; 150: 700–703.

10. Zargar SA, Kochhar R, Nagi B, et al. Ingestion of strong corrosive alkalis: spectrum of injury to upper gastrointestinal tract and natural history. American Journal of Gastroenterology 1992; 87: 337–341.

11. Zargar SA, Kochhar R, Nagi B, et al. Ingestion of corrosive acids: spectrum of injury to upper gastrointestinal tract and natural history. Gastroenterology 1989; 97: 702–707.

12. Moulin D, Bertrand JM, Buts JP, et al. Upper airway lesions in children after accidental ingestion of caustic substances. Journal of Pediatrics 1985; 106: 408–410.

13. Scott JC, Jones B, Eisele DW, et al. Caustic ingestion injuries of the upper aerodigestive tract. Laryngoscope 1992; 102: 1–8.

14. Crain EF, Gershel JC, Mezey AP. Caustic ingestions: symptoms as predictors of esophageal injury. American Journal of Diseases of Childhood 1984; 138: 863–865.

15. Gaudreault P, Parent M, McGuigan MA, et al. Predictability of esophageal injury from symptoms and signs: a study of caustic ingestion in 378 children. Pediatrics 1983; 71: 767–770.

16. Christesen HB. Prediction of complications following unintentional caustic ingestion in children. Is endoscopy always necessary? Acta Pediatrica 1995; 84(10): 1177–1182.

17. Muhlendahl KE, Oberdisse U, Krienke EG. Local injuries by accidental ingestions of corrosive substances by children. Archives of Toxicology 1978; 39: 299–314.

18. Ray JR, Meyers W, Lawton BR. The natural history of liquid lye ingestion: rationale for aggressive surgical approach. Archives of Surgery 1974; 109: 436–439.

19. Zitnik RS, Burchell HB, Shepherd JT. Hemodynamic effects of inhalation of ammonia in man. American Journal of Cardiology 1969; 24: 187–190.

20. Lin CH, Yang JY. Chemical burn with cresol intoxication and multiple organ failure. Burns 1992; 18: 162–166.

21. Middlekamp JN, Ferguson TB, Roper CL, et al. The management and problems of caustic burns in children. Journal of Thoracic and Cardiovascular Surgery 1969; 57: 341–347.

22. Hawkins DB, Demeter MJ, Barness TE. Caustic ingestions: controversies in management – a review of 214 cases. Laryngoscope 1980; 90: 98–109.

23. Anderson KD, Rouse TM, Randolph JG. A controlled trial of corticosteroids in children with corrosive injury of the esophagus. New England Journal of Medicine 1990; 323: 637–640.

24. Webb WR, Koutras P, Eckker RR, et al. An evaluation of steroids and antibiotics in caustic burns of the esophagus. Annals of Thoracic Surgery 1970; 9: 95–102.

25. Cannon S, Chandler JR. Corrosive burns of the esophagus: analysis of 100 patients. Eye Ear Nose Throat Monthly 1963; 42: 35–44.

26. Isolauri J, Markkula H. Lye ingestion and carcinoma of the esophagus. Acta Chirurgica Scandinavica 1989; 155: 269–271.

27. Chung RS, DenBesten L. Fibreoptic endoscopy in the treatment of corrosive injury of the stomach. Archives of Surgery 1975; 110: 725–728.

28. Mansson I. Diagnosis of acute corrosive lesions of the esophagus. Journal of Laryngology and Otology 1978; 92: 499–503.

29. Rumack BH, Burrington JD. Caustic ingestions: a rational look at diluents. Clinical Toxicology 1977; 11: 27–34.

30. Howell JM, Dalsey WC, Hartsell FW, et al. Steroids for the treatment of corrosive esophageal injury: a statistical analysis of past studies. American Journal of Emergency Medicine 1992; 10: 421–425.

31. Oakes DD, Sherck JP, Mark JB 1982 Lye ingestion: clinical patterns and therapeutic implications. Journal of Thoracic and Cardiovascular Surgery 83: 194–204.

29.16 Hydrofluoric acid

Andis Graudins • Sam Alfred

ESSENTIALS

1 Patients and medical staff are often unaware of the presence of hydrofluoric acid (HF) in household cleaning products.

2 Topical HF exposures may result in the gradual onset of severe local pain out of proportion to any clinical signs evident on presentation.

3 Patients may not relate their dermal symptoms to HF exposure due to the delay in onset of pain that occurs with domestic low concentration preparations.

4 Systemic toxicity may be life-threatening and is expected following dermal burns caused by high concentration solutions or involving body surface areas of greater than 5%, and following significant inhalations or ingestions.

5 Systemic toxicity is typically manifest as severe hypocalcaemia, hypomagnesaemia, hyperkalaemia and ventricular arrhythmias.

6 Ingestion and inhalation of HF may also result in significant gastrointestinal or respiratory burns.

Introduction

The inorganic acid of fluoride, hydrofluoric acid (HF), is a moderately corrosive chemical widely used in industry for the etching of glass, metal and stone, and in the preparation of silicon computer chips. HF is also a common constituent of rust and scale removers, car wheel cleaners, brick cleaners and solder flux mixtures. These products may be for either commercial or home use and are often found in containers with inadequate labelling in regard to the potential toxicity. Concentrations of commercially available HF may vary from 50 to 100%. Products containing HF for domestic use generally have a concentration of less than 10% but higher concentration products may be obtained illicitly for home use.

The most common route of accidental exposure to HF is topical.[1-3] This may occur when high-concentration HF leaks through damaged gloves in the industrial setting or when HF products are used in the home without gloves. Massive topical HF exposure and inhalational exposure to HF may also occur in the industrial setting.[4-7] Finally, ingestion of HF products may occur accidentally in the home in the paediatric age group or as a result of deliberate self-harm in adults.[8,9]

Pathophysiology

HF is a relatively weak acid with less corrosive effects than other stronger acids such as hydrochloric or sulphuric. In particular, low concentrations of HF (<20%) may result in little or no perceptible corrosive injury to the skin immediately following exposure. This is due to the relatively small dissociation constant ($pK_a = 3.8$), which limits the concentration of free hydrogen ions on the skin surface.[2,3,8] As HF tends to remain in an undissociated, neutral state its ability to penetrate through the skin into deeper tissues is enhanced. Gradual dissociation of HF producing free fluoride ions in the tissues leads to local tissue injury characterized by liquefactive necrosis rather than the coagulative necrosis more commonly associated with acid burns.[2,3] As the concentration of HF increases so does the potential for corrosive injury.[3,10] Nevertheless, chemical burns may result from exposures to dilute (<5%) solutions of HF, and fatal systemic poisoning has resulted from relatively small (<5% total body surface area (BSA)) burns caused by more concentrated solutions.[6,11-14]

The primary mechanism of tissue damage resulting from exposure to HF is related to fluoride toxicity following on from dissociation of the acid in exposed tissues.[2,3] A number of pathological mechanisms may be involved in both local and systemic fluoride poisoning. Fluoride binds divalent cations, especially calcium and magnesium, to form insoluble fluoride salts. The resulting hypocalcaemia and hypomagnesaemia may have profound local and systemic effects on cellular and organ functions. Fluoride is a cellular poison. It inhibits both aerobic and anaerobic metabolic enzyme systems and interferes with cellular respiration.[6,7] Fluoride also interferes with Na^+/K^+ ATPase activity and opens calcium-dependent potassium channels in cell membranes, resulting in the leak of potassium into the extracellular space with the potential for systemic hyperkalaemia.[1,15] Precipitation of calcium may also interfere with calcium-dependent clotting factors, resulting in coagulopathy.[16] Finally, exposure to HF may produce direct corrosive injury.

Fatal systemic fluoride poisonings have also been reported following inhalational and gastrointestinal (GI) exposures.[5,6] Once absorbed, fluoride ions are distributed to virtually every tissue and organ resulting in widespread disruption of organ function. Fluoride is slowly eliminated in the urine and elevations of urinary fluoride excretion can be detected following exposure to HF although these do not correlate with clinical toxicity.[3,17]

Clinical features

Exposure to HF in the industrial setting is usually recognized as such and patients will often have been decontaminated and had topical therapy applied prior to arrival at hospital. They are also likely to be in possession of appropriate information in the form of material safety data sheets. Acute dermal exposures in the domestic setting may present a more difficult diagnostic dilemma. Domestic product labels may be incomplete and offer no advice regarding the use of protective apparel such as gloves.[18] Additionally, the onset of the signs and symptoms of HF injury may be delayed after exposure to low concentration domestic products and the patient may not recognize that the symptoms are related to chemical exposure.[3,18]

Highly concentrated (>70%) HF contains enough free hydrogen ions to produce a burning sensation on the skin providing some degree of warning of an acute exposure with symptom onset within 1–2 h.[1,10] However, low concentrations of HF (<10%), found in products such as over-the-counter rust removers, often produce no symptoms at the time of contact and patients can present with gradually increasing pain from 6 to 12 h following exposure.[1,19]

The primary presenting complaint of acute topical HF injury is pain out of all proportion to any physical signs. HF exposure should always be considered in this situation. The pain is usually described as a tingling sensation that progresses to a burning pain and, then to a typical deep, throbbing and severe pain.[1,10,19–21]

Visible evidence of HF burns also follows a fairly common pattern. Initially, the burn site is erythematous and may be oedematous. As tissue injury progresses, the site becomes pale and blanched, progressing to a classical silvery grey appearance.[2,22] Local vesiculation and frank tissue necrosis may ensue. This process can progress over several days in untreated patients, resulting in the development of deep ulceration and extensive tissue loss.

Dermal exposure to HF commonly occurs on the hands or feet with relatively small areas of the skin being exposed. Systemic fluoride poisoning is rarely a problem under these circumstances. The risk of systemic toxicity increases with the percentage of BSA exposed to HF and the concentration of HF.[3] In general, if more than 3–5% BSA has been exposed to HF, there is a risk of hypocalcaemia.[3,23] Systemic fluoride toxicity is more likely following large dermal exposures, ingestion or inhalation of HF.[3,23,24]

Systemic fluoride toxicity is manifest by various effects, the most lethal of which are the severe electrolyte abnormalities produced by direct interaction with fluoride or effects on cell membranes and cellular enzyme systems.[3,6,7,15] Hypocalcaemia is due to the complexing of calcium by fluoride ions. Hypomagnesaemia may also occur. However, the primary cause of the lethal arrhythmias (refractory ventricular tachycardia, ventricular fibrillation and pulseless idioventricular rhythm) is the development of hyperkalaemia.[8,15] Patients with systemic fluoride poisoning also develop a significant metabolic acidosis.[3,8] This is the result of fluoride interference with intracellular metabolism. The systemic manifestations of significant hypocalcaemia include carpopedal spasm, hyperreflexia, tetany and coagulopathy.[16] Headache, paraesthesiae and visual complaints may be noted. In severe cases coma, seizures, shock and dysrhythmias often precede death.

Fluoride inhalation is associated with pulmonary injury, including the development of non-cardiogenic pulmonary oedema, adult respiratory distress syndrome (ARDS) and the potential for systemic fluoride toxicity.[3,5,25]

Clinical investigation

No investigations are necessary following dermal exposures to dilute domestic preparations involving less than 5% of BSA. Following significant dermal exposures to HF or any ingestion or inhalational exposure, serum electrolytes including magnesium and calcium, baseline coagulation studies and a 12-lead ECG (looking for evidence of hypocalcaemia or hyperkalaemia) are indicated. A chest radiograph should be performed in any patient with respiratory symptoms or severe systemic toxicity.

Treatment

All patients with significant dermal HF exposures (>5% BSA, exposure to concentrated industrial preparations) or any ingestion or inhalation exposures should have continuous cardiac monitoring and intravenous access established on arrival.

The initial management of an acute topical HF exposure is thorough skin decontamination with a water flush. This ideally should be performed as a first-aid measure as soon as possible following the exposure as the delayed presentation of most patients makes it unlikely that significant amounts of HF still remain on the surface of the skin. Pre-hospital use of hexafluorine preparations offers no benefit in terms of local burn minimization or prevention of systemic toxicity when compared to water irrigation of exposed surfaces.[26–28] Other first-aid measures in the work place for known or suspected HF burns include topical treatments such as calcium gluconate gel (2.5–10%) or soaks with quaternary ammonium salts such as benzalkonium or benzethonium chloride. Topical therapies are intended to form insoluble complexes with any surface fluoride ion thus preventing tissue penetration and minimizing deeper injury. Topical therapy is probably of little value once fluoride ions penetrate to deeper tissues but should be initiated on presentation to the emergency department (ED). Experimental evidence suggests that improved calcium penetration and burn control may occur with iontophoretic enhancement of divalent cation delivery; however, these observations have not yet been validated in the clinical setting.[29] Calcium gluconate gel can be applied to the hand in a rubber glove. It may provide relief to some patients with low concentration HF exposures to the digits. In most cases, topical therapy is a temporizing measure until more invasive methods of calcium administration can be employed. If calcium gluconate gel is not readily available, a 4.8% preparation can be rapidly prepared by mixing one ampoule of calcium gluconate injection BP in 10 g of KY jelly.

The definitive treatment of dermal HF burns involves the administration of calcium gluconate into the tissues affected by the exposure.[1–3,10,20,30–32] This may be achieved by a number of methods; direct tissue infiltration, regional intravenous infusion using a Bier's block technique and intra-arterial infusion.[1–3,10,20,30–32] The choice of method depends upon the site and concentration of HF involved.

Direct injection of approximately 0.5 mL per square centimetre of 10% calcium gluconate solution at the burn site can be considered in areas with little skin tension such as the trunk, forearms and legs. A small needle (25 gauge) should be used to minimize discomfort and care should be taken to infiltrate into, around and beneath the burn area as completely as possible. Only calcium gluconate should be used for local infiltration as calcium chloride is more concentrated and produces direct injury when injected into tissues.[3,32]

HF burns to the hands are relatively common. In view of the lack of loose tissues in the digits, direct dermal injection may be extremely painful and only small amounts of calcium gluconate may be injected. Additionally, the introduction of hyperosmolar calcium solutions to these limited tissues spaces may exacerbate oedema and result in vascular compromise.[1,2] HF may also penetrate beneath the fingernails. In the past, removal of fingernails was advocated to allow for injection of calcium gluconate into the nail bed.[32,33] Fortunately, the advent of focused, parenteral calcium administration techniques to the affected limb have meant that nail removal is rarely, if ever indicated.

Two techniques are available for direct injection of calcium gluconate into digital HF burns. The first is intra-arterial infusion of calcium gluconate. This technique involves inserting an arterial canula into the radial (for burns of the thumb, index and middle fingers) or brachial artery (for more extensive hand involvement) and slowly infusing a dilute solution of calcium gluconate utilizing an infusion pump. This allows the calcium to be delivered to the affected tissues through the vascular supply and avoids the pain and tissue distension associated with direct injection.[20,33,34] A typical dose is 10–20 mL of 10% calcium gluconate in 50–100 mL of dextrose, 5% in water infused over 4 h and repeated as necessary. The endpoint for therapy is the absence of pain. The number of intra-arterial infusions required for pain relief may vary from one to four or five, and depends on the concentration of HF to which exposure occurred. There is case report level evidence for the use of continuous infusions.[19,35]

Regional intravenous calcium gluconate infusion using a Bier's block technique has also been employed in the treatment of HF burns to the limbs.[10,30,36] Success has been observed for digital, hand and forearm exposures as well as for exposures to the leg.[10,30,36] The technique is similar to that described by Bier for regional limb anaesthesia and has the advantages of relative simplicity and of not requiring arterial cannulation.[37] An intravenous cannula is inserted in the dorsum of the hand of the affected limb and the arm is raised to exsanguinate the superficial venous system. A pneumatic tourniquet is applied to the upper arm and inflated to a pressure 100 mmHg above systolic blood pressure. Ten to 15 mL of 10% calcium gluconate is diluted to a total volume of 50 mL with normal saline and injected via the cannula into the ischaemic arm. The tourniquet is sequentially released after 20 to 25 min.[10] Pain relief is usually apparent within 30 min of tourniquet release.

There have been no controlled studies comparing any of these techniques in the treatment of HF burns. However, intra-arterial calcium infusion appears to be a better technique for distal digital exposures, particularly in cases where exposure has been to high concentrations (>20%) or where multiple digits are involved.[10] Intra-arterial infusion of calcium has the advantages of more focal provision of calcium to the site of digital exposures and the potential for multiple infusions in patients with ongoing pain. If the intravenous route is selected as the primary therapy and is unsuccessful following one treatment, intra-arterial calcium infusion should then be used. The use of intra-arterial magnesium sulphate in place of calcium gluconate has resulted in tissue necrosis requiring surgical debridement in a small case series and cannot be recommended.[38]

It is sometimes difficult to determine whether ongoing pain at the exposure site is due to continued tissue destruction from fluoride still present in the tissues, or to established tissue damage. This is particularly the case with patients who have had digital exposures to high concentrations of HF and received multiple infusions of intra-arterial calcium which do not seem to produce further pain relief. It also applies to patients who present more than 24 h post-exposure with ongoing pain despite calcium therapy. In both instances, failure to achieve pain relief with repeated infusions of calcium gluconate suggests that pain may be related to established tissue damage rather than ongoing tissue destruction.

Ocular HF exposures can result in serious consequences if left untreated. Patients should be treated as for other chemical exposures to the eye with copious saline irrigation, and local anaesthetic drops for pain relief. Calcium gluconate (10–20 mL/L) may be added to saline irrigation fluid although animal studies suggest that calcium gluconate eye drops are no better than copious irrigation with normal saline and may, in fact, result in delayed corneal healing.[39] Clinical case reports of calcium gluconate eye drop use suggest that this treatment is not harmful but controlled studies are lacking.[40,41]

Systemic fluoride poisoning resulting from HF ingestion, inhalation or significant dermal exposures is potentially life-threatening. Patients with HF ingestion should receive rapid GI decontamination. Aspiration of HF through a small bore nasogastric tube may limit absorption if the patient presents within an hour of ingestion. Calcium or magnesium-containing antacids can complex intragastric HF and prevent some systemic absorption of fluoride ions, although any benefit is likely to be marginal at best.[42] Endoscopy should be performed following HF ingestion as soon as the patient is clinically stable to assess the extent of any upper GI corrosive injury.[1] Nebulized calcium gluconate has been administered acutely to patients following HF inhalation.[5,43] Serum calcium, magnesium and potassium levels should be closely monitored. Intravenous calcium and magnesium replacement should be commenced prior to any fall in serum Ca^{2+} or Mg^{2+} concentrations and replacement doses may be guided by the calculated dose of fluoride ingested. Large amounts of calcium (200–300 mmol) have been used in severe cases of systemic HF poisoning with hypocalcaemia.[3,8,13] Hyperkalaemia may be recognized on the 12-lead ECG, but close monitoring of serum potassium levels is warranted. Hyperkalaemia in systemic fluoride poisoning is resistant to standard measures of potassium reduction, such as insulin, glucose and bicarbonate infusions. Ventricular arrhythmias associated with systemic fluoride poisoning are refractory to cardioversion and defibrillation, and may not respond to antiarrhythmic agents.[15] Haemodialysis is indicated for severe or refractory hypocalcaemia, hyperkalaemia or clinical toxicity (e.g. arrhythmias) and may be useful for the removal of fluoride ions.[3,7] Calcium and magnesium monitoring and replacement should continue during this procedure.

Disposition

Patients with minor dermal exposures in whom ED treatment produces complete resolution of symptoms may be discharged home with follow-up arranged within 24 h or should pain return. Those patients in whom tissue damage is evident require referral to a plastic or hand surgeon.

Patients at risk of systemic fluoride poisoning (exposure to high concentration solutions, greater than 5% BSA burns, inhalations and ingestions) require admission to an intensive care unit for ongoing monitoring and management of the electrolyte disturbances and other complications of systemic toxicity.

All patients with eye exposures require early ophthalmological referral.

Controversies

❶ Relative value of intra-arterial versus regional intravenous calcium gluconate administration.

❷ Role of iontophoretic enhancement of calcium delivery.

References

1. Salzman M, O'Malley RN. Updates on the evaluation and management of caustic exposures. Emergency Medical Clinics of North America 2007; 25: 459–476.
2. Burd A. Hydrofluoric acid-revisited. Burns 2004; 30: 720–722.
3. Dunser MW, Ohlbauer M, Rieder J, et al. Critical care management of major hydrofluoric acid burns: a case report, review of the literature, and recommendations for therapy. Burns 2004; 30: 391–398.
4. Blodgett DW, Suruda AJ, Crouch BI. Fatal unintentional occupational poisonings by hydrofluoric acid in the U.S. American Journal of Indian Medicine 2001; 40: 215–220.
5. Kono K, Watanabe T, Dote T, et al. Successful treatments of lung injury and skin burn due to hydrofluoric acid exposure. International Archives of Occupational and Environmental Health 2007; 73(Suppl): S93–S97.
6. Caravati EM. Acute hydrofluoric acid exposure. American Journal of Emergency Medicine 1988; 6: 143–150.
7. Bjornhagen V, Hojer J, Karlson-Stiber C, et al. Hydrofluoric acid induced burns and life threatening systemic poisoning – favourable outcome after haemodialysis. Journal of Toxicology – Clinical Toxicology 2003; 41(6): 855–860.
8. Chan BS, Duggin GG. Survival after a massive hydrofluoric acid ingestion. Journal of Toxicology – Clinical Toxicology 1997; 35: 307–309.
9. Holtstege C, Baer A, Brady WJ. The electrocardiographic toxidrome: the ECG presentation of hydrofluoric acid ingestion. American Journal of Emergency Medicine 2004; 23: 171–176.
10. Graudins A, Burns MJ, Aaron CK. Regional intravenous infusion of calcium gluconate for hydrofluoric acid burns of the upper extremity. Annals of Emergency Medicine 1997; 30: 604–607.
11. Chan KM, Svancarek WP, Creer M. Fatality due to acute hydrofluoric acid exposure. Journal of Toxicology – Clinical Toxicology 1987; 25: 333–339.
12. Manoguerra AS, Neuman TS. Fatal poisoning from acute HF ingestion. American Journal of Emergency Medicine 1988; 4: 362.
13. Mayer TG, Gross PL. Fatal systemic fluorosis due to hydrofluoric acid burns. Annals of Emergency Medicine 1985; 14: 149–153.
14. Bordelon BM, Saffle JR, Morris SE. Systemic fluoride toxicity in a child with hydrofluoric acid burns: case report. Journal of Trauma 1993; 34: 437–439.
15. Cummings CC, McIvor ME. Fluoride-induced hyperkalemia: the role of Ca++ dependent K+ channels. American Journal of Emergency Medicine 1988; 6: 1.
16. Auguilera IM, Vaughan RS. Calcium and the anaesthetist. Anaesthesia 2000; 55: 779–790.
17. Saady JJ, Rose CS. A case of non-fatal sodium fluoride ingestion. Journal of Analytical Toxicology 1988; 12: 270–271.
18. Smith MA. A hand burn from unmarked hydrofluoric acid [letter]. Medical Journal of Australia 1992; 157: 431.
19. Siegel DC, Heard JM. Intra-arterial calcium infusion for hydrofluoric acid burns. Aviation Space and Environmental Medicine 1992; 63: 206–211.
20. Vance MV, Curry SC, Kunkel DB, et al. Digital hydrofluoric acid burns: treatment with intra arterial calcium infusion. Annals of Emergency Medicine 1986; 15: 890–896.
21. Wilkes GJ. Intravenous regional calcium gluconate for hydrofluoric acid burns of the digits. Emergency Medicine 1993; 5: 149–244.
22. Anderson WJ, Anderson JR. Hydrofluoric acid burns of the hand: mechanism of injury and treatment. Journal of Hand Surgery [Am] 1988; 13: 52–57.
23. Mullett T, Zoeller T, Bingham H, et al. Fatal hydrofluoric acid cutaneous exposure with refractory ventricular fibrillation. Journal of Burn Care Rehabilitation 1987; 8: 216–219.
24. Sadove R, Hainsworth D, Van Meter W. Total body immersion in hydrofluoric acid. Southern Medical Journal 1990; 83: 698–700.
25. Watson AA, Oliver JS, Thorpe JW. Accidental death due to inhalation of hydrofluoric acid. Medicine, Science and the Law 1973; 13: 277–279.
26. Hojer J, Personne M, Hulten P, Ludwigs U. Topical treatments for hydrofluoric acid burns: a blind controlled experimental study. Journal of Toxicology – Clinical Toxicology 2002; 40(7): 861–866.
27. Hojer J, Personnes M, Hulten P, Ludwigs U. Existing evidence does not support the use of Hexafluorine (letter). Journal of Toxicology – Clinical Toxicology 2003; 41(7): 1033–1034.
28. Hulten P, Hojer J, Ludwigs U, Janson A. Hexafluorine vs standard decontamination to reduce systemic toxicity after dermal exposure to hydrofluoric acid. Journal of Toxicology – Clinical Toxicology 2004; 42(4): 355–361.
29. Yamashita M, Yamashita M, Suzuki M, et al. Iontophoretic delivery of calcium for experimental hydrofluoric acid burns. Critical Care Medicine 2001; 29(8): 1575–1578.
30. Ryan JM, McCarthy GM, Plunkett PK. Regional intravenous calcium – an effective method of treating hydrofluoric acid burns to limb peripheries. Journal of Accident and Emergency Medicine 1997; 14: 401–404.
31. Murao M. Studies on the treatment of hydrofluoric acid burn. Bulletin of the Osaka Medical College 1989; 35: 39–48.
32. Bracken WM, Cuppage F, McLaury RL, et al. Comparative effectiveness of topical treatments for hydrofluoric acid burns. Journal of Occupational Medicine 1985; 27: 733–739.
33. Trevino MA, Herrmann GH, Sprout WL. Treatment of severe hydrofluoric acid exposures. Journal of Occupational Medicine 1983; 25: 861–863.
34. Kohnlein HE, Achinger R. A new method of treatment of HF burns of the extremities. Chirurgie Plastica 1982; 6: 298.
35. Lin TM, Tsai CC, Lin SD, Lai CS. Continuous intra-arterial infusion therapy in hydrofluoric acid burns. Journal of Occupational and Environmental Medicine 2000; 42(9): 892–897.
36. Henry JA, Hla KK. Intravenous regional calcium gluconate perfusion for hydrofluoric acid burns. Journal of Toxicology – Clinical Toxicology 1992; 30: 203–207.
37. Bier A. Concerning a new method of local anaesthesia of the extremities. Archiv fur Klinische Chirurgia 1908; 86: 123.
38. Vance M, Curry S, Gerkin R, et al. An update on the treatment of digital hydrofluoric acid burns with intra-arterial infusion techniques. Veterinary and Human Toxicology 1986; 28: 486.
39. Beiran I, Miller B, Bentur Y. The efficacy of calcium gluconate in ocular hydrofluoric acid burns. Human and Experimental Toxicology 1997; 16: 223–228.
40. Bentur Y, Tannenbaum S, Yaffe Y, Halpert M. The role of calcium gluconate in the treatment of hydrofluoric acid eye burn. Annals of Emergency Medicine 1993; 22: 1488–1490.
41. Rubinfeld RS, Silbert DI, Arentsen JJ, Laibson PR. Ocular hydrofluoric acid burns. American Journal of Ophthalmology 1992; 114: 420–423.
42. Heard K, Delgado J. Oral decontamination with calcium or magnesium salts does not improve survival following hydrofluoric acid ingestion. Journal of Toxicology – Clinical Toxicology 2003; 41(6): 789–792.
43. Lee DC, Wiley JFD, Synder JWD. Treatment of inhalational exposure to hydrofluoric acid with nebulized calcium gluconate [letter]. Journal of Occupational Medicine 1993; 35: 470.

29.17 Pesticides

Darren M. Roberts

ESSENTIALS

1 Acute pesticide poisoning is an important cause of morbidity and mortality worldwide.

2 The toxicity of even 'slightly hazardous' pesticides is sometimes significant. Moderate-to-highly toxic pesticides may have a case-fatality rate of between 5 and 70%.

3 Ingestion of the concentrated formulations (i.e. agricultural rather than domestic products) leads to much worse outcomes.

4 Many pesticides have a delayed onset of effect. All patients with oral exposure should be monitored for a minimum of 6–12 h post-ingestion.

5 Resuscitation and supportive care are priorities in management of acute pesticide poisoning. Patients manifesting significant toxicity require prolonged admission, preferably in an intensive care unit.

6 The specific antidotes for anticholinesterase pesticide poisoning are atropine and pralidoxime. These should be administered as soon as possible and titrated to effect.

7 The mortality from acute paraquat poisoning is high and due to multiorgan failure or progressive pulmonary fibrosis. Ingestion of as little as 20 mL is sufficient to cause death. No satisfactory treatments have been identified.

8 The mechanism of toxicity of glyphosate-containing herbicides is probably due to the surfactant and leads to multiorgan toxicity and acidosis. Treatment is supportive.

Introduction

Pesticide poisoning occurs worldwide. Poisoning may occur due to either acute (intentional self-poisoning) or chronic (such as occupational) exposures. Acute poisoning is of more importance to the emergency physician and is the focus of this chapter.

A pesticide is any chemical used for the control of a plant or animal, which encompasses hundreds of chemicals. They can be sub-classified in terms of their intended target, the most common being insecticides, herbicides (selective or non-selective), fungicides, rodenticides and nematocides. Other methods for classification that have been used include mechanism of action and chemical structure.

Worldwide, pesticides are the most important cause of death from acute self-poisoning.[1] As with pharmaceutical poisoning, the toxicity of pesticides varies between individual compounds but, in general, pesticides are intrinsically more toxic than pharmaceuticals.[2,3] However, not all pesticide exposures lead to significant clinical toxicity. In Australasia, most acute pesticide exposures are accidental and the majority of patients do not require admission to hospital.

An accurate risk assessment is necessary for the proper management of patients with acute pesticide poisoning. This considers the dose ingested, time since ingestion, clinical features, patient factors and available medical facilities.[4] If a patient presents to a facility that is unable to provide sufficient medical and nursing care or does not have ready access to necessary antidotes, then arrangements should be made to rapidly and safely transport the patient to a healthcare facility where this is available.[5]

Due to the low incidence, pesticide poisoning is not always considered in the differential diagnosis. A number of case reports from Australia have described a delay in the diagnosis of significant pesticide poisoning because it was not considered initially.[6–8] These delays did not appear to adversely affect patient outcomes, but they highlight the importance for clinicians to be familiar with the clinical features of pesticide poisoning.[6]

This chapter primarily focuses on agrochemicals used in Australasia, in particular insecticides (organophosphorus pesticides (OPs) and carbamates) and herbicides (glyphosate and paraquat).

Aetiology, pathogenesis and pathology

Acute pesticide poisoning requiring admission to hospital and ongoing care usually occurs following acute intentional self-poisoning. Significant toxicity may also occur with accidental (e.g. storage of a pesticide in a milk carton) or criminal exposures.

The pathophysiology of acute pesticide poisoning, and therefore the clinical manifestations, vary widely between individual compounds. Many pesticides induce multisystem toxicity due to interactions with a number of physiological systems. The mechanism of toxicity in humans is discussed below for each pesticide; often it bears little relation to the mechanism of action in the target pest.

For many pesticides, the mechanism of toxicity is poorly described which usually means that less information is available to guide management of these exposures; however, it is an active area of research.[9]

It should be noted that proprietary pesticide products often contain other co-formulants, in particular hydrocarbon-based solvents. Herbicide products also contain surfactants to enhance herbicide penetration into the plant.[10]

Epidemiology

Acute pesticide poisoning is a major issue in developing countries of the Asia–Pacific region and OPs are considered the most important cause of death from acute poisoning worldwide.[11] In developed countries, however, the incidence of severe pesticide poisoning is relatively low. In rural areas, the incidence of severe pesticide poisoning may be higher compared to urban regions due to easier access.

Prevention

Primary exposures

Restriction of the availability of pesticides by regulatory authorities may decrease the overall mortality.[12] In Australia, for example, pesticides with a high case fatality such as paraquat, organochlorines and parathion are heavily regulated so poison exposures are increasingly rare. Proper storage, handling and use of pesticides can prevent accidental exposures.

Secondary exposures or nosocomial poisoning

There is much concern regarding the risk of nosocomial poisoning to staff and family members who are exposed to patients with acute pesticide poisoning, in particular OPs. Few cases of secondary poisoning, if any, have been confirmed by abnormal cholinesterase activities. While mild symptoms such as nausea, dizziness, weakness and headache have been reported in staff, these resolved after exposure to fresh air and were probably due to inhalation of the hydrocarbon solvent. Universal precautions using nitrile gloves are most likely to provide sufficient protection for staff members.[13,14] Dermal decontamination is necessary. Wash pesticide spills from the patient with soap and water and remove and discard contaminated clothes, shoes and other leather materials.

ANTICHOLINESTERASE PESTICIDES

Anticholinesterase pesticides are among the most widely used types of pesticides and include organophosphorus (organophosphate, OP, OGP) and carbamate compounds. In Australasia, the most commonly encountered anticholinesterase compounds are chlorpyrifos, dimethoate, fenthion, malathion (maldison), diazinon and propoxur (carbamate).[6,15]

The relationship between exposure and clinical toxicity is poorly defined and therefore all exposures should be observed and treated as significant.[6,15] Deliberate self-poisoning by ingestion is the scenario most likely to result in severe toxicity. Carbamates are generally less toxic and produce toxicity of a shorter duration than OPs. However, severe toxicity and death occur with some carbamates, in particular carbosulfan and carbofuran.[16–19]

Mechanism of toxicity

The effects of anticholinesterase compounds on human physiology are multiple, complex and incompletely described. Inhibition of acetylcholinesterase (AChE), thus preventing the hydrolysis of acetylcholine, is considered the most important mechanism.[20,21] Accumulation of acetylcholine at cholinergic synapses interferes with systemic nervous function, producing a range of clinical manifestations which are known as the acute cholinergic crisis (Table 29.17.1).

Inhibition of other esterases contributes to the clinical manifestations of acute poisoning. Inhibition of neuropathy target esterase leads to organophosphorus-induced delayed polyneuropathy (Table 29.17.1).[22]

Enzyme inhibition by an anticholinesterase compound is potentially reversible. In the case of OP-inhibited AChE, the enzyme can undergo spontaneous reactivation resulting in normal enzymatic function. But a proportion of inhibited AChE undergoes irreversible inhibition ('ageing') and enzyme resynthesis is required for restoration of nervous function. The rate of these competing reactions varies more than 10-fold between individual OPs.[20,23] This influences the clinical manifestations and response to antidotes, which reactivate inhibited AChE. Due to structural differences between carbamates and OPs there is spontaneous reactivation of carbamate-inhibited AChE and ageing does not occur.[23]

Marked differences in the clinical manifestations of acute anticholinergic poisoning from different compounds are observed.[20,21,24–26] This may reflect the variability in potency of enzyme inhibition,[20,27] physiological adaptations following prolonged stimulation,[20,23,26] pharmacokinetic factors,[20,23,24] additional

mechanisms of toxicity such as oxidative stress,[28] inter-patient differences[24,39] or a complex interplay of a number of these and other unknown factors.[20,25,28]

Clinical features

The initial manifestation of acute anticholinesterase poisoning is the acute cholinergic crisis (Table 29.17.1). The duration and manifestations of the acute cholinergic crisis vary between individual anticholinesterase compounds, as mentioned above.[20,21,24–26]

Gastrointestinal symptoms are most prevalent following oral exposures, probably a result of high pesticide concentrations in the gut prior to absorption, and the hydrocarbon solvent.[6] Tachycardia does not always appear to correlate with hypotension or pneumonia;[6] instead it may be secondary to catecholamine release from the adrenal medulla under nicotinic stimulation.[29]

Differential diagnosis

In situations where the history is not forthcoming, the differential diagnosis is broad and includes other toxins (clonidine, opioids, dopamine antagonists such as chlorpromazine or haloperidol), funnel web spider envenoming and pontine haemorrhage.

Clinical investigation

The diagnosis and management of acute anticholinesterase poisoning is primarily clinical but measurement of cholinesterase activity can assist. The reference ranges are wide due to the large inter-individual variability in baseline AChE and butyrylcholinesterase (BChE, plasma cholinesterase, pseudocholinesterase) activities.[23,31] Cholinesterase inhibition is generally noted prior to clinical effects.[23,32] AChE and BChE are generally depressed within 6 h, although enzyme inhibition may progress until 12–24 h post-ingestion.[33] AChE or BChE activity, if <80% of the lower reference range, indicates significant anticholinesterase exposure.[26,31,33] Patients in whom cholinesterase activity is higher might still have been exposed, but to a minimal degree only.

BChE inhibition is a sensitive biomarker of anticholinesterase exposure but has no relation to the *severity* of poisoning

Table 29.17.1   Clinical manifestations and treatment of acute anticholinesterase poisoning[5,20,21,22,43,45]

Clinical manifestations		Specific treatments for the routine management of acute anticholinesterase poisoning	Endpoints for titration
Acute cholinergic crisis	Markers of significant poisoning[Σ]		
• *Muscarinic features*: diarrhoea, urinary frequency, miosis, bradycardia, bronchorrhoea and bronchoconstriction, emesis, lacrimation, salivation (DUMBELS) and hypotension. Cardiac arrhythmias have also been reported.	Bradycardia, bronchorrhoea or bronchospasm, hypotension	*Atropine*. Initially 1–3 mg i.v. for adults. If endpoints are not achieved by 3–5 min, double the dose i.v. Continue to double the dose every 3–5 min until atropinization has been achieved. Large doses (hundreds of mg) may be required. Maintain atropinization by infusion, commencing with 10–20% of the loading dose every hour.	Clear chest on auscultation with resolution of bronchorrhea[§] and heart rate >80/min. Regular clinical observations are necessary to ensure that atropinization is achieved without toxicity (delirium, hyperthermia and ileus)
• *Nicotinic features*: fasciculations and muscle weakness which may progress to paralysis and respiratory failure*, mydriasis, tachycardia, and hypertension.	Muscle weakness, e.g. difficulty mobilizing or a decrease in forced vital capacity, progressing to respiratory failure requiring ventilatory support	*Intubation and ventilation, oximes* (for OPs only). The oxime used in Australasia for acute OP poisoning is pralidoxime. According to the WHO, the following is recommended for pralidoxime chloride: [#] intravenous loading dose of 30 mg/kg over 20 min, followed by an infusion of 8 mg/kg/h. In adults this approximates a 2 g loading dose, then 500 mg/h.	Administer as an infusion until recovery (12 h after atropine ceased or once BChE is noted to increase).
• *Central nervous system*: altered level of consciousness, respiratory failure* and seizures; the relative contribution of cholinergic and other neurotransmitters is not well characterized.	Altered mental status, respiratory failure and seizures	*Intubation and ventilation, benzodiazepines*. Administer i.v. as required for agitation or seizures, for example 5–10 mg diazepam, lorazepam 2–4 mg, or midazolam 5–10 mg.	Termination of agitation and/or seizures
• OP-induced delayed polyneuropathy: Characterized by demyelination of long nerves, where 1–3 weeks after an acute exposure there is neurological dysfunction, particularly motor but also sensory, which may be chronic or recurrent.		Supportive care and rehabilitation	Return of independent function

i.v., intravenously; BChE, butyrylcholinesterase; OP, organophosphates.
[Σ]A guide for identifying patients with a significant exposure. This classification is intended to guide clinical management by identifying patients who require close observation and specific treatments rather than for prognostication.
[§]Focal crepitations and/or wheeze may be noted when there has been pulmonary aspiration.
*Respiratory failure occurs due to centrally and/or peripherally mediated mechanisms. It may manifest either during the acute cholinergic crisis (Type I paralysis) or suddenly during an apparent recovery phase (intermediate syndrome, or type II paralysis). Weakness of neck flexors is an early sign of significant muscle weakness.[25,26] Intermediate syndrome was noted in 5% of all patients in an Australian series,[6] similar to that reported in China (7%)[85] and India(3%).[86]
[#]Pralidoxime is marketed as various salts which should be converted into an equivalent dose of pralidoxime chloride (1 g of pralidoxime iodide is equivalent to 650 mg of pralidoxime chloride).

because the affinity of anticholinesterase compounds for BChE is highly variable and differs to that of AChE.[23,30,32,34] Serial measurements of BChE may be useful for confirming systemic elimination of the anticholinesterase compounds. Once BChE activity starts to increase (the rate of this depends on hepatic function) it suggests that the plasma concentration of the anticholinesterase compound is negligible.[5]

Erythrocyte AChE is structurally similar to synaptic AChE and their activities change similarly in response to exogenous inhibition. The degree of AChE inhibition appears to correlate with severity of OP poisoning and it is considered the most useful biomarker of severity. In severe clinical toxicity, erythrocyte AChE activity is less than 20% of normal.[21,23,35] Serial measurements of erythrocyte AChE activity can be useful for confirming the efficacy of oximes. If AChE activity normalizes following initiation of oximes, it suggests that ageing has not occurred and that the dose of oximes is sufficient.

Cholinesterase mixing tests have been used clinically in patients with acute OP poisoning to titrate the oxime regimen.[36] In one method, the patient's plasma is mixed with an equal volume of non-poisoned donor (control) plasma. If BChE activity in the mixed sample is less than the mean of the samples from the patient and control, it suggests that free anticholinesterase compounds are present.[36] It has been suggested that a decrease in cholinesterase activity in

mixing studies is an indication to increase the dose of oximes although the AChE response to oximes is probably a more useful parameter to guide oxime dosing. Despite being widely used, neither of these approaches to monitor therapy have been demonstrated to improve outcome.

Arterial blood gases and routine blood laboratory analyses are recommended for measuring metabolic and respiratory derangements; hypokalaemia secondary to vomiting and diarrhoea is not uncommon.

Criteria for diagnosis

Acute anticholinesterase poisoning is diagnosed on the basis of a history of exposure and development of characteristic clinical features (Table 29.17.1). Therefore, a high index of clinical suspicion is necessary. Since the correlation between intent, dose and severity of toxicity appears to be poor,[6,15] and the clinical manifestations between individual compounds differ,[24] each exposure requires a thorough review.

The onset of clinical toxicity is variable; however, the majority of patients who will develop severe toxicity are symptomatic within 6 h. Patients remaining asymptomatic for 12 h post-ingestion are unlikely to develop significant clinical toxicity.[5,21,37] A possible exception is highly lipophilic compounds such as fenthion. These may produce only subtle cholinergic features initially but then go on to cause progressive muscle weakness over a number of days, including respiratory failure, requiring ventilatory support.[24,26]

Where there is doubt regarding the diagnosis or significance of an OP exposure, quantification of BChE or AChE activity is helpful if available. BChE is particularly useful because it is more widely available and a sensitive marker of exposure.[23,27,32,38]

Treatment

Resuscitation and early considerations

As with all acute poisonings, initial management begins with immediate assessment and management of disturbances in airway, breathing and circulation. Because suxamethonium is metabolized by BChE, this agent should not be used for intubation of patients with acute anticholinesterase poisoning because the duration of paralysis will be prolonged by many hours.[39] Continuous clinical monitoring, including pulse oximetry, cardiac monitoring and blood pressure are required. Intravenous vasopressors should be used for hypotension not responding to fluid loading because hypotension is often due to a decrease in systemic vascular resistance.

Although the amount ingested as per history appears to be a poor predictor of the amount absorbed,[32,40] all patients with intentional poisoning who are symptomatic should be managed in a centre with access to intensive care facilities. Oral decontamination with activated charcoal has been recommended for patients presenting within 1–2 h of ingestion;[41] however, a recent randomized controlled study demonstrated that this was not beneficial.[42]

During the immediate assessment and resuscitation of the patient, all patients should undergo some degree of dermal decontamination. The removal and discarding of exposed clothing will reduce further anticholinesterase exposure.

Subsequent interventions depend on changes in clinical observations during continuous monitoring. Antidotal therapy should be administered rapidly, as outlined in Table 29.17.1. The acute cholinergic syndrome is potentially reversible with adequate doses of atropine. Oximes such as pralidoxime may reverse muscle weakness or paralysis if administered promptly. Established OP-induced delayed polyneuropathy (OPIDP) does not respond to antidotes; instead supportive care is the priority.[5,43]

Mild clinical toxicity and dermal exposures

Patients who present with a history of accidental poisoning who are asymptomatic or mildly symptomatic (limited to GI symptoms), often do not require hospital admission. Management priorities for these patients are rapid triage, a detailed risk assessment and consideration of forensic implications. If the exposure is trivial, the patient does not need medical review and can be observed at home or in the workplace. Other patients should be decontaminated and monitored clinically for a minimum of 6–12 h. If available, cholinesterase activity should be measured to confirm whether the exposure is significant. A normal cholinesterase activity at 6 h post-exposure may be sufficient to exclude a significant oral exposure, although this approach has not been sufficiently assessed.[5]

Patients with a single acute dermal exposure rarely develop significant clinical effects and probably do not require medical assessment. Volunteer studies document that the risk of significant clinical toxicity from a dermal exposure is far below that of an oral exposure. Although the rate of anticholinesterase absorption across the skin is slower than across the gut, patients who are asymptomatic at 12 h are unlikely to develop toxicity. Such patients should be given instructions to present for medical review if there is a significant worsening of signs and symptoms. If there is significant concern regarding a dermal exposure, testing for changes in cholinesterase activity is recommended.[5]

Moderate-to-severe clinical toxicity

Patients with moderate-to-severe anticholinesterase poisoning experience prolonged and complicated hospital admissions. Close observation is required to monitor for a rapid clinical deterioration, even if there is apparent recovery from the acute cholinergic crisis.[25,44] Therefore, following resuscitation, these patients require ongoing management in an intensive care unit (ICU).[6,43,44] Priorities post-admission to ICU include careful titration of antidotes and supportive care, including ventilation and inotropes/vasopressors.[43]

Antidotes

The three most widely used classes of antidotes are muscarinic antagonists (usually atropine), oximes (usually pralidoxime in Australasia) and benzodiazepines.[5] The indications and dosing regimen of these specific antidotes are described in Table 29.17.1.

Antimuscarinic agents

Atropine is the most widely used antimuscarinic agent. It is carefully titrated to reverse muscarinic effects and has no effect on the neuromuscular junction and muscle weakness.[43,45]

Oximes

Oximes are used to reverse neuromuscular blockade by reactivating the inhibited AChE before ageing occurs and should therefore be administered as early as possible.[20]

Evidence supporting the efficacy of oximes and the dosing regimen is limited and their role in therapy is controversial.[46] Much of the controversy relates to issues with study design and low dosing regimens. Recent meta-analyses point to the limited data supporting the use of oximes.[47,48] However, the outcomes of these meta-analyses are questionable because they fail to account for the heterogeneity of the studies or the adequacy of their designs.[46]

More recently, a randomized controlled trial concluded that high doses of pralidoxime iodide are effective, although further studies were recommended.[49] In this study, all patients received an initial bolus of 2 g pralidoxime iodide followed by either 24 g/day for 48 h, then 1 g every 4 h until recovery (high dose) or the 1 g every 4 h (lower dose) until recovery.

Because carbamate-inhibited AChE does not undergo ageing, the role for oximes appears limited. However, it remains controversial given that data have been presented to suggest that oximes may increase the reactivation of carbamate-inhibited AChE,[50,51] although not consistently.[52] Oximes appear to increase carbaryl toxicity for reasons that are not understood. Despite the lack of clinical data, it is not unreasonable for oximes to be administered to patients with an unknown exposure and evidence of AChE inhibition.[5,53]

On the basis of a few reasonably conducted studies and clinical experience, oximes are recommended for use in patients with significant OP poisoning.[5,20]

Benzodiazepines

Benzodiazepines are recommended for use in patients with agitation or seizures.[45] It is proposed that early use of benzodiazepines may prevent cognitive deficits or improve the central control of respiration preventing the need for intubation; however, this has not yet been sufficiently studied.

Prognosis

The mortality in patients with anticholinesterase poisoning is variable, which may reflect differences in degree of exposure, reporting, resources, genetics or the types of compounds encountered.[54–56] However, the mortality is generally high at greater than 10%,[11] compared to a mortality of less than 0.5% for pharmaceuticals.[57]

Various tools are proposed to classify the severity of OP poisoning,[54,58–60] but few have been widely adopted or validated. Generalized approaches to prognostication in OP poisoning are difficult given that individual compounds vary markedly in the onset, severity and manifestations of clinical toxicity.[24] Further, they are not often useful for guiding management.[5]

In the case of dermal exposures, the potential for toxicity is poorly defined but prognosis appears favourable.

PARAQUAT (BIPYRIDYL HERBICIDES)

Paraquat is a non-selective contact herbicide and is considered one of the most toxic pesticides available. The mortality from acute poisoning is high, varying between 50 and 90%.[61] Fortunately, cases of acute paraquat poisoning are increasingly rare in developed countries due to regulation of availability. However, paraquat continues to be an important cause of death in developing countries around Asia, where it is widely used in subsistence farming.

Diquat is another bipyridyl herbicide that is more widely available in Australasia.

Mechanism of toxicity

Oral exposures to paraquat are most likely to lead to poisoning. Because paraquat formulations are highly irritating (and potentially corrosive), GI toxicity occurs with all oral exposures.

Paraquat is rapidly absorbed and distributed to all tissues. Free oxygen radicals are generated and non-specifically damage the lipid membrane of cells, inducing cellular toxicity and death. The extent of dysfunction depends on the concentration of paraquat at the cellular level and the efficiency of protective mechanisms such as intracellular glutathione which is a free radical scavenger. Following an exposure of only 10–20 mL of the 20%w/v solution, these protective mechanisms are overwhelmed leading to multisystem toxicity and death within 24–48 h.

Paraquat displays specific toxicity in the lung and kidney due to active uptake in type II pneumocytes and renal tubular cells. Because paraquat concentrates in these cells they are more affected by oxidative damage than other cells. Therefore, in the event of a smaller exposure where multisystem toxicity does not occur, progressive renal and respiratory failure may occur. Pulmonary effects are characterized by an initial pneumonitis, followed by neutrophil infiltration with ongoing inflammation and progressive pulmonary fibrosis. Progressive renal impairment decreases the excretion of paraquat and prolongs toxicity. Death normally occurs due to pulmonary fibrosis a number of weeks post-ingestion.

The free oxygen radicals generated by paraquat require oxygen, and supplemental inspired oxygen may exacerbate pulmonary toxicity.

Diquat does not concentrate in the pneumocytes as readily as paraquat. Therefore, if the patient survives the acute phase of multiorgan dysfunction, delayed pulmonary fibrosis is less likely to occur.

Clinical features

Severe GI toxicity including vomiting and diarrhoea is the initial manifestation of acute paraquat poisoning. Necrosis of the oral mucosa is often noted about 12 h post-ingestion; it has been reported in patients who drink the paraquat solution without swallowing, despite the brief contact time.

Patients ingesting more than 20 mL are likely to develop severe poisoning with multisystem toxicity. This manifests as pneumonitis, hypotension, hepatitis, acute renal failure and severe diarrhoea. Oesophageal perforation with extensive subcutaneous emphysema may also occur due to the corrosive effects of the formulation. Death within 48 h of ingestion is expected.

Patients ingesting less than 20 mL are less likely to die so quickly. Instead, the clinical course of these exposures is characterized by increasing dyspnoea and hypoxia until death. Death from respiratory failure due to pulmonary fibrosis has been reported a number of months post-ingestion. This is associated with various degrees of hepatic and renal impairment.[62]

Differential diagnosis

Acute paraquat poisoning may resemble sepsis or poisoning with another cellular poison, such as phosphine, colchicine or iron.

Clinical investigation

A range of investigations have been proposed and tested in patients with acute paraquat poisoning. Because outcomes from paraquat poisoning are so poor, their principal role is to more accurately define prognosis.

Initial investigations aim to confirm significant exposure to paraquat and the easiest method to do this is by the dithionite urine test. This involves the addition of 1 mL of a 1% sodium dithionite solution to 10 mL of urine. A blue colour change indicates paraquat ingestion, the darker the blue, the higher the concentration. If the test is negative on urine passed 6 h after ingestion, a significant exposure is unlikely.

The concentration of paraquat can be quantified in plasma and graphed on a nomogram to determine the chance of survival or death. A number of similar nomograms have been developed.[61] It is sometimes difficult to locate laboratories able to measure paraquat concentrations and the turn-around time may be too long for the test to be clinically useful.

Other investigations may be useful to determine the evolution of toxicity in other organ systems. Serial arterial blood gas measurements and chest X-rays demonstrate progression of the pneumonitis and pulmonary fibrosis.

Criteria for diagnosis

A diagnosis of paraquat poisoning is made on the basis of a history of exposure and the clinical symptoms, so a high index of clinical suspicion is required. The urinary dithionite test is a simple and quick method for confirming (or hopefully excluding) paraquat poisoning.

Treatment

Because death is reported following ingestion of as little as 10–20 mL, all exposures should be treated as significant and observed in hospital for 6 h post-ingestion so a dithionate urinary test can be conducted. Patients should be treated symptomatically, including intravenous fluids.

Systemic exposure to paraquat may be decreased by either reducing absorption or increasing clearance. Both Fuller's earth and activated charcoal have been advocated to decrease absorption. There are no data to suggest which is more effective and neither has been demonstrated to improve outcomes.[42,63]

Methods for increasing clearance have also been disappointing. While haemoperfusion increases paraquat elimination and reduces lethality in dogs, it is ineffective if commenced more than a few hours post-ingestion due to paraquat's rapid distribution.[64]

Treatment with antioxidants (e.g. vitamin C, vitamin E, acetylcysteine) has also been proposed but inadequately studied. There has been much research into the effect of immunosuppression (e.g. cyclophosphamide and corticosteroids). Initial studies were promising but not conclusive,[61] and while a subsequent study reported benefit from this treatment,[65] it was later criticized because of serious concerns with the study design.[66] The role of immunosuppression and antioxidants in the treatment of acute paraquat poisoning requires more research.

Despite these fairly disappointing results it is obvious that, in the absence of treatment, the majority of patients will die. This has led some clinicians to treat patients with a number of these treatments concurrently (e.g. activated charcoal, acetylcysteine, vitamins C and E, immunosuppression and either haemodialysis or haemoperfusion) in the hope that there will be a favourable outcome. The choice of whether to commence this treatment is largely a personal one and requires discussion with the patient and family. Such a treatment regimen is probably reasonable in patients with a faintly positive dithionite urinary test. However, it seems unlikely to be of assistance to patients in whom this test is strongly positive, or those with evolving multi-organ dysfunction. Instead, palliation should be the priority, including oxygen for hypoxia and morphine for dyspnoea and oropharyngeal or abdominal pain.

Prognosis

Much research has focused on the evaluation of markers of prognosis in patients with acute paraquat poisoning. Two predictors of death are well established: the dose ingested or the plasma concentration of paraquat, relative to the time of poisoning.[61] These require an accurate history and access to an appropriate laboratory. Direct markers of paraquat-induced organ toxicity that allow earlier prognostication might assist with determining which patients should be treated, palliated or discharged with confidence that harm will not occur.[61]

Alternative markers of prognosis have also been explored, although few have been validated. These include measurement of the respiratory index, temporal changes in haematological or biochemical measures such as creatinine, and pulmonary surfactants.[61]

GLYPHOSATE

Glyphosate is a non-selective herbicide that acts by inhibiting the enzymatic synthesis of aromatic amino acids in plants. This target enzyme is not present in humans. Both ready-to-use (~1–5%) and concentrated (~30–50%) formulations requiring dilution are available.

Glyphosate is absorbed from the GI tract and does not penetrate the skin to a significant extent. Respiratory, ocular and dermal symptoms may occur following occupational use but are usually of minor severity.[67] Ingestion is the most significant route of exposure in clinical toxicology.

Mechanism of toxicity

The mechanism of toxicity of glyphosate-containing herbicides in humans has not been adequately described. Experimentally, there appears to be minimal (if any) mammalian toxicity from glyphosate itself.[67,69] Toxicity has been largely attributed to surfactant co-formulants. Polyoxyethyleneamine (POEA; tallow amine) is the most common surfactant formulated in these products.

Poisoning is more severe following ingestion of concentrated formulations. This may reflect either the total dose ingested, or direct effects of the highly irritating compounds present in these products. Gastrointestinal corrosion is reported with high doses of the concentrated solutions.[70,71]

Patients with severe poisoning manifest multisystem effects. This suggests that glyphosate-containing herbicides may be non-specific in their action, or that they interfere with physiological functions that are common to a number of systems. Proposed mechanisms include disruption of cellular membranes and uncoupling of oxidative phosphorylation, although these may be inter-related.[72,73]

Clinical features

Abdominal pain with nausea, vomiting and/or diarrhoea, are the most common manifestations of acute poisoning. These may be mild and self-resolving, but in severe poisoning there may be inflammation, ulceration or infarction. Severe diarrhoea may also occur and vomiting may be recurrent, leading to dehydration.[70–72,74–77]

With more severe poisoning, hypotension, renal and hepatic dysfunction, pulmonary oedema or pneumonitis, altered level of consciousness and acidosis are reported. It is not understood which of these clinical features reflect primary or secondary toxic effects of the glyphosate-containing herbicides. These effects may be transient or severe, progressing over 12–72 h to shock and death.[71,72,74–77] Some patients who subsequently died demonstrated minimal symptoms on admission.[77]

Differential diagnosis

The differential diagnoses are wide, including any poisoning or medical condition associated with GI symptomatology and progressive multisystem toxicity.

Clinical investigation

There are no specific clinical investigations to guide management.

Targeted laboratory and radiological investigations should be conducted in patients demonstrating anything more than mild GI symptoms. Serial blood gases may be useful for detection of metabolic disequilibria.

An assay for quantifying glyphosate is not available for clinical use. Since the relationship between blood concentration and clinical outcomes has not been determined, this does not appear to be a useful investigation.

Endoscopic investigations may be useful in assessing for erosions or ulceration, particularly following exposures to the concentrated formulation.[70,71,74,75]

Criteria for diagnosis

The principal criterion for diagnosis of acute poisoning with a glyphosate-containing herbicide is a history of exposure. Therefore, a high index of suspicion is necessary for diagnosis. A number of clinical criteria for the classification of severity have been suggested, but none have been validated.[71,72,74,77]

Treatment

All patients presenting with a history of acute ingestion should be observed for a minimum of 6 h. Patients reporting a history of intentional ingestion and GI symptoms should be observed for at least 24 h given that clinical toxicity may progress.

Treatment of acute poisoning with glyphosate-containing herbicides is empiric. All patients should receive prompt resuscitation and supportive care. Oral-activated charcoal may be given if the patient presents within 1–2 h of ingestion,[41] although a recent randomized controlled trial did not support its efficacy for pesticides in general.[42] Intravenous fluids should be administered to replace GI losses and haemodynamic monitoring is recommended. Biochemical and acid–base abnormalities should be corrected where possible.

No specific antidote has been proposed or tested for the treatment of acute poisoning with glyphosate-containing herbicides. This relates largely to the unknown mechanism of toxicity of these products.

Survival in two patients with severe poisoning was attributed to haemodialysis,[78] however other patients have died despite this treatment.[74,76,79] Early initiation of haemodialysis may be required to optimize outcomes, although the efficacy of haemodialysis for poison removal has not been determined.

Prognosis

All intentional exposures should be considered significant. Retrospective studies have suggested a correlation between increasing dose and severe poisoning and death.[71,75,76]

Mortality from acute poisoning with glyphosate-containing herbicides has been estimated at 10.1% (38/377 patients).[72] This incidence was derived from pooled data in the literature, mostly from retrospective studies in tertiary centres, so there is the potential for a referral bias. Prospective studies in secondary hospitals suggest that the mortality is lower, around 3.5%.[77]

Tools for estimating prognosis in acute poisoning with glyphosate-containing herbicides have not been described in detail. Patients developing marked non-specific organ toxicity (e.g. renal failure, pulmonary

oedema, sedation, arrhythmias) are more likely to die.[76] Patients with more extensive erosions of the upper GI tract developed more severe systemic poisoning and required prolonged admission.[70]

Controversies

❶ Anticholinesterase pesticides

- Significance of other potential mechanisms of toxicity.

- Dosing, efficacy and indications for oxime therapy (including the relative efficacy of individual oximes).

- Role of other proposed antidotes and treatments including alpha-2 adrenergic receptor agonists (e.g. clonidine),[45] BChE replacement therapy,[45,80] gastric lavage,[81] extracorporeal blood purification,[82] magnesium sulphate,[45,83] organophosphorus hydrolases[45] and blood alkalinization with sodium bicarbonate.[84]

- Importance of regulatory restrictions on 'highly toxic' anticholinesterase agents in decreasing mortality.

❷ Paraquat

- Efficacy of immunosuppression, antioxidants and enhanced elimination on outcomes.

❸ Glyphosate

- The relative importance of glyphosate and other co-formulants on the development of poisoning.

- Clinical and analytical predictors of the development of significant poisoning.

References

1. Eddleston M, Phillips MR. Self poisoning with pesticides. British Medical Journal 2004; 328(7430): 42–44.
2. Eddleston M, Sudarshan K, Senthilkumaran M, et al. Patterns of hospital transfer for self-poisoned patients in rural Sri Lanka: implications for estimating the incidence of self-poisoning in the developing world. Bulletin of the World Health Organization 2006; 84(4): 276–282

3. Eddleston M, Karalliedde L, Buckley N, et al. Pesticide poisoning in the developing world – a minimum pesticides list. Lancet 2002; 360: 1163–1167.

4. Daly FFS, Little M, Murray L. A risk assessment based approach to the management of acute poisoning. Emergency Medical Journal 2006; 23: 396–399.

5. Roberts DM, Aaron CK. Management of acute organophosphorus pesticide poisoning. British Medical Journal 2007; 334(7594): 629–634.

6. Roberts DM, Fraser JF, Buckley NA, et al. Experiences of anticholinesterase pesticide poisonings in an Australian Tertiary Hospital. Anaesthesia .Intensive Care 2005; 33(4): 469–476.

7. Hollis GJ. Organophosphate poisoning versus brainstem stroke. Medical Journal of Australia 1999; 170(12): 596–597.

8. Teague B, Peter JV, O'Fathartaigh M, et al. An unusual cause for cardiac arrest. Critical Care Resuscitation 1999; 1(4): 362–365.

9. Buckley NA, Karalliedde L, Dawson A. Where is the evidence for treatments used in pesticide poisoning? Is clinical toxicology fiddling while the developing world burns? Journal of Toxicology, Clinical Toxicology 2004; 42(1): 113–116.

10. Tominack RL. Herbicide formulations. Journal of Toxicology – Clinical.Toxicology 2000; 8(2): 129–135.

11. Eddleston M. Patterns and problems of deliberate self-poisoning in the developing world. Quarterly Journal of Medicine 2000; 93(11): 715–731.

12. Roberts DM, Karunarathna A, Buckley NA, et al. Influence of pesticide regulation on acute poisoning deaths in Sri Lanka. Bulletin of the World Health Organization 2003; 81(11): 789–798.

13. Roberts D, Senarathna L. Secondary contamination in organophosphate poisoning. Quarterly Journal of Medicine 2004; 97(10): 697–698.

14. Little M, Murray L. Consensus statement: risk of nosocomial organophosphate poisoning in emergency departments. Emergency Medicine of Australasia 2004; 16(5–6): 456–458.

15. Emerson GM, Gray NM, Jelinek GA, et al. Organophosphate poisoning in Perth, Western Australia, 1987–1996. Journal of Emergency Medicine 1999; 17(2): 273–277.

16. Yang CC, Deng JF. Pattern of acute pesticide poisonings in Taiwan. Journal of Toxicology, Clinical Toxicology 2003; 41(4): 523.

17. Ameno K, Lee S-K, In S-W, et al. Blood carbofuran concentrations in suicidal ingestion cases. Forensic Science International 2001; 116(1): 59–61.

18. Paul N, Mannathukkaran TJ. Intermediate syndrome following carbamate poisoning. Clinical Toxicology 2005; 43(7): 867–868.

19. Yang P-Y, Tsao TCY, Lin J-L, et al. Carbofuran-induced delayed neuropathy. Journal of Toxicology – Clinical Toxicology 2000;38(1): 43–46.

20. Eyer P. The role of oximes in the management of organophosphorus pesticide poisoning. Toxicology Review 2003; 22(3): 165–190.

21. Namba T. Cholinesterase inhibition by organophosphorus compounds and its clinical effects. Bulletin of World Health Organisation 1971; 44: 289–307.

22. Lotti M, Moretto A. Organophosphate-induced delayed polyneuropathy. Toxicology Review 2005; 24(1): 37–49.

23. Lotti M. Cholinesterase inhibition: complexities in interpretation. Clinical Chemistry 1995; 41(12): 1814–1818.

24. Eddleston M, Eyer P, Worek F, et al. Differences between organophosphorus insecticides in human self-poisoning: a prospective cohort study. Lancet 2005; 366: 1452–1459.

25. Karalliedde L, Baker D, Marrs TC. Organophosphate-induced intermediate syndrome: aetiology and relationships with myopathy. Toxicology Review 2006; 25(1): 1–14.

26. Eddleston M, Mohamed F, Davies JOJ, et al. Respiratory failure in acute organophosphorus pesticide self-poisoning. Quarterly Journal of Medicine 2006; 99(8): 513–522.

27. Worek F, Diepold C, Eyer P. Dimethylphosphoryl-inhibited human cholinesterases: inhibition, reactivation, and aging kinetics. Archives of Toxicology 1999; 73(1): 7–14.

28. Venkatesh S, Kavitha ML, Zachariah A. Progression of type I to type II paralysis in acute organophosphorus poisoning: is oxidative stress significant? Archives of Toxicology 2006; 80(6): 354–361.

29. Petroianu G, Ruefer R. Poisoning with organophosphorous compounds. Emergency Medicine (Fremantle) 2001; 13: 258–260.

30. Carlock LL, Chen WL, Gordon EB, et al. Regulating and assessing risks of cholinesterase-inhibiting pesticides: divergent approaches and interpretations. Journal of Toxicology, Environmental and Health B Critical Review 1999; 2(2): 105–160.

31. Cochran RC, Kishiyama J, Aldous C. Chlorpyrifos: Hazard assessment based on a review of the effects of short-term and long-term exposure in animals and humans. Food Chemical Toxicology 1995; 33(2): 165–172.

32. Nolan RJ, Rick DL, Freshour NL. Chlorpyrifos: pharmacokinetics in human volunteers. Toxicology and Applied Pharmacology 1984; 73: 8–15.

33. Solecki R, Davies L, Dellarco V, et al. Guidance on setting of acute reference dose (ARFD) for pesticides. Food Chemical Toxicology 2005; 43(11): 1569–1593.

34. Nutenko I, Taitelman U. Affinity of organophosphate insecticides to acetylcholinesterase compared to plasma cholinesterase [abstract]. Journal of Toxicology – Clinical Toxicology 1999; 37(5): 662.

35. Thiermann H, Szinicz L, Eyer P, et al. Correlation between red blood cell acetylcholinesterase activity and neuromuscular transmission in organophosphate poisoning. Chemico-Biological Interactions 2005; 157–158: 345–347.

36. Dawson A, Buckley N, Whyte I. What target pralidoxime concentration? Journal of Toxicology – Clinical Toxicology 1997; 35(2): 227–228.

37. Bardin PG, van Eeden SF, Moolman JA, et al. Organophosphate and carbamate poisoning. Archives of Internal Medicine 1994; 154(13): 1433–1441.

38. Amitai G, Moorad D, Adani R, Doctor BP. Inhibition of acetylcholinesterase and butyrylcholinesterase by chlorpyrifos-oxon. Biochemical Pharmacology 1998; 56(3): 293–299.

39. Sener EB, Ustun E, Kocamanoglu S, Tur A. Prolonged apnea following succinylcholine administration in undiagnosed acute organophosphate poisoning. Acta Anaesthesiology Scandinavica 2002; 46(8): 1046–1048.

40. Eyer F, Meischner V, Kiderlen D, et al. Human parathion poisoning: a toxicokinetic analysis. Toxicological Review 2003; 22(3): 143–163.

41. Chyka PA, Seger D, Krenzelok EP, Vale JA. American Academy of Clinical Toxicology, European Association of Poisons Centres and Clinical Toxicologists. Position paper: single-dose activated charcoal. Clinical Toxicology 2005; 43(2): 61–87.

42. Eddleston M, Juszczak E, Buckley NA, et al. Randomised controlled trial multiple dose activated charcoal in acute self-poisoning. Lancet 2008; 371: 579–587.

43. Eddleston M, Dawson A, Karalliedde L, et al. Early management after self-poisoning with an organophosphorus or carbamate pesticide – a treatment protocol for junior doctors. Critical Care 2004; 8: R391–R397.

44. Sungur M, Güven M. Intensive care management of organophosphate insecticide poisoning. Critical Care 2001; 5(4): 211–215.

45. Eddleston M, Singh S, Buckley N. Organophosphorus poisoning (acute). Clinical Evidence 2005; (13): 1744–1755.

46. Buckley NA, Eddleston M, Szinicz L. Oximes for acute organophosphate pesticide poisoning. The Cochrane Database Syst Rev 2005; 25(1): CD005085.

47. Peter JV, Moran JL, Graham P. Oxime therapy and outcomes in human organophosphate poisoning: an evaluation using meta-analytic techniques. Critical Care Medicine 2006; 34(2): 502–510.

48. Rahimi R, Nikfar S, Abdollahi M. Increased morbidity and mortality in acute human organophosphate-poisoned patients treated by oximes: a meta-analysis of clinical trials. Human & Experimental Toxicology 2006; 25(3): 157–162.

49. Pawar KS, Bhoite RR, Pillay CP, et al. Continuous pralidoxime infusion versus repeated bolus injection to treat organophosphorus pesticide poisoning: a randomised controlled trial. Lancet 2006; 368: 2136–2141.

50. Dawson RM, Poretski M. Carbamylated acetylcholinesterase: acceleration of decarbamylation by bispyridinium oximes. Biochemical Pharmacology 1985; 34(24): 4337–4340.

51. Harris LW, Talbot BG, Lennox WJ, Anderson DR. The relationship between oxime-induced reactivation of carbamylated acetylcholinesterase and antidotal efficacy against carbamate intoxication. Toxicology and Applied Pharmacology 1989; 98(1): 128–133.

52. Dawson RM. Oxime effects on the rate constants of carbamylation and decarbamylation of acetylcholinesterase for pyridostigmine, physostigmine and insecticidal carbamates. Neurochemistry International 1995; 26(6): 643–654.

53. Lifshitz M, Rotenberg M, Sofer S, et al. Carbamate poisoning and oxime treatment in children: a clinical and laboratory study. Pediatrics 1994; 93(4): 652–655.

54. Karalliedde L, Feldman S, Henry J, Marrs T, eds. Organophosphates and health. London: Imperial College Press; 2001.

55. Costa LG, Cole TB, Furlong CE. Polymorphisms of paraoxonase (PON1) and their significance in clinical toxicology of organophosphates. Journal of Toxicology – Clinical Toxicology 2003; 41(1): 37–45.

56. Allebrandt KV, Souza RL, Chautard-Freire-Maia EA. Variability of the paraoxonase gene (PON1) in Euro- and Afro-Brazilians. Toxicology and Applied Pharmacology 2002; 180(3): 151–156.

57. Gunnell D, Ho D, Murray V. Medical management of deliberate drug overdose: a neglected area for suicide prevention? Journal of Emergency Medicine 2004; 21(1): 35–38.

58. Bardin PG, van Eeden SF. Organophosphate poisoning: grading the severity and comparing treatment between atropine and glycopyrrolate. Critical Care Medicine 1990; 18(9): 956–960.

59. Senanayake N, de Silva HJ, Karalliedde L. A scale to assess severity in organophosphorus intoxication: POP scale. Human & Experimental Toxicology 1993; 12: 297–299.

60. Lee P, Tai DYH. Clinical features of patients with acute organophosphate poisoning requiring intensive care. Intensive Care Medicine 2001; 27: 694–699.

61. Eddleston M, Wilks MF, Buckley NA. Prospects for treatment of paraquat-induced lung fibrosis with immunosuppressive drugs and the need for better prediction of outcome: a systematic review. Quarterly Journal of Medicine 2003; 96(11): 809–824.

62. Bismuth C, Garnier R, Baud FJ, et al. Paraquat poisoning. An overview of the current status. Drug Safety 1990; 5(4): 243–251.

63. Fountain JS. Gastrointestinal decontamination following paraquat ingestion. New Zealand Medical Journal. 2000; 113(1118): 406–407.

64. Pond SM, Rivory LP, Hampson EC, Roberts MS. Kinetics of toxic doses of paraquat and the effects of hemoperfusion in the dog. Journal of Toxicology – Clinical Toxicology 1993; 31(2): 229–246.

65. Lin JL, Lin-Tan DT, Chen KH, Huang WH. Repeated pulse of methylprednisolone and cyclophosphamide with continuous dexamethasone therapy for patients with severe paraquat poisoning. Critical Care Medicine 2006; 34(2): 368–373.

66. Gunawardena G, Roberts DM, Buckley NA. Randomized control trial of immunosuppression in paraquat poisoning. Critical Care Medicine 2007; 35(1): 330–331.

67. Goldstein DA, Acquavella JF, Mannion RM, Farmer DR. An analysis of glyphosate data from the California Environmental Protection Agency Pesticide Illness Surveillance Program. Journal of Toxicology – Clinical Toxicology 2002; 40(7): 885–892.

68. Williams GM, Kroes R, Munro IC. Safety evaluation and risk assessment of the herbicide Roundup and its active ingredient, glyphosate, for humans. Regulatory Toxicology and Pharmacology 2000; 31(2 Pt 1): 117–165.

69. IPCS. Environmental health criteria 159 Glyphosate. World Health Organization; Geneva: 1994.

70. Chang C-Y, Peng Y-C, Hung D-Z, et al. Clinical impact of upper gastrointestinal tract injuries in glyphosate-surfactant oral intoxication. Human and Experimental Toxicology 1999;18(8): 475–478.

71. Tominack RL, Yang GY, Tsai WJ, et al. Taiwan National Poison Center survey of glyphosate-surfactant herbicide

ingestions. Journal of Toxicology – Clinical Toxicology 1991; 29(1): 91–109.

72. Bradberry SM, Proudfoot AT, Vale JA. Glyphosate poisoning. Toxicological Review 2004; 23(3): 159–167.

73. Peixoto F. Comparative effects of the Roundup and glyphosate on mitochondrial oxidative phosphorylation. Chemosphere. 2005; 61(8): 1115–1122.

74. Talbot AR, Shiaw MH, Huang JS, et al. Acute poisoning with a glyphosate-surfactant herbicide ('Roundup'): a review of 93 cases. Human and Experimental Toxicology 1991; 10(1): 1–8.

75. Sawada Y, Nagai Y, Ueyama M, Yamamoto I. Probable toxicity of surface-active agent in commercial herbicide containing glyphosate. Lancet 1988; 1(8580): 299.

76. Lee H-L, Chen K-W, Chi C-H, et al. Clinical presentations and prognostic factors of a glyphosate-surfactant herbicide intoxication: a review of 131 cases. Academic Emergency Medicine 2000; 7(8): 906–910.

77. Roberts DM, Buckley NA. Acute intentional self-poisoning with glyphosate-containing herbicides. Clinical Toxicology 2006; 44(4): 414.

78. Moon JM, Min YI, Chun BJ. Can early hemodialysis affect the outcome of the ingestion of glyphosate herbicide? Clinical Toxicology 2006; 44(3): 329–332.

79. Stella J, Ryan M. Glyphosate herbicide formulation: a potentially lethal ingestion. Emergency Medicine Australasia 2004; 16(3): 235–239.

80. Güven M, Sungur M, Eser B, et al. The effects of fresh frozen plasma on cholinesterase levels and outcomes in patients with organophosphate poisoning. Journal of Toxicology – Clinical Toxicology 2004; 42(5): 617–623.

81. Li Y, Yu X, Wang Z, et al. Gastric lavage in acute organophosphorus pesticide poisoning (GLAOP) – a randomised controlled trial of multiple vs. single gastric lavage in unselected acute organophosphorus pesticide poisoning. BMC Emergency Medicine 2006; 6: 10.

82. Roberts DM, Ai P, Kaiyuan Z, Buckley NA. Extracorporeal blood purification for acute organophosphorus pesticide poisoning. Journal of Intensive Care Medicine 2007; 22(2): 124–126.

83. Pajoumand A, Shadnia S, Rezaie A, et al. Benefits of magnesium sulfate in the management of acute human poisoning by organophosphorus insecticides. Human and Experimental Toxicology 2004; 23(12): 565–569.

84. Roberts D, Buckley NA. Alkalinisation for organophosphorus pesticide poisoning. Cochrane Database Systemic Review 2005; (1): CD004897.

85. Fengsheng H, Haibing X, Fukuang Q. Intermediate myasthenia syndrome following acute organophosphate poisoning – an analysis of 21 cases. Human & Experimental Toxicology 1998; 17: 40–45.

86. Samuel J, Thomas K, Jeyaseelan L, et al. Incidence of intermediate syndrome in organophosphorous poisoning. Journal of Association of .Physicians of India 1995; 43(5): 321–323.

29.18 Ethanol and other alcohols

David McCoubrie

ESSENTIALS

1 Ethanol is a major cause of morbidity, mortality and emergency department (ED) presentation in most western societies. Presentations may result from acute intoxication, withdrawal or medical complications of chronic ethanol ingestion.

2 Ethanol causes central nervous system (CNS) depression that can be synergistic with other CNS depressants and is potentially lethal without supportive care.

3 Ethanol withdrawal has a mortality of 5% and may require inpatient management.

4 Wernicke's encephalopathy is a clinical diagnosis and requires prompt recognition and treatment with thiamine.

5 Methanol and ethylene glycol, the toxic alcohols, are potentially lethal when ingested even in relatively small volumes.

6 Methanol and ethylene glycol largely exert their toxic effects through the production of organic acid metabolites.

7 An elevated anion gap metabolic acidosis is the hallmark of toxic alcohol poisoning.

8 Osmolar gap has a poor sensitivity and is incapable of excluding toxic alcohol ingestion.

Introduction

Alcohols are hydrocarbons that contain a hydroxyl (OH) group. Ethanol, a two-carbon primary alcohol, is the most commonly used recreational drug in Australasia and elsewhere in the Western world. Ethanol misuse is a major cause of mortality and morbidity both directly and indirectly and EDs deal with the results on a daily basis. It was estimated that in 1997, 3290 Australians died from injury due to high risk drinking and there were 72 302 hospitalizations.[1] In excess of 30% of all ED presentations are deemed to be ethanol related.

The complications of chronic alcohol consumption contribute to the development of a number of medical and surgical emergencies many of which are dealt with elsewhere in this text. This chapter confines its discussion to acute ethanol intoxication, ethanol withdrawal and two other important ethanol specific emergency presentations – Wernicke's encephalopathy and alcoholic ketoacidosis.

A number of other alcohols, although far less frequently implicated in ED presentation than ethanol, are metabolized to form toxic organic acids and produce life-threatening clinical syndromes. These alcohols include methanol and ethylene glycol and are termed 'toxic alcohols'. Early recognition and intervention can prevent significant morbidity and mortality.

ETHANOL

Pharmacology

Ethanol is a small molecule that is rapidly and almost completely absorbed from the stomach and small intestine. Ethanol is both water and lipid soluble and rapidly crosses lipid membranes to distribute uniformly throughout the total body water. Ethanol is principally eliminated by hepatic metabolism with smaller amounts (5–10%) excreted unchanged by the kidneys, lungs and in sweat.

Ethanol is oxidized by cytosolic and microsomal cytochrome P450 (2EI and 1A2) alcohol dehydrogenases (ADH) to acetaldehyde, which in turn is metabolized by aldehyde dehydrogenase to acetate. Acetate is converted to acetyl-CoA and enters the Krebs cycle to be finally metabolized to carbon dioxide and water. Entry of acetyl-CoA in the Krebs cycle is dependent on adequate thiamine stores.[2] Importantly, the ADH system is saturated at relatively low blood ethanol concentrations, which results in blood ethanol elimination moving from first-order to zero-order kinetics. The rate of ethanol metabolism in non-tolerant adults is approximately 10 g/h and blood ethanol levels fall by about 0.02 g/dL/h.[3] An alternative pathway for ethanol metabolism is via the microsomal ethanol oxidizing system, the activity of which increased in response to chronic alcohol exposure. Metabolism by this route is relatively important at very high blood ethanol concentrations and in chronic alcoholics.

The mechanism of action of ethanol is poorly understood. However, ethanol acts as a central nervous system (CNS) depressant, at least partially by enhancing the effect of GABA at GABA-A receptors. Tolerance to the CNS depressant effect develops with chronic exposure.

Clinical presentation

Acute ethanol intoxication

The clinical features associated with acute ethanol intoxication predominantly relate to the CNS and progress with increasing blood alcohol level, although there is remarkable inter-individual variation, most commonly as a function of tolerance. Initial features include a sense of wellbeing, increased self-confidence and disinhibition. With increasing blood concentrations, impaired judgement, impaired coordination and emotional lability develop. At very high concentrations, ethanol can cause coma, respiratory depression, loss of airway protective reflexes and even death.

Presentation to the ED is usually as a result of the social and behavioural consequences of the alteration in higher CNS functions. Ethanol is frequently implicated in trauma, drowning, violence, self-harm, domestic and sexual abuse, and other acute social and psychiatric emergencies. Ethanol is a common co-ingestant in deliberate self poisoning. Less commonly the emergency presentation is a direct result of the CNS depressant effects of ethanol.

Table 29.18.1 Differential diagnosis of acute ethanol intoxication
Encephalopathy   • Hepatic   • Wernicke's
Head injury
Hypo-/hyperthermia
Intracranial infarction or haemorrhage
Metabolic   • Hypoglycaemia   • Hyponatraemia   • Hypoxia   • Hypocarbia
Overdose or other toxin
Post-ictal state
Psychosis
Sepsis

Many other important medical and surgical conditions that cause altered mental status may be incorrectly ascribed to ethanol intoxication or coexist with ethanol intoxication. Table 29.18.1 lists an (incomplete) differential diagnosis.

In the absence of a clear history, the diagnosis of ethanol intoxication is only confirmed upon determination of a breath or blood ethanol concentration. Because ethanol consumption is so ubiquitous, a positive reading does not exclude coexisting pathology.

Ethanol withdrawal syndrome

A withdrawal syndrome usually develops within 6–24 h of cessation or reduction in ethanol consumption in dependent individuals.[4] Symptoms can begin any time after the blood ethanol concentration begins to fall and blood ethanol is frequently still measurable in withdrawing patients. The duration of the syndrome may be from 2 to 7 days. Although the pathophysiology is not well understood, the syndrome presents as unopposed sympathetic and CNS stimulation. It is associated with a mortality of 5% and early clinical recognition of this syndrome is important.[4]

Patients may present to the ED already in withdrawal after deliberately abstaining from alcohol or after stopping drinking due to intercurrent illness or lack of funds to buy alcohol. Alternatively, ethanol-dependent patients may begin to withdraw

whilst being treated in the ED, particularly where their stay is prolonged.

Clinical features of mild ethanol withdrawal are those of mild autonomic hyperactivity and include nausea, anorexia, coarse tremor, tachycardia, hypertension, hyper-reflexia, insomnia and anxiety.[5] In more severe cases, the patient goes on to develop more pronounced anxiety, insomnia, irritability, tremor, tachycardia, hyper-reflexia, hypertension, fever, visual hallucinations, decreased seizure threshold and finally delirium. Symptoms usually peak by 50 h.[6] Delirium tremens represents the extreme end of the spectrum of ethanol withdrawal. It is an uncommon but potentially lethal complication.

Wernicke's encephalopathy

This is an acute neuropsychiatric syndrome that develops in certain alcohol-dependent individuals as a result of thiamine deficiency. It is a spectrum disorder that is classically described as a triad of:

• oculomotor disturbance (usually nystagmus and ocular palsies)
• abnormal mentation (usually confusion)
• ataxia.[7]

In up to 20% of cases, the signs and symptoms of the classic triad are not evident at presentation. Less common presentations include stupor, hypothermia, cardiovascular instability, seizures, visual disturbances, hallucinations and alterations in behaviour. In extremis the condition may present with hyperthermia, hypertonia, spastic paresis, dyskinesias and coma.[8]

Wernicke's encephalopathy is a clinical diagnosis and constitutes a medical emergency with significant morbidity and a mortality of 10–20 % if left untreated. For this reason, the emergency physician must maintain high index of suspicion in patients with long-term heavy ethanol intake.

Alcoholic ketoacidosis

Alcoholic ketoacidosis (AKA), also termed alcoholic acidosis, is an often unrecognized potentially life-threatening medical condition that develops in the alcoholic patient in response to starvation. The normal response to starvation is increased gluconeogenesis from pyruvate. In the alcoholic patient, pyruvate is preferentially converted to lactate. In response, fatty-acid metabolism is increased as an alternative source of energy, resulting in the production of acetyl-CoA and acetoacetate, which in turn is reduced to β-hydroxybutyrate (BOHB), producing the ketoacidotic state.

Patients with AKA usually present with a history of prolonged heavy alcohol misuse preceding a bout of particularly excessive intake, which has been terminated several days earlier by nausea, severe vomiting and abdominal pain.[9-11] There may be a history of previous episodes requiring brief admissions with labels of 'query pancreatitis' or 'alcoholic gastritis'.[12] Examination usually reveals tachypnoea, tachycardia, hypotension and diffuse epigastric tenderness on palpation. In contrast to patients with diabetic ketoacidosis, mental status is usually normal. The presence of an altered mental state should prompt consideration of other causes especially hypoglycaemia and acute ethanol intoxication.

Toxic alcohol poisoning is an important differential diagnosis. Toxic alcohol acidosis does not produce ketosis and in contrast does cause significant alteration to conscious state, visual symptoms (methanol) and renal failure/crystalluria (ethylene glycol).[12]

Clinical investigation

The excretion of ethanol by the lungs, although relatively unimportant in terms of ethanol elimination, obeys Henry's law, i.e. the ratio between the concentration of ethanol in the alveolar air and blood is constant. This allows breath sampling of ethanol to reliably estimate blood ethanol concentration.

Most non-tolerant adults would be expected to develop some impairment of higher functions at blood ethanol concentrations in the range of 0.025–0.05 mg/dL (5–11 mmol/L) and to develop significant CNS depression in the range of 0.25–0.4 mg/L (55–88 mmol/L).

In a patient presenting with acute intoxication, no investigations may be necessary; however, blood or breath ethanol levels (BAL) are frequently useful to confirm the diagnosis. A BAL of zero is highly significant in a patient with an altered level of consciousness, as ethanol intoxication is excluded, and other diagnoses need to be considered. A positive blood ethanol level does not exclude alternative diagnoses.

Other investigations should be performed as clinically indicated in an effort to exclude coexisting pathologies and alternative diagnoses as detailed above.

In the patient with AKA, bedside investigations reveal a low/normal glucose, low or absent breath ethanol and urinary ketones (these may be low or absent due to the inability of bedside assays to detect all ketone moieties, especially BOHB). Laboratory investigation will reveal an anion gap (AG) acidosis (this may be severe with AG > 30) and mild hyperlactaemia insufficient to account for the AG.[12]

Treatment

Acute ethanol intoxication

Severe ethanol intoxication with CNS depression is life-threatening but a good outcome is assured by timely institution of supportive care. In particular, attention may need to be given to the airway and ventilation. Hypotension generally responds to intravenous crystalloid infusion. The blood sugar level must be checked and normoglycaemia maintained. Intravenous thiamine should be administered, particularly to those with chronic ethanol abuse. There is no specific antidote to ethanol intoxication.

Less severe ethanol intoxication presents a management challenge to the emergency physician when it results in a combative or violent patient threatening harm to self or staff, or threatening to discharge against medical advice. Such patients frequently require chemical sedation with titrated doses of intravenous benzodiazepines or butyrophenones in order to facilitate assessment and observation, ensure safety for patient and staff and prevent unsafe discharge.

Ethanol withdrawal

The key to management of this condition is early recognition and institution of adequate dosing of benzodiazepines. Very large doses of benzodiazepines may be required to control symptoms. The risk and likely severity of ethanol withdrawal can usually be anticipated if an accurate history of alcohol intake and previous withdrawals is obtained. Coexisting conditions should be managed on their own merits. It is important to exclude hypoglycaemia and correct if present. Thiamine 100 mg

(preferably intravenously) should be immediately given to any chronic alcoholic patient who presents with or develops an altered mental status.

The management of ethanol withdrawal in the ED or observation ward is greatly facilitated by the use of ethanol withdrawal charts. These charts facilitate recognition of the first signs of ethanol withdrawal and timely administration of benzodiazepines in adequate doses. An example of such a chart is shown in Figure 29.18.1. Benzodiazepine, usually diazepam, administration is titrated to the clinical features of withdrawal. The total dose required to manage withdrawal is highly variable. Benzodiazepines are usually given orally but can be administered intravenously to the uncooperative or severely withdrawing patient. With extreme withdrawal, refractory to benzodiazepines, small aliquots of ethanol may need to be prescribed.

Wernicke's encephalopathy

As Wernicke's encephalopathy is a clinical diagnosis with high mortality if untreated, any known or suspected alcoholic patient who presents with altered mental status should receive thiamine 100 mg i.v. during the initial assessment. Recommended thiamine dosing in patients with suspected Wernicke's is more aggressive with 500 mg i.v. (over 30 min) three times per day for 2–3 days reducing to 250 mg once daily (i.v. or i.m.) for 3–5 days if a response is observed.[8] Parenteral administration is vital as thiamine is poorly absorbed orally. If dextrose administration is required, it must follow thiamine replacement as it may acutely worsen the neurological status of the thiamine-deficient patient. Magnesium is a co-factor for thiamine-dependent transketolase and so any magnesium deficiency should be corrected.[13]

Alcoholic ketoacidosis

Initial resuscitation should include administration of adequate volumes of crystalloids to treat hypovolaemia followed by thiamine and infusion of dextrose containing fluids. Potassium and magnesium supplementation should be given according to serum electrolyte results. Administration of dextrose, usually an infusion of 5% dextrose, is essential as it stimulates insulin release, inhibits glucagon release and

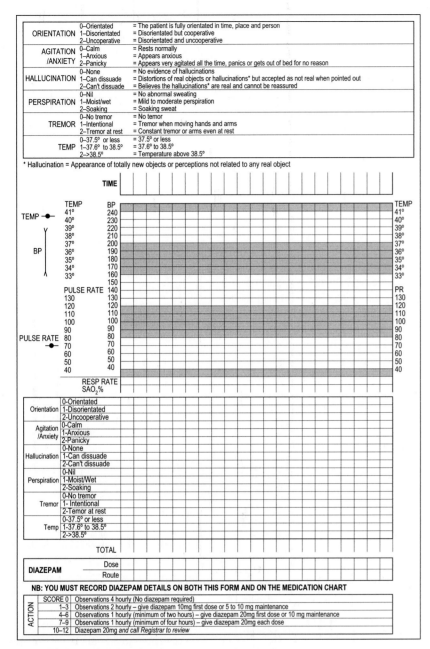

ORIENTATION	0–Orientated	= The patient is fully orientated in time, place and person	
	1–Disorientated	= Disorientated but cooperative	
	2–Uncooperative	= Disorientated and uncooperative	
AGITATION /ANXIETY	0–Calm	= Rests normally	
	1–Anxious	= Appears anxious	
	2–Panicky	= Appears very agitated all the time, panics or gets out of bed for no reason	
HALLUCINATION	0–None	= No evidence of hallucinations	
	1–Can dissuade	= Distortions of real objects or hallucinations* but accepted as not real when pointed out	
	2–Can't dissuade	= Believes the hallucinations* are real and cannot be reassured	
PERSPIRATION	0–Nil	= No abnormal sweating	
	1–Moist/wet	= Mild to moderate perspiration	
	2–Soaking	= Soaking sweat	
TREMOR	0–No tremor	= No tremor	
	1–Intentional	= Tremor when moving hands and arms	
	2–Tremor at rest	= Constant tremor or arms even at rest	
TEMP	0–37.5° or less	= 37.5° or less	
	1–37.6° to 38.5°	= 37.6° to 38.5°	
	2–>38.5°	= Temperature above 38.5°	

* Hallucination = Appearance of totally new objects or perceptions not related to any real object

Fig. 29.18.1 Alcohol withdrawal chart.

so inhibits fatty acid oxidation. Thiamine facilitates entry of pyruvate into the Krebs cycle. Administration of insulin or bicarbonate is not necessary.[14]

Fluid, electrolyte and acid–base status should be closely monitored and further therapy tailored to the clinical response. Careful evaluation and treatment of the coexisting medical disorders is essential.

Disposition

The disposition of many ethanol-intoxicated patients presenting to the ED is determined by the associated medical, surgical, psychiatric or social issues. Ethanol-intoxicated patients should only be discharged from the ED when their subsequent safety can be ensured. Discharge into the care of a competent relative or friend is sometimes appropriate. Other patients, particularly if aggressive or neurologically impaired, require admission to a safe environment until such time as the intoxication resolves and they can be reassessed. An observation ward attached to the ED may be the most appropriate place if available. More severely intoxicated patients requiring airway control and support of ventilation should be admitted to the intensive care unit.

Patients in ethanol withdrawal may require admission for management of the precipitating medical or surgical illness. For those patients who wish to complete withdrawal with a view to abstinence, the remainder of the withdrawal may be managed in a general medical ward, specialized medical or non-medical detoxification centre, or at home. Medical detoxification is mandatory where a severe withdrawal syndrome is anticipated. In any case, ongoing psychosocial support will be required and it is important for EDs to have a good knowledge of the locally available drug and alcohol services to ensure appropriate referral.

Patients with Wernicke's encephalopathy should be admitted for ongoing care and thiamine and magnesium supplementation. The ophthalmoplegia and nystagmus usually have a good response to thiamine within hours to days. Ataxia and mental changes improve more slowly if at all and have a poorer prognosis. Up to 50% of cases will show no response despite thiamine therapy.[13]

Patients with ethanol-induced ketoacidosis also require admission for ongoing dextrose and thiamine, monitoring of fluids and electrolytes and management of the precipitating medical condition. Mortality from ethanol-induced ketoacidosis per se is rare with early recognition and treatment, but death may occur as a result of the underlying medical condition, particularly if unrecognized.

Ideally, any patient with an ethanol-related presentation should be offered referral to drug and alcohol rehabilitation services for counselling.

TOXIC ALCOHOLS

Epidemiology

Both methanol and ethylene glycol poisoning are extremely rare in Australasia. This is primarily due to their limited availability.

Methanol is found in model aeroplane fuel and laboratory solvents. There is no methanol in 'methylated spirits' sold in Australia (this is in fact pure ethanol with bittering agents to minimize palatability). Methanol is more freely available in other countries where it is found in household cleaning agents and windshield de-icer. Mass poisoning incidents are reported following incorrect distillation of ethanol.

Ethylene glycol is most commonly encountered as a constituent of radiator antifreeze or coolant. It is also found in hydraulic fluids and solvent preparations. Significant poisoning in Australasia almost always occurs following deliberate ingestion.

Toxicology

Methanol and ethylene glycol are both small molecules that are rapidly absorbed from the gastrointestinal (GI) tract with a volume of distribution that approximates total body water (0.6 L/kg). Toxic alcohols are oxidized initially by hepatic cytosolic and microsomal alcohol dehydrogenases (ADH) and then further metabolized by aldehyde dehydrogenase into acidic moieties. Methanol is metabolized initially to form formaldehyde and then to formic acid. Ethylene glycol is metabolized to glycoaldehyde and then to glycolate, glyoxylate and oxylate. The plasma half-lives of the toxic alcohols are appreciably increased in the presence of ethanol because ethanol has a much higher affinity for ADH: four times that of methanol and eight times that of ethylene glycol. As a result, the presence of ethanol greatly delays the onset of clinical and biochemical features of toxicity.

Methanol toxicity is mediated through the formation of formic acid. Formic acid binds to cytochrome oxidase resulting in impairment of cellular respiration. Its half-life is prolonged (up to 20 h) and its metabolism is dependent on the presence of tetrahydrofolate. The presence of systemic acidosis enhances the movement of formic acid intracellularly. The initial acidosis is secondary to formic acid; however, as cellular respiration is disturbed and toxicity progresses a concurrent lactic acidosis is usually evident.[15] Accumulation of formic acid manifests as increasing AG acidosis, gastrointestinal and neurological toxicities.

Ethylene glycol itself is a direct irritant to the GI tract and has CNS depressant effects similar to those of ethanol. The major toxicity is mediated through the acid metabolites, glycolate and oxylate.[16] Oxalate complexes with calcium, leading to crystal deposition chiefly in the renal tubules and the CNS. Myocardium and lungs can also be affected. In addition, these acids appear to be inherently toxic.[16] Complexing with calcium produces systemic hypocalcaemia and may manifest with prolongation of the QT interval. A profound AG acidosis develops and is principally attributed to glycolic acid accumulation although a concurrent lactic acidosis (type B) also contributes.

Toxic doses

The lethal dose of methanol is conservatively estimated as 0.5–1.0 mL/kg of a 100% solution.[17] Clinical toxicity and visual sequelae may be seen with smaller doses, perhaps as little as 0.25 mL/kg.

The lethal dose of ethylene glycol is thought to be in the order of 1.0 mL/kg of a 100% solution.[16]

Clinical features

Methanol

Initially mild CNS depression typical of ethanol intoxication is evident. A latent period (6–24 h) is classically observed during which time the patient may appear asymptomatic. Progressive ophthalmic, GI and CNS symptoms may then develop. Hyperpnoea is usually observed secondary to the metabolic acidosis. Progressive obtundation leading to coma and seizures heralds the onset of cerebral oedema and signifies poorer prognosis.[18] Those who recover from serious CNS toxicity can display extrapyramidal movement disorders.[19] Retinal toxicity may be irreversible in up to a third of cases.[18]

Ethylene glycol

The progression of clinical features following ingestion of ethylene glycol is described in three stages: neurological, cardiopulmonary and renal. These stages are artificial and toxicity may progress in a rapid manner with concurrent toxicities being observed. Initially an intoxication syndrome analogous to ethanol occurs along with nausea and vomiting due to mucosal irritation. A progressively severe AG acidosis with renal failure and hypocalcaemia is characteristic. Crystalluria may be observed. With severe poisoning, renal failure progresses rapidly. Central nervous system depression is observed with severe manifestations including seizures, coma and cerebral oedema. Hyperpnoea occurs secondary to the metabolic acidosis.

Clinical investigation

Direct assay of methanol or ethylene glycol concentrations in serum is rarely readily available. In the absence of direct assays, the ability to exclude a potentially lethal toxic alcohol ingestion at presentation is limited. The combination of an osmolar gap (OG) and a wide AG acidosis is highly suggestive of either methanol or ethylene glycol intoxication. However a normal OG does not exclude toxic alcohol ingestion. In the presence of a profound acidotic state it is possible that a toxic alcohol has been largely metabolized and thus no longer sufficiently present to raise the OG. Additionally, baseline OGs may vary from −14 to +10 between individuals and so a 'normal' OG may mask a large occult increase representing a potentially lethal ingestion.[19] Similarly a normal AG at presentation is not sufficient to exclude toxic alcohol ingestion. Early in the clinical course an AG may be normal, only to develop rapidly as metabolism progresses. This is particularly so in the presence of ethanol where the onset of an AG acidosis will be delayed until the ethanol itself has been preferentially metabolized.

Falls in serum bicarbonate and arterial pH correlate well with levels of toxic organic acid metabolites in the circulation and in the absence of direct assays are their chief surrogate markers.[16,20] In this context, it is common practice to exclude toxic ingestion where there is a normal venous bicarbonate (>20) 8 h after the serum or breath ethanol has been documented as undetectable.[21,22]

When available in a clinically useful timeframe direct assays may shorten hospital assessment times especially with accidental exposures. The interpretation of serum methanol and ethylene glycol concentrations requires consideration of time since ingestion, ethanol co-ingestion and acid–base status.

Treatment

The definitive care for methanol and ethylene glycol ingestions is dialysis with concurrent ADH blockade therapy. All cases of deliberate self poisonings with a toxic alcohol need to be managed in a facility with easy access to dialysis if clinical intoxication becomes apparent. ADH blockade therapy can impede the progression of clinical toxicity and permit safe transfer to an appropriate facility.

Alcohol dehydrogenase blockade

Blockade of ADH can be achieved by the administration of either ethanol or the specific ADH antagonist fomepizole (not currently available in Australasia). These agents prevent metabolism of toxic alcohols and the accumulation of their organic acid metabolites. ADH blockade significantly increases the half-life of parent toxic alcohols and in Australasia does not represent definitive care. However, fomepizole can be used in isolation to treat toxic alcohol ingestions where sufficient supplies exist for lengthy therapy and serial levels can be obtained and tracked into safe ranges.[16]

Ethanol therapy can be initiated with a loading dose of 8 mL/kg of 10% ethanol intravenously or 1.8 mL/kg of 43% ethanol orally (equivalent to 3 × 40 mL shots of vodka in a 70 kg adult). Maintenance therapy requires an infusion of 1–2 mL/h of 10% ethanol or 0.2–0.4 mL/h of 43% ethanol orally (equivalent to one 40 mL shot of vodka each hour in a 70 kg adult). The ethanol concentration should be maintained in the range of 100–150 mg/dL (22–33 mmol/L) by careful titration of maintenance administration guided by frequent blood ethanol concentrations.

Haemodialysis

Haemodialysis represents definitive care for confirmed toxic alcohol ingestions. It effectively removes parent toxic alcohols and their acidic metabolites. Lactate free and bicarbonate buffered dialysates may assist the correction of acidaemia. Commonly accepted indications for haemodialysis are listed in Table 29.18.2. Endpoints for haemodialysis are listed in Table 29.18.3. Ethanol is also rapidly cleared by dialysis and ethanol infusion rates need to be increased (usually doubled) during haemodialysis.

Table 29.18.2   Indications for haemodialysis in toxic alcohol poisoning[15,16]
Severe metabolic acidosis (pH<7.25)
Renal failure (ethylene glycol)
History of a large toxic alcohol ingestion and osmolar gap >10 mmol/L
Visual symptoms (methanol)
Ethylene glycol or methanol levels >50 mg/dL (if available)

Table 29.18.3   Endpoints for haemodialysis in toxic alcohol poisoning[15,16]
Correction of acidosis
Osmolar gap <10 mmol/L
Ethylene glycol or methanol level <20 mg/dL (if available)

Supportive care and co-factor therapy

Folinic or folic acid administration is recommended in methanol poisoning (folinic acid 2 mg/kg i.v. qid) to aid in endogenous metabolism of formic acid.[16] Pyridoxine and thiamine supplementation is recommended in ethylene glycol poisoning when the patient is thought to be deplete (e.g. alcoholics), again to aid endogenous metabolism of the pathogenic acids.

In methanol poisoning, systemic acidaemia enhances the movement of formic acid into the intracellular compartment. Correction with intravenous bicarbonate if pH < 7.3 is recommended.[16]

Calcium replacement in ethylene glycol poisoning is contentious given that it may promote calcium oxalate crystal formation. Consequentially, calcium should only be replaced if there is symptomatic hypocalcaemia (including prolongation of the QT interval) or intractable seizures.

Prognosis

Prompt ADH blockade therapy and dialysis ensures an excellent outcome in toxic ingestions who present before the development of established end-organ toxicity. Delayed diagnosis and treatment is associated with death and permanent neurological and renal sequelae, including blindness in the case of methanol poisoning.

Controversies

❶ It has been suggested that EDs could play a pivotal role in reducing ethanol-related morbidity by adopting procedures to detect and refer individuals who misuse ethanol. A number of centres have successfully done trial screening and brief intervention strategies for hazardous ethanol consumption.[23,24]

❷ It is unclear whether fomezipole provides sufficient advantages over ethanol as an ADH blocker in toxic alcohol poisoning so as to justify the expense of importing and stocking it in Australasia.

❸ Co-factor therapy in toxic alcohol poisoning is of unproven efficacy; however, there are few contraindications to their administration.

References

1. Alcohol in Australia: Issues and Strategies. A background paper to the National Alcohol Strategy: A plan for Action 2001 to 2004. Commonwealth of Australia; 2001.
2. Abdulla A, Badawy B. The metabolism of alcohol. Clinical and Endocrinological Metabolism 1978; 7: 247–252.
3. Brennan DF, Bertzelos S, Reed R, et al. Ethanol elimination rates in an ED population. American Journal of Emergency Medicine 1995; 13: 276–280.
4. Adinoff B, Bone GH, Linnoila M. Acute ethanol poisoning and the ethanol withdrawal syndrome. Medical Toxicology 1988; 3: 172–196.
5. Turner RC, Lichstein PR, Peden JG, et al. Alcohol withdrawal syndromes: a review of pathophysiology, clinical presentation and treatment. Journal of General Internal Medicine 1989; 4: 432–444.
6. Berk WA, Todd K. Relationship of abstinence to the presentation and peak intensity of signs and alcohol withdrawal. Annals of Emergency Medicine 1993; 22: 339–345.
7. Reuler JB, Girard DE, Cooney TG. Current concepts. Wernicke's encephalopathy. New England Journal of Medicine 1985; 312: 1035–1039.
8. Sechi G, Serra A. Wernicke's encephalopathy: new clinical settings and recent advances in diagnosis and management. Lancet Neurology 2007; 6: 442–455.
9. Levy LJ, Duga J, Girgis M, et al. Ketoacidosis associated with alcoholism in non-diabetic subjects. Annals of Internal Medicine 1973; 78: 213–219.
10. Cooperman MT, Davidoff F, Spark R, et al. Clinical studies of alcoholic ketoacidosis. Diabetes 1974; 23: 433–439.
11. Fulop K, Hoberman HD. Alcoholic ketosis. Diabetes 1975; 24: 785–790.
12. McGuire LC, Cruickshank AM, Munro PT. Alcoholic ketoacidosis. Emergency Medicine Journal 2006; 23: 417–420.
13. Zuburan C, Fernandes JG, Rodnight R, et al. Wernicke–Korsakoff syndrome. Postgraduate Medical Journal 1997; 73: 27.

14. Fulop M. Alcoholic ketoacidosis. Endocrinological and Metabolic Clinics of North America 1993; 22: 209–219.
15. Barceloux DG, Bond GR, Krenzelok EP, et al. American Academy of Clinical Toxicology Ad Hoc Committee on the Treatment Guidelines for Methanol Poisoning. American Academy of Clinical Toxicology practice guidelines on the treatment of methanol poisoning. Journal of Toxicology Clinical Toxicology 2002; 40(4): 415–446.
16. Barceloux DG, Krenzelok EK, Olson K, et al. American Academy of Clinical Toxicology practice guidelines on the treatment of ethylene glycol poisoning. Journal of Toxicology – Clinical Toxicology 1999; 37(5): 537–560.
17. Jakobsen D, McMartin KE. Methanol and ethylene glycol poisonings: mechanism of toxicity, clinical course, diagnosis and treatment. Medical Toxicology 1986; 1: 309–334.
18. Naraqui S, Dethlefs RF, Slobodniuk RA. An outbreak of acute methyl alcohol intoxication. Australia & New Zealand Journal of Medicine 1979; 9: 65–68.
19. Hoffman RS, Smilkstein MJ, Howland MA, et al. Osmol gaps revisited: normal values and limitations. Journal Toxicology Clinical Toxicology 1993; 31: 81–93.
20. Sejersted OM, Jakobsen D. Formate concentrations in plasma from patients poisoned with methanol. Acta Medica Scandinavica 1983; 1213: 105–110.
21. Jolliff HA, Dart RC, Bogan GM, et al. Can the diagnosis of ethylene glycol toxicity be made without serum EG levels and osmolality values? (abstract). Journal of Toxicology –Clinical Toxicology 2000; 38(5): 539–540.
22. Murray L, Daly FFS, Little M, Cadogan M, eds. Toxicology handbook. Sydney: Elsevier; 2007.
23. Huntley JS, Blain C, Hood S, et al. Improving detection of alcohol misuse in patients presenting to an accident and emergency department. Emergency Medicine Journal 2001; 18: 99–104.
24. Hungerford DW, Pollock DA, Todd KT. Acceptability of emergency department-based screening and brief intervention for alcohol problems. Academic Emergency Medicine 2000; 7: 1383–1392.

29.19 Carbon monoxide

Nick Buckley

ESSENTIALS

1 Carbon monoxide is the commonest agent used in completed suicides by poisoning in Australia and the UK.

2 Carbon monoxide is produced by incomplete combustion and is found in car exhaust, faulty heaters, fires and in industrial settings.

3 Carbon monoxide poisoning may result in significant long-term neuropsychological sequelae.

4 Oxygen increases the elimination of carbon monoxide – and the extent of increase is proportional to the inspired oxygen pressure.

5 The optimal mode of oxygen delivery to improve clinical outcomes remains controversial.

Introduction

Carbon monoxide (CO) poisoning is an important cause of mortality and morbidity from poisoning. Immediate resuscitation including 100% oxygen therapy is essential, and the long-term results of most patients will be good with this simple intervention. It is unclear whether any additional intervention will reduce the low but important risk of serious long-term neurological damage.

Aetiology, pathophysiology and pathology

Carbon monoxide is a colourless, odourless, tasteless and non-irritant gas, produced by incomplete combustion of hydrocarbons.[1]

Small amounts are also produced endogenously by normal metabolic processes. The most common sources of significant exposure are car exhausts, cigarette smoke, fires and faulty home heaters and barbecues. Catalytic converters reduce the production of carbon monoxide and are in all cars manufactured in the last decade or two. Carboxyhaemoglobin (COHb) concentrations in cigarette smokers range as high as 10%.

The pathophysiology of CO exposure is complex and incompletely understood. Upon exposure, CO binds to haemoglobin with an affinity 210 times that of oxygen, thereby decreasing the oxygen-carrying capacity of blood. CO can also produce injury by several other mechanisms, including direct disruption of cellular oxidative processes, binding to myoglobin and cytochrome oxidases and causing peroxidation of brain lipids.[1] However, the end result is tissue hypoxia, leading to varying degrees of end-organ damage and eventually death. The severity of poisoning is a function of the duration of exposure, the ambient concentration of CO and the underlying health status of the exposed individual. Although useful for diagnosis when detected, the initial COHb level correlates poorly with outcome.[2]

Epidemiology

Poisoning with CO is an important cause of unintentional and intentional injury worldwide. In the USA alone, an estimated 1000–2000 accidental deaths due to CO exposure occur each year, resulting from an estimated 40 000 exposures.[3] In Australia and the UK it is the most common agent in completed suicide by poisoning.

Prevention

Prevention of environmental or occupational exposure is possible by use of CO air monitors. COHb concentrations are increased for any given inspired CO concentration if the person is exercising or at high altitudes (increased breathing rate and pulmonary blood flow). These considerations are relevant to acceptable levels of exposure.

The introduction of catalytic converters has reduced CO production in vehicle exhaust, and this in turn appears to be leading to a reduction in fatal suicidal poisoning in some countries.[4,5]

Clinical features

The signs and symptoms of acute carbon monoxide poisoning are shown in Table 29.19.1[6] and correlate well with the maximum COHb concentration. Initial symptoms are non-specific and probably predominantly due to compensatory mechanisms to maintain tissue oxygen delivery to vital organs (e.g. tachycardia, headache, dizziness, gastrointestinal symptoms). Signs with more severe toxicity directly reflect tissue hypoxia with central nervous and cardiovascular toxicity being the most critical manifestations. Death results rapidly when impaired oxygenation of the heart prevents the compensatory increase in cardiac output. The skin is classically cherry pink although severely ill patients are often pale or cyanosed. Preexisting cerebral or cardiovascular disease, anaemia and volume depletion or cardiac failure increases toxicity (for a given COHb). These people all have a reduced ability to compensate by increasing cardiac output or redistributing blood supply to vital organs.

Due to low oxygen pressures, the high affinity of fetal haemoglobin for CO, and the much longer half-life of CO in the fetal circulation, the fetus is particularly susceptible to CO poisoning. The outcome of

Table 29.19.1 Typical clinical symptoms and signs relative to COHb (normal = 0.5%)[6]

COHb (%)	Symptoms and signs
<10	Nil (commonly found in smokers)
10–20	Nil or vague non-descript symptoms
30–40	Headache, tachycardia, confusion, weakness, nausea, vomiting, collapse
50–60	Coma, convulsions, Cheyne–Stokes breathing, arrhythmias, ECG changes
70–80	Circulatory and ventilatory failure, cardiac arrest, death

significant CO poisoning in the mother is often fetal death or neurological damage.

Delayed or persistent neuropsychiatric sequelae occur, largely confined to those who have loss of consciousness at some stage.[7,8] Long-term follow-up is necessary as more subtle defects can develop or become apparent over a few weeks to months. The most common problems encountered are depressed mood (even in those accidentally exposed) and difficulty with higher intellectual functions (especially short-term memory and concentration).[7,8] More severe problems include parkinsonism and speech problems. Neuropsychological testing may detect subtle defects not apparent on crude mini-mental state testing. The incidence of sequelae depends on the definition used – major deficits are relatively uncommon but neuropsychiatric complaints related to memory or concentration may occur in as many as 25–50% of patients with a loss of consciousness.[7,8]

Differential diagnosis

In suicide attempts, the diagnosis of CO poisoning is generally apparent from the circumstances when the person is found. The major diagnostic issue is whether there is some other deliberate self-poisoning as this is extremely common. In unconscious patients, the ECG, paracetamol concentration and electrolytes should be reviewed with this possibility in mind.[6]

A large proportion of victims of smoke inhalation also have cyanide poisoning. This rarely leads to a change in management (due to problems with administering the cyanide antidotes in this setting) but should be suspected when CNS effects are out of proportion with COHb concentrations and if there is a marked lactic acidosis.

Clinical investigation

Blood gases and oximetry

Most pulse oximeters do not measure COHb but merely the ratio of oxyHb to deoxyHb. Thus they may give very misleading results in the setting of CO poisoning. Blood gases with a co-oximeter are required to quantify COHb. COHb concentrations (plus or minus a back calculation based on estimated half-life since removal) provide

a rough guide to the extent of exposure. However, it is difficult to accurately estimate the oxygen dose received pre-hospital and therefore the half-life. There is also substantial variability between individuals in the extent they are able to compensate for high COHb. Therefore, the correlation with acute and long-term clinical effects is not good. COHb may confirm (or possibly exclude) the diagnosis but should not be used to estimate long-term prognosis.

ECG

Patients should have a baseline ECG (electrocardiogram), repeated 6 h later, and ECG monitoring for at least 24 h and cardiac enzymes if the initial ECG is abnormal. The most important signs seen are those of cardiac ischaemia and these are identical to those seen in coronary artery disease.

Biochemistry

Cardiac enzymes should be measured when there is severe clinical toxicity or ECG changes. Metabolic acidosis, predominantly due to lactate will provide an indication of tissue hypoxia. Electrolytes (sodium, potassium, magnesium) should be measured as low concentrations of any of these may exacerbate cardiac toxicity. S100B concentrations, indicating acute neurological injury, have the potential to be useful in estimating neurological damage but further validation is required before they can be related to long-term severity in this setting.[9,10]

Criteria for diagnosis

A high COHb (>15%) with typical symptoms or signs confirms the diagnosis of acute CO poisoning.

In some parts of the world it is common to attribute many non-specific presentations to chronic carbon monoxide exposure, often despite COHb concentrations that are normal or within the range of those seen in 'healthy' smokers. There are no agreed on criteria for making a diagnosis of chronic carbon monoxide poisoning, but the diagnosis should not be seriously entertained without confirmation of high ambient CO concentrations in the proposed environmental source.

Treatment

Initial management is directed towards securing the airway and stabilizing respiration and circulation. If there is impaired consciousness, ensure the airway is maintained with intubation if necessary. The comatose patient should be placed on a cardiac monitor, a 12-lead ECG performed, an intravenous line inserted and blood drawn for full blood count, electrolytes, lactate, COHb, blood sugar and cardiac enzymes. If awake, the patient should be reassured and discouraged from activity, for muscle activity will increase oxygen demand.[6]

Metabolic acidosis should not be treated directly unless the acidosis itself contributes to toxicity (pH < 7.0). It should respond to improved oxygenation and ventilation and the net effect of acidosis on oxygen delivery is probably beneficial.

Oxygen

This decreases the biological half-life substantially from 4 h in ambient air to approximately 40 min in a 100% oxygen atmosphere (Fig. 29.19.1).[6] 100% oxygen should be administered with mechanically assisted ventilation if necessary. In patients able to tolerate it, continuous positive airway pressure by mask may allow 100%

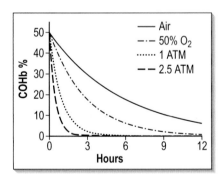

Fig. 29.19.1 Approximate decline in COHb from 50% according to the inspired oxygen concentration and pressure.

oxygen delivery without intubation. Four to six hours of 100% normobaric oxygen will remove over 90% of the carbon monoxide. If the only available oxygen delivery device is a Hudson mask, it should be remembered that at a flow rate of 15 L/min no more than 60% oxygen is delivered. At these concentrations the half-life of CO is still around 90 min and a longer period of oxygen may be required for severe poisonings (Fig. 29.19.1). Oxygen toxicity is unlikely with less than 24 h treatment but the risk increases with increasing exposure.

When immediately available, hyperbaric oxygen (HBO) should be considered for patients with serious CO poisoning. Oxygen at 2–3 atmospheres will further reduce the half-life of COHb to about 20 min (Fig. 29.19.1) but more importantly it causes very rapid reversal of tissue hypoxia due to oxygenation of tissue from oxygen dissolved in the plasma.

Controversy exists on the benefits, risks and indications for HBO (see controversies below). Indications for HBO commonly used by hyperbaric facilities are simply those factors that indicate a higher risk of long-term neuropsychiatric sequelae.[7,8] These include:

- loss of consciousness at anytime during or following exposure
- abnormal neuropsychiatric testing or neurological signs
- pregnancy.

Complications of HBO therapy[7,8] include:

- decompression sickness
- rupture of tympanic membranes
- damaged sinuses
- oxygen toxicity
- problems due to lack of monitoring.

Other treatments

Animal models suggest possible benefits from use of allopurinol and N-acetylcysteine to protect against oxidative damage during hypoxic/reperfusion injury.[11] Numerous experimental (i.e. never used in humans) agents have also been suggested. Their use cannot be recommended outside of clinical trials; however, they may be a more logical treatment to prevent neurological damage from reactive oxygen species than hyperbaric oxygen.

Controversies

❶ The major controversy is about the benefits, risks and indications for HBO – and resolving this 'clinical uncertainty' with further trials will likely be frustrated by some extremely certain HBO clinicians.[12] There have been eight HBO randomized clinical trials (RCTs) reporting very conflicting outcomes. Some have concluded that HBO is harmful[13] and others that it is beneficial.[14] A systematic review found no evidence for benefit from a combined analysis of the trials.[7,8] It also found empiric evidence of multiple biases that operated to inflate the benefit of HBO in two positive trials. In contrast, the interpretation of negative trials was hampered by low rates of follow-up, unusual interventions for control patients and inclusion of less severely poisoned patients.

❷ In centres with a chamber, the use of HBO, when it can be given rapidly and safely, may be justifiable based on the biological rationale that it is the most efficient means of rapidly increasing oxygen delivery and removing carbon monoxide. However, transferring patients between hospitals for delayed use of HBO, particularly over long distances, is not justifiable on current evidence from RCTs, animal studies[15,16] or the known pathophysiology of CO.

References

1. Weaver LK. Carbon monoxide poisoning. Critical Care Clinic 1999; 15(2): 297–317.
2. Seger D, Welch L. Carbon monoxide controversies: neuropsychologic testing, mechanism of toxicity, and hyperbaric oxygen. Annals of Emergency Medicine 1994; 24(2): 242–248.
3. Hampson NB. Emergency department visits for carbon monoxide poisoning in the Pacific Northwest. Journal of Emergency Medicine 1998; 16(5): 695–698.
4. Amos T, Appleby L, Kiernan K. Changes in rates of suicide by car exhaust asphyxiation in England and Wales. Psychological Medicine 2001; 31(5): 935–939.
5. Mott JA, Wolfe MI, Alverson CJ, et al. National vehicle emissions policies and practices and declining US carbon monoxide-related mortality. Journal of American Medical Association 2002; 288(8): 988–995.
6. Buckley NA, Dawson AH, Whyte IM. Hypertox. Assessment and Treatment of Poisoning. http://curriculum.toxicology.wikispaces.net/2.2.9.1.1+Carbon+monoxide. 2006 (accessed 4 September 2008).
7. Buckley NA, Isbister GK, Stokes B, et al. Hyperbaric oxygen for carbon monoxide poisoning : a systematic review and critical analysis of the evidence. Toxicological Review 2005; 24(2): 75–92.
8. Juurlink D, Buckley N, Stanbrook M, et al. Hyperbaric oxygen for carbon monoxide poisoning. Cochrane Database Systematic Review 2005; (1): CD002041.
9. Brvar M, Mozina M, Osredkar J, et al. Prognostic value of S100B protein in carbon monoxide-poisoned rats. Critical Care Medicine 2004; 32(10): 2128–2130.
10. Brvar M, Mozina H, Osredkar J, et al. The potential value of the protein S-100B level as a criterion for hyperbaric oxygen treatment and prognostic marker in carbon monoxide poisoned patients. Resuscitation 2003; 56(1): 105–109.
11. Omaye ST. Metabolic modulation of carbon monoxide toxicity. Toxicology 2002; 180(2): 139–150.
12. Buckley NA, Isbister GK, Juurlink DN. Hyperbaric oxygen for carbon monoxide poisoning : evidence versus opinion. Toxicological Review 2005; 24(3): 159–160.
13. Scheinkestel CD, Bailey M, Myles PS, et al. Hyperbaric or normobaric oxygen for acute carbon monoxide poisoning: a randomised controlled clinical trial. Medical Journal of Australia 1999; 170(5): 203–210.
14. Weaver LK, Hopkins RO, Chan KJ, et al. Hyperbaric oxygen for acute carbon monoxide poisoning. New England Journal of Medicine 2002; 347(14): 1057–1067.
15. Bunc M, Luzar B, Finderle Z, et al. Immediate oxygen therapy prevents brain cell injury in carbon monoxide poisoned rats without loss of consciousness. Toxicology 2006; 225(2–3): 138–141.
16. Brvar M, Finderle Z, Suput D, et al. S100B protein in conscious carbon monoxide-poisoned rats treated with normobaric or hyperbaric oxygen. Critical Care Medicine 2006; 34(8): 2228–2230.

30.1 Snakebite

Geoffrey Isbister

ESSENTIALS

1 Australia has some of the most medically important venomous snakes in the world. All are elapids (front-fanged). New Zealand has no snakes of medical importance.

2 All patients giving a history of possible snakebite should be assessed and observed for at least 12h to rule out envenoming.

3 Most fatalities occur within hours of the bite from initial cardiac arrest and multiorgan failure. Delayed deaths are now uncommon and mainly due to major haemorrhage from the venom-induced consumption coagulopathy from brown snake, the tiger snake group or taipans.

4 Pressure bandaging and immobilization appears to be an effective first-aid measure if applied early and the patient remains immobile. However, this is rarely done except in snake handlers.

5 Australian snakes are difficult to identify and treatment should be based only on expert identification of snakes, the clinical syndrome or a snake venom detection kit in an envenomed patient.

6 Antivenom is indicated for all patients with clinical or laboratory evidence of envenoming. CSL Ltd. makes antivenoms for brown snake, black snake, tiger snake, taipan and death adder, as well as a polyvalent antivenom containing antivenoms to all five.

7 Antivenom should be given early and then sufficient time allowed for recovery, especially of venom-induced consumption coagulopathy which takes 6–18h to recovery.

8 CSL antivenom is a horse-derived F(ab')$_2$ antibody and is associated with early allergic reactions in about 25% of cases, although severe anaphylaxis occurs in only 5%. Premedication is not recommended but adrenaline should be immediately available for treatment of anaphylaxis.

Introduction

Australia has a number of venomous snakes with some of the most potent venoms in the world. All the medically important snakes are elapids (front-fanged), although bites occur from colubrids and non-venomous snakes. New Zealand has no snakes of medical importance. The risk of significant coagulopathy and uncommonly death, even after apparently trivial contact with Australian snakes, remains and must be appreciated by healthcare workers.

Epidemiology

It is thought that approximately 3000 human snakebites occur annually in Australia but this figure is difficult to estimate and depends on how many suspected bites, non-venomous bites and non-envenomed cases are included. The number of envenomed cases is far less and probably in the order of 100 to 300 each year; the majority of which occur in rural and regional areas. Snakebite deaths continue to occur (about 1 to 4 per year) and are usually a result of early cardiac arrest in brown snakebites or major haemorrhage in coagulopathic patients.

The commonest clinical manifestation is coagulopathy which occurs in about three-quarters of envenomed cases, about half from brown snakes and half from the tiger snake group. Neurotoxicity and myotoxicity are now uncommon and mechanical ventilation is rarely required for treatment. The types of snakes causing major envenoming differ across Australia. Exotic snakebite remains a problem from snakes in zoos and an unknown number of illegally kept snakes, but hospital presentations are rare.

Prevention

Most snakebites are preventable and result from snake handling or interference with snakes in the wild, sometimes in the setting of alcohol consumption. Ideally, snakes should be left alone in the wild and those working with or keeping snakes should have appropriate training and licenses. Simple precautions such as wearing thick long pants and boots when walking in the bush or when working with snakes can prevent many bites due to the short length of Australian snake fangs. Snake handlers should carry and maintain first-aid kits that include at least four broad elastic bandages (15 cm; e.g. Ace®) and have practised applying the bandage. If exotic snakes are being held (including Australasian snakes out of their geographical distribution), appropriate antivenoms should be available.

Clinical features and toxinology

Envenoming results when venom is injected subcutaneously and reaches the systemic circulation. Whether or not a snakebite results in envenoming depends on a number of factors including fang length, average venom yield of the snake, effectiveness of the bite and bite site. Recent studies have suggested that only a small amount of the injected venom actually reaches the systemic circulation.[1]

Most snakebites do not result in envenoming because either insufficient venom reaches the systemic circulation or the snake is non-venomous. Envenoming is characterized by local and systemic effects, although Australasian elapids rarely cause major local effects such as necrosis and haemorrhage. The clinical features of envenoming depend on the particular toxins present in each snake's venom but non-specific systemic effects (nausea, vomiting, headache, abdominal pain, diarrhoea and diaphoresis) occur in most cases. The major clinical syndromes are coagulopathy, neurotoxicity, myotoxicity and renal impairment. Severe envenoming can result in early collapse associated with dizziness, loss of consciousness, apnoea and hypotension. In the majority of cases there is spontaneous recovery over 5 to 15 min, but in some cases this does not occur and multiorgan failure and death ensue if resuscitation is delayed.

The medically important Australian snakes and their associated clinical effects are listed in Table 30.1.1.

Coagulopathy

Venom-induced consumption coagulopathy (VICC)

This is the commonest and most important clinical effect in Australian snake envenoming. Venom-induced consumption coagulopathy (VICC) results from a pro-thrombin activator in the snake venom converting prothrombin (factor II) to thrombin which leads to consumption of fibrinogen, massive increases in fibrinogen degradation products and consumption of factors V and VIII due to thrombin activation. Most dangerous Australian snakes contain such a prothrombin activator including brown snakes, snakes in the tiger snake group and taipans. Venom-induced consumption coagulopathy develops rapidly within 15 to 60 min and the onset may coincide with the initial collapse seen with major envenoming by brown snakes and taipans. Recovery usually takes 12 to 18 h.[2]

Table 30.1.1 Summary of clinical effects, diagnosis and antivenom requirements for envenoming by major Australian snakes				
Snake type	Major clinical effect	Other clinical effects	VDK	Antivenom requirements
Brown snakes	VICC	Often asymptomatic; mild thrombocytopenia or rarely thrombotic microangiopathy (microangiopathic haemolytic anaemia, thrombocytopenia and renal failure)	+ve brown	2 vials brown snake antivenom
Tiger snake group[1]	VICC	Non-specific systemic effects, myotoxicity and neurotoxicity[2]	+ve tiger	2 vials tiger snake antivenom
Red-bellied black snake	Non-specific systemic effects	Anticoagulant coagulopathy and mild myotoxicity	+ve black[3] (eastern Australia)	1 vial of tiger or black snake antivenom
Death adder	Neurotoxicity	Non-specific systemic effects	+ve death adder	1 vial of death adder antivenom
Taipan	VICC and neurotoxicity	Non-specific systemic effects	+ve taipan (northern Australia)	3 vials of taipan antivenom
Mulga snake[4]	Myotoxicity	Non-specific systemic effects and an anticoagulant coagulopathy	VDK +ve black (not eastern seaboard)	1 vial of black snake antivenom

[1]This group includes tiger snakes (Notechis sp.) which occur in southern Australia, rough-scaled or Clarence River tiger snake (Tropidechus carinatus) occurring in northern NSW and Queensland and Hoplocephalus spp. (broad-headed, pale-headed and Stephen's banded snake) also occurring in mid- and north-eastern Australia.
[2]Myotoxicity and neurotoxicity have a much slower onset compared to VICC and may only manifest if treatment is delayed.
[3]Often positive in wells 1 and 3 (tiger and black).
[4]Collett's snake causes similar effects and is treated the same but almost exclusively occurs in snake handlers.

Anticoagulant coagulopathy

This occurs with Mulga and Collett's snake, and in about half of red-bellied black snake envenomings. It is unlikely to result in haemorrhage and of itself is rarely of clinical importance. However, anticoagulant coagulopathy is a marker of significant envenoming and is rapidly reversed with antivenom.

Neurotoxicity

Paralysis is a classic effect of snakebite and is due to either presynaptic or postsynaptic neurotoxins. Presynaptic neurotoxins disrupt neurotransmitter release from the terminal axon and are associated with cellular damage. This type of neurotoxicity does not respond to antivenom treatment and takes days to weeks to resolve. Postsynaptic neurotoxins competitively block acetylcholine receptors and this type of neurotoxicity is reported to be reversed by antivenom. Neurotoxic envenoming manifests as a progressive descending flaccid paralysis. The first sign is usually ptosis followed by facial and bulbar involvement and progressing to paralysis of the extraocular muscles, respiratory muscles and peripheral weakness in severe cases.

Myotoxicity

Some Australian snakes contain myotoxins that cause damage to skeletal muscles resulting in local and/or generalized muscle pain, tenderness and weakness, associated with a rapidly rising creatine kinase and myoglobinuria. In rare severe cases, secondary renal impairment can occur.

Renal damage

Renal impairment or acute renal failure can occur secondary to severe myolysis, in association with thrombotic microangiopathy or, more rarely and to a minor degree, in isolation with brown snake envenoming. Thrombotic microangiopathy occurs in a small proportion of brown snakebites and is characterized by severe thrombocytopenia worse 3 to 4 days after the bite, acute renal failure often lasting 2 to 8 weeks and requiring dialysis, and microangiopathic haemolytic anaemia. This is also reported less commonly with taipan and tiger snakebites.

Local effects

Local effects vary from minimal effects with brown snakebites to local pain, swelling and occasionally tissue injury following black and tiger snakebites.

Most fatalities occur within hours of the bite from initial cardiac arrest and multiorgan failure. Delayed deaths are now uncommon and mainly due to major haemorrhage from the VICC from brown snake, the tiger snake group or taipan. Respiratory failure from neurotoxicity remains a problem in Papua New Guinea where there continue to be large numbers of cases, mainly taipan bites, and a shortage of both antivenom and resources for mechanical ventilation.

Treatment

First aid

Australian snake venoms appear to be absorbed via the lymphatic system so absorption is likely to be increased by movement and exercise. The aim of first aid is to minimize movement of venom to the systemic circulation. This is achieved by a pressure bandage (elastic bandage such as ACE®) being applied over the bite site and then covering the whole limb with a similar pressure to that used for a limb sprain. The bitten limb must be immobilized as well as the whole patient, or the first aid is ineffective.[3] Immobilization consists of splinting and complete prevention of movement or exercise of the bitten part. It has been shown that movement of all limbs, not just the affected one, needs to be minimized for optimal effect.[4] Transport should be brought to the patient and walking must be avoided. Prompt, properly applied first aid probably prevents significant absorption of venom for many hours although there is only anecdotal evidence to support this. Pressure bandaging is clearly impractical for bites that are not on the limbs but direct pressure with a pad and immobilization may be useful. The bite site should not be washed so that it can be swabbed for venom detection.

First aid must eventually be removed but this should take place in a resuscitation area of a facility with the means to definitively treat envenoming. The first aid is removed when:

- thorough clinical and laboratory assessment fail to demonstrate any evidence of envenoming. In these patients, further clinical and laboratory evaluation for suspected envenoming is needed following removal of the bandage
- there is definite clinical or laboratory evidence of envenoming. The bandage is removed after commencement of treatment with intravenous antivenom. Although there is no evidence of any difference in outcome related to timing, removal of bandaging halfway through the initial dose of antivenom is commonly recommended.

Initial assessment and treatment

Figure 30.1.1 provides a simple approach to the management of suspected and envenomed snakebite patients. The patient is managed in an area with full resuscitation facilities. Assessment and management proceed simultaneously. The airway, breathing and circulation are assessed and stabilized. The majority of patients are not critically unwell and can have a focused neurological examination for early signs of paralysis (e.g. ptosis, drooling), examination of draining lymph nodes and general examination for signs of bleeding (oozing from the bite site, gum bleeds). Intravenous access should be established and intravenous fluids commenced.

Further management

Two major diagnostic and risk assessment issues exist for snakebite:

- whether or not the patient is envenomed;
- in patients with envenoming, which snake is responsible and therefore which antivenom should be administered.

The majority of patients are not envenomed, but all patients must initially be assessed as if they are potentially envenomed. Asymptomatic patients, particularly those seen early after a brown snakebite, may still be severely envenomed with VICC. The diagnosis of envenoming is made on history, examination and the clinical investigations listed below. Although systemic envenoming can be ambiguous in patients with mild envenoming, the following definitions are useful for determining whether patients require antivenom:

- VICC is defined as an elevated international normalized ratio (INR) or prothrombin time (PT) associated with an elevated D-dimer. A low or unrecordable fibrinogen will also occur but is not required for the diagnosis. In the majority of cases there is complete consumption with unrecordable PT/INR, activated partial thromboplastin time (aPTT) and undetectable fibrinogen and the decision to give antivenom is straightforward. Milder forms of coagulopathy may occur with elevated D-dimer and only minimally elevated INR. Antivenom is still indicated in most cases but these can be discussed with a clinical toxicologist.

- Neurotoxicity is defined as at least ptosis, but usually progresses without antivenom to include bulbar palsy, extra-ocular ophthalmoplegia, respiratory muscle paralysis and limb paralysis.
- Myotoxicity is defined as local or generalized myalgia and/or muscle weakness in association with an elevated creatine kinase.
- Non-specific systemic features include nausea, vomiting, abdominal pain, diarrhoea, diaphoresis and headache and may in some cases be an indication for antivenom depending on the type of snake.

If there is no evidence of envenoming after clinical assessment and initial laboratory testing the first-aid bandage can be removed. The patient requires ongoing close observation including repeated investigations one hour after bandage removal, and at 6 and 12 h after the bite (see Figure 30.1.1).

If the patient is envenomed then management must proceed with antivenom. A small number of patients present in extremis, usually following collapse and in cardiac arrest and should have antivenom administered immediately as part of advanced life support.

The next step is to determine the snake group responsible for the envenoming in order to allow the administration of the appropriate monovalent antivenom. This is done taking into account:

- local geographical information on the potential snake species that could be responsible
- clinical syndrome (see Table 30.1.1)
- snake venom detection kit (SVDK).

In the majority of cases a combination of these three factors allows determination of

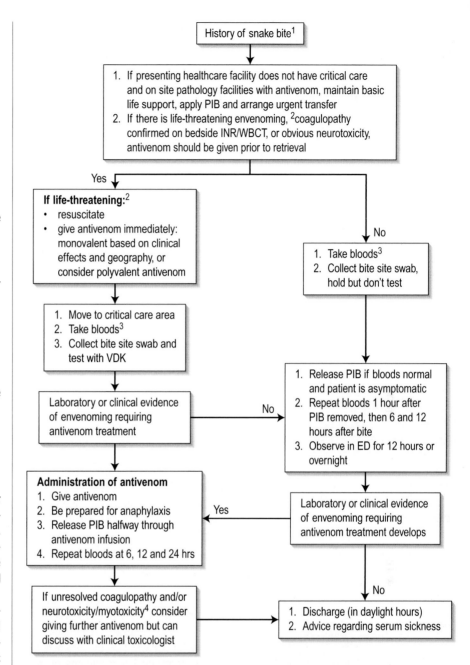

Figure 30.1.1 Early management of snakebite (modified from Therapeutic Guidelines Emergency Medicine, March 2008 with permission)
[1]A toxicologist can be contacted at anytime via the Poison Information Centre 131126.
[2]Cardiac arrest, respiratory failure secondary to paralysis or major haemorrhage (intracranial, major gastrointestinal or other life-threatening bleeding).
[3]Blood tests include: coagulation tests (INR/PT, aPTT, D-dimer, fibrinogen), FBC and blood film for fragments red cells, EUC, CK and LDH.
[4]Any improvement in coagulation studies such as measurable but still abnormal aPTT or PT after 6 h is sufficient evidence of resolving coagulopathy. Neurotoxicity and myotoxicity are usually irreversible and further antivenom is unlikely to help.
PIB, pressure immobilization bandaging; INR, international normalized ratio; WBCT, whole blood clotting time; ED, Emergency Department.

the correct monovalent snake antivenom required. If it is unclear which snake is involved then one vial of polyvalent antivenom should be administered. This contains sufficient antivenom for an initial dose for all types of snakes. In some parts of Australia, such as Victoria and Perth, a combination of brown and tiger snake antivenom can be administered in preference to polyvalent. In Tasmania only tiger snake antivenom is required.

Administration of antivenom

Snake antivenom should be administered by the intravenous route after being diluted 1 in 10 with normal saline or Hartmann's solution and administered over 15 min. In patients with cardiac arrest or life-threatening effects, undiluted antivenom may be administered more rapidly.

The initial dose of antivenom for children is the same as for adults and is provided in Table 30.1.1. Further doses are usually not required and recovery is determined by the reversibility of effects and the time it takes for recovery once venom is neutralized. The benefits of antivenom are listed in Table 30.1.2, which underlines the

Table 30.1.2 The benefits of antivenom for different effects of envenoming (Modified from Therapeutic Guidelines Emergency Medicine, March 2008 with permission)	
Clinical effect	**Benefit**
Venom-induced consumption coagulopathy (VICC)	Appears to neutralize toxin effect allowing clotting factors to be resynthesized and clotting to recover over 6 to 18 hours
Anticoagulant coagulopathy	Neutralizes a toxin inhibitor of coagulation with immediate improvement in coagulation studies
Neurotoxicity	Neutralizes toxin in the intravascular compartment and will prevent further development of neurotoxicity but will not reverse neurotoxic effects already present
Myolysis/ rhabdomyolysis	Neutralizes myotoxins and will prevent further muscle injury but will not reverse effects
Local effects	Unlikely to reverse any already developed local effects
Renal damage	Unlikely to have an effect

Generalized systemic effects: nausea, vomiting, headache, abdominal pain, diarrhoea and diaphoresis.
Rapidly reverses non-specific effects and is a useful indication of antivenom binding venom components.

importance of waiting for recovery after antivenom administration, particularly with VICC.[5] Although there is controversy over the dose of antivenom, recent studies have demonstrated that previously recommended large doses are not required. For brown snake envenoming an initial dose of two vials binds all venom and sufficient time must then be allowed for resynthesis of clotting factors.[1,2]

Premedication for snake antivenom administration has previously been controversial but is no longer recommended in Australia. One randomized controlled trial suggested that adrenaline was an effective premedication for snake antivenom.[6] However, the trial was for an antivenom with a much higher reaction rate and was too small to assess the safety of adrenaline.[7] Promethazine has been shown to be ineffective as a premedication,[8] and often leads to drowsiness that makes neurological assessment difficult. Immediate-type hypersensitivity reactions occur in about a quarter of antivenom administrations in Australia, but are only severe (mainly hypotension) in 5% of administrations.[9] Reactions are more common with tiger snake antivenom and polyvalent antivenom compared to brown snake antivenom. Antivenom should always be administered in a critical care area with readily available adrenaline, intravenous fluids and resuscitation equipment.

The frequency of delayed-type reactions to antivenom or serum sickness is probably higher than acute reactions and likely to depend on the amount of horse protein administered. All patients given antivenom should be warned of serum sickness and a course of oral steroids (prednisolone 50 mg/day for 5 days) may be considered in patients receiving large amounts of antivenom. However, there is no evidence that prophylactic corticosteroids will reduce the risk of serum sickness. A similar course of steroids should be used for treatment in patients who re-present with serum sickness.

Other treatments

Tetanus prophylaxis should be given as appropriate but local wound care is rarely required with Australasian snakes due to minimal local effects.

Preliminary clinical studies have shown that the use of fresh frozen plasma (FFP) appears to speed the recovery of VICC if administered early (after antivenom), but whether the decreased risk of bleeding is large enough to balance the risk of blood products remains unclear. Previously the theoretical concern was that the administration of clotting factors would worsen the consumptive process, but there is no evidence to support this. Until further evidence is available FFP should be reserved for patients with coagulopathy and active bleeding.

Clinical investigation

Assessment of the potentially envenomed requires the following investigations to be performed, usually serially:

- coagulation profile: prothrombin time (PT) or international normalized ratio (INR), activated partial thromboplastin time (aPTT), cross-linked fibrinogen degradation products or D-dimers and fibrinogen
- full blood count including a blood film looking for fragments, red cells and evidence of haemolysis
- urea, creatinine, electrolytes, creatine kinase and lactate dehydrogenase
- blood group and cross-match
- snake venom detection kit (SVDK): a swab should be taken from the bite site
- Urinalysis.

Snake venom detection kit

It is important to note that the SVDK is designed to confirm which major snake group is responsible and therefore which antivenom to be given. It does not confirm or exclude envenoming and should only be included in the assessment of envenomed patients. It is best done by laboratory staff. In all patients with suspected snake envenoming a bite site swab must be collected and stored. The bandage should not be removed to swab the wound: a window should be cut to obtain access. Controversy remains as to whether this should be tested immediately or left to be tested if the patient becomes envenomed.

In non-envenomed patients the SVDK has a high false positive rate, especially in the brown snake well. This is even more problematic for urine testing so a bite site swab is preferred if available. A positive VDK on urine does not indicate systemic toxicity and in asymptomatic patients with normal laboratory studies this is most likely a false positive. The test should not be done on blood. If the snake responsible for the bite accompanies the patient, a swab of the fangs can be tested except that this may require considerable dilution because it will be too concentrated and overwhelms the SVDK with all wells changing colour.

Disposition

Patients with suspected snakebite but no evidence of envenoming one hour after the removal of first aid may be admitted to an observation area. Blood tests including coagulation studies and a creatine kinase (CK) should be repeated at 1 and 6h after first aid is removed and be observed for 12 h or overnight (Fig. 30.1.1). Envenomed patients requiring ventilatory support should have continued management in ICU, but patients with coagulopathy only

are commonly managed in ED observation wards.

Controversies

❶ The initial antivenom dose appears to be less than previously recommended. Excessive dosing of antivenom is a result of insufficient time being allowed for VICC to recover after venom binding by antivenom.

❷ Although factor replacement appears to speed the recovery of VICC, whether the decreased risk of bleeding is large enough to balance the risk of blood products remains unclear.

References

1. Isbister GK, O'Leary MA, Schneider JJ, et al. Efficacy of antivenom against the procoagulant effect of Australian brown snake (Pseudonaja sp.) venom: In vivo and in vitro studies. Toxicon 2007; 49: 57–67.
2. Isbister GK, Williams V, Brown SG, et al. Clinically applicable laboratory end-points for treating snakebite coagulopathy. Pathology 2006; 38: 568–572.
3. Sutherland SK, Coulter AR, Harris RD. Rationalisation of first-aid measures for elapid snake bite. Lancet 1979; 1: 183–186.
4. Howarth DM, Southee AE, Whyte IM. Lymphatic flow rates and first-aid in simulated peripheral snake or spider envenomation. Medical Journal 1994; 161: 695–700.
5. Isbister GK. Snake bite: a current approach to management. Australian Prescribing 2006; 29: 125–129.
6. Premawardhena AP, de Silva CE, Fonseka MMD, et al. Low dose subcutaneous adrenaline to prevent acute adverse reactions to antivenom serum in people bitten by snakes: randomised, placebo controlled trial. British Medical Journal 1999; 318: 1041–1043.
7. Lalloo DG, Theakston RD. Snake antivenoms. Journal of Toxicology: Clinical Toxicology. 2003; 41: 277–290.
8. Fan HW, Marcopito LF, Cardoso JL, et al. Sequential randomised and double blind trial of promethazine prophylaxis against early anaphylactic reactions to antivenom for bothrops snake bites. British Medical Journal 1999; 318: 1451–1452.
9. Isbister GK, Brown SG, MacDonald E, et al. Australian Snakebite Project Investigators. Current use of Australian snake antivenoms and frequency of immediate-type hypersensitivity reactions and anaphylaxis. Medical Journal Australia. 2008 Apr 21;188(8):473–476.

30.2 Spider bite

Geoffrey Isbister

ESSENTIALS

1 Australasia has a number of venomous spiders but the majority of bites cause only minor problems.

2 Fatalities have been recorded in Australia after bites by the redback and the funnel web spiders (FWS).

3 Redback spider (a widow spider) bite is the most common cause of medically significant human envenoming in Australia. It can cause severe and persistent pain, and less often systemic effects.

4 Australia appears to have the highest rate of widow spider envenoming (latrodectism) in the world.

5 Funnel web spider bite can cause life-threatening neurotoxic envenoming.

6 Redback antivenom is a horse-derived F(ab')₂ antivenom and causes relatively few allergic reactions (5%). The antivenom can be given intramuscularly or intravenously and the initial dose should be two vials.

7 Antivenom to the FWS is rabbit serum based and so less antigenic. No premedication is necessary and it is given intravenously.

Introduction

Australasia is home to a variety of spiders as well as some species that have been introduced, probably including the redback spider. The majority of spiders have small jaws which are too small to penetrate human skin. Larger spiders with toxic venom, and habits and distribution that promote human encounters, can cause medically significant envenoming. Although there are over 2000 characterized species of spiders in Australia, a much smaller group is responsible for the majority of human bites with six families of spiders being responsible for over 80% of bites.[1] Spiders commonly responsible for human bites include huntsman spiders (*Sparassidae*), orb weaving spiders (*Araneidae*), white-tail spiders (*Lampona* spp.), redback spiders and the closely related *Steatoda* spp. (*Theridiidae*), wolf spiders (*Lycosidae*) and jumping spiders (*Salticidae*).[1] Fatalities have occurred in Australia after being bitten by the redback and the funnel web spider (FWS).[2]

Redback spider (*Latrodectus hasselti*)

Distribution and taxonomy

The redback spider is a member of the widow group of spiders (*Latrodectus* spp.). The widow spider group is the single most medically important group of spiders worldwide and belongs to the family of comb-footed spiders (*Theridiidae*). Widow spiders are distributed throughout the world and thrive in urban environments, ensuring that they frequently come into contact with humans. There are probably around 40 species, including the North American black widow (*Latrodectus mactans*), the Australian redback (*L. hasselti*), the New Zealand katipo (*L. katipo*) and the brown widow (*L. geometricus*), which is found on most continents including Australia. All species produce venom with similar properties although the clinical syndrome (latrodectism) appears to differ in some cases. Australia probably has the highest rate of latrodectism in the world, with at least 2000 definite bites per annum. New Zealand reports few cases of envenoming by its widow spider, the katipo. There is at least one other important genus of spiders in this family, *Steatoda* spp., that is responsible for human envenoming. They are black spiders with the same body shape and size as widow spiders, but without the red markings.

Venom

The components toxic to humans in the venom of widow spiders are α-latrotoxins that cause massive release of neurotransmitters and deplete synaptic vesicles at nerve endings. Recent work based on in vitro effects suggests that all widow spiders have a similar toxin.[3] However, although the effects of the toxin are well understood at the cellular level it remains unclear how it produces the clinical syndrome.

Epidemiology

Most bites occur when the spider is disturbed in human-made objects, such as clothes, shoes, gloves, furniture, building materials and sheds. The majority of bites are on extremities and occur during the warmer months of the year. There were at least 13 deaths in Australia prior to the introduction of antivenom. High reported mortality rates in other countries such as the USA are likely to be overestimates due to reporting bias.

Clinical features

The majority of patients bitten develop some effects from redback spider bites with pain being the most common and important symptom. Systemic effects occur in about a third of cases. Initially the bite may be painless, or may feel like a pinprick or a burning sensation. The pain then increases over the first hour and may radiate proximally to the regional lymph nodes or the chest or abdomen. Localized sweating and less commonly piloerection may occur and are virtually pathognomonic of latrodectism. Regional and distant sweating is also common, and bilateral below knee sweating can occur. Systemic effects include malaise, lethargy, nausea and vomiting and headache. A summary of the clinical effects is listed in Table 30.2.1, including less common effects. Pain and systemic effects persist for 1 to 4 days.[4] Delayed effects or effects persisting for days to weeks have been reported but it

Table 30.2.1 Clinical features of redback spider bite (Reproduced with permission from Therapeutic Guidelines Emergency Medicine 2008)

Local and regional effects
- Local pain: increasing pain at the bite site over minutes to hours, which can last for days
- Radiating pain: from the bite site to the proximal limb, trunk or local lymph nodes
- Local sweating
- Regional sweating: unusual distributions of diaphoresis, e.g. bilateral below knee diaphoresis
- Less common effects: piloerection, local erythema, fang marks (5%)

Systemic effects
- Nausea, vomiting and headache
- Malaise and lethargy
- Remote or generalized pain
- Abdominal, back or chest pain
- Less common effects: hypertension, irritability and agitation,[1] fever, paraesthesia or patchy paralysis, muscle spasms, priapism

[1]More common with paediatric cases.

is unclear in many cases whether the effects are a consequence of the spider bite.

Diagnosis

The diagnosis is clinical and based on history, typically one of persistent increasing pain that can radiate, and may be associated with local sweating. There are no tests to confirm latrodectism. As the bite may not be felt, doctors should suspect the condition in circumstances where patients have been working in sheds, potting plants, or where contact with widow spiders is possible.

Treatment

First aid

Local application of ice has been recommended although its efficacy remains unproven. Warm compresses provide relief in some cases. Pressure-immobilization bandaging is not appropriate.

Analgesia

Adequate analgesia is an important part of the treatment of redback spider bite. Paracetamol and/or non-steroidal anti-inflammatories and/or oral opioids should be used initially, although intravenous opioids may be required if the pain does not respond. Failure to respond to intravenous opioids is frequently reported and further research is required to define the most appropriate analgesia in redback spider bite.

Antivenom therapy

Antivenom is regarded as the primary treatment for redback spider bite. Despite it conventionally being given by the intramuscular (i.m.) route there has been increased use by the intravenous (i.v.) route. Two randomized controlled trials have shown no difference between i.v. and i.m. antivenom administration and the median dose used in both trials was two vials.[5] Fears that i.v. antivenom results in a higher rate of reactions are not founded yet and the reaction rate with diluted i.v. administration is similar to that with i.m. antivenom.[6] It is therefore reasonable to administer redback antivenom by either i.m. injection or slow i.v. infusion (diluted in 100 mL normal saline and given over 15 min). The initial dose should be two vials and premedication is not recommended. Repeat doses of antivenom are sometimes used and reassessment is appropriate after a period of 2 h. However, it is important that ongoing analgesia is also given to the patient. As for all antivenoms, the dose for children is the same as for adults.

Steatoda species (Cupboard or button spiders)

There have been a number of reports of bites by *Steatoda* spp., mainly in Australia.[7] They appear to cause a similar syndrome to latrodectism with persistent local pain but fewer systemic features. In vitro studies of these spiders' venom demonstrate that they cause similar but far less potent effects compared to α-latrotoxin. These studies also demonstrate in vitro neutralization of *Steatoda* venom with redback antivenom.[8] The majority of bites by this group of spiders cause only minor effects, although the patient may have annoying pain for a period of hours.[7] Uncommonly, they can cause more severe and persistent pain, similar to widow spiders. In the latter case it is postulated that redback antivenom may be an appropriate treatment.[7]

Funnel web spider (*Atrax* and *Hadronyche* Species)

Distribution and taxonomy

At least 39 species of funnel web spiders (FWS) occur along the east coast of Australia, including Tasmania and Adelaide. However, only six species occurring from Southern NSW to Southern Queensland have been associated with significant envenoming – Sydney FWS (*Atrax robustus*), the Southern Tree FWS (*Hadronyche cerberea*), the Northern Tree FWS (*H. formidabilis*), the Blue Mountains FWS (*H. versuta*), the Toowoomba or Darling Downs FWS (*H. infensa*) and the Port Macquarie FWS (*H.* sp 14).[9] Historical records suggest there is an increase in bites by other species in the last few decades compared to most

bites being due to the Sydney FWS in the past. This may be due to increasing population density in the area of distribution of *Hadronyche* species. Funnel web spiders are burrowing spiders and most encounters with humans occur when males are out looking for mates.

Venom

The males have a more potent venom than the females and only males have been reported to cause significant illness in humans.[10] The important toxins in human envenoming appears to be δ-atracotoxins which have been isolated from the venom of a number of species of FWS.[10] These are low-molecular-weight neurotoxins that prevent inactivation of sodium channels. The main effect of the neurotoxin is an autonomic storm that can be predominantly sympathetic or parasympathetic, or mixed in effect, associated with initial excitation at neuromuscular junctions, followed by paralysis.[10]

Epidemiology

Although there are a large number of suspected FWS bites each year, severe envenoming is rare and only 5 to 10 cases requiring antivenom occur annually.[9] Many definite bites by FWS do not result in envenoming (dry bites) and the frequency of non-envenoming varies between species.[9] In addition, many cases are a result of other big black spiders that appear to be FWS and are not collected or identified.

Clinical features

The initial bite is painful due to the size of the fangs and fang marks are usually present. Severe envenoming develops rapidly and usually occurs within 30 min.[9] Initial effects include paraesthesia (local, distal extremities and perioral), local fasciculations, tongue fasciculations and non-specific systemic effects (nausea, vomiting and abdominal pain). Autonomic features are typical of systemic envenoming with hypersalivation, lacrimation and generalized sweating. Other autonomic features can include miosis, mydriasis, tachycardia or bradycardia and hypertension. Initially, the patient is usually agitated and anxious with decreased level of consciousness and coma

developing as late signs.[9] Non-cardiogenic pulmonary oedema may develop, and is thought to result from venom-induced capillary leakage. Prior to antivenom treatment this occurred early, but is now more commonly reported as a delayed effect.

Diagnosis

As with redback spider bite the diagnosis is clinical.

Treatment

First aid

Pressure-immobilization is the recommended first aid and if not applied at the scene, it should be applied in hospital on arrival.

Supportive treatment

With the introduction of antivenom therapy the requirement for intensive care therapy is less common. Attention to basic resuscitation is essential, but usually does not require more than i.v. fluid therapy after assessment and stabilization of the airway and ventilation. Atropine can be used to treat cholinergic features, but this is not a substitute for antivenom. The use of inotropes and other pharmacological agents is unnecessary except in the rare instance of delayed presentation with severe envenoming not responding to antivenom. If pulmonary oedema occurs, this can be treated with diuretics and continuous positive airways pressure ventilation in association with antivenom therapy.

Antivenom therapy

Definitive treatment is venom neutralization with specific FWS antivenom. The antivenom is derived from rabbit serum and appears to be less antigenic to humans than horse serum antivenoms with a low reaction rate (<2%).[9] Premedication is not recommended but antivenom must be administered in a critical care area with adrenaline available. Antivenom is indicated for systemic envenoming as defined above. Initially, two vials should be given (four if severe), and repeated every 15 min if there is no improvement. Delayed serum sickness reactions have been reported in at least one case.[9]

Mouse spiders (*Missulena* spp.)

Another group of spiders, the mouse spiders (*Missulena* spp.), are rarely reported to cause similar effects to FWSs.[11] These spiders belong to the family *Actinopodidae*, and occur in most parts of Australia. Most bites are by wandering male spiders and do not cause any major effects. The initial bite causes pain and fang marks, due to the size of the fangs. There is one report of a bite by the Eastern mouse spider (*Missulena bradleyi*) that caused a syndrome similar to funnel web envenoming in a 19-month-old child.[11] Recent work on the venom of the Eastern mouse spider has demonstrated that the venom causes similar effects in vitro to FWS venom, and it is neutralized in vitro by funnel web antivenom.[12] However, all other reported cases have caused only local effects and less commonly local neurotoxic effects and/or mild non-specific systemic effects.[11]

Other Australasian spiders

There are a number of other Australian spiders that can and do cause human bites. In the majority of cases they cause only minor effects and symptomatic treatment is all that is required. In a large study of definite spider bites there were no cases of necrotic lesions or allergic reactions, suggesting these effects are either rare or do not occur.[1] The incidence of secondary infection is also low, and occurred in less than 1% of cases in the same study.[1]

Necrotic arachnidism

Necrotic arachnidism is generally defined as necrotic lesions or ulcers that occur following a spider bite and are a result of venom effects. Significant skin necrosis following bites from recluse spiders (*Loxosceles* species) is well reported in many parts of the world.[13] *Loxosceles rufescens* has been introduced to South Australia and has been responsible for a few bites, but there is no evidence that it has spread beyond this distribution.

The white-tailed spider (*Lampona cylindrata/murina* group) has been implicated in the development of necrotic arachnidism. However, recent studies show that this is not the case, with 130 definite bites by these spiders causing no cases of necrotic lesions.[14]

Other spiders have been implicated in this condition, including wolf spiders, sac spiders and the black house spiders, but there is similarly little evidence to support this and prospective cases of definite bites by these groups of spiders have not demonstrated necrotic lesions.[1] Table 30.2.2 provides an approach to the patient with a skin ulcer attributed to a spider bite.

An approach to the patient with spider bite

The first step is to take a careful history so as to determine whether the case is a definite spider bite or only a suspected spider bite. The diagnosis of definite spider bite requires sighting of the spider at the time of the bite and usually some initial symptoms such as local pain. If there is no history of bite or no spider was seen, then other diagnoses must be excluded. This is particularly important in persons presenting with ulcers or skin lesions with suspected spider bites (Table 30.2.2). It is important in these cases that appropriate investigations are done and the case treated as a necrotic ulcer of unknown aetiology. In the majority of these cases an infective cause is found, although less commonly they are a result of pyoderma gangrenosum or a vasculitis.[15]

If the patient has a definite history of a spider bite and has either captured the spider or has a good description of the spider, a simple approach can be taken. Health professionals should not attempt to identify spiders beyond the following simple classification:

Table 30.2.2 An approach to the investigation and diagnosis of necrotic skin ulcers presenting as suspected spider bites (From: Isbister, GK. Spider bite. Australian Doctor 2004 with permission)

A. Establish whether or not there is a history of spider bite

Clear history of spider bite (better if spider is caught):
- Refer to information on definite spider bites

No history of spider bite:
- Investigation should focus on the clinical findings: ulcer or skin lesion
- Provisional diagnosis of a suspected spider bite is inappropriate

B. Clinical history and examination

Important considerations:
- Features suggestive of infection, malignant processes or vasculitis
- Underlying disease processes: diabetes, vascular disease
- Environmental exposure: soil, chemical, infective
- Prescription medications
- History of minor trauma
- Specific historical information about the ulcer can assist in differentiating some conditions:
  - Painful or painless
  - Duration and time of progression
  - Preceding lesion

C. Investigations

Skin biopsy:
- Microbiology: contact microbiology laboratory prior to collecting specimens so that appropriate material and transport conditions are used for fungi, *Mycobacterium* spp. and unusual bacteria
- Histopathology

Laboratory investigations: may be important for underlying conditions (autoimmune conditions, vasculitis), including, but not be limited to:
- Biochemistry (including liver and renal function tests)
- Full blood count and coagulation studies
- Autoimmune screening tests, cryoglobulins

Imaging:
- Chest radiography
- Colonoscopy
- Vascular function studies of lower limbs

D. Treatment

Local wound management
Treatment based on definite diagnosis or established pathology
Investigation and treatment of underlying conditions may be important, (e.g. pyoderma gangrenosum or diabetes mellitus)

E. Follow-up and monitoring

The diagnosis may take weeks or months to be established, so patients must have ongoing follow-up.
Continuing management: coordinated with multiple specialties involved

- redback spider
- moderate to large black spider that is potentially a FWS in Eastern Australia
- all other spiders.

The majority of redback spiders are likely to be identified correctly and with supporting clinical features this diagnosis is usually straightforward. The second group is only important in regions where FWS are known to occur and cause significant effects (east coast of Australia from Southern Queensland to Southern NSW). If the spider is large and black then the patient should be managed as a FWS. Pressure-immobilization is the appropriate first-aid measure. Once in the emergency department (ED) they should be observed for at least 2 h after the pressure mobilization has been released or after the bite in a patient without first aid. If the patient is asymptomatic at this time, they can be safely discharged. No attempt should be made to identify the spider because the distinction between some FWS and the less significant trapdoor spiders is impossible for non-experts.

The third group includes all other spiders. Despite previous concerns about particular spiders, such as the badged huntsman (*Neosparassus* spp.) and white-tail spiders, all other spiders are very unlikely to cause more than minor effects.[1]

Patients can be reassured, their tetanus status confirmed and updated, if required, and symptomatic treatment with ice and analgesia can be offered. These patients do not need to be observed in hospital.

Controversies

❶ The optimal route of administration of redback spider antivenom remains problematic with no evidence to support the i.v. over the i.m. route. However, pharmacokinetic studies demonstrate that antivenom is only detectable in blood after i.v. administration making it difficult to interpret the clinical studies. A placebo randomized controlled trial of redback antivenom is now underway.

References

1. Isbister GK, Gray MR. A prospective study of 750 definite spider bites, with expert spider identification. Quarterly Journal of Medicine 2002; 95: 723–731.
2. Isbister GK. Spider bite: a current approach to management. Australian Prescribing 2006; 29: 154–156.
3. Graudins A, Padula M, Broady K, et al. Red-back spider (Latrodectus hasselti) antivenom prevents the toxicity of widow spider venoms. Annals of Emergency Medicine 2001; 37: 154–160.
4. Isbister GK, Gray MR. Latrodectism: a prospective cohort study of bites by formally identified redback spiders. Medical Journal of Australia 2003; 179: 88–91.
5. Ellis RM, Sprivulis PC, Jelinek GA, et al. A double-blind, randomized trial of intravenous versus intramuscular antivenom for Red-back spider envenoming. Emergency Medicine Australasia 2005; 17: 152–156.
6. Isbister GK. Safety of i.v. administration of redback spider antivenom. Internal Medicine Journal 2007; 37: 820–822.
7. Isbister GK, Gray MR. Effects of envenoming by comb-footed spiders of the genera Steatoda and Achaearanea (family Theridiidae: Araneae) in Australia. Journal of Toxicology: Clinical Toxicology 2003; 41: 809–819.
8. Graudins A, Gunja N, Broady KW, et al. Clinical and in vitro evidence for the efficacy of Australian red-back spider (Latrodectus hasselti) antivenom in the treatment of envenomation by a Cupboard spider (Steatoda grossa). Toxicon: 2002; 40: 767–775.
9. Isbister GK, Gray MR, Balit CR, et al. Funnel-web spider bite: a systematic review of recorded clinical cases. Medical Journal of Australia 2005; 182: 407–411.
10. Nicholson GM, Graudins A. Spiders of medical importance in the Asia-Pacific: Atracotoxin, latrotoxin and related spider neurotoxins. Clinical and Experimental Pharmacology and Physiology 2002; 29: 785–794.
11. Isbister GK. Mouse spider bites (Missulena spp.) and their medical importance. A systematic review. Medical Journal of Australia 2004; 80: 225–227.
12. Rash LD, Birinyi-Strachan LC, Nicholson GM, et al. Neurotoxic activity of venom from the Australian Eastern mouse spider (Missulena bradleyi) involves modulation of sodium channel gating. British Journal of Pharmacology 2000; 130: 1817–1824.
13. Swanson DL, Vetter RS. Bites of brown recluse spiders and suspected necrotic arachnidism. New England Journal of Medicine 2005; 352: 700–707.
14. Isbister GK, Gray MR. White-tail spider bite: a prospective study of 130 definite bites by Lampona species. Medical Journal of Australia 2003; 179: 199–202.
15. Isbister GK, Whyte IM. Suspected white-tail spider bite and necrotic ulcers. Internal Medicine Journal 2004; 34: 38–44.

30.3 Marine envenoming and poisoning

Mark Little

ESSENTIALS

1 The management of jellyfish stings includes the provision of basic life support, application of vinegar to the sting site (for tropical jellyfish stings) and transporting the patient to a hospital. Supportive and symptomatic care is adequate for most patients. Hot water treatment is recommended for bluebottle (*Physalia* sp.) stings. Box jellyfish antivenom is available, but is rarely required.

2 The management of sea-snake envenoming is the same as for that by terrestrial snakes. If sea-snake antivenom is unavailable, then tiger-snake antivenom can be used.

3 Blue-ringed octopus and cone-shell envenoming can present with a rapid onset of flaccid paralysis. Pressure-immobilization bandaging and supportive care are indicated.

4 The management of a fish spine injury includes immersion of the limb in hot water, regional analgesia and wound care. Antivenom is available for stonefish envenoming.

Introduction

Australia's coastline provides a habitat to numerous creatures with the potential to envenom. Although many of these envenomings cause only discomfort, some have the potential to cause death.

Jellyfish envenoming

Every summer many thousands of people are stung by jellyfish, resulting in painful stings. Fortunately, only the box jellyfish (*Chironex fleckeri*) and the species of jellyfish responsible for Irukandji syndrome have been documented to cause deaths. Approximately 70 deaths have been attributed to *Chironex* in Australian waters, and children are particularly prone to a fatal outcome.[1] The last ten *Chironex fleckeri* deaths in the Northern Territory have been children. *Chiropsalmus quadrigatus* is closely related to the box jellyfish, and although no deaths have been recorded, serious envenoming may occur and recommended management is as for *Chironex*.

Two deaths have been attributed to the Irukandji syndrome in North Queensland.

First aid

First aid for all non-tropical Australian jellyfish stings consists of removing the tentacles.[2] Vinegar is not recommended due to concerns that it may increase firing of undischarged nematocysts. For non-tropical blue bottle (*Physalia* sp.) stings hot water has been demonstrated to reduce pain[3]. It should be applied as hot as can be tolerated, ensuring the patients do not burn themselves. For other non-tropical jellyfish stings, ice is recommended as first aid, although the evidence for this is minimal.[2]

First aid for jellyfish stings in tropical Australia involves local application of vinegar to inactivate undischarged nematocysts. However, vinegar will not inactivate venom from discharged nematocysts and will not reduce pain.[1,4] Vinegar should be applied liberally for at least 30 s. Pressure immobilization bandages are no longer recommended.[2]

Box jellyfish envenoming

The box jellyfish, also known as the sea wasp (*Chironex fleckeri*), is found in the tropical, particularly shallow coastal and estuarine, waters of northern Australia, predominantly between November and April. In this environment the jellyfish may be extremely difficult to see and the sudden severe pain of a sting may be the first indication of its presence. Tentacles are often still adherent to the victim's skin on removal from the water. These tentacles have a typical banded, ladder appearance and leave similar marks on the skin. The venom has numerous effects, including cardiotoxicity and dermatonecrosis. Shock and loss of consciousness from cardiorespiratory depression may occur and victims, especially children, have died within minutes of being stung. However, in a prospective study of jellyfish stings presenting to the

Royal Darwin Hospital over a 12-month period, of 23 patients with nematocyst proven *Chironex fleckeri* sting, only one required parenteral analgesia and none received antivenom.[5]

Chironex stings can be prevented by avoiding swimming in their known habitat during the dangerous months of the year, usually November to April but varying depending on the region, swimming within netted areas on beaches (mainly in Queensland), the wearing of lycra protective suits or pantyhose when swimming and entering the water slowly as the jellyfish may take evasive action to avoid a swimmer.

Treatment

- Remove the victim from the water.
- Commence CPR if indicated and continue until adequate antivenom is administered.
- Apply vinegar to the affected areas for at least 30 s.
- Scrape off adherent tentacles.
- Box jellyfish antivenom is indicated if:
  - severe pain not relieved by parenteral opiates
  - any cardiorespiratory compromise, including arrythmias.

Box jellyfish antivenom is preferably given diluted 1 in 10 in normal saline by slow intravenous (i.v.) injection, but may also be given by paramedics or surf lifesavers by intramuscular (i.m.) injection (3 ampoules). In cardiac arrest the use of up to 6 ampoules given consecutively undiluted has been advocated.[4] Premedication is not recommended because allergic reactions are uncommon.

- Animal work has suggested some benefit in adding magnesium to the treatment regime and this should be considered in unstable patients not responding to antivenom.[6]
- General and supportive management, usually in an ICU.
- Treat sting as a burn. Watch for and treat any secondary infection.
- A delayed hypersensitivity rash may develop 1–2 weeks after the sting and responds to corticosteroid cream.

Irukandji syndrome

The Irukandji jellyfish (*Carukia barnesi*) consists of a bell measuring only 2 cm across,

but with tentacles up to 75 cm in length. It is found in waters north of Geraldton, Western Australia and Mackay, Queensland. This jellyfish is almost invisible in the water. It was first captured in 1961 in Cairns by Dr Jack Barnes, who proved this jellyfish was responsible for the Irukandji syndrome by reproducing the symptoms by stinging himself, his 9-year-old son and the local lifeguard.[7] All three were taken to hospital for treatment! Evidence is emerging that more than one jellyfish species may be responsible for this syndrome.

Patients with Irukandji syndrome often have minimal symptoms at the time of the sting. After a latent period of approximately half an hour the 'Irukandji syndrome' may develop, with clinical features that include vomiting, abdominal, chest and back pain, sweats, blood pressure lability, and tachycardia.[8,9] Occasionally these cases go on to develop pulmonary oedema. Pulmonary oedema usually occurs within 10 h of a sting but can occur within 3 h. All patients developing cardiac dysfunction have ongoing pain. There have now been two deaths from Irukandji syndrome, although these were as a result of cerebral haemorrhage rather than pulmonary oedema.[10]

Treatment

Vinegar is recommended as first aid.[2] These patients are in pain and may require large doses of opioids to relieve their symptoms. In a review of 62 cases of Irukandji syndrome presenting to Cairns hospitals in one year, 38 required parenteral analgesia.[8] Fentanyl has been recommended. Patients should be observed in hospital for 6 h after their last dose of opioid and, if asymptomatic, may then be discharged. Those patients who go on to develop pulmonary oedema usually require intensive care admission for supportive care of ventilation and blood pressure. Global cardiac hypokinesis has been documented in this situation and inotropes may be necessary. Intravenous magnesium has been advocated in assisting the management of patients with ongoing symptoms.[11] There is no available antivenom.

Sea snake envenoming

Sea snakes are readily distinguished from terrestrial snakes by their flat oar-like tail.

It is important to remember that terrestrial snakes may also take to the water, but swim on the surface. Sea snakes, like terrestrial snakes, are air-breathing reptiles and in Australia are found in tropical or temperate waters. They do not survive long out of water but bites have been recorded from handling animals that have been washed ashore.

The bite of a sea snake typically causes minimal pain,[1,9] in contrast to fish stings which tend to cause intense pain. Symptoms include progressive muscle pain and tenderness, with pain and stiffness on passive movement. Neuromuscular paralysis and rhabdomyolysis are common, but coagulopathy is rare.[9] Fortunately, as for terrestrial snakes, most bitten victims are not envenomed.

Treatment

- Apply pressure-immobilization bandaging.
- Antivenom and resuscitative facilities should be available before pressure-immobilization bandaging is removed.
- Give antivenom if there is clinical or biochemical evidence of envenoming. Specific sea snake antivenom is preferred but, if unavailable, tiger snake antivenom is an alternative.[4]
- One ampoule of sea snake antivenom (1000 units), or alternatively, 3 ampoules of tiger snake antivenom, is diluted 1 in 10 with crystalloid and infused over 30 min. Further doses may be required and, as with any antivenom, the dose is titrated to effect. Polyvalent antivenom could be used.
- Supportive care including airway management, ventilatory assistance and treatment of rhabdomyolysis may be required.
- If the patient is asymptomatic after 4 h without first-aid measures being instituted, envenoming is unlikely. As with terrestrial snakebite, it is recommended that patients with confirmed or suspected sea snake bite be observed for a minimum of 12 h prior to discharge.

Note: CSL venom detection kit (VDK) does not detect sea snake venom.

Blue-ringed octopus envenoming

This small octopus, which may weigh only 10–100 g and measure 12–20 cm across the tentacles, is common along the Australian coastline. It is normally brown in colour, but the characteristic bright blue rings become apparent when the animal is agitated. Humans are at risk of envenoming when they disturb the animal. There are two documented deaths from the blue-ringed octopus (*Hapalochlaena maculosa*) in Australia,[1] and several other cases of potentially fatal envenoming that were successfully managed. The active component of the venom, maculotoxin, is similar or identical to tetrodotoxin. It acts as a paralyzing agent by preventing conduction in motor nerves via sodium channel blockade.[9] Death occurs from respiratory failure due to paralysis. The bite is typically painless, but a small lesion with bleeding may occasionally be visible. There is a spectrum of envenoming, from no symptoms to localized neurology to rapid onset of paralysis, during which time the patient remains conscious until succumbing to the effects of hypoxia.

Treatment

- Apply pressure-immobilization bandaging after washing the bite site.
- Institute supportive management, which may include artificial ventilation with sedation and inotropes for up to 12 h, as required.
- Antivenom is not available.

Patients who are asymptomatic 6 h after a bite may be discharged home safely.

Cone-shell envenoming

Of the many species of cone shell, about 18 have been implicated in human envenoming. The sole Australian fatality reported was caused by *Conus geographus* in 1936.[12] The cone shell animal injects venom from a radular tooth harpoon carried on a proboscis that protrudes from the narrow end of the shell. The venom consists of peptitoxins called conotoxins. Pain is usually felt at the site of the bite and, in serious envenoming, evidence of muscular weakness may rapidly develop and occasionally progress to respiratory paralysis.

Treatment

- Apply pressure-immobilization bandaging.

- Be prepared to commence expired air resuscitation.
- Supportive ventilation and sedation may be required.
- Antivenom is not available.
- Clinical recovery has been documented after 4 h of assisted ventilation.

Stonefish envenoming

Although the stonefish (*Synanceia* sp.) has caused deaths elsewhere, there are no confirmed Australian fatalities,[1] although Sutherland reports the death of an Army doctor on Thursday Island in 1915.[9] The stonefish possesses 13 dorsal fin spines, each with paired venom glands. These spines become erect when the fish is trodden on and venom is discharged deep into the wound. The venom has neurotoxic, myotoxic, vascular and myocardial effects. Because of their excellent camouflage stonefish are not often seen, and the first indication of their presence may be the excruciating pain of a sting.

Treatment

- Immerse the limb in hot (approximately 40–45°C) water.[1,4] Scalding may be prevented by placing the unaffected limb in the water as well.
- Pressure-immobilization bandaging is not indicated as it is likely to exacerbate the intense pain.
- Opioid analgesics are often ineffective. Regional anaesthesia with bupivacaine may be required.
- Stonefish antivenom, 1 ampoule (2000 units) per two puncture wounds via i.m. or i.v. injection should be given if there is significant envenoming.[4]
- Debride the wound. Consider radiography to exclude retained foreign body.
- Tetanus prophylaxis should be given if indicated.
- Contaminated wounds may require appropriate antibiotic treatment.

Management of other venomous fish stings

The following generalizations may apply to the management of any fish spine wound:

- The appropriate first aid is immersion of the affected limb in hot (40–45°C) water. Scalding may be prevented by placing the unaffected limb in the water as well.

- Pressure-immobilization bandaging is not indicated.
- Regional nerve blockade is preferable to local infiltration.
- Radiography should be considered to exclude retained foreign body. This is much less common with fish spine injuries than with sea urchin spines.
- Wound debridement may be necessary.
- Consider appropriate antibiotics for contaminated wounds.
- Tetanus prophylaxis should be given if indicated.
- If the wound fails to heal or becomes infected then a retained foreign body is likely.

Stingray injury

Stingrays possess a barbed spine with an enveloping integumentary sheath and associated venom glands on the tail. Human injury usually occurs from slashing of the tail when the animal is trodden on. Three deaths have been documented in Australia as a result of stingray injury, the last occurring in 2006. All died from penetrating cardiac wounds.[1,13] In one of these cases, cardiac tamponade occurred 5 days post injury, secondary to myonecrosis of myocardium at the site of the wound. Part of the spine is not infrequently left in the wound. Injury occurs from both direct trauma and envenoming. Treatment is symptomatic and as for any fish spine injury, no antivenom is available.

Ciguatera poisoning

Ciguatera poisoning is caused by eating tropical fish contaminated with ciguatoxin, a lipid-soluble toxin that accumulates up the food chain. The toxin originates in dynoflagellate algae. Humans are exposed to the toxin when they eat contaminated fish. The toxin is heat stable and, therefore, not inactivated by cooking. There is no test that will readily detect it in fish. In Australia, ciguatoxic fish are particularly found between Mackay and Cairns, but also occur around Fraser Island, Rockhampton, Groote Eylandt and Gove.

Poisoning is characterized by an acute gastrointestinal illness and a subsequent neurological illness classically involving reversal of heat and cold sensation.[9] Gastrointestinal and neurological symptoms usually begin within 1 and 24 h of eating contaminated fish. Gastrointestinal symptoms include nausea, vomiting, abdominal pain and diarrhoea, and neurological symptoms include myalgia, paraesthesiae, a burning sensation on contact with cold, mood disorders and disturbance of balance. Alcohol classically exacerbates symptoms, which may recur on eating contaminated fish. Treatment is supportive. A recent randomized controlled trial has demonstrated no benefit in using mannitol.[14]

Scombroid poisoning

Scombroid poisoning is an allergic-type reaction to a toxin that develops in the flesh of fish after they have been landed. It typically occurs from eating the flesh of mackerel, bonito and tuna. If the fish is not immediately refrigerated upon being caught, micro-organisms may break down histidine in the flesh to form histamine-like substances. Following the ingestion of fish containing this toxin, the features of histamine ingestion appear, including an urticarial rash with associated weakness and lethargy. Associated features may include bronchospasm, diarrhoea and vomiting. Less severe reactions may be treated with antihistamines but more severe reactions should be treated as for anaphylaxis.[15]

Paralytic shellfish poisoning

Paralytic shellfish poisoning is similar to ciguatera in that it occurs as a result of the concentration of a toxin produced by a dynoflagellate microorganism. The toxin, known as saxitoxin, becomes concentrated in the flesh of bivalve molluscs and has similar effects to tetrodotoxin. Treatment is supportive. Death may result from respiratory failure in untreated cases.[9]

Tetrodotoxin poisoning

Tetrodotoxin (TTX) is a paralytic toxin that occurs in the flesh, skin and viscera of puffer fish. Tetrodotoxin acts by selectively blocking voltage-sensitive sodium channels and thus preventing conduction in motor and sensory nerves. In Australia, TTX poisoning is rare and usually occurs in those who do not know the puffer fish to be poisonous. In Japan, where such fish are a delicacy called 'fugu', numerous cases and deaths occur every year. Toxicity usually manifests soon after eating the fish, with typical features including perioral paraesthesiae followed by numbness of the mouth, tongue and face, and then widespread paralysis. Severe cases can progress to death from respiratory failure. Management is supportive as there is no antidote.[1,9] All cases should be admitted for observation until peak clinical effects have passed. It is extremely unlikely that life-threatening effects will occur after 24 h in patients who have not already developed severe effects.[16]

Controversies

❶ The biology and venoms of potentially lethal Australian jellyfish remain poorly understood. Further basic research in this area is needed to help prevent and treat envenomings more effectively.

❷ Many of the current recommendations for first aid and treatment of marine envenomings and poisonings are based on anecdotal experience. Quality research into identifying the most effective treatment for many marine envenomings and poisonings is required.

❸ The most effective first aid for jellyfish stings, particularly in tropical Australia, remains controversial. A recent laboratory study demonstrated that heat inactivates box jellyfish venom and the role of hot showers in first aid merits further investigation.[17]

References

1. Williamson JA, Fenner PJ, Burnett JW, Rifkin JF (eds). Venomous and Poisonous Marine Animals – a Medical and Biological Handbook. Sydney: University of New South Wales Press; 1996.

2. Australian Resuscitation Council guideline 8.9.6: Envenomation – Jellyfish Stings. http://www.resus.org.au (Accessed 31st January 2008).

3. Loten C, Stokes B, Worsley D, et al. A randomised trial of hot water (45°C) immersion versus ice packs for pain relief in bluebottle stings. Medical Journal of Australia 2006; 184: 329–330.

4. White J. CSL Antivenom Handbook. Melbourne: CSL Ltd.; 1995.

5. O'Rielly G, Isbister GK, Lawrie PM, et al. Prospective study of jellyfish stings from tropical Australia, including the major box jellyfish Chironex fleckeri. Medical Journal of Australia 2001; 175: 652–655.

6. Ramasamy S, Isbister GK Seymour JE, et al. The in vivo cardiovascular effects of box jellyfish Chironex fleckeri venom in rats: efficacy of pre treatment with antivenom, verapamil and magnesium sulphate. Toxicon 2004; 43: 685–690.

7. Barnes J. Cause and effect in Irukandji stingings. Medical Journal of Australia 1964; 177: 654–655.

8. Little M, Mulcahy R. A year's experience of Irukandji envenoming in far north Queensland. Medical Journal of Australia 1998; 169: 638–641.

9. Sutherland SK, Tibballs J (eds). Australian Animal Toxins, 2nd edn. Melbourne: Oxford University Press; 2001.

10. Fenner PJ, Hadok JC. Fatal envenomation by jellyfish causing Irukandji syndrome. Medical Journal of Australia 2002; 177: 362–363.

11. Corkeron M, Pereira P, MacKrocanis C. Early experience with magnesium administration in Irukandji Syndrome. Anaesthetic Intensive Care 2004; 32: 666–669.

12. Flecker H. Cone shell mollusc poisoning with report of a fatal case. Medical Journal of Australia 1936; 1: 464–466.

13. Fenner PJ, Williamson JA, Skinner RA. Fatal and non-fatal stingray envenomation. Medical Journal of Australia 1989; 151: 621–625

14. Schnorf H, Tauarii M, Cundy T. Ciguatera fish poisoning: a double blinded randomised trial of mannitol therapy. Neurology 2002; 58: 873–880.

15. Smart DR. Scombroid poisoning: a report of seven cases involving the Western Australian salmon Arripis truttaceus. Medical Journal of Australia 1992; 157: 748–751.

16. Isbister GK, Son J, Wang F, et al. Puffer fish poisoning: a potentially life-threatening condition. Medical Journal of Australia 2002; 177: 650–653.

17. Carrette TJ, Cullen P, Little M, et al. Temperature effects on box jellyfish venom: a possible treatment for envenomed patients? Medical Journal of Australia 2002; 177: 654–655.

TOXINOLOGY

Index